AF802882

Greenfield's Neuropathology

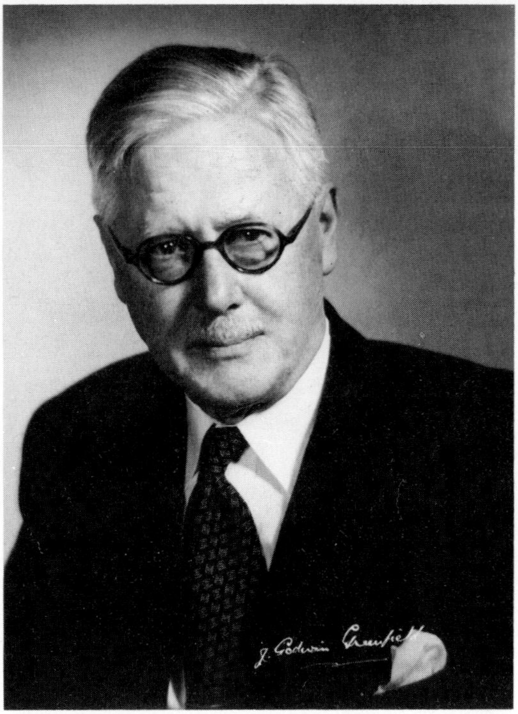

J. G. Greenfield, MD, FRCP, LLD
(1884–1958)

Born in Edinburgh, Scotland. Graduated in Medicine at Edinburgh University 1908. House physician (1910) subsequently Pathologist to the National Hospital, Queen Square 1914–1949 and Dean of the Medical School 1923–1943. Visiting Professor National Institutes of Health, Bethesda 1954–1958. Founder of the Neuropathological Club (now the British Neuropathological Society) and Editor of the first edition of this book, 1958.

Greenfield's
Neuropathology

Fourth Edition

Edited by

J. Hume Adams PhD, MBChB, FRCP, FRCPath
Professor of Neuropathology, University of Glasgow and Institute of Neurological Sciences, Southern General Hospital, Glasgow

J.A.N. Corsellis FRCP, FRCPath, FRCPsych
Emeritus Professor of Neuropathology, University of London
Honorary Consultant Neuropathologist, Bethlem Royal and Maudsley Hospitals, London and Runwell Hospital, Wickford, Essex

L.W. Duchen MD, PhD, DSc, FRCP, FRCPath
Professor of Neuropathology, Institute of Neurology
Honorary Consultant Neuropathologist, The National Hospital for Nervous Diseases, Queen Square, London

A Wiley-Medical Publication

John Wiley & Sons
New York

© Edward Arnold (Publishers) Ltd, 1984

First published 1958

Fourth edition 1984

Published in the USA by Wiley-Medical,
a division of
John Wiley & Sons, Inc., New York

Library of Congress Cataloging in Publication Data
Greenfield, J. Godwin (Joseph Godwin) 1884–1958.
Greenfield's Neuropathology.
(A Wiley Medical Publication)
Includes Bibliographies and Index.
1. Nervous System—Diseases. I. Adams, J. Hume.
II. Title. III. Title: Neuropathology.
IV. Series.
(DNLM: 1. Nervous System Diseases—Pathology.
WL 100 G812N)
RC 347.G73 1985 616.8′047 84–21923
ISBN 0–471–82307–4

All Rights Reserved. No part of this publication may be reproduced, stored in a retrieval system, or transmitted, in any form or by any means, electronic, mechanical, photo-copying, recording or otherwise, without the prior permission of the publishers.

Printed in Great Britain

Contributors

J. Hume Adams, PhD, MBChB, FRCP, FRCPath
Professor of Neuropathology, University of Glasgow and Institute of Neurological Sciences, Southern General Hospital, Glasgow

Ingrid V. Allen, MD, DSc, FRCPath
Professor of Neuropathology, Neuropathology Laboratory, Department of Pathology, Queen's University, Belfast

J.B. Brierley, MD, FRCPath, FRCPsych
Formerly Scientific Officer (Clinical), MRC Laboratories, Woodmansterne Road, Carshalton, Surrey

Betty Brownell, BA, MB, BCh, BAO, FRCPath
Consultant Neuropathologist, Department of Neuropathology, Frenchay Hospital, Bristol

J.A.N. Corsellis, FRCP, FRCPath, FRCPsych
Emeritus Professor of Neuropathology, University of London:
Honorary Consultant Neuropathologist, Bethlem Royal and Maudsley Hospitals, London and Runwell Hospital, Wickford, Essex

L.W. Duchen, MD, PhD, DSc, FRCP, FRCPath
Professor of Neuropathology, Institute of Neurology
Honorary Consultant Neuropathologist, The National Hospital for Nervous Diseases, Queen Square, London

D.I. Graham, PhD, MB, BCh, MRCP, FRCPath
Professor of Neuropathology, University of Glasgow:
Honorary Consultant in Neuropathology Institute of Neurological Sciences, Southern General Hospital, Glasgow

D.G.F. Harriman, MD, FRCP, FRCPath
Reader in Neuropathology, University of Leeds:
Honorary Consultant Neuropathologist, The General Infirmary, Leeds

J. Trevor Hughes, MA, DPhil, MD, FRCP(Lond and Ed), FRCPath
Clinical Lecturer in Neuropathology and Fellow of Green College, University of Oxford:
Consultant Neuropathologist, The Radcliffe Infirmary, Oxford

Jean M. Jacobs, BSc, PhD
Lecturer in Neuropathology, Institute of Neurology, The National Hospital for Nervous Diseases, Queen Square, London

R.H.M. King, PhD, MSc, BSc
Lecturer, Department of Neurological Science, Royal Free Hospital School of Medicine, London

Brian D. Lake, BSc, PhD, FRCPath
Reader in Histochemistry, Department of Histopathology, Hospital for Sick Children and Institute of Child Health, Great Ormond Street, London

D.N. Landon, BSc, MB, BS, MRCS, LRCP
Reader in Neurocytology, Institute of Neurology, The National Hospital for Nervous Diseases, Queen Square, London

Jeanne-Claudie Larroche, MD
Maître de Recherches au CNRS
Hôpital Port-Royal, Paris, France

Pamela M. Le Quesne, DM, BSc, FRCP
Member MRC Toxicology Unit; Honorary Consultant Neurologist, Department of Neurological Studies, The Middlesex Hospital, London

B.S. Meldrum, PhD, MB, BChir
Reader in Experimental Neurology, Department of Neurology, Institute of Psychiatry, London

J. Douglas Miller, MD, PhD, FRCS, FACS, FRCP
Professor of Surgical Neurology, University of Edinburgh at the Western General Hospital, Edinburgh

D.R. Oppenheimer, MA, DM, FRCPath
Formerly University Lecturer and Honorary Consultant in Neuropathology, The Radcliffe Infirmary, Oxford: and Fellow of Trinity College, Oxford

F. Scaravilli, MD, PhD
Senior Lecturer in Neuropathology, Institute of Neurology, The National Hospital for Nervous Diseases, Queen Square, London

P.K. Thomas, DSc, MD, FRCP
Professor of Neurology in the University of London at the Royal Free Hospital School of Medicine and the Institute of Neurology, London

A.H. Tomlinson, MA, D.Phil, FRCPath
Formerly at the Virology Laboratory, Public Health Laboratory, John Radcliffe Hospital, Oxford

B.E. Tomlinson, CBE, MD, FRCP, FRCPath
Professor of Pathology and Consultant Pathologist, Department of Pathology, Newcastle General Hospital, Newcastle upon Tyne

C.S. Treip, MA, MD, PhD, FRCPath
University Lecturer in Pathology and Fellow of Wolfson College, Cambridge.
Honorary Consultant in Neuropathology, Addenbrooke's Hospital, Cambridge

Roy O. Weller, BSc, PhD, MD, FRCPath
Professor of Neuropathology in the University of Southampton at the Department of Pathology (Neuropathology), Southampton General Hospital, Southampton

Preface to the fourth edition

More than 25 years have passed since the publication of the first edition of Neuropathology, which, since the second edition in 1963, has been known as Greenfield's Neuropathology in recognition of the pioneering work of Dr Greenfield at the National Hospital for Nervous Diseases, Queen Square. The fundamental approach and the format of the book remain true to the Greenfield tradition which was established in the first edition but the subject has inevitably enlarged and changed reflecting the rapid developments which are taking place in all branches of the neurosciences. Many of the chapters have been completely rewritten and there is now a greater emphasis on ultrastructure and biochemistry. A new generation of neuropathologist contributors has been joined by specialists in clinical fields and in other laboratory disciplines to provide what we think are up-to-date and authoritative surveys of their topics. To bring in the new does not necessitate discarding the old and much of the irreplaceable expertise expressed by the original authorship has been retained. Many of the recent discoveries in neurobiology have yet to be applied to the clinical and neuropathological study of man and the subject inevitably continues to grow. This is reflected in the size of the book which has grown with each edition but it is still contained within a single volume and this has unfortunately led to the omission of some of the historical aspects of the subject. Although the personal links with J.G. Greenfield himself are now not strong, many of the contributors were students of his fellow authors Blackwood, Meyer, McMenemey, Norman and Dorothy Russell who together with Greenfield laid the foundations of Neuropathology in Great Britain.

JHA
JANC
LWD

Acknowledgements

Individual acknowledgements are made where possible throughout the text. Special thanks are due to Professor D.G. McDowall, University of Leeds; Mr Alwyn Brown, MRC Toxicology Laboratories Carshalton; Dr Seth Love and Mr J.A. Mills, Institute of Neurology, and Mrs V.V. Smith, Institute of Child Health. The photograph of Dr J.G. Greenfield was provided by Mr H. Prentice, The National Hospital, Queen Square. Many more people have made important contributions towards the preparation of this book than can be thanked individually. Our gratitude to the many friends and colleagues who have provided illustrative material is very considerable. In many hospitals and universities, to which Neuropathology laboratories are affiliated, loyal and tolerant secretarial, technical and photographic staff have given invaluable expert support to the contributors. Thanks are due in particular to our secretaries, Mrs E. Daniell, Miss Jean Pegrum, Mrs E. Perkins, Mrs Joan Rubython; to Miss Gillian Clarke for much expert editorial help and to Mr P.J. Price and Miss Barbara Koster of Edward Arnold for their help in overcoming the many problems which arose in the production of this volume.

JHA
JANC
LWD

Contents

Frontispiece ii
Preface vii

1 **General pathology of neurons and neuroglia** *L. W. Duchen* 1
2 **The pathophysiology of raised intracranial pressure** *J. Douglas Miller and J. Hume Adams* 53
3 **Head injury** *J. Hume Adams* 85
4 **Hypoxia and vascular disorders of the central nervous system** *J. B. Brierley and D. I. Graham* 125
5 **Spontaneous intracranial haemorrhage** *Roy O. Weller* 208
6 **Bacterial infections of the central nervous system** *D. G. F. Harriman* 236
7 **Virus diseases of the central nervous system** *Betty Brownell and A. H. Tomlinson* 260
8 **Parasitic and fungal infections of the nervous system** *F. Scaravilli* 304
9 **Demyelinating diseases** *Ingrid V. Allen* 338
10 **Malformations of the nervous system** *Jeanne-Claudie Larroche* 385
11 **Perinatal brain damage** *Jeanne-Claudie Larroche* 451
12 **Lysosomal enzyme deficiencies** *Brian D. Lake* 491
13 **Nutritional deficiencies and metabolic disorders** *L. W. Duchen and Jean M. Jacobs* 573
14 **Toxic disorders of the nervous system** *Jean M. Jacobs and Pamela M. Le Quesne* 627
15 **Diseases of the basal ganglia, cerebellum and motor neurons** *D. R. Oppenheimer* 699
16 **The hypothalamus and pituitary gland** *C. S. Treip* 748
17 **Disorders of the spine and spinal cord** *J. Trevor Hughes* 779
18 **Diseases of the peripheral nerves** *P. K. Thomas, D. N. Landon and R. H. M. King* 807
19 **Epilepsy** *B. S. Meldrum and J. A. N. Corsellis* 921
20 **Ageing and the dementias** *B. E. Tomlinson and J. A. N. Corsellis* 951
21 **Diseases of muscle** *D. G. F. Harriman* 1026

Index 1097

1

General pathology of neurons and neuroglia

L.W. Duchen

Neuropathology, as surveyed in this volume, deals mainly with morphological aspects of the study of diseases of the nervous system. The foundations of this science were established in the nineteenth century by the pioneer neurohistologists in France, Germany and Spain, many whom combined clinical neuropsychiatric practice with laboratory investigation. Greenfield (1958) and subsequently Greenfield and Meyer (1963) and Blackwood (1976) briefly reviewed the historical development of neuropathology.

The complexity of structure and composition of the nervous system necessitates a wide range of technical methods for its microscopic study. Each component has some method of staining most appropriate for its visualization, and the importance of each method varies in different pathological conditions. The methods applied to the study of cases with complex neurological disease which may have required many hours of clinical investigation should be the most appropriate for each individual case. Obviously, therefore, the details of the clinical history of a case under study need to be known. As complete a post-mortem examination of the nervous system as is possible should be the aim in every case. Widespread sampling of tissues should be a routine procedure, so that the examination will include not only different areas of the brain and spinal cord but also nerve roots, sensory and autonomic ganglia, peripheral nerves, muscles, visceral innervation and sensory receptor organs. The brain should normally be fixed intact. Indiscriminate slicing of the fresh unfixed brain may preclude further useful study but it is possible to obtain fresh brain tissue without compromising later histological study. For example, a cut through one frontal lobe anterior to the lateral ventricle will provide a good sample of cortex and white matter. In diseases affecting the brain symmetrically, a mid-sagittal division will provide one hemisphere for histological examination while the other can be studied by techniques requiring unfixed tissue. This type of combined approach enables advances in neurobiology to become applicable to the study of human neurological disease. The application of electron microscopy to human clinical neuropathology remains a considerable, perhaps intractable, problem. The rapid development of post-mortem artefact due to autolytic changes, the disruption of membranes and the consequent impairment of adequate fixation and staining make it difficult to apply criteria for significant pathological change even when the period between death and fixation is reduced to 3 to 4 hours. Only the most stable, and metabolically therefore the most inactive, constituents can be identified with certainty in post-mortem electron micrographs. Nevertheless, electron microscopy of post-mortem tissue has made important contributions to our understanding of the pathogenesis of neurological disease and could be used more widely and routinely when the material is suitable.

Brain weight

The weight of the brain is a useful measure of its pathological state. Fixation in 10 per cent formalin usually causes a small but variable increase in weight while fixation in 30 per cent formalin leads to a small decrease. Brain weight is related to age, height and sex, and many tables have been published giving the normal range. A recent extensive survey (Dekaban and Sadowsky, 1978) was based on recorded fresh unfixed weights from more than 2700 male and nearly 2000 female patients dying with histologically normal brains. Brain weight was correlated with height, weight, age and sex, and it was found that in males brain weight is almost 10 per cent greater than in females of similar age. The largest rate of increase occurs between birth and 3 years, the maximum weight is in young adults around the 19th year and there is a progressive decline after 45–50 years of age. Lowest values occur after 86 years, when brain weight is about 11 per cent lower than the maximum. Average brain weights for males are 380 g at birth; 970 g at 1 year; 1120 g at 2 years; 1300 g at 5 years; 1400 g at 10; 1450 g at 19–21; 1430 g at 50; 1370 g at 60 and 1330 g at 80. In females the maximum is 1340 g at age 18, which declines to 1140 g at 80.

The neuron

The great variety of shapes and sizes of nerve cells makes it difficult, if not impossible, to define the morphological characteristics of a typical neuron. The identification of alterations in the morphology of neurons is one of the cornerstones of neuropathology and it is useful to compare suspected alterations in pathological states with control material of the same type of cell. Some features are common to all nerve cells, large or small. Nuclei tend to be rounded in section—i.e. they are spherical (Fig. 1.1)—and on electron microscopy can be seen to be bounded by a double membrane which in places is fused to form nuclear pores or diaphragms. Often, and usually in the large neurons such as large pyramidal (Betz) cells of motor cortex and Purkinje* cells of cerebellum, there is a large prominent, nearly central, nucleolus. Typically, neuronal nuclei lie in the centre of the cell body, and displacement to the periphery may be evidence of pathology. However, the nucleus may be normally eccentric in some neurons such as in the cells of Clarke's column of the spinal cord and in neurosecretory cells of the hypothalamus. Nuclei may also seem to be displaced by perikaryal accumulation of lipofuscin pigment and

* In view of its common usage the spelling Purkinje has been retained instead of the more correct form, Purkyně.

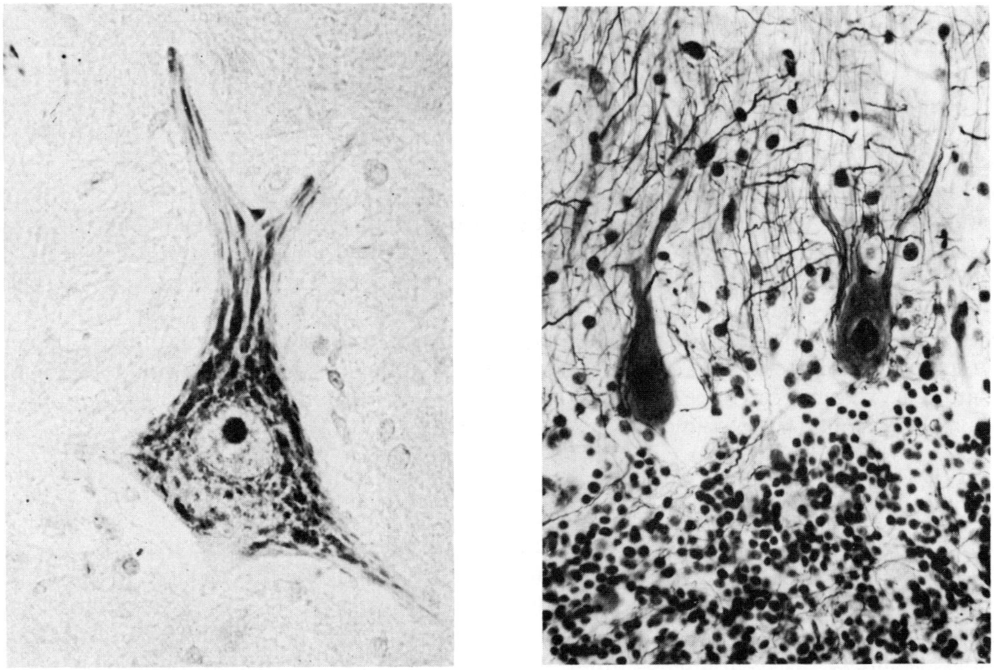

a b

Fig. 1.1 Normal neurons. (**a**) Anterior horn cell from lumbar spinal cord. Note the central round nucleus, prominent nucleolus, and Nissl bodies in the perikaryon extending into dendrites but absent from the axon hillock and axon. Thionin (Nissl's method) × 550. (**b**) Cerebellar cortex showing two Purkinje cells with their dendrites extending up into the molecular layer. Axons from basket cells surround the cells and pass up the dendrites. Bielschowsky silver impregnation × 400.

in normal cells of the substantia nigra or locus ceruleus where there is abundant perikaryal neuromelanin. In small neurons such as cerebellar granule cells the nucleus forms the major constituent of the cell body. The sex chromatin, characteristically larger in females, was described in nerve cells of the cat where it forms a juxtanucleolar mass (Barr and Bertram, 1949). In other species, including man, it may be seen as attached to the internal aspect of the nuclear membrane.

Perikaryal constituents vary in amount and in proportion among neurons but most elements are common to all nerve cells. As in other cell types actively synthesizing protein, neuronal perikarya are rich in ribosomes (composed of ribonucleic acid) which may be grouped in polysomes or arranged along stacks of membrane in parallel array (the rough endoplasmic reticulum) forming Nissl bodies or granules (Fig. 1.1). These granules are readily visible with light microscopy and are stainable with haematoxylin and with basic aniline dyes such as cresyl fast violet or thionin which also stain the nucleolus. The presence and distribution of Nissl granules throughout the perikaryon or the more diffuse basophilia produced by free ribosomes is of importance because abnormalities in these components of the cell occur under pathological conditions. Normally ribosomes are absent from the axon but they are found in dendrites.

In addition to the stacks of organized rough endoplasmic reticulum there are other perikaryal organelles which include arrays of agranular (smooth) endoplasmic reticulum, often lying close to the nucleus and forming the Golgi apparatus, abundant mitochondria, smooth as well as coated vesicles, multivesicular bodies, neurofilaments and neurotubules (Fig. 1.2). Lipofuscin granules and, in specific sites, neuromelanin granules are other normal constituents. The normal electron microscopic structure of nerve cells has been reviewed by Peters, Palay and Webster (1976). With light microscopy the use of silver impregnation techniques in either paraffin or frozen sections adds very greatly to the extent of neuronal visualization. Neuronal processes and perikarya rich in neurofilaments are readily stainable in paraffin sections by methods such as those of Palmgren (1948) and Marsland, Glees and Erikson (1954), while the Golgi silver technique (as used and modified by Valverde, 1970, and Ramon-Moliner, 1970) in thick sections gives the most extensive picture of the neuron and is particularly valuable in the assessment of the size of the dendritic arborization and the density of dendritic spines.

The density of the perikaryon varies considerably among neurons, with both light and electron microscopy, giving rise to the terms 'large light' and 'small dark' cells. This is particularly apparent in sensory ganglia where the large light cells have prominent well-ordered stacks of rough endoplasmic reticulum forming Nissl granules widely separated from each other by cytoplasm containing abundant neurofilaments and microtubules and dense organelles (see Lieberman, 1976). Small dark cells have more closely packed ribosomes, mostly free or in packets, and few well-organized Nissl granules. The cells of autonomic ganglia differ in many respects from neurons of the CNS. A comprehensive account of structure and function of adrenergic neurons has been given by Burnstock and Costa (1975).

Synaptic morphology was reviewed by D.G. Jones (1975) and by Peters, Palay and Webster (1976) and can, for convenience, be divided into symmetrical types in which densities are present on both pre- and postsynaptic membranes and asymmetrical where the postsynaptic density is the more prominent. The characteristic organelles of the axonal terminal are synaptic vesicles (Fig. 1.3) which are agranular (clear) or dense-cored in type. Agranular vesicles may be spherical with a diameter of 40–50 nm or somewhat flattened or ellipsoidal, depending to some extent on the type of fixative used. The association of flattened vesicles with symmetrical synapses and their neurophysiological correlates points towards an inhibitory function in these synapses while the spherical vesicles are the preponderant type in excitatory synapses as at the neuromuscular junction. Dense-cored vesicles of 40–60 nm diameter are considered to be sites of storage of noradrenaline. Larger dense-cored vesicles of 80–90 nm diameter are found throughout the central nervous system and in peripheral autonomic fibres but their functional correlate is uncertain. Other constituents associated with the transmitter function of neurons include neurosecretory vesicles which are much larger than other synaptic vesicles, up to 300 nm in diameter, and are found in the neurons of the supraoptic and paraventricular nuclei and their terminals in the neurohypophysis. At a light microscopic level these vesicles correspond to the stainable

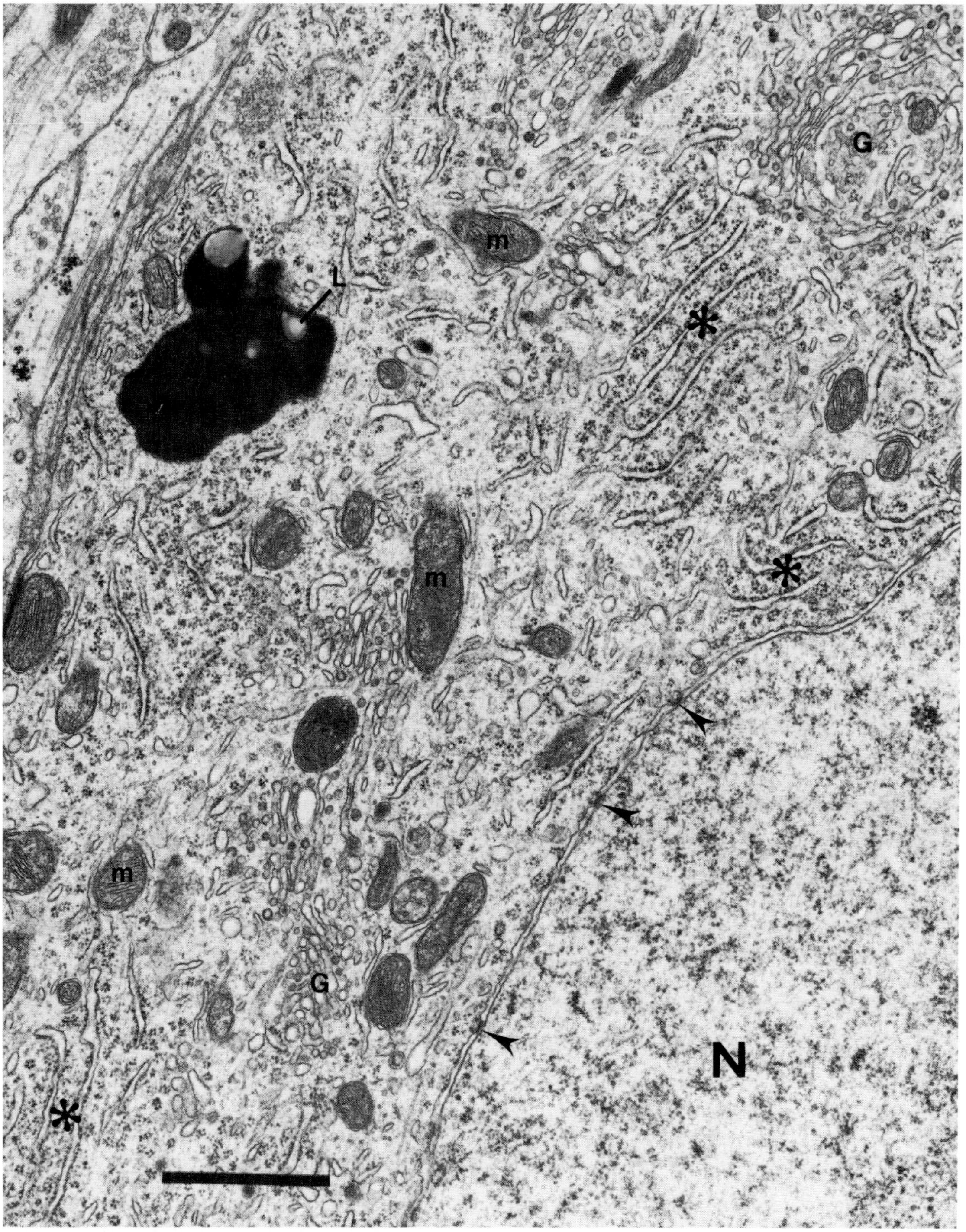

Fig. 1.2 Electron micrograph of part of an anterior horn cell of the spinal cord of a normal rat. The nucleus (N) is bounded by a double membrane which is fused at the nuclear pores (arrowheads). In the perikaryon the parallel arrays of rough endoplasmic reticulum (✱) correspond to the Nissl bodies seen by light microscopy. There are abundant polysomes (small groups of ribosomes), mitochondria (m) and cisternae of smooth endoplasmic reticulum forming the Golgi apparatus (G). Occasional microtubules and one lipofuscin inclusion (L) are also shown. Bar = 1 μm. (Preparation by Dr Jean M. Jacobs).

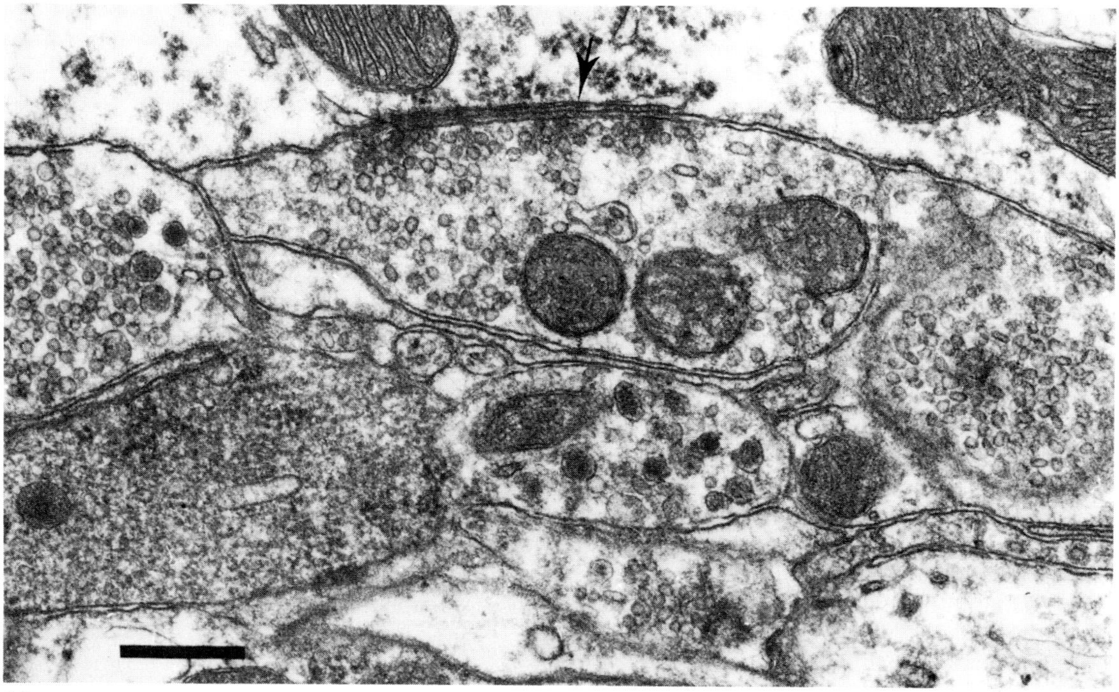

(a)

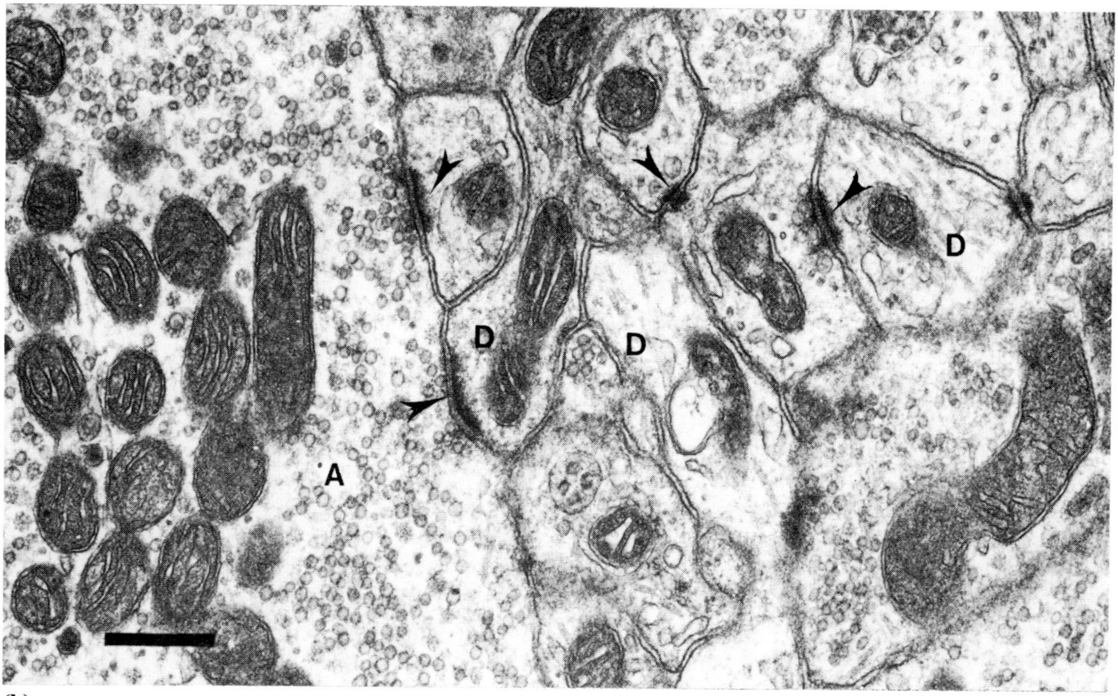

(b)

Fig. 1.3 Electron micrographs showing nerve terminals and synapses. (**a**) Several axonal terminals are seen containing synaptic vesicles which have a varied morphology. Some are round and clear, others are round and have a dense core. Clear but elliptical vesicles are also shown. One synapse (arrow) on the perikaryal membrane of an anterior horn cell has an associated flattened cisterna lying close to the postsynaptic membrane. Bar $= 0.5\,\mu m$. (**b**) In the cerebellar granule cell layer a large axonal terminal (A) of a mossy fibre contains abundant mitochondria and clear rounded synaptic vesicles. Several dendritic profiles (D) and synapses (arrowheads) are shown; in some there is a prominent postsynaptic density but in others pre- and postsynaptic densities are of similar thickness. Bar $= 0.5\,\mu m$. (Preparations by Dr Jean M. Jacobs) neurosecretory material demonstrable by the Gomori chrome alum haematoxylin stain and contain the hormones oxytocin and vasopressin and their carrier proteins.

A great deal of interest attaches to the functional relationships between vesicles, neurotransmitters and the mechanism of transmitter release from nerve terminals. Much discussion has centred on the problems as they present at the neuromuscular junction, where the physiological studies of Katz and his collaborators established the quantal nature of transmitter release (see Katz, 1969). The question as to whether this release is by exocytosis from vesicles or by some other mechanism controlling acetylcholine release from a cytoplasmic pool has been discussed by Israel, Dunant and Manaranche (1979) and by Ceccarelli and Hurlbut (1980). It seems that although a proportion (estimated at about 40 per cent) of transmitter is present within vesicles and that an exocytotic process does occur, it is by no means certain that quantal transmitter release is by exocytosis or is derived from vesicles.

The correlation between neuronal structure, the identification of neurotransmitter function of identified neurons and their pathology is still a new field (see Iversen, 1982). The putative transmitters include gamma-aminobutyric acid (GABA), glycine, glutamic acid, acetylcholine, dopamine, noradrenaline, adrenaline, 5-hydroxytryptamine and histamine. Methods for the localization of these transmitters, particularly in nerve terminals, may rely more on identification of synthesizing enzymes such as glutamic acid decarboxylase, choline acetyltransferase or tyrosine hydroxylase than of the transmitter substance itself. Other hormone-like, rather than transmitter, substances include oxytocin and vasopressin, while recently identified neuropeptides seem likely to act as modulators of neuronal activity rather than as neurotransmitters and include the opioid peptides, substance P, hypothalamic releasing factors, gut hormones and pituitary peptides. These peptides can be localized by immunocytochemical methods (see Chan-Palay and Palay, 1982; Gaspar et al., 1983; Pearson, 1983) which can also be applied to receptor localization. Clearly, methods for the identification of transmitters are set to make great contributions to the understanding of neurological disease.

The use of monoclonal antibody techniques, developed by Köhler and Milstein (1975), has greatly facilitated the exact localization of antigens in the nervous system and these methods are now being applied to the identification and characterization of cells, both neuronal and glial. Neuronal cell markers, localizable by immunocytochemical techniques (fluorescence or immunoperoxidase) include neurofilament polypeptide (Anderton et al., 1980; Yen and Fields, 1981), and the antibodies A2B5 (Eisenbarth, Walsh and Nirenberg, 1979), A4 and 38D7. Other methods for the identification of neurons are tetanus toxin binding and the visualization of neuron-specific enolase. These cell markers are already making great contributions to neurobiological research, particularly for identification of cells in tissue culture, and their applicability to problems of human neurological disease is apparent (see Kennedy, 1982).

Artefact

Artefact occurs all too readily at various stages of neurohistological preparation and may cause errors of interpretation. *Post mortem* autolysis seems to be less of a problem in the central nervous system than in other viscera, at least for light microscopy, and reasonable histological staining can be obtained even several days after death, provided refrigeration has been adequate. The autolytic changes which develop after brain death has occurred but with the patient maintained with life-supporting systems may be a major obstacle to useful histological study. After only 24 hours on a respirator, changes resemble hypoxic cell damage. Longer periods on artificial ventilation after brain death lead to failure of the brain to become adequately fixed and hardened in formalin and renders detailed histological study useless. The 'respirator brain' is considered in more detail in Chapter 4.

Other artefactual changes have been reviewed by Blackwood (1976) and include the formation of 'mucocytes' (Buscaino bodies) in the white matter. These 'metachromatic bodies' were studied by Smith (1949). They occur only in some cases, and are seen in frozen sections as well as paraffin- and celloidin-embedded tissue. Separation of cell layers from each other is also artefactual and affects particularly the granule cell and molecular layers of cerebellum and the hippocampus in paraffin-embedded blocks. These are probably akin to the perineuronal and perivascular spaces which appear in paraffin sections and are shrinkage artefacts occurring during tissue processing. They can be partially avoided by prolonging the duration of each stage of dehydration, clearing and impregnation with paraffin wax and by celloidin embedding. Fixation artefact is also probably the cause of 'selective granule cell necrosis' in which the granule cell layer of cerebellar cortex appears pale grey or whitish macroscopically and the cells fail to stain adequately. The exact cause is not known, perhaps being autolytic, but it is a very rare occurrence when brains are fixed in a stronger formalin solution (20–30%) than in general use and the volume of formalin relative to brain is adequate (i.e. 6 litres or more of formalin).

Shrunken dark neurons have been clearly demonstrated to be artefactual (Cammermeyer, 1960, 1961; Brown, 1977) and are caused by pressure on unfixed brain tissue. They are irregular in outline, the apical dendrite has a twisted, corkscrew-like appearance, the nucleus and cytoplasm stain darkly and Nissl bodies cannot be identified (Fig. 1.4). There may also be a perinuclear halo. The presence of dark neurons is often a problem, particularly in biopsy specimens of cortex and in experimental animal material in which brain tissue is handled in the fresh state and subjected to pressure. The artefact can be prevented or at least reduced by minimizing handling of the brain when fresh and unfixed. In experimental animals the use of perfusion-fixation and leaving the brain untouched in the skull for several hours before removal helps to prevent artefact.

Artefactual changes are easily induced during removal and handling of the spinal cord, which, if bent or kinked sharply before fixation, may develop swellings which may resemble intrinsic tumours. The cord should therefore not be subjected to pressure and should be kept as straight

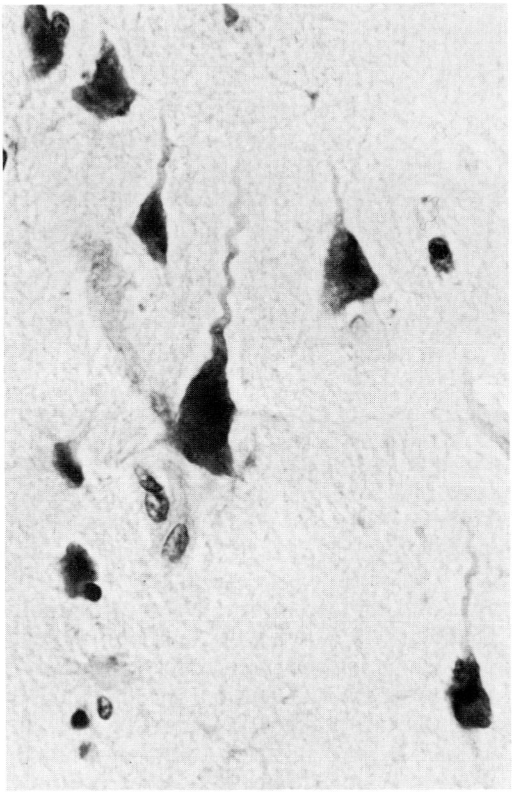

Fig. 1.4 Artefactually shrunken neurons near the cut edge of a cortical biopsy. These cells are darkly stained and the apical dendrite has a twisted corkscrew-like appearance. Haematoxylin and van Gieson ×400.

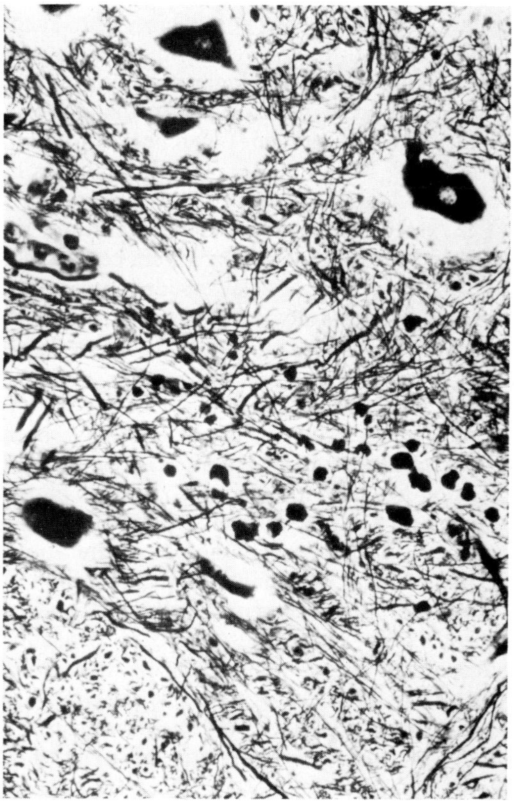

Fig. 1.5 Argyrophilic bodies in the spinal cord are shown in grey matter close to several anterior horn cells. Paraffin section of lumbar spinal cord of a patient without neurological disease. Glees silver impregnation ×160.

as possible until placed in fixative in a suitable container.

Argyrophilic bodies in the spinal cord

Argyrophilic bodies (Fig. 1.5) up to 30 μm in diameter are a constant finding in the anterior horns of the grey matter of the spinal cord in adults (Smith, 1955). Their nature is uncertain but because of their ubiquity they are not considered to be indicative of any specific pathology in spite of their resemblance to axonal retraction balls.

General pathology of the neuron

Hypoxic neuronal damage

One of the commonest forms of injury to neurons is that caused by hypoxia, this term being used to cover a wide range of underlying physiological disturbances such as arrested or impaired blood flow, reduced oxygen tension in circulating blood or toxic factors. Furthermore, because of the dependence of the neuron on glucose as its main metabolic substrate, hypoglycaemia of whatever cause can induce morphological changes similar to those caused by hypoxia due to the neuron's inability to utilize oxygen (Lawrence, Meyer and Nevin, 1942; Meyer, 1963). The mechanisms of these disturbances are discussed in Chapter 4.

The early neuropathological literature referred to Nissl's acute cell or severe cell disease but these terms have been superseded. For details of the older terminology the reader may refer to the previous editions of this book or to Spielmeyer (1922).

The sequence and time-course of events following hypoxic injury to the neuron have been well defined in experimental animals. The use of perfusion-fixation and delayed removal of the brain has allowed the differentiation between artefactual and significant pathological alterations and in particular has facilitated the definition of the early stages of hypoxic cell damage (see Brown, 1977). The earliest stage of ischaemic neuronal pathology was named *microvacuolation* by Brown and Brierley (1966). The cell (Fig. 1.6) may be normal in size or only slightly shrunken, and the nucleus also only slightly shrunken while the perikaryon is vacuolated. The majority of vacuoles (which are up to about 2 μm in diameter) are swollen mitochondria, while some may be due to dilatations of endoplasmic reticulum or of other intracytoplasmic organelles (Fig. 1.7). Microvacuolation has been identified in hippocampal and cortical neurons in the rat after only 5–15 minutes of hypoxia. In the rhesus monkey microvacuolation has been observed within 15 minutes of severe hypotension and 30 minutes of hypoglycaemia, and Brierley (unpublished) has identified the changes in the brain of a human case dying 1 hour after cardiac arrest. Microvacuolation can, however, only rarely be identified in man because of early autolytic changes. Microvacuolation occurs earlier and seems to persist for a shorter time in small neurons than in

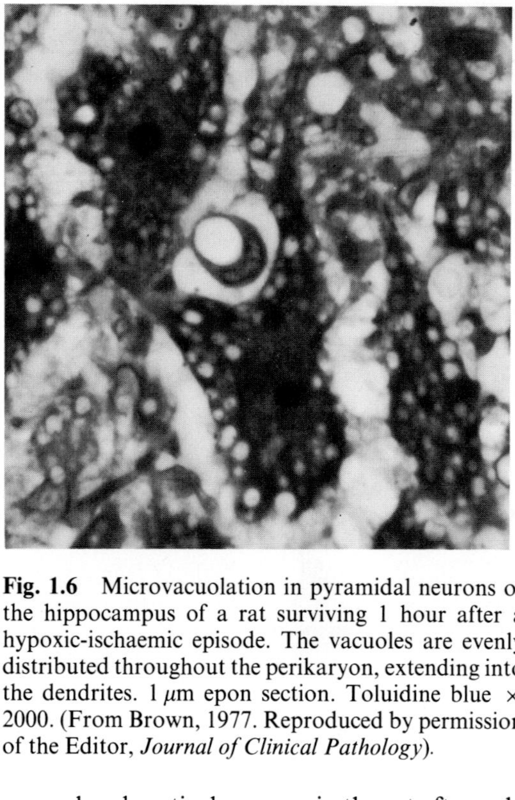

Fig. 1.6 Microvacuolation in pyramidal neurons of the hippocampus of a rat surviving 1 hour after a hypoxic-ischaemic episode. The vacuoles are evenly distributed throughout the perikaryon, extending into the dendrites. 1 μm epon section. Toluidine blue × 2000. (From Brown, 1977. Reproduced by permission of the Editor, *Journal of Clinical Pathology*).

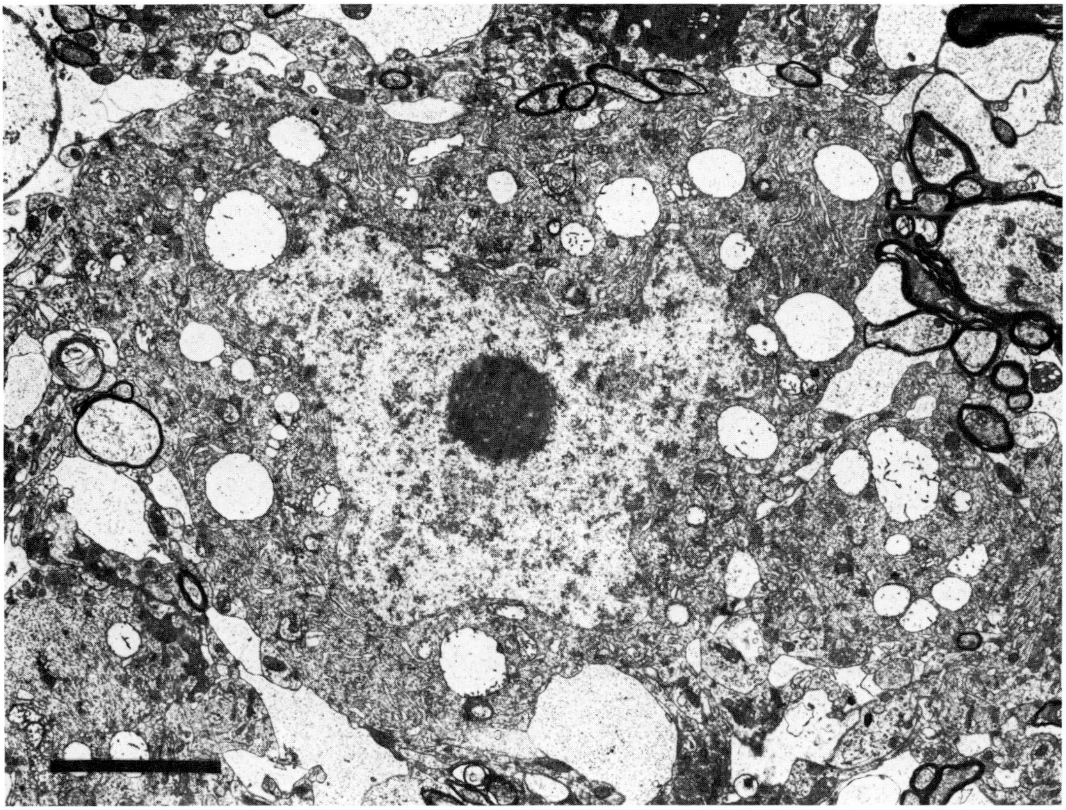

Fig. 1.7 Electron micrograph showing microvacuolation of a pyramidal cell of the hippocampus of a rat as in Fig. 1.6. Swollen mitochondria with disorganized cristae lie within a cytoplasm of increased electron density. The nucleus is irregular in shape. Bar = 5 μm. (Preparation by A. W. Brown).

large in which it has been seen for up to 4 hours after the ischaemic-hypoxic insult.

The stage termed *ischaemic cell change* (Fig. 1.8) develops as a gradual transition from the stage of microvacuolation to one in which the neuron is shrunken, staining darkly with cresyl violet, its cytoplasm becoming markedly eosinophilic and containing finely granular dispersed Nissl substance. The nucleus is also shrunken and often triangular and darkly staining, and the nucleolus may be eosinophilic. Luxol fast blue stains nucleus and cytoplasm bright blue to dark mauve. Electron microscopy has shown increased electron density of the cytoplasm which contains degenerating but usually identifiable organelles and remnants of microvacuoles. A later stage in the ischaemic cell process is the appearance of *incrustations* which stain darkly in most preparations (Fig. 1.9), and are seen on the perikaryon and dendrites. Electron microscopy has shown incrustations to be electron-dense profiles of neuronal cytoplasm, including some derived from the dendrites, formed into projections from the cell surface which is indented and distorted by clear swollen astrocytic processes (Fig. 1.10). Ischaemic cells with incrustations are found as early as 30 minutes in the rat and 90 minutes in the monkey after the hypoxic episode, and they may persist for 48 hours. As Greenfield pointed out (1958) the cells with incrustations are haphazardly distributed, in some areas almost every cell being affected, while in other cases or in other areas in the same case none is seen, although there may be other evidence of hypoxic damage.

A later stage of neuronal morphology observed after a hypoxic ischaemic insult is *homogenizing cell change* (Fig. 1.11). This was first described in Purkinje cells by Spielmeyer (1922) who considered that it was not necessarily due to ischaemia since he observed it in association with infectious and toxic disorders, and Greenfield (1958) believed it to be due to a less severe or less

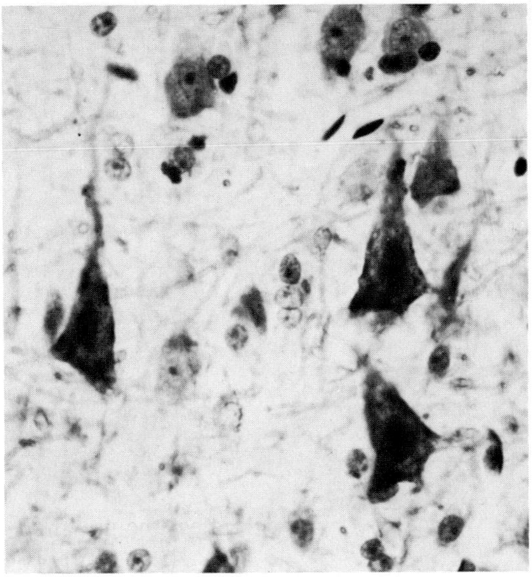

Fig. 1.8 Ischaemic cell change in pyramidal neurons in the cortex of a rhesus monkey 3 hours after a hypotensive episode. The cell bodies are shrunken and the nuclei triangular and darkly stained. Celloidin. Luxol fast blue–cresyl violet ×600. (From Brown, 1977. Reproduced by permission of the Editor, *Journal of Clinical Pathology*).

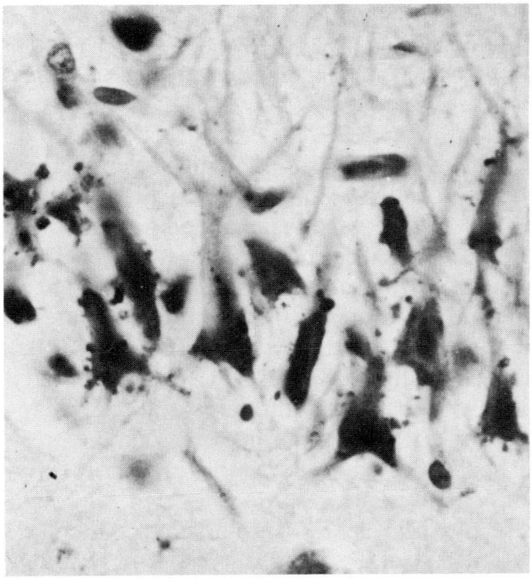

Fig. 1.9 Ischaemic cell change with incrustations is seen in hippocampal neurons of a rat surviving 24 hours after a hypoxic-ischaemic episode. The small dense incrustations project from the cell surfaces. Cresyl violet ×640. (From Brown, 1977. Reproduced by permission of the Editor, *Journal of Clinical Pathology*).

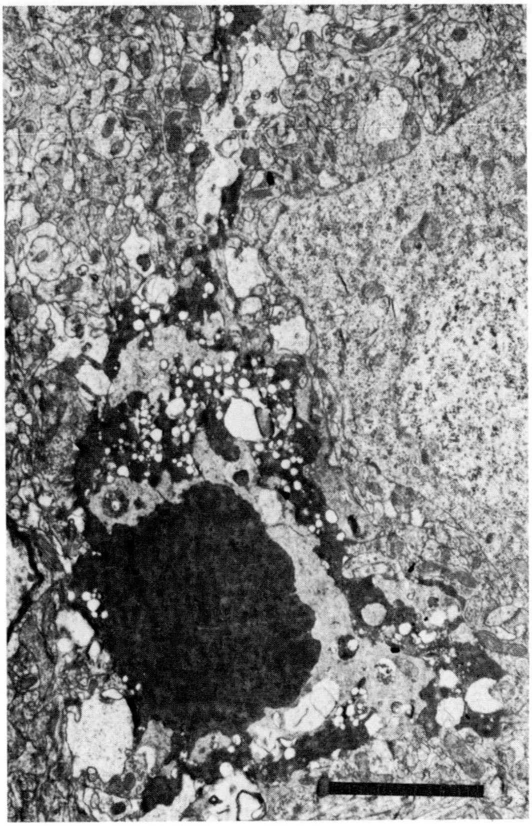

Fig. 1.10 Electron micrograph of a neuron from a rat as in Fig. 1.9. The incrustations are shown to be electron-dense portions of perikaryon and dendrites distorted by swollen astrocytic profiles. Bar = 4 μm. (From Brown, 1977. Reproduced by permission of the Editor, *Journal of Clinical Pathology*).

prolonged hypoxia and to develop at a rather later stage than the other, acute, hypoxic cell changes. However, homogenizing cell change has been seen after a few hours' survival in the rat and primate, and in man and experimental animals may persist for 10 days or more. The cytoplasm is uniformly structureless and eosinophilic while with aniline dyes it may be unstained or yellowish. The nucleus is shrunken and granular or fragmented. Electron microscopy shows evidence of more advanced degeneration with decreased electron density of the nucleus and rupture of the nuclear membranes, dense cytoplasmic organelles and patches of homogeneous, finely granular material at the periphery of the cell. Homogenizing cell change is not confined to Purkinje cells but can be seen in neurons of all vulnerable regions. The end-

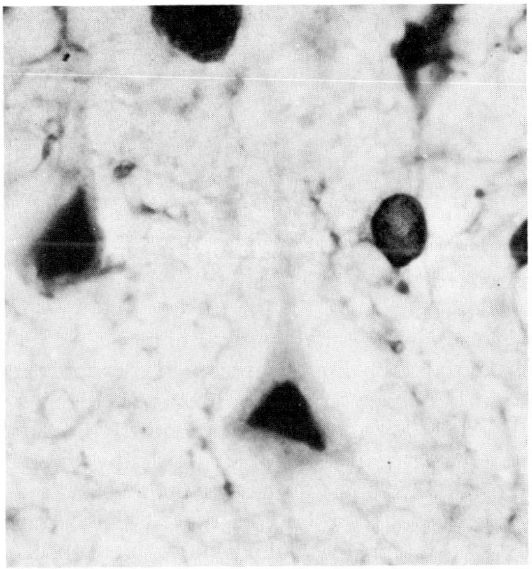

Fig. 1.11 Homogenizing cell change in pyramidal neurons of the cortex of a rat as in Fig. 1.9. The cell is shrunken and no Nissl bodies are demonstrable. The nucleus is densely stained and triangular. Luxol fast blue–cresyl violet × 1300. (From Brown, 1977. Reproduced by permission of the Editor, *Journal of Clinical Pathology*).

stage of hypoxic cell damage is a shrunken pyknotic and fragmented nucleus without recognizable cytoplasm.

Other aspects of hypoxic damage—particularly the glial reaction—are dealt with under other headings in this chapter and in Chapter 4. However, the glial and vascular endothelial reactions are of importance when estimating the time of survival after hypoxic neuronal damage. Astrocytic processes become swollen early in the course of ischaemic neuronal damage and contribute to the deformation of neuronal outlines and the formation of incrustations. An increase in numbers of microglial cells begins within 2 days, and early neuronophagy (i.e. phagocytosis of necrotic neurons) may begin about the same time.

Neuronophagy

When nerve cells undergo rapid death it is common to find their cell body and proximal dendrites invaded by phagocytic cells. When the necrotic process is very acute, as in poliomyelitis, the earliest invading cells may be polymorphonuclear leucocytes, but in later stages the great majority of the phagocytes appear to be derived from either the microglia or macrophages. It is characteristic of poliomyelitis to see groups of these cells, indicating the positions of dead neurons (Fig. 1.12a). When the necrosis of nerve cells is less acute than in poliomyelitis the microglial cells are less numerous and often form a capsule round the cell body or invade it at a few places only (Fig. 1.12b). For this process the term 'neuronophagy', which was given by classical writers, is apt and descriptive. True neuronophagy by microglial cells must be distinguished from *satellitosis*, which is mainly a reaction of oligodendroglia. In the former case the nerve cell is undergoing dissolution, while in the latter case it shows much less evidence of degeneration. Neuronophagy is specially common in all forms of encephalomyelitis which affect the grey matter, and it may be that the manner of death of the neuron has a special chemotactic attraction for microglial cells.

Neuronophagy may be seen in the white matter in childhood involving nerve cells which have failed to reach the cortex in their developmental migration. A very characteristic appearance may be seen in the neuronophagy of Purkinje cells. Here the microglial phagocytes are grouped not only round the cell body but also along the dendrites in the molecular layer where the normal paucity of nuclei makes their increase very obvious. A shrub-like arrangement of cell bodies and short processes is thus formed to which Spielmeyer gave the name Gliastrauchwerk (glial shrub formation). This was first described in typhus fever, but is also seen, affecting few or many Purkinje cells, in some forms of virus encephalitis and also in non-inflammatory processes, for example in the cerebellar degeneration associated with carcinoma.

Other forms of neuronal degeneration

Degeneration and loss of nerve cells is characteristic of many neurological diseases and a discussion of the localization of neuronal loss and its associated pathology is dealt with in many sections of this volume. In many cases with system degenerations, shrinkage ('simple atrophy') of neurons is the principal pathological change. Examples of disease characterized by neuronal atrophy include motor neuron disease, Huntington's chorea, Friedreich's ataxia and multiple system atrophy. The neuronal degeneration is accompanied by breakdown of the axon and its myelin sheath, giving rise to tract degeneration. If the pace of neuronal loss is very slow, there will be little or no evidence at any one time of axonal fragmentation or sudanophilic lipid except for the presence of breakdown products of myelin stainable by the Marchi technique and also by the presence of reactive astrocytic gliosis.

In certain situations neuronal degeneration is associated with the formation of axonal swellings which are packed with dense bodies, degenerated organelles, filaments or tubules. Purkinje cells of the cerebellum characteristically show an axonal swelling, commonly known as a 'torpedo' (Fig.1.13), during the course of slowly progressive degeneration (but not during acute hypoxic changes). Swellings on the proximal axonal segments of spinal anterior horn cells have been observed in cases of human motor neuron disease (Carpenter, 1968) in a canine form of anterior horn cell degeneration (Cork et al.,

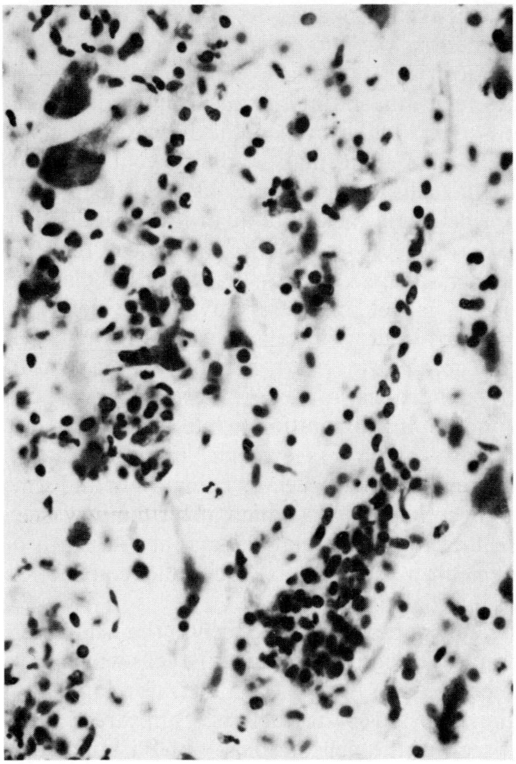

(a)

Fig. 1.12 (**a**) Section of motor cortex from a case dying of acute poliomyelitis. Invading polymorphs and macrophages mark the sites of necrotic large pyramidal cells. Celloidin. Cresyl violet × 350.

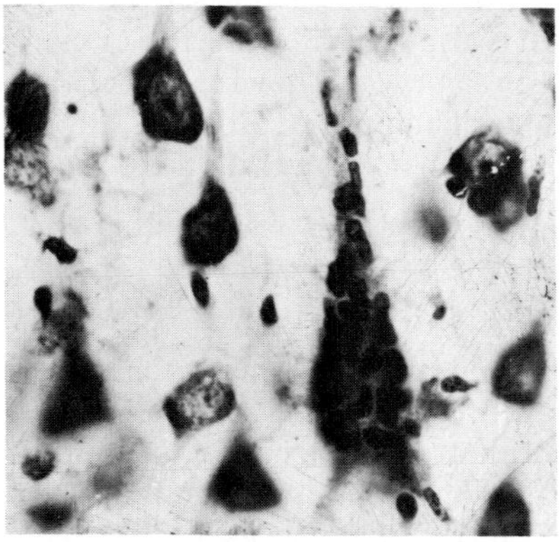

(b)

Fig. 1.12 (**b**) Section of hippocampus of *M. mulatta* surviving 7 days after a hypoxic episode. A pyramidal neuron is surrounded by microglia, the process of neuronophagy. Celloidin. Cresyl violet × 1100 (Preparation by Dr J.B. Brierley)

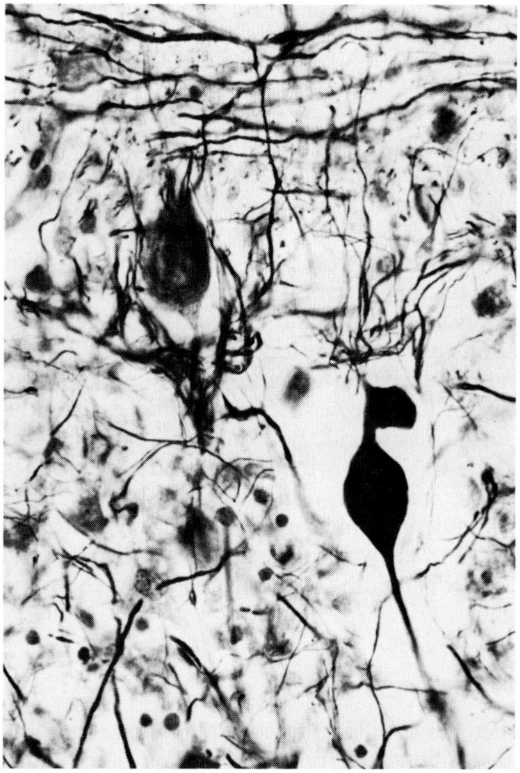

Fig. 1.13 Section of cerebellum from a case of Creutzfeldt–Jakob disease. A swelling ('torpedo') on the axon of a Purkinje cell indicates degeneration of that neuron. Glees silver impregnation × 400.

1979) and in experimental animals given imidodiproprionitrile (Chou and Hartmann, 1964). Aggregations of neurofilaments have also been found in neuronal perikarya and axons after experimental administration of Vinca alkaloids and colchicine. The fact that these compounds cause disruption of neurotubules and impair axonal flow suggests that disturbances of axonal flow and transport may underlie the formation of axonal spheroids.

Vacuolation of neurons is found in several conditions and should perhaps also be regarded as relatively non-specific. It occurs in kuru (Klatzo, Gajdusek and Zigas, 1959) and Creutzfeldt-Jakob disease (CJD) in man and in scrapie in the sheep (Beck, Daniel and Parry, 1964). Vacuolation of neurons is also found in animals experimentally inoculated with material from cases of kuru (Beck et al., 1975). A somewhat different form of vacuolation is seen in neurons of the brain stem and spinal cord (Fig. 1.14) in

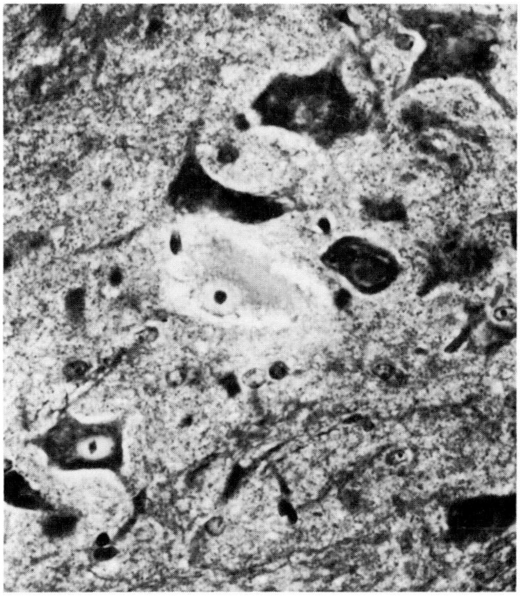

Fig. 1.14 Sections of cervical spinal cord of a *wobbler* mouse. One degenerating ventral horn cell is vacuolated and its nucleus is eccentric. Luxol fast blue-cresyl violet × 350.

the hereditary form of motor neuron disease in the mouse (the mutant *wobbler*). Here the vacuoles appear to arise from distensions of endoplasmic reticulum which then coalesce, ultimately totally destroying the cell (Duchen, Strich and Falconer, 1968; Andrews and Maxwell, 1969; Duchen, 1978).

Binucleated or multinucleated nerve cells have been observed in a number of normal and pathological situations (reviewed by Greenfield and Meyer, 1963). It is generally accepted that the mature neuron is postmitotic but there is evidence that some nuclear division does occur under pathological conditions. Binucleation of neurons may be a rare and non-specific reaction to injury (Beck et al., 1975).

Iron in the nervous system

Incrustation of nerve cells with haematoxyphilic granules (Fig. 1.15) is found in areas of old infarction or, perhaps more characteristically, in areas damaged during perinatal birth injury (see Urich, 1976). The ferrugination of nerve cells confers a positive Prussian blue reaction for iron and also a positive von Kossa reaction for calcium. The presence of calcium as well as of iron has been confirmed by electron-probe analysis of the deposits by Leestma and Martin (1968), who also identified phosphorus and traces of sulphur as well as of other elements.

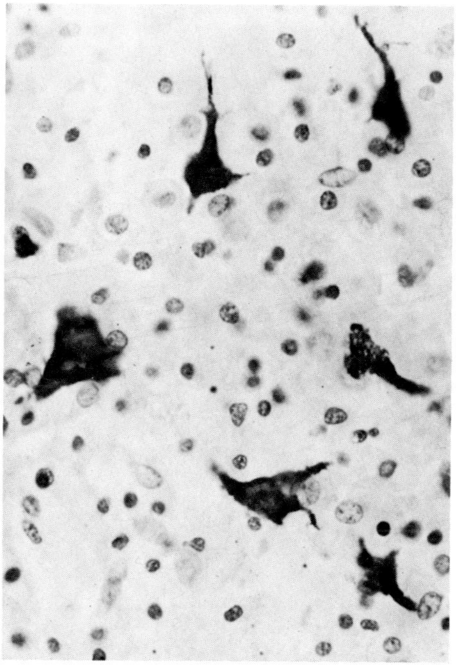

Fig. 1.15 Ferrugination (incrustation with iron and calcium) of neurons in an old ischaemic area of cortex. Haematoxylin and van Gieson × 350.

Deposits of pigment in the globus pallidus are characteristically found in cases with the Hallervorden–Spatz syndrome and in the putamen in striatonigral degeneration. This pigment, which imparts a yellow-brown colour to the tissue macroscopically, gives a positive reaction for iron and also a positive PAS reaction, and is associated with lipid. Granules of pigment may be within nerve cells, but as there is great neuronal loss, most of the pigment is found within microglia and astrocytes.

Haemosiderin deposition after subarachnoid haemorrhage imparts an orange-yellow pigmentation to the meninges, particularly over the base of the brain. This may be visible for a very long time after the haemorrhage, while pigmentation at the site of cortical contusions may also remain permanently. Very extensive haemosiderosis of brain and spinal cord occurs as a complication of hemispherectomy, an operation used for the treatment of infantile hemiplegia with epilepsy. Repeated bleeding into the hemispherectomy cavity leads to infiltration by iron pigment into all surfaces exposed to CSF and encystment of the blood within the cavity. Glial cell hyperplasia and collagenous fibrous tissue may obliterate the ependyma and obstruct foramina, particularly the foramen of Munro on the unoperated side leading to dilatation of the remaining lateral ventricle. The clinical complications of hemispherectomy have been reviewed by Wilson (1970) and the pathology described by Ulrich, Isler and Vassalli (1965) and Oppenheimer and Griffith (1966). A recent modification of the hemispherectomy operation proposed by Adams (1983) may prevent the development of haemosiderosis in the future.

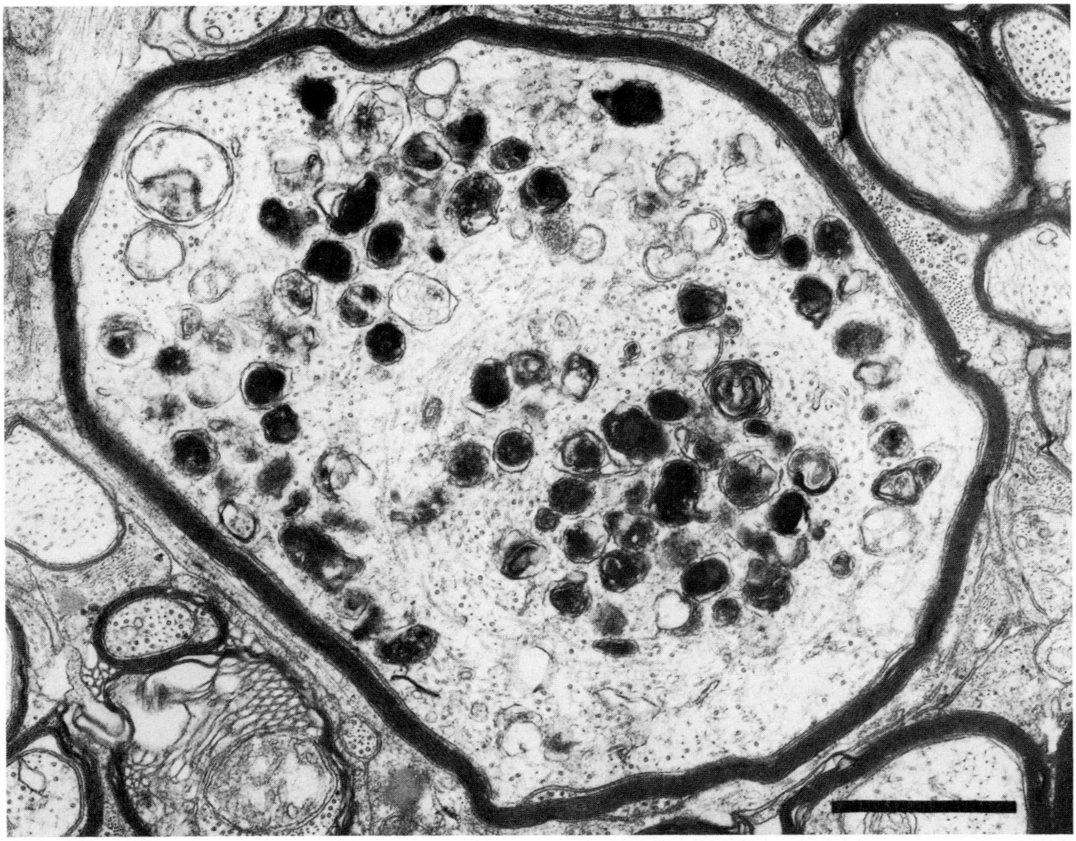

Fig. 1.16 An early stage of nerve fibre degeneration in the CNS. This electron micrograph shows the accumulation of dense bodies, filaments and tubules in the degenerating axon while the myelin sheath is still intact. Bar = 1 μm. (Preparation by Dr Jean M. Jacobs).

Anterograde (wallerian) degeneration in the central nervous system

Degeneration of the entire arborization of a neuron, dendrites, axon and axonal branches, inevitably follows necrosis of the neuronal cell body and its nucleus. The loss of the entire projection of a neuron is a common occurrence, perhaps most frequently seen as a consequence of cortical infarction. Degeneration of part of an axon, with its myelin sheath, will follow its separation from the cell body. This process has been most studied in the peripheral nervous system, and is known as wallerian degeneration following Waller's (1850) original description of the changes he observed after cutting the glossopharyngeal and hypoglossal nerves in the frog, but the same term can be applied to anterograde degeneration in the central nervous system. In the CNS probably the commonest cause of axonal damage is infarction affecting white matter but other situations where axons may be damaged leaving neuronal perikarya intact include trauma, tumours and haemorrhage. Wallerian degeneration in central and peripheral nervous systems share many similarities (see Chapter 18).

Lampert and Cressman (1966) studied tract degeneration in the dorsal column of rats after myelotomy, and Vaughn, Hinds and Skoff (1970) and Vaughn and Pease (1970) studied wallerian degeneration in the optic nerve of the rat. Abnormalities in axons severed from their neuronal perikarya precede changes in the myelin sheath. Within 4 days the whole length of axon degenerates and there appear multiple fusiform swellings of increased electron density and packed with neurofilaments or tubules, vesicular elements and degenerating mitochondria. These organelles soon lose their definition and only granular amorphous debris remains (Fig. 1.16). Light microscopic changes, demonstrable with silver methods, show axonal fragmentation which, with longer survival, progresses so that the argyrophilic fragments become smaller (Fig. 1.17). Various silver impregnation methods have been developed particularly for the demonstration of degenerating axons (Nauta and Gygax, 1954) or degenerating terminals (Fink and Heimer, 1967). Most axonal debris disappears from degenerating tracts within about a month.

The sequence of events in nerve terminals severed from their parent neuron has been much studied (e.g. Brodal and Grant, 1962). Silver impregnation shows densely argyrophilic terminals as blobs or rings—degenerating *boutons terminaux* (Fig. 1.18). Electron microscopy shows a loss of definition of organelles, aggregations of dense bodies and degenerating mitochondria and collections of neurofilaments. In certain situations, such as in the terminals of degenerating Purkinje cell axons (Fig. 1.19), there are usually masses of neurofilaments and little else (Janota, 1974). Colonnier (1964) and Bodian (1971) among others studied the fate of degenerating axonal terminals. The terminals remain attached to the postsynaptic membranes with their thickenings and become invaginated into glial or dendritic profiles. Both astrocytic and microglial cells are involved in the removal of degenerated terminals which disappear within a few days, long before axons and myelin sheaths are removed.

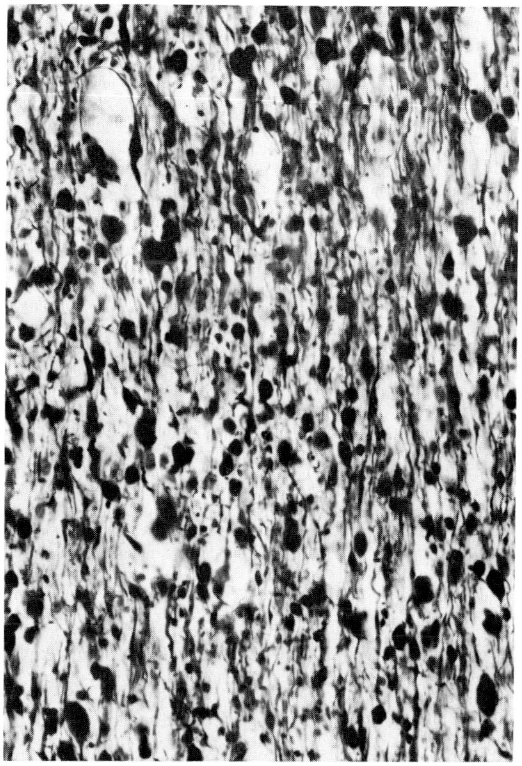

Fig. 1.17 Degenerating nerve fibres in white matter near an infarct of 10 days' duration. Silver impregnation shows the axons broken up into argyrophilic fragments. Glees' method × 300.

Myelin sheaths become collapsed and the lam-

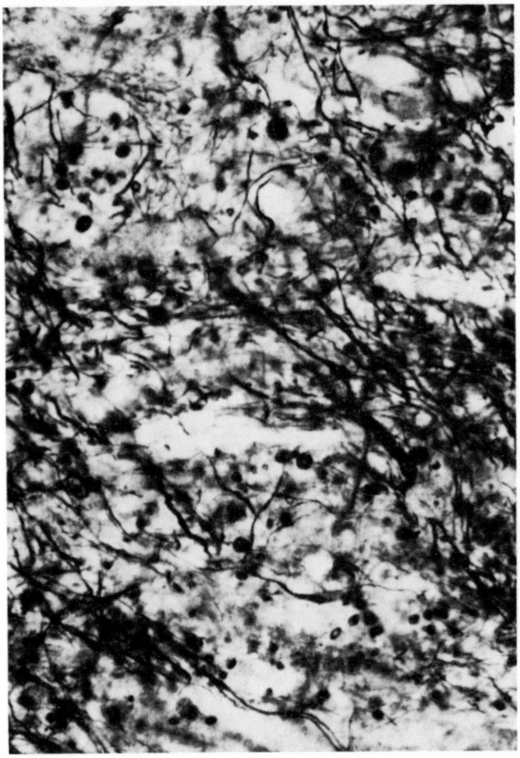

Fig. 1.18 Dentate nucleus in a case with extensive recent infarction of cerebellar cortex. Densely argyrophilic rings or granules indicate degenerating terminals. Glees silver impregnation × 400.

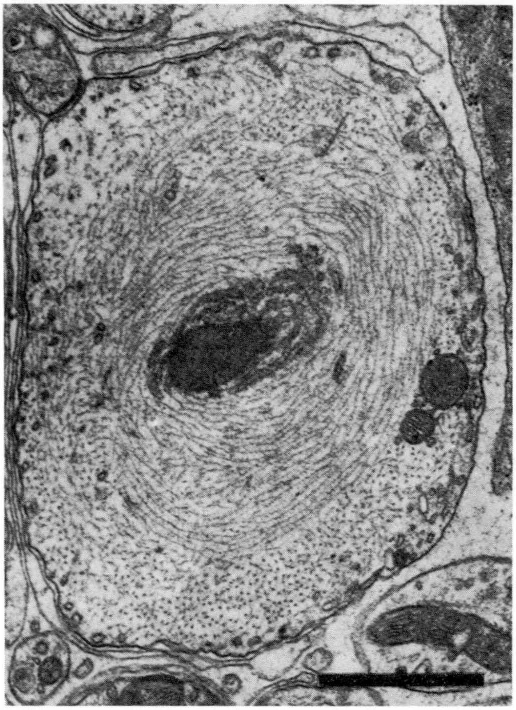

Fig. 1.19 Degenerating terminal of a Purkinje cell of a cat 4 days after cerebellar cortical ablation. There is a marked accumulation of neurofilaments. A few mitochondria and vesicles remain near the axolemma. Bar = 1 μm. (Preparation by Dr I. Janota).

ellae become loose but the myelin sheath may remain intact for up to 52 days. At the site of injury axonal and myelin changes are exaggerated and take place more rapidly. Lampert and Cressman (1966) observed few macrophages containing debris in tract degeneration far from the site of the lesion and noted that astrocytes proliferated and contained myelin fragments. Vaughn and his co-workers (Vaughn, Hinds and Skoff, 1970) observed multipotential glial cells which engulfed myelin and axonal debris and incorporated them into phagolysosomes. They also observed that some astrocytes became phagocytic. With light microscopy the myelin sheaths lose their regular smooth outline and become broken up into ovoids which are readily demonstrable by staining methods for myelin in paraffin sections (Fig. 1.20) or in frozen sections. As the degeneration of myelin progresses, ovoids become broken down into smaller globules. The biochemical aspects of myelin degradation in wallerian degeneration are reviewed by Davison and Thompson (1981). Breakdown of myelin into simpler lipids begins only after 100 days (McCaman and Robins, 1959).

Histological techniques which yield useful information on the state of myelin breakdown include the use of fat-soluble dyes such as Sudan IV, Sudan black or oil-red O in frozen sections, and also the Marchi technique which demonstrates the products of myelin degeneration by osmium tetroxide after the staining of normal myelin is prevented by mordanting in potassium dichromate solution (see Smith, 1951, 1956a, b).

Daniel and Strich (1969) studied Wallerian degeneration in baboon spinal cord where ascending tract degeneration in the posterior columns was initiated by cutting dorsal nerve roots. They found that myelin sheaths break up into ellipsoids within 48 hours but retain the staining properties of normal myelin for many weeks. Increased cellularity in the degenerating tracts was due to the greater number of astrocytes and there were mitotic figures within 10 days. They

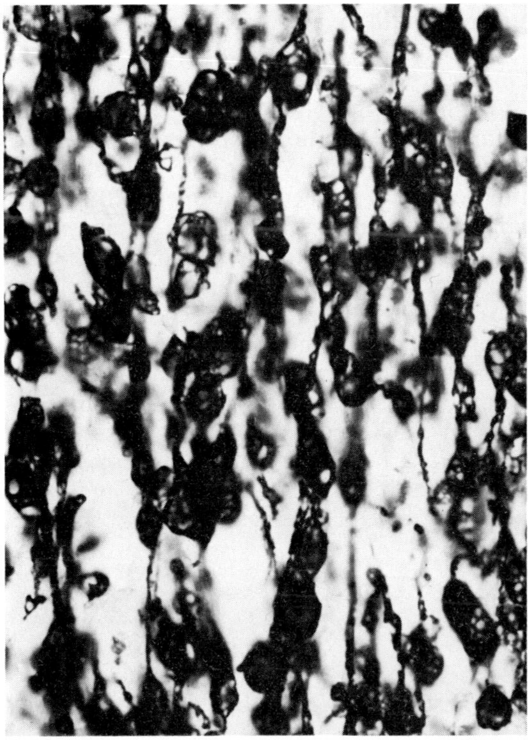

Fig. 1.20 Degenerating myelinated fibres in superior cerebellar peduncle 10 days after infarction of the dentate nucleus. Myelin sheaths are broken up into ovoids. Luxol fast blue–cresyl violet × 400.

noted a remarkable absence of any microglial or macrophage reaction, and lipid phagocytes (fat granule cells) were seen only after 7–8 weeks. In the late stages there were numerous plump astrocytes with only slight fibrous gliosis 1 year after injury but fat granule cells remained visible for many months.

The earliest Marchi-stainable material appears in the CNS within a few days of the onset of wallerian degeneration but for some time is not contained within macrophages. In the early stages the reaction is obtainable only by block impregnation with Marchi fluid and the stainable material is readily removed from the tissues by formalin (Smith, Strich and Sharp, 1956). Later, as the products of degeneration are taken up by macrophages and astrocytes, the characteristics of the Marchi-positive material change and it becomes resistant to prolonged formalin fixation (Strich, 1968).

There is a striking contrast between the peripheral and central nervous systems in the rate at which nerve fibres break down and products of degeneration are removed (Daniel and Strich, 1969). In peripheral nerve, perhaps as a result of the increased permeability of the perineurium after injury and the greater accessibility to circulating macrophages, the breakdown of myelin is rapid and most of the breakdown products are removed within weeks. In contrast, the process of tract degeneration in the CNS is very much slower, lipid-laden cells demonstrable by the Marchi technique (Fig. 1.21) remaining *in situ* for many months or even several years.

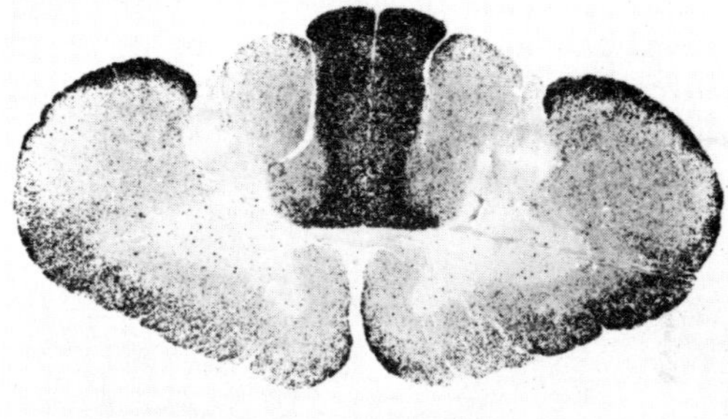

Fig. 1.21 Frozen section of cervical (C8) spinal cord after destruction of the lower thoracic cord by metastatic carcinoma. Products of myelin degeneration in ascending tracts are stained black by the Marchi method. × 6.

Time course of anterograde degeneration

It has been known since the work of Cajal (1928) that axonal degeneration takes place at different rates depending on a number of variables (van Crevel and Verhaart, 1963a, b). Axonal degeneration occurs more rapidly in larger calibre fibres than smaller, in younger as opposed to older animals, and in mammals as compared with cold-blooded animals such as amphibia. In young mammals, large axons show varicosities within 30 hours (Cajal, 1928) while at 4–5 days they become broken up into fragments. Thinner fibres may show the earliest abnormalities only after 10 days. Products of axonal degeneration in the CNS persist and are demonstrable by appropriate techniques for up to 6 months but this varies greatly according to the system under study, and probably the optimal survival time for the use of the Nauta–Gygax technique is much longer than for the Fink–Heimer.

Transneuronal degeneration

Changes occur in neurons when fibres afferent to them are lost. Foix, Chavany and Hillemand (1926) used the term 'trans-synaptic degeneration' for the process because it occurs as a result of loss of synaptic input upon a cell. It seems that the rate at which transneuronal degeneration occurs differs somewhat according to age, proceeding at a slower pace with increasing age. The proportion of a synaptic input lost also seems to be of importance; the more afferents lost, the more likely it is that transneuronal changes will take place.

Transneuronal degeneration has been observed at many sites (see Cowan, 1970). Its occurrence is well known in the lateral geniculate body (Fig. 1.22) after loss of an eye, or lesions of the retina, optic nerve or optic tract (see Kupfer, 1965a, b); in the mamillary body after a lesion of the fornix; in gracile and cuneate nuclei following loss of sensory fibres in the posterior columns of the spinal cord; and in pontine nuclei following leucotomy lesions which interrupt fibres of the prefrontopontine tract (Beck, 1950). In the adult brain the deafferented neurons slowly become atrophied, with the atrophy affecting nucleus, nucleolus and perikaryon with a loss of Nissl bodies (Fig. 1.23). Neuronal cell loss and reactive gliosis occur later (Matthews, Cowan and Powell, 1960; Matthews, 1964). In young experimental animals there are more rapidly developing degenerative changes in neurons and earlier cell loss (Torvik, 1956; Matthews and Powell, 1962).

A different morphological type of transneuronal degeneration occurs in the cells of the inferior olivary nucleus (Fig. 1.24) particularly after lesions of the central tegmental tract. Olivary neurons undergo an initial irregular hypertrophy associated with vacuolation of the cytoplasm during the first few months after the lesion (most commonly an ischaemic infarct within the brain stem or dentate nucleus) together with astrocytic hyperplasia and fibrillary gliosis, but later the nerve cells atrophy and disappear (Gautier and Blackwood, 1961; Sohn and Levine, 1971). Hypertrophy of the olives was also found by Verhaart and Voogd (1962) in the cat 8 months after experimental ablation of the cerebellum and dentate nuclei. In man, olivary hypertrophy, frequently associated with palatal myoclonus, is quite a common lesion (Sohn and Levine, 1971) when the clinical material is derived mainly from an elderly population with many cases surviving for long periods after infarcts.

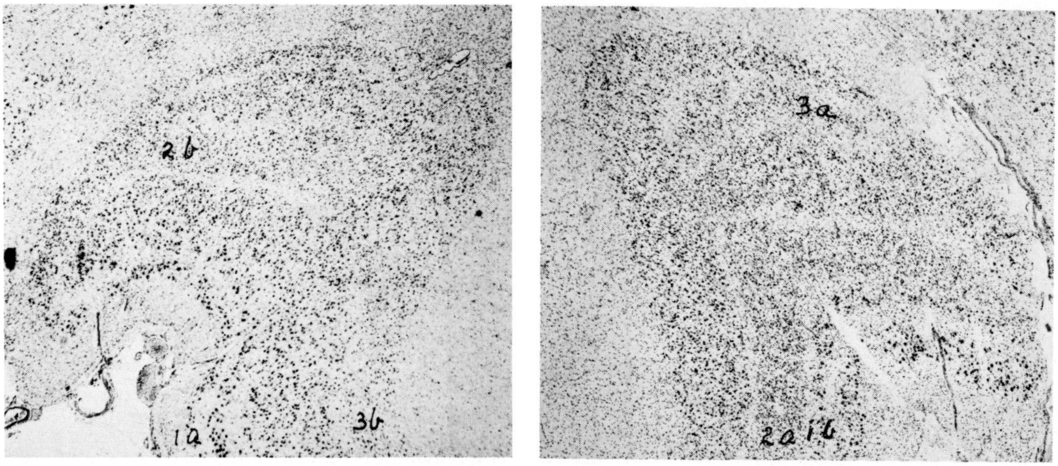

a b

Fig. 1.22 Transneuronal degeneration in lateral geniculate bodies resulting from the loss of the right eye. (**a**) Left side. Atrophy of layers 1a, 2b and 3b. (**b**) Right side. Atrophy of layers 1b, 2a and 3a. Celloidin. Thionin × 10.

The phenomenon of transneuronal degeneration probably plays a part in the slow progression of some 'system degenerations' (see Chapter 15). It may occur as a second-order degeneration at a very late stage after the initial neuronal atrophy. An example of this may be seen in late cerebellar cortical atrophy developing secondary

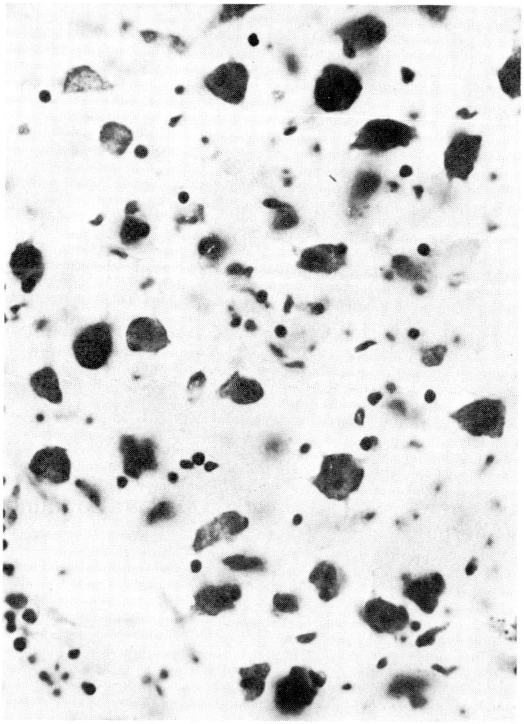

(a)

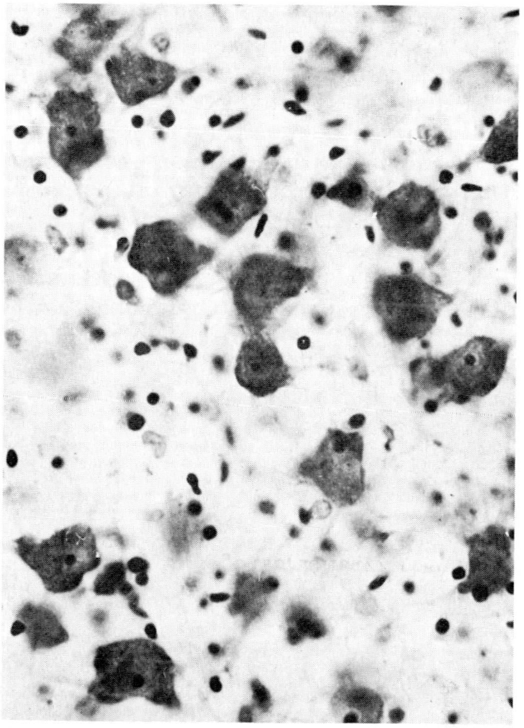

(b)

Fig. 1.23 (**a**) Transneuronal atrophy of pontine neurons in a case where leucotomy had caused a long-standing degeneration of the prefrontopontine tract. Nuclei, nucleoli and perikarya are shrunken compared with normal pontine neurons in (**b**). Celloidin. Cresyl violet × 150. (Preparation by Mrs Elisabeth Beck).

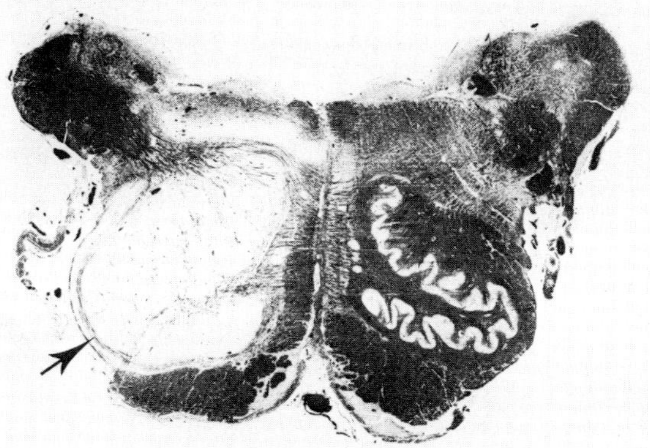

(a)

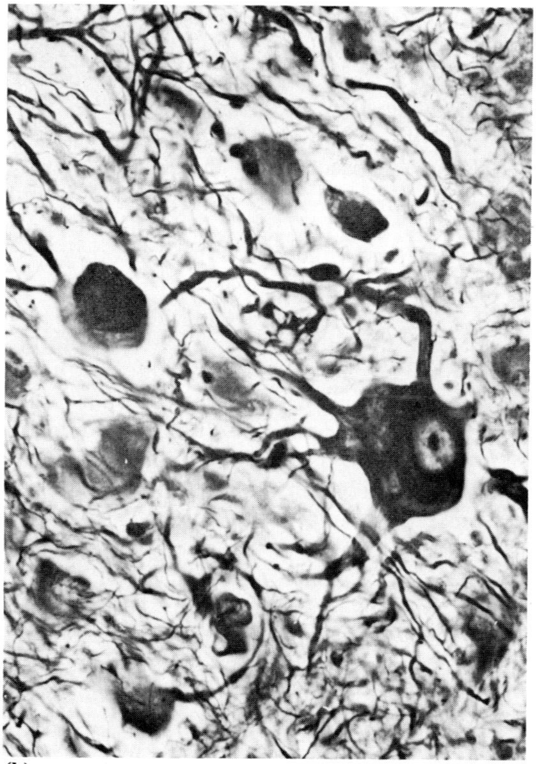

(b)

Fig. 1.24 (**a**) Hypertrophy of the left inferior olivary nucleus (arrow) in a case with infarction involving the central tegmental tract. Celloidin. Loyez myelin stain × 4 reduced to 85%. (From Gautier and Blackwood, 1961. Reproduced by permission of the Editor, *Brain*). (**b**) Hypertrophied and vacuolated neurons in a hypertrophied inferior olive. Palmgren silver impregnation × 400. (Preparation by Dr I. Janota) to a transneuronal loss of neurons in pontine nuclei after corticopontine fibres are destroyed. It is also known that transneuronal degeneration may occur in a retrograde fashion—i.e. changes occur in cells that project on to other neurons which have degenerated (reviewed by Cowan, 1970). Examples of this are known to occur in the visual pathways where retinal ganglion cell degeneration has followed long-standing lesions of optic radiation or calcarine cortex in man (Haddock and Berlin, 1950) and experimental animals (van Buren, 1963).

Chromatolysis

The term 'chromatolysis' is here used synonymously with 'central chromatolysis' and 'the axonal reaction'. None of these names is entirely suitable to describe a process in the neuronal cell body that is a reaction to injury of its axon, first observed by Nissl (1892) and since studied by many authors (see Lieberman, 1971; Torvik, 1976). Although much of the literature concerns the changes studied in experimental animals, the findings are applicable to human neuropathology in which observations on clinical material have yielded much valuable information.

Injury to the axon causes a series of changes in the neuronal perikaryon, which (taking a pyramidal cell as an example) include all or some of the following (Fig. 1.25): the cell body becomes rounded; the Nissl bodies in the central part of the perikaryon become broken up and disappear, leaving only a peripheral rim of cytoplasmic RNA; the central part of the cell is pale, slightly pink with cresyl violet and homogeneously eosinophilic; the nucleus is displaced to the periphery of the cell and may be closely applied to the cell membrane, even distorting its outline; the nucleus may become indented or reniform, the indented surface facing into the cell cytoplasm; the nucleolus may be enlarged. With electron microscopy (Fig. 1.26) the chromatolytic central part of the neuron contains abundant smooth endoplasmic reticulum, dense bodies, stacks of Golgi membranes, vesicles and neurofilaments (Pannese, 1963; Barron et al., 1970; Zelena, 1971). Typically the nuclear membrane is deeply infolded. Most of these alterations are seen also in sensory ganglion cells (see Lieberman, 1971) and sympathetic neurons (Matthews and Raisman, 1972).

Other changes occurring as a result of axonal

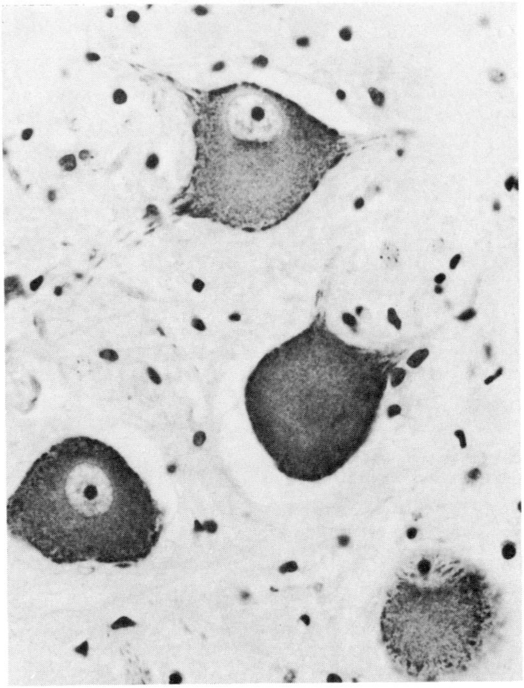

Fig. 1.25 Chromatolysis in anterior horn cells of lumbar cord in a case with long-standing peripheral neuropathy. Note the rounded shape of the neurons, eccentric nuclei, the loss of Nissl bodies from the central part of the cell and their persistence at its periphery. Cresyl violet ×350.

injury include the detachment of afferent synapses observed in axotomized sympathetic ganglion cells by Matthews and Nelson (1975) and in the hypoglossal nucleus of the rat (see Watson, 1974), proliferation of microglial cells and astrocytic hyperplasia around axotomized facial or hypoglossal neurons (Cammermeyer, 1955; Watson, 1974), alterations in cell metabolism (Watson, 1968) and changes in the physiological responsiveness of the cell (Kuno and Llinas, 1970).

There are exceptions to the above description. Some neurons (e.g. Purkinje cells) fail to show chromatolytic changes when their axons are cut. Others, such as the neurons of the facial nucleus of the mouse, show increased cytoplasmic basophilia rather than the expected decrease (Torvik and Heding, 1967). There may be differences among species and there are certainly differences between neuronal systems in the same animal. One example is that a chromatolytic reaction in the sensory ganglion cell develops if the peri-

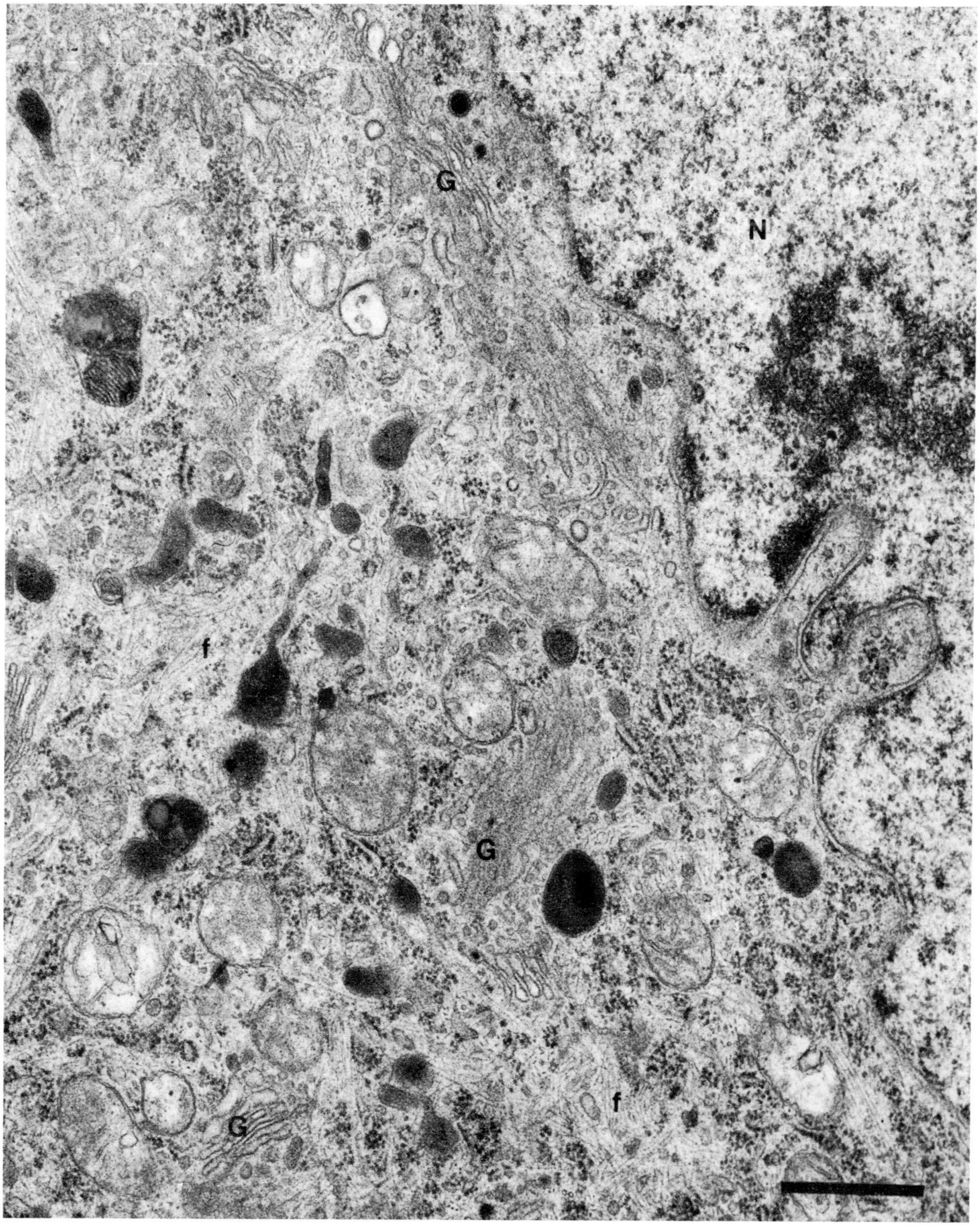

Fig. 1.26 Electron micrograph of sensory ganglion cell showing characteristics of chromatolysis in a *Sprawling* mouse. The nucleus (N) is indented. The perikaryon lacks Nissl bodies but contains many dense bodies, mitochondria, abundant Golgi cisternae (G) and numerous filaments (f) coursing between the organelles. Bar $= 0.5\,\mu m$.

pheral 'axonal' branch is cut but not if the lesion affects the central branch. Furthermore, the axonal reaction occurs where the axon is demyelinated but not interrupted. It has also been observed that axonal sprouting induced by blocking neuromuscular transmission with botulinum toxin (Duchen and Strich, 1968; Duchen, 1970) is accompanied by the neuronal metabolic changes characteristic of chromatolysis (Watson, 1969). Another strange anomaly has been observed in the mutant mouse *Sprawling* in which sensory ganglion cells show the morphological characteristics of chromatolysis in the absence of axonal injury but as a developmental abnormality (Duchen, 1975; Duchen and Scaravilli, 1977). The appearance of chromatolysis is also characteristic of pellagra (see Chapter 13), being visible in neurons in very many regions of the CNS and unlikely to be due to axonal damage.

A number of factors influence the development of chromatolysis and its outcome. The time after injury at which cell changes are recognizable varies greatly, beginning within 24 hours in the facial nucleus of the mouse. Changes may persist for many months. It is a common finding in anterior horn cells of the spinal cord in cases of Guillain-Barré syndrome or other forms of peripheral neuropathy with prolonged survival. As with other reactions to injury in the nervous system, age exerts a considerable influence, neuronal changes taking place more rapidly in young animals than in adults and progressing to total disintegration of the cell. The end-result of chromatolysis varies in different systems, and those cells whose axons project out of the CNS into the peripheral nerves seem most likely to sustain axonal regeneration—cells which include motor neurons of brain stem and spinal cord, sensory ganglion cells, intermediolateral column cells of the sympathetic outflow and cells of the supraoptic and paraventricular nuclei which project into the neurohypophysis (see Daniel and Prichard, 1975). However, neurons whose projections lie entirely within the CNS tend eventually to degenerate. Thus Meyer, Beck and McLardy (1947) observed progressive neuronal loss and reactive gliosis in the dorsomedial nucleus of the thalamus in cases with long survival after prefrontal leucotomy, while extensive studies in experimental animals in which localized cortical ablations have been made has led to the identification of the thalamic nuclear connections with the various regions of cortex.

An important factor in determining the effects on the cell of injury to its axon is the distance of a lesion from the perikaryon. The closer to the cell the injury is, the more severe the outcome with the likelihood of eventual neuronal degeneration. The presence of proximal axonal collateral branches arising between cell body and injury seems to prevent or delay the appearance of chromatolysis and confers a more favourable outcome. Hypophysectomy, pituitary stalk sec-

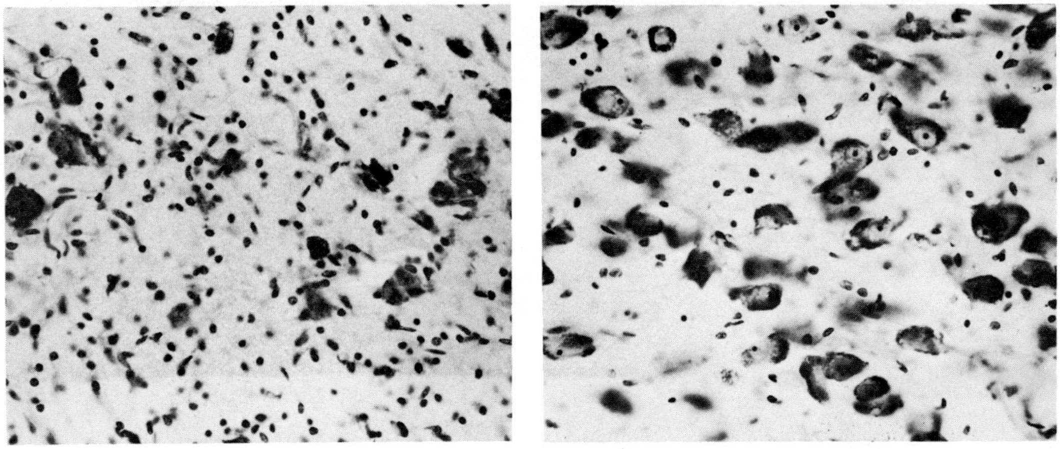

(a) **(b)**

Fig. 1.27 (**a**) Retrograde degeneration in the supraoptic nuclei of the hypothalamus after destruction of the neurohypophysis and pituitary stalk by metastatic carcinoma. Note loss of neurons and marked gliosis compared with normal supraoptic nucleus (**b**). Celloidin. Cresyl violet × 260. (From Duchen, 1966. Reproduced with permission of the Editor, *Journal of Pathology*).

tion or destruction of the neurohypophysis by metastatic carcinoma affects cells of the supraoptic and paraventricular neurons, the severity of effects varying according to the level of the transection of hypothalamohypophyseal fibres. The closer this is to the hypothalamus the more complete the loss of neurons (Fig. 1.27) while in more distal lesions, surviving neurons may show axonal regeneration (see Duchen, 1966; Daniel and Prichard, 1975; and see also Chapter 16).

Recovery of the neuronal Nissl bodies and survival of the cell is more likely to take place when axons are allowed to regenerate and reinnervate their target cells. In peripheral nerves recovery is more likely after crush injury than after complete transection but in young animals both types of injury lead to extensive cell loss (Torvik, 1976).

Special pathology of neurons

Some neuronal disease states are characterized by the presence of inclusions which often imply a specific diagnosis and are readily recognizable. Although each of these changes in neuronal morphology is described in detail in the relevant section of this volume, it seems appropriate to include brief descriptions and illustrations in this introductory chapter.

Alzheimer's neurofibrillary degeneration

A characteristic neuronal abnormality in Alzheimer's disease and senile dementia of the Alzheimer type is the presence of neurofibrillary tangles within the cytoplasm. These are demonstrable by silver impregnation techniques in frozen or paraffin sections and appear as thick black bands, likened to skeins of thread lying parallel to each other or interweaving and forming a basketwork (Fig. 1.28). Often (probably a late stage) the nucleus and cytoplasm fail to stain, giving the tangles the appearance of a racquet or triangle. In the hippocampal pyramidal cells, where these changes are common, the tangles give a tapering or flame-shaped outline to the cell. In many instances, the neurofibrillary tangles have staining properties of amyloid, particularly in hippocampal neurons. Electron microscopy (see Wisniewski et al., 1983) has shown the tangles to be composed of paired filaments, each about 10 nm in diameter, with a space of about 20 nm between them and wound in a helical fashion crossing at 80 nm intervals. Neurofibrillary tangles are also found in the brain stem in postencephalitic Parkinsonism and in the Parkinson–dementia complex, in the cortex of the brains of boxers (Corsellis, Bruton and Freeman-Browne, 1973) and in cases of Down's syndrome surviving into adulthood. Under experimental conditions such as the administration of aluminium, argyrophilic tangles are found but are composed of masses of single filaments.

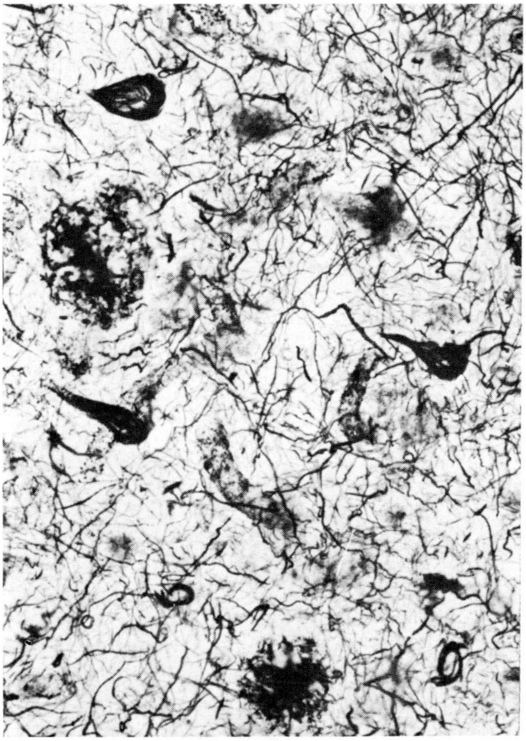

Fig. 1.28 Frozen section of cortex in Alzheimer's disease. Several degenerating neurons contain thick argyrophilic neurofibrillary tangles. There are also two neuritic plaques. Von Braunmühl silver impregnation ×400.

Granulovacuolar degeneration

Small inclusions, consisting of a central haematoxyphilic body (0.5–1.5 μm diameter) and surrounded by a vacuolar space up to 5 μm diameter, are found most commonly in pyramidal cells of the hippocampus (Fig. 1.29). An affected cell may contain several inclusions. Although granulovacuolar degeneration is commonly seen in the brains of elderly non-demented people, the change is usually present in only a small proportion of hippocampal neurons and granules are few in number in individual cells. With increasing dementia an increasing number of cells are affected and granules are more numerous. The pathological changes associated with dementia are discussed in detail in Chapter 20.

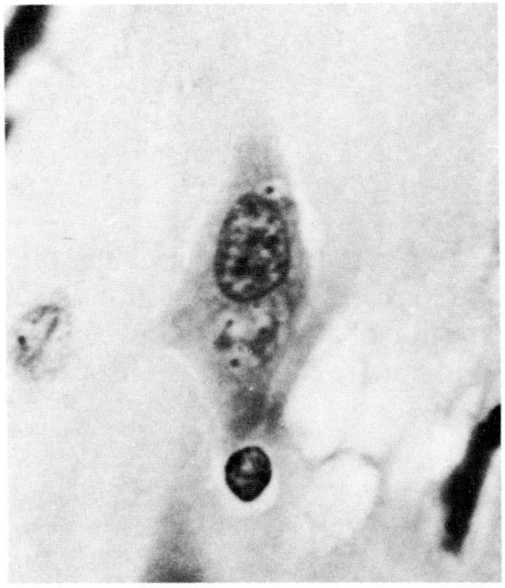

Fig. 1.29 Granulovacuolar degeneration in a pyramidal cell of the hippocampus in a case with dementia. Darkly stained cytoplasmic granules are each surrounded by a clear space. Haematoxylin and eosin × 640.

Swelling and argyrophilic inclusions in Pick's disease

A distinctive type of degeneration in Pick's disease is swelling of cortical neurons. The nucleus in the affected call may be displaced to the periphery while the cytoplasm is ballooned, usually lacks Nissl bodies and stains in a hyaline eosinophilic manner (Fig. 1.30a). These swollen cells

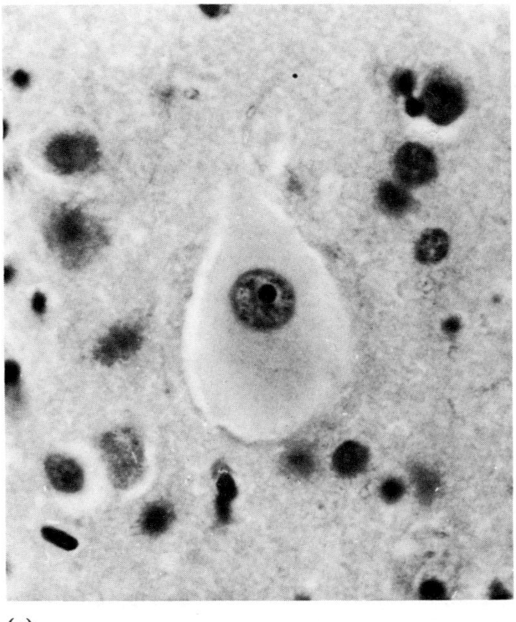

(a)

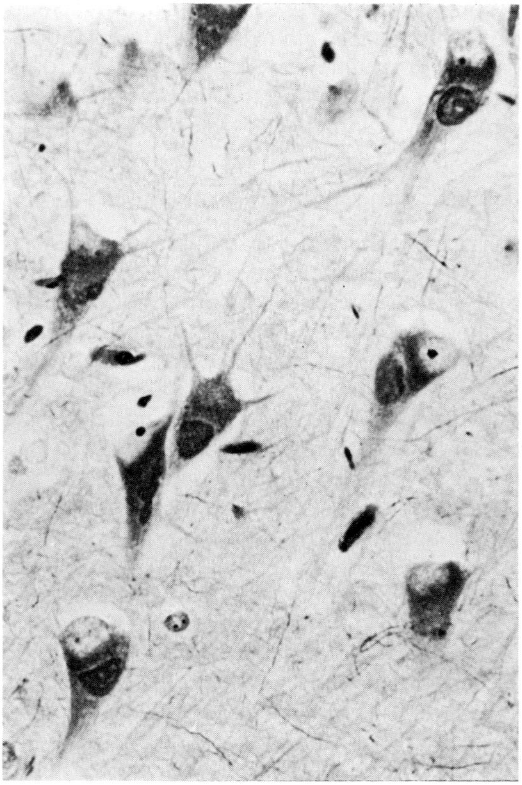

(b)

Fig. 1.30 Neuronal abnormalities in Pick's disease. (**a**) A swollen cell in frontal cortex. The cytoplasm is homogeneously pale and eosinophilic, and lacks Nissl bodies. Haematoxylin and eosin ×640. (**b**) Neurons in the hippocampus contain densely argyrophilic inclusions in the cytoplasm. Von Braunmühl ×400.

closely resemble chromatolytic neurons, which some think they are. They may be neurons which are showing a reaction to axonal injury in the early stages of the disease since in cases with very long histories they may be absent or very few in number, suggesting that these swollen cells eventually disappear (Cummings and Duchen, 1981). Electron microscopy has shown the swollen cytoplasm to be packed with neurofilaments and tubules. Argyrophilic Pick bodies are somewhat different with light microscopy, being demonstrable as fairly well-defined, rounded bodies (Fig 1.30b). The neuronal cytoplasm may be almost completely filled by one of these bodies. Electron microscopy shows these also to consist of masses of tubules and filaments.

Bunina bodies

These cytoplasmic inclusions (Bunina, 1962) consist of small, single or multiple eosinophilic structures which are rounded, elongated or ribbon-like. They have been seen in spinal neurons in amyotrophic lateral sclerosis (Hart et al., 1977) as well as in Betz cells, but Iwata and Hirano (1979) consider them as non-specific.

Lafora bodies

Lafora (1923) described cytoplasmic inclusions in a case of myoclonus epilepsy. These are rounded, concentric bodies with a central basophilic core and a peripheral, paler rim (Fig. 1.31). The core is composed of masses of filaments, and stains strongly with the PAS reaction and metachromatically with cresyl violet (see Harriman and Millar, 1955). They may also be found in axonal or dendritic processes and, probably after degeneration of the neuron, lying freely in the neuropil.

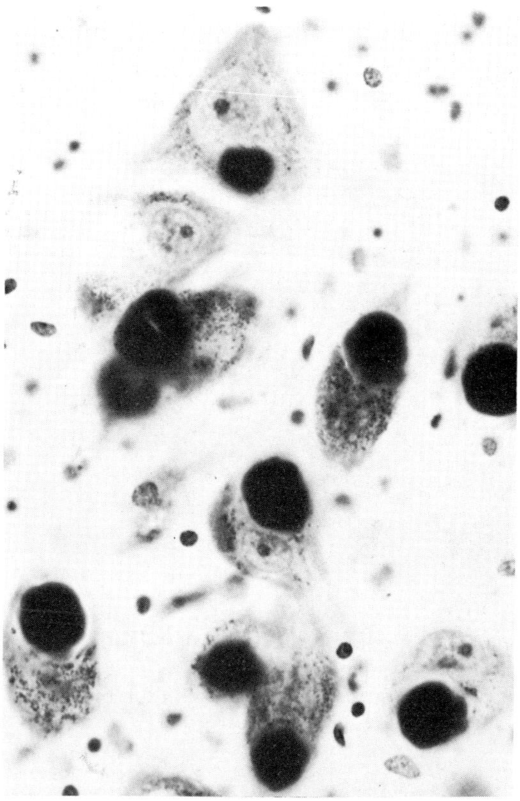

Fig. 1.31 Lafora bodies in neurons of the substantia nigra in a case of myoclonus epilepsy. These rounded inclusions are stained intensely by the periodic acid–Schiff reaction. ×400.

Lewy bodies

Cytoplasmic inclusions, mainly though not exclusively in the pigmented nuclei of the brain stem and characteristic of Parkinson's disease, take the form of eosinophilic hyaline bodies often with a central core and a surrounding pale peripheral rim (Fig. 1.32). They may be single or multiple in an affected neuron. Greenfield and Bosanquet (1953) showed them to be stainable with phloxine-tartrazine and by Giemsa's stain but the eosinophilia of the hyaline core makes them readily seen in routine haematoxylin and eosin preparations. Electron microscopy (Duffy and Tennyson, 1965) has shown the Lewy body to consist of a dense central mass of filaments and granules with a looser, less dense periphery of radiating filaments. The relationship of Lewy bodies to Parkinson's disease and their distribution is discussed in Chapter 15.

Marinesco bodies

Intranuclear inclusions described by Marinesco (see Janota, 1979), which are acidophilic and about the size of a nucleolus or a little larger, occur especially in pigmented cells of the brain stem but can be more widely dispersed. They are increasingly common with increasing age and have been found by careful study in the majority of cases over 21 years of age (Yuen and Baxter, 1963). Their electron microscopic structure is of

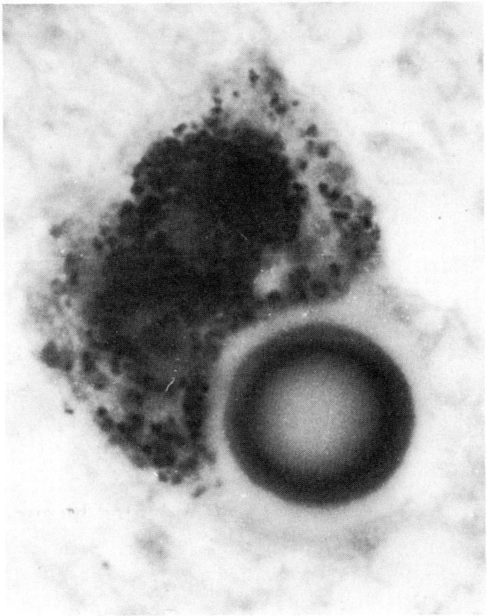

Fig. 1.32 Lewy body in Parkinson's disease. The rounded concentric hyaline inclusion lies in the cytoplasm of a pigmented neuron in locus ceruleus. Phloxine-tartrazine ×1700. (Preparation by Dr D.R. Oppenheimer).

a meshwork of fibrils or filaments about 10–12 nm diameter. It is generally considered that Marinesco bodies have no pathological significance though Janota's (1979) case suggests that at least in some rare instances they may be implicated in the pathogenesis of neurological disease.

Inclusions in lysosomal enzyme deficiencies

A variety of characteristic inclusions is found in the lysosomal enzyme deficiency states. With each recognized deficiency the morphology of the inclusion depends on the nature of the material accumulated which in turn depends on the metabolic disturbance present. The storage of material may affect neurons primarily or white matter as in the leucodystrophies. The morphology and biochemistry of the inclusions are discussed in Chapter 12.

Neuronal inclusions in viral infections

Although inclusions are common findings in viral diseases of the nervous system they may be few and far between, requiring prolonged and careful search, and indeed might not be present in some undoubted cases. Furthermore, occasional neurons may contain inclusions without definite evidence of viral infection. The most common type of inclusion is intranuclear in position and it may be found in neurons or glial cells in infections such as poliomyelitis, herpes simplex encephalitis or subacute sclerosing panencephalitis. In rabies the characteristic inclusion is the Negri body (Fig. 1.33), an intracytoplasmic granular, oval inclusion, eosinophilic and stainable with Giemsa's method. These inclusions should be sought in the brains of test animals (mice) after inoculation of suspect human material. The viral infections of the nervous system are discussed in Chapter 7.

Fig. 1.33 Negri body in rabies. The oval inclusion (arrow) lies in the cytoplasm of a Purkinje cell. Giemsa ×640.

The glial cells

The glial elements of the nervous system include the neuroglia, derived from neuroectodermal 'spongioblasts', and the microglia. The neuroglia, sometimes known as macroglia, consist of the astrocytes, oligodendroglia and ependymal cells. The many reviews of the development and function of glial cells include those by Penfield (1932), Windle (1958), De Robertis and Carrea (1965), Stewart and Rosenberg (1979) and Sears (1982).

Astrocytes

Astrocytes are classified as *protoplasmic* or *fibrous* forms (Figs. 1.34 and 1.35), the former being largely confined to grey matter and the latter to white matter. With light microscopy both types of astrocyte have a rounded or oval nucleus about 7–10 μm diameter with rather homogeneous chromatin. Electron microscopy (Fig. 1.36) shows the nuclei of fibrous astrocytes as somewhat irregular in shape, those of the protoplasmic forms being more rounded. Although appropriate light microscopic techniques show fine fibrils in fibrous astrocytes, electron microscopy has demonstrated that both types contain typical 7–9 nm glial filaments. The outlines of the perikarya differ, in that fibrous astrocytes have a smoother outline while those of the protoplasmic form are irregular as if indented by surrounding structures. The perikaryon of the astrocyte has a low electron density with few

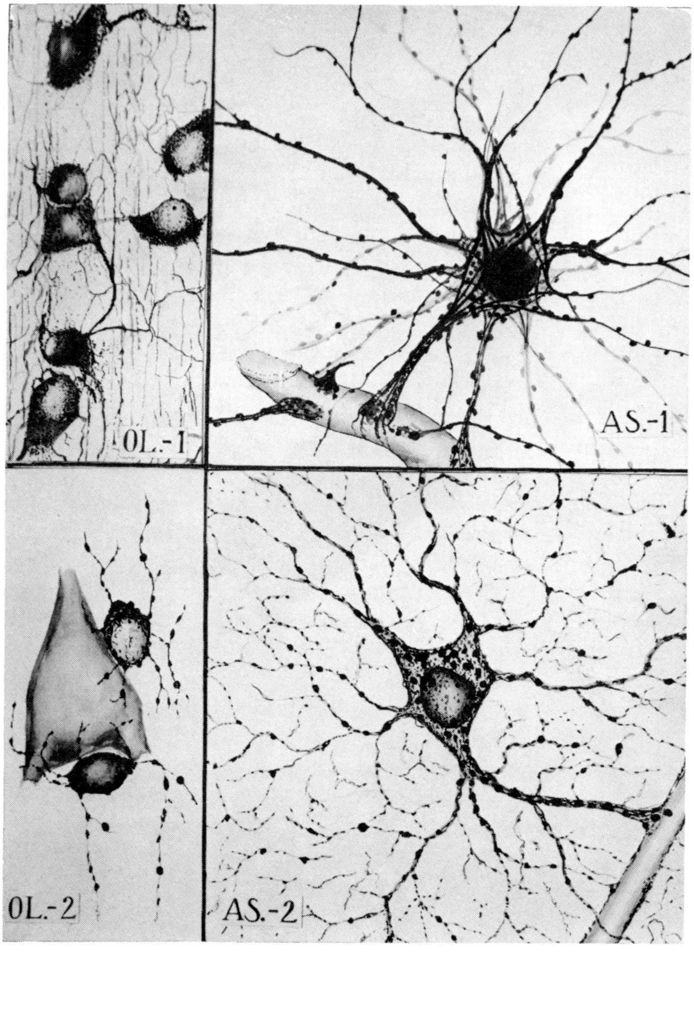

Fig. 1.34 Types of neuroglial cell. AS-1: fibrous astrocyte. AS-2: protoplasmic astrocyte. OL-1: interfascicular oligodendroglia. OL-2: satellite oligodendrocytes. (From Penfield, 1932. Reproduced by permission)

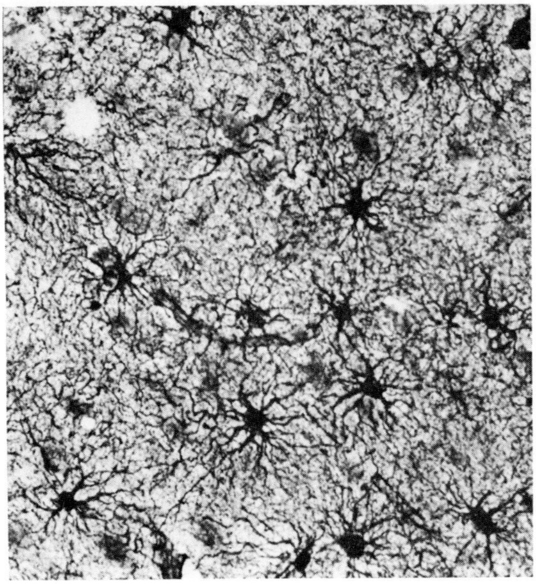

a

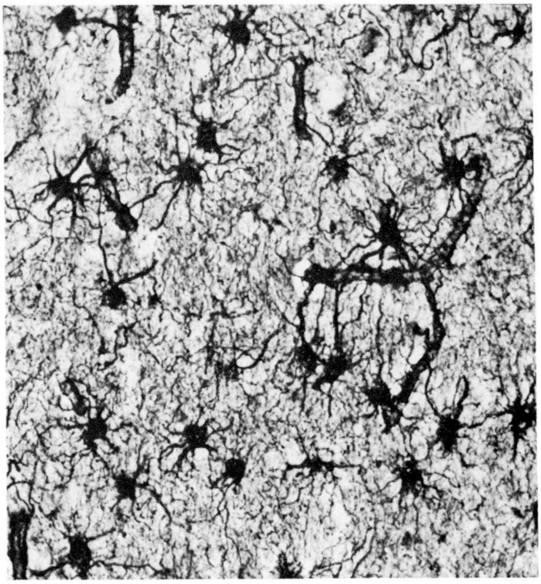

b

Fig. 1.35 Normal astrocytes. (**a**) Protoplasmic. (**b**) Fibrous astrocytes in the cortex. Cajal's gold sublimate × 280.

elongated mitochondria and scanty rough endoplasmic reticulum and Golgi membranes. Glycogen granules are found in the perikarya and processes of astrocytes. Microtubules are numerous in young fibrous astrocytes and decrease with age, whereas filaments increase with age. Microtubules are not found in protoplasmic types. The demonstration of astrocytes in sections for light microscopy is best achieved with special staining methods. In frozen sections Cajal's gold sublimate (see Fig. 1.35) or del Rio-Hortega's silver carbonate methods show the radiating branching processes which may be seen to be attached to the external surface of small blood vessels by a foot process. Capillaries are almost completely surrounded by a layer of foot processes attached to the basal lamina around the vessel (Fig. 1.37). In paraffin sections the method of Holzer and Mallory's phosphotungstic acid–haematoxylin (PTAH) method (Fig. 1.38) are useful though sometimes capricious. In material undergoing rapid fixation such as biopsies or perfusion-fixed animal brains astrocytes often remain unstained by these methods whereas brain tissue fixed only after some *post mortem* delay may show much better astrocyte staining. A disadvantage of the PTAH method is that myelin is also stained. A useful method for demonstrating glial fibres is the use of polarized light which shows them as birefringent fine processes distinguishable from collagen without much difficulty.

Fibrous astrocyes are present throughout the central nervous system. In certain regions of grey matter protoplasmic forms predominate and fibrous astrocytes are found only around the larger vessels. These regions include the 3rd, 4th and 5th layers of the cortex, the caudate nucleus (except beneath the ependyma),the putamen and the substantia gelatinosa Rolandi. The globus pallidus contains fibrous astrocytes in the bundles of myelinated nerve fibres which traverse it and around the blood vessels. There is a thick feltwork of glial fibres in subependymal tissue especially marked around the aqueduct, in the 4th ventricle and in the central canal of the spinal cord. There is also always a layer of subpial glial fibres (Fig. 1.39) in the cortex and spinal cord. With increasing age there are more glial fibres in these situations while in the inferior olives there is always, even in young adult brains, a dense meshwork of glial fibres not necessarily associated with cell degeneration or cell loss. The astrocytes of the cerebral and cerebellar white matter normally form only a loose meshwork which is not prominent in Holzer or PTAH preparations. Protoplasmic astrocytes form one of the group of glial cells which are satellites to

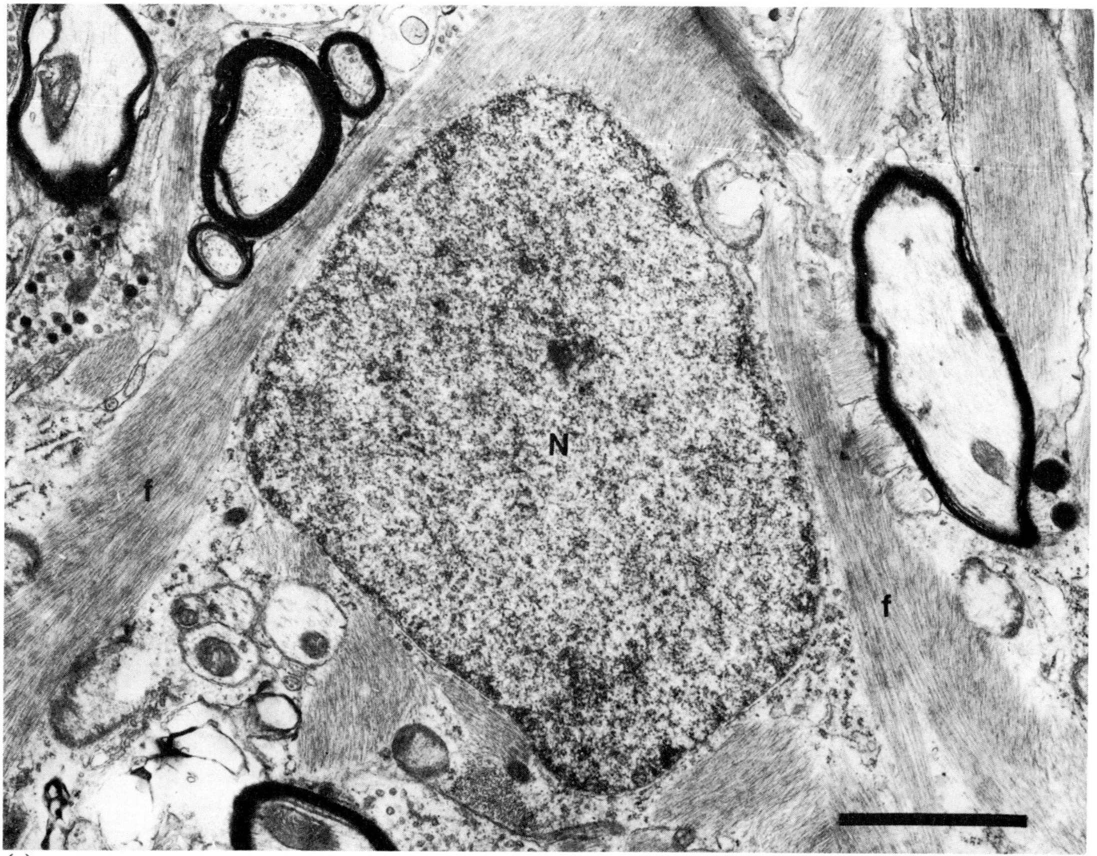

(a)

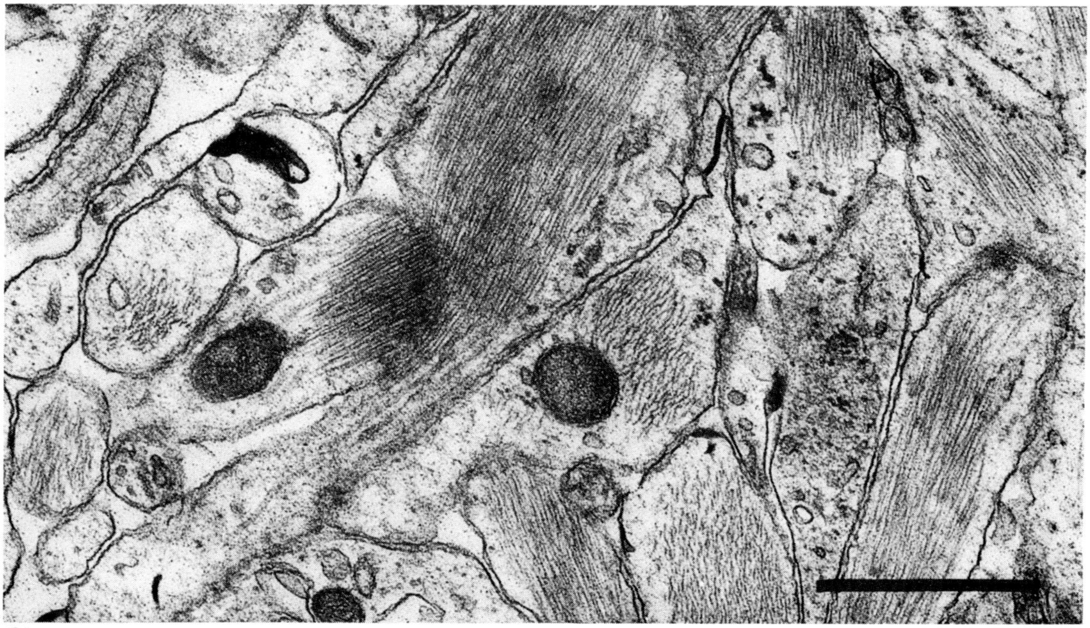

(b)

Fig. 1.36 (**a**) Electron micrograph showing an astrocyte in a cortical biopsy. The nucleus (N) contains finely granular, evenly dispersed chromatin. Bundles of filaments (f) lie in the cytoplasm. Bar = 5 μm. (**b**) Profiles containing astrocytic glial filaments. Granules of glycogen are also shown. Bar = 1 μm.

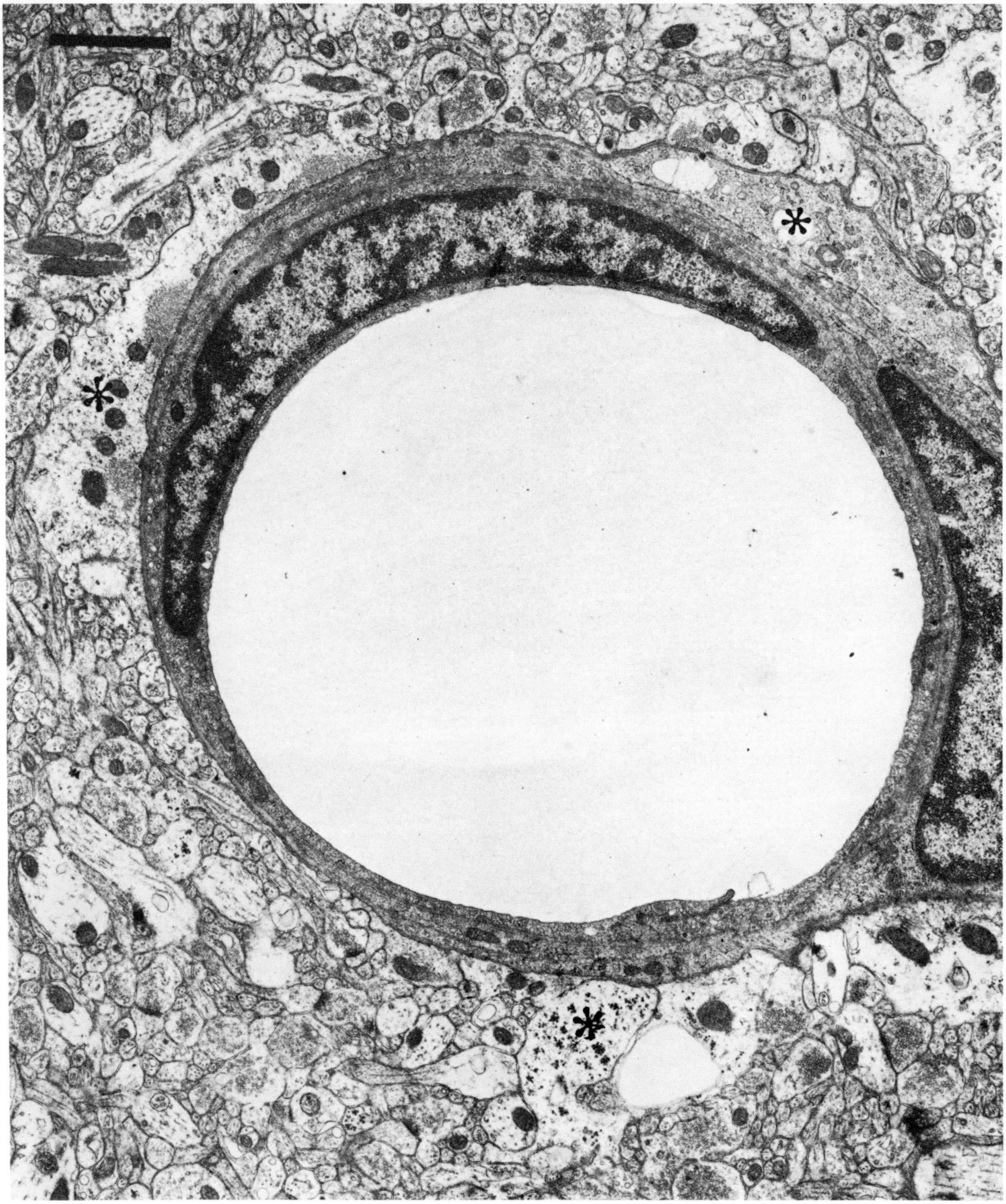

Fig. 1.37 Electron micrograph showing attachment of astrocytes to the basal lamina around a cerebral capillary. Astrocytic processes (✻) contain filaments or granules of glycogen. Bar $= 2\,\mu m$.

neuronal perikarya and their processes tend to be thin and flat and closely invest neurons and their processes except at synapses.

In the cerebellar cortex the granular layer contains only protoplasmic astrocytes while in molecular layer the Bergmann astrocytes, fibrous in type (also known as Golgi epithelial cells), lie in the same plane as the Purkinje cells

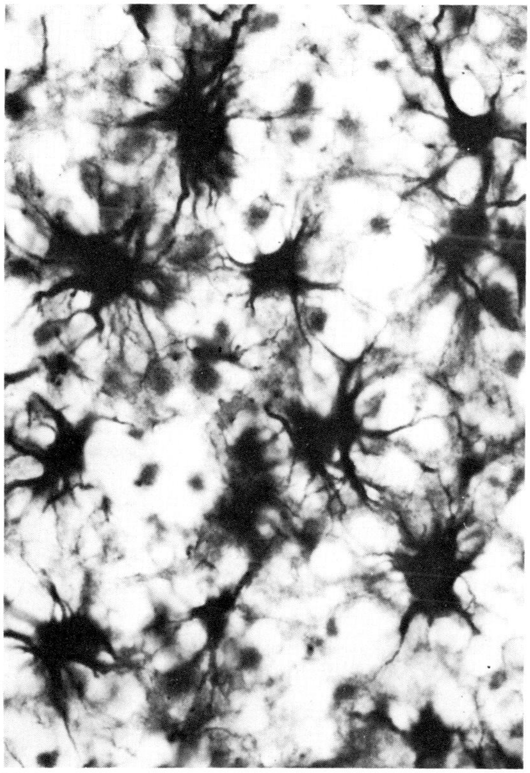

(a)

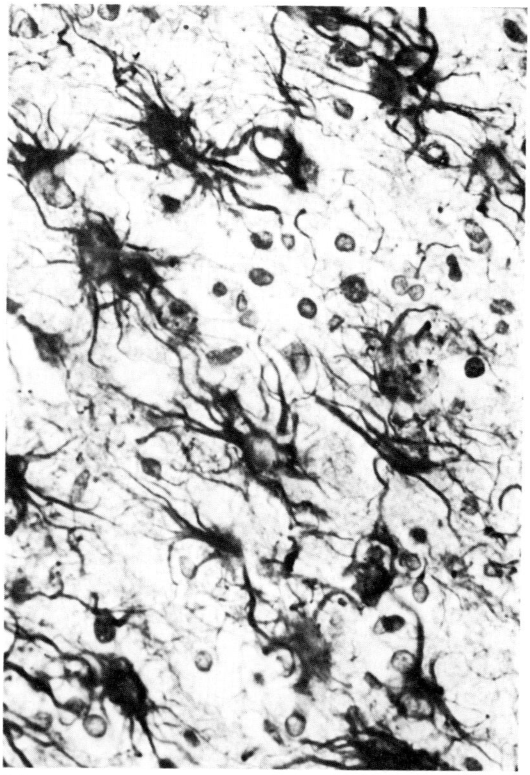

(b)

Fig. 1.38 Hypertrophy and hyperplasia of protoplasmic astrocytes in the cortex in Creutzfeldt-Jakob disease. (**a**) Cajal's gold sublimate ×400. (**b**) Holzer's method ×400.

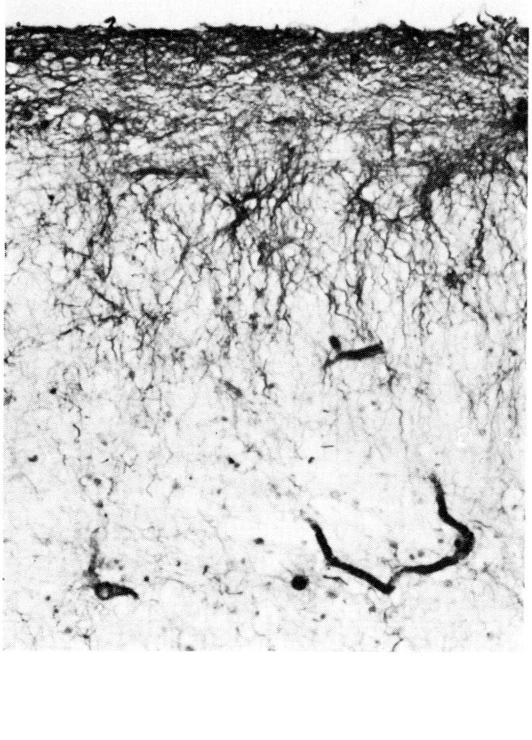

usually as a layer one cell in thickness. Processes from the Bergmann cells radiate through the molecular layer perpendicular to the surface and are attached by footplates to the pia.

In most astrocytes the nucleus is normally diploid. In a study of Bergmann astrocytes, Mann and Yates (1979) found tetraploid cells only in the human and chimpanzee cerebellum.

Functional properties of astrocytes

Although astrocytes clearly play a structurally supportive role in the central nervous system we now have abundant evidence that this is not their only function, and there may be specialized subclasses of astrocytes performing different functions. During fetal development, the radial glia are of importance in guiding migrating neurons to their permanent positions in the cortex of both

Fig. 1.39 Subpial astrocytic fibres in the spinal cord of an elderly patient without neurological disease. Holzer's method ×160.

cerebrum and cerebellum (Rakic, 1971, 1972). An insulating role for astrocytes is suggested by electron microscopy (Peters, Palay and Webster, 1976), which shows astrocytic processes tending to surround and isolate the synaptic surfaces of neurons particularly in the anterior horns and the substantia gelatinosa of the spinal cord and in the cerebellum (see Palay and Chan-Palay, 1974). Purkinje cells tend to be closely surrounded by processes derived from Bergmann astrocytes while processes of the velate astrocytes (i.e. having veil-like processes) in the granule cell layer surround the glomeruli and separate them from each other.

Functional relationships between neurons and astrocytes have been postulated because of their close structural relationships as well as from biochemical evidence (see Orkand, 1982). Neuronal activity is accompanied by a marked increase in extracellular K^+ concentration. Astrocytic glial cells could be of importance in the regulation of the ionic composition of extracellular fluid since they are known to be selectively permeable to K^+, taking up this ion avidly (Hertz, 1978), and it has been postulated that K^+ may be distributed among astrocytes through gap junctions between their processes.

Other metabolic roles for astrocytes concern Ca^{2+}, which has been observed in these cells (Gambetti et al., 1975), and neurotransmitters GABA, glutamate and amines (see Hertz, 1977). Glial cells are known to be capable of taking up neurotransmitters. In the peripheral nervous system Schwann cells may take up and release acetylcholine as a concomitant of axonal terminal degeneration (Miledi and Stefani, 1970), and glial cells may behave similarly in the CNS. The reaction of astrocytes to kainic acid, a structural analogue of glutamic acid, added to organotypic cerebellar culture (Renkawek, Matyja and Mossakowski, 1982) is in keeping with the astrocyte's ability to take up glutamate, as is the presence of glutamine synthetase (Martinez-Hernandez, Bell and Norenberg, 1977). This latter enzyme is localized in, and restricted to, astrocytes and could facilitate the return of glutamine to neurons by taking up and converting glutamate released during neuronal activity.

The enzyme cytochemistry of normal astrocytes has been extensively studied (see Oehmichen, 1980). Friede (1962) showed that there is normally little oxidative enzyme activity. Succinic dehydrogenase, DPN and TPN-diaphorase and cytochrome oxidase activity were hardly demonstrable except in ependyma, which showed strong DPN-diaphorase activity. These observations were confirmed by other authors. Koenig and Barron (1963) observed glutamate dehydrogenase activity. Glycogen-synthesizing enzymes, such as phosphorylase, can be correlated with the presence of glycogen in astrocytic processes on electron microscopy. Schmechel, Marangos and Brightman (1978) studied the localization of various forms of enolase (2-phospho-D-glycerate hydrolase) and found that one of the isoenzymes, termed a non-neuronal enolase, could be a specific marker enzyme of astrocytes. Immunocytochemistry showed its presence in astrocytic perivascular and subpial processes.

Astrocytic fibrils have, in recent years, been shown to consist of an acidic protein which has been characterized, purified and used as an antigen. It is now generally accepted that glial fibrillary acidic protein (GFAP) is a major component of astrocyte filaments, and is chemically and immunologically distinct from other proteins of filamentous or tubular origin (reviewed by Eng and DeArmond, 1983). The use of immunocytochemical (direct immunofluorescence or immunoperoxidase) techniques has greatly facilitated research in diagnostic neuropathology, particularly in the identification of human tumours (see DeArmond, Eng and Rubinstein, 1980), in the study of experimental tumours as demonstrated by Vandenberg et al. (1976) and in neuro-ontogeny. Embryonic cells, such as the radial glia, and cells in tissue culture can now be identified by the presence of GFAP, and have enabled plasticity in the development of glial cells to be recognized with certainty. Raff, Miller and Noble (1983) showed in tissue culture by the use of a double labelling technique (GFAP antibody and the monoclonal antibody A2B5) that a glial precursor may develop into either an astrocyte or an oligodendrocyte depending on the conditions of culture.

Plasticity in glial cell proliferation was demonstrated by Privat, Valat and Fulcrand (1981) who showed with tritiated thymidine labelling that primitive glioblasts developed into different types of glial cell under different conditions. The absence of axons led to a reduction in oligodendrocyte formation and an absence of the astrocyte proliferation ('myelination gliosis') that usually accompanies myelination.

Reaction of astrocytes to injury

Astrocytes show changes in response to almost every type of injury or disease in the central nervous system. Their reactions may take the form of degeneration, hypertrophy or hyperplasia. It does not seem that there are significant differences between protoplasmic and fibrous astrocytes in their responses to injury, and in all the progressive reactions abundant glial fibrils, demonstrable by anti-GFAP antibody, are formed.

In anoxic-ischaemic insults to the brain, astrocytes undergo degeneration in areas of complete infarction but are less vulnerable than neurons since at the margins of lesions, astrocytes survive where neurons die. There is very little information in the literature on the vulnerability of glial cells to hypoxia, but Collewijn and Schadé (1965) studied the size of astrocytes using freeze-substitution techniques and glial staining and found that 10 minutes of experimentally induced cardiac arrest caused shrinkage of astrocyte cell bodies to about a quarter of their normal size while oligodendrocytes increased in size by a third. They also found that astrocytes were smaller at 20°C than at 37°C.

Degenerative changes in astrocytes include cytoplasmic swelling, the disintegration of their processes into granules and the appearance of lipid droplets in the cytoplasm. The disintegration of processes was named *clasmatodendrosis* (breaking up of branches) by Cajal. The nucleus becomes pyknotic, undergoes karyorrhexis and eventually disappears.

Hypertrophy and hyperplasia of astrocytes (see Fig. 1.40) are common findings. Loss of neurons from any cause, breakdown of myelin or injury to nerve fibres, is followed by an increase in the number of astrocytes and, with increasing survival times, a progressive increase in the formation of glial fibres. In some instances the astrocytic hypertrophy and hyperplasia seem out of proportion to the degree of neuronal or axonal and myelin loss. Characteristically, intensely gliotic tissue is firmer than normal and tends to appear grey and translucent as in plaques of multiple sclerosis. Glial fibrils also form a dense meshwork around old softenings and line syringomyelic cavities. In any neuropathological study, therefore, one of the surest indicators of abnormality in the CNS is the finding of excessive numbers of astrocytes and their fibres.

For many years it was considered that astrocytes did not undergo mitosis but proliferated amitotically. This is now known not to be the case. Lapham (1962) found an increase in size and doubling of DNA content of astrocytic nuclei, using microspectrophotometry, but did not see mitotic figures among reactive astrocytes in human *post mortem* material. Cavanagh and Lewis (1969) and Cavanagh (1970) identified mitotic figures in astrocytes reacting around needle tracks in the rat brain. Bignami and Ralston (1969) found astrocytes in mitosis in experimental Wallerian degeneration in the CNS. The most conclusive evidence for the occurrence of mitosis in astrocytes has been provided by Latov et al. (1979) who showed, by combining autoradiography of tritiated thymidine-labelled nuclei and GFAP staining, that astrocytic fibrils and radio-labelled nuclei occurred in the same cell. Proliferation of astrocytes may take place soon after injury, Cavanagh (1970) finding the mitotic index at its maximum 2–3 days after a needle wound in the rat brain. The distribution of chromosomes in the metaphase stage of mitosis of astrocytes is particularly characteristic (Fig. 1.40) and can often be seen around tumours in biopsy material as well as in experimental animals, for example in the pituicytes of the neurohypophysis of rats given hypertonic saline (Duchen, 1962).

Hypertrophy of astrocytes is seen in acute as well as in chronic processes. In oedematous white matter (Fig. 1.41) such as around an abscess or tumour the astrocytes become enlarged and rounded and have an eosinophilic homogeneous cytoplasm with a rather poorly defined outline and sometimes containing a few granules or vacuoles. The nucleus is often slightly enlarged, lies eccentrically, close to the edge of the cytoplasm and there may be two nuclei in the cell. These cells are known as *reactive* or *gemistocytic* (swollen-bodied) astrocytes. They are strongly stained by immunoperoxidase methods for GFAP (Fig. 1.42). Resolution of acute lesions and of white matter oedema is followed by shrinkage of these cells and the extensive formation of glial fibres, leaving a permanently abnormal gliotic tissue as an indicator of previous damage.

Evidence for proliferation of astrocytes may be seen in the cortex, especially in conditions such as subacute sclerosing panencephalitis in which the evidence for neuronal loss may not be

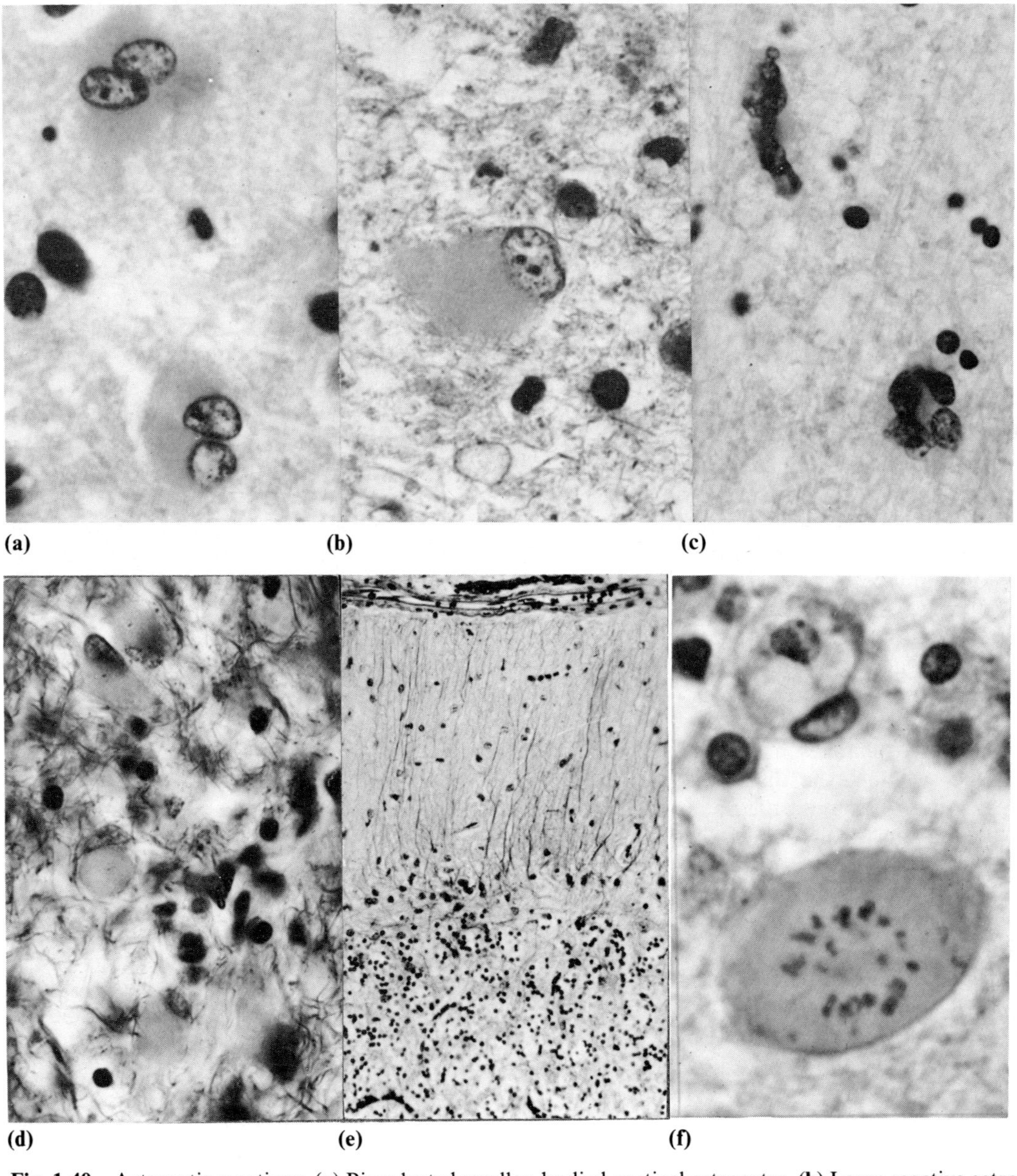

Fig. 1.40 Astrocytic reactions. (**a**) Binucleated swollen-bodied cortical astrocytes. (**b**) Large reactive astrocyte in white matter. (**c**) Irregular multinucleation of astrocytes in oedematous white matter around an abscess. (**d**) Swelling and hyperplasia of astrocytes with fibre formation in diffuse sclerosis. (**e**) Isomorphous gliosis in molecular layer of cerebellar cortex. (**f**) Mitotic figure in astrocyte in white matter. (**a**)–(**e**) PTAH. (f) Haematoxylin and van Gieson.

readily detected (Fig. 1.43). Nuclei of astrocytes may be seen in pairs or groups of four or more, indicating previous nerve cell death.

In chronic, slowly progressive conditions such as leucodystrophy or in oedematous white matter of long-standing, the astrocytic cells may become markedly enlarged (see Fig. 1.40). The cytoplasm is rounded and eosinophilic, measuring 25 μm in diameter or more and showing few processes.

The immediate factors stimulating hypertrophy and hyperplasia of astrocytes when there has

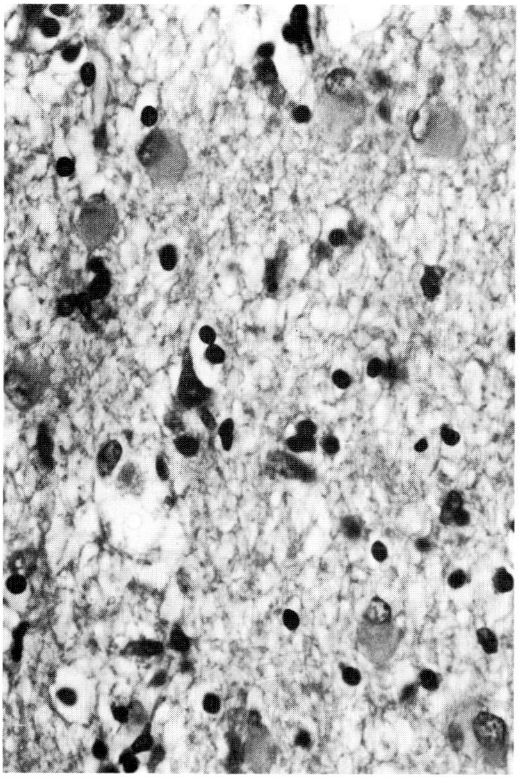

Fig. 1.41 Oedematous white matter showing numerous reactive astrocytes. These reactive cells have abundant homogeneous eosinophilic cytoplasm. PTAH ×350.

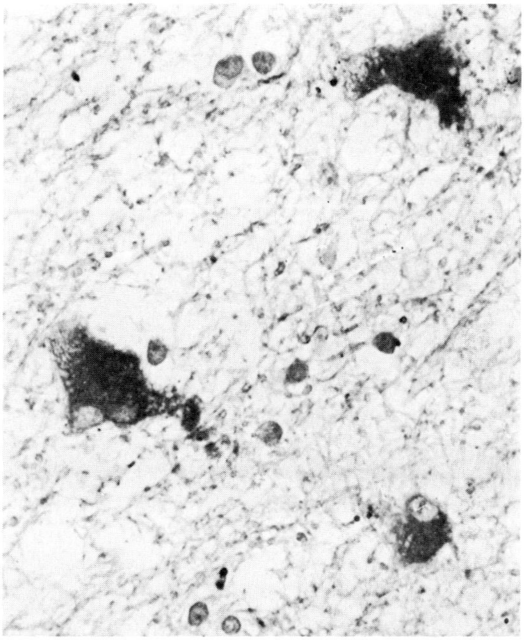

Fig. 1.42 Reactive astrocytes in oedematous white matter. The cytoplasm of these cells is strongly positive for GFAP by immunoperoxidase staining. ×400.

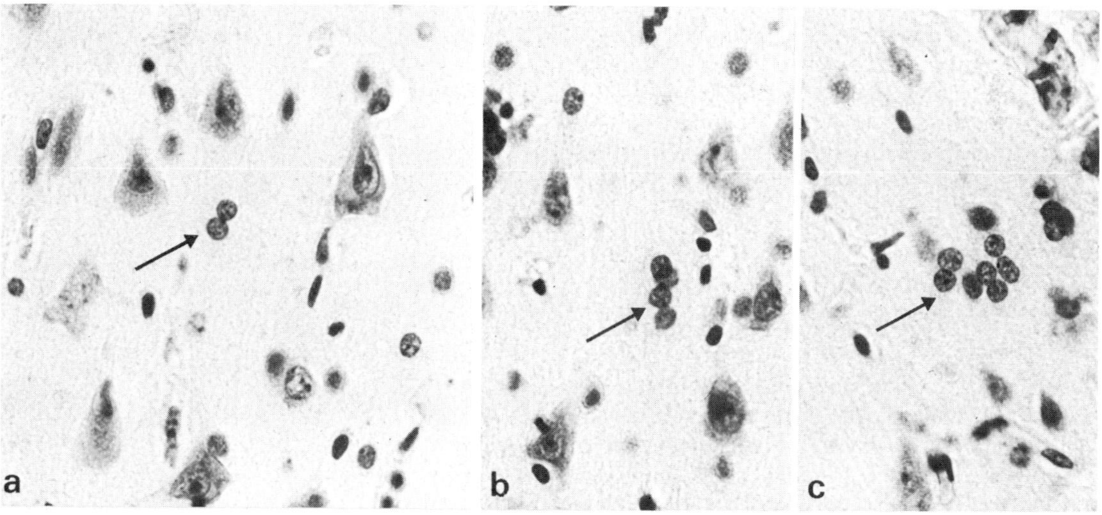

Fig. 1.43 Cerebral cortex in a case of subacute encephalitis from a region where loss of nerve cells was not obvious nor was there perivascular cuffing. In (**a**) there are two, in (**b**) four and in (**c**) a pair and five astrocyte nuclei close together (arrows). This is evidence of astrocytic hyperplasia. Celloidin. Haematoxylin and van Gieson. ×440.

been a breakdown of CNS tissue or a demyelinating process or oedema have received considerable attention. The experimental approach in which astrocytes are maintained in tissue culture (see Raff et al., 1983) lends itself particularly to the study of their reactions to growth factors. Sheffield and Kim (1977) added soluble myelin basic protein to cultures of astrocytes and found evidence to suggest an increase in cell proliferation. This experiment was an attempt to mimic the effects of demyelinating lesions which are accompanied by glial cell hyperplasia. In another experiment Hanson and Partlow (1980) added cell-free supernatant produced from sonicated neurons and found a marked increase in astrocytic uptake of ^{3}H-labelled thymidine, an effect not produced by intact neurons. These findings suggest that soluble fractions derived from nerve cells, axoplasm and myelin are capable of stimulating astrocytic proliferation. Kimelberg, Narumi and Bourke (1978) studied enzyme activities of cultured glial cells derived from young rat brains and found that an increase in sodium and potassium ATPase, bicarbonate-stimulated ATPase and carbonic anhydrase activity reflected glial proliferation. The addition of cyclic-AMP and its analogues caused a marked alteration of cell morphology accentuating astrocyte characteristics with the formation of cell processes.

The activity of enzymes in reactive astrocytes differs from that in normal resting cells and suggests that their metabolism may become permanently altered. Enzymes which are normally scarcely demonstrable (e.g. DPNH-tetrazolium reductase and succinic dehydrogenase) are greatly increased (Friede, 1962), and there is also an early increase in phosphorylase activity and generally increased activity of all oxidoreductases (see Oehmichen, 1980).

Rosenthal fibres

These bodies are formed in the perikarya and processes of astrocytes. They appear as homogeneous, hyaline, eosinophilic structures which may be rounded, oval or elongated and club-shaped and vary greatly in size, being on the average about 10 μm in diameter and up to 40 μm in length. They are remarkably stable and are not removed from sections by vigorous treatment with fat solvents such as ether or chloroform although Sudan black staining methods reveal some lipid component in them. Staining with Mallory's PTAH demonstrates these bodies well, giving them a red to purple colour, the larger bodies showing a purple core with a red periphery. Electron microscopy shows finely granular material in the centre with glial fibrils embedded in the periphery. With GFAP-immunoperoxidase methods the central part of the Rosenthal fibre remains unstained while a rim of GFAP staining can usually be demonstrated (Janzer and Friede, 1981). These bodies are found in a variety of circumstances which include any long-standing intense fibrillary gliosis such as around syringomyelic cavities or tumours; within slowly growing astrocytomas, particularly in the cerebellum or optic nerve; and invariably in Alexander's disease (see Chapter 9). There is some evidence that nickel is capable of inducing the formation of Rosenthal fibres. Kress et al. (1981) found a heavy deposition of these bodies around nickel wire implanted experimentally into rat brain.

Corpora amylacea

Corpora amylacea are spherical bodies (Fig. 1.44) with an average diameter of 15 μm which

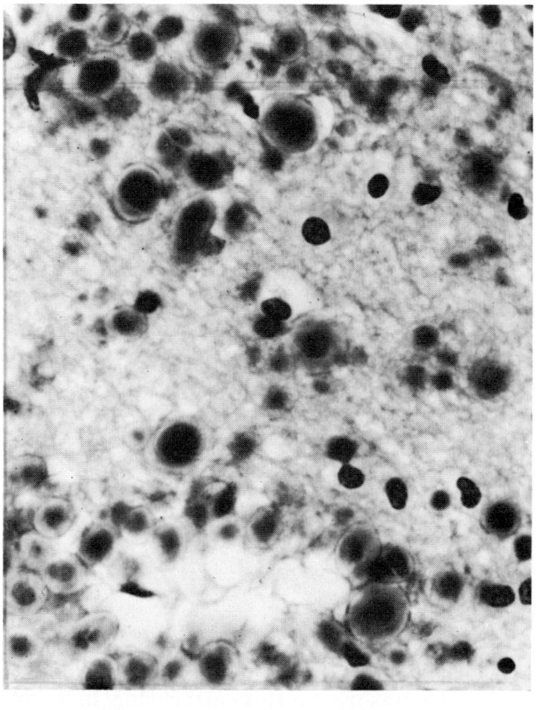

Fig. 1.44 Corpora amylacea. Celloidin. Haematoxylin and eosin $\times 630$.

are often found in the grey matter close to the pia or around blood vessels in the white matter of the brain and cord. They are more numerous in older persons and are particularly numerous in degenerative conditions such as motor neuron disease or when there is much atrophy. They contain an amorphous basophilic material, sometimes with a deeper staining central core. They stain positively with iodine, methyl violet, PAS, and with Best's stain for glycogen and are metachromatic with toluidine blue. Ramsay (1965) showed electron microscopically that they are intracytoplasmic bodies, forming swellings in the processes of fibrous astrocytes. They represent a non-specific degenerative change and contain a glycogen-like substance to which phosphate and sulphate groups are bound (Stam and Roukema, 1973).

Oligodendrocytes

Oligodendroglial cells, the myelin-forming cells of the central nervous system, are seen in routine sections stained with haematoxylin and eosin (Fig. 1.45) as having small dark, rounded nuclei which in size and appearance resemble those of lymphocytes. Their perikaryon and processes are stainable with difficulty by silver impregnation and show few protoplasmic expansions. In the white matter these cells are seen mainly as *interfascicular glia* while in grey matter they form one type of *perineuronal satellite* cell (see Fig. 1.34) as well as being in relation to myelin sheaths. The interfascicular cells lie in rows in longitudinal array between myelinated fibres. The perineuronal cells are commonly seen around the pyramidal cells of the cortex and the large cells of the basal ganglia. They are rarely found around anterior horn cells in the spinal cord, motor neurons in the brain stem, or in the precentral gyrus, nor in relation to Purkinje cells. They may multiply in degenerative conditions of neurons though this is uncertain since six or more cells may be seen around a neuron under what appear to be normal conditions.

The relationship between oligodendrocytes and the myelin sheaths of the central nervous system was established by Bunge and his coworkers (see Bunge, 1968) and it seems clear that each oligodendrocyte sends out processes which form internodes on many nearby axons (Fig. 1.46). Electron microscopy shows (Fig. 1.47) a moderately dense perikaryon, rich in cisternae of Golgi apparatus, rather inconspicuous mitochondria and abundant rough endoplasmic reticulum with many ribosomes. In young animals the actively developing and myelin-forming oligodendrocytes are larger and lighter than in the mature well-myelinated white matter of the adult where the cells become progressively darker. The sparse perikaryon contains no glial fibrils and is not stained by methods demonstrating GFAP. Oligodendroglial processes contain abundant microtubules but no intermediate filaments. The cell membrane can sometimes be seen in close apposition to myelinated fibres and it may be apparent in some electron micrographs that the myelin sheath is derived from that cell. Recent work on oligodendrocyte development (reviewed by Bunge, 1982) shows that the presence of axons is necessary for their proliferation and that they express galactocerebroside as a surface antigen and specific cell marker. Questions concerning the capacity of mature oligodendroglia to proliferate and repair myelin after injury are of wide

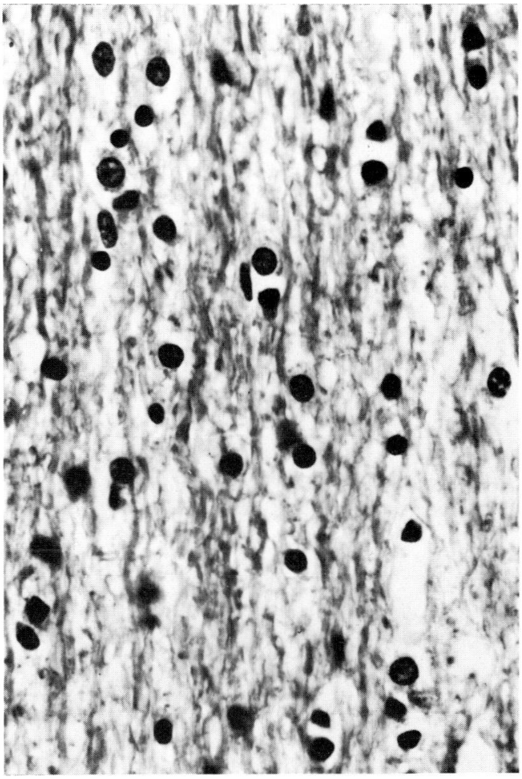

Fig. 1.45 Oligodendroglia in normal white matter. Note their rounded darkly stained nuclei. Haematoxylin and eosin ×400.

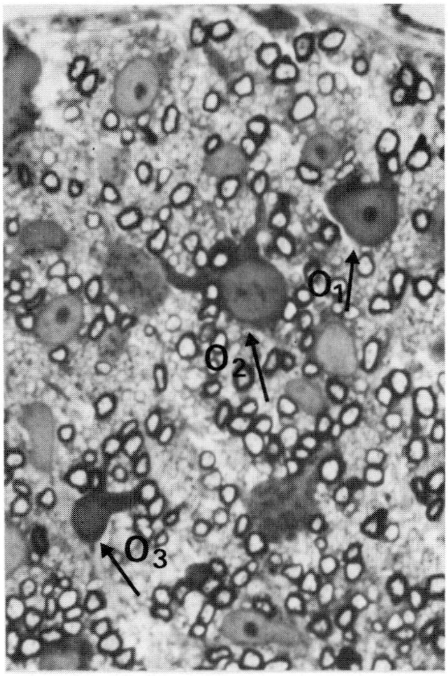

Fig. 1.46 Transverse section of white matter of spinal cord of a 5-day-old kitten. Myelin sheaths appear as darkly stained rings. Three oligodendrocytes (O_1, O_2 and O_3) are shown, each displaying processes that appear related to myelinated axons. 1 μm epon section. Toluidine blue × 1200. (Reproduced by courtesy of Dr R.P. Bunge)

Fig. 1.47 Electron micrograph showing an oligodendrocyte and its relationship to myelinated axons in the optic nerve of a rat. The nucleus is irregular in outline and chromatin is clumped beneath the nuclear membrane. The cytoplasm is compact and electron-dense and contains abundant rough endoplasmic reticulum, Golgi membranes, mitochondria and ribosomes. Bar = 2 μm. (Preparation by Dr Jean M. Jacobs)

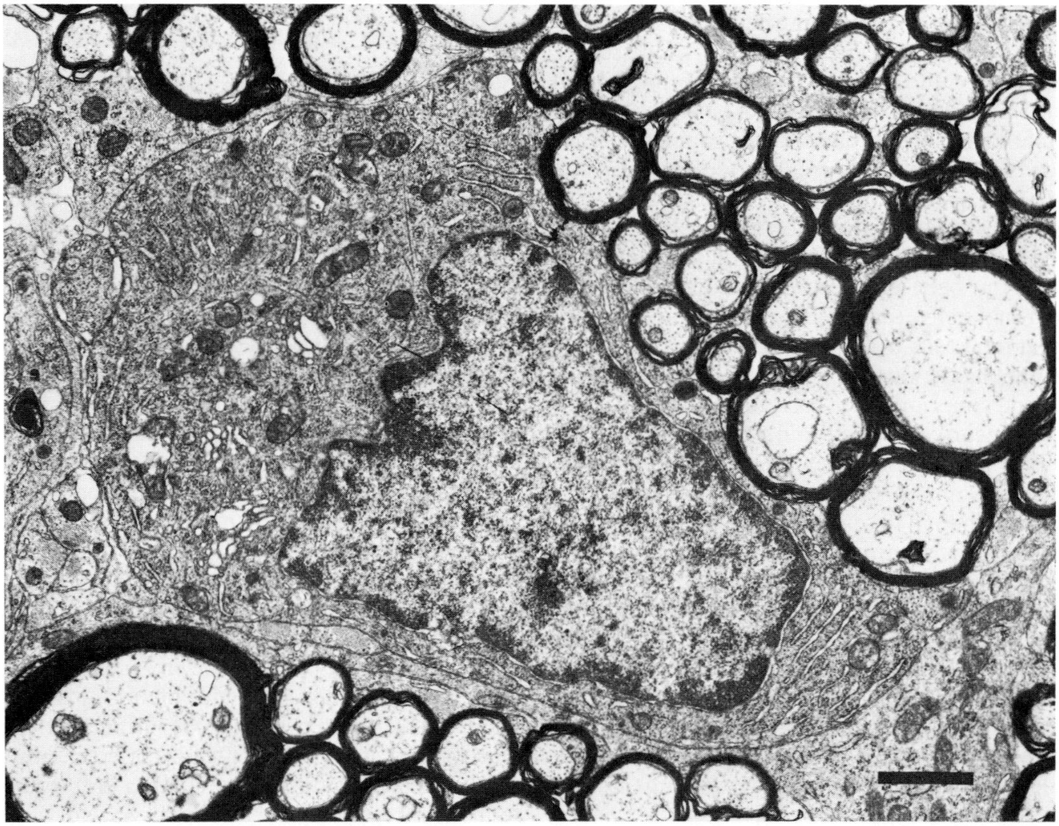

importance in relation to the demyelinating diseases (Chapter 9).

Ependyma

The ependymal lining of the ventricles and central canal of the spinal cord is derived from neuroectoderm, and during fetal development may be several cell layers in thickness. The appearance of the ependyma varies from place to place within the ventricular system ranging from low cuboidal to rather taller columnar cells lining the third ventricle and its recesses near the hypothalamus and hypophyseal recesses. Tall cells with long tapering processes which may extend through to the outer surface of the brain are known as tanycytes, and various neuroendocrine or ionic transport functions have been speculatively ascribed to them.

The ventricular surface of the ependyma is normally uninterrupted. Cilia project from this surface of the cell and originate from basal bodies, the blepharoplasts, which can be stained by PTAH. With the electron microscope the cilia have the characteristic nine pairs of microtubules surrounding a central pair and the basal body is surrounded by fine filaments and finely granular material (Peters, Palay and Webster, 1976). Each ependymal cell is attached to a layer of dense material similar to basal lamina which merges with astrocytic glial processes underlying the ependyma. The ependymal cell nuclei are regularly oval or rounded. Between adjacent cells there are several types of junction—*gap junctions*, *zonulae adhaerentes* and *zonulae occludentes*—but the ependyma does not prevent the passage of particles such as peroxidase or of dyes.

With increasing age there may be a progressive loss of cilia. It also seems that the mature ependyma has little if any capacity for proliferation and regeneration, and once the surface is broken it probably is not reconstituted. The central canal of the spinal cord is often encroached on, or filled by, an ingrowth of glial fibres among which groups of ependymal cells will be seen. When that occurs in the aqueduct, which is narrow and forms a natural bottleneck in the cerebrospinal fluid pathway, occlusion may result in obstruction to the flow of cerebrospinal fluid. It has been considered that the ependymal cells are particularly vulnerable to mumps virus (see Johnson, 1980).

Beneath the ependyma there is normally a layer of 'subependymal glia'. These are astrocytes which lie in compact groups and have the capacity for proliferation. In this region there are normally abundant glial fibrillary processes.

The most commonly seen pathological change in the ependyma is *granular ependymitis* which may develop after any inflammation but was best known as a characteristic feature of neurosyphilis. The macroscopic appearance of granular ependymitis is of tiny clear granules looking like drops of water. They are best seen in the floor of the fourth ventricle but occur throughout the ventricular system. Microscopically these granules consist of collections of astrocytes with fibrils which may or may not be covered by a layer of ependyma and which may have a row or small nests or acini of ependymal cells beneath (Fig. 1.48). The appearances suggest that the overgrowth of glial fibres has burst through the ependymal lining, but the process may also be the result of breaks occurring in the ependyma due to ventricular dilatation. In experimental hydrocephalus, Weller, Wisniewski and Shulman (1971) found that the ependyma became disrupted and that the underlying white matter showed evidence of damage. If intraventricular pressure returned to normal the continuity of the ependyma seemed to be re-established with residual subependymal loss of nerve fibres and gliosis. In more long-standing conditions such as chronic meningovascular syphilis the ependyma may be covered by a pad of neuroglial tissue, giving it a matt appearance.

Microglia

The identification of the group of cells now known as microglia and their separation from the neuroglial astrocytes and oligodendrocytes stemmed from the studies of Robertson (1900) and del Rio-Hortega (1919, 1932) and was based on metallic impregnation techniques. Since that time many studies of the nature and origin of microglia have been reported (see reviews by Oehmichen, 1980, 1982; Ling, 1981) and there is no doubt that these cells have phagocytic properties and contribute to the central nervous system's macrophage response to injury.

Intrinsic (resting) microglia within the normal nervous system comprise about 4–5 per cent of glia. The macrophages derived from extrinsic sources after injury would correspond to wan-

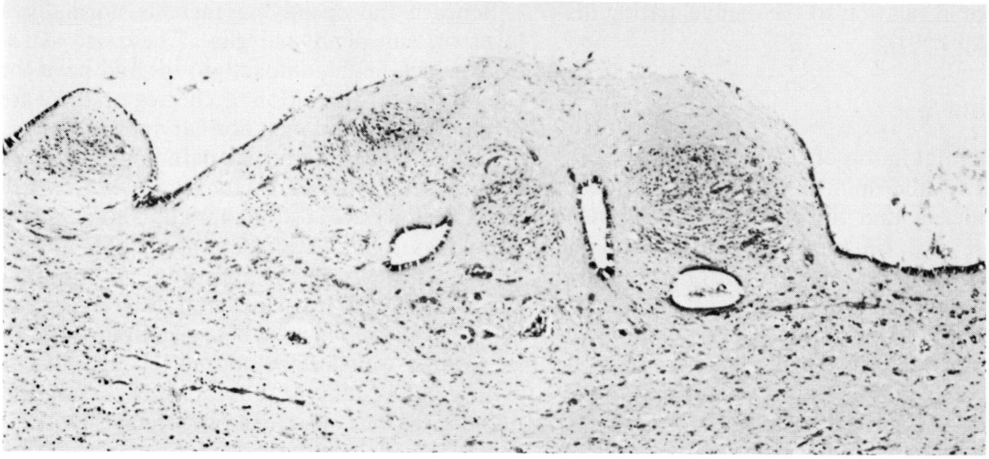

Fig. 1.48 Granular ependymitis in the lateral ventricle. The ependyma, partly deficient, is elevated over aggregations of astrocytes. Small nests of ependymal cells are seen beneath the glial cells. Haematoxylin and eosin × 50.

dering or amoeboid cells of other tissues, and many studies have shown that macrophages may invade damaged CNS tissue from blood vessel walls or from the blood itself (e.g. Konigsmark and Sidman, 1963; Cammermeyer, 1970; Kitamura, 1980; Brierley and Brown, 1982a, b).

In routinely stained sections of normal brain, microglial cells can be identified by their nuclei which are rather hyperchromatic and elongated measuring about 10 × 3 μm. With silver staining in frozen sections (Weil and Davenport, 1933) or paraffin sections (Scott, 1971) thin short processes with fine lateral projections are visible. In grey matter these cells may lie free or may be perineuronal or perivascular satellites. In white matter most occur around vessels. With electron microscopy (Fig. 1.49) the oval or elongated nucleus shows coarse clumps of chromatin, giving it a darker appearance than astrocyte or oligodendrocyte nuclei. The cytoplasm forms a thin rim around the nucleus, has an irregular shape and contains abundant granular endoplasmic reticulum with long cisternae and prominent Golgi apparatus. Characteristically the cell contains dense bodies, lipofuscin and multivesicular bodies. These inclusions are more prominent than in other glial cells. Enzyme histochemical staining (Oehmichen, 1980) shows little of significance

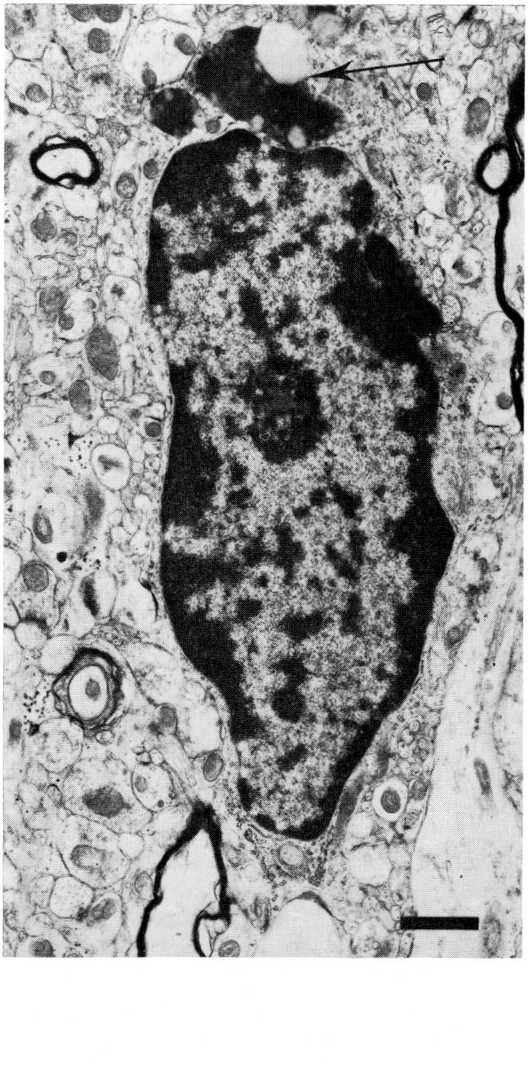

Fig. 1.49 Electron micrograph of a microglial cell. The nucleus is elongated and chromatin arranged in coarse clumps. Cytoplasm is scanty and contains lipofuscin (arrow). Bar = 2 μm.

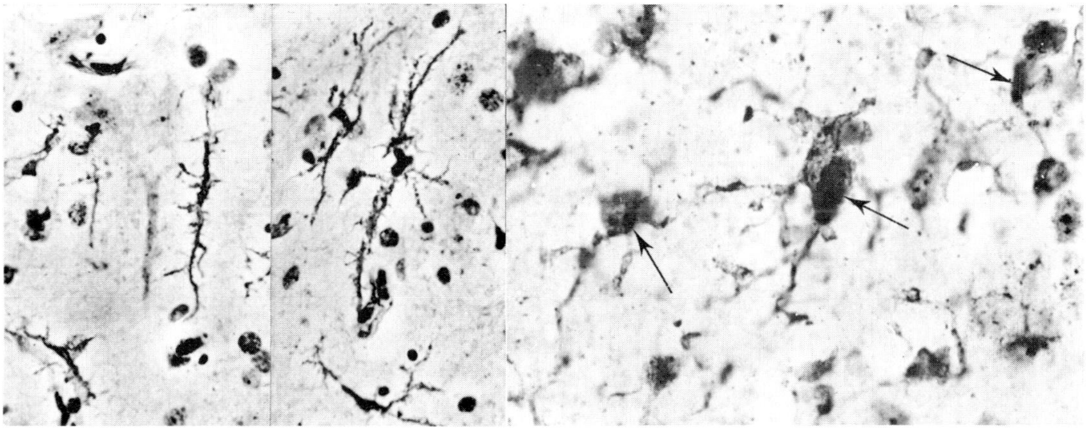

a b c

Fig. 1.50 Microglial reactions. Rod cell (**a**) and triradiate cell (**b**) in cerebral cortex in general paresis. Silver carbonate ×400. (**c**) Molecular layer of cerebellum in a case of kuru. Microglia are enlarged and contain droplets of lipid (arrows). Processes are becoming shortened and thickened. Frozen section stained with oil red O (for fat) and Penfield's method for microglia ×450. (Preparation by Mrs Elisabeth Beck).

except some acid phosphatase activity. The reactions to injury include hyperplasia and hypertrophy, the latter developing as the cell accumulates products of tissue breakdown. The conditions under which microglial reaction is found cover the whole gamut of neuropathology ranging from a mild proliferation around chromatolytic neurons (Watson, 1974) through the removal of degenerating terminals to the invasion of totally necrotic brain as in an infarct or contusion.

Reactive microglia (Fig. 1.50) tend to become rounded and their processes shorten. The characteristic lipid phagocyte is a spherical cell, distended by fat droplets and containing a small rounded nucleus close to the cell membrane (Fig. 1.51) and showing strong acid phosphatase and oxidoreductase activity (Oehmichen, 1980). Many names have been applied to this cell such as *compound granular corpuscle*, *fat granule cell*, *foamy cell* or, in German, the *Gitterzell* (=lattice cell). *Lipid phagocyte* or *macrophage* seem the most acceptable names.

Much attention has been given in the literature to the origin of microglia, under both normal and abnormal conditions. Some, including Kitamura (1980), believe that intrinsic microglia do not contribute to macrophage formation and that all fully developed macrophages are derived from circulating mononuclear leucocytes. The

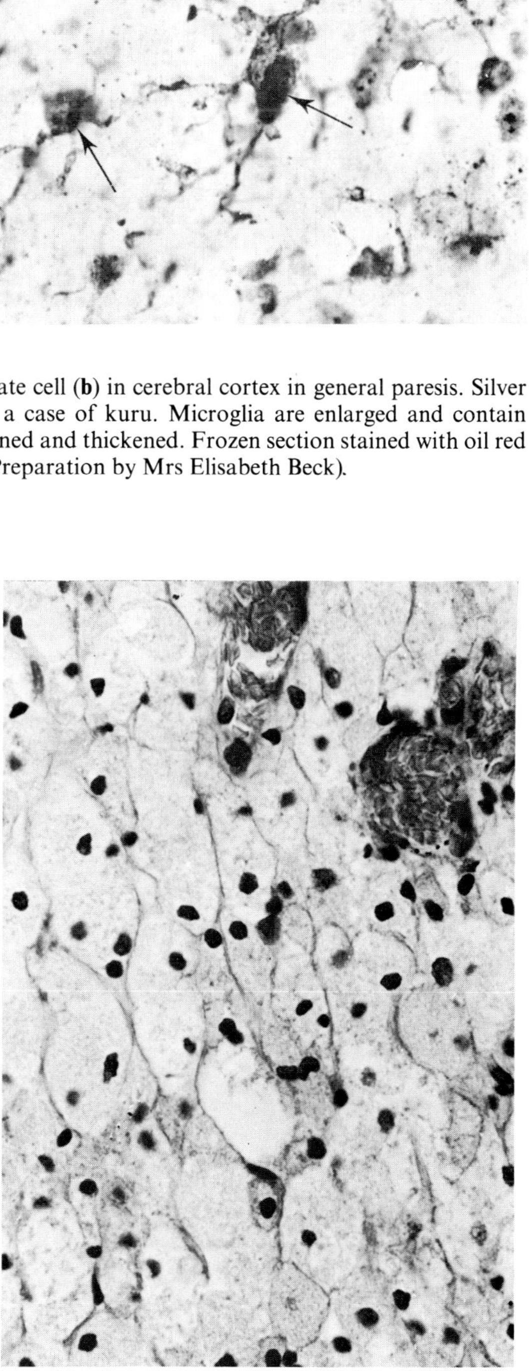

Fig. 1.51 Lipid phagocytes in an area of necrosis 18 months old in the spinal cord. Haematoxylin and van Gieson ×400.

studies of Brierley and Brown (1982a, b) show that selective neuronal necrosis without tissue breakdown or haemorrhage causes activation of microglia to form rod cells with phagocytic properties but only a minority of these cells become lipid phagocytes. When infarction or some other form of brain destruction occurs, adventitial cells (probably fibroblasts) derived from the remaining larger vessels proliferate by mitotic division and give rise to typical lipid phagocytes. Whether it is the physical breakdown of tissue, the biochemical composition of products of degeneration or its quantity that underlies the differences in microglial response and morphology is not clear. In any area of brain necrosis, lipid phagocytes persist for a long time (see Fig. 1.51) and tend to lie around vessels. Clumps of microglial cells (*glial stars*) containing 10–20 small nuclei may be the only evidence of damage or cell loss either after physical injury to axons (Strich, 1961; Oppenheimer, 1968) or after viral infections (Fig. 1.52).

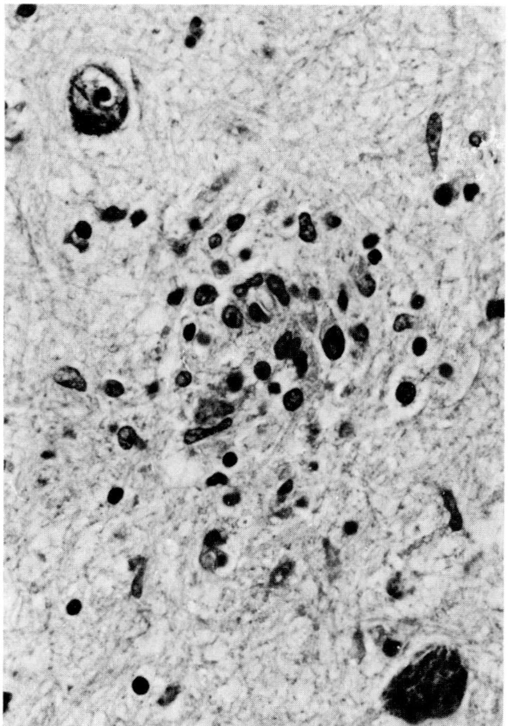

Fig. 1.52 A glial 'star' composed of microglial cells and astrocytes marks the site of loss of a nerve cell. Haematoxylin and van Gieson ×400.

Effects of x-irradiation on the nervous system

Ionizing radiation causes the ejection by x-rays of orbital electrons from molecules, producing direct injury to macromolecules and, particularly in the presence of oxygen, to the formation of peroxide or superoxide free radicals, among others, from water. Injury to macromolecules, of which DNA is the most vulnerable, may result also indirectly from subsequent interactions with the aqueous free radicals. Much of the early experimental work on radiation effects on the nervous system was done with enormous doses of x-rays, and the rapidly developing cell necrosis, brain haemorrhages and breakdown of the blood–brain barrier bear little relationship to the damage seen after the clinical use of irradiation. The principal biological sequelae after irradiation are those mediated by its effects on cell division, and these may include: delay of the cell cycle by inhibition of mitosis after DNA synthesis; cell death during or after one or several mitotic divisions; or non-lethal damage to chromosomes (see Little, 1968). The dose of x-rays usually used in clinical tumour therapy is below the level which causes immediate cell death and the dosage is fractionated to minimize tissue damage. Tissues with a high rate of cell turnover and renewal, such as the intestinal epithelium, are the most sensitive to radiation. The nervous system, with a low rate of cell turnover confined to glial and endothelial cells, has been considered to be among the more radioresistant tissues of the body. However, many cases of damage due to x-irradiation have been reported which, together with the reports on the experimental use of irradiation including experimental teratology, form an extensive literature.

The delayed effects of radiation on the central nervous system may be divided into early or late types. Early delayed effects have been described particularly in patients in whom the brain stem and spinal cord have been included in the beam of radiation directed at extraneural tumours, most commonly those in the head and neck. These early delayed changes have been observed within 2 weeks after irradiation (A. Jones, 1964) and may be transient, presenting with Lhermitte's sign. Progressive cord or brain stem damage with a fatal outcome was reported by Monro and Mair (1968) beginning at 6 weeks and by Lampert and Davis (1964) at 13 weeks post-irradiation. In these cases the damage was mainly to white matter and the descriptions emphasized demyelination resembling an acute plaque of multiple sclerosis, although there was also axonal breakdown. Several of Palmer's (1972) cases surviving 5 months had no clinical manifestations but pathological study showed myelin pallor, fibrous thickening of vessels or focal 'vasculitis' in the spinal cord. In experimental animals the effects of x-irradiation on the spinal cord vary, depending on strain, age, dose of radiation and the level of cord exposed to the beam of x-rays (see Hopewell, 1979; van der Kogel, 1979). In the cervical cord the principal changes are demyelination and necrosis of white matter. In the lumbosacral region the main damage is to nerve roots. Mastaglia et al. (1976) examined single myelinated fibres teased from the spinal cord of rats after irradiation and found breakdown of paranodal myelin or nodal widening beginning as soon as 2 weeks postradiation and becoming more prominent over 2 months. Later, paranodal breakdown was less frequent and nodal widening more prominent. With increasing survival time the presence of increasing numbers of thinly myelinated fibres suggested remyelination. These findings offer an explanation for the early delayed spinal lesions including transient myelopathy, though they do not explain the late delayed progressive necrotizing lesions.

The late delayed effects are well described by Rubinstein (1972) in cerebral tumour patients receiving radiotherapy and in experimental animals by van der Kogel (1979). In these late cases the radionecrosis may present as an acutely developing space-occupying lesion and tends to affect white more than grey matter, the white matter. Microscopically (Fig. 1.53) the striking pathological features are a coagulative necrosis of all elements, with little or no reaction, and abnormal vessels. The vessels show changes poorly demarcated from the underlying white matter. Microscopically (Fig. 1.53) the striking pathological features are a coagulative necrosis of all elements, with little or no reaction, and abnormal vessels. The vessels show changes which have given rise to the theory of the ischaemic pathogenesis of radionecrosis (Pennybacker and Russell, 1948). There is fibrinoid or hyaline change of their walls with endothelial proliferation and perivascular fibrosis. Vessels may be surrounded by extravasated fibrinoid material which permeates adjacent brain tissue and occasionally there may be extensive deposition of material, giving the staining reactions for amyloid (Mandybur and Gore, 1969). Reactive swollen astrocytes, many with bizarre abnormal nuclei, are also seen.

In the rat spinal cord (van der Kogel, 1979) the latent period for the development of late delayed lesions decreases with increasing dose of x-rays. Late changes include vascular telangiectases, haemorrhages and haemorrhagic infarction.

The pathogenesis of the late delayed radiation injury to the central nervous system is not entirely clear. Cells with the greatest turnover (i.e. vascular endothelial cells and glia) are the cells most likely to be damaged by irradiation. The turnover of glial cells in the spinal cord has been shown to be slow (Hornsey, Myers and Warren, 1982) but glial cell populations change after irradiation, a decrease in numbers of astrocytes and oligodendrocytes after 1 month being followed by a rise and then subsequently by a rapid fall prior to the occurrence of necrosis (Hubbard and Hopewell, 1979). The appearance of vascular lesions is accelerated, in experimental animals, by hypertension which itself is known to cause an increase in the turnover of endothelial cells.

Fast-neutron irradiation has also been implicated in late delayed radionecrosis. The case reported by Manz, Woolley and Ornitz (1979) developed brain stem necrosis 10 months postradiation and two other cases are recorded with latent periods of 9 and 19 months respectively.

X-irradiation in low or therapeutic dosage causes little damage to normal peripheral nerves although lumbar nerve roots of the rat show demyelination and necrosis with doses above 2000 rad (van der Kogel, 1979). However, in conditions causing Schwann cell proliferation, irradiation suppresses this proliferation (Cavanagh, 1968) and leads to subsequent impairment of recovery such as from the effects of botulinum toxin where axonal growth and myelination are required (Gomez, Duchen and Hornsey, 1982) and from crush injury (Love, 1983) when Schwann cell proliferation seems to be necessary for adequate myelination of regenerated axons.

Tumours in the nervous system after x-irradiation

A number of reports implicate previous use of x-irradiation in the development of tumours.

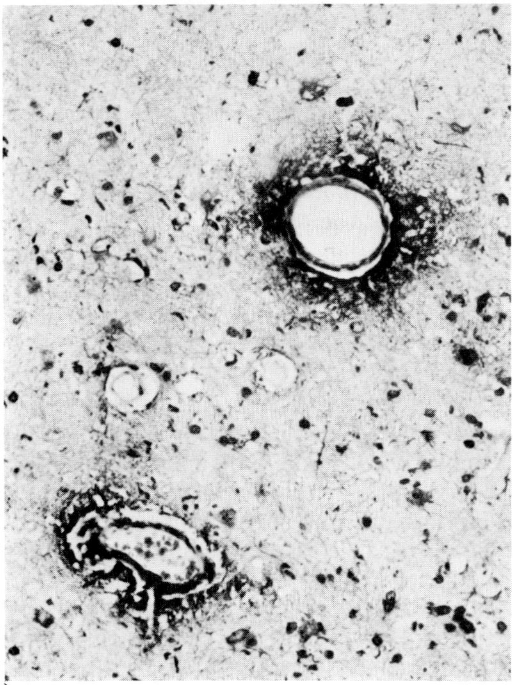

(a)

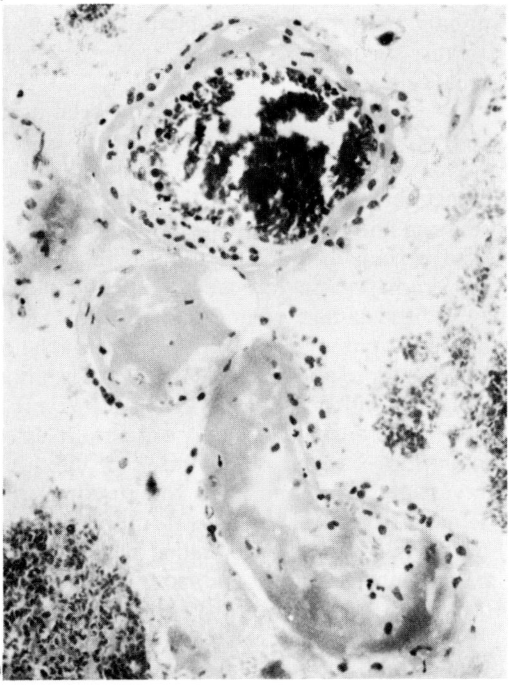

(b)

Fig. 1.53 Radionecrosis in temporal lobe 18 months after irradiation of carcinoma of external auditory meatus. (**a**) Perivascular exudation of fibrin and rarefaction and oedema of brain tissue. PTAH ×150. (**b**) Amorphous hyaline material resembling amyloid in vessel walls. Haematoxylin and eosin ×150.

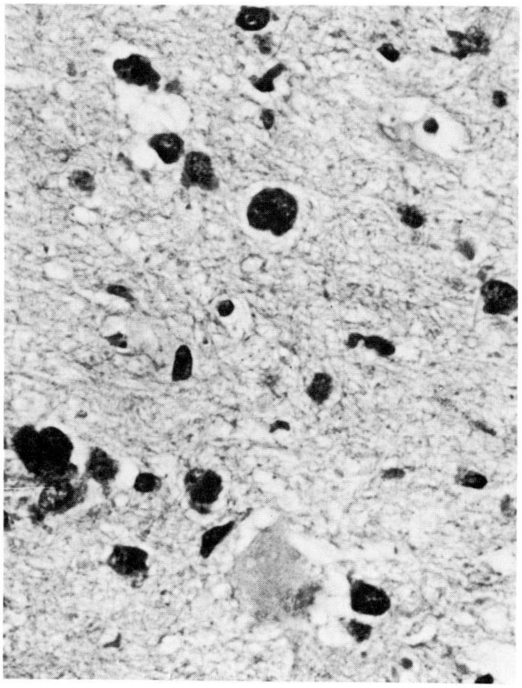

(c)

Fig. 1.53 (**c**) Reactive astrocytes, glial cells with large abnormal nuclei and a binucleated cell. Haematoxylin and eosin ×400.

These include sarcomas in the region of the pituitary fossa after irradiation of pituitary adenomas (Waltz and Brownell, 1966) and sarcomas in the meninges after radiotherapy of primary brain or optic nerve gliomas.

Meningiomas have occurred with greater than expected frequency and at an earlier age in people who received low-dosage scalp irradiation for fungal infections (Beller, Feinsod and Sahar, 1972).

The development of benign and malignant peripheral nerve sheath tumours after irradiation has been reported in man and animals. Foley et al. (1980) described malignant nerve sheath tumours developing more than 20 years after irradiation. Van der Kogel (1979) described proliferative Schwann cell changes and frankly malignant nerve sheath tumours developing in rats which survived irradiation for more than a year. These animals had received less than 2000 rad to the lumbosacral region of the cord and the tumours of the nerve roots contrasted with the necrosis which occurred after higher doses.

Laser irradiation

If a laser beam of sufficient intensity is focused on the skull of an animal it will die instantaneously, death being due to a sudden rise in intracranial pressure due to vaporization of the brain under the bone which absorbs the energy (Hayes, Fox and Stein, 1967). At lower intensities there is a circumscribed area of coagulation necrosis (Lampert, Fox and Earle, 1966) surrounded by a zone of oedema.

Alpha-particle radiation

The effects of alpha-particle radiation on the brain have proved interesting. Tissue is damaged according to the amount of energy absorbed, and this is greatest at the greatest depth of particle penetration (Malis et al., 1960). Therefore irradiation with alpha particles produces a thin straight line of necrosis with a zone of partial damage above it. A marked growth of nerve fibres, which become myelinated, takes place across the gap (Rose et al., 1960; Maxwell and Kruger, 1964; Estable-Puig et al., 1965). This is one of the few situations where regeneration or at least nerve growth can be studied in the adult central nervous system.

Ultrasound

Focused ultrasound waves may produce a circumscribed lesion in the brain especially in the white matter, the tissue in the path of the beam remaining apparently normal (Åstrom et al., 1961). The beam must be applied through a burr hole in the skull because the high ultrasonic absorption of bone results in much heat and secondary damage to surrounding tissues (Lynn and Putnam, 1944). There is necrosis of the target area, with fragmentation and severing of the nerve fibres and blood vessels though with little haemorrhage. This kind of lesion has been used as an alternative to frontal leucotomy in psychiatric patients. On post-mortem examination of 25 such cases, Nelson, Lindstrom and Haymaker (1959) found degrees of tissue damage varying from slight astrocytic reaction and questionable myelin damage to large areas of necrosis in the white matter surrounded by a zone of demyelination. In cases where the dura had been accidentally opened, laminar cortical necrosis was also seen. The central core of the lesion in the white matter was remarkable in that it sometimes showed no dissolution even several weeks after treatment.

References

Adams, C.B.T. (1983). Hemispherectomy—a modification. *Journal of Neurology, Neurosurgery and Psychiatry* **46,** 617–19.

Anderton, B.H., Thorpe, R., Cohen, J., Selvendran, S. and Woodhams, P. (1980). Specific localization by immunofluorescence of 10 nm filament polypeptides. *Journal of Neurocytology* **9,** 835–44.

Andrews, J.M. and Maxwell, D.S. (1969). Motor neuron diseases in animals. In *Motor Neuron Diseases* (Eds. Norris, F.H. and Kurland, L.T.). Grune and Stratton, New York, pp. 369–85.

Åstrom, K.E., Bell, E., Ballantine, H.T. and Heidensleben, E. (1961). An experimental neuropathological study of the effect of high-frequency focused ultrasound on the brain of the cat. *Journal of Neuropathology and Experimental Neurology* **20,** 484–520.

Barr, M.L. and Bertram, L.F. (1949). A morphological distinction between neurones of the male and female and the behaviour of the nucleolar satellite during accelerated nucleoprotein synthesis. *Nature (London)* **163,** 676–7.

Barron, K.D., Daniels, A.C., Chiang, T.Y. and Doolin, P.F. (1970). Fine structure of chromatolytic feline motoneurons. *Experimental and Molecular Pathology* **12,** 46–57.

Beck, E. (1950). The origin, course and termination of the prefronto-pontine tract in the human brain. *Brain* **73,** 368–91.

Beck, E., Bak, I.J., Christ, J.F., Gajdusek, D.C., Gibbs, C.J. and Hassler, R. (1975). Experimental kuru in the spider monkey. Histopathological and ultrastructural studies of the brain during early stages of incubation. *Brain* **98,** 595–612.

Beck, E., Daniel, P.M. and Parry, H.B. (1964). Degeneration of the cerebellar and hypothalamo-neurohypophysial systems in sheep with scrapie; and its relationship to human system degenerations. *Brain* **87,** 153–76.

Beller, A.J., Feinsod, M. and Sahar, A. (1972). The possible relationship between small dose irradiation to the scalp and intracranial meningiomas. *Neurochirurgia* **15,** 135–43.

Bignami, A. and Ralston, H.J. (1969). The cellular reaction to Wallerian degeneration in the central nervous system of the cat. *Brain Research* **13,** 444–61.

Blackwood, W. (1976). Normal structure and general pathology of the nerve cell and neuroglia. In *Greenfield's Neuropathology*, 3rd edn (Eds. Blackwood, W. and Corsellis, J.A.N.). Edward Arnold, London, pp. 1–42.

Bodian, D. (1971). Presynaptic organelles and junctional integrity. *Journal of Cell Biology* **48,** 707–11.

Brierley, J.B. and Brown, A.W. (1982a). The origin of lipid phagocytes in the central nervous system. I. The intrinsic microglia. *Journal of Comparative Neurology* **211,** 397–406.

Brierley, J.B. and Brown, A.W. (1982b). The origin of lipid phagocytes in the central nervous system. II. The adventitia of blood vessels. *Journal of Comparative Neurology* **211,** 407–17.

Brodal, A. and Grant, G. (1962). Morphology and temporal course of degeneration in cerebellar mossy fibers following transection of spinocerebellar tracts in the cat. *Experimental Neurology* **5,** 67–87.

Brown, A.W. (1977). Structural abnormalities in neurones. *Journal of Clinical Pathology* **30,** Suppl. (Royal College of Pathologists) 11, 155–69.

Brown, A.W. and Brierley, J.B. (1966). Evidence for early anoxic-ischaemic cell damage in the rat brain. *Experientia* **22,** 546–7.

Bunge, R.P. (1968). Glial cells and the central myelin sheath. *Physiological Reviews* **48,** 197–251.

Bunge, R.P. (1982). Cellular and non-cellular influences on myelin-forming cells. In *Neuronal-Glial Cell Interrelationships*. (Ed. Sears, T.A.) Springer, Berlin. pp. 115–30.

Bunina, T.L. (1962). On intracellular inclusions in familial amyotrophic lateral sclerosis. *Korsakov Journal of Neurology and Psychiatry* **62,** 1293–9.

van Buren, J.M. (1963). Transsynaptic retrograde degeneration in the visual system of primates. *Journal of Neurology, Neurosurgery and Psychiatry* **26,** 402–9.

Burnstock, G. and Costa, M. (1975). *Adrenergic Neurons*. Chapman and Hall, London.

Cajal, S. Ramon y (1928). *Degeneration and Regeneration of the Nervous System* (Translated by R.M. May). Oxford University Press, London.

Cammermeyer, J. (1955). Astroglial changes during retrograde atrophy of nucleus facialis in mice. *Journal of Comparative Neurology* **102,** 133–50.

Cammermeyer, J. (1960). The post-mortem origin and mechanism of neuronal hyperchromatosis and nuclear pyknosis. *Experimental Neurology* **2,** 379–405.

Cammermeyer, J. (1961). The importance of avoiding 'dark' neurons in experimental neuropathology. *Acta Neuropathologica* **1,** 245–270.

Cammermeyer, J. (1970). The life history of the microglial cell: a light microscopic study. In *Neurosciences Research*, vol. 3 (Eds. Ehrenpreis, S. and Solnitzky, O.C.) Academic Press, New York, pp. 43–129.

Carpenter, S. (1968). Proximal axonal enlargement in motor neuron disease. *Neurology* **18,** 841–51.

Cavanagh, J.B. (1968). Effects of x-irradiation on the proliferation of cells in peripheral nerve during Wallerian degeneration in the rat. *British Journal of Radiology* **41,** 275–82.

Cavanagh, J.B. (1970). The proliferation of astrocytes around a needle wound in the rat's brain. *Journal of Anatomy* **106,** 471–87.

Cavanagh, J.B. and Lewis, P.D. (1969). Perfusion-fixation, colchicine and mitotic activity in the adult rat brain. *Journal of Anatomy* **104,** 341–50.

Ceccarelli, B. and Hurlbut, W.P. (1980). The vesicle hypothesis of the release of quanta of acetylcholine. *Physiological Reviews* **60,** 396–441.

Chan-Palay, V. and Palay, S.L. (Eds.) (1982). *Cytochemical Methods in Neuroanatomy*. Liss, New York.

Chou, S.M. and Hartmann, H.A. (1964). Axonal lesions and waltzing syndrome after IDPN administration in rats. *Acta Neuropathologica* **3,** 428–50.

Collewijn, H. and Schadé, J.P. (1965). Changes in the size of astrocytes and oligodendrocytes during anoxia, hypothermia and spreading depression. In *Progress in Brain Research*, vol. 15 (Eds. De Robertis, E.D.P. and Carrea, R.). Elsevier, Amsterdam, pp. 184–95.

Colonnier, M. (1964). Experimental degeneration in the cerebral cortex. *Journal of Anatomy* **98,** 47–53.

Cork, L.C., Griffin, J.W., Munnell, J.F., Lorenz, M.D., Adams, R.J. and Price, D.L. (1979). Hereditary canine spinal muscular atrophy. *Journal of Neuropathology and Experimental Neurology* **38,** 209–21.

Corsellis, J.A.N., Bruton, C.J. and Freeman-Browne, D. (1973). The aftermath of boxing. *Psychological Medicine* **3,** 270–303.

Cowan, W.M. (1970). Anterograde and retrograde transneuronal degeneration in the central and peripheral nervous system. In *Contemporary Research Methods in Neuroanatomy* (Eds. Nauta,

W.J.H. and Ebbesson, S.O.E.). Springer, Berlin, pp. 217–51.

van Crevel, H. and Verhaart, W.J.C. (1963a). The rate of secondary degeneration in the central nervous system. I. The pyramidal tract of the cat. *Journal of Anatomy* **97,** 429–49.

van Crevel, H. and Verhaart, W.J.C. (1963b). The rate of secondary degeneration in the central nervous system. II. The optic nerve of the cat. *Journal of Anatomy* **97,** 451–64.

Cummings, J.L. and Duchen, L.W. (1981). Kluver-Bucy syndrome in Pick disease: clinical and pathologic correlations. *Neurology* **31,** 1415–22.

Daniel, P.M. and Prichard, M.M.L. (1975). Studies of the hypothalamus and pituitary gland: with special reference to the effects of transection of the pituitary stalk. *Acta endocrinologica* **80,** Suppl. 201, 1–216.

Daniel, P.M. and Strich, S.J. (1969). Histological observations on Wallerian degeneration in the spinal cord of the baboon, *Papiopapio. Acta neuropathologica* **12,** 314–28.

Davison, A.N. and Thompson, R.H.S. (1981). *The Molecular Basis of Neuropathology*. Edward Arnold, London.

DeArmond, S.J., Eng, L.F. and Rubinstein, L.J. (1980). The application of glial fibrillary acidic (GFA) protein immunohistochemistry in neurooncology. *Pathology Research and Practice* **168,** 374–94.

Dekaban, A.S. and Sadowsky, D. (1978). Changes in brain weights during the span of human life: relation of brain weights to body heights and body weights. *Annals of Neurology* **4,** 345–56.

De Robertis, E.D.P. and Carrea, R. (Eds.) (1965). *Biology of Neuroglia. Progress in Brain Research*, vol. 15. Elsevier, Amsterdam.

Duchen, L.W. (1962). The effect of ingestion of hypertonic saline on the pituitary gland in the rat: a morphological study of the pars intermedia and posterior lobe. *Journal of Endocrinology* **25,** 161–8.

Duchen, L.W. (1966). Metastatic carcinoma in the pituitary and hypothalamus. *Journal of Pathology and Bacteriology* **191,** 347–55.

Duchen, L.W. (1970). Changes in the motor innervation and cholinesterase localization induced by botulinum toxin in skeletal muscle of the mouse: differences between fast and slow muscles. *Journal of Neurology, Neurosurgery and Psychiatry* **33,** 40–54.

Duchen, L.W. (1975). *Sprawling*: a new mutant mouse with failure of myelination of sensory axons and a deficiency of muscle spindles. *Neuropathology and Applied Neurobiology* **1,** 89–101.

Duchen, L.W. (1978). Motor neuron diseases in man and animals. *Investigative and Cell Pathology* **1,** 249–62.

Duchen, L.W. and Scaravilli, F. (1977). Quantitative and electron microscopic studies of sensory ganglion cells of the Sprawling mouse. *Journal of Neurocytology* **6,** 465–81.

Duchen, L.W. and Strich, S.J. (1968). The effects of botulinum toxin on the pattern of innervation of skeletal muscle in the mouse. *Quarterly Journal of Experimental Physiology* **53,** 84–9.

Duchen, L.W., Strich, S.J. and Falconer, D.S. (1968). An hereditary motor neurone disease with progressive denervation of muscle in the mouse: the mutant 'wobbler'. *Journal of Neurology, Neurosurgery and Psychiatry* **31,** 535–42.

Duffy, P.E. and Tennyson, V.M. (1965). Phase and electron microscopic observations of Lewy bodies and melanin granules in the substantia nigra and locus ceruleus in Parkinson's disease. *Journal of Neuropathology and Experimental Neurology* **24,** 398–414.

Eisenbarth, G.S., Walsh, F.S. and Nirenberg, M. (1979). Monoclonal antibody to a plasma membrane antigen of neurons. *Proceedings of the National Academy of Sciences of the USA* **76,** 4913–17.

Eng, L.F. and DeArmond, S.J. (1983). Immunochemistry of the glial fibrillary acidic protein. In *Progress in Neuropathology*, vol. 5 (Ed. Zimmerman, H.). Raven Press, New York, pp. 19–39.

Estable-Puig, J.F., de Estable, R.F., Tobias, C. and Haymaker, W. (1965). Degeneration and regeneration of myelinated fibers in the cerebral and cerebellar cortex following damage from ionizing particle radiation. *Acta Neuropathologica* **4,** 175–90.

Fink, R.P. and Heimer, L. (1967). Two methods for selective silver impregnation of degenerating axons and their synaptic endings in the central nervous system. *Brain Research* **4,** 369–74.

Foix, C., Chavany, J.A. and Hillemand, P. (1926). Le syndrome myoclonique de la calotte. Etude anatomo-clinique du nystagmus du voile et des myoclonies rythmiques associées oculaires, faciales etc. *Revue Neurologique* **1,** 942–57.

Foley, K.M., Woodruff, J.M., Ellis, F.T. and Posner, J.B. (1980). Radiation-induced malignant and atypical peripheral nerve sheath tumors. *Annals of Neurology* **7,** 311–18.

Friede, R.L. (1962). The cytochemistry of normal and reactive astrocytes. *Journal of Neuropathology and Experimental Neurology* **21,** 471–8.

Gambetti, P., Erulkar, S., Somlyo, A.P. and Gonatas, N.K. (1975). Calcium-containing structures in vertebrate glial cells, ultrastructural and microprobe analysis. *Journal of Cell Biology* **64,** 322–30.

Gaspar, P., Berger, B., Gay, M., Hamon, M., Cesselin, F., Vigny, A. et al. (1983). Tyrosine hydroxylase and methionine-enkephalin in the human mesencephalon. *Journal of the Neurological Sciences* **58,** 247–67.

Gautier, J.C. and Blackwood, W. (1961). Enlargement of the inferior olivary nucleus in association with lesions of the central tegmental tract or dentate nucleus. *Brain* **84,** 349–61.

Gomez, S., Duchen, L.W. and Hornsey, S. (1982). Effects of x-irradiation on axonal sprouting induced by botulinum toxin. *Neuroscience* **7,** 1023–36.

Greenfield, J.G. (1958). General pathology of the nerve cell and neuroglia. In *Neuropathology*. Edward Arnold, London, pp. 1–66.

Greenfield, J.G. and Bosanquet, F.D. (1953). The brain-stem lesions in Parkinsonism. *Journal of Neurology, Neurosurgery and Psychiatry* **16,** 213–26.

Greenfield, J.G. and Meyer, A. (1963). General pathology of the nerve cell and neuroglia. In *Greenfield's Neuropathology*, 2nd edn (Eds. Norman, R.M., Blackwood, W., Meyer, A., McMenemey, W.H. and Russell, Dorothy S.). Edward Arnold, London, pp. 1–70.

Haddock, J.N. and Berlin L. (1950). Trans-synaptic degeneration in the visual system. *Archives of Neurology and Psychiatry* **64,** 66–73.

Hanson, G.R. and Partlow, L.M. (1980). A comparison of two factors affecting the proliferation of non-neuronal (glial) cells in vitro. *Brain Research* **192,** 371–81.

Harriman, D.G.F. and Millar, J.D.H. (1955). Progressive familial myoclonic epilepsy in three families: its clinical features and pathological basis. *Brain* **78,** 325–49.

Hart, M.N., Cancilla, P.A., Frommes, S. and Hirano, A. (1977). Anterior horn cell degeneration and Bunina-type inclusions associated with dementia. *Acta Neuropathologica* **38,** 225–8.

Hayes, J.R., Fox, J.L. and Stein, M.N. (1967). The effects of laser irradiation on the central nervous system. I. Preliminary studies. *Journal of Neuropathology and Experimental Neurology* **26,** 250–8.

Hertz, L. (1977). Drug-induced alterations of ion distribution at the cellular level of the central nervous system. *Pharmacological Reviews* **29,** 35–65.

Hertz, L. (1978). An intense potassium uptake into astrocytes, its further enhancement by high concentrations of potassium and its possible involvement in potassium homeostasis at the cellular level. *Brain Research* **145,** 202–8.

Hopewell, J.W. (1979). Late radiation damage to the central nervous system: a radiobiological interpretation. *Neuropathology and Applied Neurobiology* **5,** 329–43.

Hornsey, S., Myers, R. and Warren, P. (1982). Residual injury in the spinal cord after treatment with X-rays and neutrons. *British Journal of Radiology* **55,** 516–19.

Hubbard, B.M. and Hopewell, J.W. (1979). Changes in the neuroglial cell populations of the rat spinal cord after local x-irradiation. *British Journal of Radiology* **52,** 816–21.

Israel, M., Dunant, Y. and Manaranche, R. (1979). The present status of the vesicular hypothesis. *Progress in Neurobiology* **13,** 237–75.

Iversen, L.L. (1982). Neurotransmitters and CNS disease. *Lancet* **2,** 914–18.

Iwata, M. and Hirano, A. (1979). Current problems in the pathology of amyotrophic lateral sclerosis. In *Progress in Neuropathology*, vol. 4 (Ed. Zimmerman, H.M.). Grune and Stratton, New York, pp. 277–98.

Janota, I. (1974). Neurofibrillary change in the terminal parts of Purkyne cell axons in the dentate nucleus of the cerebellum following destructive cortical lesions in the cerebellar hemisphere in the cat. An electron microscopic study. *Journal of the Neurological Sciences* **22,** 367–73.

Janota, I. (1979). Widespread intranuclear neuronal corpuscles (Marinesco bodies) associated with a familial spinal degeneration with cranial and peripheral nerve involvement. *Neuropathology and Applied Neurobiology* **5,** 311–17.

Janzer, R.C. and Friede, R.L. (1981). Do Rosenthal fibers contain glial fibrillary acid protein? *Acta Neuropathologica* **55,** 75–6.

Johnson, R.T. (1980). Selective vulnerability of neural cells to viral infections. *Brain* **103,** 447–72.

Jones, A. (1964). Transient radiation myelopathy. *British Journal of Radiology* **37,** 727–44.

Jones, D.G. (1975). *Synapses and Synaptosomes*, Chapman and Hall, London.

Katz, B. (1969). *The Release of Neural Transmitter Substances*. University Press, Liverpool.

Kennedy, P.G.E. (1982). Neural cell markers and their applications to neurology. *Journal of Neuroimmunology* **2,** 35–53.

Kimelberg, H.K., Narumi, S. and Bourke, R.S. (1978). Enzymatic and morphological properties of primary rat brain astrocyte cultures and enzyme development in vivo. *Brain Research* **153,** 55–7.

Kitamura, T. (1980). Dynamic aspects of glial reactions in altered brains. *Pathology Research and Practice* **168,** 301–43.

Klatzo, I., Gajdusek, C.D. and Zigas, V. (1959). Pathology of kuru. *Laboratory Investigation* **8,** 799–847.

Koenig, H. and Barron, K.D. (1963). Reactive gliosis—a histochemical study. *Journal of Neuropathology and Experimental Neurology* **22,** 336 (Abstract).

van der Kogel, A.J. (1979). *Late Effects of Radiation on the Spinal Cord*. Radiobiological Institute of the Organization for Health Research TNO, Rijswijk, The Netherlands.

Köhler, G. and Milstein, C. (1975). Continuous cultures of fused cells secreting antibody of predefined specificity. *Nature (London)* **256,** 495–7.

Konigsmark, B.W. and Sidman, R.L. (1963). Origin of brain macrophages in the mouse. *Journal of Neuropathology and Experimental Neurology* **22,** 643–76.

Kress, Y., Gaskin, F., Horoupian, D. and Brosnan, C. (1981). Nickel induction of Rosenthal fibers in rat brain. *Brain Research* **210,** 419–25.

Kuno, M. and Llinas, R. (1970). Enhancement of synaptic transmission by dendritic potentials in chromatolysed motoneurones of the cat. *Journal of Physiology* **210,** 807–21.

Kupfer, C. (1965a). The laminar pattern and distribution of cell size in the lateral geniculate nucleus of man. *Journal of Neuropathology and Experimental Neurology* **24,** 645–52.

Kupfer, C. (1965b). The distribution of cell size in the lateral geniculate nucleus of man following transneuronal cell atrophy. *Journal of Neuropathology and Experimental Neurology* **24,** 653–61.

Lafora, G.R. (1923). Les myoclonies et les corps amylacés dans les cellules nerveuses. *Revue Neurologique* **2,** 399–413.

Lampert, P.W. and Cressman, M.R. (1966). Fine structural changes of myelin sheaths after axonal degeneration in the spinal cord of rats. *American Journal of Pathology* **49,** 1139–55.

Lampert, P.W. and Davis, R.L. (1964). Delayed effects of radiation on the human central nervous system. *Neurology* **14,** 912–17.

Lampert, P.W., Fox, J.L. and Earle, K.M. (1966). Cerebral edema after laser radiation. An electron microscopic study. *Journal of Neuropathology and Experimental Neurology* **25,** 531–41.

Lapham, L.W. (1962). Cytological and cytochemical studies of neuroglia. I: a study of the problem of amitosis in reactive protoplasmic astrocytes. *American Journal of Pathology* **41,** 1–21.

Latov, N., Nilaver, G., Zimmerman, E.A., Johnson, W.G., Silverman, A.-J., Defendini, R. and Cote, L. (1979). Fibrillary astrocytes proliferate in response to brain injury. *Developmental Biology* **72,** 381–4.

Lawrence, R.D., Meyer, A. and Nevin, S. (1942). The pathological changes in the brain in fatal hypoglycaemia. *Quarterly Journal of Medicine* **11,** 181–202.

Leestma, J.E. and Martin, E. (1968). An electron probe and histochemical study of the 'ferruginated' neuron. *Archives of Pathology* **122,** 597–605.

Lieberman, A.R. (1971). The axon reaction: a review of the principal features of perikaryal responses to axon injury. *International Review of Neurobiology* **14,** 50–124.

Lieberman, A.R. (1976). Sensory ganglia. In *The Peripheral Nerve* (Ed. Landon, D.N.). Chapman and Hall, London, pp. 188–287.

Ling, E.-A. (1981). The origin and nature of microglia. In *Advances in Cellular Neurobiology* vol. 2 (Eds. Fedoroff, S. and Hertz, L). Academic Press, New York, pp. 33–82.

Little, J.B. (1968). Cellular effects of ionizing radiation. *New England Journal of Medicine* **278,** 308–15; 369–76.

Love, S. (1983). An experimental study of peripheral nerve regeneration after x-irradiation. *Brain* **106,** 39–54.

Lynn, J.G. and Putnam, T.J. (1944). Histology of cerebral lesions produced by focused ultrasound. *American Journal of Pathology* **20,** 637–49.

McCaman, R.E. and Robins, E. (1959). Quantitative biochemical studies of Wallerian degeneration in the peripheral and central nervous systems. I. Chemical constituents. II. Twelve enzymes. *Journal of Neurochemistry* **5,** 18–42.

Malis, L.I., Baker, C.P., Kruger, L. and Rose, J.E. (1960). Effects of heavy, ionizing monoenergetic particles on the cerebral cortex. *Journal of Comparative Neurology* **115,** 219–41.

Mandybur, T.I. and Gore, I. (1969). Amyloid in late post-irradiation necrosis of brain. *Neurology* **19,** 983–92.

Mann, D.M.A. and Yates, P.O. (1979). A quantitative study of the glia of the Purkinje cell layer of the cerebellum in mammals. *Neuropathology and Applied Neurobiology* **5,** 71–6.

Manz, H.J., Woolley, P.V. and Ornitz, R.D. (1979). Delayed radiation necrosis of brainstem related to fast neutron beam irradiation. *Cancer* **44,** 473–9.

Marsland, T.A., Glees, P. and Erikson, L.B. (1954). Modification of the Glees silver impregnation for paraffin sections. *Journal of Neuropathology and Experimental Neurology* **13,** 587–91.

Martinez-Hernandez, A., Bell, K.P. and Norenberg, M.D. (1977). Glutamine synthetase: glial localization in brain. *Science* **195,** 1356–8.

Mastaglia, F.L., McDonald, W.I., Watson, J.V. and Yogendran, K. (1976). Effects of x-irradiation on the spinal cord: an experimental study of the morphological changes in central nerve fibres. *Brain* **99,** 101–22.

Matthews, M.R. (1964). Further observations on transneuronal degeneration in the lateral geniculate nucleus of the macaque monkey. *Journal of Anatomy* **98,** 225–63.

Matthews, M.R., Cowan, W.M. and Powell, T.P.S. (1960). Transneuronal degeneration in the lateral geniculate nucleus of the macaque monkey. *Journal of Anatomy* **94,** 145–69.

Matthews, M.R. and Nelson, V.H. (1975). Detachment of structurally intact nerve endings from chromatolytic neurones of rat superior cervical ganglion during the depression of synaptic transmission induced by post-ganglionic axotomy. *Journal of Physiology* **245,** 91–135.

Matthews, M.R. and Powell, T.P.S. (1962). Some observations on transneuronal degeneration in the olfactory bulb of the rabbit. *Journal of Anatomy* **96,** 89–102.

Matthews, M.R. and Raisman, G. (1972). A light and electron microscopic study of the cellular response to axonal injury in the superior cervical ganglion of the rat. *Proceedings of the Royal Society of London*, Series B **181,** 43–79.

Maxwell, D.S. and Kruger, L. (1964). Electron microscopy of radiation-induced laminar lesions in the cerebral cortex of the rat. In *Response of the Nervous System to Ionizing Radiation* (Eds. Haley, T.J. and Snider, R.S.). Little, Brown, Boston, pp. 54–83.

Meyer, A. (1963). Anoxic poisons and the problem of selective vulnerability. In *Greenfield's Neuropathology*, 2nd edn (Eds. Norman, R.M., Blackwood, W., Meyer, A., McMenemey, W.H., and Russell, Dorothy S.). Edward Arnold, London, pp. 237–61.

Meyer, A., Beck, E. and McLardy, T. (1947). Prefrontal leucotomy: a neuro-anatomical report. *Brain* **70,** 18–49.

Miledi, R. and Stefani, E. (1970). Miniature potentials in denervated slow muscle fibres of the frog. *Journal of Physiology* **209,** 179–86.

Monro, P. and Mair, W.G.P. (1968). Radiation effect on the human central nervous system 14 weeks after x-radiation. *Acta Neuropathologica* **11,** 267–74.

Nauta, W.J.H. and Gygax, P.A. (1954). Silver impregnation of degenerating axons in the central nervous system. A modified technic. *Stain Technology* **29,** 91–3.

Nelson, E., Lindstrom, P.L. and Haymaker, W. (1959). Pathological effects of ultrasound on the human brain. A study of 25 cases in which ultrasonic irradiation was used as a lobotomy procedure. *Journal of Neuropathology and Experimental Neurology* **18,** 489–508.

Nissl, F. (1892). Über die Veränderungen der Ganglienzellen am Facialiskern des Kaninchens nach Ausreissung der Nerven. *Allgemeine Zeitschrift für Psychiatrie* **48,** 197–8.

Oehmichen, M. (1980). Enzyme-histochemical differentiation of neuroglia and microglia: a contribution to the cytogenesis of microglia and globoid cells. *Pathology Research and Practice* **168,** 344–73.

Oehmichen, M. (1982). Functional properties of microglia. In *Recent Advances in Neuropathology* vol. 2 (Eds. Smith, W.T. and Cavanagh, J.B.). Churchill Livingstone, Edinburgh, pp. 83–107.

Oppenheimer, D.R. (1968). Microscopic lesions in the brain following head injury. *Journal of Neurology, Neurosurgery and Psychiatry* **31,** 299–306.

Oppenheimer, D.R. and Griffith, H.B. (1966). Persistent intracranial bleeding as a complication of hemispherectomy. *Journal of Neurology, Neurosurgery and Psychiatry* **29,** 229–40.

Orkand, R.R. (1982). Signalling between neuronal and glial cells. In *Neuronal–Glial Cell Interrelationships* (Ed. Sears, T.A.). Springer, Berlin, pp. 147–58.

Palay, S.L. and Chan-Palay, V. (1974). *Cerebellar Cortex. Cytology and Organization.* Springer, Berlin, p. 61.

Palmer, J.J. (1972). Radiation myelopathy. *Brain* **95,** 109–22.

Palmgren, A. (1948). A rapid method for selective silver staining of nerve fibres and nerve endings in mounted paraffin sections. *Acta Zoologica (Stockholm)* **29,** 377–92.

Pannese, E. (1963). Investigations on the ultrastructural changes of the spinal ganglion neurons in the course of axon regeneration and cell hypertrophy. *Zeitschrift für Zellforschung und mikroskopische Anatomie* **61,** 561–86.

Pearson, J. (1983). Neurotransmitter immunocytochemistry in the study of human development, anatomy and pathology. In *Progress of Neuropathology*, vol. 5 (Ed. Zimmerman, H.M.). Raven Press, New York, pp. 41–97.

Penfield, W. (1932). Neuroglia: normal and pathological. In *Penfield's Cytology and Cellular Pathology of the Nervous System*, vol. 2. Hoeber, New York, pp. 423–79.

Pennybacker, J. and Russell, D.S. (1948). Necrosis of the brain due to radiation therapy: clinical and pathological observations. *Journal of Neurology, Neurosurgery and Psychiatry* **11,** 183–98.

Peters, A., Palay, S.L. and Webster, H.deF. (1976). *The Fine Structure of the Nervous System*, 2nd edn. Saunders, Philadelphia.

Privat, A., Valat, J. and Fulcrand, J. (1981). Proliferation of neuroglial cell lines in the degenerating optic nerve of young rats. *Journal of Neuropathology and Experimental Neurology* **40,** 46–60.

Raff, M.C., Miller, R.H. and Noble, M. (1983). A glial progenitor cell that develops in vitro into an astrocyte or an oligodendrocyte depending on culture medium. *Nature (London)* **303,** 390–6.

Raff, M.C., Abney, E.R., Cohen, J., Lindsay, R. and Noble, M. (1983). Two types of astrocytes in cultures of developing rat white matter: differences in morphology, surface gangliosides, and growth characteristics. *Journal of Neuroscience* **3,** 1289–1300.

Rakic, P. (1971). Neuron–glia relationship during

granule cell migration in developing cerebellar cortex. A Golgi and electron microscopic study in *Macacus rhesus*. *Journal of Comparative Neurology* **141**, 283–312.

Rakic, P. (1972). Mode of cell migration to the superficial layers of fetal monkey neocortex. *Journal of Comparative Neurology* **145**, 61–84.

Ramon-Moliner, E. (1970). The Golgi-Cox technique. In *Contemporary Research Methods in Neuroanatomy* (Ed. Nauta, W.J.H. and Ebbesson, S.O.E.). Springer, Berlin, pp. 32–55.

Ramsay, H.J. (1965). Ultrastructure of corpora amylacea. *Journal of Neuropathology and Experimental Neurology* **24**, 25–39.

Renkawek, K., Matyja, E. and Mossakowski, M.J. (1982). Glial fibrillary changes induced by kainic acid in organotypic culture of rat cerebellum. *Journal of the Neurological Sciences* **53**, 321–30.

del Rio-Hortega, P. (1919). El tercer elemento de los centros nerviosos. I. La microglia. II. Intervencion de la microglia en los procesos patologicas. III. Naturaleza probable de la microglia. *Boletin de la Sociedad española de biologia* **9**, 69–120.

del Rio-Hortega, P. (1932). Microglia. In *Penfield's Cytology and Cellular Pathology of the Nervous System*, vol. 2. Hoeber, New York, pp. 483–534.

Robertson, W.F. (1900). A microscopic demonstration of the normal and pathological histology of mesoglia cells. *Journal of Mental Science* **46**, 724.

Rose, J.E., Malis, L.I., Kruger, L. and Baker, C.P. (1960). Effects of heavy ionizing monoenergetic particles on the cerebral cortex. *Journal of Comparative Neurology* **115**, 243–96.

Rubinstein, L.J. (1972). Tumors of the central nervous system. *Atlas of Tumor Pathology*, Fascicle 6. Armed Forces Institute of Pathology, Washington, pp. 349–60.

Schmechel, D., Marangos, P. and Brightman, M. (1978). Brain enolases as specific markers of neuronal and glial cells. *Science* **199**, 313–15.

Scott, T. (1971). A rapid silver impregnation technique for oligodendrocytes, microglia and astrocytes. *Journal of Clinical Pathology* **24**, 578–80.

Sears, T.A. (Ed.) (1982). *Neuronal-Glial Cell Interrelationships*. Springer, Berlin.

Sheffield, W.D. and Kim, S.U. (1977). Myelin basic protein causes proliferation of lymphocytes and astrocytes in vitro. *Brain Research* **132**, 580–4.

Smith, M.C. (1949). Metachromatic bodies in the brain. *Journal of Neurology, Neurosurgery and Psychiatry* **12**, 100–10.

Smith, M.C. (1951). The use of Marchi staining in the later stages of human tract degeneration. *Journal of Neurology, Neurosurgery and Psychiatry* **14**, 222–5.

Smith, M.C. (1955). Argyrophile bodies in the human spinal cord. *Journal of Neurology, Neurosurgery and Psychiatry* **18**, 13–16.

Smith, M.C. (1956a). Observations on the extended use of the Marchi method. *Journal of Neurology, Neurosurgery and Psychiatry* **19**, 67–78.

Smith, M.C. (1956b). The recognition and prevention of artefacts of the Marchi method. *Journal of Neurology, Neurosurgery and Psychiatry* **19**, 74–83.

Smith, M.C., Strich, S.J. and Sharp, P. (1956). The value of the Marchi method for staining tissue stored in formalin for prolonged periods. *Journal of Neurology, Neurosurgery and Psychiatry* **19**, 62–4.

Sohn, D. and Levine, S. (1971). Hypertrophy of the olives: a report on 43 cases. In *Progress in Neuropathology*, vol. 1 (Ed. Zimmerman, H.M.). Grune and Stratton, New York, pp. 202–17.

Spielmeyer, W. (1922). *Histopathologie des Nervensystems*. Springer, Berlin.

Stam, F.C. and Roukema, P.A. (1973). Histochemical and biochemical aspects of corpora amylacea. *Acta Neuropathologica* **25**, 95–102.

Stewart, R.M. and Rosenberg, R.N. (1979). Physiology of glia: glial-neuronal interactions. *International Review of Neurobiology* **21**, 275–309.

Strich, S.J. (1961). Shearing of nerve fibres as a cause of brain damage due to head injury: a pathological study of twenty cases. *Lancet* **2**, 443–8.

Strich, S.J. (1968). Notes on the use of the Marchi method for staining degenerating myelin in the peripheral and central nervous system. *Journal of Neurology, Neurosurgery and Psychiatry* **31**, 110–14.

Torvik, A. (1956). Transneuronal changes in the inferior olive and pontine nuclei in kittens. *Journal of Neuropathology and Experimental Neurology* **15**, 119–45.

Torvik, A. (1976). Central chromatolysis and the axon reaction: a reappraisal. *Neuropathology and Applied Neurobiology* **2**, 423–32.

Torvik, A. and Heding, A. (1967). Histological studies on the effect of actinomycin D on retrograde nerve cell reaction in the facial nucleus of mice. *Acta Neuropathologica* **9**, 146–57.

Ulrich, J., Isler, W., and Vassalli, L. (1965). L'effet d'hémorrhagies leptoméningées répétées sur le système nerveux. *Revue Neurologique* **112**, 466–71.

Urich, H. (1976). Malformations of the nervous system, perinatal damage and related conditions in early life. In *Greenfield's Neuropathology*, 3rd edn (Eds. Blackwood, W. and Corsellis, J.A.N.). Edward Arnold, London, pp. 361–469.

Valverde, F. (1970). The Golgi method. A tool for comparative structural analyses. In *Contemporary Research Methods in Neuroanatomy* (Eds. Nauta, W.J.H. and Ebbesson, S.O.E.). Springer, Berlin, pp. 12–31.

Vandenberg, S.R., Ludwin, S.K., Herman, M.M. and Bignami, A. (1976). In vitro astrocytic differentiation from embryoid bodies of an experimental mouse testicular teratoma. *American Journal of Pathology* **83,** 197–212.

Vaughn, J.E., Hinds, P.L. and Skoff, R.P. (1970). Electron microscopic studies of Wallerian degeneration in rat optic nerves. I. The multipotential glia. *Journal of Comparative Neurology* **140,** 175–206.

Vaughn, J.E. and Pease, D.C. (1970). Electron microscopic studies of Wallerian degeneration in rat optic nerves. II. Astrocytes, oligodendrocytes and adventitial cells. *Journal of Comparative Neurology* **140,** 207–26.

Verhaart, W.J.C. and Voogd, J. (1962). Hypertrophy of the inferior olives in the cat. *Journal of Neuropathology and Experimental Neurology* **21,** 92–104.

Waller, A. (1850). Experiments on the section of the glossopharyngeal and hypoglossal nerves of the frog, and observations of the alterations produced thereby in the structure of their primitive fibres. *Philosophical Transactions of the Royal Society of London* **140,** 423–69.

Waltz, T.A. and Brownell, B. (1966). Sarcoma: a possible late result of effective radiation therapy for pituitary adenoma. Report of two cases. *Journal of Neurosurgery* **24,** 901–7.

Watson, W.E. (1968). Observations on the nucleolar and total cell body nucleic acid of injured nerve cells. *Journal of Physiology* **196,** 655–76.

Watson, W.E. (1969). The response of motor neurones to intramuscular injection of botulinum toxin. *Journal of Physiology* **202,** 611–30.

Watson, W.E. (1974). Cellular responses to axotomy and to related procedures. *British Medical Bulletin* **30,** 112–15.

Weil, A. and Davenport, H.A. (1933). Staining of oligodendroglia and microglia in celloidin sections. *Archives of Neurology and Psychiatry* **30,** 175–8.

Weller, R.O., Wisniewski, H. and Shulman, K. (1971). Experimental hydrocephalus in young dogs: histological and ultrastructural study of the brain tissue damage. *Journal of Neuropathology and Experimental Neurology* **30,** 613–27.

Wilson, P.J.E. (1970). Cerebral hemispherectomy for infantile hemiplegia. *Brain* **93,** 147–80.

Windle, W.F. (1958). *Biology of Neuroglia.* Thomas, Springfield.

Wisniewski, H.M., Merz, G.S., Merz, P.A., Wen, G.Y. and Iqbal, K. (1983). Morphology and biochemistry of neuronal paired helical filaments and amyloid fibers in humans and animals. In *Progress in Neuropathology*, vol. 5 (Ed. Zimmerman, H.). Raven Press, New York, pp. 139–50.

Yen, S.H. and Fields, K.L. (1981). Antibodies to neurofilament glial filament and fibroblast intermediate filament proteins bind to different cell types of the nervous system. *Journal of Cell Biology* **88,** 115–26.

Yuen, P. and Baxter, D.W. (1963). The morphology of Marinesco bodies (paranucleolar corpuscles) in the melanin pigmented nuclei in the brainstem. *Journal of Neurology, Neurosurgery and Psychiatry* **26,** 178–83.

Zelena, J. (1971). Neurofilaments and microtubules in sensory neurons after peripheral nerve section. *Zeitschrift für Zellforschung und Mikroskopische Anatomie* **117,** 191–211.

2

The pathophysiology of raised intracranial pressure

J. Douglas Miller and J. Hume Adams

Thinking on raised intracranial pressure (ICP) was for long based on the Monro (1783)-Kellie (1824) doctrine which, in essence, states that once the fontanelles and sutures have closed the intracranial contents consist of incompressible brain and blood within a rigid, unyielding skull. This concept had, however, to be modified to take the cerebrospinal fluid (CSF) into account (Burrows, 1846). In defining the four clinical stages of 'cerebral compression', Duret (1878) and Kocher (1901) promoted the important concept of *spatial compensation* whereby, as an intracranial mass lesion increases in size, a compensatory reduction of other intracranial contents can for a time modify or prevent an increase in ICP. Once this capacity has become exhausted, ICP must rise, slowly at first but then rapidly to levels approaching that of arterial pressure. Other milestones in thinking about the interrelationships of intracranial CSF and blood volume, and ICP were the studies of Weed and McKibben (1919), Weed (1929), Weed and Flexner (1933), and the several papers of the Evans-Ryder group in Cincinnati (Evans, 1956; Ryder et al., 1952a, b, 1953).

In experimental studies on brain compression in monkeys Langfitt and his group (Weinstein, Langfitt and Kassell, 1964; Langfitt, Kassell and Weinstein, 1965; Langfitt, Weinstein and Kassell, 1965; Langfitt, 1969) defined stages similar to those described by Duret and Kocher, and established the importance of *cerebral vasomotor paralysis* in the end-stage in patients with intracranial expanding lesions when intrinsic vasomotor tone is lost in arteries and arterioles, capillaries and veins are distended, ICP becomes equal to systemic arterial pressure, cerebral blood flow ceases and brain death occurs.

Many intracranial processes—tumour, abscess, haematoma, recent infarction, oedema—eventually produce an increase in ICP and often do not threaten life until then, and an important factor contributing to the effective size of many expanding lesions is associated brain swelling. Most intracranial expanding lesions are localized and produce distortion and herniation of the brain, leading frequently to differences in pressure (i.e. **pressure gradients**) between the supratentorial and infratentorial compartments of the skull by occlusion of the subarachnoid space at the tentorial incisura, or between the intracranial compartment and the spinal subarachnoid space by obliteration of the subarachnoid space at the foramen magnum. It was not until the existence of these pressure gradients was recognized (Browder and Meyers, 1936, 1938; Smyth and Henderson, 1938; Langfitt et al., 1964a, b) that it was appreciated that CSF pressure on lumbar puncture could be normal in a patient with a raised ICP.

Although the processes of raised ICP and distortion of the brain can be defined separately as they are here, they act in concert in individual cases, each process contributing to the dynamic sum of the pathophysiological changes experienced by the patient. As a generalization, *the more slowly* a focal lesion expands, the more likely it is to produce displacement of the brain without an early increase in ICP, since intrinsic compensatory mechanisms—particularly a reduction in the volume of CSF—can operate at their maximum efficiency, and it is in such cases that distortion and herniation of the brain are most pronounced. In contrast, if the focal lesion is *expanding rapidly*, the more likely it is that distortion of the brain will be accompanied by a high ICP, and it is in such cases that brain death not infrequently supervenes before much distortion and herniation can occur. The age of the patient is an important modifying factor: if there is pre-existing cerebral atrophy and a corresponding increase in the volume of CSF as is seen in elderly patients, compensatory capacity is potentially greater than in a younger individual. Furthermore, in an infant, the skull may expand. Even when ICP is normal in the presence of a slowly expanding mass lesion, however, a marginal increase in the volume of any of the intracranial contents, for example the vasodilatation that occurs during sleep, is likely to result in an increase in ICP because of volume–pressure relationships (see below).

Our aim in this chapter is to describe the mechanisms by which ICP can be increased and the harm that this can do to the brain, its blood supply and the rest of the body. The various patterns of distortion and herniation of the brain will be described and the interactions between them and ICP defined in physiological and pathological terms.

Genesis of raised intracranial pressure

Intracranial pressure is the pressure of the CSF within the cranial cavity. It is normally equal throughout the craniospinal axis when the patient is recumbent and the same reference point used. In the upright position intracranial CSF pressure falls to or below zero and lumbar CSF pressure increases. As indicated above, if there is a block to the free circulation of CSF at the tentorial hiatus or the cisterna magna, transient or lasting *pressure gradients* can develop in which ICP may considerably exceed lumbar CSF pressure (Langfitt et al., 1964a).

Intracranial pressure may be measured within the CSF from the lateral ventricle, the cranial subarachnoid space, the cisterna magna or the lumbar subarachnoid space. It may also be measured by transducers placed in the cranial subdural and extradural spaces. The latter must be regarded as approximations of CSF pressure but with modern pressure-detection equipment CSF pressure is fairly accurately transduced across the arachnoid and dural membranes (Lundberg, 1960; Hulme and Cooper, 1966; Jacobson and Rothballer, 1967; Coroneos et al., 1973; Vries, Becker and Young, 1973; Symon and Dorsch, 1975; Levin, 1977; Miller, 1978; Mendelow et al., 1983).

Normal intracranial pressure

The pressure in the CSF has a pulsatile quality at two different frequencies—one synchronous with the arterial pulse wave due to the beat by beat change of intracranial blood volume, while the other is slower, synchronous with respiration and caused by changes in intrathoracic and central venous pressure (Key and Retzius, 1875; Dunbar, Guthrie and Karpell, 1966; Laitinen, 1968; Bradley, 1970). As mean ICP rises the amplitude of the arterial component of CSF pressure increases, while the respiratory or venous component becomes relatively less apparent. For this reason *mean* ICP is defined as the diastolic pressure plus one-third of the pulse pressure (Brock and Hartung, 1972).

The normal range of CSF pressure is 0–1.3 kPa (0–10 mmHg). In practice, however, the upper limit in patients undergoing continuous monitoring of ICP is usually taken as 2 kPa (15 mmHg) in adults, while in very young children the upper limit of normal may be very much lower; e.g. 0.65 kPa (5 mmHg) in a 5-year-old child and 0.4 kPa (3 mmHg) in the newborn (Welch, 1980).

Elevated intracranial pressure

The normal upper limit of ICP is transiently exceeded every time a person coughs or strains. It becomes important only when the increase is sustained for a minute or more. With some 20 years' experience of continuous monitoring of ICP, the clinical significance of certain threshold levels for brain function in different pathological conditions has become well recognized. In patients with intracranial expanding lesions mild elevations of ICP in the range of 2–3 kPa (15–21.5 mmHg) are well tolerated and do not in themselves suggest a need for any therapy specifically aimed at reducing it. Elevation of mean ICP to 4 kPa (30 mmHg) must be regarded as moderate intracranial hypertension requiring therapy, and any increase above 5 kPa (37.5 mmHg) is severe intracranial hypertension that is virtually always associated with diminution of cerebral electrical activity and usually with signs of cerebral ischaemia (Miller, Stanek and Langfitt, 1972; Johnston and Jennett, 1973; Greenberg, Mayer and Becker, 1976; Miller et al., 1977, 1981). Intracranial pressure higher than 8 kPa (60 mmHg) is almost invariably a prelude to death in patients with intracranial expanding lesions and head injury. On the other hand, when intracranial hypertension is unassociated with distortion of the brain such as in benign intracranial hypertension or communicating hydrocephalus, increased ICP is better tolerated by the brain for brief periods even up to levels of 10 kPa (75 mmHg) (Johnston and Paterson, 1974).

Waves of increased intracranial pressure

Elevations of ICP are rarely sustained for long and in most instances take the form of *pressure waves* (Guillaume and Janny, 1951; Ecker, 1955). Lundberg (1960), on the basis of his extensive experience, defined two main types of pressure wave. The first and clinically most significant type is the plateau wave or **A-wave** in which ICP increases abruptly and spontaneously from a baseline little above normal, and rises exponentially until the mean pressure exceeds 6.7 kPa (50 mmHg); there is then a steady elevation of pressure lasting between 5 and 20 minutes, rarely longer, and then an equally abrupt and spontaneous reduction of pressure to the baseline level. This form of pressure wave is most often seen in patients with intracranial expanding lesions and obstructive hydrocephalus. When the wave is at its height the patient's condition is frequently worse, ranging from a feeling of fullness in the head with headache and flushing of the face to frank neurological deterioration sometimes with decerebrate rigidity. These waves are thought to result from *cerebrovascular vasodilatation* when the capacity for spatial compensation is reduced (Ingvar and Lundberg, 1961; Risberg, Lundberg and Ingvar, 1969). They occur most frequently at night when rapid eye movement sleep or carbon dioxide retention are likely to cause a relaxation of the cerebral vessels and an increase in cerebral blood volume (Hulme and Cooper, 1966; Marshall, Smith and Shapiro, 1978).

The most frequent type of pressure wave, although of less adverse clinical significance, is the **B-wave**. This is a sharply peaked wave in which mean ICP rises from a variable baseline to a level 2.7–4.0 kPa (20–30 mmHg) higher, and then falls abruptly with no intervening period of sustained intracranial hypertension. This type of wave occurs once or twice per minute in patients who have periodic respiration. It has therefore been related directly to changes in end-tidal and arterial P_{CO_2}. B-waves are also seen, however, in patients on artificial ventilation in whom arterial P_{CO_2} is constant. Other factors must therefore contribute to these waves, but the source is thought to be in changes in cerebrovascular tone and cerebral blood volume (Miller, 1975a).

Changes in brain water, cerebrospinal fluid and intracranial blood volume

Variations in the volume of the normal intracranial constituents and interactions between them are crucial factors in the genesis of ICP.

Brain water This is volumetrically the most important constituent of brain tissue, the average water content being 75 per cent. Cerebral oedema is dealt with later in this chapter but, defined as an increase in the volume of the brain due to an increase in its water content, it occurs frequently around focal expanding lesions in the brain and may be a major factor contributing to their effective size.

Cerebrospinal fluid The total volume of CSF in the normal adult is about 140 ml. Its rate of absorption is sensitively linked to changes in ICP and its volume can fall rapidly during surges of intracranial hypertension.

Intracranial blood volume Changes in the calibre of arterial vessels are important for the regulation of cerebral blood flow but the important vessels contributing to changes in cerebral blood volume—and therefore referred to as *capacitance vessels*—are the capillaries, venules and cerebral veins prior to their entry into the dural venous sinuses (Bedford, 1935; Cairns, 1939). Admission of blood to the cranial cavity depends on the arterial resistance, and factors that reduce this, such as hypercapnia and hypoxaemia, thereby increase cerebral blood volume. The calibre of veins draining the brain and, therefore, cerebral blood volume may also be influenced by sympathetic nervous activity (D'Alecy, 1972). Most rapid alterations in ICP stem from changes in cerebral blood volume. The extent of the alteration in pressure is not simply a function of the extent of the change of the volume of blood in the system, however, since it is related also to overall pressure–volume relationships.

Intracranial pressure–volume relationships

Clinical and experimental observations on the relationship between intracranial expanding lesions and ICP have emphasized the importance of intracranial pressure–volume relationships (Flexner, Clark and Weed, 1932; Masserman, 1935). The basic example of this is obtained when the volume of a mass lesion, usually an inflatable balloon in an experimental animal, is plotted against the ICP (Langfitt, Kassell and Weinstein, 1965; Langfitt, Weinstein and Kassell, 1965; Nakatani and Ommaya, 1975). During initial inflation of the balloon there is little persisting change in ICP but once the balloon attains a certain threshold, ICP begins to increase, rising more and more steeply with each increment of volume, thus defining an exponential relationship between balloon volume and ICP. This is known as the **intracranial pressure–volume curve** (Fig. 2.1). The threshold volume was at first

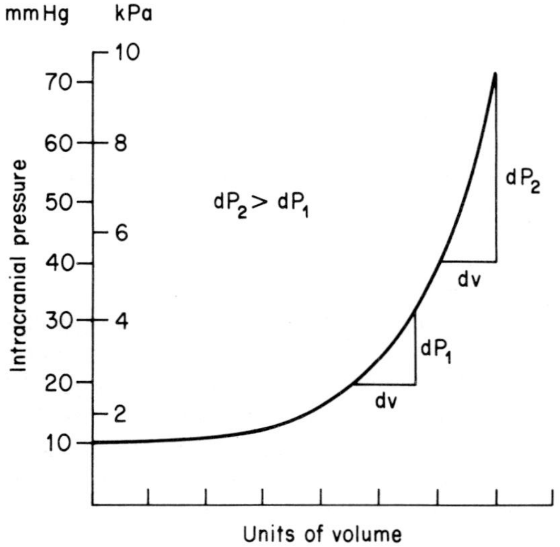

Fig. 2.1 Theoretical intracranial pressure–volume curve. As volume increases and ICP rises, uniform increments of volume (dv) produce progressively larger increases in ICP (dP_1 and dP_2). Increases or decreases in volume cause correspondingly greater changes in ICP on the steep part of the curve.

sidered simply to be a measure of the total displaceable volume of blood and CSF in the cranial cavity but this cannot be entirely so for the threshold volume varies with the speed of expansion of the balloon. The more rapidly it expands, the sooner ICP begins to rise. Intracranial pressure, however, cannot rise indefinitely, its upper limit being the level of arterial blood pressure.

Although this model of intracranial pressure–volume relationships is an oversimplification, it has proved useful as an explanation for phenomena observed clinically. In a patient with a progressively expanding intracranial mass lesion, ICP eventually increases. Once this increase has begun and the steep part of the pressure–volume curve is approached, the patient is very vulnerable to any subsequent increase in volume of any of the intracranial constituents (blood, CSF or brain water) (Miller, 1975a). Thus cerebral vasodilatation in a patient with an intracranial expanding lesion is a much more serious event than in a normal individual. Sudden neurological deterioration in a patient with a brain tumour is often ascribed to haemorrhage within the tumour, but it is more likely to be due to an increase in the volume of any of the intracranial constituents, when the steep part of the pressure–volume curve has already been reached (Fig. 2.1). The usual cause of an abrupt increase in cerebral blood volume is arterial vasodilatation and/or venous obstruction.

The effects of raised intracranial pressure

During severe intracranial hypertension, ICP rises towards the level of the arterial blood pressure. The latter may rise ahead of the increasing ICP and so the patient sustains extremely high levels of arterial hypertension, the systolic pressure sometimes exceeding 300 mmHg (Cushing, 1901, 1902, 1903). If ICP attains the level of the arterial pressure, however, the effects are dramatic and disastrous: neurological function ceases abruptly, the pupils become fixed and unresponsive to light, brain-stem reflexes disappear, and no motor response can be obtained from the face or upper limbs. Angiography at this time will show that contrast medium will not enter the cranial cavity (Riishede and Ethelberg, 1953; Pribram, 1961; Troupp and Heiskanen, 1963; Langfitt and Kassell, 1966). Measurements of cerebral blood flow will confirm a complete arrest of the circulation of blood in the cerebral hemispheres (Balslev-Jørgensen et al., 1972). This is a dramatic illustration of the fact that the difference between arterial and intracranial pressure is equivalent to the **cerebral perfusion pressure**, and that when this is reduced to zero cerebral blood flow ceases.

Prior to the production of brain death by severe intracranial hypertension, however, lesser degrees of increased ICP may be responsible for varying levels of cerebral ischaemia. The relationship between ICP and cerebral blood flow is central to the understanding of the clinical effects of intracranial hypertension. Strictly speaking, cerebral perfusion pressure is the difference in pressure between arteries entering the cranial subarachnoid space and veins leaving it. Arterial pressure recorded directly from cerebral arteries is the same as the blood pressure recorded in the brachial artery (Ferguson, 1972). Under conditions of increased intracranial CSF pressure, pressure within cerebral veins increases, remaining 0.25–0.5 kPa (2–4 mmHg) higher than CSF pressure. If this did not occur, the veins would collapse (Yada, Nakagawa and Tsuru, 1973; Johnston and Rowan, 1974). This small pressure difference is maintained by a variable constriction of the extreme end of the venous system prior to its entry into the pressure-protected dural venous sinuses, functioning as a Starling resistor (Starling, 1896; Wright, 1938; Permutt and Riley, 1963). Within the venous sinus there is a considerable pressure gradient, ranging from nearly level with ICP at the anterior end of the superior sagittal sinus to atmospheric or central venous pressure (whichever is the higher) at the torcular and in the jugular venous system (Shulman and Verdier, 1967; Johnston and Rowan, 1974; Martins, Kobrine and Larsen, 1974). This distal pressure gradient between ICP and systemic venous pressure is important for the regulation of absorption of CSF (Levine, Povlishock and Becker, 1982). Proximal to the sinuses, however, *the difference between arterial pressure and ICP* becomes a useful approximation of the cerebral perfusion pressure.

The relationship between cerebral perfusion pressure and cerebral blood flow and the phenomenon of **autoregulation** (see Chapter 3) has been widely studied under experimental and clinical conditions (Harper, 1966; Miller, Stanek and Langfitt, 1972, 1973; Johnston et al., 1972, 1973; Symon et al., 1973). Experimentally, when the cerebral circulation is intact, a steady reduction in cerebral perfusion pressure produces only a slight change in cerebral blood flow until a threshold level of about 8 kPa (60 mmHg) is reached. This process in which compensatory cerebral arterial and arteriolar vasodilatation occurs is termed autoregulation. Up to this point it matters little whether the perfusion pressure is reduced by arterial hypotension or by intracranial hypertension. Beyond this point, however, there is a major difference. With haemorrhagic arterial hypotension, cerebral blood flow begins to fall with any further reduction in perfusion pressure below 8 kPa (60 mmHg). If arterial hypotension is drug-induced, however, or is produced by haemorrhage after a chemical or surgical sympathectomy, perfusion pressure can fall to as low as 5.3 kPa (40 mmHg) before cerebral ischaemia begins (Fitch, MacKenzie and Harper, 1975). This difference in pressure thresholds for ischaemia is ascribed to sympathetic vasoconstriction of the proximal extraparenchymal and major cerebral vessels during haemorrhagic hypotension (Harper et al., 1972). When perfusion pressure falls to below 2.7 kPa (20 mmHg) as a result of reduced arterial pressure, cerebral blood flow virtually ceases. When perfusion pressure is reduced by intracranial hypertension, normal levels of cerebral blood flow are maintained provided the arterial pressure is normal or elevated until the perfusion pressure falls to 5.3 kPa (40 mmHg); there is then a progressive decrease in flow as perfusion pressure falls to zero, but cerebral blood flow does not cease completely until there is no perfusion pressure.

Because of the compensatory increases in arterial pressure that can occur during intracranial hypertension, cerebral blood flow may still be maintained at normal or near-normal levels even when the ICP is greater than 8 kPa (60 mmHg). The key pressure is the perfusion pressure. These findings have been obtained under ideal experimental conditions, and may therefore not be the same in patients because *autoregulation may be impaired in the presence of acute brain damage* resulting, for example, from a head injury or an acute stroke (Fieschi et al., 1968; Enevoldsen et al., 1976); it may also be impaired in the vicinity of an expanding lesion (Palvolgyi, 1969). Thus impairment of autoregulation is the likely explanation for the failure of patients with acute brain damage or other expanding lesion to tolerate increases in ICP in excess of 5 kPa (37.5 mmHg) that do not normally reduce perfusion pressure to critical levels. The essential link between the level of ICP and clinically observed neurological dysfunction or depression of cerebral electrical activity appears to be the cerebral circulation. When cerebral blood flow is reduced below 40 per cent of its normal value, cerebral electrical activity ceases. At blood flows below 30 per cent of normal, the concentration of extracellular potassium increases in the affected brain: as potassium leaves the cell, calcium enters, and irreversible structural damage to neural elements occurs (Bourke et al., 1975; Astrup et al., 1977; Astrup, 1982).

The pathology of intracranial expanding lesions

Several different yet related factors have to be taken into account when a mass lesion within the cranial cavity starts to expand. The first is distortion of the adjacent brain (Walsh and Schettini, 1976); because of its viscoelastic properties brain tissue adjacent to the mass will flow away from it—i.e. there is axial movement of the brain in addition to the more conventional displacements. Schettini and Walsh (1973) have shown that when a pressure sensitive transducer is driven downwards to indent the surface of the brain, the pressure recorded on the face of the transducer diminishes as the brain accommodates the distorting mass. But while this might suggest that the local properties of brain tissue can contribute to the prevention of a rise in ICP, *the major factor responsible for spatial compensation is a reduction in the volume of intracranial CSF.*

The basic sequence of events, therefore, is local deformity, a reduced volume of CSF, shift and distortion of the brain and eventually, in the intact skull, the appearance of *internal herniae—i.e. displacement of brain tissue from one intracranial compartment into another, or into the spinal canal* (Fig. 2.2). These in turn lead to the development of pressure gradients between compartments because of obliteration of the subarachnoid space and cisterns, and secondary vascular complications such as haemorrhage and ischaemic brain damage (Moore and Stern, 1938; Weinstein et al., 1968).

Supratentorial expanding lesions

As an intrinsic lesion in a cerebral hemisphere—usually a tumour, a haematoma, a recent infarct or an abscess—expands, so also does the hemisphere: the surface of the brain is pressed against the unyielding dura, gyri are flattened, sulci are

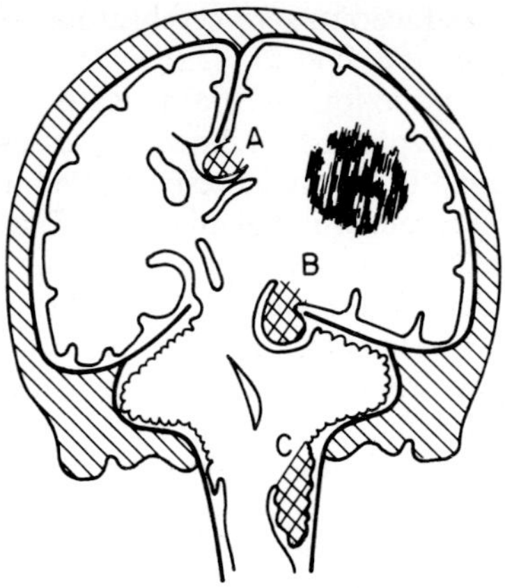

Fig. 2.2 Diagrammatic representation of distortion and herniation of the brain caused by a tumour in a cerebral hemisphere. The midline and the lateral ventricles are displaced, and varying degrees of supracallosal (A), tentorial (B) and tonsillar (C) herniation are produced.

narrowed and, as CSF is displaced from the subarachnoid space, the surface of the brain becomes dry. The lateral ventricle on the side of the lesion and the third ventricle become reduced in size and there is a **lateral shift** of the midline structures, viz. the pericallosal arteries, the interventricular septum and the third ventricle away from the lesion (Fig. 2.3). Obliteration of the contralateral foramen of Monro may lead to enlargement of the contralateral lateral ventricle (Fig. 2.3), and this occurrence is closely related to the development of increased ICP. The sylvian fissure is narrowed and the lesser wing of the sphenoid bone may produce a groove on the inferior surface of the frontal lobe. The floor of the third ventricle is displaced into the basal cisterns and the mamillary bodies become wedged into a narrowed interpeduncular fossa. At autopsy the dura may be so tense that it is difficult to incise it without damaging the underlying cortex. Lindenberg (1955) suggested that there may be sufficient compression of the terminal branches of the cerebral arteries to produce ischaemic cortical necrosis in the depths of sulci, but it seems more likely that reduced perfusion pressure in a patient with a high ICP is the major factor contributing to these perisulcal infarcts (Janzer and Friede, 1979).

While this sequence of events may occur with any expanding lesion within a cerebral hemisphere, certain displacements are selectively affected by the site of the lesion. Thus, an expanding lesion in the frontal lobe will produce displacement of the free margin of the anterior part of the falx; the posterior part of the falx, however, is rarely displaced laterally because it is firmly tethered at this level. Furthermore, a lesion in a temporal lobe will produce selectively severe shift of the third ventricle and will displace upwards the Sylvian fissure and the branches of the middle cerebral artery which it contains.

The next stage is the development of **internal herniae**, viz. displacement of brain tissue from one intracranial compartment to another.

Supracallosal hernia (*subfalcine or cingulate hernia*) The ipsilateral cingulate gyrus herniates under the free edge of the falx and produces selective displacement of the pericallosal arteries away from the midline (Fig. 2.3). Because the posterior end of the falx is firmly tethered in position, a posterior supracallosal hernia can occur only after there has been downward displacement of the roof of the ipsilateral ventricle. A wedge of pressure necrosis may occur along the groove where the cingulate gyrus comes in contact with the falx (Fig. 2.4). If, as a result of treatment, the brain returns to its normal shape this wedge of necrosis can be taken as being indicative of previous herniation (Fig. 2.4). The shift and herniation may, however, become severe enough to compromise the circulation through the pericallosal arteries leading to more extensive infarction in the territories which they supply, resulting in weakness or sensory loss in one or both legs.

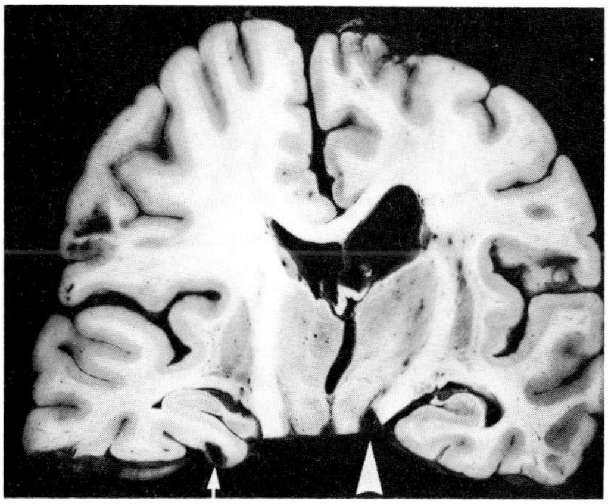

Fig. 2.3 Lateral shift. There is displacement of the midline structures to the right, a supracallosal hernia, enlargement of the contralateral lateral ventricle, haemorrhagic pressure necrosis in relation to a tentorial hernia on the left (arrow) and haemorrhagic necrosis in the contralateral cerebral peduncle (arrowhead). (Reproduced, with permission, from Miller and Adams, 1972).

Tentorial hernia (*uncal or lateral transtentorial hernia*) The uncus and the medial part of the

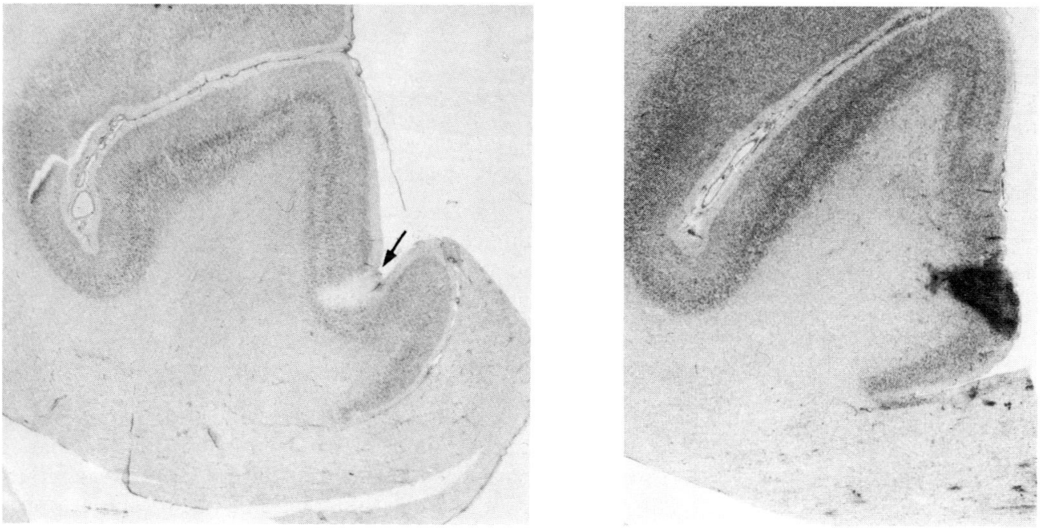

(a) **(b)**

Fig. 2.4 Pressure necrosis in cingulate gyrus. (**a**) Recent rarefaction necrosis (arrow) in relation to a supracallosal hernia. (**b**) Densely cellular wedge indicative of a previous supracallosal hernia (patient survived comatose for 2 weeks after evacuation of a subdural haematoma). Cresyl violet, both ×4. (Reproduced, with permission: (**a**) from Adams, 1975; (**b**) from Adams and Graham, 1976).

parahippocampal gyrus herniate medially and downwards through the tentorial incisura (Fig. 2.5). The width of the hernia varies widely, this being related to some extent to variation in size of the tentorial incisura (Corsellis, 1958) as well as to the size and site of the mass lesion. This type of hernia may occur in association with any supratentorial expanding lesion but is usually most pronounced when it is in the temporal lobe. As the parahippocampal gyrus herniates, the midbrain is narrowed in its transverse axis, the aqueduct is compressed and the contralateral cerebral peduncle is pushed against the opposite free edge of the tentorium (see Fig. 2.3). The *ipsilateral oculomotor nerve* becomes compressed between the petroclinoid ligament or the free edge of the tentorium and the posterior cerebral artery. The resulting paralysis of the oculomotor nerve produces ptosis, dilatation of the pupil with loss of the direct response to light shone in the affected eye and the consensual response to light shone in the opposite eye; there is loss of upward and medial movement of the eye and in its resting position it deviates laterally due to the unopposed action of the sixth cranial nerve. *Dilatation of the pupil* is the earliest consistent sign of a tentorial hernia and may occur before there is any impairment of consciousness (Meyer, 1920; Vincent, David and Thiebaut, 1936; Jefferson, 1938; Reid and Cone, 1939; Sunderland, 1958; Jennett and Stern, 1960; Finney and Walker, 1962). The nerve is at first only flattened where it is compressed and angulated over the posterior cerebral artery but there is often ultimately haemorrhage into it (Fig. 2.6).

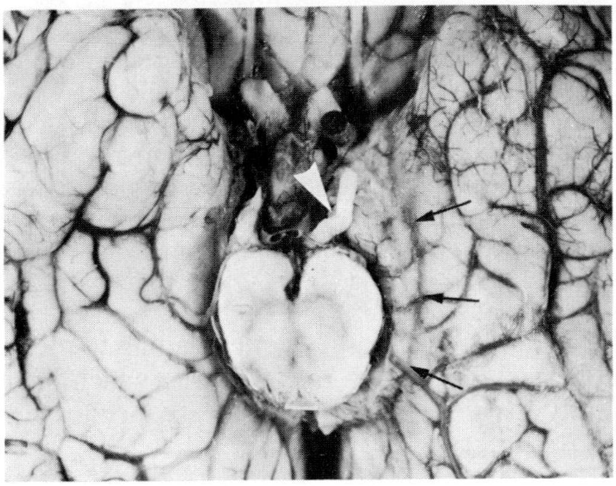

Fig. 2.5 Tentorial hernia. There is a deep groove (arrows) in the left parahippocampal gyrus, and there is flattening and angulation of the ipsilateral oculomotor nerve (arrowhead).

As the hernia enlarges, a wedge of necrosis often accompanied by haemorrhage appears along the line of the groove in the parahippocampal gyrus (Fig. 2.7), and compression of the contralateral cerebral peduncle against the free edge of the tentorium (Kernohan and Woltman, 1929) may lead to infarction with or without haemorrhage in the dorsal part of the peduncle and the adjacent tegmentum (Fig. 2.8). This will produce weakness followed by extensor rigidity in the limbs ipsilateral to the expanding lesion. A large hernia will produce a distinct groove on the upper surface of the adjacent cerebellar hemisphere.

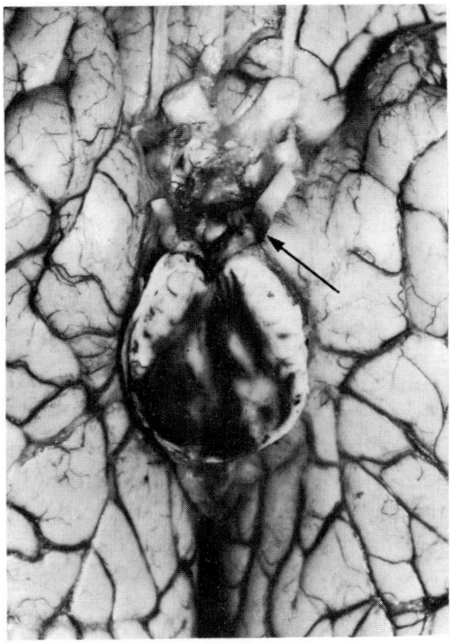

Fig. 2.6 Tentorial hernia. The groove in the parahippocampal gyrus is less obvious than in Fig. 2.5 but there is focal haemorrhage into the ipsilateral oculomotor nerve (arrow) and there is severe secondary haemorrhage into the brain stem. (Reproduced, with permission, from Adams, 1975).

Because some degree of shift and herniation of brain can occur during the period of spatial compensation without ICP becoming significantly high, it may be difficult to establish *post mortem* if the ICP has been high during life. Adams and Graham (1976) have suggested that the pathognomonic feature of a high ICP due to a supratentorial expanding lesion is the presence—best seen in coronal sections of the

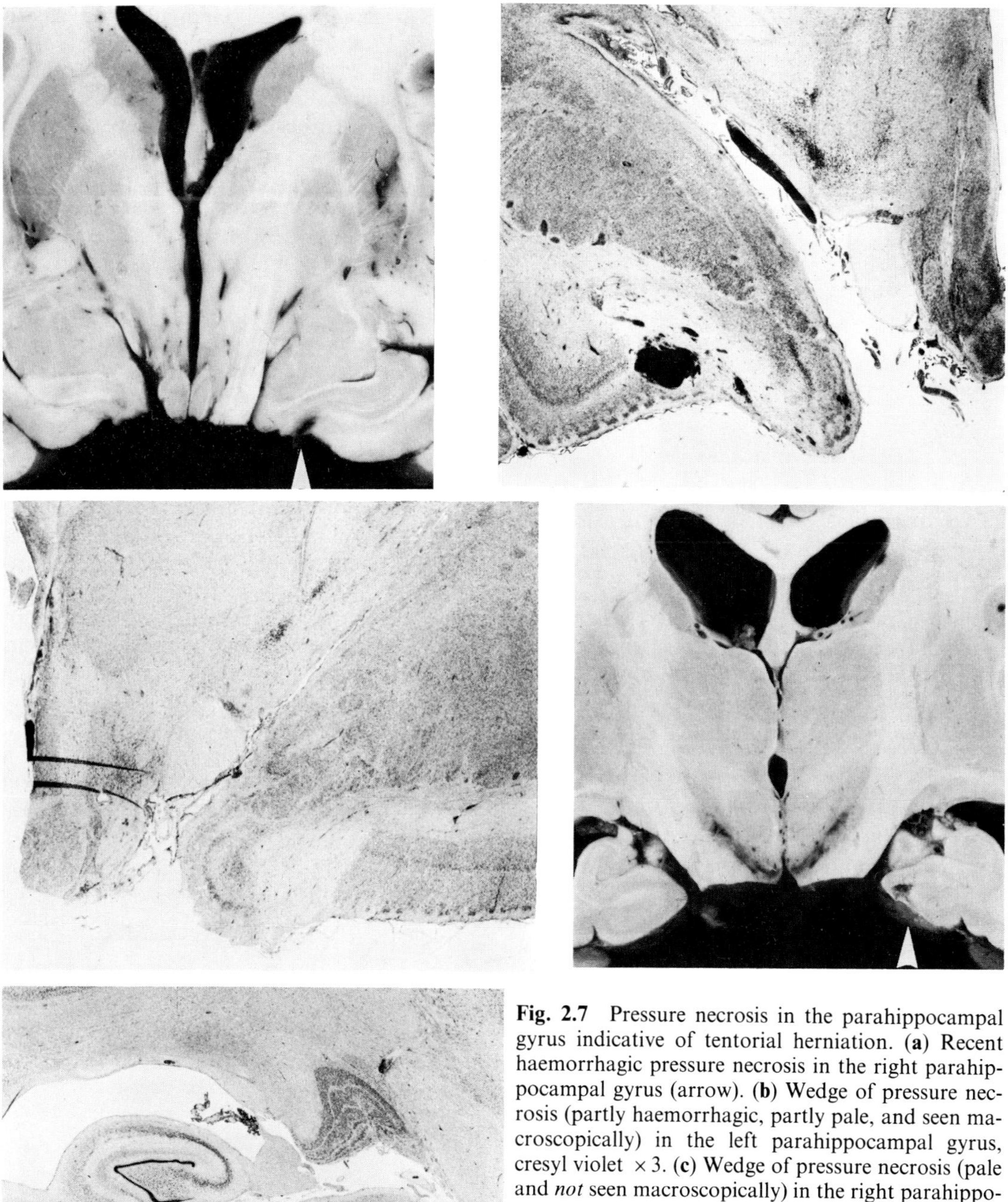

(a) (b) (c) (d)

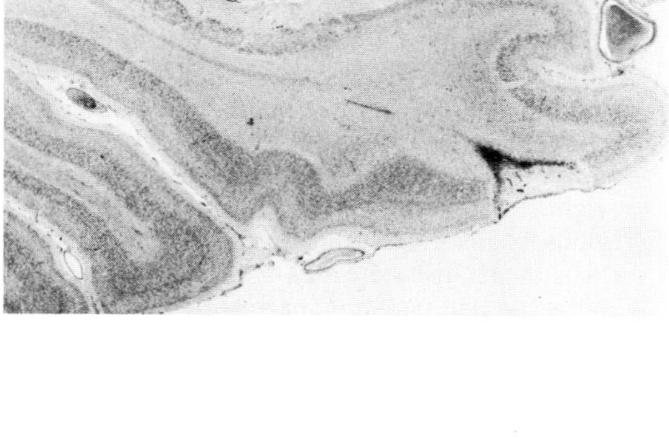

(e)

Fig. 2.7 Pressure necrosis in the parahippocampal gyrus indicative of tentorial herniation. (**a**) Recent haemorrhagic pressure necrosis in the right parahippocampal gyrus (arrow). (**b**) Wedge of pressure necrosis (partly haemorrhagic, partly pale, and seen macroscopically) in the left parahippocampal gyrus, cresyl violet × 3. (**c**) Wedge of pressure necrosis (pale and *not* seen macroscopically) in the right parahippocampal gyrus, cresyl violet × 3. (**d**) Small cystic lesion (arrow) in the right parahippocampal gyrus indicative of previous tentorial herniation (patient survived vegetative for 3 months after evacuation of a subdural haematoma). (**e**) Wedge of long-standing pressure necrosis in the left parahippocampal gyrus indicative of previous tentorial herniation (patient survived vegetative for 6 weeks after evacuation of an intracerebral haematoma. Cresyl violet × 3. (All reproduced, with permission, from Adams and Graham, 1976).

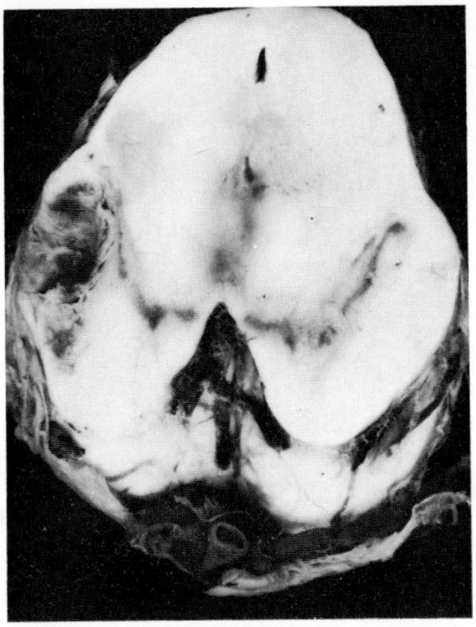

Fig. 2.8 Haemorrhagic necrosis in the lateral part of the cerebral peduncle contralateral to an expanding lesion. (Same case as Fig. 2.3.)

brain—of a wedge of pressure necrosis in one or both parahippocampal gyri. Pressure necrosis of this type was seen in every patient known to have had an ICP of more than 5.3 kPa (40 mmHg) during life, in most of the patients with an ICP between 2.7 and 5.3 kPa (20 and 40 mmHg) and in no patient with an ICP of less than 2.7 kPa (20 mmHg). When the pressure necrosis is haemorrhagic it can be identified macroscopically but if there is no haemorrhage it may only be identifiable microscopically (see Fig. 2.7). A past episode of tentorial herniation associated with a high ICP can be recognized by the presence of a small organized wedge of pressure necrosis in the parahippocampal gyrus (see Fig. 2.7). Lindenberg (1955) has also emphasized the importance of local pressure necrosis in the parahippocampal gyri: this can be distinguished from a herniation contusion (see p. 91) by its more lateral situation.

As already indicated, a tentorial hernia will eventually cause obliteration of the subarachnoid space at the tentorial incisura leading to a CSF pressure differential between the supratentorial and infratentorial compartments, and it may be that pressure necrosis in one or both parahippocampal gyri can be equated with a pressure differential. When such a pressure gradient exists, any process which causes an increase in ICP will increase the gradient thus adding to the driving force producing tentorial herniation.

This mechanism has been modelled in experiments by Fitch and McDowall (1971) and Miller (1975b) in which an intracranial balloon is gradually inflated to the point where a pressure gradient has just begun to develop between the lateral ventricle and the cisterna magna. At this time dilatation of the pupil ipsilateral to the balloon begins to occur. If inflation of the balloon is now stopped so that the size of the mass lesion remains the same, and an agent which causes cerebral vasodilatation (such as halothane or carbon dioxide) is administered to the animal, there is an increase in supratentorial pressure without an equivalent increase in infratentorial pressure and dilatation of the pupil becomes complete. Studies in patients with head injury and with intracranial tumours (Smyth and Henderson, 1938; Kaufmann and Clark, 1970) have shown that transtentorial pressure gradients are not uncommon, and when present they are frequently accompanied by the clinical signs of tentorial herniation. Any increase in the pressure gradient is commonly associated with an abrupt worsening of the patient's neurological status such as the onset of decerebrate rigidity. The expansion of a supratentorial mass lesion may therefore be responsible for initiating tentorial herniation and establishing the beginnings of a transtentorial pressure gradient. Thereafter any process which would normally produce a diffuse

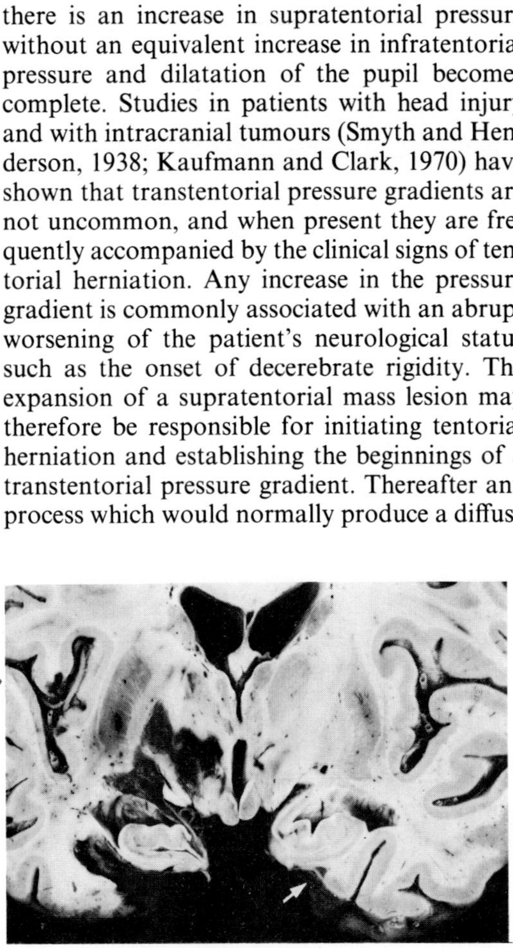

Fig. 2.9 Infarction in territory supplied by the left anterior choroidal artery—the internal segment of the globus pallidus, the adjacent internal capsule and the optic tract. There is also a large wedge-shaped infarct in the left parahippocampal gyrus and a small one in the right parahippocampal gyrus (arrow) indicative of previous bilateral tentorial herniation. Patient survived in a vegetative state for 4 weeks after the evacuation of a left acute subdural haematoma.

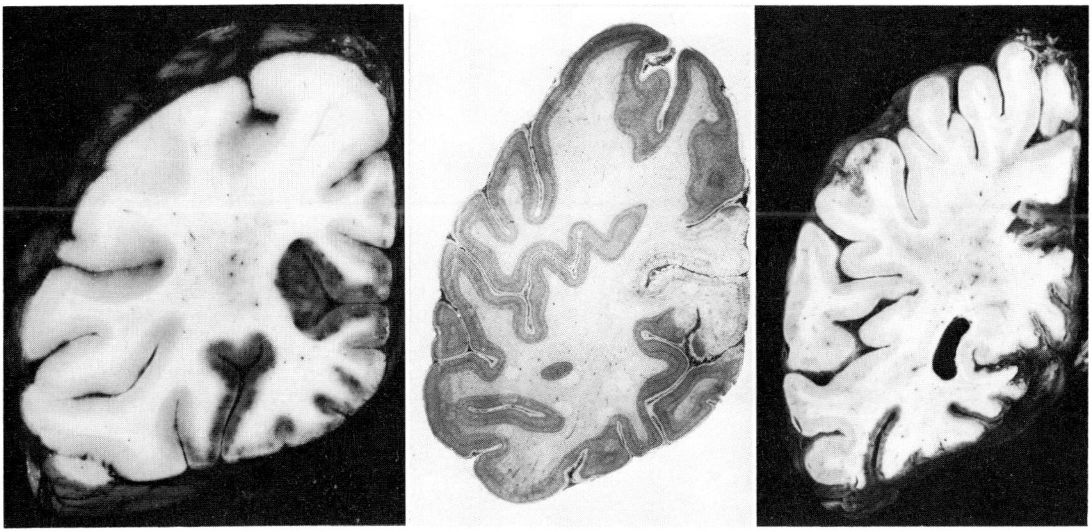

a b c

Fig. 2.10 Infarction in the territory supplied by the posterior cerebral artery. (**a**) Recent haemorrhagic infarction involving the medial and inferior surfaces of the left occipital lobe. (**b**) Recent pale infarction (not identifiable macroscopically) affecting the medial surface of the left occipital lobe in a patient who died shortly after evacuation of an extradural haematoma. Cresyl violet ×2. (**c**) Previous infarction—now shrunken and granular—involving the medial and inferior surfaces of the left occipital lobe (patient survived in a vegetative state for 4 weeks after evacuation of a subdural haematoma). ((**b**) Reproduced with permission, from Adams and Graham, 1976).

increase in intracranial pressure will increase the tentorial pressure gradient and accentuate the process of herniation. A further factor which may contribute to a high ICP in these circumstances is the development of hydrocephalus due to obstruction of the flow of CSF from the lateral ventricles to the third and fourth ventricles. The foramen of Monro may be blocked and the aqueduct narrowed by lateral midline shift.

Other sequelae of raised ICP and tentorial herniation include the *compression of arteries*: thus compression of an anterior choroidal artery may lead to infarction in the medial part of the globus pallidus, in the internal capsule and in the optic tract (Fig. 2.9); compression of a posterior cerebral artery—the artery most commonly affected—may lead to infarction in the thalamus, in the temporal lobe including the hippocampus, and in the cortex on the medial and inferior surfaces of the occipital lobe (Fig. 2.10); and compression of a superior cerebellar artery may lead to infarction in the superior part of the cerebellum. Infarction in the cortex of the occipital lobe and in the cerebellum is often intensely haemorrhagic but on occasions it can only be identified microscopically (Fig. 2.10). These circulatory disturbances usually occur on the same side as the hernia but they may also be bilateral and occasionally they are restricted to the other hemisphere (Adams and Graham, 1976).

Central transtentorial herniation This is brought about by caudal displacement of the diencephalon and the rostral brain stem, may be preceded by a lateral transtentorial hernia, and occurs particularly in response to frontal and parietal lesions or to bilateral expanding lesions. If ICP increases rapidly in association with lesions of this type, both parahippocampal gyri may herniate through the tentorial incisura, leading to the formation of a *circular* or *ring hernia* (Fig. 2.11). This type of hernia is most evident posteriorly and results in compression of the tectal plate: the clinical manifestations of such a hernia are therefore bilateral ptosis and failure of upward gaze, followed by loss of the pupillary light response.

Minor degrees of caudal displacement are less easy to identify, even in a properly fixed brain, than the lateral shifts already described, but when such central herniation is established the mamillary bodies are displaced backwards and

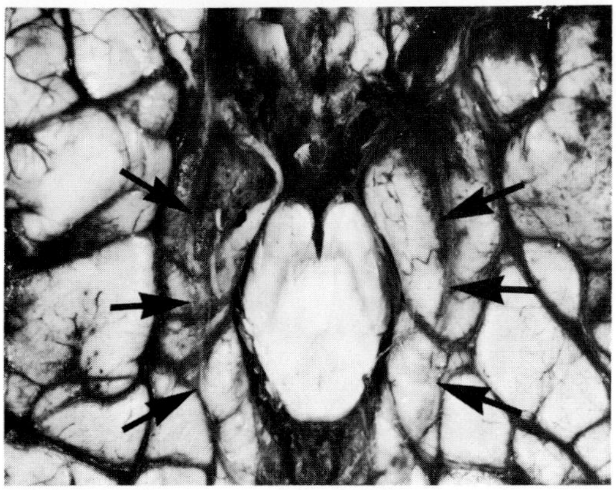

Fig. 2.11 Bilateral tentorial ('ring') herniae. Deep grooves (arrows) are present in both parahippocampal gyri and there is narrowing of the midbrain.

downwards, the pituitary stalk is compressed, and the posterior part of the floor of the third ventricle comes to lie below the level of the tentorial incisura. Focal infarction may occur in the mamillary bodies, and in the anterior lobe of the pituitary gland due to impairment of blood flow through the long hypothalamohypophyseal portal vessels. The caudal shift causes distortion of the thalamus and elongation of individual neurons (Fig. 2.12), and even more elongation and angulation of the oculomotor nerves than occurs with lateral transtentorial herniation: this is often bilateral. Infarction in the territories supplied by the anterior choroidal, posterior cerebral and superior cerebellar arteries is again a frequent occurrence. Decerebrate rigidity and loss of consciousness are common, at least partly because of distortion of the rostral brain stem, and the blood pressure becomes elevated as a result of increased sympathetic activity. The important area in the brain stem associated with this type of arterial hypertension appears to be the floor of the fourth ventricle and the nucleus of the tractus solitarius, especially on the left side (Hoff and Reis, 1970; Fein, 1982). Depression of the heart rate and changes in respiration are also common (Cushing, 1903; Howell, 1959; Thompson and Malina, 1959).

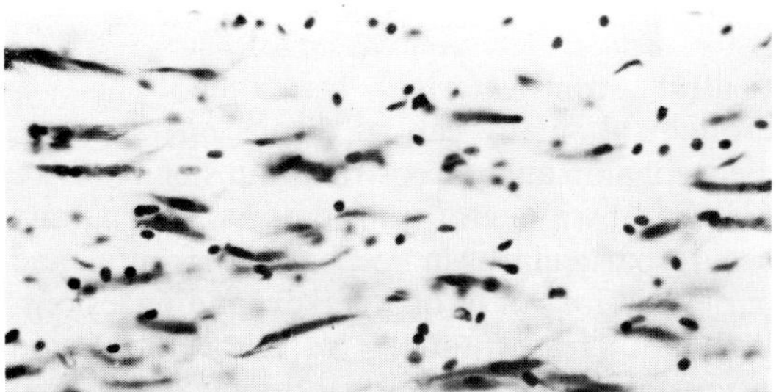

Fig. 2.12 Elongated neurons in the thalamus brought about by distortion of the brain. Cresyl violet ×250.

Haemorrhage and infarction in the midbrain and pons This is a common and often a terminal event in patients with supratentorial expanding lesions, a high ICP and tentorial herniation (Fig. 2.13). Emphasis is usually placed on the occurrence of haemorrhage since this is obvious macroscopically, but microscopical examination often shows ischaemic infarction to be as important as frank haemorrhage (Fig. 2.14). Both types of lesion occur mainly adjacent to the mid-

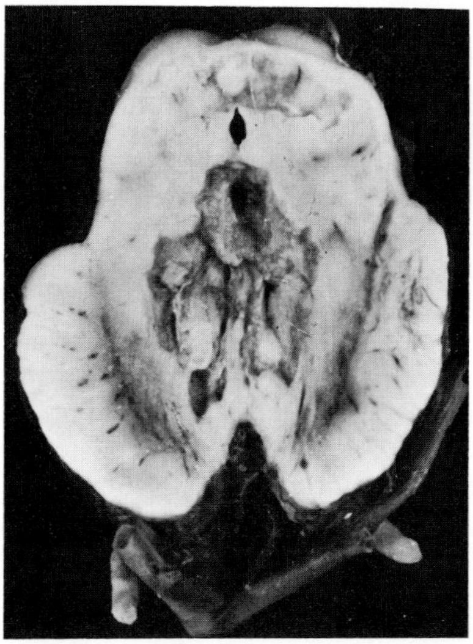

Fig. 2.13 Secondary damage in the brain stem. The acute changes are shown in Fig. 2.6. If the patient survives, the affected tissue comes to be represented by a discoloured partly cystic lesion in the midbrain (this patient survived vegetative for 8 weeks after the evacuation of an acute subdural haematoma).

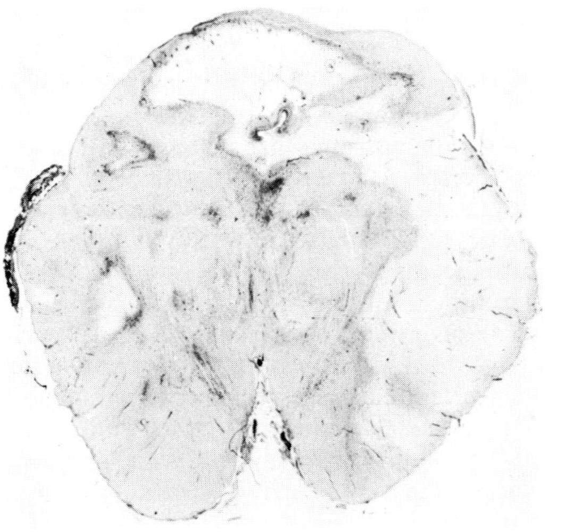

Fig. 2.14 Secondary damage in the brain stem. There is extensive pale infarction that was not apparent macroscopically. Cresyl violet ×2 reduced to 85%. (Reproduced, with permission, from Adams, 1975).

line, in the tegmentum of the midbrain and in the tegmental and basal parts of the pons. First described by Duret (1878) there has always been considerable controversy as to the pathogenesis of the haemorrhage and the ischaemic damage. The most important factors are likely to be caudal displacement and anteroposterior elongation of the rostral brain stem, and relative immobility of the basilar artery. As the displacement continues, the arteries which arise from the basilar artery and supply the rostral brain stem are stretched. This in turn leads to shearing strain, spasm and infarction or haemorrhage (Johnson and Yates, 1956; Hassler, 1967). According to Klintworth (1965, 1966) the propensity to bleed into the brain stem may be increased when a high ICP and axial brain-stem shift are suddenly reduced so that there is an increase in blood flow in the previously ischaemic brain stem.

Tonsillar hernia (*foraminal impaction, cerebellar cone*) Downward displacement of the cerebellar tonsils through the foramen magnum may also occur in association with a supratentorial space-occupying lesion. Because of the considerable variations in the normal configuration of the cerebellar tonsils, a tonsillar hernia secondary to an intracranial expanding lesion can be said to be present only if there is haemorrhagic necrosis at their tips, and a groove on the ventral surface of the medulla when it has been compressed against the anterior edge of the foramen magnum (Fig. 2.15). The distortion of the spinomedullary junction associated with tonsillar herniation can result in apnoea with preservation of consciousness. More usually, however, tonsillar herniation is the sequel to a series of intracranial events, at least one of which has already been responsible for loss of consciousness, and usually there are other abnormal neurological signs, such as decerebrate rigidity and impairment of brainstem reflexes before apnoea appears. Where the tonsillar hernia is due to an expanding lesion in the posterior fossa, however, apnoea may occur in isolation.

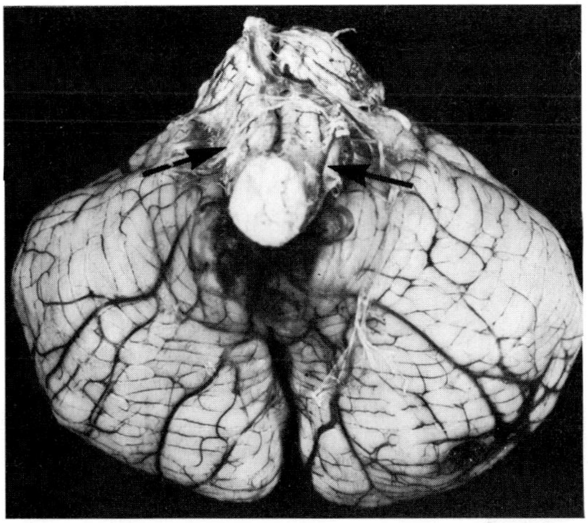

Fig. 2.15 Tonsillar hernia. The tips of the tonsils are haemorrhagic and there is a groove (arrows) on the ventral surface of the medulla oblongata.

Extracerebral lesions An essentially similar sequence of events to that already described occurs in association with supratentorial extracerebral expanding lesions such as extradural or subdural haematoma, or a tumour arising from the meninges. One difference is that convolutional flattening associated with acute subdural haematoma is restricted to the contralateral hemisphere (see p. 95). With a meningioma there is often destruction of adjacent brain tissue, which also contributes to spatial compensation.

Diffuse brain swelling When ICP is high because of diffuse brain swelling, the ventricles become small but remain symmetrical and there is no lateral shift of the midline structures. Bilateral tentorial herniae may occur, their size depending to some extent on the rate of brain swelling and the size of the tentorial incisura. Caudal displacement of the diencephalon and brain stem (i.e. a central transtentorial hernia) is the major factor contributing to a fatal outcome.

Infratentorial expanding lesions

Hydrocephalus is the commonest abnormality associated with mass lesions in the posterior fossa, whether they be in the fourth ventricle, in the cerebellum or extracerebellar. When the lesion is not in the midline, the aqueduct and fourth ventricle are compressed and displaced to the other side. Tonsillar herniation tends to be more severe than with a supratentorial expanding lesion. Occasionally the posterior inferior cerebellar arteries may be so compressed that infarction occurs in the inferior part of one or both cerebellar hemispheres. Herniation of the cerebellum may also occur in an upward direction—the so-called *reversed tentorial hernia*: if the lesion is expanding very slowly, upward herniation of the superior vermis of the cerebellum can produce considerable distortion of the temporal lobes.

Other effects

Bony changes These tend to occur only if ICP has been high for a considerable period of time. In adults the dorsum sellae is the first structure to be affected. At first there is loss of detail of the cortex (lamina dura) anteriorly at the lower part of the dorsum. With the passage of time the bony changes in the dorsum may be more extensive and the floor of the pituitary fossa may also become involved. These changes may be attributed to downward pressure on the diaphragma sellae: certainly a deeply cupped diaphragma is often seen *post mortem* in patients with slowly expanding intracranial lesions. Pressure effects on the floor of the sella may be accentuated when the subarachnoid space extends into the sella turcica—the so-called *empty sella syndrome*. Cerebral cortex may also extrude through the dura mater to produce small pot-holes in bone, particularly in the middle cranial fossa (Fig. 2.16) and ultimately there may be considerable erosion of the orbital plates and the lesser wings of the sphenoid bone (Fig. 2.16).

In infants and in children up to about 10 years old, an early sign of raised ICP is separation of the sutures at the vault. There is also enlargement

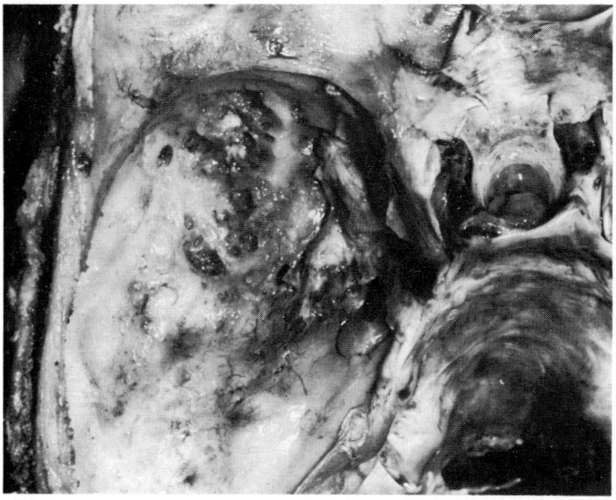

(a)

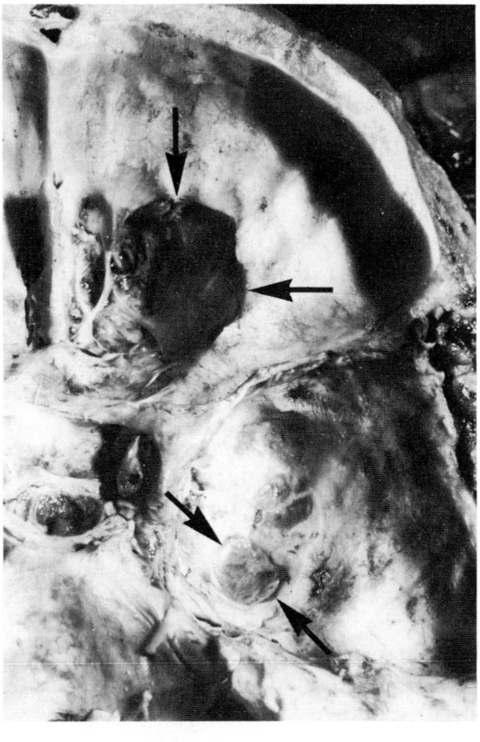

(b)

Fig. 2.16 Bony changes. (**a**) There are many small pits in the floor of the left middle cranial fossa—patient with metastatic carcinoma in cerebral hemisphere. (**b**) There is extensive erosion of bone (arrows) in the right anterior and middle cranial fossae—patient with a glioma of some 4 years' duration. ((**b**) Reproduced, with permission, from Miller and Adams 1972) of the skull, thinning of the bones of the vault and prominence of the convolutional impressions.

External herniae These occur when there is a defect—usually surgical—in the skull. They may simply amount to protrusion of small 'nubbins' of cortex through burr holes but if an external decompression has been undertaken, a large part of the cerebral hemisphere may herniate through the defect in the calvaria. Associated with this there is often haemorrhagic pressure necrosis at the edge of the hernia, swelling of the adjacent brain due to venous obstruction at the margins of the bony defect, and ultimately there may be extensive necrosis of the herniated cortex and white matter.

Hydrocephalus

Hydrocephalus denotes an **increased volume of CSF** within the cranial cavity. Its occurrence in relation to various specific pathological processes is discussed in Chapter 10 but this section is aimed at presenting a brief general review of the subject.

Definitions

Various types of hydrocephalus have been defined. In **internal** hydrocephalus the increased volume of CSF is within the ventricular system and in general the term hydrocephalus is usually employed to denote internal hydrocephalus. In **external** hydrocephalus the excess CSF is in the subarachnoid space over the surface of the brain. If CSF can flow freely from the ventricles to the subarachnoid space, the hydrocephalus is said to be **communicating**; if it cannot, it is **non-communicating**. **Active** hydrocephalus is associated with progressive enlargement of the ventricular system and an increased intraventricular pressure; in **arrested** hydrocephalus intraventricular pressure has returned to normal and there is no longer a stimulus for further ventricular enlargement. As will become apparent below (p. 70), however, patients with arrested hydrocephalus may be unduly susceptible to any further apparently minor increase in the volume of the intracranial contents. Hydrocephalus **ex vacuo** or **compensatory** hydrocephalus is characterized by an increase in the volume of CSF under normal pressure that is compensatory to loss of brain tissue: the hydrocephalus will be diffuse if it is secondary to generalized cerebral atrophy, or focal if secondary to localized loss of brain tissue (e.g. an old shrunken infarct). The term **occult** hydrocephalus is sometimes used when there are no signs or symptoms of intracranial hypertension.

Formation and absorption of cerebrospinal fluid

Numerous comprehensive reviews on this subject with extensive bibliographies have been published in recent years (Davson, 1972; Milhorat, 1972, 1975; Welch, 1975; Bradbury, 1979; Fishman, 1980) and only the salient features will be summarized here. The normal volume of CSF in the adult is about 140 ml and in normal conditions about 20 ml per hour is produced and absorbed. The bulk is secreted by the choroid plexus which is formed as a result of invagination of the ependyma into the ventricles by the blood vessels of the pia mater. The epithelium of the choroid plexus is composed of a single row of cuboidal cells folded into villi and, since their ventricular surface has a brush border composed of microvilli, it closely resembles other epithelia noted for fluid transport. The *formation of CSF by the choroid plexus involves two distinct processes*—filtration through the fenestrated capillaries of the choroid plexus into its interstitial spaces that is dependent on hydrostatic pressure, followed by active secretion by the epithelium. Both pinocytosis and vesicular transport have been observed in the epithelium (Brightman, 1975). There also seems little doubt that there are extrachoroidal sources for the bulk formation of CSF, but according to Milhorat (1975) work aimed at demonstrating its secretion by ependymal cells has involved such drastic experimental procedures that judgement concerning the validity of the findings must be reserved, while Fishman (1980) has indicated that there are no data available to establish the relative contributions of choroidal and extrachoroidal sources. The rate of formation of CSF remains constant over a wide range of circumstances but seems to be related most closely to the overall cerebral metabolic rate. Its rate of production is not reduced by intracranial hypertension until this is severe enough to reduce cerebral blood flow (Sahar, Hochwald and Ransohoff, 1970).

Cerebrospinal fluid circulates slowly throughout the ventricular system, leaves it by way of the *exit foramina* in the fourth ventricle—the midline foramen of Magendie and the lateral foramina of Luschka—and flows over the surface of the brain and the spinal cord in the subarachnoid space to be absorbed at the arachnoidal granulations. These are small herniations of the arachnoid that protrude into the lumina of the major intracranial venous sinuses and penetrate the dura of spinal root sleeves into small spinal veins (Fishman, 1980). This absorption is through variable-aperture one-way valves within the arachnoid granulations and is directly proportional to the pressure difference between CSF and the dural venous sinuses (Welch and Friedman, 1960; Welch and Pollay, 1961; Rubin et al., 1966; Cutler et al., 1968; Davson, Hollingsworth and Segal, 1970; Lorenzo, Page and Watters, 1970; Martins, 1973). Since pressure in the posterior venous sinuses does not increase substantially during intracranial hypertension, a considerable pressure gradient can build up in these areas. Tripathi (1974) and Levine, Povlishock and Becker (1982) have shown that the pathway for absorption of CSF consists of microvesicles that enlarge and may link to form open channels as the pressure gradient increases. Thus absorption of CSF can be rapidly increased in patients with intracranial expanding lesions, this making a major contribution to spatial compensation: as already indicated (p. 58) one of the striking features in a patient dying as a result of such a lesion is a flattened, dry brain because of obliteration of the subarachnoid space, and small ventricles.

The extent to which CSF is normally reabsorbed transependymally is not established but it is an important process in obstructive hydrocephalus.

The pathogenesis of ventricular enlargement

This remains a controversial issue which is not yet fully understood apart from the inevitable enlargement brought about by a reduction in the volume of brain tissue (Russell, 1949). With acute experimental obstruction to the flow of CSF, the cerebral ventricles dilate within a few hours (Milhorat, 1972, 1975; Pickard, 1982) and the surface of the brain becomes flattened. This enlargement occurs at the expense of the white matter despite the fact that CSF flows into the periventricular white matter causing interstitial oedema leading to an increase in its water and sodium content (Fishman and Greer, 1963; Milhorat, 1972). In a series of experiments in young rabbits and young dogs in which hydrocephalus was produced by the injection of silicone oils into the cisterna magna, Weller and Wisniewski (1969), Wisniewski, Weller and Terry (1969) and Weller et al. (1971) have shown that as the ventricles enlarge in the early stages there is disruption of the ependyma, and both interstitial oedema and destruction of nerve fibres in periventricular white matter. By 80 days, when the hydrocephalus is arrested, there is re-establishment of a continuous but flattened ependymal lining: periventricular oedema is reduced but there is a decrease in axons and an increase in fibrous astrocytic processes. Essentially similar features have been found in biopsies from young children with infantile hydrocephalus (Weller and Shulman, 1972). In man the presence of

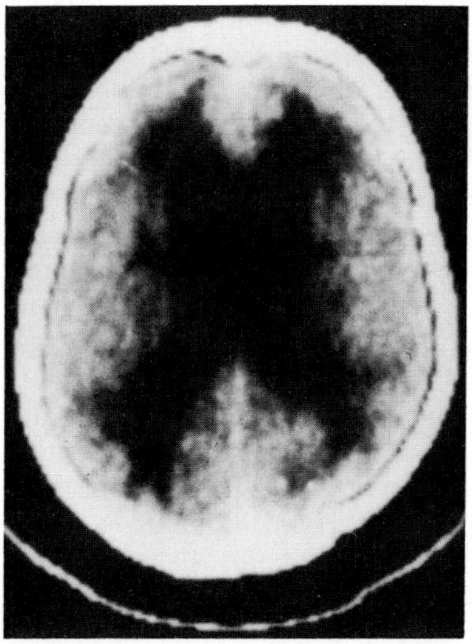

Fig. 2.17 Acute hydrocephalus. CT scan showing enlarged ventricles and reduced density in the periventricular white matter (interstitial oedema). (Courtesy of Dr Peter Macpherson, Institute of Neurological Sciences, Glasgow).

interstitial oedema in association with acute obstructive hydrocephalus is shown by reduced density of the periventricular white matter in CT scans (Fig. 2.17). At this stage ventricular drainage may result in a rapid reduction in the size of the ventricles (Fig. 2.18) but the mechanism which allows of this rapid restoration of the width of the cerebral mantle remains unexplained. The available evidence suggests that in man, unless complete intraventricular obstruction to the free flow of CSF leads to a very high ICP and fatal compression of the brain stem, active hydrocephalus may ultimately become arrested. In that event the intraventricular pressure returns to normal and there is no further stimulus for continuing ventricular enlargement: this infers that a new equilibrium has been reached between the production and absorption of CSF, and if the hydrocephalus is obstructive this increased absorption must be transependymal. It has been suggested by Hakim (1972, 1977) that this increased transependymal absorption of CSF is related to the increased area of the ventricular surface, and by Weller et al. (1971) to defects in the ependyma or functionally abnormal flattened ependymal cells.

The pathogenesis of hydrocephalus in man

As emphasized by Dorothy Russell (1949) many years ago, the most important cause of hydrocephalus is obstruction to the free flow of CSF. The abnormality may be congenital (Chapter 10) or acquired, and it is the site of the lesion, not its size, that matters. Thus, a very small lesion in a vulnerable site (e.g. in or adjacent to the midbrain aqueduct) is of much greater importance in this respect than a large tumour in an occipital or frontal lobe. The nature of the lesion is also relatively unimportant—it may be a tumour, a haematoma, an abscess, a granuloma or a recent swollen infarct. Or the cause may be some inflammatory process—microbiological (e.g. tuberculous meningitis) or sterile (e.g. blood in the subarachnoid space)—leading to obliteration of the CSF pathways usually at particularly vulnerable sites such as the exit foramina from the fourth ventricle or the subarachnoid space around the midbrain at the level of the tentorium. Furthermore, expanding lesions in the posterior fossa almost invariably produce rapidly progressive obstructive hydrocephalus. Many of the rarer causes of hydrocephalus also affect the structures in the posterior fossa, such as gliosis of the aqueduct, ectasia and tortuosity of the basilar artery, Paget's disease affecting the base of the skull, and the Chiari malformations.

In essence, the ventricular system *proximal* to the obstruction enlarges. Thus if there is obstruction at one foramen of Monro, one lateral ventricle enlarges; if it is within the third ventricle, both lateral ventricles enlarge; if it is at the level of the aqueduct, the third and lateral ventricles enlarge; and if it is at the level of the exit fora-

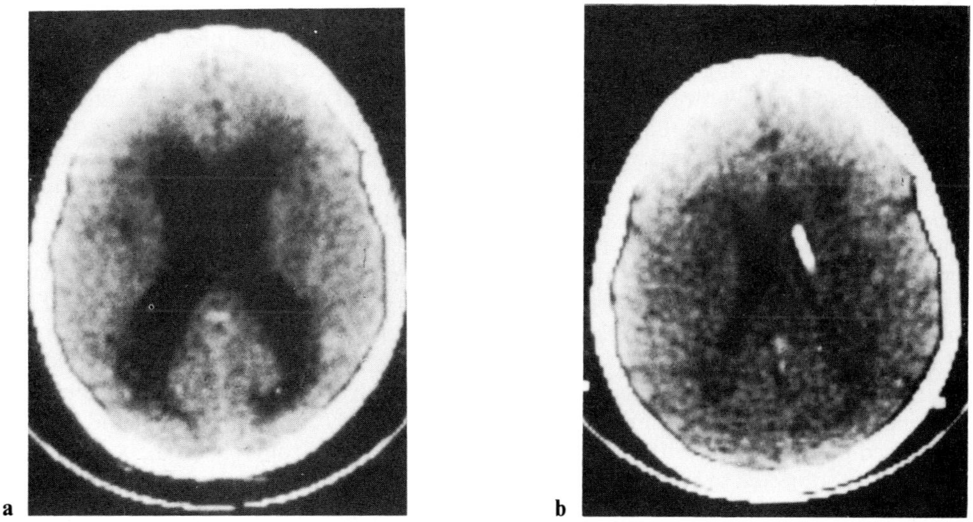

Fig. 2.18 Hydrocephalus. CT scan (**a**) before and (**b**) after ventricular drainage. Note the difference in the widths of the cerebral mantle. (Courtesy of Dr Peter Macpherson, Institute of Neurological Sciences, Glasgow).

mina, the entire ventricular system enlarges. Thus radiological studies are of the utmost importance in cases of hydrocephalus to assess whether it is communicating or non-communicating in type, and, if the former, where the obstruction lies.

Theoretically, hydrocephalus could also be produced by increased production or by decreased absorption of CSF. The former probably does not occur if the choroid plexus is normal but Eisenberg, McComb and Lorenzo (1974) have shown that increased production may occur in association with a papillary tumour of the choroid plexus. In patients with this type of tumour, however, hydrocephalus may also be the result of desquamation of tumour cells with some associated subarachnoid haemorrhage, the irritant effects of which cause obliteration of the subarachnoid space (Russell, 1949).

Impaired absorption of CSF is a possible but as yet unproven cause of communicating hydrocephalus. Ellington and Margolis (1969) found a variable degree of distension of the arachnoidal granulations with red cells after subarachnoid haemorrhage and suggested that this might be a cause of hydrocephalus, while the known association of hydrocephalus in some patients with spinal schwannomas or meningiomas has led to the suggestion that the arachnoidal granulations may become occluded by substances derived from the spinal tumours. Impaired cerebral venous drainage brought about by venous thrombosis may be a cause of intracranial hypertension, but according to Russell (1949) and Milhorat (1972) there is no proof that it is a cause of hydrocephalus in the acute stage. Thrombosis of the superior sagittal sinus, however, may well lead to cerebral infarction (p. 189) and the ventricles will enlarge later as the infarcted tissue shrinks.

Normal pressure hydrocephalus This is the term most commonly used for a syndrome characterized by chronic hydrocephalus and a clinical triad consisting of progressive dementia, gait disturbance and urinary incontinence or urgency (Adams et al., 1965; Hakim and Adams, 1965). The mean CSF pressure at lumbar puncture is not raised but if patients with this type of hydrocephalus are subjected to continuous monitoring of ICP, episodes of moderate intracranial hypertension can be demonstrated (Symon and Dorsch, 1975; Symon and Hinzpeter, 1977; Pickard et al., 1980), particularly during sleep. A more appropriate term for this type of hydrocephalus may therefore be *intermittent hydrocephalus*. In some cases there is a known possible antecedent cause, such as a cyst in the third ventricle (Adams et al., 1965), head injury (Hakim and Adams, 1965) or subarachnoid haemorrhage (Symon and Dorsch, 1975), but in others—so-called *idiopathic normal pressure hydrocephalus*—no known cause may be found even after *post-mortem* examination. On the basis of the demonstration of episodes of intracranial hypertension, and the studies of Lorenzo, Bresnan and Barlow (1974) and Hussey, Schauzer and Katzman (1970) using ventriculolumbar perfusion and constant lumbar perfusion of mock CSF, it now seems clear that in patients with idiopathic 'normal pressure hydrocephalus' CSF absorption mechanisms are often impaired. They may show an unusually large rise in pressure in response to the infusion of a volume of mock CSF for which a normal individual could easily compensate. Symon and Dorsch's (1975) view is that the absorption of CSF is defective at some level: this leads to ventricular enlargement but as the syndrome progresses a new equilibrium is reached between the production and absorption of CSF. Di Rocco et al. (1977) have demonstrated leptomeningeal fibrosis, disruption of the ependymal lining of the ventricular system and perivascular demyelination and spongiosus in patients with 'normal pressure hydrocephalus'. Once established it would appear that normal adaptive pressure–volume mechanisms are exhausted and so subsequent minor stresses to the system (e.g. transient increases of $Pa\text{CO}_2$ during sleep leading to vasodilatation and a consequent increase in cerebral blood volume) result in an exaggerated increase in ICP. The special importance of 'normal pressure hydrocephalus', however, is that it may be the underlying mechanism in a small proportion of patients presenting with dementia (Marsden and Harrison, 1972) and that the clinical state of these patients may be improved by a ventricular shunt (Fisher, 1977; Hughes et al., 1978).

The term *normal volume hydrocephalus* has been used by Engel, Carmel and Chutorian (1979) for a syndrome that may occur in patients with shunt-dependent hydrocephalus in which ventricular size remains normal despite a marked increase in ventricular pressure caused by shunt malfunction. Their study of pressure–volume measurements has shown that in these patients the withdrawal of a small quantity of ventricular CSF results in a considerable fall in intraventricular pressure. These patients are therefore on the steep portion of the pressure-volume curve (see p. 56) and the ability of the intracranial contents to compensate for further increases of volume has become exhausted.

Benign intracranial hypertension

This term is used for a small group of patients in whom the symptoms and signs of raised ICP occur without a demonstrable cause. There is often papilloedema and headache, and computerized tomography or other types of neuroradiological investigation reveal that the ventricular system is not enlarged. In most cases the ventricles are smaller than normal. Since the comprehensive reviews by Foley (1955) and Johnston and Paterson (1974) much information has accrued about the pattern of elevated ICP seen in such cases and the relationship between raised ICP and papilloedema. Thus all patients with a persistent elevation of ICP over 3 kPa (21.5 mmHg) have papilloedema (Johnston and Paterson, 1974). Waves of severely increased pressure, up to 10 kPa (75 mmHg), can occur without the shattering effect on brain function that such levels of intracranial hypertension would cause in head-injured patients. Because ICP is evenly distributed throughout the craniospinal axis in this condition there are no intracranial pressure gradients, or shift or herniation of the brain.

Controversy still abounds as to the cause of this syndrome; indeed it is not yet clear whether benign intracranial hypertension represents a single clinical entity or is merely the end-point of several different disease processes, all of which cause raised ICP and none of which causes brain shift or herniation. Johnston (1973) has advanced the hypothesis that the problem is related to a failure of absorption of CSF, while Reid, Matheson and Teasdale (1980) consider that an increase in cerebral blood volume or brain water content is a more likely cause. In extensive angiographic investigations of a group of patients with benign intracranial hypertension, Janny et al. (1975) found that in half of their cases there was occlusion of at least one of the major dural venous sinuses. The term *otitic hydrocephalus* was one of the early synonyms for benign intracranial hypertension, and it may be that this represents a specific subset. With the recognition of other specific causes of diffuse elevation of ICP, such as Reye's syndrome, encephalitis and hepatitis, it is likely that other subsets of benign intracranial hypertension may be identified in the future (Chandler and Kindt, 1976; Mickell et al., 1976; Miller, 1979b).

Brain swelling and oedema

An increase in the volume of all or part of the brain is a potential complication of head injury, ischaemia, haemorrhage, tumours, infection, hypoxia and other insults. If the process is generalized, the subarachnoid space is obliterated and the ventricles are decreased in size. If localized, there is a mass effect that may considerably augment the size of the causative lesion itself; for example, a meningioma or a metastasis (Fig. 2.19). While such processes will eventually cause raised ICP, recent computer tomographic studies in patients with early post-traumatic brain swelling show that a reduction in the volume of the ventricular system is not necessarily a reliable sign of raised ICP. Absence of the third ventricle and the basal cisterns in patients with diffuse brain damage, and dilatation of the contralateral ventricle when the process is unilateral, are better indicators of the presence of intracranial hypertension (Roberson et al., 1979; Teasdale et al., 1984). The expansion of brain tissue may be due to an increase in intravascular blood volume in the brain—**congestive brain swelling**—or to an increase in the water content of brain tissue itself—**cerebral oedema**.

Congestive brain swelling

This process may occur with startling rapidity, particularly in children who have sustained a head injury (see p. 112) and in patients with traumatic acute subdural haematoma (see

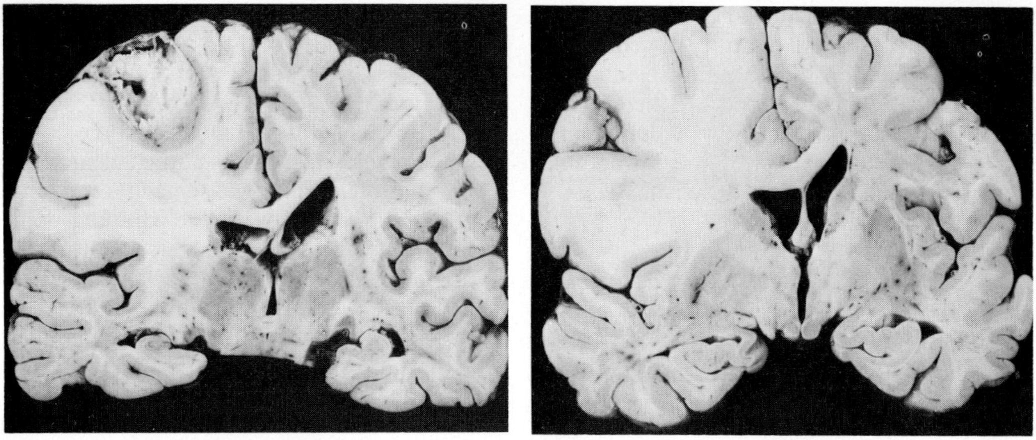

a b

Fig. 2.19 Cerebral oedema (**a**) Metastatic carcinoma in left parietal lobe. (**b**) Diffuse swelling of cerebral hemisphere anterior to the metastasis.

p. 112). The increase in cerebral blood volume is mainly in the capillary and postcapillary part of the cerebrovascular bed. In spite of its frequency, the pathophysiology of the process is not entirely clear. There has to be relaxation of arterioles to permit flooding of the vascular bed at high intravascular pressure and/or a relative constriction of the venous outflow into the more rigid dural sinuses. To what extent the subarachnoid bridging veins change passively in calibre with transmural pressure (in this situation the difference between subarachnoid venous and CSF pressure) or change calibre actively under nervous control is not established.

When congestive brain swelling occurs, the brain rapidly expands, particularly when arterial pressure is high (Leech and Miller, 1974). There is a reduction in the size of the subarachnoid space and the ventricles, and when ICP eventually rises it is often in the form of pressure waves (see p. 55). While cerebrovascular dilatation can occur as a result of clearly identifiable causes such as hypercapnia, hypoxaemia or severe elevations of arterial pressure, other instances are much less easily explained, particularly since central influences on the cerebrovascular resistance are much less well understood. Lesions or stimuli in the hypothalamus and in the medulla oblongata have been shown not only to interfere with reactivity of the cerebral circulation to physiological stimuli but also on occasions to induce a marked primary cerebral vasodilatation and elevation of ICP (Ishii, 1966; Shalit et al., 1967). When this vasodilatation is combined with arterial hypertension and loss of the capacity of the cerebral arterioles to constrict, the rapidity and severity of brain swelling is devastating. Intracranial pressure soon attains the level of systemic arterial pressure, perfusion of the brain ceases and brain death supervenes, this being the end-stage of generalized cerebral vasomotor paralysis (Langfitt, Weinstein and Kassell, 1965).

From the pathological standpoint, congestive brain swelling is a rather unsatisfactory entity since it may subside as a result of the *ante mortem* fall in blood pressure, leaving only the less specific evidence of a previous episode of a high ICP such as pressure necrosis in one or both parahippocampal gyri (see Fig. 2.7). When there is prolonged congestive brain swelling, however, vasogenic cerebral oedema (see below) supervenes, water accumulates in the extracellular space and the brain remains swollen after death.

Cerebral oedema

Cerebral oedema is an increase in brain volume due to an increased tissue water content (Fishman, 1975), but this definition does not differentiate between an intra- or extracellular location of the water. In the past, German authors distinguished between *Hirnschwellung*, where the water was intracellular, and *Hirnödem*, where the water was located in the extracellular space (Reichardt, 1911). Nowadays, however, the term 'brain swelling' is widely accepted as being synonymous with an increase in cerebral blood volume and therefore best prefaced with the term 'congestive'. Estimates of the water content of normal brain vary greatly, depending upon whether the measurements are confined to white matter or grey matter, or represent a combination of both. The normal water content of grey matter is 80 per cent of the wet weight (or 800 mg/g), while that of white matter is considerably lower at 68 per cent of wet weight (or 680 mg/g), except for the subcortical arcuate fibres where the water content approaches that of grey matter (Adachi and Feigin, 1966). Typical values in instances of cerebral oedema would be 81–82 per cent in grey matter and 76–79 per cent in white matter. The greater accumulation of water therefore occurs in white matter; this is usually apparent in brain slices (see Fig. 2.19) and on computerized tomography, both of which will show expansion of the centrum semiovale as water spreads fairly freely through the white matter of the hemisphere.

The causes of cerebral oedema are an increase in intravascular pressure, damage and increased permeability of the cerebral vascular wall and/or a decrease in plasma colloid osmotic pressure. Any of these, alone or in combination, can upset the Starling equilibrium favouring a greater net outflow of water from the vascular bed into brain tissue. In clinical practice and in the laboratory six principal varieties of oedema can be distinguished (Miller, 1979a), discussed below.

Vasogenic oedema This type of oedema occurs as a result of damage to the blood–brain barrier; water, sodium and protein molecules extravasate from blood vessels that are located principally in grey matter and the oedema fluid then moves on to accumulate in the extracellular space of the white matter. There has been considerable controversy in the past about the size of the extracellular space in the brain but it is now generally accepted that it constitutes about 13 per cent and 18 per cent of the volume of grey matter and white matter respectively (Bradbury, 1979). This type of oedema can most easily be produced experimentally by the application of intense cold to the surface of the brain (Clasen et al., 1962; Bakay and Hague, 1964; Klatzo, 1967) and it seems likely that this is the type of oedema that occurs in the vicinity of brain tumours, intracerebral haematomas, cerebral abscesses and contusions. Klatzo's view was that water and protein molecules escaped from the vascular bed via openings in the normally tight endothelial junctions of the capillary bed in the brain. It seems, however, more likely that a dramatic increase in pinocytotic activity is the explanation for the outward migration of at least the protein molecules. Using horseradish peroxidase as a marker, Petito, Schaefer and Plum (1976) have demonstrated greatly increased pinocytotic activity in the area around cerebral tumours.

This type of oedema is often a major factor contributing to the effective mass of an intracranial expanding lesion such as a glioma, a meningioma or a deposit of metastatic carcinoma (see Fig. 2.19). As indicated above, it occurs mainly in white matter, and if it has been present for some time the affected white matter often develops a pale green colour. Histological examination shows pallor of staining, and myelin sheaths which often appear abnormally swollen, vacuolated and beaded are less closely packed than in normal white matter. This stage is soon followed by the appearance of swollen (gemistocytic) astrocytes but oligodendrocytes remain of normal appearance. If oedema persists for some time, myelin begins to break down as shown by the presence of lipid phagocytes. This may occasionally progress to the development of cystic spaces in the affected white matter.

Cytotoxic oedema due to energy failure An early response of brain tissue to injury is swelling of astrocytes. If energy failure occurs there is eventually swelling of all cellular elements because of a disturbance of the pump and transport mechanisms for chloride, bicarbonate, potassium and calcium, leading to lipid peroxidization in cell membranes and then to an accumulation of intracellular water (Bourke et al., 1975; Astrup et al., 1977). This form of oedema is seen in ischaemic-hypoxic brain damage, although there may also be an element of vasogenic oedema at the margins of an infarct. In essence, however, this form of oedema is intracellular and is therefore much more prominent in grey than in white matter (O'Brien and Waltz, 1973).

Cytotoxic oedema due to poisoning Experimental oedema can be produced by the administration of hexachlorophene or triethyl tin (Torack, Terry and Zimmerman, 1960). In this special form of oedema the fluid is trapped within the myelin lamellae in the white matter.

Hydrostatic oedema Even if vascular endothelium remains intact, a sudden increase of intravascular pressure or of transmural pressure can overcome the cerebrovascular resistance, producing high-pressure flooding of the capillary bed. This can occur when arterial pressure suddenly becomes high during craniotomy, or when an intracranial mass lesion that has been causing severe intracranial hypertension is abruptly decompressed. The congestive brain swelling that occurs immediately is followed after some minutes by extravasation of protein-poor fluid into and through the extracellular space of the brain (Schutta, Kassell and Langfitt, 1968). An experimental preparation of this form of oedema was developed by Ishii et al. (1959), who inflated an intracranial balloon in experimental animals to the point of incipient tentorial herniation. After maintaining the balloon inflated for several hours, it was abruptly deflated and this was followed by severe brain swelling, closer examination of which revealed an increase in extracellular water content typical of cerebral oedema. This model has clear clinical parallels in patients suffering from acute space-occupying lesions in whom surgical decompression has been undertaken.

A particularly severe example of this form of oedema may be seen in patients with a very high ICP in whom a bony decompression is carried out, leading to rapid external herniation of the brain. A similar sequence of events has been described in subhuman primates subjected to craniectomy minutes after the experimental production of acute subdural haematoma (Adams, Graham and Gennarelli, 1982; see p. 112). Computerized tomography during life shows the marked decrease in radiodensity in the extruded brain typical of oedematous tissue.

Interstitial oedema In patients with acute obstructive hydrocephalus there is an increase in the water content of the periventricular tissues (see p. 69). With the advent of computerized tomography it is now possible to identify this abnormality during life (see Fig. 2.17). In such cases it appears that fluid under high pressure is forced through damaged ependyma into the periventricular white matter. Fishman (1975) has termed this process interstitial cerebral oedema.

Hypo-osmotic oedema It has been known since the experiments of Stern and Coxon (1964) that the infusion of distilled water into the peritoneal cavity or intravenously, and so reducing the serum osmolality, may produce diffuse expansion of the brain associated with a raised ICP, an increased tissue water content and a reduced cerebral blood flow (Meinig, Reulen and Magavly, 1973). A severe reduction in serum osmolality to less than 120 mEq/l is frequently associated in head-injured patients with diffuse cerebral oedema and elevation of ICP. Such reductions in osmolality may be the result of excessive replacement of fluid loss by intravenous dextrose/water solutions, or may be due to development of the syndrome of inappropriate secretion of antidiuretic hormone.

Spread and resolution of cerebral oedema

Klatzo (1972), Clasen et al. (1974), Hochwald et al. (1976) and Reulen et al. (1978) have investigated the factors that regulate the rate and extent of the spread of oedema fluid through the brain from a focal point by labelling with dyes or radioisotopes. Factors responsible for cerebral arterial or arteriolar vasodilatation (hypercapnia, hypoxaemia, severe arterial hypertension, hyperthermia and certain drugs) accelerate the rate of formation of oedema and the rate of spread of labelled elements of oedema fluid across the brain. Conversely, any factor that causes cerebral vasoconstriction tends to impede this process. Diffuse elevation of ICP also impedes the progress of oedema fluid across the brain. For several years it was considered that all oedema fluid passed eventually into the ventricles to be absorbed with the CSF. More recently, however, uptake of labelled protein molecules has been observed in glial cells in periventricular regions, in blood vessels in the same area, and in regional lymph nodes draining the tissues of the head and neck. It appears, therefore, that several different routes of absorption of oedema fluid exist. Double marking techniques also suggest that different constituents of the oedema fluid migrate at different rates through the extracellular space of cerebral white matter (Hahm et al., 1980). In earlier studies of vasogenic brain oedema the concept of an *oedema front* was advanced. This referred to the advancing wave of fluid that emerged from a damaged area of the brain. By labelling the protein component of the oedema fluid, the progress of the 'oedema front' could be followed over time.

The discovery that protein, water and other components pass through the extracellular space of the brain at different rates has modified some concepts of the dynamics of brain oedema. Another modifying factor is the recognition that pinocytosis occurs more commonly than previously thought. But while this may explain the emergence of larger molecules of protein into the extracellular space, increases in tissue water content do not always occur in areas of protein extravasation. While it is firmly accepted that factors which increase intracapillary pressure, and factors which reduce plasma osmotic pressure favour both the formation and spread of 'vasogenic' oedema, the exact mechanisms by which this occurs are less well understood now than it was formerly believed.

The effects of cerebral oedema

There is no firm evidence that an increase in brain water, local or generalized, can directly interfere with neuronal activity or a patient's neurological state, and Penn (1980) has convincingly demonstrated the lack of correlation between areas of cerebral oedema demonstrated by computerized tomography and the appropriate signs of focal neurological dysfunction. This may appear to conflict with a general belief that cerebral oedema is an important cause of brain dysfunction; but it does so only when it is *sufficiently severe to cause cerebral ischaemia or distortion and herniation of the brain.*

When regional cerebral blood flow is measured within areas of cerebral oedema, the flow levels are low. Several explanations have been offered for this observation. The ICP may be high enough to reduce cerebral perfusion pressure to critical levels; or lesser degrees of ICP may reduce local cerebral blood flow if autoregulation is also impaired in the oedematous area; or tissue pressure may be elevated so much above the general level of ICP that local perfusion pressure is reduced sufficiently to cause local ischaemia (Hedges et al., 1964). Unfortunately, such increases in tissue pressure have never been convincingly demonstrated. Finally, it has been pointed out that local cerebral blood flow is measured in millilitres per 100 grams of tissue per minute. If the weight of tissue is increased by water, as it is in cerebral oedema, an apparent fall in flow may in fact represent an unchanged volume of blood perfusing a greater weight of tissue. While this explanation can account for some of the observed reduction in flow found in cerebral oedema, it is not sufficient to explain the degree of cerebral ischaemia that is frequently encountered.

Papilloedema

The classic indications of raised ICP are headache, vomiting and papilloedema. Of these, headache is probably related to stretching and distortion of the dura and major intracranial vessels, the vomiting, to distortion or pressure on the floor of the fourth ventriole. Papilloedema, however, has long been regarded as a reliable index of raised ICP with the implication that when it is absent, ICP is not elevated, but this relationship requires reappraisal.

It has proved possible to produce papilloedema experimentally by the slow expansion of an intracranial mass lesion. Bordley and Cushing (1909) used injections of wax into the subdural space. Hayreh (1964) used expansion of an intracranial balloon with continuous measurement of ICP and proved conclusively the close relationship between raised ICP and papilloedema. Hayreh (1964) also showed that the development of papilloedema depended on extension of the subarachnoid space about the optic nerve into the orbit. Incision of the sheath into this space prevented papilloedema even when ICP was persistently elevated.

The swelling of the optic nerve head that characterizes papilloedema is not due to an increased water content but is thought to be due to the accumulation of axoplasm in the optic papilla consequent on blockage of axoplasmic flow from the ganglion cells along the optic nerve. The relative lack of myelin in these axons may facilitate papillary swelling when sustained intracranial hypertension compresses the optic nerve and blocks centripetal axoplasmic flow (Wittschafter, Rizzo and Smiley, 1975; Tso and Hayreh, 1977).

In patients with benign intracranial hypertension, chronic subdural haematoma and brain tumour, there is a close relationship between chronically elevated ICP and papilloedema (Johnston and Paterson, 1974; van Crevel, 1979). In acute severe head injury the position seems to be different since papilloedema (of low grade only) is found in less than 5 per cent of cases although the ICP is high in 50 per cent (Selhorst et al., 1983). It is possible that the severity of the injury disrupts axoplasmic flow, or that intracranial hypertension does not persist for a sufficient time for papilloedema to develop. Thus, while papilloedema is a valuable indicator of the presence of chronically elevated ICP, its absence in acute situations cannot be taken to mean that ICP is normal.

Systemic sequelae of raised intracranial pressure

The changes in blood pressure and heart rate that are associated with axial brain shift and raised ICP have already been referred to. The usual pattern of response is one or more surges of arterial hypertension followed by a steadily falling blood pressure that soon becomes unresponsive to central vasopressor drugs, such as dopamine. By this stage brain death has virtually always supervened and circulatory arrest will soon follow. The rise in arterial pressure is associated with increased sympathetic activity and can be blocked by local anaesthetic instilled into the cisterna magna (Cushing, 1901), or by surgical or drug-induced sympathectomy (Hoff and Mitchell, 1972; Fitch and McDowall, 1977).

Signs of myocardial dysfunction or damage are also often present in patients with raised ICP and distortion of the brain. These are electrocardiographic changes—ST segment elevation and T-wave inversion, suggestive of myocardial ischaemia—and pathological findings of subendocardial haemorrhage and widespread foci of myocardial cell necrosis (Connor, 1968). These changes can also be prevented by autonomic blockade, both sympathetic and parasympathetic, at least in experimental animals (Hawkins and Clower, 1971). In man there is also some evidence in favour of beta-sympathetic blockade as a means of preventing myocardial dysfunction. This suggests that the fall in arterial pressure that follows the Cushing reflex may be due to myocardial damage (Levett et al., 1980).

The effects of raised ICP and distortion of the brain upon respiration have also been referred to. Plum and Posner (1966) proposed that the various disorders of respiration observed in comatose patients could be associated with damage or dysfunction in particular areas of the brain. Thus, periodic respiration was associated with forebrain damage, central neurogenic hyperventilation with midbrain damage, and ataxic respiration with lower pontine or medullary damage.

After an extensive survey of the patterns of respiration observed in patients with many different types of brain damage, North and Jennett (1974, 1976) failed to confirm this proposed hierarchy of respiratory disorder. They pointed out that different respiratory patterns could be observed at different times in the same patient and concluded that while abnormalities of respiratory pattern were more frequent in patients with lower brainstem damage or dysfunction, accurate localization of brain damage according to the type of respiratory abnormality was not possible.

A further respiratory problem in patients with raised ICP and distortion of the brain is that blood is not effectively oxygenated in the lungs. Ducker (1968) and others have proposed that sympathetic overactivity is also responsible for this problem, either by affecting pulmonary capillary blood flow so as to alter the ventilation/perfusion ratio or by altering conditions in the alveolar wall. A major difficulty in substantiating these theories is that patients with raised ICP due to head injury, brain tumour or intracranial haemorrhage may have several other possible reasons for poor pulmonary oxygenation, such as aspiration, atelectasis or infection (Frost, 1977). The causes of hypoxaemia in comatose patients with raised ICP remain a matter of controversy.

The mucosa of the digestive and urogenital tracts can become haemorrhagic, eroded and ulcerated in patients with raised ICP and distortion of the brain. The most common sites are the gastric mucosa, the distal duodenum, the proximal jejunum and the urinary bladder. Cushing (1932) drew attention to the problem of acute peptic ulceration and suggested that it was related to sympathetic overactivity and increased gastric acid production. More recent studies confirm that gastric erosions are common in comatose patients with a high incidence of raised ICP. Although gastric acidity is increased, the levels are not higher than those seen in individuals with chronic peptic ulceration (Gudeman et al., 1983). The administration of histamine receptor antagonists reduces acidity in these patients, and reduces the incidence and severity of gastric haemorrhage but does not affect the incidence of gastric erosion (Halloran et al., 1980). This suggests that the cause of gastric ulceration and haemorrhage is a combination of increased gastric acidity and some other process, probably ischaemia in the mucosa, that is produced by sympathetic overactivity.

Conclusion

It should be clear from this chapter that there are few acute neurological disorders where an increase in ICP and associated distortion and herniation of the brain leading to compression of and, ultimately, structural damage in the brainstem are not as important as the primary intracranial lesion whether this be a malignant tumour, a simple tumour, a haematoma, an abscess or a recent infarct. As we have emphasized before (Miller and Adams, 1972), however, distortion and herniation of the brain cannot be equated with a high ICP: thus there may be very little distortion and herniation of the brain if the fatal increase in ICP occurs very rapidly as a result of a diffuse process such as swelling or oedema; and if ICP increases very slowly, there can be severe distortion and herniation of the brain without the ICP having attained a level to cause clinical concern. A proper understanding of the pathophysiology of a high ICP is therefore essential to all with an interest in the neurosciences, whether it be the early recognition and management of the process, or the interpretation of structural changes in the brain *post mortem*.

References

Adachi, M. and Feigin, I. (1966) Cerebral oedema and the water content of normal white matter. *Journal of Neurology, Neurosurgery and Psychiatry* **29,** 446–50.

Adams, J.H. (1975) The neuropathology of head injuries. In *Handbook of Clinical Neurology*, vol. 23 (Eds. Vinken, P.J. and Bruyn, G.W.) pp. 35–65. North Holland: Amsterdam.

Adams, J.H. and Graham, D.I. (1976) The relationship between ventricular fluid pressure and the neuropathology of raised intracranial pressure. *Neuropathology and Applied Neurobiology* **2,** 323–32.

Adams, J.H., Graham, D.I. and Gennarelli, T.A. (1982) Neuropathology of acceleration-induced head injury in the subhuman primate. In *Head Injury: Basic and Clinical Aspects* (Eds. Grossman, R.G. and Gildenberg, P.L.). pp. 141–50 Raven Press, New York.

Adams, R.D., Fisher, C.M., Hakim, S., Ojemann, R.G. and Sweet, W.H. (1965) Symptomatic occult hydrocephalus with 'normal' cerebrospinal fluid pressure. *New England Journal of Medicine* **273,** 117–26.

Astrup, J. (1982) Energy-requiring cell functions in the ischemic brain. *Journal of Neurosurgery* **56,** 482–97.

Astrup, J., Symon, L., Branston, N.M. and Lassen, N.A. (1977) Cortical evoked potentials and extracellular K^+ and H^+ at critical levels of brain ischemia. *Stroke* **8,** 52–7.

Bakay, L. and Hague, I. (1964). Morphological and chemical studies in cerebral edema. I. Cold-induced edema. *Journal of Neuropathology and Experimental Neurology* **23,** 393–418.

Balslev-Jørgensen, P., Heilbrun, M.P., Boysen, G., Rosenklint, A. and Jørgensen, E.O. (1972) Cerebral perfusion pressure correlated with regional cerebral blood flow, EEG and aortocervical arteriography in patients with severe brain disorders progressing to death. *European Neurology* **8,** 207–12.

Bedford, T.H.B. (1935) The effect of increased intracranial venous pressure on the pressure of cerebrospinal fluid. *Brain* **58,** 427–47.

Bordley, J. and Cushing, H. (1909). Observations on choked disc with especial reference to decompressive cranial operations. *Journal of the American Medical Association* **52,** 353–64.

Bourke, R.S., Kimelberg, H.K., West, C.R. and Bremer, A.M. (1975) The effect of HCO_3 on the swelling and ion uptake of monkey cerebral cortex under conditions of raised extracellular potassium. *Journal of Neurochemistry* **25,** 323–8.

Bradbury, M. (1979) *The Concept of a Blood–Brain Barrier*. John Wiley, Chichester.

Bradley, K.C. (1970) Cerebrospinal fluid pressure. *Journal of Neurology, Neurosurgery and Psychiatry* **33,** 387–97.

Brightman, M.W. (1975) Ultrastructural characteristics of adult choroid plexus. In *The Choroid Plexus in Health and Disease* (Eds. Netsky, M.G. and Shuangshoti, S.) pp. 86–112. University of Virginia Press, Charlottesville.

Brock, M. and Hartung, C. (1972) Glossary of definitions, standards and abbreviations. In *Intracranial Pressure* (Eds. Brock, M. and Dietz, H.). pp. 372–5. Springer, Berlin.

Browder, J. and Meyers, R. (1936) Observations on behavior of the systemic blood pressure, pulse and spinal fluid pressure following craniocerebral injury. *American Journal of Surgery* **31,** 403–27.

Browder, J. and Meyers, R. (1938) Behavior of systemic blood pressure, pulse rate and spinal fluid pressure associated with acute changes in intracranial pressure artificially produced. *Archives of Surgery* **36,** 1–19.

Burrows, G. (1846) *On Disorders of the Cerebral Cir-*

culation and on the Connection between Affections of the Brain and Diseases of the Heart. Longman, Brown, Green and Longman, London, pp. 55–6.

Cairns, H. (1939) Raised intracranial pressure: hydrocephalic and vascular factors. *British Journal of Surgery* **27,** 275–94.

Chandler, W.F. and Kindt, G.W. (1976) Monitoring and control of intracranial pressure in non-traumatic encephalopathies. *Surgical Neurology* **5,** 311–14.

Clasen, R.A., Cooke, P.M., Pandolfi, S., Boyd, D. and Raimondi, A.J. (1962) Experimental cerebral edema produced by focal freezing. *Journal of Neuropathology and Experimental Neurology* **21,** 579–96.

Clasen, R.A., Pandolfi, S., Laing, I. and Casey, D. (1974) Experimental study of relation of fever to cerebral edema. *Journal of Neurosurgery* **41,** 576–81.

Connor, R.C.R. (1968) Heart damage associated with intracranial lesions. *British Medical Journal* **3,** 29–31.

Coroneos, N.J., McDowall, D.G., Gibson, R.M., Pickerodt, V.W.A. and Keaney, N.P. (1973) Measurement of extradural pressure and its relationship to other intracranial pressures. *Journal of Neurology, Neurosurgery and Psychiatry* **36,** 514–22.

Corsellis, J.A.N. (1958) Individual variation in the size of the tentorial opening. *Journal of Neurology, Neurosurgery and Psychiatry* **21,** 279–83.

van Crevel, H. (1979) Papilledema, CSF pressure and CSF flow in cerebral tumors. *Journal of Neurology, Neurosurgery and Psychiatry,* **42,** 493–500.

Cushing, H. (1901) Concerning a definite regulatory mechanism of the vasomotor centre which controls blood pressure during cerebral compression. *Johns Hopkins Hospital Bulletin* **12,** 290–2.

Cushing, H. (1902) Some experimental and clinical observations concerning states of increased intracranial tension. *American Journal of Medical Science* **125,** 375–400.

Cushing, H. (1903) The blood pressure reaction of acute cerebral compression, illustrated by cases of intracranial hemorrhage. *American Journal of Medical Science* **125,** 1017–44.

Cushing, H. (1932) Peptic ulcers and the interbrain. *Surgery, Gynecology and Obstetrics* **55,** 1–34.

Cutler, R.W.P., Page, L.K., Galicich, J. and Watters, G.V. (1968) Formation and absorption of cerebrospinal fluid in man. *Brain* **91,** 707–20.

D'Alecy, L.G. (1972) Relation between sympathetic cerebral vasoconstriction and CSF pressure. *European Neurology* **6,** 180–4.

Davson, H. (1972) *Physiology of the Cerebrospinal Fluid.* Churchill, London.

Davson, H., Hollingsworth, G. and Segal, M.B. (1970) The mechanism of drainage of the cerebrospinal fluid. *Brain* **93,** 665–78.

Di Rocco, C., Di Trapani, G., Maira, G., Bentivoglio, G., Macchi, G. and Rossi, G. (1977) Anatomoclinical correlations in normotensive hydrocephalus. *Journal of the Neurological Sciences* **33,** 437–52.

Ducker, T.B. (1968) Increased intracranial pressure and pulmonary edema. *Journal of Neurosurgery* **28,** 112–17.

Dunbar, H.S., Guthrie, T.C. and Karpell, B. (1966) A study of the cerebrospinal fluid pulse wave. *Archives of Neurology* **14,** 624–30.

Duret, H. (1878) *Etudes expérimentales et cliniques sur les traumatismes cérébraux.* Paris.

Ecker, A. (1955) Irregular fluctuations of elevated cerebrospinal fluid pressure. *Archives of Neurology and Psychiatry* **74,** 641–9.

Eisenberg, H.M., McComb, J.G. and Lorenzo, A.V. (1974) Cerebrospinal fluid overproduction and hydrocephalus associated with choroid plexus papilloma. *Journal of Neurosurgery* **40,** 381–5.

Ellington, E. and Margolis, G. (1969) Block of arachnoid villus by subarachnoid haemorrhage. *Journal of Neurosurgery* **30,** 651–7.

Enevoldsen, E.M., Cold, G., Jensen, F.T. and Malmros, R. (1976) Dynamic changes in regional CBF, intraventricular pressure, CSF pH and lactate levels during the acute phase of head injury. *Journal of Neurosurgery* **44,** 191–214.

Engel, M., Carmel, P.W. and Chutorian, A.M. (1979) Increased intraventricular pressure without ventriculomegaly in children with shunts: 'normal volume' hydrocephalus. *Neurosurgery* **5,** 549–52.

Evans, J.P. (1956) Increased intracranial pressure: its physiology and management. *Surgical Clinics of North America* **36,** 233–42.

Fein, J.M. (1982) Hypertension and the central nervous system. *Clinical Neurosurgery* **29,** 666–721.

Ferguson, G.G. (1972) Direct measurement of mean and pulsatile blood pressure at operation in human intracranial saccular aneurysm. *Journal of Neurosurgery* **36,** 560–3.

Fieschi, C., Agnoli, A., Battastini, N., Bozzao, L. and Prencipe, M. (1968) Derangements of regional cerebral blood flow and of its regulatory mechanisms in acute cerebrovascular lesions. *Neurology* **18,** 1166–79.

Finney, L.A. and Walker, A.E. (1962) *Transtentorial herniation.* Thomas, Springfield.

Fisher, C.M. (1977) The clinical picture of occult hydrocephalus. *Clinical Neurosurgery* **24,** 270–84.

Fishman, R.A. (1975) Brain edema. *New England Journal of Medicine* **293,** 706–11.

Fishman, R.A. (1980) *Cerebrospinal Fluid in Diseases of the Nervous System.* Saunders, Philadelphia.

Fishman, R.A. and Greer, M. (1963) Changes in the

cerebrum associated with experimental obstructive hydrocephalus. *Archives of Neurology* **8,** 156-61.
Fitch, W. and McDowall, D.G. (1971) Effect of halothane on intracranial pressure gradients in the presence of intracranial space-occupying lesions. *British Journal of Anaesthesia* **43,** 904-12.
Fitch, W. and McDowall, D.G. (1977) Systemic vascular responses to increased intracranial pressure. *Journal of Neurology, Neurosurgery and Psychiatry* **40,** 833-42.
Fitch, W., Mackenzie, E.T. and Harper, A.M. (1975) Effects of decreasing arterial blood pressure on cerebral blood flow in the baboon. Influence of the sympathetic nervous system. *Circulation Research* **37,** 550-7.
Flexner, L.B., Clark, J.H. and Weed, L.H. (1932) The elasticity of the dural sac and its contents. *American Journal of Physiology* **101,** 292-303.
Foley, J. (1955) Benign forms of intracranial hypertension—'toxic' and otitic hydrocephalus. *Brain* **78,** 1-41.
Frost, E.A.M. (1977) Respiratory problems associated with head trauma. *Neurosurgery* **1,** 300-6.
Greenberg, R.P., Mayer, D.J. and Becker, D.P. (1976) Correlation in man of intracranial pressure and neuroelectric activity determined by multimodality evoked potentials. In *Intracranial Pressure III* (Eds. Beks, J.W.F., Bosch, D.A. and Brock, M.) pp. 58-62. Springer, Berlin.
Gudeman, S.K., Wheeler, C.B., Miller, J.D., Halloran, L.G. and Becker, D.P. (1983) Gastric secretory and mucosal injury response to severe head trauma. *Neurosurgery* **12,** 175-9.
Guillaume, J. and Janny, P. (1951) Manometrie intracranienne continue: intérêt de la méthode et premiers résultats. *Revue Neurologique* **84,** 131-42.
Hahm, H., Ferzt, R., Muller, J. and Cervos-Navarro, J. (1980) Topography of diffuse brain edema. In *Brain Edema—Pathology, Diagnosis and Therapy* (Eds. Cervos-Navarro, J. and Ferzt, R.) pp. 299-316. Raven Press, New York.
Hakim, S. (1972) Biomechanics of hydrocephalus. In *Cisternography and Hydrocephalus* (Ed. Harbert, J.C.). Thomas, Springfield, pp. 25-54.
Hakim, S. (1977) Considerations on the physics of hydrocephalus and its treatment. In *The Ocular and Cerebrospinal Fluids* (Eds. Bito, L.Z., Davson, H. and Fenstermacher, J.D.) pp. 391-9. Academic Press, New York.
Hakim, S. and Adams, R.D. (1965) The special clinical problems of symptomatic hydrocephalus with normal cerebrospinal pressure. *Journal of the Neurological Sciences* **2,** 307-27.
Halloran, L.G., Zfass, A.M., Gayle, W.E., Wheeler, C.B. and Miller, J.D. (1980) The prevention of acute gastrointestinal complications after severe head injury. *American Journal of Surgery* **139,** 44-8.
Harper, A.M. (1966) Autoregulation of cerebral blood flow: influence of arterial blood pressure on the blood flow through the cerebral cortex. *Journal of Neurology, Neurosurgery and Psychiatry* **29,** 398-403.
Harper, A.M., Deshmukh, V.D., Rowan, J.O. and Jennett, W.B. (1972) The influence of sympathetic nervous activity on cerebral blood flow. *Archives of Neurology* **27,** 1-6.
Hassler, O. (1967) Arterial pattern of human brain stem. Normal appearance and deformation in expanding supratentorial conditions. *Neurology* **17,** 368-75.
Hawkins, W.E. and Clower, B.R. (1971) Myocardial damage after head trauma and simulated intracranial haemorrhage in mice: the role of the autonomic nervous system. *Cardiovascular Research* **5,** 524-9.
Hayreh, S.S. (1964) Pathogenesis of oedema of the optic disc (papilloedema). *British Journal of Ophthalmology* **48,** 522-43.
Hedges, T.R., Weinstein, J.D., Kassell, N. and Stein, S. (1964) Cerebrovascular responses to increased intracranial pressure. *Journal of Neurosurgery* **21,** 292-7.
Hochwald, G.M., Marlin, A.E., Wald, A. and Malhan, C. (1976) Movement of water between blood, brain and CSF in cerebral edema. In *Dynamics of Brain Edema* (Eds. Pappius, H.M. and Feindel, W.) pp. 129-37. Springer, Berlin.
Hoff, J.T. and Mitchell, R.A. (1972) The effect of hypoxia on the Cushing response. In *Intracranial Pressure* (Eds. Brock, M. and Dietz, H.) pp. 205-9. Springer, Berlin.
Hoff, J.T. and Reis, D.J. (1970) Localization of regions mediating the Cushing response in the central nervous system of the cat. *Archives of Neurology* **22,** 228-40.
Howell, D.A. (1959) Upper brain stem compression and foraminal impaction with intracranial space-occupying lesions and brain swelling. *Brain* **82,** 525-50.
Hughes, C.P., Siegel, B.A., Coxe, W.S., Grado, M.H., Grubb, R.L., Coleman, R.E. and Berg, L. (1978) Adult ideopathic communicating hydrocephalus with and without shunting. *Journal of Neurology, Neurosurgery and Psychiatry* **41,** 961-71.
Hulme, A. and Cooper, R. (1966) A technique for the investigation of intracranial pressure in man. *Journal of Neurology, Neurosurgery and Psychiatry* **29,** 154-6.
Hussey, F., Schauzer, B. and Katzman, R. (1970) A simple constant infusion manometric test for measurement of CSF absorption. II. Clinical studies. *Neurology* **20,** 665-80.
Ingvar, D.H. and Lundberg, N. (1961) Paroxysmal

symptoms in intracranial hypertension studied with ventricular fluid pressure recording and EEG. *Brain* **84,** 446–59.

Ishii, S. (1966) Brain swelling. In *Head Injury* (Eds. Caveness, W.E. and Walker, A.E.) pp. 276–99. Lippincott, Philadelphia.

Ishii, S., Hayner, R., Kelly, W.A. and Evans J.P. (1959) Studies of cerebral swelling. II. Experimental cerebral swelling produced by supratentorial extradural compression. *Journal of Neurosurgery* **16,** 152–66.

Jacobson, S.A. and Rothballer, A.B. (1967) Prolonged measurement of experimental intracranial pressure using a subminiature absolute pressure transducer. *Journal of Neurosurgery* **26,** 603–8.

Janny, P., Flori, B., Jovan, J.D. and Janny, L. (1975) CSF resistance to flow as an aid to diagnosis of normal pressure hydrocephalus. In *Intracranial Pressure II* (Eds. Lundberg, N., Ponten, U. and Brock, M.) pp. 512–15. Springer, Berlin.

Janzer, R.C. and Friede, R.L. (1979) Perisulcal infarcts: lesions caused by hypotension during increased intracranial pressure. *Annals of Neurology* **6,** 399–404.

Jefferson, G. (1938) The tentorial pressure cone. *Archives of Neurology and Psychiatry* **40,** 857–76.

Jennett, W.B. and Stern, W.E. (1960) Tentorial herniation, the mid-brain and the pupil. Experimental studies in brain compression. *Journal of Neurosurgery* **17,** 598–608.

Johnson R.T. and Yates, P.O. (1956) Brain stem haemorrhages in expanding supratentorial conditions. *Acta Radiologica* **46,** 250–6.

Johnston, I. (1973) The reduced CSF absorption syndrome: a reappraisal of benign intracranial hypertension and related conditions. *Lancet* **2,** 418–20.

Johnston, I.H. and Jennett, B. (1973) The place of continuous intracranial pressure monitoring in neurosurgical practice. *Acta Neurochirurgica* **29,** 53–63.

Johnston, I. and Paterson, A. (1974) Benign intracranial hypertension. II. CSF pressure and circulation. *Brain* **97,** 301–12.

Johnston, I.H. and Rowan, J.O. (1974) Raised intracranial pressure and cerebral blood flow. 3. Venous outflow tract pressures and vascular resistances in experimental intracranial hypertension. *Journal of Neurology, Neurosurgery and Psychiatry* **37,** 392–402.

Johnston, I.H., Rowan, J.O., Harper, A.M. and Jennett, W.B. (1972) Raised intracranial pressure and cerebral blood flow. 1. Cisterna magna infusion in primates. *Journal of Neurology, Neurosurgery and Psychiatry* **35,** 285–96.

Johnston, I.H., Rowan, J.O., Harper, A.M. and Jennett, W.B. (1973) Raised intracranial pressure and cerebral blood flow. 2. Supratentorial and infratentorial mass lesions in primates. *Journal of Neurology, Neurosurgery and Psychiatry* **36,** 161–70.

Kaufmann, G.E. and Clark, K. (1970) Continuous simultaneous monitoring of intraventricular and cervical subarachnoid cerebrospinal fluid pressure to indicate the development of cerebral or tonsillar herniation. *Journal of Neurosurgery* **33,** 145–50.

Kellie, G. (1824) An account of the appearances observed in the dissection of two of three individuals presumed to have perished in the storm of the 3rd and whose bodies were discovered in the vicinity of Leith on the morning of the 4th November 1821, with some reflections on the pathology of the brain. *Transactions of the Medico-Chirurgical Society of Edinburgh* **1,** 84–169.

Kernohan, J.W. and Woltman, H.W. (1929) Incisura of the crus due to contralateral brain tumour. *Archives of Neurology and Psychiatry* **21,** 274–87.

Key, A. and Retzius, G. (1875) *Studien in der Anatomie der Nervensystems und des Bindegewebes.* Stockholm.

Klatzo, I. (1967) Neuropathological aspects of brain edema. *Journal of Neuropathology and Experimental Neurology* **26,** 1–14.

Klatzo, I. (1972) Pathophysiological aspects of brain edema. In *Steroids and Brain Edema* (Eds. Reulen, H.J. and Schurmann, K.) pp. 1–8. Springer, Berlin.

Klintworth, G.K. (1965) The pathogenesis of secondary brain stem hemorrhage as studied with an experimental model. *American Journal of Pathology* **47,** 525–36.

Klintworth, G.K. (1966) Secondary brain stem haemorrhage. *Journal of Neurology, Neurosurgery and Psychiatry* **29,** 423–5.

Kocher, T. (1901) Hirnerschütterung, Hirndruck und chirurgische Eingriffe bei Hirnerkrankungen. In *Nothnagel: Specielle Pathologie und Therapie*, vol. 9, part 3, pp. 92–134. Holder, Vienna.

Laitinen, L. (1968) Origin of arterial pulsation of cerebrospinal fluid. *Acta Neurologica Scandinavica* **44,** 168–76.

Langfitt, T.W. (1969) Increased intracranial pressure. *Clinical Neurosurgery* **16,** 436–71.

Langfitt, T.W. and Kassell, N.F. (1966) Non-filling of cerebral vessels during angiography: correlation with intracranial pressure. *Acta Neurochirurgica* **14,** 96–104.

Langfitt, T.W., Kassell, N.F. and Weinstein, J.D. (1965) Cerebral blood flow with intracranial hypertension. *Neurology* **15,** 761–73.

Langfitt, T.W., Weinstein, J.D. and Kassell, N.F. (1965) Cerebral vasomotor paralysis produced by intracranial hypertension. *Neurology* **15,** 622–41.

Langfitt, T.W., Weinstein, J.D., Kassell, N.F. and Simeone, F.A. (1964a) Transmission of increased intracranial pressure. I. Within the craniospinal axis. *Journal of Neurosurgery* **21,** 989-97.

Langfitt, T.W., Weinstein, J.D., Kassell, N.F. and Gagliardi, W. (1964b) Transmission of increased intracranial pressure. II. Within the supratentorial space. *Journal of Neurosurgery* **21,** 998-1005.

Leech, P.J. and Miller, J.D. (1974) Intracranial volume/pressure relationships during experimental brain compression in primates. I. Pressure responses to changes in ventricular volume. *Journal of Neurology, Neurosurgery and Psychiatry* **37,** 1093-8.

Levett, J.M., Johns, L.M., Replogle, R.L. and Mullan, S. (1980) Cardiovascular effects of experimental cerebral missile injury in primates. *Surgical Neurology* **13,** 59-64.

Levin, A.B. (1977) The use of a fiberoptic intracranial pressure monitor in clinical practice. *Neurosurgery* **1,** 266-71.

Levine, J.E., Povlishock, J.T. and Becker, D.P. (1982) The morphological correlates of primate cerebrospinal fluid absorption. *Brain Research* **241,** 31-41.

Lindenberg, R. (1955) Compression of brain arteries as a pathogenic factor for tissue necrosis and their areas of predilection. *Journal of Neuropathology and Experimental Neurology* **14,** 233-43.

Lorenzo, A.V., Bresnan, M.J. and Barlow, C.F. (1974) Cerebrospinal fluid absorption defect in normal pressure hydrocephalus. *Archives of Neurology* **30,** 387-93.

Lorenzo, A.V., Page, L.K. and Watters, G.V. (1970) Relationship between cerebrospinal fluid formation, absorption and pressure in human hydrocephalus. *Brain* **93,** 679-92.

Lundberg, N. (1960) Continuous recording and control of ventricular fluid pressure in neurosurgical practice. *Acta Psychiatrica et Neurologica Scandinavica* **36,** Suppl. 149, 1-193.

Marsden, C.D. and Harrison, M.J.G. (1972) Outcome of investigation of patients with presenile dementia. *British Medical Journal* **2,** 249-52.

Marshall, L.F., Smith R.W. and Shapiro, H.M. (1978) The influence of diurnal rhythms in patients with intracranial hypertension: implications for management. *Neurosurgery* **2,** 100-2.

Martins, A.N. (1973) Resistance to drainage of cerebrospinal fluid: clinical measurement and significance. *Journal of Neurology, Neurosurgery and Psychiatry* **36,** 313-18.

Martins, A.N., Kobrine, A.I. and Larsen, D.F. (1974) Pressure in the sagittal sinus during intracranial hypertension in man. *Journal of Neurosurgery* **40,** 603-8.

Masserman, J.H. (1935) Studies of the volume elasticity of the human ventriculo-subarachnoid system. *Journal of Comparative Neurology* **61,** 543-52.

Meinig, G. Reulen, H.J. and Magavly, C. (1973) Regional cerebral blood flow and cerebral perfusion pressure in global brain edema induced by water intoxication. *Acta Neurochirurgica* **29,** 1-13.

Mendelow, A.D., Rowan, J.O., Murray, L. and Kerr, A.E. (1983) A clinical comparison of subdural screw pressure measurements with ventricular pressure. *Journal of Neurosurgery* **58,** 45-50.

Meyer, A. (1920) Herniation of the brain. *Archives of Neurology and Psychiatry* **4,** 387-400.

Mickell, J.J., Cook, D.R., Reigel, D.H., Painter, M.J. and Safar, P. (1976) Intracranial pressure monitoring in Reye-Johnson syndrome. *Critical Care Medicine* **4,** 1-7.

Milhorat, T.H. (1972) *Hydrocephalus and the Cerebrospinal Fluid.* Williams and Wilkins, Baltimore.

Milhorat, T.H. (1975) The third circulation revisited. *Journal of Neurosurgery* **42,** 628-45.

Miller, J.D. (1975a) Volume and pressure in the craniospinal axis. *Clinical Neurosurgery* **22,** 76-105.

Miller, J.D. (1975b) Effects of hypercapnia on pupillary size, intracranial pressure and cerebral venous Po_2 during experimental brain compression. In *Intracranial Pressure II* (Eds. Lundberg, N., Ponten, U. and Brock, M.) pp. 444-6 Springer, Berlin.

Miller, J.D. (1978) Intracranial pressure monitoring. *British Journal of Hospital Medicine* **19,** 497-503.

Miller, J.D. (1979a) Clinical management of cerebral oedema. *British Journal of Hospital Medicine* **20,** 152-66.

Miller, J.D. (1979b) Barbiturates and raised intracranial pressure. *Annals of Neurology* **6,** 189-93.

Miller, J.D. and Adams, J.H. (1972) Physiopathology and management of increased intracranial pressure. In *Scientific Foundations of Neurology* (Eds. Critchley, M., O'Leary, J. and Jennett, B.) pp. 308-24. Heinemann Medical, London.

Miller, J.D., Stanek, A. and Langfitt, T.W. (1972) Concepts of cerebral perfusion pressure and vascular compression during intracranial hypertension. In *Progress in Brain Research*, vol. 35: *Cerebral Blood Flow* (Eds. Meyer, J.S. and Schade, J.P.). pp. 411-32. Elsevier, Amsterdam.

Miller, J.D., Stanek, A.E. and Langfitt, T.W. (1973) Cerebral blood flow regulation during experimental brain compression. *Journal of Neurosurgery* **39,** 186-96.

Miller, J.D., Becker, D.P., Ward, J.D., Sullivan, H.G., Adams, W.E. and Rosner, M.J. (1977) Significance of intracranial hypertension in severe head injury. *Journal of Neurosurgery* **47,** 503-16.

Miller, J.D., Butterworth, J.F., Gudeman, S.K., Faulkner, J.E., Choi, S.C., Selhorst, J.B. et al. (1981) Further experience in the management of severe head injury. *Journal of Neurosurgery* **54,** 289-99.

Monro, A. (1783) *Observations on the Structure and Function of the Nervous System*. Creech and Johnston, Edinburgh.

Moore, M.T. and Stern, K. (1938) Vascular lesions of the brain stem and occipital lobe occurring in association with brain tumours. *Brain* **61,** 70–81.

Nakatani, S. and Ommaya, A.K. (1975) Volume pressure curves and pial vascular pressure gradients in the Rhesus monkey. In *Intracranial Pressure II* (Eds. Lundberg, N., Ponten, U. and Brock, M.). pp. 89–96. Springer, Berlin.

North, J.B. and Jennett, S. (1974) Abnormal breathing patterns associated with acute brain damage. *Archives of Neurology* **31,** 338–44.

North, J.B. and Jennett, S. (1976) Response of ventilation and of intracranial pressure during rebreathing of carbon dioxide in patients with acute brain damage. *Brain* **99,** 169–82.

O'Brien, M.D. and Waltz, A.G. (1973) Intracranial pressure gradients caused by experimental cerebral ischemia and edema. *Stroke* **4,** 694–98.

Palvolgyi, R. (1969) Regional cerebral blood flow in patients with intracranial tumors. *Journal of Neurosurgery* **31,** 149–63.

Penn, R.D. (1980) Cerebral edema and neurological function: CT, evoked responses and clinical examination. In *Brain Edema—Pathology, Diagnosis and Therapy* (Eds. Cervos-Navarro, J. and Ferzt, R.) pp. 383–94. Raven Press, New York.

Permutt, S. and Riley, R.L. (1963) Hemodynamics of collapsible vessels with tone: the vascular waterfall. *Journal of Applied Physiology* **18,** 924–32.

Petito, C.K., Schaefer, J.A. and Plum, F. (1976) The blood brain barrier in experimental seizures. In *Dynamics of Brain Edema* (Eds. Pappins, H.M. and Feindel, W.) pp. 38–42. Springer, Berlin.

Pickard, J.D. (1982) Adult communicating hydrocephalus. *British Journal of Hospital Medicine* **27,** 35–44.

Pickard, J.D., Teasdale, G., Matheson, M., Lindsay, K., Galbraith, S., Wyper, D. and Macpherson, P. (1980) Intraventricular pressure waves—the best predictive test for shunting in normal pressure hydrocephalus. In *Intracranial Pressure IV* (Eds. Shulman, K., Marmarou, A., Miller, J.D., Becker, D.P., Hochwald, G.M. and Brock, M.) pp. 498–500. Springer, Berlin.

Plum, F. and Posner, J.B. (1966) *The Diagnosis of Stupor and Coma* (1980, 3rd edn.). Davis, Philadelphia.

Pribram, H. (1961) Angiographic appearances in acute intracranial hypertension. *Neurology* **11,** 10–21.

Reichardt, M. (1911) Über Hirnschwellung. *Zeitschrift für die gesamte Neurologie und Psychiatrie* **3,** 1–43.

Reid, A.C., Matheson, M.S. and Teasdale, G. (1980) Volume of the ventricles in benign intracranial hypertension. *Lancet* **2,** 7–8.

Reid, W.L. and Cone, W.V. (1939) The mechanism of fixed dilatation of the pupil resulting from ipsilateral cerebral compression. *Journal of the American Medical Association* **112,** 2030–4.

Reulen, H.J., Tsuyumu, M., Tack, A., Fenske, A.R. and Prioleau, G.R. (1978) Clearance of edema fluid in cerebrospinal fluid. *Journal of Neurosurgery* **48,** 754–64.

Risberg, J., Lundberg, N. and Ingvar, D.H. (1969) Regional cerebral blood volume during acute transient rises of intracranial pressure (plateau waves). *Journal of Neurosurgery* **31,** 303–10.

Riishede, J. and Ethelberg, S. (1953) Angiographic changes in sudden and severe herniation of the brain stem through the tentorial incisura. *Archives of Neurology and Psychiatry* **70,** 399–409.

Roberson, F.C., Kishore, P.R.S., Miller, J.D. Lipper, M.H. and Becker, D.P. (1979) The value of serial computerized tomography in the management of severe head injury. *Surgical Neurology* **12,** 161–7.

Rubin, R.C., Henderson, E.S., Ommaya, A.K., Walker, M.D. and Rall, D.P. (1966) The production of cerebrospinal fluid in man and its modification by acetazolamide. *Journal of Neurosurgery* **25,** 430–6.

Russell, D.S. (1949) Obervations on the pathology of hydrocephalus. *Special Report Series of the Medical Research Council, London* no. 265.

Ryder, H.W., Espey, F.F., Kimball, F.D., Penka, E.J., Rosenauer, A., Podolsky, B. and Evans, J.P. (1952a) Influence of changes in cerebral blood flow on the cerebrospinal fluid pressure. *Archives of Neurology and Psychiatry* **68,** 165–9.

Ryder, H.W., Espey, F.F., Kimball, F.D., Penka, E.J., Rosenauer, A., Podolsky, B. and Evans, J.P. (1952b) Effect of changes in systemic venous pressure on the cerebrospinal fluid pressure. *Archives of Neurology and Psychiatry* **68,** 175–9.

Ryder, H.W., Espey, F.F., Kimball, F.D., Penka, E.J., Rosenauer, A., Podolsky, B. and Evans, J.P. (1953) Mechanism of the change in cerebrospinal fluid pressure following an induced change in the volume of the fluid space. *Journal of Laboratory and Clinical Medicine* **41,** 428–35.

Sahar, A., Hochwald, G.M. and Ransohoff, J. (1970) Experimental hydrocephalus: cerebrospinal fluid formation and ventricular size as a function of intraventricular pressure. *Journal of the Neurological Sciences* **11,** 81–91.

Schettini, A. and Walsh, E.K. (1973) Pressure relaxation of the intracranial system in vivo. *American Journal of Physiology* **225,** 513–17.

Schutta, H.S., Kassell, N.F. and Langfitt, T.W. (1968) Brain swelling produced by injury and aggravated by arterial hypertension—a light and electron microscopic study. *Brain* **9,** 281–94.

Selhorst, J.B., Gudeman, S.K., Butterworth, J.F., Harbison, J.W., Miller, J.D. and Becker, D.P. (1984) Papilloedema following acute head injury. *Neurosurgery* (In press).

Shalit, M.N., Reinmuth, O.M., Shimojyo, S. and Scheinberg, P. (1967) Carbon dioxide and cerebral circulatory control. III. The effects of brain stem lesions. *Archives of Neurology* **17,** 342–53.

Shulman, K. and Verdier, G.R. (1967) Cerebral vascular resistance changes in response to cerebrospinal fluid pressure. *American Journal of Physiology* **213,** 1084–8.

Smyth, G.E. and Henderson, W.R. (1938) Observations on the cerebrospinal fluid pressure on simultaneous ventricular and lumbar punctures. *Journal of Neurology and Psychiatry* **1,** 226–37.

Starling, E.H. (1896) On the absorption of fluids from the connective tissue spaces. *Journal of Physiology* **19,** 312–26.

Stern, W.E. and Coxon, R.V. (1964) Osmolality of brain tissue and its relation to brain bulk. *American Journal of Physiology* **206,** 1–7.

Sunderland, S. (1958) The tentorial notch and complications produced by herniation through that aperture. *British Journal of Surgery* **45,** 422–38.

Symon, L. and Dorsch, N.W.C. (1975) Use of long-term intracranial pressure measurements to assess hydrocephalic patients prior to shunt surgery. *Journal of Neurosurgery* **42,** 258–73.

Symon, L. and Hinzpeter, T. (1977) The enigma of normal pressure hydrocephalus. *Clinical Neurosurgery* **24,** 285–315.

Symon, L., Pasztor, E., Dorsch, N.W.C. and Branston, N.M. (1973) Physiological responses of local areas of the cerebral circulation in experimental primates determined by the method of hydrogen clearance. *Stroke* **4,** 632–42.

Teasdale, E., Cardosa, E., Galbraith, S. and Teasdale, G. (1984) A new CT scan appearance with raised intracranial pressure in severe diffuse head injury. *Journal of Neurology, Neurosurgery and Psychiatry* **47,** 600–603.

Thompson, R.K. and Malina, S. (1959) Dynamic axial brain stem distortion as a mechanism explaining the cardiorespiratory changes in increased intracranial pressure. *Journal of Neurosurgery* **16,** 664–75.

Torack, R.M., Terry, R.D. and Zimmerman, H.M. (1960) The fine structure of cerebral fluid accumulation. II. Swelling produced by triethyltin poisoning and its comparison with that in the human brain. *American Journal of Pathology* **36,** 273–87.

Tripathi, R. (1974) Tracing the bulk outflow route of cerebrospinal fluid by transmission and scanning electron microscopy. *Brain Research* **80,** 503–11.

Troupp, H. and Heiskanen, O. (1963) Cerebral angiography in cases of extremely high intracranial pressure. *Acta Neurologica Scandinavica* **39,** 213–23.

Tso, M.O.M. and Hayreh, S.S. (1977) Optic disc edema in raised intracranial pressure. III. A pathologic study of experimental papilledema. *Archives of Ophthalmology* **95,** 1148–57.

Vincent, C., David, M. and Thiebaut, F. (1936) Le cone de pression temporal dans les tumeurs des hémisphères cérébraux. Sa symptomatologie; sa gravité; les traitements qu'il convient de lui opposer. *Revue Neurologique* **65,** 536–45.

Vries, J.K., Becker, D.P. and Young, H.F. (1973) A subarachnoid screw for monitoring intracranial pressure. *Journal of Neurosurgery* **39,** 416–19.

Walsh, E.K. and Schettini, A. (1976) Elastic behavior of brain tissue in vivo. *American Journal of Physiology* **230,** 1058–62.

Weed, L.H. (1929) Some limitations of the Monro–Kellie hypothesis. *Archives of Surgery* **18,** 1049–68.

Weed, L.H. and Flexner, L.B. (1933) The relations of the intracranial pressures. *American Journal of Physiology* **105,** 266–72.

Weed, L.H. and McKibben, P.S. (1919) Pressure changes in cerebrospinal fluid following intravenous injection of solutions of various concentrations. *American Journal of Physiology* **48,** 512–30.

Weinstein, J.D., Langfitt, T.W. and Kassell, N.F. (1964) Vasopressor response to increased intracranial pressure. *Neurology* **14,** 1118–31.

Weinstein, J.D., Langfitt, T.W., Bruno, L., Zaren, H.A. and Jackson, J.L.F. (1968) Experimental study of patterns of brain distortion and ischemia produced by an intracranial mass. *Journal of Neurosurgery* **28,** 513–21.

Welch, K. (1975) The principles of physiology of the cerebrospinal fluid in relation to hydrocephalus including normal pressure hydrocephalus. In *Advances in Neurology*, vol. 13 (Ed. Friedlander, W.J.) pp. 247–332. Raven Press, New York.

Welch, K. (1980) The intracranial pressure in infants. *Journal of Neurosurgery* **52,** 693–9.

Welch, K. and Friedman, V. (1960) The cerebrospinal fluid valves. *Brain* **83,** 454–69.

Welch, K. and Pollay, M. (1961) Perfusion of particles through arachnoid villi of the monkey. *American Journal of Physiology* **201,** 651–4.

Weller, R.O. and Shulman, K. (1972) Infantile hydrocephalus: clinical, histological and ultrastructural study of brain damage. *Journal of Neurosurgery* **36,** 255–65.

Weller, R.O. and Wisniewski, H. (1969) Histological and ultrastructural changes with experimental hydrocephalus in adult rabbits. *Brain* **92,** 819–28.

Weller, R.O., Wisniewski, H., Shulman, K. and Terry, R.D. (1971) Experimental hydrocephalus in young dogs: histological and ultrastructural study of the brain tissue damage. *Journal of Neuropathology and Experimental Neurology* **30,** 613–24.

Wisniewski, H., Weller, R.O. and Terry, R.D. (1969)

Experimental hydrocephalus produced by the subarachnoid infusion of oil. *Journal of Neurosurgery* **31,** 10–14.
Wittschafter, J.D., Rizzo, F.J. and Smiley, B.C. (1975) Optic nerve axoplasm and papilledema. *Survey of Ophthalmology* **20,** 157–89.
Wright, R.D. (1938) Experimental observations on increased intracranial pressure. *Australian and New Zealand Journal of Surgery* **7,** 215–35.
Yada, K., Nakagawa, Y. and Tsuru, M. (1973) Circulatory disturbance of the venous system during experimental intracranial hypertension. *Journal of Neurosurgery* **39,** 723–9.

3

Head injury

J. Hume Adams

Sabina Strich (1976) wrote in the previous edition of Greenfield's *Neuropathology* 'On looking through the literature on head injuries, it becomes clear that there has been very little new since 1900'. At that time few, if any, would have seriously challenged that assertion. Since then, however, there have been many new developments. Thus—as will become apparent below—all of the major types of brain damage that occur in man as a result of a non-missile head injury have been reproduced in subhuman primates by acceleration of the head without anything striking the head; there is a greater awareness of the clinicopathological entity diffuse axonal injury, attention to which was first drawn by Strich in 1956, and there is increasing evidence that this type of brain damage is the most important single factor governing the outcome in anyone who sustains a non-missile head injury; there is a better understanding of the pathogenesis of cerebral contusions; the importance of hypoxic brain damage and diffuse brain swelling is being increasingly recognized; and the importance of diffuse axonal injury and hypoxic brain damage in the pathogenesis of severe disability and the vegetative state after non-missile head injury has recently been underlined. There is therefore a real need for clinicians and pathologists—including forensic pathologists—with an interest in head injury to become acquainted with recent developments in this field because many of the more subtle types of brain damage may be easily overlooked *post mortem* unless their existence is known, particularly since some can only be seen microscopically. Thus death may still be certified as being due to cerebral contusions and fracture of the skull when neither may have been the cause even of the patient's being unconscious.

There are two basic types of head injury: blunt or non-missile injury, and missile head injury. The former will be dealt with first.

Non-missile head injury

The problem

Brain damage occurring as a result of a non-missile head injury has long been a particular problem facing society. A particularly distressing feature is that many people who sustain such injuries are adolescent or in early adult life, and if thereafter they remain severely or moderately disabled, as defined by Jennett and Bond (1975), they are likely to require care in institutions or from their families for many years. Even if physical disability is not severe, intellectual or psychological problems or changes in personality may impose a great strain on their family and friends (Brooks and McKinlay, 1983).

The precise incidence of head injury is difficult to define but according to Jennett and Teasdale (1981) there are each year in Britain 9 deaths from head injury per 100 000 population: they account for 1 per cent of all deaths, a quarter of deaths from trauma, and almost half of those caused by road traffic accidents. Corresponding figures in other countries may well be higher (Caveness, 1979; Anderson and McLaurin,

1980), and preliminary results from studies in central Virginia and in San Diego indicate that deaths from head injury in these regions each year amount to about 24 per 100 000 population (Jennett and Teasdale, 1981). In a recent report Simpson et al. (1981) concluded that in South Australia and New South Wales there are some 25 deaths from head injury per 100 000 population per year. In a survey of severe head injuries in representative areas of the UK, the USA and Holland, Jennett et al. (1977) found that between 1 and 5 per cent remained vegetative and between 5 and 18 per cent severely disabled 6 months after their injury. The accumulating population of disabled survivors from head injury results in an estimated prevalence in the UK of 150 per 100 000 population with major persisting handicap—i.e. about 700 000 individuals (*Lancet*, 1983). One family in 300 has a member with such a disability.

It is because of figures like these that it is difficult to overemphasize the importance of non-missile head injury. Attempts at prevention must clearly continue to be pursued but so also must the identification of at least potentially avoidable factors contributing to brain damage such as the delayed recognition of intracranial haematoma (Galbraith, 1976; Jennett and Carlin, 1978; Seelig et al., 1981). Thus neuropathologists have much to offer in the field of head injury: their task is not simply to define the cause of death but to identify the sequence of events leading to the fatal outcome and so to contribute to the recognition of such avoidable factors.

Experimental models of head injury

The mechanisms of brain damage in head injury are complex but in any head injury physical forces affect and may damage the brain. The aims of experimental models of head injury have been to reproduce, by conditions that simulate real-life situations, the types of brain damage that occur in man, and to identify the types of force that produce the brain damage. The pathogenesis of many of the types of brain damage caused by non-missile head injury will be discussed in the appropriate sections that follow, but in the experimental field many investigations have been based on the pioneering work of Denny-Brown and Russell (1941) in subhuman primates. They were able to reproduce the clinical state of concussion by delivering controlled blows to the freely movable head by a calibrated pendulum, a situation similar to the common clinical one of an impact to a head which is free to move. Denny-Brown and Russell (1941) also established that acceleration of the head was a vital factor in the production of concussion since it was much more difficult to produce if the head was fixed. Prolonged coma in the absence of intracranial haematoma—a frequent occurrence in severe head injury (Gennarelli et al., 1982b)—was not produced. The importance of acceleration/deceleration impulses was emphasized by Holbourn (1945) who was convinced that during rotational movement of the head shear strains would be produced in the brain because of brain lag, whilst Pudenz and Shelden (1946) and Ommaya (1966) demonstrated swirling and gliding of the cerebral convolutions when the head was free to move after an impact. There has been a tendency in the past to place particular emphasis on either acceleration *or* deceleration of the head in the pathogenesis of brain damage; both, however, produce essentially similar effects and occur in greater or lesser degree in all types of non-missile head injury apart from those due to crushing of the skull.

The subhuman primate has remained the animal of choice in experimental models of head injury because brain structure, angulation of the brain/brain stem/spinal cord, and head to brain/mass ratio are similar to those in man. In experimental studies using subhuman primates, increasing attention has been paid to head injuries with minimum direct impact (Ommaya, Faas and Yarnell, 1968; Unterharnscheidt and Higgins, 1969; Ommaya and Corrao, 1970; Gennarelli, Thibault and Ommaya, 1971, 1972; Ommaya and Hirsch, 1971) and it has come to be appreciated that the principal mechanisms in head injury can be reduced to two categories of input—*contact phenomena* and *acceleration* (Ommaya and Gennarelli, 1974; Gennarelli et al., 1982b). Contact phenomena result from an object striking the head and, as will be seen below, consist of local effects such as laceration of the scalp, fracture of the skull, extradural haematoma and some types of cerebral contusion. Contact phenomena also generate shock waves at the site of impact that travel through the skull and through the brain which may in turn produce fracture of the base of the skull, contusions remote from the site of impact and intracerebral haemorrhage. Acceleration, in contrast, results from head movement in the instant after an injury and leads to pressure gradients within the skull and brain as well as shear, tensile and compressive strains (Dawson et al., 1980). As will be seen below, such inertial (i.e. non-impact) phenomena, are responsible for the two most important types of damage encountered in non-missile head injury in man (Gennarelli et al., 1982b)—acute subdural haematoma resulting from tearing of subdural bridging veins, and diffuse damage to axons which can be attributed mainly to shear or tensile strain generated in the brain at the moment of injury.

In recent years major advances have been made in the understanding of the pathogenesis of brain damage in non-missile head injury as a result of the development of head-accelerating devices so designed as to allow of the delivery of controlled and reproducible acceleration to the head without there being any impact to the head. In experiments on squirrel monkeys Ommaya and Gennarelli (1974) established that **translational acceleration** (i.e. moving the head from posterior to anterior along a straight line) did not produce concussion whereas **angular acceleration** (rotational) with a centre of rotation in the lower cervical spine readily did so. With the aim of studying in greater detail the effects of angular acceleration in larger subhuman primates, a device was then developed (Abel, Gennarelli and Segawa, 1978; Gennarelli et al, 1982a) which allowed of angular acceleration of the head through 60 degrees in the sagittal plane. This was called the **Penn 1 device** (Gennarelli, 1983). At low and moderate acceleration levels transient cerebral concussion, with or without contusions, was readily produced (Gennarelli et al., 1979; Adams, Graham and Gennarelli, 1982). Attempts to produce more severe concussion by using a higher acceleration were not successful because, within a few hours of injury, the animals died from acute subdural haematoma because of rupture of the parasagittal bridging veins. After a review of the mechanics it became clear that the subdural bridging veins were strain rate sensitive; i.e. they were sensitive not only to stretching but also to the rate at which they were stretched (Gennarelli and Thibault, 1982). The model was then modified to allow the acceleration impulse to act over a longer period of time (Gennarelli et al., 1982c; Gennarelli, 1983): with this **Penn 2 device** rupture of the bridging veins did not occur and, for the first time in an experimental model, prolonged traumatic coma in the absence of an intracranial expanding lesion and a high intracranial pressure was produced. Subsequent histological studies established that the structural basis of this was diffuse damage to axons. With these devices all of the major types of brain damage seen in man as a result of a non-missile head injury have now been produced in the subhuman primate by pure inertial (i.e. non-impact) controlled angular acceleration of the head. Thus nothing needs to strike the head, nor the head to strike anything, to produce brain damage in head injury—what matters is the acceleration/deceleration conditions that exist at the moment of injury.

Classification of brain damage

This has to take into account two extremes: the patient who remains unconscious from the moment of impact until death; and the patient who is apparently normal shortly after the initial injury but who, as a result of a complication, lapses into fatal coma. Even an apparently trivial head injury may set in motion a series of events leading to a fatal outcome unless their onset is recognized early and, where feasible, appropriate treatment instituted. Emphasis in the past has therefore tended to be placed on *primary* or immediate impact damage, and *secondary* damage or complications of the original injury (Adams and Graham, 1972; Adams, 1975; Adams et al., 1980a; Jennett and Teasdale, 1981; Adams, Gennarelli and Graham, 1982).

There is, however, a trend for clinicians (Gennarelli et al., 1982b; Gennarelli, 1983) and pathologists (Adams, Graham and Gennarelli, 1983; Adams and Graham, 1984) to classify brain damage as **focal** or **diffuse.** *Focal damage* includes cerebral contusions, intracranial haematoma, the various types of secondary brain damage—including haemorrhage and infarction in the brain stem—that can be produced by intracranial expanding lesions, as well as infection and other less commonly encountered lesions such as pontomedullary tears and avulsion of the pituitary stalk and cranial nerves. *Diffuse brain damage* is fundamentally different and exists in four principal forms (Adams and Graham, 1984): three of these are encountered in patients who survive long enough to reach hospital—diffuse axonal injury, hypoxic brain damage and diffuse brain swelling; the fourth, however, appears to be virtually restricted to patients who die within a very short time of their injury and consists of multiple small haemorrhages throughout the brain. These types of brain damage, when sufficiently severe, cause coma not by compression of the brain stem but by diffuse injury to the cerebral hemispheres and/or the brain stem (Gennarelli, 1983). In an unconscious patient without any evidence of intracranial haematoma—a situation that occurs in almost 50 per cent of patients who have sustained a non-missile head injury (Gennarelli, 1983)—it is usually concluded that the patient has sustained diffuse brain damage but its precise type is rarely identifiable during life. It may also be difficult to define *post mortem* unless the brain is properly fixed prior to dissection and appropriate histological studies are undertaken.

Lesions of the scalp and skull

The scalp is often lacerated or bruised at the time of head injury and such lesions are the best indication of the site of impact. Other important features of lacerations are that they may bleed copiously and be a potential route for the entry of infection.

The presence of a fracture of the skull indicates that the impact has had considerable force but many patients with a fracture may have no evidence of brain damage and make a smooth and uneventful recovery, whilst in the consecutive series of 151 fatal head injuries in a neurosurgical unit analysed by Adams et al. (1980a) 19 per cent of the patients did not have a fracture of the skull. Thus there may be a tendency to exaggerate their importance, but patients with a fracture of the skull have a much higher incidence of intracranial haematoma (Teasdale and Galbraith, 1981) than those who do not have a fracture. Impact against a flat surface will produce *fissure* fractures which often extend into the base of the skull, whilst impact against a smaller or irregular object will produce a more localized fracture which is often *depressed*—i.e. the fragments of the inner table of the skull are depressed by at least the thickness of the skull (Jennett and Teasdale, 1981). A depressed fracture is said to be *compound* if there is an associated laceration of the scalp, and *penetrating* if there is also a tear in the dura. Fractures of the base of the skull are evidence of severe impact and because they often pass through the middle ear or the anterior cranial fossa, producing in some cases a cerebrospinal fluid otorrhoea or rhinorrhoea, they may open up potential channels for later infection (see p. 98). According to Robinson (1970), aerocele occurs in almost one-third of patients with rhinorrhoea. When the impact has been particularly severe there may be a *'hinge'* fracture extending across the base of the skull, usually in the region of the posterior part of the pituitary fossa or the rostral part of the clivus, and the adjacent squamous parts of the temporal bones.

The term *contrecoup* fracture is sometimes used to describe fractures located at a distance from the point of impact and *not* direct extensions of the fracture originating at the point of impact. They occur principally in the roofs of the orbits and the ethmoid plates in association with a fall on the occiput (Hirsch and Kaufman, 1975). *Growing* fractures occur in infancy; the dura is so firmly attached to the skull in this age group that it is readily torn in association with a fracture resulting in the interposition of soft tissue and meninges between the edges of the fracture. Stein and Tenner (1972) have emphasized that brain tissue protruding into the fracture may prevent it from healing and indeed enlarge it. As a result there may, some months after the injury, be a protruding swelling consisting mainly of brain tissue at the site of the fracture.

Focal brain damage in non-missile head injury

Cerebral contusions

These are common in non-missile head injury, and have been considered their hallmark. Nevertheless, patients, particularly those with diffuse brain damage, may die as a result of a head injury with minimal or even no contusions. The appearances of contusions, however, are so characteristic that it can often be stated categorically that a patient has sustained a head injury recently or some time in the past. A distinction is sometimes made between *contusions* and *lacerations*: in the former the pia-arachnoid is not breached, but with lacerations the pia arachnoid and the underlying brain are torn.

Contusions characteristically occur at the crests of gyri but not all contusions are immediately apparent on external examination of the brain because they may be restricted to the

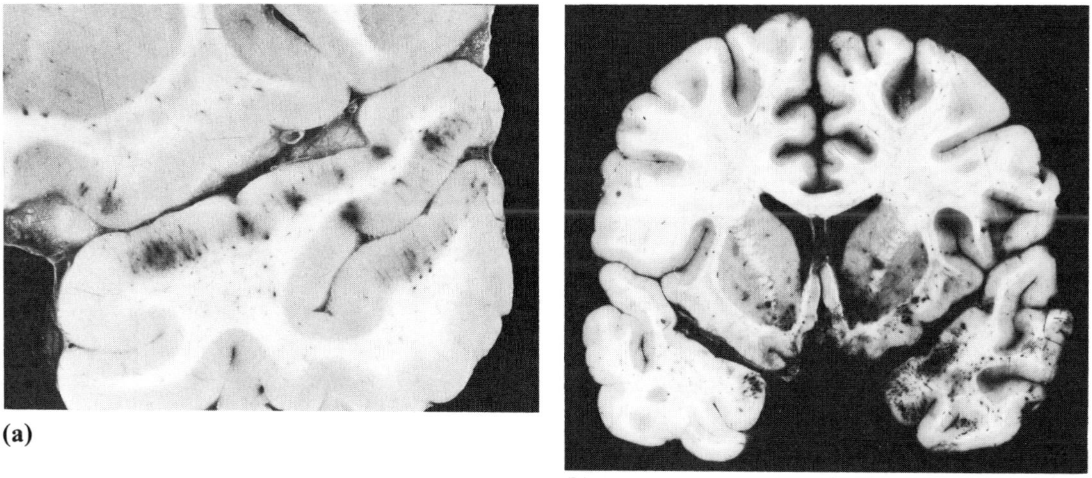

(a) (b)

Fig. 3.1 Contusions. (*a*) Early contusions taking the form of essentially linear perivascular haemorrhages in the cortex. (**b**) More severe recent contusions and haemorrhage. Both patients were said to have died within minutes of road traffic accidents.

deeper layers of the cortex, with or without involvement of the adjacent white matter. In the early stages they are characterized by groups of punctate haemorrhages or streaks of haemorrhage at right angles to the cortical surface (Fig. 3.1a); that they can occur very rapidly is shown by the fact that contusions of this type may be very obvious in patients said to have died instantaneously (Fig. 3.1b). Thereafter haemorrhage becomes more extensive and blood often permeates into the digitate white matter (Fig. 3.2). With the passage of time these acute contusions come to be represented by shrunken—often brown because of the persistence of haemosiderin—scars at the crests of gyri (Fig. 3.3); they can thus be distinguished from foci of old ischaemic damage which are almost invariably more severe within the depths of sulci. Contusions present similar features in all age groups apart from early infancy (Lindenberg and Freytag, 1969); non-missile head injury in this age group produces tears—often apparent macro-

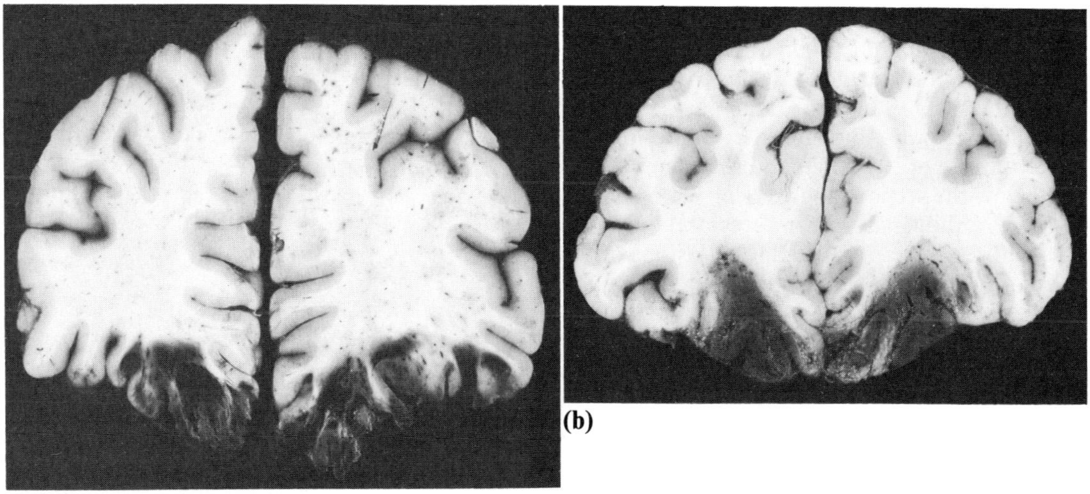

(b)

(a)

Fig. 3.2 Contusions on the orbital surfaces of the frontal lobes extending into the adjacent white matter (**a**) A patient who survived for 9 hours after a head injury. (**b**) More clearly demarcated contusions in a patient who survived for 23 days after a head injury.

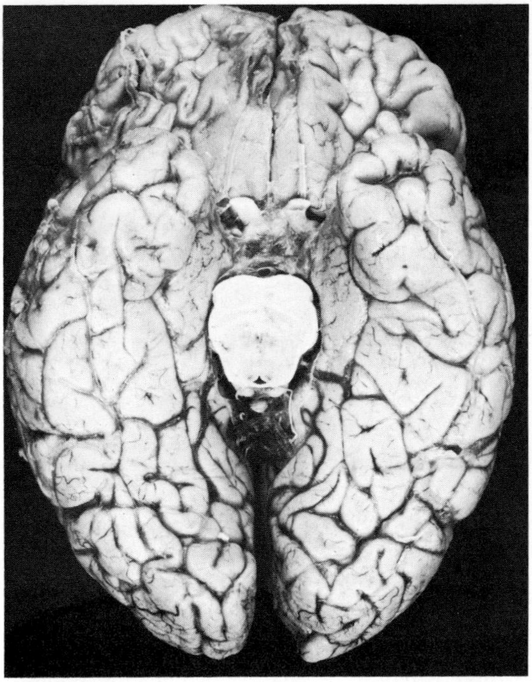

Fig. 3.3 Old contusions in the frontal and temporal lobes in a patient who had made a good recovery from a head injury sustained more than 50 years previously. (Reproduced, with permission, from Adams, Gennarelli and Graham, 1982).

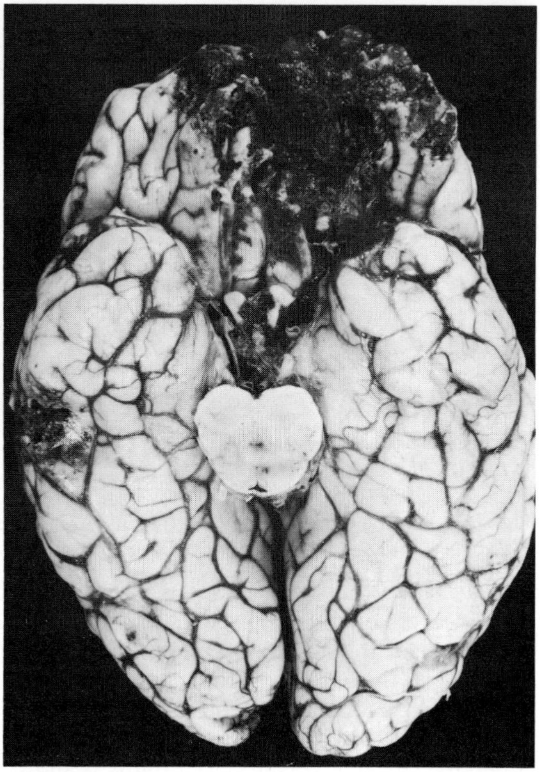

Fig. 3.4 Recent contusions in the frontal and temporal lobes. (Reproduced, with permission, from Adams, 1975).

scopically—in the subcortical white matter and in the outer layers of the cortex, particularly in the frontal and temporal lobes.

Contusions have a very characteristic distribution whatever the site of the original injury. Thus they affect particularly the frontal poles, the orbital surfaces of the frontal lobes (Fig. 3.4), the temporal poles, the lateral and inferior surfaces of the temporal lobes and the cortex above and below the sylvian fissures (Fig. 3.5). The last of these, although common, are rarely identifiable before the brain is sliced. Contusions of the parietal and occipital lobes and of the cerebellum are uncommon unless they are directly related to a fracture of the skull. A precisely similar distribution (Fig. 3.6) is seen in subhuman primates subjected to angular acceleration of the head (Adams, Graham and Gennarelli, 1982). In the acute stage there is frequently some swelling of brain tissue adjacent to contusions (Fig. 3.27); contusions and swelling may therefore influence the early clinical state, but, because contusions are essentially a focal type of brain damage in

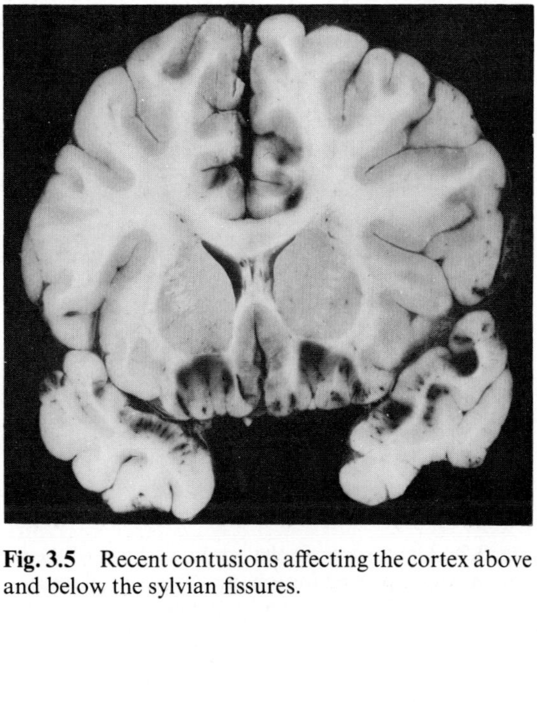

Fig. 3.5 Recent contusions affecting the cortex above and below the sylvian fissures.

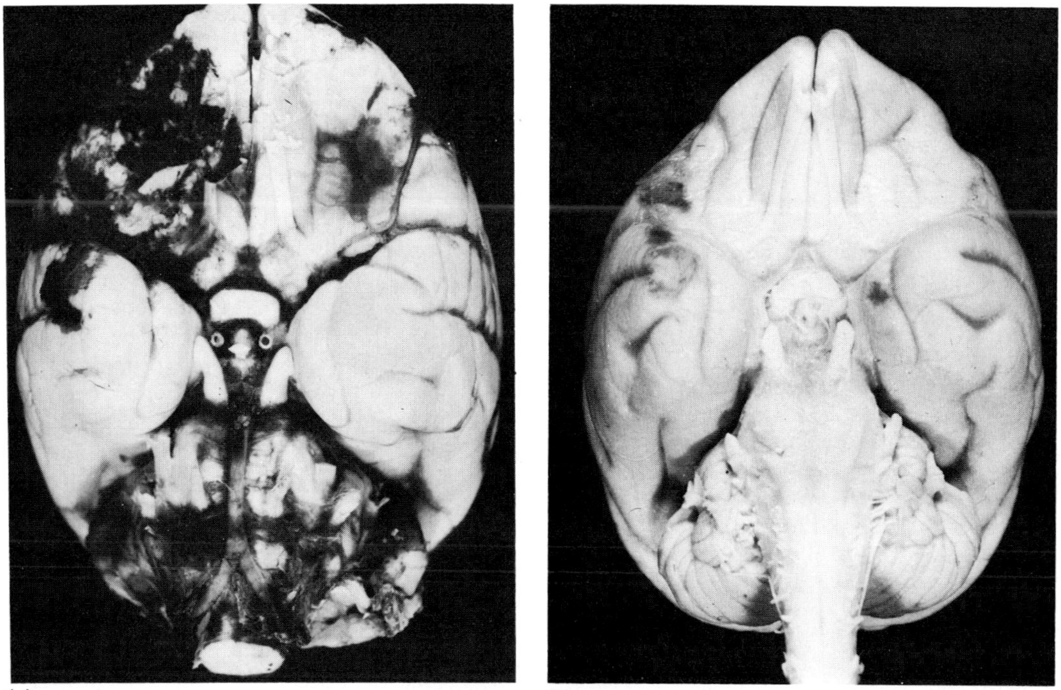

(a) **(b)**

Fig. 3.6 Contusions in the frontal and temporal lobes, caused by acceleration of the head in subhuman primates. (**a**) Recent. (**b**) Old. (Reproduced with permission, from Adams, Graham and Gennarelli, 1983).

regions relatively unimportant to immediate survival, patients and subhuman primates with quite severe contusions may make a smooth and uneventful recovery if there are no other types of brain damage, or complications in the form of intracranial haematoma. Healed contusions were reported as an incidental finding in 2.5 per cent of 2000 consecutive necropsies in a general hospital by Welte (1948).

Contusions have been the subject of detailed and comprehensive studies for many years (Krauland, 1950; Gurdjian, Webster and Lissner, 1955; Lindenberg and Freytag, 1957, 1960; Lindenberg, 1971; Adams et al., 1980b), and numerous subdivisions have been defined. *Fracture contusions* occur at the site of a fracture and tend to be particularly severe in the frontal lobes in association with fractures in the anterior fossa. *Coup contusions* occur at the site of impact in the absence of a fracture; they tend to be more severe in relation to a blow to the stationary head than when the moving head is suddenly decelerated (Lindenberg, 1971) and their size depends on the size of the area of the skull between the striking object and the skull. *Contrecoup contusions* occur in the brain diametrically opposite to the point of impact; they occur more in relation to sudden deceleration of the head than to a blow, and the classic example is a fall on the occiput resulting in severe contusions in and adjacent to the frontal and temporal poles. *Herniation contusions* occur where the parahippocampal gyri and the cerebellar tonsils are impacted against the edge of the tentorium and the foramen magnum respectively at the time of injury; they are more frequently observed in association with missile injuries (Freytag, 1963b) but they may also occur with non-missile injuries. Lindenberg and Freytag (1960) introduced the term *gliding contusions*—and this name has stood the test of time although *parasagittal contusions* might be a more appropriate term—to describe focal haemorrhage in the cortex and subjacent white matter at the superior margins of the cerebral hemispheres (Fig. 3.7); gliding contusions tend to be bilateral, are not infrequently symmetrical, and are sometimes restricted to the white matter macroscopically although histological examination will almost always show some involvement of the cortex. They may become quite large as haematomas develop in relation to them in the parasagittal white matter. The term *intermediary*

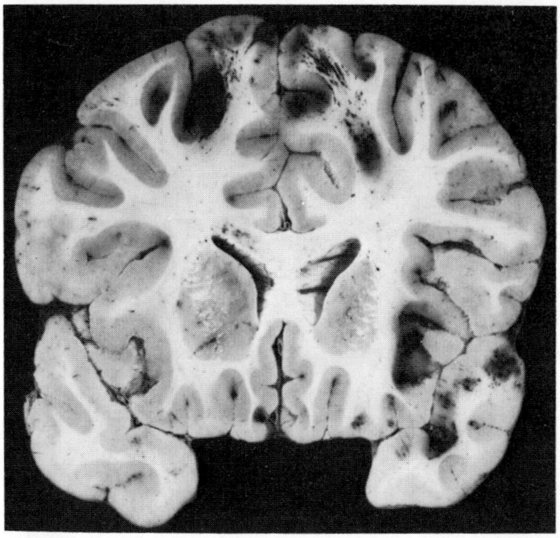

Fig. 3.7 Bilateral parasagittal 'gliding' contusions. Other contusions are seen adjacent to the right sylvian fissure.

coup contusions has been used by Lindenberg (1971) for single or multiple 'contusion haemorrhages' in the deeper structures of the brain, such as the white matter, the corpus callosum, the basal ganglia, the hypothalamus and the brain stem, on the basis that they are as much directly related to the injury as are contusions affecting the surface of the brain. The logic of this cannot be refuted but in the present account the term 'contusion' is restricted to a lesion that involves (or at least comes close to) the surface of the cerebral hemispheres or the cerebellum, whilst deeper lesions, also directly attributable to injury, are considered to be part of diffuse brain damage and hence of greater clinical significance.

Much of what has been written on cerebral contusions, albeit instructive and informative, has been based on subjective impressions. Adams et al. (1980b) have therefore attempted to develop a quantitative approach to cerebral contusions by introducing the concept of a *contusion index*. This index is based on the extent and depth of contusions in various regions of the brain, and for each region is derived from the product of the extent and depth of contusional damage. Because there is frequently a zone of pale rarefaction necrosis that cannot be identified macroscopically deep to the haemorrhagic part of a contusion, the regional indices had to be based on microscopical studies since this related zone of pallor was considered to be part of the contusion. Using this technique, individual contusion indices can be derived for the frontal, temporal, parietal and occipital lobes; the cortex above and below the sylvian fissures; and the cerebellum. It is then possible to derive a total contusion index for an individual brain, mean contusion indices for specific anatomical locators, and mean total contusion indices for a series of cases or for subsets. The results of this albeit preliminary study on a consecutive series of 151 brains showed clearly that contusions are most severe in the frontal and temporal lobes and that there is slightly more severe involvement of the frontal lobes. The next most severely affected region is the cortex above and below the sylvian fissures, whilst contusions tend to be minimal in the occipital and parietal lobes and in the cerebellum except in direct relationship to a fracture of the skull. A similar distribution of contusions has been observed in subhuman primates subjected to acceleration of the head (Adams, Graham and Gennarelli, 1982).

An analysis of cases with localizing fractures produced no evidence to suggest that contusions were more severe in the contralateral than in the ipsilateral hemisphere, whilst in patients with frontal or occipital fractures contusions were more severe in the frontal lobes. Thus whilst contusions can be most severe diametrically opposite the point of impact (i.e. contrecoup contusions), particularly in relation to falls on the occiput, it does not follow that because the most severe contusions are in a particular region of the brain, the impact occurred in the diametrically opposite part of the skull. One criticism of this conclusion is that Adams et al. (1980b) failed to exclude fracture contusions when comparing frontal and occipital impacts, since according to Dawson et al. (1980) fracture contusions are not relevant to the coup/contrecoup mechanism. This study, however, established that contusions are more severe in patients with a fracture of the skull than in those who do not have a fracture, and are less severe in patients with diffuse axonal injury (see p. 100) than in patients without this type of brain damage. There was no difference in the severity of contusions in patients who had or had not experienced a lucid interval.

Structural changes In patients who die almost immediately after a head injury a contusion is composed essentially of perivascular haemorrhage, hence the linear disposition of the haemorrhage that is often apparent macroscopically (see Fig. 3.1a). Blood then extends into the adjacent cortex where neurons in the affected region undergo necrosis as shown by the presence of ischaemic cell change. Haemorrhage may also extend into the white matter. There are then reactive changes in the form of proliferation of capillaries, astrocytes and microglia. The dead tissue is ultimately removed and the contusion comes to be represented by a shrunken and gliosed, rather fenestrated, scar often containing residual haemosiderin-filled macrophages (Fig. 3.8). An old contusion tends to be triangular in shape, its broad base being at the crest of a gyrus and its apex in the digitate white matter.

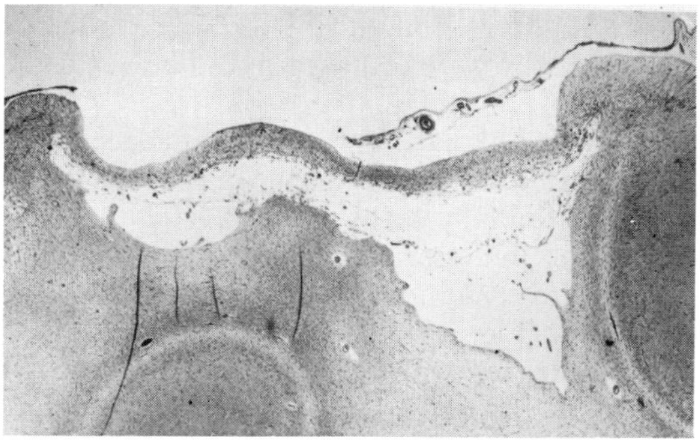

Fig. 3.8 Old contusion from a head injury sustained 5 years before death. There is a wedge-shaped defect in the cortex at the crest of a gyrus. Reticulin stain × 23 reduced to 90 per cent.

Pathogenesis This has always been a controversial issue but the subject has recently been reappraised and fully reviewed by Dawson et al. (1980). In the course of a fall the head rotates through approximately 90 degrees and gravitational torque acting on the body causes downward acceleration of the head in excess of that due to gravity. This leads to brain lag towards the trailing cranial surface, where the protective layer of cerebrospinal fluid is reduced. At impact the skull's acceleration and rotation are abruptly halted but the brain continues in motion because of its rotational inertia—the gliding motion of the brain in relation to the skull referred to by Holbourn (1943, 1945). Shearing stress develops where this rotational gliding is hindered—hence the frequency of contusions adjacent to the frontal and temporal poles where the brain comes in contact with a rough and irregular bony surface. At impact, contrecoup compressive stress may occur, this being contributed to by loss of cerebrospinal fluid consequent upon brain lag. The effect of this process is to thicken the protective layer of cerebrospinal fluid over the brain at the point of impact, a fact which helps to account for the absence of coup contusions in moving head impacts unless a fracture occurs at the site of impact. Attachments of the brain to the dura also interfere with the rotational gliding motion of the brain at impact and this explains the occurrence of gliding contusions in the parasagittal regions where the brain is relatively adherent to the dura. The importance of rotation in the production of gliding contusions has also been emphasized by Voigt, Lowenheilm and Ljung (1977). In resting head impacts there is neither brain lag nor an abnormal distribution of cerebrospinal fluid, this accounting for the usual absence of contrecoup contusions in these circumstances.

Gennarelli et al. (1982a) have stressed that contusions are mainly impact-related phenomena and it is therefore not surprising, as indicated above, that they are significantly more severe in patients with a fracture of the skull than in those who do not have a fracture. In their earlier experiments on acceleration injury in subhuman primates, impact phenomena occurred at short-duration high-acceleration levels with the Penn 1 device (see p. 87) that were sufficient to cause fracture of the skull and contusions of the brain (Adams, Graham and Gennarelli, 1982). As in man, the contusions occurred particularly at the frontal and temporal poles (Gennarelli et al., 1979). Their depth and surface extent increased as the mechanical input to the head increased. It appeared that the extent of contusions was primarily determined by the immediate traumatic event but that the depth of a contusion could increase with time. As the mechanical input increased, contusions at the frontal pole occurred before contusions at the temporal pole.

Intracranial haemorrhage

This is a common complication of a non-missile head injury and is the commonest cause of clinical deterioration and death in patients who have experienced a lucid interval after their injury (Reilly et al., 1975). It is the event as a result of which even an apparently trivial head injury can become a threat to life, and in a series of patients in whom it was judged that death might have been prevented by more effective management, almost two-thirds were found to have an intracranial haematoma (Jennett and Carlin, 1978). The majority of patients who develop intracranial haematoma have a fracture of the skull (Teasdale and Galbraith, 1981). It has in the past tended to be assumed that the main effects of an intracranial haematoma are delayed until it is large enough to cause distortion and herniation of the brain and raised intracranial pressure. Routine CT scanning of head-injured patients has, however, shown that intracranial haematomas are often present before they produce clinical deterioration and may even be present in a patient who would not previously have been suspected of having this complication (Teasdale and Galbraith, 1981). This raises the possibility that progressive swelling in the underlying hemisphere (see p. 112) may contribute materially to the failure of spatial compensation (see Chapter 2) to accommodate the expanding lesion. It would therefore appear that haemorrhage usually begins at the time of injury—i.e. it is a *primary* event—but the clinical presentation is usually that of a *complication* because of the interval between the onset of haemorrhage and the appearance of the clinical features of an intracranial expanding lesion. When this interval is more than 24 hours, the haematoma is said to be 'delayed' (Baratham and Dennyson, 1972). In most cases it seems likely that this is due to slow enlargement of the haematoma but, in a series of 50 patients in whom the initial CT scan did not show a haematoma, Snoek et al. (1979) found that a new haematoma had developed in 15 patients who were subjected to a second CT scan because of clinical deterioration. The pathogenesis of these delayed haematomas is not known.

In traumatic intracranial haemorrhage, there may be bleeding into the extradural, subdural or subarachnoid spaces, into the brain, or into the ventricles. Some degree of subarachnoid haemorrhage is common in association with contusions, and intraventricular haemorrhage is a frequent occurrence in patients with diffuse axonal injury (see p. 103) but extradural, subdural and intracerebral haematomas are the usual causes of expanding intracranial lesions. Because of the frequency with which intracerebral and subdural haematomas occur together (a 'burst' lobe), perhaps the most useful classification is to consider the haematomas as being **extradural** or **intradural.** Even this simple classification presents certain problems because in more than one-third of extradural haematomas there may also be an intradural haematoma (Jamieson and Yelland, 1968).

Extradural haematoma This occurs in approximately 2 per cent of all types of head injury (Lindenberg, 1971). In fatal head injuries extradural haematoma is found in between 5 per cent (Maloney and Whatmore, 1969) and 15 per cent (Freytag, 1963a) of cases. A fracture of the skull is present in the great majority of patients (Jamieson and Yelland, 1968) but it is well recognized that extradural haematoma can occur in children in the absence of a fracture. In the cases reported by Mazza et al. (1982), however, some of the children thought not to have a fracture radiologically were found to have one at operation.

This type of haemorrhage takes place from meningeal vessels, and as the haematoma enlarges it gradually strips the dura from the skull to form a circumscribed ovoid mass (Fig. 3.9a) that progressively indents and flattens the adjacent brain (Fig. 3.9b). Because the initial injury may be apparently trivial and the patient experiences a lucid interval, there is frequently little or only minimal evidence of other types of brain damage. On the other hand, extradural haematoma may occur also in patients with other types of brain damage and for this reason some patients may have been unconscious from the time of the original injury. Classically the haematoma occurs as a result of tearing of a middle meningeal artery in the region of the squamous part of the temporal bone where the bone is thin and easily fractured, but in some 20–30 per cent of cases the haematoma occurs elsewhere (Lewin, 1949; McKissock et al., 1960); for example, in the frontal and parietal regions or in the posterior fossa. Occasionally, extradural haematoma is bilateral (Maurer and Mayfield, 1965).

Intradural haematoma This takes three forms: 'pure' subdural haematoma brought about by rupture of the veins that bridge the subdural space where they connect the superior surface of the cerebral hemispheres to the sagittal sinus; 'pure' intracerebral haematoma that is presumably brought about by the rupture of intrinsic cerebral vessels at the time of head injury; and a combination of these—blood in the subdural

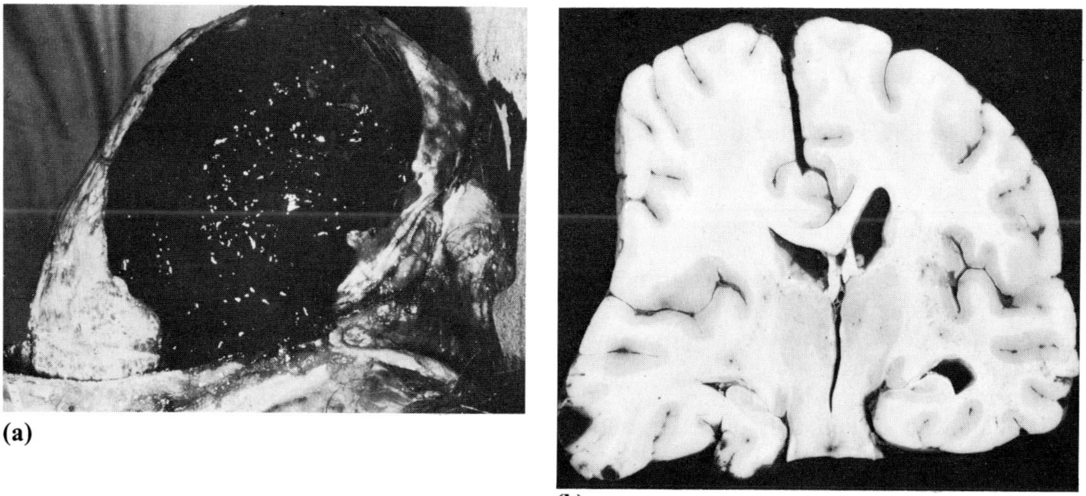

(a) (b)

Fig. 3.9 Extradural haematoma. (**a**) Ovoid circumscribed mass of blood on the outer surface of the dura. (**b**) Distortion and displacement of the brain produced by the haematoma.

space, contusions on the surface of the brain and an adjacent intracerebral haematoma, this frequently being referred to as a 'burst' lobe.

Subdural haematoma Because 'pure' subdural haematoma is brought about by rupture of the bridging veins, there may be very little evidence of other brain damage—indeed a subdural haematoma may be caused by a whiplash injury when there is no impact to the head (Ommaya and Yarnell, 1969). The haematoma may develop very rapidly or over a period of several hours. Because the blood can spread freely throughout the subdural space, it tends to cover the entire hemisphere, with the result that a subdural haematoma is more extensive than an extradural haematoma.

Subdural haematomas have in the past been defined as **acute, subacute** or **chronic** but there is no uniformity of nomenclature (Jennett and Teasdale, 1981) and attempts to age the haematoma on the basis of histological studies, although actively pursued by Lindenberg (1971), have in the author's experience not proved very satisfactory. There is also no experimental model whereby the process can be studied. Neurosurgical opinion is hardening towards classifying subdural haematomas as *acute* when the haematoma is composed of clotted blood, as *subacute* when there is a mixture of clotted and fluid blood, and as *chronic* when the haematoma is fluid (Cameron, 1978; Jennett and Teasdale, 1981). The blood is clotted for at least 48 hours and sometimes several days; thereafter there is a mixture of blood clot and fluid blood; and after about 3 weeks no clot remains. Despite the presence of an acute or subacute haematoma and distortion of the brain, the gyral and sulcal pattern on the side of the haematoma is well preserved whilst there is marked flattening of the convolutions in the contralateral hemisphere. This is because the subdural blood is in contact with both gyri and sulci, and therefore exerts uniform compression on the subjacent brain (Dawson et al., 1980). As will be shown below, there is a significant correlation between acute subdural haematoma and swelling of the ipsilateral cerebral hemisphere.

The biomechanics of 'pure' acute subdural haematoma have recently been reviewed by Gennarelli and Thibault (1982). In their clinical studies they were able to identify patients with acute subdural haematoma where rupture of the bridging veins was judged to be the primary pathological process; in 72 per cent of these cases the head injury had been produced by a fall or an assault, whereas in only 24 per cent the cause had been a road traffic accident. These figures are in marked contrast to patients without mass lesions who had been unconscious for more than 24 hours (i.e. patients with diffuse brain damage, see p. 100), when 89 per cent were road traffic accidents and only 10 per cent falls and assaults. Experimental studies on acceleration of the head in subhuman primates have helped to clarify the situation. In animals subjected to the Penn 1 device (see p. 87) there was an admixture of concussion and acute subdural haematoma. Increasing the acceleration and maintaining a constant duration led to increasingly severe injury up to acute and rapidly fatal subdural haematoma. On the other hand, acute subdural haematoma did not occur with the Penn 2 device (see p. 87) where the duration of acceleration was increased. This indicates that bridging veins are more liable to tear when the acceleration (or deceleration) is applied rapidly than when acceleration (or deceleration) occurs more slowly. This accords with the finding of a significantly high incidence of acute subdural haematoma in individuals who sustain falls or are assaulted, because these types of injury are associated with a very high rate of acceleration or deceleration. In contrast, in road traffic accidents the deceleration rate is much slower.

Chronic subdural haematoma may present weeks or months after a head injury that may have seemed at the time to have been trivial. The precise pathogenesis of chronic subdural haematoma is not clear, since it is now known from CT scanning that small acute subdural haematomas normally resolve spontaneously and do not progress to a chronic subdural haematoma (Dolinskas et al., 1979). The haematoma becomes encapsulated in a membrane (Fig. 3.10) and slowly increases in size, possibly as a result of repeated small haemorrhages into it, until it becomes large enough to produce symptoms attributable to distortion of the brain and raised intracranial pressure (Fig. 3.11). Because chronic subdural haematoma is particularly common in older age groups in whom there may already be some cerebral atrophy, and because the haematoma expands fairly slowly, the period of spatial compensation (see p. 53) may be so long that the cerebral hemispheres may be severely distorted (Fig. 3.11) before there is any significant increase in intracranial pressure. In untreated cases, however, death is often attributable to brain damage secondary to increased intracranial pressure and compression of the brain stem although apparently incidental chronic subdural haematomas may occasionally be encountered *post mortem* in elderly individuals. Chronic subdural haematoma is not infrequently bilateral.

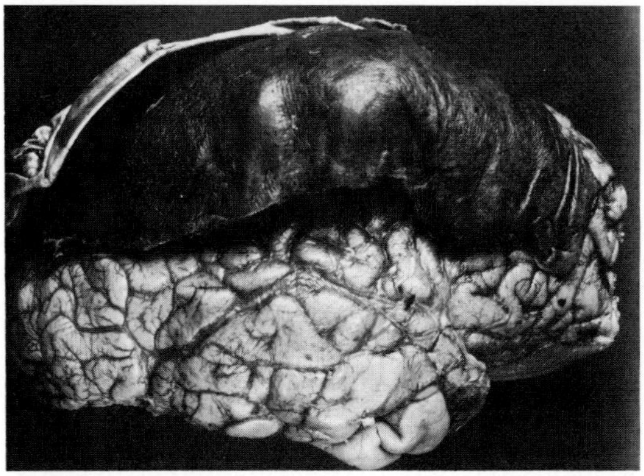

Fig. 3.10 Chronic subdural haematoma. The haematoma is encapsulated and not attached to the dura or the arachnoid.

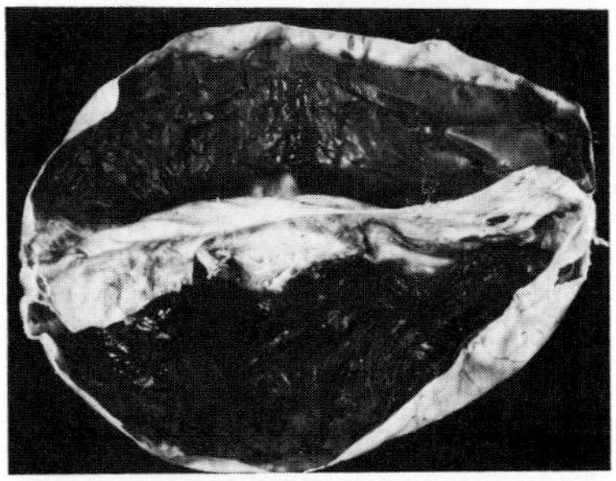

(a)

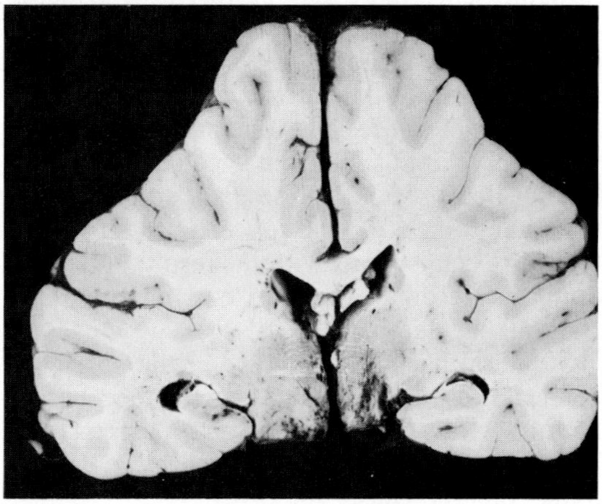

(b)

Fig. 3.11 Chronic subdural haematoma. (**a**) Bilateral encapsulated haematomas. (**b**) Distortion of the brain and secondary haemorrhagic infarction in the brain stem and thalamus produced by the haematomas.

Intracerebral haematoma 'Pure' intracerebral haematomas in head injury are haematomas not in contact with the surface of the brain. They are often multiple and, although they are said to be most common in the frontal and temporal regions (Jennett and Teasdale, 1981), they may occur deep within the hemispheres (Fig. 3.12). Their precise pathogenesis is not clear but it seems likely that they are caused by the direct rupture of intrinsic cerebral vessels at the time of injury and they may therefore be related to the multiple small haemorrhages that are seen in patients dying very rapidly after a head injury because of diffuse brain damage (see p. 113). Of the various types of traumatic intracranial haematoma, it is the intracerebral type that is most

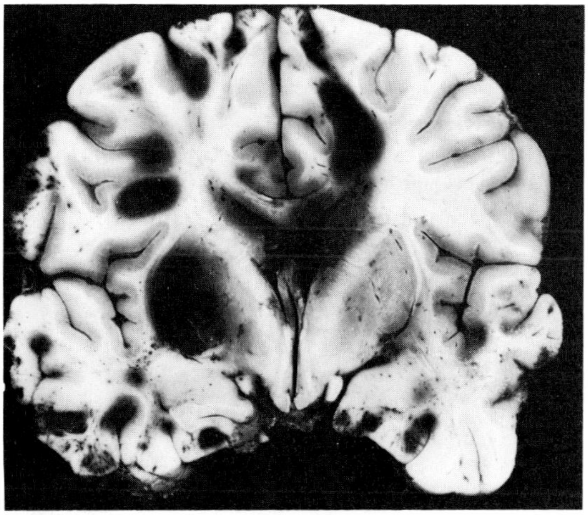

Fig. 3.12 Intracerebral haematoma. Numerous haematomas are present in both cerebral hemispheres.

likely to be 'delayed'—the so-called delayed traumatic apoplexy of Bollinger.

A fall may be precipitated by spontaneous intracranial haemorrhage, and may be severe enough to produce a fracture of the skull, cerebral contusions and intracranial haemorrhage. The interpretation of the findings *post mortem* can be difficult or even impossible and much depends on the site of the haematoma, particularly if it is solitary, when the possibility of a ruptured aneurysm or pre-existing hypertension has to be borne in mind. Even when all the possibilities have been taken into consideration, it may still be difficult to reach a final conclusion.

Burst lobe This is a convenient term to describe the coexistence of cerebral contusions, blood in the subdural space caused by haemorrhage from superficial cortical vessels, and a haematoma in the white matter deep to the contusions. Because contusions tend to be most severe in the frontal and temporal poles, these are also the usual sites for a burst lobe (Fig. 3.13).

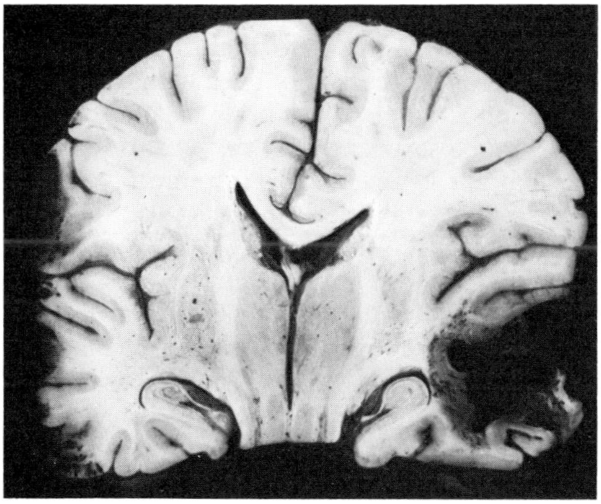

Fig. 3.13 Burst lobe. The haematoma in the right temporal lobe was in continuity with an acute subdural haematoma. Contusions in the left cerebral hemisphere are restricted to the crests of gyri.

Subdural haematoma in infancy There may be a history of a traumatic delivery or of a fall on the head. This is also the commonest type of intracranial injury found in infants subjected to non-accidental injury, and when such a haematoma is found it is advisable to look for other evidence of injury and undertake a skeletal survey. A frequent clinical sign is enlargement of the head. The haematoma may contain some blood clot but often it is chronic and consists of encapsulated xanthochromic fluid. This is sometimes referred to as a **subdural hygroma.** The latter term is, however, also used to denote a collection of clear cerebrospinal fluid in the subdural space that is thought to occur as a result of a defect in the arachnoid caused by some type of trauma. The fluid leaks into the subdural space from which it cannot be reabsorbed.

Brain damage secondary to raised intracranial pressure

This subject has been dealt with in Chapter 2 where various factors, including the importance of direct measurement of intracranial pressure, have been emphasized. A high intracranial pressure with associated distortion, shift and herniation of the brain is common in head injury, and in the series of 151 consecutive fatal head injuries reported by Adams et al. (1980a) there was evidence that the intracranial pressure had been high in 125 (83 per cent) of patients. The usual causes were intracranial haematoma or brain swelling, and in the great majority of the 125 cases there was secondary haemorrhage and/or infarction in the rostral brain stem. It might therefore be suspected that this type of damage to the brain stem would be a common cause of the vegetative state or severe disability after head injury but, in a series of 32 patients who died more than 1 month after a non-missile head injury and who had been classified clinically as being vegetative or severely disabled (Jennett and Bond, 1975), there was not one case where the clinical state could be attributed solely to secondary damage in the brain stem (Graham et al., 1983). The principal structural abnormalities identified were diffuse axonal injury (see p. 100) and hypoxic brain damage (see p. 109) or combinations of these with or without secondary damage in the brain stem.

Infection

Meningitis is a well recognized complication of a non-missile head injury and is usually due to the spread of micro-organisms through an open fracture of the calvaria or through a perhaps unrecognized fracture of the base of the skull bringing the subarachnoid space into continuity with major air sinuses. The latter is often associated with a cerebrospinal fluid rhinorrhoea or otorrhoea, or an aerocele. If there is a small defect in the dura at the base of the skull, meningitis may be delayed for many months or even years (Jennett and Teasdale, 1981); a small traumatic fistula may also be a cause of recurrent episodes of meningitis. Subdural or intracerebral abscess is a less common complication of non-missile head injury but in penetrating head injury (see p. 118) infective material may be carried directly into the cranial cavity.

Other types of focal brain damage

Pontomedullary rent This consists of a tear in the brain stem at the junction between the pons and medulla. In severe instances there may be complete avulsion of the medulla from the pons (Hardman, 1979). In less severe examples, haemorrhages extend rostrally from the pontomedullary junction into the tegmentum of the pons (Lindenberg and Freytag, 1970). There is often an associated ring fracture of the base of the skull or dislocation and/or fracture of the first or second cervical vertebra (Lindenberg and Freytag, 1970), and it has been suggested that severe hyperextension of the head is an important factor in the pathogenesis of these rents (Leestma, Kalelkar and Teas, 1983). Ring fractures and pontomedullary rents have also been produced at very high acceleration levels (Adams, Graham and Gennarelli, 1982) in subhuman primates by the Penn 1 device (see p. 87). Despite a wide experience, the present author has not seen one instance of pontomedullary rent in patients who have survived their injury long enough to be admitted to hospital. This accords with previous reports—indeed all 21 patients described by Lindenberg and Freytag (1970) were dead on arrival at hospital.

Recently, however, Pilz, Strohecker and Grobovschek (1982) have described two patients with subtotal pontomedullary rents (Fig. 3.14) who survived 8 days and 26 days respectively after being involved in road traffic accidents. Both had clinical features suggestive of primary damage in the brain stem, and in each patient there were clearly defined tears at the pontomedullary junction associated with which there were well-established reactive changes. There is

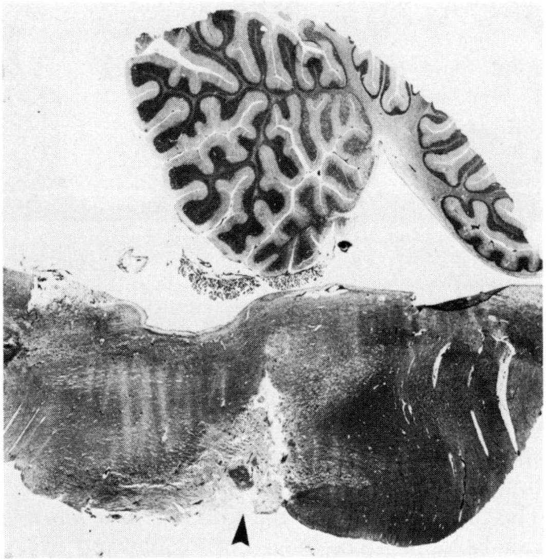

Fig. 3.14 Pontomedullary rent. There is a subtotal wedge-shaped rent (arrow) between the pons and the medulla. This patient survived for 26 days after a head injury, and there were established reactive changes in the walls of the rent. Luxol fast blue-cresyl violet ×2 reduced to 90 per cent.

therefore little doubt that these lesions occurred at the time of the injury and it would appear that this is one—and possibly the only—type of primary damage to the brain stem that may occur in isolation (see p. 114).

Cranial nerves Almost any of the cranial nerves may be damaged at the time of injury: the frequency of occurrence is difficult to define but the overall incidence is probably not of great significance. Loss of a sense of smell is not uncommon after head injury (Jennett and Teasdale, 1981), and this is not surprising in view of the relative severity of contusions affecting the undersurfaces of the frontal lobes and the frequency of fractures in the anterior cranial fossa. The optic nerve may also be damaged, usually in the canal where there may be an associated orbital or anterior fossa fracture (Jennett and Teasdale, 1981). Haemorrhagic, ischaemic and shearing lesions have been found *post mortem* (Crompton, 1970). In patients with a fracture of the petrous bone the seventh and eighth cranial nerves may be damaged.

Hypothalamus The types of damage that can occur in the hypothalamus and pituitary gland have been reviewed by Treip (1970) and there is no doubt that the pituitary stalk may occasionally be torn at the time of head injury, this leading to infarction in the anterior lobe of the pituitary gland (Adams, Daniel and Prichard, 1966). Most of the damage sustained by the hypothalamus and the pituitary stalk in patients with fatal non-missile head injury is, however, secondary to raised intracranial pressure leading to distortion and compression of these structures.

Corpus callosum Particular attention has been drawn to lesions in the corpus callosum by Lindenberg et al. (1955) and by Komatsu et al. (1979) but it is not clear from these publications how many of the patients with lesions in the corpus callosum also had diffuse axonal injury (see p. 100). Other causes for lesions in the corpus callosum include ischaemic damage in the territory supplied by the pericallosal arteries usually secondary to a supracallosal hernia (see p. 59), and fat embolism.

Vascular lesions Though uncommon, there are certain clearly defined vascular abnormalities which are of importance in any consideration of head injury. *Traumatic thrombosis of the internal carotid artery* is an occasional complication of an injury to the neck (Adams and Graham, 1967; Hardman, 1979; Adams, Gennarelli and Graham, 1982). The pathogenesis of the thrombosis is not always clear but one precipitating mechanism is dissection in the wall of the internal carotid artery in the neck (Fig. 3.15), and it has been suggested that the dissection may be caused by stretching of the artery when the neck is hyperextended at the time of injury. Subsequent thrombosis, with or without propagation of thrombus into the major intracranial arteries, may lead to a massive cerebral infarct. The clinical picture is usually that of the appearance of hemiplegia some hours after the injury.

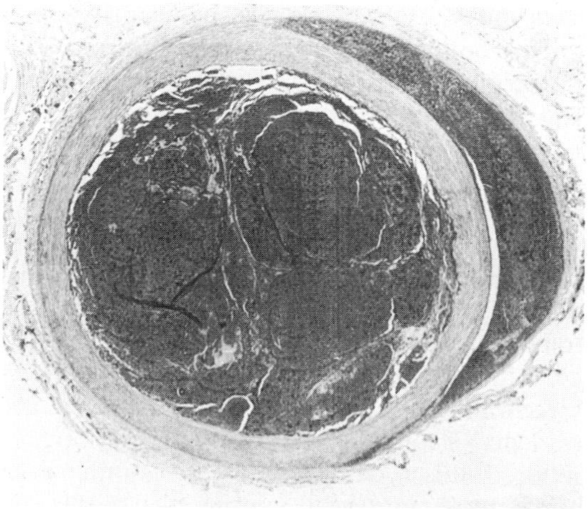

Fig. 3.15 Traumatic thrombosis of an internal carotid artery. Note the dissection in the wall of the artery. (Reproduced, with permission, from Adams and Graham, 1967)

Traumatic rupture of the vertebral artery (Cameron and Mant, 1972; Adams, Gennarelli and Graham, 1982; Harland, Pitts and Watson, 1983) is being increasingly recognized. A bruise or laceration below and behind one ear is almost invariably present and in some cases there is a fracture of the transverse process of the first cervical vertebra. The precise mechanism of the haemorrhage is not clearly understood but it would appear that the vertebral artery in relation to the transverse process of the first cervical vertebra ruptures and this is followed by massive subarachnoid haemorrhage. Most cases die very soon after injury and the striking feature *post mortem* is severe and extensive subarachnoid haemorrhage, particularly in the posterior fossa. Death may be attributed to rapid tonsillar herniation leading to respiratory arrest (see p. 65).

Caroticocavernous fistula is another rare sequel of head injury (see p. 227).

Diffuse brain damage in head injury

The concept of diffuse brain damage in patients who have sustained a non-missile head injury is not new. Thus, Symonds (1940, 1962) has long emphasized its importance as being the cause not only of 'instantaneous loss of cerebral function so frequently observed after head injury' but also of many of the long-continued disturbances of consciousness often followed by residual symptoms in patients who were rendered unconscious at the moment of injury. Diffuse brain damage was also the dominant theme in the early experimental work of Denny-Brown and Russell (1941) and, more recently, in a comprehensive clinical study Gennarelli et al. (1982b) have emphasized that immediate prolonged unconsciousness unaccompanied by an intracranial mass lesion occurs in almost half of severely head injured patients and is associated with 35 per cent of all head injury deaths. Furthermore, Gronwall and Wrightson (1974) have produced evidence strongly suggestive of persisting, if mild, diffuse damage in the brain after apparently minor head injuries even if this evidence can be obtained only by inducing a mild degree of cerebral hypoxia (Ewing et al., 1980).

Diffuse brain damage is more difficult to define and delineate than the more obvious focal types of damage because macroscopic abnormalities may appear minimal or even trivial, whilst much of it can only be recognized microscopically even when the brain has been properly fixed prior to dissection. There are four principal types of diffuse brain damage: of these, three are seen frequently in patients who survive their injury long enough to be admitted to hospital—diffuse axonal injury, hypoxic brain damage and brain swelling; the fourth—multiple petechial haemorrhages in various parts of the brain—seems to be restricted to patients who die very soon after their head injury (Tomlinson, 1970), but multiple intracerebral haematomas (see p. 97) presumably have a similar pathogenesis.

Diffuse axonal injury

Patients who sustain severe diffuse axonal injury are unconscious from the moment of impact, do not experience a lucid interval, and remain unconscious, vegetative or at least severely disabled until death (Adams et al., 1982). Their clinical state has been referred to in the past as primary brain stem injury, but although there is damage to the brain stem in diffuse axonal injury, it is always accompanied by evidence of diffuse brain damage.

Strich (1956) was the first to define clearly the occurrence of 'diffuse degeneration of the cerebral white matter' in a series of patients with severe post-traumatic dementia. This type of brain damage resulting from head injury is now widely recognized, although it has been referred to by other authors under different names—shearing injury (Strich, 1961, 1969, 1970; Peerless and Rewcastle, 1967), diffuse damage to white matter of immediate impact type (Adams et al., 1977) and diffuse white matter shearing injury (Zimmerman et al., 1978). The structural basis of 'inner cerebral trauma' described by Grcevic (1982) is probably the same. Jennett and Plum (1972) believe that diffuse damage to white matter is the commonest cause of the vegetative state after head injury. Strich has always taken the view that diffuse damage to white matter is brought about by the shearing of nerve fibres at the moment of injury but others have contended that it is secondary to hypoxic or ischaemic brain damage, cerebral oedema or secondary damage to the brain stem resulting from an intracranial expanding lesion (Jellinger and Seitelberger, 1970; Jellinger, 1977; Peters and Rothemund, 1977).

Clinicopathological studies undertaken by Adams et al. (1977, 1982) have endorsed Strich's views and have defined the time-course of the structural abnormalities in white matter. Similar structural abnormalities have now been produced in subhuman primates using the Penn 2 device (see p. 87) without there being any increase in intracranial pressure or episode of hypoxia (Adams, Gennarelli and Graham, 1982; Gennarelli et al., 1982c); as a result of these experiments the pathogenesis of this type of brain damage now seems clear, and the most appropriate term by which to refer to it is *diffuse axonal injury*.

Fig. 3.16 Diffuse axonal injury—lesions in the corpus callosum. (**a**) There is an acute haemorrhagic lesion to the right of the midline; there is also a small haematoma in the right hippocampus (6 days' survival). (**b**) Multiple small haemorrhagic foci in and adjacent to the midline (5 days' survival). (**c**) Similar lesion in a subhuman primate after acceleration of the head (24 hours' survival). (**d**) In addition to a haemorrhagic lesion

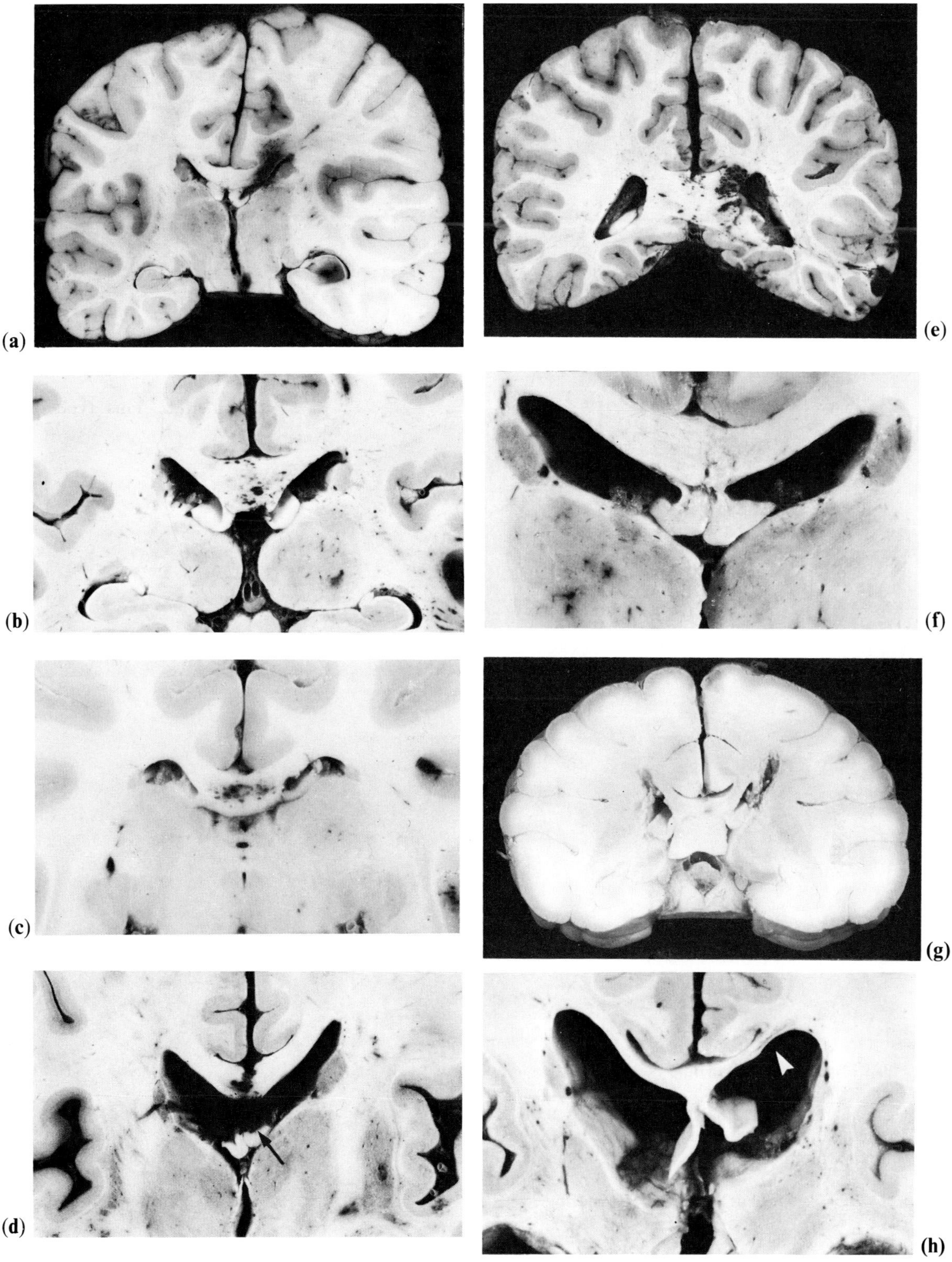
(a) (b) (c) (d) (e) (f) (g) (h)

Fig. 3.16 (continued) in the corpus callosum, the interventricular septum is ruptured and there are small foci of haemorrhage in the fornix (arrow) (10 days' survival). (**e**) Haemorrhagic lesion accentuated in the lateral part of the splenium (5 days' survival). (**f**) Disintegrating non-haemorrhagic lesion (12 weeks' survival). (**g**) Small discoloured focus in a subhuman primate after acceleration of the head (7 weeks' survival). (**h**) Shrunken cystic lesion (arrow)—cf. (**a**) (21 months' survival. (**a** and **h** reproduced, with permission, from: **a,** Adams, 1975; **h**, Adams et al., 1977.)

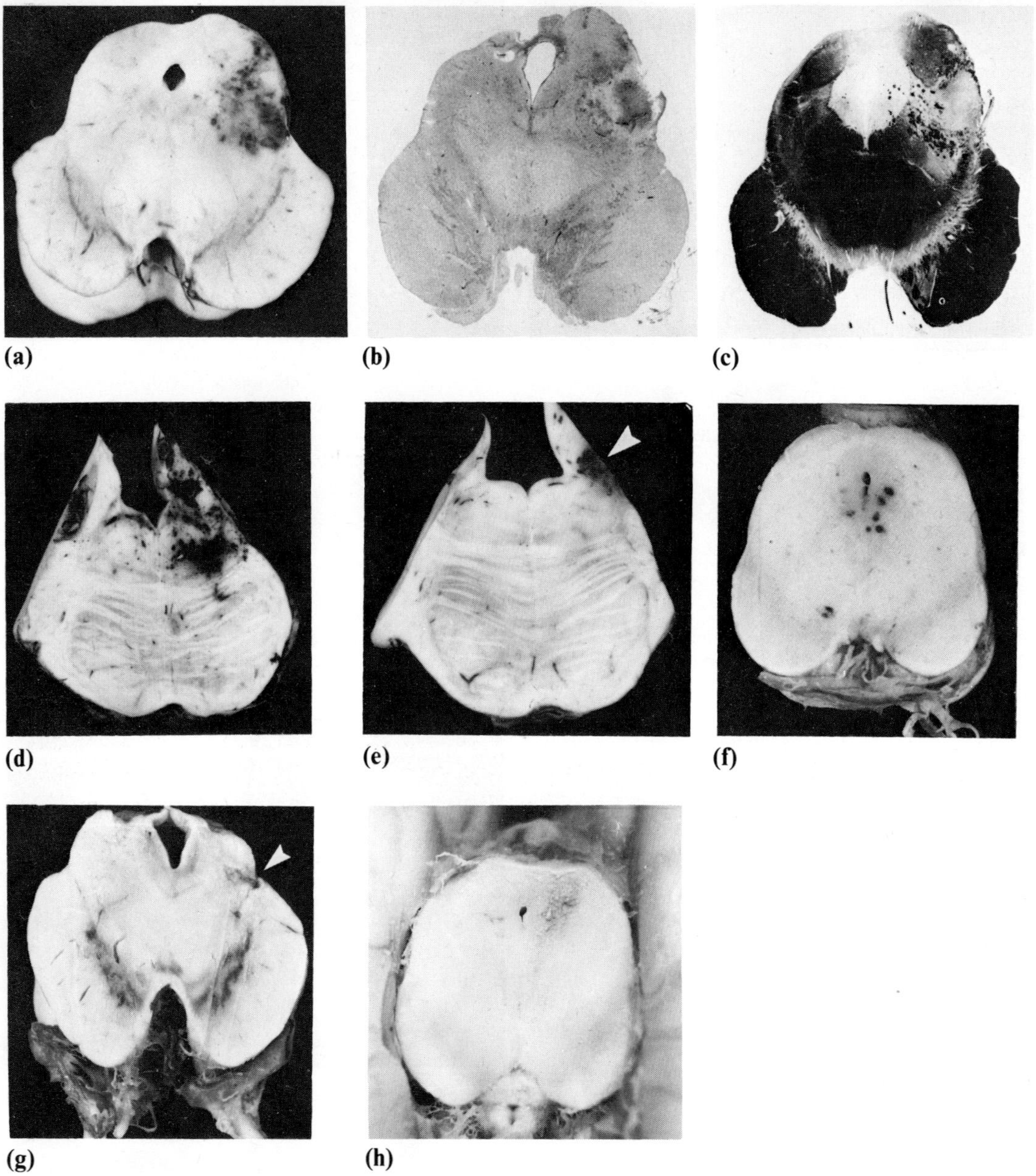

Fig. 3.17 Diffuse axonal injury—lesions in the dorsolateral quadrant of the rostral brain stem. (**a**) Well-defined haemorrhagic lesion in the midbrain (12 days' survival). (**b**) Same lesion. Cresyl violet. (**c**) Same lesion. Heidenhain. (**d**) Large haemorrhagic lesion in the rostral pons (5 days' survival). (**e**) Small haemorrhagic lesion (arrow) centred on the superior cerebellar peduncle (2 days' survival). (**f**) Small haemorrhages in midbrain of subhuman primate after acceleration of the head (24 hours' survival). (**g**) Old shrunken lesion (arrow) in midbrain (9 months' survival). (**h**) Granular lesion in midbrain of subhuman primate after acceleration of the head (7 weeks' survival). (**a, d, f, g** reproduced, with permission, from: **a** and **g**, Adams, 1975; **d**, Adams et al., 1977; **f**, Gennarelli et al., 1982c.)

Structural abnormalities There are three distinctive features in the pathology of diffuse axonal injury in its most severe form: (1) a focal lesion in the corpus callosum, (2) focal lesions in the dorsolateral quadrant or quadrants of the rostral brain stem adjacent to the superior cerebellar peduncles, and (3) diffuse damage to axons. Because the first two of these can usually be identified macroscopically, it is generally easy to make the diagnosis of diffuse axonal injury *post mortem* provided the brain has been properly fixed prior to dissection, but the diffuse damage to axons can only be seen microscopically. It is, however, becoming increasingly apparent that not all of these abnormalities occur in patients who sustain less severe diffuse axonal injury.

The appearances of the individual lesions depend on the length of survival after injury.

Corpus callosum In the early stages after injury (hours to days) the focal lesion in the corpus callosum is typically haemorrhagic. Although often measuring not more than 2–3 mm across, the lesions usually extend over an anteroposterior distance of several centimetres. They generally occur in the inferior part of the corpus callosum and on one or other side of the midline (Fig. 3.16a); they may, however, extend to the midline (Figs 3.16b and c) to involve the interventricular septum (which is often ruptured and may therefore be the cause of the not infrequently associated intraventricular haemorrhage) and the fornix (Fig. 3.16d). Haemorrhagic lesions are sometimes restricted to the splenium where they are frequently bilateral, particularly affecting its lateral margins (Fig. 3.16e). After some days the lesion becomes rather granular and less easy to identify macroscopically (Figs 3.16f and g), and with the passage of time comes ultimately to be represented by a shrunken, and sometimes cystic, focus (Fig. 3.16h).

Histological studies have established that the haemorrhage is first perivascular and then extends into the adjacent tissue. Numerous axonal retraction balls are soon seen adjacent to the focal lesions. There are then the usual reactive changes of microglial, astrocytic and capillary endothelial proliferation, the appearance of lipid phagocytes, and the progressive removal of the damaged tissue. The end-stage is a rarified lesion traversed by astrocytic fibres among which there are haemosiderin-containing macrophages.

Brain stem The lesions in the dorsolateral quadrant of the rostral brain stem follow an essentially similar course. In patients of short survival they are usually haemorrhagic, when they can be readily identified macroscopically in the dorsolateral part of the midbrain and the rostral pons, almost always involving the superior cerebellar peduncle (Figs 3.17a–f). When bilateral, one lesion is usually larger than the other.

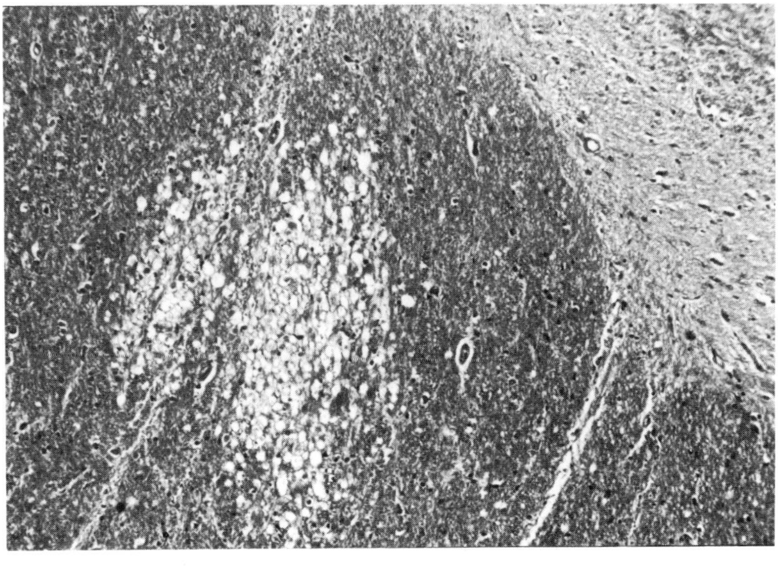

Fig. 3.18 Diffuse axonal injury. Rarefied lesion in superior cerebellar peduncle (3 days' survival). Haematoxylin and eosin × 100. (Reproduced, with permission, from Adams, 1975.)

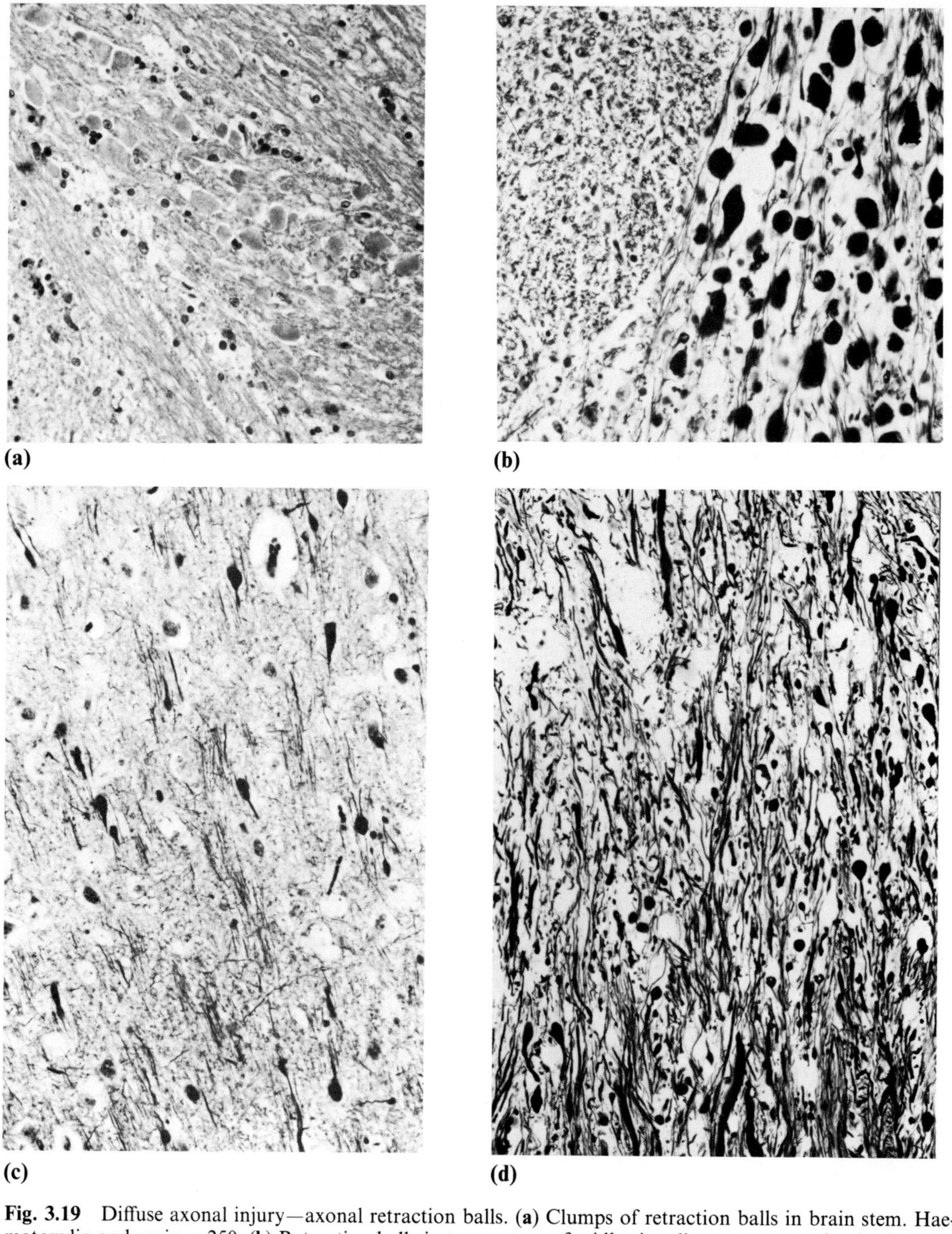

(a) **(b)** **(c)** **(d)**

Fig. 3.19 Diffuse axonal injury—axonal retraction balls. (**a**) Clumps of retraction balls in brain stem. Haematoxylin and eosin ×250. (**b**) Retraction balls in tegmentum of midbrain, all on axons running in the same direction. Palmgren ×400. (**c**) Retraction balls in the parasagittal white matter. Palmgren ×250. (**d**) Retraction balls in the parasagittal white matter in a subhuman primate after acceleration of the head. Palmgren ×100 (**e**) Axonal retraction balls in the corpus callosum. Palmgren ×400. (**f**) Axonal retraction balls in the thalamus. Palmgren ×250. (**g**) Axonal retraction balls in the central tegmental tract. Palmgren × 250. (**h**) Irregularly beaded axon in the corpus callosum. Palmgren ×400. (**a–h** reduced to 90%.)

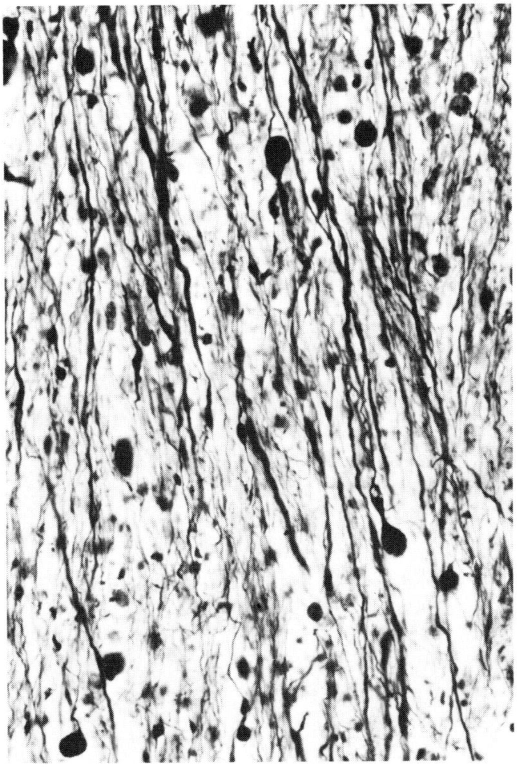

(e)

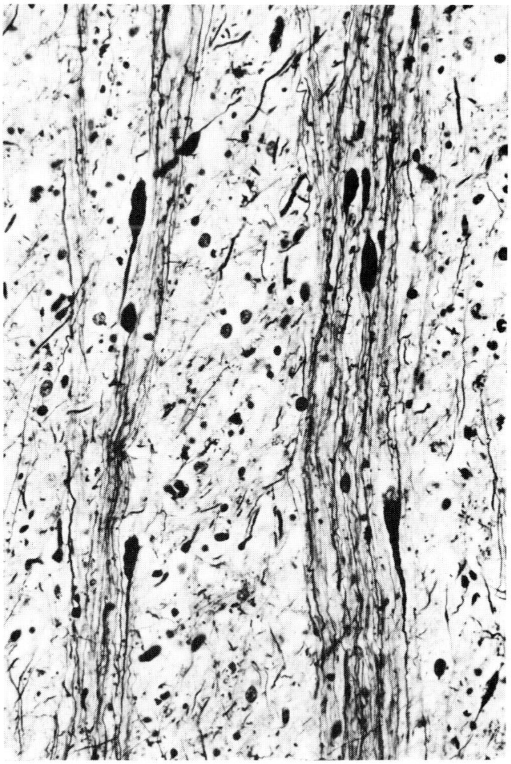

(f)

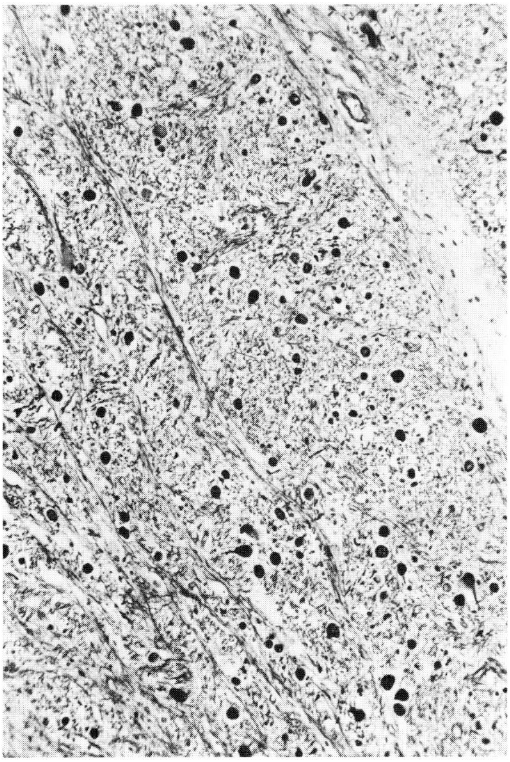

(g)

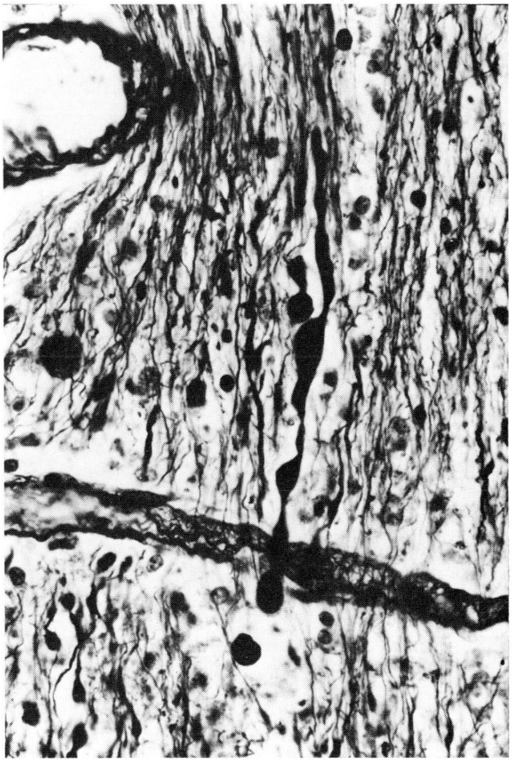

(h)

With the passage of time these focal lesions become brown and often rather granular, and are ultimately represented by shrunken, sometimes cystic, scars (Figs 3.17g and h). The sequence of histological changes is similar to that described above for the corpus callosum but on occasion, particularly if the lesion is small, it is represented in the early stages by a rarefied and coarsely vacuolated focus in which haemorrhage is absent or minimal (Fig. 3.18) that can only be identified microscopically.

Because the lesions in the corpus callosum and in the dorsolateral quadrant(s) of the rostral brain stem are often small, it is not surprising that pathologists may think that they are of no great significance. When both are present, however, the patient has almost certainly sustained diffuse axonal injury.

Diffuse damage to axons In patients of short (days) survival this is shown by the presence of large numbers of eosinophilic (Fig. 3.19a) and argyrophilic swellings on nerve fibres (Fig. 3.19b)—the retraction balls of Cajal (1959)—in the white matter of the cerebral hemispheres, the cerebellum and the brain stem. Their distribution is not uniform or symmetrical but they occur particularly in the subcortical parasagittal white matter (Figs 3.19c and d), in the corpus callosum remote from the focal lesions referred to above (Fig. 3.19e), in the fornix, in the internal capsule and deep grey matter (Fig. 3.19f), in the external capsule adjacent to the outer limits of the caudate nucleus and in cerebellar folia dorsal to the dentate nuclei. Various tracts in the brain stem are involved but, as has been emphasized by Strich (1976), there is often particularly severe but asymmetrical involvement of the corticospinal tracts, the medial lemnisci, the medial longitudinal bundles and the central tegmental tracts (Fig. 3.19g). It is quite common to find large numbers of retraction balls in nerve fibres running in one direction, and none in an immediately adjacent tract running in a different direction (Fig. 3.19b). In addition to typical retraction balls, there may be coarse varicosities on axons (Fig. 3.19h).

After a few weeks the most striking abnormality is the presence of vast numbers of small clusters of microglia throughout the white matter of the cerebral hemispheres, the cerebellum and the brain stem (Fig. 3.20). By this stage the damaged axons have become fragmented and the myelin sheaths broken up, with the result that axonal retraction balls are rarely identifiable. After 2–3 months wallerian-type degeneration (Fig. 3.21) becomes easy to detect, particularly with the Marchi method (Strich, 1968). This is often particularly conspicuous in the medial lemnisci and in the pyramidal tracts throughout the brain stem and the spinal cord, but it can also be identified in the white matter of the cerebral hemispheres including subcortical white matter and the internal capsules (Adams, 1975). By this time there is usually some reduced bulk and increased consistency of the white matter of the cerebral hemispheres, thinning of the corpus callosum, and compensatory enlargement of the ventricular system (Fig. 3.22).

Any other type of brain damage due to non-missile head injury may occur in association with

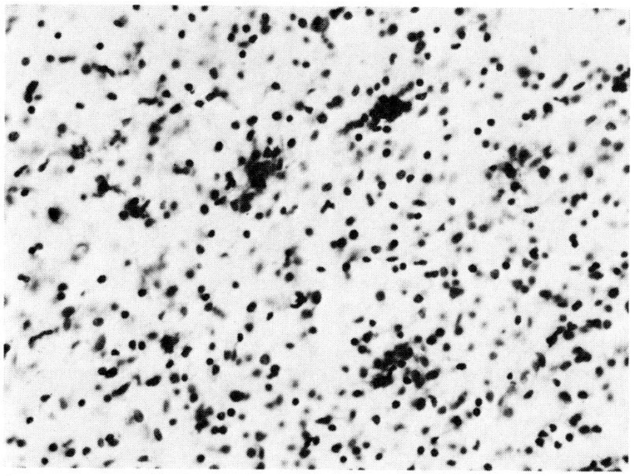

(a)

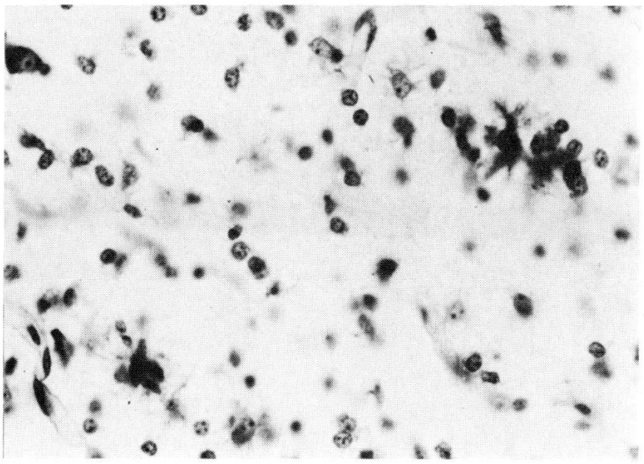

(b)

Fig. 3.20 Diffuse axonal injury—clusters of microglia in the white matter. (**a**) In man. Cresyl violet ×100 reduced to 80%. (**b**) In a subhuman primate after acceleration of the head. Cresyl violet ×200 reduced to 80%. (Both reproduced, with permission, from Adams, Graham and Gennarelli, 1983.)

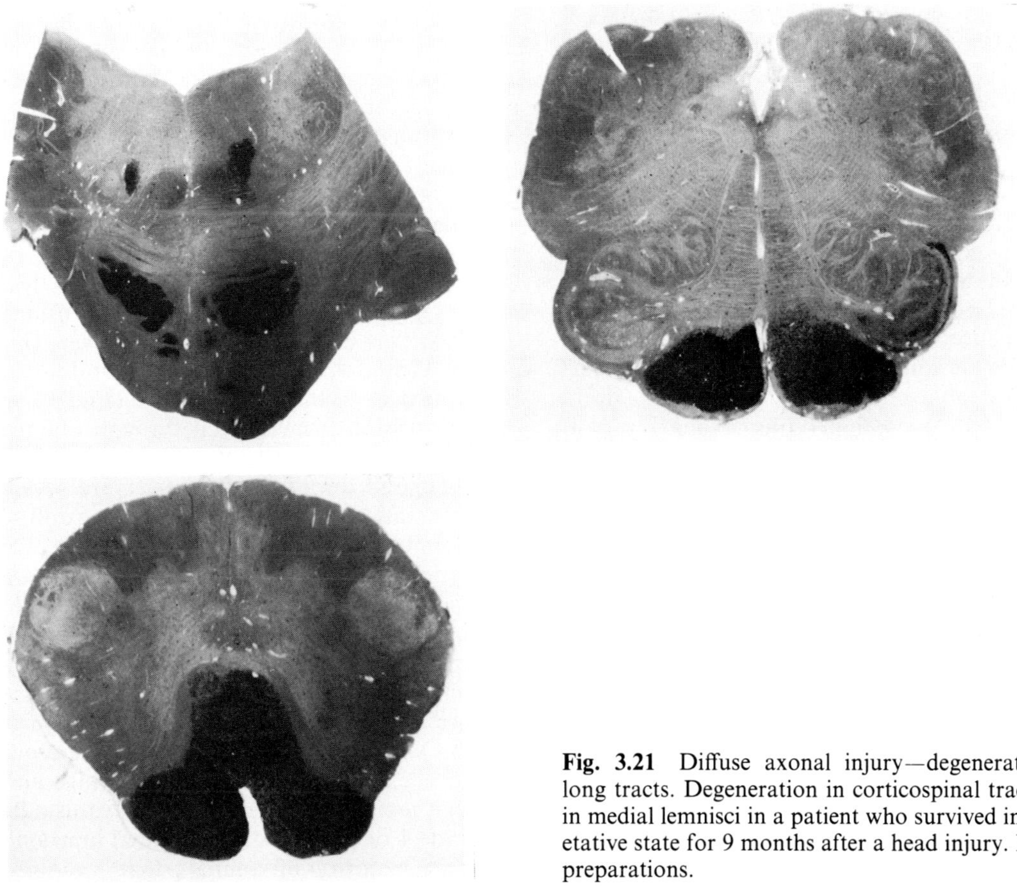

Fig. 3.21 Diffuse axonal injury—degeneration of long tracts. Degeneration in corticospinal tracts and in medial lemnisci in a patient who survived in a vegetative state for 9 months after a head injury. Marchi preparations.

diffuse axonal injury, but in a recent analysis of 177 fatal head injuries including 45 cases of diffuse axonal injury (Adams et al., 1982) there was in the latter a statistically significant lower incidence of cerebral contusions, intracranial haematoma and evidence of a high intracranial pressure. Brain swelling and hypoxic brain damage were not statistically different in the two groups. In the patients with diffuse axonal injury there was also a statistically significant lower incidence of lucid interval, fracture of the skull and falls, and a higher incidence of head injury due to road traffic accidents. Although contusions tend to be minor in patients and subhuman primates with diffuse axonal injury, gliding contusions are often prominent as are small haematomas deep in the cerebral hemispheres and in the Ammon's horns (see Figs 3.16a and 3.23).

Diffuse axonal injury in subhuman primates In the earlier series of experiments undertaken by Gennarelli and his group in Philadelphia using

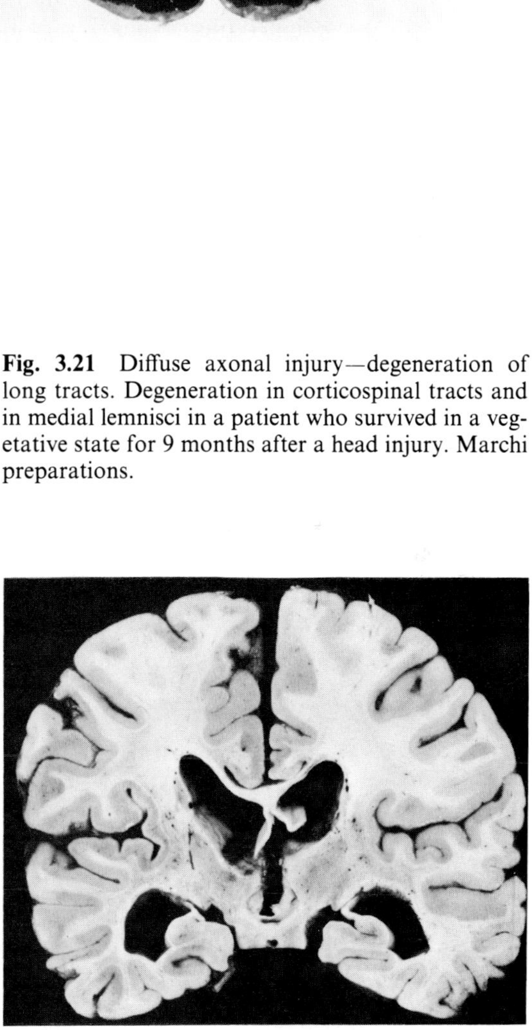

Fig. 3.22 Diffuse axonal injury. Enlargement of the ventricular system in a patient who survived in a vegetative state for 21 months after a head injury. The corpus callosum is narrowed.

the Penn 1 device (see p. 87), all of the focal types of brain damage encountered in non-missile head injury in man were produced (Adams, Graham and Gennarelli, 1982). Prolonged traumatic unconsciousness in the absence of an intracranial expanding lesion was, however, not produced. When the model was modified to allow of acceleration of the head in the oblique and lateral planes as well as sagittal, and when the duration of the acceleration was increased—the Penn 2 device (see p. 87)—prolonged traumatic coma was produced in the absence of an intracranial expanding lesion (Gennarelli et al., 1982c). The structural abnormalities in these brains were identical to those seen in diffuse axonal injury in man: these consisted of focal lesions in the corpus callosum (see Figs 3.16c and g) and in the dorsolateral quadrant of the rostral brain stem (see Figs 3.17f and h), and microscopical evidence of diffuse damage to axons (see Figs 3.19d and 3.20b).

In this experimental situation it was possible to define three grades of diffuse axonal injury (Gennarelli et al., 1982c). In grade 1 structural abnormalities were restricted to axonal retraction balls or small clusters of microglia in the white matter, in grade 2 there was also a focal lesion in the corpus callosum, whilst in grade 3 there was in addition a focal lesion in the dorsolateral quadrant of the rostral brain stem. As in man, axonal damage was particularly conspicuous in the parasagittal white matter of the cerebral hemispheres, in the corpus callosum, in the superior cerebellar peduncles, in the medial lemnisci, in the medial longitudinal bundles, in the central tegmental tracts and in the corticospinal tracts in the brain stem. So far no subhuman primate has been kept alive long enough to allow of the demonstration of wallerian degeneration.

In these experiments there were occasional mild conventional contusions and small amounts of blood in the subarachnoid and subdural spaces. On the other hand, gliding contusions (see p. 91) were conspicuous and there were frequently haematomas deep in the cerebral hemispheres similar to those seen in man (Fig. 3.23). The progression from sagittal through oblique to lateral angular acceleration was associated with increased duration of coma, more severe post-traumatic disability and more severe diffuse axonal injury. Furthermore, as the degree of traumatic coma increased from transient to severe, both the incidence and the severity of diffuse axonal injury increased, the latter in proportion to the duration of the coma. There was also a close correlation between outcome and the presence and severity of diffuse axonal injury: when the animal made a good recovery there was no evidence of diffuse axonal injury, whilst animals that remained moderately disabled usually had grade 1 or grade 2 diffuse axonal injury; in the great majority of animals that remained severely disabled or in persistent coma until death, the structural abnormalities were those of grade 3. Diffuse axonal injury was most readily

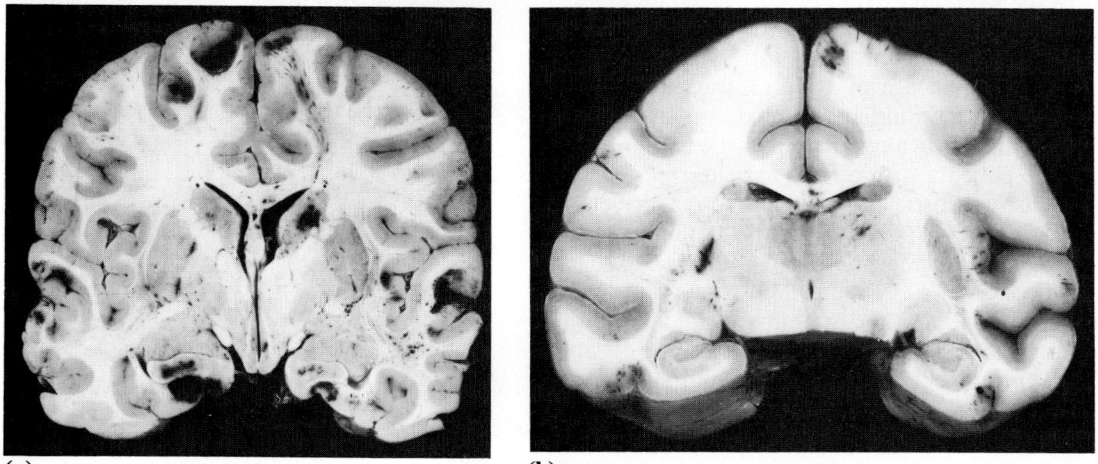

(a) **(b)**

Fig. 3.23 Diffuse axonal injury. (**a**) Gliding contusions, haemorrhagic focus in basal ganglia and a lesion in the corpus callosum (5 days' survival). (**b**) Similar abnormalities in a subhuman primate after acceleration of the head (48 hours' survival).

produced by lateral acceleration of the head and this correlated highly with the production of severe traumatic coma, poor neurological recovery and the occurrence and severity of diffuse axonal injury. This is the first experimental model of head injury that has produced prolonged traumatic coma in the absence of an intracranial expanding lesion, a situation frequently encountered in man, and it has established that this type of brain damage can occur without anything striking the head.

This accords well with the clinicopathological findings in man (Adams et al., 1982): if the acceleration/deceleration is short, as occurs in falls, the principal findings are subdural haematoma and contusions; if it is of longer duration, as occurs in road traffic accidents, diffuse axonal injury is more likely to be produced. Because traumatic coma occurred instantaneously in the subhuman primates described by Gennarelli et al. (1982c), and because none of the 45 human cases of diffuse axonal injury described by Adams et al. (1982) experienced a lucid interval in contrast to the 42 per cent of patients found not to have diffuse axonal injury who did experience a lucid interval, there now seems no reasonable doubt that diffuse axonal injury occurs at the moment of injury and that it is related to shear and tensile strains in axons. The fact that the lesions in the corpus callosum and in the dorsolateral quadrant in the rostral brain stem are often haemorrhagic suggests that these strains can also produce rupture of small vessels. It further seems likely that diffuse axonal injury is the most important single factor contributing to the severity of brain damage and to the outcome in any patient who sustains a non-missile head injury because it occurs at the moment of injury, and that it is the pathological substrate of many of the neurological sequelae—even mild (Gronwall and Wrightson, 1974)—that may occur after head injury.

Relatively little attention appears to have been paid to the identification of less severe degrees of diffuse axonal injury in man. Certainly on the basis of the experiments referred to above it would seem inevitable that grade 1 and grade 2 diffuse axonal injury should occur. Oppenheimer (1968), however, has shown that occasional clusters of microglia can be found in patients dying from some unrelated cause soon after a minor head injury; Clark (1974) also has drawn attention to the frequent occurrence of such clusters in the white matter in patients dying as a result of a head injury; and Povlishock et al. (1983) have identified occasional axonal retraction balls in cats subjected to minor head injury. In this connection it should be noted that the author has recently encountered several head injuries where death was attributable principally to an acute intracranial haematoma but in which there were scattered axonal retraction balls in the parasagittal white matter, and one patient who survived for 3 weeks with a fracture-dislocation in the cervical region in whom there had also been clinical evidence of a mild head injury where scattered microglial clusters were observed in the cerebral white matter. It may therefore be that less severe grades of diffuse axonal injury have in general failed to be recognized in the past. This is a field that requires further study.

Hypoxic brain damage

It has long been recognized that hypoxic-ischaemic brain damage up to and including frank infarction is common in patients dying as a result of a non-missile head injury (Helfand, 1939; Evans and Scheinker, 1943, 1945; Maloney and Whatmore, 1969; Graham and Adams, 1971; Jennett et al., 1973). In a consecutive series of 151 fatal head injuries subjected to a detailed neuropathological analysis reported by Graham, Adams and Doyle (1978), however, there was an unexpectedly high incidence of hypoxic brain damage. This is probably not as surprising as at first thought since even quite severe hypoxic damage of short duration cannot be recognized macroscopically even after the brain has been properly fixed and dissected. This underlines Strich's observation (1976) that statements about brain damage due to head injury based on naked eye appearances alone are very misleading. The highest incidence of hypoxic damage was observed in the Ammon's horns (80 per cent) and in the basal ganglia (79 per cent) but much of this could be at least partly attributed to raised intracranial pressure and a compromised circulation through one or both posterior cerebral arteries (see Chapter 2). The cerebellum was also involved (44 per cent) but, even after infarction of the medial occipital cortex of the type attributed to an impaired circulation through the posterior cerebral artery in association with a tentorial hernia (see Chapter 2) had been excluded, hypoxic damage was observed in the cerebral cortex in 46 per cent of cases: this was assessed as being severe in 41 per cent, moderately severe in 50 per cent and mild in 9 per cent of the affected cases.

The hypoxic damage in the cerebral cortex took several forms. In the commonest type it was centred on the *boundary zones* between the major cerebral arterial territories (Fig. 3.24), particularly between the anterior and middle cerebral arterial territories, and in the majority of the cases it was bilateral. The next most common pattern was *diffuse damage* in the cortex of both cerebral hemispheres (Fig. 3.25) whilst in the third and smallest group it was centred on the territories supplied by the anterior and/or middle cerebral arteries. The pathogenesis of this type

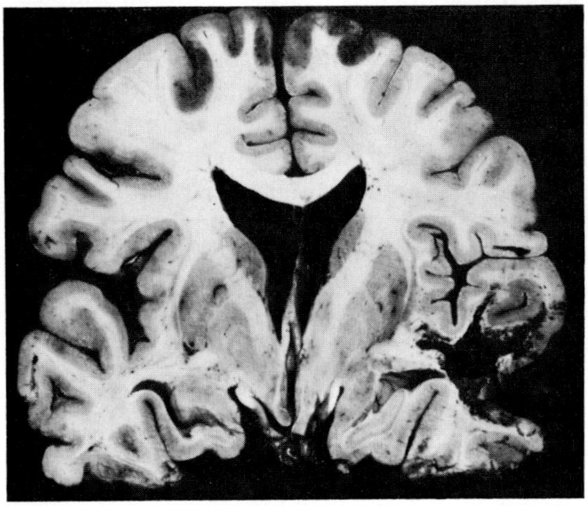

(a)

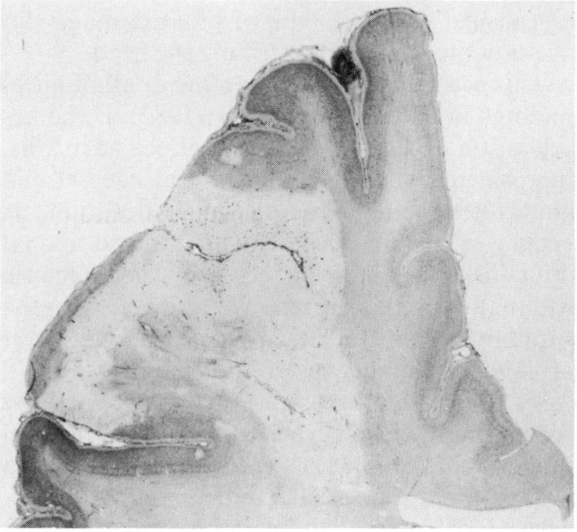

(b)

Fig. 3.24 Hypoxic brain damage. (**a**) Bilateral haemorrhagic infarction in the cerebral cortex at the dorsal angle of each hemisphere, i.e. in the boundary zones between the anterior and middle cerebral arterial territories. There is also a 'burst' temporal lobe. (**b**) Large wedge-shaped infarct barely recognizable macroscopically. Cresyl violet ×1. (Both reproduced, with permission, from Adams, 1975).

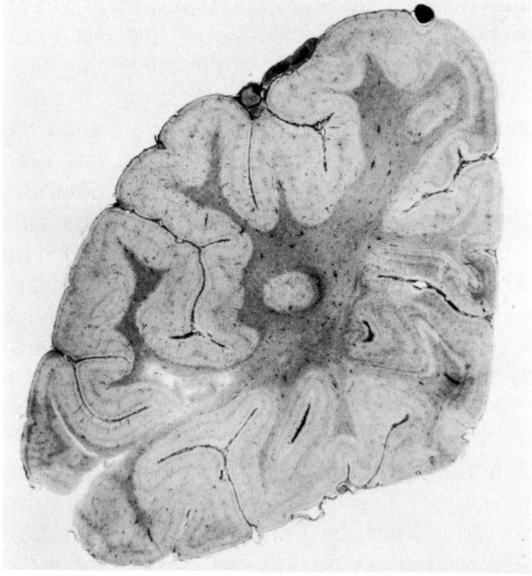

(a)

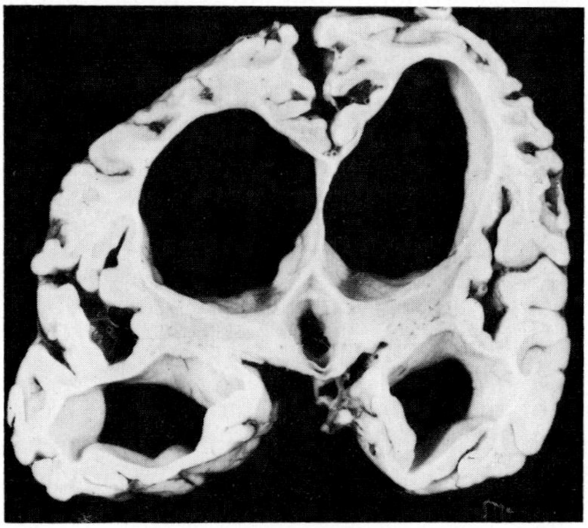

(b)

Fig. 3.25 Hypoxic brain damage. (**a**) Diffuse neuronal necrosis in an occipital lobe: the necrosis was not apparent macroscopically. Cresyl violet ×1. (**b**) Old hypoxic brain damage in a patient who survived in a vegetative state for 4 years after a head injury.

of brain damage is not yet fully understood but in the series described by Graham, Adams and Doyle (1978) it was significantly more common in patients who had sustained a known clinical episode of hypoxia (defined as a systolic blood pressure of less than 80 mmHg for at least 15 minutes or a $Pa\text{O}_2$ of 6.7 kPa (50 mmHg) at some time after the injury) than in those who had not. It was also commoner in patients who had experienced a high intracranial pressure during life. Nevertheless the high incidence of damage to the cerebral cortex in arterial boundary zones suggests that perfusion failure due to a transient reduction in cerebral blood flow is at least a contributing factor (see Chapter 4), whilst in some of the patients who sustained diffuse hypoxic damage there was either a known episode of cardiac arrest or status epilepticus. Intracranial arterial spasm is accepted as occurring in patients who have sustained a head injury (Wilkins and Odom, 1970), whilst Macpherson and Graham (1978) have established that there is a statistically significant correlation between hypoxic brain damage in head injury and angiographic evidence of arterial spasm. Precisely when this hypoxic brain damage occurs is also in doubt but it seems likely from the study by Graham, Adams, and Doyle (1978) that it occurs fairly soon after injury. There is therefore no doubt that an insufficient supply of oxygen to the brain is common in patients who have sustained a head injury; this has also been emphasized by Strich (1976) and by Jennett (1984). Hypoxic damage in the neocortex (Fig. 3.26a) has been observed in only a small proportion of subhuman primates subjected to acceleration of the head (Adams, Graham and Gennarelli, 1982); this is not surprising because blood pressure and arterial oxygenation were monitored. There was, however, a high incidence of lesions in the hippocampus, these usually taking the form of focal neuronal necrosis with or without haemorrhage (Fig. 3.26b) and with subsequent loss of nerve cells and reactive changes in the distal part of the Sommer sector and in the adjacent entorhinal region. The pathogenesis of this type of damage has not yet been established.

Brain swelling

That brain swelling occurs frequently in association with head injury and may be a major factor

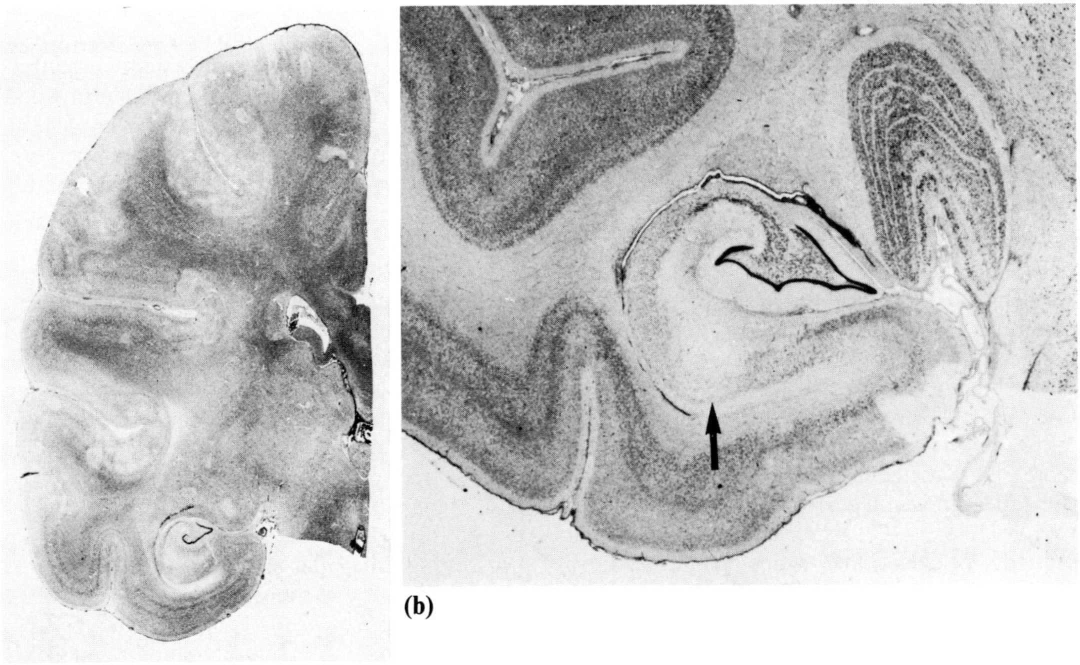

(b)

(a)

Fig. 3.26 Hypoxic brain damage in a subhuman primate after acceleration of the head. (**a**) Multiple foci of neuronal necrosis. Haematoxylin and eosin ×2. (**b**) Focus of neuronal necrosis (arrow) in the hippocampus. Cresyl violet ×3.

contributing to an increase in intracranial pressure is not in doubt, but its pathogenesis and the extent to which it is due to cerebral vasodilatation (i.e. congestive brain swelling) or to cerebral oedema (i.e. an increase in tissue water content) are not yet clear. The subject of swelling and oedema is discussed in greater detail in Chapter 2, but three principal types of brain swelling are encountered in patients who have sustained a head injury—swelling adjacent to contusions, diffuse swelling of one cerebral hemisphere and diffuse swelling of both cerebral hemispheres.

Swelling of white matter adjacent to contusions is a frequent occurrence (Fig. 3.27). Adjacent to the physically disrupted and necrotic tissue there is a zone of damaged vessels with increased

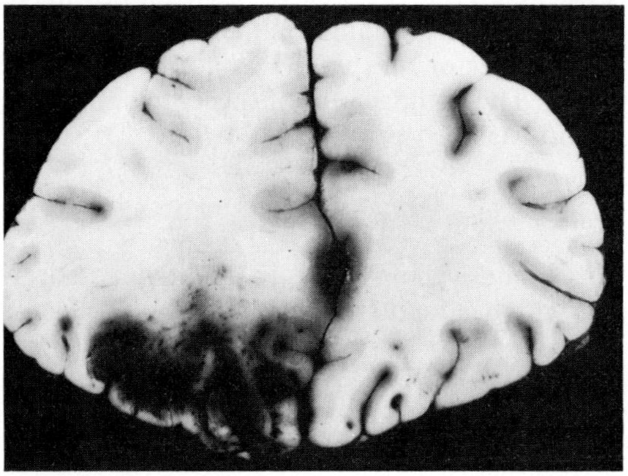

Fig. 3.27 Brain swelling in relation to contusions. (Reproduced, with permission, from Adams et al., 1980a).

permeability at capillary level and loss of normal physiological regulation at arteriolar level (Miller and Corales, 1981), the circumstances being very similar to those produced by the application of intense cold to the surface of the brain and the subsequent flow of oedema fluid into the adjacent white matter. The water content of brain tissue around cerebral contusions is increased (Tornheim and McLaurin, 1978) and this type of oedema corresponds to that referred to by Klatzo (1979) as vasogenic. A similar sequence of events may occur around an intracerebral haematoma.

Diffuse brain swelling is more difficult to account for; according to Miller and Corales (1981) the crucial evidence that it is due to cerebral oedema is lacking despite the fact that extravasation of horseradish peroxidase into extracellular spaces in the brain has been demonstrated shortly after experimental head injury in cats (Povlishock et al., 1978). In these experiments it appeared that horseradish peroxidase crossed the blood–brain barrier as a result of increased pinocytosis rather than because of any breakdown of the blood–brain barrier at tight junctions. Diffuse swelling of one cerebral hemisphere is most often seen in association with an ipsilateral acute subdural haematoma (Adams et al., 1980a): when the haematoma is evacuated the brain simply expands to fill the space so created (Fig. 3.28a), a situation similar to that created by Langfitt, Weinstein and Kassell (1965) in their experimental studies and attributed by them to engorgement of a non-reactive vascular bed secondary to cerebral ischaemia produced by a high intracranial pressure. The extent to which ischaemia contributes to this vasomotor paralysis remains in some doubt but this type of brain swelling can occur very soon after the occurrence of subdural haematoma. This has been clearly demonstrated by Adams, Graham and Gennerelli (1982) in their experimental studies on subhuman primates with the Penn 1 device (see p. 87). Acute subdural haematoma due to rupture of the bridging veins was readily produced with this device: if a craniectomy was undertaken within minutes to evacuate the haematoma with the aim of reducing intracranial pressure, the brain tissue simply herniated through the craniectomy (Fig. 3.28b). Because it is difficult to conceive of cerebral oedema occurring so rapidly, there can be little doubt that this type of swelling is due in the first instance to vasodilatation with or without significant pre-existing ischaemia. If this state persists, however, it seems likely that subsequent breakdown of the blood–brain barrier may lead to cerebral oedema: this, however, has not yet been established. Indeed it has been suggested in patients in whom subdural haematoma does not declare itself clinically until 2 or 3 days after the injury, that progressive development of brain swelling is more likely to be the cause of clinical deterioration and an increase in intracranial pressure than is enlargement of the haematoma itself (Miller and Corales, 1981).

Diffuse swelling of the entire brain (Fig. 3.29) occurs mainly in children and adolescents (Adams, Gennarelli and Graham, 1982); its pathogenesis is also obscure but it may be contributed to by early epilepsy (Adams, 1975). Its presence is indicated during life by the demon-

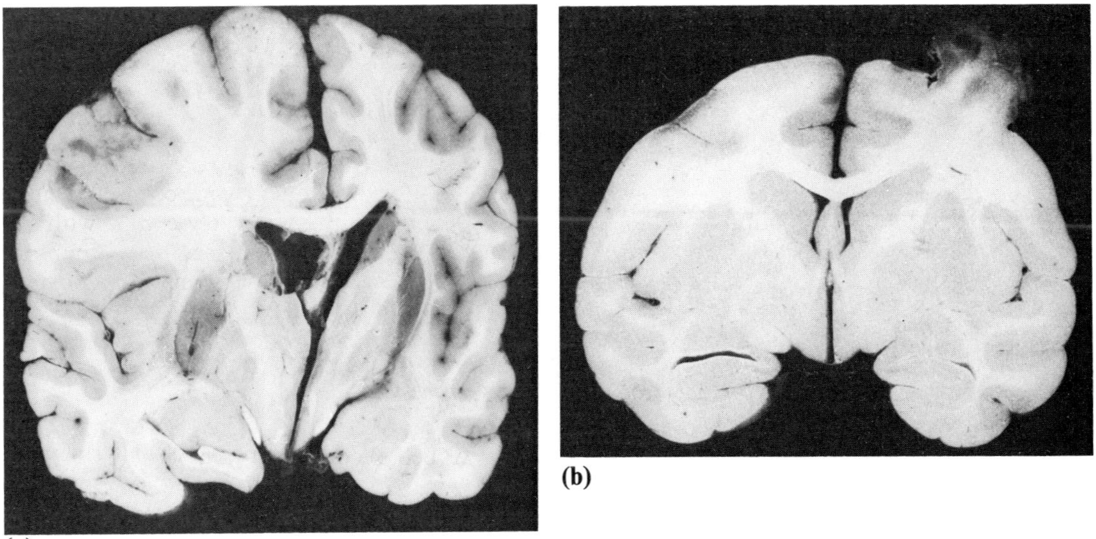

(a) (b)

Fig. 3.28 Brain swelling. (**a**) Diffuse swelling of the left cerebral hemisphere on the same side as an acute subdural haematoma that had been evacuated. (**b**) Swelling of the right cerebral hemisphere of a subhuman primate after acceleration of the head: brain tissue herniated through the craniectomy undertaken to evacuate an acute subdural haematoma. (**a** and **b** reproduced, with permission, from: **a**, Adams et al., 1980a; **b**, Adams, Gennarelli and Graham, 1982).

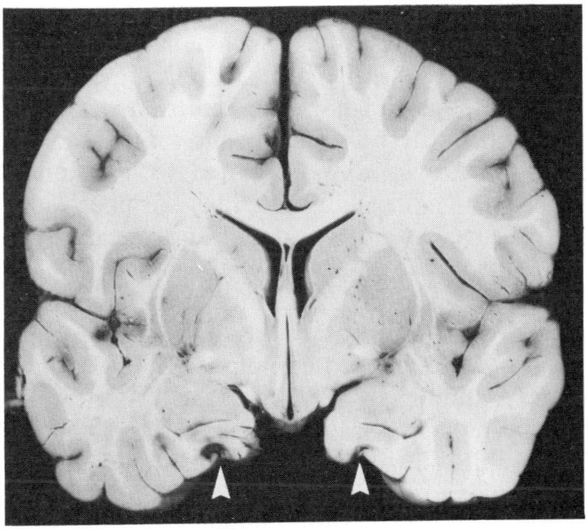

Fig. 3.29 Brain swelling. Diffuse swelling of both cerebral hemispheres in a 5-year-old child who survived for 30 hours after a head injury. Note the absence of contusions and the presence of bilateral tentorial herniae (arrows).

stration of small symmetrical ventricles and occlusion of the basal cisterns on computerized tomography (Teasdale et al., 1984). This problem has been studied in considerable detail by Bruce et al. (1981) and by Zimmerman et al. (1978). Some of the children with diffuse brain swelling had experienced a lucid interval whilst others had not, and the available evidence suggests that the diffuse swelling is brought about by an increase in cerebral blood volume. If this persists, it seems again possible that true cerebral oedema will subsequently occur. One of the problems facing pathologists in assessing the presence of diffuse brain swelling *post mortem* on the basis of convolutional flattening, obliteration of sulci and small symmetrical ventricles is that brain swelling occurs after the onset of brain stem death (Adams, 1976) and after death (Sarwar and McCormick, 1978).

Multiple small haemorrhages in the brain

These are seen most frequently and are probably restricted to patients who die very soon after head injury—i.e. they must be classified as a type of primary brain damage. Indeed it is remarkable how conspicuous they can be in patients who are reported as having died 'instantaneously' (Fig. 3.30). Their importance has been emphasized by Tomlinson (1970) who has suggested that they are indicative of damage of a type and distribution which is incompatible with life; this is also the author's experience. Many of these haemorrhages can be identified macroscopically, but many more can be seen microscopically when they take the form of periarterial, perivenous or

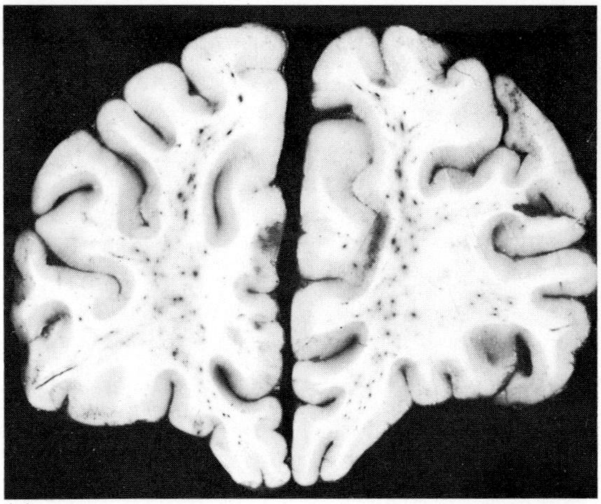

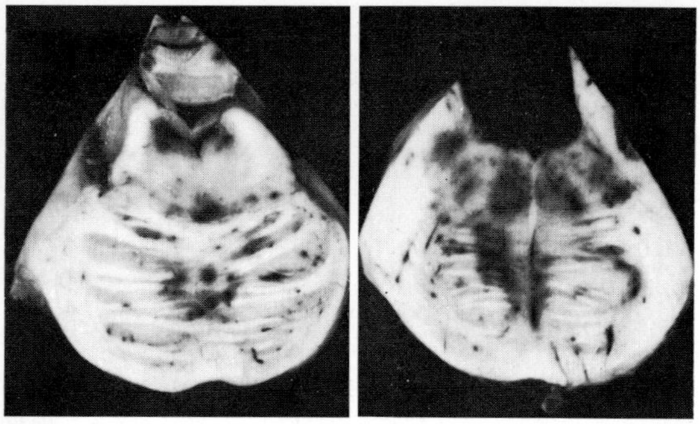

(b)

(a)

Fig. 3.30 Multiple small haemorrhages in the brain. (**a**) 30 minutes' survival). (**b**) Less than 10 minutes' survival.

pericapillary haemorrhage. They can occur in any part of the brain but they tend to be particularly conspicious in the white matter of the anterior parts of the frontal and temporal lobes, in and adjacent to the thalamus, and in the brain stem. In the brain stem they are particularly numerous in the subependymal tissues around the aqueduct and in the floor of the rostral part of the fourth ventricle; they occur rarely in the caudal pons or medulla (Tomlinson, 1970; Strich, 1976). They have been referred to as primary brain stem haemorrhages by Tomlinson (1970) but in the author's experience they are more appropriately considered as a primary type of diffuse brain damage in view of their wide distribution throughout the cerebral hemispheres as well as the brain stem.

Haemorrhages of this type may be seen in the corpus callosum and in the dorsolateral quadrant of the rostral brain stem but, unlike typical examples of diffuse axonal injury, they are neither restricted to, nor particularly severe in, these sites. Because this type of brain damage has not been produced by acceleration of the head in subhuman primates, the mechanism of their occurrence has not been established; it may, however, be further evidence that various structures in the brain—like the subdural bridging veins (see p. 96) and axons (see p. 109)—have different responses to acceleration/deceleration impulses.

Primary brain stem damage in head injury This has long been a controversial issue and clinicians have tended to use the term 'primary brain stem injury' for patients who are unconscious from the moment of injury and who do not have an intracranial expanding lesion. Various types of primary damage to the brain stem have been referred to above—pontomedullary rents, focal lesions in the dorsolateral part of the rostral brain stem and multiple petechial haemorrhages. In the author's experience the only type of primary damage to the brain stem that occurs in isolation is the pontomedullary rent; these are rare and are usually associated with instantaneous death although there may very occasionally be survival for some days if the rent is partial (Pilz, Strohecker and Grobovschek, 1982). The other types of primary damage to the brain stem are part of a diffuse process affecting many regions of the brain. Rosenblum et al. (1981), however, found what they interpreted as primary lesions in the midbrain in 23 of a series of 35 fatal head injuries. Most of the lesions they illustrate are similar to those that occur in diffuse axonal injury, but the neuropathological findings they report are inadequate to allow of a full appraisal of this interesting study and it could be that the cases reported by them are examples of diffuse axonal injury with lesions in the corpus callosum and histological evidence of widespread damage to axons. Rosenblum et al. (1981) also place considerable emphasis on the fact that secondary damage to the brain stem is usually a terminal event and is therefore relatively fresh at autopsy. This, however, is not necessarily so since patients with secondary damage in the brain stem not infrequently survive for days or even weeks after an intracranial expanding lesion has been evacuated (see p. 64).

Thus on the basis of comprehensive clinico-neuropathological studies on patients who are unconscious from the moment of injury, and on the results obtained from the Philadelphia model with the Penn 2 device (see p. 108), there is increasing evidence to support the earlier contention of Mitchell and Adams (1973) that the pathological substrate of so-called primary brain stem damage is diffuse axonal injury.

Concussion and its structural basis have also long been controversial issues although the importance of acceleration forces was established by Denny-Brown and Russell as long ago as 1941. It was, however, not until 1974 that Ommaya and Gennarelli established that angular acceleration of the head is of much greater importance in the production of concussion than is translational acceleration (see p. 87). The controversy will doubtless continue but it seems increasingly that the substrate of concussion is diffuse brain damage and not some focal lesion in a particular region of the brain. Now that diffuse axonal injury similar to that which has long been known to occur in man has been produced in subhuman primates, and it has been shown that there is a close correlation between the duration of coma and neurological signs and the severity of axonal damage (Gennarelli, 1983), the concept that concussion is brought about by minor degrees of diffuse axonal injury is attractive.

Fat embolism Some patients who sustain a head injury also have multiple injuries, including limb and other fractures. They are therefore at risk of developing systemic fat embolism. Indeed fulminating fat embolism is a well recognized, if uncommon, cause of rapid progressive neurological deterioration in such a patient without an acute intracranial expanding lesion (Adams et al., 1980a). The subject of fat embolism is dealt with in Chapter 4 but it is important for pathologists to appreciate that classic petechial haemorrhages may be absent despite the presence of extensive fat embolism. In patients with multiple injuries, therefore, the brain has to be screened routinely for fat embolism.

Outcome after head injury

Most patients who sustain a head injury make a good recovery. Others remain moderately or severely disabled or remain in the vegetative state (Jennett and Plum, 1972; Jennett and Bond, 1975; Jennett and Teasdale, 1981). Pathologists can only define the types of brain damage that occur in fatal cases, and it might therefore be thought that they have little to contribute to the understanding and management of patients who sustain a head injury. This is not so because it is only by detailed post-mortem studies that the sequence of events leading to the fatal outcome can be established, and that at least potentially preventable factors can be identified. Furthermore, it is only as a result of such studies that clinicians can have some insight into the types of structural changes responsible for persistent disability after head injury, since it seems inevitable that these must be similar to but less severe than those identified in fatal cases.

Severe disability and the vegetative state

The underlying basis of severe brain damage after head injury has been fully and comprehensively studied by Jellinger and Seitelberger (1969, 1970), by Jellinger (1977), and by many other authors including Peters and Rothemund (1977) and Grcevic (1977) where a comprehensive bibliography will be found. Jellinger and Seitelberger have emphasized the frequency of abnormalities in the rostral brain stem, intracranial haematoma, brain swelling, and respiratory and circulatory distress, and consider that the morphology of this type of post-traumatic encephalopathy is on the whole dominated by secondary traumatic lesions and their sequelae. In his series of 80 cases of prolonged unconsciousness after head injury, Jellinger (1977) observed that by far the commonest finding (86.3 per cent of cases) was secondary damage to the brain stem although there was also a high incidence of hypoxic brain damage. Peters and Rothemund (1977) also take the view that the determining factor in traumatic vegetative (or, as they are sometimes called, apallic) states is the occurrence of transtentorial herniation. These conclusions are at variance with those of Strich (1969) and Graham et al. (1983). The former has always placed particular emphasis on the presence of diffuse brain damage in patients who remain vegetative after head injury and on her failure to identify any case of prolonged post-traumatic coma where damage was confined to the brain stem. In the comprehensive neuropathological assessment undertaken by Graham et al. (1983) of 35 patients who remained vegetative or severely disabled for more than 1 month after a non-missile head injury, diffuse axonal injury was found in 22 cases: in two of these cases there was also moderate to severe hypoxic brain damage and in three midline lesions in the brain stem of the type classically associated with raised intracranial pressure and tentorial herniation. There was moderate to severe hypoxic brain damage in 16 cases, and in eight of these there was also damage of secondary type in the brain stem. There was not one case where damage was confined to the brain stem; this suggests that patients with intracranial expanding lesions who develop tentorial herniation and other secondary types of brain damage, such as infarction in the diencephalon, in the brain stem and in the occipital cortex, rarely survive for more than a few weeks after the episode of secondary brain damage.

This therefore remains a somewhat controversial field that is in need of further study. There are problems of nomenclature and in the interpretation of the pathogenesis of lesions in the brain stem although the structural abnormalities indicative of diffuse axonal injury (see p. 100) are becoming increasingly clearly defined. Certainly in the author's experience diffuse axonal injury is the commonest cause of the persistent vegetative state, whilst in experimental studies in subhuman primates diffuse axonal injury has been the pathological substrate for post-traumatic coma and severe disability. There seems therefore to be increasing evidence from clinicopathological and experimental studies that the commonest causes of the vegetative state and severe disability after head injury—at least in patients who survive their injury for more than 1 month—are diffuse axonal injury and hypoxic brain damage. Because it is well established that patients with quite severe types of focal brain damage may make a very good recovery provided that appropriate treatment where applicable is instituted early, it seems likely that persistent disability after head injury is attributable more to diffuse than to focal brain damage.

Post-traumatic epilepsy

The underlying pathology and electrophysiology of post-traumatic epilepsy are not well understood but a clear distinction has been made between *early* epilepsy (occurring during the first week after injury) and *late* epilepsy (Jennett, Teather and Bennie, 1973; Jennett, 1974, 1975). In almost half the patients in whom late epilepsy eventually develops, the first fit is delayed for a year or more, but the occurrence of early epilepsy considerably enhances the risk of late epilepsy. In adults early epilepsy seldom occurs except in association with prolonged post-traumatic amnesia, depressed fracture of the skull or intracranial haematoma, but it occurs more commonly in young children and only in them does it complicate trivial injuries. The particular significance of early epilepsy in young children is that it may progress rapidly to status epilepticus which, if not rapidly and adequately controlled, may lead to the occurrence of varying degrees of irreversible hypoxic brain damage (see Chapter 4). According to Jennett and Teasdale (1981) late traumatic epilepsy is by far the most frequent delayed complication of a non-missile head injury, and the risk is higher in patients who have had an intracranial haematoma, a compound depressed fracture or early epilepsy.

The incidence of late epilepsy is much higher after missile head injuries than after non-missile head injuries (about 40 per cent compared with 5 per cent), and the incidence has remained the same from one war to another in spite of marked improvement over decades in patient transport, surgical techniques, medical management and the prophylactic use of anticonvulsants (Caveness et al., 1979). These authors found a highly significant relationship between the degree of focal brain destruction and the liability to epilepsy. This liability is enhanced when the focal damage is associated with prolonged loss of consciousness, the latter being taken as a clinical indication of diffuse as well as focal brain damage (Caveness, 1979). The close relationship between the degree of focal brain damage and epilepsy, however, tends to suggest that the most important cause of post-traumatic epilepsy in any type of head injury is focal brain damage.

Progressive neurological disease

This aspect of head injury has been reviewed by Strich (1969, 1976) who, despite the occasional striking association between a head injury and the onset of neurological disease, finds many of the cases reported unconvincing. Diseases in which the possibility of a connection with head injury has been reported include Alzheimer's disease (Corsellis and Brierley, 1959; Hollander and Strich, 1970), Pick's disease (McMenemey, Grant and Behrman, 1965), Parkinson's disease (Grimberg, 1934), motor neuron disease, and Creutzfeldt–Jakob disease (Behrman, Mandybur and McMenemey, 1962). It has, however, to be accepted that a direct correlation between any of these diseases and a previous head injury remains to be established.

Subarachnoid haemorrhage occurs frequently in all types of head injury and the consequent obliteration of the subarachnoid space as blood is organized is a recognized cause of normal pressure hydrocephalus, and this may lead to dementia (see Chapter 2). There are, however, other causes of enlargement of the ventricles in patients who survive for some time after a severe head injury, such as a reduction in the mass of the brain due to diffuse axonal injury or hypoxic brain damage. Recently Meyers et al. (1983) have suggested, on the basis of serial CT scans, that early enlargement of the ventricles after closed head injury is due to obstruction to the flow of CSF, and that late enlargement is contributed to by diffuse axonal injury and hypoxic brain damage.

It is well recognized that persons subjected to large numbers of concussive or subconcussive blows, such as boxers, sometimes develop neurological signs and progressive dementia (Martland, 1928; Critchley, 1957; Mawdsley and Ferguson, 1963). The condition, often referred to as the *punch-drunk syndrome*, may come on years after the last injury, affects amateur as well as professional boxers and is more likely to develop in boxers with long careers who have been dazed if not knocked out on many occasions. Corsellis, Bruton and Freeman-Browne (1973) have analysed the abnormalities in the brains of 15 ex-boxers. They found a characteristic pattern of brain damage, the principal features of which were abnormalities in the septum pellucidum with enlargement of the cavum, and fenestration of the leaves of the interventricular septum (Fig. 3.31). In some cases, there was thinning of the adjacent fornices and corpus callosum, scarring and neuronal loss in the cerebellum, degeneration of the substantia nigra as shown by loss of neurons and pigment, and the presence of numerous neurofibrillary tangles (Fig. 3.32) diffusely throughout the cerebral cortex and the brain stem. These tangles broadly conformed to the topographic pattern found in Alzheimer's disease but showed a distinct predilection for the medial temporal grey matter. In contrast to the very numerous tangles there was a remarkable sparsity or, in most cases, a total absence of senile plaques (see Chapter 20).

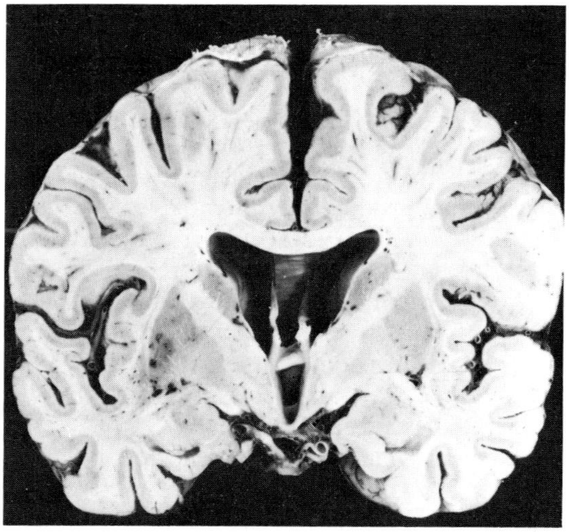

Fig. 3.31 Well-known boxer, died aged 83. There is cerebral atrophy, enlargement of the ventricular system, and a wide cavum with torn walls in the interventricular septum.

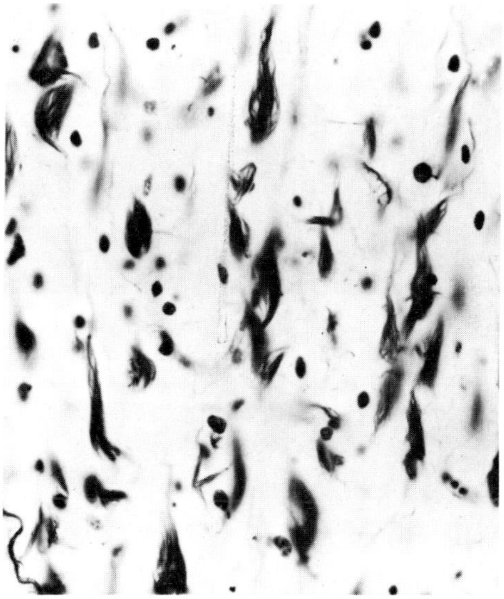

Fig. 3.32 Professional boxer. There are abundant neurofibrillary tangles in the cortex of the temporal lobe. Bielschowsky ×325.

Missile head injury

These are injuries produced by various types of object which fall or are propelled through the air. Small flying objects which have a high kinetic energy may produce considerable local damage but little rotational injury because there will be little movement of the head (Strich, 1976). The size of the wound produced depends on factors such as the mass, shape and velocity of the missile, and the direction of the impact. The injury may be classified as depressed, penetrating or perforating (Lindenberg, 1971).

In *depressed* injuries the missile does not enter the cranial cavity but produces a depressed fracture of the skull and subjacent fracture contusions. Brain damage is therefore focal and consciousness is frequently lost only briefly or not at all. Clinical examination may be misleading because the scalp laceration may not lie directly over the fracture, or an apparently intact outer table may conceal a depression of the inner table of the skull.

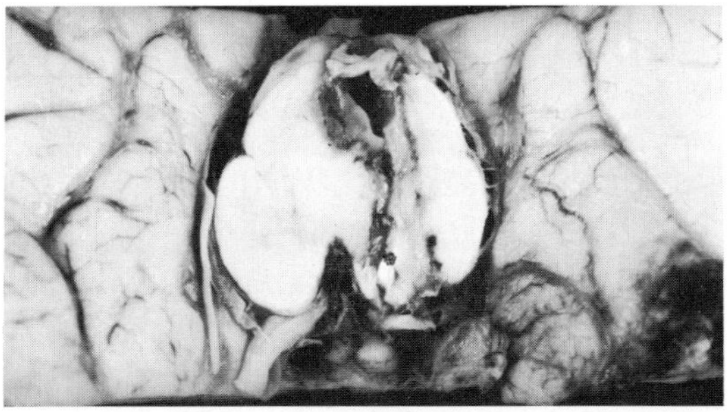

Fig. 3.33 Missile head injury. In this case the tip of a toy sword had penetrated directly into the midbrain.

In *penetrating* injuries the object enters the cranial cavity but does not pass through it. If the object is small and sharp, such as a nail, there may be very little direct injury to the skull or the brain: this damage may only too easily escape clinical detection if the missile is no longer embedded in the skull. Brain damage is again focal and there is often no history of loss of consciousness. Not infrequently patients with a penetrating missile, such as a screw driver, are admitted to a neurosurgical unit with the missile still in position and the patient fully conscious. Occasionally, however, the missile may penetrate deeply enough to damage some vital structure (Fig. 3.33). With penetrating head injuries there is a high risk of infection, frequently in the form of an abscess (Fig. 3.34), rather than meningitis.

In a *perforating* injury the object, usually a bullet, traverses the cranial cavity and leaves through an exit wound. Brain damage is often severe but a high-velocity bullet may on occasion pass through the head without knocking the victim down or causing impairment of consciousness (Strich, 1976). The exit wound in the skull is characteristically larger than the entry wound. Bullets of low velocity cause more damage at the site of entry and rarely pass completely through the skull; the bullet, however, may ricochet from the skull and traverse the brain in various directions (Freytag, 1963b). Injuries from low-

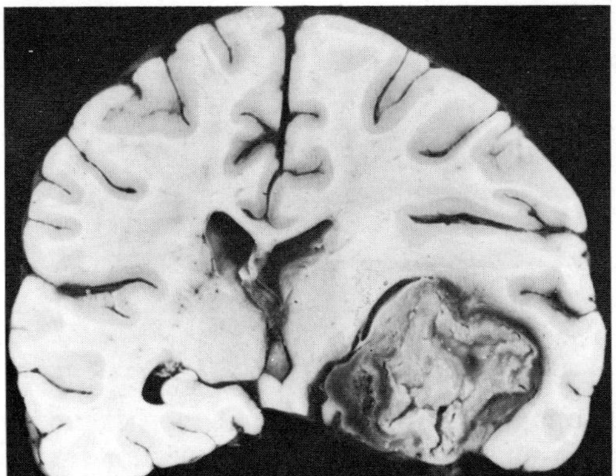

(a)

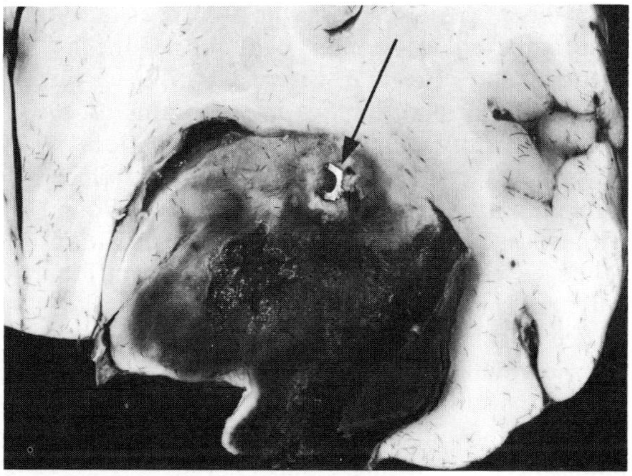

(b)

Fig. 3.34 Missile head injury. (**a**) Abscess in the right temporal lobe. (**b**) Air gun pellet (arrow) in the wall of the abscess. The abscess presented 21 months after the original injury.

velocity missiles tend to be complicated by fragments of bone, scalp and sometimes clothing driven into the brain (Sights, 1969), resulting in severe laceration of the brain with damage to blood vessels causing haemorrhage and necrosis (Freytag, 1963b). According to Freytag (1963b) most wound canals correspond to the size of the bullet and are of even diameter throughout their length (Fig. 3.35). In some cases, however, because of severe fracturing of the bone at the entry site, the canal near the entrance wound appears larger than near the exit wound because of laceration of the surrounding tissues by bony fragments. A cross-section of the wound canal may show three different zones (Lindenberg, 1971): a central zone containing brain tissue and blood, an intermediate band of tissue necrosis, and a marginal slightly discoloured zone. Radial displacement forces from the bullet track frequently cause remote contusions affecting the frontal and temporal poles and the undersurface of the cerebellum. Contrecoup fractures (see p. 88) may also occur in the orbital plates.

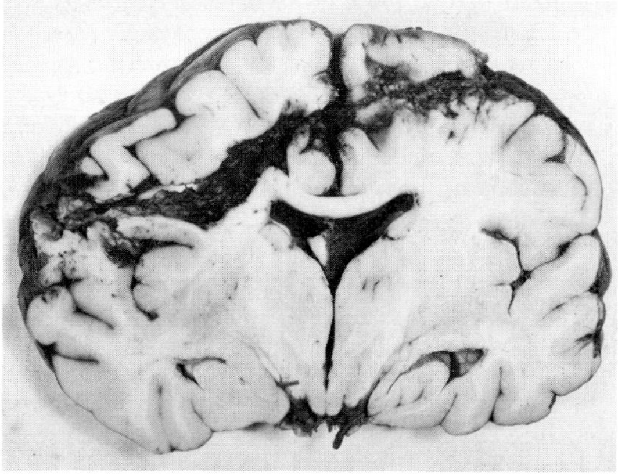

Fig. 3.35 Missile head injury. Track of bullet wound through brain.

In a histological analysis of the brains of 24 patients dying as a result of craniocerebral missile injury, Campbell et al. (1958) observed thrombosis and necrosis of small blood vessels, haemorrhage and oedema, swollen and varicose axons, and many other non-specific changes. In recent studies on experimental missile injuries, Allen, Scott and Tanner (1982) and Allen et al. (1983) found extensive subarachnoid, intraventricular and subependymal haemorrhage. There were also perivascular ring haemorrhages, oedema and blood vessels surrounded by zones of decreased or increased staining intensity both close to and away from the missile track. They also reported what they consider to be a more specific abnormality—selective swelling of astrocytes that was more evident in grey than in white matter. Adjacent neurons, oligodendrocytes, pericytes and endothelial cells appeared normal.

Bullet wounds to the head are usually rapidly fatal, only 10 per cent of the 254 cases described by Freytag (1963b) surviving for more than 24 hours. Only 10 patients survived for more than 7 days. In patients who do survive there is, as in all types of penetrating and perforating missile injury, a high risk of infection and epilepsy.

References

Abel, J., Gennarelli, T.A. and Segawa, H. (1978) Incidence and severity of cerebral concussion in the rhesus monkey following sagittal plane angular acceleration. In *Proceedings of the 22nd Stapp Car Crash Conference*, pp. 35–53. Society of Automotive Engineers, New York.

Adams, J.H. (1975) The neuropathology of head injuries. In *Handbook of Clinical Neurology*, vol. 23, *Injuries to the brain and Skull*, part 1 (Eds. Vinken, P.J. and Bruyn, G.W.), pp. 35–65. American Elsevier, New York.

Adams, J.H. (1976) The 'respirator brain'. *Archives of Neurology* **33,** 589.

Adams, J.H., Daniel, P.M. and Prichard, M.M.L. (1966) Transection of the pituitary stalk in man: anatomical changes in the pituitary glands in 21 patients. *Journal of Neurology, Neurosurgery and Psychiatry* **29,** 545–55.

Adams, J.H., Gennarelli, T.A. and Graham, D.I. (1982) Brain damage in non-missile head injury: observations in man and subhuman primates. In *Recent Advances in Neuropathology, 2* (Eds. Smith, W.T. and Cavanagh, J.B.), pp. 165–90. Churchill Livingstone, Edinburgh, London. Melbourne and New York.

Adams, J.H. and Graham, D.I. (1967) Twelve cases of fatal cerebral infarction due to arterial occlusion in the absence of atheromatous stenosis or embolism. *Journal of Neurology, Neurosurgery and Psychiatry* **30,** 479–88.

Adams, J.H. and Graham, D.I. (1972) The pathology of blunt head injuries. In *Scientific Foundations of Neurology* (Eds. Critchley, M., O'Leary, J.L. and Jennett, B.), pp. 478–91. Heinemann Medical, London.

Adams, J.H. and Graham, D.I. (1984) Diffuse brain

damage in non-missile head injury. In *Recent Advances in Histopathology* vol. 12, pp 241–57 (Eds. Anthony, P.P. and MacSween, R.N.M.). Churchill Livingstone, Edinburgh.

Adams, J.H., Graham, D.I. and Gennarelli, T.A. (1982) Neuropathology of acceleration-induced head injury in the subhuman primate. In *Head Injury: Basic and Clinical Aspects* (Eds. Grossman, R.G. and Gildenberg, P.L.), pp. 141–50. Raven Press, New York.

Adams, J.H., Graham, D.I. and Gennarelli, T.A. (1983) Head injury in man and experimental animals—neuropathology. *Acta Neurochirurgica* Suppl. 32, 15–30.

Adams, J.H., Mitchell, D.E., Graham, D.I. and Doyle, D. (1977) Diffuse brain damage of immediate impact type. *Brain* **100,** 489–502.

Adams, J.H., Graham, D.I., Scott, G., Parker, L.S. and Doyle, D. (1980a) Brain damage in non-missile head injury. *Journal of Clinical Pathology* **33,** 1132–45.

Adams, J.H., Scott, G., Parker, L.S., Graham, D.I. and Doyle, D. (1980b) The contusion index: a quantitative approach to cerebral contusions in head injury. *Neuropathology and Applied Neurobiology* **6,** 319–24.

Adams, J.H., Graham, D.I., Murray, L.S. and Scott, G. (1982) Diffuse axonal injury due to non-missile head injury in humans: an analysis of 45 cases. *Annals of Neurology* **12,** 557–63.

Allen, I.V., Scott, R. and Tanner, J.A. (1982) Experimental high velocity missile head injury. *Injury* **14,** 183–93.

Allen, I.V., Kirk, J., Maynard, R.L., Cooper, G.K., Scott, R. and Crockard, A. (1983) An ultrastructural study of experimental high velocity penetrating head injury. *Acta Neuropathologica* **59,** 277–82.

Anderson, D.W. and McLaurin, R.L. (1980) Report on the national head and spinal cord injury survey conducted for the National Institute of Neurological and Communicative Disorders. *Journal of Neurosurgery* **53,** Suppl., S1–S43.

Baratham, G. and Dennyson, W.G. (1972) Delayed traumatic intracranial haemorrhage. *Journal of Neurology, Neurosurgery and Psychiatry* **25,** 698–706.

Behrman, S., Mandybur, T. and McMenemey, W.H. (1962) Un cas de maladie Creutzfeldt-Jakob à la suite d'un traumatisme cérébral. *Revue Neurologique* **107,** 453–9.

Brooks, D.N. and McKinlay, W. (1983) Personality and behavioural change after severe blunt head injury—a relative's view. *Journal of Neurology, Neurosurgery and Psychiatry* **46,** 336–44.

Bruce, D.A., Alavi, A., Bilaniuk, L., Kolinskas, C., Obrist, W. and Uzzell, B. (1981) Diffuse cerebral swelling following head injuries in children: the syndrome of 'malignant brain edema'. *Journal of Neurosurgery* **54,** 170–8.

Cajal, S.Ramony (1959) *Degeneration and Regeneration of the Nervous System*, vol. 2 (translated and edited by May, R.M.). Hafner, New York.

Cameron, J.M. and Mant, A.K. (1972) Fatal subarachnoid haemorrhage associated with cervical trauma. *Medicine, Science and the Law* **12,** 66–70.

Cameron, M.N. (1978) Chronic subdural haematoma: a review of 114 cases. *Journal of Neurology, Neurosurgery and Psychiatry* **41,** 834–9.

Campbell, E.H., Kuhlenbeck, R.L., Cavenaugh, R.L. and Nielsen, A.E. (1958) Clinicopathological aspects of fatal missile-caused craniocerebral injuries. In: *Surgery in World War II, Neurosurgery* **1,** 335–99.

Caveness, W.F. (1979) Incidence of craniocerebral trauma in the United States in 1976 with trend from 1970 to 1975. In *Advances in Neurology*, vol 22, *Complications of Nervous System Trauma* (Eds. Thompson, R.A. and Green, J.R.), pp. 1–3. Raven Press, New York.

Caveness, W.F., Meirowsky, A.M., Rish, B.L., Mohr, J.P., Kistler, J.P., Dillon, J.D. et al. (1979) The nature of post-traumatic epilepsy. *Journal of Neurosurgery* **50,** 545–53.

Clark, J.M. (1974) Distribution of microglial clusters in the brain after head injury. *Journal of Neurology, Neurosurgery and Psychiatry* **37,** 463–74.

Corsellis, J.A.N. and Brierley, J.B. (1959) Observations on the pathology of insidious dementia following head injury. *Journal of Mental Science* **105,** 714–20.

Corsellis, J.A.N., Bruton, C.J. and Freeman-Browne, D. (1973) The aftermath of boxing. *Psychological Medicine* **3,** 270–303.

Critchley, M. (1957) Medical aspects of boxing particularly from a neurological standpoint. *British Medical Journal* **1,** 357–66.

Crompton, M.R. (1970) Visual lesions in closed head injury. *Brain* **93,** 785–92.

Dawson, S.L., Hirsch, C.S., Lucas, F.V. and Sebek, B.A. (1980) The contrecoup phenomenon: reappraisal of a classic problem. *Human Pathology* **11,** 155–66.

Denny-Brown, J.P. and Russell, W.R. (1941) Experimental cerebral concussion. *Brain* **64,** 93–164.

Dolinskas, C.S., Zimmerman, R.A., Bilaniuk, L.T. and Gennarelli, T.A. (1979) Computed tomography of post-traumatic extracerebral hematomas. *Journal of Trauma* **19,** 163–9.

Evans, J.P. and Scheinker, I.M. (1943) Histological studies of the brain following head trauma. *Archives of Neurology and Psychiatry* **50,** 258–78.

Evans, J.P. and Scheinker, I.M. (1945) Histological studies of the brain following head trauma. *Research Publications of the Association for Research in Mental and Nervous Disease* **24,** 254–74.

Ewing, R., McCarthy, D., Gronwall, D. and Wrightson, P. (1980) Persisting effects of minor head injury observable during hypoxic stress. *Journal of Clinical Neuropsychology* **2,** 147–55.

Freytag, E. (1963a) Autopsy findings in head injuries from blunt forces. *Archives of Pathology* **75,** 402–13.

Freytag, E. (1963b) Autopsy findings in head injuries from firearms. *Archives of Pathology* **76,** 215–25.

Galbraith, S. (1976) Misdiagnosis and delayed diagnosis in traumatic intracranial haematoma. *British Medical Journal* **1,** 1438–9.

Gennarelli, T.A. (1983) Head injury in man and experimental animals—clinical aspects. *Acta Neurochirurgica* Suppl. 32, 1–13.

Gennarelli, T.A. and Thibault, L.E. (1982) Biomechanics of acute subdural hematoma. *Journal of Trauma* **22,** 680–6.

Gennarelli, T.A., Thibault, L. and Ommaya, A.K. (1971) Comparison of linear and rotational acceleration in experimental cerebral concussion. In *Proceedings of the 16th Stapp Car Crash Conference*, pp. 797–803. Society of Automotive Engineers, New York.

Gennarelli, T.A., Thibault, L. and Ommaya, A.K. (1972) Pathophysiologic responses to rotational and translational acceleration of the head. In *Proceedings of the 16th Stapp Car Crash Conference*, pp. 296–308. Society of Automotive Engineers, New York.

Gennarelli, T.A., Abel, J.M., Adams, J.H. and Graham, D.I. (1979) Differential tolerance of frontal and temporal lobes to contusion induced by angular acceleration. In *Proceedings of the 23rd Stapp Car Conference*, pp. 561–86. Society of Automotive Engineers, New York.

Gennarelli, T.A., Segawa, H., Wald, U., Czernicki, Z., Marsh, K. and Thompson, C. (1982a) Physiological response to angular acceleration of the head. In *Head Injury: Basic and Clinical Aspects* (Eds. Grossman, R.G. and Gildenberg, P.L.), pp. 129–40. Raven Press, New York.

Gennarelli, T.A., Spielman, G.M., Langfitt, T.W., Gildenberg, P.L., Harrington, T., Jane, J.A. et al. (1982b) Influence of the type of intracranial lesion on outcome from severe head injury. *Journal of Neurosurgery* **56,** 26–36.

Gennarelli, T.A., Thibault, L.E., Adams, J.H., Graham, D.I., Thompson, C.J. and Marcincin, R.P. (1982c) Diffuse axonal injury and traumatic coma in the primate. *Annals of Neurology* **12,** 564–74.

Graham, D.I. and Adams, J.H. (1971) Ischaemic brain damage in fatal head injuries. *Lancet* **1,** 265–6.

Graham, D.I., Adams, J.H. and Doyle, D. (1978) Ischaemic brain damage in fatal non-missile head injuries. *Journal of the Neurological Sciences* **39,** 213–34.

Graham, D.I., McLellan, D., Adams, J.H., Doyle, D., Kerr, A. and Murray, L.S. (1983) The neuropathology of severe disability after head injury. *Acta Neurochirurgica* Suppl. **32,** 65–7.

Grčević, N. (1977) Neuropathological correlates of supratentorial lesions in traumatic and nontraumatic apallic syndrome. In *The Apallic Syndrome* (Eds. Ore, G.D., Gerstenbrand, F., Lucking, C.H., Peters, G. and Peters, U.H.), pp. 109–13. Springer, Berlin.

Grčević, N. (1982) Topography and pathogenic mechanisms of lesions in 'inner cerebral trauma'. *Rad jug. Akad. Znan. Umj. Od. med. Nauke* **402/18,** 265–331.

Grimberg, L. (1934) Paralysis agitans and trauma. *Journal of Nervous and Mental Diseases* **79,** 14–42.

Gronwall, D. and Wrightson, P. (1974) Delayed recovery of intellectual function after minor head injuries. *Lancet* **2,** 605–9.

Gurdjian, E.S., Webster, J.E. and Lissner, H.R. (1955) Observations on the mechanism of brain concussion, contusion and laceration. *Surgery, Gynecology and Obstetrics* **101,** 680–90.

Hardman, J.M. (1979) The pathology of traumatic brain injuries. In *Advances in Neurology*, vol. 22, *Complications of Nervous System Trauma* (Eds. Thompson, R.A. and Green, J.R.), pp. 15–50. Raven Press, New York.

Harland, W.A., Pitts, J.F. and Watson, A.A. (1983) Subarachnoid haemorrhage due to upper cervical trauma. *Journal of Clinical Pathology* **36,** 1335–41.

Helfand, M. (1939) Cerebral lesions due to vasomotor disturbances following brain trauma. *Journal of Nervous and Mental Diseases* **90,** 157–79.

Hirsch, C.S. and Kaufman, B. (1975) Contrecoup skull fractures. *Journal of Neurosurgery* **42,** 530–4.

Holbourn, A.H.S. (1943) Mechanics of head injuries. *Lancet* **2,** 438–41.

Holbourn, A.H.S. (1945) The mechanics of brain injuries. *British Medical Bulletin* **3,** 147–9.

Hollander, D. and Strich, S.J. (1970) Atypical Alzheimer's disease with congophilic angiopathy presenting with dementia of acute onset. In *Alzheimer's Disease and Related Conditions*, Ciba Foundation Symposium (Eds. Wolstenholme, G.E.W. and O'Connor, M.), pp. 105–24. Churchill, London.

Jamieson, K.G. and Yelland, J.D.N. (1968) Extradural hematoma: report of 167 cases. *Journal of Neurosurgery* **29,** 13–23.

Jellinger, K. (1977) Pathology and pathogenesis of apallic syndromes following closed head injuries. In *The Apallic Syndrome* (Eds. Ore, G.D., Gerstenbrand, F., Lucking, C.H., Peters, G. and Peters, U.H.), pp. 88–103. Springer, Berlin.

Jellinger, K. and Seitelberger, F. (1969) Protracted

post-traumatic encephalopathy. In *The Late Effects of Head Injury* (Eds. Walker, A.E., Caveness, W.F. and Critchley, M.), pp. 168–81. Thomas, Springfield.

Jellinger, K. and Seitelberger, F. (1970) Protracted post-traumatic encephalopathy: pathology, pathogenesis and clinical implications. *Journal of the Neurological Sciences* **10,** 51–94.

Jennett, B. (1974) Early traumatic epilepsy. *Archives of Neurology* **30,** 394–8.

Jennett, B. (1975) *Epilepsy after Non-Missile Head Injuries*, 2nd edn. Heinemann Medical, London.

Jennett, B. and Bond, M. (1975) Assessment of outcome after severe brain damage: a practical scale. *Lancet* **1,** 480–4.

Jennett, B. and Carlin, J. (1978) Preventable mortality and morbidity after head injury. *Injury* **10,** 31–9.

Jennett, B. and Plum, F. (1972) Persistent vegetative state after brain damage. *Lancet* **1,** 734–7.

Jennett, B. and Teasdale, G. (1981) *Management of Head Injuries*. Davis, Philadelphia.

Jennett, B., Graham, D.I., Adams, J.H. and Johnston, I.H. (1973) Ischemic damage after fatal blunt head injury. In *Cerebral Vascular Diseases, Eighth Conference* (Eds. McDowell, F.H. and Brennan, R.W.), pp. 163–70. Grune and Stratton, New York.

Jennett, B., Teather, D. and Bennie, S. (1973) Epilepsy after head injury. *Lancet* **2,** 652–3.

Jennett, B., Teasdale, G., Galbraith, S., Pickard, J., Grant, H., Braakman, R. et al. (1977). Severe head injuries in three countries. *Journal of Neurology, Neurosurgery and Psychiatry* **40,** 291–8.

Jennett, S. (1984) Pulmonary function in the head-injured patient. In *Head Injuries and Anaesthesia* (Eds. Fitch, W. and Barker, J.). Elsevier/North-Holland, Amsterdam. In press.

Klatzo, I. (1979) Cerebral oedema and ischaemia. In *Recent Advances in Neuropathology*, 1 (Eds. Smith, W.T. and Cavanagh, J.B.), pp. 27–39. Churchill Livingstone, Edinburgh, London and New York.

Komatsu, S., Sato, T., Kagawa, S., Mori, T. and Hamiki, T. (1979) Traumatic lesions of the corpus callosum. *Neurosurgery* **5,** 32–5.

Krauland, W. (1950) Über Hirnschaden durch stumpfe Gewalt. *Deutsche Zeitschrift für Nervenheilkunde* **163,** 265–328.

Lancet (1983) Caring for the disabled after head injury **2,** 948–9.

Langfitt, T.W., Weinstein, J.D. and Kassell, N.F. (1965) Cerebral vasomotor paralysis produced by intracranial hypertension. *Neurology* **15,** 622–41.

Leestma, J.E., Kalelkar, M.B. and Teas, S. (1983) Pontomedullary avulsion associated with cervical hyperextension. *Acta Neurochirurgica* Suppl. **32,** 69–73.

Lewin, W. (1949) Acute subdural and extradural haematoma in closed head injury. *Annals of the Royal College of Surgeons of England* **5,** 240–74.

Lindenberg, R. (1971) Trauma of meninges and brain. In *Pathology of the Nervous System*, vol. 2 (Ed. Minckler, J.), pp. 1705–65. McGraw Hill, New York.

Lindenberg, R. and Freytag, E. (1957) Morphology of cerebral contusions. *Archives of Pathology* **63,** 23–42.

Lindenberg, R. and Freytag, E. (1960) A mechanism of cerebral contusions: a pathologic–anatomic study. *Archives of Pathology* **69,** 440–69.

Lindenberg, R. and Freytag, E. (1969) Morphology of brain lesions from blunt trauma in infancy. *Archives of Pathology* **87,** 298–305.

Lindenberg, R. and Freytag, E. (1970) Brainstem lesions of traumatic hyperextension of the head. *Archives of Pathology* **90,** 509–15.

Lindenberg, R., Fisher, R., Durlacher, S.H., Lovitt, W.V. and Freytag, E. (1955) Lesions of the corpus callosum following blunt mechanical trauma to the head. *American Journal of Pathology* **31,** 297–317.

McKissock, W., Taylor, J.C., Bloom, W.H. and Till, K. (1960) Extradural haematoma: observations on 125 cases. *Lancet* **2,** 167–72.

McMenemey, W.H., Grant, H.C. and Behrman, S. (1965) Two examples of 'presenile dementia' (Pick's disease and Stern–Garcin syndrome) with a history of trauma. *Archiv für Psychiatrie und Nervenkrankheiten* **208,** 162–76.

Macpherson, P. and Graham, D.I. (1978) Correlation between angiographic findings and the ischaemia of head injury. *Journal of Neurology, Neurosurgery and Psychiatry* **41,** 122–7.

Maloney, A.J.F. and Whatmore, W.J. (1969) Clinical and pathological observations in fatal head injuries—a 5-year study of 172 cases. *British Journal of Surgery* **56,** 23–51.

Martland, H.S. (1928) Punch drunk. *Journal of the American Medical Association* **91,** 1103–7.

Maurer, J.J. and Mayfield, F. H. (1965) Acute bilateral extradural hematomas. *Journal of Neurosurgery* **23,** 63.

Mawdsley, C. and Ferguson, F.R. (1963) Neurological disease in boxers. *Lancet*, **2,** 795–801.

Mazza, C., Pasqualin, A., Ferriotti, G. and da Pian, R. (1982) Traumatic extradural haematoma in children. *Acta Neurochirurgica* **65,** 67–80.

Meyers, C.A., Levin, H.S., Eisenberg, H.M. and Guinto, F.C. (1983) Early versus late lateral ventricular enlargement following closed head injury. *Journal of Neurology, Neurosurgery and Psychiatry* **46,** 1092–7.

Miller, J.D. and Corales, R.L. (1981) Brain edema as a result of head injury: fact or fallacy. In *Brain Edema* (Eds. de Vlieger, M., de Lange, S.A. and Beks, J.W.S.), pp. 99–115. Wiley, New York.

Mitchell, D.E. and Adams, J.H. (1973) Primary focal impact to the brain stem in blunt head injuries: does it exist? *Lancet* **2,** 215–18.

Ommaya, A.K. (1966) Trauma to the nervous system: a clinical and experimental study. *Annals of the Royal College of Surgeons of England* **39,** 317–47.

Ommaya, A.K. and Corrao, P.G. (1970) Pathologic biomechanics of central nervous system injury in head impact and whiplash trauma. In *Accident Pathology* (Ed. Brinkhous, K.M.), pp. 160–81. US Government Printing Office, Washington DC.

Ommaya, A.K., Faas, F. and Yarnell, P. (1968) Whiplash injury and brain damage. *Journal of the American Medical Association* **204,** 285–9.

Ommaya, A.K. and Gennarelli, T.A. (1974) Cerebral concussion and traumatic unconsciousness: correlation of experimental and clinical observations on blunt head injuries. *Brain* **97,** 633–54.

Ommaya, A.K. and Hirsch, A.E. (1971) Tolerance for cerebral concussion from head impact and whiplash in primates. *Journal of Biomechanics* **4,** 13–23.

Ommaya, A.K. and Yarnell, P. (1969)) Subdural haematoma after whiplash injury. *Lancet* **2,** 237–9.

Oppenheimer, D.R. (1968) Microscopic lesions in the brain following head injury. *Journal of Neurology, Neurosurgery and Psychiatry* **31,** 299–306.

Peerless, S.J. and Rewcastle, N.B. (1967) Shear injuries of the brain. *Canadian Medical Association Journal* **96,** 577–82.

Peters, G. and Rothemund, E. (1977) Neuropathology of the traumatic apallic syndrome. In *The Apallic Syndrome* (Eds. Ore, G.D., Gerstenbrand, F., Lucking, C.H., Peters, G. and Peters, U.H.), pp. 78–87. Springer, Berlin.

Pilz, P., Strohecker, J. and Grobovschek, M. (1982) Survival after pontomedullary tear. *Journal of Neurology, Neurosurgery and Psychiatry* **45,** 422–7.

Povlishock, J.T., Becker, D.P., Sullivan, H.G. and Miller, J.D. (1978) Vascular permeability alterations to horseradish peroxidase in experimental brain injury. *Brain Research* **153,** 223–39.

Povlishock, J.T., Becker, D.P., Cheng, C.L.Y. and Vaughan, C.W. (1983) Axonal change in minor head injury. *Journal of Neuropathology and Experimental Neurology* **42,** 225–42.

Pudenz, R.H. and Shelden, C.H. (1946) The lucite calvarium: a method for direct observation of the brain. II. Cranial trauma and brain motion. *Journal of Neurosurgery* **3,** 487–505.

Reilly, P.L., Graham, D.I., Adams, J.H. and Jennett, B. (1975) Patients with head injury who talk and die. *Lancet* **2,** 375–7.

Robinson, R.G. (1970) Cerebrospinal fluid rhinorrhoea, meningitis and pneumocephalus due to non-missile injuries. *Australian and New Zealand Journal of Surgery* **39,** 328–44.

Rosenblum, W.I., Greenberg, R.P., Seelig, J.M. and Becker, D.P. (1981) Midbrain lesions: frequent and significant prognostic features in closed head injury. *Neurosurgery* **9,** 613–20.

Sarwar, M. and McCormick, W.F. (1978) Decrease in ventricular and sulcal size after death. *Radiology* **127,** 409–11.

Seelig, J.M., Becker, D.P., Miller, J.D., Greenberg, R.P., Ward, J.D. and Choi, S.C. (1981) Traumatic acute subdural haematoma. *New England Journal of Medicine* **304,** 1511–18.

Sights, W.P. (1969) Ballistic analysis of shot gun injuries to the central nervous system. *Journal of Neurosurgery* **31,** 25–33.

Simpson, D., Antonio, J.B., North, J.B., Ring, I.T., Selecki, B.R. and Sewell, M.F. (1981) Fatal injuries of the head and spine. Epidemiological studies in New South Wales and South Australia. *Medical Journal of Australia* **2,** 660–4.

Snoek, J., Jennett, B., Adams, J.H., Graham, D.I. and Doyle, D. (1979) Computerised tomography after recent severe head injury in patients without acute intracranial haematoma. *Journal of Neurology, Neurosurgery and Psychiatry* **42,** 215–25.

Stein, B.M. and Tenner, M.S. (1972) Enlargement of skull fracture in childhood due to cerebral herniation. *Archives of Neurology* **26,** 137–43.

Strich, S.J. (1956) Diffuse degeneration of the cerebral white matter in severe dementia following head injury. *Journal of Neurology, Neurosurgery and Psychiatry* **19,** 163–85.

Strich, S.J. (1961) Shearing of nerve fibres as a cause of brain damage due to head injury. *Lancet* **2,** 443–8.

Strich, S.J. (1968) Notes on the Marchi method for staining degenerating myelin in the peripheral and central nervous system. *Journal of Neurology, Neurosurgery and Psychiatry* **31,** 110–14.

Strich, S.J. (1969) The pathology of brain damage due to blunt head injuries. In *The Late Effects of Head Injury* (Eds. Walker, A.E., Caveness, W.F. and Critchley, M.), pp. 501–24. Thomas, Springfield, Illinois.

Strich, S.J. (1970) Lesions in the cerebral hemispheres after blunt head injury. In *The Pathology of Trauma* (Eds. Sevitt, S. and Stoner, H.B.), *Journal of Clinical Pathology* **23,** Suppl. (Royal College of Pathologists) 4, 166–71.

Strich, S.J. (1976) Cerebral trauma. In *Greenfield's Neuropathology*, 3rd edn (Eds. Blackwood, W. and Corsellis, J.A.N.), pp. 327–60. Edward Arnold, London.

Symonds, C.P. (1940) Concussion and contusion of the brain. In *Injuries of the Skull, Brain and Spinal Cord* (Ed. Brock, S.), pp. 71–115. Baillière, London.

Symonds, C. (1962) Concussion and its sequelae. *Lancet* **1,** 1-5.

Teasdale, G.M. and Galbraith, S. (1981) Acute traumatic intracranial hematomas. In *Progress in Neurological Surgery*, vol. 10 (Eds. Krayenbuhl, H., Maspes, P.E. and Sweet, W.H.), pp. 252-90. Karger, Basel.

Teasdale, E., Cardoso, E., Galbraith, S. and Teasdale, G. (1984). CT scan in severe diffuse head injury: physiological and clinical correlations. *Journal of Neurology, Neurosurgery and Psychiatry* **47,** 600-603.

Tomlinson, B.E. (1970) Brain-stem lesions after head injury. In *The Pathology of Trauma* (Eds. Sevitt, S. and Stoner, H.B.), *Journal of Clinical Pathology* **23,** Suppl. (Royal College of Pathologists) **4,** 154-65.

Tornheim, P.A. and McLaurin, R.L. (1978) Effect of dexamethasone on cerebral edema from cranial impact in the cat. *Journal of Neurosurgery* **48,** 220-7.

Treip, C.S. (1970) Hypothalamic and pituitary injury. In *The Pathology of Trauma* (Eds. Sevitt, S. and Stoner, H.B.), *Journal of Clinical Pathology* **23,** Suppl. (Royal College of Pathologists), 4, 154-65.

Unterharnscheidt, F. and Higgins, L.S. (1969) Traumatic lesions of the brain and spinal cord due to non-deforming angular acceleration of the head. *Texas Reports on Biology and Medicine* **27,** 127-66.

Voigt, G.E., Lowenheilm, P. and Ljung, C.B.A. (1977) Rotational cerebral injuries near the superior margin of the brain. *Acta Neuropathologica* **39,** 201-9.

Welte, E. (1948) Über die Zusammenhänge zwischen anatomischem Befund und Klinischem Bild bei Rindenprellungsherden nach stumpfen Schädeltrauma. *Archiv für Psychiatrie und Nervenkrankheiten* **179,** 243-315.

Wilkins, R.H. and Odom, G.L. (1970) Intracranial arterial spasm associated with craniocerebral trauma. *Journal of Neurosurgery* **32,** 626-33.

Zimmerman, R.A., Larissa, T., Bilaniuk, L.T. and Gennarelli, T.A. (1978) Computed tomography of shearing injuries of the cerebral white matter. *Radiology* **127,** 393-6.

4

Hypoxia and vascular disorders of the central nervous system

J.B. Brierley and D.I. Graham

The aim of the first part of this chapter is to provide a reasonably comprehensive account of the general and local effects on the brain of a reduction in the supply or utilization of oxygen and substrate. The main forms of cerebral damage resulting from these disturbances are cerebral infarction, with its important immediate or delayed effects, and selective neuronal necrosis (the ischaemic cell process). The principal pathophysiological mechanisms underlying these changes are discussed. The second part consists of an account of the more common cerebrovascular disorders apart from intracranial haemorrhage and its effects on the brain, which are considered in Chapter 5.

The term *hypoxic* rather than *ischaemic* will be used even though it is likely that much of this type of brain damage is due to reduced cerebral perfusion; a reduced oxygen content of the blood may, however, potentiate any physiological stress. There are many causes of irreversible hypoxic brain damage but they can be divided into three principal types. First, those due to a deficiency of oxygen and/or glucose (both essential for maintaining the viability of the nervous system); second, those due to an inadequate blood flow (disorders of the cardiovascular system); and third, those in which there is a combination of metabolic and cardiovascular factors. The neuropathology of all three may be the same.

The energy requirements of the brain demand adequate supplies of oxygen and glucose. Normally, about 90 per cent of the energy needed for the transmission of electrical impulses and the maintenance of ionic gradients across cell membranes is obtained from the oxidation of glucose. As neither of these substances is stored in the brain, it is inevitably susceptible to their deficiency. Considerable clinical evidence suggests that certain areas of the brain survive for only a few minutes if the oxygen supply is reduced below a critical level.

Irreversible hypoxic damage may occur as a consequence of such diverse conditions as respiratory obstruction, lung and heart disease, shock, epilepsy, hypoglycaemia, carbon monoxide poisoning, cardiac arrest, an episode of severe hypotension or a variety of anaesthetic accidents. The ultimate degree of neurological recovery is determined by the severity of the initial stress and whether adequate resuscitation was begun before brain damage had become irreversible. Crises of this kind are not uncommon in clinical practice, yet the critical duration of hypoxia representing the threshold between recovery and permanent brain damage in man remains controversial. Physiological monitoring is minimal or absent in these acute situations, the obvious priority being resuscitation. There is also a paucity of systematic neuropathological studies of fatal cases.

Hypoxia and the central nervous system

Whatever the circumstances, the final common denominators of hypoxic brain damage are a reduced content of oxygen or glucose in the blood and a reduced blood flow to the brain—

usually in combination. Each is provided by the functions of respiration and circulation, some aspects of which must be considered before the neuropathology of hypoxic brain damage is described.

Respiration

At sea level the atmospheric pressure is 101.3 kPa (760 mmHg) of which the partial pressure of oxygen is 19.9 kPa (149 mmHg). The stream of oxygen from the atmosphere to the neuronal mitochondria can be envisaged as a cascade over five successive steps (Fig. 4.1). Within the pulmonary alveoli the oxygen tension is reduced to 14 kPa (105 mmHg) because of the presence of carbon dioxide and water vapour. The small difference between the oxygen tensions in alveoli (14 kPa, 105 mmHg) and arterial blood (12.8 kPa, 96 mmHg) is not due to restricted diffusion from one to the other, but to venous admixture from bronchopulmonary veins and to a few pulmonary arteriovenous shunts. Oxygen tension falls largely in capillaries and is about 4.5 kPa (34 mmHg) in the veins and venous sinuses of the brain.

Because of the close coupling between cerebral function and the production of adenosine triphosphate (ATP), the overall energy metabolism of the brain can be deduced from the amount of oxygen or glucose consumed. In many studies in normal adult resting subjects the cerebral metabolic rate for oxygen (CMR O_2) has been derived from blood flow and arteriovenous differences of between 3.2 and 3.8 ml O_2/100 g per minute. Higher values (5.1 ml O_2/100 g per minute) are found in children.

The oxygen content of blood falls from 19.6 ml/dl to 12.9 ml/dl while passing through the brain, so 6.7 ml of O_2/dl blood are used to meet the requirements of brain oxidative metabolism. Carbon dioxide content rises from 48.2 ml/dl in arterial blood to 54.8 ml/dl in the internal jugular vein, so the brain produces 6.6 ml CO_2/dl blood. Thus the respiratory quotient (CO_2/O_2) of the brain is almost unity, indicating that glucose is virtually the sole source of energy by oxidation.

Signs of cerebral hypoxia appear when the arterial oxygen tension ($Pa{O_2}$) falls below 6.7 kPa (50 mmHg), when there is a rapid loss of critical judgement, progressive impairment of performance and clouding of consciousness leading to unconsciousness at a $Pa{O_2}$ of about 4.0 kPa (30 mmHg) and a cerebral venous $P{O_2}$ below 2.6 kPa (20 mmHg) (Ernsting, 1966). The precise relationships between symptoms and signs and the cerebral energy state in hypoxia have not been defined in man. Considerable information, however, is now available from animal experiments (see Siesjö, 1978).

More recently, in a primate model developed from that of Levine (1960), Brierley et al. (1980) found that if arterial oxygenation was lowered progressively (normal blood flow being maintained), metabolism and function were affected

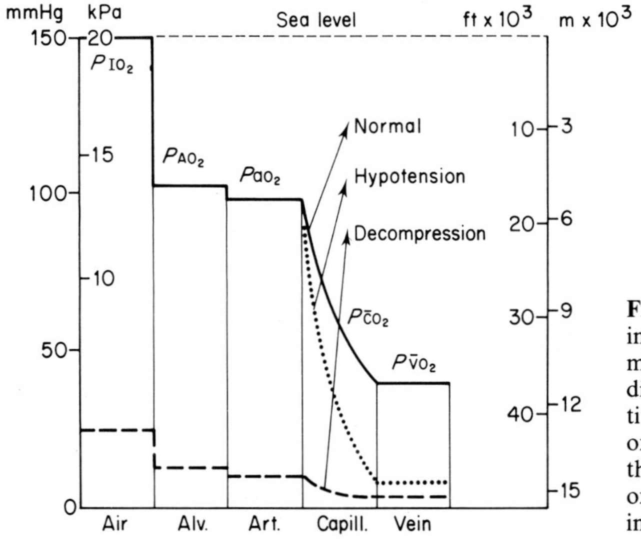

Fig. 4.1 The decrease in oxygen tension from inspired air to venous blood ('oxygen cascade'; modified from Luft and Finkelstein, 1968). Ordinate = PO_2 (mmHg) and corresponding altitudes (feet and metres). Hypotension—venous oxygen tension is low as a result of reduced flow through the capillary bed. Decompression—oxygen tension is reduced at each step from inspired air to venous blood.

only when Pa_{O_2} was reduced from 2.8 to 3.2 kPa (21 to 24 mmHg) for at least 8 minutes. Hypoxia of this severity was associated with an isoelectric EEG and the production of brain damage. It should be stressed, however, that the primate brain is able to tolerate a Pa_{O_2} of about 3.3 kPa (25 mmHg) without the EEG being affected and without brain damage as long as a normal cerebral perfusion, even *via* one single common carotid artery, is maintained.

Circulation

The normal adult brain receives about 15 per cent of the cardiac output even though the brain accounts for only 2.5 per cent of the body weight; i.e. the mean blood flow to the brain is about 50 ml/100 g per minute in the adult and about twice as high in children aged 6 years because of their higher respiratory rate (McIlwain and Bachelard, 1971). Flow within grey matter (80–100 ml/100 g per minute) is higher than that in white (20–25 ml/100 g per minute), reflecting the greater metabolic activity and vasculature of grey matter.

The relationship between perfusion pressure and cerebral blood flow is critical for the outcome in situations as diverse as shock, surgery under hypotension and raised intracranial pressure. This relationship is governed primarily by *autoregulation* of cerebral blood flow, which is the intrinsic tendency of the brain brought about by arteriolar dilatation or constriction to maintain a relatively constant blood flow in response to moderate variations in perfusion pressure (Lassen, 1959). There are defined upper and lower limits of arterial blood pressure over which autoregulation can maintain a normal cerebral blood flow in man (8.7–18.7 kPa; 65–140 mmHg). At the lower limit the vessels are dilated, the autoregulatory mechanism fails and flow falls as the pressure decreases. Symptoms of cerebral ischaemia do not develop immediately since the brain can extract more oxygen. At the upper limit cerebral vasoconstriction cannot be sustained and the blood flow increases. This is the upper limit or the 'breakthrough' of autoregulation. Any factor altering the ability of the cerebral vessels to constrict or dilate interferes with autoregulation. As perfusion pressure falls, vasodilatation is greatest in the anastomotic vessels along the arterial boundary zones (Brierley et al., 1969), which are the first regions in which flow is reduced to a critical level.

The rate of blood flow through the brain depends upon two factors: the pressure difference, known as the *cerebral perfusion pressure*, between arteries and veins; and the *cerebrovascular resistance* of the intervening vessels. The latter is determined by the intracranial pressure (< 0.7 kPa (5 mmHg) normally), the viscosity of the blood and the tone of the smooth muscle in the vessel walls. This muscle tone is influenced by the intracranial pressure, the tensions of oxygen and carbon dioxide in the blood and also its pH. As the pressure inside the cerebral veins is only slightly greater than that of the cerebrospinal fluid or intracranial pressure, the cerebral perfusion pressure is commonly regarded as the difference between systemic arterial pressure and the *intracranial pressure*. The interactions between these two pressures are complex and a critical point is reached when the intracranial pressure rises to within about 5.9 kPa (44 mmHg) of the mean systemic arterial pressure, after which cerebral blood flow falls.

The maintenance of normal overall brain blood flow ('volume flow') depends on cardiac output, systemic blood pressure and peripheral vascular resistance. Thus the supply of oxygen and substrate may be compromised by impaired action of the heart, by stenosis of supplying vessels down to arteriolar level and by any rise in central venous pressure. At normal blood pressure the internal cross-sectional area of an artery must be reduced by up to 90 per cent before blood flow is impaired (Tindall et al., 1962; Brice, Dowsett and Lowe, 1964). On the other hand, a considerably smaller degree of stenosis can lead to a reduction in blood flow if the blood pressure falls. There is also evidence from angiographic studies (Kuhn, 1962) that the 'velocity flow' of the blood in the vertebrobasilar system is less than that in the carotid arterial system, an observation which may be relevant to the more severe involvement of the posterior parts of the cerebral hemispheres in most types of brain hypoxia.

Cerebral energy supply

Energy is produced in the brain almost entirely from the oxidative metabolism of glucose. This energy is needed for the synthesis of large molecules, transport mechanisms, the maintenance of membrane potentials and neurotransmitter metabolism. The amount of glucose consumed is very high (0.3 mmol per minute; 60 mg per minute), reflecting the inability of the brain to make use of other substrates.

Oxidative metabolism of glucose yields energy in the form of high-energy phosphate compounds, the most important of which is ATP. The metabolism of one molecule of glucose produces 38 molecules of ATP. When the supply of oxygen is so low that metabolism changes to a largely anaerobic form and glucose is partially oxidized to lactic acid, only some 5 per cent of potential energy within the molecule is available. The possibility that substrates other than glucose (e.g. ketone bodies) may support energy production in the brain has been discusssed recently (see Siesjö, 1978).

Terminology

Anoxia implies an absence of oxygen in the pulmonary alveoli. In *hypoxia* alveolar oxygen tension is reduced, leading to a corresponding hypoxaemia. *Ischaemia* implies an arrest of flow within the whole or some part of the circulation; *oligaemia* implies a reduced blood flow. *Consumptive hypoxia* occurs when the oxygen requirements of hyperactive neurons exceed the available supply. *Asphyxia* is usually taken to mean suffocation (Van Liere and Stickney, 1963).

The categories of brain hypoxia

Brain damage does not result from either uncomplicated hypoxic hypoxia or uncomplicated anaemic hypoxia (with the clear exception of carbon monoxide poisoning). Commonly, at least two aetiological factors are involved in any one case, but in most brain damage is due to reduced perfusion pressure. The most complex states are febrile convulsions and status epilepticus. Other categories include those due to poisoning of brain respiratory enzymes (histotoxic hypoxia) and the lack of the chief metabolic substrate, glucose (hypoglycaemia). Thus the following classification of brain hypoxia is based on Barcroft (1925) and takes account of the views of Van Liere and Stickney (1963), Luft (1965) and Brierley (1976).

Stagnant hypoxia (ischaemic and oligaemic)

Ischaemic The brain or some part of it is deprived of its blood supply.
Oligaemic The brain or some part of it receives a reduced supply of blood.

Anoxic and hypoxic hypoxia

Anoxia In the absence of oxygen in the pulmonary alveoli, there is anoxaemia and a little later anoxia in brain tissue.
Hypoxia A reduced oxygen tension in the alveoli leads to brain tissue hypoxia through the medium of hypoxaemia.

Anaemic hypoxia

Because of a reduced haemoglobin content, the oxygen content of the blood is reduced while oxygen saturation and tension may be normal. This situation may be brought about by restoration of plasma volume after blood loss, and by anaemia. There is no evidence that uncomplicated anaemic hypoxia can lead to brain damage.

Carbon monoxide poisoning, by reducing the amount of circulating haemoglobin available to combine with oxygen, is the only example of anaemic hypoxia known to produce hypoxic damage in grey and white matter.

Histotoxic hypoxia (Peters and Van Slyke, 1932)

The oxygen tension and content of arterial blood are normal while those in cerebral venous blood are raised because the poisoning of brain respiratory enzymes (e.g. by cyanide) results in a failure to utilize oxygen.

Hypoglycaemia

In spite of a normal arterial oxygen tension the brain is unable to utilize oxygen because of a deficiency of glucose (oxyachrestia; Lawrence, Meyer and Nevin, 1942).

Structural changes resulting from hypoxia

Nerve cells are more vulnerable to oxygen deficiency than oligodendroglia and astrocytes, while the microglia and the blood vessels are least vulnerable (Jacob, 1963).

Neurons of the phylogenetically older portions of the nervous system are more resistant than the newer. The grey matter of the spinal cord and most of that in the adult brain stem may be undamaged in the presence of almost total destruction of the cerebral cortex. In contrast, the brain stem in children is more vulnerable. After any episode of hypoxia, structural damage may be limited to nerve cells (*selective neuronal necrosis*) but if more severe, may also involve glia, nerve fibres and blood vessels. This level of damage also constitutes an infarct which is described later in this chapter.

Alterations in neurons

The identification of neuronal alterations unequivocally attributable to hypoxia is critically dependent upon satisfactory fixation of tissue. This is because certain stages in the course of hypoxic neuronal damage can be confused with artefact (see Chapter 1). In the human brain, histological artefact may be due to autolysis, the rate of cooling of the body, the slow penetration of fixative and the processing of the tissue.

The use of perfusion-fixation has permitted the identification, with the light microscope, of neuronal alterations in the primate brain 20 minutes after an episode of controlled hypoxia. Evidence from experimental primates is combined with that from the human brain in the following descriptions of the neuronal alterations due to hypoxia.

Whilst immersion-fixation of the brain will obscure the earliest stages of hypoxic neuronal abnormalities because of histological artefact, the later stages of the same process after a survival of days or weeks are easily recognizable as a loss of nerve cells and a developing gliomesodermal reaction.

Although the neuronal alterations in types of hypoxia are relatively stereotyped, they vary greatly in their distribution, and so characteristic patterns can be recognized. The adequate delineation of the consequences of hypoxia demands the examination of numerous large blocks which include representative regions of the cortex including the arterial boundary zones, the hippocampus at at least two levels, the basal ganglia, the brain stem, the spinal cord, and both cerebellar hemispheres and the vermis.

The ischaemic cell process This begins with early and subtle alterations in the neuron and ends with its disappearance. It can be encountered in many situations other than circulatory arrest. In the latter instance, however, it can be initiated only if there is an early restoration of blood flow. Studies in experimental primates and in selected human material have shown that the time-course of this alteration is constant for neurons according to their site and size.

Given optimal histology, the interval between a hypoxic episode and death can be determined with reasonable accuracy in the brain of an experimental animal. In the human brain, however, prediction will be less accurate since all factors relevant to fixation cannot be controlled.

The earliest stage of the ischaemic cell process is *microvacuolation* (Brown and Brierley, 1966; Brierley, Brown and Meldrum, 1971a, b). The stage of simple *ischaemic cell change* follows that of microvacuolation. The succeeding stages are *ischaemic cell change with incrustations*, and finally *homogenizing cell change* (Brown, 1977) and eventual disappearance of the neuron (see Chapter 1).

Associated glial and mesodermal reactions

Whilst the time-course of the neuronal alterations following a critical period of hypoxia of any type is rapid, the greater part of the astrocytic and the whole of the microglial and mesodermal reactions take place after neurons have been irreversibly damaged (i.e. after the stage of microvacuolation) and may continue for months. These reactions are proportional to the extent of neuronal destruction. Thus, if selective neuronal necrosis is mild, the gliomesodermal reaction is also mild; if it is severe, the reaction is intense and the tissue comes ultimately to be represented by firm shrunken scar (sclerosis) in certain laminae of the neocortex and certain zones of the hippocampus. When hypoxic damage attains the level of infarction, astrocytic and gliomesodermal reactions are restricted to the periphery of the necrotic regions and to zones around viable vessels within the infarct. When the damage is less severe, fibre-forming astrocytes proliferate and their processes, together with collagen and reticulin fibres derived from mesodermal sources, contribute to the formation of a gliomesodermal network within which occasional neurons may survive.

Alterations in the *oligodendrocytes* within a region of hypoxic damage are slight and seldom more than the 'acute swelling' described by Penfield and Cone (1926). This type of cell change is non-specific and may be artefactual, as it is seldom seen in comparable regions of hypoxic damage in the brains of experimental primates fixed by perfusion.

The intrinsic or indigenous *microglia*, where hypoxic damage is purely neuronal, are transformed into rod cells (Stäbchenzellen) which are characteristically orientated at right angles to the pial surface of the neocortex, radially within the hippocampus and in the molecular layer of the cerebellum, and more or less haphazardly in the basal ganglia and brain stem. Rod cells are often more apparent than neuronal loss when this is minor (e.g. in the Ammon's horn and in the cerebellum). After a survival of 2 or 3 days, fine lipid droplets may be seen in their cytoplasm and a little later division by mitosis takes place (Brierley and Brown, 1982a). The daughter cells develop into typical lipid phagocytes which may have no obvious relationship to nerve cells and are probably involved in the removal of myelin debris. Others lying close to dead neurons divide by mitosis, so the original contour of the nerve cell becomes outlined by a capsule of microglial cells and lipid phagocytes.

When hypoxic damage is restricted to nerve cells, the blood vessels may be entirely normal and there is no evidence of escape of any haematogenous elements into the tissue. After infarction only the peripheral arteries may be preserved and the fibroblasts in their adventitia are the source of lipid phagocytes (Brierley and Brown, 1982b). Similar lipid phagocytes are also derived from the pia mater.

Lipid phagocytes do not migrate actively from the sites of their formation and the pattern of their distribution after long survival mirrors the original destruction of tissue (Fig. 4.2).

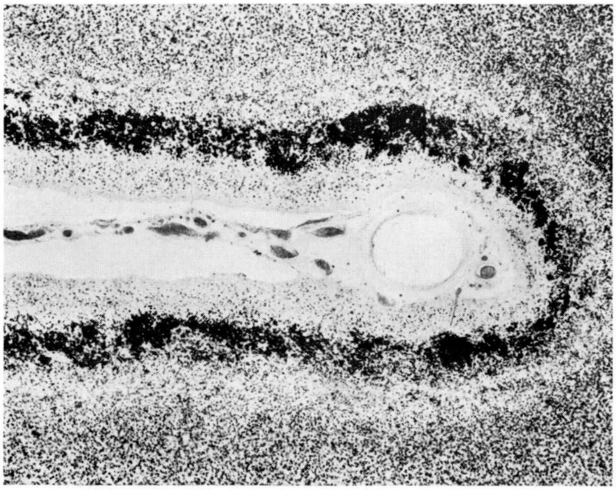

Fig. 4.2 Male, aged 17 years, dying 9 months after cardiac arrest. Occipital lobe showing laminar disposition of lipid phagocytes. Celloidin; Marchi × 15.

Associated changes in white matter

Hypoxic damage when restricted to a small proportion of a vulnerable neuronal population causes only limited destruction of the intrinsic nerve fibres and no primary alteration in the surrounding white matter. With increasing neuronal destruction some pallor of myelin staining is seen in the adjacent white matter. Within a day or so, however, rod cells become conspicuous in the affected region, and after a week or more lipid phagocytes can be identified. In the extreme situation of subtotal cortical destruction (a rare sequel of circulatory arrest) virtually the whole of each centrum semiovale is occupied by lipid phagocytes with some accumulation around blood vessels. After long survival, wallerian degeneration may be seen in the corticospinal tracts as a consequence of neuronal destruction in the precentral gyri (Fig. 4.3). White matter damage may be seen after cardiac arrest, hypoglycaemia, neonatal hypoxaemia, and carbon disulphide and sodium nitrite intoxication (Brucher, 1967).

Primary hypoxic alterations in white matter may be diffuse or focal. When diffuse there is loss of myelin in each centrum semiovale, spreading

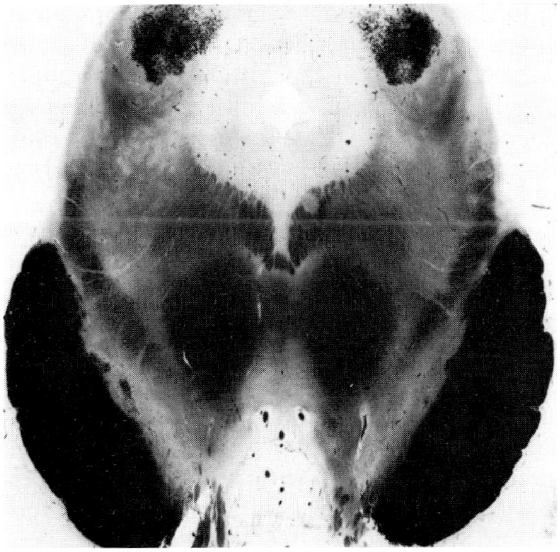

Fig. 4.3 Male, aged 17 years, dying 9 months after cardiac arrest. Midbrain. Marchi-positive staining in cerebral peduncles indicates wallerian degeneration in tracts descending from neurons destroyed at higher levels. Celloidin; Marchi.

from the periventricular region into the digitate white matter but usually sparing the subcortical U-fibres. The corpus callosum, anterior commissure and the white matter of the cerebellum may also be involved. Sometimes there is relative preservation of myelin around blood vessels giving a speckled or 'thrush breast' appearance. After survival of a few days, the region of myelin destruction presents a spongy and often finely cystic texture; in cases with longer survival, the small cysts may become confluent to form larger ones which may be visible to the naked eye.

Focal damage appears as more or less circumscribed lesions within which destruction of myelin and axons is virtually complete with a corresponding population of lipid phagocytes.

'Selective vulnerability' within the brain—morphological aspects

The neuropathological consequences of hypoxia depend on the number of cellular elements involved and the survival time. Although differences between nerve cells in their susceptibility to a lack of oxygen were appreciated by the end of the last century, the elaboration of the concept of selective vulnerability to hypoxia has been due, in particular, to Spielmeyer (1925), Scholz (1953, 1963) and Meyer (1936, 1956, 1963).

The pattern of 'selective vulnerability'

In its classic form this is seen after an episode of cardiorespiratory arrest. Recently it has been suggested that the concept of selective vulnerability is also applicable in instances of focal ischaemia. For example, evidence of neuronal necrosis may be limited to certain layers of the cortex after occlusion of the middle cerebral artery in man, and also in the rat (Brown and Brierley, 1968), the gerbil (Levy, Brierley and Plum, 1975) and the primate (Little, Sundt and Kerr, 1974). In the four-vessel occlusion model in the rat (Pulsinelli, Brierley and Plum, 1982) there is a greater reduction of cerebral blood flow in the deeper than in the more superficial layers of the cortex (Pulsinelli, Levy and Duffy, 1982), these changes corresponding to evidence of selective neuronal necrosis in layers three, five and six. However, in this particular model of hypoxia–ischaemia the time-course of the ischaemic cell process is markedly retarded compared with other models and man.

Neocortex Damage is usually greater in the parietal and occipital lobes and decreases towards the temporal and frontal poles. Damage is commonly greater in the depths and sides of sulci than over the crests of gyri. Among the cortical layers the third is the most vulnerable, and the fifth and sixth are somewhat less; the second and fourth layers are the most resistant.

Allocortex The convexities of the *parahippocampal gyri* with the islets of Calleja on their dorsal surfaces are remarkably resistant to hypoxia. The entorhinal region and subiculum are often involved in continuity with ischaemic damage in the latter. Within the hippocampus (Ammon's horn), the Sommer sector (CA 1) and the end folium (CA 3 to CA 4) are the most vulnerable, whilst CA 2 is often referred to as the 'resistant zone'. The fascia dentata (dentate gyrus) is the least vulnerable zone of the hippocampus.

Basal ganglia In the *striatum* ischaemic alterations are most frequent within the outer halves of the head and body of the caudate nucleus and in the outer half of the putamen. In each, the small polymorphic cells are more vulnerable than the larger pyramidal elements. In addition to the special case of carbon monoxide intoxication (see p. 145) damage in the *pallidum* may occur in all types of hypoxia. There is no evidence for an intrinsic difference between the vulnerabilities of the two segments. Primary hypoxic damage in the *thalamus* is commonest in the anterior nuclear complex, followed by the dorsomedial nuclei (parvocellular portions) and the lateral angles of the ventrolateral nuclei. Involvement of the centromedian nuclei is infrequent whilst the sensory relay nuclei, together with the midline and intralaminar nuclei, may be regarded as the most resistant in the thalamus. Alterations in the geniculate bodies are also unusual, and when present usually involve the lateral geniculate body. In the *amygdaloid nucleus* the more superficial or corticomedial portion is resistant and the deeper or basolateral portion is relatively vulnerable; damage in the latter is usually associated with severe ischaemic changes in the hippocampus.

The supraoptic, paraventricular and lateral nuclei of the *hypothalamus* are very rarely affected by hypoxia. Alterations in the mamillary bodies are rare in adults but frequent in infants and young children.

In the adult *brain stem* the reticular zones of the substantia nigra, the inferior colliculi and the inferior olives are relatively vulnerable. In infants and young children there may be additional ischaemic alterations in the oculomotor nuclei, the spinal nuclei of the fifth nerves, the cochlear and vestibular nuclei, the nuclei ambigui, and the gracile and cuneati nuclei in the lower medulla.

In the *cerebellar cortex* the Purkinje and basket cells are most vulnerable, followed by the granule cells whilst the Golgi cells are the most resistant. Alterations in the dentate nuclei and in the roof nuclei are usually considerably less than those in the Purkinje cells.

Arterial boundary zones (border zones) As a consequence of a rapid and considerable reduction in cerebral perfusion pressure as occurs with hypotension, hypoxic brain damage may be restricted to the arterial boundary zones (originally termed 'watersheds') in the neocortex and cerebellum (see Fig. 4.11). Experimental studies in primates have shown that, in the absence of hypoxaemia or a significant reduction of blood pH, ischaemic brain damage accentuated along the arterial boundary zones can be induced by reducing the cerebral perfusion pressure to 3.3 kPa (25 mmHg) and the maintenance of an isoelectric EEG for at least 15 minutes. Under these conditions vasodilatation is maximal, cerebral blood flow is pressure dependent, and, as a result of the unique anatomy of the cortical arterial supply, flow is first reduced to a critical level along the boundary zones (Brierley and Excell, 1966; Brierley et al., 1969; Meldrum and Brierley, 1969).

A similar pattern of ischaemic brain damage has been induced by Brierley et al. (1980) in lightly anaesthetized baboons spontaneously breathing an oxygen nitrogen mixture with a $Pa\text{O}_2$ of between 2.9 and 3.3 kPa (22 and 25 mmHg) for some 20 minutes before occluding one and then the other common carotid artery. This pattern of brain damage has also been induced in baboons with renovascular hypertension submitted to halothane-induced hypotension (Fitch et al., 1978), and after the intracarotid injection of air (Meldrum and Brierley, 1971).

This pattern of damage has been described in man after dental anaesthesia in a semi-recumbent position (Brierley and Miller, 1966), after the overzealous treatment of malignant hypertension by antihypertensive agents (Graham, 1975) and in the brains of patients dying from non-missile head injuries (Graham, Adams and Doyle, 1978).

When ischaemic brain damage occurs along the arterial boundary zones, the critical factor is a reduction in the availability of tissue oxygen, usually because of a local reduction in cerebral blood flow. The vulnerability of the arterial boundary zones is a consequence of the anastomosis of small vessels with their counterparts from adjacent arterial fields. Once the capacity for autoregulation of blood flow is lost as a result of some combination of reduced perfusion pressure and hypoxaemia, oxygen falls to a critical level in those parts of the arterial territories that are most remote from the parent stems (i.e. along the boundary zones).

The influence of maturity on hypoxic brain damage Hypoxic brain damage in the fetus and newborn infant accounts for a high proportion of children with cerebral palsy, mental retardation and epilepsy (see Chapter 11).

Periventricular leucomalacia is the common hypoxic lesion in the preterm brain. It is widely accepted as being due to failure of perfusion along the boundary zones between the centripetal and centrifugal arteries within the brain (Takashima and Tanaka, 1978). Probably prolonged apnoea or peripheral circulatory failure in the preterm infant may lead to severe hypotension: autoregulation of cerebral blood flow becomes deranged and cerebral hypoxia develops.

The pattern of hypoxic brain damage seen after birth asphyxia in the term infant is variable, and includes damage to the cortex, the white matter, the basal ganglia, the cerebellum and the brain stem (Wigglesworth and Pape, 1978). The several patterns of brain damage are similar to those that can be produced in fetal monkeys (see Myers, 1977). From these studies it is evident that many factors other than hypoxia determine the range and severity of brain lesions in preterm and term infant brains.

Only recently has a suitable model of perinatal hypoxic damage in the small laboratory animal become available. In the Levine preparation in 7-day-old postnatal rats, Rice, Vannucci and Brierley (1981) induced severe hypoxic neuronal damage on the same side as the ligated common carotid artery in 90 per cent. In contrast to the pattern of damage in adult animals, there was in the immature rats also necrosis of white matter spreading out from myelinogenic foci. The evolution of the hypoxic neuronal change and the associated gliomesodermal reaction were more rapid than in the adult.

Categories of brain hypoxia

Stagnant hypoxia

There are two types: ischaemic and oligaemic. In both the brain or some part of it is either deprived of (ischaemic) or receives a reduced (oligaemic) supply of blood.

Ischaemic hypoxia—localized If the blood flow through an artery is arrested, an *infarct* will develop that may affect an entire arterial territory or only part of it. If a middle cerebral artery is occluded and there is no collateral inflow, a massive infarct is the inevitable result. Usually, however, there is some collateral circulation by way of the anterior and posterior cerebral arteries with the result that the blood flow through only part of the middle cerebral arterial territory falls below the level necessary to maintain tissue viability. The resulting infarct is usually of the central type but if the collateral inflow from the anterior cerebral territory exceeds that from the posterior cerebral, the infarct 'moves' towards the latter territory. Occasionally the collateral circulation may be so adequate that the infarct is limited to the basal ganglia and the internal capsule. These structures, unlike the cortex, will be spared if the occlusion lies distal to the origin of the penetrating and ganglionic branches of the major cerebral arteries.

Factors influencing the size of an infarct, especially in the cortex, include the functional efficiency of superficial cortical anastomotic vessels (Hutchinson and Yates, 1961; Baker, Dahl and Sandler, 1963) and the configuration of the circle of Willis. The latter is anatomically 'normal' in only some 50 per cent of adults (Alpers, 1959), with an even higher incidence of anatomical variation in patients with cerebral infarcts *post mortem* (Alpers and Berry, 1963; Riggs and Rupp, 1963). Other factors include disease of the major neck arteries (Hutchinson and Yates, 1961) and the level of systemic blood pressure. If all of these are normal, the cortical infarct will be small; if one or more are abnormal, the lesion will be large.

The blood supply to the basal ganglia and the deep white matter is critical because the penetrating and ganglionic branches of the major cerebral arteries are end-arteries. This implies that proximal occlusion of a large cerebral artery will produce a deeply placed infarct as retrograde flow from adjacent anastomotic channels is limited. In the healthy subhuman primate, division of the proximal middle cerebral artery results in an infarct that may be limited to the internal capsule (Symon and Brierley, 1976). In many other experimental models of focal ischaemia the lesions have been larger, affecting cortex, white matter and basal ganglia (Molinari and Laurent, 1976; Waltz, 1979), emphasizing the importance of two factors in the pathogenesis of cerebral infarction in man, viz. some impairment of cardiac function with a reduction in cerebral blood flow and some degree of stenotic and/or occlusive vascular disease. Therefore in an autopsy on a patient who has died with a cerebral infarct the heart, major neck arteries and circle of Willis must be examined.

Ischaemic hypoxia—generalized The sequence of events following abrupt and total interruption of the human cerebral circulation was described by Rossen, Kabat and Anderson (1943). Five seconds after inflation of a pneumatic pressure cuff around the neck, the eyes became fixed in the midline, the visual fields narrowed sometimes to the point of blindness, and consciousness was lost at the sixth second. From the start of nitrogen overbreathing (anoxic anoxia) consciousness is lost at 17–20 seconds. The period of 6 seconds represents the oxygen reserve of the tissue whilst the additional 11–14 seconds represent the circulation time between heart and brain and the time required for the blood to become desaturated.

Cessation of circulation to the brain occurs only in the event of systemic circulatory arrest, and, if not deliberate, as in open heart surgery under hypothermia, is usually due to cardiac asystole or ventricular fibrillation and is most commonly a complication of surgery under general anaesthesia at normal body temperature. Cardiac arrest accounted for 212 deaths in the series of 517 151 anaesthetics (i.e. 1 in 2384) surveyed by Stephenson, Reid and Hinton (1953) and for 199 deaths in the series of 600 000 (i.e. 1 in 3018) reported by Beecher and Todd (1954), both series coming from the USA. Corresponding figures for the UK are not available because such cases are registered only as 'anaesthetic deaths'. Milstein (1956) estimated cardiac arrest related to surgery to be the cause of about 300 deaths per year in the UK. According to Wylie (1975) the number of such deaths in England and Wales had fallen to 100 per annum by 1970. The incidence is slightly higher in males than in females (6:4) and 20 per cent of all cases occur during the first decade of life. Whilst the nature of the anaesthetic agent may influence the frequency of cardiac arrest there is no convincing evidence that any one anaesthetic is associated with a specific neuropathological picture.

The prognosis is good in patients who, after resuscitation, regain consciousness quickly with complete neurological recovery. However, many remain unconscious and die within 24 hours of the cardiac arrest (see Willoughby and Leach, 1974). Modern methods of resuscitation have influenced the outcome, not only reducing the mortality but also causing an increasing number of cases who unfortunately survive with permanent brain damage (Brierley et al., 1971; Jennett and Plum, 1972). There is an increasing awareness that if the eventual outcome of patients in coma could be predicted accurately within hours of a cardiac arrest, resuscitative measures could be concentrated on those with a reasonable chance of recovery. Outcome has therefore been correlated with duration of coma, the presence or absence of brain stem reflexes, and with the EEG (Prior, 1979), evoked cortical responses and cerebral blood flow.

In man, cardiac arrest is an emergency, so its precise duration is seldom known and serial records even of heart rate and blood pressure before and after the event are virtually non-existent. Cardiac arrest may be preceded, and is often initiated, by a period of hypoxaemia which may reduce cardiac output and cerebral blood flow. Eventually, sinus rhythm is usually restored, either spontaneously after defibrillation or following internal or external cardiac massage. Even then some time may elapse before cardiac output returns to a normal level. In each case the period of true circulatory arrest and the preceding and the succeeding periods of reduced blood flow will vary. This will be reflected in the ultimate neuropathological picture. If circulatory arrest starts and ends abruptly, and lasts more than 3–4 minutes at normal body temperature, brain damage will be generalized throughout the neocortex and the cerebellum but variable in the basal ganglia. If a shorter period of circulatory arrest was preceded and/or followed by appreciable periods of reduced cerebral blood flow, the neuropathological alterations within at least the neocortex and cerebellum will be accentuated along the arterial boundary zones.

Macroscopic appearances of the brain These depend on the severity of the initial neuronal destruction and on the survival time. Within the first 36–48 hours the brain may appear entirely normal macroscopically. After a few days there is often macroscopic evidence of an episode of severe hypoxic brain damage. This is most clearly seen in the hippocampus and in the neocortex where there may be loss of definition and some granularity in the Sommer sector (CA 1) and within the cortical ribbon.

With longer survival there may be an appreciable reduction in the weight of the brain, some milky opacity of the leptomeninges, and evidence of atrophy of the cortical gyri and cerebellar folia, all of which may have a more or less granular surface. In coronal slices ventricular enlargement is slight after survival for a few weeks but may be considerable when it is months or years (Fig. 4.4). With increasing survival the width of the cortical ribbon is reduced, parti-

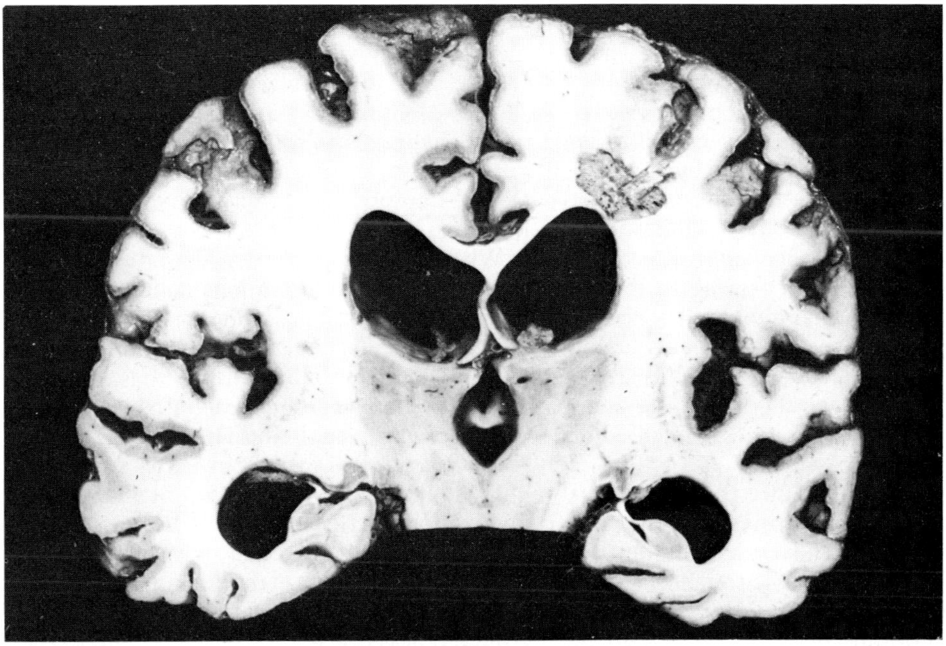

Fig. 4.4 Male, aged 48 years, dying 5 months after cardiac arrest. Brain slice showing cortical necrosis and enlargement of third and lateral ventricles.

cularly in the parietal and occipital lobes. An intracortical band of necrosis of variable width is often visible: this may appear grey and gelatinous or take the form of an apparently empty slit separating the outer and inner layers of the cortex, or the whole cortex, from the white matter (Fig. 4.5). Whilst the parahippocampal gyri are usually well preserved, the hippocampi may be shrunken and a crescentic slit seen within each Sommer sector (Fig. 4.6).

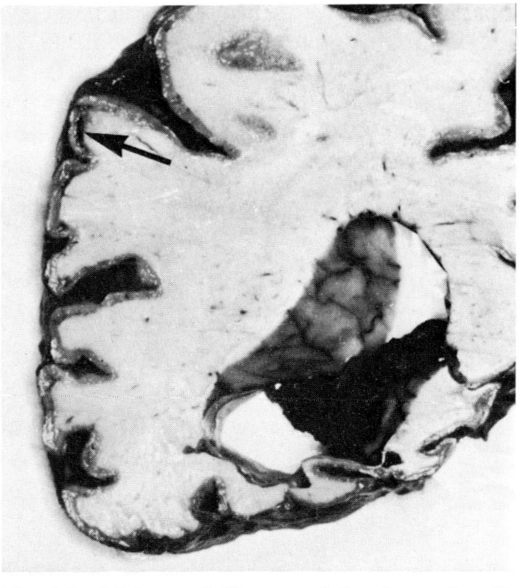

Fig. 4.5 Male, aged 58 years, dying 5 months after cardiac arrest. Brain slice showing slit (arrow) at junction between cortex and white matter.

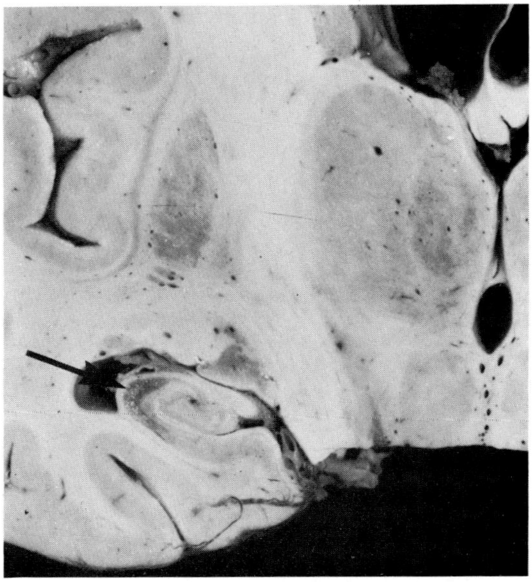

Fig. 4.6 Same case as Fig. 4.5. The Sommer sector—CA 1 (arrow)—of the hippocampus appears as a crescent of spongy tissue.

Macroscopic changes in the basal ganglia are unusual if survival is less than 36 hours. Thereafter there may be patchy discoloration in the outer half of the head and body of the caudate nucleus and in the upper third of the putamen. With the passage of time the affected regions become pale and shrunken. Even when neocortical destruction is severe the thalami may appear normal macroscopically when survival is only a few weeks. With increasing survival the thalami gradually shrink and each pulvinar may become narrow and wedge-shaped. In the amygdaloid nuclei, the corticomedial portions usually appear normal while the basolateral portions may show variable shrinkage and sometimes focal discoloration.

In the adult brain stem, after protracted survival, there may be some shrinkage of the pons, medullary pyramids and olives. In the infant and young child it may be possible to detect shrinkage and discoloration in the inferior colliculi, the spinal nuclei of the fifth nerves, and in the gracile and cuneate nuclei.

Macroscopic alterations may be identifiable in the cerebellum after survival of more than 4 days and take the form of softening of the deeper folia over the dorsal aspects and posterior borders of the hemispheres and vermis. After survival for weeks or months the damaged folia are sclerotic, the central white matter is reduced, and the dentate nuclei appear shrunken and grey-brown in colour.

Microscopic appearances The involvement of the 'selectively vulnerable' regions of the brain can be seen to its fullest extent in certain instances of circulatory arrest. The neuropathological changes have been described by Weinberger, Gibbon and Gibbon (1940), Neubuerger (1954), Lapresle and Milhaud (1962) and Brierley et al. (1971).

When survival is from a few hours to a few days, microscopic alterations contrast with the macroscopic normality of the brain. They consist of ischaemic cell change and the earliest stages of glial and mesodermal reactions.

In the human *neocortex* microvacuolation may be seen in small and large pyramidal neurons after survival for 1 hour. After survival for 4–12 hours, typical ischaemic cell change, with and without incrustations, and also early homogenizing change are readily identifiable. Damage is usually greatest in the parietal and occipital lobes and decreases towards the temporal and frontal poles (Fig. 4.7).

With increasing length of survival, the loss of neurons is accompanied by a gliomesodermal reaction, the picture ranging from minor necrosis within a single lamina up to almost total cortical destruction. In exceptional cases total destruction of the fifth and sixth cortical layers results in virtual isolation of the outer neocortical layers from the subjacent white matter. In spite of the apparent normality of the neurons in these layers, the EEG is isoelectric (Brierley et al., 1971).

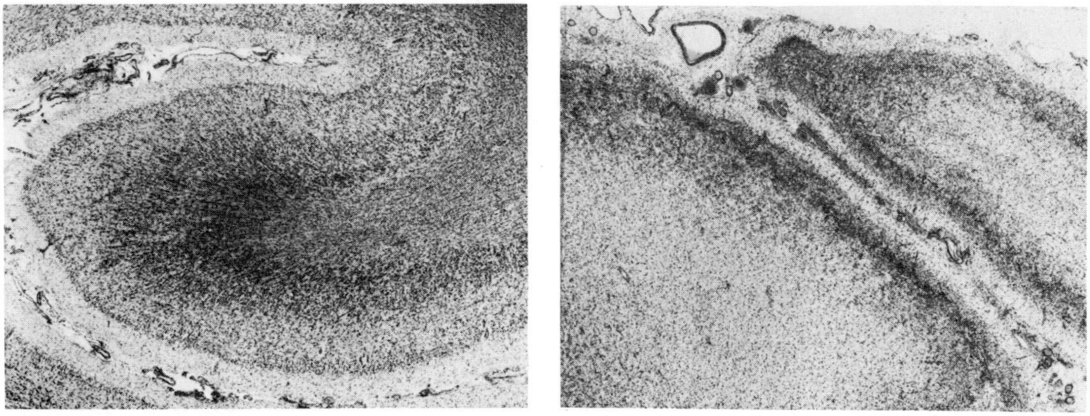

(a) **(b)**

Fig. 4.7 Male, aged 17 years, dying 9 months after cardiac arrest. (**a**) Frontal cortex showing relative preservation of cytoarchitecture over the crest of a gyrus. Celloidin; cresyl violet × 11. (**b**) Occipital lobe showing gross narrowing of the cortex and marked gliomesodermal proliferation in layer 3. Celloidin; cresyl violet × 11.

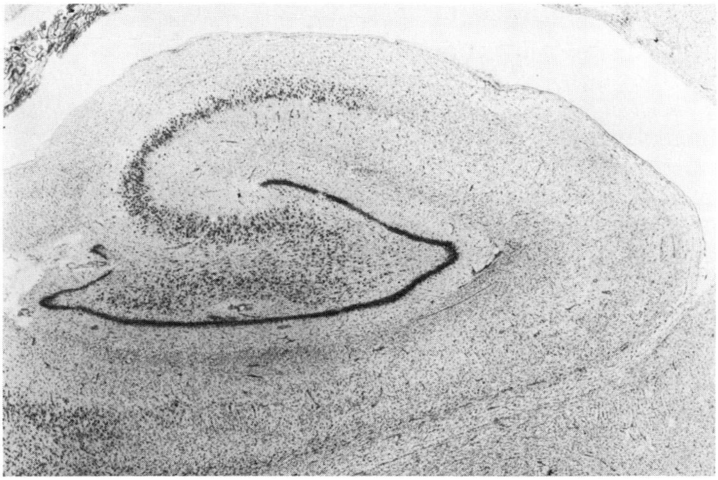

Fig. 4.8 Male, aged 49 years, dying 7 months after cardiac arrest. Hippocampus showing almost total loss of neurons in CA 1 (Sommer sector) and relative preservation in CA 2, and CA 3 and 4 (end folium). Celloidin; cresyl violet × 9.

The *hippocampus* may show ischaemic damage (Fig. 4.8) but total infarction of the Sommer sector and of the end folium is rare. When damage is minor, a few rod cells lie within a loose network of glial fibres which are particularly well developed in the end folium.

In the *amygdaloid nucleus* ischaemic alterations most frequently involve the basolateral portion, and this part may be considerably shrunken with a corresponding expansion of the tip of the inferior horn of the ventricle.

Involvement of the *caudate nucleus and putamen* is common but not invariable. It ranges from destruction of smaller neurons along the upper borders (Fig. 4.9) to total necrosis with cyst formation after long survival.

Ischaemic damage in the *globus pallidus* is also inconstant and may affect either or both segments up to the level of infarction.

The anterior and dorsomedial nuclei of the *thalamus* are usually diffusely damaged, whilst ischaemic damage in the ventrolateral nuclei is limited to the upper part. Even when ischaemic damage is severe and extensive in the cortex, alterations in the thalami are only moderate and infarction has not been described. Neocortical damage, in cases of long survival, will add some element of retrograde degeneration in the thalamic projection nuclei.

Damage in the *subthalamic nucleus* is not uncommon and the ensuing gliomesodermal reaction contrasts sharply with the surrounding white matter.

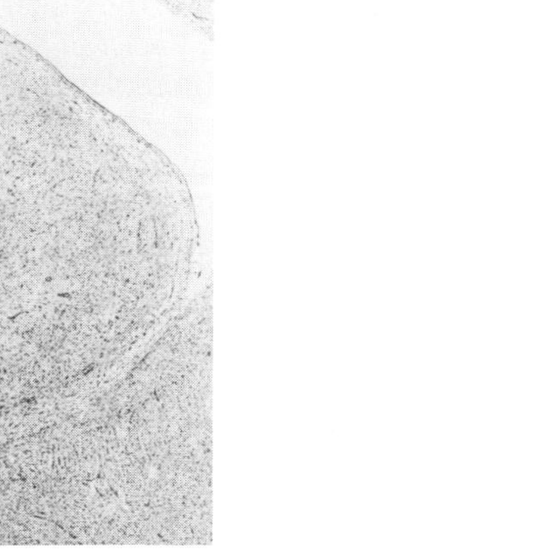

Fig. 4.9 Female, aged 56 years, dying 2 weeks after cardiac arrest. Basal ganglia. There is patchy neuronal loss with gliomesodermal proliferation in the putamen. Celloidin; cresyl violet × 18.

In the *hypothalamus* ischaemic alterations are seen occasionally in the mamillary bodies of adults and frequently in those of infants and young children.

The influence of age on the pattern of the ischaemic alterations due to circulatory arrest can be seen most clearly in the *brain stem*. In the adult, changes are usually restricted to the reticular zone of the substantia nigra, the inferior colliculi and the inferior olives. In infants and young children there is often additional involvement of the nucleus of the third nerve, the superior olive, the motor and the spinal nuclei of the fifth nerve, the vestibular nuclear complex, nucleus solitarius, and the cuneate and gracile nuclei (Fig. 4.10). This pattern of damage in brain stem nuclei closely resembles that observed in the infant monkey after neonatal asphyxia (Ranck and Windle, 1959).

In contrast, involvement of the same brain stem nuclei is more rarely seen in the adult (Neubuerger, 1954; Gilles, 1963; Lindenberg, 1963; Brierley et al., 1971).

In the *cerebellum* involvement of Purkinje cells may be restricted to the depths of some sulci with an increase in the glial shrubwork, or may be widespread and associated with some thinning of the granule layers. The dorsal aspects of the hemispheres and the superior vermis are more affected than the ventral aspects of the hemispheres and the inferior vermis.

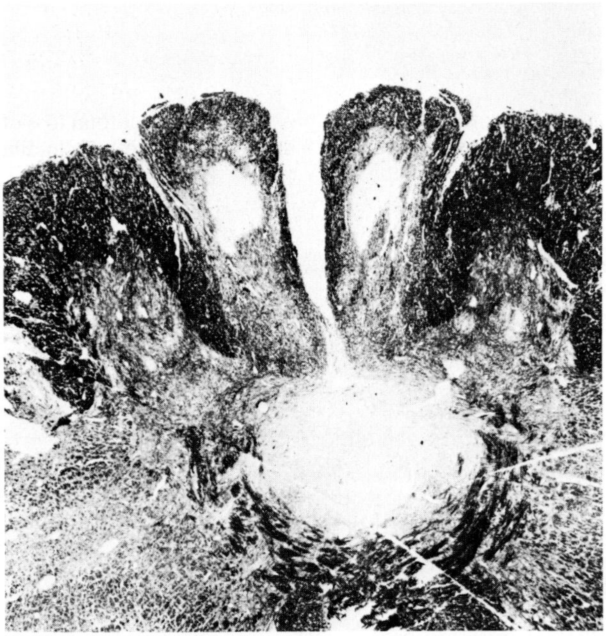

Fig. 4.10 Male, aged 2½ years, dying 30 days after cardiac arrest. Lower medulla showing discrete necrosis in each nucleus gracilis. Celloidin; Heidenhain × 11.

Experimental studies Attempts to arrest the cerebral circulation in normothermic experimental animals have been numerous but often incomplete because of the brain's extensive protective collateral circulation (Hoff, Grenell and Fulton, 1945). Whilst the blood flow through the carotid and vertebral arteries has been arrested in various ways, it has proved much more difficult to eliminate inflow from the spinal arteries.

The principal methods used to arrest cerebral blood flow have been reviewed by Brierley (1980) who considered that recent studies in experimental animals fell into three main groups. In the first group brain ischaemia was produced in paralysed, mechanically ventilated animals by a combination of an inflated cuff to occlude the major neck arteries and drug-induced hypotension to eliminate inflow through the collateral vessels (Nemoto et al., 1977). From such studies (entailing intensive care of the animals) it was concluded that the ischaemic threshold of the brain in the Rhesus monkey is about 15 minutes, a figure virtually the same as that found by Miller and Myers (1970). In the second group a combination of major arterial occlusion and drug-induced hypotension was used (Hossmann and Sato, 1970; Hossmann and Zimmermann, 1974). In the studies reported by Hossmann, cerebral circulatory arrest for up to 60 minutes was followed by some recovery of neuronal function as shown by the return of an abnormal EEG and considerable restoration of brain energy metabolism. From such findings it has been concluded that the brain can tolerate a much longer period of ischaemia than thought previously (Schneider,

1963). In the third group of experiments cerebral circulation was arrested by raising the pressure of the cerebrospinal fluid above that of the systolic blood pressure (Brierley, Ljunggren and Siesjö, 1975; Marshall et al., 1975) with the production of ischaemic cell change in the cerebral cortex and hippocampus after 10–15 minutes.

The neuropathology of circulatory arrest cannot be divorced from consideration of the clinically all-important question—what period of circulatory arrest can the brain tolerate before it is damaged? Attempts to define such a threshold have been reviewed by Hoff, Grenell and Fulton (1945), Meyer (1963) and Brierley (1976). There was endorsement of the traditional view, epitomized by Schneider (1961), that complete recovery without neurological or histological damage cannot occur after a complete arrest of cerebral circulation of more than 4–5 minutes. If, however, subsequent cardiac insufficiency can be averted or minimized, the period may be increased to 8 minutes (Schneider, 1961).

In contrast to this view it has been claimed that cerebral circulatory arrest for up to 1 hour in the cat (Hossmann and Sato, 1970) and in the Rhesus monkey (Hossmann and Zimmermann, 1974) can be followed by unequivocal signs of neuronal recovery. The recovery of neuronal function described in these experiments, however, amounted to the return of an abnormal EEG and the pyramidal response. The ability of these animals to resume breathing spontaneously and to appear normal neurologically was not recorded nor has any conventional systematic neuropathological examination been reported. Furthermore, Hirsch et al. (1975) failed to confirm the findings of Hossmann and Sato (1970) and attributed recovery after such protracted ischaemia to the protective effects of anaesthesia and hypothermia. As already noted, when neuropathological changes have been demonstrated, the ischaemic threshold, at least in the Rhesus monkey, is about 15 minutes (Nemoto et al., 1977), a figure similar to the 14- to 15-minute threshold established by Miller and Myers (1970) and by Wolin, Massopust and Taslitz (1971).

Several studies have suggested that incomplete ischaemia (a cerebral blood flow of less than 10 per cent of normal) is more harmful than complete ischaemia. Explanations for this apparent anomaly include inadequate recirculation after ischaemia (Hossmann and Kleihues, 1973), the progressive accumulation of lactic acid during incomplete ischaemia with the continued supply of glucose (Siemkowicz and Hansen, 1978), and damage to membranes from free radicals that are produced during hypoxia but not during anoxia (see Siesjö, 1981). The issue remains unresolved if only because models and the duration of ischaemia vary widely and there are discrepancies between biochemical and electrophysiological criteria of recovery. The contention that incomplete is more harmful than complete cerebral ischaemia rests upon acute experiments in rodents, and there are no survival studies in primates.

Oligaemic hypoxia—localized A reduction of blood flow in all or part of an arterial territory is usually due to a combination of systemic hypotension and stenosis. Provided that thrombosis and embolism can be excluded, such local oligaemia is a not uncommon cause of ischaemic brain damage, and if blood flow is sufficiently impaired the outcome will be an infarct involving grey and white matter.

Oligaemic hypoxia—generalized Global oligaemia implies some reduction in the overall flow of blood through the brain. Subsequent neuropathological alterations, if any, are determined by the oxygenation of the blood, the rate at which blood flow was reduced, the lowest level attained and its duration, and also by the rate at which normal brain blood flow was restored. In any one case brain damage will conform to one of the three patterns described by Adams et al. (1966).

1. Ischaemic alterations are concentrated along the arterial boundary zones of the cerebral cortex and cerebellum (Fig. 4.11) and are variable in the basal ganglia.

The boundary zone pattern of ischaemic brain damage is usually seen after a conscious subject has collapsed as a result of some sudden reduction in cardiac output or when an episode of anoxaemia or hypoxaemia has led to impaired myocardial activity.

Meyer (1953) first regarded that localized necrosis of grey and white matter along the boundary zones between major arterial territories was the result of a sudden fall in blood pressure. Earlier Wolf and Siris (1937) had illustrated symmetrical necrosis in the boundary zones between the anterior and middle cerebral arteries

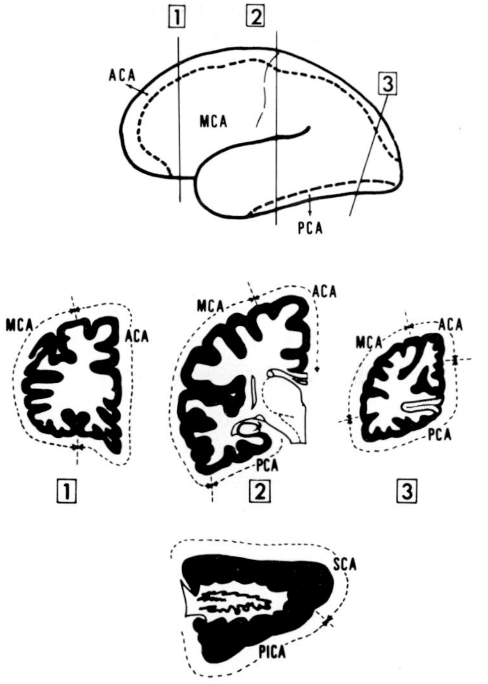

Fig. 4.11 The arterial territories of the human cerebrum and cerebellum. ACA, anterior cerebral artery; MCA, middle cerebral artery; PCA, posterior cerebral artery; SCA, superior cerebellar artery; PICA, posterior inferior cerebellar artery.

(although these were not recognized as such) in four neurosurgical patients operated on in the sitting position. Serial blood pressure readings gave evidence of abrupt arterial hypotension. These observations have been confirmed and extended by Zülch (1953), Zülch and Behrend (1961), and Romanul and Abramowicz (1964).

The neocortex around the parieto-occipital sulci, representing the boundary zone between the territories of the anterior, middle and posterior cerebral arteries, is the most vulnerable portion of the boundary zones since it is most remote from the origin of each major artery. Minimal boundary zone lesions are most likely to occur in this region whilst larger lesions spread anteriorly along the anterior/middle cerebral artery and/or the middle/posterior cerebral artery boundary zones. In the former, involvement of the pre- and postcentral gyri is not unusual, but extension around the frontal pole on to the orbital surface is exceptional. The middle/posterior cerebral artery boundary zone passing forwards and downwards into the temporal lobe is rarely involved to its full extent.

Boundary zone lesions in the neocortex vary widely. A minor lesion may appear as a crescent of ischaemic nerve cells or gliomesodermal reaction (Fig. 4.12). Larger lesions may take the form of typical laminar necrosis (Fig. 4.13)

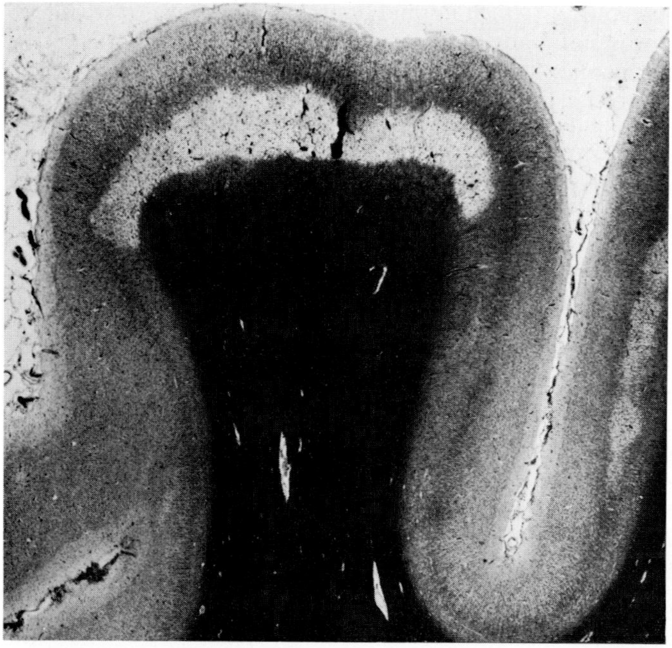

Fig. 4.12 Male, aged 46 years, dying 5 weeks after a severe hypotensive episode. Second frontal gyrus showing necrosis of deeper cortical layers. Celloidin; Heidenhain × 9.

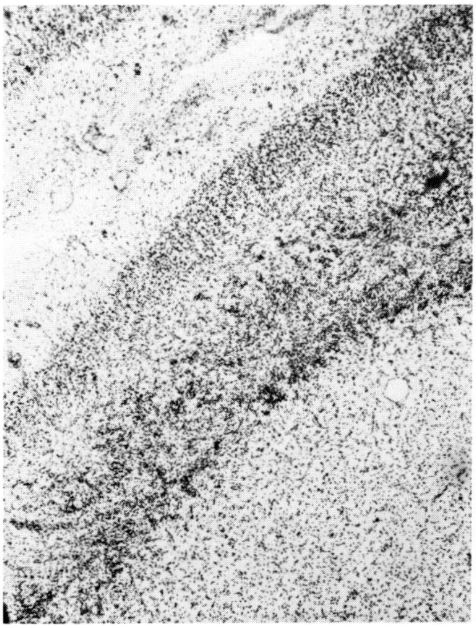

Fig. 4.13 Female, aged 46 years, dying 2 months after an episode of circulatory collapse under general anaesthesia. Occipital lobe showing gliomesodermal reaction in deeper layers of cortex. Celloidin; cresyl violet × 8.

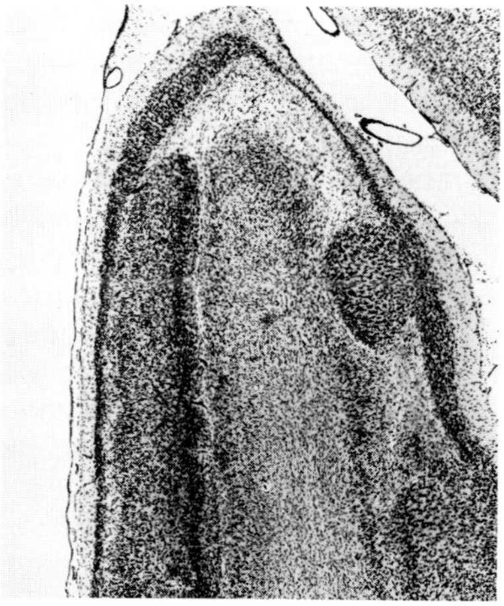

Fig. 4.15 *Macaca mulatta*. Subatmospheric decompression with secondary hypotension. Occipital lobe showing irregular loss of cortical neurons with preservation of islands of normal cells. Celloidin; cresyl violet × 10.

within which islands of normal neurons may be preserved. Major lesions may involve all layers over a wide area (Fig. 4.14) or may be irregular with islands of preserved nerve cells within the lesion (Fig. 4.15). Boundary zone lesions may or may not be haemorrhagic (Fig. 4.16). Involvement of the white matter is not uncommon and when present is often associated with large irregular cortical lesions. The damaged white matter takes the form of a wedge, the apex pointing towards the lateral ventricles.

Although Coceani and Gloor (1966) stated that in *Macaca mulatta* '... the hippocampus definitely lies on the watershed between the car-

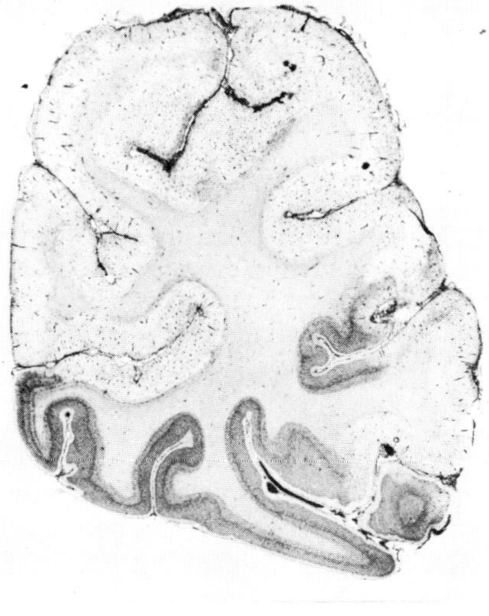

Fig. 4.14 Male, aged 17 years, dying 6 days after an episode of cardiorespiratory arrest. Occipital lobe showing complete necrosis of the cortex of the medial and lateral surfaces. There is sparing of the inferior surface. Celloidin; cresyl violet × 2.

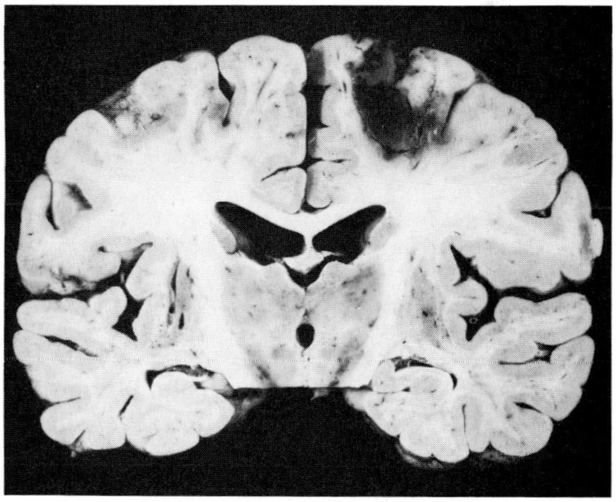

Fig. 4.16 Female, aged 63 years, dying 5 days after episode of severe hypotension. There is haemorrhagic infarction of the sides and depths of the right superior frontal sulcus in the boundary zone between the anterior and middle cerebral arteries.

otid and vertebrobasilar arterial territories . . .' it is seldom involved in this species or in man when major boundary zone lesions are present in the cerebrum and cerebellum.

Ischaemic alterations in the basal ganglia cannot be regarded as boundary zone lesions because there are virtually no important anastomoses between the several arterial territories (Vander Eecken, 1959). They must be attributed to a critical reduction in blood flow through the capillary bed. While neocortical boundary zone lesions may occur in the absence of ischaemic lesions in the basal ganglia, the converse is very rare. Damage in the putamen is usually in the upper part of the anterior third whilst the outer and the inner segments of the globus pallidus are equally involved. Alterations in the thalamus and amygdaloid nucleus are rare.

In the cerebellum the minimal lesion along the boundary zone between the territories supplied by the superior and the posterior inferior cerebellar arteries (see Fig. 4.11) occurs in the depths of the cortex adjacent to the central white matter. Larger lesions are triangular in vertical section with their apices deep and their bases along the posterior border (Fig. 4.17).

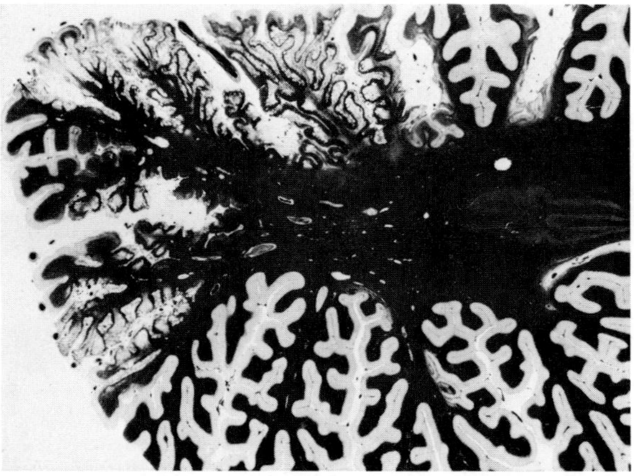

Fig. 4.17 Male, aged 61 years, dying 7 months after a severe hypotensive episode. Cerebellum showing necrotic folia at boundary zone between superior and posterior inferior cerebellar arteries. Celloidin; PTAH × 1.25.

2. Ischaemic changes are generalized in the cortex of the cerebrum and cerebellum, minor or absent in the hippocampi, and often severe in the thalami. Reports of this pattern of damage are few and the patients were usually under anaesthesia. Probably the generalized brain damage is due to hypotension (sometimes postural) of relatively slow onset and of long duration. A slowly falling perfusion pressure within a fully dilated vascular bed may reduce flow to a critical level in the brain as a whole and not just along the boundary zones.

In the first reported instance of this distribution of ischaemic alterations (Brierley and Cooper, 1962) neuronal loss was laminar or pseudolaminar in the cortex (Fig. 4.18), decreasing from the occipital lobes forwards. It was minor in the hippocampi, absent in the caudate and lentiform nuclei but considerable in the thalami. Loss of neurons was slight and patchy in the reticular zone of the substantia nigra and in the olives but severe among Purkinje cells. Similar neuropathological findings were reported in four cases by Adams et al. (1966).

3. Ischaemic alterations are generalized in the cortex of cerebrum and cerebellum but with variable accentuation along the arterial boundary zones. The hippocampi are usually spared and there is patchy damage in the basal ganglia. This pattern is seen when a conscious subject collapses after brief cardiac arrest (followed by cardiac massage) or some postoperative hypotension. It was also seen as a consequence of subatmospheric decompression in the cats of Altmann and Schubothe (1942) and in the two baboons of Brierley and Nicholson (1969). It has not been produced in experimental primates as a consequence of hypotension uncomplicated by hypoxaemia. The physiological basis for this pattern of brain damage remains undefined but an initial abrupt reduction in blood flow followed by a reduced overall flow of hypoxaemic blood is probable.

As the neuropathology of this group of cases includes the features of groups (1) and (2) in varying proportions, a separate description is

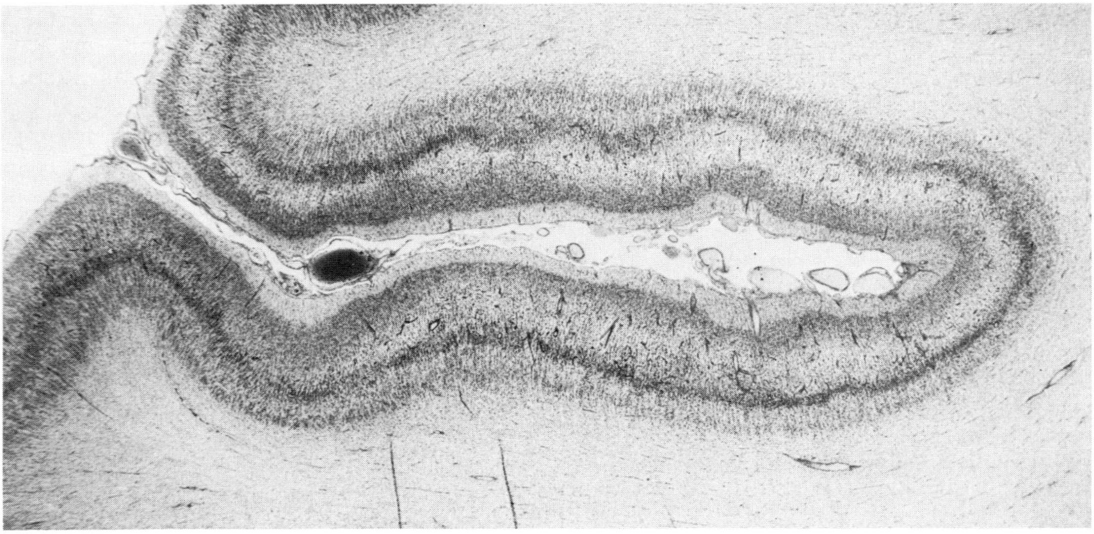

Fig. 4.18 Female, aged 24 years, dying 8 days after a period of sustained moderate hypotension. Occipital lobe showing neuronal loss and gliomesodermal proliferation in third layer. Celloidin; cresyl violet × 11.

not merited. Five typical cases have been presented by Adams et al. (1966), and a single case by Brierley and Miller (1966).

In the clinical situation a reduction in cerebral perfusion pressure, while arterial oxygenation remains normal, is virtually confined to the technique of hypotensive anaesthesia with controlled ventilation, particularly if there is head-up tilt. Other factors that may result in brain damage after a period of relatively moderate hypotension are some degree of hypoxaemia, some pre-existing vascular disease (particularly atheroma of the extra- and/or intracranial arteries and hypertensive arteriosclerosis) and also variations in the configuration of the circle of Willis. The frequency of these complications of reduced cerebral blood flow due to systemic hypotension is largely responsible for the observation that hypoxic brain damage along the arterial boundary zones is the most common neuropathological outcome of hypoxia in all its forms.

Anoxic and hypoxic hypoxia

Anoxic hypoxia This term implies that the blood leaving the lungs is devoid of oxygen. It occurs if atmospheric pressure falls to zero when pressurization fails in the vehicle of an astronaut orbiting in space or within his space suit while he is outside the vehicle; if there is complete obstruction of the respiratory tract above the tracheal bifurcation (as in accidental or suicidal hanging); if respiration is arrested after disease or injury to the spinal cord; after crush injuries of the thorax; and after the arrest of alveolar oxygen exchange due to the inhalation of inert gases or to drowning.

Experimental studies The physiological events in each of these situations have not been documented, but the anoxia due to the inhalation of pure nitrogen by conscious volunteers has been studied by Gastaut, Fischgold and Meyer (1961), Gastaut et al. (1961) and Ernsting (1963). After 15–16 seconds of nitrogen overventilation (which rapidly induces anoxaemia), Ernsting (1963) observed that there was low-voltage activity in the EEG at 11–13 cycles per second and that consciousness was lost at 17–20 seconds. The subsequent course of events has been demonstrated by studies in experimental animals. Swann and Brucer (1949) exposed dogs to pure nitrogen and observed hyperventilation, cyanosis and convulsions within the first minute. Bradycardia supervened with heart failure and a falling blood pressure. Apnoea occurred at the third minute and the blood pressure was 0.7–2.7 kPa (5–20 mmHg) at the fifth minute. Survival after 5.5 minutes was possible only if administration of oxygen was combined with external cardiac massage. If resuscitation was delayed until 6.5 minutes, brain damage was evident.

More recently the effects of anoxia have been studied in anaesthetized, mechanically ventilated and physiologically monitored dogs (Snyder et al., 1979). After occluding the trachea, mean arterial blood pressure rose initially before declining gradually: the EEG became slower, and 15–30 seconds before mean arterial pressure became zero the EEG became isoelectric. Seven minutes later cardiopulmonary resuscitation was instituted. Ischaemic brain damage was found in the neocortex (often with a laminar distribution), in the basal ganglia, the thalamus and cerebellum.

It is evident that in the human subject or experimental animal, pure anoxaemia will be complicated by some degree of circulatory failure and therefore cannot alone produce brain damage. If resuscitation is successful and brain damage is eventually proved, this must be ascribed to a combination of anoxaemia and a reduced cerebral blood flow. This combination, for reasons already elaborated (see p. 139), is likely to lead to ischaemic alterations along the arterial boundary zones. Thus any delineation of purely anoxic brain damage is not, as yet, justified.

Hypoxic hypoxia This term implies some reduction in the oxygen tension of arterial blood as a consequence of a lowered oxygen content of the inspired air (high altitudes, failure of pressurization in aircraft, inhalation of air mixed with inert gases including anaesthetics) or of impairment of pulmonary function.

Many attempts have been made to define a 'critical' level of blood oxygenation in man below which brain damage will occur. Campbell (1965) considered 4.0 kPa (30 mmHg) to be the critical arterial oxygen tension when the corresponding brain venous oxygen tension would be in the range 2.3–2.5 kPa (17–19 mmHg) (Luft, 1965). However, Gray and Horner (1970) could not confirm these values and showed that oxygen tensions as low as 1.0 kPa (7.5 mmHg) in arterial and 0.3 kPa (2.0 mmHg) in venous blood were compatible with survival without clinical evidence of brain damage. Lübbers (1966), however, has stressed that even venous oxygen tension is not a reliable index of brain tissue hypoxia, as a local tissue oxygen tension of 0.13 kPa (1.0 mmHg) or less can be recorded by appropriate electrodes on the brain of a normal experimental animal.

The concept of an oxygen tension 'critical' for the production of brain damage also assumes that in the human subject or experimental animal such a level can be sustained without any alteration in cerebral blood flow, long enough to be the sole cause of irreversible neuronal damage. In the literature of so-called hypoxic brain damage in man, virtually all reports fail to document blood pressure and heart rate during the period of hypoxaemia. Nevertheless, Scholz (1952, 1957) and Buchner (1957) considered that oligaemia resulted in alterations in the cerebral and cerebellar cortex and in the hippocampus whilst damage in the striatum, pallidum and subthalamic nucleus was the consequence of hypoxaemia. Although both patterns of hypoxic brain damage exist, their physiological bases remain elusive.

Experimental studies Experiments in primates have provided answers to the questions (1) can uncomplicated hypoxaemia produce brain damage, and (2) are the 'cortical' and 'basal ganglia' patterns of brain damage regularly associated with oligaemia and hypoxaemia respectively?

1. The exposure of primates to subatmospheric decompression in a decompression chamber provides a model for hypoxia (Brierley and Nicholson, 1969; Blagbrough, Brierley and Nicholson, 1973). Using this model it has been shown that, in the brains of baboons and Rhesus monkeys, damage in the cerebral and cerebellar cortex is concentrated along arterial boundary zones but is inconstant and variable in the basal ganglia. The involvement of the arterial boundary zones indicated that some reduction in cerebral perfusion followed the initial hypoxaemia. Bradycardia occurred towards the end of the decompression, when respiration was greatly slowed. Physiological events during the critical period before apnoea were not recorded so neither a 'final' circulatory crisis nor the formation of gaseous embolism could be excluded (p. 145).

As the limit of tolerance to profound hypoxia (decompression) was indicated by respiratory failure, it was necessary to record physiological data before and after 'the last breath'. Brierley et al. (1978) achieved this in lightly anaesthetized and spontaneously breathing baboons and monkeys which inhaled at ambient pressure 3.2% oxygen in nitrogen (equivalent to an altitude of 37 500 feet) from air and after pre-exposure to 14% oxygen (equivalent to an altitude of 10 000 feet). Each hypoxic exposure to 3.2% oxygen ended in a typical cardiorespiratory crisis. As blood pressure fell, breathing stopped and the EEG became isoelectric. Mechanical ventilation, begun soon after the 'last breath', usually allowed recovery of the heart, spontaneous respiration and the EEG. Brain damage was rare and occurred along boundary zones and in the basal ganglia. The response to such profound hypoxia was different between the two species of animal and this was thought to be due to the different altitudes of their natural habitats.

The contrast between the frequency and severity of the brain damage following subatmospheric decompression and its rarity when the same levels of hypoxia were produced by the inhalation of nitrogen/oxygen mixtures at normal atmospheric pressure may be explained by studies of air embolism. It is known that after accidental air embolism in man (Brion, Psimaras and Gallissot, 1974) and its experimental induction in subhuman primates (Naquet and Vigouroux, 1966; Meldrum and Brierley, 1971; Brion et al., 1974) ischaemic damage occurs along the arterial boundary zones of the cerebrum and the cerebellum and is variable in the basal ganglia. Thus the neuropathology of gaseous embolism may be virtually indistinguishable from that due to reduced cerebral blood flow combined with hypoxaemia. It is highly likely, therefore, that gaseous embolism was a major factor in the aetiology of the brain damage seen after subatmospheric decompression. This possibility could only be excluded if similar decompressions were carried out with Doppler monitoring for gas bubbles, in the neck arteries, and full physiological monitoring. On the other hand, Fryer (1969) emphasized that damage consistent with gaseous embolism had been described in only a few human cases of subatmospheric decompression.

Evidently the pattern of brain damage when seen in profound hypoxia is indistinguishable from that seen after oligaemic hypoxia, underlining the fact that systemic hypoxia can bring about brain damage only through the medium of a secondary reduction in perfusion pressure. The animals employed in these various experiments were healthy and had normal systemic and cerebral vessels; in a human subject exposed to hypoxia, the usual initial increase in cerebral blood flow may be so restricted by cerebrovascular disease that hypoxic damage may ensue.

2. Scholz (1952, 1957) and Buchner (1957) considered that damage in the cortex of the cerebrum and cerebellum was a consequence of oligaemia and damage in the basal ganglia was due to hypoxaemia. Both patterns were seen when systemic hypotension was combined with normal arterial oxygenation (oligaemic hypoxia) in primates (Brierley et al., 1969). These experimental studies showed that hypoxic and oligaemic hypoxia can each lead to the 'cortical' and 'basal ganglia' patterns of damage and both are likely to have anatomical rather than physiological explanations.

The critical contribution of oligaemia secondary to hypoxaemia in the production of brain damage was supported by the observations of Brown and Brierley (1968) in rats exposed intermittently to nitrogen. Brain damage occurred only when a considerable bradycardia developed towards the end of each period of hypoxia. The evidence now available from many experimental studies is in line with the conclusion of Schneider (1961) that 'ischaemia is the last common path of all forms of hypoxia'. Thus the neuropathology of hypoxic hypoxia is that of oligaemic hypoxia.

Anaemic hypoxia

Carbon monoxide intoxication Carbon monoxide (CO) gives rise to anaemic hypoxia because its affinity for the ferrous haem of haemoglobin is about 250 times that for oxygen. The remaining normal haemoglobin has a normal oxygen saturation and blood oxygen tension is normal but the oxygen content is reduced. Furthermore, the dissociation curve of oxyhaemoglobin is shifted to the left and so less oxygen is available to the tissues at a particular oxygen tension. The affinity of carbon monoxide for the iron of cytochrome oxidase and cytochrome P450 implies the possibility of an additional histotoxic element.

Garland and Pearce (1967) described four personal cases and also presented a comprehensive review of the neurological complications of CO poisoning. They emphasized the rarity of clinical evidence of permanent brain damage among the many survivors of exposure to carbon monoxide. They also made the important observation that no combination of neurological and psychiatric symptoms can be regarded as specific for CO intoxication since all may be encountered after cardiac arrest, hypoglycaemia, closed head injury, air embolism or hepatic encephalopathy.

When death occurs within a few hours of poisoning, the blood, brain, muscles, skin and viscera show the pink-red colour characteristic of carboxyhaemoglobin. The brain and leptomeninges are usually congested. Haemorrhages are frequent and may be either petechial, with a predilection for the white matter and the corpus callosum in particular, or large and without preferential sites. Alterations in the basal ganglia, unless haemorrhagic, are seldom recognizable if survival is less than 24 hours.

When death is delayed there is the usual relationship between survival time and macroscopic alterations. When survival is 48 hours or more, brain weight may be increased as a result of swelling. Macroscopic inspection may then show petechial haemorrhages and early necrosis in the globus pallidus, the hippocampus and sometimes in the reticular zone of the substantia nigra. This localization was first described by Hiller (1924); the microscopic description was provided by Meyer (1926). Meyer (1963) pointed out that the pallidal necrosis could also be the sequel of cyanide intoxication and of anaesthetic accidents. Furthermore, after CO intoxication the globus pallidus may be normal (Hsü and Ch'eng, 1938; Lapresle and Fardeau, 1967).

The typical pallidal lesions become well circumscribed macroscopic infarcts after survival of 48 hours or even less (Fig. 4.19) and are not always symmetrical. Thereafter there is the usual proliferation of microglia followed by the appearance of lipid phagocytes, fibre-forming astrocytes and blood vessels in the central zone with a well-circumscribed peripheral capsule of gliomesodermal elements enclosing the products of tissue breakdown. The lesion, more commonly seen in the anterior and upper portion of the inner segment of the globus pallidus, may extend upwards into the internal capsule and into the external segment and sometimes downwards into the sublentiform region. When survival is long, haemosiderin may be seen in lipid phagocytes and pseudocalcium deposits around the larger blood vessels.

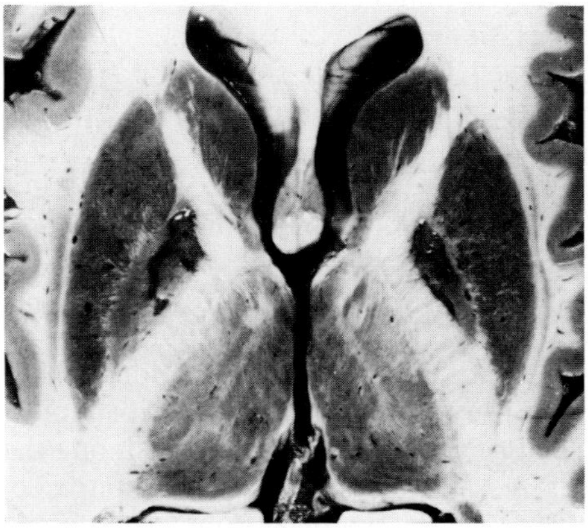

Fig. 4.19 Male, aged 48 years, dying 9 months after carbon monoxide intoxication. Horizontal brain slice showing irregular necrosis with cyst formation in each globus pallidus.

A minimal pallidal lesion may be no more than an irregular slit at the junction between the inner segment and the internal capsule, and this can be missed if serial sections are not studied (Lapresle and Fardeau, 1967).

Hypoxic necrosis may also be seen in the cerebral cortex. This may be focal and often perivascular, or appear as a laminar necrosis of the third and sometimes the second layers or only the fifth and sixth layers. Similar alterations may involve the hippocampus and the Purkinje cells of the cerebellum. In a case surviving 16 years (Meyer, 1926), the cerebral hemispheres, particularly in the frontal and occipital lobes, presented the picture of granular atrophy in the form of irregular focal loss of neurons, gliosis and irregular retraction of the surface (Fig. 4.20). A similar case was described by Raskin and Mullaney (1940).

Poursines, Alliez and Toga (1956) reported a 33-year-old woman who lived for 26 days after a suicidal attempt by exposure to illuminating gas. There was necrosis in each globus pallidus and along arterial boundary zones, particularly those between the anterior and middle cerebral arterial territories. These boundary zone lesions suggest that there had been a fall in cerebral perfusion pressure (see p. 139) but cardiac and respiratory data are lacking. The observation of Neubuerger and Clarke (1945) in which patchy infarction of the myocardium was seen in a case surviving for 13 days after CO poisoning suggests that the level of circulating carboxyhaemoglobin may not be the only cause of brain damage, and that it might be contributed to by additional hypoxaemia or reduced cerebral blood flow.

Alterations in the *white matter* are a common and often conspicuous result of CO intoxication. Their extent is not necessarily proportional to the damage in grey matter, so the latter may even

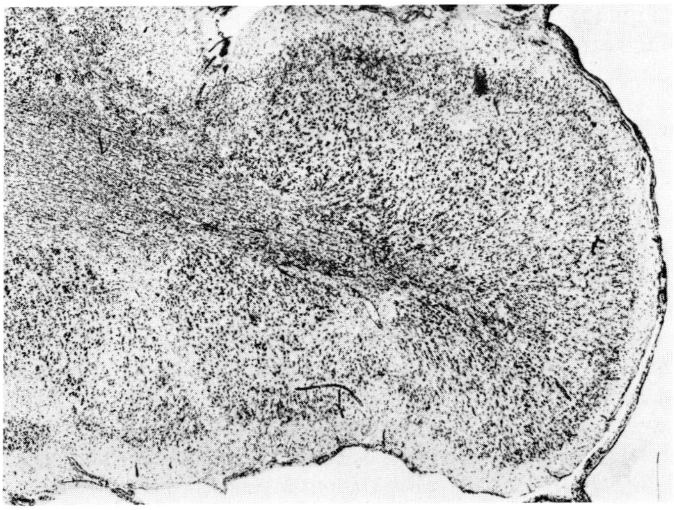

Fig. 4.20 Carbon monoxide poisoning, 16 years' survival. Focal loss of nerve cells with subsequent gliosis in cerebral cortex and white matter. Cresyl violet × 20.

appear normal when there is extensive myelin breakdown. White matter damage can take three forms:

1. Discrete, usually perivascular foci of myelin destruction may occur throughout the white matter of the corpus callosum, the internal and external capsules and the optic tracts. Similar foci, sometimes haemorrhagic, may occur beneath the ependyma.
2. Generalized destruction of myelinated fibres that may extend from the frontal to the temporal and occipital poles with some periventricular accentuation. In the corpus callosum there may be a butterfly-like distribution of myelin damage in the coronal plane. Usually there is sparing of the subcortical U-fibres and of a narrow subependymal zone. Within each centrum semiovale a gliomesodermal reaction provides a sharp demarcation between normal and abnormal tissue.
3. Pallor of myelin staining or frank demyelination taking the form of plaques which may or may not be confluent. The plaques occur in the posterior and deeper parts of the central white matter and are unusual in the commissures, the subcortical U-fibres, the internal and external capsules and the optic pathways. Microscopically the plaques show a more or less spongy texture, a relative sparing of myelin sheaths around blood vessels and sometimes concentric demyelination similar to that described by Balò (1928). There is relative preservation of the axis cylinders. Eventually the accumulation of lipid phagocytes is associated with the proliferation of fibre-forming astrocytes which are more numerous around the periphery of the plaque than at its centre.

Lapresle and Fardeau (1966) analysed white matter damage in 16 cases. In a well-illustrated report they suggested that alterations of type 1 occurred in patients who had been comatose from the outset and died within 1 week. Lesions of type 2 were usually seen in those with an unremitting coma ending in death after 9–140 days. Similar instances were described by Neubuerger and Clarke (1945) and Brucher (1967). Lesions of type 3, first described by Grinkler (1925), are usually associated with a biphasic clinical picture, and Jacob (1939) suggested that such degeneration in white rather than in grey matter was the pathological substrate in those patients in whom delayed neuropsychiatric symptoms followed the initial intoxication. Similar cases were described by Hsü and Ch'eng (1938), six by Lapresle and Fardeau (1966) and two by Vuia (1967).

Experimental studies One of the earliest was that of Ferraro and Morrison (1928), who found in rabbits that neuronal alterations were more frequent in the hippocampus than in the globus pallidus. On the other hand, Meyer (1928) observed pallidal softenings in all of nine cats exposed to CO whilst the hippocampus was involved in only one. Meyer (1932) showed that exposure to CO resulted in a purely pallidal necrosis in the dog whilst in the rabbit and guinea-pig there was also equal involvement of the cerebral cortex, the hippocampus and the cerebellum.

Yant et al. (1934) studied the effects of rapid asphyxiation by CO in the dog (death at the end of an exposure of 20–30 minutes) and also slow CO asphyxiation (death at 16–165 days). In animals surviving days and weeks there was loss of neurons with a gliomesodermal reaction in the cerebral cortex and the corpus striatum. Diffuse demyelination was seen in animals surviving more than a few days.

Lewey and Drabkin (1944) exposed dogs to CO for 5.5 hours a day, for 6 days a week and for 11 weeks. Abnormal ECGs were noted in some. After a survival of 3 months small foci of necrosis were seen in the cerebral cortex, the globus pallidus, the white matter and the brain stem. Ehrich, Bellet and Lewey (1944) analysed the ECGs in the dogs of Lewey and Drabkin (1944) and also described and illustrated focal haemorrhagic and necrotic lesions in the myocardium in those animals in which carboxyhaemoglobin exceeded 75 per cent for 1 hour or more. This single experimental study confirmed earlier observations and also drew attention to the fact that CO can damage heart muscle and thereby add an element of oligaemia to hypoxia of anaemic type.

Studies by Meyer (1933) and van Bogaert, Dallemagne and Wegria (1938) in the monkey failed to reveal any neuropathological abnormality, in contrast to those of Ginsberg, Myers and McDonagh (1974) who exposed 19 physiologically monitored juvenile Rhesus monkeys to mixtures containing 0.2% or 0.3% CO plus normal amounts of oxygen for periods of 60-325 minutes. A carboxyhaemoglobin level of 72–77 per cent was maintained throughout the exposure. Some degree of hypotension occurred in all animals, respiration was not depressed and cardiac arrhythmias were common. The EEG was slowed progressively and there were intermittent isoelectric periods in 12 animals. Fourteen animals survived the exposure for from 2 weeks to 5 months. Three showed severe neurological disability, three mild disability and eight appeared normal.

In the brains of all of the animals damage to white matter was the salient feature. This was usually symmetrical and more marked anteriorly. The destruction of myelin was either diffuse or in the form of plaques. The cerebral cortex, cerebellum, brain stem and spinal cord were stated to be normal and alterations in the globus pallidus and hippocampus were seen in less than one-fifth of the brains. More recently it has been shown that the severity of damage to the white matter correlates with the reduction in blood pressure but not with the duration of CO inhalation, carboxyhaemoglobin level, fall in pH or bicarbonate (Preziosi et al., 1970; Okeda et al., 1981).

The pathogenesis of CO encephalopathy has been reviewed recently by Ginsberg (1979). In addition to the high affinity of CO for the ferrous haem of haemoglobin and its binding to brain cytochromes, vascular mechanisms have been postulated in the pathogenesis of the damage to white matter.

In conclusion, many studies have underlined the overall importance of systemic circulatory factors, whilst the concentration of damage in white matter may be due to a local cytotoxic effect of CO with an additional moderate reduction in blood flow. Ginsberg (1979) has suggested that the latter combination may be responsible for the clinical syndrome of delayed neurological deterioration following exposure to CO.

Histotoxic hypoxia

Cyanide The histotoxic effects of the cyanide ion are due to the inhibition of cytochrome oxidase, the terminal enzyme in the respiratory electron transport chain which utilizes the oxygen derived from the dissociation of oxyhaemoglobin. Cyanide probably combines reversibly with the iron (ferric haem) of cytochrome oxidase. It does not combine with circulating haemoglobin but only with methaemoglobin. The latter may be formed *in vivo* when sodium nitrite is given in the treatment of cyanide intoxication and *post mortem* as a breakdown product of haemoglobin. There is no essential difference between the neuropathological effects of sodium and potassium cyanide, hydrocyanic acid and cyanogen chloride.

In acute intoxication, death from respiratory failure ensues rapidly and is often preceded by convulsions. The brain shows no more than hyperaemia and, occasionally, petechial, subarachnoid and subdural haemorrhages; there are no significant microscopic alterations.

Only a few human cases with delayed death

have been described. That of Lambert (1919) was a man aged 40 dying 16 days after the accidental inhalation of hydrocyanic acid gas. There was coma for the first 3 days with frequent convulsions. Macroscopically there were small haemorrhages in the white matter of the cerebrum and cerebellum. Microscopically there was a conspicuous loss of Purkinje cells in the cerebellum and gliosis in the cerebral cortex. Haymaker, Ginzler and Ferguson (1952) suggested that a single case might have been reported first by Schmorl (1920) and subsequently by Edelmann (1921). This was a man dying 36 hours after accidental exposure to hydrocyanic acid. There was general hyperaemia and a symmetrical haemorrhagic softening in each globus pallidus with ring haemorrhages, hyaline thrombi in vessels and 'regressive' changes in nerve cells.

Experimental studies These have shown that cyanide can damage myelin sheaths after administration by any route. Grey matter may also be damaged when cardiorespiratory complications and epilepsy occur.

Demyelination was described after cyanide poisoning in the dog and rabbit (Meyer, 1933), in the cat and monkey (Ferraro, 1933), in the monkey (Hurst, 1940), in the rat (Hicks, 1950a) and in the dog (Haymaker, Ginzler and Ferguson, 1952). In these studies damage to white matter was seen in subcortical structures including the corpus callosum, and Ferraro (1933) considered that the lesions resembled multiple sclerosis. Neuronal abnormalities described in all these studies with the exception of Hicks, 1950a) were probably non-specific and due to the use of immersion-fixation. The ischaemic neuronal alterations described by Hicks (1950a) in perfusion-fixed material were probably due to a combination of coma, apnoea and severe convulsions.

Levine and Stypulkowski (1959) examined the brain damage due to cyanide after unilateral ligature of a common carotid artery in rats. The animals were killed 2–4 days later and their brains were fixed by immersion. In grey matter, alterations were restricted to the side of carotid ligature but demyelination was always symmetrical in the corpus callosum and its radiations, and in the hippocampal and anterior commissures. Levine and Stypulkowski concluded that, in a normal animal exposed to cyanide, the involvement of grey matter (usually a concomitant of severe intoxication) was most probably due to the accompanying ischaemia and/or hypoxic hypoxia. The symmetry of damage to white matter in the presence of unilateral ischaemia was attributed to symmetrical maximal metabolic depression.

The important study of Hirano, Levine and Zimmermann (1967), also in the rat, showed that the earliest alteration (after 1–2 hours) in the fine structure of white matter was swelling of axis cylinders within which mitochondria were expanded and their cristae more or less disorganized. At this stage, myelin sheaths, glial elements and the extracellular space all appeared normal. Damage to myelin was only appreciable during a later or reactive phase.

Brierley, Brown and Calverley (1976) in a light microscopic study gave sodium cyanide to rats by slow intravenous infusion. After *in vivo* perfusion-fixation, damage to white matter, particularly the corpus callosum, was seen in six of 19 animals and grey matter additionally in only one. In the latter animal bradycardia, epileptic seizures and hypotension were particularly marked and neuronal damage was attributed to the secondary effects of cyanide on the circulation. The earliest alteration in white matter was a pallor of myelin staining associated with fragmentation of the nuclei of oligodendrocytes. In a recent study in physiologically monitored, lightly anaesthetized and spontaneously breathing monkeys (Brierley et al., 1977) sodium cyanide was given by intravenous infusion. The animals were killed by *in vivo* perfusion-fixation. Brain damage was seen in only four of 11 animals. It involved digitate white matter but spared the commissures in all four, and in one animal there was a striking pallor of staining in the optic tracts. Ischaemic cell change was restricted to the striatum of a single animal in which there had been a period of bradycardia, hypotension and raised central venous pressure. It was concluded that in the Rhesus monkey, as in the rat, there is no evidence to support the occurrence of hypoxic neuronal damage of purely histotoxic type.

Azides Sodium azide (NaN_3) inhibits the action of cytochrome oxidase, and its ability to depress the respiration of cerebral cortex has been demonstrated *in vitro*. The experimental studies of Hurst (1942) in the monkey and of Hicks (1950b) and Környey (1963) in the rat showed that myelinated fibres, as well as nerve cells, could be damaged.

Whilst there are no neuropathological reports of azide intoxication in man, Mettler and Sax (1972) have described cerebellar damage as a consequence of the intravenous injection of sodium azide in Rhesus monkeys. A single injection produced hyperventilation, pupillary dilatation, a fall in blood pressure to about 3.3 kPa (25 mmHg) and a convulsion. Animals that recovered exhibited ataxia, and neuropathological examinations showed that alterations, confined to the cerebellum, ranged from almost complete decortication to minor cortical damage in the depths of sulci around the horizontal fissures. As this region is a cerebellar arterial boundary zone it was recognized that the cytotoxic effects of azide could not be separated from the considerable hypotension that it may induce.

Hypoglycaemia

Hypoglycaemia may lead to damage in the human brain when the associated coma is irreversible (i.e. when it does not respond to the administration of glucose). In relation to brain damage, Meyer (1963) stated that 'the findings in the literature show some variation, but there is no doubt that they closely resemble those which occur in other types of anoxia'. It is well known, however, that hypoglycaemic coma may be accompanied or followed by some depression of cardiovascular or respiratory function, epileptic seizures or raised intracranial pressure, each of which may contribute to the structural damage. The ability of uncomplicated hypoglycaemia to initiate the ischaemic cell process in the brains of experimental primates has been demonstrated only recently (see below). The situations in which hypoglycaemia may occur are diverse and have been classified by Marks and Rose (1965) on the basis of aetiology and of clinical presentation.

Neuropathological descriptions of the brain damage attributed to hypoglycaemia in man have been derived from (1) patients dying after insulin shock therapy for psychoses; (2) diabetic patients developing irreversible coma after treatment with insulin; (3) rare instances of islet cell tumours of the pancreas (insulinoma); (4) rare instances of attempted suicide by injection of insulin; (5) examples of idiopathic hypoglycaemia in infants; and (6) occasional instances of 'white liver' disease in infants with proved hypoglycaemia (as in two of the 12 cases of Cullity and Kakulas (1970)). A patient with unilateral carotid artery occlusion/stenosis may develop a hemiparesis in the presence of a moderate hypoglycaemia (Meyer and Portnoy, 1958; Portnoy, 1965).

When survival is short the intact and sliced brain may appear normal. Brain swelling is unusual (Lawrence, Meyer and Nevin, 1942; Brierley, 1965; Vital et al., 1967). In cases surviving for days/weeks there is laminar granularity in the cortex and in the hippocampus. Dilated ventricles, cortical atrophy and shrinkage of the hippocampi are marked only when survival is more than a few months. In a personal (JBB) case (attempted suicide by the injection of insulin) who survived demented for 16 years, the brain weighed only 700 g. In addition to general cortical atrophy the first, second and third temporal gyri on each side were reduced to paper-thin membranes whilst the parahippocampal gyri were intact and the hippocampi showed only moderate sclerosis.

As in all types of hypoxic brain damage, histological abnormalities depend on the duration of survival, ranging from ischaemic cell change to neuronal loss and a gliomesodermal reaction. In the cerebral cortex, neuronal damage is almost invariable and, although sometimes focal, is more usually laminar (Fig. 4.21) with an em-

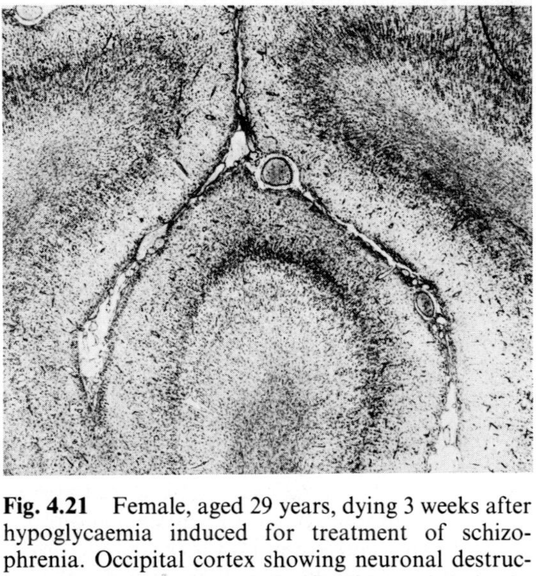

Fig. 4.21 Female, aged 29 years, dying 3 weeks after hypoglycaemia induced for treatment of schizophrenia. Occipital cortex showing neuronal destruction and gliomesodermal proliferation, largely in the outer layers. Celloidin; cresyl violet × 6.5.

phasis on the third and fifth layers. Occasionally necrosis of all layers may be seen, particularly in the posterior half of the brain, but usually with a relative preservation of the visual cortex. Demyelination, diffuse rather than focal, may accompany the cortical damage (Richardson and Russell, 1952). Also, normal myelin staining may be associated with widespread fibrillary gliosis in the white matter, as in two of the six cases of Lawrence, Meyer and Nevin (1942).

The hippocampi usually show typical hypoxic necrosis (Fig. 4.22), sometimes approaching the level of infarction. Among subcortical structures the almost total necrosis of the striatum seen in the third case of Lawrence, Meyer and Nevin (1942) was probably exceptional, as this structure was normal in the three cases of Vital et al. (1967) and showed only minor or moderate damage in six of the eight cases of Brierley (1965). Involvement of the globus pallidus is unusual and is usually only moderate in the thalamus. In the cerebellum damage to Purkinje cells is appreciably less than in other types of hypoxia (Meyer, 1963). In the brain stem neuronal alterations are usually slight.

Experimental studies Most of these have been carried out in subhuman primates; the brains were usually removed with minimal delay and fixed by immersion, so histological artefacts most probably account for the very diverse abnormalities in neurons that have been reported.

The long-term neurological and neuropathological effects of uncomplicated insulin-induced hypoglycaemia in physiologically monitored Rhesus monkeys were studied by Kahn and Myers (1971) and Myers and Kahn (1971). Blood glucose fell to 1.1 mmol/l (20 mg/dl) after 1.5–3 hours. This level was maintained for 4–10 hours in 11 animals and was terminated by the intravenous injection of glucose. In the seven animals with persisting neurological impairment, convulsions occurred during the recovery phase in five. Neuropathological alterations consisted of loss of neurons and a gliomesodermal reaction in the striatum, the neocortex and the hippocampus in decreasing order of frequency.

In an attempt to define the early stages of the neuronal alterations due to uncomplicated hypoglycaemia in the monkey under light pentobarbitone anaesthesia, Meldrum, Horton and

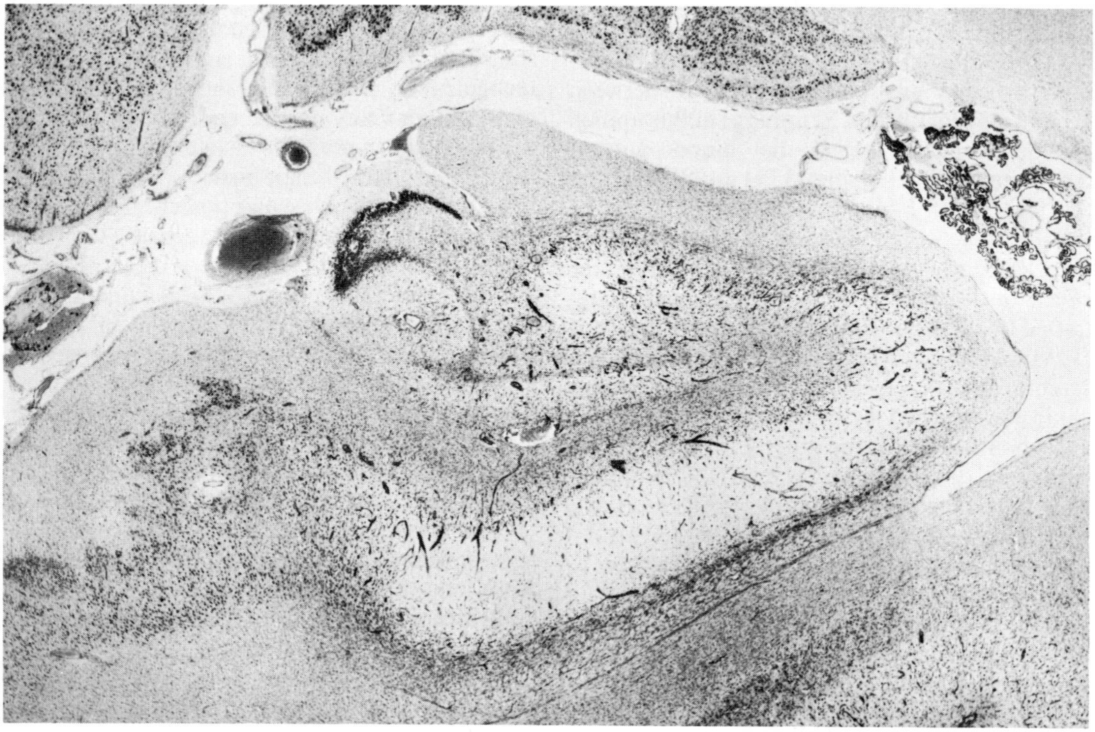

Fig. 4.22 Same case as Fig. 4.21. Hippocampus, showing almost total neuronal destruction in CA 1 (Sommer sector), and CA 3 and CA 4 (end folium), with relative preservation of CA 2. Celloidin; cresyl violet × 10.

Brierley (1971) monitored brain arterial and venous blood gas tensions, pH and glucose. The ECG, EEG and somatosensory evoked potentials were also recorded. Hypoglycaemia was induced in 15 animals by the intravenous injection of insulin over periods of 2–7 hours and was terminated after 2–8 hours by the injection of glucose. The brains were fixed by *in vivo* perfusion after survival for 30 minutes to 15 hours.

Neuropathological alterations seen in eight animals (Brierley, Brown and Meldrum, 1971a, b) consisted of ischaemic cell change at the stage of microvacuolation after survival for half an hour, and then of typical ischaemic cell change without and later with incrustations. In seven animals the neocortex was diffusely involved but with an emphasis on the occipital and parietal regions. The hippocampi, the corpora striata and the cerebellar Purkinje cells were involved in one animal. In these animals blood glucose was below 1.1 mmol/l (20 mg/dl) for more than 2 hours, there was no epileptic activity, blood pressure and oxygenation were well maintained, and there was no rise in intracranial pressure and no post-mortem evidence of brain swelling. In the eighth animal damage was concentrated along the cortical arterial boundary zones. The cerebral perfusion pressure had fallen to between 3.7 and 4.3 kPa (28 and 32 mmHg) in this animal for 30 minutes whilst the blood glucose did not fall below 1.9 mmol/l (34 mg/dl). Neither this degree of hypoglycaemia nor the hypotension alone would have resulted in brain damage. Evidently one factor can potentiate the effects of the other. This conclusion is also supported by the experiments of Meyer and Portnoy (1958) in the cat. After occlusion of one middle cerebral artery, localized neurological signs could be obtained by inducing hypoglycaemia and abolished by giving glucose. Whilst the experiments of Kahn and Myers (1971) and of Meldrum, Horton and Brierley (1971) indicate that blood glucose must fall to 1.1 mmol/l (20 mg/dl) if uncomplicated hypoglycaemia is to produce brain damage, a higher level of blood glucose if combined with hypotension, hypoxaemia or epileptic activity may have the same outcome.

It should now be apparent that ischaemic cell change is the consequence of every type of hypoxia as well as hypoglycaemia. While physiologically inappropriate in the latter situation, the term 'hypoxia' is justified because of the neuronal alterations observed.

'Selective vulnerability' within the brain—anatomical, physiological and metabolic aspects

Those regions of the brain that are selectively vulnerable to hypoxia in its widest sense have already been described. Only global brain ischaemia, as brought about by cardiac arrest, can lead to typical alterations in most of the vulnerable regions in many cases (see p. 133). An overall reduction in cerebral blood flow, with or without hypoxaemia, results in ischaemic lesions along arterial boundary zones which must also be regarded as regions of selective vulnerability.

There is a wide variation in the number of the selectively vulnerable regions involved in any one case. In the great majority there is sparing of the anterior horn cells of the spinal cord, the motor nuclei of the brain stem and the principal nuclei of the hypothalamus. Although the higher and more recently evolved regions of the telencephalon are most vulnerable, hypoxic damage is never complete in the neocortex. Even in instances of the 'apallic state' lamination is usually recognizable in the frontal lobes and each lamina may contain many normal neurons.

Two major hypotheses have been advanced to explain the characteristic distribution of hypoxic brain damage: the 'vascular theory' (Spielmeyer, 1925); and the concept of 'pathoclisis' (Vogt and Vogt, 1937), which postulated local physicochemical factors as a basis for local vulnerability. The vascular theory invoked anatomical factors such as the length and tortuosity of a particular artery and also physiological factors such as vasospasm and stasis. The arguments for and against the vascular theory were reviewed by Scholz (1963) and A. Meyer (1963). The normality of the hippocampus after an episode of hypotension in man, while major lesions may be present along the neocortical arterial boundary zones, implies that anatomical vascular factors alone cannot account for the sparing of the hippocampus when blood flow is greatly reduced. Neither can they explain why typical hypoxic alterations do occur when a normal or only slightly reduced blood flow is complicated by some reduction in blood oxygen or glucose content.

Scholz (1963) noted that the vascular theory could not explain the neuropathological changes seen in the cerebellum, '... the Purkinje cells are those most vulnerable to hypoxia, they are followed by the granular cells whereas the Golgi cells are the most resistant. This scale of vulnerability can hardly be explained by differences in vascularisation as suggested by Uchimura (1928) ...', an argument applicable to other regions of the brain. Apparent confirmation of the role of a vascular factor in the genesis of hypoxic brain damage was advanced by Lindenberg (1955, 1963) who claimed that selective vulnerability could be attributed to compression of arteries by a presumably invariable posthypoxic brain swelling. In order that intracranial pressure should exceed that within arteries he stated that '... acute lowering of systemic arterial pressure is a pre-requisite for such compression ...' (Lindenberg, 1963). Evidence for such hypotension and the corresponding levels of intracranial pressure have not been published. This hypothesis ignores the fact that intracranial pressure is sustained by cerebral perfusion pressure and can only exceed it in rare agonal states. It is demonstrable, in the experimental primate with a posthypoxic rise in intracranial pressure, that a sudden hypotensive episode produces an immediate and parallel fall in intracranial pressure (Brierley, Meldrum and Brown, 1971). Scholz (1963) pointed out that vascular compression could not explain the vulnerability of special fields in a structure such as the hippocampus, and Brierley (1961) and Brierley et al. (1971) have established that posthypoxic brain swelling is by no means an invariable occurrence and that typical hypoxic alterations occur in the vulnerable regions in its absence. Furthermore, when such swelling does occur, it does not give rise to the major internal herniae and brain stem haemorrhages so often associated with acute intracranial expanding lesions.

The local physicochemical properties postulated by the theory of pathoclisis have proved hard to isolate and define, and of those investigated none is related with certainty to damage in a particular region. Thus the demonstration by Maske (1955) of a high concentration of zinc in the hippocampi of animals was confirmed in human post-mortem material by Friede (1966) using the histochemical method of Timm (1958). The concentration of the metal is high in CA 2 and CA 3 and low in CA 1. McLardy (1962) demonstrated that the zinc is concentrated not in the cell bodies of CA 2 and CA 3 but in the terminations of the mossy fibres derived from the cells of the dentate gyrus. A parallel distribution of lactic dehydrogenase in these regions led Friede (1966) to speculate that high levels of the enzyme may imply an improved capacity for anaerobic glycolysis and thus an increased ability to survive hypoxia.

Further evidence for metabolic differentiation within the hippocampus was provided by Coggeshall and MacLean (1958) who found, in mice, that a single dose of 3-acetylpyridine, a nicotinic acid analogue, resulted in partial or complete loss of neurons in the zinc-rich zones CA 2 and CA 3. Whilst there is increasing evidence to show that physicochemical differences do exist in the hippocampus and that some are coincident with the distribution of hypoxic damage, it is not yet possible to say which are causally related to the phenomenon of selective damage. A biochemical approach to the latter was initiated by Kato and Lowry (1973), who found considerable differences in the enzyme patterns of cell bodies of different neuronal populations (e.g. cortical, hippocampal, cerebellar), using quantitative microchemical techniques.

Irreversible brain damage in the vulnerable areas has been attributed to levels of brain lactic acid in excess of 20 μmol/g (Myers, 1979; Rehncrona, Rosen and Siesjö, 1981). Lactacidosis, however, is not an invariable accompaniment of the various categories of hypoxia and therefore cannot qualify as a major, and particularly a selective, determinant of cell damage. Furthermore, there is no apparent correlation between deterioration of cellular energy metabolism and the development of irreversible cell damage identifiable microscopically.

In the search for a common mechanism of neuronal damage, increasing attention has been paid to events occurring in the period of posthypoxic recirculation. There is no doubt that ion homoeostasis is disturbed and that there is release of potassium and an influx of calcium into neurons. Mitochondrial function may be disturbed by the accumulation of free fatty acids, some of the metabolites of which having the characteristics of free radicals and being therefore potentially toxic. A working hypothesis has been developed by Siesjö (1981) whereby a disturbed calcium homoeostasis, the associated activation of phospholipases, and an accumulation of free fatty acids could, singly or in combination, account for cell damage. It has therefore been proposed that the vulnerability of certain cells to the ischaemic cell process may be due to an abnormal local influx of calcium but this has not yet been demonstrated in any population of vulnerable neurons.

A number of studies indicate that neuronal injury indistinguishable from ischaemic cell change can be induced in susceptible nerve cells by exceptionally enhanced neuronal activity (Meldrum and Brierley, 1973; Blennow et al., 1978). Since seizure activity augments cerebral energy consumption, a failure of the supply of energy to keep pace with its utilization is likely to be an important factor in the genesis of epileptic brain damage. However, the finding that brain damage can be lessened by reducing the available oxygen or glucose implies that energy consumption cannot be the sole mechanism. Although Ingvar and Siesjö (1981) conclude that cellular injury in seizures is unlikely to be due to a mismatching of local metabolism and blood flow, studies using kainic acid (Nadler, Perry and Cotman, 1978; Ben-Ari, Tremblay and Ottersen, 1980) have suggested that such mismatching can be a pathogenic factor. Celik et al. (1982) found a marked increase in the measured rate of glucose utilization in parts of the limbic system, such as the hippocampus and the septal nuclei, unaccompanied by significant changes in local blood flow. Similar results were obtained by Lothman and Collins (1981), who found that kainic acid selectively enhanced local metabolic rate without producing irreversible damage in limbic structures. There is therefore some evidence that increased neuronal activity may enhance susceptibility to hypoxia and that degrees of metabolic and functional activity, not pathogenic *per se*, may become so when supplies of substrate and oxygen are limited.

A further factor that may determine the pattern of selective vulnerability to hypoxia-ischaemia is the influence of immaturity (Rice, Vannucci and Brierley, 1981; Welsh, Vannucci and Brierley, 1982). In these experiments 7-day-old rats were subjected to unilateral carotid artery ligation and exposed to 8% oxygen at 37°C for 3.5 hours. Brain damage, seen in 90 per cent of the survivors, consisted of a columnar distribution of hypoxic damage within the cortex supplied by the middle cerebral artery corresponding to the columns seen in autoradiographs using the $[^{14}C]$deoxyglucose technique (Pulsinelli and Duffy, 1979) and by the method of reduced nicotinamide adenine dinucleotide fluorescence (Welsh, O'Connor and Langfitt, 1977). These metabolic columns are thought to represent reversible disturbances in regional metabolism since severe cerebral hypoxia-ischaemia in experimental animals and man usually produces irreversible neuronal damage with a laminar distribution. In contrast to adult animals, the pattern of cortical damage is columnar in immature rats, with little or no suggestion of selective laminar vulnerability (Rice, Vannucci and Brierley, 1981). It is likely that in the immature cortex metabolic differences between laminae have not yet developed, so the pattern of damage reflects vascular architecture, the width and height of the columns depending upon the anatomy of the penetrating arterioles.

The development by Levine (1960) of a preparation in the rat in which unilateral anoxic-ischaemic damage occurs in 80 per cent of animals, enabled the results of histo- and cytochemical techniques to be compared with those of conventional neurohistology. It had been hoped that the earliest alterations in the vulnerable regions could be defined in biochemical terms. The first 5 years of such studies were reviewed by Spector (1965) and it is evident that all workers were in more or less close agreement with the view of Becker (1963) that, where anoxic-ischaemic damage is concerned, in standard preparations detectable abnormalities before 12 hours are rare. It was claimed that histochemical techniques could define a 'biochemical lesion' before any derived from conventional histological techniques (MacDonald and Spector, 1963).

Employing *in vivo* perfusion-fixation of the rat Levine preparation, Brown and Brierley (1966, 1968) showed that microvacuolation was the earliest stage of ischaemic cell change and could be recognized in animals perfused immediately after 5 and 15 minutes intermittent exposure to nitrogen (Brown and Brierley, 1973). The conclusion is inescapable that if a 'biochemical lesion' does precede that revealed by the light microscope in optimally fixed material, it must be demonstrated not after a survival of hours when neuronal damage is far advanced and irreversible but within the first few minutes of survival. Until cytochemical studies employing light and electron microscopes have been deployed within this brief period, the local metabolic factors responsible for selective vulnerability will remain elusive.

The respirator brain

This term is synonymous with 'brain death' which '... occurs when irreversible damage to the cerebral hemispheres and brain stem is so severe that the nervous system can no longer maintain internal homoeostasis', (Plum, 1972) and the patient is apnoeic even if hypercapnia is allowed to develop. After the start of mechanical ventilation, systemic circulatory failure develops within a few days or occasionally a few weeks. The EEG is isoelectric throughout and although spinal reflexes may remain, brain stem reflexes are abolished. Such total failure of brain function is usually brought about by the arrest of cerebral circulation due to gross brain swelling and may be confirmed by the failure of contrast medium to enter the skull in the course of angiography (Heiskanen, 1964).

In the absence of circulation the dead brain undergoes a process of *in vivo* autolysis and at autopsy the brain may be increased in weight: its consistency is semifluid and it hardens poorly or not at all in formalin. The tissue is discoloured and there is loss of definition between grey and white matter and disintegration of tissue, particularly in the deep grey matter of the cerebrum and in the cerebellum. Fragments of the latter may be found along the spinal cord. Histologically, there is vacuolation of neuronal cytoplasm and poor staining of neuronal nuclei. In such circumstances any evidence of ischaemic cell change, or of a gliomesodermal reaction in the brain, must be interpreted as having preceded the onset of brain death. These changes are particularly severe within the Purkinje and granule cells of the cerebellum (Matakas, Cervos-Navarro and Schneider, 1973; Walker, Diamond and Moseley, 1975).

Complications of hypoxic brain damage

Swelling

It is well known that subjects dying within 48 hours of a systemic hypoxic stress, such as cardiac arrest, hypoglycaemia or status epilepticus, may show the pathological features of brain swelling. These include flattening of the cortical convolutions and of the cerebellar folia, internal herniae and small ventricles. The swelling is rarely enough to produce infarction in the territories supplied by the posterior cerebral arteries or secondary damage in the brain stem. It is to be stressed that in ultrastructural studies of grey matter neurons are not swollen at any stage and there is no evidence of increase in the extracellular space but there is progressive swelling of astrocytic processes (Brown, 1977). In white matter, on the other hand, there is a true expansion of the extracellular space. The pathogenesis of this type of brain swelling is therefore undecided.

There is ample clinical evidence to indicate that death from postischaemic brain swelling is greatest 2–4 days after occlusion of the internal carotid artery (Bounds et al., 1981). It was severe enough to produce brain shift, tentorial herniation and secondary haemorrhages in the brain stem.

In regions of infarction, experimental studies have shown that vascular permeability to horseradish peroxidase occurs almost immediately, and its extent and severity correlate with the ischaemic damage (Petito, 1979a). This early increase in permeability to horseradish peroxidase is due to enhanced micropinocytosis, the interendothelial junctions always remaining tight. These studies suggest that in the first few hours after vascular occlusion the blood–brain barrier remains intact, while leakage of horseradish peroxidase after a few hours represents passive diffusion through necrotic vessel walls.

Various biogenic amines have been considered responsible for changes in the permeability of the blood–brain barrier, but the major factor is whether or not there is reperfusion of the ischaemic area. Reperfusion could occur either through the main stem of the artery of supply, as after breakdown of an embolus, or through the collateral circulation at the edge of the ischaemic area. Both of these mechanisms have been suggested as a cause of 'haemorrhagic', as distinct from 'non-haemorrhagic', cerebral infarction (Kamijyo, Garcia and Cooper, 1977). However, reperfusion alone cannot account for haemorrhagic infarcts as these are so rare in experimental animals when circulation has been restored by removal of a clip or ligature and subsequent microscopic examination shows virtually total destruction of all vascular elements within the core of the infarct. The mechanism responsible for the apparent sealing of vessels at the periphery of an infarct remains obscure.

Epilepsy

Although epileptic seizures are uncommon in patients surviving cardiorespiratory arrest, epilepsy is a common complication of other types of cerebral hypoxia. Early in the resuscitation after cardiorespiratory arrest, Prior (1979) found EEG evidence of epileptiform activity in about 30 per cent of cases. Among patients with post-anoxic epilepsy, a few recovered without, or with minimal, evidence of residual brain damage. The majority died without regaining consciousness. Epileptiform EEG discharges continuing for several days after resuscitation were suggestive of brain damage. Epileptic seizures are generally considered to be an uncommon symptom of focal cerebral ischaemia, and an incidence of 10–30 per cent has been reported (see Cocito, Favale and Reni, 1982).

Meldrum and Brierley (1973) have shown that status epilepticus induced by the alkaloid bicuculline in baboons leads to ischaemic neuronal changes in the selectively vulnerable regions of the neocortex, the hippocampus, the basal ganglia and the cerebellum, similar to that seen in man (Meyer, Beck and Shepherd, 1955; Meyer, 1963). This posthypoxic epilepsy may add an element of secondary damage when it takes the form of status epilepticus rather than discrete seizures.

The no-reflow phenomenon

This phenomenon implies that impaired vascular reperfusion after hypoxic stress is the principal cause of hypoxic damage in brain which might otherwise have been normal. Alternatively, it may occur only in brains which have already suffered primary irreversible ischaemic damage and then as a further increment. There is now sufficient evidence (Levy, Brierley and Plum, 1975; Levy et al., 1975; Little, Kerr and Sundt, 1975) to indicate that impaired reperfusion (no-reflow) plays little if any part in the pathogenesis of global ischaemic brain damage. A failure of reperfusion at a local vascular level may imperil additional neurons (Ames, 1973).

Thresholds of ischaemia

Studies of focal ischaemia have shown that if arterial oxygenation remains normal, there is a close association between reduced cerebral blood flow and disturbances in cerebral function. As flow is reduced, a progressive sequence of events justifies the concept of 'thresholds of ischaemia'. In general, cerebral dysfunction first becomes evident after a 50 per cent reduction in flow. After occlusion of the middle cerebral artery in baboons and when cerebral blood flow is about 30 per cent of normal, the EEG becomes isoelectric and evoked potentials are lost (Branston et al., 1974; Astrup et al., 1977). At levels of about 12–15 per cent of normal there is release of potassium, but biochemical evidence of irreversible brain damage occurs only when flow is reduced to about 10 per cent of normal (see Astrup, 1982).

There is therefore an upper threshold of electrical failure and a lower one of failure of energy and the ion pump. Between these thresholds the ischaemic brain is electrically silent with a normal or only slightly increased potassium content. This situation characterizes a ring of tissue—the *penumbra*—around a core of irreversibly damaged brain (an infarct) in which energy failure and ion pump failure have developed (Astrup, Siesjö and Symon, 1981). The penumbra may remain unchanged for several hours as long as there is sufficient collateral blood supply. The tissue, while non-functioning, is still viable and capable of full recovery.

Vascular disorders of the central nervous system

D. I. Graham and J. B. Brierley

Applied anatomy and physiology

Arterial blood supply

The brain is supplied with blood through the internal carotid and the vertebral arteries which anastomose at the base of the brain via the circle of Willis. From this circle arteries arise as (1) paramedian vessels perforating the base of the brain to supply structures near the midline, (2) short circumferential vessels supplying the thalamus, lentiform nuclei and other basal ganglia, and (3) long circumferential anterior, middle and posterior cerebral arteries and their branches supplying principally the cortex and underlying white matter (Yates, 1976a).

The study of occlusive vascular disease has emphasized the importance of the collateral circulation. When a major vessel in the neck is occluded, the anatomical connections between the internal and external carotid arteries and between the vertebrobasilar and the carotid circulations become apparent (Meyer and Loeb, 1965). However, for cerebral blood flow to be adequate after occlusion of an internal carotid artery, not only must the collateral circulation be normal but also the circle of Willis so that retrograde flow can develop through the ophthalmic artery. Thus the circle of Willis plays a vital role in readjusting blood flow to the brain following occlusion of a major vessel in the neck. Its classic configuration has been described by Alpers, Berry and Paddison (1959) but this pattern is seen in less than half of all adults (Riggs and Rupp, 1963). Most variations are of little clinical importance though certain configurations such as hypoplasia of the proximal anterior cerebral artery or of the anterior or posterior communicating arteries may prevent the establishment of an adequate collateral blood supply. Another important collateral circulation comprises anastomoses between the anterior, middle and posterior cerebral arteries on the surface of the brain (Vander Eecken and Adams, 1953). Whilst the neocortex has an important collateral circulation, deeper structures, including the basal ganglia, are generally supplied by non-anastomosing penetrating vessels. However, important arterial anastomoses between central and peripheral systems within the brain may be found near the angle of the lateral ventricle where the lateral striate vessels contribute a substantial branch to the postcentral gyrus in 4 per cent of cases (Cole, 1967).

The major arteries supplying the brain stem and the cerebellum are derived from the vertebrobasilar system. These comprise (1) paramedian branches from the basilar artery, (2) short circumferential branches and (3) long circumferential arteries such as the superior, anterior and posterior inferior cerebellar arteries. Whereas the vertebral arteries are often asymmetrical, and sometimes remarkably so, anomalies of the basilar artery are relatively rare. Anomalies of the cerebellar arteries are more common, usually taking the form of hypoplasia. There are ipsi- and bilateral anastomoses between the cortical branches of the cerebellar arteries, and also between branches of the superior cerebellar and posterior cerebral arteries. In the pons, the paramedian arteries supplying the ventromedial portion of the brain stem have no significant anastomosis with each other across the midline or with other arteries supplying the brain stem. The ventrolateral portion of the midbrain and pons are supplied by the short circumferential arteries but there is disagreement about the blood supply to the tegmentum as defined by injection techniques and the extent of infarction after vascular occlusion (Foix and Hillemand, 1926; Kubik and Adams, 1946; Atkinson, 1949; Biemond, 1951).

The blood supply to the spinal cord is considered in Chapter 17.

Venous drainage

The veins of the cerebrum vary in size, number and length. The superficial veins either lie beside arteries within sulci or they cross gyri. The majority drain via the superior sagittal and transverse sinuses into the internal jugular veins. Veins from the basal ganglia and deep white matter enter the internal cerebral veins which join to form the vein of Galen, which drains into the straight sinus. The dural sinuses communicate with the extracranial veins via the vascular channels in the diploë of the bones of the skull. Emissary veins connect the dural venous sinuses with extracranial veins. Other anastomoses connect veins of the posterior fossa, vertebral plexuses and the systemic venous system.

The veins of the pons and medulla form a superficial plexus that drains into the inferior petrosal and sigmoid sinuses. The venous drainage of the spinal cord corresponds mainly to the arterial supply. There are, however, many venous tributaries both within and around the cord and, although variable and frequently duplicated, they constitute a single median spinal vein posteriorly.

Epidemiology of vascular disorders of the central nervous system

Mortality figures when analysed for factors such as country of origin, race and climate reveal differences in the incidence of stroke (Kurtzke, 1969). For example, in England and Wales during this century there has been a decreasing death rate from cerebral haemorrhage and an increase in that from cerebral infarction (Yates, 1964). Many of the difficulties inherent in historical surveys have been reduced by prospective epidemiological investigations of cerebrovascular disease such as that undertaken during the last two decades at Framingham, Massachusetts (Shurtleff, 1970; Gordon, Sorlie and Kannel, 1971; Kannel, 1976).

Cerebrovascular disorders are a major cause of admission to hospital and account for much of the residual disability after an acute stroke. This major health problem, according to Wolf and Kannel (1982), accounts for 500 000 new patients in the USA with stroke each year; about half of these die. Strokes account for some 10 per cent of all deaths and, of those who survive, about 50 per cent are severely disabled, only 10 per cent returning to normal activity (Gresham et al., 1979). The incidence of stroke rises rapidly with increasing age, some 80 per cent of cases occurring in patients over 65 (Kannel et al., 1976). Nevertheless, strokes do occur in neonates (Barmada, Moossy and Shuman, 1979), infants and children (Schoenberg, Mellinger and Schoenberg, 1978), and young adults (see Marshall, 1982).

About 75 per cent of strokes are due to cerebral infarction (atherothrombosis in 60 per cent, cerebral embolism in 10 per cent and cerebral lacunae in 5 per cent), whilst 15 per cent are due to haemorrhage (subarachnoid in 10 per cent, and intracerebral in 5 per cent). In about 10 per cent of cases the patient presents with a transient ischaemic attack (see p. 181).

A number of premorbid factors presaging stroke have been identified. Some are related to the development of atheroma and hypertension, the most important predisposing factors, whilst others are heart disease and diabetes mellitus (Wolf and Kannel, 1982). The incidence of stroke is six times higher in hypertensives than in normotensive individuals of the same age. Some 50 per cent occur in the 20 per cent of the adult population that is hypertensive. Hypertension is common in the elderly, an age group particularly liable to stroke. About 75 per cent of patients who have had a stroke have one or more signs of cardiac failure, atrial fibrillation or an enlarged heart. Statistically patients with coronary artery disease have a two- to five-fold increased risk of stroke. Cerebral infarcts are from two to four times more common in diabetics than in non-diabetic patients of the same age and sex (Wolf and Kannel, 1982).

Compared with hypertension, heart disease and diabetes mellitus, other factors that increase the risk of stroke are relatively minor (Wolf and Kannel, 1982). Some have been classed as personal attributes, others as due to environment and the remainder as due to life styles that predispose to cerebrovascular disorder. Among personal attributes are a family history, obesity, haemoglobin level, the haematocrit and the level of low-density lipids in blood. The important environmental considerations include climate, the drinking water (whether hard or soft), occupation, stress, diet and cigarette smoking. In addition, stroke has been associated with the use of oral contraceptives and identified as a sequel of open heart and cardiopulmonary bypass surgery.

Cerebral infarction

A cerebral infarct is defined as a volume of tissue within which all cell bodies (neuronal and glial), blood vessels (arteries, veins and capillaries) and nerve fibres (myelinated and non-myelinated) have undergone necrosis as a result of a critical reduction in blood supply. This last may be due to either an *arrest* (ischaemia) or a critical *reduction* (oligaemia) in blood flow (see p. 128). Circulatory arrest may be either permanent or for a period beyond the ischaemic threshold for each structural element. The thresholds will be influenced by the availability of oxygen and glucose. The principal causes of infarction are arterial occlusion by thrombus formation or embolism, spasm occurring in association with subarachnoid haemorrhage and a failure of cerebral perfusion.

Infarcts range in size from a few millimetres (recognizable only histologically) (see Fig. 4.43) to those affecting an entire arterial territory as a result of occlusion close to its origin from the circle of Willis. It is particularly in the larger infarcts that white as well as grey matter is involved (Figs 4.23 to 4.28).

Macroscopic appearances of the brain These depend upon the size of the lesion and the survival time. In the fresh specimen larger recent infarcts are swollen (greater in white than in grey matter) and hyperaemic, and are also soft to palpation. In

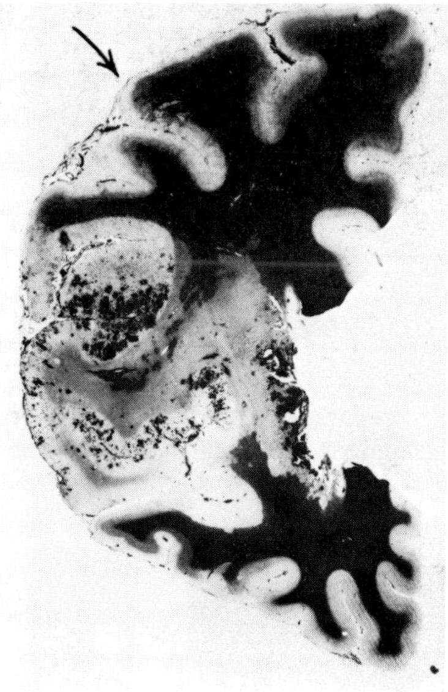

Fig. 4.24 Myelin preparation of Fig. 4.23. Note the sharp edge to the necrotic white matter which does not stain. In some places only the subcortical U-fibres are necrotic; in other places the deep white matter is damaged. Note the older lesion (arrow).

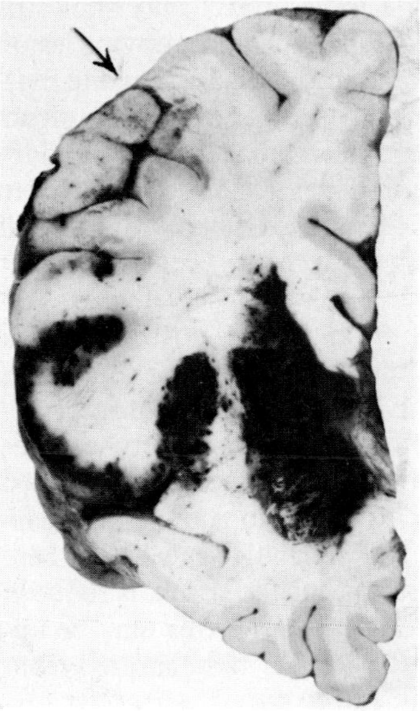

Fig. 4.23 Coronal section of frontal lobe. In the lower part of the picture there is recent haemorrhagic infarction (cortex more than white matter). The affected tissue is swollen and the demarcation between cortex and white matter is ill-defined. In the upper part of the picture (arrow) there is an older lesion of about 6 week's duration.

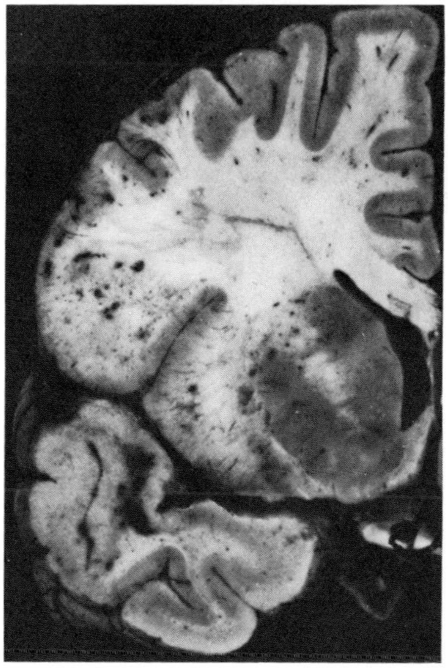

Fig. 4.25 Coronal section at level of anterior basal ganglia. There is extensive infarction due to embolic occlusion of the middle cerebral artery of 3 weeks' duration. The necrotic grey matter, which is friable, is not clearly defined from the white matter. In the centrum semiovale the edge of the necrotic white matter is clearly visible. The inferomedial half of the corpus callosum (supplied by the recurrent artery of Heubner) is not necrotic.

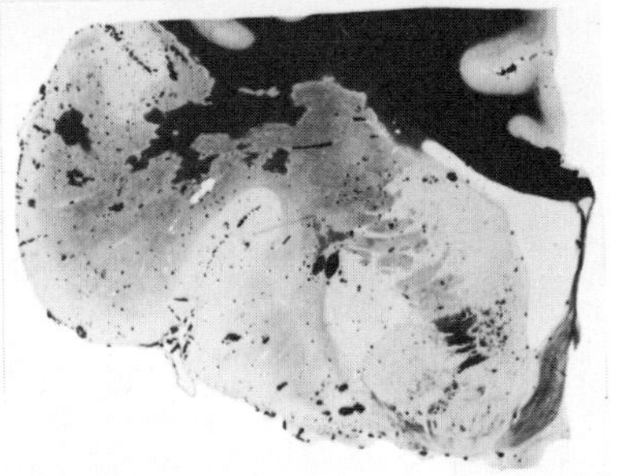

Fig. 4.26 Myelin preparation of middle part of Fig. 4.25. Note the sharp edge to the necrotic white matter.

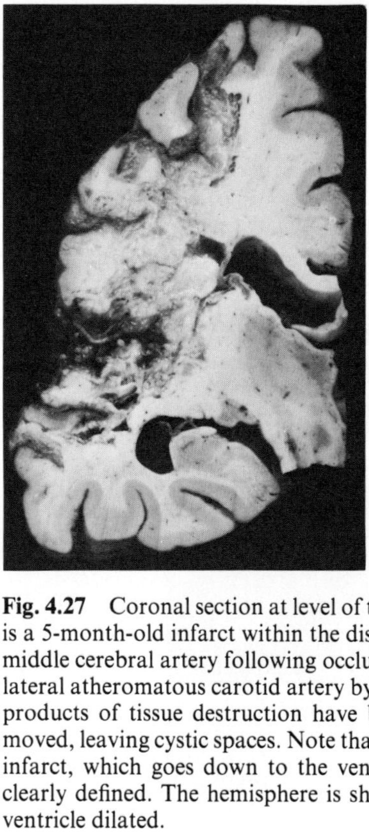

Fig. 4.27 Coronal section at level of thalamus. There is a 5-month-old infarct within the distribution of the middle cerebral artery following occlusion of the ipsilateral atheromatous carotid artery by thrombus. The products of tissue destruction have been largely removed, leaving cystic spaces. Note that the edge of the infarct, which goes down to the ventricular wall, is clearly defined. The hemisphere is shrunken and the ventricle dilated.

fixed preparations the hyperaemia may be less apparent, and in slices there is diminished structural definition but also a more marked distinction between infarcted and normal tissue. Haemorrhages ranging from discrete to apparently confluent may be seen in grey and white matter (*haemorrhagic infarction*). They may be entirely absent (*non-haemorrhagic infarction*).

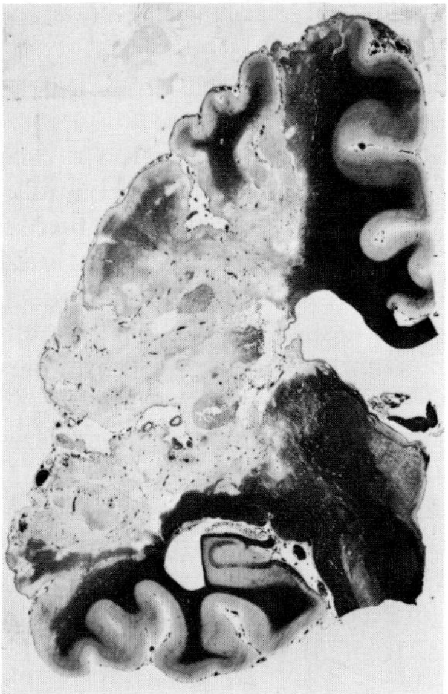

Fig. 4.28 Myelin preparation showing well-defined margin of the infarct corresponding to that seen in Fig. 4.27. Celloidin; Loyez.

When survival is 24 hours or more a hemisphere containing a large infarct may show the features associated with a space-occupying lesion as a result of oedema in the adjacent white matter. Thus, there may be a shift of midline structures, typical internal herniae and secondary brain stem haemorrhages (see Fig. 4.37) (van Trotsenburg and Vinken, 1966; Adams and Graham, 1967). Swelling of a recent cerebellar infarct may cause hydrocephalus by acting as an acute expanding lesion in the posterior fossa (Graham and Adams, 1972). Within a few weeks the swelling within and around an infarct decreases and the infarcted grey matter becomes soft and granular. White matter also shrinks, becomes rubbery on palpation and is increasingly demarcated from normal tissue. Later there is further shrinkage so that the cortex is reduced to a narrow structureless band: this may be apposed to white matter or may be separated from it by an apparently empty cyst or slit. Cyst formation is frequent in the basal ganglia (see Fig. 4.38) in the brain stem and in subcortical white matter. Total infarction of the hippocampus is rare, and when seen it is always at a posterior level and may be restricted to CA 1. In the cerebellum an old infarct may appear either as a region in which there has been loss of tissue possibly with cyst formation or as a region of cortex in which there has been gross shrinkage (folial or lobular sclerosis).

Microscopic appearances of the brain Brain that has undergone recent infarction may show irregular pallor of staining and the histological appearances are those of *coagulative necrosis* affecting all tissue elements. Within grey matter the outlines of dead neurons are recognizable, their cytoplasm is intensely eosinophilic and usually contains numerous, often large, vacuoles, and the nucleus stains poorly with haematoxylin. This picture, which is recognizable within the first 4–6 hours, is followed by one of decreasing stainability of nucleus and cytoplasm until a barely detectable ghost cell is all that remains (Fig. 4.29). Incrustations are not seen in

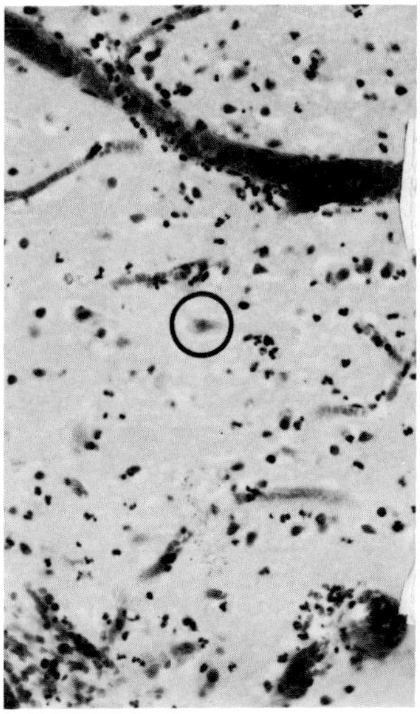

Fig. 4.29 Recent infarction of grey matter showing polymorphonuclear leucocytes migrating from the dilated blood vessels into the necrotic parenchyma. The circle encloses a dead nerve cell. Celloidin; haematoxylin and van Gieson × 195.

the central region of the infarct but occur frequently at its edges. Their absence in the central region, together with the absence of any evidence of selective vulnerability (e.g. between cortical layers or neuronal types (p. 131)), indicate that the alterations observed are not those of the ischaemic cell process (Chapter 1) but are those characteristic of brain death (p. 151, and see Chapter 1). Ultrastructural studies in the cat have shown that there is swelling of astrocytic cytoplasm and processes 30 minutes after complete and permanent cerebral ischaemia (Kalimo et al., 1977). By about 12 hours the spongy appearance of the neuropil is due to a combination of the swelling of astrocytic processes and of axis cylinders. There is enlargement of oligodendroglial nuclei and swelling of their cytoplasm by 4–6 hours. Disintegration of microglia can be seen after 24 hours (Brierley and Brown, 1982b). Within the capillary bed there is electron microscopic evidence of early necrosis and swelling of endothelial cells in subhuman primates (Garcia, Cox and Hudgins, 1971). After 2 days the capillary bed can no longer be identified (Brierley and Brown, 1982b). Larger vessels—arteries and veins—on the other hand, can be identified after up to 4–5 weeks in the centre of an infarct.

Within white matter, pallor of myelin staining and swelling of axons and myelin sheaths develop between 16 and 24 hours. A sharp and often very irregular line of demarcation between normal and abnormal myelin also appears early (Fig. 4.30). Over the next 12–24 hours these appearances intensify and axons and myelin sheaths begin to disintegrate.

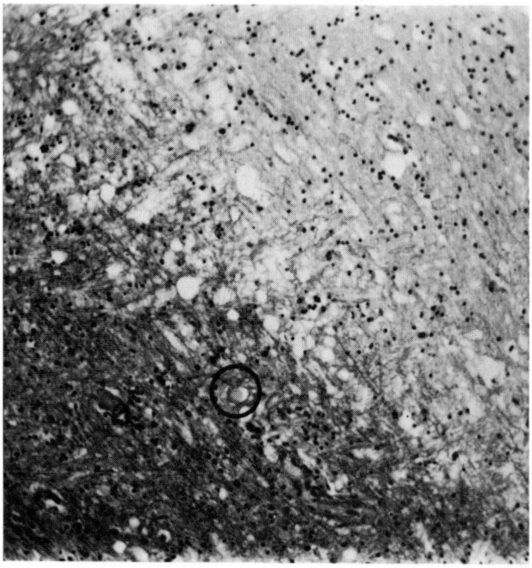

Fig. 4.30 Edge of recent infarct. The infarcted white matter in the upper right-hand side of the picture shows coagulative necrosis and stains poorly. At the margin of the lesion the myelin sheaths are distended and sometimes contain a swollen axon (circle). Celloidin; haematoxylin and van Gieson × 100.

In a haemorrhagic infarct there are variable numbers of diapedetic haemorrhages in grey and white matter (Fig. 4.31).

Whilst infiltration by polymorphonuclear leucocytes is prominent at the edge of an infarct at 24 hours (see Fig. 4.29), they are seldom numerous in the central regions at any time. Experimental studies of non-haemorrhagic infarcts have shown that the first evidence of phagocytic activity is seen in the fibroblasts of the vascular adventitia at 2 days (Brierley and Brown, 1982b). These cells divide mitotically, 'round up' and migrate from the vessel wall and at 5–7 days take the form of typical more or less circular/cylindrical phagocytes (Fig. 4.32). The breakdown products of neuronal cytoplasm and of myelin were seen by electron microscopy from 5 days onwards in these cells. By light microscopy many of these cells already contain sudanophilic and crystalline anisotropic material (Fig. 4.33). At no stage were leucocytes seen within the infarct. Konigsmark and Sidman (1963) from a study of stab wounds in the mouse brain concluded that phagocytes were derived from circulating monocytes. This may account for the appearance of mononuclear phagocytes in infarcts in the human brain after 4 or 5 days. Thus in an infarct the microglia are destroyed and the two sources of lipid phagocytes are circulating monocytes and the adventitial fibroblasts in the walls of remaining blood vessels. In a haemorrhagic infarct red blood corpuscles disintegrate and the phagocytes contain material staining positively with Prussian blue.

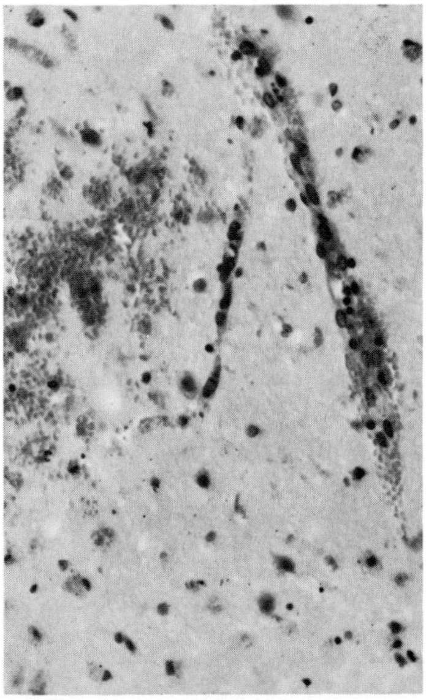

Fig. 4.31 Recent infarction of grey matter showing swelling of the capillary endothelium and diapedetic haemorrhage. Celloidin; haematoxylin and van Gieson × 195.

Combined light and electron microscopic studies of experimental infarction have provided no evidence that macrophages can penetrate the thickened walls of the residual vessels (the capillary bed having been destroyed). Degeneration of the phagocytes *in situ* was first seen at 10 days in the rat, and at 32 days the paucity of phagocytes in large cystic spaces in the primate indicated that most had disappeared. Those that remained were degenerate (Brierley and Brown, 1982b).

The end-result of phagocytic activity is the creation of cysts (Fig. 4.34). At the periphery of the infarct there is both hypertrophy and proliferation of fibre-forming and gemistocytic astrocytes; some are binucleated. Proliferation of the adventitial fibroblast is largely responsible for the thickening of the walls of remaining blood vessels and the laying down of reticulin and collagen at 7 days (Brierley and Brown, 1982b). At the same time there is the first evidence of newly formed capillaries (Garcia and Kamijyo, 1974). It is the combination of these processes that leads to increasing thickness of the gliomesodermal cyst wall. After some months the picture is one of large and small cysts that may appear either empty or contain variable numbers of lipid phagocytes. The walls of some cysts are orange-brown in colour because of blood pigments. The outer wall of a cyst or slit in the cerebral cortex may consist of the pia and the heavily gliosed first layer of the cortex, but sometimes even the latter may be absent. The wall is then formed of pia mater, from which a small number of delicate collagen fibrils pass towards the surviving blood vessels near the margin of the cyst.

Types of vascular disorder

Atheroma (atherosclerosis)

Atheroma is the commonest and most important disease of the arteries in people living in developed countries, and is a major cause of illness and death from coronary heart disease, cerebral infarction and ischaemia of the lower limbs. It is

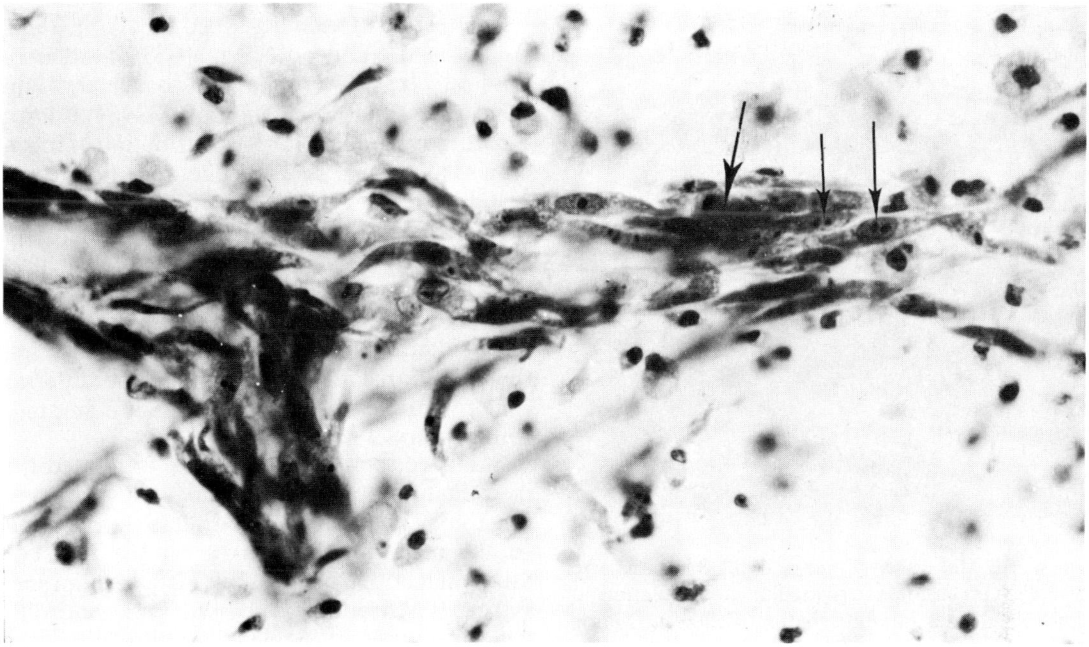

(a)

a

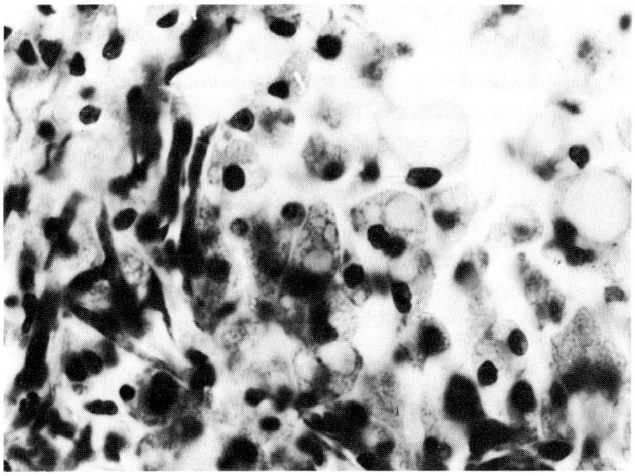

(b)

Fig. 4.32 *Macaca mulatta.* Perfusion-fixation 7 days after severe hypotension. (**a**) Boundary zone lesion showing proliferation of fusiform cells derived from vascular adventitia. The nuclei contain two centrosomes (small arrows). Mitotic division (large arrow) gives rise to lipid phagocytes. Celloidin; cresyl violet and Luxol fast blue × 1300. (**b**) Lipid phagocytes in a cortical boundary zone lesion. The cytoplasm is variably foamy and vacuolated. Celloidin; cresyl violet and Luxol fast blue × 900.

characterized by focal thickening of the intima (plaques) due to the deposition of lipids and the formation of fibrous tissue. Even though atheroma is almost always present to some extent in the middle aged and elderly, the process may start at a much earlier age since fatty streaks are commonly seen in the large vessels of children and young adults. The earliest lesions recognizable as atheroma are found in the aorta and large arteries of young adults in atheroma-prone communities. Eccentrically situated plaques enlarge, thicken and may become confluent. Eventually, in addition to stenosis, there are complications such as ulceration, the formation of mural thrombus and the deposition of calcium. At this stage the lesions are no longer restricted to the intima but involve the media, so the vessel wall is weakened and an aneurysm may develop.

Atheroma of the arteries to the brain is no different from that in the aorta and other major arteries. Whilst the pathogenesis of atheroma is not fully understood, a number of predisposing factors are recognized. These have already been noted in relation to stroke and the several risk factors are clearly synergistic.

Various methods of grading atheroma in ar-

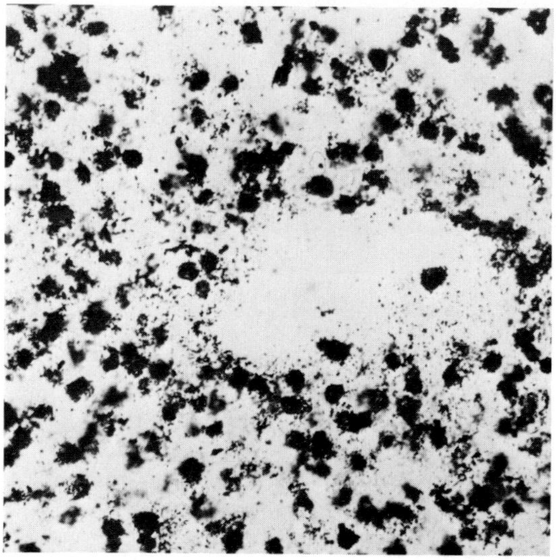

Fig. 4.33 Male, aged 42 years, dying 8 months after severe hypotension. Perivascular accumulation of lipid phagocytes in white matter. Celloidin; Marchi × 450.

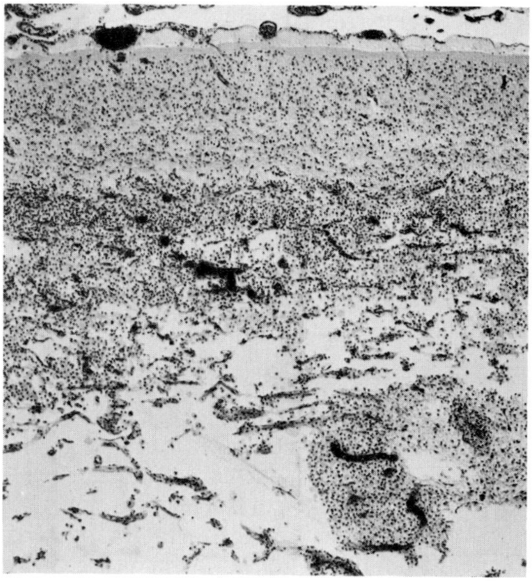

Fig. 4.34 Six-week-old cerebral infarct. The superficial layers of the cortex have survived. The rest of the cortex and the underlying white matter are largely replaced by spaces filled with fluid and traversed by blood vessels. Groups of phagocytes are also present. Celloidin; haematoxylin and eosin × 30.

terial trees have been described (Wolkoff, 1933; Adams and Vander Eecken, 1953). Studies of unselected cases were made by Baker and Iannone (1959) and Resch and Baker (1964) using a quantitative grading for the distribution of intracranial atheroma. The most commonly affected vessels were the internal carotid arteries, the basilar artery at its bifurcation and in its middle and lower parts, the middle and posterior cerebral and the vertebral arteries. Certain vessels appeared to be spared. These included the posterior inferior and superior cerebellar arteries, the posterior communicating and the anterior cerebral arteries distal to the anterior communicating artery.

Standard scoring systems have facilitated the investigation of the aetiology of cerebral atheroma. Thus, as already discussed in relation to the causation of strokes on the basis of atheroma, both hypertension (Fisher et al., 1965; Baker, Resch and Loewenson, 1969) and diabetes (Grunnet, 1963) have been recognized as important predisposing factors. Furthermore, in over 5000 consecutive autopsies Flora et al. (1968) found that atheroma of the cerebral arteries was less common in females than in males dying between the ages of 40 and 60 years. After the sixth decade the frequency increased more rapidly in females so that after the age of 65 the amount of atheroma was equal in the two sexes. Geographical studies have also compared different groups within a single country and populations of different countries (Baker et al., 1967; Williams, Resch and Loewenson, 1969).

Although atheroma of cerebral arteries is clearly implicated in the pathogenesis of cerebral infarction in man, a suitable experimental model has only recently become available. Spontaneously hypertensive rats (Okamoto, 1969) develop severe arterial fatty lesions within 6 months of being fed a hypercholesterolaemic diet. In substrains of the same rats the animals were even more likely to develop fatty lesions on a diet containing 20 per cent suet, 5 per cent cholesterol and 2 per cent cholic acid when compared with normotensive rats fed a similar diet for 3 months. In the stroke-prone strain of the spontaneously hypertensive rat (Yamori et al., 1976), fed a similar hypercholesterolaemic diet with 1 per cent salt in the drinking water, the amount of fat deposited in the basal cerebral arteries was found to be related to arterial blood pressure, the level of serum cholesterol, and the age and strain of the rat used. The level of blood pressure was considered to be the most important factor. It has been shown in the Rhesus monkey fed a diet with a high cholesterol and fat content that widespread atheroma develops (Taylor et al., 1962). Armstrong and Warner (1971) found in a group of Rhesus monkeys given a diet containing 1.2 per cent cholesterol and 40 per cent of total calories for 17 months that there was moderate to marked atheroma in the terminal internal carotid arteries, traces in the basal arteries but none in the branches of the circle of Willis.

Evidently it has not been possible to produce in any experimental animal the pattern and severity of atheroma of the cerebral arteries seen in man. This failure may be due to the absence of sustained hypertension, the damping effect of cerebrospinal fluid arterial pulsation and the presence of only a single elastic lamina. It is possible that there are differences between this diet-induced atheroma in the Rhesus monkey and that found in man (Woolf, 1978). In monkeys fed an atherogenic diet for 20 months, Heistad et al. (1980) found that cerebral blood flow and vascular resistance were similar in normal and atheromatous monkeys. Moderate hypotension did not decrease cerebral blood flow but the vasodilator response to hypercapnia was impaired in the animals with atheroma. There were fibrofatty plaques with necrosis and calcification in the common and internal carotid arteries but only fatty streaks in the intracranial arteries.

Stenosis and occlusion of the extracranial and intracranial arteries

It has long been known that ischaemic lesions, particularly in the distribution of the middle cerebral artery, may be secondary to disease of the internal carotid arteries in the neck (Hultquist, 1942; Fisher, 1951). More recently the importance of disease of the cervical vertebral arteries has been stressed (Hutchinson and Yates, 1956, 1957, 1961; McGee, McPhedran and Hoffman, 1962). These studies emphasized that when atheroma affects one of the four main arteries to the brain it is likely to affect the others to a varying degree.

Internal carotid artery

Thromboembolic occlusion of this artery was found in 2 and 4 per cent in an unselected group of autopsies (Choi and Crampton, 1961; Schwartz and Mitchell, 1961) and in 5.2 per cent by Torvik and Jorgensen (1964). The incidence of carotid occlusion increased with age, in men, but it was about the same in women of all age groups.

Thrombus due to atheroma (Fig. 4.35) is the commonest cause of occlusion of the internal carotid artery (Torvik and Jorgensen, 1964; Castaigne et al., 1970). As atheroma is most common in the carotid sinus, so also is thrombosis (Hutchinson and Yates, 1961; Lhermitte, Gautier and Derouesne, 1966). Thrombus, however, may form at sites that are only minimally affected by atheroma.

The size of the cerebral infarct due to occlusion of one carotid artery depends on the efficiency of the collateral circulation and on whether the thrombus extends into the circle of Willis (Torvik and Jorgensen, 1966). It is known that thrombus can spread from the sinus to the upper end of the internal carotid artery in hours (Castaigne et al., 1970) or weeks (Torvik and Jorgensen, 1964).

Occlusion of the carotid arteries by embolism is much less common than by thrombosis, the commonest site being the upper end of the internal carotid artery. Torvik and Jorgensen (1964) found that eight out of 43 recent occlusions were embolic, an incidence similar to that reported by Castaigne et al. (1970).

Whilst there is a strong association between carotid occlusion and cerebral infarction, that between cerebral ischaemia and carotid stenosis (Fig. 4.36) is less clear, particularly as carotico-vertebral stenosis is no more frequent at autopsy in cases of stroke than in a random population (Hutchinson and Yates, 1957; Schwartz and Mitchell, 1961; McGee, McPhedran and Hoffman, 1962).

Russell and Cranston (1961) showed that the pressure in the ophthalmic artery fell only when stenosis was almost complete. Similarly, Brice, Dowsett and Lowe (1964) found that blood flow through the internal carotid artery in man does not fall until the lumen of the vessel is reduced to 2–4 mm^2 (i.e. by 80–90 per cent). Thus only a small proportion of radiologically demonstrable stenotic lesions of the major neck arteries give rise to symptoms. When symptoms occur in patients with mild stenosis or ulceration of the carotid artery they are probably due to the formation of mural thrombi and embolism. The observation of small emboli in the retinal circu-

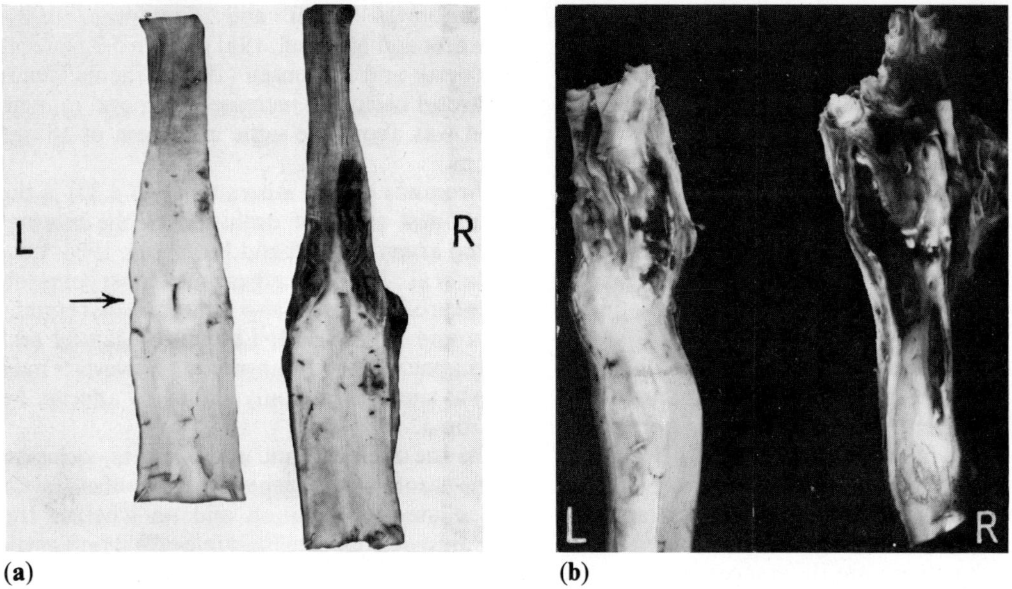

Fig. 4.35 (**a**) Carotid arteries from the neck of a male aged 61 years. The common and internal carotid arteries have been opened longitudinally. The arrow indicates the origin of the internal carotid artery. On the left there is atheromatous thickening of the intima in this region and on the right there is adherent thrombus that extends into the internal carotid artery. (**b**) Carotid arteries from neck of a male, aged 62 years. Both common carotid arteries showed a ring of calcification and atheroma at their points of bifurcation. On the left the internal carotid, which has been opened up, is atheromatous with adherent thrombus. On the right side, about 2.5 cm above its origin, the internal carotid is almost completely occluded by old pale thrombus. Below this, recent reddish thrombus extends downwards into the lumen of the common carotid artery.

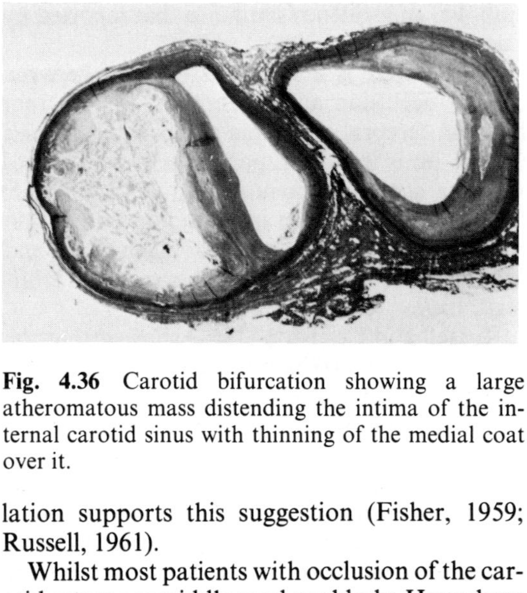

Fig. 4.36 Carotid bifurcation showing a large atheromatous mass distending the intima of the internal carotid sinus with thinning of the medial coat over it.

lation supports this suggestion (Fisher, 1959; Russell, 1961).

Whilst most patients with occlusion of the carotid artery are middle aged or elderly, Humphrey and Newton (1960) found increasing evidence of its occurrence in young adults. Trauma was the commonest factor, accounting for almost one-half of the cases. Others included subarachnoid haemorrhage, syphilis and tuberculosis, blood dyscrasias and the aortic arch syndrome. The internal carotid arteries may sustain accidental trauma (Hughes and Brownell, 1968), particularly in view of their close relationship to the anterior aspects of the transverse processes of the vertebrae. A hemiplegia occurring some hours or days after an injury to the head or neck may not always be due to intracranial haemorrhage but rather to extension of thrombus from the site of injury into the stem of the middle cerebral artery. Sindermann, Bechinger and Dichgans (1970) established that in patients under 40 years of age with a stroke, non-atheromatous occlusion of the intracranial vessels is more likely than that of the cervical portion of the internal carotid artery. Carotid occlusion in the absence of atheromatous stenosis or embolism may also occur (Adams and Graham, 1967).

In general, five patterns of ischaemic brain damage can be identified following occlusion or stenosis of an internal carotid artery: (1) massive infarction involving the entire distribution of the middle (Figs 4.37 and 4.38), and sometimes

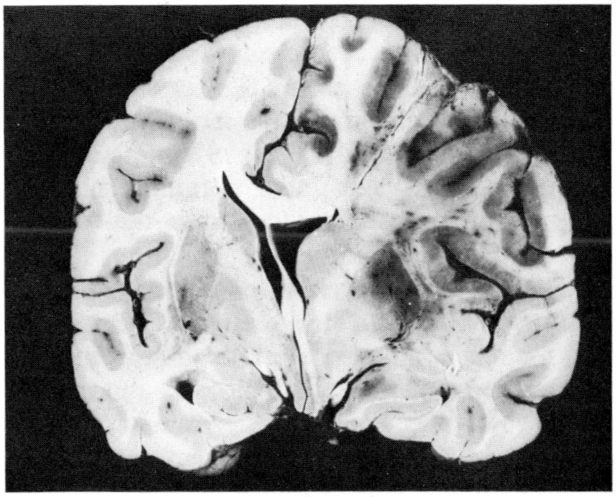

Fig. 4.37 Male, aged 70 years, dying 7 days after the onset of a left hemiplegia. There is a large swollen infarct in the territories supplied by the right anterior and middle cerebral arteries due to occlusion of the ipsilateral internal carotid artery. Note the shift of the midline structures to the left and the supracallosal hernia. There was a tentorial hernia and secondary haemorrhage into the brain stem.

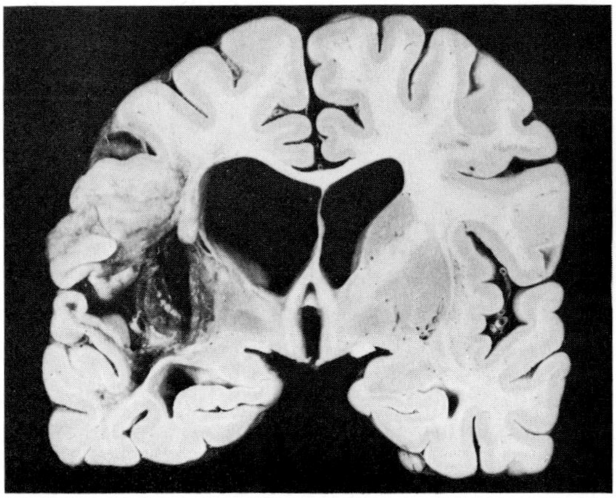

Fig. 4.38 Female, aged 73 years, dying 6 months after the onset of a right hemiplegia. There is an old infarct in the central distribution of the left middle cerebral artery. The proximal part of the left common carotid artery was occluded by old thrombus superimposed upon atheroma.

within that of the anterior cerebral artery (infarcts of this type accounted for 55 per cent of the series of Torvik and Jorgensen (1966)); (2) infarction of the cortex around the sylvian fissure, with or without involvement of the basal ganglia and internal capsule; (3) infarction restricted to the internal capsule (the so-called 'capsular infarct'); (4) small infarcts within the white matter supplied by the peripheral branches of the middle cerebral artery (Hultquist, 1942); and (5) infarction along the boundary zone between the territories of the anterior and middle cerebral arteries (Zülch, 1961) and, less commonly, between the territories of the posterior and middle cerebral arteries.

Permanent occlusion or major stenosis of one or more of the large arteries in the neck may be symptomless. This has been shown even if both internal carotid arteries are occluded (Wrigley, Sheldon and Whitty, 1967). Doniger (1963) described a patient who made a good recovery from a stroke even though both internal carotid arteries in the neck and the basilar artery were occluded.

Subclavian artery

Disease of the subclavian and innominate arteries accounts for only a minority of cerebral infarcts in spite of a high incidence of atheroma in these arteries in patients over the age of 66 years (Battacharji, Hutchinson and McCall, 1967). Occlusion of these vessels by complicated atheroma has been described in a group of patients with transient ischaemic attacks (Callow et al., 1968). Trauma or an underlying cervical rib may contribute to the occlusion.

Obstruction of the subclavian and innominate arteries is of importance because of the part it plays in causing the *subclavian steal syndrome* (Reivich et al., 1961). If occlusion is proximal to the origin of the vertebral artery, the blood supply to the arm depends on retrograde flow in the latter, thus 'stealing' blood from the basilar artery and the circle of Willis. Exercise of the arm muscles, with up to a fourfold increase of blood flow, may precipitate cerebral ischaemia. A similar reversal of flow via the ophthalmic artery may occur after occlusion of an external carotid artery. Similarly, if the common carotid artery is occluded, retrograde flow down the internal carotid may extend into the external carotid artery and its territory. Within the skull similar 'steal' conditions may exist after infarction when the cerebral vessels are fully dilated.

Vertebrobasilar system

The vertebral artery ascends through the foramina in the transverse processes of the upper six cervical vertebrae before curving behind the lateral mass of the atlas to enter the skull through the foramen magnum. It then joins the vessel of the opposite side to form the basilar artery. These vessels are difficult to examine, and only a limited number of post-mortem studies are available in which the vertebral arteries have been examined in detail.

Full autopsy studies have been reported by Hutchinson and Yates (1961), Fisher et al. (1965) and Mitchell and Schwartz (1965). In their 145 cases, Battacharji, Hutchinson and McCall (1967) found that the vertebral artery was occluded in 30 and the basilar in 3. A detailed study was carried out by Castaigne et al. (1973) on 44 cases: in 35 cases occlusion was due to the formation of thrombus on an atheromatous plaque, in 4 it was ascribed to embolism from the heart and in 5 no cause was established. Thrombus was most common when stenosis was severe, and in 12 cases developed between the second cervical vertebra and the lower end of the basilar artery, in 4 at the proximal end of the vertebral artery and in 1 within its course through the transverse processes. Like Hutchinson and Yates (1961), Castaigne et al. (1973) noted that after occlusion of the proximal vertebral artery, thrombus very rarely extended throughout its full length.

In the cervical portions of the vertebral arteries in the middle aged and elderly, distortion due to osteoarthritis may be considerable (Fig. 4.39) and together with atheroma may be sufficient to cause obstruction after certain movements of the neck (Hutchinson and Yates, 1956; Easton and Sherman, 1977). The most common sites of compression by osteophytes are at the fourth/fifth and fifth/sixth cervical articulations (Sheehan, Baur and Meyer, 1960). Many of the patients developing a stroke after cervical manipulation are young, and vertebrobasilar insufficiency may be due to such factors as abnormalities of the spine, congenital asymmetry of the vessels, hyperextension of the neck, and other abrupt movements of the head during the manipulation itself (Sherman, Hart and Easton, 1981). Vertebrobasilar insufficiency may also occur in association with subluxation of the atlantoaxial joint in rheumatoid arthritis (Jones and Kaufmann, 1976) and may occur if one vertebral artery becomes stenosed or occluded, the other artery being congenitally small.

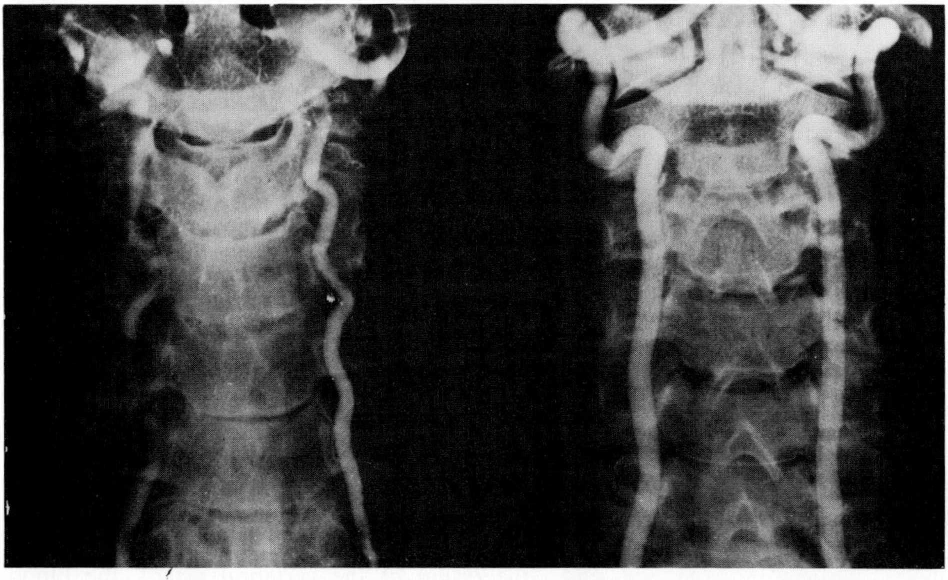

Fig. 4.39 Post-mortem angiography of vertebral arteries. Normal appearances are shown in the illustration on the right. In the illustration on the left there is distortion by osteoarthritic change and stenosis by atheroma.

The vertebral arteries may be damaged during assisted cephalic and breech presentations, all of which involve twisting and traction of the neck. Yates (1959) reported bruising and haemorrhagic dissection of the vertebral arteries in 42 per cent of 250 cases of neonatal death. The significance of hindbrain ischaemia in failure to initiate cardiorespiratory function at birth is obvious, but in survivors there may be poor suckling, extraocular palsies, inner ear deafness and other disabilities referable to damage in the vertebrobasilar territory.

Occlusion of the basilar artery was studied by Kubik and Adams (1946) and Biemond (1951) who found that thrombosis on the basis of atheroma was the most common cause (Fig. 4.40). This was confirmed by Castaigne et al. (1973) who found a retrograde thrombus in four of 18 cases and an anterograde extension of the thrombus in seven. There were two examples of emboli passing from either the basilar or the vertebral artery into the posterior cerebral circulation. Spontaneous occlusion of the vertebrobasilar arterial system has also been described (Graham and Adams, 1972).

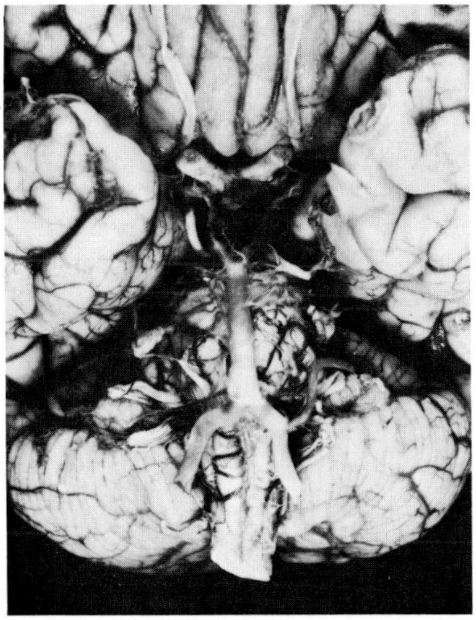

Fig. 4.40 Male, aged 55 years, a known hypertensive, dying 4 weeks after the onset of the 'locked-in' syndrome. There is occlusion of an atheromatous basilar artery by thrombus.

Vertigo and nystagmus are common in vertebrobasilar insufficiency, and are often associated with cranial nerve palsies, dysarthria and dysphagia. There may be hemiparesis or hemisensory loss. If the basilar artery is occluded, coma, flaccid quadriplegia and a bulbar palsy develop rapidly. Other cases develop the 'locked-in' syndrome in which a conscious mute patient is completely paralysed apart from some eye movements (Nordgren et al., 1971; Hawkes, 1974). The pathological basis is extensive infarction of the ventral pons, which interrupts the corticospinal and corticobulbar tracts, the medial lemniscus and some of the centres that control eye movement.

If the short paramedian branches of the basilar artery (including the lateral artery of the medulla) are occluded (usually unilaterally (Fig. 4.41)), the patient may present with a sixth, seventh or twelfth cranial nerve palsy with contralateral hemiplegia and sensory loss. Infarcts may also be present in the cerebellar cortex, in the distribution of the short circumferential arteries of the brain stem, and in the territories of one or both posterior cerebral arteries. Occlusion of the long circumferential branches gives rise to signs and symptoms referable to the cerebellum and/or the brain stem.

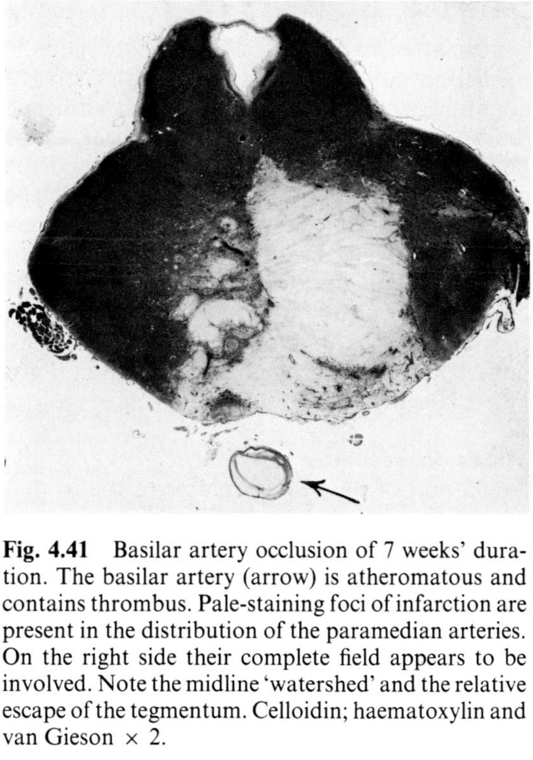

Fig. 4.41 Basilar artery occlusion of 7 weeks' duration. The basilar artery (arrow) is atheromatous and contains thrombus. Pale-staining foci of infarction are present in the distribution of the paramedian arteries. On the right side their complete field appears to be involved. Note the midline 'watershed' and the relative escape of the tegmentum. Celloidin; haematoxylin and van Gieson × 2.

Occlusion of certain intracranial arteries

As the arteries of the central nervous system have a fairly constant anatomical distribution (McCormick and Schochet, 1976), occlusion of the trunk or of one or more of the larger branches produces a relatively constant neurological deficit (Beevor, 1908; Stopford, 1915, 1917; Abbie, 1934). Adams (1943) gave a detailed list of the arterial distribution to the cerebellum, and Critchley and Schuster (1933) and Atkinson (1949) described the branches of the basilar artery. The clinical syndromes resulting from arterial occlusion were reviewed by Tichy (1949) and by Kiloh (1953).

Anterior cerebral artery The principal field supplied by this artery is the cortex and subjacent white matter (to a depth of about 25 mm) on the medial surface of the frontal lobe with a strip of about the same width along the dorsal surface of the frontal and parietal lobes as far back as the parieto-occipital fissure; also the genu and the anterior four-fifths of the corpus callosum. The recurrent artery of Heubner is a proximal branch passing through the anterior perforated substance to supply the lower part of the head of the caudate nucleus, the lower and anterior part of the putamen, the anterior part of the globus pallidus and the adjacent portion of the anterior limb of the internal capsule.

Middle cerebral artery This artery supplies the lateral part of the orbital surface of the frontal lobe, the temporal pole, the insula and the convexity of the cerebral hemisphere, except the strip supplied by the anterior cerebral artery, the lateral surface of the occipital lobe, including its pole, and a strip along the inferolateral border of the temporal lobe (see Fig. 4.11). It also supplies the subjacent white matter and the superior half of both limbs of the internal capsule and the optic radiation where it lies lateral to the occipital horn. It also supplies the caudate nucleus (except the inferior portion of its head, and its tail), the putamen (except the lower part of its frontal pole) and the lateral segment of the globus pallidus.

This vessel is more often occluded than any other cerebral artery. In a pathological study of 47 infarcts within its distribution in 41 patients, Lhermitte, Gautier and Derouesne (1970) found that in 20 of 31 cases there was permanent occlusion of the middle cerebral artery associated with occlusion of the internal carotid artery. Embolism was of major importance, occurring in 20 of the 31 cases with permanent occlusion of the middle cerebral artery, and in an additional 8 there was evidence of transient embolism. They concluded that intracranial arterial disease very rarely accounts for occlusion of the middle cerebral artery, the usual cause being disease of either the internal carotid artery or the heart.

Posterior cerebral artery Although usually seen as a branch of the basilar artery, this artery develops as a continuation of the posterior communicating artery; it originates therefore as a branch of the carotid artery (Abbie, 1934; Williams, 1936).

The principal field of supply of the posterior cerebral artery is the inferior surface and adjacent inferolateral border of the hemisphere behind the temporal pole, the medial surface of the occipital lobe, excluding the pole itself (posterior end of area 17), and the underlying white matter. It also supplies the mamillary body, the subthalamic nucleus, the posterior half of the thalamus including the geniculate bodies, the posterior half of the hippocampal formation, the posterior two-thirds of the cerebral peduncle, and portions of the substantia nigra, red nucleus and superior cerebellar peduncle.

Infarction within the distribution of the posterior cerebral artery is not uncommon as an incidental finding at post-mortem in the elderly. If the whole artery is occluded there will be homonymous hemianopia with macular sparing and often hemiparesis and disturbance of sensation. If the dominant hemisphere is involved, there will be alexia (Foix and Masson, 1923).

Granular atrophy of the cortex After removing the pia arachnoid, the affected surface of the brain resembles that of a kidney with 'granular atrophy' (Fig. 4.42). The condition is rare, and often bilaterally symmetrical. Pentschew (1933) found that it was usually limited to the middle frontal gyrus and to the parieto-occipital convolutions. In certain cases of thromboangiitis obliterans, Lindenberg and Spatz (1939) found a paramedian sickle-shaped zone of granular atrophy extending from the frontal pole over the vertex to the occipital pole and sometimes on to the inferior surface of the hemisphere from the occipital to the temporal pole. This distribution represents the boundary zones between the cortical fields of the major cerebral arteries.

Microscopically, each depression in the cortex overlies a cone-shaped gliomesodermal scar with its base at the cortical surface (Fig. 4.43). Narrowing of small cortical arteries and arterioles in

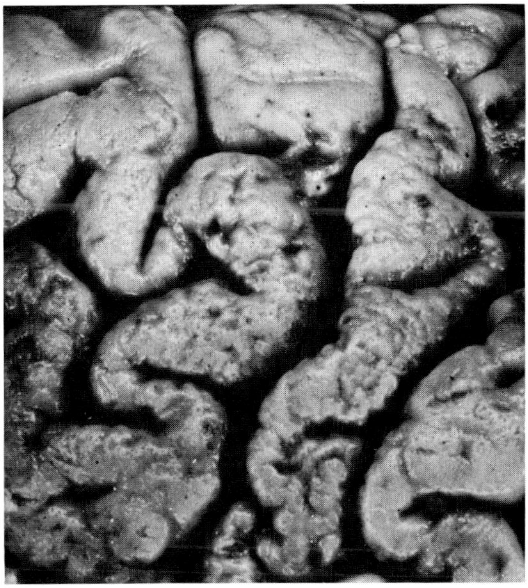

Fig. 4.42 Granular atrophy of the cortex. Lateral aspect of the left cerebral hemisphere after removal of the leptomeninges. Note the numerous depressions of the surface.

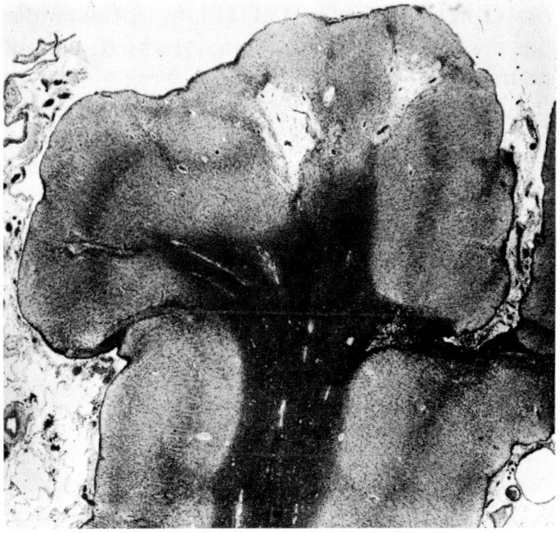

Fig. 4.43 Region of granular atrophy from the same case as Fig. 4.42; a man aged 37 with chronic endarteritis of uncertain type. Note the thickened and narrowed arteries in the leptomeninges and the numerous depressions in the cortex which are associated with the 'softenings' and scars that run in at right angles to the surface. Celloidin; PTAH × 9.

association with hypertension, or thromboangiitis obliterans, has been reported. Pentschew (1933) observed it as a sequel of carbon monoxide poisoning.

Anterior choroidal artery This artery supplies the pyriform cortex, the posteromedial border of the anterior commissure, part of the head and most of the tail of the caudate nucleus, the posteromedial part of the amygdaloid nucleus, the medial segment of the globus pallidus, the lateral part of the lateral geniculate body, the optic tract, the middle third of the cerebral peduncle, the subthalamic region, the posterior two-thirds of the posterior limb of the internal capsule, the beginning of the optic radiation, the antero-inferior parts of the fascia dentata, the anterior half of the hippocampus (including the uncus) and the choroid plexus.

Proven cases of occlusion of the anterior choroidal artery are rare (Abbie, 1933), and the anterior half of the hippocampus is seldom involved.

Superior cerebellar artery This artery supplies the dorsolateral portions of the caudal midbrain and the cranial part of the pons, the superior cerebellar peduncle, part of the dentate nucleus and part of the cortex of the superior surface of the cerebellar hemisphere.

Occlusion of this artery is rare. Cases due to atheroma (Guillain, Bertrand and Peron, 1928; Russell, 1931), atheroma and syphilis (Davison, Goodhart and Savitsky, 1935) and embolism (Freeman and Jaffe, 1941) have been reported.

Anterior inferior cerebellar artery This artery supplies the lateral portion of the tegmentum of the caudal pons, the inferior part of the middle cerebellar peduncle, the inferior cerebellar peduncle, the flocculus and the anterior part of the lower surface of the lateral lobes of the cerebellar hemispheres.

Damage to this artery was considered by Atkinson (1949) to be the principal cause of death following operative removal of an acoustic schwannoma. Proven cases of occlusion of this artery, secondary to atheroma, are extremely rare (Goodhart and Davison, 1936; Adams, 1943).

Posterior inferior cerebellar artery This artery supplies a wedge of tissue in the dorsolateral quadrant of the medulla extending vertically from just above the level of the cuneate and gracile nuclei to the upper border of the medulla. It also supplies the inferior cerebellar peduncle, the inferior vermis, the lower surface of the cerebellar hemisphere, the dentate nucleus, and the roof of the fourth ventricle and its choroid plexus.

Ischaemic lesions occur more frequently in the distribution of this than of any other cerebellar artery. There may be thrombosis of the vertebral artery (Fisher, Karnes and Kubik, 1961) without occlusion of the posterior inferior cerebellar artery.

Hypertension and the brain

The pathophysiology of the cerebral circulation in hypertension It has been known for over 30 years that the absolute value for cerebral blood flow of 50 ml/100 g per minute is the same in hypertensive and normotensive subjects (Kety et al., 1948) and also in normotensive and hypertensive baboons (Strandgaard et al., 1974, 1975). One of the earliest indications of a shift to the right of the autoregulatory curve of cerebral blood flow in hypertension (Fig. 4.44) was reported by Finnerty, Witkin and Fazekas (1954) who found that, during hexamethonium-induced hypotension, hypertensive patients developed symptoms of cerebral ischaemia at a

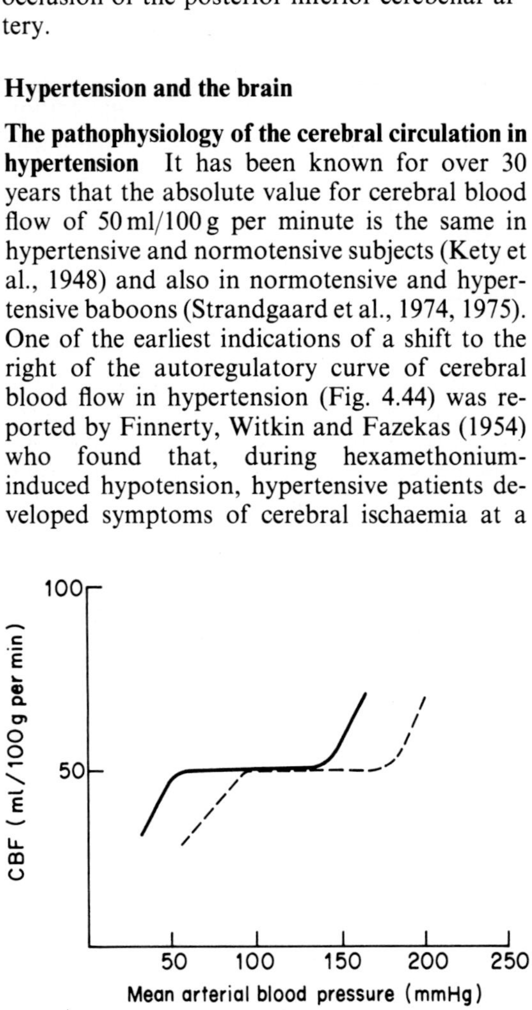

Fig. 4.44 Diagrammatic representation of the relationship between cerebral blood flow (CBF) and mean arterial blood pressure in normotensive and hypertensive subjects. Note the 'shift to the right' of the autoregulatory curve in hypertensive subjects. —— normotensive subjects; ----- hypertensive subjects.

higher level of blood pressure than did normotensive subjects. That is to say, hypertensive patients are more susceptible to cerebral ischaemia because they are less able to compensate for a fall in blood pressure. A similar resetting of the lower limit of autoregulation of cerebral blood flow has been found in baboons with untreated renovascular hypertension (Jones and Strandgaard, 1975), and in spontaneously hypertensive (Fujishima and Omae, 1976) and in renovascular hypertensive rats (Barry et al., 1982). The degree of shift depended on the duration of hypertension (Jones et al., 1976; Strandgaard, 1976).

The upper limit of autoregulation in the hypertensive baboon is raised to between 21.3 and 24 kPa (160 and 180 mmHg) mean arterial blood pressure (Strandgaard et al., 1975). It is probable that there is a similar adaptation in chronically hypertensive patients who may tolerate remarkably high blood pressures without developing hypertensive encephalopathy (Strandgaard et al., 1975), implying that the alterations in their blood vessels increase tolerance to high blood pressure (Folkow, 1971).

Hypertensive patients are vulnerable to cerebral ischaemia during periods of hypotension. Thus, antihypertensive agents may themselves reduce the blood pressure to a level which, though normal, will lead to a fall in the cerebral blood flow. Jackson et al. (1976), for example, has described six elderly patients who developed neurological symptoms within a week of starting treatment, and Graham (1975) has described two patients who suffered brain damage due to antihypertensive therapy: there was infarction along the boundary zones between the territories of the major cerebral arteries. More recently, Ledingham and Rajagopalan (1979) have described ten patients with malignant hypertension who developed acute neurological signs when the blood pressure was lowered rapidly. In six the lowest pressures recorded were within the normal range. Three died and at autopsy ischaemic brain damage was again found along the arterial boundary zones. Hulse, Taylor and Dillon (1979) have reported three children with severe hypertension who became blind during hypotensive treatment, one also developing a transverse myelopathy. Though firm evidence was lacking, it was felt that in all of these patients a relative drug-induced hypotension had contributed to infarction of the retina, the optic nerves and the spinal cord.

Pathological changes in hypertension In addition to abnormal cerebrovascular physiology, hypertension produces pathological alterations in the brain (see Gautier, 1976). The principal lesions comprise aggravation of atheroma, hyaline arteriosclerosis, lacunae, multi-infarct dementia, hypertensive encephalopathy, Binswanger's disease and intracerebral haemorrhage (see Chapter 5).

Aggravation of atheroma There is considerable evidence that atheroma of the systemic and particularly of the larger cerebral vessels is aggravated by hypertension (Fisher et al., 1965; Baker, Resch and Loewenson, 1969). In normotensive subjects atheroma does not usually affect vessels less than 2 mm in diameter, such as those supplying the basal ganglia and pons (Adams and Fisher, 1961). In severe chronic hypertension, however, atheroma can be found in the penetrating arteries of the internal capsule, the basal ganglia and the pons (Adams, 1957). Multiple stenoses recognizable in angiograms, and as yellow flecks on the leptomeningeal vessels at autopsy are almost pathognomonic of severe long-standing hypertension. In some hypertensive patients a series of ladder-like yellow or orange bars on the vertebral and basilar arteries is said to be characteristic (Arab, 1957).

Hyaline arteriosclerosis Within large and medium-sized arteries hypertension first produces hypertrophy of smooth muscle and the elastica (Fig. 4.45). The latter becomes thickened and there is reduplication towards the intima. These changes occur in both the elderly and in long-standing hypertensives, and give way to fibrous replacement of muscle whilst elastic tissue may break up and undergo partial absorption. The arterial walls are thickened and more rigid, their lumina are dilated and the vessels become longer and tortuous.

In vessels of 1 mm diameter or less, in addition to hypertrophy of the media, the intima becomes thickened by a concentric increase in connective tissue. In the smallest arteries the intimal change predominates and may result in narrowing of the lumen, in contrast to the dilatation seen in the large arteries. There may be hyaline thickening of arterioles (hyaline arteriosclerosis) which gradually extends over the whole circumference, and when severe replaces all structures except the

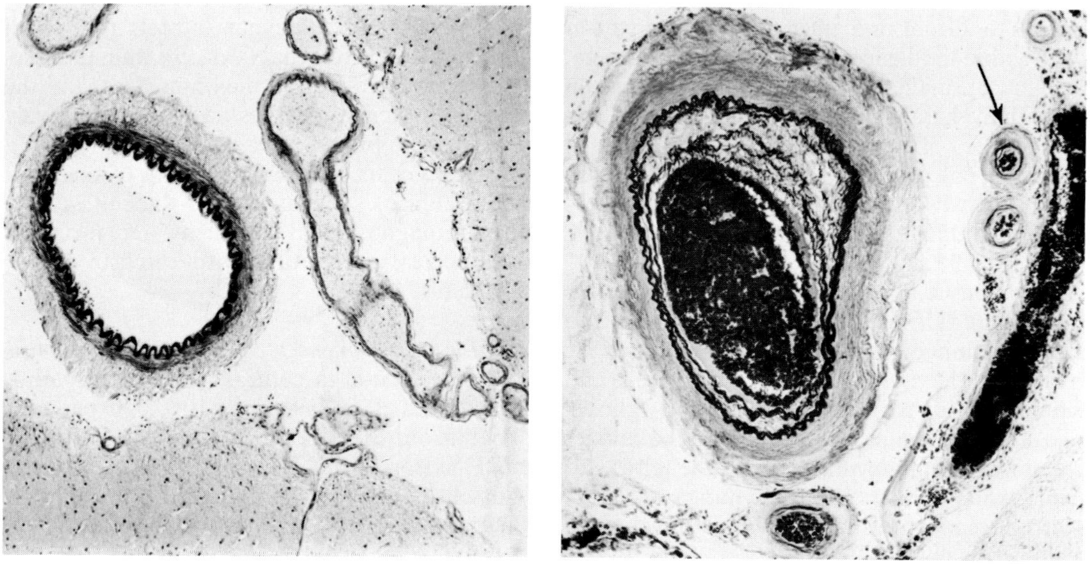

(a) **(b)**

Fig. 4.45 (**a**) Normal arteries and arterioles lying in a sulcus of the brain. Note the internal elastic lamina, the dark-staining muscularis, no external elastic lamina and the small amount of adventitia. Celloidin; Weigert's elastic—van Gieson × 64. (**b**) Hypertensive vascular disease. Arteries and arterioles in a cerebral sulcus (patient aged 51 years, blood pressure 190/125 mmHg, heart weight 470 g). The artery shows hypertrophy of the media, adventitial fibrosis, and eccentric splitting and duplication of the elastic lamina. The arterioles (arrow) show an increase in the thickness of the media and adventitia. Celloidin; Weigert's elastic × 100.

endothelium. This latter change, however, is also seen in the elderly. Other lesions, such as lipohyalinosis—acute arterial distension with atheroma—have also been described (Fisher, 1972).

Cook and Yates (1972) measured the thickness of the media of cerebral and renal arteries fixed when distended to their normal diameter *in vivo*. They found that the ratio between thickness of the media and the cross-sectional diameter could be defined for a vessel of given luminal size, the ratio being lower for cerebral than for renal arteries. In hypertensive subjects the ratio increased in both types of arteries irrespective of their calibre. These findings differed somewhat from those of Russell (1963) who found an increase in the luminal diameter of the middle and anterior cerebral arteries of hypertensive subjects but a decrease in lumen and increase in wall thickness in small penetrating arteries of the brain. Recent morphometric studies have shown a statistically significant increase of media/radius ratio in the cerebral vessels in spontaneously hypertensive rats (Nordborg and Johansson, 1980).

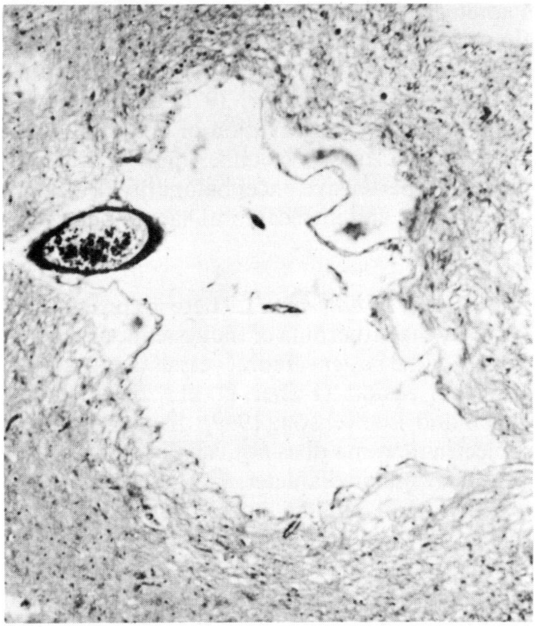

Fig. 4.46 État lacunaire. Small artery lying at one side of the space that its spiralled course now occupies.

Lacunae These are small cavities, measuring from 3 to 20 mm in diameter, occurring principally within the diencephalon and the brain stem. Lacunae of smaller diameter are commonly seen beneath the basal ganglia in the ageing brain and also in cases of cerebral atrophy. According to Fisher (1965) some 90 per cent of lacunae are associated with hypertension. They may, however, be found in 9 per cent of normotensive subjects (Cole and Yates, 1968).

They consist of expanded perivascular spaces (Fig. 4.46). There is irregular rarefaction and disintegration of the parenchyma around the vessel, and the cavity contains very few cells and is limited by a narrow border of fibrillary gliosis. The term 'état lacunaire' is used when the cavities are numerous in grey matter, and the term 'état criblé, when similar cavities are numerous in the centrum semiovale and other richly myelinated regions (Blackwood, 1958).

Cole and Yates (1968) suggested that lacunae are '... the result of spiralled elongations of small intracerebral arteries under the effects of raised blood pressure' (Fig. 4.47). On the other hand, lacunae have been attributed to occlusive vascular disease. For example, the smaller lesions appeared to be due to lipohyalinosis (Fisher, 1969, 1972) and the larger to atheroma (Fisher, 1965, 1979) or emboli (Fisher, 1979).

The question of lacunar infarcts (i.e. small perivascular infarcts that lie deep within the cerebral hemispheres and in the brain stem) and the associated lacunar strokes has been extensively reviewed by Fisher, (1982) and Mohr (1982). Their importance lies in the nature of the associated clinical syndromes, the difficulties they pose in diagnosis and treatment, and their epidemiological correlation with cerebrovascular disorders.

Multi-infarct dementia The incidence of this type of dementia in clinical surveys and pathological studies ranges from 10 to 20 per cent (Tomlinson, Blessed and Roth, 1968; Marsden and Harrison, 1972). It is due to multiple infarcts (Corsellis, 1962) and is discussed more fully in Chapter 20.

Malignant hypertension and hypertensive encephalopathy The term 'hypertensive encephalopathy' was introduced by Oppenheimer and Fishberg (1928) to describe a sudden rise of blood pressure, usually preceded by severe headache and followed by convulsions and coma and various neurological abnormalities. The

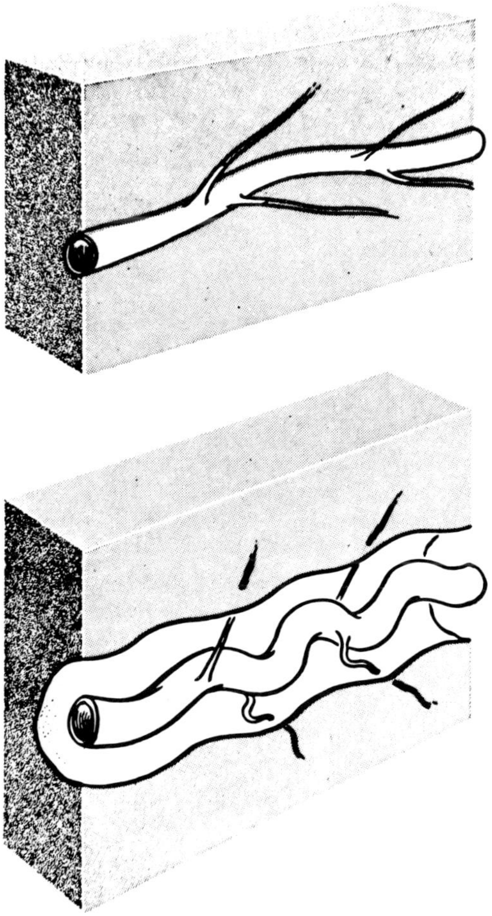

Fig. 4.47 Diagram illustrating the changes in intracerebral arteries that bring about the condition of 'état lacunaire'—elongation, dilatation and spiralling of the artery with distortion of branches and separation from brain tissue.

condition is rare and may complicate acute glomerulonephritis, toxaemia of pregnancy and 'malignant' hypertension. Whilst various alterations have been described in the brains of patients with 'malignant' hypertension (Oppenheimer and Fishberg, 1928; Rosenberg, 1940; Feigin and Prose, 1959) it is only recently that a comprehensive clinicopathological study has been undertaken in 20 cases (Chester et al., 1978). At autopsy the brains were not significantly heavier than those of controls. Multiple petechial haemorrhages were seen in eight cases and, in general, atheroma of the circle of Willis was severe. Characteristically, there was fibrinoid necrosis of the walls of arterioles and small arteries (Fig. 4.48); this was variable in 13 and absent in seven and in all the controls. In 12 of the cases histological evidence of fibrin thrombi was found, and in all 20 there were both focal and segmental irregularities of the walls of arterioles and small arteries. Multiple microscopic infarcts were commonly seen in the basis pontis. Fewer were present in the basal ganglia, in the white matter of the cerebral hemispheres and in the spinal cord. The severity and extent of these lesions correlated with the magnitude of the neurological deficits and the degree of hypertension. Chester et al. (1978) concluded that hypertensive encephalopathy is characterized by fibrinoid nec-

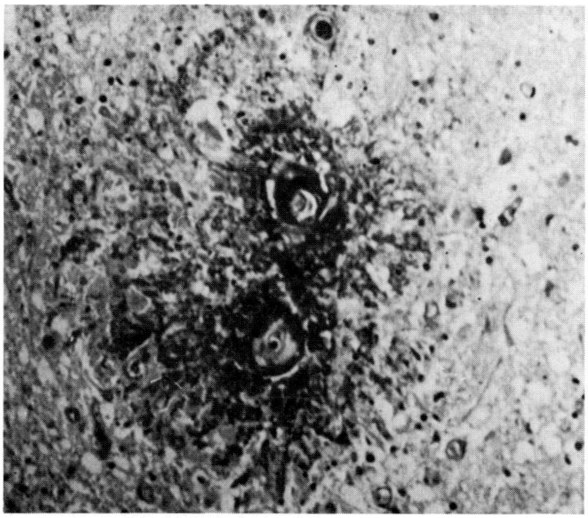

Fig. 4.48 Malignant hypertension. Two branches of a small intracerebral artery showing necrosis of their walls and fibrinous exudate. The surrounding brain shows early rarefaction and dissolution.

rosis, fibrin thrombi and microinfarcts. Similar histological findings have been seen in systemic lupus erythematosus (Johnson and Richardson, 1968) but without concentration in the basis pontis.

The pathogenesis of hypertensive encephalopathy remains uncertain. Although severe hypertension is accepted as the underlying cause, its mode of action is disputed. On the one hand the encephalopathy has been attributed to 'spasm' of the cerebral vessels (Byrom, 1954; Meyer, Waltz and Gotoh, 1960; Dinsdale, Robertson and Chiang, 1974), and on the other to excessive vasodilatation, damage to the blood-brain barrier and cerebral hyperaemia—the breakthrough hypothesis (MacKenzie et al.,

1976; Auer, 1978). Indeed Byrom (1974, 1976) has adopted this view.

Evidence for the breakthrough hypothesis comes from various sources. It has, for example, been shown in experimental hypertension that there is an upper limit to autoregulation beyond which cerebral blood flow increases passively as blood pressure rises. This has been shown in the baboon (Strandgaard et al., 1974, 1976) and in man (Skinhoj and Strandgaard, 1973; Johannson, Strandgaard and Lassen, 1974). Most studies have shown that extreme hypertension is associated with an abnormally high cerebral blood flow, strongly suggesting marked vasodilatation (MacKenzie et al., 1976). It was concluded that forced dilatation of the smaller cerebral vessels in response to hypertension is the essential basis of hypertensive encephalopathy as originally suggested by Lassen and Agnoli (1973).

The blood–brain barrier in acutely induced experimental hypertension has been studied extensively. Haggendal and Johannson (1972a, b) suggested that the increased permeability to Evans blue might be due to overstretching of the vessel walls, but recent studies have failed to identify either destruction of endothelial cells or opening of interendothelial tight junctions. The principal mechanism of increased permeability has been identified as enhanced pinocytosis (Nag, Robertson and Dinsdale, 1977). In view of this evidence the concept of hypertensive encephalopathy as a breakthrough in autoregulation because of forced cerebral hyperperfusion is now superseding the earlier hypothesis of vasospasm.

Subcortical arteriosclerotic encephalopathy of Binswanger This rare disorder is now believed to be associated with hypertension. Since the initial description of 'encephalitis sub-corticalis chronica progressiva' in eight patients (Binswanger, 1894), further clinical and neuropathological descriptions have been published (Olszewski, 1962; Burger, Burch and Kunze, 1976; Caplan and Schoene, 1978; Janota, 1981). The condition generally starts between the ages of 50 and 60 years and is characterized by a slowly developing dementia, focal neurological deficits including pseudobulbar palsy, and also psychiatric disturbances. Evolution is remorseless over some 3–5 years.

Pathologically the disease is characterized by focal and diffuse loss of myelin with associated reactive changes in the deep white matter of the cerebral hemispheres, the subcortical arcuate fibres being largely spared. The changes are most severe in the occipital and temporal lobes with relative sparing of the frontal lobes. In severe cases there may be almost complete loss of the white matter of an affected lobe with compensatory ventricular dilatation. In some cases the margins of myelin destruction are sharply delineated like plaques of multiple sclerosis. Microscopy reveals rarefaction of tissue, lipid phagocytes and a fibrillary gliosis. The demyelination is thought to be due to reduced perfusion on the basis of hyaline arteriosclerosis and atheroma affecting not only the large vessels of the circle of Willis but also the small penetrating vessels (Caplan and Schoene, 1978). These vascular changes, although not diagnostic, have been interpreted as a form of hypertensive vascular disease. The characteristic structural changes have, however, been seen in normotensive individuals (Caplan and Schoene, 1978; Loizou, Jefferson and Smith, 1982).

Experimental models have greatly enhanced understanding of the pathogenesis and the effects of a high blood pressure (see Yamori, 1979). Spontaneous hypertension in the rat is comparable to other forms of experimentally induced chronic hypertension and represents the closest analogue of essential hypertension in man (Okamoto, 1969; Yamori, 1979). By selective inbreeding a stroke-prone strain of hypertensive rat has been produced in which cerebral lesions are particularly likely to develop (80 per cent in males over 100 days of age; 60 per cent in females over 150 days). In young animals blood pressure increases rapidly to 240 mmHg, and they die of a stroke from a few days to 24 weeks after the onset of symptoms. The pathology of the cerebrovascular lesions in such animals (Hazama et al., 1976) includes focal infarcts, massive intracerebral haemorrhage and various arterial changes closely resembling those seen in hypertensive man.

Studies in the monkey have assessed the role of hypertension in the genesis of cardiovascular disease in animals fed either an atherogenic or a non-atherogenic diet (Hollander et al., 1976, 1977). During a 15-month period half of the group of hypertensive animals on the atherogenic diet developed cardiovascular disease leading to heart failure, myocardial infarction, stroke and sudden death. At autopsy these animals had both hypertensive and atheromatous heart disease. The cerebrovascular complications of hypertension included hypertensive encephalopathy, transient ischaemic attacks and haemorrhagic stroke. In contrast, hypertensive animals fed a low-cholesterol diet did not develop complicated atheroma and normotensive animals fed a hypercholesterolaemic diet developed mild atheroma of only the major coronary arteries.

Cerebral embolism

Blood flow through the brain and spinal cord may be arrested by emboli which, according to their size, become impacted in arteries, arterioles and capillaries. Emboli reaching the brain through the internal carotid arteries are usually arrested within the distribution of the middle cerebral artery.

During the last 30 years there has been an increasing awareness of the importance of embolism. It is estimated that about 60 per cent of acute strokes in the USA are of embolic origin (Meyer, 1982). This high incidence appears to be at variance with the figure of 10 per cent derived from the Framingham study (Kannel, 1976). In the latter, however, the incidence may have been underestimated and some strokes ascribed to atheroma were in fact of embolic origin. The importance of cerebral embolism has been emphasized by various autopsy studies. For example, Adams and Vander Eecken (1953) and Torvik and Jorgensen (1966) considered that 50 per cent of cerebral infarcts were embolic in origin, and a possible source of emboli was found in 58 per cent of 581 cases (McCall and Fletcher, 1975).

Cerebral emboli may arise as a result of valvular and ischaemic heart disease, and atheroma of the large arteries in the neck. They may also consist of air, nitrogen or fat (see McDowell, 1972).

Embolism of cardiac origin

Rheumatic valvular disease and myocardial infarction are the major sources of cerebral emboli in adults (Vost, Wolochow and Howell, 1964; Blackwood et al., 1969; Easton and Sherman, 1980). It has been estimated that 10–20 per cent of patients with rheumatic heart disease develop signs of embolism, some 40 per cent of which affect the brain. Patients with mitral stenosis or incompetence are particularly at risk when there is atrial fibrillation. There is a high incidence of cerebral infarction in patients with ischaemic heart disease (Vost, Wolochow and Howell, 1964; McCall and Fletcher, 1975). In a recent study, Thompson and Robinson (1978) found that 1.7 per cent of 783 consecutive patients with myocardial infarction had had a stroke, and the probability of a stroke was related to the amount of myocardial damage. Two-thirds of cerebral emboli develop within the first 3 weeks of an acute myocardial infarction. Cerebral infarction in a patient with a myocardial infarct may be due to hypotension (p. 139) and is not necessarily embolic.

Rarer sources of cardiac emboli include a prolapsing mitral valve (Barnett et al., 1976), cardiac myxoma, and cardiomyopathy, particularly in association with congestive heart failure or arrhythmias (Easton and Sherman, 1980). A further source is non-bacterial thrombotic endocarditis. This is most frequent in association with the cachexia of advanced chronic illness in the elderly, particularly malignant disease. Cerebral embolism often complicates subacute infective endocarditis and may even be a presenting symptom. In older patients cerebral embolism is increasingly due to conditions such as calcific aortic stenosis.

Paradoxical embolism occurs when material passes through an atrial septal defect to enter the systemic circulation. About 4 per cent of cerebral emboli are of this type (Thompson and Evans, 1930; McCall and Fletcher, 1975). Paradoxical embolism is normally prevented by the flap which closes the foramen ovale, since pressure is higher in the left than in the right atrium. Paradoxical embolism occurs when this pressure gradient is reversed as in pulmonary embolism and chronic pulmonary hypertension.

Brain damage due to embolism during cardiac surgery, especially mitral valvotomy, first described by Bjork and Hultquist (1960), remains a serious potential complication (Branthwaite, 1972; Aberg, 1974). More recently, open heart surgery with cardiopulmonary bypass has created new sources of cerebral emboli which include not only the pump oxygenator but also diseased heart tissue, air trapped in the heart during surgery, fat from bone marrow and particles of silicone (antifoam).

The neuropathological findings in 46 patients

dying after open heart surgery were reported in detail by Brierley (1963, 1967). In only nine patients was the brain normal. Brain damage due to embolism was common, being due to a thrombus in the ligated stump of anomalous vessels, air, fat, antifoam agents and calcified debris from valves. Brain damage due to circulatory arrest or moderate hypotension was attributed to the blood flow being reduced by faulty or inadequate cerebral perfusion by the pump oxygenator.

The emboli responsible for small cortical infarcts may be difficult to identify in autopsy material because they may be lysed *in situ* as shown by serial angiography (Dalal et al., 1965). Also, because blood flow is restored through the area of ischaemia, the infarct is often haemorrhagic.

Atheromatous embolism

Occlusion of small arteries (Fig. 4.49) by such emboli with accompanying infarction may be found *post mortem* (Soloway and Aronson, 1964; McDonald, 1967). In some patients, multiple cerebral infarcts are due to disseminated atheromatous emboli (Sturgill and Netsky, 1963).

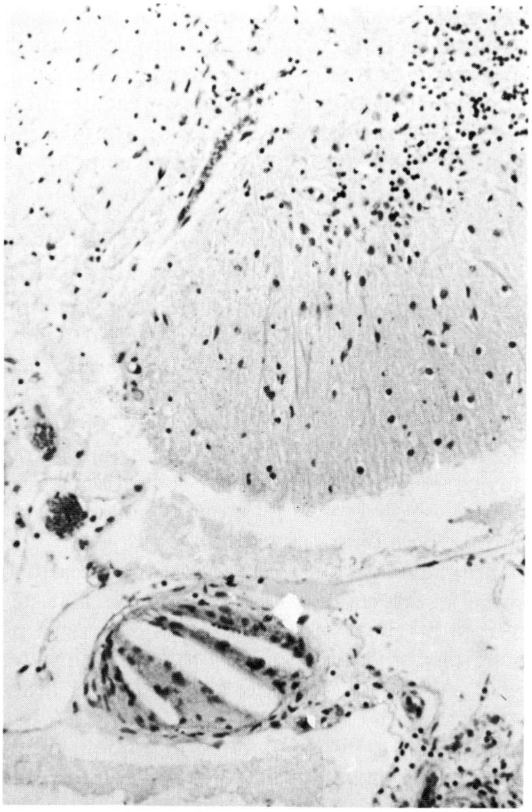

Fig. 4.49 Embolism of small cerebellar artery by three crystals of atheromatous debris. Small old infarct of nearby cortex.

Cerebral fat embolism

Fat emboli can be demonstrated in the lungs of some 90–100 per cent of patients with fractures. They may also occur in pancreatitis, prolonged treatment with steroids, burns, trauma to subcutaneous tissues or to fatty viscera and when bones are transected to give access to organs such as the heart. Intravascular fat embolism is therefore common whilst the syndrome of fat embolism is rare (Szabo, 1970) and is associated only with fractures of the limb and limb girdles.

At the site of fracture, fat from the marrow enters damaged veins in the form of small globules. If sufficiently numerous, some will not be trapped in the pulmonary circulation and enter the systemic circulation as a potential source of embolism (Watson, 1970). According to Sevitt (1962) gross pulmonary fat embolism may not necessarily cause symptoms or death.

The neuropathology of cerebral fat embolism has recently been reviewed (Kamenar and Burger, 1980). In cases of fulminating fat embolism dying within a day or two of an injury, the brain may appear entirely normal macroscopically. More characteristically, in patients surviving 3–4 days, the white matter of the brain is diffusely studded with petechial haemorrhages of pericapillary, ring and ball type (Fig. 4.50). Many fat

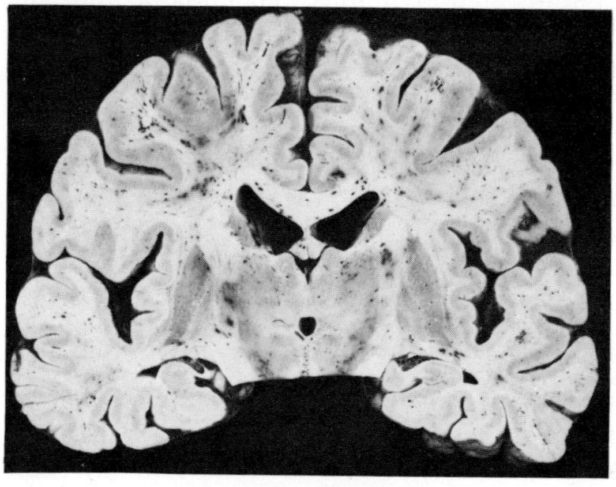

Fig. 4.50 Female, aged 78 years, dying 5 days after sustaining fracture of femur. There are multiple petechial haemorrhages due to fat embolism in the white matter of the cerebral hemispheres.

globules are visible and sometimes the capillary walls are necrotic. There may be foci of myelin pallor, or perivascular infarcts infiltrated by polymorphonuclear leucocytes. In grey matter, fat globules are equally numerous, but haemorrhages and tissue damage do not occur. This is because in grey matter the capillaries are individually short and anastomoses are frequent. In white matter the capillaries are long and anastomoses are few, so after embolism endothelial damage is more likely.

After survival of several days alterations may be found in grey matter. In a case surviving a week (Neubürger, 1925) there were multiple foci of necrosis chiefly in the deeper layers of the cortex and also in the cerebellum. Fat globules were present in the capillaries of both altered and normal brain. In a case surviving 12 days Winkelman (1942) found small infarcts of varying ages in the deeper layers of the cortex, in the white matter especially of the frontal lobes, and in the brain stem especially in the pons. When survival was from 3 months to 7 years there was gross atrophy of the cerebral white matter (McTaggart and Neubuerger, 1970; von Hochstetter and Friede, 1977). In contrast, changes in grey matter were minimal, consisting of scattered foci of neuronal loss.

Cerebral fat embolism has also been observed in the brains of patients after open heart surgery (see p. 178) and after the use of methylmethacrylic bone cement (Adams et al., 1972).

Air embolism

Air may enter the circulation during abortion; after trauma, cardiac and pulmonary surgery, artificial pneumothorax, self-inflicted or surgical venesection in the neck, and venous and arterial catheterization; and during neurosurgical operations with the patient in the sitting position and during subatmospheric decompression (Menkin and Schwartzman, 1977). If the volume of air is small, there may be no clinical sequelae; if large, it is rapidly mixed with blood in the heart to produce a frothy fluid which will enter the coronary and the systemic circulations. The amount of air required to cause major symptoms, and possibly death, in the human adult has been estimated to be between 300 and 500 ml (see McDowell, 1972). Death is probably due to a combination of pulmonary and cardiac dysfunction rather than to cerebral air embolism itself. The prognosis after air embolism is, however, much better than after fat embolism. If the patient survives the first 10–15 minutes, the danger has largely passed. Severe neurological deficits may completely disappear within hours or days, although mental disturbance may persist (Menkin and Schwartzman, 1977).

The procedures to be taken at autopsy when air embolism is suspected have been detailed (Taylor, 1952). When death occurs within a few minutes, air is largely in the veins, there are no haemorrhages and the brain is normal. In a case surviving 55 hours (Neubürger, 1925), cortical damage took the form of small, perivascular, foci of neuronal damage and of laminar necrosis. Lhermitte and Barrelet (1934) found marked changes in the cortex but none in the white matter in a patient dying of pneumonia some weeks after air embolism. There was a spongy state in the outer layers of the cerebal cortex and scattered, small, irregularly shaped foci from which all nerve and glial cells had disappeared.

An accentuation of ischaemic damage along cortical arterial boundary zones after accidental air embolism in man was first described by Ameuille, L'Hermitte and Krudelski (1935) and confirmed by Brion, Psimaras and Gallissot (1974). Thus the neuropathology of air embolism may be virtually indistinguishable from that due to a combination of reduced cerebral blood flow and hypoxaemia. In some cases, however, cerebral alterations consist of perivascular foci of ischaemic neuronal damage which may be single, multiple or confluent. They are often outlined by a narrow zone of pallor of staining so that larger lesions have a characteristically 'geographical' outline (Brion, Psimaras and Gallissot, 1974).

Nitrogen embolism (hyperbaric and hypobaric decompression sickness)

Hyperbaric decompression This is brought about by the reduction of an elevated (hyperbaric) atmospheric pressure to a normal level. The hyperbaric environment is common to underwater divers and to workers in caissons. Decompression is necessary before ascent to the surface, and if carried out slowly according to recommended practice there are no adverse effects. If too rapid, symptoms of caisson disease may appear with damage, particularly to the spinal cord, and even death.

At any given atmospheric pressure inspired

gases dissolve in blood, tissue fluids and fat. Nitrogen is particularly soluble in fat. If the subject then passes too rapidly from a high to normal pressure, the dissolved gases come out of solution. Whereas oxygen and carbon dioxide are rapidly reabsorbed, nitrogen tends to form small bubbles which may coalesce. In addition to causing damage where they form, 'the bends' develop when the bubbles collect around joints and the 'chokes' when they develop within the interstitial tissues of the lungs. Bubbles of nitrogen may appear in the blood stream. At autopsy on patients surviving for only a short time the brain and spinal cord are intensely congested and there may be haemorrhages. After longer survival multiple small infarcts may be seen, particularly in the upper levels of the thoracic cord. In the affected segments ischaemic damage is essentially restricted to white matter, most commonly in the central portion of each posterior column (Haymaker, 1957). A similar distribution of lesions has been reported by Palmer et al. (1981) in a patient who died 12 days after making an almost complete functional recovery from spinal decompression sickness. According to Haymaker (1957) the lesions in the spinal cord are due to bubbles of nitrogen that appear in the blood stream after the drop in atmospheric pressure, together with embarrassment of the venous circulation of the cord by gas bubbles arising in the epidural and/or retroperitoneal fat.

Hypobaric decompression This is the reduction of atmospheric pressure from normal (sea level) to a lower (hypobaric) level as at high altitude or in a hypobaric decompression chamber. If decompression is slow enough there are no adverse effects, but if not there may be symptoms, brain damage and even death.

There are only a few reports detailing the neuropathological findings in subjects dying either from exposure to simulated high altitude in decompression chambers (Haymaker and Davison, 1950; Haymaker and Johnston, 1955) or after high-altitude flights (Haymaker and Johnston, 1955; Haymaker, Johnston and Downey, 1956). Characteristically, there are multiple foci of ischaemic damage accentuated in the grey matter of the cerebral hemispheres, the cerebellum and the brain stem. There is relative sparing of the spinal cord, though in some cases the findings were similar to those described in caisson disease (Haymaker and Johnston, 1955; Haymaker, Johnston and Downey, 1956). The lesions have been attributed to a combination of gaseous and fat embolism, and circulatory collapse.

Experimental studies on cerebral embolism These have been undertaken using atheroma, fat, air and nitrogen. There is often a disturbance of the blood–brain barrier leading to vasogenic oedema and a raised intracranial pressure.

It has been shown that the aggregation of platelets can induce the formation of thrombus and precipitate thromboembolism (Hovig, 1970), as, for example, after the intravascular injection of prostaglandin E_2 and arachidonic acid (Furlow and Bass, 1976). Nevertheless, it has been difficult to identify platelet thrombi within cerebral infarcts. This apparent discrepancy was explored by Petito (1979b) after unilateral carotid artery occlusion with systemic hypoxia in the rat. After recovery of up to 2 hours the brains were examined by light and electron microscopy. Platelet thrombi were seen only in areas of infarction and not in areas of selective neuronal necrosis. This suggested that platelet thrombi were secondary to and not the cause of the infarction.

Atheromatous emboli consist of thrombus and cholesterol crystals. The effects of cholesterol emboli have been studied in rats by their infusion into one carotid artery (Steiner, Rail and Rose, 1980). Blood flow was reduced to only a limited extent in small vessels and there was no tendency for thrombus to form. However, when material derived from plaques of human atheroma was injected into a common carotid artery in the rabbit, intravascular thrombus formation (Jeynes and Warren, 1982) was seen, suggesting that the effects of atheromatous emboli may be related to their capacity to induce thrombus formation.

The intravascular injection of relatively small numbers of radioactively labelled microspheres has been used to measure global or local cerebral blood flow at the end of an acute experiment. The number of microspheres injected is determined by the sensitivity of the detection system and it is assumed that such emboli do not appreciably affect local vascular reactivity. Furthermore, the possibility that embolism by these small numbers of microspheres could lead to microinfarcts in surviving animals has not yet been excluded by a systematic study.

The syndrome of fat embolism and its pathogenesis have been reviewed by Szabo (1970). The use of radioisotope-labelled fat emboli and semiquantitative histological methods in rabbits has suggested that the symptoms and signs of fat embolism in man are probably due to arterial hypoxaemia rather than to the emboli. The hypoxaemia is attributed to shunting of unoxygenated blood through the lungs and the toxic action on lung tissue of unesterified fatty acids (Prys-Roberts et al., 1970).

Hallenbeck, Bove and Elliott (1975) and Hallenbeck (1976) have reproduced the spinal cord damage associated with hyperbaric decompression sickness in dogs. Measurements taken before and after a simulated dive, including cinephotomicrography, revealed that the epidural vertebral venous system and the dorsal pial vessels became blocked by bubbles in those animals that developed a neurological deficit and in which there was evidence of haemorrhage in the white matter of the spinal cord. The grey matter was normal. If venous obstruction was not demonstrable, the spinal cord was normal histologically. The appearances in the cord were attributed to venous stasis and infarction. All segments of the cord could be involved, but there was a predilection for the cervical and dorsal regions. Lesions were seen in the brain stem in two animals, and in all the cerebral and cerebellar hemispheres were spared. Neither acute pulmonary hypertension nor central venous congestion was an important factor.

On the other hand the lesions produced in the spinal cord of goats (Palmer, Blakemore and Greenwood, 1976; Palmer et al., 1978) subjected to experimental hyperbaric decompression sickness have been attributed to a combination of intra-arterial bubble formation and a reduced perfusion pressure. The sequelae of bubbles in blood have been reviewed by Elliott, Hallenbeck and Bove (1974), and include the formation of lipid emboli, sludging of red blood cells and platelet aggregation. The importance of these vascular events has been confirmed by Palmer and Blakemore (1980). It has recently been suggested that damage to the spinal cord is due not to such secondary emboli but to bubbles that develop at a local pressure sufficiently high to exceed the perfusion pressure and thus occlude blood flow (Hills and James, 1982).

Experimental studies have made a considerable contribution to the understanding of the nature and pathogenesis of the brain damage due to air embolism. Spielmeyer (1913) injected air into one carotid artery in the monkey, and demonstrated oval or triangular areas of typical ischaemic neuronal damage. From direct observations of the pial vessels in the baboon, Naquet and Vigouroux (1966) concluded that, after carotid injection, air bubbles were initially distributed throughout the territory of the internal carotid artery without there being any evidence of vasospasm. If the volume of air was sufficient there could be cortical circulatory arrest for up to 3 minutes and marked slowing of, or even an isoelectric, EEG (Meldrum, Papy and Vigouroux, 1971; Brierley and Meldrum, 1974). The latter authors concluded that the period of circulatory arrest was too short to be responsible for the observed lesions and, in the absence of systemic hypotension, '... persistence of air within the vascular bed of the boundary zones after it has been cleared from the central arterial territories is the cause of the localised ischaemia producing focal lesions'.

Experimental studies of hypobaric decompression have already been described (p. 144).

Transient ischaemic attacks

Transient ischaemic attacks are fully reversible neurological deficits usually lasting for no more than a few minutes, but occasionally up to 24 hours.

Clinically, they represent an advance warning of cerebral infarction. Estimates of the risk of subsequent permanent stroke range from 13 per cent (Fields et al., 1970) to 50 per cent (Acheson and Hutchinson, 1964). The chance of developing cerebral infarction within 5 years of an attack is approximately 30 per cent (Toole et al., 1975), whilst most develop within 6 months.

Pathological studies suggest that there is little reason to believe that the pathogenesis of most attacks differs from that of small cerebral infarcts and haemorrhages (Yates, 1976b). It is generally believed that repeated attacks are due to ischaemia rather than haemorrhage, and three causes may act singly or in combination: first, emboli arising from abnormalities of the heart and large arteries in the neck; second, changes in the composition of the circulating blood (p. 186); and third, changes in cardiac output and cerebral perfusion. Thus the pathogenesis resembles that of cerebral infarction (Wolf and Kannel, 1982).

Less common varieties of cerebral arterial disorders

Fibromuscular dysplasia

First described in the renal arteries (Leadbetter and Burkland, 1938), fibromuscular dysplasia is characterized by areas of fibrous and muscular thickening of the intima alternating with aneurysmal dilatations to give a 'string of beads' appearance in an arteriogram. Since its first description in the internal carotid artery (Connett and Lausche, 1965) it has been identified with increasing frequency. Affected vessels include either singly or in combination the internal carotid arteries and the vertebral arteries. The external carotid arteries may also be affected. Involvement of the intracranial arteries is rare. Most patients are women over the age of 50 years; the condition is bilateral in 75 per cent, and in 25 per cent there is an associated congenital aneurysm. The condition has been fully reviewed by Mettinger (1982) and by Mettinger and Ericson (1982).

The aortic arch syndrome

This name is given to a combination of clinical signs and symptoms due to progressive narrowing of the aortic arch and the origins of the innominate artery, the left common carotid and the left subclavian arteries (Fig. 4.51). It is known by many other names, including 'pulseless disease', aortic arch arteritis and Takayasu's arteritis.

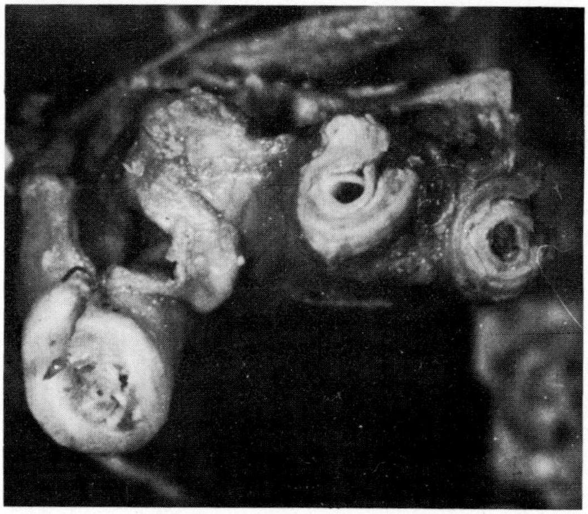

Fig. 4.51 Takayasu's arteritis. Vessels arising from the arch of the aorta showing great thickening of arterial walls and occlusion of lumina. The innominate artery is on the left.

For example, the aortic arch syndrome was first thought to be a neurological entity due to a panarteritic granulomatous process, and leading to marked scarring of the vessel walls and thrombus formation. The early cases were described in young Oriental women but the condition has now been identified in older women and men throughout the world and vessels other than the aorta and its branches are affected. In many instances the condition is due to a specific disease process (see Bernsmeier and Held, 1972). Other inflammatory conditions may give rise to the aortic arch syndrome, including thromboangiitis obliterans (Buerger's disease), collagen disorders including polyarteritis nodosa, giant cell arteritis, syphilis and tuberculosis. It has also been attributed to congenital variations of the vessels, to trauma and to embolism.

Acute carotid arteritis

Now rare, this condition was seen in children and young adults in the preantibiotic era. The inflammation may arise from retropharyngeal tissues and lymph nodes in the neck and from septic occlusion of the cavernous sinus (Mathew et al., 1971). Within the vessel the inflammation is non-specific and its site depends upon the site of the primary inflammation.

Endarteritis obliterans

In meningovascular syphilis, tuberculous leptomeningitis and subacute or chronic pyogenic leptomeningitis it is not uncommon to find thickening of the walls of arteries and veins (Fig. 4.52). The intima is separated concentrically or eccentrically from the internal elastic lamina by a cellular infiltrate composed at first of monocytes and lymphocytes. In syphilis, plasma cells are usually present and eosinophil leucocytes are common. The cellular infiltrate may be replaced by fibroblasts, collagen and fine elastic fibrils lying internal to the elastic lamina, which itself remains intact. The media may be normal or may show slight inflammatory cell infiltration or fibrosis. The adventitia is thickened, by inflammatory cells or fibrous tissue.

Endarteritis obliterans is no more than a reaction of arteries to systemic bacterial infection

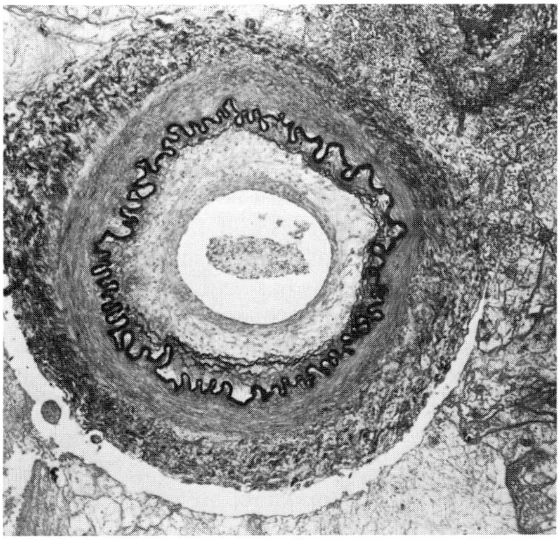

Fig. 4.52 Endarteritis obliterans. Note the artery at the base of the brain, taken from a case of pneumococcal leptomeningitis, treated with sulpha drugs for 1 month. Fibrinous exudate is present round the vessel which shows a thickened adventitia, an intact internal elastic membrane and concentric intimal thickening. Fine elastic fibres are visible in the depths of the intimal wall. An adjacent artery, in the upper right-hand side of the picture, shows necrosis and cellular infiltration of its wall. Paraffin; Weigert's elastic—van Gieson × 57.

of several types (Chapter 6). It is most probably due to an irritant acting on the vessels from without, as exemplified by those spinal anaesthetics which may be complicated by delayed paraplegia. In addition to fibrous thickening and obliteration of the fluid spaces of the pia arachnoid (arachnoiditis) up to the base of the brain, there are often alterations that are marked in the arteries but less so in the veins.

In the patient reported by Brain and Russell (1937), paralysis developed 1 month after spinal anaesthesia, and death occurred 3.5 months later. At autopsy there was an endophlebitis and a necrotizing panarteritis of the pial and perforating arterioles of the lumbar cord with extensive infarction of the grey and white matter. In the cases of Greenfield, Rickards and Manning (1955) paralysis developed about 7, 8 and 24 weeks after the anaesthetic and death occurred about 5, 1 and 1 week later respectively. At autopsy vascular changes were restricted to the leptomeningeal vessels of the lower thoracic and lumbosacral segments of the cord. In the arteries there was adventitial fibrosis, fibrous replacement of the media, rupture, thickening or reduplication of the elastica, and fibrous thickening (usually concentric) of the intima. Coagulative necrosis was seen in one small artery and thrombosis in another. The walls of the veins were partially or wholly replaced by fibrous tissue. These changes were attributed to the anaesthetic itself or to an associated substance.

In order to assess the possible contribution of a substance other than the anaesthetic agent itself, Hurst (1955) injected a number of detergents and antiseptics in high dilution into the cisterna magna of monkeys. He found that many of these, although chemically dissimilar, damaged the subpial and subependymal tissues of the brain and spinal cord. They produced cellular proliferation and fibrosis in the pia arachnoid, and necrosis of the media and often of the adventitia of the leptomeningeal arteries with subsequent intimal thickening. The end-result was therefore similar to that described in man. Hurst (1955) considered that the experimental lesions were due to the direct irritative action of the non-anaesthetic chemicals tested.

Moyamoya disease

This is a condition seen predominantly in young women in whom cerebral angiography shows an unusual net-like appearance of small blood vessels (resembling a puff of smoke) at the base of the brain. The disease at first thought to be confined to the Japanese has now been reported from other parts of the world, yet with a preponderance in the Japanese (see Nishimoto and Takeuchi, 1972).

Pathological studies have not contributed materially to an understanding of the disease. In the case described by Carlson, Harvey and Loop (1973) there was arteriographic evidence of bilateral stenosis of the upper ends of the internal carotid arteries, telangiectasis of the vessels in the diencephalon and dural anastomoses with the external carotid artery. The principal histological abnormality was a focal absence or atrophy of the internal elastic lamina in most arteries of the circle of Willis and its branches.

The aetiology of moyamoya disease is obscure but two major hypotheses have been advanced. The first is that it is a true congenital vascular malformation. The second is that the abnormal angiographic appearances represent a collateral circulation developing in response to acquired stenosis of the internal carotid arteries. The features of moyamoya disease have been seen angiographically in association with a number of acquired conditions, including atheroma (O'Sullivan et al., 1977), tuberculous meningitis, cerebral embolism (Numaguchi et al., 1976), sickle cell disease (Merkel et al., 1978), neurofibromatosis and after irradiation.

Collagen disorders

Polyarteritis nodosa This acute, or subacute, disease of the walls of medium-sized and small arteries and arterioles is characterized by multiple foci of subendothelial 'oedema' followed by fibrinoid or hyaline necrosis of the media, destruction of the internal elastic lamina and infiltration of all coats by inflammatory cells (Fig. 4.53). These changes may affect the whole

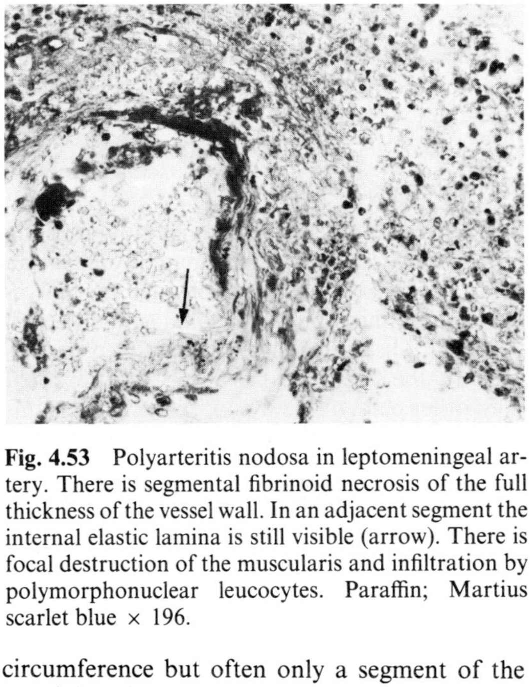

Fig. 4.53 Polyarteritis nodosa in leptomeningeal artery. There is segmental fibrinoid necrosis of the full thickness of the vessel wall. In an adjacent segment the internal elastic lamina is still visible (arrow). There is focal destruction of the muscularis and infiltration by polymorphonuclear leucocytes. Paraffin; Martius scarlet blue × 196.

circumference but often only a segment of the arterial wall. The cellular infiltration is most abundant in the adventitia and is composed of neutrophil leucocytes, lymphocytes, large mononuclear cells and eosinophil leucocytes. Vascular damage may involve the endothelium leading to occlusion by secondary thrombosis. Sometimes damage is so severe that nodular dilatation, aneurysm formation or rupture may occur. In the healing or healed stage the arteries show concentric or eccentric subendothelial fibrosis. The internal elastic lamina is partially or wholly fragmented or destroyed, the media is more or less replaced by fibrous tissue, and there is slight fibrous thickening of the adventitia. The vascular lesions are most common in the kidneys, heart, splanchnic region, brain, spinal cord, nerves and muscle. The pathogenesis of the disease is not known but hypersensitivity to micro-organisms, drugs or autoantigens has been suggested.

The vascular changes seen in muscle and in the nervous system are believed to be identical to those encountered in other organs. Polyarteritis nodosa affects the central nervous system in 10–20 per cent of cases, the peripheral nervous system in 20–50 per cent and muscle in 40–80 per cent. The symptoms and signs are protean though certain clinical patterns can be recognized (see Goetz, 1980).

At autopsy the pial and intracerebral arteries may appear beaded because of aneurysmal dilatation. Rupture of these aneurysms is uncommon but subarachnoid haemorrhage is the presenting feature in some 5 per cent. Characteristically, there are multiple infarcts and haemorrhage, particularly in the cortex, the basal ganglia, the white matter and the brain stem. Whilst these may well be due to the arteritic process, it should be remembered that many patients suffer severe terminal hypertension and so some alterations may be due to hypertensive encephalopathy (Roger, Poursines and Roger, 1955).

Wegener's granulomatosis This is a fatal systemic disease in which granulomas and multiple foci of arteritis develop in the respiratory tract, the kidneys and other organs, including the nervous system (see Stern, 1980). In a series of 56 autopsies Walton (1958) found that the peripheral nervous system was involved in 29 per cent and the brain and meninges in 7 per cent. In contrast, Drachman (1963) found involvement of the nervous and neuromuscular systems in 56 of 105 cases in the literature. The clinical features are protean but ocular manifestations are common. The nervous system may be involved by extension of the granulomatous process from the nasal cavity and paranasal sinuses, by the development of granulomatous lesions remote from the upper respiratory tract, and by a vasculitis affecting the vasa nervorum in cases presenting with peripheral neuropathy (Chapter 18). Drachman (1963) discussed the similarity between Wegener's granulomatosis and involvement of the nervous system by other granulomatous and arteritic diseases, including polyarteritis nodosa. It has been suggested that the midline granuloma (Stewart's syndrome) is a localized form of Wegener's granulomatosis (Blatt et al., 1959; Anderson, Jamieson and Jefferson, 1975).

Systemic lupus erythematosus Like rheumatic fever, scleroderma and polyarteritis nodosa, this multisystem disease is regarded as a connective tissue disorder. It occurs most frequently in adolescent and young women and may run an acute or sometimes a more prolonged course with death usually from renal failure within months or a few years. Affected organs include skin, kidneys, endocardium and the serous membranes. Microscopic changes are most marked in vessels less than 100 μm diameter and consist of acute fibrinoid necrosis and marked thickening with minimal inflammatory cell infiltration. Some vessels are occluded by thrombi with corresponding microinfarcts. These changes do not, however, account for all features of the disease. Immunopathological mechanisms, and in particular the deposition of immune complexes, are thought to account for the kidney lesions (Cochrane and Koffler, 1973) but remain unproven within the nervous system although deposits of immune complex have been identified in the choroid plexus of patients with neurological manifestations of the illness (see Richardson, 1980).

The neuropathological features in 54 cases of systemic lupus erythematosus were reviewed by Berry and Hodges (1965). No gross abnormalities were seen in 48 per cent, and in 37 per cent there were multiple foci of infarction, particularly in the cerebral cortex and the subcortical grey matter. Focal haemorrhages were seen in 7 per cent and there was granular atrophy of the cortex in a further 7 per cent. Histologically the features ranged from acute fibrinoid necrosis of vessels to cystic encephalopathy. However, as noted by Berry (1971), 'Despite neurologic involvement clinically, there often is a disconcerting lack of gross and even microscopic findings in the nervous system on post-mortem examination'.

Rheumatic fever Most of the lesions in the central nervous system, in both the acute and the chronic phases of rheumatic fever, are either non-specific or are due directly to the associated heart disease. Some lesions are certainly due to embolism, some to local thrombosis and some to cardiac insufficiency (Yates, 1976a).

Giant cell or temporal arteritis

This subacute inflammatory arterial disease of unknown aetiology usually occurs in patients of either sex over the age of 55 years. It often involves the superficial temporal arteries, which become swollen, tender, tortuous and nodular; pulsation is usually diminished or lost and the artery may eventually shrink and become hard. The disease is not limited to the temporal arteries and almost all larger arteries, including the aorta, have been found to be involved. Among medium- and smaller-sized arteries, those of particular importance are the coronary arteries and the ophthalmic arteries and their branches including the ciliary arteries and the central artery of the retina (see Goodwin, 1980). The cervical portions of the internal carotid and vertebral arteries are frequently involved, the intracranial arteries to a lesser extent and those of the spinal cord least of all.

Histologically there is a panarteritis that may be multifocal or involve the whole length of the vessel. Initially there is intimal proliferation which, in the active stage of the disease, often consists of an inner thicker zone composed of loosely packed cellular fibrous tissue with a mucoid intercellular substance, and an outer thinner part of vascular granulomatous tissue infiltrated by a variable number of mononuclear cells, plasma cells and a few neutrophil polymorphs. Eosinophil leucocytes are uncommon, in contrast to polyarteritis nodosa. The internal elastic lamina of the media is always severely but irregularly fragmented. The media is infiltrated by small and large mononuclear cells, some of 'epithelioid' type. Giant cells of either Langhans or foreign body type (10–100 μm diameter) are almost invariably present, either in the media close to the damaged internal elastic lamina or in the adjacent intima (Fig. 4.54). Occasionally, small foci of fibrinoid necrosis are seen. A lesser degree of inflammatory cell proliferation with giant cells is also present in the adventitia (Harrison, 1948; Heptinstall, Porter and Barkley, 1954). With healing there is fibrous scarring of the media and occasionally aneurysm formation. In some cases the vessels are occluded by organizing thrombus.

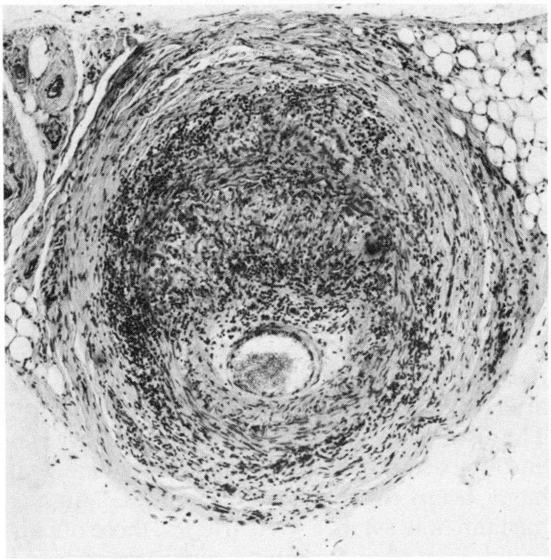

Fig. 4.54 Giant cell arteritis. Ciliary artery of the eye, showing intimal proliferation and cellular infiltration, including multinucleated giant cells close to the irregularly damaged internal elastic lamina. There is mononuclear infiltration of the media and, to a lesser extent, of the adventitia. Celloidin; haematoxylin—van Gieson × 64.

It has been estimated that some 25–30 per cent of patients with temporal arteritis develop neurological complications. This high incidence must be set against the apparent absence of arteritic changes in the intracranial vessels. It has been suggested, therefore, that many of the symptoms are due to emboli arising from the neck arteries.

The temporal vessels remain the most popular site for biopsy, largely because of their accessibility. It should be stressed, however, that a negative biopsy does not exclude a diagnosis of giant cell arteritis, if only because of its focal nature. On the other hand, it is possible to make a histological diagnosis in biopsies taken from arteries that appear clinically normal.

Thromboangiitis obliterans (Winiwarter–Buerger's disease)

This is a disease of the arteries and veins of unknown aetiology characteristically affecting the limbs of young males who are heavy smokers. Since its original description it has become known that the disease may affect vessels throughout the body and there is now considerable evidence to justify its recognition as a distinct disease process (see Parker and Schwartzman, 1980). Nevertheless the existence of a cerebral form remains uncertain. The essential problem lies in making a distinction between cases of thromboangiitis obliterans and other vascular diseases including embolism. It may well be that the diagnosis of thromboangiitis obliterans can only be made with certainty after an autopsy that includes examination of the vessels of the limbs.

Blood diseases

Polycythaemia Whether primary or secondary to cardiac and pulmonary disease, there is an increase in the number of red cells and thus an increased red cell mass, haematocrit and blood volume. Consequently, there is a tendency for both arteries and veins to become occluded.

Predictably, transient ischaemic attacks, cerebral infarction and cerebral haemorrhage are all recognized complications of polycythaemia (Millikan, Siekert and Whisnant, 1960; Silverstein, Gilbert and Wasserman, 1962). The importance of cerebrovascular disease in polycythaemia was further emphasized by Chievitz and Thiede (1962), who found that cerebral infarction was the cause of death in 15 per cent of patients and cerebral haemorrhage in 4 per cent.

Direct measurement of cerebral blood flow has shown that it is reduced when high viscosity occurs in polycythaemia (Thomas et al., 1977a; Paulson, Henriksen and Smith, 1979) and in patients with a high 'normal haematocrit' (Thomas et al., 1977b). Not surprisingly, patients with a 'high normal haemoglobin and haematocrit' are more likely to develop ischaemic brain damage. Kannel et al. (1972), for example, showed that a haemoglobin level greater than 15 g/dl in men and 14 g/dl in women doubled the risk. This was later confirmed when it was shown that, by keeping the haematocrit below 0.46 dl/dl, the risk of vascular complications was greatly reduced (Pearson and Wetherley-Mein, 1978; Tohgi et al., 1978).

Thrombotic thrombocytopenic purpura This rare disease, first described by Moschowitz (1925), is characterized by fever, purpura, haemolytic anaemia and thrombocytopenia. The kidneys are commonly affected and the nervous system is said to be involved in 90 per cent of cases (Silverstein, 1968). It runs a rapid course and death usually supervenes within a few days or weeks. It is rather more common in adolescents and young adults than in the elderly.

The pathology was reviewed by Adams, Cammermeyer and Fitzgerald (1948). At necropsy there are no specific macroscopic alterations but histologically there is widespread occlusion of small vessels by granular or hyaline eosinophilic material (possibly fibrin and/or platelets) (Fig. 4.55) which may be undergoing organization. Within the brain the lesions, virtually confined to grey matter, consist of hyperplasia of endothelial and probably of adventitial cells of terminal arterioles and capillaries with increase in their overall diameter. Sometimes the vessel wall is necrotic and the lumen is occluded by acidophilic material. There is, however, a striking disparity between alterations that are marked in the vessels but slight in the surrounding tissue. Numerous small cerebral infarcts and petechial haemorrhages are common, but larger areas of haemorrhage and infarction have been described.

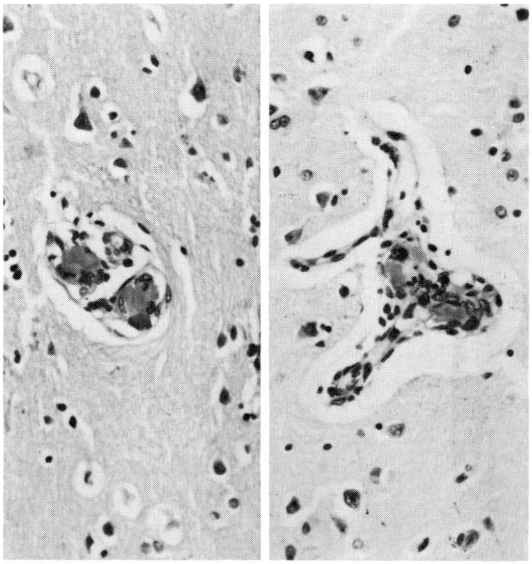

Fig. 4.55 Thrombotic microangiopathy. Hyaline eosinophilic thrombus obstructs the dilated lumen at the arteriolocapillary junction zone. There is endothelial hyperplasia. The adjacent grey matter of the brain does not show any noticeable abnormality (apart from artefact due to shrinkage). Paraffin; haematoxylin and eosin × 200. (Reproduced by courtesy of Prof. W. Symmers.)

The aetiology is not known, but the possibility that immunological mechanisms may play a part was suggested by Symmers (1956) in a case of thrombotic microangiopathy associated with acute haemorrhagic leucoencephalitis and sensitivity to oxophenarsine. A somewhat similar condition has been described in diabetic ketoacidosis (Timperley, Preston and Ward, 1974).

Sickle cell anaemia and other haemoglobinopathies The nervous system is affected in about 25 per cent of patients with sickle cell disease. Stroke and other syndromes are more frequent in the disease than in the general population (Portnoy and Herion, 1972; Wood, 1978). According to Boros and Weiner (1979) the main cause of cerebral and systemic damage is the occlusion of small vessels by sickled cells, but thrombosis of large vessels, massive intracranial haemorrhage, meningitis and fat embolism may also occur. Patients may also present with an acute spinal cord syndrome. The interrelationships between red blood cell deformability, haemoglobin oxygenation, viscosity and blood flow determine the site of vascular occlusion in the disease (Klug, Lessin and Radice, 1974). In a single case of a 7-year-old boy recorded by Merkel et al. (1978) angiography showed a moyamoya appearance (p. 183) that at autopsy was shown to be due to severe occlusive vascular disease of the upper ends of the internal carotid arteries and the circle of Willis.

The nervous system may also be involved in patients with thalassaemia (Boros and Weiner, 1979).

Macroglobulinaemia Neurological complications occur in some 20–50 per cent of patients with Waldenström's macroglobulinaemia (see Abramsky, 1980). These include subarachnoid haemorrhage, hypoxic encephalopathy, myelopathy and neuropathy. The pathogenesis is complex and includes abnormalities of the clotting mechanisms with a marked tendency to bleed, and increased blood viscosity. Other factors, particularly within the peripheral nervous system, may include lymphoma, amyloidosis and the deposition of immune complexes.

Oral contraceptives and cerebral infarction

Attention was drawn in the early 1960s (Family Planning Association, 1962) to the occurrence of cerebrovascular disorders in young women taking oral contraceptives. Further evidence was provided by Illis et al. (1965) and the relationship seemed to be proven when Bickerstaff and Holmes (1967) found a fivefold increase in the incidence of stroke in a group of 25 young women taking oral contraceptives. In contrast, however, Jennett and Cross (1967) found no such relationship in a group of non-pregnant women with carotid strokes, but later the studies by Vessey and Doll (1969) and the Collaborative Group for the Study of Stroke in Young Women (1973) led to the conclusion that there was a six- to ninefold increased risk of cerebral infarction in young women taking oral contraceptives. Several authors have noted the frequency with which this group of patients present with vertebrobasilar artery ischaemia.

The pathogenesis of strokes associated with the use of oral contraceptives is not clear but a direct effect on vessels is regarded as less likely than a hypercoagulable state related to the oestrogen content of the preparation itself and to the increased platelet adhesiveness that it engenders.

Cerebral infarction associated with pregnancy and the puerperium

The association between stroke and pregnancy and the puerperium is well recognized but fortunately uncommon. In the past it has been ascribed to cerebral thrombophlebitis, and this may be the cause in some cases (Carroll, Leak and Lee, 1966). Recent studies, however, have shown other causes, including occlusion of the cerebral arteries (Cross, Castro and Jennett, 1968) and paradoxical embolism, some secondary to occult embolism from the aorta and heart. Although arterial disease such as atheroma might be modified in some way by hormonal changes in pregnancy and the puerperium, it is thought that the association is not due to vessel disease *per se* but to an increased thrombotic tendency, including enhanced platelet adhesiveness.

Granulomatous angiitis

This uncommon form of vasculitis in the brain and spinal cord is characterized by the infiltration and obliteration of small arteries and veins by a granulomatous inflammatory process (Cravioto and Feigin, 1959; Kolodny et al., 1968). Whilst it shares the basic features of a vasculitis, Burger, Burch and Vogel (1976) consider that its clinicopathological features enable it to be distinguished from other types of angiitis. An infectious aetiology had long been suspected but was only confirmed when Reyes et al. (1976) reported virus-like particles and a granulomatous angiitis in the brain of a 67-year-old woman dying after 5 months of progressive multiple neurological abnormalities. Electron microscopy of formalin-fixed material revealed intranuclear inclusions resembling herpesvirus. The precise aetiology, however, remains uncertain because Arthur and Margolis (1977) have reported mycoplasma-like structures in granulomatous angiitis of the nervous system whilst Rosenblum, Hadfield and Young (1978) have reported a case of granulomatous angiitis following herpes zoster infection.

Miscellaneous cerebral arterial disorders

Intracranial occlusive vascular disease has been recorded secondary to irradiation (Darmody, Thomas and Gurdjian, 1967; Painter, Chutorian and Hilal, 1975), in association with addiction to heroin (Brust and Richter, 1976), as a complication of inflammatory bowel disease (Mayeux and Fahn, 1978; Schneiderman, Sharpe and Sutton, 1979), in association with migraine (Castaldo, Anderson and Reeves, 1982), in patients with inherited disorders of connective tissue (Herrero, 1980) and in familial oculoleptomeningeal amyloidosis (Goren, Steinberg and Farboody, 1980). Congophilic angiopathy may be seen in demented patients and be associated with multiple infarcts and senile plaques (Chapter 20).

Thrombosis of the veins and dural sinuses of the brain

This may be primary (non-infectious) or secondary to pyogenic infection.

Primary thrombosis

Aseptic thrombosis may complicate malnutrition, dehydration, heart disease usually with congestive cardiac failure, trauma, pregnancy and the puerperium, the postoperative state (excluding intracranial surgery), haematological disorders such as sickle cell anaemia, haemolytic anaemia, paroxysmal nocturnal haemoglobinuria, leukaemia and polycythaemia, the use of oral contraceptives, abortion and inflammatory bowel disease (Kalbag and Woolf, 1972). The superior sagittal sinus is most commonly involved often with extension into the cerebral veins and/or the transverse and lateral sinuses.

The incidence of intracranial venous thrombosis, though unknown, may be more frequent than previously realized. Its aetiology is also uncertain. In some of the associated conditions there is hypercoagulability of the blood, as in pregnancy, the puerperium, certain postoperative states and in various blood disorders. Also, the circulation may be slowed (dehydration or congestive cardiac failure) and there is the further possibility of retrograde venous embolism. Anatomical continuity has been demonstrated in man between the uterovaginal veins, the vertebral veins, the intracranial veins and the dural venous sinuses (Batson, 1940). It is therefore possible that during a period of high intra-abdominal pressure a small embolus might pass from the pelvic into the intracranial veins and dural venous sinuses by this route to form a nidus for a larger thrombus (Martin, 1941). Such an embolus could easily arise from one of the thrombosed veins normally found in the pelvis after parturition or abortion.

Localized thrombus formation is unlikely to impair the venous drainage of the brain or lead to permanent damage because of the abundant collateral circulation. On the other hand, when both a sinus and a portion of its tributaries are obstructed by thrombus, there will be serious interference with venous drainage (Fig. 4.56). The affected cortex and underlying white matter become congested, swollen and haemorrhagic (Fig. 4.57) leading to *venous infarction*. Haemorrhages, mainly in the white matter, range from petechial to large and are associated with some subarachnoid haemorrhage. To the naked eye, recently thrombosed venous channels are distended and bluish in colour. Necrotic cortex and white matter disintegrate rapidly, leaving tissue that is shrunken, cystic and yellowish-brown in colour. Thrombus in sinuses and veins is rapidly organized and recanalized, so it may be difficult to prove its existence after macroscopic and microscopic examinations.

The clinical features have been discussed by Krayenbuhl (1967) and Kalbag and Woolf (1972).

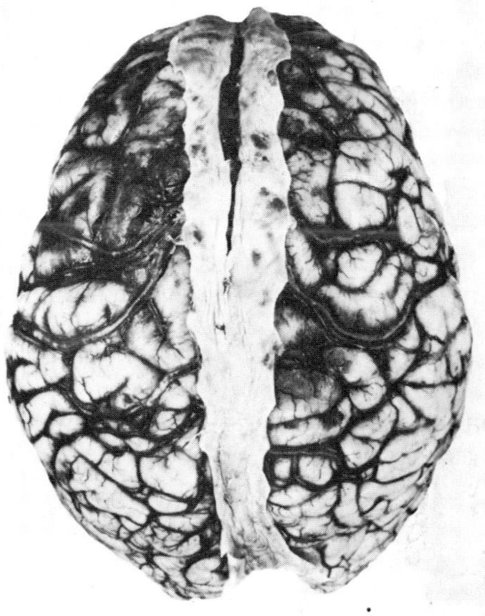

Fig. 4.56 Thrombosis of the superior sagittal sinus, and thrombophlebitis of the cortical veins which are distended by partly pale, partly dark thrombus. Note the marked perivascular subarachnoid haemorrhage. Clinically 3 days' duration. Puerperal woman with breast abscess.

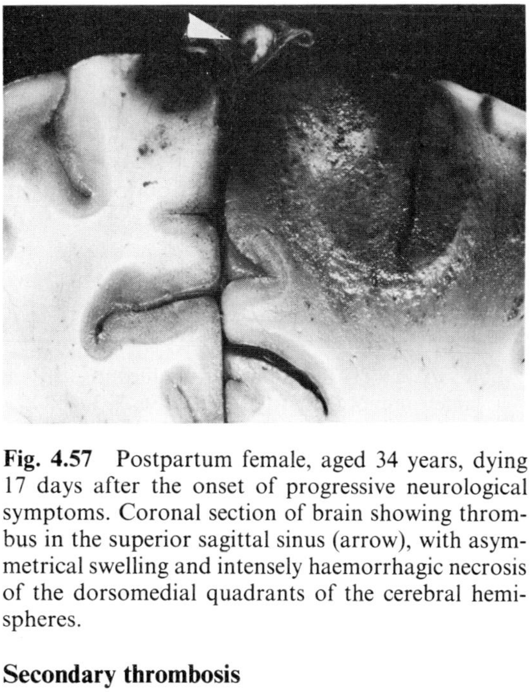

Fig. 4.57 Postpartum female, aged 34 years, dying 17 days after the onset of progressive neurological symptoms. Coronal section of brain showing thrombus in the superior sagittal sinus (arrow), with asymmetrical swelling and intensely haemorrhagic necrosis of the dorsomedial quadrants of the cerebral hemispheres.

Secondary thrombosis

This is most often found as a complication of pyogenic infection. Examples include spread of infection to the superior sagittal sinus from the frontal air sinuses and to the lateral sinuses from the mastoid air spaces or the middle ear. Secondary thrombosis may also follow subdural abscess, pyogenic infection of the face (especially the eyes, nose, cheeks and the upper jaw) and infection of the cavernous sinus. Thrombus may spread from the focus of infection into the sinus, or the sinus wall may itself become inflamed. The thrombus may not appear infected, but if it is, it may fragment to give rise to pyaemia and abscesses.

Lateral sinus thrombosis This commonly occurs secondary to otitis media and mastoiditis, and may or may not be septic. If there is no communication between the right and left lateral sinuses and the torcular, thrombosis of the left lateral sinus may obstruct the venous return from the basal ganglia via the great vein of Galen and straight sinus, resulting in infarction of the basal ganglia.

In the few cases that have been examined *post mortem*, the lateral sinus has always been thrombosed, sometimes with extension into the torcular (Foley, 1955). In a critical review Symonds (1956) concluded that the venous obstruction caused swelling of the brain and intracranial hypertension without ventricular dilatation. The sixth nerve palsies were attributed to their compression in the inferior petrosal sinuses. However, further detailed post-mortem studies are necessary in this condition (otitic hydrocephalus), with particular attention to the extent of the thrombus, the pattern of anastomosis at the torcular and the condition of the inferior petrosal sinus.

Cavernous sinus thrombosis This is usually secondary to pyogenic infection within the central part of the face, the nose and related soft tissues. The thrombus usually becomes infected, and in untreated cases purulent leptomeningitis is commonly present at the time of death. The facial and ophthalmic veins are often thrombosed and there is swelling of the soft tissues of the orbit with proptosis. Haemorrhages are found in the retina. It has been suggested that paralyses of the sixth and, less commonly, of the third and fourth cranial nerves are due to thrombosis of vasa nervorum.

Thrombosis of internal cerebral veins This, in children, may be primary in the veins or secondary to thrombosis of the dural sinuses. It may develop with or without pyogenic infection. The result is a haemorrhagic infarct in part or the whole of the field of venous drainage, including the septum pellucidum, the corpus striatum, the thalamus, the ventral portion of the corpus callosum, the medial aspects of the occipital lobe and the superomedial surface of the cerebellum on each side (Ehlers and Courville, 1936). Kalbag and Woolf (1972) and Norman (1958) considered that occlusion of cerebral veins at birth or in the first year of life could be an important factor in the pathogenesis of cerebral palsy (see Chapter 11).

References

Abbie, A. A. (1933) Clinical significance of the anterior choroidal artery. *Brain* **56,** 233–46.

Abbie, A. A. (1934) The morphology of the forebrain arteries, with special reference to the evolution of the basal ganglia. *Journal of Anatomy* **68,** 433–70.

Aberg, T. (1974) Effect of open heart surgery on intellectual function. *Scandinavian Journal of Thoracic and Cardiovascular Surgery*, Suppl. 15, 1–63.

Abramsky, O. (1980) Neurologic manifestations of macroglobulinemia. In *Handbook of Clinical Neurology. Neurological manifestations of systemic diseases*, vol. 39, part II (Eds. Vinken, P. J. and Bruyn, E. W.), pp. 181–99, North-Holland, Amsterdam.

Acheson, J. and Hutchinson, E. C. (1964) Observations on the natural history of transient cerebral ischaemia. *Lancet* **2,** 871–4.

Adams, J. H. and Graham, D. I. (1967) Twelve cases of fatal cerebral infarction due to arterial occlusion in the absence of atheromatous stenosis or embolism. *Journal of Neurology, Neurosurgery and Psychiatry* **30,** 479–88.

Adams, J. H., Brierley, J. B., Connor, R. C. R. and Treip, C. S. (1966) The effects of systemic hypotension upon the human brain. Clinical and neuropathological observations in 11 cases. *Brain* **89,** 235–68.

Adams, J. H., Graham, D. I., Mills, E. and Sprunt, T. G. (1972) Fat embolism and cerebral infarction after use of methylmethacrylic cement. *British Medical Journal* **3,** 740–1.

Adams, R. D. (1943) Occlusion of anterior inferior cerebellar artery. *Archives of Neurology and Psychiatry* **49,** 765–70.

Adams, R. D. (1957) Pathology of cerebral vascular disease. B. Cranial cerebral lesions. In *Princeton Conferences on Cerebrovascular Disease*, 2nd edn, (Ed. Millikan, C. H.), p. 23. Grune and Stratton, New York.

Adams, R. D., Cammermeyer, J. and Fitzgerald, P. J. (1948) Neuropathological aspects of thrombocytic acro-angiotherombosis; clinico-anatomical study of generalized platelet thrombosis. *Journal of Neurology, Neurosurgery and Psychiatry* **11,** 27–43.

Adams, R. D. and Fisher, C. M. (1961) Pathology of cerebral arterial occlusion. In *Pathogenesis and Treatment of Cerebrovascular Disease* (Ed. Fields, W. S.), pp. 126–42. Thomas, Springfield, Ill.

Adams, R. D. and Vander Eecken, H. M. (1953) Vascular diseases of brain. *Annual Review of Medicine* **4,** 213–52.

Alpers, B. J. (1959) Compensatory mechanisms in occlusive vascular disease of the brain. *Archives of Neurology* **1,** 531–4.

Alpers, B. J. and Berry, R. G. (1963) Circle of Willis in cerebral vascular disorders. *Archives of Neurology* **8,** 398–402.

Alpers, B. J., Berry, R. G. and Paddison, R. M. (1959) Anatomical studies of the circle of Willis in normal brain. *Archives of Neurology and Psychiatry* **81,** 409–18.

Altmann, H. W. and Schubothe, H. (1942) Funktionelle und organische Schädigungen des Zentralnervensystems der Katze im unter Druck Experiment. *Beiträge zur pathologischen Anatomie und zur allgemeinen Pathologie* **107,** 3–116.

Ames, A. (1973) Discussion, in Symposium on the threshold and mechanism of anoxic-ischemic brain injury. *Archives of Neurology* **29,** 364–6.

Ameuille, P., L'Hermitte, J. and Krudelski, E. (1935) Embolie gazeuse consécutive à une insufflation pleurale. Ramollissement cérébral massif. *Revue Neurologique* **63,** 867–76.

Anderson, J. M., Jamieson, D. G. and Jefferson, J. M. (1975) Non-healing granuloma and the nervous system. *Quarterly Journal of Medicine* **44,** 309–23.

Arab, A. (1957) L'artériosclerose cérébrale scalariforme hypertensive. *Psychiatrie und Neurologie (Basel)* **134,** 175–93.

Armstrong, M. L. and Warner, E. D. (1971) Morphology and distribution of diet-induced atherosclerosis in Rhesus monkeys. *Archives of Pathology* **92,** 395–401.

Arthur, G. and Margolis, G. (1977) Mycoplasma-like structures in granulomatous angiitis of the cerebral nervous system. *Archives of Pathology and Laboratory Medicine* **101,** 382–7.

Astrup, J. (1982) Energy-requiring cell functions in the ischemic brain. Their critical supply and possible inhibition in protective therapy. *Journal of Neurosurgery* **56,** 482–97.

Astrup, J., Siesjö, B. K. and Symon, L. (1981) Thresholds in cerebral ischemia—the ischemic penumbra. *Stroke* **12,** 723–5.

Astrup, J., Symon, L., Branston, N. M. and Lassen, N. A. (1977) Cortical evoked potential and extracellular K^+ and H^+ at critical levels of brain ischemia. *Stroke* **8,** 51–7.

Atkinson, W. J. (1949) Anterior inferior cerebellar artery, its variations, pontine distribution and significance in surgery of cerebello-pontine angle tumours. *Journal of Neurology, Neurosurgery and Psychiatry* **12,** 137–51.

Auer, L. M. (1978) The pathogenesis of hypertensive encephalopathy. *Acta Neurochirurgica* Suppl. 27.

Baker, A. B., Dahl, E. and Sandler, B. (1963) Cerebrovascular disease: etiologic factors in cerebral infarction. *Neurology* **13,** 445–54.

Baker, A. B. and Iannone, A. (1959) Cerebrovascular disease. 1. The large arteries of the circle of Willis. *Neurology* **9,** 321–32.

Baker, A. B., Resch, J. A. and Loewenson, R. B. (1969) Hypertension and cerebral atherosclerosis. *Circulation* **39,** 701–10.

Baker, A. B., Flora, G. C., Resch, J. A. and Loewenson, R. (1967) The geographic pathology of atherosclerosis: a review of the literature with some personal observations on cerebral atherosclerosis. *Journal of Chronic Diseases* **20,** 685–706.

Balò, J. (1928) Encephalitis periaxialis concentrica. *Archives of Neurology and Psychiatry* **19,** 242–64.

Barcroft, J. (1925) *The Respiratory Functions of the Blood.* Part 1. *Lessons from High Altitudes.* Cambridge University Press, London.

Barmada, M. A., Moossy, J. and Shuman, R. M. (1979) Cerebral infarcts with arterial occlusion in neonates. *Annals of Neurology* **6,** 495–502.

Barnett, H. J. M., Jones, M. W., Boughner, D. R. and Kostuk, W. J. (1976) Cerebral ischemic events associated with prolapsing mitral valve. *Archives of Neurology* **33,** 777–82.

Barry, D. I., Strandgaard, S., Graham, D. I., Braendstrup, O., Svendsen, U. G., Vorstrup, S. et al. (1982) Cerebral blood flow in rats with renal and spontaneous hypertension: resetting of lower limit of autoregulation. *Journal of Cerebral Blood Flow and Metabolism* **2,** 347–53.

Batson, O. V. (1940) Function of vertebral veins and their role in spread of metastases. *Annals of Surgery* **112,** 138–49.

Battacharji, S. K., Hutchinson, E. C. and McCall, A. J. (1967) Stenosis and occlusion of vessels in cerebral infarction. *British Medical Journal* **2,** 270–4.

Becker, N. H. (1963) Cytochemical studies in cerebral hypoxia. In *Selective Vulnerability of the Brain in Hypoxaemia* (Eds Schadé, J. P. and McMenemey, W. H.), pp. 317–25. Blackwell Scientific, Oxford.

Beecher, H. K. and Todd, D. P. (1954) A study of the deaths associated with anesthesia and surgery. *American Lecture Series*, no. 254. Thomas, Springfield Illinois.

Beevor, C. E. (1908) On the distribution of the different arteries supplying the human brain. *Philosophical Transactions of the Royal Society of London* Series B, **200,** 1–55.

Ben-Ari, Y., Tremblay, E. and Ottersen, O. P. (1980) Injections of kainic acid into the amygdaloid complex of the rat: an electrographic, clinical and histological study in relation to the pathology of epilepsy. *Neuroscience* **5,** 515–28.

Bernsmeier, A. and Held, K. (1972) The aortic arch syndrome. In *Handbook of Clinical Neurology. Vascular Diseases of the Nervous System*, part II, vol. 12 (Eds Vinken, P. J. and Bruyn, G. W.), pp. 398–421. North-Holland, Amsterdam.

Berry, R. G. (1971) Lupus erythematosus. In *Pathology of the Nervous System* (Ed. Minckler, J.), pp. 1482–8. McGraw-Hill, New York.

Berry, R. G. and Hodges, J. H. (1965) Nervous system involvement in systemic lupus erythematosus. *Transactions of the American Neurological Association* **90,** 231–3.

Bickerstaff, E. R. and Holmes, J. M. (1967) Cerebral arterial insufficiency and oral contraceptives. *British Medical Journal* **1,** 726–9.

Biemond, A. (1951) Thrombosis of the basilar artery and the vascularization of the brain stem. *Brain* **74,** 300–17.

Binswanger, O. (1894) Die Abgrenzung der allgemeinen progressiven Paralyse. *Klinische Wochenschrift* **31,** 1180–6.

Bjork, V. O. and Hultquist, G. (1960) Brain damage in children after deep hypothermia for open-heart surgery. *Thorax* **15,** 284–91.

Blackwood, W. (1958) Vascular disease of the central nervous system. In *Neuropathology* (Eds Greenfield, J. G., Blackwood, W. and McMenemey, W. H., Meyer, A. and Norman, R. M.), pp. 67–131. Edward Arnold, London.

Blackwood, W., Hallpike, J. F., Kocen, R. S. and Mair, W. G. P. (1969) Atheromatous disease of the carotid arterial system and embolism from the heart in cerebral infarction: a morbid anatomical study. *Brain* **92,** 897–910.

Blagbrough, A. E., Brierley, J. B. and Nicholson, A. N. (1973) Behavioural and neurological disturbances associated with hypoxic brain damage. *Journal of the Neurological Sciences* **18,** 475–88.

Blatt, I. M., Seltzer, H. S., Rubin, P., Furstenberg, A. C., Maxwell, J. H. and Schull, W. J. (1959) Fatal granulomatosis of the respiratory tract (lethal midline granuloma—Wegener's granulomatosis). *Archives of Otolaryngology* **70,** 707–57.

Blennow, G., Brierley, J. B., Meldrum, B. S. and Siesjö, B. K. (1978) Epileptic brain damage. The role of systemic factors that modify cerebral energy metabolism. *Brain* **101,** 687–700.

van Bogaert, L., Dallemagne, M. J. and Wegria, R. (1938) Recherche sur le besoin d'oxgène chronique et aigu chez *Macacus rhesus*. Absence de lésions expérimentales des centres nerveux après intoxication par l'oxyde carbone, le nitrite de soude et l'appauvrissement de l'air en oxygène. *Archives Internationales de Médecine Expérimentale* **13,** 335–78.

Boros, L. and Weiner, W. J. (1979) Sickle cell anemia and other hemoglobinopathies. In *Handbook of Clinical Neurology. Manifestations of Systemic Diseases*, part I, vol. 38 (Eds Vinken, P. J. and Bruyn, G. W.), pp. 35–51. North-Holland, Amsterdam.

Bounds, J. V., Wiebers, D. O., Whisnant, J. P. and Okazaki, H. (1981) Mechanisms and timing of deaths from cerebral infarction. *Stroke* **12,** 474–77.

Brain, W. R. and Russell, D. S. (1937) Myelomalacia following spinal anaesthesia. *Proceedings of the Royal Society of Medicine* **30,** 1024–30.

Branston, N. M., Symon, L., Crockard, H. A. and Pasztor, E. (1974) Relationship between the cortical evoked potential and local cortical blood flow following acute middle cerebral artery occlusion in the baboon. *Experimental Neurology* **45,** 195–208.

Branthwaite, M. A. (1972) Neurological damage related to open-heart surgery. *Thorax* **27,** 748–53.

Brice, T. G., Dowsett, D. J. and Lowe, R. D. (1964) The effect of constriction on carotid blood flow and pressure gradient. *Lancet* **1,** 84–5.

Brierley, J. B. (1961) Some neuropathological contributions to problems of hypoxia. In *Cerebral Anoxia and the Electroencephalogram* (Eds Gastaut, H. and Meyer, J. S.), pp. 164–71. Thomas, Springfield, Illinois.

Brierley, J. B. (1963) Neuropathological findings in patients dying after open-heart surgery. *Thorax* **18,** 291–304.

Brierley, J. B. (1965) The influence of brain swelling, age and hypotension upon the pattern of cerebral damage in hypoxia. In *Proceedings of the 5th International Congress of Neuropathology*, Zurich. Excerpta Medica International Congress Series, no. 100, pp. 21–8.

Brierley, J. B. (1967) Brain damage complicating open-heart surgery: a neuropathological study of 46 patients. *Proceedings of the Royal Society of Medicine* **60,** 858–9.

Brierley, J. B. (1976) Cerebral hypoxia. In *Greenfield's Neuropathology* 3rd edn. (Eds Blackwood, W. and Corsellis, J. A. N.), pp. 43–85. Edward Arnold, London.

Brierley, J. B. (1980) Hypoxic brain damage. In *Animal Models of Neurological Disease* (Eds Rose, F. C. and Behan, P. O.), pp. 338–46. Pitman Medical, Tunbridge Wells.

Brierley, J. B. and Brown, A. W. (1982a) The origin of lipid phagocytes in the central nervous system. I. The intrinsic microglia. *Journal of Comparative Neurology* **211,** 397–406: (1982b) The origin of lipid phagocytes in the central nervous system. II. The adventitia of blood vessels. *Journal of Comparative Neurology* **211,** 407–17.

Brierley, J. B., Brown, A. W. and Calverley, J. (1976) Cyanide intoxication in the rat: physiological and neuropathological aspects. *Journal of Neurology, Neurosurgery and Psychiatry* **39,** 129–40.

Brierley, J. B., Brown, A. W. and Meldrum, B. S. (1971a) The nature and time course of the neuronal alterations resulting from oligaemia and hypoglycaemia in the brain of *Macaca mulatta*. *Brain Research* **25,** 483–99.

Brierley, J. B., Brown, A. W. and Meldrum, B. S. (1971b) The neuropathology of insulin-induced hypoglycaemia in a primate (*M. mulatta*); topography and cellular nature. In *Brain Hypoxia* (Eds Brierley, J. B. and Meldrum, B. S.), Clinics in Developmental Medicine 39/40, pp. 225–9. Spastics International Medical Publications/Heinemann Medical, London.

Brierley, J. B. and Cooper, J. E. (1962) Cerebral complications of hypotensive anaesthesia in a healthy adult. *Journal of Neurology, Neurosurgery and Psychiatry* **25,** 24–30.

Brierley, J. B. and Excell, B. J. (1966) The effects of profound systemic hypotension upon the brain of *M. rhesus*. Physiological and pathological observations. *Brain* **89,** 269–98.

Brierley, J. B., Ljunggren, B. and Siesjö, B. K. (1975) Neuropathological alterations in rat brain after complete ischaemia due to raised intracranial pressure. In *Intracranial Pressure II* (Eds Lundberg, N., Ponten, U. and Brock, M.), pp. 166–71. Springer, Berlin.

Brierley, J. B. and Meldrum, B. S. (1974) The nature and distribution of brain damage due to air embolism. In *L'Embolie Gazeuse du Systèmie Carotidien* (Eds Arfel, G. and Naquet, R.), pp. 180–3. Doin, Editeurs, Paris.

Brierley, J. B., Meldrum, B. S. and Brown, A. W. (1971) Post-hypoxic brain swelling: physiological and anatomical aspects. In *Brain Hypoxia*, Clinics in Developmental Medicine 39/40 (Eds Brierley, J. B. and Meldrum, B. S.), pp. 136–43. Spastics International Medical Publications/ Heinemann Medical, London.

Brierley, J. B. and Miller, A. A. (1966) Fatal brain damage after dental anaesthesia. Its nature, aetiology and prevention. *Lancet* **2,** 869–73.

Brierley, J. B. and Nicholson, A. N. (1969) Neuropathological correlates of neurological impairment following prolonged decompression. *Aerospace Medicine* **40,** 148–52.

Brierley, J. B., Brown, A. W., Excell, B. J. and Meldrum, B. S. (1969) Brain damage in the Rhesus monkey resulting from profound arterial hypotension. I. Its nature, distribution and general physiological correlates. *Brain Research* **13,** 68–100.

Brierley, J. B., Adams, J. H., Graham, D. I. and Simpson, J. A. (1971) Neocortical death after cardiac arrest. *Lancet* **2,** 560–5.

Brierley, J. B., Prior, P. F., Calverley, J. and Brown, A. W. (1977) Cyanide intoxication in *Macaca mulatta*. Physiological and neuropathological aspects. *Journal of the Neurological Sciences* **31,** 133–7.

Brierley, J. B., Prior, P. F., Calverley, J. and Brown, A. W. (1978) Profound hypoxia in *Papio anubis* and *Macaca mulatta*—physiological and neuropathological effects. I. Abrupt exposure following normoxia. II. Abrupt exposure following moderate hyoxia. *Journal of the Neurological Sciences* **37,** 1–29.

Brierley, J. B., Prior, P. F., Calverley, J., Jackson, S. J. and Brown, A. W. (1980) The pathogenesis of ischaemic neuronal damage along the cerebral arterial boundary zones in *Papio anubis*. *Brain* **103,** 929–65.

Brion, S., Psimaras, A. and Gallissot, M. C. (1974) Neuropathologie de l'embolie gazeuse humaine au cours de la chirurgie cardiaque. In *L'Embolie Gazeuse du Systèmie Carotidien* (Eds Arfel, G. and Naquet, R.), pp. 194–8. Doin, Paris.

Brion, S., Psimaras, A., Mikol, J. and Gallissot, M. C. (1974) Étude neuropathologique de l'embolie gazeuse experimentale. In *L'Embolie Gazeuse du Systèmie Carotidien* (Eds Arfel, G. and Naquet, R.), pp. 175–9. Doin, Paris.

Brown, A. W. (1977) Structural abnormalities in neurones. *Journal of Clinical Pathology* **30,** Supplement (Royal College of Pathologists) **11,** 155–69.

Brown, A. W. and Brierley, J. B. (1966) Evidence for early anoxic-ischaemic cell damage in the rat brain. *Experientia* **22,** 546–7.

Brown, A. W. and Brierley, J. B. (1968) The nature, distribution and earliest stages of anoxic-ischaemic nerve cell damage in the rat brain as defined by the optical microscope. *British Journal of Experimental Pathology* **49,** 87–106.

Brown, A. W. and Brierley, J. B. (1973) The earliest alterations in rat neurones after anoxia-ischaemia. *Acta Neuropathologica* **23,** 9–22.

Brucher, J. M. (1967) Neuropathological problems posed by carbon monoxide poisoning and anoxia. In *Carbon Monoxide Poisoning* (Eds Bour, H. and Ledingham, I. McA.), *Progress in Brain Research*, vol. 24, pp. 75–100. Elsevier, Amsterdam.

Brust, J. C. M. and Richter, R. W. (1976) Stroke associated with addiction to heroin. *Journal of Neurology, Neurosurgery and Psychiatry* **39,** 194–9.

Buchner, F. (1957) Die pathologie der cellulären und geweblichen Oxydationen. In *Handbuch der allgemeinen Pathologie*, Band 4/2, pp. 569–668. Springer, Berlin.

Burger, P. C., Burch, J. G. and Kunze, U. (1976) Subcortical arteriosclerotic encephalopathy (Binswanger's disease). *Stroke* **7,** 626–31.

Burger, P. C., Burch, J. G. and Vogel, F. S. (1976) Granulomatous angiitis. An unusual etiology of stroke. *Stroke* **8,** 29–35.

Byrom, F. B. (1954) Pathogenesis of hypertensive encephalopathy and its relation to the malignant phase of hypertension. Experimental evidence from the hypertensive rat. *Lancet* **2,** 201–11.

Byrom, F. B. (1974) The evolution of acute hypertensive arterial disease. *Progress in Cardiovascular Diseases* **17,** 31–7.

Byrom, F. B. (1976) Tension and the artery. The experimental elimination of pseudo-uraemia and malignant nephrosclerosis. *Clinical Science* **51,** Suppl. 3, 3S–11S.

Callow, A. D., Moran, J. M., Kahn, P. C. and Deterling, R. A. (1968) Patterns of atherosclerosis of extracranial cerebral arteries. *Annals of the New York Academy of Sciences* **149,** 974–88.

Campbell, E. J. M. (1965) Respiratory failure. *British Medical Journal* **1,** 1451–60.

Caplan, L. R. and Schoene, W. C. (1978) Clinical features of subcortical arteriosclerotic encephalopathy (Binswanger disease). *Neurology* **28,** 1206–15.

Carlson, C. B., Harvey, F. H. and Loop, J. (1973) Progressive alternating hemiplegia in early childhood with basal arterial stenosis and telangiectasia (moya moya syndrome). *Neurology* **23,** 734–44.

Carroll, J. D., Leak, D. and Lee, H. A. (1966) Cerebral thrombophlebitis in pregnancy and in the puerperium. *Quarterly Journal of Medicine* **35,** 347–68.

Castaigne, P., Lhermitte, F., Gautier, J.-C., Escourolle, R. and Derouesné, C. (1970) Internal carotid artery occlusion. A study of 61 instances in fifty patients with post mortem data. *Brain* **93,** 231–58.

Castaigne, P., Lhermitte, F., Gautier, J. C., Escourolle, R., Desrouesné, C., der Agopian, P. and Popa, C. (1973) Arterial occlusions in the vertebrobasilar system. A study of 44 patients with post mortem data. *Brain* **96,** 133–54.

Castaldo, J. E., Anderson, M. and Reeves, A. G. (1982) Middle cerebral artery occlusion with migraine. *Stroke* **13,** 308–11.

Celik, G., Graham, D. I., Kelly, P. A. T. and McCulloch, J. (1982) Kainic acid administration and the relationship between local cerebral glucose utilization and local blood flow. In *Cerebral Blood Flow: Effects of Nerves and Neurotransmitters* (Eds Heistad, D. D. and Marcus, L.), pp. 249–55. Elsevier/North-Holland, Amsterdam.

Chester, E. M., Agamanolis, D. P., Banker, B. Q. and Victor, M. (1978) Hypertensive encephalopathy: a clincopathologic study of 20 cases. *Neurology* **28,** 928–39.

Chievitz, E. and Thiede, T. (1962) Complications and causes of death in polycythemia vera. *Acta Medica Scandinavica* **172,** 513–23.

Choi, S. S. and Crampton, A. (1961) Atherosclerosis of arteries of neck. Post mortem angiographic and pathologic study. *Archives of Pathology* **72,** 379–85.

Coceani, F. and Gloor, P. (1966) The distribution of the internal carotid circulation in the brain of the Macaque monkey (*Macaca mulatta*). *Journal of Comparative Neurology* **128,** 419–28.

Cochrane, C. G. and Koffler, D. (1973) Immune complex disease in experimental animals and man. *Advances in Immunology* **16,** 185–264.

Cocito, L., Favale, E. and Reni, L. (1982) Epileptic seizures in cerebral arterial occlusive disease. *Stroke* **13,** 189–95.

Coggeshall, R. E. and MacLean, P. D. (1958) Hippocampal lesions following administration of 3-acetylpyridine. *Proceedings of the Society for Experimental Biology and Medicine* **98,** 687–9.

Cole, F. M. (1967) A variation in the course and distribution of the 'lateral striate artery'. *Journal of Anatomy* **102,** 125–8.

Cole, F. M. and Yates, P. O. (1968) Comparative incidence of cerebrovascular lesions in normotensive and hypertensive patients. *Neurology* **18,** 255–9.

Collaborative Group for the Study of Stroke in Young Women (1973) Oral contraception and increased risk of cerebral ischaemia or thrombosis. *New England Journal of Medicine* **288,** 871–8.

Connett, M. C. and Lausche, J. M. (1965) Fibromuscular hyperplasia of the internal carotid artery. Report of a case. *Annals of Surgery* **162,** 59–62.

Cook, T. A. and Yates, P. O. (1972) A histometric study of cerebral and renal arteries in normotensives and chronic hypertensives. *Journal of Pathology* **108,** 129–35.

Corsellis, J. A. N. (1962) *Mental Illness and the Ageing Brain*. Oxford University Press, London.

Cravioto, H. and Feigin, I. (1959) Non-infectious granulomatous angiitis with a predilection for the nervous system. *Neurology* **9**, 599–609.

Critchley, M. and Schuster, P. (1933) Beiträge zur Anatomie und Pathologie der Arteria cerebelli superior. *Zeitschrift für die gesamte Neurologie und Psychiatrie* **144**, 681–741.

Cross, J. N., Castro, P. O. and Jennett, W. B. (1968) Cerebral strokes associated with pregnancy and the puerperium. *British Medical Journal* **2**, 214–18.

Cullity, G. J. and Kakulas, B. A. (1970) Encephalopathy and fatty degeneration of the viscera: an evaluation. *Brain* **93**, 77–88.

Dalal, P. M., Shah, P. M., Sheth, S. C. and Deshpande, C. K. (1965) Cerebral embolism. Angiographic observations on spontaneous clot lysis. *Lancet* **1**, 61–4.

Darmody, W. R., Thomas, L. M. and Gurdjian, E. S. (1967) Post irradiation vascular insufficiency syndrome. *Neurology* **17**, 1190–2.

Davison, C., Goodhart, S. P. and Savitsky, N. (1935) Syndrome of superior cerebellar artery and its branches. *Archives of Neurology and Psychiatry* **33**, 1143–74.

Dinsdale, H. B., Robertson, D. M. and Chiang, T. Y. (1974) Cerebral blood flow in acute hypertension. *Archives of Neurology* **31**, 80–7.

Doniger, D. E. (1963) Bilateral complete carotid and basilar artery occlusion in a patient with minimal deficit. *Neurology* **13**, 673–8.

Drachman, D. A. (1963) Neurological complications of Wegener's granulomatosis. *Neurology* **8**, 145–55.

Easton, J. D. and Sherman, D. G. (1977) Cervical manipulation and stroke. *Stroke* **8**, 594–7.

Easton, J. D. and Sherman, D. G. (1980) Management of cerebral embolism of cardiac origin. *Stroke* **11**, 433–42.

Edelmann, F. (1921) Ein Beitrag zur Vergiftung mit gasformiger Blausäure insbesondere zu den dabei auftretenden Gehirnveränderungen. *Deutsche Zeitschrift für Nervenheilkunde* **72**, 259–87.

Ehlers, H. and Courville, C. B. (1936) Thrombosis of internal cerebral veins in infancy and childhood: review of literature and report of 5 cases. *Journal of Pediatrics* **8**, 600–23.

Ehrich, W. E., Bellet, S. and Lewey, F. H. (1944) Cardiac changes from CO poisoning. *American Journal of the Medical Sciences* **208**, 511–23.

Elliott, D. H., Hallenbeck, J. M. and Bove, A. A. (1974) Acute decompression sickness. *Lancet* **2**, 1193–9.

Ernsting, J. (1963) Some effects of brief profound anoxia upon the cerebral nervous system. In *Selective Vulnerability of the Brain in Hypoxaemia* (Eds Schadé, J. P. and McMenemey, W. M.), pp. 41–5. Blackwell Scientific, Oxford.

Ernsting, J. (1966) The effects of hypoxia upon human performance and the electroencephalogram. In *Oxygen Measurements in Blood and Tissues* (Eds Payne, J. P. and Hill, D. W.), pp. 245–59. Churchill, London.

Family Planning Association (1962) Contraindications to oral contraception. *British Medical Journal* **2**, 315–16.

Feigin, I. and Prose, P. (1959) Hypertensive fibrinoid arteries of the brain and gross cerebral hemorrhage. A form of 'hyalinosis'. *Archives of Neurology* **1**, 98–110.

Ferraro, A. (1933) Experimental toxic encephalomyelopathy. (Diffuse sclerosis following subcutaneous injections of potassium cyanide.) *Psychiatric Quarterly* **7**, 267–83.

Ferraro, A. and Morrison, R. (1928) Illuminating gas poisoning. An experimental study of the lesions of the nervous system in acute and chronic stages. *Psychiatric Quarterly* **2**, 506–41.

Fields, W. S., Maslenikov, V., Meyer, J. S., Hass, W. K., Remington, R. D. and MacDonald, M. (1970) Joint study of extracranial arterial occlusion. Progress report of prognosis following surgery or non-surgical treatment for transient cerebral ischaemic attacks and cerebral carotid artery lesions. *Journal of the American Medical Association* **211**, 1993–2003.

Finnerty, F. H., Witkin, L. and Fazekas, J. F. (1954) Cerebral hemodynamics during cerebral ischemia induced by hypotension. *Journal of Clinical Investigation* **33**, 1227–32.

Fisher, C. M. (1951) Occlusion of internal carotid artery. *Archives of Neurology and Psychiatry* **65**, 346–77.

Fisher, C. M. (1959) Observations of the fundus oculi in transient monocular blindness. *Neurology* **9**, 333–47.

Fisher, C. M. (1965) Lacunes: small, deep cerebral infarcts. *Neurology* **15**, 774–84.

Fisher, C. M. (1969) The arterial lesions underlying lacunes. *Acta Neuropathologica* **12**, 1–15.

Fisher, C. M. (1972) Cerebral miliary aneurysms in hypertension. *American Journal of Pathology* **66**, 313–30.

Fisher, C. M. (1979) Capsular infarcts: the underlying vascular lesions. *Archives of Neurology* **36**, 65–73.

Fisher, C. M. (1982) Lacunar strokes and infarcts: a review. *Neurology* **32**, 871–6.

Fisher, C. M., Karnes, W. E. and Kubik, C. S. (1961) Lateral medullary infarction—the pattern of vascular occlusion. *Journal of Neuropathology and Experimental Neurology* **20**, 323–79.

Fisher, C. M., Gore, I., Okabe, N. and White P. D. (1965) Atherosclerosis of the carotid and vertebral arteries—extracranial and intracranial. *Journal of Neuropathology and Experimental Neurology* **24**, 455–76.

Fitch, W., Jones, J. V., Graham, D. I., MacKenzie, E. T. and Harper, A. M. (1978) Effects of hypotension induced by halothane on the cerebral circulation in baboons with experimental renovascular hypertension. *British Journal of Anaesthesia* **50,** 119–25.

Flora, G. C., Baker, A. B., Loewenson, R. B. and Klassen, A. C. (1968) A comparative study of cerebral atherosclerosis in males and females. *Circulation* **38,** 859–69.

Foix, C. and Hillemand, P. (1926) Contribution à l'étude des ramolissments protrubérantiels. *Revue de médecine* **43,** 287–305.

Foix, C. and Masson, A. (1923) Le syndrome de l'artère cerebrale postérieure. *Presse médicale* **31,** 361–5.

Foley, J. (1955) Benign forms of intracranial hypertension—'tonic' and 'otitic' hydrocephalus. *Brain* **78,** 1–41.

Folkow, B. (1971) The haemodynamic consequences of adaptive structural changes of the resistance vessels in hypertension. *Clinical Science* **41,** 1–12.

Freeman, W. and Jaffe, D. (1941) Occlusion of superior cerebellar artery: report on case with necropsy. *Archives of Neurology and Psychiatry* **46,** 115–26.

Friede, R. L. (1966) The histochemical architecture of the Ammon horn as related to its selective vulnerability. *Acta Neuropathologica* **6,** 1–13.

Fryer, D. I. (1969) *Sub-atmospheric Decompression Sickness in Man*, pp. 1–343. Advisory Group for Aerospace Research and Development, NATO Publ. Technician Series, Slough.

Fujishima, M. and Omae, T. (1976) Lower limit of cerebral autoregulation in normotensive and spontaneously hypertensive rats. *Experientia* **32,** 1019–21.

Furlow, T. W. and Bass, N. H. (1976) Arachidonate-induced cerebrovascular occlusion in the rat. The role of platelets and aspirin in stroke. *Neurology* **26,** 297–304.

Garcia, J. H., Cox, J. V. and Hudgins, W. R. (1971) Ultrastructure of the microvasculature in experimental cerebral infarction. *Acta Neuropathologica* **18,** 273–85.

Garcia, J. H. and Kamijyo, Y. (1974) Cerebral infarction. Evaluation of histopathological changes after occlusion of a middle cerebral artery in primates. *Journal of Neuropathology and Experimental Neurology* **33,** 408–21.

Garland, H. and Pearce, J. (1967) Neurological complications of carbon monoxide poisoning. *Quarterly Journal of Medicine* **36,** 445–55.

Gastaut, H., Fischgold, H. and Meyer, J. S. (1961) Conclusions of the International Colloquium on Anoxia and the EEG. In *Cerebral Anoxia and the Encephalogram* (Eds Gastaut, H. and Meyer, J. S.), pp. 599–617. Thomas, Springfield, Illinois.

Gastaut, H., Bostem, F., Fernandez-Guardiola, A., Naquet, R. and Gibson, W. (1961) Hypoxic activation of the EEG by nitrogen inhalation. I. Preliminary observations in generalized epilepsy. In *Cerebral Anoxia and the Encephalogram* (Eds Gastaut, H. and Meyer, J. S.), pp. 343–54. Thomas, Springfield, Illinois.

Gautier, J. C. (1976) Cerebral ischaemia in hypertension. In *Cerebral Arterial Disease* (Ed. Russell, R. W. R.), pp. 181–209. Churchill Livingstone, Edinburgh.

Gilles, F. H. (1963) Selective symmetrical neuronal necrosis of certain brain stem tegmental nuclei in temporary cardiac standstill. *Journal of Neuropathology and Experimental Neurology* **22,** 319.

Ginsberg, M. D. (1979) Delayed neurological deterioration following hypoxia. In *Cerebral Hypoxia and its Consequences. Advances in Neurology*, vol. 26, (Eds Fahn, S., Davis, J. N. and Rowland, L. P.), pp. 21–44. Raven Press, New York.

Ginsberg, M. D., Myers, R. E. and McDonagh, B. F. (1974) Experimental carbon monoxide encephalopathy in the primate. II. Clinical aspects. Neuropathology and physiologic correlation. *Archives of Neurology* **30,** 209–16.

Goetz, C. G. (1980) Polyarteritis nodosa. In *Handbook of Clinical Neurology. Neurological Manifestations of Systemic Diseases*, part II, vol. 39 (Eds Vinken, P. J. and Bruyn, G. W.), pp. 295–311. North-Holland, Amsterdam.

Goodhart, S. P. and Davison, C. (1936) Syndrome of posterior inferior and anterior inferior cerebellar arteries and their branches. *Archives of Neurology and Psychiatry* **35,** 501–24.

Goodwin, J. A. (1980) Temporal arteritis. In *Handbook of Clinical Neurology. Neurological Manifestations of Systemic Diseases*, part II, vol. 39 (Eds Vinken, P. J. and Bruyn, G. W.), pp. 313–42. North-Holland, Amsterdam.

Gordon, T., Sorlie, P. and Kannel, W. B. (1971) An epidemiological investigation of cardiovascular disease, coronary heart disease, atherothrombotic brain infarction, intermittent claudication. A multivariate analysis of some factors related to their incidence. *The Framingham Study—16 Year Follow-up*. US Government Printing Office, Washington DC.

Goren, H., Steinberg, M. C. and Farboody, G. H. (1980) Familial oculoleptomeningeal amyloidosis. *Brain* **103,** 473–95.

Graham, D. I. (1975) Ischaemic brain damage of cerebral perfusion failure type after treatment of severe hypertension. *British Medical Journal* **4,** 739.

Graham, D. I. and Adams, H. (1972) 'Idiopathic' thrombosis in the vertebrobasilar arterial system in young men. *British Medical Journal* **1,** 20–8.

Graham, D. I., Adams, J. H. and Doyle, D. (1978) Ischaemic brain damage in fatal non-missile head injuries. *Journal of the Neurological Sciences* **39,** 213–34.

Gray, F. D. and Horner, G. H. (1970) Survival following extreme hypoxemia. *Journal of the American Medical Association* **211,** 1815–17.

Greenfield, J. G., Rickards, A. G. and Manning, G. B. (1955) Pathology of paraplegia occurring as delayed sequela of spinal anaesthesia, with special reference to vascular changes. *Journal of Pathology and Bacteriology* **69,** 97–107.

Gresham, G. E., Phillips, T. F., Wolf, P. A. McNamara, P. M., Kannel, W. B. and Dawber, T. R. (1979) Epidemiologic profile of long-term stroke disability: the Framingham study. *Archives of Physical Medicine and Rehabilitation* **60,** 487–91.

Grinkler, R. R. (1925) Über einen Fall von Leuchtgasvergiftung mit doppelseitiger Pallidumerweichung und schwerer Degeneration des tieferen Grosshirn Marklagers. *Zeitschrift für die gesamte Neurologie und Psychiatrie* **98,** 433–56.

Grunnet, M. L. (1963) Cerebrovascular disease: diabetes and cerebral atherosclerosis. *Neurology* **13,** 486–91.

Guillain, G., Bertrand, I. and Peron, N. (1928) Le syndrome de l'artère cérébelleuse supérieure. *Revue Neurologique* **2,** 835–43.

Haggendal, E. and Johansson, B. (1972a) On the pathophysiology of the increased cerebrovascular permeability in acute arterial hypertension in cats. *Acta Neurologica Scandinavica* **48,** 265–70.

Haggendal, E. and Johansson, B. (1972b) Effects of increased intravascular pressure on the blood brain barrier to protein in dogs. *Acta Neurologica Scandinavica* **48,** 271–5.

Hallenbeck, J. M. (1976) Cinephotomicrography of dog spinal vessels during cord-damaging decompression sickness. *Neurology* **26,** 190–9.

Hallenbeck, J. M., Bove, A. A. and Elliott, D. H. (1975) Mechanisms underlying spinal cord damage in decompression sickness. *Neurology* **25,** 308–16.

Harrison, C. V. (1948) Giant-cell or temporal arteritis: a review. *Journal of Clinical Pathology* **1,** 197–211.

Hawkes, C. H. (1974) 'Locked-in' syndrome: report of seven cases. *British Medical Journal* **4,** 379–82.

Haymaker, W. (1957) Decompression sickness. In *Handbuch der speziellen pathologischen Anatomie und Histologie* (Eds Lubarsch, O., Henke, F. and Rössle, R.), pp. 1600–72. Springer, Berlin.

Haymaker, W. and Davison, C. (1950) Fatalities resulting from exposure to simulated high altitudes in decompression chambers. A clinico-pathological study of five cases. *Journal of Neuropathology and Experimental Neurology* **9,** 29–59.

Haymaker, W., Ginzler, A. M. and Ferguson, R. L. (1952) Residual neuropathological effects of cyanide poisoning. A study of the central nervous system of 23 dogs exposed to cyanide compounds. *Military Surgeon* **111,** 231–46.

Haymaker, W. and Johnston, A. D. (1955) Pathology of decompression sickness. A comparison of the lesions in airmen with those in caisson workers and divers. *Military Medicine* **117,** 285–306.

Haymaker, W., Johnston, A. D. and Downey, V. M. (1956) Fatal decompression sickness during jet aircraft flight. *Journal of Aviation Medicine* **27,** 2–17.

Hazama, F., Amano, S., Haebara, H., Yamori, Y. and Okamoto, K. (1976) Pathology and pathogenesis of cerebrovascular lesions in spontaneously hypertensive rats. In *The Cerebral Vessel Wall* (Eds Cervos-Navarro, J., Betz, E., Matakas, F. and Wullenweber, R.), pp. 245–52. Raven Press, New York.

Heiskanen, O. (1964) Cerebral circulatory arrest caused by acute increase of intracranial pressure. A clinical and roentgenological study of 25 cases. *Acta Neurologica Scandinavica* **40,** Suppl. 17, 1–57.

Heistad, D. D., Marcus, M. L., Piegors, D. J. and Armstrong, M. L. (1980) Regulation of cerebral blood flow in atherosclerotic monkeys. *American Journal of Physiology* **239** (Heart Circ. Physiol. 8), H539–H544.

Heptinstall, R. H., Porter, K. H. and Barkley, H. (1954) Giant-cell (temporal) arteritis. *Journal of Pathology and Bacteriology* **67,** 507–19.

Herrero, F. A. (1980) Neurological manifestations of heritable connective tissue disorders. In *Handbook of Clinical Neurology. Neurological Manifestations of Systemic Diseases*, part II, vol. 39 (Eds Vinken, P. J. and Bruyn, G. W.), pp. 379–418. North-Holland, Amsterdam.

Hicks, S. P. (1950a) Brain metabolism *in vivo*. I. The distribution of lesions caused by cyanide poisoning, insulin hypoglycemia, asphyxia in nitrogen and fluoroacetate poisoning in rats. *Archives of Pathology* **49,** 111–37.

Hicks, S. P. (1950b) Brain metabolism *in vivo*. II. The distribution of lesions caused by azide, malonitrile, plasmocid and dinitrophenol poisoning in rats. *Archives of Pathology* **50,** 545–61.

Hiller, F. (1924) Ueber die krankhaften Veränderungen in Zentralnervensystem nach Kohlenoxydvergiftung. *Zeitschrift für die gesamte Neurologie und Psychiatrie* **93,** 594–646.

Hills, B. A. and James, P. B. (1982) Spinal decompression sickness: mechanical studies and a model. *Undersea Biomedical Research* **9,** 185–201.

Hirano, A., Levine, S. and Zimmermann, H. M. (1967) Experimental cyanide encephalopathy. Electron microscopic observations of early lesions in white matter. *Journal of Neuropathology and Experimental Neurology* **26,** 200–13.

Hirsch, H., Oberdorster, G., Zimmer, R., Benner, K. V. and Lang, R. (1975) The recovery of the electrocorticogram of normotensive canine brains after complete ischemia. *Archiv für Psychiatrie und Nervenkrankheiten* **221,** 171-9.

von Hochstetter, A. R. and Friede, R. L. (1977) Residual lesions of cerebral fat embolism. *Journal of Neurology* **216,** 227-33.

Hoff, E. C., Grenell, R. G. and Fulton, J. F. (1945) Histopathology of the central nervous system after exposure to high altitudes, hypoglycemia and other conditions associated with central anoxia. *Medicine* **24,** 161-217.

Hollander, W., Madoff, I., Paddock, J. and Kirkpatrick, B. (1976) Aggravation of atherosclerosis by hypertension in a subhuman primate model with coarctation of the aorta. *Circulation Research* **38,** Suppl. 11, 63-72.

Hollander, W., Prusty, S., Kirkpatrick, B., Paddock, J. and Nagraj, S. (1977) Role of hypertension in ischemic heart disease and cerebral vascular disease in the Cynomolgus monkey with coarctation of the aorta. *Circulation Research* **40,** Suppl 1, 1-70-1-83.

Hossmann, K. A. and Kleihues, P. (1973) Reversibility of ischemic brain damage. *Archives of Neurology* **29,** 375-82.

Hossman, K. A. and Sato, K. (1970) Recovery of neuronal function after prolonged cerebral ischemia. *Science* **168,** 375-6.

Hossmann, K. A. and Zimmermann, V. (1974) Resuscitation of the monkey brain after 1 hour complete ischemia. I. Physiological and morphological observations. *Brain Research* **81,** 59-74.

Hovig, T. (1970) The role of platelets in thrombosis. *Thrombosis et Diathesis Haemorrhagica* **42,** Suppl., 137-53.

Hsü, Y. K. and Ch'eng, Y. L. (1938) Cerebral subcortical myelopathy in carbon monoxide poisoning. *Brain* **61,** 384-92.

Hughes, J. T. and Brownell, B. (1968) Traumatic thrombosis of the internal carotid artery in the neck. *Journal of Neurology, Neurosurgery and Psychiatry* **31,** 307-14.

Hulse, J. A., Taylor, D. S. I. and Dillon, M. J. (1979) Blindness and paraplegia in severe childhood hypertension. *Lancet* **2,** 553-6.

Hultquist, G. T. (1942) *Über Thrombose und Embolie der Arteria Carotidis und hierbei vorkommende Gehirnveränderungen.* Fisher, Jena, Stockholm.

Humphrey, J. G. and Newton, T. H. (1960) Internal carotid artery occlusion in young adults. *Brain* **83,** 565-78.

Hurst, E. W. (1940) Experimental demyelination of the central nervous system. I. The encephalopathy produced by potassium cyanide. *Australian Journal of Experimental Biology and Medical Science* **18,** 201-23.

Hurst, E. W. (1942) Experimental demyelination of the central nervous system. 3. Poisoning with potassium cyanide, sodium azide, hydroxylamine, narcotics, carbon monoxide, etc. *Australian Journal of Experimental Biology and Medical Science* **20,** 297-312.

Hurst, E. W. (1955) Adhesive arachnoiditis and vascular blockage caused by detergents and other chemical irritants: experimental study. *Journal of Pathology and Bacteriology* **70,** 167-78.

Hutchinson, E. C. and Yates, P. O. (1956) The cervical portion of the vertebral artery: a clinico-pathological study. *Brain* **79,** 319-31.

Hutchinson, E. C. and Yates, P. O. (1957) Carotico-vertebral stenosis. *Lancet* **1,** 2-8.

Hutchinson, E. C. and Yates, P. O. (1961) *Cerebral Infarction: the Role of Stenosis of the Extracranial Cerebral Arteries.* Special Report Series of the Medical Research Council, London, no. 300. HMSO, London.

Illis, L., Kocen, R. S., McDonald, W. I. and Mondkar, V. P. (1965) Oral contraceptives and carotid artery occlusion. *British Medical Journal* **2,** 1164-6.

Ingvar, M. and Siesjö, B. K. (1981) Cell damage in sustained seizures: role of local cerebral blood flow and local metabolic rate. *Journal of Cerebral Blood Flow and Metabolism* **1,** Suppl. 1, S98-S99.

Jackson, G., Mahon, W., Pierscianowski, T. A. and Condon, J. (1976) Inappropriate antihypertensive therapy in the elderly. *Lancet* **2,** 1317-18.

Jacob, H. (1939) Über die diffuse Hemisphärenmarkerkrankung nach Kohlenoxydvergiftung bei Fällen mit klinisch intervallärer Verlaufsform. *Zeitschrift für die gesamte Neurologie und Psychiatrie* **167,** 161-79.

Jacob, H. (1963) CNS tissue and cellular pathology in hypoxaemic states. In *Selective Vulnerability of the Brain in Hypoxaemia* (Eds Schadé, J. P. and McMenemey, W. H.), pp. 153-63. Blackwell Scientific, Oxford.

Janota, I. (1981) Dementia, deep white matter damage and hypertension: 'Binswanger's disease'. *Psychological Medicine* **11,** 39-48.

Jennett, B. and Plum, F. (1972) Persistent vegetative state after brain damage: a syndrome in search of a name. *Lancet* **1,** 734-7.

Jennett, W. B. and Cross, J. N. (1967) Influence of pregnancy and oral contraception on the incidence of strokes in women of childbearing age. *Lancet* **1,** 1019-23.

Jeynes, B. J. and Warren, B. A. (1982) Cerebral atheroembolism. An animal model. *Stroke* **13,** 312-18.

Johansson, B., Strandgaard, S. and Lassen, N. A. (1974) On the pathogenesis of hypertensive encephalopathy: the hypertensive 'breakthrough' of autoregulation of cerebral blood flow with forced vasodilation, flow increase and blood-brain-barrier damage. *Circulation Research* Suppl. 34/35, 1.167–1.171.

Johnson, R. T. and Richardson, E. P. (1968) The neurological manifestation of systemic lupus erythematosus: a clinical pathological study of 24 cases and review of the literature. *Medicine* **47,** 337–69.

Jones, J. V., Fitch, W., Mackenzie, E. T., Strandgaard, S. and Harper, A. M. (1976) Lower limit of cerebral blood flow autoregulation in experimental renovascular hypertension in the baboon. *Circulation Research* **39,** 555–7.

Jones, J. V. and Strandgaard, S. (1975) Cerebral autoregulation in chronically hypertensive baboons. *Journal of Physiology* **250,** 16P–17P.

Jones, M. W. and Kaufmann, J. C. E. (1976) Vertebrobasilar artery insufficiency in rheumatoid atlantoaxial subluxation. *Journal of Neurology, Neurosurgery and Psychiatry* **39,** 122–8.

Kahn, K. J. and Myers, R. E. (1971) Insulin-induced hypoglycaemia in the non-human primate. I. Clinical consequences. In *Brain Hypoxia* (Eds Brierley, J. B. and Meldrum, B. S.), Clinics in Developmental Medicine 39/40, pp. 185–94. Spastics International Medical Publications/Heinemann Medical, London.

Kalbag, R. M. and Woolf, A. L. (1972) Thrombosis and thrombophlebitis of cerebral veins and dural sinuses. In *Handbook of Clinical Neurology. Vascular Diseases of the Nervous System*, vol. 12 (Eds Vinken, P. J. and Bruyn, G. W.), pp. 422–46. North-Holland, Amsterdam.

Kalimo, H., Garcia, J. H., Kamijyo, Y., Tanaka, J. and Trump, B. F. (1977). The ultrastructure of 'brain death'. II. Electron microscopy of feline cortex after complete ischemia. *Virchows Archiv. B. Cell Pathology* **25,** 207–20.

Kamenar, E. and Burger, P. C. (1980) Cerebral fat embolism: a neuropathological study of a microembolic state. *Stroke* **11,** 477–84.

Kamijyo, Y., Garcia, J. H. and Cooper, J. (1977) Temporary regional cerebral ischemia in the cat. A model of hemorrhagic and subcortical infarction. *Journal of Neuropathology and Experimental Neurology* **36,** 338–50.

Kannel, W. B. (1976) Epidemiology of cerebrovascular disease. In *Cerebral Arterial Disease* (Ed. Russell, R. W. R.), pp. 1–23. Churchill Livingstone, Edinburgh.

Kannel, W. B., Dawber, T. R., Sorlie, P. and Wolf, P. A. (1976) Components of blood pressure and risk of atherothrombotic brain infarction: the Framingham study. *Stroke* **7,** 327–31.

Kannel, W. B., Gordon, T., Wolf, P. A. and McNamara, P. (1972) Hemoglobin and the risk of cerebral infarction: the Framingham study. *Stroke* **3,** 409–20.

Kato, T. and Lowry, O. H. (1973) Enzymes of energy-containing systems in individual mammalian nerve cell bodies. *Journal of Neurochemistry* **20,** 151–63.

Kety, S. S., Hafkenschiel, J. H., Jeffers, W. A., Leopold, I. H. and Shenkin, H. A. (1948) The blood flow, vascular resistance and oxygen consumption of the brain in essential hypertension. *Journal of Clinical Investigation* **57,** 511–14.

Kiloh, L. G. (1953) Syndromes of arteries of brain and spinal cord. *Postgraduate Medical Journal* **29,** 65–74, 119–28.

Klug, P. P., Lessin, L. S. and Radice, P. (1974) Rheologic aspects of sickle cell disease. *Archives of Internal Medicine* **133,** 577–90.

Kolodny, E. H., Rebeiz, J. J., Caveness, V. S. and Richardson, E. P. (1968) Granulomatous angiitis of the central nervous system. *Archives of Neurology* **19,** 510–24.

Konigsmark, B. W. and Sidman, R. L. (1963) Origin of brain macrophages in the mouse. *Journal of Neuropathology and Experimental Neurology* **22,** 643–76.

Kornyey, S. (1963) Patterns of CNS vulnerability to CO, cyanide and other poisoning. In *Selective Vulnerability of the Brain in Hypoxaemia* (Eds Schadé, J. P. and McMenemey, W. M.), pp. 165–76. Blackwell Scientific, Oxford.

Krayenbuhl, H. (1967) Cerebral venous and sinus thrombosis. *Clinical Neurosurgery* **14,** 1–24.

Kubik, C. S. and Adams, R. D. (1946) Occlusion of the basilar artery—a clinical and pathological study. *Brain* **69,** 73–121.

Kuhn, R. A. (1962) The speed of cerebral circulation. *New England Journal of Medicine* **267,** 689–95.

Kurtzke, J. F. (1969) *Epidemiology of Cerebrovascular Disease*. Springer, Berlin.

Lambert, S. W. (1919) Poisoning by hydrocyanic acid gas with special reference to its effects upon the brain. *Neurology Bulletin* **2,** 93–105.

Lapresle, J. and Fardeau, M. (1966) Les leucoencéphalopathies de l'intoxication oxycarbonée. Étude de seize observations anatomocliniques. *Acta Neuropathologica* **6,** 327–48.

Lapresle, J. and Fardeau, M. (1967) The central nervous system and carbon monoxide poisoning. II. Anatomical study of brain lesions following intoxication with carbon monoxide (22 cases). In *Carbon Monoxide Poisoning* (Eds Bour, H. and Ledingham, I. McA.), *Progress in Brain Research*, vol. 24, pp. 31–74. Elsevier, Amsterdam.

Lapresle, J. and Milhaud, M. (1962) Lésions du système nerveux central après arrêt circulatoire. Étude de 10 cas. *Presse médicale* **70,** 429–32.

Lassen, N. A. (1959) Cerebral blood flow and oxygen consumption in man. *Physiological Reviews* **39,** 183–238.

Lassen, N. A. and Agnoli, A. (1973) The upper limit of autoregulation of cerebral blood flow: on the pathogenesis of hypertensive encephalopathy. *Scandinavian Journal of Clinical and Laboratory Investigation* **30,** 113–16.

Lawrence, R. D., Meyer, A. and Nevin, S. (1942) The pathological changes in the brain in fatal hypoglycemia. *Quarterly Journal of Medicine* **11,** 181–202.

Leadbetter, W. F. and Burkland, C. E. (1938) Hypertension in unilateral renal disease. *Journal of Urology* **39,** 611–26.

Ledingham, J. G. G. and Rajagopalan, B. (1979) Cerebral complications in the treatment of accelerated hypertension. *Quarterly Journal of Medicine* **48,** 25–41.

Levine, S. (1960) Anoxic-ischemic encephalopathy in rats. *American Journal of Pathology* **36,** 1–17.

Levine, S. and Stypulkowski, W. (1959). Effect of ischemia on cyanide encephalopathy. *Neurology* **9,** 407–44.

Levy, D. E., Brierley, J. B. and Plum, F. (1975) Ischaemic brain damage in the gerbil in the absence of 'no-reflow'. *Journal of Neurology, Neurosurgery and Psychiatry* **38,** 1197–205.

Levy, D. E., Brierley, J. B., Silverman, D. G. and Plum, F. (1975) Brief hypoxia-ischemia initially damages cerebral neurons. *Archives of Neurology* **32,** 450–6.

Lewey, F. H. and Drabkin, D. L. (1944) Experimental chronic carbon monoxide poisoning of dogs. *American Journal of the Medical Sciences* **208,** 502–11.

Lhermitte, J. and Barrelet (1934) Embolie gazeuse cérébrale d'origine péripherique. Étude anatomique. *Revue Neurologique* **2,** 851–7.

Lhermitte, F., Gautier, J. C. and Derouesné, C. (1966) Anatomopathologie et physiopathologie des sténoses carotidiennes. *Revue Neurologique* **115,** 641–72.

Lhermitte, F., Gautier, J. C. and Derouesné, C. (1970) Nature of occlusions of the middle cerebral artery. *Neurology* **20,** 82–8.

Lindenberg, R. (1955) Compression of brain arteries as a pathogenic factor for tissue necrosis and their areas of predilection. *Journal of Neuropathology and Experimental Neurology* **14,** 223–43.

Lindenberg, R. (1963) Patterns of CNS vulnerability in acute hypoxaemia, including anaesthetic accidents. In *Selective Vulnerability of the Brain in Hypoxaemia* (Eds Schadé, J. P. and McMenemey, W. H.), pp. 184–209. Blackwell Scientific, Oxford.

Lindenberg, R. and Spatz, H. (1939) Über die Thromboendarteriitis obliterans der Hirngefässe (cerebrale form der v. Winiwarter-Buergerschen Krankheit). *Virchows Archiv für pathologische Anatomie und Physiologie* **305,** 531–57.

Little, J. R., Kerr, F. W. L. and Sundt, T. M. (1975) Microcirculatory obstruction in focal cerebral ischemia. Relationship to neuronal alterations. *Mayo Clinic Proceedings* **50,** 264–70.

Little, J. R., Sundt, T. M. and Kerr, F. W. L. (1974) Neuronal alterations in developing cortical infarction. An experimental study in monkeys. *Journal of Neurosurgery* **39,** 186–98.

Loizou, L. A., Jefferson, J. M. and Smith W. T. (1982) Subcortical arteriosclerotic encephalopathy (Binswanger's type) and cortical infarcts in a young normotensive patient. *Journal of Neurology, Neurosurgery and Psychiatry* **45,** 409–17.

Lothman, E. W. and Collins, R. C. (1981) Kainic acid induced limbic seizures: metabolic, behavioral, electroencephalographic and neuropathological correlates. *Brain Research* **218,** 299–318.

Lübbers, D. W. (1966) The oxygen pressure field of the brain and its significance for the normal and critical oxygen supply of the brain. In *Oxygen Transport in Blood and Tissue* (Eds Lübbers, D. W., Luft, V. C., Thews, G. and Witzleb, E.), pp. 124–39. Thieme, Stuttgart.

Luft, V. C. (1965) Aviation physiology—the effects of altitude. In *Handbook of Physiology*, Section 3, Respiration, vol. II, pp. 1099–145. American Physiological Society, Washington DC.

Luft, V. C. and Finkelstein, S. (1968) Hypoxia: a clinical-physiological approach. *Aerospace Medicine* **39,** 105–10.

McCall, A. J. and Fletcher, P. J. H. (1975) Pathology. In *Strokes. Natural History, Pathology and Surgical Treatment* (Eds Hutchinson, E. C. and Acheson, E. J.), pp. 36–105. Saunders, London.

McCormick, W. F. and Schochet, S. S. (1976) *Atlas of Cerebrovascular Disease*, Saunders, Philadelphia.

MacDonald, M. and Spector, R. G. (1963) The influence of anoxia on respiratory enzymes in rat brain. *British Journal of Experimental Pathology* **44,** 11–15.

McDonald, W. I. (1967) Recurrent cholesterol embolism as a cause of fluctuating cerebral symptoms. *Journal of Neurology, Neurosurgery and Psychiatry* **30,** 489–96.

McDowell, F. H. (1972) Cerebral embolism. In *Handbook of Clinical Neurology. Vascular Diseases of the Nervous System*, vol. II (Eds Vinken, P. J. and Bruyn, G. W.), pp. 386–414. North-Holland, Amsterdam.

McGee, D. A., McPhedran, R. S. and Hoffman, H. J. (1962) Carotid and vertebral artery disease. A clinicopathological survey of 70 cases. *Neurology* **12,** 848–59.

McIlwain, H. and Bachelard, H. S. (1971) *Biochemistry and the Central Nervous System*, 4th edn. Churchill Livingstone, Edinburgh.

MacKenzie, E. T., Strandgaard, S., Graham, D. I., Jones, J. V., Harper, A. M. and Farrar, J. K. (1976) Effects of acutely induced hypertension in cats on pial arteriolar calibre, local cerebral blood flow and the blood–brain barrier. *Circulation Research* **39,** 33–9.

McLardy, T. (1962) Zinc enzymes and the hippocampal mossy fibre system. *Nature* **194,** 300–2.

McTaggart, D. M. and Neubuerger, K. T. (1970). Cerebral fat embolism: pathologic changes in the brain after survival of 7 years. *Acta Neuropathologica* **15,** 183–7.

Marks, V. and Rose, F. C. (1965) *Hypoglycaemia.* Blackwell Scientific, Oxford.

Marsden, C. D. and Harrison, M. J. G. (1972) Outcome of investigation of patients with presenile dementia. *British Medical Journal* **2,** 249–52.

Marshall, J. (1982) The cause and prognosis of strokes in people under 50 years. *Journal of the Neurological Sciences* **53,** 473–88.

Marshall, L. F., Graham, D. I., Durity, F., Lounsbury, R., Welsh, F. and Langfitt, T. W. (1975) Experimental cerebral oligemia and ischemia produced by intracranial hypertension. Part 2. Brain morphology. *Journal of Neurosurgery* **43,** 318–22.

Martin, J. P. (1941) Thrombosis in superior longitudinal sinus following childbirth. *British Medical Journal* **2,** 537–40.

Maske, H. (1955) Über den topochemischen Nachweis von Zink in Ammonshorn verschiedenen Säugetiere. *Naturwissenschaften* **42,** 424.

Matakas, F., Cervos-Navarro, J. and Schneider, H. (1973) Experimental brain death. I. Morphology and fine structure of the brain. *Journal of Neurology, Neurosurgery and Psychiatry* **36,** 497–508.

Mathew, N. T., Abraham, J., Taori, G. M. and Gopalakrishma, V. I. (1971) Internal carotid artery occlusion in cavernous sinus thrombosis. *Archives of Neurology* **24,** 11–16.

Mayeux, R. and Fahn, S. (1978) Strokes, and ulcerative colitis. *Neurology* **28,** 571–4.

Meldrum, B. S. and Brierley, J. B. (1969) Brain damage in the Rhesus monkey resulting from profound arterial hypotension. II. Changes in the spontaneous and evoked electrical activity of the neocortex. *Brain Research* **13,** 101–18.

Meldrum, B. S. and Brierley, J. B. (1971) Circulatory factors and cerebral boundary zone lesions. In *Brain Hypoxia* (Eds Brierley, J. B. and Meldrum, B. S.), Clinics in Developmental Medicine, no. 39/40, pp. 20–33. Spastics International Medical Publications/Heinemann Medical, London.

Meldrum, B. S. and Brierley, J. B. (1973) Prolonged epileptic seizures in primates: ischemic cell change and its relation to vital physiological events. *Archives of Neurology* **28,** 10–17.

Meldrum, B. S., Horton, R. W. and Brierley, J. B. (1971) Insulin-induced hypoglycaemia in the primate: relationship between physiological changes and neuropathology. In *Brain Hypoxia* (Eds Brierley, J. B. and Meldrum, B. S.), Clinics in Developmental Medicine 39/40, pp. 207–24. Spastics International Medical Publishers/Heinemann Medical, London.

Meldrum, B. S., Papy, J. J. and Vigouroux, R. A. (1971) Intracarotid air embolism in the baboon: effects on cerebral blood flow and the electroencephalogram. *Brain Research* **25,** 305–15.

Menkin, M. and Schwartzman, R. J. (1977) Cerebral air embolism. Report of five cases and review of the literature. *Archives of Neurology* **34,** 168–70.

Merkel, K. H. H., Ginsberg, P. L., Parker, J. D. and Post, M. J. D. (1978) Cerebrovascular disease in sickle cell anemia: a clinical, pathological and radiological correlation. *Stroke* **9,** 45–52.

Mettinger, K. L. (1982) Fibromuscular dysplasia and the brain. II. Current concept of the disease. *Stroke* **13,** 53–8.

Mettinger, K. L. and Ericson, K. (1982) Fibromuscular dysplasia and the brain. Observations on angiographic, clinical and genetic characteristics. *Stroke* **13,** 46–52.

Mettler, F. A. and Sax, D. S. (1972) Cerebellar arterial degeneration due to acute azide poisoning. *Brain* **95,** 505–16.

Meyer, A. (1926) Ueber die Wirkung der Kohlenoxydvergiftung auf das Zentralnervensystem. *Zeitschrift für die gesamte Neurologie und Psychiatrie* **100,** 201–47.

Meyer, A. (1928) Über das Verhalten des Hemisphärenmarks bei der menschlichen Kohlenoxydvergiftung. *Zeitschrift für die gesamte Neurologie und Psychiatrie* **112,** 172–82.

Meyer, A. (1932) Experimentelle Vergiftungsstudien. II. Vergleichende phylogenetische Untersuchungen Über Kohlenoxydvergiftung des Gehirns. *Zeitschrift für die gesamte Neurologie und Psychiatrie* **139,** 422–3.

Meyer, A. (1933) Experimentelle Vergiftungsstudien. III. Über Gehirnveränderungen bei experimenteller Blausäurevergiftung. *Zeischrift für gesamte Neurologie und Psychiatrie* **143,** 333–48.

Meyer, A. (1936) The selective regional vulnerability of the brain and its relation to psychiatric problems. *Proceedings of the Royal Society of Medicine* **29,** 1175–81.

Meyer, A. (1956) Neuropathological aspects of anoxia. *Proceedings of the Royal Society of Medicine* **49,** 619–22.

Meyer, A. (1963) Anoxias, intoxications and metabolic disorders. In *Greenfield's Neuropathology* (Eds Blackwood, W., McMenemey, W. H., Meyer, A. and Russell, D. S.), 2nd edn, pp. 235–87. Williams and Wilkins, Baltimore, Maryland.

Meyer, A., Beck, E. and Shepherd, M. (1955) Unusually severe lesions in the brain following status epilepticus. *Journal of Neurology, Neurosurgery and Psychiatry* **18,** 24–33.

Meyer, J. E. (1953) Über die Lokalisation fruhkindlicher Hirnschaden in arteriellen Grenzgebieten.

Archiv für Psychiatrie und Nervenkrankheiten **190,** 328–41.
Meyer, J. S. (1982) Course prognosis and medical management of patients with acute stroke. In *Diagnosis and Management of Stroke and TIAs* (Eds Meyer, J. S. and Shaw, T.), pp. 155–72. Addison-Wesley, London.
Meyer, J. S. and Loeb, C. (1965) *Strokes due to Vertebro-Basilar Disease.* Thomas, Springfield, Illinois.
Meyer, J. S. and Portnoy, H. D. (1958) Localized cerebral hypoglycemia simulating stroke. A clinical and experimental study. *Neurology* **8,** 601–14.
Meyer, J. S., Waltz, A. G. and Gotoh, F. (1960) Pathogenesis of cerebral vasospasm in hypertensive encephalopathy. II. The nature of increased irritability of smooth muscle of pial arterioles in renal hypertension. *Neurology* **10,** 859–67.
Miller, J. R. and Myers, R. E. (1970) Neurological effects of systemic circulatory arrest in the monkey. *Neurology* **20,** 715–24.
Millikan, C. H., Siekert, R. G. and Whisnant, J. P. (1960) Intermittent carotid and vertebrobasilar insufficiency associated with polycythemia. *Neurology* **10,** 188–96.
Milstein, B. B. (1956) Cardiac arrest and resuscitation. *Annals of the Royal College of Surgeons of England* **19,** 69–87.
Mitchell, J. R. A. and Schwartz, C. J. (1965) *Arterial Disease.* Blackwell, Oxford.
Mohr, J. P. (1982) Lacunes. *Stroke* **13,** 3–11.
Molinari, G. F. and Laurent, J. P. (1976) A classification of experimental models of brain ischemia. *Stroke* **7,** 14–17.
Moschowitz, E. (1925) An acute febrile pleiochromic anemia with hyaline thrombosis of the terminal arterioles and capillaries. *Archives of Internal Medicine* **36,** 89–93.
Myers, R. E. (1977) Experimental models of perinatal brain damage: relevance to human pathology. In *Intrauterine Asphyxia and the Developing Fetal Brain* (Ed. Gluck, L.), pp. 37–97. Year Book Medical, Chicago.
Myers, R. E. (1979) A unitary theory of causation of anoxic and hypoxic brain pathology. In *Cerebral Hypoxia and its Consequences. Advances in Neurology,* vol. 26 (Eds Fahn, S., Davis, J. N. and Rowland, L. P.), pp. 195–213. Raven Press, New York.
Myers, R. E. and Kahn, K. J. (1971) Insulin-induced hypoglycaemia in the non-human primate. II. Long-term neuropathological consequences. In *Brain Hypoxia* (Eds. Brierley, J. B. and Meldrum, B. S.), Clinics in Developmental Medicine, no. 39/40, pp. 195–206. Spastics International Medical Publications/Heinemann Medical, London.
Nadler, J. V., Perry, B. W. and Cotman, C. W. (1978) Preferential vulnerability of hippocampus to intraventricular kainic acid. In *Kainic Acid as a Tool in Neurobiology* (Eds McGeer, G., Olney, J. W. and McGeer, P. L.), pp. 219–39. Raven Press, New York.
Nag, S., Robertson, D. M. and Dinsdale, H. B. (1977) Cerebral cortical changes in acute experimental hypertension. An ultrastructural study. *Laboratory Investigation* **36,** 105–61.
Naquet, R. and Vigouroux, R. A. (1966) Embolies expérimentales pour voie carotidienne chez le babouin (*Papio-papio*). *Revue Neurologique* **144,** 339–60.
Nemoto, E. M., Bleyaert, A. L., Stezoski, S. W., Moossy, J., Rao, G. R. and Safar, P. (1977) Global brain ischemia: a reproducible monkey model. *Stroke* **8,** 558–64.
Neubürger, K. T. (1925) Ueber cerebrale Fett und Luftembolie. *Zeitschrift für die gesamte Neurologie und Psychiatrie* **95,** 278–318.
60.
Neubuerger, K. T. and Clarke, E. R. (1945) Subacute carbon monoxide poisoning with cerebral myelinopathy and multiple myocardial necroses. *Rocky Mountain Medical Journal* **42,** 29–34.
Neubürger, K. T. (1925) Über cerebrale fett und luftembolie. *Zeitschrift für die Gesamte Neurologie und Psychiatrie* **95,** 278–318.
Nishimoto, A. and Takeuchi, S. (1972) Moyamoya disease: abnormal cerebrovascular network in the cerebral basal region. In *Handbook of Clinical Neurology. Vascular Diseases of the Nervous System,* vol. 12 (Eds. Vinken, P. J. and Bruyn, G. W.), pp. 352–83. North-Holland, Amsterdam.
Nordborg, C. and Johansson, B. B. (1980) Morphometric study on cerebral vessels in spontaneously hypertensive rats. *Stroke* **11,** 266–70.
Nordgren, R. E., Markesbery, W. R., Fukuda, K. and Reeves, A. G. (1971) Seven cases of cerebromedullospinal disconnection: the 'locked-in' syndrome. *Neurology* **21,** 1140–8.
Norman, R. M. (1958). Malformations of the nervous system, birth injury and diseases of early life. In *Neuropathology* (Eds Greenfield, J. G., Blackwood, W. McMenemey, W. H. and Meyer, A.), pp. 300–407. Edward Arnold, London.
Numaguchi, Y., Balsys, R., Marc, J. A. and O'Brien, M. S. (1976) Some observations in progressive arterial occlusions in children and young adolescents (Moya moya disease). *Surgical Neurology* **6,** 293–300.
Okamoto, K. (1969) Spontaneous hypertension in rats. In *International Review of Experimental Pathology,* vol. VII (Eds Richter, G. W. and Epstein, M. A.), pp. 227–70. Academic Press, New York and London.
Okeda, R., Funata, N., Takano, T., Miyazaki, Y., Higashino, F., Yokoyama, K. and Manabe, M.

(1981) The pathogenesis of carbon monoxide encephalopathy in the acute phase—physical and morphological correlation. *Acta Neuropathologica* **54,** 1–10.

Olszewski, J. (1962) Subcortical arteriosclerotic encephalopathy. *World Neurology* **3,** 359–75.

Oppenheimer, B. S. and Fishberg, A. M. (1928) Hypertensive encephalopathy. *Archives of Internal Medicine* **41,** 264–78.

O'Sullivan, D. J., Lim, G. H. K., Darveniza, P. and Coffey, G. L. (1977) Multiple progressive intracranial arterial occlusions ('moya moya' disease). *Journal of Neurology, Neurosurgery and Psychiatry* **40,** 853–60.

Painter, M. J., Chutorian, A. M. and Hilal, S. K. (1975) Cerebrovasculopathy following irradiation in childhood. *Neurology* **25,** 189–94.

Palmer, A. C. and Blakemore, W. F. (1980) Neuropathology of experimental decompression (goats). In *Proceedings of the 5th Annual Scientific Meeting of the European Undersea Biomedical Society,* (Ed. Grimstad, J.) pp. 153–6. European Undersea Biomedical Society.

Palmer, A. C., Blakemore, W. F. and Greenwood, A. G. (1976) Neuropathology of experimental decompression sickness (dysbarism) in the goat. *Neuropathology and Applied Neurobiology* **2,** 145–56.

Palmer, A. C., Blakemore, W. F., Payne, J. E. and Sillence, A. (1978) Decompression sickness in the goat: nature of brain and spinal cord lesions at 48 hours. *Undersea Biomedical Research* **5,** 275–86.

Palmer, A. C., Calder, I. M., McCallum, R. I. and Mastaglia, F. L. (1981) Spinal cord degeneration in a case of 'recovered' spinal decompression sickness. *British Medical Journal* **283,** 888.

Parker, J. C. and Schwartzman, R. J. (1980) Cerebral thromboangiitis obliterans. In *Handbook of Clinical Neurology. Neurological Manifestations of Systemic Disease,* vol. 39 (Eds Vinken, P. J. and Bruyn, G. W.), pp. 201–11. North-Holland, Amsterdam.

Paulson, O. B., Henriksen, L. and Smith, R. J. (1979) The effect of hemodilution on cerebral blood flow and blood gases in patients with polycythemia. *Acta Neurologica Scandinavica* **60,** Suppl. 72, 588–9.

Pearson, T. C. and Wetherley-Mein, G. (1978) Vascular occlusive episodes and venous haematocrit in primary proliferative polycythaemia. *Lancet* **2,** 1219–22.

Penfield, W. and Cone, W. (1926) Acute swelling of oligodendroglia. A specific type of neuroglia change. *Archives of Neurology and Psychiatry* **16,** 131–53.

Pentschew, A. (1933) Die granuläre Atrophie der Grosshirnrinde. *Archiv für Psychiatrie* **101,** 80–136.

Peters, J. P. and Van Slyke, D. D. (1932) Hemoglobin and oxygen. In *Quantitative Clinical Chemistry,* vol. 1, pp. 518–62. Williams and Wilkins, Baltimore, Maryland.

Petito, C. K. (1979a) Early and late mechanisms of increased vascular permeability following experimental cerebral infarction. *Journal of Neuropathology and Experimental Neurology* **38,** 222–34.

Petito, C. K. (1979b) Platelet thrombi in experimental cerebral infarction. *Stroke* **10,** 192–6.

Plum, F. (1972) Organic disturbances of consciousness. In *Scientific Foundations of Neurology* (Eds Critchley, M., O'Leary, J. L. and Jennett, B.), pp. 193–201. Heinemann Medical, London.

Portnoy, B. A. and Herion, J. C. (1972) Neurological manifestations in sickle cell disease, with a review of the literature and emphasis on the prevalence of hemiplegia. *Annals of Internal Medicine* **76,** 643–52.

Portnoy, H. D. (1965) Transient 'ischemic' attacks produced by carotid stenosis and hypoglycemia. *Neurology* **15,** 830–2.

Poursines, Y., Alliez, J. and Toga, M. (1956) Etude des lésions corticales d'un cas d'intoxication oxycarbonée. *Revue Neurologique* **94,** 731–5.

Preziosi, T. J., Lindenberg, R., Levy, D. and Christenson, M. (1970) An experimental investigation in animals of the functional and morphologic effects of single and repeated exposures to high and low concentrations of carbon monoxide. *Annals of the New York Academy of Sciences* **174,** 369–84.

Prior, P. F. (1979) Monitoring in the intensive care unit. In *Monitoring Cerebral Function,* pp. 165–204. Elsevier/North-Holland Biomedical Press, Amsterdam.

Prys-Roberts, C., Greenbaum, R., Nunn, J. F. and Kelman, G. R. (1970) Disturbances of pulmonary function in patients with fat embolism. *Journal of Clinical Pathology* **23,** Suppl. 4, 143–9.

Pulsinelli, W. A., Brierley, J. B. and Plum, F. (1982) Temporal profile of neuronal damage in a model of transient forebrain ischemia. *Annals of Neurology* **11,** 491–8.

Pulsinelli, W. A. and Duffy, T. E. (1979) Local cerebral glucose metabolism during controlled hypoxemia in rats. *Science* **204,** 626–9.

Pulsinelli, W. A., Levy, D. E. and Duffy, T. E. (1982) Regional cerebral blood flow and glucose metabolism following transient forebrain ischemia. *Annals of Neurology* **11,** 499–509.

Ranck, J. B. and Windle, W. F. (1959) Brain damage in the monkey, Macaca mulatta, by asphyxia neonatorum. *Experimental Neurology* **1,** 130–54.

Raskin, N. and Mullaney, O. C. (1940) The mental and neurological sequelae of carbon monoxide asphyxia in a case observed for 15 years. *Journal of Nervous and Mental Disease* **92,** 640–59.

Rehncrona, S., Rosen, I. and Siesjö, B. K. (1981) Brain

lactic acidosis and ischemic cell damage: 1. Biochemistry and neurophysiology. *Journal of Cerebral Blood Flow and Metabolism* **1,** 297–311.

Reivich, M., Holling, H. E., Roberts, B. and Toole, J. F. (1961) Reversal of blood flow through the vertebral artery and its effect on cerebral circulation. *New England Journal of Medicine* **265,** 878–85.

Resch, J. A. and Baker, A. B. (1964) Etiologic mechanisms in cerebral atherosclerosis. *Archives of Neurology* **10,** 617–28.

Reyes, M. G., Fresco, R., Chokroverty, S. and Salud, E. Q. (1976) Virus-like particles in granulomatous angiitis of the central nervous system. *Neurology* **26,** 797–9.

Rice, J. E., Vannucci, R. C. and Brierley, J. B. (1981) The influence of immaturity on hypoxic-ischemic brain damage in the rat. *Annals of Neurology* **9,** 131–41.

Richardson, E. P. (1980) Systemic lupus erythematosus. In *Handbook of Clinical Neurology. Neurological Manifestations of Systemic Diseases*, vol. 39 (Eds Vinken, P. J. and Bruyn, G. W.), pp. 283–93. North-Holland, Amsterdam.

Richardson, J. E. and Russell, D. S. (1952) Cerebral disease due to functioning islet-cell tumours, with pathological reports. *Lancet* **2,** 1054–9.

Riggs, H. E. and Rupp, C. (1963) Variation in the form of circle of Willis. *Archives of Neurology* **8,** 8–14.

Roger, B., Poursines, Y. and Roger, J. (1955) Les aspects neurologiques de la périartérite nœuds. *Revue Neurologique* **92,** 430–64.

Romanul, F. C. A. and Abramowicz, A. (1964) Changes in brain and pial vessels in arterial border zones. *Archives of Neurology* **11,** 40–65.

Rosenberg, E. F. (1940) The brain in malignant hypertension. A clinicopathologic study. *Archives of Internal Medicine* **65,** 545–86.

Rosenblum, W. I., Hadfield, M. G. and Young, H. F. (1978) Granulomatous angiitis with preceding varicella zoster. *Annals of Neurology* **3,** 374–5.

Rossen, R., Kabat, H. and Anderson, J. P. (1943) Acute arrest of cerebral circulation in man. *Archives of Neurology and Psychiatry* **50,** 510–28.

Russell, C. K. (1931) Syndrome of brachium conjunctivum and tractus spinothalamicus. *Archives of Neurology and Psychiatry* **25,** 1003–10.

Russell, R. W. R. (1961) Observations on the retinal blood vessels in monocular blindness. *Lancet* **2,** 1422–8.

Russell, R. W. R. (1963) Observations on intracerebral aneurysms. *Brain* **86,** 425–42.

Russell, R. W. R. and Cranston, W. I. (1961) Ophthalmodynamometry in carotid artery disease. *Journal of Neurology, Neurosurgery and Psychiatry* **24,** 281–6.

Schmorl, (1920) Demonstrationen. 3. Gehirn bei Blausäurevergiftung. *Münchener medizinische Wochenschrift* **67,** 913.

Schneider, M. (1961) Survival and revival of the brain in anoxia and ischaemia. In *Cerebral Anoxia and the Electroencephalogram* (Eds Gastaut, H. and Meyer, J. S.), pp. 134–43. Thomas, Springfield, Illinois.

Schneider, M. (1963) Critical blood pressure in the cerebral circulation. In *Selective Vulnerability of the Brain in Hypoxaemia* (Eds Schadé, J. P. and McMenemey, W. M.), pp. 7–20. Blackwell, Oxford.

Schneiderman, J. H., Sharpe, J. A. and Sutton, D. M. C. (1979) Cerebral and retinal vascular complications of inflammatory bowel disease. *Annals of Neurology* **5,** 331–7.

Schoenberg, B. S., Mellinger, J. F. and Schoenberg, D. G. (1978) Cerebrovascular disease in infants and children: a study of incidence, clinical features and survival. *Neurology* **28,** 763–8.

Scholz, W. (1952) Les nécroses parenchymateuses électives par hypoxémie et oligémie et leur expression topistique. *Proceedings of the First International Congress of Neuropathology (Rome)*, vol. 1, pp. 321–46. Rosenberg and Sellier, Torino.

Scholz, W. (1953) Selective neuronal necrosis and its topistic patterns in hypoxemia and oligemia. *Journal of Neuropathology and Experimental Neurology* **12,** 249–61.

Scholz, W. (1957) An nervösesystemegebundene (topistische) Kreislaufschäden. In *Handbuch der speziellen pathologischen Anatomie und Histologie* XIII/I (Eds Lubarsch, O., Henke, F. and Rössle, R.), Bandteil B. pp. 1326–83. Springer, Berlin.

Scholz, W. (1963) Topistic lesion. In *Selective Vulnerability of the Brain in Hypoxaemia* (Eds Schadé, J. P. and McMenemey, W. M.), pp. 257–67. Blackwell Scientific, Oxford.

Schwartz, C. J. and Mitchell, J. R. A. (1961) Atheroma of the carotid and vertebral arterial systems. *British Medical Journal* **2,** 1057–63.

Sevitt, S. (1962) *Fat Embolism*. Butterworths, London.

Sheehan, S., Bauer, R. D. and Meyer, J. S. (1960) Vertebral artery compression in cervical spondylosis. *Neurology* **10,** 968–86.

Sherman, D. D., Hart, R. G. and Easton, J. D. (1981) Abrupt change in head position and cerebral infarction. *Stroke* **12,** 2–6.

Shurtleff, D. (1970) An epidemiological investigation of cardiovascular disease. Some characteristics related to the incidence of cardiovascular disease and death. *The Framingham Study: 16 Year Follow-up*, Section 26. US Government Printing Office, Washington DC.

Siemkowicz, E. and Hansen, A. J. (1978) Clinical restitution following cerebral ischemia in hypo-, normo- and hyperglycemic rats. *Acta Neurologica Scandinavica* **58,** 1–8.

Siesjö, B. K. (1978) *Brain Energy Metabolism*. Wiley, Chichester.

Siesjö, B. K. (1981) Cell damage in the brain: a speculative synthesis. *Journal of Cerebral Blood Flow and Metabolism* **1,** 155–85.

Silverstein, A. (1968) Thrombotic thrombocytopenic purpura. The initial neurologic manifestations. *Archives of Neurology* **18,** 358–62.

Silverstein, A., Gilbert, H. and Wasserman, L. P. (1962) Neurologic complications of polycythemia. *Annals of Internal Medicine* **57,** 909–16.

Sindermann, F., Bechinger, D. and Dichgans, J. (1970) Occlusions of the internal carotid artery compared with those of the middle cerebral artery. *Brain* **93,** 199–210.

Skinhoj, E. and Strandgaard, S. (1973) Pathogenesis of hypertensive encephalopathy. *Lancet* **1,** 461–2.

Snyder, B. D., Ramirez-Lassepas, M., Sukhum, P., Fryd, D. and Sung, J. H. (1979) Failure of thiopental to modify global anoxic injury. *Stroke* **10,** 135–41.

Soloway, H. B. and Aronson, S. M. (1964) Atheromatous emboli to central nervous system. Report of 16 cases. *Archives of Neurology* **11,** 657–67.

Spector, R. G. (1965) Enzyme chemistry of anoxic brain injury. In *Neurohistochemistry* (Ed. Adams, C. W. M.), pp. 547–57. Elsevier, Amsterdam.

Spielmeyer, W. (1913) Über die anatomischen Folgen der Luftembolie. In *Gehirn Verhandlungen des Deutschen Kongresses für innere Medizin* **30,** 359–65.

Spielmeyer, W. (1925) Zur Pathogenese örtlich elektiven Gehirnveränderungen. *Zeitschrift für die gesamte Neurologie und Psychiatrie* **99,** 756–76.

Steiner, T. J., Rail, D. L. H. and Rose, F. C. (1980) Cholesterol crystal embolization in rat brain: a model for atheroembolic cerebral infarction. *Stroke* **11,** 184–9.

Stephenson, H. E., Reid, L. C. and Hinton, J. W. (1953) Some common denominators in 1200 cases of cardiac arrest. *Annals of Surgery* **137,** 731–44.

Stern, G. (1980) Wegener's granulomatosis. In *Handbook of Clinical Neurology. Neurological manifestations of Systemic Diseases*, vol. 39 (Eds. Vinken, P. J. and Bruyn, G. W.), pp. 343–5. North-Holland, Amsterdam.

Stopford, J. S. B. (1915) The arteries of the pons and medulla oblongata. *Journal of Anatomy and Physiology* **50,** 131–64.

Stopford, J. S. B. (1917) The arteries of the pons and medulla oblongata. Part III. Clinical applications of parts I and II. *Journal of Anatomy and Physiology* **51,** 250–77.

Strandgaard, S. (1976) Autoregulation of cerebral blood flow in hypertensive patients: the modifying influence of prolonged antihypertensive treatment on the tolerance to acute drug induced hypotension. *Circulation* **53,** 720–7.

Strandgaard, S., MacKenzie, E. T., Sengupta, D., Rowan, J. O., Lassen, N. A. and Harper, A. M. (1974) Upper limit of autoregulation of cerebral blood flow in the baboon. *Circulation Research* **34,** 435–40.

Strandgaard, S., Jones, J. V., MacKenzie, E. T. and Harper, A. M. (1975) Upper limit of cerebral blood flow autoregulation in experimental renovascular hypertension in the baboon. *Circulation Research* **37,** 164–7.

Strandgaard, S., MacKenzie, E. T., Jones, J. V. and Harper, A. M. (1976) Studies on the cerebral circulation of the baboon in acutely induced hypertension. *Stroke* **7,** 287–90.

Sturgill, B. C. and Netsky, M. G. (1963) Cerebral infarction by atheromatous emboli. *Archives of Pathology* **76,** 189–96.

Swann, H. G. and Brucer, M. (1949) The cardiorespiratory and biochemical events during rapid hypoxic death. I. Fulminating hypoxia. *Texas Reports on Biology and Medicine* **7,** 511–38.

Symmers, W. StC. (1956) Thrombotic microangiopathy (thrombotic thrombocytopenic purpura) associated with acute haemorrhagic leucoencephalitis and sensitivity to oxophenarsine. *Brain* **79,** 511–21.

Symon, L. and Brierley, J. B. (1976) Morphological changes in cerebral blood vessels in chronic ischemic infarction: flow correlation obtained by the hydrogen clearance method. In *The Cerebral Vessel Wall* (Eds Cervos-Navarro, J., Betz, E., Matakas, F. and Wullenweber, R.), pp. 165–74. Raven Press, New York.

Symonds, C. (1956) Otitic hydrocephalus. *Neurology* **6,** 681–5.

Szabo, G. (1970) The syndrome of fat embolism and its origin. *Journal of Clinical Pathology* **23,** Suppl. 4, 123–31.

Takashima, S. and Tanaka, K. (1978) Development of cerebrovascular architecture and its relationship to periventricular leukomalacia. *Archives of Neurology* **35,** 11–16.

Taylor, C. B., Cox, G. E., Manalo-Estrella, P., Southworth, J., Patton, D. E. and Cathcart, C. (1962) Atherosclerosis in Rhesus monkeys. II. Arterial lesions associated with hypercholesterolemia induced by dietary fat and cholesterol. *Archives of Pathology* **74,** 16–34.

Taylor, J. E. D. (1952) Post-mortem diagnosis of air embolism by radiography. *British Medical Journal* **1,** 890–3.

Thomas, D. J., du Boulay, G. H., Marshall, J., Pearson, T. C., Russell, R. W. R., Symon, L. et al. (1977a) Cerebral blood flow in polycythaemia. *Lancet* **2,** 161–3.

Thomas, D. J., du Boulay, G. H., Marshall, J., Pearson, T.C., Russell, R.W.R., Symon, L. et al. (1977b) Effect of haematocrit on cerebral blood flow. *Lancet* **2**, 941–3.

Thompson, P.L. and Robinson, J.S. (1978) Stroke after acute myocardial infarction: relation to infarct size. *British Medical Journal* **2**, 457–9.

Thompson, T. and Evans, W. (1930) Paradoxical embolism. *Quarterly Journal of Medince* **23**, 135–50.

Tichy, F. (1949) Syndromes of cerebral arteries. *Archives of Pathology* **48**, 475–88.

Timm, F. (1958) Zur Histochemie des Ammonshorngebietes. *Zeitschrift für Zellforschung und mikroskopische Anatomie* **48**, 548–55.

Timperley, W.R., Preston, F.E. and Ward, J.D. (1974) Cerebral intravascular coagulation in diabetic ketoacidosis. *Lancet* **1**, 952–6.

Tindall, G.T., Odom, G.L., Cupp, H.B. and Dillon, M.L. (1962) Studies on carotid artery flow and pressure: observations in 18 patients during graded occlusion of proximal carotid artery. *Journal of Neurosurgery* **19**, 917–23.

Tohgi, H., Yamanouchi, H., Murakami, M. and Kameyama, M. (1978) Importance of the hematocrit as a risk factor in cerebral infarction. *Stroke* **9**, 369–74.

Tomlinson, B.E., Blessed, G. and Roth, M. (1968) Observations on the brains of non-demented old people. *Journal of the Neurological Sciences* **7**, 331–56.

Toole, J.F., Janeway, R., Choi, K., Cordell, R., Davis, C., Johnston, F. and Miller, H.S. (1975) Transient ischemic attacks due to atherosclerosis. *Archives of Neurology* **32**, 5–12.

Torvik, A. and Jorgensen, L. (1964) Thrombotic and embolic occlusions of the carotid arteries in an autopsy material. I. Prevalence, location and associated diseases. *Journal of the Neurological Sciences* **1**, 24–39.

Torvik, A. and Jorgensen, L. (1966) Thrombotic and embolic occlusions of the carotid arteries in an autopsy series. II. Cerebral lesions and clinical course. *Journal of the Neurological Sciences* **3**, 410–32.

van Trotsenburg, L. and Vinken, P.J. (1966) Fatal cerebral infarction simulating an acute expanding lesion. *Journal of Neurology, Neurosurgery and Psychiatry* **29**, 241–3.

Uchimura, J. (1928) Zur Pathogenese der örtlich elektiven Ammonshornerkrankung. *Zeitschrift für die gesamte Neurologie und Psychiatrie* **114**, 567–601.

Van Liere, E.J. and Stickney, J.C. (1963) *Hypoxia.* University of Chicago Press, Chicago.

Vander Eecken, H.M. (1959) *The Anastomoses between the Leptomeningeal Arteries of the Brain.* Thomas, Springfield, Illinois.

Vander Eecken, H.M. and Adams, R.D. (1953) The anatomy and functional significance of the meningeal arterial anastomoses of the human brain. *Journal of Neuropathology and Experimental Neurology* **12**, 132–57.

Vessey, M.P. and Doll, R. (1969) Investigation of relation between use of oral contraceptives and thromboembolic disease. A further report. *British Medical Journal* **2**, 651–7.

Vital, C.I., Picard, J., Arné, L., Aubertin, J., Fenelon, J. and Mouton, L. (1967) Étude anatomoclinique de 3 cas d'encéphalopathie hypoglycémique (dont un après sulfamidotherapie). *Diabète* **12F**, 291–6.

Vogt, C. and Vogt, O. (1937) Sitz und Wesen der Krankheiten im Lichte der topistischen Hirnforschung und des Variierens der Tiere. *Journal für Psychologie und Neurologie* **47**, 237–457.

Vost, A., Wolochow, D.A. and Howell, D.A. (1964) Incidence of infarcts of the brain in heart disease. *Journal of Pathology and Bacteriology* **88**, 463–70.

Vuia, O. (1967) Leucoencephalopathie sous-corticale par intoxication au CO. *Acta Neuropathologica* **7**, 305–14.

Walker, A.E., Diamond, E.L. and Moseley, J. (1975) The neuropathological findings in irreversible coma. A critique of the 'respirator brain'. *Journal of Neuropathology and Experimental Neurology* **34**, 295–323.

Walton, E.W. (1958) Giant cell granuloma of the respiratory tract (Wegener's granulomatosis). *British Medical Journal* **2**, 265–70.

Waltz, A.G. (1979) Clinical relevance of models of cerebral ischemia. *Stroke* **10**, 211–13.

Watson, A.J. (1970) Genesis of fat emboli. *Journal of Clinical Pathology* **23**, Suppl. 4, 132–42.

Weinberger, L.M., Gibbon, M.H. and Gibbon, J.H. (1940) Temporary arrest of the circulation to the central nervous system. II. Pathologic effects. *Archives of Neurology and Psychiatry* **43**, 961–86.

Welsh, F.A., O'Connor, M.J. and Langfitt, T.W. (1977) Regions of cerebral ischemia located by pyridine nucleotide fluorescence. *Science* **198**, 951–3.

Welsh, F.A., Vannucci, R.C. and Brierley, J.B. (1982) Columnar alterations of NADH fluorescence during hypoxia-ischemia in immature rat brain. *Journal of Cerebral Blood Flow and Metabolism* **2**, 221–8.

Wigglesworth, J.S. and Pape, K.E. (1978) An integrated model for haemorrhage and ischaemic lesions in the newborn brain. *Early Human Development* **2**, 179–99.

Williams, A.O., Resch, J.A. and Loewenson, R.B. (1969) Cerebral atherosclerosis—a comparative autopsy study between Nigerian Negroes and American Negroes and Caucasians. *Neurology* **19**, 205–10.

Williams, D.J. (1936) The origin of the posterior cerebral artery. *Brain* **59**, 175–80.

Willoughby, J. O. and Leach, B. G. (1974) Relation of neurological findings after cardiac arrest to outcome. *British Medical Journal* **3,** 437–9.

Winkelman, N. W. (1942) Cerebral fat embolism: clinico-pathologic study of 2 cases. *Archives of Neurology and Psychiatry* **47,** 57–76.

Wolf, A. and Siris, J. (1937) Acute non-traumatic encephalomalacia complicating neurosurgical operations in the sitting position. *Bulletin of the Neurological Institute of New York* **6,** 42–61.

Wolf, P. and Kannel, W. (1982) Controllable risk factors for stroke: preventive implications of trends in stroke mortality. In *Diagnosis and Management of Stroke and TIAs* (Eds Meyer, J. S. and Shaw, T.), pp. 25–61. Addison-Wesley, London.

Wolin, L. R., Massopust, L. C. and Taslitz, N. (1971) Tolerance to arrest of cerebral circulation in the Rhesus monkey. *Experimental Neurology* **30,** 103.

Wolkoff, K. (1933) Über Atherosklerose der Gehirnarterien. *Beiträge zur pathologischen Anatomie und zur allgemeinen Pathologie* **91,** 515–52.

Wood, D. H. (1978) Cerebrovascular complications of sickle cell anemia. *Stroke* **9,** 73–5.

Woolf, N. (1978) The pathogenesis of atherosclerosis. In *Recent Advances in Histopathology*, vol. 10 (Eds Anthony, P. P. and Woolf, N.), pp. 45–67. Churchill Livingstone, Edinburgh.

Wrigley, P. F. M., Sheldon, P. and Whitty, C. W. M. (1967) Normal cerebral function with bilateral carotid occlusion. *British Medical Journal* **1,** 93–4.

Wylie, W. D. (1975) 'There, but for the Grace of God ...' *Annals of the Royal College of Surgeons of England* **56,** 171–80.

Yamori, Y. (1979) Experimental models of hypertension as a tool for the control and prevention of clinical hypertension. In *Arterial Hypertension* (Eds Gross, F. and Robertson, J. I. S.), pp. 209–26. Pitman Medical, Tunbridge Wells.

Yamori, Y., Horie, R., Sato, M. and Fukase, M. (1976) Hypertension as an important factor for cerebrovascular atherogenesis in rats. *Stroke* **7,** 120–5.

Yant, W. P., Chornyak, J., Schrenk, H. H., Patty, F. A. and Sayers, R. R. (1934) Studies in asphyxia. *Public Health Bulletin* no. **211,** 1–61.

Yates, P. O. (1959) Birth trauma in the vertebral arteries. *Archives of Disease in Childhood* **34,** 436–41.

Yates, P. O. (1964) A change in the pattern of cerebrovascular disease. *Lancet* **1,** 65–9.

Yates, P. O. (1976a) Vascular disease of the central nervous system. In *Greenfield's Neuropathology* (Eds Blackwood, W. and Corsellis, J. A. N.), 2nd edn, pp. 86–147. Edward Arnold, London.

Yates, P. O. (1976b) The pathogenesis of transient ischaemic attacks. In *Stroke* (Eds Gillingham, F. J., Mawdley, C. and Williams, A. E.), pp. 178–87. Churchill Livingstone, Edinburgh.

Zülch, K. J. (1953) Neue Befunde und Deutungen aus der Gefässpathologie des Hirns und Rückenmarks. *Zentralblatt für allgemeine Pathologie und pathologische Anatomie* **90,** 402.

Zülch, K. J. (1961) Die Pathogenese von Massenblutung und Erweichung unter besonderen Berücksichtigung klinischer Gesichtespunkte. *Acta Neurochirurgica*, Suppl. 7, 51–117.

Zülch, K. J. and Behrend, R. C. H. (1961) The pathogenesis and topography of anoxia, hypoxia, and ischemia of the brain in man. In *Cerebral Anoxia and the Electroencephalogram* (Eds Gastaut, H. and Meyer, J. S.), pp. 144–63. Thomas, Springfield, Illinois.

5

Spontaneous intracranial haemorrhage

R.O.Weller

Haemorrhage into the intracranial cavity may occur as a result of a recognizable event such as trauma, or hypoxia at birth, or it may be spontaneous. Extradural, subdural and intracranial haemorrhages due to trauma are discussed in Chapter 3, and the subependymal and intraventricular haemorrhages in premature infants associated with birth hypoxia are reviewed in Chapter 11.

Spontaneous intracranial haemorrhage falls into two major categories: (1) **intracerebral haemorrhage,** or haemorrhage into the cerebellum or brain stem, which occurs usually as a complication of hypertension; and (2) **subarachnoid haemorrhage,** due for the most part to rupture of a saccular aneurysm. The less common causes of spontaneous intracranial haemorrhage will be discussed later in this chapter.

Incidence and sites of spontaneous intracranial haemorrhage

There are two major events which have affected the incidence and detection of intracranial haemorrhage during the last decade. First, control of hypertension in the population has led to a reduction in cerebrovascular disease including intracerebral haemorrhage (Soltero et al., 1978; Co-operative Group, 1982; Tanaka et al., 1982; Nicholls and Johansen, 1983) but not to a decrease in the incidence of subarachnoid haemorrhage (Phillips et al., 1980). Secondly, the development of computerized axial tomography (CT scanning) and its use in the investigation of patients with strokes has allowed more accurate clinical evaluation of the primary pathology, thus enabling haematomas to be clearly distinguished from cerebral infarcts (Tanaka et al., 1982; Ojemann and Heros, 1983).

Detailed follow-up programmes, such as the Framingham Study (Sacco et al., 1982) over a period of 26 years, give an indication of the relative incidence of different types of stroke and their mortality rates. Among a population of 5209 men and women who were between 30 and 62 years of age on entry to the Study, there were 394 strokes in 26 years (198 in men and 196 in women). The distribution, with 30-day mortality figures in parentheses, was:

Atherothrombotic cerebral infarction	57%	(15%)
Cerebral embolus	16%	(46%)
Intracerebral haemorrhage	4%	(82%)
Subarachnoid haemorrhage	10%	(46%)
Transient ischaemic attacks	10%	
Stroke from other causes	3%	

The mean age range in this study for all strokes was 60–70 years, and hypertension was a major contributory factor. Of recurrent strokes, 65 per cent were atherothrombotic cerebral infarction but the recurrence rate was reduced by treatment of hypertension, particularly in men. Intracranial haemorrhage, both intracerebral and subarachnoid, had a high mortality at 30 days. Although reported mortality rates differ according to the period and population surveyed, among stroke patients the high mortality of intracranial haemorrhage is in general higher than in other types of stroke (Matsumoto et al., 1973).

The two major causes of death in spontaneous intracerebral haemorrhage are rupture into the ventricles and brain stem compression due to transtentorial herniation from an expanding cerebral mass (see Chapter 2), whereas early death from subarachnoid haemorrhage is usually a result of widespread cerebral infarction or concomitant intracerebral haemorrhage.

In the pre-CT scan era, when the precise diagnosis was often confirmed only at autopsy, the high mortality of intracerebral haemorrhage in particular led to an overestimate of the incidence of intracerebral haemorrhage among stroke patients. CT scanning, however, has allowed better evaluation of the incidence of intracerebral haemorrhage and its differentiation from infarction; it has also shown a higher proportion of small intracerebral haemorrhages and a lower mortality rate than was previously estimated in post-mortem studies (Douglas and Haerer, 1982).

Detailed post-mortem records of The London Hospital (D.S. Russell, 1954) and of the National Hospital for Nervous Diseases in London (as set out in Table 5.1 and in previous editions of this book), give valuable information about the relative incidence of spontaneous haemorrhage in different parts of the brain in patient populations prior to the widespread treatment of hypertension. Russell (1954) excluded all varieties in which trauma played a part, and all neonatal haemorrhages. She recorded only cases in which there were significantly large haematomas (in the brain stem of 1.5 cm diameter or more, in the cerebrum 3 cm or more).

The London Hospital is a general hospital and the National Hospital for Nervous Diseases is a neurological hospital, and this probably accounts for the greater frequency of hypertensive cases, blood diseases and mycotic aneurysms in The London Hospital figures. In 3.5–4 per cent of cases, the cause of the haemorrhage was not found. Some of these were probably due to saccular aneurysms or to small cryptic venous or arteriovenous malformations, such as those described by Crawford and Russell (1956), which were destroyed by the haemorrhage.

Hypertensive cerebrovascular disease

There are widespread changes throughout the body in patients with hypertension. Cardiomegaly, particularly with left ventricular hypertrophy, is a feature of long-standing hypertension and, in the absence of valvular disease, or cardiomyopathy, a significant increase in the weight and size of the heart suggests the presence of hypertension. In long-standing benign hypertension there is an increase in atherosclerosis affecting the larger blood vessels, including the carotid and intracranial cerebral arteries (Evans, 1965). In addition, the smaller arteries and arterioles in the kidney and brain show changes which are an accentuation of the thickening and hyalinization of blood vessel walls which occur with age (Russell, 1963; Heptinstall, 1983). The malignant phase of hypertension is characterized by endothelial cell damage and fibrinoid necrosis of arteriolar walls (Sinclair, Antonovych and Mostofi, 1976).

Blood vessel changes in hypertension are usually most severe in the kidneys, and depend upon the time course and the severity of the hypertension. There is little detectable change in the early stages of benign hypertension but in long-standing hypertension there is arteriosclerosis of the arcuate vessels in the kidney with fibrous thickening of the intima and a reduction in their lumina. Fraying and splitting of the internal elastic lamina are seen and some thickening of the media may be observed (Heptinstall, 1983). There is thickening of the intima and duplication of the elastic lamina in interlobar arteries. Arterioles, less than 100 μm in diameter, exhibit intimal thickening with hyalinization of the subintimal regions and some medial hypertrophy. This hyaline arteriolar sclerosis is, in effect, an accentuation of an ageing change in these vessels. Arteries and arterioles within the brain are also affected by hypertension but although the changes are similar to those in the kidney, they are usually not so severe (Russell, 1963; Evans, 1965).

Inspection of a brain at autopsy from a young normotensive patient reveals thin-walled cerebral arteries on the surface; the vessels are usually collapsed and blood can be seen through the translucent walls. In hypertensive patients, however, the major vessels of the circle of Willis are usually atherosclerotic, fibrotic and often increased in diameter; they remain rigidly open and do not collapse in the same way as normal

Table 5.1 Causes of spontaneous intracranial haemorrhage as determined from post-mortem records.

The London Hospital, 1912–52 (D. S. Russell, 1954)*		
Hypertensive		232
Basal ganglia	151	
Cerebral white matter	21	
Subcortical (cerebrum)	4	
Meninges	6	
Pons and midbrain	32	
Cerebellum	18	
Defects of cerebral arteries (92 cases with saccular aneurysms)		96
Blood diseases		36
Acute leukaemia	15	
Thrombocytopenia	13	
Aplastic anaemia	3	
Other anaemias	3	
Erythrocythaemia	1	
Haemophilia	1	
Mycotic aneurysm		28
Vascular hamartoma		21
Telangiectasis	0	
Multiple cavernous angioma	1	
Arteriovenous malformation ('angioma')	20	
Arteritis (no aneurysm)		13
Pyaemia	10	
Associated purulent leptomeningitis	3	
Neoplasm		9
Arterial degeneration (no cardiovascular hypertrophy)		7
Various		3
Cause not found		16
*The National Hospital, Queen Square, 1909–69**		
Hypertensive		143
Cerebrum	113	
Pons	12	
Cerebellum	13	
Pons and cerebellum	5	
Saccular (berry) aneurysm		246
Patients with a single aneurysm	200	
Patients with multiple aneurysms	46	
In the 246 patients there were 302 aneurysms distributed as follows:		
Internal carotid in cavernous sinus	4	
Junction of terminal portion of internal carotid and its branches	106	
Junction of anterior cerebral and anterior communicating	82	
Middle cerebral at first major branching	73	
Basilar artery and its branches	17	
Vertebral	8	
Anterior cerebral at distal points of branching	5	
Junction of internal carotid and ophthalmic artery	6	
Trigeminal artery (basilar/internal carotid)	1	
Blood diseases		2
Mycotic aneurysm		1
Vascular hamartoma		25
Telangiectasis (cerebellar)	2	
Arteriovenous malformation ('angioma') (cerebral 19, cerebellar 4)	23	
Four of these arteriovenous malformations also had saccular aneurysms, 1, 2, 3 and 4 in number respectively. In one case rupture of an aneurysm was the cause of death. These are not included among the saccular aneurysms.		
Haemorrhage into a neoplasm		14
Cause not found		18

* Excludes any in which trauma played a part and all neonatal haemorrhages. Includes only cases with significantly large haemorrhages (diameter 1.5 cm or more in brain stem or 3 cm or more in cerebrum).

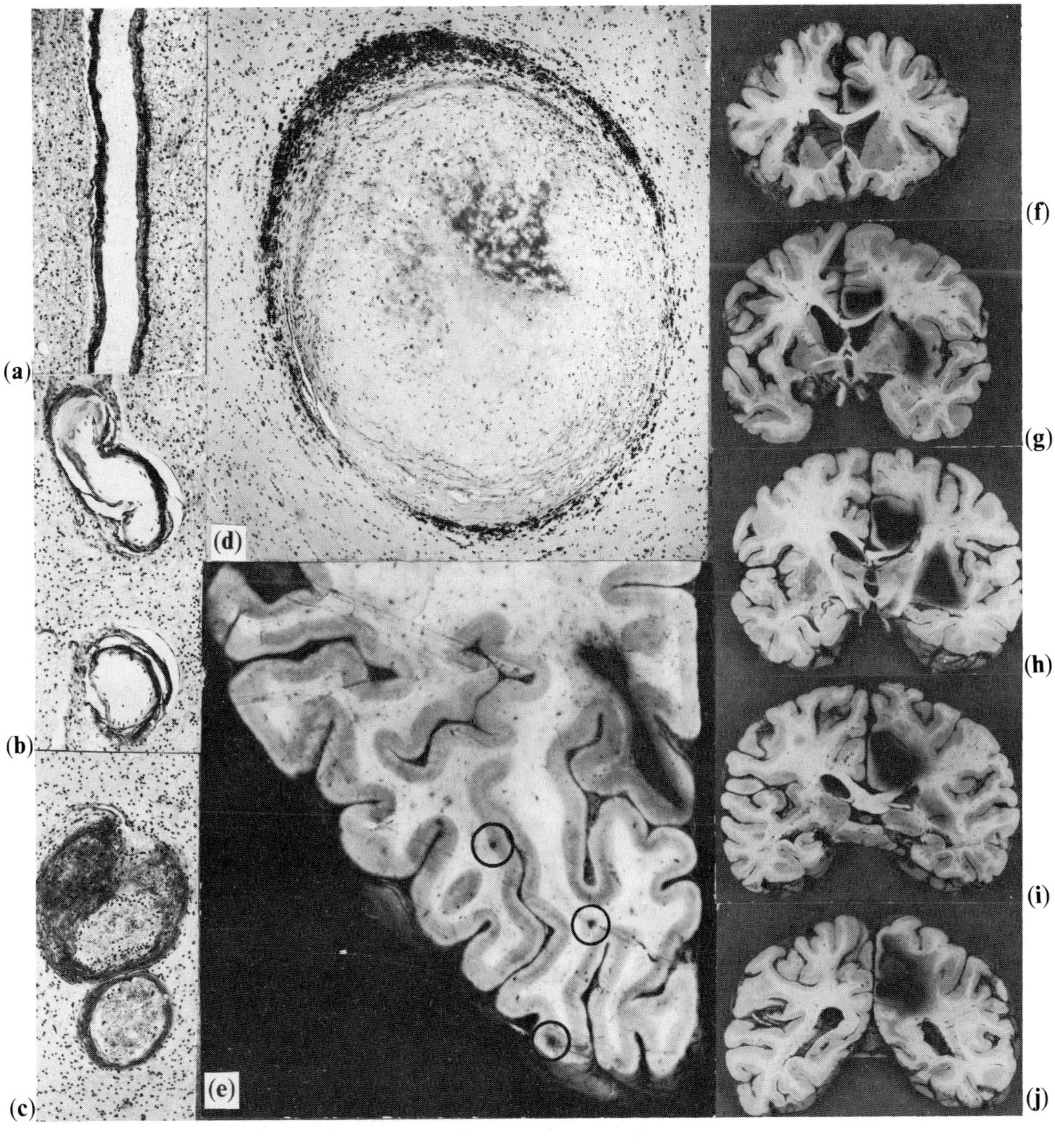

Fig. 5.1 Hypertensive vascular disease. These pictures illustrate the progressively more severe lesions which may be found in this condition. (**a**) to (**d**) are from one brain, (**e**) is from a different case and (**f**) to (**j**) are from a third case. (**a**) Small artery in the superficial cerebral white matter, showing hypertrophy of the muscle in the media, from a man aged 59 (blood pressure 240/160, heart weight 550 g) who died from uraemia. Small frontal and occipital haemorrhages were present. Celloidin; haematoxylin and van Gieson × 40. (**b**) Another small artery in the superficial white matter, showing fibrosis of the vessel wall. × 40. (**c**) Small arteries in the superficial white matter, showing degeneration of the wall and aneurysmal dilatation. In the lower vessel, the wall is necrotic but the lumen contains fluid blood. In the upper vessel the wall is necrotic and dilated but otherwise intact; the lumen is partly occluded by thrombus. A patent capillary is visible in the upper part of the picture; its lumen is in continuity with the residual lumen of the artery. × 40. (**d**) Microscopic appearance of a haemorrhagic lesion in the cortex, similar to those in (**e**). The wall of the original artery is necrotic and there has been haemorrhage into the surrounding tissue. The lumen is completely filled with old thrombus. Around this 'false aneurysm' there are macrophages containing haemosiderin, which appear dark in colour. × 50. (**e**) Horizontal section of the occipital lobe in a male aged 53 (blood pressure 250/150) with left ventricular hypertrophy. Small punctate haemorrhages (circles) are seen in the cortex and white matter. There is a slit-haematoma (upper right) involving the junction between the cortex and white matter, at which many miliary aneurysms are seen. (**f–j**) Coronal slices of the cerebral hemispheres of a patient aged 51 (blood pressure 190/125, heart weight 470 g), showing several recent haematomas (clinically 10 days' duration) in the white matter of the cingulate gyrus and the putamen. The cingulate haemorrhage measures 9 cm anteroposteriorly; an area of old haemorrhagic softening is present in the left corpus striatum.

young arteries. Even the smaller branches in the cerebral sulci have stiffened walls and retain their circular profiles when sectioned. Histologically, the changes in the larger intracranial arteries are indistinguishable from atherosclerosis.

Changes in the vessels within brain tissue are most marked in hypertensive patients over the age of 50. Again, many of the changes appear to be an accentuation of age changes in these arteries (Russell, 1963). In the normal brain, small arteries and arterioles are thin walled and the arterioles are composed of up to three layers of smooth muscle and an incomplete internal elastic lamina (Roggendorf, Cervós-Navarro and Iglesias Rozas, 1981). The veins have very thin walls and larger lumina than the arteries. In hypertension, changes are seen in the small arteries and arterioles 50–300 μm in diameter. There is hypertrophy of the muscle in the media (Fig. 5.1a) (Cook and Yates, 1972) but in long-standing hypertension, particularly in older patients, the vessels become fibrotic and thickened (Fig. 5.1b). Hyaline change occurs in the subendothelial regions and in the media of vessels within the brain and in the smaller arteries in the meninges (Ziegler, 1972) as a result of an increase in thickness of the endothelial and smooth muscle basement membranes and due to the deposition of serum proteins in vessel walls (Amano, 1977; Roggendorf, Cervós-Navarro and Iglesias Rozas, 1981). Many of the changes affect only segments of a vessel or only part of its circumference. There may also be necrosis of vessel walls with aneurysmal dilatation, perivascular haemorrhage or thrombotic occlusion of the lumen (Fig. 5.1c–e). The changes differ from atherosclerosis of the larger arteries because there is little or no deposition of lipid within the small arteries and arterioles. As elsewhere in the body, elongation and tortuosity of the arteries in the brain accompany fibrosis of the vessel walls in ageing and in hypertension (Fig. 5.2).

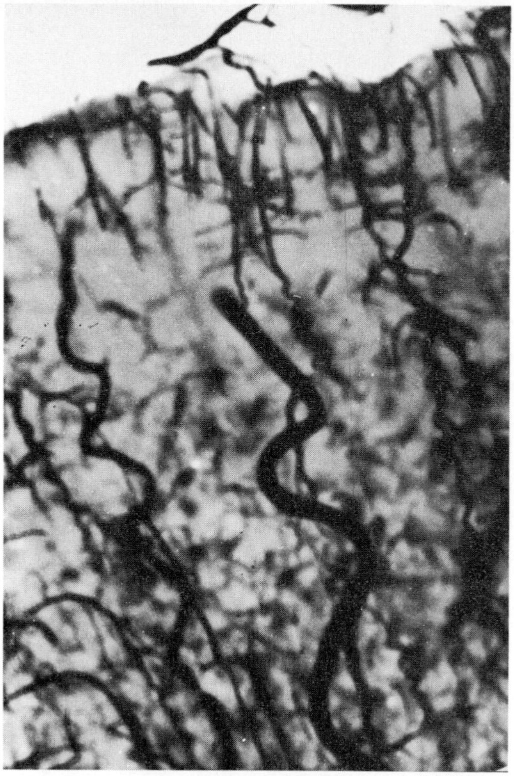

Fig. 5.2 Cleared thick section of cerebral cortex, showing arterial spiralling that occurs particularly in young hypertensive people. Injected specimen × 10. (Courtesy of Professor P.O. Yates)

Miliary aneurysms (microaneurysms) in hypertension

Since these structures were first postulated by Charcot and Bouchard in 1868, there has been much discussion about their existence, origin and role in hypertensive intracerebral haemorrhage. Injection of radio-opaque material into the cerebral arteries of hypertensive and normotensive patients *post mortem* (Russell, 1963; Cole and Yates, 1967a, b) allows of the radiological identification and subsequent histological examination of these miliary aneurysms. They occur on small arteries 100–300 μm in diameter and are seen as outpouchings of the vessel walls (Fig. 5.3), often partly filled by thrombus (Fig. 5.4). Such aneurysms are rare under the age of 50 years (Fig. 5.5) and occur most commonly in the brains of hypertensive patients. They should, however, be distinguished from pseudoaneurysms which are due to blood accumulating around a vessel (see Fig. 5.1d) rather than to dilatation of the vessel lumen (Cole and Yates, 1967c).

In detailed surveys of the distribution of true miliary aneurysms in hypertensive brains, Russell (1963) and Cole and Yates (1967a) showed that miliary aneurysms were most commonly located in the putamen, pallidum and thalamus but were also present in the caudate nucleus, internal capsule, centrum semiovale and cortical

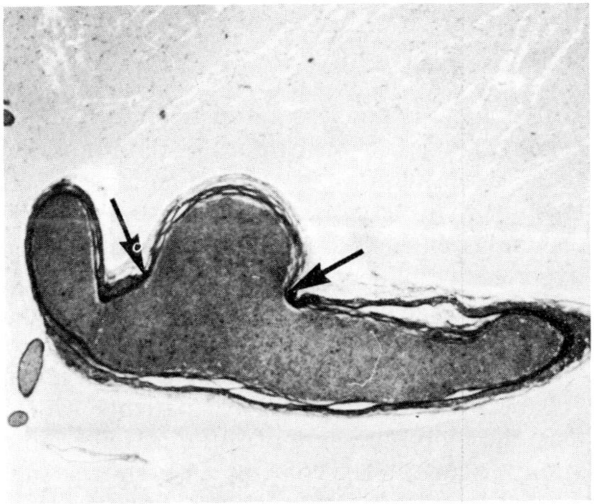

Fig. 5.3 Miliary aneurysm. Small artery with aneurysm filled by gelatin cast. Arrows indicate points at which the medial coat and the internal elastic lamina stop at the base of the sac which is formed of collagen only. (Courtesy of Professor P.O. Yates)

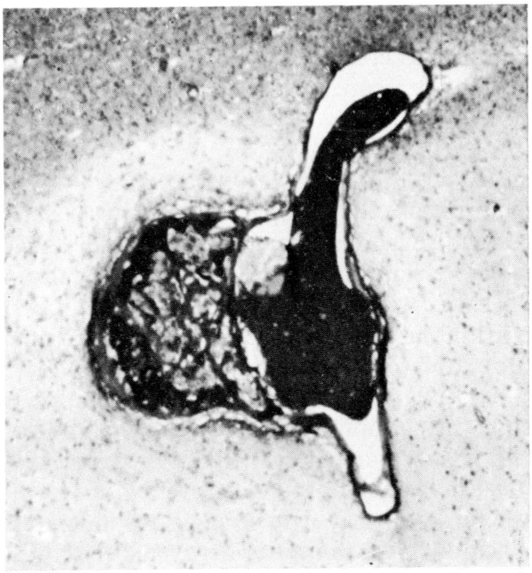

Fig. 5.4 Miliary aneurysm. Small intracerebral artery with aneurysm sac on the left side partially occluded by organizing thrombus. (Lumen of vessel contains shrunken gelatin cast.) (Courtesy of Professor P.O. Yates)

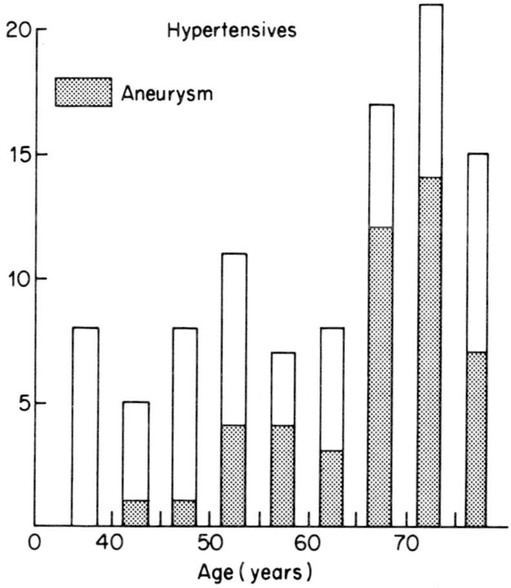

Fig. 5.5 The incidence of miliary aneurysms (microaneurysms) at various ages in the brains of 100 hypertensive people. (Courtesy of Professor P.O. Yates)

grey matter. Miliary aneurysms were identified in 71 per cent of hypertensive patients in the 65- to 69-year age group (Cole and Yates, 1967a). The aneurysms were often seen at branches of vessels and were multiple on some arteries. They occurred mainly on the lateral branches of the striate arteries or on the penetrating vessels in the cerebral cortex. Histological examination showed that the walls of the aneurysms are fibrous and thin (see Figs. 5.3 and 5.4), and lacking in smooth muscle or elastic lamina. Small haemorrhages, haemosiderin-laden macrophages and gliosis are seen in the brain tissue surrounding the aneurysms.

The implication of rupture of miliary aneurysms as the cause of intracerebral haemorrhage comes from the observation that the miliary aneurysms are concentrated in the central grey matter, the subcortical regions and in the internal capsules; these are all regions of the brain in which small and massive cerebral haemorrhages usually occur (Cole and Yates, 1967a, b). Some miliary aneurysms were observed in the brains of normotensive patients but not in the numbers in which they appeared in older hypertensives (see Fig. 5.5) (Russell, 1963; Cole and Yates, 1967a). This suggests that the aneurysms form as part of the wear and tear process during ageing and that this is accentuated by hypertension. Miliary aneurysms also occur in the brains of hypertensive rats (Amano, 1977).

Changes in arterioles in malignant hypertension

Patients with severely elevated diastolic blood pressure of 130 mmHg or more may develop papilloedema, retinal haemorrhages and hypertensive encephalopathy (Healton et al., 1982). Autoregulation of the cerebral circulation may fail (Strandgaard, 1978) and hypertensive encephalopathy may ensue. In such patients there are severe vascular changes with fibrinoid necrosis and thrombotic occlusion of arterioles within the brain (Fig. 5.6) (Chester et al. 1978).

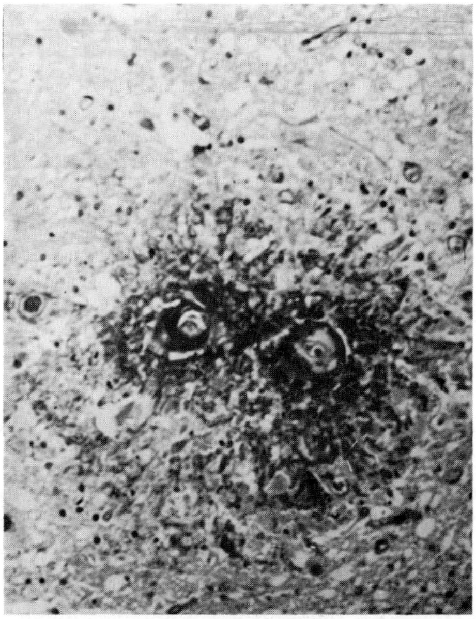

Fig. 5.6 Malignant hypertension. Two branches of a small artery, showing necrosis of their walls and fibrinous exudate. The surrounding brain is necrotic and oedematous. (Courtesy of Professor P.O. Yates)

Similar changes are seen in the kidneys in the 1–7 per cent of patients who pass into the malignant phase of hypertension (Heptinstall, 1983). Immunocytochemical studies have shown that IgG, complement, fibrinogen and albumin are all present in areas of fibrinoid necrosis in arteriolar walls (Paronetto, 1965). Intimal thickening with narrowing of vessels may be seen, and Sinclair, Antonovych and Mostofi (1976) suggest that the vessel changes are caused by endothelial cell damage leading to increased permeability and the leak of serum proteins and erythrocytes into the intima. Intimal thickening by the proliferation of myointimal cells is part of the healing and scarring process in the vessel wall.

Pathological changes in the brain in hypertension

Just as there is no clear-cut distinction between ageing changes in the arteries in the brain and their accentuation in long-standing hypertension, there is considerable overlap between changes seen in brain tissue in ageing and in hypertensive patients. There are, however, certain lesions in which hypertension is the most frequent precursor disease.

Cole and Yates (1968) conducted a survey of 100 brains from hypertensive patients with a diastolic blood pressure of 110 mmHg or more and 100 age-matched controls. They showed that cerebrovascular lesions were twice as common in hypertensive patients as in those with normal blood pressure. Hypertensives had a greater number of infarcts and haemorrhages, and there was an almost invariable association of massive intracerebral haemorrhage with hypertension. Many small haemorrhages occurred in the brains of hypertensive patients but the number of infarcts was only slightly increased in the brains of hypertensives compared with those with a normal blood pressure.

Lacunae

The brains of older people, but more especially those with hypertension, characteristically have small holes which can be seen macroscopically in the basal ganglia and white matter. Their appearance in the basal ganglia (*état lacunaire*) and in the white matter (*état criblé*) appear to have no correlation with large haemorrhages or large infarcts despite their prominence in patients with hypertension (Cole and Yates, 1968). Microscopically, lacunae may be smooth-walled cysts with a vessel in the centre or they may be small cystic infarcts or haemorrhagic cavities. There has been much discussion regarding the origin of lacunae and confusion has arisen over their precise definition. Fisher (1969), in a detailed study of serial sections of brain, showed that many lacunae were small infarcts, and he demonstrated segmental vessel disease and thrombotic occlusion in the region of the lacunae. Hughes (1965), on the other hand, proposed that lacunae around blood vessels were caused by elongation of the vessel and pulsatile trauma to the surrounding brain. The presence of haemosiderin-containing macrophages in many lacunae suggested that they could also be caused by small haemorrhages (Cole and Yates, 1968).

Frequently, a lacuna has a relatively normal vessel in its centre and an expanded perivascular space which is traversed by reticulin fibres. On the other hand, giant lacunae (Poirier, 1983), which may be up to several millimetres in diameter, appear to be empty. It is probable that lacunae within the basal ganglia of older individuals and those with hypertension have multiple origins. Some are small infarcts recognizable by the presence of macrophages within the lacunae, and others may be due to small haemorrhages; those around relatively normal vessels are true *état lacunaire* (Cole and Yates, 1968), and may be a reflection of atrophy of the surrounding brain due to infarcts in the vicinity. Widening of perivascular spaces is seen in other diseases and even in infants with hydrocephalus in whom there has been destruction and a reduction in volume of cerebral white matter (Weller and Williams, 1975).

Intracerebral haemorrhage

Patients with hypertension present clinically with a variety of neurological symptoms and signs (Ziegler, 1972); headaches are common and seizures may occur. Focal neurological deficits due to small infarcts, or haemorrhages in the brain, are a feature of hypertension, and there may also be visual disturbances with papilloedema and retinal haemorrhages.

Intracerebral haematomas in hypertensive patients show a wide range in size. Small perivascular collections of blood (see Fig. 5.1c) or accumulations of haemosiderin-containing macrophages (Fig. 5.7) are frequently found in the brains of hypertensive patients. In addition to the small haematomas, slit-haematomas several centimetres in length may be found in the deep cortex and white matter of hypertensive patients (see Fig. 5.1e) (Cole and Yates, 1967b). Haematomas several centimetres in diameter (see Fig. 5.1f–j) are not always fatal (Rudick, 1981). They may be multiple but are frequently sited in the basal ganglia (Douglas and Haerer, 1982) in hypertensive patients. Lobar haemorrhages in the white matter (see Fig. 5.1i and j) do occur in hypertensive patients, but may also be found in the absence of hypertension or as a complication of haematological disorders, arteriovenous malformations or metastatic tumours (Ropper and Davis, 1980). Small haemorrhages in the basal ganglia (Fig. 5.8) may cause little displacement of brain and little destruction of brain tissue but massive haemorrhages in the basal ganglia or thalamus (Fig. 5.9) may rupture into the ventricles (Weisberg, 1979) or through the cerebral hemispheres into the subdural space (Schwartz, 1972). The majority of massive intracerebral haemorrhages occur in hypertensive patients but they may also be seen in normotensive individuals (Weisberg, 1979).

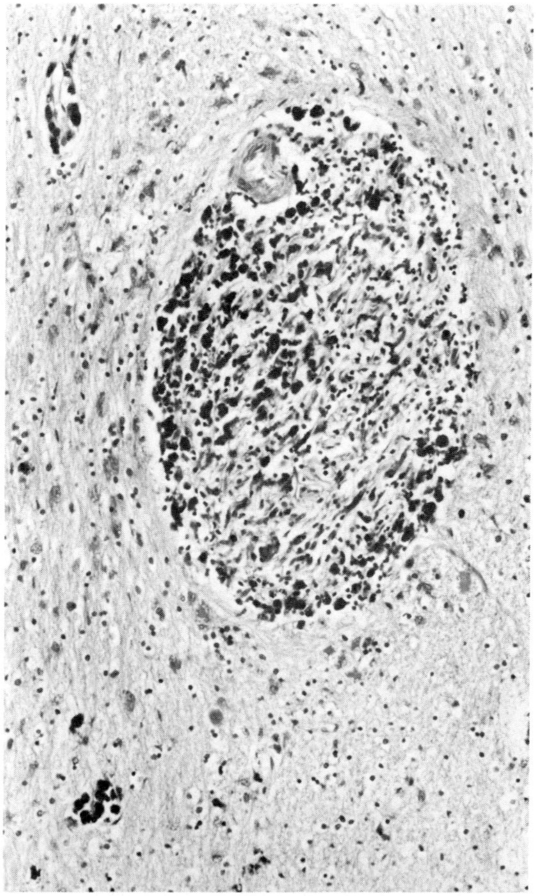

Fig. 5.7 Small perivascular haemorrhage. An accumulation of haemosiderin-containing macrophages (darkly staining) is seen around a vessel (top left). Haematoxylin and eosin × 160.

There have been many surveys which have demonstrated the value of CT scans in the precise diagnosis of cerebral haemorrhage. Douglas and Haerer (1982) investigated 70 patients with intracerebral haemorrhage; 80 per cent had proven hypertension and there was an early mortality

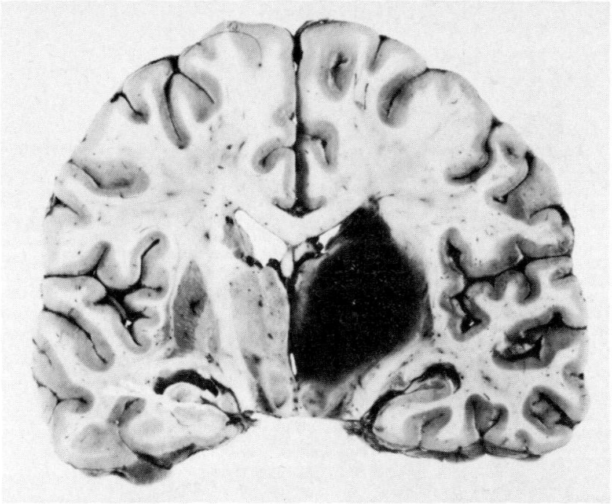

Fig. 5.8 Hypertensive intracerebral haemorrhage. A relatively small recent haematoma involves the thalamus, the internal capsule and the lentiform nucleus on the right. There is little displacement of the brain. (Courtesy of Dr I. Janota)

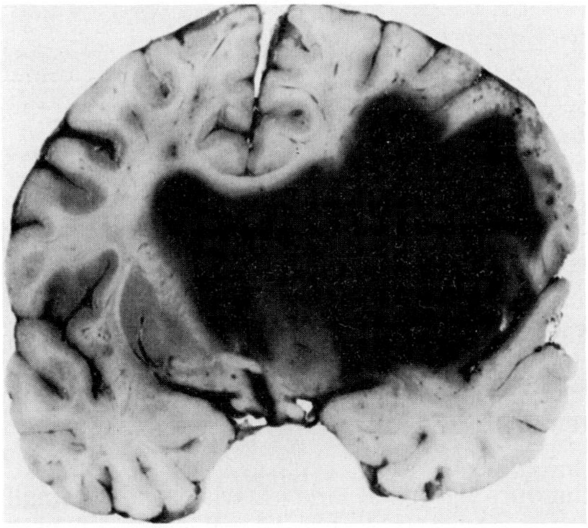

Fig. 5.9 Hypertensive intracerebral haemorrhage. A massive recent haemorrhage has occurred in the area of the right basal ganglia and has ruptured into the lateral ventricles. There is displacement of the midline towards the left.

rate of 40 per cent. They excluded from this survey subarachnoid haemorrhage, arteriovenous malformation and haemorrhagic infarcts, and concluded that those patients who survive a primary hypertensive intracerebral haemorrhage have a good prognosis and are not likely to rebleed. The age range was 30–70 years but this may have been influenced by the age incidence of hypertension in the population studied. Of the intracerebral haematomas, 44 per cent were more than 5 cm in diameter and the prognosis was worse if they were large and when there was extension into the ventricles. Sixty-three per cent of the haematomas were in the basal ganglia or thalamus, 23 per cent were lobar haemorrhages, 11 per cent were in the cerebellum and 3 per cent were in the brain stem. The early mortality rate for haemorrhage into the cerebral hemispheres was between 30 and 40 per cent depending upon the site, whereas cerebellar haemorrhage carried a 50 per cent mortality rate; the two patients with brain stem haemorrhage died. The mortality rate in patients with acute cerebellar haemorrhage is lower in those who are treated by evacuation of the haematoma (Chin and Carney, 1983), but in 60 per cent of untreated cerebellar haemorrhages the course is progressive, death being due to compression of the brain stem (Little, Tubman and Etheir, 1978). Hypertension was an antecedent factor in 70 per cent of the cerebellar haemorrhages reviewed by Little, Tubman and Etheir (1978).

Pathological studies (see Table 5.1) confirm the relatively high incidence of haemorrhage into the basal ganglia in hypertensive patients but also emphasize the occurrence of haemorrhage into the brain stem and cerebellum. If the patient dies immediately or within a few hours of an intracerebral haemorrhage, the blood clot forms a dark red mass displacing the surrounding brain tissue and even the whole hemisphere (see Fig. 5.9). When the haematoma extends into the ventricles, blood may escape from the fourth ventricle and spread into the subarachnoid space around the brain stem. Large haematomas may cause herniation of the parahippocampal gyrus through the opening of the tentorium cerebelli, leading to secondary haemorrhage in the midbrain. Primary haemorrhages into the midbrain or pons usually cause extensive tissue damage and have a 60 per cent mortality (Nakajima, 1983). Cerebellar haematomas may result in brain stem compression by their mass effect or from herniation of the cerebellar tonsils through the foramen magnum.

A patient may survive the initial haemorrhage, especially if the haematoma is small and in a cerebral hemisphere. Gradually, the haematoma turns brown and becomes a soft semiliquid granular mass. After several years, all that remains is a cyst with brown or orange stained walls—the so-called *apoplectic cyst*.

Histologically, there is sharp demarcation of a recent haematoma from the surrounding brain. Within the first 24 hours, dead and disrupted neurons and glia are observed in the tissue immediately adjacent to the blood clot. Also at this time the adjacent tissue starts to swell because of the cerebral oedema. During the next few days and weeks increasing numbers of monocytes and macrophages invade the edges of the haematoma and the surrounding brain tissue. The coiled remains of dead or hypocellular arteries may be seen in the tissue at this time, and may be mistaken for parts of an arteriovenous malformation. Once the haematoma has been present for a week or more the inflammatory reaction with macrophages and reactive astrocytes in the tissue surrounding the haemorrhage is similar to that seen adjacent to an infarct. One major difference, however, is the presence of large amounts of blood and, later, blood pigment within macrophages and astrocytes around the haematoma. Several years after the haemorrhage, the wall of the residual cyst is gliotic, and haemosiderin is present within macrophages and within the cytoplasm of many of the astrocytes.

Pathogenesis of intracerebral haemorrhage The presence of miliary aneurysms (Charcot-Bouchard aneurysms) at the major sites of haemorrhage into the cerebral hemispheres and brain stem and their increased incidence in hypertensive patients (Russell, 1963; Cole and Yates, 1967a; Nakajima, 1983) suggest that the haemorrhage may be the result of rupture of such aneurysms.

Takebayashi and Kaneko (1983) examined the lenticulostriate arteries around and within intracerebral haematomas at surgery and *post mortem*. They identified ruptured arteries in 50 per cent of cases. In patients with large and fatal haematomas it appeared that larger arteries (500–700 μm in diameter) were ruptured, whereas smaller vessels (less than 300 μm in diameter) ruptured to form the smaller haematomas that could be evacuated surgically. Rupture of a miliary aneurysm was identified in only 2 out of 61 ruptures of vessels in their series (Takebayashi and Kaneko, 1983), but histological examination of the damaged vessels showed that in the other 59 vessels the site of rupture was at or near a bifurcation. Breaks in the elastic lamina, medial fibrosis and intimal thickening were seen in many of the smaller arteries. These observations suggest that weakening of the wall of small blood vessels in hypertension, particularly by the replacement of smooth muscle by fibrous tissue or by necrosis, may result in rupture of vessels with or without the prior formation of a microaneurysm. It is still not clear, however, why certain arteries such as the branches of the lenticulostriate arteries are particularly prone to rupture. The site of intracerebral haemorrhage in hypertensive rats is similar to that observed in man, and Yamori et al. (1976) have suggested that the recurrent branching of the lenticulostriate arteries in both species may be a factor in the induction of vessel wall changes and in haemorrhage.

Hypertensive encephalopathy

In the majority of patients with hypertension brain damage, including infarction and haemorrhage, accompanies long-term and variable elevation of the blood pressure. Hypertensive encephalopathy, however, supervenes in a small proportion of cases, particularly in previously normotensive patients who suffer a severe acute elevation of blood pressure as in eclampsia or acute nephritis; it may also accompany the accelerated malignant phase of hypertension (Dinsdale, 1982). Clinically, hypertensive encephalopathy presents with severe headaches, drowsiness, vomiting, convulsions, focal neurological signs or coma (Rail and Perkin, 1980). The diastolic pressure is raised to 130 mmHg or more, and papilloedema with retinal haemorrhages may be seen (Healton et al., 1982). On CT scan (Rail and Perkin, 1980) there is evidence of cerebral oedema with areas of low attenuation in the white matter involving mainly the superior and posterior parts of the cerebral hemispheres. These changes usually resolve within 3 months of treatment.

Pathological studies have shown that patients dying in the acute stages of hypertensive encephalopathy have an increased brain weight with flattening of the cerebral gyri, reduction in the size of the ventricles and oedema of the white matter (Feigin and Popoff, 1963; Adachi et al., 1966; Dinsdale, 1982). Petechial haemorrhages and fibrinoid necrosis of the walls of small arteries are also seen. Oedema may not be present if patients survive the acute stages (Dinsdale, 1982) but fibrinoid necrosis of the vessel walls persists and may be most severe in the brain stem (Chester et al., 1978).

Experimental studies have shown that hypertensive encephalopathy is associated with a high cerebral blood flow and breakdown of the blood–brain barrier with consequent cerebral oedema (Nag, Robertson and Dinsdale, 1977; Strandgaard, 1978; Johansson and Linder, 1981). In man, the cerebral oedema is increased by hypercapnia (Skinhip and Strandgaard, 1973). Normally, cerebrovascular autoregulation ensures that a constant blood flow in brain tissue is maintained by varying the calibre of the smallest resistance vessels (i.e. the arteries and arterioles). If the blood pressure is raised to 40–60 per cent above the normal level in very sudden or prolonged hypertension, autoregulation fails and cerebral blood flow increases. After initial vasoconstriction there is vasodilatation, blood–brain barrier dysfunction, cerebral oedema and hypertensive encephalopathy (Strandgaard, 1978).

Dementia and Binswanger's disease

Dementia, often with focal neurological signs and stepwise deterioration, is a well recognized occurrence in hypertensive patients as multi-infarct dementia (Hachinski, Lassen and Marshall, 1974). This type of dementia, however, is not restricted to patients with hypertension (see Chapter 20). The infarcts, in most cases, are the result of multiple small emboli arising from the heart or the carotid arteries. Examination of the brain in such cases reveals infarcts of varying size and age in the cortex and white matter.

In a minority of patients with dementia and hypertension, there is diffuse damage in the deep white matter of the cerebral hemispheres, due to infarction. The cortex, in contrast, is well preserved (Janota, 1981). This type of involvement of the brain was recognized by Binswanger (1894) and has been known as the chronic progressive subcortical encephalitis of Binswanger or merely Binswanger's disease. The changes in white matter have been recognized as areas of reduced density on CT scan (Rosenberg et al., 1979; Valentine, Moseley and Kendall, 1980), and although most patients with Binswanger's disease have a history of hypertension (Caplan and Schoene, 1978) the disorder is also seen in normotensive individuals (Loizou, Jefferson and Smith, 1982).

Major pathological changes are seen in the white matter in Binswanger's disease. The cerebral white matter is grey and shrunken and may show some cavitation; the corpus callosum frequently is reduced in thickness. Histologically, there may be diffuse loss of myelin and axons from the white matter with widespread gliosis and invasion by macrophages, or clearly demarcated foci of myelin destruction in the white matter (Fig. 5.10). The extracellular space in the white matter is increased and this produces pallor of myelin staining in the deep white matter corresponding to the decreased density on the CT scan. Small arteries and arterioles within the white matter have the thickened, fibrous and hyaline walls of obliterative arteriosclerosis (Loizou, Jefferson and Smith, 1982). Although infarcts may be seen in the white matter of the cerebral hemispheres in the brain stem and in other parts of the brain, a striking feature of this disorder is the relative preservation of the cerebral cortex.

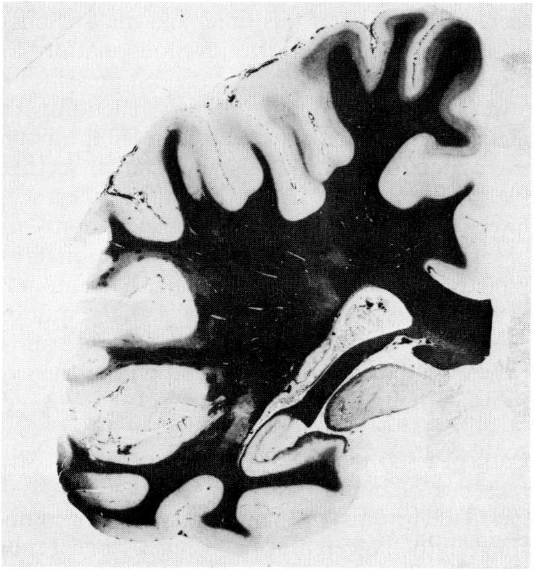

Fig. 5.10 Multiple, often clearly demarcated, foci of myelin destruction in the white matter of a hypertensive patient of the type seen in Binswanger's subcortical encephalopathy. Celloidin; Loyez.

The pathogenesis of Binswanger's disease is unclear. Janota (1981) suggests that there is poor perfusion of the deep white matter and that this may occur in patients treated for hypertension. The lower limit of autoregulation, below which cerebral blood flow is reduced, is raised in untreated or uncontrolled hypertension, and tolerance to acute hypotension is decreased in these individuals. It is in this way that some hypertensive patients may suffer reduced cerebral perfusion during treatment with hypotensive drugs (Strandgaard, 1978).

Arterial changes in experimental hypertension

Many of the changes seen in arteries and the brain in human hypertension may also be seen in spontaneously hypertensive rats, a breed obtained originally by mating a hypertensive male with a hypertensive female (Okamoto, 1969). Hypertensive cerebral lesions are seen in 8 per cent of these animals; 19 per cent suffer myocardial infarction and 39 per cent pass into a malignant phase of their hypertension. Amano (1977) studied a group of spontaneously hypertensive rats and showed that the blood pressure rose at the age of 6 weeks and stabilized at 210 mmHg at 20 weeks. Some of the animals suffered cerebral haemorrhage and infarction. Examination of the intracerebral arteries revealed hyaline change of the media which, on electron microscopy, was seen to be due to excessive thickening of the basement membrane of the endothelial cells and smooth muscle cells in addition to the deposition of cellular debris and acid mucopolysaccharides. Fibrinoid material within the walls consisted of fibrin whereas atypical fibrinoid was composed of plasma proteins. Ogata et al. (1980) examined the brains of spontaneously hypertensive rats which developed malignant hypertension at the age of 4–5 months; at the time of the study the animals were 11–15 months old. In those animals which developed abnormal diffuse neurological signs, mainly reflected in their behaviour, there were small haemorrhages in the cerebral hemispheres, multiple cystic infarcts and cerebral oedema. Fibrinoid necrosis was seen in 84 per cent of the intracerebral blood vessels in these rats and mainly involved arterioles less than 30 μm in diameter; the walls of the vessels were thick and homogeneous on microscopical examination. Microaneurysms were present within the arterial tree and perivascular lymphocytes and macrophages were seen. Some small vessels were thrombosed and there were multiple petechial haemorrhages. These changes are very similar to those described in malignant hypertension and hypertensive encephalopathy in man (Chester et al., 1978; Dinsdale, 1982).

The role of cerebral oedema in the pathogenesis of hypertensive encephalopathy has been studied in rats made hypertensive by the administration of amphetamines and bicuculline, or by the induction of renal hypertension. In these cases, and particularly in the renal hypertensives, there is extravasation of protein and fluid into the brain which corresponds to the oedema seen in human hypertensive encephalopathy (Johansson and Linder, 1981). Increased vascular permeability, however, is not a constant feature in spontaneously hypertensive rats (Limas, Westrum and Limas, 1980; Nag, Robertson and Dinsdale, 1980).

Aneurysms

The term 'aneurysm' means dilatation of an artery. In relation to the central nervous system we are concerned with:

1. Saccular (berry) aneurysms.
2. Atherosclerotic fusiform aneurysms.
3. Spontaneous and post-traumatic arteriovenous aneurysms or fistulae between the internal carotid artery and the cavernous sinus.
4. Dissecting aneurysms.
5. Mycotic aneurysms.
6. Intracerebral miliary aneurysms (microaneurysms)—see previous section.

Saccular aneurysms

Incidence Saccular aneurysms occur at the bifurcations of intracranial arteries in between 1 and 2 per cent of the population (McCormick and Nofzinger, 1965); in individuals with aneurysms they are multiple in 20–30 per cent (see Fig. 5.14) (Andrews and Spiegel, 1979).

Site Most aneurysms arise from the terminal portion of the internal carotid artery and from the major branches of the anterior portion of the circle of Willis. Although the figures in various surveys differ, approximately 40 per cent of all aneurysms are related to the intracranial portion of the internal carotid artery (usually at the junction of the internal carotid and posterior communicating arteries), 30 per cent are in the region of the anterior communicating artery, and 20 per cent are on a middle cerebral artery mainly at the proximal point(s) of branching (Fig. 5.11). Some 5–10 per cent of aneurysms are associated with the posterior cerebral arteries, with the basilar and vertebral arteries, or with other vessels in the posterior fossa (Andrews and Spiegel, 1979, 1981). Almost all saccular aneurysms arise at or very close to points of division of arteries (Crawford, 1959; Rhoton, 1980).

Age An analysis of previously published figures shows that 60 per cent of saccular aneurysms are diagnosed in patients 40–60 years of age with a peak incidence in the 50- to 60-year age group in both sexes (McCormick and Nofzinger, 1965; Andrews and Spiegel, 1979). Subarachnoid or intracerebral haemorrhage due to rupture of a saccular aneurysm also has a peak incidence in the 40- to 60-year age group (Locksley, Sahs and Knowler, 1966). Less than 10 per cent of aneurysms are encountered under the age of 30 (Andrews and Spiegel, 1979) and only about 2 per cent under 20 years of age (Patel and Richardson, 1971). Although there is a male predominance in patients under 20 years of age, the female/male ratio is 2:1 in patients over 60 years of age (Andrews and Spiegel, 1979).

Predisposing factors for saccular aneurysms No constant predisposing factor has been identified but there is an increased incidence of saccular aneurysms in certain disorders in which there is either a defect in connective tissue or blood flow through the cerebral circulation. Such disorders include fibromuscular dysplasia (Mettinger, 1982), polycystic kidney disease (Wakabayashi et al., 1983), moyamoya disease (Yabumoto et al., 1983) and coarctation of the aorta (Le Blanc et al., 1968). Perhaps one of the better documented predisposing factors for saccular aneurysms is their association with arteriovenous malformations. Between 3 and 9 per cent of patients with cerebral arteriovenous malformations have saccular aneurysms, and it is estimated that between 37 and 77 per cent of the aneurysms arise on arteries which are haemodynamically related to the arteriovenous malformation (Perret and Nishioka, 1966; Suzuki and Omuna, 1979; Hayashi et al., 1981; Miyasaka, Wolpert and Prager, 1982). Although there are reports of an increased incidence of saccular aneurysms in some families (Fox and Ko, 1980; Morooka and Waga, 1983), in the great majority of cases there is no family history.

Hypertension was considered to be an important factor in the formation of saccular aneurysms (Stehbens, 1972). However, in a more recent clinicopathological analysis of 250 patients with aneurysms, McCormick and Schmalsteig (1977) found no evidence of an increase in the incidence of hypertension over an age- and sex-matched control autopsy population. They concluded that saccular aneurysms can arise in the absence of arterial hypertension and that they also rupture in the absence of fixed hypertension. Andrews and Spiegel (1979) reached similar conclusions in their study of 350 patients, 212 of whom had aneurysms. They showed that hypertension was no more significant or prevalent in the population with aneurysms than in an age-matched general population except for females aged 18–54 years. They did show, however, that under the age of 55 years both male and female hypertensive patients are twice as likely to have multiple aneurysms as normotensive patients. With increasing age, and rising systolic and diastolic blood pressure, there was a higher incidence of multiple aneurysms in female patients.

Macroscopical appearances Aneurysms vary widely in their size and shape; some are only 1–2 mm in diameter whereas others are 5–10 mm in diameter. Giant aneurysms are those more than 2.5 cm in diameter; they are discussed below. Smaller aneurysms may be destroyed as they rupture and blood escapes into the subarachnoid space or into the cerebral hemispheres. The detection of aneurysms at post-mortem may be difficult as they may be obscured by large amounts of blood clot in the subarachnoid space or by intracerebral haematoma (Figs. 5.11 to 5.14); guidance to the site of the aneurysm from cerebral angiography or CT scan is often invaluable. Even in the absence of recent subarachnoid haemorrhage, there may be evidence of previous bleeding from an aneurysm as shown by orange discoloration of the arachnoid and surrounding brain. Many aneurysms are thin-walled, but fairly rigid berry-like pouches may

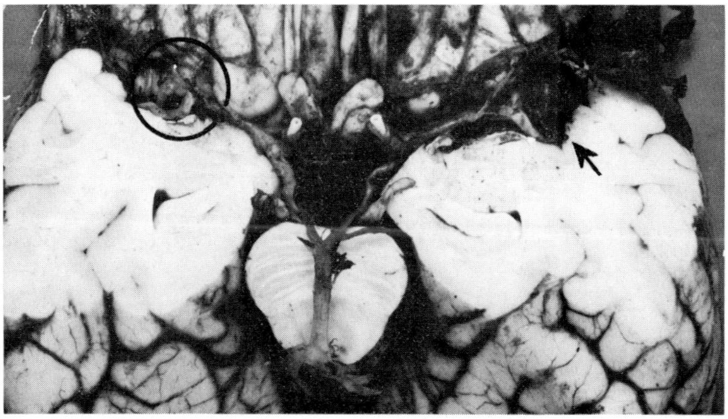

Fig. 5.11 Ruptured saccular aneurysm on the left middle cerebral artery (arrow). The blood has passed into the subarachnoid space of the insula and of the basal cisterns (from which it has been partly removed to display the aneurysm). The aneurysm is arising from the point of bifurcation of the artery in the lateral (sylvian) fissure. The corresponding point of branching of the right middle cerebral artery is ringed.

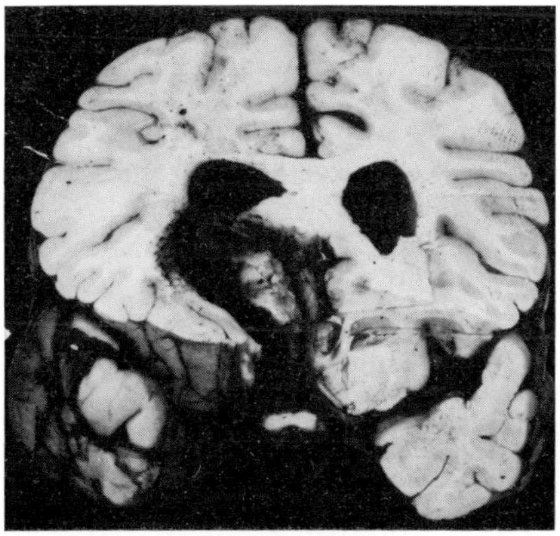

Fig. 5.12 Ruptured saccular aneurysm of the right anterior cerebral/anterior communicating artery. The blood has ploughed through the substance of the frontal lobe into the lateral ventricle.

arise from the arteries of the circle of Willis and its major branches; they also occur on the basilar and vertebral arteries or on other vessels in the posterior fossa. The walls of the aneurysm tend to be pale and opaque due to fibrous thickening. If the aneurysm has ruptured, it may be difficult to recognize, and only its frayed edges may be identifiable. In cases of massive subarachnoid haemorrhage where the site of the aneurysm has not already been established radiologically, preliminary removal of fresh blood clot and carrying out an extensive search for the aneurysm is advisable before fixing the brain because it is much more difficult to dissect fixed blood from the arteries. Not uncommonly, aneurysms on the circle of Willis bury themselves in the brain substance and do not protrude in an obvious fashion from the vessel (Rhoton, 1980). Lamellated blood clot is often seen within the lumen of larger aneurysms and occasionally may be a source of emboli into distal arteries (Fisher, Davidson and Marcus, 1980; Sakaki et al., 1980). Some aneurysms are completely fibrosed and the

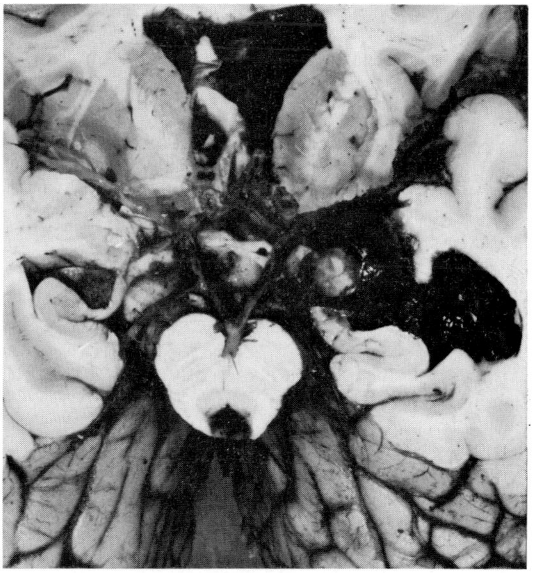

Fig. 5.13 Ruptured saccular aneurysm of the left internal carotid/posterior communicating artery. Blood has passed laterally through the choroidal fissure into the left lateral ventricle. The third ventricle, the aqueduct and the fourth ventricle were full of blood.

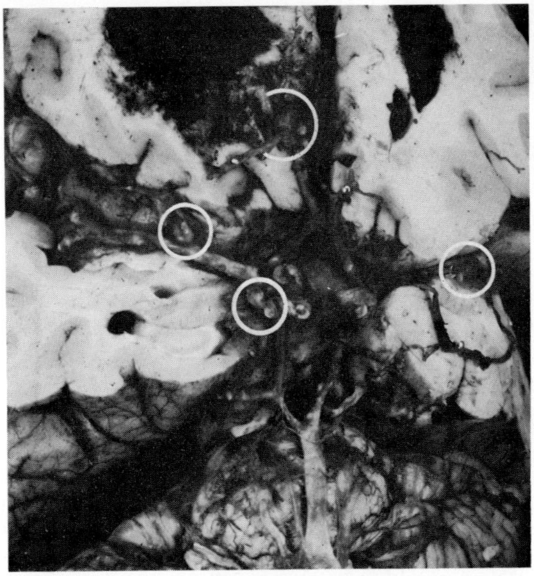

Fig. 5.14 Base of the brain in a patient with multiple saccular aneurysms (ringed). An aneurysm on the right anterior cerebral artery has bled into the substance of the right frontal lobe and into the lateral ventricle.

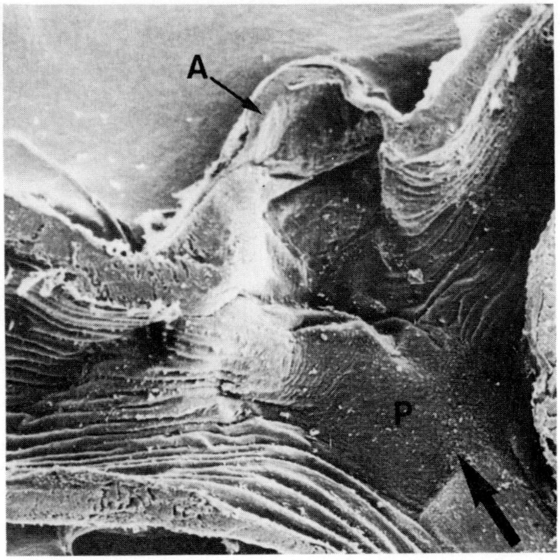

Fig. 5.15 Saccular aneurysm at a bifurcation of a middle cerebral artery. In this scanning electron micrograph, the artery and its bifurcation have been bisected longitudinally. A thin-walled aneurysm (A) less than 1 mm in diameter has formed at the bifurcation. A pad of vessel wall thickening (P) where the rugose pattern of the normal vessel wall is disturbed is seen proximal to the bifurcation. The large arrow indicates the direction of blood flow. Scanning electron micrograph; × 33. (Reproduced with permission, from Sheffield and Weller, 1980)

lumen is occluded. Calcification occurs particularly in the walls of larger aneurysms.

Microscopical appearances The relationship of saccular aneurysms to bifurcations in arteries can be seen especially when the aneurysms are still small. In Fig. 5.15, the aneurysm is a thin-walled pouch at a bifurcation; this appearance can be compared with a similar view of a normal artery (Fig. 5.16). Pads of intimal thickening proximal to the normal bifurcation and proximal to the aneurysm appear as flattened areas which have lost the rugose pattern of the vessel wall (Sheffield and Weller, 1980). The inner surface of the aneurysm is smooth, but in some cases the endothelium is incomplete and adherent blood clot may be seen (Hassler, 1972; Scanarini et al., 1978; Sheffield and Weller, 1980).

Histological sections through an aneurysm and its associated bifurcation (Figs. 5.17 and 5.18) show how the smooth muscle coat and the elastic lamina of the normal artery stop abruptly at the neck of the aneurysm. The wall of the aneurysm is composed of fibrous tissue; it varies in thickness and may show focal calcification. Fibrin and laminated blood clot may be adherent

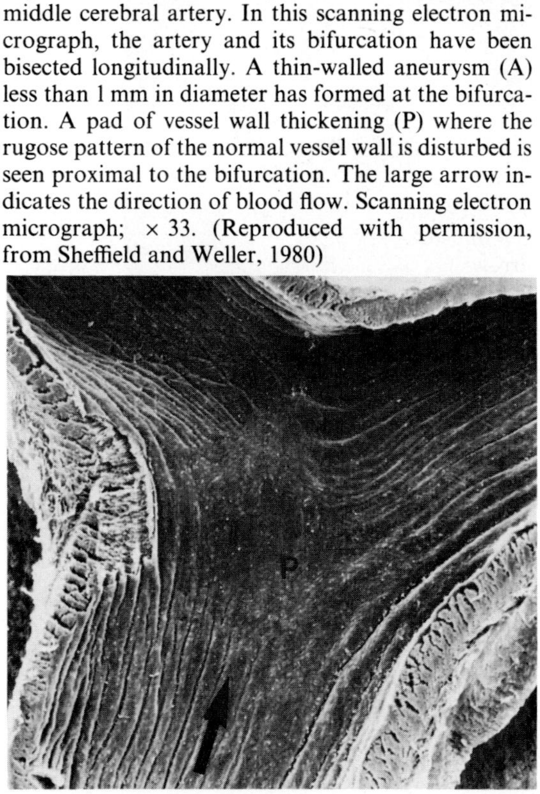

Fig. 5.16 Bifurcation of a normal middle cerebral artery from a 55-year-old male. Cut in a similar plane to Fig. 5.15, the pad of arterial wall thickening (P) is seen proximal to the bifurcation. The direction of blood flow is indicated by the arrow. Scanning electron micrograph; × 47. (Courtesy of Dr E.A. Sheffield)

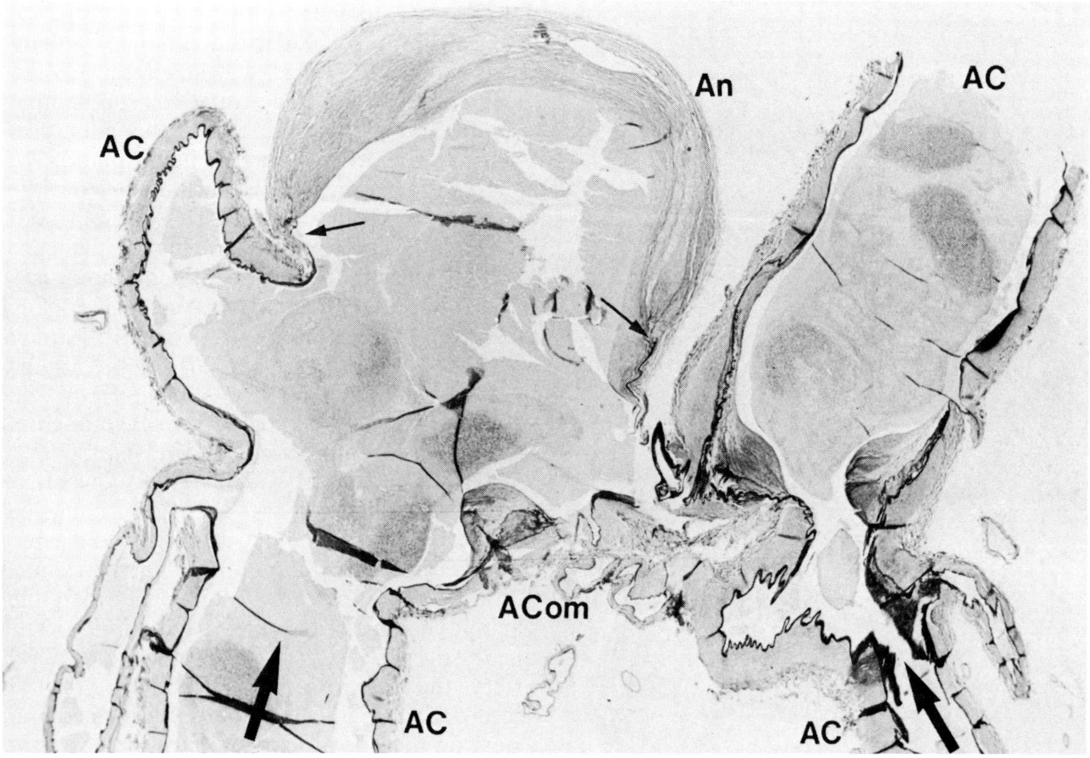

Fig. 5.17 Saccular aneurysm of the anterior communicating artery. A longitudinal section through the anterior cerebral (AC) and anterior communicating (ACom) arteries. (Direction of blood flow is indicated by the large arrows.) A saccular aneurysm (An) with a thick fibrous wall is arising from the anterior aspect of the anterior communicating artery. The internal elastic lamina (black) stops at the neck of the aneurysm (small arrows). Elastic van Gieson × 16. (Reproduced, with permission, from Weller, 1984)

to the inner surface of the unruptured aneurysm wall. Many of the features of an atherosclerotic artery (e.g. lipid-laden macrophages) may be observed within the wall of the aneurysm, and frequently there are macrophages containing haemosiderin. The walls of aneurysms which have recently ruptured may be necrotic and inflamed.

Pathogenesis of saccular aneurysms One of the most striking features of saccular aneurysms is that they occur almost exclusively at bifurcations or on curved portions of arteries (Rhoton, 1980). Histological studies of normal arteries in the circle of Willis and its major branches have shown that there is frequently a gap in the smooth muscle media at the point at which the vessel divides (Forbus, 1930; Crawford, 1959; Hassler, 1963; Stehbens, 1972; Sheffield and Weller, 1980). Similar gaps in the media occur in arteries elsewhere in the body (Hassler, 1963). The gaps in the smooth muscle coat of the artery are seen at the V-shaped distal carina, so at this point the vessel wall may be composed only of intimal endothelium, elastic lamina and a small amount of adventitial fibrous tissue (Sheffield and Weller, 1980). It is considered by most authors that aneurysms form in the region of the medial gap and for this reason saccular aneurysms have been said to be 'congenital'. The pattern of presentation of aneurysms, however, suggests that they are not congenital but that they form as a result of a combination of different factors. Why aneurysms form on some vessels and not others, and in only 1–2 per cent of the population, is not clear.

Most aneurysms present over the age of 40 years, and those in younger patients are often associated with diseases of vessels such as fibromuscular dysplasia (Mettinger, 1982) or polycystic kidney disease (Wakabayashi et al., 1983). As previously mentioned, the familial incidence of

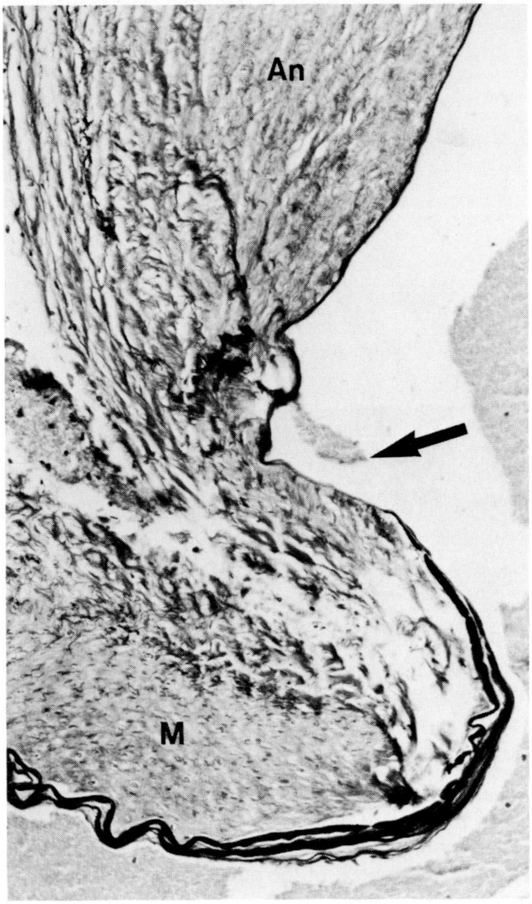

Fig. 5.18 Neck of a berry aneurysm (arrow); taken from the left side of the aneurysm in Fig. 5.17. The duplicated black-staining elastic lamina of the anterior cerebral/anterior communicating artery is seen at the bottom of the picture. M, media of artery. The thick fibrotic wall of the aneurysm (An) is devoid of smooth muscle and elastic lamina. Elastic van Gieson × 106. (Reproduced, with permission, from Weller, 1984)

aneurysms is low and this suggests that genetic factors do not play an important part in their formation.

Age changes in the artery wall due to haemodynamic stress may play a major part in the formation of aneurysms in adults. As a cerebral artery ages, fibrous intimal pads form particularly in relation to bifurcations (Hassler, 1962; Sheffield and Weller, 1980). In addition, their walls become less elastic (Sheffield and Weller, 1980). The configuration of arteriosclerotic intimal thickening probably alters the haemodynamic stress upon the bifurcations of cerebral arteries (Ferguson, 1972; Macfarlane, Canham and Roach, 1983) and, in the presence of a medial gap and a fenestrated elastic lamina (Campbell and Roach, 1981), the aneurysm forms as a fibrous pouch. The formation of aneurysms as a result of wear and tear, and the alteration of haemodynamic stresses on arterial bifurcations, could explain the higher incidence of aneurysms in older age groups and the coincidence of saccular aneurysms on vessels supplying arteriovenous malformations (Tognetti, Limoni and Testa, 1983). Some support for the importance of haemodynamic stress in the formation of saccular aneurysms comes from experimental studies. Hashimoto, Handa and Hazama (1979) and Hashimoto et al. (1980) have shown that aneurysms of the cerebral circulation could be produced in rats made hypertensive and treated with steroids and β-aminopropionitrile fumarate, but only after carotid ligation to alter the haemodynamics of the cerebral circulation. The aneurysms were formed on the anterior cerebral artery, the anterior communicating artery and the proximal segment of the posterior cerebral artery on the side of ligation, or in the posterior part of the circle of Willis if carotid ligation was bilateral.

Other factors may be important in the pathogenesis of aneurysms but the significance of observations such as the deficiency of type III collagen in the arteries of some patients with aneurysms (Neil-Dwyer et al., 1983) is, as yet, unexplained.

Subarachnoid haemorrhage and other complications of saccular aneurysms

Although subarachnoid haemorrhage, intracerebral haemorrhage, arterial vasospasm and infarction are the most dramatic complications of saccular aneurysms, neurological disorders also result from the presence of unruptured aneurysms and as a late result of subarachnoid haemorrhage.

Local effects of unruptured aneurysms Small unruptured aneurysms on the arteries around the circle of Willis often cause no neurological symptoms. In the minority of cases, however, aneurysms may compress an optic tract or the third, fourth or sixth cranial nerves and so interfere with their functions. The ophthalmic division of the fifth nerve may also be affected, leading to loss of sensation in the cutaneous area supplied by that nerve. Various well-recognized clinical syndromes occur due to the local effects of saccular aneurysms (Weller et al., 1983). When large, and particularly when embedded in the temporal lobe, saccular aneurysms may be associated with epilepsy.

Rupture of saccular aneurysms Both *subarachnoid* and *intracerebral* haemorrhage may result from rupture of a saccular aneurysm (see Figs. 5.11 to 5.13). Approximately 25 000 saccular aneurysms rupture each year in the USA and the incidence of subarachnoid haemorrhage is 11–12 per 100 000 per year (Drake, 1981). Intracerebral or intraventricular haemorrhage occurs in 15–40 per cent of patients, and is found especially in those dying within the first week (Reynolds and Shaw, 1981; Mohr et al., 1983; Wheelock et al., 1983).

Some indication of the position of ruptured aneurysms may be gained from angiograms, from the detection of a haematoma on CT scanning (Wheelock et al., 1983) or by the distribution of subarachnoid bleeding at post-mortem. Rupture of aneurysms situated on the circle of Willis tends to result in a symmetrical distribution of blood in the basal cisterns whereas bleeding from an aneurysm on a middle cerebral artery within the lateral fissures may produce an asymmetrical pattern of subarachnoid haemorrhage concentrated around the affected fissure. Bleeding from aneurysms on the anterior communicating or anterior cerebral arteries may cause blood to accumulate between the frontal lobes and to track back above the corpus callosum. Rupture of an aneurysm on a middle cerebral artery or on an anterior cerebral artery into the ventricles may produce both an intracerebral haematoma and subarachnoid haemorrhage due to the flow of blood through the ventricular system and its entry into the subarachnoid space through the foramina of Luschka on each side of the pons.

In a survey of 163 ruptured aneurysms. Crawford (1959) found that 28 per cent were on the anterior communicating artery, 12 per cent on the anterior cerebral artery and 34 per cent on the middle cerebral artery, mainly in its proximal portion. The junction of the internal carotid and posterior communicating artery was the site of the aneurysm in 18 per cent of cases, the basilar artery in 4 per cent, the posterior cerebral artery in 2 per cent and less than 1 per cent were on the vertebral and cerebellar arteries. There is considerable variation in the size of ruptured aneurysms but they are usually more than 10 mm in diameter (Wiebers, Whisnant and O'Fallon, 1981) with a range of 6–60 mm; in general, they are larger than unruptured aneurysms (range 2–10 mm) (McCormick and Acosta-Rua, 1970). Aneurysms seem to increase in size with time (Hashimoto and Handa, 1983). Although there is variation in the shape of aneurysms and the thickness of the wall at different points of the circumference, the fundus appears to be the commonest site of rupture (Crawford, 1959; Suzuki and Ohara, 1978).

Arterial spasm and cerebral ischaemia Clinically, patients may recover from the initial neurological effects of a ruptured aneurysm but then show a progressive decline in conscious level with signs of focal cerebral ischaemia. Cerebral infarction is found in some 75 per cent of patients dying during the first hospital admission for subarachnoid haemorrhage (Crompton, 1964; Drake, 1981). Angiography 3–4 days after subarachnoid haemorrhage may reveal narrowing of major cerebral arteries, especially the vessel bearing the ruptured aneurysm and those arteries surrounded by substantial blood clot. Cerebral vasospasm is most severe about 7 days after the subarachnoid haemorrhage and declines thereafter (Wilkins, 1980). In patients who have not undergone surgery for clipping of an aneurysm there is a significant relationship between the presence and degree of vasospasm and the ischaemic brain damage following subarachnoid haemorrhage (Graham, Macpherson and Pitts, 1983). An intracerebral haematoma probably increases the risk of infarction associated with vasospasm but does not, alonc, seem to cause ischaemic brain damage (Graham, Macpherson and Pitts, 1983).

Other factors, particularly during aneurysm surgery, may contribute to cerebral ischaemia in the presence of arterial vasospasm. Subarachnoid blood may decrease the ability of the cerebral circulation to compensate for moderate hypotension and this, together with secondary features such as haematoma formation, hydrocephalus or cerebral oedema, may contribute to cerebral ischaemia (Leading Article, 1983).

The cause of vasospasm is not known; no

single pharmacological agent has been identified which causes it or reverses it. Although it seems probable that blood products released from the investing clot cause the spasm, it is still difficult to explain why spasm is not usually seen for 3 days or so after the subarachnoid haemorrhage (Leading Article, 1983). Histological study of arteries following subarachnoid haemorrhage shows inflammation and necrosis of smooth muscle of the vessel walls soon after the bleed (Conway and McDonald, 1972; Smith et al., 1983), and thickening and fibrosis of the arterial walls years or months later (Hughes and Schianchi, 1978).

Perivascular haemorrhages and microinfarcts are frequently seen in the hypothalamus of patients dying soon after subarachnoid haemorrhage (Crompton, 1963). The hypothalamic lesions are in the walls of the third ventricle and involve the paraventricular nuclei (Doshi and Neil-Dwyer, 1977). There is a correlation between electrocardiographic abnormalities, focal myocardial necrosis and hypothalamic lesions in patients with subarachnoid haemorrhage (Doshi and Neil-Dwyer, 1977), and it is suggested that the high levels of circulating catecholamines in these patients may induce the focal myocardial necrosis (Neil-Dwyer et al., 1978).

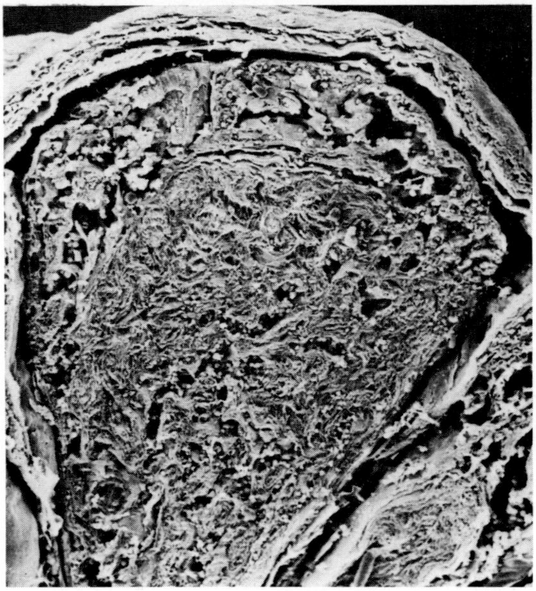

Fig. 5.19 Arachnoid granulation following subarachnoid haemorrhage. In this scanning electron micrograph the dural cap covering the granulation is seen at the top of the picture. The core of the granulation contains channels through which cerebrospinal fluid flows; these are partially filled with red blood cells. Scanning electron micrograph × 147. (Courtesy of Dr M. L. Upton)

Hydrocephalus Ventricular dilatation is a well recognized occurrence in the acute stages of subarachnoid haemorrhage, but hydrocephalus may also develop as a late complication (Pickard, 1982) (see Chapter 2). Experimental studies have shown that there is an increase in the outflow resistance and CSF pressure in rats following subarachnoid infusion of plasma or whole blood and that this is due to a decrease in transport of fluid across the epithelium of arachnoid villi (Butler et al., 1981). Heparin prevents this rise in CSF pressure and aids absorption (Blasberg, Johnson and Fenstermacher, 1981). However, direct evidence of obstruction to the CSF drainage pathways in man is sparse. In patients dying soon after subarachnoid haemorrhage, red blood cells but little fibrin are seen in the drainage channels within arachnoid granulations (Figs. 5.19 and 5.20) (Ellington and Margolis, 1969; Upton and Weller, 1984). To what extent fibrosis and obliteration of arachnoid granulations (Lorenzo, Bresnan and Barlow, 1974) or the subarachnoid space are contributory factors in late onset hydrocephalus following subarachnoid haemorrhage is uncertain (Di Rocco et al., 1977).

Giant cerebral aneurysms

Although most saccular aneurysms associated with arteries of the circle of Willis and their branches are between 2 and 20 mm in diameter, about 5 per cent of aneurysms exceed 2.5 cm in their largest diameter (Cohen et al., 1983). Many present as mass lesions and subarachnoid haemorrhage occurs in approximately one-third of cases. Giant aneurysms may arise in the posterior fossa, at the base of the cerebral hemispheres or within the lateral fissures from which they expand into the cerebral hemispheres. Spontaneous thrombosis frequently occurs within giant aneurysms (Whittle, Dorsch and Besser, 1982), and they may not be visible on angiography if the lumen is occluded. The appearances on CT scanning are those of a dense rounded lesion, and calcification may be seen in the wall of the aneurysm. Examination of giant

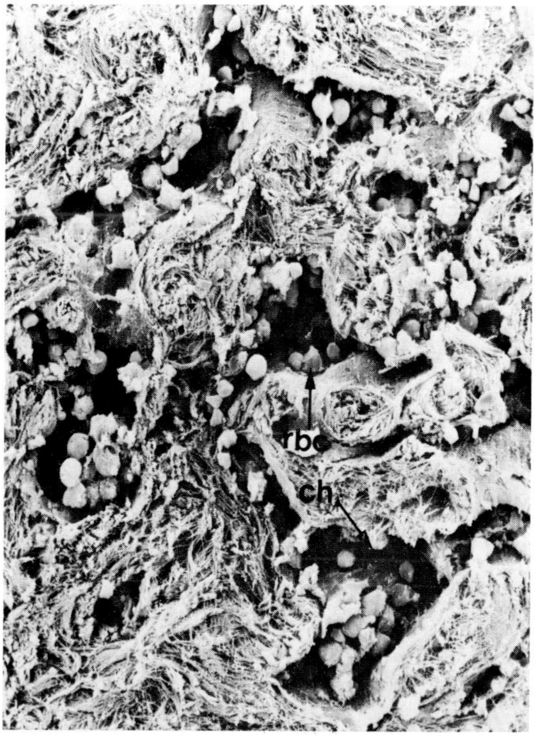

Fig. 5.20 A high power view of the central core of the arachnoid granulation in Fig. 5.19. Irregular channels (ch) separated by fibrous collagen bundles, are partially filled by red blood cells (rbc). Few, if any, strands of fibrin are seen in the channels. Scanning electron micrograph × 596. (Courtesy of Dr M. L. Upton)

aneurysms that have been removed surgically often shows that the lumen is filled with laminated thrombus and that the wall of the aneurysm is no more than a thin, often focally calcified fibrous shell. Although the blood clot may have been present for a very long time, organization does not readily occur and there is often little macrophage invasion even into the periphery of the blood clot.

Atherosclerotic fusiform aneurysms

Fusiform dilatation of the basilar or the internal carotid artery is commonly seen in patients with severe atherosclerosis. As the atherosclerosis increases in severity, the vertebral and basilar arteries of the circle of Willis not only develop atherosclerotic plaques but also the wall of the arteries may stretch because of replacement of the smooth muscle media by fibrous tissue. The lumen of the artery may be increased in size (ectasia); such an appearance is not uncommon in the basilar artery and in the intracranial part of the internal carotid arteries and the related proximal parts of the middle and anterior cerebral arteries. In many cases, the basilar artery is elongated and pursues an S-shaped course along the front of the brain stem. When the dilatation is extreme, the artery becomes a fusiform aneurysm. The supraclinoid segment of the internal carotid artery is the commonest site for such an aneurysm (Little et al., 1982) which may extend to involve the proximal segment of the middle cerebral artery; the basilar artery (Fig. 5.21) is also frequently aneurysmal (Steel, Thomas and Strollo, 1982). The main complications of fusiform aneurysms are compression of adjacent structures and transient ischaemic attacks possibly due to small emboli originating in the walls of the aneurysm (Steel, Thomas and Strollo, 1982) or due to stretching and distortion of branches of the aneurysmal artery (Hughes, 1965). Haemorrhage from a fusiform aneurysm may also occur (Little et al., 1982).

Carotid–cavernous sinus aneurysm or fistula

As the internal carotid artery enters the base of the skull, it passes into the wall of the cavernous sinus. At this point, the artery forms the S-shaped syphon of the internal carotid artery. The wall of the artery and its surrounding sympathetic nerve plexus are separated from the blood in the cavernous sinus only by a layer of endothelium. Fistulae between the carotid artery and the venous cavernous sinus may develop spontaneously, often in middle-aged women, but most follow trauma and may result from a spicule of bone piercing the artery; they may be bilateral (West, 1980). Some of the spontaneous cases are secondary to rupture of saccular aneurysms on the internal carotid artery projecting into the cavernous sinus as in Fig. 5.22. In other cases, however, angiography fails to demonstrate any predisposing lesion (Hamby, 1966). The result of arterial blood passing into the cavernous sinus is a distinctive clinical picture of unilateral pulsating exophthalmos with oedema of the eyelids and structures related to

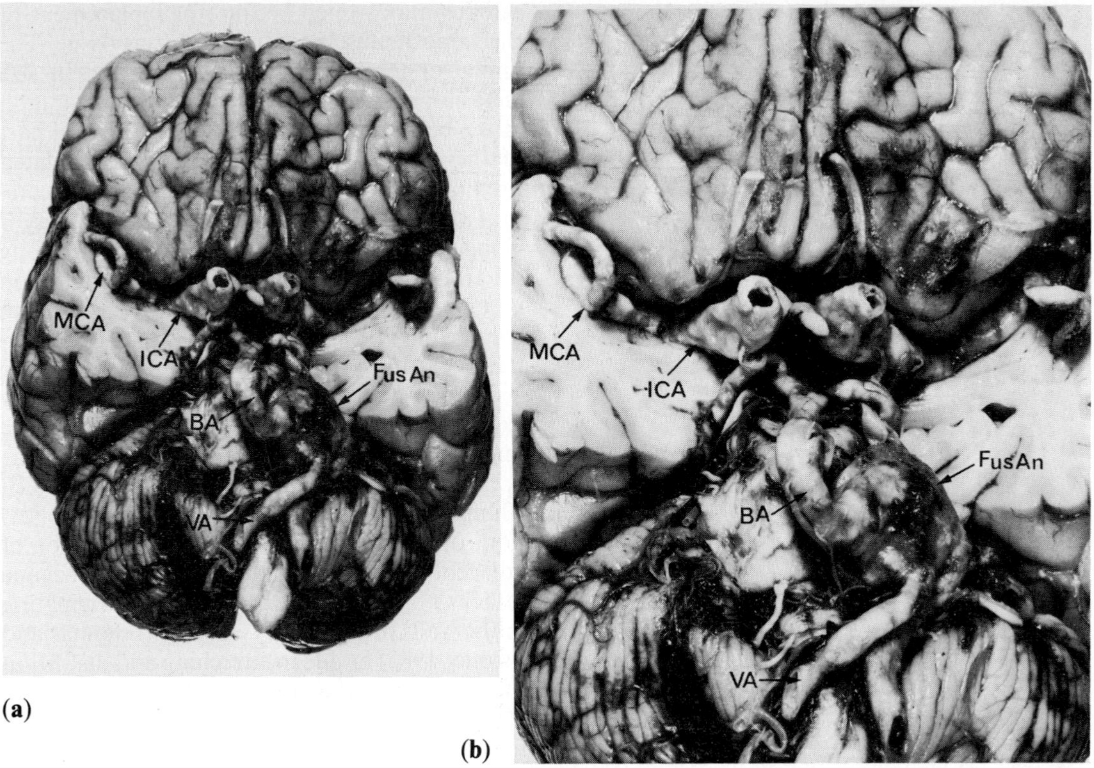

Fig. 5.21 Atherosclerotic fusiform aneurysm. (**a**) The base of the brain from a 68-year-old male, showing severe atherosclerosis of the major cerebral vessels with fusiform dilatation of the internal carotid arteries (ICA) and the basilar artery (BA). (**b**) A close-up view of the vessels at the base of the brain. The internal carotid arteries have thickened rigid walls and show aneurysmal dilatation. The middle cerebral arteries (MCA) are atherosclerotic. The basilar artery runs a serpiginous course along the front of the pons; at its lower end the artery is grossly dilated to form a fusiform aneurysm (Fus An). VA, vertebral artery.

the eye. A loud murmur can be heard on auscultation over the eye and there is usually complete or partial ophthalmoplegia on the affected side which may be due to damage to the third, fourth and sixth cranial nerves in the wall of the cavernous sinus. Thrombosis may occur within the aneurysm and occasionally spontaneous cure ensues. In most cases, carotid ligation significantly reduces the flow through the fistula.

Dissecting aneurysms of intracranial arteries

Most cases of dissecting aneurysm of intracranial arteries are a result of blunt neck or head injury (Adams et al., 1982) although they may be spontaneous or associated with fibromuscular dysplasia (Pilz and Hartjes, 1976) or polycystic kidney disease (Kulla et al., 1982). Although more frequent in the second and third decades, dissecting aneurysms do occur in younger children and may be bilateral (Nass, Hays and Chutorian, 1982). The basilar, vertebral, middle cerebral and intracranial portions of the carotid arteries are the most commonly affected vessels (Yonas et al., 1977; Berkovic et al., 1983). Dissection occurs between the intima and the media (Yonas et al., 1977; Nass, Hays and Chutorian, 1982) or between the media and the adventitia (Adams et al., 1982; Berkovic et al., 1983).

The affected vessel may be occluded and may lead to infarction in the parts of the brain supplied by the artery (Nass, Hays and Chutorian, 1982). If the dissection ruptures, it may cause subarachnoid haemorrhage (Adams et al., 1982). In those patients who survive, thrombus in the true and false lumina of the vessel becomes organized (Weller, 1984).

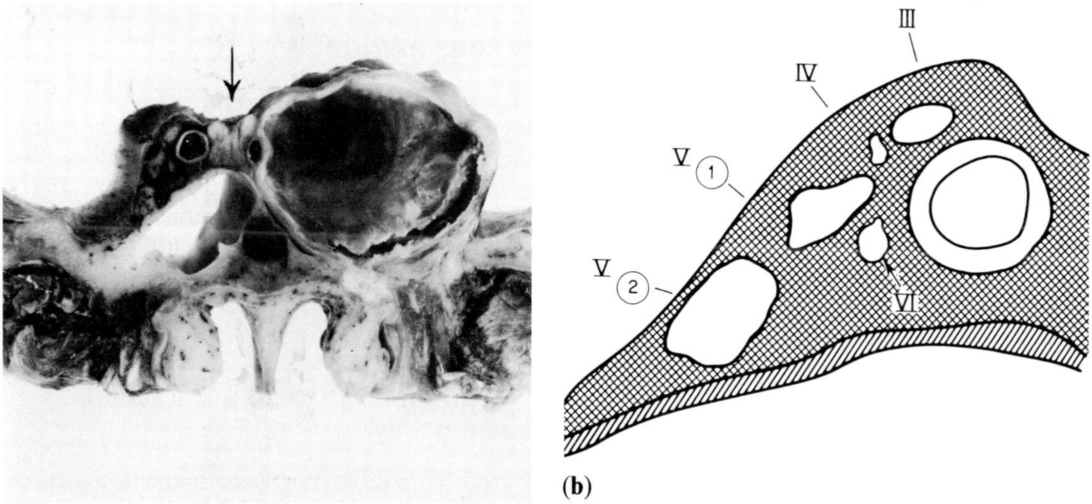

(a) (b)

Fig. 5.22 (**a**) Coronal section of the skull of a patient with an intracavernous saccular aneurysm of the right internal carotid artery. The section passes through the pituitary gland (arrow). On the left of the pituitary can be seen the normal internal carotid artery, the cavernous sinus, the third and fourth cranial nerves, two divisions of the fifth cranial nerve, and the sixth cranial nerve (see diagram (**b**)). On the right of the pituitary is the large, partly thrombosed, sac of the aneurysm. The wall of the internal carotid artery is complete at this level; the neck of the sac lay further forward. Blood, which had leaked from the aneurysm into the right sphenoidal air sinus, is visible below and medial to the sac of the aneurysm.

Bacterial and mycotic aneurysms

It has been estimated that 3 per cent of all patients with bacterial endocarditis develop small aneurysms on the distal branches of the middle, anterior and posterior cerebral arteries (Frazee, Cahan and Winter, 1980). About 65 per cent of the aneurysms rupture within the first 5 weeks of the endocarditis and account for the high mortality rate, perhaps as high as 80 per cent (Bohmfalk et al., 1978). *Streptococcus viridans* or *Staphylococcus aureus* are the common organisms involved, and the aneurysms are multiple in 20 per cent of cases (Bohmfalk et al., 1978). Bacterial aneurysms appear to form distal to the point at which the vessel is occluded by an infected embolus. Experimental studies suggest that organisms spread from the embolus, and within 24 hours there is inflammation and necrosis of the vessel wall and aneurysmal dilatation; inflammation is often most severe in the adventitia (Molinari et al., 1973).

Fungal (mycotic) aneurysms may also form on the distal branches of cerebral arteries. Commonly seen on the smaller branches of the middle cerebral artery, fungal aneurysms are multiple and usually measure 1–2 mm in diameter (Horten et al., 1976). Fungal emboli from the heart or fungal meningitis are the commonest causes; Aspergillus is the usual organism involved. The nasal sinuses or endocarditis are a frequent source of infection, and rupture of the aneurysm with extensive haemorrhage and disruption of brain tissue commonly occurs.

Histologically, necrosis and inflammation of the vessel wall are seen with fungal hyphae growing within it (Weller, 1984).

Arteriovenous malformations and cavernous angiomas

Arteriovenous malformations most commonly present in the second to fourth decade with recurrent subarachnoid or intracerebral haemorrhage (Graf, Peret and Torner, 1983). The cerebral hemispheres are the commonest site for these developmental abnormalities. They appear as tangled masses of vessels on the surface of the brain or deep within a hemisphere. Histologically, arteriovenous malformations are seen as dilated, often poorly formed, arterial and venous vessels surrounded by gliotic brain tissue containing haemosiderin resulting from previous bleeds (Russell and Rubinstein, 1977). The association of arteriovenous malformations with saccular aneurysms has already been mentioned, but these malformations are themselves an important cause of subarachnoid and intracerebral haemorrhage (Crawford and Russell, 1956). The smaller lesions are commonly supplied by the middle cerebral artery; they tend to bleed but subarachnoid haemorrhage from an arteriovenous malformation is rarely accompanied by vasospasm (Parkinson and Bachers, 1980). Occasionally, arteriovenous malformations regress spontaneously—probably due to widespread thrombosis of the component vessels (Wakai et al., 1983).

Venous malformations in the brain may be very large and occasionally they present with sudden haemorrhage (Cabanes et al., 1979).

Cavernous angiomas occur in the brain, often in the cerebral white matter and, although they may not be visualized on angiography, they enhance on a CT scan (Pozzati et al., 1980); they may be multiple. Most present in the third to fifth decade but they also produce symptoms in children. Giobini and Morello (1978) found in their series that 23 per cent of patients with cavernous angiomas presented with intracranial bleeding, 38 per cent with epilepsy, 28 per cent with headache and 12 per cent with focal neurological disturbance. Histologically, these lesions are seen as vascular malformations rather than true tumours (Russell and Rubinstein, 1977). They are composed of dilated abnormal vascular channels crowded together with little or no intervening brain tissue. Gliosis of the surrounding brain is often seen and blood pigment may be present as evidence of previous haemorrhage.

Uncommon causes of intracranial haemorrhage

Intracerebral haemorrhage (which is often multifocal), or subarachnoid haemorrhage, may present as a complication of anticoagulation, clotting disorders such as leukaemia, thrombotic thrombocytopenic purpura, sickle cell disease or amyloid angiopathy (McCormick and Rosenfield, 1973; Almani and Awid, 1982).

Primary and metastatic tumours in the brain account for some 10 per cent of all spontaneous intracranial haemorrhages (Scott, 1975). Mandybur (1977) has estimated that significant haemorrhage is a complication of 14 per cent of metastatic tumours in the brain but only 0.8 per cent of gliomas. Metastases from choriocarcinoma, malignant melanoma and bronchial carcinoma are most prone to bleed spontaneously. There are a few reports of meningiomas (Modesti, Binet and Collins, 1976) and acoustic neuromas (Yonemitsu et al., 1983) causing intracranial haemorrhage but this is a rare complication.

Neoplastic aneurysms may form in a way analogous to bacterial aneurysms and cause intracranial haemorrhage (Ho, 1982). There is segmental destruction of vessel walls by tumour cells derived from emboli in the vessels and bleeding may occur from the aneurysmal dilatations of the involved vessels.

References

Adachi, M., Rosenblum, W.I. and Feigin, I. (1966) Hypertensive disease and cerebral oedema. *Journal of Neurology, Neurosurgery and Psychiatry* **29,** 451–5.

Adams, H.P., Aschenbrener, C.A., Kassell, N.F., Ansbacher, L. and Cornell, S.H. (1982) Intracranial hemorrhage produced by spontaneous dissecting intracranial aneurysm. *Archives of Neurology* **39,** 773–5.

Almani, W.S. and Awid, A.S. (1982) Spontaneous

intracranial bleeding in hemorrhagic diathesis. *Surgical Neurology* **17**, 137–40.

Amano, S. (1977) Vascular changes in the brain of spontaneously hypertensive rats: hyaline and fibrinoid degeneration. *Journal of Pathology* **121,** 119–28.

Andrews, R.J. and Spiegel, P.K. (1979) Intracranial aneurysms: age, sex, blood pressure and multiplicity in an unselected series of patients. *Journal of Neurosurgery* **51,** 27–32.

Andrews, R.J. and Spiegel, P.K. (1981) Intracranial aneurysms: characteristics of aneurysms by site, with special reference to anterior communicating artery aneurysms. *Surgical Neurology* **16,** 122–6.

Berkovic, S.F., Spokes, R.L., Anderson, R. McD. and Bladin, P.F. (1983) Basilar artery dissection. *Journal of Neurology, Neurosurgery and Psychiatry* **46**, 126–9.

Binswanger, O. (1894) Die Abgrenzung der allgemeinen progressiven Paralyse. *Klinische Wochenschrift* **31,** 1180–6.

Blasberg, R., Johnson, D. and Fenstermacher, J. (1981) Absorption resistance of cerebrospinal fluid after subarachnoid hemorrhage in the monkey; effects of heparin. *Neurosurgery* **9**, 686–91.

Bohmfalk, G.L., Story, J.L., Wissinger, J.P. and Brown, W.E. (1978) Bacterial intracranial aneurysm. *Journal of Neurosurgery* **48**, 369–82.

Butler, A.B., Maffeo, C.J., Johnson, R.N. and Bass, N.H. (1981) Alteration of CSF outflow in acute subarachnoid hemorrhage; effect of blood components on outflow resistance and vesicular transport of CSF in arachnoid villus endothelium. In *Cerebral Microcirculation and Metabolism* (Eds. Cervós-Navarro, J. and Fritschka, E.), pp. 409–14. Raven Press, New York.

Cabanes, J., Blasco, R., García, M. and Tamarit, L. (1979) Cerebral venous angioma. *Surgical Neurology* **11**, 385–9.

Campbell, G.J. and Roach, M.R. (1981) Fenestration in the internal elastic lamina at bifurcations of human cerebral arteries. *Stroke* **12,** 489–96.

Caplan, L.R. and Schoene, W.C. (1978) Clinical features of subcortical arteriosclerotic encephalopathy (Binswanger disease). *Neurology* **28,** 1206–15.

Charcot, J.-M. and Bouchard, C. (1868) Nouvelles recherches sur la pathogénie de l'hémorrhagie cérébrale. *Archives de Physiologie Normale et de Pathologie* **1,** 110–27, 643–65.

Chester, E.M., Agamandis, D.P., Banker, B.Q. and Victor, M. (1978) Hypertensive encephalopathy: a clinicopathologic study of 20 cases. *Neurology* **28,** 928–39.

Chin, D. and Carney, P. (1983) Acute cerebellar hemorrhage with brainstem compression in contrast with benign cerebellar hemorrhage. *Surgical Neurology* **19,** 406–9.

Cohen, A.R., Aleksic, S., Budzilovich, G.N., Pinto, R.S. and Flamm, E.S. (1983) Giant intracranial aneurysm presenting as a posterior fossa mass. *Surgical Neurology* **20,** 160–4.

Cole, F.M. and Yates, P.O. (1967a) The occurrence and significance of intracerebral microaneurysms. *Journal of Pathology and Bacteriology* **93,** 393–411.

Cole, F.M. and Yates, P.O. (1976b) Intracerebral microaneurysms and small cerebrovascular lesions. *Brain* **90,** 759–68.

Cole, F.M. and Yates, P.O. (1967c) Pseudoaneurysm in relationship to massive cerebral haemorrhage. *Journal of Neurology, Neurosurgery and Psychiatry* **30,** 61–6.

Cole, F.M. and Yates, P.O. (1968) Comparative incidence of cerebrovascular lesions in normotensive and hypertensive patients. *Neurology* **18,** 255–9.

Conway, L.W. and McDonald, L.W. (1972) Structural changes of the intradural arteries following subarachnoid hemorrhage. *Journal of Neurosurgery* **37,** 715–23.

Cook, T.A. and Yates, P.O. (1972) A histometric study of cerebral and renal arteries in normotensives and chronic hypertensives. *Journal of Pathology* **108,** 129–35.

Co-operative Group (1982) Five-year findings of the hypertension detection and follow up programme. III. Reduction in stroke incidence among persons with high blood pressure. *Journal of the American Medical Association* **247,** 633–8.

Crawford, J.V. and Russell, D.S. (1956) Cryptic arteriovenous and venous hamartomas of brain. *Journal of Neurology, Neurosurgery and Psychiatry* **19,** 1–11.

Crawford, T. (1959) Some observations on the pathogenesis and natural history of intracranial saccular aneurysms. *Journal of Neurology, Neurosurgery and Psychiatry* **22,** 259–66.

Crompton, M.R. (1963) Hypothalamic lesions following rupture of berry aneurysms. *Brain* **86,** 301–14.

Crompton, M.R. (1964) Cerebral infarction following rupture of cerebral artery aneurysm. *Brain* **87,** 263–79.

Dinsdale, H.B. (1982) Hypertensive encephalopathy. *Stroke* **13,** 717–19.

Doshi, R. and Neil-Dwyer, G. (1977) Hypothalamic and myocardial lesions after subarachnoid haemorrhage. *Journal of Neurology, Neurosurgery and Psychiatry* **40,** 821–6.

Douglas, M.A. and Haerer, A.F. (1982) Long-term prognosis of hypertensive intracerebral hemorrhage. *Stroke* **13,** 488–91.

Drake, C.G. (1981) Management of cerebral aneurysm. *Stroke* **12,** 273–83.

Ellington, E. and Margolis, G. (1969) Block of arachnoid villus by subarachnoid hemorrhage. *Journal of Neurosurgery* **30,** 651–7.

Evans, P.H. (1965) Relation of longstanding blood-pressure levels to atherosclerosis. *Lancet* **1,** 516–19.

Feigin, I. and Popoff, N. (1963) Neuropathological changes late in cerebral edema: the relationship to trauma, hypertensive disease and Binswanger's encephalopathy. *Journal of Neuropathology and Experimental Neurology* **22,** 500–11.

Ferguson, G.G. (1972) Physical factors in the initiation growth and rupture of human intracranial saccular aneurysms. *Journal of Neurosurgery* **37,** 666–77.

Fisher, C.M. (1969) The arterial lesions underlying lacunes. *Acta Neuropathologica* **12,** 1–15.

Fisher, M., Davidson, R.I. and Marcus, E.M. (1980) Transient focal cerebral ischemia as a presenting manifestation of unruptured cerebral aneurysms. *Annals of Neurology* **8,** 367–72.

Forbus, W.D. (1930) On the origin of miliary aneurysms of the superficial cerebral arteries. *Bulletin of the Johns Hopkins Hospital* **47,** 239–84.

Fox, J.L. and Ko, J.P. (1980) Familial intracranial aneurysms. Six cases among 13 siblings. *Journal of Neurosurgery* **52,** 501–3.

Frazee, J.G., Cahan, L.D. and Winter, J. (1980) Bacterial intracranial aneurysms. *Journal of Neurosurgery* **53,** 633–41.

Giobini, S. and Morello, G. (1978) Cavernous angiomas of the brain: account of fourteen personal cases and review of the literature. *Acta Neurochirugica* **40,** 61–82.

Graf, C.J., Perret, G.E. and Torner, J.C. (1983) Bleeding from cerebral arteriovenous malformations as part of their natural history. *Journal of Neurosurgery* **58,** 331–7.

Graham, D.I., Macpherson, P. and Pitts, L.H. (1983) Correlation between angiographic vasospasm, hematoma, and ischemic brain damage following SAH. *Journal of Neurosurgery* **59,** 223–30.

Hachinski, V.C., Lassen, N.A. and Marshall, J. (1974) Multi-infarct dementia. A cause of mental retardation in the elderly. *Lancet* **2,** 207–10.

Hamby, W.B. (1966) *Carotid-Cavernous Fistula.* Thomas, Springfield, Illinois.

Hashimoto, N. and Handa, H. (1983) The size of cerebral aneurysms in relation to repeated rupture. *Surgical Neurology* **19,** 107–11.

Hashimoto, N., Handa, H. and Hazama, F. (1979) Experimentally induced cerebral aneurysms in rats. III. Pathology. *Surgical Neurology* **11,** 299–304.

Hashimoto, N., Handa, H., Nagata, I. and Hazama, F. (1980) Experimentally induced cerebral aneurysms in rats. V. Relation of hemodynamics in the circle of Willis to formation of aneurysms. *Surgical Neurology* **13,** 41–5.

Hassler, O. (1962) Physiological intima cushions in the large cerebral arteries of young individuals. 2. location. *Acta Pathologica et Microbiologica Scandinavica* **55,** 28–30.

Hassler, O. (1963) Media defects in human arteries. *Angiology* **14,** 368–71.

Hassler, O. (1972) Scanning electron microscopy of saccular intracranial aneurysms. *American Journal of Pathology* **68,** 511–20.

Hayashi, S., Arimoto, T., Hakura, T., Fujii, T., Nishiguchi, T. and Komai, N. (1981) The association of intracranial aneurysms and arteriovenous malformation of the brain. *Journal of Neurosurgery* **55,** 971–5.

Healton, E.B., Brust, J.C., Feinfeld, D.A. and Thomas, G.E. (1982) Hypertensive encephalopathy and the neurologic manifestations of malignant hypertension. *Neurology* **32,** 127–32.

Heptinstall, R.H. (1983) *Pathology of the Kidney* 3rd edn. vol. 1, pp. 202–218. Little, Brown, Boston.

Ho, K.-L. (1982) Neoplastic aneurysm and intracranial hemorrhage. *Cancer* **50,** 2935–40.

Horten, B.C., Abbott, G.F. and Porro, R.S. (1976) Fungal aneurysms of intracranial vessels. *Archives of Neurology* **33,** 577–9.

Hughes, J.T. and Schianchi, P.M. (1978) Cerebral artery spasm. A histological study at necropsy of the blood vessels in cases of subarachnoid hemorrhage. *Journal of Neurosurgery* **48,** 515–25.

Hughes, W. (1965) Origin of lacunes. *Lancet* **2,** 19–21.

Janota, I. (1981) Dementia, deep white matter damage and hypertension 'Binswanger's disease'. *Psychological Medicine* **11,** 39–48.

Johansson, B.B. and Linder, L.-E. (1981) Hypertension and brain oedema: an experimental study on acute and chronic hypertension in the rat. *Journal of Neurology, Neurosurgery and Psychiatry* **44,** 402–6.

Kulla, L., Deymeer, F., Smith, T.W., Weiner, M. and Mullins, T.F. (1982) Intracranial dissecting and saccular aneurysms in polycystic kidney disease. *Archives of Neurology* **39,** 776–8.

Leading Article (1983) *Lancet* **1,** 141–3.

Le Blanc, F.E., Charrette, E.P., Dobell, A.R.C. and Branch, C.L. (1968) Neurological complications of aortic co-arctation. *Canadian Medical Association Journal* **99,** 299–303.

Limas, C., Westrum, B. and Limas, C.J. (1980) The evolution of vascular changes in the spontaneously hypertensive rat. *American Journal of Pathology* **98,** 357–84.

Little, J.R., Tubman, D.E. and Etheir, R. (1978) Cerebellar hemorrhage in adults. Diagnosis by computerized tomography. *Journal of Neurosurgery* **48,** 575–9.

Little, J.R., St Louis, P., Weinstein, M. and Dohn, D.F. (1982) Giant fusiform aneurysm of the cerebral arteries. *Stroke* **12,** 183–8.

Locksley, H.B., Sahs, A.L. and Knowler, L. (1966) Report on the Co-operative Study of intracranial aneurysms and subarachnoid hemorrhage. II. General survey of cases in the Central Registry and characteristics of the sample population. *Journal of Neurosurgery* **24,** 922–32.

Loizou, L.A., Jefferson, J.M. and Smith, W.T. (1982) Subcortical arteriosclerotic encephalopathy (Binswanger's type) and cortical infarcts in a young normotensive patient. *Journal of Neurology, Neurosurgery and Psychiatry* **45,** 409–17.

Lorenzo, A.V., Bresnan, M.J. and Barlow, C.F. (1974) Cerebrospinal fluid absorption deficit in normal pressure hydrocephalus. *Archives of Neurology* **30,** 387–93.

McCormick, W.F. and Acosta-Rua, G.J. (1970) The size of intracranial saccular aneurysms. An autopsy study. *Journal of Neurosurgery* **33,** 422–7.

McCormick, W.F. and Nofzinger, J.D. (1965) Saccular intracranial aneurysms (an autopsy study). *Journal of Neurosurgery* **22,** 155–9.

McCormick, W.F. and Rosenfield, D.B. (1973) Massive brain hemorrhage: a review of 144 cases and an examination of their causes. *Stroke* **4,** 946–54.

McCormick, W.F. and Schmalsteig, E.J. (1977) The relationship of arterial hypertension to intracranial aneurysms. *Archives of Neurology* **34,** 285–7.

Macfarlane, T.W.R., Canham, P.B. and Roach, M.R. (1983) Shape changes at the apex of isolated human cerebral bifurcations with changes in transmural pressure. *Stroke* **14,** 70–6.

Mandybur, T.I. (1977) Intracranial hemorrhage caused by metastatic tumors. *Neurology* **27,** 650–5.

Matsumoto, N., Whisnant, J.P., Kunand, L.T. and Okazaki, H. (1973) Natural history of stroke in Rochester, Minnesota, 1955 through 1969: an extension of a previous study, 1945 through 1954. *Stroke* **4,** 20–9.

Mettinger, K.L. (1982) Fibromuscular dysplasia and the brain. II. Current concept of the disease. *Stroke* **13,** 53–8.

Miyasaka, K., Wolpert, S.M. and Prager, R.J. (1982) The association of cerebral aneurysms, infundibula and intracranial arteriovenous malformations. *Stroke* **13,** 196–203.

Modesti, L.M., Binet, E.F. and Collins, G.H. (1976) Meningiomas causing spontaneous intracranial hematomas. *Journal of Neurosurgery* **45,** 437–41.

Mohr, G., Ferguson, G., Khan, M., Mallow, D., Watts, R., Benoit, B. and Weir, B. (1983) Intraventricular hemorrhage from ruptured aneurysm. Retrospective analysis of 91 cases. *Journal of Neurosurgery* **58,** 482–7.

Molinari, G.F., Smith, L., Goldstein, M.N. and Satran, R. (1973) Pathogenesis of cerebral mycotic aneurysms. *Neurology* **23,** 325–32.

Morooka, Y. and Waga, S. (1983) Familial intracranial aneurysms: report of four families. *Surgical Neurology* **19,** 260–2.

Nag, S., Robertson, D.M. and Dinsdale, H.B. (1977) Cerebral cortical changes in experimental hypertension. An ultrastructural study. *Laboratory Investigation* **36,** 150–61.

Nag, S., Robertson, D.M. and Dinsdale, H.B. (1980) Morphological changes in spontaneously hypertensive rats. *Acta Neuropathologica* **52,** 27–34.

Nakajima, K. (1983) Clinicopathological study of pontine hemorrhages. *Stroke* **14,** 485–93.

Nass, R., Hays, A. and Chutorian, A. (1982) Intracranial dissecting aneurysms in childhood. *Stroke* **13,** 204–7.

Neil-Dwyer, G., Walter, P., Cruickshank, J.M., Doshi, B. and O'Gorman, P. (1978) Effect of propranolol and phentolamine on myocardial necrosis after subarachnoid haemorrhage. *British Medical Journal* **2,** 990–2.

Neil-Dwyer, G., Bartlett, J.R., Nicholls, A.C., Narcisi, P. and Pope, F.M. (1983) Collagen deficiency and ruptured cerebral aneurysms. A clinical and biochemical study. *Journal of Neurosurgery* **59,** 16–20.

Nicholls, E.S. and Johansen, H.L. (1983) Implications of changing trends in cerebrovascular and ischemic heart disease mortality. *Stroke* **14,** 153–6.

Ogata, J., Fujishima, M., Tamaki, K., Nakatomi, Y., Ishitsuka, T. and Omae, T. (1980) Stroke-prone spontaneously hypertensive rats as an experimental model of malignant hypertension. 1. A light- and electron-microscopic study of the brain. *Acta Neuropathologica* **51,** 179–84.

Ojemann, R.G. and Heros, R.C. (1983) Spontaneous brain hemorrhage. *Stroke* **14,** 458–75.

Okamoto, H. (1969) Spontaneous hypertension in rats. *International Review of Experimental Pathology* **7,** 227–70.

Parkinson, D. and Bachers, G. (1980) Arteriovenous malformations. Summary of 100 consecutive supratentorial cases. *Journal of Neurosurgery* **53,** 285–99.

Paronetto, F. (1965) Immunocytochemical observations on the vascular necrosis and renal glomerular lesions of malignant nephrosclerosis. *American Journal of Pathology* **46,** 901–15.

Patel, A.N. and Richardson, A.E. (1971) Ruptured intracranial aneurysms in the first two decades of life. A study of 58 patients. *Journal of Neurosurgery* **35,** 571–6.

Perret, G. and Nishioka, H. (1966) Report on the co-operative study of intracranial aneurysms and subarachnoid hemorrhage. VI. Arteriovenous malformations. An analysis of 545 cases of cranio-cerebral arteriovenous malformations and fistulae reported to the co-operative study. *Journal of Neurosurgery* **25,** 467–90.

Phillips, L.H., Whisnant, J.P., O'Fallon, W.M. and Sundt T.M. Jr (1980) The unchanging pattern of subarachnoid hemorrhage in a community. *Neurology* **30,** 1034–40.

Pickard, J.D. (1982) Adult communicating hydrocephalus. *British Journal of Hospital Medicine* **27,** 35–44.

Pilz, P. and Hartjes, H.J. (1976) Fibromuscular dysplasia and multiple dissecting aneurysms of intracranial arteries. A further cause of Moyamoya syndrome. *Stroke* **7,** 393–8.

Poirier, J. (1983) Giant cerebral lacuna due to dilatation of the perivascular space: a case report. *Clinical Neuropathology* **2,** 138–40.

Pozzati, E., Padovani, R., Morrone, B., Finizio, F. and Gaist, G. (1980) Cerebral cavernous angiomas in children. *Journal of Neurosurgery* **53,** 826–32.

Rail, D.L. and Perkin, G.D. (1980) Computerized tomographic appearance of hypertensive encephalopathy. *Archives of Neurology* **37,** 310–11.

Reynolds, A.F. and Shaw, C.M. (1981) Bleeding patterns from ruptured intracranial aneurysms: an autopsy series of 205 patients. *Surgical Neurology* **15,** 232–5.

Rhoton, A.L. (1980) Anatomy of saccular aneurysms. *Surgical Neurology* **14,** 59–66.

Di Rocco, C., Di Trapani, G., Maira, G., Bentivoglio, M., Macchi, G. and Rossi, G.F. (1977) Anatomo-clinical correlations in normotensive hydrocephalus. *Journal of the Neurological Sciences* **33,** 437–52.

Roggendorf, W., Cervós-Navarro, J. and Iglesias Rozas, J.R. (1981) Contractile elements of human brain vessels in chronic hypertension. In *Cerebral Microcirculation and Metabolism* (Eds. Cervós-Navarro, J. and Fritschka, E.), pp. 443–53. Raven Press, New York.

Ropper, A.H. and Davis, K.R. (1980) Lobar cerebral hemorrhages: acute clinical syndromes in 26 cases. *Annals of Neurology* **8,** 141–7.

Rosenberg, G.A., Kornfeld, M., Stovring, J. and Bicknell, J.M. (1979) Subcortical arteriosclerotic encephalopathy (Binswanger): computerized tomography. *Neurology* **29,** 1102–06.

Rudick, R.A. (1981) Asymptomatic intracerebral hematoma as an incidental finding. *Archives of Neurology* **38,** 396.

Russell, D.S. (1954) Discussion: The pathology of spontaneous intracranial haemorrhage. *Proceedings of the Royal Society of Medicine* **47,** 689–704.

Russell, D.S. and Rubinstein, L.J. (1977) *Pathology of Tumours of the Nervous System*, 4th edn. Edward Arnold, London.

Russell, R.W.R. (1963) Observations on intracerebral aneurysms. *Brain* **86,** 425–42.

Sacco, R.L., Wolf, P.A., Kannel, W.B. and McNamara, P.M. (1982) Survival and recurrence following stroke. The Framingham Study. *Stroke* **13,** 290–5.

Sakaki, T., Kinugawa, K., Tanigake, T., Miyamoto, S., Kyoi, K. and Utsumi, S. (1980) Embolism from intracranial aneurysms. *Journal of Neurosurgery* **53,** 300–4.

Scanarini, M., Mingrino, S., Zuccarello, M. and Trincia, G. (1978) Scanning electron microscopy (SEM) of biopsy specimens of ruptured intracranial saccular aneurysms. *Acta Neuropathologica* **44,** 131–4.

Schwartz, P. (1972) Apoplectic lesions of the brain in adults. In *Handbook of Clinical Neurology*, vol. 11 (Eds. Vinken, P.J. and Bruyn, G.W.), pp. 578–659. North-Holland, Amsterdam.

Scott, M. (1975) Spontaneous intracerebral hematoma caused by cerebral neoplasms. Report of eight verified cases. *Journal of Neurosurgery* **42,** 338–92.

Sheffield, E.A. and Weller, R.O. (1980) Age changes at cerebral artery bifurcations and the pathogenesis of berry aneurysms. *Journal of the Neurological Sciences* **46,** 341–52.

Sinclair, R.A., Antonovych, T.T. and Mostofi, F.K. (1976) Renal proliferative arteriopathies and associated glomerular changes. *Human Pathology* **7,** 565–88.

Skinhip, E. and Strandgaard, S. (1973) Pathogenesis of hypertensive encephalopathy. *Lancet* **1,** 461–2.

Smith, R.R., Clower, B.R., Peeler, D.F. and Yoshioka, J. (1983) The angiopathy of subarachnoid hemorrhage: angiographic and morphologic correlates. *Stroke* **14,** 240–5.

Soltero, I., Lin, K., Cooper, R., Stamler, J. and Garside, D. (1978) Trends in mortality from cerebrovascular disease in the United States, 1960 to 1975. *Stroke* **9,** 549–58.

Stehbens, W.E. (1972) *Pathology of the Cerebral Blood Vessels.* Mosby, St Louis.

Steel, J.G., Thomas, H.A. and Strollo, P.J. (1982) Fusiform basilar aneurysm as a cause of embolic stroke. *Stroke* **13,** 712–16.

Strandgaard, S. (1978) Autoregulation of cerebral circulation in hypertension. *Acta Neurologica Scandinavica* **57,** Suppl. 66, 1–82.

Suzuki, J. and Ohara, H. (1978) Clinicopathological study of cerebral aneurysms. Origin, rupture, repair and growth. *Journal of Neurosurgery* **48,** 505–14.

Suzuki, J. and Omuna, T. (1979) Intracranial aneurysms associated with arteriovenous malformations. *Journal of Neurosurgery* **50,** 742–6.

Takebayashi, S. and Kaneko, M. (1983) Electron microscopic studies of ruptured arteries in hypertensive intracerebral hemorrhage. *Stroke* **14,** 28–36.

Tanaka, H., Tanaka, Y., Hayashi, M., Ueda, Y.,

Date, C., Baba, T. et al. (1982) Secular trends in mortality for cerebrovascular diseases in Japan 1960 to 1979. *Stroke* **13,** 574–81.

Tognetti, F., Limoni, P. and Testa, C. (1983) Aneurysm growth and hemodynamic stress. *Surgical Neurology* **20,** 74–8.

Upton, M. and Weller, R.O. (1984) The morphology of human arachnoid granulations. (In preparation.)

Valentine, A.R., Moseley, I.F. and Kendall, B.E. (1980) White matter abnormality in cerebral atrophy: clinicoradiological correlations. *Journal of Neurology, Neurosurgery and Psychiatry* **43,** 139–42.

Wakabayashi, T., Fujita, S., Ohbora, Y., Suyama, T., Tamaki, N. and Matsumoto, S. (1983) Polycystic kidney disease and intracranial aneurysms. *Journal of Neurosurgery* **58,** 488–91.

Wakai, S., Chen, C.-H., Wu, K.-Y. and Chiu, C.-W. (1983) Spontaneous regression of a cerebral arteriovenous malformation. Report of a case and review of the literature. *Archives of Neurology* **40,** 377–80.

Weisberg, L.A. (1979) Computerized tomography in intracranial hemorrhage. *Archives of Neurology* **36,** 422–6.

Weller, R.O. (1984) Colour *Atlas of Neuropathology.* Harvey Miller and Oxford University Press, Oxford.

Weller, R.O. and Williams, B.N. (1975) Cerebral biopsy and assessment of brain damage in hydrocephalus. *Archives of Disease in Childhood* **50,** 763–8.

Weller, R.O., Swash, M., McLellan, D.L. and Scholtz, C.L. (1983) *Clinical Neuropathology.* Springer, Berlin.

West, C.G.H. (1980) Bilateral carotid–cavernous fistulae: a review. *Surgical Neurology* **13,** 85–90.

Wheelock, B., Weir, B., Watts, R., Mohr, G., Khan, M., Hunter, M. et al. (1983) Timing of surgery for intracranial hematomas due to aneurysm rupture. *Journal of Neurosurgery* **58,** 476–81.

Whittle, I.R., Dorsch, N.W. and Besser, M. (1982) Spontaneous thrombosis in giant intracranial aneurysms. *Journal of Neurology, Neurosurgery and Psychiatry* **45,** 1040–7.

Wiebers, D.O., Whisnant, J.P. and O'Fallon, W.M. (1981) The natural history of unruptured aneurysms. *New England Journal of Medicine* **304,** 696–9.

Wilkins, R.H. (Ed.) (1980) *Cerebral Arterial Spasm.* Williams and Wilkins, Baltimore.

Yabumoto, M., Funahashi, K., Fujii, T., Hayashi, S. and Komai, N. (1983) Moyamoya disease associated with intracranial aneurysm. *Surgical Neurology* **20,** 20–4.

Yamori, Y., Horie, R., Handa, H., Sato, M. and Fukase, M. (1976) Pathogenic similarity of strokes in stroke-prone spontaneously hypertensive rats and humans. *Stroke* **7,** 46–53.

Yonas, H., Agamanolis, D., Takaoka, Y. and White, R.J. (1977) Dissecting intracranial aneurysms. *Surgical Neurology* **8,** 407–15.

Yonemitsu, T., Niizuma, H., Kodama, N., Fujiwara, S. and Suzuki, J. (1983) Acoustic neurinoma presenting as subarachnoid hemorrhage. *Surgical Neurology* **20,** 125–30.

Ziegler, D.K. (1972) Hypertensive vascular diseases of the brain. In *Handbook of Clinical Neurology.* Vol. 11 (Eds. Vinken, P.J. and Bruyn, G.W.) North-Holland, Amsterdam. pp. 552–77.

6

Bacterial infections of the central nervous system

D.G.F. Harriman

The central nervous system is well shielded from bacteria by anatomical structures and capillary barriers, but once organisms have gained entry they proliferate more easily than elsewhere. The natural immunity of the CNS is comparatively ineffective, so non-pathogenic bacteria become pathogenic and weak pathogens become virulent. When that immunity is further impaired, opportunist infections by rarely encountered bacteria, viruses or fungi are permitted. Such agents rarely if ever invade the CNS unless the body's immunity is depressed by, for example, cytotoxic drugs or disease.

Allergy, now more often referred to as a hypersensitivity state, has long been considered to play an important part in some infections, as for example the caseation necrosis in tuberculosis which is ascribed to a delayed hypersensitivity reaction to *Mycobacterium tuberculosis.* This type of reaction does not seem to be important in many other infections, whereas other forms of immunoreaction or their lack play a part in every infection.

The cellular reactions which develop in the course of bacterial infections form only part of the immune reaction but are still vital in histological diagnosis. The histological demonstration of organisms is of more limited value, but can be helpful, for example, in meningococcal meningitis when intracellular diplococci can be demonstrated. Sometimes *post-mortem* cultures succeed when those taken during the course of clinical investigation have been inhibited by antibiotic therapy. Close attention should be paid to the types of cells in the inflammatory exudate—whether polymorphs, lymphocytes, histiocytes, plasma cells or macrophages—so as not to be misled by the more limited perivascular cellular reactions induced by necrosis, infarction or the earlier stages of demyelinating disease. The cells seen in non-infective exudates are mainly lymphocytes and macrophages.

The inflammatory response of the central nervous system to bacteria, if not resolved, is followed by repair but less effectively than in other organs. The best repair in the CNS is induced by purulent infections: thus there may be a complete return to normal after successful treatment of an acute bacterial meningitis. An abscess is eventually surrounded by a fibrous capsule even though poor in comparion to that of a renal or pulmonary abscess. Haematomas stimulate a mild fibrotic reaction, tissue necrosis little or none. There are two reasons for ineffective repair in the CNS. First, there are relatively few fibroblasts in the CNS, with the result that reactive fibrosis is confined to the vascular adventitia and to the meninges. Secondly, astrocytes within a region of infection are prone to destruction; those that survive at the periphery multiply and form a zone of gliosis outside the thin capsule, and this is of little value in hindering the spread of infection.

Bacterial immunology

The increasing recognition of the important part played by cellular and humoral reactions in disease has led to a greater understanding of the pathogenesis of infection of the CNS (Leibowitz and Hughes, 1983). Immunology explains how the same organism may produce, in different individuals, mild, recurrent or fatal disease, or none at all. The CNS is at a disadvantage when it comes to admitting or producing antibodies because serum proteins are unable to diffuse easily into its substance. In the cerebrospinal fluid IgG and IgA are present but IgM cannot be detected, presumably because of its greater molecular weight. Complexes of antigen (bacterial or otherwise) and antibody are likely to be formed whenever there is an immune response of humoral type. Antigen–antibody complexes are sometimes produced within blood vessels, with resultant damage. Because their formation does not depend on tissue antibody, the fibrinoid necrosis that results is no less common in the brain than elsewhere, and this mechanism explains the arteritis that may develop in tuberculous meningitis or rarely in other forms of infection of the CNS.

Two further bacteria that are important in infection of the brain are associated with immune complex disease—*Treponema pallidum*, and the staphylococcus that infects atrioventricular shunts. The nephritis that follows is of the immune complex type. Immune complexes play an important part in all infections by activating the complement system, by attracting polymorphs, lymphocytes, macrophages, and by recognizing their receptors and becoming bound to them. Knowledge in this area is growing fast and the neuropathologist may be asked to identify with as much precision as possible the cells taking part in the different types of inflammatory exudate. Help is provided by the immunoperoxidase techniques on paraffin or fresh-frozen sections.

Anatomy

Some structural features of the CNS play a role in the pathogenesis of infection. The shield of bony and fibrous membranes is overcome at times by the transport of organisms from the scalp or face by the emissary veins, or by the diploic veins which anastomose in the skull and have external venous connections as well as internal ones to venous sinuses. In chronic infections such as osteomyelitis it may be impossible to discover how organisms gain access to the interior of the skull. The dura mater, its two layers fused over the brain but remaining separate in the vertebral canal, is a valuable barrier and may prevent the spread of infection through it indefinitely. The external cellular layer of the arachnoid also provides a check to the infection in both directions, and the pia mater, delicate though it appears, inhibits the spread of infection from the subarachnoid space to the cerebral cortex and vice versa. Separate infections can therefore occur in four sites—*epidural*, *subdural*, *subarachnoid* and *within the brain*.

Two anatomical barriers to infection are visible only at a microscopical level: the **blood–brain** and the **blood–CSF barriers.** These are formed by capillaries whose permeability is similar to that of the capillaries of the proximal renal tubules. The barrier is effective against water-soluble polar compounds, but lipid-soluble compounds cross readily. It has been speculated that this may prevent the invasion of some types of micro-organisms or their toxins, but the efficacy of the barrier may itself be damaged by established infection.

Cerebral oedema and infections

Cerebral oedema is dealt with in Chapter 2. Bacterial infections may produce vasogenic oedema (Fishman, 1978), and the causative agents include powerful bacterial toxins, such as those produced by *Clostridium botulinum*, *Cl. tetani* and *Corynebacterium diphtheriae*. Other similar toxins include streptolysin O, the staphylococcal alpha-toxin and those of *Shigella dysenteriae*, *Bacillus anthracis* and *Haemophilus pertussis*. Although the toxin of *S. dysenteriae* is not specific for the CNS, it may act on cerebral blood vessels directly and produce oedema. Unexplained cerebral oedema therefore requires microbiological examination of potential sources, especially the lungs, gastrointestinal and renal tracts, and should be done at an early stage before oedema becomes irreversible.

Routes of invasion

Despite the protection given by skin, bone, meninges and vascular barriers, bacteria still manage to enter the intracranial cavity and vertebral canal. Organisms must reach the CNS in one of two ways: via the blood stream or by extension from local sources.

Few bacteria regularly invade the blood by penetrating an epithelium, unlike many viruses which nearly always do. Bacteria multiply extracellularly in the blood stream and release toxins, and so are associated with severe disease, whilst viruses are usually carried passively in the blood, and when multiplying within cells do not release toxins. Bacteria commonly encountered in the CNS as a result of septicaemia are the pneumococcus, the meningococcus and the streptococcus. One organism which is almost invariably present in the blood of an affected patient but never invades the CNS is *Mycobacterium leprae* which is carried by mononuclear cells in the blood for long periods. The reason for the inability of the mononuclears to cross the blood–brain barrier is not understood. Another and less frequent method by which the CNS is invaded through the blood stream is by septic emboli. These originate in the heart from valvular vegetations, or in the lung, from infected veins within foci of chronic infection. In the brain the emboli may form mycotic aneurysms (see pp. 229, 246) or cause single or multiple infarcts or abscesses.

Infections spreading from local sources erode bone, especially where it is thin, or gain entry by transmission along anastomotic venous channels, through fractures or separated sutures, or along cranial nerves. Infection can gain access to the interior of the skull as a result of osteomyelitis affecting the full thickness of the calvaria, but more frequently infections pass through the thin bone covering an infected middle ear or mastoid process or through the wall of an air sinus, this being betrayed by a perforation, sometimes very small, in the bone. Such defects can also be congenital. Transmission through bony ostia or along cranial nerves is more often inferred than seen, for the organism may leave no trace of its passage.

Another route of infection to the CNS has been introduced recently by the use of ventriculoatrial or ventriculoperitoneal shunts in the treatment of hydrocephalus. Catheters may remain *in situ* for years without any complications, but some become obstructed or infected and need to be revised. 'If infection occurs it is introduced at the time of insertion, and late infections are missed early ones' (Bayston, 1982). The organism best looked for in the shunt reservoir or the valve is often *Staphylococcus albus* and is cultured with difficulty. Complications include meningitis, ventriculitis, endocarditis, septicaemia and shunt nephritis.

Pyogenic infections

Epidural suppurations and granulomas

Skull Infections of the intracranial epidural space usually take the form of a small flattened abscess, for the dura develops increasingly strong adhesion to the bone throughout life and becomes more difficult to detach. The adhesion of the dura to the bone confines the abscess, which is usually found over infected thin-walled frontal or mastoid sinuses, but they can also follow osteomyelitis of thicker parts of the skull. An *epidural abscess* may even follow a glancing blow to the head, allowing osteomyelitis to develop superficially and slowly. Infections of air sinuses other than frontal and mastoid are unlikely to give rise to an epidural abscess: they more often spread *through* the adherent dura to infect the subdural or subarachnoid spaces.

Spine In contrast to the skull, there is a considerable amount of space between the loose inner layer of dura and the vertebral column to accommodate epidural infection which is therefore much commoner here than in the intracranial cavity. The source of infection is usually osteomyelitis of the thoracic or lumbar vertebrae, often the consequence of trivial skin sepsis. The patient develops extreme pain in his back with paraparesis, and when the spine is palpated focal tenderness is found. This is an acute emergency which can be treated successfuly if recognized in time, but if compression of the cord by the abscess continues long enough, thrombosis of spinal vessels may ensue, particularly in one of the major radicular arteries, this leading to infarction of the spinal cord and a permanent paraplegia.

Abscesses in the spinal epidural space can be localized or widely spread depending on the development of fibrous adhesions, and are caused most often by *Staph. aureus*, or sometimes by *Salmonella typhi.* Subacute and chronic infections produce not an abscess but a widespread *granuloma* attached to and involving the dura, infiltrated by lymphocytes and mononuclear cells, and extending over many segments. Small pockets of pus may persist in it. The infection may be so protracted before it compresses the cord that the original infective focus is no longer obvious. Spinal cord compression can be relieved by simple laminectomy. The pachymeningitis can be very indolent and extensive, as in a patient whose sacral infection has spread along the whole length of the vertebral column, enclosing small staphylococcal abscesses en route, invading the posterior fossa and presenting clinically with cranial nerve palsies. Pleural empyema, subphrenic abscess and perinephric abscess may extend into the spinal epidural space by means of the intervertebral foramina, but spread of infection in the opposite direction is extremely rare. Pachymeningitis is not confined to pyogenic organisms; it occurs also in tuberculosis, and syphilis should be excluded as a cause.

Subdural infections

Infection of the subdural space may occasionally be localized by adhesions to form an abscess, but the wide extent of this potential space and the relative avascularity of its walls are such that pus, once formed in it, normally spreads too rapidly for effective adhesions to develop. It is then no longer an abscess but a *subdural empyema*. Eventually pus may loculate, forming multiple abscesses (Fig. 6.1). Infections in the paranasal air sinuses and cranial osteomyelitis are the usual sources of infection which may reach the space by direct extension or by way of veins. Other recognized causes are a compound fracture of the skull and, rarely, a complication of

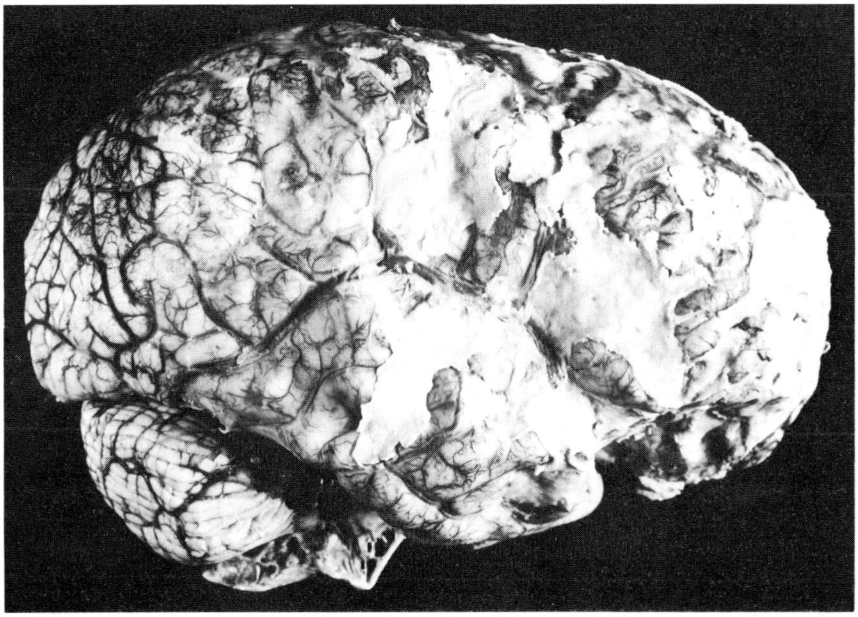

(a)

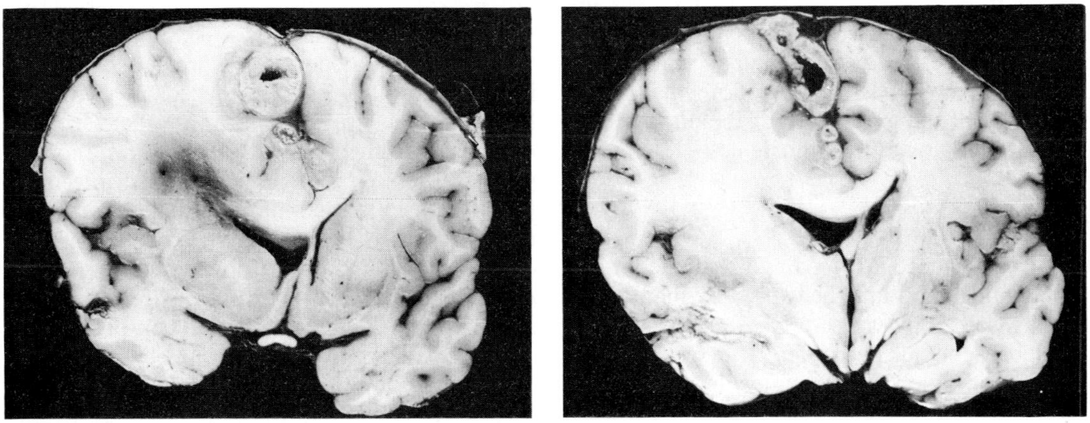

(b)

Fig. 6.1 Subdural empyema. (**a**) The pus is clearly on the surface of the arachnoid and not within the subarachnoid space. (**b**) Loculated collections of pus in the subdural space have led to the formation of multiple abscesses.

acute purulent meningitis in neonates. Frontal sinusitis may cause thrombophlebitis of the anterior part of the superior sagittal sinus, infection then spreading to the subdural space bilaterally. The circular and petrosal sinuses may be infected from the sphenoid air sinus, and both middle fossae may then be involved. The spread of subdural empyema far from the original focus is to be expected. Pus is not infrequently bilateral, covering vertex, falx and base. The veins and venous sinuses need to be examined with care when trying to discover the method of spread. Collections of pus in inaccessible sites make surgical drainage very difficult. Antibiotics have little chance of reaching the empyema via the circulation, and craniotomies are, of necessity, extensive. The causative organisms tend to be virulent pathogens—staphylococci and streptococci—so it is not surprising that the mortality is high.

Histopathology As there is virtually no capillary bed in the arachnoid, a layer of pus in the subdural space excites a granulation tissue and inflammatory reaction in the dura, and an inflammatory cell reaction alone in the subarachnoid space. In acute and severe infections the pus is not hindered from diffusing widely. In chronic infections adhesions do develop through the pia-arachnoid to the cortical surface, and occasionally small perforating arteries undergo thrombosis to produce small cortical infarcts. The adhesions do little to hinder spread of pus, but small abscesses are enmeshed in the adhesions and form, in time, a larger localized capsulated subdural abscess. The end-result of a successfully treated or of a small spontaneously resolved empyema is nothing more than focal thickening of the inner layer of the dura, a rare incidental finding at post-mortem.

Leptomeningitis

Usually shortened to 'meningitis', infection of the leptomeninges may be caused by many bacteria as well as by viruses, fungi and protozoa. The subarachnoid space offers little resistance to infection and the CSF facilitates its spread over the brain and spinal cord and into the ventricles. Although the pial vascular bed allows the ready passage of leucocytes, there are no capillaries in the arachnoid space itself and the rate of access of polymorphs may be insufficient for an early infection to be abolished. Whatever the reason, virulent organisms invading the subarachnoid space can cause death within a few hours, and bacteria that are non-pathogenic elsewhere may be responsible for severe illness.

The *organism* most often responsible for meningitis varies with the age of the patient. Meningitis is not infrequent in the neonatal period, when it is usually due to Gram-negative organisms, particularly *Escherichia coli*. Neonatal meningitis presents particular difficulties: early signs are non-specific and may be overlooked, diagnosis may be too late, host defence is relatively incompetent, and Gram-negative organisms are difficult to treat. In infants antibiotics pass into the CSF with difficulty, so effective doses are also toxic. In young children bacteria from the respiratory tract are the commonest cause, especially *Haemophilus influenzae*, and in adolescence and adult life the meningococcus and pneumococcus are the most frequently encountered. The recent emergence of strains of pneumococcus resistant not only to penicillin but also to several other antibiotics is giving rise to concern (Radetsky et al., 1981). A long list of other bacteria may cause meningitis from time to time, including the rare but serious infections by *Bacillus anthracis*, *Brucella abortus*, *Salmonella typhi* and *Listeria monocytogenes*. The last-named causes meningitis or meningoencephalitis, apparently in two separate age groups—either neonatal or in adults over 40—but because its isolation and culture are difficult it may be responsible for more infections than are apparent at the present time. The organism is found in many domestic and wild animals.

Meningitis may develop in previously healthy individuals, but is often preceded by a viral infection of the upper respiratory tract, such as influenza. It may also occur in immunosuppressed individuals as an opportunist infection. The organism is then more often than not bacterial. Among the Gram-negative organisms that complicate neurosurgical procedures, *Pseudomonas aeruginosa* is the most feared, and the same group of organisms tend to complicate leucopenia. Meningitis due to *L. monocytogenes* not infrequently complicates the lymphomas and cytotoxic drug therapy, but streptococcal meningitis tends to follow splenectomy.

Meningococcal meningitis If any one organism can be considered more dangerous and more difficult to eradicate than another, it is the meningococcus *Neisseria meningitidis*. It is over 40 years since adequate antimicrobial treatment became available, and in the early days it was hoped that there would be an end to recurrent epidemics of cerebrospinal fever with its high mortality. But epidemics continue in many parts of the world, and are by no means confined to areas of poverty or poor hygiene. Peltola et al. (1982) have described three epidemics in the five countries of Scandinavia in 1970–1979; 3000 patients were affected, of whom 250 died. This happened despite the availability of prompt treatment, intensive care and effective vaccines. The organism now shows increased resistance to sulphonamides, but it is still sensitive to penicillin. Slack (1982), in a careful epidemiological study of the disease in England and Wales, has shown that there is no real evidence of a significant reduction in mortality: 170 deaths in 1959, 205 in 1973 and 96 in 1978. In a study of individual cases, she formed the opinion that although treatment was started promptly once the condition was diagnosed, it was not early enough. A febrile patient with a purpuric rash or meningeal signs demands immediate intravenous antibiotic therapy. In overwhelming infection medullary compression due to tonsillar herniation may occur within a few hours.

In the majority of infections, however, the person becomes a healthy carrier. In the carrier state the organisms are matched by antibody-forming cells, counteracting both protein and polysaccharide antigens. The unsuspected carrier is of great importance in the spread of disease, which is by droplet infection of the upper respiratory tract. From there the meningococci will enter the blood stream and, unless defeated by the immune system, will produce an infection varying in severity from the Waterhouse–Friderichsen syndrome to acute meningitis or an insidious subacute infection liable to dangerous complications. The acute disease may develop with extraordinary rapidity, starting with headache and followed by fits and deep coma within a few hours.

The autopsy in meningitis Although most fatal cases of menigitis are the direct result of primary infection by an organism, meningitis may also be a complication of trauma, operations or malformations of the CNS. The exposed neuroplaque in meningomyelocoele, for example, provides easy access of bacteria to the meninges, and at post-mortem thick pus will be found covering the spinal cord and brain and lining the ventricles. A simple midline occipital fistula may be responsible. Postoperative infection in neurosurgical procedures is rare, but appears to have a slightly higher incidence in some centres after the trans-sphenoidal approach to the pituitary gland.

In head injury, infection is a hazard of open wounds, of compound or depressed fractures, of suture separation, and particularly of fractures of the base of the skull which allow access of organisms in air sinuses or in the middle ears to the cranial cavity (see Chapter 3). An unusual and curious cause of localized meningitis is infection of a cortical infarct which becomes covered by pus.

The post-mortem examination in hyperacute disease may disclose adrenal haemorrhage, centrilobular necrosis of the liver or disseminated intravascular coagulation. If the infection is from a local source it may be found in the scalp, cranium, air sinuses or middle ear, but if blood-borne it can be difficult or impossible to trace. When death occurs within 24 hours there is no pus in the meninges: but they are deeply congested, so much so as to suggest subarachnoid haemorrhage. The congestion and oedema may be such that they resemble the congested form of brain death that occurs during prolonged assisted ventilation. Death in hyperacute meningitis may be due not only to the meningococcus but also to one of the rare pathogens, such as anthrax. Survival for 2 days or longer allows the migration of leucocytes, and the entire brain, vertex and base will be enveloped by pus—creamy, yellow or green depending on the responsible organism. The diagnosis of pyogenic meningitis is now obvious and it is worth noting that the delicate arachnoid is able to confine the pus to the subarachnoid space. It is very rare for pus to become subdural, where it will spread easily as an empyema. A knife gently scraped over the arachnoid surface will not disturb the meningeal exudate. If the patient dies at a stage intermediate between the hyperacute phase and fully developed purulent meningitis, pus is visible only as cloudiness in the basal cisterns and as thin creamy lines alongside cortical meningeal veins.

The brain shows the usual signs of oedema, and yet when it is sectioned the ventricles may already be slightly enlarged rather than compressed. The ventricular CSF is purulent because of ventriculitis. The ependyma and the subependymal region are deeply congested and often covered by flakes of pus. The choroid plexus is similarly affected. The aqueduct and fourth ventricle may contain thick pus, a potential cause of obstructive hydrocephalus. It is rare for any change to be noted in the periventricular tissue or cortex, but when the patient survives for some days petechiae (especially in meningococcal meningitis), congestion or minute softenings can sometimes be recognized. Survival for a matter of weeks, or months, perhaps following a cryptic initial infection, inevitably is accompanied by hydrocephalus and slightly more obvious cortical infarcts. Such complications often permit indefinite survival, but with neurological deficit.

Histopathology At the acute stage the meningeal exudate is composed entirely of polymorphs. Bacteria are both intracellular and extracellular. Involvement of small meningeal arteries or veins is rare initially but the exudate is often accompanied by wisps of fibrin. The contrast between the appearance of the meninges and that of the underlying cortex is remarkable: few if any polymorphs enter the cortical perivascular spaces. But the cortex is oedematous, as shown by large artificial perineuronal spaces and a spongiform ground substance. Neuronal cytoplasm is often acidophilic. In the meninges at the hyperacute highly congested phase the exudate is very sparse but organisms are numerous.

After some days the polymorphonuclear leucocytes are less numerous, and lymphocytes and a few plasma cells appear in the exudate. There is more fibrin, and macrophages are formed.

A small number of blood vessels in the exudate may now show fibrinoid necrosis and thrombosis. Some cells of the exudate enter the outer cortical perivascular spaces, and subpial microglia proliferate. Vascular thrombosis results in small foci of cortical necrosis. The exudate covering the ventricular wall denudes it of ependyma, and mild subependymal perivascular infiltration occurs. When similar changes develop in the aqueduct the purulent exudate that it contains inspissates and may organize. Obstruction here or at the exit foramina of the fourth ventricle will lead to hydrocephalus, but the existence alone of an extensive meningeal exudate may itself have the same result.

Complications In subacute and chronic infections, especially those due to the meningococcus, the meningeal exudate does not resolve completely and is focally organized. Complications are virtually inevitable. Thickening of the meninges loculating the CSF will produce *communicating hydrocephalus* by blocking the basal cisterns. The same process of fibrous organization around the spinal cord can cause *infarction* by compression or thrombosis. The meningeal thickening around the cord is similar to 'progressive spinal arachnoiditis', a rare complication of spinal anaesthesia of obscure origin possibly due to bacteria of low virulence. It must be distinguished from meningeal fibrosis and loculation due to non-infective chemical irritation, to which the meninges are sensitive. There may be an interval of several months before paraplegia ensues from spinal complications.

Encysted collections of fluid may develop over the surface of the hemisphere (*cystic arachnoiditis*), and, if numerous or large enough, may cause significant compression. They have to be distinguished from developmental *arachnoid cysts*, some of which are lined by a simple epithelium and are likely to be derived from ectopic glial nests (Jabukiac, Dunsmore and Beckett, 1968).

The resolution of old cortical infarcts in chronic meningitis will lead, in the course of time, to cortical atrophy and *compensatory hydrocephalus*. Other complications of meningitis include *cranial neuritis*, especially of the auditory nerves which is an important cause of nerve deafness in children.

Subdural effusions (Fig. 6.2) clear or blood-stained, are a more frequent complication than was formerly thought, especially in infants. They are often large enough to require surgery and are usually explained by the formation of a valvular tear in the arachnoid. It is not clear how the tears are formed. One suggestion is that they result from necrosis around an arteritic meningeal vessel. The demonstration that ^{131}I human serum albumin enters a subdural effusion after intravenous injection (Rabe, 1967) means that some of the effusion comes from plasma, and indeed the protein content is high. In infancy only 5 per cent follow meningitis, 40 per cent are traumatic and the remainder are of unknown aetiology (Till, 1968). Some effusions (*hygromas*) form a membrane (Fig. 6.2)

Subdural empyema may also complicate chronic meningitis but, contrary to expectation,

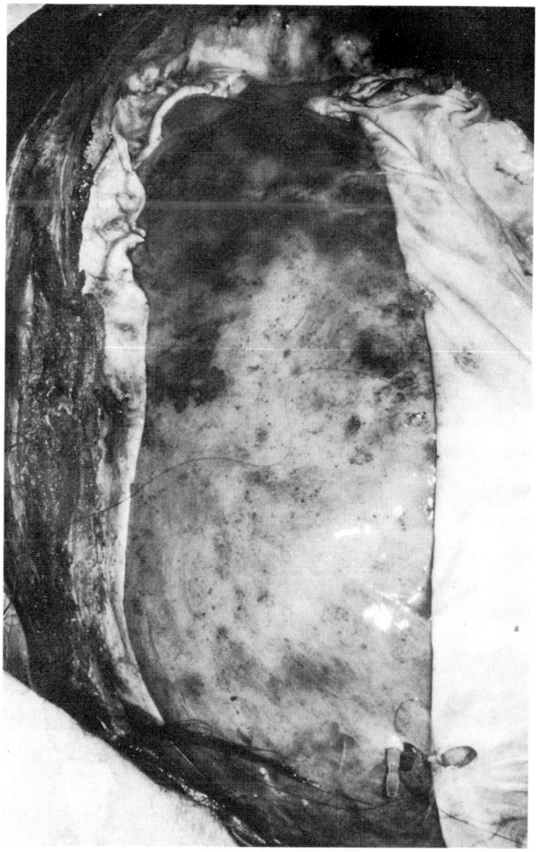

Fig. 6.2 Subdural hygroma at autopsy in a girl of 11 years. Fresh haemorrhage has occurred in the frontal part above. Elsewhere the thin sac containing clear fluid is pale. The dura, lightly adherent to the hygroma, has been reflected superiorly.

is rarer than effusion. A very rare sequel is diffuse necrosis of the subcortical white matter (Buchan and Alvord, 1969) due to venous sinus occlusion.

Recurrent meningitis is usually due to a defect in the dura on the base of the skull secondary to a head injury (see p. 98), or to a congenital sinus or fistula, usually in the midline on the patient's back.

Brain abscess

Brain abscesses might be expected to have become rare; their incidence has fallen, but they are still frequently encountered in neurosurgical practice. The mortality rate was in the region of 40 per cent for 25 years until 1980, but recently has been as low as 14 per cent (Smith and Hendrick, 1983). Curiously, experience in China from 1952 to 1972, using only ultrasound, exploratory needles and the clinical features, resulted in a significantly improved mortality of 22 per cent in 400 cases (Yang, 1981). The efficient use of antibiotics, good localization by CT scan and the use of modern microbiological techniques have all contributed to fewer 'sterile' cultures and to improved treatment.

An abscess is treated either by simple drainage or by excision, and chemotherapy must be used immediately without waiting for the bacteriological report. Knowledge of the source of the abscess is useful; for example, an abscess derived from an air sinus—usually the frontal—may well be due to *Streptococcus milleri*, which is penicillin-sensitive, but an abscess resulting from dental infection may contain an obligate anaerobe (Leading Article, 1978).

As in the case of leptomeningitis, the *source of infection* producing a brain abscess may be local or blood-borne. Passage through the blood stream may be due to bacteraemia or septicaemia, but there must be occasions when organisms reaching the brain capillaries are prevented by the blood-brain barrier from entering the brain. Bacteria will sometimes cause an abscess if local resistance is reduced, as for example in congenital cyanotic heart disease. Kagawa et al. (1983) reviewed 62 such cases, and found a peak incidence between the ages of 4 and 7 years; only one-fifth were multiple. The overall mortality was 37 per cent, but when aspiration alone without excision was adopted there were no further deaths.

A rare familial disorder, *chronic granulomatous disease*, predisposes to recurrent infections including staphylococcal cerebral abscess in children. It is due to a deficiency of nicotinamide adenine dinucleotide in leucocytes with the result that they are unable to digest organisms, and is associated with hypergammaglobulinaemia.

Staphylococcal septic foci in the skin and osteomyelitis, rare sources of blood-borne infection, tend to produce solitary rather than multiple abscesses. One or other may be the source of solitary parietal lobe abscesses whose origin usually remains undetected. The infective focus may have healed, for the development of solitary metastic abscesses appears to be unduly slow.

An important source of metastatic infection is the lung, where chronic sepsis—especially bronchiectasis—may eventually result in brain abscesses. These are usually in the middle cerebral arterial territory, suggesting that they are due to septic emboli from infected pulmonary veins. In the same manner, septic emboli may arise from vegetations of infective endocarditis.

Locally derived brain abscesses occur more frequently than metastatic, are nearly always single and are a less formidable neurosurgical challenge. For many years a chronically infected middle ear has been considered the commonest source, and still is because of the continuing neglect of chronic and recurrent discharge from the middle ear. Adhesion between the petrous temporal bone and the temporal lobe or the cerebellum leads to abscess in these common sites. Chronic mastoid infection may have a similar end result. Chronic sinusitis, especially of the frontal and paranasal air sinuses, subacute or chronic pyogenic meningitis, septic foci on the scalp or face have all been the source of cerebral abscess. In infants and children malformations are a frequent pathway, especially meningomyelocele, encephalocele and sinuses connecting the exterior to the spinal or cerebral meninges. In the case of trauma, failure to prevent the passage of infection through fractures (especially of the base) or merely separation of sutures, may end in abscess. Even minor trauma, such as a blow to the scalp, can produce indolent local infection, osteomyelitis and abscess. Finally, mention must be made of dental sepsis, generally to be a local source of infection because the associated abscess occurs in a frontal lobe. The route taken by the organisms is obscure, but the same ones are found in both sites, usually an anaerobe, supporting local rather than blood spread.

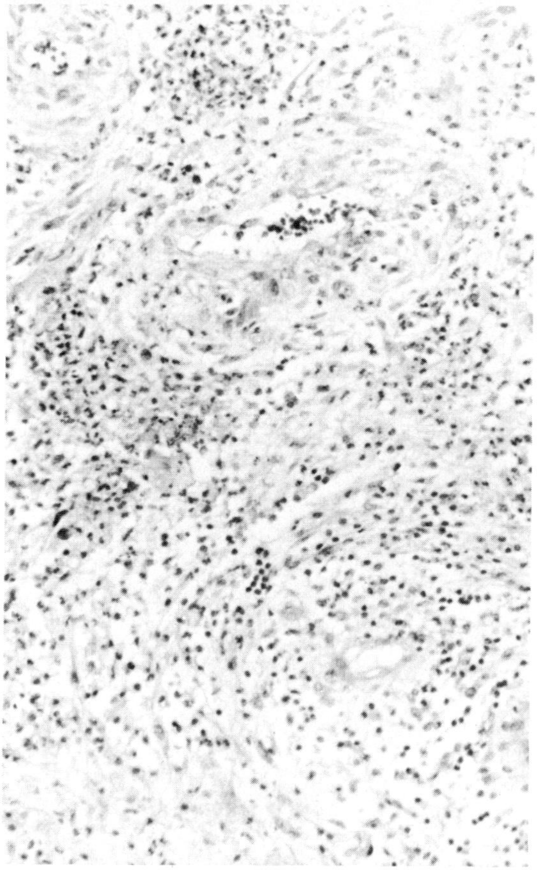

Fig. 6.3 Suppurative encephalitis. Infiltration of leucocytes, chiefly polymorphs, and small pockets of pus. Vascular endothelium is swollen and there is capillary proliferation. Haematoxylin and eosin × 208.

Site of abscess formation The frontal, temporal and parietal lobes have already been mentioned, as well as the cerebellum. These are the commoner sites, but abscesses may occur anywhere, always with a decided preference for the less vascular white matter. The presence of metastatic abscesses in white matter is understandable, but local infection as from the middle ear must always traverse cortex before it reaches white matter. Appropriate sections through the meninges and cortex show their adhesion to dura through which infection must have travelled, and a healed or healing track in the grey matter leading to the abscess can sometimes be found. Clearly the greater capillary density of the grey matter helps to overcome infection there.

Development of abscess The first event on the arrival of bacteria in cortex or white matter is the migration of polymorphs from local capillaries, whose endothelium becomes swollen, and the formation of an area of *suppurative encephalitis* (Fig. 6.3). Astrocytes swell and start to proliferate, polymorphs gather into microscopical foci, microglia are mobilized, and the tissue becomes oedematous, haemorrhagic and undergoes necrosis. The cellular proliferation described is no more than moderate except for leucocytic exudation, and perivascular spaces in the vicinity become cuffed with polymorphs and lympho-

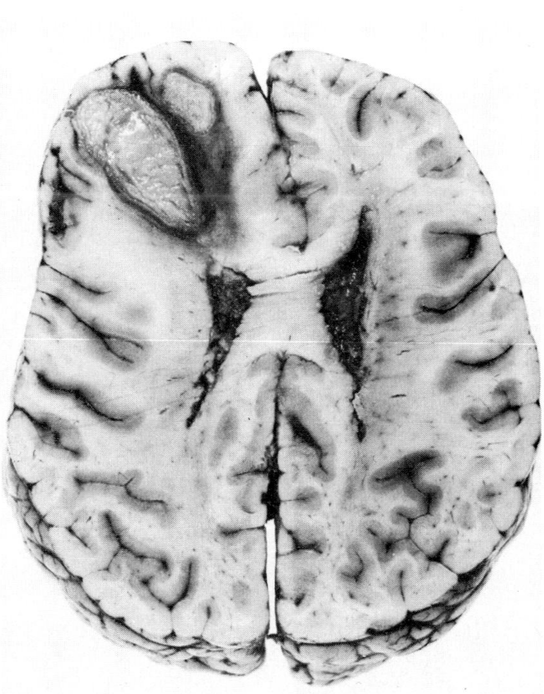

Fig. 6.4 Multilocular abscess in the white matter of the frontal lobe, with a well defined capsule. It followed the drainage of a retro-orbital abscess in a boy of 17 years. Clinically silent for a month, it caused widespread cerebral oedema. He died on admission to hospital.

cytes. The number of foam cells formed before coalescence of the microabscesses into a single abscess in the white matter is variable. An abscess may vary greatly in size, is usually oval, and in any one plane may appear multiple but serial cuts will often reveal that it is solitary but locular (Fig. 6.4). The white matter around the abscess, at least in the earlier stages, contains fresh foci of suppurative encephalitis and micro-abscesses; in their further development they may coalesce with the main abscess, enlarging it and forming loculi. Rupture into a ventricle is common, causing ventriculitis; the pus may spread in the CSF or be thick enough to be confined to an angle by adhesions. The capsule of the abscess is at first poorly defined, but as time passes it becomes firmer and can be stripped easily from the surrounding oedematous white matter. The oedema around an abscess, like that extending widely from a long-established meningioma is often widespread, giving the white matter a delicate light green tint.

Microscopically the wall or capsule of a cerebral abscess varies with its age (Fig. 6.5). In the earlier stages the pus is confined by a narrow irregular layer of inflammatory granulation tissue, infiltrated by polymorphs, lymphocytes and some macrophages. The cells spread into the surrounding oedematous white matter. In some places the young capsule is very thin or even deficient. At a later stage, more fibroblasts appear and outside this gliosis begins. The astrocytes in the oedematous white mater are gemistocytic in type. Plasma cells accompany the lymphocytes in the wall. Further development consists of fibroblastic proliferation and condensation to a fibrous capsule, and outside this fibrillary gliosis with lessening of leucocytic infiltration.

The thickness of the collagenous capsule varies in different parts of the abscess, so its area is not accurately estimated by measuring the wall. Individual variation in reaction, depending on age and immunity, makes the traditional rule of thumb that thickness increases by 1 mm per month unreliable, but it is a rough guide in the first 2 or 3 months.

In former days neurosurgeons found that Thorotrast (a proprietary preparation of thorium dioxide) injected into the abscess for radiography promoted encapsulation, but stopped using it when its safety was questioned. Twenty years later there were rare reports of carcinoma following its use. Some neuroradiologists believe that iophendylate injection (Myodil) is just as effective in promoting fibrosis. In rare cases, an abscess may heal entirely by natural means, forming a mass of collagen, but still potentially epileptogenic.

The chief differences between cerebral and other visceral abscess are thus: (1) the small supply of fibrocytes and the consequent slow and limited encapsulation; (2) poor local immunity; and (3) the danger of spreading oedema. The neuroglial reaction also is slow and has little value in confining the infection; in fact, the astrocytes are often destroyed by the abscess and gliosis is impaired.

Septic embolism Septic emboli from lung or infected valvular vegetations may not only be responsible for metastatic cerebral abscesses, but also may lodge in small cerebral arteries, infect-

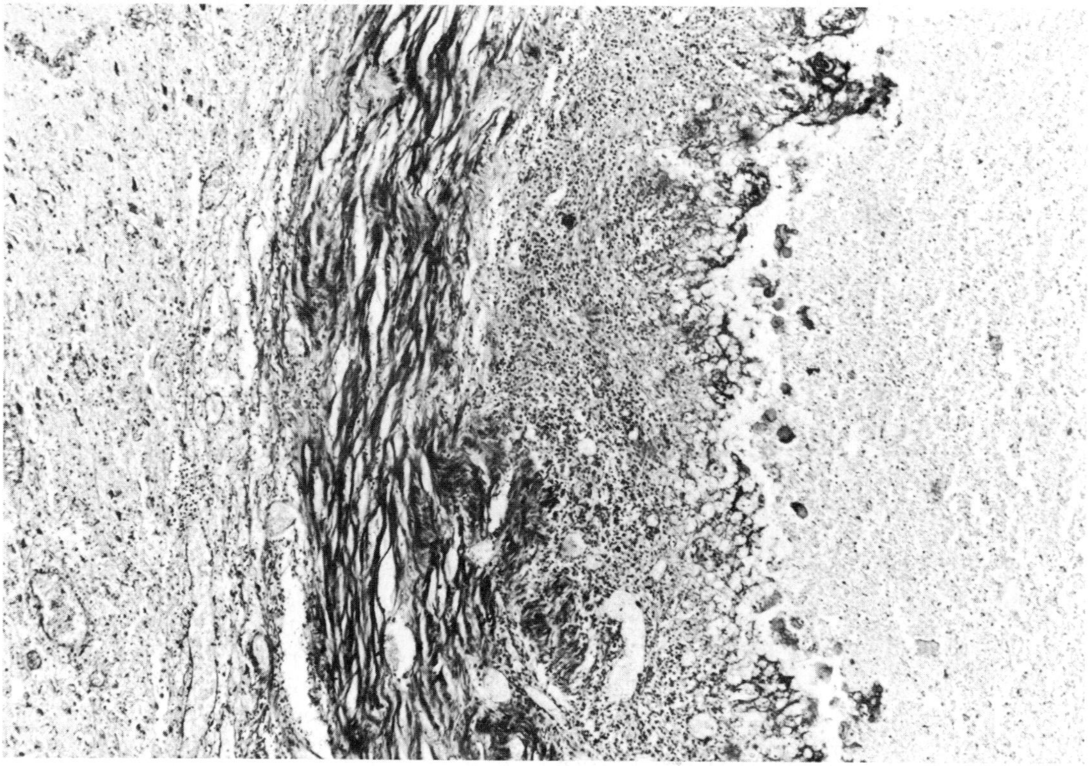

Fig. 6.5 Capsule of the abscess shown in Fig. 6.4. From right to left, pus including few calcified bodies, granulation tissue, fibrous capsule and gliosis in white matter. PTAH × 80 reduced to 90%.

ing and weakening their walls so that mycotic aneurysms result.* The aneurysms enlarge and rupture, or cause multiple coalescent infarcts. It is not always easy to distinguish septic from aseptic emboli as both may attract leucocytes; but septic emboli are more often multiple, they are more heavily infiltrated by neutrophils, and organisms can usually be stained within them.

Changes in the CSF

Since the previous edition of *Greenfield's Neuropathology* was published, Système International (SI) units have been generally accepted, but the old units have not disappeared. SI units applicable to normal CSF, with corresponding former values, are: cells 0–8 × 10^6/l; protein 0.1–0.45 g/l (formerly 10–45 mg/100 ml); chlorides as NaCl, 120–128 mmol/l (700–750 mg/100 ml); and glucose 2.5–4.8 mmol/l (45–85 mg/100 ml).

Lumbar puncture is employed less often in diagnosis today because of advances in neuroradiology, but remains essential in the precise diagnosis and follow-up of infections of the CNS. In bacterial infections, changes in the CSF vary with the site of sepsis.

If the subarachnoid space is involved there are always changes in cell count and protein level, and *subdural infection* frequently has a similar but less drastic effect. Cerebral abscess produces variable changes, but in *cranial epidural abscess* the CSF is usually normal.

Spinal epidural granulomas, on the other hand, affect the spinal fluid, by blocking the subarachnoid space. The free flow of CSF is hindered, and if the circulation is obstructed blood oozes out of the vessels (Froin–Nonne syndrome). The fluid is then yellowish-red and has a high protein content in the more extreme cases. The pus from a spinal epidural abscess may gravitate to the

* In this context the term 'mycotic' is used in the general sense of micro-organisms, although the original Greek, *mykes*, means mushroom.

epidural lumbar theca, from which it may be aspirated—by design or inadvertently. Its thick creamy consistency distinguishes it from the most purulent of cerebrospinal fluids. If a mixture of normal CSF and epidural pus is obtained it can be distinguished from purulent meningitis by normal levels of glucose and chlorides, despite a large content of leucocytes and organisms.

In *purulent meningitis* the most important characteristics of the fluid, apart from the increased pressure, are (1) its tendency to form a stringy fibrinous coagulum; (2) the lowering or absence of glucose; and (3) the presence of bacteria in the centrifuged deposit. The traditional explanation for the low glucose level—glycolysis by bacterial growth—has not yet been convincingly displaced. The cell count can be very high, over 1000–2000 × 10^6/l polymorphs. In late cases and in some subacute infections the count is comparatively low and may contain a varying proportion of lymphocytes and mononuclears, including plasma cells. The protein rises in proportion to the cell count. Glucose always falls rapidly and often disappears completely from the fluid. The chlorides also may fall to 111 mmol/l (650 mg/100 ml) or below. In meningococcal meningitis, when diplococci are scanty and, as is usual, intracellular, they are best demonstrated by Gram's stain counterstained by methyl green pyronin: the cocci are a brilliant red against the green (or purple) of the nucleus.

In *cerebral abscess* the changes in the fluid vary with the location of the abscess, but attempts to culture organisms from the CSF are, more often than not, unsuccessful. The cells are not all polymorphs; these form about 25 per cent of the total. There are no more than 50 × 10^6/l, and the protein is in the region of 1.0 g/l. There is no coagulum, and glucose and chlorides are normal. If, however, the abscess is close to the meningeal surface or to a ventricle, or has ruptured into a ventricle, the fluid becomes purulent. Obviously this can be misinterpreted as meningitis, but the fluid is different. There is no coagulum, it contains over 1.8 mmol/l glucose and there are no bacteria in the centrifuged deposit. All variations between these two characteristic types of fluid may be found. The mere presence of polymorphs in the CSF does not necessarily indicate infection; they may also be a reaction to necrosis in a tumour, to infarction or to blood in the subarachnoid space. The formation of a fibrin coagulum is the rule in meningitis, but rare in other conditions.

Tuberculous infection

The histopathology of tuberculosis of the central nervous system has changed but little since specific chemotherapy became available, but at least in developed countries tuberculous meningitis is no longer seen in large numbers of children. Primary infections are now more common in adults. In the UK, immigrants (who form 5 per cent of the population) are more susceptible than others. As an illustration, there were 17 cases of tuberculous meningitis over a 5-year period in Leicester, of whom 15 were Asian (Swart, Briggs, and Millac, 1981). These authors reported a fall from 400 cases per year in England and Wales in the mid-1960s to a current figure of about 100. This represents only 1 per cent of all cases of tuberculosis, and the mortality rate is high at 30 per cent. Tuberculosis of the CNS also occurs in patients whose immunity is impaired by autoimmune disease, chemotherapy or steroid treatment—it is an important opportunist infection. Curiously, it is rare as a complication of the acquired immunodeficiency syndrome (Waterson, 1983), which predisposes mainly to viral and fungal infections. In this syndrome immunity is impaired by T-cell dysfunction.

The present failure to eliminate tuberculous meningitis is partly due to new diagnostic difficulties (Parsons, 1982). The presentation on admission tends no longer to include the classic features of photophobia, fever, headache, vomiting and neck stiffness; meningitis develops late. A normal ESR, a negative Mantoux test and a history of BCG vaccination do not exclude the diagnosis. CT scans are helpful but only in the later stages when a basal exudate, a tuberculoma, hydrocephalus or infarcts have formed.

The usual strains of *M. tuberculosis* to infect man (the human and bovine) never reach the central nervous system directly. The *portals of entry* are either the respiratory or the alimentary tract, where the primary lesion is formed. The lipid-coated bacteria are carried to a lymph node where they proliferate slowly to cause caseation, a form of cellular necrosis whose thick creamy consistency is responsible for the name.

Caseation also occurs at the site of primary infection. Depending on the immune response and the number of bacteria, either no further spread will occur or it takes place via the thoracic duct into the blood stream. Delay before vascular dissemination varies greatly—it may be a week or many years. The effect of blood spread is also variable, resulting in scattered tubercles or the familiar widespread miliary tuberculosis. As in the case of purulent infections, tuberculosis may infect the epidural or subdural spaces, the leptomeninges or the neural tissue.

Epidural tuberculosis This is very rare in the cranial cavity, virtually only originating from otitis media. It is better known in the vertebral canal arising in a tuberculous infection in vertebrae. Spinal column tuberculosis is still a major cause of back pain in the developing countries. The infection starts in the cancellous bone, causing a tuberculous granuloma which destroys both bone cortex and the intervertebral disc (which can resist pyogenic but not tuberculous infection). The granuloma enters and extends widely in the epidural space, eventually compressing the spinal cord or causing thrombosis of one of the major radicular arteries.

Subdural tuberculous infection There is only one form of tuberculous infection in the subdural space that deserves separate mention, and that is the rare *tuberculoma en plaque*. Fairly large flattened or nodular masses adhere to the dura and to the leptomeninges. Often adhesions develop to the cortex, which may be invaded. Miliary tubercles may sometimes be found on the dura on the floor of the skull—a useful diagnostic sign in tuberculous meningitis.

Meningeal tuberculomas A well known medical dictionary defines a tuberculoma as a 'tuberculous abscess'. It is not. It is a mass of tuberculous granulation tissue in which bacilli are very sparse, having been contained by the body's immune system. It begins to resemble an abscess only when it undergoes necrosis and forms acellular, caseous, non-purulent material.

Isolated tuberculomas of varying size are occasionally found in the leptomeninges, and may later give rise to generalized tuberculous meningitis. Single tuberculomas may also occur in the brain (discussed later in this chapter), and can be large and compressive, measuring up to 7 or 8 cm in diameter. Multiple small meningeal tuberculomas, a few millimetres in diameter, are not uncommon at necropsy in patients who die of tuberculosis without clinical evidence of intracranial disease. They are often associated with small cerebral tuberculomas, also asymptomatic.

Tuberculous meningitis

This relatively common form of meningitis responds well to antibiotic and chemotherapy if treatment is started early, but if diagnosis is delayed it is liable to result in fatal complications or to leave the patient severely handicapped. The drugs used in treatment are themselves toxic and require careful monitoring. The vestibular and auditory damage provoked by streptomycin is well known.

Tuberculous meningitis is no longer a disease predominantly of young children, but occurs at any age. Access of tubercle bacilli to the meninges is presumably by spread from the primary complex, pulmonary or intestinal. In former days when miliary tuberculosis was common, 80 per cent of cases developed tuberculous meningitis; but this could develop also in the absence of miliary spread. Rich (1951), in an elaboration of earlier work, showed that these apparently conflicting events could be explained by postulating that a small tuberculoma first developed in the cortex bordering the meninges. Meningitis did not occur until the tuberculoma discharged into the subarachnoid space, producing a violent reaction in the sensitized (Mantoux-positive) patient. This explanation may not always be correct, as widespread inflammatory tuberculous meningitis can be found when the Mantoux reaction is negative, and in the presence of impaired immunity. It is true that at necropsy careful examination of the brain will nearly always reveal a 'Rich's focus' or more than one which could have discharged bacilli into the CSF (Fig. 6.6). Tuberculomas in the choroid plexus have also been suggested as a source, but examination of the plexuses usually reveals miliary tubercles similar in age to those in the subarachnoid space.

The *gross appearance* of the brain in tuberculous meningitis is usually characteristic (Fig. 6.6). There may be a slight grey-green opacity of the meninges over the cerebral convexity but a much thicker green exudate fills the basal cisterns, covers the front of the pons and enters the sylvian fissures and cisterna magna. The spinal cord is also enveloped. Tubercles are not easy to find in the exudate, but can sometimes be seen under the lips of the sylvian fissures and near the

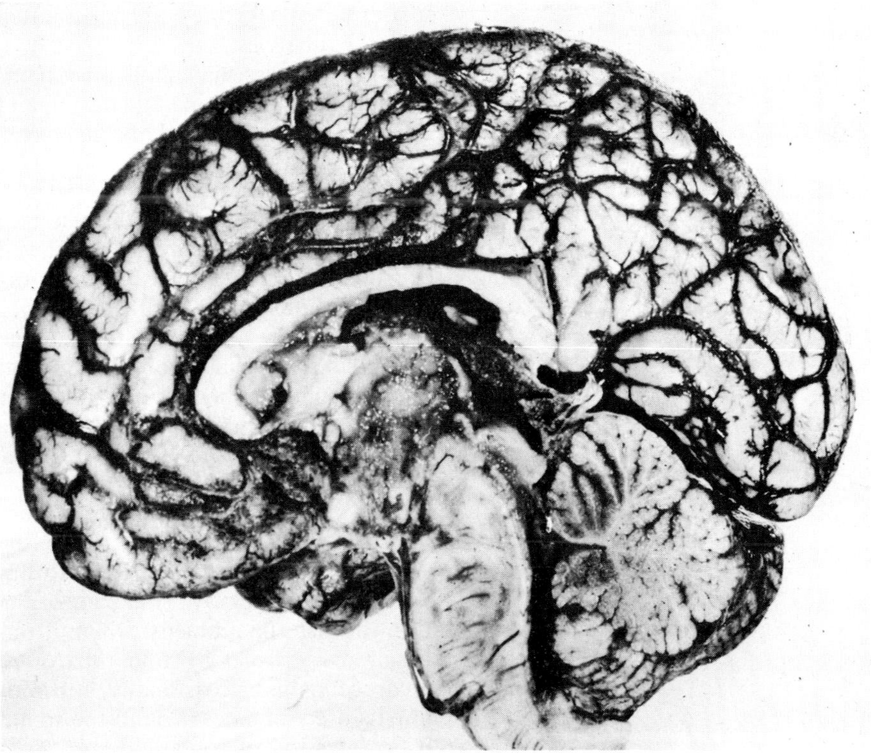

(a)

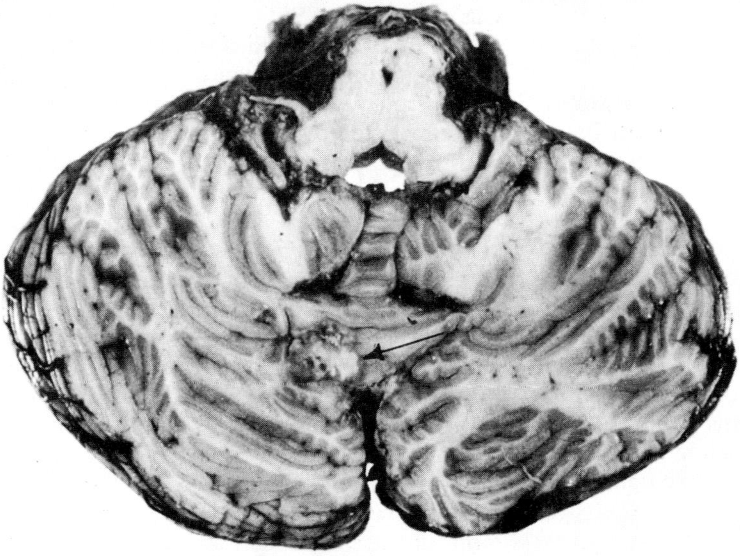

(b)

Fig. 6.6 Tuberculous meningitis. (**a**) View of the medial surface of the brain. The basal cistern is filled with exudate, and glistening tubercles are seen on the walls of the dilated ventricle and septum pellucidum. (**b**) Rich's focus (arrow).

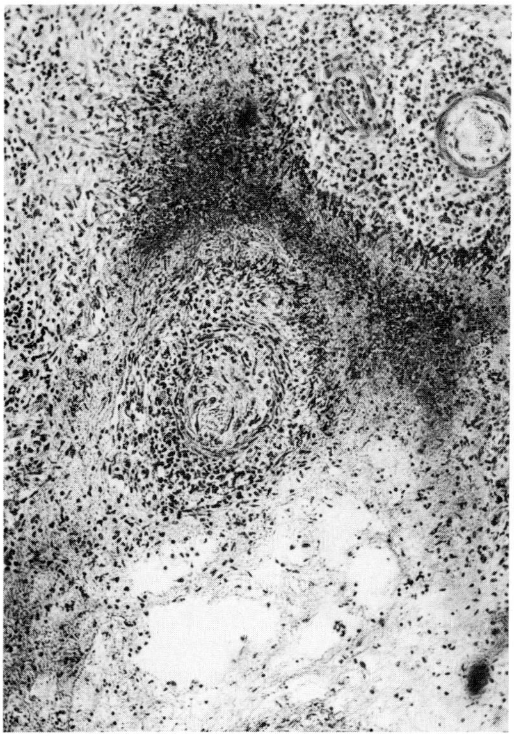

Fig. 6.7 Tuberculous meningitis, showing an area of caseation and a small inflamed and thrombosed meningeal artery. Note the absence of Langhans giant cells.

pre- and postcentral veins over the convexity. Here they must not be confused with arachnoid granulations. As mentioned earlier, the floor of the skull should be included in the search. Histology is always required to confirm a suspected diagnosis.

The thickness of the exudate depends to some extent on the duration of the meningitis, but in rare cases it is focal, limited to a small area of the brain surface and sparing the base. The reason for this is usually an adjacent or underlying tuberculoma in the brain or meninges.

Microscopically in cases which have lasted for a few weeks the meningeal exudate consists of lymphocytes, plasma cells and epitheloid cells lying in a matrix of degenerate and partly caseated fibrin (Fig. 6.7). Giant-celled tuberculous nodules can be seen in this exudate, but are often scanty and may be absent. The degree of cellular exudate and of caseation varies from case to case. It is often concentrated around the meningeal vessels. The mycobacterium may be abundant or scanty. In the latter case they are most often found within the tubercles.

The meningeal arteries may show an inflammatory reaction in the adventitia and media, and often in the intima, or subintimal fibrous hyperplasia may occur as in Heubner's arteritis (see p. 255). Inflammation in arteries and veins may proceed to fibrinoid necrosis with resulting thrombosis and multiple infarcts within the basal ganglia because of involvement of the perforating vessels. The outer laminae of the cerebral cortex and some of the superficial folia of the cerebellum show microglial proliferation and there is usually some lymphocytic infiltration of the entering veins. Small tuberculous nodules are not uncommonly seen near to these, but widespread involvement of the cortex is rare.

In streptomycin-treated patients dying more than 10 weeks after the onset of the illness, the exudate is more fibrous and may even be ligneous. It is especially thick over the base of the brain and in the cisterna ambiens, where it obstructs the circulation of CSF and thus often leads to hydrocephalus. Occasionally, tuberculous meningitis predominates around the spinal cord with compression of roots and cord by a thick exudate (Dastur and Wadia, 1969).

Changes in the CSF The importance of early diagnosis of tuberculous meningitis cannot be overemphasized. The typical cerebrospinal fluid in tuberculous meningitis is under increased pressure, often over 300 mm. It is clear or very slightly opalescent, and on standing a fine cobweb coagulum forms in it. The cell count is usually between 50 and 200 cells $\times 10^6$/l, and consists chiefly of lymphocytes with plasma cells and other large mononuclear cells; neutrophil polymorphs may also be present in considerable numbers. The total protein is only moderately increased in the early stages, but as the disease progresses it often exceeds 2 g/l. The glucose almost always falls to 1.2–1.6 mmol or lower but is rarely completely absent. The chlorides fall progressively and often very considerably so that levels below 100 mmol/l of NaCl are not uncommon. In the early stages, however, they may be in the region of 120 mmol/l NaCl. They are therefore less reliable than the level of glucose in diagnosis. The mycobacterium may be found either in a spread of the coagulum or in the centrifuged deposit. The proportion of cases in which tubercle bacilli can be found varies with the technique but with care may exceed 90 per cent. Guinea-pig injection and culture of the deposit are even more reliable. Staff handling potentially infective material must take the usual precautions.

The chief diseases which may cause difficulty in the differential diagnosis are various forms of meningoencephalitis due to viruses, cerebral abscess, and subacute and chronic meningitis due to organisms other than *M. tuberculosis* (e.g. cryptococci). Viral meningitis and cerebral abscess are most easily distinguished by the normal level of glucose and, usually, of chlorides in these conditions and by the absence of a typical coagulum, although this rarely may form in poliomyelitis and other virus infections. The nature of the cell count and the presence of organisms are the most valuable criteria in distinguishing tuberculous from other forms of ingravescent meningitis. But these very seldom come into question on clinical grounds.

Some patients who show all the signs of an incipient meningitis, and in whom tuberculous meningitis is suspected, have a normal CSF apart from a raised cell count up to $300 \times 10^6/1$. Although tubercle bacilli have never been shown in the CSF, these patients are sometimes later found to have a tuberculoma. The condition has been referred to as *serous tuberculous meningitis*, and carries a good prognosis.

Tuberculomas of the brain and spinal cord

Tuberculous granulomas were formerly a very common form of intracranial tumour and remain far from rare in areas where tuberculosis is rife (Dastur and Desai 1965). Cerebellar tuberculomas were at one time the most frequent form of intracranial mass in children and the cerebellum is still the commonest site. Supratentorial tuberculomas often cease to enlarge after a time and may become calcified in their outer parts, but cerebellar masses less often become quiescent. It is rather more common to find multiple than single intracerebral tuberculomas (Fig. 6.8). They may form round or oval masses or may have a more lobular shape from the fusion of several smaller nodules. On section the centre is necrotic but firm and of a creamy colour. The capsule, which may be from 1 to 3 mm in thickness, is grey, gelatinous and rather tough, and a narrow zone of grey gliosis surrounds it. There is much less external softening than around cerebral abscesses. A tuberculoma can often be separated cleanly from the brain tissue at operation, but before streptomycin was available this procedure was almost always followed by tuberculous meningitis.

Microscopically the capsule of an intracerebral tuberculoma contains varying proportions of collagenous tissue and giant-celled tubercles, enclosing caseous material (Fig. 6.8). Outside the capsule there is a zone of gliosis in which large spider-like astrocytes with thick processes are often found. There is a varying amount of lymphocytic infiltration of the vessel walls in the neighbourhood. In long-standing cases the capsule becomes more fibrous and loses more or less completely its tubercles and inflammatory infiltrations. At this stage calcification is often present, especially in the outer parts of the necrotic centre, and bone may be formed in occasional cases.

Tuberculous abscess True abscesses of the brain, as opposed to tuberculomas, have been described but are very rare. Tubercle bacilli are very numerous in the pus which forms; eventually a capsule develops similar to that produced by pyogenic organisms, devoid of systematized follicles. A solitary abscess has been reported (Bannister, 1970) (Fig. 6.9), but those previously described have been multiple. All have to be distinguished from pseudoabscesses formed by the liquefaction of caseous material in tuberculomas. In true abscesses the absence of the usual granulomatous reaction to the tubercle bacilli suggests the failure of an immune mechanism.

Sarcoidosis (Schaumann's disease)

Sarcoidosis has been recognized for many years as the most usual cause of the syndrome of uveoparotitis. The facial nerve is often involved in its course in or near the parotid gland. Sarcoid granulomas are conventionally distinguished from tubercles by the absence of necrosis, but now van Maarsseveen et al. (1983) state that necrosis of individual cells and fibrinoid vascular necrosis can be found in a substantial number of affected lymph nodes. Many cases have now been reported in which sarcoidosis has affected the meninges, brain or spinal cord. It may also involve skeletal muscle (see Chapter 21). Only a few have also shown uveoparotitis, and others a spread of disease to the lungs, spleen or bones. In a small

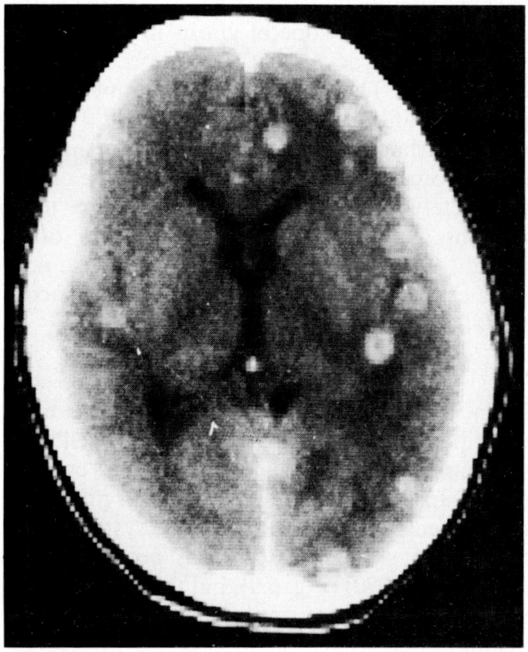

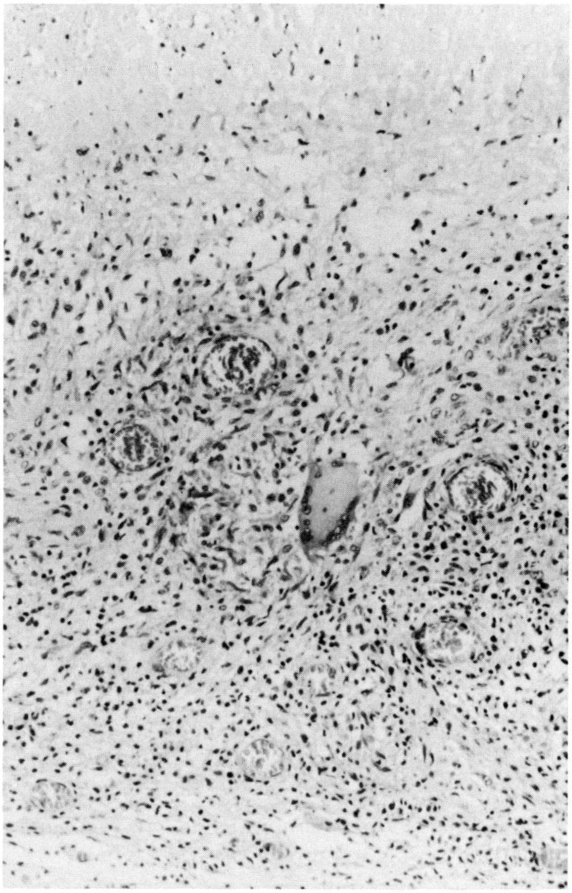

(a) **(b)**

Fig. 6.8 (**a**) CT scan showing numerous cerebral tuberculomas with caseous centres. Enhanced. (Courtesy of Dr I. Holland.) (**b**) Biopsy of one of the lesions. The 'capsule' of tuberculous granulation tissue merges into caseous material (above). Haematoxylin and eosin × 208 reduced to 75%. (Courtesy of Dr P.B. Hamal.)

number of cases the disease has apparently been confined to the cranial cavity.

The diagnosis of sarcoidosis depends on clinical evidence (e.g. diabetes insipidus or papilloedema complicating the uveoparotid syndrome) and on investigations such as the serum calcium level, Kveim and Mantoux reactions or lymph node biopsy. The disease is frequently self-limited, but necropsy reports of CNS involvement are available (Herring and Urich, 1969). In the majority the disease has been localized in one of two situations: (1) the leptomeninges, most often over the base of the brain and in the posterior fossa; (2) the infundibulum and the floor and anterior part of the walls of the third ventricle (Fig. 6.10). The optic nerves and chiasma may also be invaded. Cerebral nodules of sarcoid granulomas have been described (Karnik, 1982). The perivascular spaces of the vessels in the basal ganglia and pons may be distended with granuloma, with little invasion of the meninges, or there may be a similar perivascular invasion of the cerebral and cerebellar cortex with lesions in the overlying meninges. Rarely, the spinal cord may be infiltrated by granulomas overshadowing meningeal involvement.

Electron microscopy has rarely been possible in cerebral sarcoidosis. Trombley, Mirra and Miles (1981) obtained biopsies from three female patients and found the same features of subplasmalemmal linear densities and cytoplasmic projections like villi in the epitheloid and multi-

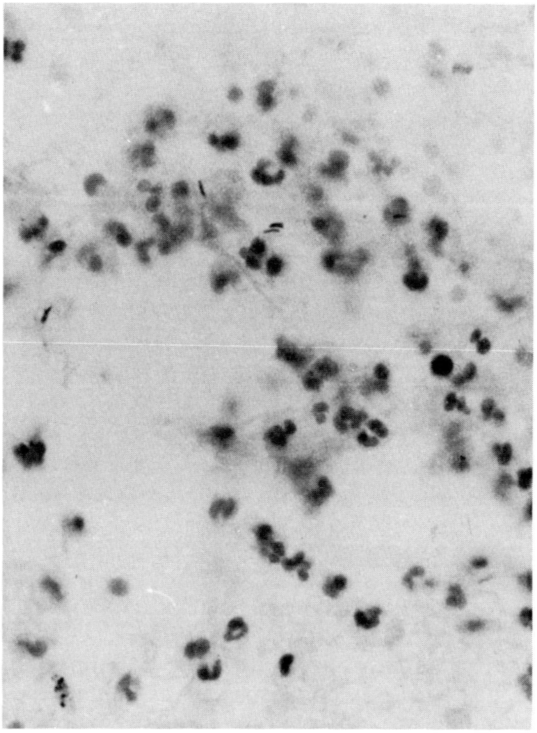
(a)

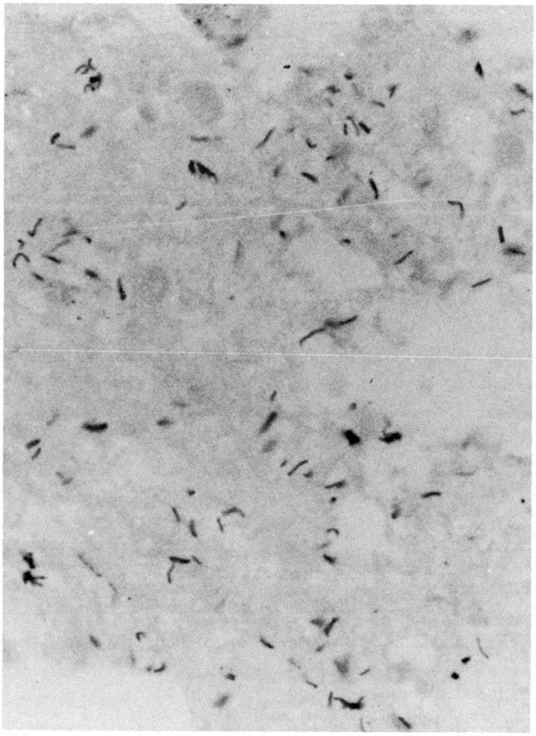
(b)

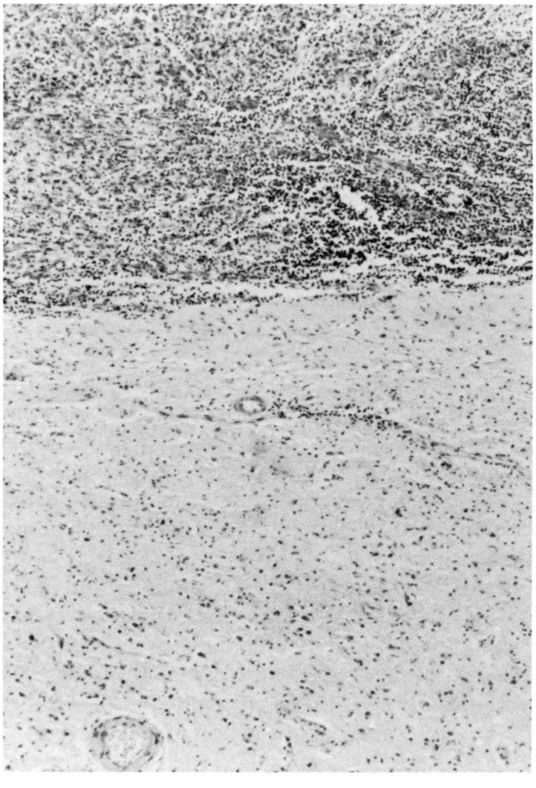
(c)

Fig. 6.9 Tuberculous abscess in a white male aged 55 years. (**a**) The first cerebral biopsy disclosed small pockets of polymorphs and a few tubercle bacilli. Ziehl–Neilsen × 530. (**b**) A second biopsy 1 month later included caseous material with numerous acid-fast bacilli. Ziehl–Nielsen × 840. (**c**) At autopsy 1 year later the abscess cavity (top) was filled with macrophages containing barium sulphate. There was neither a fibrous capsule nor tuberculous granulation tissue. Haematoxylin and eosin × 50.

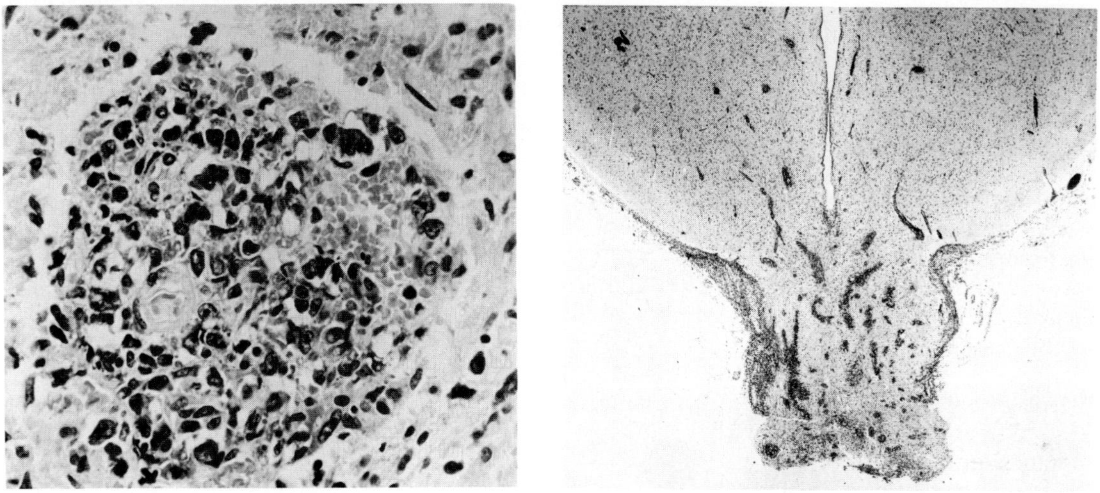

(a) (b)

Fig. 6.10 Sarcoidosis. (**a**) Mainly perivascular infiltration of the hypothalamus. (**b**) Infiltration of the basal meninges and infundibular region.

nucleate cells as occur in the same cells (of the macrophage series) in visceral sarcoid. Multinucleate cells may be small and scarce in the neural tissue and reticulin is less abundant than in sarcoid lesions elsewhere, but these differences are not basic. The *granulomas* are often perivascular, and even within the brain may be confined to perivascular spaces (Fig. 6.10). Granulomas in the floor of the third ventricle may not be recognized as sarcoid lesions unless more typical lesions are found in other organs.

The course of intracranial disease is usually slow and there may be clinical remission or arrest of progress, but some cases are fatal within a few weeks. When the disease is limited to the meninges the symptoms are usually those of hydrocephalus or cranial nerve palsies. When the infundibulum and the floor of the third ventricle are invaded, diabetes insipidus or other signs of hypothalamic dysfunction may result. Direct invasion of the optic chiasma or nerves will lead to hemianopia or blindness.

Neurosyphilis

Neurosyphilis presents clinically in three main groups: asymptomatic, meningovascular and parenchymatous (Catterall, 1977). In the first the histopathology is unknown, and microscopy of the active phases of the second and third groups ceased 40 years ago. Some forms, such as cerebral gummas, have virtually disappeared. Today, neuropathologists are very unlikely to encounter the inflammatory exudative lesions of neurosyphilis. The incidence of all forms has fallen, yet there is a rise in the number of cases of early infectious syphilis, especially in homosexual men. Early treatment of known cases reduces the number of patients who develop neurosyphilis, and undetected cases will naturally respond to large doses of penicillin given incidentally for other infections. The present account of neurosyphilis is therefore abbreviated, but a full account by Greenfield is available in the first two editions of this textbook.

Primary and secondary stages

Neurosyphilis is not confined to the tertiary stage, for lumbar punctures taken during the primary and secondary stages show that, in a significant proportion of cases, the treponeme invades the meninges during the first 2 years after primary infection. Asymptomatic neurosyphilis occurs in 10 per cent of primary infections and 30 per cent of secondary syphilis (Manu and Varade, 1982). The evidence for this is provided by surveys of the results of lumbar puncture. The criteria for diagnosis are positive fluorescent treponemal antibody absorption tests in blood and CSF, and more than 12 white blood cells $\times 10^6/1$ and over 0.5 g/1 protein in the CSF. A rise in lymphocytes is the first change to occur and the cell count is a reliable indicator of response to treatment when it falls. The pathology of the asymptomatic form of neurosyphilis is often assumed to be that of a mild meningovascular affection but this may not be true. It is known from lumbar punctures that evidence of parenchymatous syphilis may be present for months before symptoms and signs develop. The fact that the prognosis of asymptomatic neurosyphilis is excellent means that the inflammatory processes in meninges and brain can resolve without trace.

Meningovascular neurosyphilis The classification of neurosyphilis into meningovascular and parenchymatous forms is convenient but the two types are not completely exclusive. Some degree of meningovascular involvement is usually found in paretic dementia (general paralysis of the insane), and minor cortical changes are the rule in meningovascular syphilis. The classification does no more than emphasize the predominant site.

The meningitic element in meningovascular syphilis is that of chronic inflammation, diffuse or localized to the base of the brain. Lymphocytes and a few plasma cells intermingle within fibrous tissue. Occasionally the pia is weakened or destroyed, thus allowing bundles of fibrillary astrocytes to project from the cortex into the subarachnoid space. Miliary gummas may be found in the thickened meninges, superficially resembling miliary tubercles by containing histiocytes, giant cells and focal necrosis, but differing from them by the form of the necrosis. In tubercles necrosis affects cells only, and caseous material contains no reticulin; in syphilis, connective tissue becomes necrotic, whilst reticulin survives and can be demonstrated in gummas generally.

Syphilitic meningitis may be virtually confined to the spinal cord, and is then traditionally referred to as *spinal arachnoiditis*. Or the infection may be confined to the cervical region, where the pia arachnoid and both layers of the dura are thickened, adherent and encircle the cord. When it was described in the latter half of the nineteenth century it was named pachymeningitis cervicalis hypertrophica, even though it was not a purely dural infection.

The vascular element of meningovascular syphilis (referred to as Heubner's arteritis) consists of crescentric fibrous and eventually collagenous thickening of the intima (endarteritis obliterans), and corresponding thinning of the media. The elastic lamina remains intact. Lymphocytes and plasma cells infiltrate the adventitia, which is also thickened, and penetrate the media. The vasa vasorum are cuffed by the inflammatory cells (Fig. 6.11). Although the changes are due to inflammation the residual effect on the artery when the inflammation has abated is so like natural atherosclerosis that the two conditions become indistinguishable. Arteritis is seen in large and medium-sized vessels, but the fully developed lesion is rare. When ischaemic lesions occur in the brain or spinal cord in meningovascular syphilis, meningeal arteritis is responsible. The most frequent complications are, however, cranial nerve palsies and hydrocephalus, both due to meningeal fibrosis.

Nowadays syphilitic meningitis runs a benign course and remission occurs within a few weeks without treatment. The full-blown picture of meningovascular syphilis is rarely fatal, and its course is also benign despite mental changes.

Parenchymatous neurosyphilis

Tabes dorsalis Parenchymatous syphilitic disease of the spinal cord differs from that of the brain, and the reason for the difference is not clear. There is meningeal thickening with a variable inflammatory element, degeneration of dorsal nerve roots and degeneration of the posterior columns in the spinal cord, especially at lower thoracic and lumbosacral levels (Fig. 6.12). In long-standing tabes the posterior column degeneration is so marked as to present an excavated dorsal surface, giving the disease its name. Sometimes degeneration is most obvious in the cervical region. Obersteiner and Redlich (1894) considered that the pathology of tabes could be explained by inflammation and fibrosis of the dorsal nerve roots, especially where the root pierces the pia mater. Opponents of this theory point out that meningovascular syphilis does not cause degeneration of posterior nerve roots, but it may be more accurate to consider that it may do so and transform meningovascular syphilis into tabes dorsalis. Nageotte (1894) held that the main lesion was in the 'radicular' nerve—that part of the spinal nerve root lying between the dorsal root ganglion and the subarachnoid space. The root is here within a dural sleeve, where he found inflammation.

Tabes dorsalis is still occasionally seen at

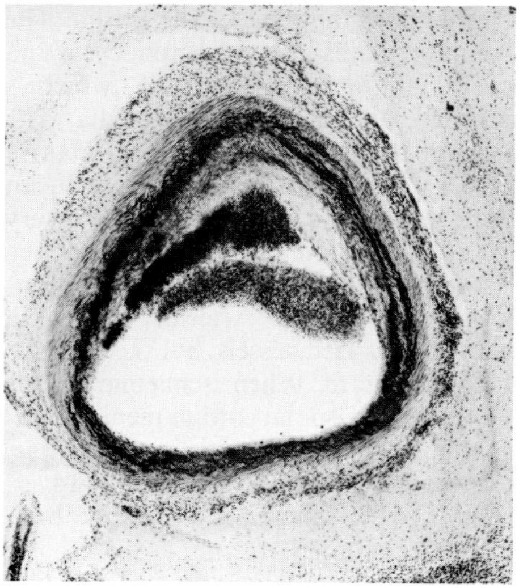

(a)

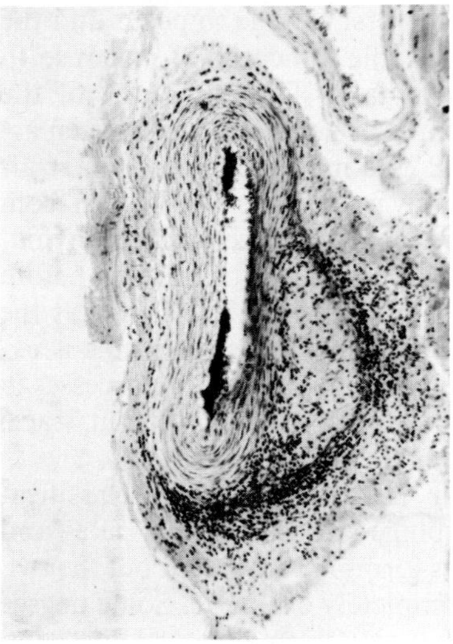

(b)

Fig. 6.11 Syphilitic arteritis. (**a**) Heubner's arteritis in a vessel on the surface of the cerebellum. There is infiltration and thickening of the adventitia, thinning of the media, duplication of the elastica and proliferation of the intima. Elastin. (**b**) A small gumma in the wall of the anterior spinal artery. Haematoxylin and van Gieson.

Fig. 6.12 Tabes dorsalis. The subtotal degeneration of the posterior columns and their excavation are clearly seen. Loyez × 10 reduced to 95%.

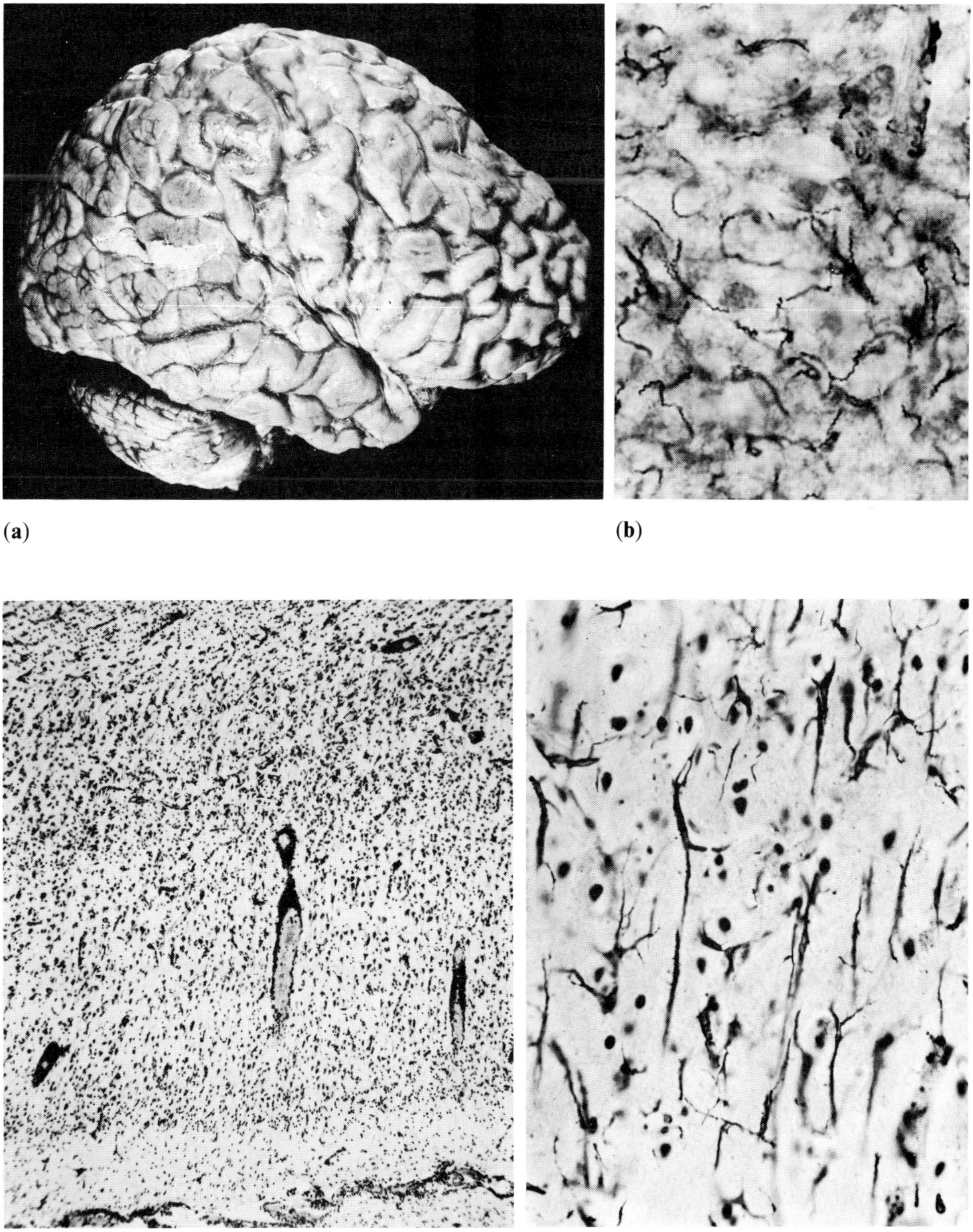

(**a**) (**b**) (**c**) (**d**)

Fig. 6.13 Paretic dementia. (**a**) External surface of the brain, showing thickening of the arachnoid and atrophy of the frontal convolutions. (**b**) Treponemas in cortex. Jahnel's silver method. (**c**) Low power view of the cortex, showing loss of definition of the cell layers and perivascular infiltration. Nissl × 50. (**d**) Rod cell forms of microglia. Silver carbonate × 1400.

post-mortem, but with all traces of inflammation gone.

Paretic dementia (general paralysis of the insane) In former days the severely affected patient dying after several years of dementia showed characteristic changes in the brain. It was shrunken and firm, and covered with a remarkably thick and opaque pia arachnoid (Fig. 6.13), tending to conceal gyral atrophy. This was most marked frontally, decreasing towards the occipital poles. The ventricles were much dilated and the fine ground-glass appearance of the ependyma, especially in the floor of the fourth ventricle, betrayed extensive granular ependymitis.

Some cases of general paralysis of the insane (GPI) came to necropsy at a much earlier stage of the disease, with little to see grossly except perhaps ependymal granulations. On *microscopical examination*, however, at both stages there was meningeal thickening, and loss of the normal laminar pattern in the cortex (Fig. 6.13). Scattered neurons had disappeared; others were degenerate or shrunken, with reactive proliferation of astrocytes and microglia. The microglial proliferation was striking (Fig. 6.13): the cells became hypertophied and elongated, and impregnated with iron so that they were easily demonstrated by Perl's stain. The blue-stained cells were first called rod cells by Nissl. Vessels in the meninges showed some degree of inflammation, and in the cortex there was perivascular cuffing by lymphocytes and plasma cells. There was a high proportion of plasma cells in GPI, in both cortex and meninges, but none of the changes was specific. Confirmation of the diagnosis could be provided only by staining the treponeme with a specific silver impregnation.

Several forms of subacute encephalitis resemble GPI histologically.

At the present time GPI is seen by pathologists only in the healed stage. Two cases examined in the author's laboratory, clinically and neurologically confirmed, showed no meningeal thickening, no atrophic or obstructive hydrocephalus, and no signs of inflammation microscopically. In a few areas there was patchy neuronal loss and reactive gliosis. Not unexpectedly, treponemes were not demonstrated.

Congenital neurosyphilis

This in active form must be almost as rare at autopsy as GPI. Congenital infection results in invasion of the CNS at different times: in early pregnancy it produces malformation, in early postnatal life meningovascular syphilis, and thereafter juvenile congenital GPI from 6 to 21 years. Juvenile congenital tabes dorsalis is much less common. The most frequent manifestation of congenital syphilis is said to be perceptive deafness.

References

Bannister, C. M. (1970) A tuberculous abscess of the brain. Case report. *Journal of Neurosurgery* **33,** 203–6.

Bayston, R. (1982) Postoperative infections in shunts for hydrocephalus (letter). *British Medical Journal* **285,** 1117.

Buchan, G.C. and Alvord, E.C. (1969) Diffuse necrosis of subcortical white matter associated with bacterial meningitis. *Neurology* **19,** 1–9.

Catterall, R.D. (1977) Neurosyphilis. *British Journal of Hospital Medicine* **17,** 585–604.

Dastur, D.K. and Wadia, N.H. (1969) Spinal meningitis with radiculo-myelopathy. 2. Pathology and pathogenesis. *Journal of the Neurological Sciences* **8,** 261–97.

Dastur, H.M. and Desai, A.D. (1965) A comparative study of brain tuberculomas and gliomas based on 107 case records of each. *Brain* **88,** 375–96.

Fishman, R.A. (1978) The pathophysiology and treatment of brain oedema. In *Recent Advances in Clinical Neurology—2* (Eds. Matthews, W.B. and Glaser, G.H.), pp. 119–27. Churchill Livingstone, Edinburgh.

Herring, A.B. and Urich, H. (1969) Sarcoidosis of the central nervous system. *Journal of the Neurological Sciences* **9,** 405–22.

Jabukiac, P., Dunsmore, R.H. and Beckett, S.R. (1968) Supratentorial brain cysts. *Journal of Neurosurgery* **28,** 129–36.

Kagawa, M., Takeshita, M., Yato, S. and Kitamura, K. (1983) Brain abscess in congenital cyanotic heart disease. *Journal of Neurosurgery* **58,** 913–17.

Karnik, A.S. (1982) Nodular cerebral sarcoidosis simulating metastatic carcinoma. *Archives of Internal Medicine* **142,** 385–6.

Leading Article (1978) Chemotherapy of brain abscess. *Lancet* **2,** 1081-2.

Leibowitz, S. and Hughes, R.A.C. (1983) *Immunology of the Nervous System.* Edward Arnold, London.

van Maarsseveen, A.M.C. Th., Veldhuizen, R.W., Stam, J., Alons, C.L. and Mullink, H. (1983) A quantitative histomorphologic analysis of lymph node granulomas in sarcoidosis in relation to radiological stage I and II. *Journal of Pathology* **139,** 441-53.

Manu, P. and Varade, W. (1982) Penicillin therapy for asymptomatic neurosyphilis: in-patient, intravenous or out-patient intramuscular? (letter) *Lancet* **2,** 924-5.

Nageotte, J. (1894) La lésion primitive du tabes. *Bulletin de la Société d'Anatomie de Paris* **69,** 808-20.

Obersteiner, H. and Redlich, E. (1894) Über Wesen und Pathogenese der tabischen Hinterstrangsdegeneration. *Arbeit aus dem Institut für Anatomie und Physiologie des Zentralnerven systems und der Wiener Universität* **2,** 158-72.

Parsons, M. (1982) Diagnoses not to be missed. Tuberculous meningitis. *British Journal of Hospital Medicine* **27,** 682-4.

Peltola, H., Jonsdottir, K., Lystad, A., Sievers, C.J. and Kallings, I. (1982) Meningococcal disease in Scandinavia. *British Medical Journal* **284,** 1618-21.

Rabe, E.F. (1967) Subdural effusions in infants. *Pediatric Clinics of North America* **14,** 831-50.

Radetsky, M.S., Istre, G.R., Johansen, T.L., Parmelee, S.W., Laver, B.A., Wiesenthal, A.M. et al. (1981) Multiply resistant pneumococcus causing meningitis: its epidemiology within a day-case centre. *Lancet* **2,** 771-3.

Rich, A.R. (1951) *The Pathogenesis of Tuberculosis*, 2nd edn. Blackwell Scientific, Oxford.

Slack, J. (1982) Deaths from meningococcal infection in England and Wales in 1978. *Journal of the Royal College of Physicians of London* **16,** 40-4.

Smith, H.P. and Hendrick, E.B. (1983) Subdural empyema and epidural abscess in children. *Journal of Neurosurgery* **58,** 392-7.

Swart, S., Briggs, R.S. and Millac, P.A. (1981) Tuberculous meningitis in Asian patients. *Lancet* **2,** 15-16.

Till, K. (1968) Subdural haematoma and effusion in infancy. *British Medical Journal* **3,** 400-2.

Trombley, I.K., Mirra, S.S. and Miles, M.L. (1981) An electron microscopic study of central nervous system sarcoidosis. *Ultrastructural Pathology* **2,** 257-67.

Waterson, A.P. (1983) Acquired immune deficiency syndrome. *British Medical Journal* **286,** 743-6.

Yang, S. (1981) Brain abscess: a review of 400 cases. *Journal of Neurosurgery* **55,** 794-9.

7

Virus diseases of the central nervous system

Betty Brownell and A.H. Tomlinson

There are few subjects in neuropathology in which, during the past two decades, more advances in understanding have been made than in virus infections of the nervous system. This is due to several factors: virus infection steadily becomes more significant and serious as bacterial diseases are prevented or cured; immunosuppression in the course of treatment for transplant rejection or malignant disease has allowed new forms of virus disease to develop; laboratory techniques such as electron microscopy and antibody labelling in tissue sections have led to greatly enhanced diagnostic accuracy; the availability of a range of antiviral agents has made diagnosis and pathogenesis of virus disease of the nervous system a matter of considerable clinical importance and urgency; finally the suitability of small laboratory animals as models for human diseases caused by a number of virus groups has greatly increased our knowledge of how viruses in the central nervous system cause the particular clinical syndromes associated with such infections.

Types of virus disease

Virus infections of the nervous system fall into five broad categories depending on the sites of infection, which determine the nature of the pathological lesions, and, in turn, the clinical presentation. Although there are cases which have features common to more than one category, it will be convenient here to discuss the diseases under the headings: (1) meningitis, (2) encephalomyelitis, (3) acute postinfectious encephalitis, (4) acute infective encephalitis and (5) subacute encephalitis.

Viral meningitis, in which the infection is confined to the leptomeninges—with no involvement of the underlying nervous tissue—is usually benign, resolves spontaneously and, in sharp contrast to the serious nature of bacterial meningitis, rarely leaves sequelae. In modern Western countries this is the commonest type of viral infection of the nervous system. Mumps virus is a constant common cause but in epidemic years an enterovirus may be the most frequent agent.

In **encephalomyelitis,** although there are signs of meningism and a pleocytosis in the cerebrospinal fluid ((CSF), the main pathological process is a lytic infection of neurons in the anterior horns of the spinal cord, in the motor nuclei of the brain stem and, to a minor degree, in the motor cortex of the cerebrum. The rest of the cerebrum and cerebellum is spared. The symptoms are those of a lower motor neuron paralysis which may range from mild weakness of a single limb to complete respiratory paralysis or the frequently fatal 'bulbar' palsies. In the past, polioviruses were the cause of large epidemics and they are still prevalent in countries where vaccination is not employed, but in areas of good vaccination, sporadic, and occasionally epidemic, poliomyelitis is caused by other enteroviruses (Sabin, 1981).

Acute postinfectious encephalitis (postvaccinial encephalitis), may follow measles, chickenpox, rubella or mumps and also vaccination against smallpox or rabies, and has the clinical signs and symptoms of a brain infection sometimes leading to coma and death. It is not, however, possible to isolate virus from the brain of such cases and the principal histological features—perivascular cuffing and demyelination—suggest an immunological pathogenesis.

World wide, the most common viral infection of the nervous system is **acute infective encepha-**

litis, which is characterized by infection and destruction of neurons and glial cells. The resulting inflammatory response produces neuronophagia, gliosis, infiltration by mononuclear cells and oedema of the brain. The severity of the lesions and the distribution between cerebrum, brain stem, cerebellum and, sometimes, spinal cord depend on the infecting virus—members of the herpes group, rabies, the arboviruses and some others. The clinical picture usually includes fever, altered consciousness and focal neurological signs, and the outcome ranges from complete recovery through varying degrees of mental or physical sequelae to death.

The **subacute encephalitides,** in which the illness lasts for months or years, are infections of the brain by a group of ill-assorted agents. Subacute sclerosing panencephalitis is caused by measles (and, very rarely, rubella) virus reactivated years after the primary infection. Progressive multifocal leucoencephalopathy is the result of an opportunistic infection in the brain of an immunocompromised host by a virus which normally infects, without obvious illness, much of the human population. Kuru and Creutzfeldt-Jakob disease are distinguished from all other encephalitides by spongiform degeneration of the brain, by the nature of the infecting agent, which is unlike any other virus, and by the length of the incubation period following natural or experimental infection.

Virus biology

The peculiar properties of viruses distinguish them from all other parasites and have a profound influence on the way they produce disease and on the host defences mounted against them. The distinguishing features are: (1) their small size, 20–300 nm; (2) the fact that a virus contains only one type of nucleic acid, DNA or RNA; and (3) their lack of metabolic activity except when inside a host cell.

The basic composition of a virus particle, or *virion*, is a core of nucleic acid, single or double-stranded, surrounded by protein units, capsomeres, and the combined nucleic acid–protein structure is called the nucleocapsid. The nucleocapsids of some genera of viruses (e.g. adenovirus and enterovirus) are naked but in other genera (e.g. myxovirus and the herpes group) they are surrounded by an envelope composed of protein, glycoprotein and lipid, usually viral in origin but sometimes containing elements of host material.

Viruses replicate only within living cells and the first step in the process is chance collision of the virion with a receptor site on the host cell surface where it is absorbed and the nucleocapsid enters the cell. The complex process of producing more infective virus varies considerably between the different groups but the basic pattern is common. The viral nucleic acid, using host sources of energy, carbon and nitrogen compounds, directs the synthesis of new viral nucleic acid and protein which are assembled into virions, within the nucleus in the case of a DNA virus such as herpes or in the cytoplasm for poliovirus. Release of complete infective virus from the cells occurs either by rupture of the cell and its immediate death, as occurs with poliovirus, or more commonly by a process of virus budding out from the cell membrane which, as observed in tissue culture, may continue for many hours before cell death.

The process just described, a *lytic infection*, is the commonest interaction between virus and host cell, but there are two other responses—*latent infection* and *transformation*. All the herpes group of viruses can, after a primary infection, go latent and be reactivated months or years later. Herpes simplex is known to go latent in trigeminal, sacral and some autonomic ganglia, and latency in the central system is suspected. Varicella-zoster virus can be latent in cranial and dorsal root ganglia. The Epstein-Barr virus is found latent in circulating B-lymphocytes, and cytomegalovirus exhibits latency though the site is undetermined—probably lymphoid tissue. Measles and rubella viruses are known to persist in latent form in the brain.

In the process of *transformation*, first observed with cultured mouse cells infected by polyomavirus, the majority of cells suffer a lytic infection and die but a small proportion are transformed so that they grow more rapidly than normal cells, will grow in multilayered colonies and have less exacting nutritional requirements—in fact, have become like tumour cells. Natural and experimental infections with papovaviruses, adenoviruses, herpesviruses and retroviruses produce tumours in rodents and some monkeys but in man the only firm associations of virus and tumour are those of Epstein-Barr virus with the Burkitt lymphoma and with nasopharyngeal carcinoma.

Virus particles contain proteins both in their capsids and in any envelope, and these envelope proteins may appear in the membranes of virus-infected cells so that each of these components acts as an antigen to the infected host and usually elicits an immune response. Antibody acquired after a previous infection, or vaccination, appears to be the main defence against reinfection. IgA antibody in secretions of the respiratory tract, tears, saliva or in the gut will combine with viral surface protein and 'neutralize' infectivity. Circulating antibody, IgG or IgM, restricts blood-borne dissemination of virus from the primary site of infection to other target organs, as for example the spread of poliovirus from the gut to the CNS. By neutralizing extracellular virus, antibody in tissue spaces can prevent the spread of infection from one cell to another, but those viruses which can fuse cell membranes, such as the herpes group and measles virus, beat this defence by reaching the next cell without ever being exposed to antibody. An immune response of special interest is the appearance within the brain of plasma cells producing antibody to a current virus infection—cells which can be identified by labelled antiglobulins as producing alpha, mu or gamma heavy chains, and kappa or delta light chains. Measurement of antibody in CSF at a concentration exceeding that produced by serum leakage has proved a useful diagnostic technique.

In the termination of viral infections the cell-mediated immune response is at least as important as humoral antibody. Sensitized T-lymphocytes, natural killer cells and lymphokine-activated macrophages can kill virus-infected cells without the aid of antibody, and there are also T-cells which show antibody-mediated cytotoxicity as well as the phagocytosis by macrophages which is antibody-dependent. Inadequate cell-mediated immunity, due either to disease or to immunosuppressive drugs, is an important element in the pathogenesis of progressive multifocal leucoencephalopathy, and certain cases of encephalitis caused by measles, varicella-zoster and cytomegaloviruses.

In contrast, active cell-mediated immune responses play a part in two virus-associated neurological disorders. The lymphocytes of patients with postinfectious encephalomyelitis and Guillain–Barré syndrome (which is often associated with a virus infection) are known to be stimulated *in vitro* by myelin basic protein or peripheral nerve protein, and the histopathology shows that the demyelination is mediated by lymphocytes. Similar conditions can be produced in animals by immunizing with the appropriate protein, but how a natural virus infection sensitizes lymphocytes to the proteins of nervous tissue is yet to be explained.

Viruses rarely survive long in the environment. Pox viruses can, however, survive in separated scabs for some months, enteroviruses and hepatitis A virus can persist for a while in sewage, and arthropod-borne viruses survive in biting insects, but the majority of viruses must pass direct from host to host. The commonest route of entry is through the mucous membrane of the respiratory or gastrointestinal tracts, where, if the virus is not neutralized by secretory IgA antibody, it infects and multiplies in the cells of first contact, spreads to local lymphatic tissue and often to the blood stream. Rabies virus, herpesvirus simiae and all the arboviruses gain access through the skin as a result of the bite of an animal or insect and, almost certainly, first multiply in local tissues—rabies virus, for example, grows in muscle cells.

All natural virus infections of the central nervous system begin with local virus growth in non-neural tissue from which it spreads—pre-existing antibody and phagocytic cells permitting—by the neural or haematogenous route to the brain or cord. Direct spread to the limbic system of the brain via olfactory receptor cells and the olfactory nerve has long been considered as a mode of entry for viruses and, experimentally, herpes, polio and rabies can be shown to infect by this route, but there is little evidence that this process occurs naturally in man.

The transmission of herpesvirus, rabies and polioviruses by the neural route in experimental animals is well established but for some time there has been debate about the mechanism. In 1923 Marinesco and Dragonesco favoured movement in perineural spaces and lymphatics while Goodpasture and Teague suggested growth in axon cylinders, and much later Johnson (1964) observed, in a mouse model, herpesvirus progressively infecting Schwann cells. It is now known that viruses cannot grow in axon cylinders, remote from the metabolic activity of the perikaryon, but electron microscopy has revealed their presence in transit, and dynamic studies have shown adequate flow of axoplasm to account for virus movement both centripetally and centrifugally. Other studies have demonstrated that transport of virus from the periphery to ganglia occurs faster than sequential growth of virus in Schwann cells. Axonal flow therefore appears to be the main vehicle in the neural route carrying, for example, herpes or varicella-zoster virus to ganglia where they may become latent, or carrying reactivated virus from ganglia to the periphery.

The majority, however, of viruses which cause infection of the central nervous system gain access via the blood stream. The enteroviruses (polio, coxsackie and echoviruses) measles, mumps, adenoviruses, lymphocytic choriomeningitis virus and the arboviruses all give rise to a viraemia following establishment and growth at the site of entry. Particles (viruses included) are cleared from the blood by the reticuloendothelial system, so if the viraemia is to persist virus must be protected or replaced. Measles virus certainly, and mumps virus probably, enter and grow in lymphocytes. Poliovirus, after initial establishment in the nasopharynx, infects and grows for some time in lymphoid tissue of the gut; many arboviruses grow in spleen or lymph nodes and some of them in the endothelium of small vessels, thus maintaining the viraemia. At one time the blood–brain barrier was thought to exclude blood-borne virus from the CNS, but means of access have now been discovered: thus distemper virus has been seen to be carried into perivascular spaces inside lymphocytes; some viruses infecting glial cells adjacent to undamaged small vessels may traverse the endothelium by pinocytosis; and yet others may grow in, and so through, endothelial cells. The route to the CSF is less speculative because the small vessels of the choroid plexus have fenestrated endothelial cells which allow virus access to the epithelium of the choroid plexus but not direct leakage between endothelial cell junctions out to the fluid. Growth in the epithelial cells causes seeding into the CSF.

By using labelled antibodies it has been possible to determine the susceptibility of different cell populations in the CNS to individual viruses, and Johnson (1980) has summarized the findings in experimental animals. For the human subject there is less information but some pattern is apparent. Coxsackie, echo and mumps viruses frequently infect the meninges but rarely neurons. Polioviruses sometimes cause only meningeal symptoms but more frequently infect neurons, but only motor neurons, leaving sensory paths untouched. In contrast, rabies infects only neurons, and initially only sensory neurons, so in the early stages of the disease motor functions and mental alertness are unaffected. Once established in the brain, herpes simplex virus infects all types of cell and its distribution in the limbic system and the temporal lobes produces a disease which starts with behavioural change, aphasia or clouded consciousness before the appearance of focal signs. A further specialization is shown by JC virus which, growing only in oligodendrocytes, causes the demyelination of progressive multifocal leucoencephalopathy. The reasons for this selectivity of viruses infecting the nervous system remain a fascinating unsolved problem.

Whereas the pathogenesis of many viral infections is explained by cell destruction or the consequences of the inflammatory response, an interesting pathogenic mechanism hinted at, but so far little explored, is the ability of some viruses to produce a persistent infection which suppresses 'luxury functions' without killing the cells. Oldstone, Holmstoen and Welsh (1977) found that lymphocytic choriomeningitis virus suppressed the acetylcholine enzymes of cultured neuroblastoma cells; paramyxovirus infections suppressed the beta-adrenergic receptors of cultured glioma cells (Koschel and Muenzel, 1980); and an *in vivo* effect of rabies virus on the activity of acetylcholine receptors in rat brain was noted by Tsiang, Ermine and Marcovistz (1982).

The biology of viruses is fully described by Luria et al. (1978), general mechanisms of microbial pathogeneses by Mims (1977) and viral infections of the nervous system are comprehensively surveyed by Johnson (1982). A good atlas of virus morphology has been published by Madeley (1972).

The necropsy

The pathologist, when called upon to make a tissue diagnosis of a virus disease of the central nervous system, whether at necropsy or biopsy, should be fully aware of helpful diagnostic procedures and should not neglect, at the outset, to procure suitable tissue and retain it by methods appropriate to subsequent virological examination. In addition to the routine examination of formalin-fixed tissue, investigation for virus disease should always include (when possible) the provision of fresh material for virus culture, glutaraldehyde-fixed tissue for electron microscopy, and fresh or frozen tissue to supply cryostat sections for examination by labelled antibody techniques to demonstrate the presence of virus antigen. The introduction of the immunoperoxidase technique, by which, if suitable antiserum is available, virus antigen can be demonstrated in paraffin wax sections of tissue which has been fixed in formalin, was a great advance and has led to a situation in which a diagnosis may often be made retrospectively on stored tissue. Information obtained by this method, however, depends very much on the stability of the virus antigen and on the strength of the antiserum, and the method cannot be relied upon to demonstrate all types of virus. In some cases the fluorescent antibody technique, carried out on frozen sections, provides a much better chance of identifying virus in tissue.

All the above comments apply equally to biopsy and necropsy tissue. At a post-mortem examination, the pathologist also has the opportunity to obtain a sample of CSF for virus antibody levels, and, if this is taken, a post-mortem blood sample should also be obtained. It should not be forgotten that in many virus diseases of the central nervous system there may be virus in the respiratory and gastrointestinal tracts, and suitable samples should also be obtained at post-mortem and submitted for virological investigation. Finally, on the subject of necropsy in virus diseases, suitable precautions should always be taken to prevent infection. Necropsies on cases of certain virus diseases are not permitted in the UK except under laboratory conditions defined in the Code of Practice (Department of Health and Social Security et al., 1978). The examination of brain tissue in suspected cases of Creutzfeldt–Jakob disease has also been the subject of a special report (Department of Health and Social Security, 1981) in which specific recommendations concerning the sterilization of instruments and apparatus are made.

General pathological features of virus disease of the central nervous system

The reactions of the meninges, brain and spinal cord to infection by viruses are somewhat stereotyped and, with a few important exceptions, tend to be similar in all forms of virus disease. They vary, however, both in the emphasis on one or other type of reaction and in their distribution throughout the central nervous system.

Macroscopical appearance

In a patient who has died as a result of an acute virus infection of the nervous system, the brain and spinal cord may appear normal macroscopically, particularly if death occurs in the early stages of the disease. There may, however, be slight meningeal opacity or vascular congestion, generalized or localized swelling in the brain or spinal cord, and slight or severe softening of nervous tissue. In general, the macroscopic changes found at autopsy are neither very helpful nor very significant unless complicating factors are present such as the sequelae of hypoxia, or of severe brain swelling and herniation. Exceptions are the brain in herpes simplex encephalitis and the spinal cord in poliomyelitis when a positive diagnosis can often be made on macroscopical examination.

Microscopical appearances

Inflammatory cell infiltration This is almost always present and may be the most conspicuous histological abnormality (Fig. 7.1a). Even in those types of viral disease in which some parts of the brain are selectively and severely involved, cellular infiltration is usually seen diffusely throughout the brain and, often, the spinal cord. The components of the cellular exudate vary according to the stage of the disease and the nature of the infection. In the earliest stages of some acute forms of encephalitis, the cellular infiltrate may consist largely of polymorphonuclear leucocytes, but this is by no means true of all types of acute viral infection. At a later stage in these infections, and indeed at all stages in many of the conditions under discussion, the exudate consists almost entirely of lymphocytes, plasma cells and large mononuclear cells. Inflammatory cell infiltration of the leptomeninges, whether by polymorphs or mononuclear cells, is not usually very severe although it is likely to be universal and not confined to any particular region. A more significant and characteristic feature than meningitis is the presence of *perivascular cuffing* (Fig. 7.1a). A single layer of mononuclear cells in the Virchow–Robin spaces of small venules, and thicker cuffs of lymphocytes round the larger vessels, are particularly

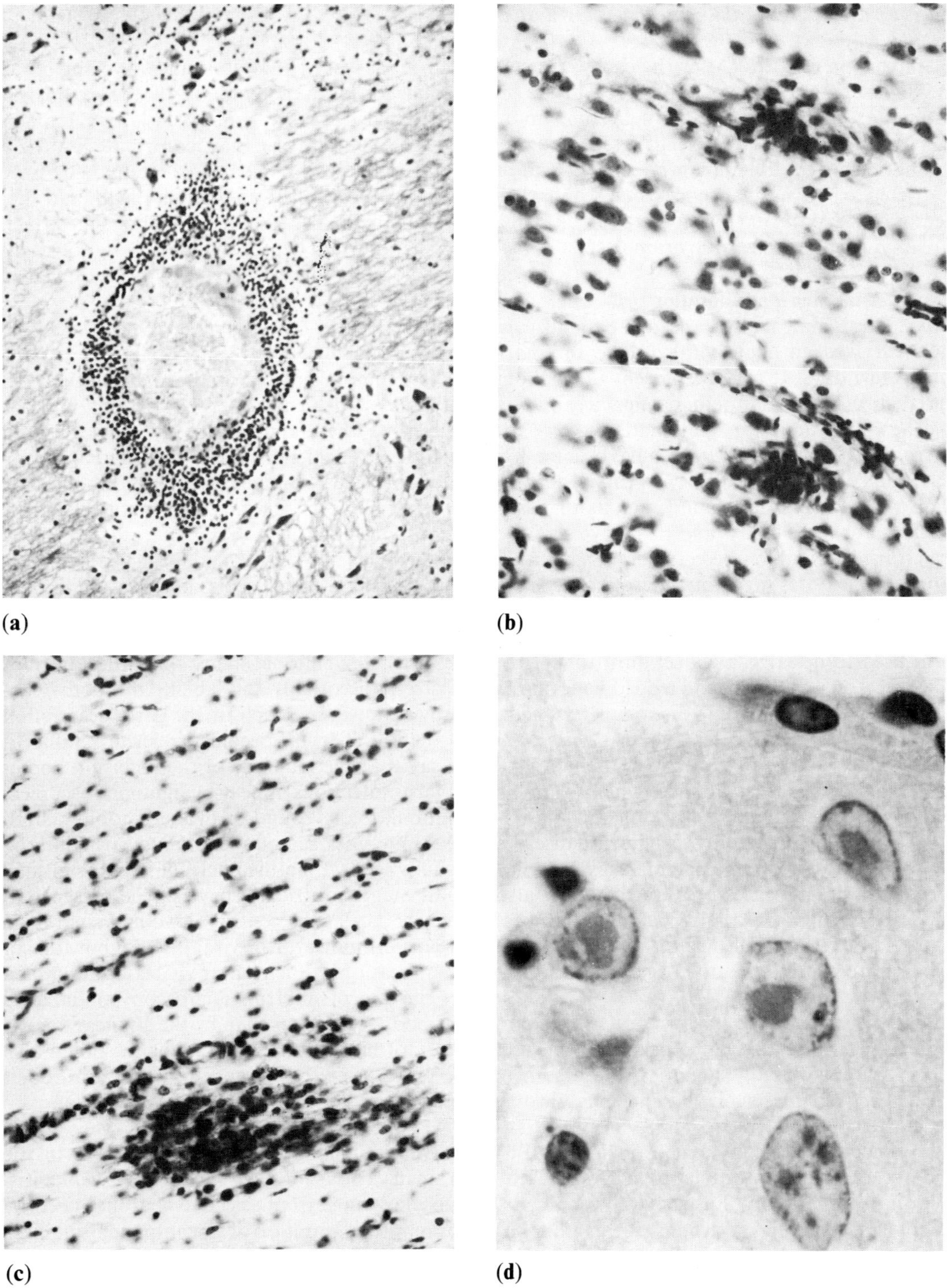

Fig. 7.1 General features of virus infection of the central nervous system. (**a**) Perivascular cuffing in a case of acute necrotizing encephalitis. Note the mononuclear cells around a fairly large vessel in the pons. Haematoxylin and eosin × 150. (**b**) Neuronophagia in a case of subacute sclerosing panencephalitis. Two neurons in the cerebral cortex are obscured by microglia. Cresyl violet × 250. (**c**) Microglial star in a case of acute necrotizing encephalitis. Note the large aggregate of microglial cells in the white matter in the brain stem. There is also diffuse hypertrophy of microglia. Cresyl violet × 250. (**d**) Intranuclear inclusion bodies in a case of acute necrotizing encephalitis. Three neuronal nuclei contain inclusion bodies. Haematoxylin and eosin × 1200. (**a**–**c** reproduced, with permission, from Adams, 1973.)

characteristic features. After the early stages of the disease, plasma cells are included in the inflammatory infiltrate and may become more numerous round the vessels. If tissue necrosis has not occurred, inflammatory cells tend to be restricted to perivascular spaces, but, if and when necrosis has occurred, leucocytes of all types stream out into the necrotic brain tissue.

Hyperplasia and proliferation of microglial cells This is almost always seen in patients who have survived an acute viral disease for more than a few days. It may be present throughout the cerebrum and hindbrain, particularly involving the cortex and deep grey matter, where the microglial cells can be seen to have become hypertrophied to form rod cells. Microglial activity is also intense in and around regions of tissue destruction where many lipid phagocytes will be seen if the survival has been long enough. Other important features involving microglial cells are neuronophagia (Fig. 7.1b) and the formation of microglial stars (Fig. 7.1c). *Neuronophagia* is the term used to describe a collection of hypertrophied microglial cells around a dead neuron, the latter often being difficult to distinguish. It therefore occurs in grey matter, whereas *microglial stars*, which consist of collections of hypertrophied microglial cells, are seen mainly in the white matter. Although neuronophagia and microglial stars are commonly seen in viral diseases of the central nervous system, they are not specific to viral diseases because they may also be seen in hypoxic brain damage, cerebral trauma and neuronal degenerations of unknown aetiology (e.g. motor neuron disease).

Astrocytosis Reactive astrocytes are commonly seen where tissue necrosis has occurred, the appearances being similar to those seen in other reactive states such as ischaemia, chronic oedema etc. In subacute forms of encephalitis—e.g. subacute sclerosing panencephalitis (SSPE) and progressive multifocal leucoencephalopathy (PML)—proliferation of astrocytes with the development of large hypertrophic forms is an important feature, and in long-standing cases fibrous gliosis is a significant finding.

Changes in neurons These are frequently present but are non-specific and in individual cases may be due to terminal hypoxia, or the result of brain swelling. Such non-specific changes as loss of Nissl substance, swelling of the perikaryon and eosinophilia of the cytoplasm have been described, but it should be remembered that autolysis may contribute to these changes, especially in cases where patients have been maintained for any length of time on life-support machines. One neuronal change which is an important feature in the spongiform encephalopathies is the presence of cytoplasmic vacuolation.

Inclusion bodies The presence of inclusion bodies is an important feature in many of the viral diseases of the central nervous system, and the bodies may be found in neurons, astrocytes and oligodendroglial cells (Fig. 7.1d). The majority are intranuclear, but intracytoplasmic bodies are also seen, one of the most important being the Negri body of rabies.

Much has been written about the appearances and staining characteristics of inclusion bodies, and they have been classified into various types according to their light microscopical appearances by conventional stains. Since the advent of electron microscopy and labelled antibody techniques, however, much of the early description of these bodies has become irrelevant. Suffice it to say that the majority of the inclusion bodies of virus infections appear by light microscopical examination as round or oval eosinophilic bodies, sometimes surrounded by a clear halo, and usually seen within the nuclei of neurons or glial cells, mainly oligodendrocytes. The presence of such bodies in the central nervous system is an important indicator of viral disease, but further identification of their nature is better attempted by the use of electron microscopy or labelled antibody techniques than by the application of a range of histopathological stains. It should also be noted that the absence of inclusion bodies does not exclude a viral aetiology.

Necrosis This is an important feature in the brain in various forms of acute viral encephalitis, and may range from selective neuronal necrosis to complete infarction of all components of large areas of neural tissue. Necrosis may have a characteristic distribution as in herpes simplex encephalitis, or it may be widespread in the central nervous system as in St Louis encephalitis. The incidence and the distribution of necrosis may also be considerably influenced by terminal events. Thus selective neuronal necrosis in susceptible parts of the brain (such as the Sommer sector of the hippocampus, the Purkinje cells of the cerebellum, or various groups of neurons in the deep cerebral grey matter) are more likely to be due to terminal hypoxic changes as a result of factors such as circulatory disturbances and/or raised intracranial pressure than to the virus infection itself. When tissue necrosis has occurred as a direct result of the viral infection, the histological features resemble those of infarction, combined with those of inflammation; i.e. dead brain tissue surrounded by lipid phagocytes and inflammatory cells according to the stage of the disease. In fact, it is sometimes difficult, when examining sections from a severely involved part of the brain in, for example, acute herpes simplex virus encephalitis, to distinguish the changes from those of a recent infarct. Nevertheless, histological examination of parts of the brain remote from the area of maximum damage should show the inflammatory features characteristic of viral disease.

Demyelination Lesions in the white matter are important features in the postinfectious encephalitides. On macroscopical examination these appear as small grey areas situated around the veins, in any part of the cerebrum, hindbrain or spinal cord. The lesions are usually symmetrical, and, although more conspicuous in white matter, grey matter may also be involved. On microscopical examination, the lesions show cuffing of small veins by inflammatory cells consisting of a mixture of polymorphs, lymphocytes and plasma cells. Surrounding the cellular cuff, in a zone 1–2 mm wide, there is destruction of neural tissue in which myelin breakdown may be more prominent or more extensive than is involvement of axons. This feature has led to the inclusion of 'perivenous encephalitis' among the demyelinating diseases, but such classification appears to be of doubtful value.

Status spongiosus. This is an important pathological feature in the group of conditions known as the spongiform encephalopathies. The spongy state involves the grey matter, including cerebral cortex and central grey matter and sometimes cerebellum, and macroscopically appears as very fine microcystic degeneration. Histologically, the spongy state is associated with neuronal loss and astrocytic proliferation, although not necessarily dependent upon the severity of either.

Aseptic meningitis

In the diagnosis of meningitis, or encephalitis, the first laboratory examination is that of the CSF, and Table 7.1 gives the normal values and the range of values to be expected in different conditions. It is not possible to give precise diagnostic values, but a polymorphonuclear pleocytosis changing to one of a few hundred lymphocytes with moderately elevated protein and normal glucose levels strongly suggest viral meningitis. Specimens for virus isolation—CSF, throat swab in transport medium and faeces—should be submitted immediately, together with a specimen of serum. A second serum collected 14 days later may show, in some cases, a diagnostic rise in antibody titre, but it cannot be too strongly emphasized that virus isolation is the preferred diagnostic procedure in cases of meningitis because the commonest aetiological agents

Table 7.1 The cerebrospinal fluid

	Cells ($\times 10^6$/l)	Protein (g/l)	Glucose (mmol/l)
Normal	<4 lymphocytes	0.15–0.40	2.7–4.0
Bacterial meningitis	>2000 polymorphs	0.8–4.0	Reduced 0–2.2
Tuberculous meningitis	Initially >200 polymorphs Later 100–1000 lymphocytes	1.0–6.0	0–2.2
Viral meningitis	Initially <100 polymorphs Later >1000 lymphocytes	0.5–1.5	Normal
Encephalitis	Initially <100 polymorphs Later <500 lymphocytes	0.5–1.5	Normal

are the enteroviruses and their number (71) usually makes serological diagnosis impractical.

The genus enterovirus includes poliovirus 1, 2 and 3, six coxsackie B viruses, 24 coxsackie A viruses and 34 echoviruses, together with four new isolates, enteroviruses 68–71 (Melnick, Wenner and Phillips, 1979). The yearly totals in the Communicable Diseases Report of the UK Public Health Laboratory Service show that infections with coxsackie and echoviruses together account for most cases of aseptic meningitis but the predominant serotype changes with the year —for a summary see Christie (1980). Enterovirus infections are most frequent in the late summer and autumn. In areas where poliovirus is not controlled by vaccination a number of infections with it present as meningitis.

The second commonest cause of viral meningitis, occurring mostly early in the year, is mumps virus with or without parotitis. Russell and Donald (1958) reported a 6 per cent incidence of meningitis in an outbreak of mumps among troops, but in children as many as 50 per cent of the cases of meningitis do not have parotitis (Azimi, Cramblett and Haynes, 1969).

Schneweis (1962) distinguished two serotypes of herpes simplex virus and their differing types of disease were identified by Dowdle et al. (1967)—type 1 commonly causing labial herpes, eye infections and, rarely, encephalitis, whereas type 2 is predominantly found in genital lesions. In some adults with a genital infection, herpesvirus type 2 spreads to produce a meningitis, and virus can be recovered from the CSF (Sköldenberg, Jeansson and Wolontis, 1973). A similar meningitis can occur in neonates infected at birth and there are rare instances of meningitis in children caused by type 1 virus (Craig and Nahmias, 1973).

Pathological findings. In fatal cases of aseptic meningitis, there are no specific macroscopic abnormalities of the brain, which may, however, show evidence of secondary complications. Histological abnormalities are virtually restricted to infiltration of the leptomeninges by mononuclear inflammatory cells and perivascular cuffing spreading into the superficial layers of the cortex (see Fig. 7.5d). Evidence of inflammatory change or of neuronal necrosis in deeper parts of the brain or spinal cord is not seen in aseptic meningitis.

Encephalomyelitis

Encephalomyelitis due to polioviruses

Of this group of diseases characterized by polioclastic infection of the cord or brain stem, that caused by the polioviruses has been most thoroughly investigated. Prior to about 1890 the term 'infantile paralysis' or Heine's 'Kinderlähmung' was applied to a sporadic disease of children under the age of 5 years, which began with a short fever to be followed by pain in the back or limbs and then muscular weakness or paralysis. In contrast to that sporadic pattern, Medin in 1890 (cited by Paul, 1971) described an outbreak of 44 cases in Sweden; in 1894 Calverly (cited by Paul, 1971) recorded a group of 132 cases in Vermont, USA, and Wickman (1907), describing an epidemic of 1031 cases, established the person-to-person spread, as with other infectious diseases, and noted that children and youngsters were affected as well as infants. By the beginning of this century the natural history of 'infantile paralysis' was changing.

Landsteiner and Popper, in 1909, demonstrated the transmission of poliomyelitis to a monkey by injecting into its brain a bacteria-free suspension of spinal cord from a fatal case, but it was years later before the three serotypes, without cross-immunity, were defined. For many years research was concentrated entirely on the neurotropic properties of the virus until in the early 1930s Trask and Paul confirmed the work of Kling, showing that virus can be found in the pharynx and the gut of patients (Paul, 1971). With the realization of the enteric nature of the infection the pathogenesis and epidemiology of poliomyelitis became clearer. Poliovirus in a new host first multiplies in the oropharynx and then spreads to the mucosa of the ileum and to Peyer's patches (Bodian, 1959), but further extension to the CNS is an infrequent event. It is estimated that for every case there are 50–500 people with an enteric infection (Nathanson and Martin, 1979), the exact ratio depending on the strain of virus and the herd immunity. Virus is present in the throat for about 10 days but persists in the faeces for from 3 weeks up to 2–3 months.

The mechanism of spread to the CNS is still not fully understood but in most cases it is by way of the blood stream. The viraemia observed in human cases by Bodian and Paffenbarger (1954) was confirmed by Horstmann, McCollum and Mascola (1954) who also showed that in monkeys the short-lived viraemia preceded the paralysis by 6 days. Although it is known that circulating antibody does not prevent the growth of virus in the gut, a large-scale controlled trial showed that prophylactic gamma-globulin protected most of the recipients from paralytic poliomyelitis (Hammon et al., 1953), indicating the importance of viraemia for infection of the CNS. Circulating antibody does not, however, always prevent paralysis in monkeys (Craig and Brown, 1959) or in man (Fox, 1980), so there still remains the possibility of transmission to the CNS by the autonomic nervous system. In fatal cases it is possible to isolate virus from spinal cord or brain for some days after the onset of paralysis but, because the virus is seldom found in the lumbar CSF during life, culture of this fluid is not diagnostically useful. After natural infection or oral polio vaccine (live attenuated virus) secretory IgA protects the oropharynx and the gut so that the virus is less likely to produce any infection even in the gut.

In regions of the world where hygiene is poor all infants are infected early in life and a few develop paralysis, but all produce antibodies so that older children and adults are immune and epidemics do not occur. Some years ago it was supposed that paralytic poliomyelitis was rare in such countries but lameness surveys have shown an incidence similar to that of the USA in the epidemic years 1944–1954 (Horstmann, 1982).

Rising standards of hygiene in the developed countries delayed first infection to later in life, resulting in epidemic, rather than endemic, disease until the advent of vaccines changed the pattern. In 1952 the incidence of paralytic polio in the USA was 13.7 per 100 000 population, and by 1981 the figure was 0.003 per 100 000. There are, however, a very small number of vaccine-associated cases. From 1969 to 1981 in the USA 312 million doses of oral polio vaccine were given and there were 99 cases of vaccine-associated paralysis—37 in recipients and 62 in contacts (Moore et al., 1982).

Paralytic disease indistinguishable from classic poliomyelitis can also be produced by at least 19 other enteroviruses and six have been isolated from the spinal cord of fatal cases in whom the structural changes in the cord were typical of poliomyelitis—coxsackieviruses A4, A7 and B3, echoviruses 2 and 9 and enterovirus 71 (Sabin, 1981). Enterovirus 71 caused an epidemic in Bulgaria with 147 patients showing bulbar or spinal paralysis and 44 deaths (Chumakov et al., 1979). In populations which are well vaccinated the possibility of poliomyelitis caused by viruses other than polio must always be kept in mind.

In children with immunodeficiencies poliovirus and echovirus can produce an atypical persistent meningoencephalitis (Davis et al., 1977; Wilfert et al., 1977).

Pathological findings. The pathological changes found at necropsy in a patient who has had poliomyelitis will obviously vary considerably with the stage of the disease process. If death occurs in the acute stage of the disease, the central nervous system may show no macroscopical abnormalities, but in very severe cases it may be just possible to detect vascular congestion, haemorrhage, or necrosis in the anterior grey horns of the spinal cord or in the dorsal medulla. In cases coming to necropsy months or years after the initial infection it is generally possible to detect atrophy of the affected anterior spinal nerve roots which will appear grey and shrunken, and there may also be a corresponding reduction in size of the associated anterior grey horn at the relevant level of the spinal cord.

Microscopically, in the early stages, there will be diffuse lymphocytic infiltration of the spinal leptomeninges. In the first few days, lymphocytic infiltration is present in the anterior horns of the spinal cord and there may also be a reaction of polymorphonuclear leucocytes. After the first few days, the inflammatory cells will be accompanied by hypertrophied microglial cells, and, as necrosis of the motor cells takes place, the characteristic features of neuronophagia and microglial nodules will appear (Fig. 7.2a). In severe cases, dying within the first few weeks of the illness, the inflammatory and glial cell reactions are so intense that the normal anatomy of the cord grey matter may be obscured (Fig. 7.2b).

At a later stage, the intense cellular infiltration becomes less dominant and neuronophagia is the most prominent feature. Microglial cell reaction remains a noticeable feature and may be present long after the effect of the virus upon the neurons has ceased. During the early stages of the illness, inclusion bodies may be found in anterior horn cells, but their presence is not a prominent feature in poliomyelitis.

In cases which come to necropsy long after the

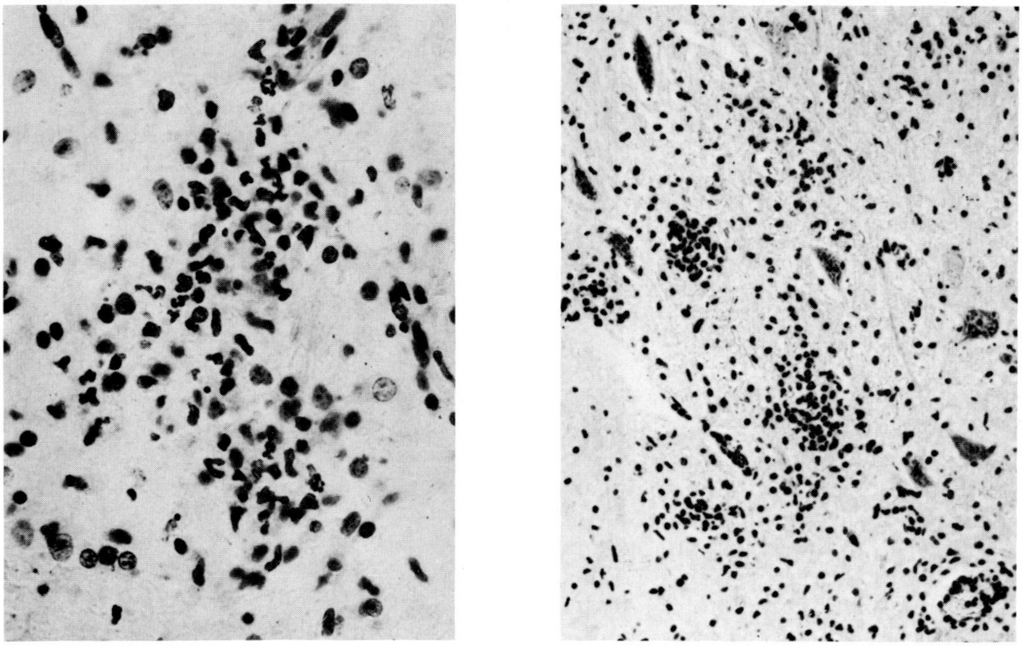

(a) **(b)**

Fig. 7.2 Poliomyelitis. Ventral horns of the spinal cord in the acute stage. **(a)** Very early neuronophagia with many polymorphonuclear leucocytes. **(b)** Slightly later stage of established neuronophagia without leucocytes. Note the normal appearance of some neurons.

acute disease, it is always possible to find changes in the spinal cord or medulla if paralysis has been present. The most obvious change is loss of neurons in the anterior horns of the spinal cord, loss of myelinated fibres in this region, and atrophy of the appropriate anterior spinal nerve roots. The lesions found generally correlate well with the clinical localization of paralysis, and examination of appropriate muscles supplied by the diseased spinal segments will demonstrate the presence of long-standing denervation atrophy.

Distribution of lesions. In severe cases which are fatal at an early stage, lesions may be very widespread indeed, and may even involve parts of the nervous system not generally thought to be affected by this group of viruses (for example, the central grey matter of the cerebrum, the pons and the cerebellum). The brunt of the disease, however, almost always falls upon the spinal cord and medulla, and in the cord the most severe lesions are generally found in the anterior two-thirds of the grey matter. The lesions may vary from level to level and are often conspicuously asymmetrical. Within the cord, the most severely involved levels are usually the cervical and lumbar enlargements, and the lower sacral segments are generally spared. In severely involved segments, there appears to be a tendency for the cell loss to be greatest in more medially placed cell groups, this being possibly a function of their slightly poorer blood supply, with hypoxia adding to the neurotropic effect of the virus.

In cases of bulbar poliomyelitis, dense cellular infiltrations are seen in relation to most of the nuclei of the motor cranial nerves, with eventual neuronophagia. The nerve cells of sensory nuclei are usually unaffected, and this also applies to the sensory neurons of the spinal posterior root ganglia. Infiltration by inflammatory cells and neuronal necrosis are generally present in the cortex of the precentral gyrus, the rest of the cerebral cortex being generally spared. In early fatal cases, infiltration by inflammatory cells, glial proliferation and neuronal necrosis may be found in many areas of the deep central grey matter of the cerebrum, the midbrain, pons and medulla and in the cerebellum, either cortex or dentate nuclei.

Encephalomyelitis due to varicella-zoster virus

Herpes zoster is a disease characterized by a crop of vesicles in the dermatome of a sensory nerve, usually preceded for 4 or 5 days by malaise and pain. Fresh crops of vesicles may occur for 7 days and then begin to dry up, frequently leaving scars and some postherpetic pain, which in patients over 40 years of age may persist for months. The dermatome of any sensory nerve may be attacked, but those most frequently affected are of the fifth cranial and third to tenth thoracic (Hope-Simpson, 1965). Occasionally, the sensory symptoms are accompanied by motor signs and, rarely, by an acute myelitis (Greenberg, 1970; Hogan and Krigman, 1973).

Elucidation of the natural history of zoster has been a slow process. Head and Campbell (1900) documented the inflammation, necrosis and haemorrhage in dorsal root ganglia which accompany zoster, and von Bókay (1909) postulated an infectious agent common to zoster and chickenpox, to be supported by Netter and Urbain (1926) who showed that the antibodies which appear after the two diseases cross-react. Only after the virus had been grown in tissue culture by Weller and Stoddard (1952) was it possible to prove conclusively that chickenpox and zoster are caused by the same virus—a member of the herpes group identical in appearance with herpes simplex virus, but biologically and antigenically distinct.

Hope-Simpson (1965), after a detailed epidemiological study, was able to delineate clearly the theory of latency which had been developing. Chickenpox is a primary infection in which the virus, after invading the nasopharynx is blood-borne to produce skin vesicles, whence it can travel in sensory nerves to spinal or cranial ganglia—just as herpes simplex virus can be shown to travel in the nerves of experimental animals. The virus goes latent in the ganglia to reactivate in later life when immunity, both humoral (Tomlinson and MacCallum, 1970) and cellular (Miller, 1980), has declined. Immunosuppression by diseases such as the reticuloses or by cytotoxic drugs tends to trigger the onset of zoster. Following reactivation in the ganglia virus spreads centrifugally in sensory nerves to the skin and its presence in ganglion and nerve has been shown by electron microscopy and immunofluorescence (Esiri and Tomlinson, 1972). In addition, centripetal spread can affect the dorsal nerve roots and the anterior horns, producing myelitis.

Pathological findings. The pathological changes in zoster infection are usually limited to the dorsal root ganglia or to the ganglion of a sensory cranial nerve, the nerve root close to the affected ganglia, and the skin. As has been noted above, the most frequently involved dermatomes are those of the fifth cranial and the third to the tenth thoracic nerves (Hope-Simpson, 1965) but cervical ganglia are also often affected. Generally one ganglion is most severely involved, but less severe changes can usually be found in the immediately adjacent ganglia. When the trigeminal ganglion is affected, it is usually in the part which is related to the ophthalmic division. Otic and geniculate zoster also occurs.

If an autopsy is performed on a case dying in the acute stage, the typical vesicular skin eruption may still be present. In such cases, virus particles may be found in epidermal cells by electron microscopical examination, and varicella-zoster virus may be isolated from the skin lesions.

The macroscopical findings, in acute cases, will be initially observed on exposing the spinal cord (or trigeminal ganglion), when the maximally affected ganglion will appear swollen and congested. The spinal cord itself may also be swollen over a few segments adjacent to the ganglion.

Microscopically, there is intense inflammation, almost exclusively lymphocytic, within the affected ganglion. This may be associated with necrosis which, in severe cases, may be massive and involve the entire ganglion, the appearances resembling those of an infarct. Small blood vessels may show necrosis of the walls, and it is not uncommon to find thrombosis in such vessels. The sensory nerve cells of the affected ganglion show degenerative changes, including loss of Nissl granules, eosinophilia of the cytoplasm and neuronophagia (Fig. 7.3a). Inflammation may extend for a short distance into the posterior nerve root and also into the posterior grey horn of the spinal cord at the root entry zone.

In most patients who die during or soon after the acute stage of the disease, abnormalities will be seen within the spinal cord at the level of the affected ganglia. In addition to the inflammation already described in the dorsal horn near the posterior root entry zone, changes may be seen in the anterior horn which are similar to those of

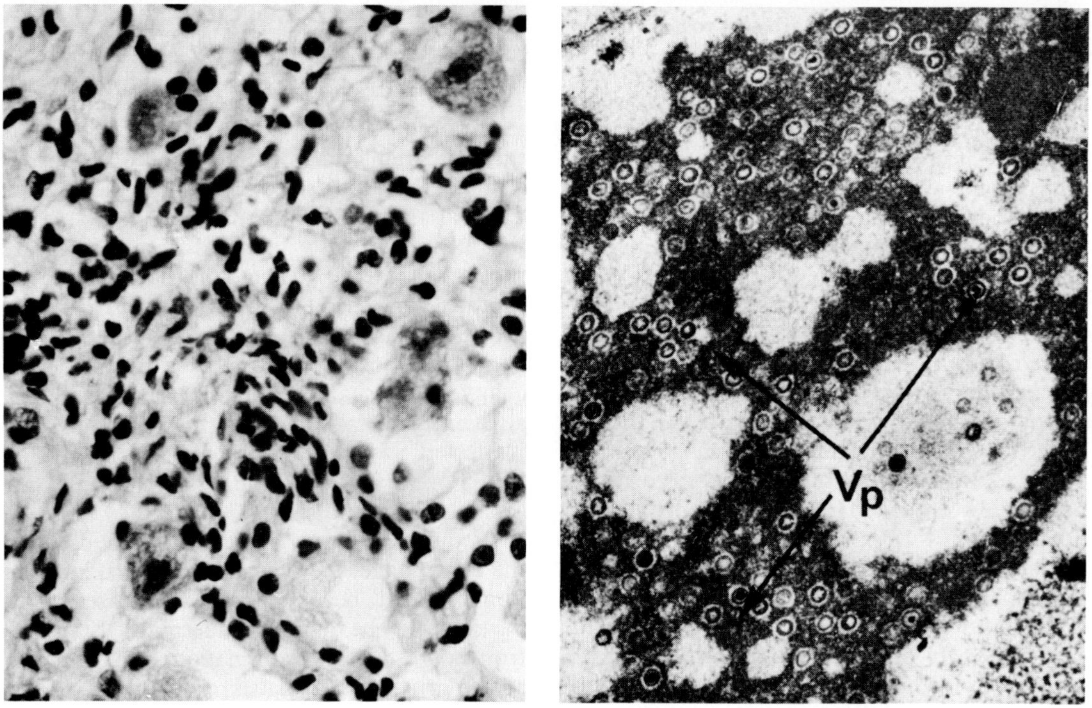

(a) (b)

Fig. 7.3 Herpes zoster. (**a**) Neuronal necrosis and infiltration by inflammatory cells in sensory ganglion. Haematoxylin and eosin × 500. (**b**) Part of a neuron containing numerous immature varicella-zoster virus particles (VP). × 20 000 (Reproduced, with permission, from Esiri and Tomlinson, 1972.)

infection by poliovirus—namely, central chromatolysis in motor neurons, neuronophagia, microglial cell proliferation and perivascular cuffing by lymphocytes. Such changes may also be seen involving Clarke's column.

In cases of trigeminal zoster infection, the pathological changes in the ganglion are similar to those described in spinal ganglia. The brain stem may also be involved, as in the case of the spinal cord, with evidence of lymphocytic infiltration and neuronal degeneration found within the neural tissue of the pons. Arteritis occasionally develops in large arteries, and this may lead to extensive infarction of neural tissue (Linneman and Alvira, 1980; Doyle, Gibson and Dolman, 1982).

In both spinal and cranial zoster infections, inclusion bodies are rarely seen in routine paraffin sections, and the attempted identification of virus particles by electron microscopy or labelled antibody techniques has so far not proved very successful. Esiri and Tomlinson (1972) have, however, identified varicella-zoster virus by electron microscopy and immunofluorescence in an acute case of trigeminal zoster infection, thus illustrating that, if suitable preparations are made and reliable techniques applied, the virus can be detected (Fig. 7.3b). It is suggested that electron microscopy and labelled antibody techniques are more useful than culture for examining post-mortem tissue because of the fact that this virus is particularly labile.

Acute encephalitis

The acute encephalitides fall into two categories not always easily distinguished on clinical grounds but clearly separated by their pathology—the postinfectious and the infective necrotizing types.

Postinfectious, or perivenous demyelinating, encephalitis

The diseases measles, mumps, varicella, rubella, smallpox and vaccinia are occasionally complicated by the sudden onset of encephalitis and a similar condition can follow the administration of Pasteur's rabies vaccine. Post-measles encephalitis is typical of the group and has been especially closely studied. Miller (1964) surveyed 53 000 cases of measles seen in general practice in England and Wales and noted an incidence of encephalitis of 1.2 per 1000 cases. Scott (1967) reported a similar incidence in the USA and he described the clinical picture as a sudden deterioration in a patient who has begun to recover from measles, with high fever, headache, vomiting, convulsions leading to coma and, sometimes, focal neurological signs. The modal time of onset is 5 days after the rash but it may be as late as 25 days: rarely, onset precedes the rash. The mortality is about 10 per cent, and of the survivors over a quarter have permanent neurological defects. In countries where it is assiduously used, vaccine has so reduced the incidence of measles that encephalitis is rare, but because the vaccine is a live virus, encephalitis occurred in 1 in a million vaccinees in the USA during 1963–1971 (Landrigan and Witte, 1973).

With only two exceptions, all attempts to isolate measles virus from CSF or brain in cases of acute encephalitis have been unsuccessful, and all the evidence points to an immunological mechanism for the demyelination. The two isolations were made from atypical cases of measles encephalitis (ter Meulen et al., 1972; Purdham and Batty, 1974).

As noted above, mumps virus commonly causes meningitis, and virus is found in the CSF, so in those rarer cases where encephalitis ensues it is not always clear whether it is infective or postinfectious, but a proportion of the fatalities are certainly due to perivenous demyelinating encephalitis (Hart and Earle, 1975).

In children neurological complications of chickenpox occur in about 1 per 1000 cases and cerebellar ataxia accounts for most of these, but postinfectious encephalitis is infrequent (Takashima and Becker, 1979). Neurological complications of rubella have an incidence of 1 in 20 000, and some of these cases are perivenous encephalitis.

The eradication of smallpox has ended the prophylactic use of vaccine and with it postvaccinial encephalitis, but for many years this complication was a serious hazard. Christie (1980) quotes the incidence in different episodes as varying between 1 in 6300 and 1 in 150 000 vaccinees. The onset was an abrupt elevation of temperature, neck rigidity, often clouding of consciousness, and movement disorders (Spillane and Wells, 1964). The pathology of the condition has been fully described by de Vries (1960).

From the earliest days of its use the administration of Pasteur's rabies vaccine was occasionally followed by an encephalopathy which, if fatal, proved to be a perivenous demyelinating disease. Initially rabies virus was thought to be responsible but Rivers and Schwentker (1935) showed that a similar disease could be produced by injecting only rabbit brain into monkeys. This experimental allergic encephalitis has been much studied as a model for naturally occurring demyelinating disease, and Paterson (1960) showed that it could be transferred passively by lymph node cells. An attack on myelin by sensitized lymphocytes appears to be the pathogenic mechanism of all postinfectious encephalitides, though how virus infection sensitizes lymphocytes to myelin is not yet known.

At present there are no specific laboratory tests to aid in the clinical diagnosis of postinfectious encephalitis. The pathological changes in this condition are described in Chapter 9.

Acute infective encephalitis

In contrast to the postinfectious type, the acute infective encephalitides are clearly due to damage caused by the growth of virus in cells of the brain and by the ensuing inflammatory reaction. Human cases are mostly caused by viruses of three groups. First are the herpes viruses which naturally infect only man and which can go latent in human tissue and show later reactivation. There are rare human infections with a simian herpesvirus. Secondly, rabies is a rhabdovirus which naturally infects mammals, wild and domestic, and is only incidentally spread to man when he is bitten by the natural host. Thirdly, there is the large group of arthropod-borne viruses of which each species has a limited natural range of hosts, small mammals or birds, between which it is transmitted by biting insects and occasionally by the same insects to man.

Apart from the above groups, adenoviruses and enteroviruses are occasionally the cause of acute encephalitis.

Herpes simplex virus encephalitis. In temperate parts of the world, herpes simplex virus (HSV) is the commonest cause of sporadic acute encephalitis.

Although the association of virus and disease

had been postulated earlier, it was Smith, Lennette and Reames (1941) who first reported a case of clinical encephalitis which, at necropsy, proved to have an acute necrotizing encephalitis with typical inclusion bodies and from which herpes simplex virus was isolated. van Bogaert, Radermecker and Devos (1955) defined acute necrotizing encephalitis as a clinical and pathological entity, and by 1962 Bennett, ZuRhein and Roberts had found 59 such cases in the literature. The clinical features and the diagnosis of herpes simplex encephalitis have been well reviewed by Illis and Gostling (1972).

Initially the clinical features are indefinite, so early diagnosis is difficult. Often personality changes, drowsiness and speech difficulties are the first signs, with or without fever and headache. As the disease progresses, consciousness is clouded and the patient may become comatose. Focal neurological signs do not occur in all cases but some have a hemiparesis, and unilateral seizures have been reported in 39 per cent of patients at onset and 64 per cent of all patients at some stage (Olson et al., 1967). A few patients present with a mild diffuse encephalitis, diagnosed from the presence of antibody in CSF, and make a good spontaneous recovery; for most cases, however, the prognosis is poor. Longson and Bailey (1977) assembled the findings of seven surveys of the literature which showed that the mortality of the untreated disease was 51–76 per cent and that although a few, even untreated, survive with no residual defects, many survivors have serious physical or mental disabilities. Miller and Ross (1968) confirmed earlier reports that the prognosis in children is better than in adults.

The incidence of this encephalitis is difficult to assess, but Longson (1979) has suggested 50 cases per year in England and Wales, and Johnson (1982) has postulated 1000–2000 cases per year in the USA.

Laboratory diagnosis. Raised intracranial pressure and the danger of coning may preclude lumbar puncture; if, however, a puncture is performed, a lymphocytosis and a moderate rise in protein in the CSF usually eventually indicate the presence of encephalitis although at onset the findings may be unremarkable. The cell count usually rises to $100–400 \times 10^6$ cells/l and the protein to 0·5–1·5 g/l, whereas the glucose level remains normal (Illis and Gostling, 1972). Early identification of the aetiological agent is as difficult as the clinical diagnosis because the presence of cutaneous herpetic lesions has no relevance, virus is very rarely found in the CSF (once in more than 50 cases in the writers' experience) and the wide dissemination of herpetic infection in the population means that the presence of serum antibody does not help in the diagnosis. Successful immunofluorescence staining of virus antigen in cells of the CSF was reported by Dayan and Stokes (1973) but their results have not been confirmed.

A diagnosis by isolating virus from tissue obtained at brain biopsy was first described by MacCallum, Potter and Edwards (1964), and Johnson, Olson and Buescher (1968) concluded that such a procedure is the only certain method of making the early diagnosis necessary before starting treatment with toxic antiviral agents. When biopsy tissue is available a tentative diagnosis can often be made rapidly by histopathological examination of tissue smears or sections (Adams and Miller, 1973) and a specific diagnosis can be achieved within 2–3 hours by the immunofluorescence technique (Flewett, 1973; Tomlinson, Chinn and MacCallum, 1974). Now that computer-assisted tomography can diagnose tumours and abscesses (and, though not so effectively, encephalitis), and less toxic drugs are available for therapy, there is a need for a non-invasive diagnostic technique. Many, though not all, patients produce serum antibody in high titre but MacCallum, Chinn and Gostling (1974) showed that antibody is also produced within the CNS and that comparison of serum and CSF titres, with appropriate controls, can provide a specific diagnosis 14–21 days after onset; the technique has been refined by Klapper, Laing and Longson (1981) so that in some patients the diagnosis can be established in less than 10 days.

The sensitivity and specificity of various diagnostic procedures have been assessed by Nahmias et al. (1982), who assembled the findings in 206 patients, all of whom had been biopsied for suspected HSV encephalitis. Of the 113 brain samples from which herpesvirus was isolated, 56 per cent showed evidence of HSV infection by histopathology, 70 per cent by immunofluorescence and 45 per cent by electron microscopy, and these techniques showed apparent false positives in 14 per cent, 9 per cent and 2 per cent respectively of samples from which virus was not isolated. Of those 113 patients, 72 per cent showed diagnostic rises in serum antibody titre and 94 per cent in CSF titre. Surprisingly, these authors did not employ a second antibody or concentration of albumin as a control on leakage of serum to CSF.

Pathogenesis. The pathogenesis of herpes encephalitis has long been the subject of speculation and, despite much work on the human disease and animal models, the route of virus to the brain is not yet defined. Virus can reach the brain by (1) the blood stream, (2) neural pathways or (3) the olfactory route through the cribriform plate as discussed by Johnson and Mims (1968). Except in the case of a generalized infection of neonates, there is no evidence that herpes simplex virus is spread in the blood stream.

Spread along nerves, first mooted by Goodpasture and Teague (1923), has been proven by subsequent work (Johnson, 1964; Wildy, 1967; Kristensson et al., 1978) and it now seems certain that the transit is in axon cylinders (Hill, Field and Roome, 1972; Cook and Stevens, 1973). The nasal mucosa offers a peculiar route of entry for viruses because the ends of olfactory rods are exposed and cuffs of arachnoid, not covered by dura, pass through the cribriform plate into the mucosa. Johnson (1982) has summarized the experimental evidence for the passage of dyes and of polio, West Nile and rabies viruses from nose to olfactory bulbs. There is, however, little evidence that this route is important in any natural disease.

In polio and rabies, virus is known to replicate at a peripheral site before reaching the CNS, but most patients with HSV encephalitis do not have a recognized peripheral infection, and the problem is complicated by the phenomenon of latency. The throat or mouth are the commonest sites for a primary herpes infection, most often in the first decade of life; primary genital infections occur in young adults (Juel-Jensen and MacCallum, 1972). Recurrent lesions can occur at or near the site of the primary infection; the involvement of sensory ganglia in this process was shown by Carton (1953), who noted that section of a sensory root precipitated herpes in the dermatome provided that the distal nerve was intact. Bastian et al. (1972) were the first of several groups to show that herpesvirus can be reactivated *in vitro* from sensory ganglia, and evidence that the reactivation is in neurons was produced by Cook, Bastone and Stevens (1974) and by McLennan and Derby (1980). After a primary infection human patients acquire antibody and retain it indefinitely.

Many patients with herpes simplex encephalitis have no history of previous infection whilst others are known to suffer from recurrent cold sores. In their series of 76 cases, Nahmias et al. (1982) found 23 patients without and 53 with antibody at the onset of the disease. If cases without pre-existing antibody are primary infections some peripheral site of infection might be expected but none is consistently found—Longson (personal communication) has isolated herpesvirus from the nasopharynx of occasional patients, but not consistently.

The virus which infects the brain of a patient with antibody at the onset of encephalitis presumably comes from a site of latency, and although the trigeminal ganglion is an obvious source there are no direct pathways from the fifth nerve nuclei in the pons to the limbic system. Furthermore, any virus found in the pons (never very much) appears later than in more rostral sites (Esiri, 1982a). Reactivation in the trigeminal ganglion and spread via a branch of the ophthalmic division to the dura of the middle and anterior fossae is a mechanism suggested by Davis and Johnson (1979), but as meningitis is not a prominent feature this, too, seems improbable. Another unsupported possibility is that virus, reactivated in the trigeminal ganglion, spreads to the nasal mucosa and thence by the olfactory route to the amygdaloid nuclei and the limbic system.

There have been few systematic studies of the olfactory tract in HSV encephalitis, but Dinn (1979, 1980) did find virus in the tract in 4 out of 4 cases and Esiri (1982a) found it in 9 out of 15 cases; whether virus was spreading centripetally or centrifugally is not known, but Tomlinson and Esiri (1983) showed that in mice virus can travel from the olfactory tracts to the limbic system. These observations are consonant with Esiri's theory (1982a, b) that in some cases the encephalitis may originate from virus latent in the brain. Sporadic latency in the brains of mice by wild-type HSV has been shown by Cook and Stevens (1976), Cabrera et al. (1980) and by Kastrukoff et al. (1981), and a more consistent latency of temperature-sensitive mutants was found by Watson et al. (1980). Using nucleic acid hybridization techniques, Sequiera et al. (1979) and Fraser et al. (1981) claim to have detected parts of the HSV genome in the brains of patients not suffering from encephalitis. Neither group defined precisely the areas of brain examined nor did they demonstrate *in vitro* reactivation.

It seems possible, therefore, that some cases of HSV encephalitis arise from virus which has been latent in the brain following entry by the olfactory route. The pathogenesis of those cases which appear to be primary infections remains obscure.

Pathological findings. These are highly characteristic, the distinctive feature being widespread and usually asymmetrical necrosis, particularly in the temporal lobes (Hughes, 1969; Adams and Miller, 1973) (Figs. 7.4 and 7.5). On macroscopical examination of the sliced fixed brain there is usually generalized swelling, but one hemisphere is likely to be more affected than the other (Fig. 7.4a). Areas of necrosis are visible to naked eye examination, and those parts of the cerebrum

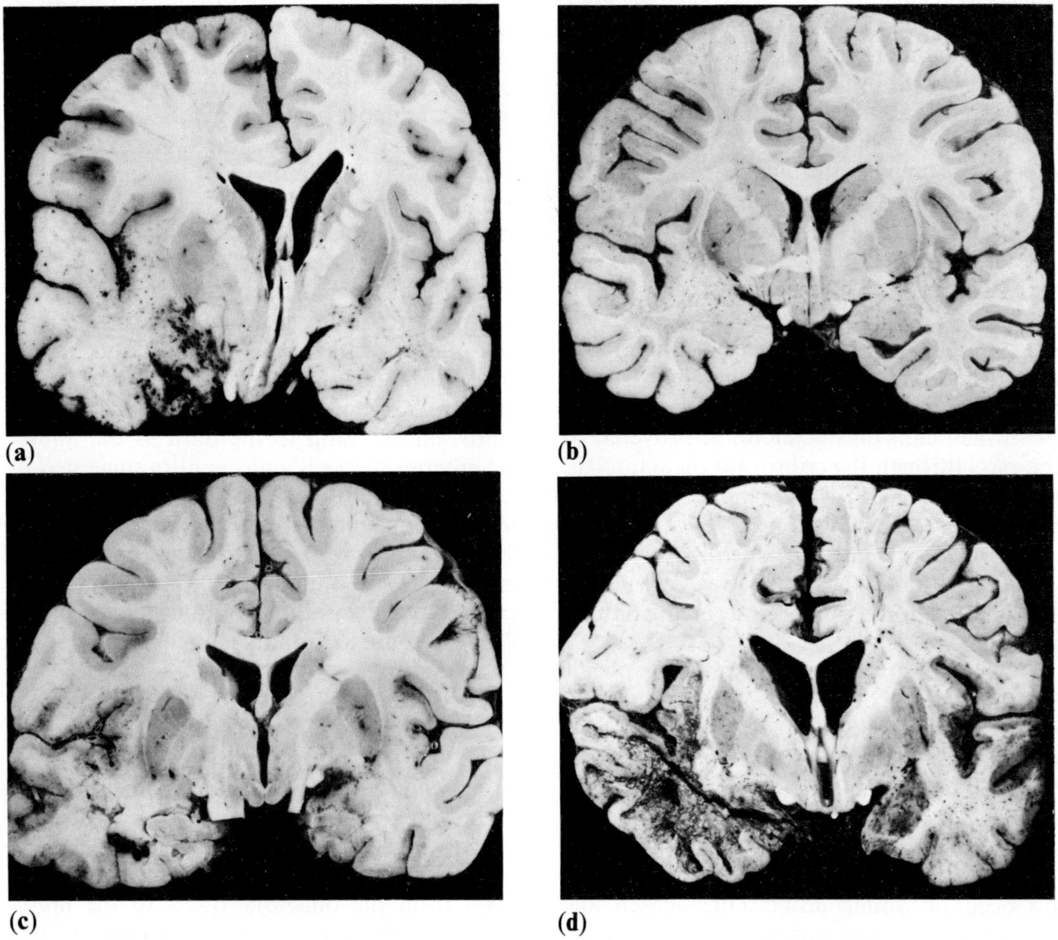

Fig. 7.4 Herpes simplex virus encephalitis. (**a**) Short survival. The left temporal lobe is swollen and necrotic and its medial part is focally haemorrhagic. The midline structures are shifted to the right and there are tentorial and supracallosal (subfalcine) herniae. (**b**) Short survival. In this case there is no focal haemorrhage or midline shift. Necrosis was more severe in the left hemisphere. Note the loss of definition between cortex and white matter in the medial part of the left temporal lobe compared with the right temporal lobe. (**c**) A few weeks' survival. The abnormal tissue in the more severely affected left hemisphere (temporal lobe, insula and cingulate gyrus) is beginning to disintegrate. Similar but much less severe abnormalities are seen in the right parahippocampal gyrus and in the insula. (**d**) Several weeks' survival. The abnormal regions are now cystic. Note the extensive cavitation in the left temporal lobe and insula compared with the much smaller lesions in the right hemisphere. Necrosis is also clearly seen in the cingulate gyri (from Adams 1973). (**a, b, d** reproduced, with permission, from: **a** and **d**, Adams, 1973; **b**, Adams and Miller, 1973.)

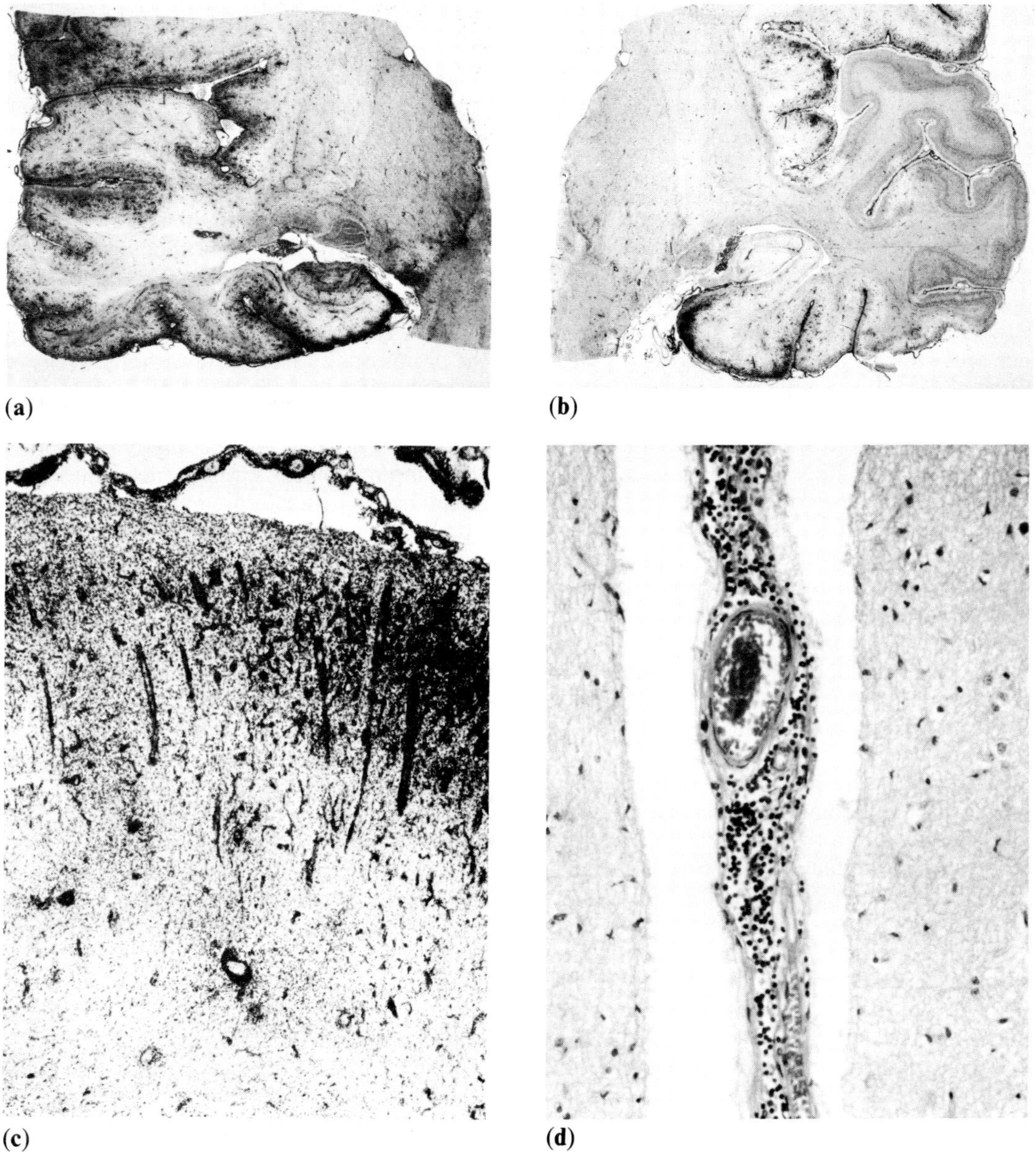

Fig. 7.5 (**a**) Herpes simplex encephalitis (a few weeks' survival). Photomicrograph of left temporal lobe to show total necrosis of the cortex of the left temporal lobe, the insula, and the adjacent part of the inferior frontal gyrus. Cresyl violet. (**b**) Same case as (**a**). In the right temporal lobe, necrosis is much less extensive than on the left, being restricted principally to the parahippocampal, fusiform and inferior temporal gyri and to the insula. Cresyl violet. (**c**) Herpes simplex encephalitis. Reactive changes—perivascular cuffing and microglial proliferation—are most conspicuous immediately deep to the pia and around vessels. Cresyl violet × 25. (**d**) Aseptic meningitis. Vascular congestion, and infiltration of leptomeninges by lymphocytes. Note normal underlying cortex. Haematoxylin and eosin × 200 reduced to 95%. (**a–c** reproduced, with permission, from Adams, 1973.)

worst affected include the anterior parts of the parahippocampal, the fusiform and the inferior and middle temporal gyri, and the posterior orbital cortex; necrosis may also extend through the superior temporal gyrus to become continuous with necrosis in the insula. The necrosis is not restricted to the neocortex but involves the white matter, the hippocampus, the amygdaloid nucleus and the putamen. If one hemisphere is less severely affected, necrosis may be restricted to the parahippocampal and fusiform gyri and the adjacent part of the inferior temporal gyrus. Other areas fairly consistently affected by necrosis are the insulae and the cingulate gyri, often bilaterally (Fig. 7.4d).

Examination of the brain from a patient who has died in the acute stage of the disease generally reveals all the sequelae of severe brain swelling with features attributable to the asymmetrical nature of the disease process (Fig. 7.4a). There is likely to be severe compression of the ventricles, a shift of the midline structures and a subtentorial hernia of the medial part of the severely affected temporal lobe. Midbrain compression and haemorrhages are frequently present, these being the ultimate cause of death in many of the cases.

The changes seen on microscopical examination will vary somewhat, according to the stage of the disease, and in the early stages are essentially those of rarefaction necrosis associated with a diffuse meningoencephalitis, the inflammatory reaction being characteristically intensified in and adjacent to the necrotic tissue (Fig. 7.5a, b, c). If the patient survives for a week or two, disintegration of the dead tissue occurs and microscopical examination now shows intense reactive changes in and around the necrotic tissue in the form of microglial hyperplasia, going on to the formation of large numbers of lipid phagocytes with abundant lymphocytes and plasma cells in the meninges and around vessels (Fig. 7.5c). Vessel walls themselves may show necrotizing changes, and may be infiltrated by polymorphonuclear leucocytes, which may also be seen in the necrotic brain tissue. At the same time, however, there may still be parts of the brain in which apparently more recent rarefaction necrosis is taking place, suggesting that the virus may spread progressively or in an episodic way to susceptible parts of the brain.

In addition to necrosis and inflammation in the neural tissue, there is always a typical diffuse meningoencephalitis as shown by infiltration of the leptomeninges by lymphocytes, plasma cells and large mononuclear cells, perivascular cuffing, neuronophagia and diffuse microglial hyperplasia (Fig. 7.5c). Intranuclear inclusion bodies occur, but they are by no means common or easy to detect, and, as with brain biopsy, the most reliable means of identifying the virus within the brain tissue is by labelled antibody techniques (Tomlinson, Chinn and MacCallum, 1974) (Fig. 7.6a and b). In a study of autopsy material from 29 fatal cases, Esiri (1982a) found virus antigen in the brains of all cases dying within 3 weeks of onset, most abundant in the first week. In her cases, virus antigen was usually present in both cerebral hemispheres, but mainly concentrated in the temporal lobes. Virus particles may also be found by electron microscopical examination, as even though the post-mortem tissue does not provide a good sample for ultrastructural examination, the virus particles appear to be relatively resistant to autolytic changes (Fig. 7.6c). However, because of the size of samples which can be examined, electron microscopical examination is less likely to yield positive information than is that of labelled antibody techniques which can be applied to much larger areas of affected brain.

In patients who have survived an attack of herpes simplex virus for weeks, months or years, pathological examination of the brain will usually again reveal the characteristic distribution of the lesions; i.e. asymmetrical damage, with the temporal lobes maximally affected. The affected tissue will be shrunken, with destruction of cortex and often underlying cyst formation. Severe cavitation with almost complete destruction of one temporal lobe may be seen, and there may be resultant degeneration of descending white matter tracts.

Histological examination of cases of long survival shows fibrous gliosis in affected regions, often with persistence of some microglial proliferation and lymphocytic infiltration. Virus antigen is not likely to be found in the brain of patients dying more than 3 weeks after the onset of the disease (Esiri, 1982a), and it has also been found that, in cases which have been treated with antiviral agents, virus antigen is unlikely to be found at necropsy (Nahmias et al., 1982).

Encephalitis due to other herpes viruses. Primary infection with varicella-zoster virus

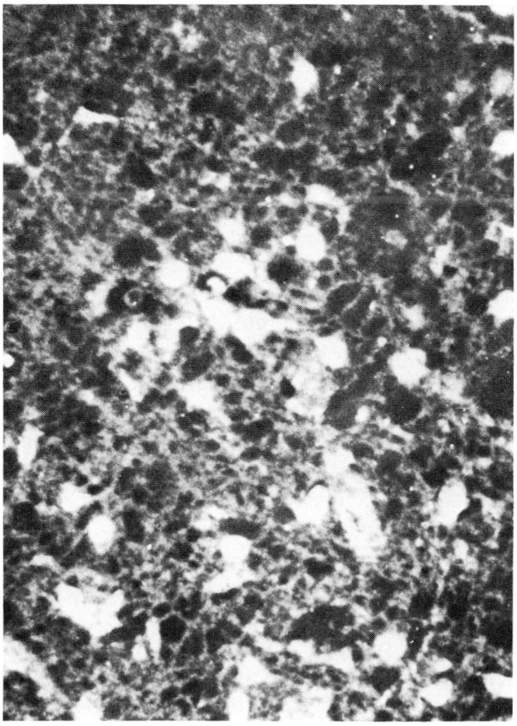

(a)

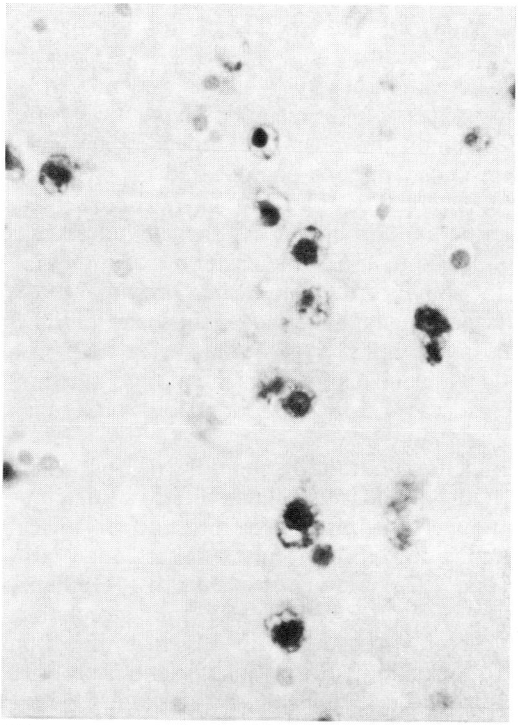

(b)

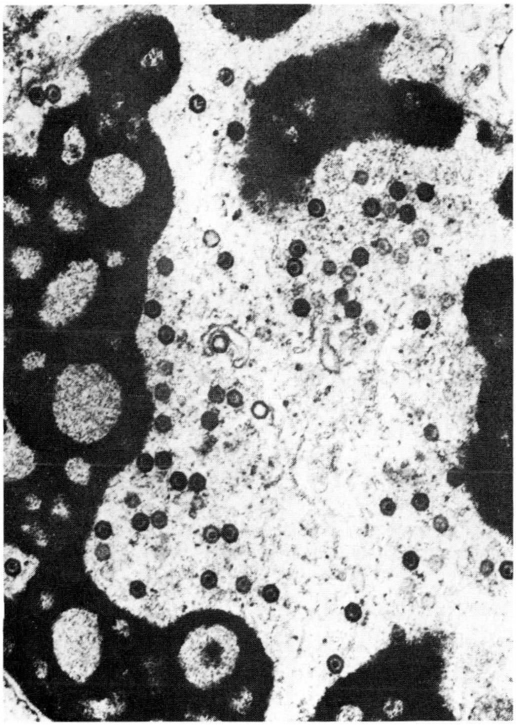

(c)

Fig. 7.6 Herpes simplex encephalitis. (**a**) Immunofluorescent staining of viral antigen in a section of cerebral tissue. × 200 reduced to 90%. (**b**) Immunoperoxidase preparation showing viral antigen in a paraffin section of post-mortem brain tissue from temporal lobe. Intranuclear inclusion bodies show positive staining. × 500 reduced to 95 per cent. (**c**) Electron micrograph showing part of a neuron containing virus particles within the nucleus. × 25 300 reduced to 90%. (**c** kindly provided by Professor R.O. Weller.)

causes chickenpox, usually in children, and all the evidence—epidemiological and histopathological—indicates that zoster is the consequence of reactivation of virus which has been latent in sensory ganglia, but reactivation *in vitro* has not been demonstrated as with herpes simplex virus. Chickenpox may be complicated by postinfectious encephalitis or by Reye's syndrome (Miller, Stanton and Gibbon, 1956; Appelbaum, Kreps and Sunshine, 1962), and zoster by inflammation of the spinal cord or brain stem proximal to the infected ganglia. True encephalitis is rare. Infection of the brain by varicella-zoster virus in a child with leukaemia and in an adult with Hodgkin's disease has been reported by McCormick et al. (1969).

Infection with the Epstein–Barr virus, which in young adults is usually manifest as infectious mononucleosis, rarely gives rise to neurological complications (Silverstein, Steinberg and Nathanson, 1972). Transverse myelitis, Guillain–Barré syndrome, Bell's palsy and encephalitis have been associated with EB virus infection (Grose et al., 1975) but insufficient necropsies have been done to establish the pattern of encephalitis.

Cytomegalovirus infections also have been associated with the Guillain–Barré syndrome (Leonard and Tobin, 1971; Schmitz and Enders, 1977) but this virus has only rarely been conclusively shown to cause acute encephalitis (Phillips et al., 1977). The neurological disease most frequently caused by cytomegalovirus follows intrauterine infection. The pathological changes in this disorder are described in Chapter 10.

Herpesvirus B (herpesvirus simiae) may cause human infection in which case the pathological findings are those of transverse myelitis, ascending myelitis and/or acute encephalitis (Sabin and Wright, 1934; Hull, 1973). Macroscopically the essential pathological features are those of acute multifocal necrotizing encephalitis with abundant inflammatory cells. Inclusion bodies have not been observed in cases examined.

Rabies

This unusual type of human encephalitis with a unique clinical presentation and consistently fatal outcome has for centuries been associated with the bite of a rabid animal.

Virus is introduced from infected saliva by a bite, by contact with abrasions or through mucous surfaces, and infection has been acquired by the respiratory route in bat-infested caves. When the infecting incident can be identified—not always possible—the incubation period in man varies from 15 days to a year, with a mode of 40 days (Nicholson, 1983), which is a variability unique among infectious diseases. The incubation period is shorter in children and in patients with bites on the head. The onset is of malaise, headache and fever, sometimes with nausea and diarrhoea and occasionally paraesthesia at the site of the bite. After this prodrome the disease may develop either as *furious* or *dumb* rabies. In the former, fasciculation, convulsions, meningism and cerebellar signs progress to death in 3–5 days and the hyperexcitability, which causes pharyngeal spasm in about half the patients, is the cause of hydrophobia. About 20 per cent of patients have dumb (paralytic) rabies with paresis of a limb or an ascending paralysis like the Guillain–Barré syndrome (Chopra et al., 1980) and a duration of up to 11 days. With either type, death is usually due to myocarditis or cardiorespiratory disturbance.

Rabies virus is a rhabdovirus, 150 × 100 nm, but frequently pleomorphic; it contains single-stranded RNA and is of a single major antigen type, though there are minor antigenic variants (Schneider, 1982). There are five rabies-related viruses, from insects and rodents, whose importance in human disease is not yet known (Shope, 1982). The virus is found world-wide except for Australia, Great Britain, Japan and New Zealand where sea frontiers have facilitated control. The virus naturally infects wild carnivores, and in the past the dog has been the commonest source of human infection and still is in India and south-east Asia. Now, with dogs controlled or vaccinated, the skunk is the main reservoir in the USA and the fox in Europe; the mongoose is the reservoir in South Africa and vampire bats infect many cattle and some humans in South America. Surprisingly, some insectivorous and fruit-eating bats also carry the virus. Fifty per cent of rabid dogs do not excrete virus in their saliva but in those that do it begins some days before symptoms, and secretion for several months by asymptomatic dogs has been observed (Fekadu, 1975).

Murphy et al. (1973a) studied the spread of rabies virus following intramuscular injection into experimental animals. Virus first replicated in myocytes and spread to neuromuscular and neurotendinal spindles and thence along axons to sensory ganglia and spinal cord. Schwann, endoneurial and satellite cells were not infected. In these animals virus reached the brain in 3–5 days and by 5 days had spread centrifugally to retina and cornea, to nerve endings associated with hair roots, to taste buds and salivary glands, and to viscera and myocardium (Murphy et al., 1973b), thus confirming the work of Dean, Evans and McClure (1963) who had shown that neurectomy prevented spread of infection from limb to brain and that denervation of the salivary gland largely prevented excretion of virus. It appears that the length of the incubation period is dependent on the time taken for replication at the site of infection and the progression to nerve endings because transit thence to the brain is rapid (Baer and Cleary, 1972). The pathogenesis of human disease is thought to follow the pattern just described but the long and variable incubation is not adequately explained.

Just how the infection produces such a profound functional disturbance of the CNS without morphological evidence of cell destruction or inflammatory response is a mystery but Tsiang, Ermine and Marcovistz (1982) have found a hint—the binding capacity of acetylcholine receptors in the rat brain was reduced twofold by rabies infection.

Laboratory confirmation of rabies during life is by isolation of virus from saliva, by immunofluorescence demonstration of antigen in corneal cells or in the nerves of hair follicles, and by detection of rising titres of antibody. *Post mortem*, the search for Negri bodies can also be used. For a full discussion of diagnostic techniques, see Johnson (1979).

In most Western countries all work with rabies cases and virus is controlled by regulations on dangerous pathogens; e.g. for the UK, the *Code of Practice* (Department of Health and Social Security et al., 1978).

Pathological findings. Macroscopical examination of the brain does not usually reveal any external abnormality. Histologically, the changes are those of a polioencephalomyelitis (Dupont and Earle, 1965) with inflammatory changes occurring predominantly in the grey matter. Perivascular cuffing by lymphocytes and plasma cells is present and microglial hyperplasia and neuronophagia may be present, but the

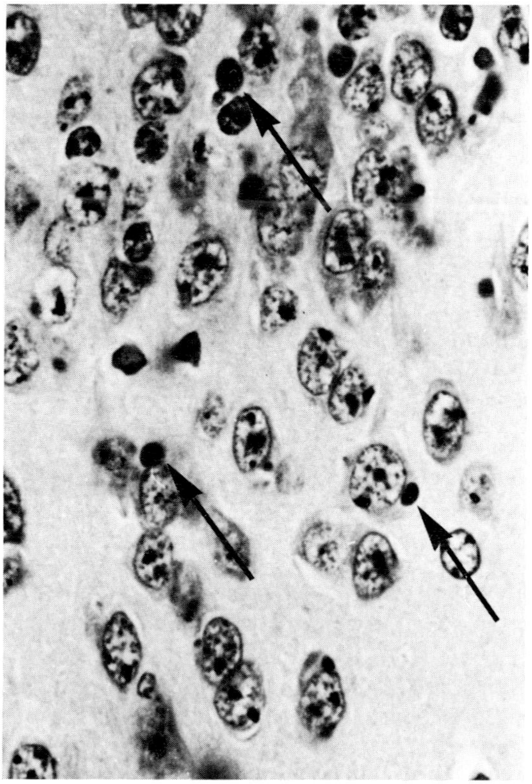

Fig. 7.7 Rabies. Intracytoplasmic Negri bodies within cortical neurons of a mouse. Mann's stain × 500.

pathognomonic histological feature of rabies is the *Negri body* (Fig. 7.7).

These bodies, which are not found in every case, are usually most numerous in the pyramidal cells of the hippocampus but they are also common in the cerebral cortex and in Purkinje cells. They are more abundant and larger in cases surviving for more than 4 or 5 days, and may be difficult to find in patients who succumb during the first 48 hours. The Negri body is a sharply defined, rounded or oval, eosinophilic neuronal cytoplasmic inclusion measuring 1–7 μm across. They may lie anywhere in the cytoplasm of the cell body or its dendrites and more than one may be seen in a single cell. The largest bodies are seen in the pyramidal cells of the hippocampus, in the adjacent temporal cortex and in the Purkinje cells. When present in motor neurons of the spinal cord, they may also be very large. The nature of the Negri body has been somewhat of a mystery in the past, and Negri (1903) originally considered that they represented a stage in the life cycle of a protozoal parasite. The introduction of immunofluorescent staining, however, has resulted in the identification of rabies virus antigen within Negri bodies by the fluorescent antibody technique, and ultrastructural examination has revealed virus particles (De Brito, Araujo and Tiriba, 1973).

Another form of inclusion body, the lyssa body, has also been described in rabies (Dupont and Earle, 1965). These appear by light microscopy as simple acidophilic cytoplasmic inclusions and have been thought to be non-specific, but electron microscopy has revealed that they are identical to Negri bodies (Sung et al., 1976) and it is therefore suggested that the term lyssa body should no longer be used.

Evidence of an inflammatory reaction to the presence of either type of body may be entirely lacking, scanty or florid (Lindenberg and Haymaker, 1982). When florid, the appearances are those of a severe polioencephalomyelitis, including acute as well as chronic inflammatory cells, and hyperplasia of both microglia and astrocytes.

In the paralytic form of rabies, the most striking pathological changes are seen in the spinal cord (Chopra et al., 1980). There may be lymphocytic leptomeningeal infiltration, and the cord shows neuronal degeneration in the anterior horns, with more or less severe inflammatory cell infiltration and proliferation of microglial cells. Dorsal root ganglia are also involved, showing degeneration of neurons with inflammatory infiltration (Tangchai and Vejjajiva, 1971). Lumbar and lower dorsal segments of the cord appear to be the most commonly involved, being probably related to the site at which the subject was bitten.

The brain stem and cerebrum also show inflammatory cell infiltration in paralytic rabies, and cases with clinical bulbar involvement show neuronophagia and microglial nodules. Negri bodies are generally present, being most consistently found in the Purkinje cells and in the pyramidal neurons of the hippocampus (Chopra et al., 1980).

Peripheral nerves relevant to the site of the bite generally show degenerative changes and infiltration by inflammatory cells (Tangchai and Vejjajiva, 1971; Maton, Pollard and Newsom Davis, 1976), and segmental demyelination and remyelination have also been found in teased peripheral nerve preparations (Chopra et al., 1980).

Myocarditis is a well recognized complication of rabies (Ross and Armentrout, 1962; Cheetham et al., 1970; Cohen et al., 1976) and may be found at post-mortem. Although the heart may appear normal macroscopically, histological examination may show necrosis of muscle fibres, with infiltration by lymphocytes, histiocytes and occasional neutrophils. It should be noted, however, that necropsies on cases of suspected rabies may not be performed in the UK except in specially designated centres (Department of Health and Social Security et al., 1978).

Acute encephalitis caused by arboviruses

Of the 500 or more viruses known to have a life-cycle alternating between a vertebrate and an arthropod host, only 18 species (in five taxa) regularly cause encephalitis in man. All contain RNA.

In the alphaviruses, Eastern, Western and Venezuelan equine encephalitis viruses are all spread by mosquitoes, with birds as the principal hosts for the first two and horses and small mammals for the Venezuelan virus. Within the flavivirus group, the five of the St Louis complex circulate between mosquitoes and birds whereas six are tick-borne with birds or small mammals as their main hosts. Two bunyaviruses infect small mammals and mosquitoes, and the one encephalitogenic reovirus is tick-borne.

These viruses all multiply within the vertebrate host and at some stage cause a viraemia from which the haematophagous arthropod is infected and the virus then undergoes a further multiplication cycle. There is a time lapse of up to 14 days, depending on temperature, season and other factors, before the arthropod's bite is infective. Man is only incidentally infected and the species of mosquito infecting him, or spreading infection from man to man, may be different from that in the natural cycle. There is some evidence that in the vertebrate host arboviruses first multiply at the site of the bite and their spread to the CNS is certainly blood-borne. The natural history of the encephalitogenic arboviruses is discussed by Johnson (1982).

To make a laboratory diagnosis, virus can be isolated in suckling mice by injecting blood taken during the patient's viraemic phase, but as the viraemia is short-lived, this attempt is rarely successful. Virus is more readily isolated from the brain or spinal cord of fatal cases. Diagnosis is more usually made by looking for rising titres of antibody in spaced sera. Diagnostic procedures are fully described by Shope and Sather (1979).

Pathological findings in Eastern, Western and Venezuelan equine encephalitis. The pathology in Eastern and in Western encephalitis is similar, but as the clinical disease is more fulminant in the former, the pathological changes are more acute (Lindenberg and Haymaker, 1982). Macroscopically the brain is congested and swollen, and microscopically there is a severe meningoencephalitis, polymorphonuclear leucocytes being prominent in the acute stage. There is also an acute vasculitis with necrosis of, and fibrin deposition in, vessel walls. There are many areas of tissue necrosis, and selective neuronal necrosis with neuronophagia is common. No part of the brain may be spared although in some cases the cerebrum is most severely involved, whereas in other cases the brunt of the disease falls upon the brain stem.

In both Eastern and Western equine virus encephalitis, the spinal cord is generally spared, but, when affected, the lesions are generally limited to the upper cervical region. This may help to distinguish virus infections due to these agents from other forms of acute encephalitis.

The Venezuelan type of equine encephalitis is most severe in children, and 75 per cent of all fatal cases have been children under 5 years of age (Johnson, 1982). The pathological changes in this condition are those of a mild encephalomyelitis in which the inflammation is most prominent in the putamen and in the cerebral white matter (Haymaker, 1961).

Pathological findings in St Louis encephalitis. As in many other forms of acute encephalitis, the brains in fatal cases may show no specific abnormalities. However, Reyes et al. (1981) found, in an examination of 14 patients who died during an epidemic in northern Illinois in 1975, that all cases showed perivascular cuffing or infiltration by lymphocytes, histiocytes, plasma cells and occasional polymorphonuclear leucocytes around venules, veins, arterioles and small arteries. All cases showed histiocytes or lymphocytes invading the leptomeninges, and perivascular cellular infiltration was present in a majority of cases. Proliferation of microglial cells was also found, often in the form of microglial nodules. The distribution of the lesions is predominantly cerebral, with basal ganglia, cerebral cortex and cerebral white matter being the commonest sites, although no part of the central nervous system is likely to be spared. In the study by Reyes et al. (1981), neuritic plaques and neurofibrillary tangles were seen in three out of ten cases, but although occasional hyaline intranuclear inclusion bodies were present in one case, no viral antigen was detected by immunofluorescence in any of the cases examined.

In a comparison between Western equine and St Louis encephalitis, Leech and Harris (1977) found that inflammatory cell infiltration was much more prominent and widespread in St Louis encephalitis, whereas the Western equine type was characterized by more extensive necrosis but less inflammation.

Pathological findings in encephalitis due to tick-borne viruses. The pathological changes in the nervous system of infection due to this group of viruses are not specifically distinguishable. In general they consist of any or all of the features of virus encephalitis already described under the heading of general changes—i.e. varying degrees of neuronal necrosis in the cerebral cortex and basal ganglia, the brain stem, cerebellum and spinal cord. The neuronal necrosis is accompanied by infiltration by inflammatory cells, perivascular cuffing and glial hyperplasia of varying severity.

Subacute encephalitis

The subacute measles encephalitides

Measles virus is now known to be the cause of two forms of subacute encephalitis quite distinct from the acute postinfectious encephalitis referred to above (p. 272).

Subacute sclerosing panencephalitis

A form of subacute encephalitis with intranuclear inclusion bodies in brain cells was described by Dawson (1933), and after further cases had been reported by van Bogaert (1945), Greenfield (1950) correlated their findings and introduced the now accepted name of subacute sclerosing panencephalitis. This is predominantly a disease of children characterized by the insidious onset of behavioural changes, mental deterioration followed by myoclonus, ataxia and, sometimes, seizures. Vision may be affected, and after a period of stupor the patient dies. The age of onset ranges from 2 to 21 years with a mean of 7 years, and about half the patients are known to have had measles before the age of 2 years (Jabbour et al., 1972; Modlin et al., 1977). The patients are not febrile and neither the blood picture nor the findings in the CSF are indicative of infection, but the consistent finding of intranuclear inclusion bodies suggests the presence of a virus. All attempts to implicate a virus were negative until Bouteille et al. (1965) found, by electron microscopy, nucleocapsids of a paramyxovirus within the inclusion bodies and Connolly et al. (1967) showed that patients with the disease have high titres of measles antibody in serum and CSF, and that measles antigen demonstrable by immunofluorescence is present in neurons and glial cells. Final confirmation was provided by a novel technique (Horta-Barbosa et al., 1969; Payne, Baublis and Habashi 1969). Viable brain tissue was cultured and then cocultivated with HeLa or monkey kidney cells in which measles virus was found by immunofluorescence or haemadsorption techniques. They found (and others have confirmed) that cell-free virus can be isolated from the cultures of the brains of some patients, but not from all. The presence of measles-specific IgM antibody in serum and CSF (Connolly, Haire and Hadden, 1971; Kiessling et al., 1977) points to a release of antigen from a persistent infection.

Subacute sclerosing panencephalitis (SSPE) is, therefore, a slow infection by measles virus reactivated many years after an attack of measles, and two main theories of pathogenesis have been invoked. The first theory postulated SSPE strains different from measles virus but there is no evidence of clustering of cases as would occur if there were peculiar strains. Furthermore, many comparisons of the biological and biochemical features of viruses isolated from SSPE and from measles have failed to show consistent differences (Choppin, 1981). The second postulate was of a defective immune response but antibody, both IgG and IgM, is produced in abundance and there is no evidence of cellular immunodeficiency (Agnarsdóttir, 1977). Patients with subacute sclerosing panencephalitis do, however, fail to produce antibody to the virus protein M necessary for the release of free measles virus (Hall, Lamb and Choppin, 1979), most probably because brain cells do not permit the production of M antigen (Hall and Choppin, 1979). Despite much theorizing (Johnson, 1982) there is still no wholly satisfactory explanation of the long latency and the slow evolution of the disease.

Pathological findings. As the length of survival in this condition varies considerably from case to case, the pathological findings will depend to some extent on the stage of the disease at which death supervenes. In cases of short duration the brain may appear normal on macroscopical examination but in long-standing cases it may be atrophic and abnormally firm. On slicing the brain, the macroscopical appearances may again be normal or show a full range of abnormalities depending on the stage. In cases with a relatively short history, changes are usually confined to the white matter which may appear rather granular or discoloured. Cases which have survived for many months or even years show severe and generalized cerebral atrophy affecting cortex, white matter, central grey matter and also the cerebellum.

Microscopical examination shows the features of a subacute encephalitis, again varying somewhat according to the duration of the illness (Ohya et al., 1974). In cases of relatively short duration there is generally a fairly heavy cellular infiltrate of lymphocytes and plasma cells in the leptomeninges and perivascular spaces. In the more severely affected parts of the cortex there may be considerable loss of neurons with astrocytic and microglial hyperplasia. Neuronophagia is common. Neurofibrillary degeneration of Alzheimer type has been reported by Malamud, Haymaker and Pinkerton (1950) and by Corsellis (1951). Intranuclear inclusion bodies are always present, in both oligodendroglial cells and neurons (Fig. 7.8a and b). Electron microscopical examination, even on formalin-fixed tissue, may demonstrate viral nucleocapsids (Fig. 7.8c and d).

A wide range of abnormalities may be found in the white matter, which may show only mild perivascular cuffing with lymphocytes and plasma cells or more extensive inflammatory infiltration associated with numerous hypertrophied astrocytes, with or without a diffuse fibrous gliosis. Gliosis tends to be much more conspicuous than myelin destruction, this often being particularly apparent when sections from the same case are stained for myelin and glial fibrils. Nevertheless, there are usually scattered

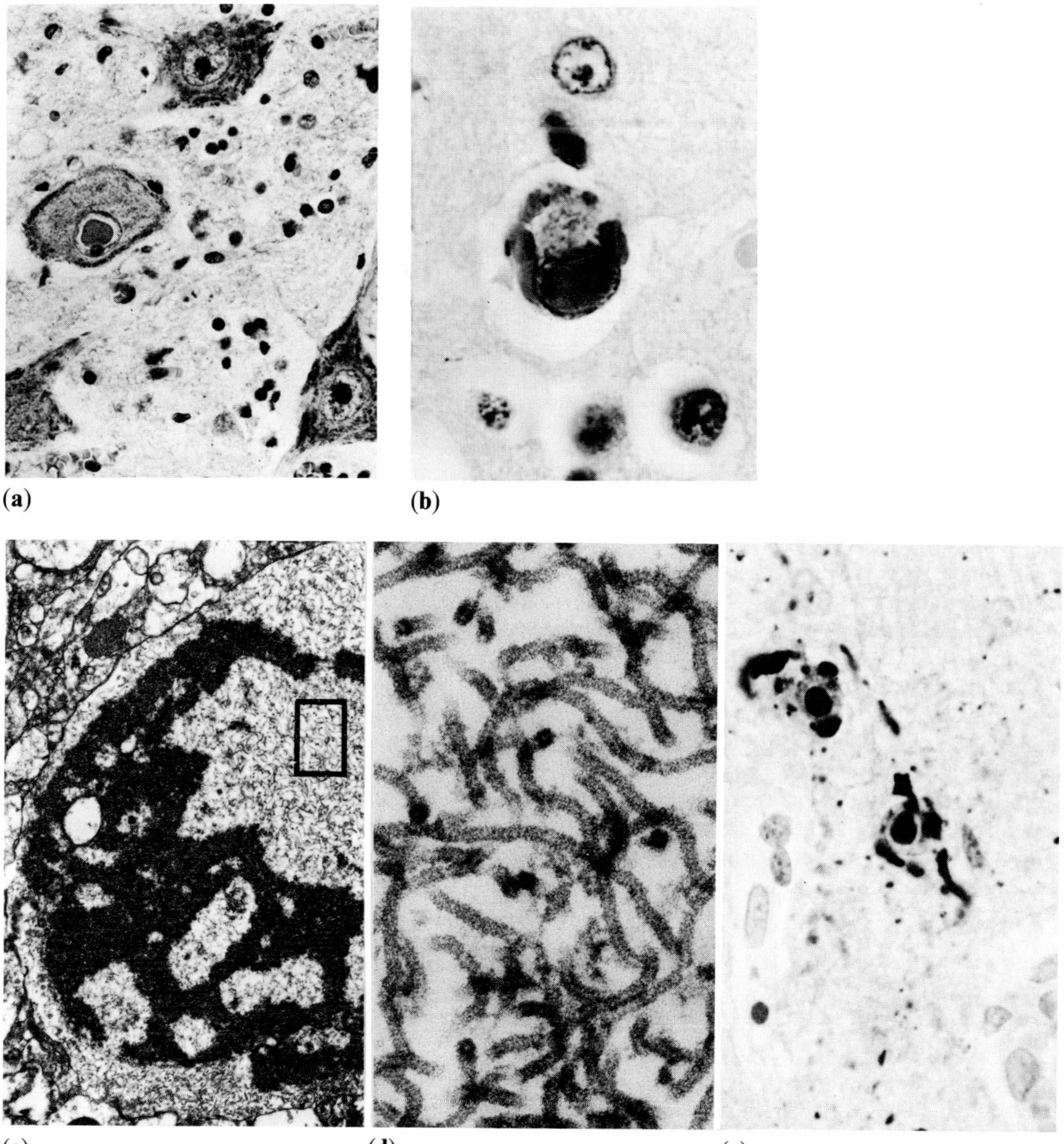

(a) (b) (c) (d) (e)

Fig. 7.8 Subacute sclerosing panencephalitis. (**a**) Inclusion body and central chromatolysis in a ventral horn neuron from the eighth cervical segment. (**b**) Intranuclear and intracytoplasmic inclusion bodies in a cortical neuron (**c, d**) Electron micrographs showing viral nucleocapsids in a nucleus from the temporal lobe. × 15 000 and 125 000. (**e**) Immunoperoxidase preparation, using measles virus antiserum, on a paraffin section of post-mortem brain, showing positive staining of viral antigen in nuclei and cytoplasm. The cells are probably neurons. × 800 reduced to 90%. (**c** and **d** kindly provided by Mrs J.E. Richmond, Central Public Health Laboratory.)

microglial cells containing sudanophilic lipid whilst areas of more complete demyelination occur occasionally.

In cases which have survived for long periods in an apparently arrested state, the histological appearances are somewhat different. There is generally severe neuronal loss in the cortex and central grey matter, and thinning of the white matter with severe gliosis. Inflammatory cells may be very scanty indeed, with no evidence of a meningitis remaining, and possibly just a few perivascular cuffs of lymphocytes in a haphazard distribution. Inclusion bodies also may be very scanty, but can usually be found if a careful search is made.

In both early and late cases the most reliable way of establishing the diagnosis is by the application of the immunoperoxidase technique to paraffin sections, using a measles antiserum (Fig. 7.8e). In a study by Esiri et al. (1981) of six cases of subacute sclerosing panencephalitis with survival rates varying from a few weeks to several years, measles virus antigen was found in all cases, though in varying amounts, tending to be more abundant in the cases with a shorter clinical history than in those with longer survival. The virus antigen was remarkably widely distributed, being present in all cases in the brain stem, basal ganglia, cerebral white matter and cortex, and not present in any case in the cerebellum. There appeared to be no single area within the brain for which the virus had a particular predilection, and it is therefore apparent that very extensive histological sampling should be made when examining the brains of such cases because the amounts of antigen may be small.

In addition to the expected changes of subacute encephalitis, and the presence of measles antigen by immunocytochemical or electron microscopical examination, histological changes due to secondary phenomena may also be seen. In particular, epileptic seizures are common in cases with long survival, and may lead to neuronal necrosis in expected sites, and anticonvulsant drugs used in the treatment of such seizures may also be responsible for further neuropathological changes. In cases with prolonged survival, examination of the brain stem and spinal cord will show degeneration of descending long tracts.

Measles inclusion body encephalitis in the immunosuppressed. This condition was first reported by Lyon (1972) in a child being treated for nephrosis. Agamanolis, Tan and Parker (1979) described the disease in an adult transplant patient, and Chadwick et al. (1982) observed the condition in a 20-year-old without recognized immunosuppression, but of the 24 cases reviewed by Agamanolis and colleagues, although the ages ranged from 2 to 52 years, most were children and the commonest underlying disease was acute lymphatic leukaemia. Many had a history of contact with measles or an actual attack from which they recovered fully and then neurological disease developed some months later. Confusion and lethargy progressed to myoclonus, focal neurological signs, seizures and death within a few weeks for 20 of the patients; four survived with severe neurological impairment. Only four of the 24 patients had pleocytosis or raised protein in the CSF, and although some had high titres of antibody in serum and CSF, as in subacute sclerosing panencephalitis, for others the titres were unremarkable, presumably depending on whether B-cell activity was spared or suppressed. Whether or not antibody is present, the brains of these patients show inclusion bodies, typical nucleocapsids, and measles antigen stainable by labelled antibody.

The laboratory can assist in the diagnosis by measurement of antibody in serum and CSF, and for cases of subacute sclerosing panencephalitis the titres are usually significant and the serum/CSF ratio less than 200:1. For the immunosuppressed, high titres are diagnostic, but little or no antibody does not exclude the diagnosis. Biopsy or post-mortem tissue, even formalin-fixed tissue, can be stained by immunofluorescence (Drysdale et al., 1976) or immunoperoxidase (Esiri et al., 1981) techniques to give a firm diagnosis.

Pathological findings. The external appearance of the brain in such cases may be normal, and certainly does not show the severe swelling and necrosis associated with most of the acute viral encephalitides. Examination of the fixed brain in slices may or may not show focal abnormalities such as areas of softening or discoloration in the cortex or white matter (Fig. 7.9a), and as a general rule the diagnosis of this condition can be made only on histological examination. This may also be difficult on initial examination, as infiltration by inflammatory cells may be almost entirely lacking and the presence of inclusion

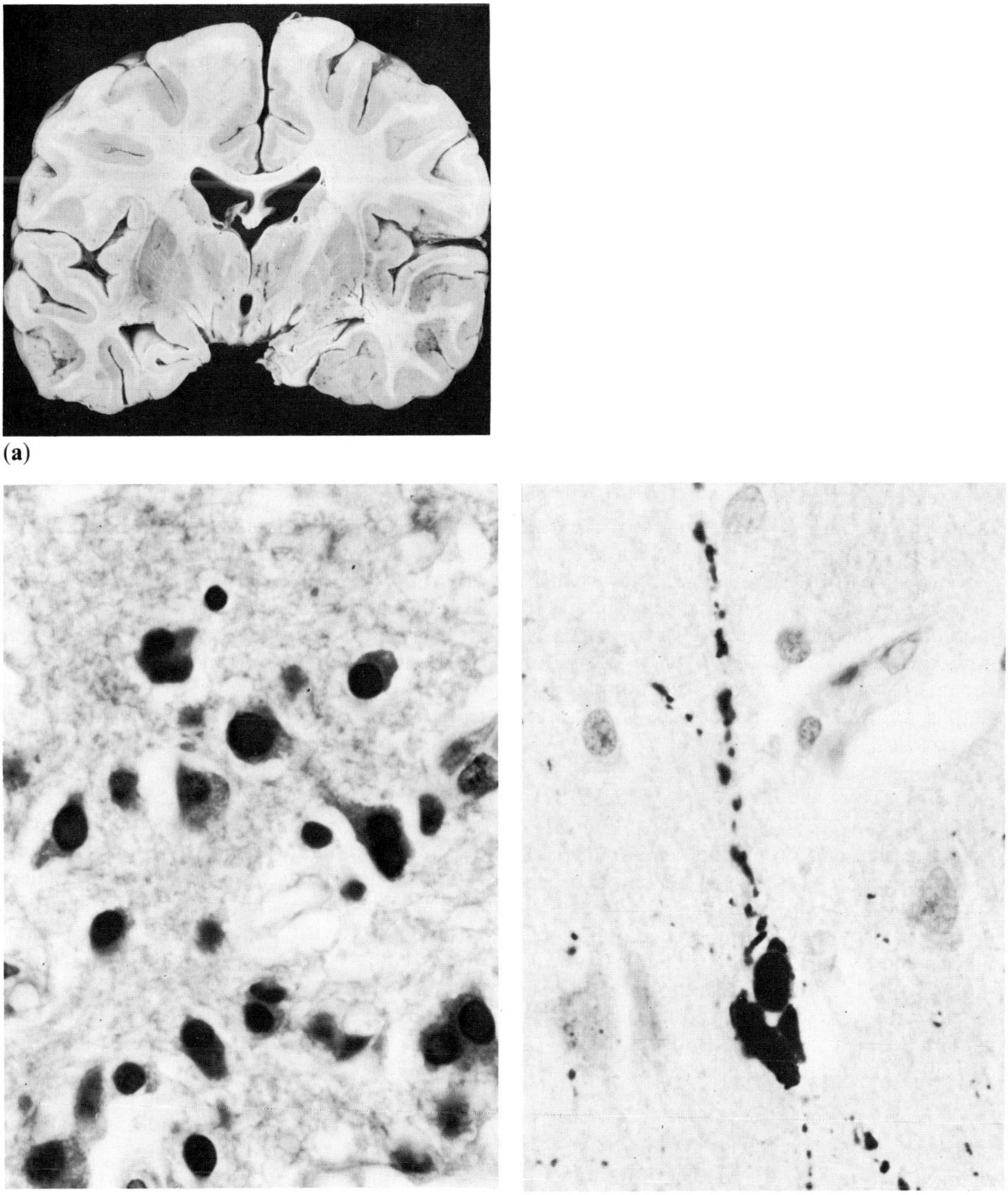

(**a**)

(**b**) (**c**)

Fig. 7.9 Measles encephalitis in immunosuppression. (**a**) Coronal slice of brain from an 8-year-old child with treated acute leukaemia, dying after a 6-week neurological illness. Note the relatively normal appearances, except for areas of congestion in the temporal lobes, maximum on the right. (**b**) Section from the cortex of the temporal lobe from the same case, showing numerous inclusion bodies but no trace of an inflammatory cell reaction. Haematoxylin and eosin × 800. (**c**) Immunoperoxidase preparation on a section from the same block as (**b**), using measles antiserum, showing the presence of measles antigen in the nucleus, cytoplasm, axons and dendrites of a cortical neuron. × 1000.

bodies may thus be missed. However, in cases where the clinical features and/or serological examination make the diagnosis of measles infection in an immunosuppressed patient the likely diagnosis, a careful search for inclusion bodies should be made on a number of representative sections. The diagnostic feature is the presence of eosinophilic, usually intranuclear, inclusion bodies situated in neurons, oligodendrocytes or apparently lying free in the tissue (Fig. 7.9b). The collections of these bodies may be remarkably focal and unattended by cellular reaction whether by inflammatory cells, microglial cells or astrocytes. In two cases examined by one of the authors (B.B.), the distribution of inclusion bodies was remarkably widespread in the cerebrum, brain stem and cerebellum, with no apparent predilection for grey or white matter. Neuronal necrosis may be seen in the worst-affected areas, but demyelination is not a feature of this condition.

The diagnosis of a measles infection can be confirmed by identifying the inclusion bodies by immunocytochemical techniques using a measles antibody (Drysdale et al., 1976) (Fig. 7.9c). Electron microscopical examination of suitable tissue samples will also demonstrate the presence of virus particles.

Progressive rubella panencephalitis

A progressive panencephalitis similar to SSPE has occurred as a late sequel of congenital rubella infection (Townsend et al., 1975; Weil et al., 1975) and also following non-congenital rubella (Lebon and Lyon, 1974). The patients have high titres of rubella antibody in serum and CSF, and rubella virus was recovered from the brain of one patient (Cremer et al., 1975). The scarcity of published cases suggests that this is a rare disease.

Pathological findings. The neuropathological changes in this rare disease are those of widespread neuronal destruction in the cerebrum, cerebellum and brain stem with perivascular lymphocytic infiltration and vasculitis with fibrinoid necrosis (Townsend et al., 1982).

Progressive multifocal leucoencephalopathy

This disease, first described by Åström, Mancall and Richardson (1958), has an insidious onset of dementia, weakness, visual loss and sometimes ataxia, which usually progresses to death within 6 months, though a few patients appear to have remissions and survive for some years. The patients are usually of middle age and are generally suffering from an underlying condition which affects their immune competence—e.g. Hodgkin's disease, leukaemia, lymphoma, sarcoid, tuberculosis and cancer (Richardson, 1961)—or are receiving immunosuppressive therapy (Legrain et al., 1974; ZuRhein and Varakis, 1974). A small number of patients do not have any underlying disease or recognized immune deficiency (Walker, 1978). The multiplicity of symptoms is a reflection of the multifocal demyelination apparent at necropsy. There are no abnormalities in the CSF to aid the diagnosis, which can only be confirmed by examining tissue from biopsy or necropsy.

The first indication of a viral aetiology was the discovery by ZuRhein and Chou (1965) of arrays of virus-like particles 30 nm in diameter within the inclusion bodies in oligodendrocytes. No virus was isolated in the common tissue cultures or by animal inoculation but Padgett et al. (1971) reported the isolation of a virus *post mortem* from the brain of a patient, JC, by using cultures of human fetal glial cells. This virus, named JC (not to be confused with the agent of Creutzfeldt–Jakob disease) was of the papova group, but was not SV40 of monkeys, polyoma virus of mice nor a human wart virus. Coincidentally, a similar virus, BK, was isolated from the urine of a renal transplant patient (Gardner et al., 1971) and later SV40 virus was isolated from the brains of two patients with progressive multifocal leucoencephalopathy (Weiner et al., 1972). These three are members of the genus polyomavirus; they are the only ones known to infect humans; they have species-specific antigens and a small amount of common antigen (Penney and Narayan, 1973) and all produce tumours in hamster brains.

Infections with JC and BK viruses are widespread. Surveys have found antibody to JC virus in 27 per cent of 9-year-old children, and in 65 per cent at 14 years rising to 80 per cent later (Padgett and Walker, 1973) whereas antibody to BK is acquired earlier, reaching 73 per cent in 4- to 6-year-old children (Gardner, 1973). Polyoma-viruses have been found in the urine of 13 per cent of transplant patients (Coleman, Gardner and Field, 1973) and viruses JC or BK were found in the urine of 1 per cent of 1235 pregnant women surveyed by Coleman et al. (1980). It appears, therefore, that infection with these viruses acquired early in life is reactivated by any interference with the immune function such as pregnancy or the use of immunosuppressive drugs.

BK virus has not so far been implicated in PML; SV40 virus, known from surveys to cause infrequent human infection, has been found in only two cases and the majority of cases fully investigated (over 30) have been due to JC virus. Willoughby et al. (1980) showed that although the lymphocytes in patients with progressive multifocal leucoencephalopathy have a generally reduced response to mitogens, the migration inhibition response is specifically reduced to JC virus. It is not known whether PML is the consequence of a primary infection in an immune compromised patient or whether the immunosuppressive underlying disease causes a reactivation peculiar to oligodendrocytes. While the cellular response is depressed, patients with PML produce high titres of antibody. As virions are found profusely in oligodendrocytes, rarely in astrocytes and never in neurons, and immunofluorescent staining shows many antigen-containing cells round the lesions (Narayan et al., 1973), it is apparent that the disease results from the failure of infected oligodendrocytes to maintain myelination.

The diagnosis is made by finding characteristic arrays of virions, supported by immune-electron microscopy, or by immunofluorescence staining of tissue sections. Antibody measurements are rarely helpful and culture of the viruses involved is very slow and tedious.

Pathological findings. The brain may appear perfectly normal externally but there may be some cortical atrophy. In the sliced fixed brain the most characteristic macroscopic feature is the presence of multiple grey foci distributed throughout the white matter of the cerebrum and, to a lesser extent, the cerebellum and brain stem (Fig. 7.10a). Lesions may also be present in grey matter, but here they are less conspicuous to the naked eye. Some of the lesions have appearances similar to those of the plaques seen in multiple sclerosis, but in some cases the lesions may be large and confluent, and these can appear as areas of softening, necrosis or even cystic change (Adams and Short, 1965). Microscopical examination shows multiple, sometimes confluent, foci of demyelination (Fig. 7.10b). At first sight, the most striking cytological feature in and around the lesions is the presence of enlarged abnormal astrocytes, which are often multinucleate and have numerous large processes. A few chronic inflammatory cells, mainly lymphocytes, may also be present in relation to the lesion, but the most important pathological finding is the presence of intranuclear inclusions, which may be basophilic or eosinophilic, mainly found within large swollen oligodendrocytes (Fig. 7.10c). These cells are not seen in the centre of large confluent lesions but they are numerous at the periphery of the demyelinated areas and in the immediately adjacent brain.

Although the lesions of PML are characteristically described as demyelination, the sparing of axons is only relative and the central part of larger lesions may exhibit frank necrosis with a phagocytic reaction indistinguishable from that seen in an infarct. In such cases there is usually widespread hypertrophy of microglial cells. The diagnosis of PML may be confirmed, if appropriate antiserum is available, by immunofluorescent or immunoperoxidase techniques, demonstrating that the inclusion bodies contain virus antigen (Fig. 7.10d). In a study of 46 autopsied cases by Budka and Shah (1982), using cross-reacting anti-SV40 virus sera, antigen was found in 32 cases. Positive staining was mainly seen in the large swollen oligodendrocytes, but was also present in some of the bizarre giant astrocytes. Electron microscopy on suitable samples, taken from near the edge of a lesion, may also confirm the presence of polyoma virus (Fig. 7.10e).

Kuru and Creutzfeldt-Jakob disease

Two subacute encephalopathies, Creutzfeldt-Jakob disease and kuru, which appear to be degenerative diseases are in fact caused by transmissible agents allied to those of scrapie and transmissible mink encephalopathy but quite unlike the common viruses.

Creutzfeldt-Jakob disease, first fully described by Jakob (1921) begins with the insidious onset of confusion, depression and altered sensation progressing in weeks or months to dementia, ataxia, sometimes cortical blindness, and bulbar palsy. In the more rapidly progressive disease the patient soon becomes akinetic and mute. Onset is usually in the sixth decade (range 27 to over 70 years) and the duration of the disease 7 months (range 1–55 months) as reported by Masters et al. (1979). The disease is world-wide, producing an average annual mortality of 0.30 per million population though in some areas, or age groups, it is over 1.0 (Brown, 1980), and the analysis of 1435 cases in the USA showed that 15 per cent of the cases were familial (Masters et al., 1979).

Kuru, first described by Gajdusek and Zigas (1957), has the features of a progressive cerebellar degeneration, sometimes with dementia, which begins with trivial inco-ordination and proceeds to gross clumsiness in walking and loss of balance. Finally, the patient cannot sit up, perform voluntary movements or speak intelligibly and dies of inanition in 12–18 months (Hornabrook, 1979). The disease is confined to a small population, the Fore people, in Papua New Guinea, and when first observed the incidence was 1 per cent of the population per year but it has declined steadily since then and all the evidence points to endocannibalism as a factor in its spread (Alpers, 1979).

Scrapie is a progressive and fatal disease of

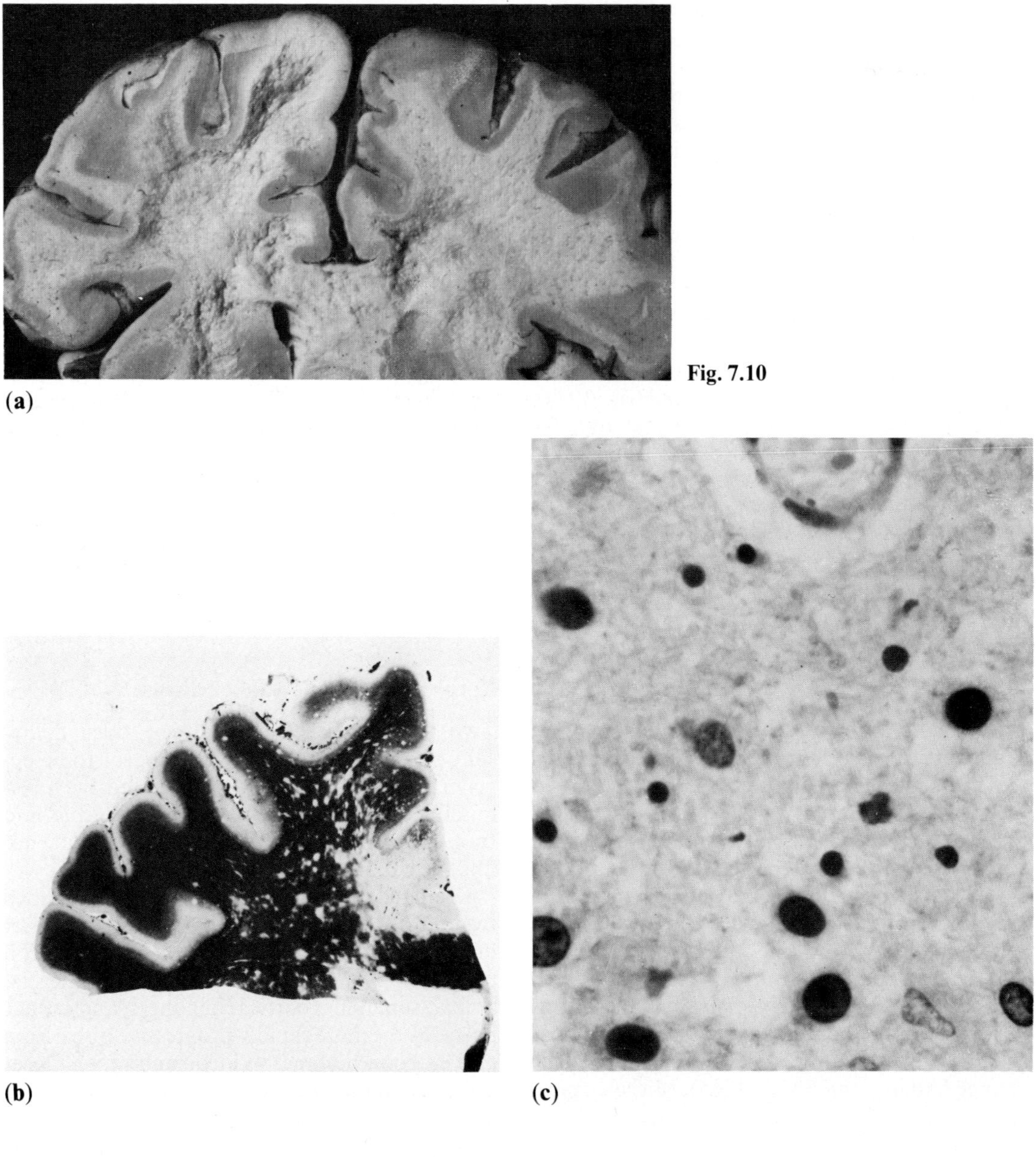

Fig. 7.10

(a)

(b)

(c)

sheep in which the pathological changes are vacuolation of neurons, spongy change in the neuropil and astrocytosis. It was shown to be experimentally transmissible from sheep to sheep (Cuillé and Chelle, 1936) and from sheep to mice (Chandler, 1961). The pathological similarities between scrapie and kuru prompted Hadlow (1959) to suggest that kuru might be transmissible, and Gajdusek, Gibbs and Alpers (1966) were able to report the transmission of kuru to chimpanzees, soon to be followed by the reported transmission of Creutzfeldt–Jakob disease (Gibbs et al., 1968).

The agent of scrapie has been more fully studied but it is probable that most of its characteristics are shared by the agents of the other two diseases. The agents can be detected only by animal inoculation, with incubation periods of 6 months to 8 years, and the ease of transmission depends on the strain of the agent and genetic factors in the animals—summarized for scrapie by Dickinson (1976) and for Creutzfeldt–Jakob disease and kuru by Gibbs, Gajdusek and Amyx (1979). Consistent transmission of Creutzfeldt–Jakob disease and kuru is possible with chimpanzees and squirrel monkeys, but erratic with other animals. The infective unit is about 30–40 nm in size but no infective particles have been recognized by electron microscopy. Infected brains show no inflammatory infiltration and there is no evidence of humoral or cellular immunity so the agents do not appear to be antigenic. Exceptional resistance to thermal and chemical disinfection is shown by the agents responsible for scrapie (Kimberlin et al., 1983) and for Creutzfeldt–Jakob disease (Brown et al., 1982), and the resistance of all three agents to ionizing and ultraviolet radiation suggests a genome size of only 65 000 daltons if it is nucleic acid, or 100 000 if it is a glycoprotein (Latarjet, 1979). There have

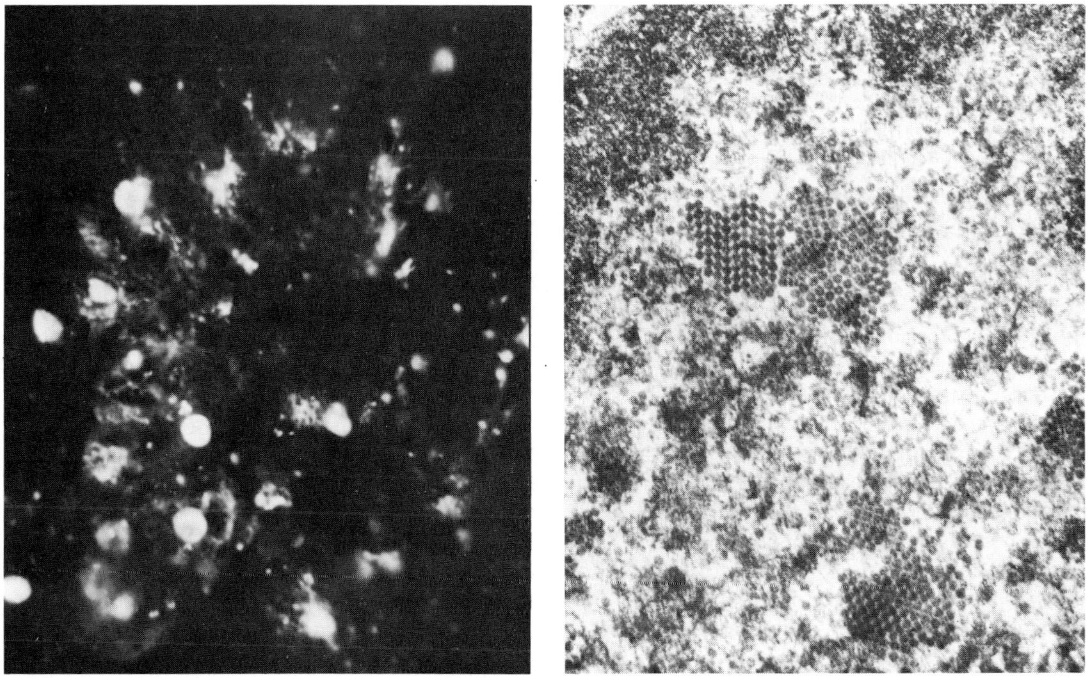

(d) **(e)**

Fig. 7.10 Progressive multifocal leucoencephalopathy. (**a**) Section of brain to show many small abnormal foci in the white matter. Some are coalescing to form larger confluent partly cystic lesions. (**b**) Posterior part of left frontal lobe. There are many small foci of demyelination in the white matter, and confluent demyelination in the cingulate gyrus. Heidenhain. (**c**) Edge of demyelinated area to show atypical oligodendroglia with large dense hyperchromatic nuclei and ill-defined intranuclear inclusion bodies. Haematoxylin and eosin × 525. (**d**) Immunofluorescence preparation on brain section, showing JC virus in brain cells stained by fluorescein conjugate. (**e**) Electron micrograph showing papova virus in a nucleus. × 45 200 reduced to 90%. (**a–c** reproduced, with permission, from Adams and Short, 1965. **d** kindly provided by Professor R.T. Johnson. **e** kindly provided by Professor R.O. Weller.)

been many theories, with rather tenuous support, for the chemical nature of these agents and the latest is a 'novel proteinaceous particle' (Prusiner, 1982).

Kuru, with its initial high incidence and cannibalism as a probable mode of spread, can reasonably be called an infectious disease. Creutzfeldt–Jakob disease, however, is an enigma. With an annual incidence of less than 1 in a million, with little evidence for case clustering and the only certain case-to-case spread being by surgery (Duffy et al., 1974; Bernoulli et al., 1977; Will and Matthews, 1982) it is difficult to understand how Creutzfeldt–Jakob disease can maintain itself. One possibility is that the agent may be widespread in the population but only a small number, particularly predisposed, are affected as with progressive multifocal leucoencephalopathy. This thesis can be tested only when a simple and cheap means of detecting infection becomes available. There is no useful microbiological diagnostic test for Creutzfeldt–Jakob disease or kuru.

Pathological findings in kuru. Pathological studies have established that the disease is restricted to the nervous system and that it is a subacute encephalopathy (Fowler and Robertson, 1959; Klatzo, Gajdusek and Zigas, 1959; Beck and Daniel, 1965; Beck et al., 1969). Macroscopically the brain may appear normal apart from some atrophy of the cerebellum, particularly in the vermis and flocculonodular lobe. Histologically the disease process involves grey matter and, though it is most severe in the cerebellum, the cerebrum is also affected. The widespread generalized changes in the cerebral hemispheres are characterized by a mild status spongiosus particularly in the limbic and paralimbic cortex and in the thalamus (Fig. 7.11a). The status spongiosus is associated with loss of neurons, and an excess of hypertrophied astrocytes and microglial cells. The latter may be in the form of rod cells, but also may take the form of lipid-laden macrophages. Neuronal loss is often severe in the central grey matter, including the caudate nuclei and the anterior and medial nuclei of the thalamus, and here, as in the other sites where grey matter is involved, there may be coarse vacuolation of neurons (Fig. 7.11b). Plaques of the type described below in the cerebellum may also be found in the grey matter of the cerebral hemispheres.

The most dramatic histological abnormalities occur in the cerebellum, particularly in the palaeocerebellum (Fig. 7.11c and d). Loss of granule cells is more conspicuous than loss of Purkinje cells although many of the latter which survive appear abnormal and have torpedo swellings in their axons and antler-like thickening of the dendrites. A particularly characteristic feature of kuru is the presence of so-called plaques (Fig. 7.11d); these are most numerous in the granule cell layer but they also occur in the molecular and Purkinje cell layers and in the subcortical white matter. Each plaque consists of a solid homogeneous core surrounded by a halo of delicate radially arranged fibrils; they are readily apparent in sections stained with haematoxylin and eosin, are strongly PAS-positive and are birefringent. These plaques, which have been found in approximately three-quarters of all cases examined (Beck and Daniel, 1979), have the staining properties and electron microscopical appearances of amyloid. No antibody activity has been identified in the plaques, and their presence is not considered to be an indicator of the pathogenesis of the disease.

Infiltration by inflammatory cells is not a feature of the histopathology of kuru, and no virus particles have been found on electron microscopic examination. Although human cases of kuru have not been subjected to detailed ultrastructural studies, the experimentally produced encephalopathy has been extensively studied in chimpanzees and spider monkeys (Lampert et al., 1969; Beck et al., 1975). In a recent study on the brains of nine spider monkeys inoculated with human kuru material, Beck et al. (1982) found that the most striking ultrastructural feature was the formation of abnormal configurations of plasma membranes (ACPMs), the numbers of which varied according to the length of incubation, with a peak at 13 weeks. It was suggested that ACPMs are due to an excessive synthesis of some membrane constituent by the cell perikaryon, and that they are the underlying cause of intracytoplasmic vacuolation, which in turn builds up to produce the histological phenomenon of status spongiosus.

For further details of the pathology of naturally occurring and experimentally produced spongiform encephalopathies, including Creutzfeldt-Jakob disease see Chapter 20.

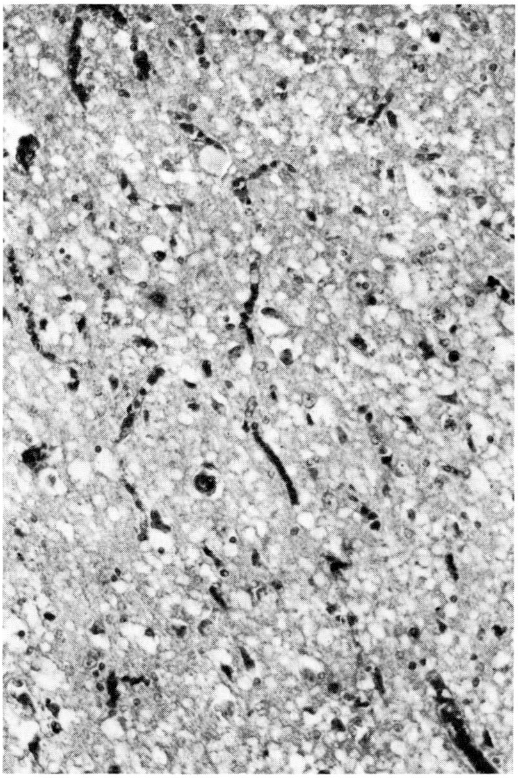

(a)

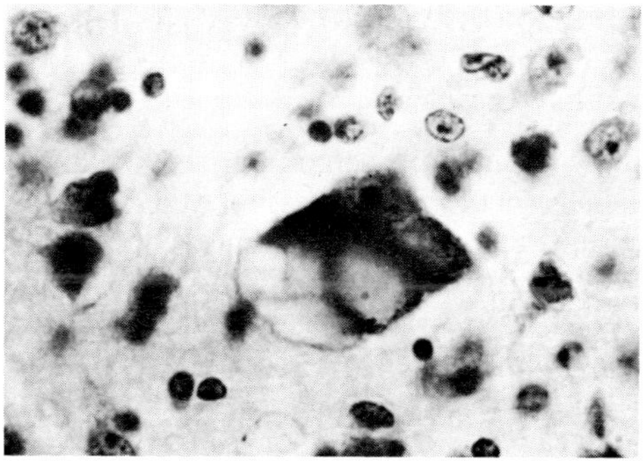

(b)

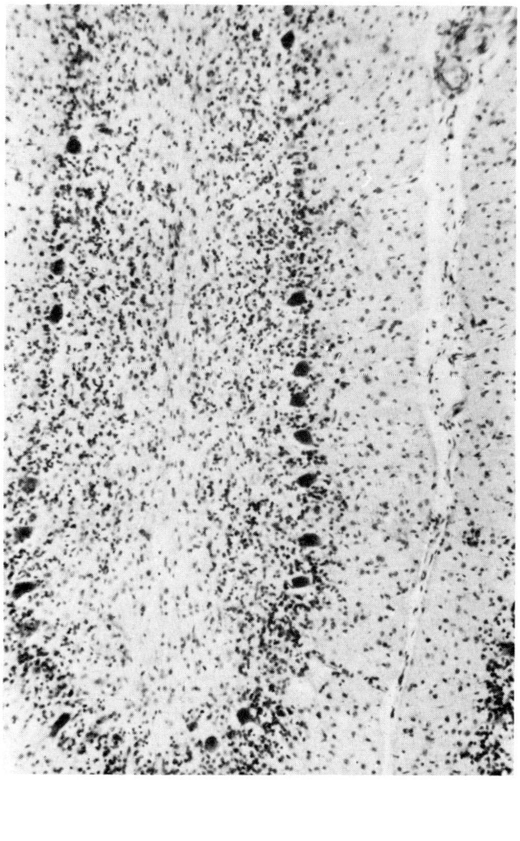

(c)

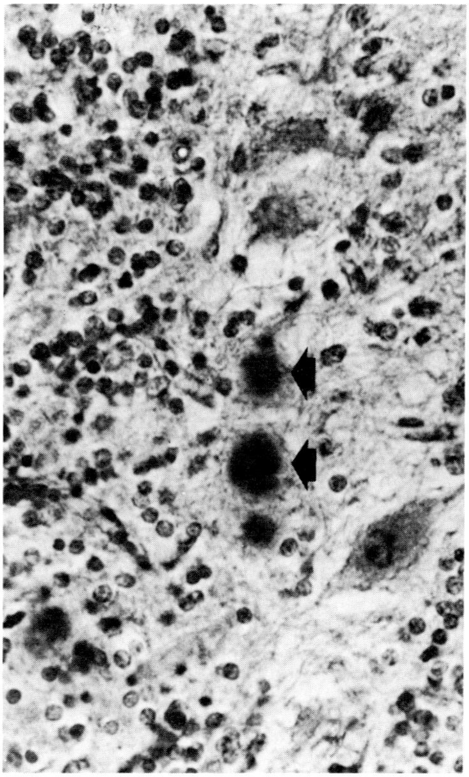

(d)

Fig. 7.11 Kuru. (**a**) Status spongiosus in cingulate gyrus. PAS × 190. (**b**) Coarse intracytoplasmic vacuolation of a large neuron in caudate nucleus. Cresyl violet × 320. (**c**) Loss of granule cells and Purkinje cells in the cerebellar vermis. Cresyl violet × 120. (**d**) Plaques in cerebellum (arrowed). PAS × 300. (Illustrations kindly provided by Professor P.M. Daniel and Mrs E. Beck.)

Encephalopathies of uncertain aetiology

Encephalitis lethargica

A form of encephalitis characterized by fever, somnolence, oculomotor palsies and signs of cerebral and meningeal irritation was observed in epidemic form in France and Austria in 1915, and was described in detail by von Economo (1917). Epidemics occurred in England in 1919 and 1920 (Parsons, 1922), and during the subsequent decade it was reported from most parts of the world but had almost disappeared by 1930. Attempts, with the limited techniques then available, to implicate a virus were unsuccessful, as were the efforts to relate the encephalitis to the contemporaneous pandemic of influenza.

In the absence of an identified aetiological agent, it is difficult to be sure that all the cases said to be encephalitis lethargica, with a somewhat varied clinical picture, were in fact a single entity, and even more difficult to identify currently diagnosed sporadic cases with the epidemic diseases of the 1920s.

Pathological findings. There are no recent descriptions of the neuropathology of this disorder, and descriptions are based on articles by von Economo (1931) and Buzzard and Greenfield (1919). The neuropathology appears to have been that of congestion and inflammation involving the grey matter of the cortex, basal ganglia and, in particular, the brain stem adjacent to the aqueduct and floor of the fourth ventricle. Microscopically, the most conspicuous abnormality was perivascular infiltration by lymphocytes and plasma cells. Inflammatory changes were found to be greatest in the midbrain, both in the tegmentum and in the substantia nigra, but they were also seen in the cerebral cortex, basal ganglia and the lower brain stem, and in many cases in the cervical segments of the spinal cord.

Lesions of neurons were present in most cases, and in particular, a specific feature was the degeneration of neurons in the substantia nigra and in the oculomotor nuclei. In cases surviving for more than 2 weeks, it was found that most of the cells of the substantia nigra had disappeared and that melanin pigment lay free in the tissues or was in the process of being absorbed by phagocytic cells. Cortical lesions were less constant but Buzzard and Greenfield (1919) found areas of astrocytic hyperplasia and intense perivascular infiltration in a patient who survived for 6 weeks.

In *postencephalitic parkinsonism* there is a severe diffuse loss of nerve cells from the substantia nigra. Some loss of nerve cells and gliosis in the lentiform nuclei and hypothalamus may also be found, and neurofibrillary changes resembling those of Alzheimer's disease can usually be seen in some of the pigmented cells of the brain stem. Postencephalitic parkinsonism is described in greater detail in Chapter 15.

Reye's syndrome

This disease, predominantly affecting children aged between 6 months and 16 years, usually develops when the patient is recovering from some illness, presumed to be of viral aetiology. The patient suddenly becomes profoundly ill with severe vomiting and lethargy, progressing to coma and major convulsions, and may die within a few days from raised intracranial pressure. Although jaundice is rare, half the patients have enlarged livers and all show evidence of liver disease (e.g. elevated serum transaminases and ammonia). Of the cases described by Reye, Morgan and Baral (1963), 80 per cent died; now the mortality is about 20 per cent (Sullivan-Bolyai and Corey, 1981) but about half the survivors may have some residual neurological or psychiatric disorder (Brunner et al., 1979). The main post-mortem findings are fatty degeneration of the liver and cerebral oedema.

In the predisposing illness more than 20 viruses have been associated with the syndrome but the principal infections are varicella (Sullivan-Bolyai, Marks and Johnston, 1980), influenza B (Corey, Rubin and Thompson, 1977) and influenza A (Halsey, Hurwitz and Micklejohn, 1980). Despite this epidemiological association, a virus is seldom isolated at the time of the Reye's syndrome and extremely rarely from the CNS. Toxic agents such as salicylates, aflatoxin and insecticides have also been associated with the syndrome, and current, rather tenuous, theories postulate the interaction of viral infection and toxin as the cause (Editorial, 1982).

Pathological findings. The neuropathology of the disorder is not very suggestive of a virus infection. Macroscopically, the brain is large, swollen and heavy, but does not appear particularly congested nor is there any evidence of meningeal opacity. On slicing the brain, the appearance is again one of very severe swelling with ventricular compression, and the white matter may be soft and oedematous. No focal lesions can be seen unless the swollen brain has herniated, in which case secondary phenomena will be visible. Cerebellar tonsillar herniation is frequently present, and there may be necrosis of the tips of the tonsils if this has occurred.

The microscopical features in the brain are those of non-specific swelling and oedema, generally without evidence of inflammatory cell infiltration or neuronal necrosis. If the patient has been kept alive on a respirator, secondary pathological changes may be present. The diagnosis in this syndrome is made on the basis of the clinical history, the finding of an abnormal liver at autopsy, and a swollen oedematous brain with no specific pathological features on light microscopy. However, ultrastructural studies have revealed neuronal abnormalities, swelling of astrocytes and myelin bleb formation (Partin et al., 1975). In a study of brain biopsy material from three cases during the acute stage of the illness and subsequently after recovery (Partin et al., 1978), mitochondrial abnormalities in neurons were found during the acute stage but not after recovery, suggesting that the neuronal damage was reversible.

Microscopical examination of the liver shows widespread, gross fatty change, and fat droplets have also been seen in renal tubular epithelium (Griffin, Keeling and Tomlinson, 1979).

Behçet's disease

This disease most commonly presents as recurrent ulceration of the mouth and genitalia accompanied by eye disease—uveitis or iridocyclitis—but a fifth of the patients may have a dangerous affection of the brain (Wolf, Schotland and Phillips, 1965). Because of the diversity of the lesions, the condition may simulate multiple sclerosis.

There have been a number of claims of viruses isolated from patients with Behçet's disease but two critical assessments (Dudgeon, 1961; Johnson and Herndon, 1974) have failed to substantiate them. If there is a Behçet's virus it has yet to be identified.

Pathological findings. The neuropathology is that of multifocal necrotizing lesions with a marked inflammatory cell reaction. Tissue necrosis may be seen in grey or white matter, and there appears to be no part of the cerebrum, cerebellum, brain stem or spinal cord which is immune from disease (Lindenberg and Haymaker, 1982). Vasculitis is considered to be the underlying lesion, but histological changes in the cerebral vessels are of a non-specific nature.

References

Adams, J.H. (1973) The neuropathology of viral infections of the nervous system. *British Journal of Hospital Medicine* **10,** 392–401.

Adams, J.H. and Miller, D. (1973) Herpes simplex encephalitis: a clinical and pathological analysis of twenty-two cases. *Postgraduate Medical Journal* **49,** 393–7.

Adams, J.H. and Short, I.A. (1965) Progressive multifocal leucoencephalopathy. *Scottish Medical Journal* **10,** 195–202.

Agamanolis, D.P., Tan, J.S. and Parker, D.L. (1979) Immunosuppressive measles encephalitis in a patient with a renal transplant. *Archives of Neurology* **36,** 686–90.

Agnarsdóttir, G. (1977) Subacute sclerosing panencephalitis. *Recent Advances in Clinical Virology,* vol. 1 (Ed. Watserson, A.P.), pp. 21–49. Churchill Livingstone, Edinburgh.

Alpers, M.P. (1979) Epidemiology and ecology of kuru. In *Slow Transmissible Diseases of the Nervous System,* vol. 1 (Eds. Prusiner, S.B. and Hadlow, W.J.), pp. 67–90. Academic Press, New York.

Appelbaum, E., Kreps, S.I. and Sunshine, A. (1962) Herpes zoster encephalitis. *American Journal of Medicine* **32,** 25–31.

Åström, K.E., Mancall, E.L. and Richardson, E.P. (1958) Progressive multifocal leukoencephalopathy. *Brain* **81,** 93–111.

Azimi, P.H., Cramblett, H.G. and Haynes, R.E. (1969) Mumps meningoencephalitis in children. *Journal of the American Medical Association* **207,** 509–12.

Baer, G.M. and Cleary, W.F. (1972) A model in mice for the pathogenesis and treatment of rabies. *Journal of Infectious Diseases* **125,** 520–7.

Bastian, F.O., Rabson, A.S., Yee, C.L. and Tralka, T.S. (1972) Herpes virus hominis—isolation from human trigeminal ganglion. *Science* **178,** 306–7.

Beck, E. and Daniel, P.M. (1965) Kuru and scrapie compared: are they examples of system degeneration? In *Slow, Latent and Temperate Virus Infections*, NINDB monograph no. 2 (Eds. Gajdusek, D.C., Gibbs, C.J.Jr and Alpers, M.), pp. 85–93. US Government Printing Office, Washington DC.

Beck, E. and Daniel, P.M. (1979) Kuru and Creutzfeldt–Jakob disease; neuropathological lesions and their significance. In *Slow Transmissible Disease of the Nervous System*, vol. 1 (Eds. Prusiner, S.B. and Hadlow, W.J.), pp. 253–70. Academic Press, New York.

Beck, E., Daniel, P.M., Alpers, M.P., Gadjusek, D.C. and Gibbs, C.J.Jr (1969) Neuropathological comparisons of experimental kuru in chimpanzees with human kuru. In *Pathogenesis and Etiology of Demyelinating Diseases:* addendum to *International Archives of Allergy* **36,** 553–62. Karger, Basel and New York.

Beck, E., Bak, I.J., Christ, J.F., Gajdusek, D.C., Gibbs, C.J.Jr and Hassler, R. (1975) Experimental kuru in the spider monkey. *Brain* **98,** 595–612.

Beck, E., Daniel, P.M., Davey, A.J., Gadjusek, D.C. and Gibbs, C.J.Jr (1982) The pathogenesis of transmissible spongiform encephalopathy. *Brain* **105,** 755–86.

Bennett, D.R., ZuRhein, G.M. and Roberts, T.S. (1962) Acute necrotizing encephalitis. *Archives of Neurology* **6,** 96–113.

Bernoulli, C., Siegfried, J., Baumgartner, G., Regli, F., Rabinowicz, T. Gajdusek, D.C. et al. (1977) Danger of accidental person-to-person transmission of Creutzfeldt–Jakob disease by surgery. *Lancet* **1,** 478–9.

Bodian, D. (1959) Poliomyelitis: pathogenesis and histopathology. In *Viral and Rickettsial Infections of Man*, 3rd edn (Eds. Rivers, T.M. and Horsfall, F.L.), pp. 479–98. Pitman Medical, London.

Bodian, D. and Paffenbarger, R.S. (1954) Poliomyelitis infection in households. Frequency of viremia and specific antibody response. *American Journal of Hygiene* **60,** 83–7.

van Bogaert, L. (1945) Une leuconecephalite sclérosante subaigue. *Journal of Neurology, Neurosurgery and Psychiatry* **8,** 101–20.

van Bogaert, L., Radermecker, J. and Devos, J. (1955) Sur une observation mortelle d'encéphalite aiguë nécrosante. *Revue Neurologique* **92,** 329–56.

von Bókay, J. (1909) Über den ätiologischen Zusammenhang der Varizellen mit gewissen Fällen von Herpes Zoster. *Wiener klinische Wochenschrift* **22,** 1323–6.

Bouteille, M., Fontaine, C., Vedrenne, C.L. and Delarue, J. (1965) Sur un cas d'encéphalite subaiguë à inclusions. Etude anatomoclinique et ultrastructurale. *Revue Neurologique* **113,** 454–8.

Brown, P. (1980) An epidemiologic critique of Creutzfeldt–Jakob disease. *Epidemiologic Reviews* **2,** 113–35.

Brown, P., Gibbs, C.J., Amyx, H.L., Kingsbury, D.T., Rohwer, R.G., Sulima, M.P. et al. (1982) Chemical disinfection of Creutzfeldt–Jakob disease virus. *New England Journal of Medicine* **306,** 1279–82.

Brunner, R.L., O'Grady, D.J., Partin, J.C., Partin, J.S. and Schubert, W.K. (1979) Neuropsychologic consequences of Reye syndrome. *Journal of Pediatrics* **95,** 706–11.

Budka, H. and Shah, K.V. (1982) Papova virus antigens in PML brains. *Journal of Neuropathology and Experimental Neurology* **41,** 366.

Buzzard, E.F. and Greenfield, J.G. (1919) Lethargic encephalitis: its sequelae and morbid anatomy. *Brain* **42,** 305–38.

Cabrera, C.V., Wohlenberg, C., Openshaw, H., Rey-Mendez, M., Puga, A. and Notkins, A.L. (1980) Herpes simplex virus DNA sequences in the CNS of latently infected mice. *Nature* (*London*) **288,** 288–90.

Carton, C.A. (1953) Effect of previous sensory loss on the appearance of herpes simplex. *Journal of Neurosurgery* **10,** 463–8.

Chadwick, D.W., Martin, S., Buxton, P.H. and Tomlinson, A.H. (1982) Measles virus and subacute neurological disease: an unusual presentation of measles inclusion body encephalitis. *Journal of Neurology, Neurosurgery and Psychiatry* **45,** 680–4.

Chandler, R.L. (1961) Encephalopathy in mice produced by inoculation with scrapie brain material. *Lancet* **1,** 1378–9.

Cheetham, H.D., Hart, J., Coghill, N.F. and Fox B. (1970) Rabies with myocarditis. *Lancet* **1,** 921–2.

Choppin, P.W. (1981) Measles virus and chronic neurological diseases. *Annals of Neurology* **9,** 17–20.

Chopra, J.S., Banerjee, A.K., Murthy, J.M.K. and Pal, S.R. (1980) Paralytic rabies: a clinico-pathological study. *Brain* **103,** 789–802.

Christie, A.B. (1980) *Infectious Diseases*, 3rd edn Churchill Livingstone, Edinburgh. [Smallpox, pp. 222–61. Lymphocytic meningitis, pp. 565–71. Enterovirus infections (Coxsackie virus and echovirus), pp. 519–40.]

Chumakov, M., Voroshilova, M., Shindarov, L., Lavrova, I., Gracheva, L., Koroleva, G. et al. (1979) Enterovirus 71 isolated from cases of epidemic poliomyelitis-like disease in Bulgaria. *Archives of Virology* **60,** 329–40.

Cohen, S.L., Gardner, S., Lanyi, C., McDonald, J.R., Ree, H., Southorn, P.A. et al. (1976) A case of rabies in man: some problems in diagnosis and management. *British Medical Journal* **1**, 1041–2.

Coleman, D.V., Gardner, S.D. and Field, A.M. (1973) Human polyomavirus infection in renal allograft recipients. *British Medical Journal* **3**, 371–5.

Coleman, D.V., Wolfendale, M.R., Daniel, R.A., Dhanjal, N.K., Gardner, S.D., Gibson, P.E. et al. (1980) A prospective study of human polyomavirus infection in pregnancy. *Journal of Infectious Diseases* **142**, 1–8.

Connolly, J.H., Allen, I.V., Hurwitz, L.J. and Millar, J.H.D. (1967) Measles-virus antibody and antigen in subacute sclerosing panencephalitis. *Lancet* **1**, 542–4.

Connolly, J.H., Haire, M. and Hadden, D.S.M. (1971) Measles immunoglobulins in subacute sclerosing panencephalitis. *British Medical Journal* **1**, 23–5.

Cook, M.L., Bastone, V.B. and Stevens, J.G. (1974) Evidence that neurons harbor latent herpes simplex virus. *Infection and Immunity* **9**, 946–51.

Cook, M.L. and Stevens, J.G. (1973) Pathogenesis of herpetic neuritis and ganglionitis in mice: evidence for intra-axonal transport of infection. *Infection and Immunity* **7**, 272–88.

Cook, M.L. and Stevens, J.G. (1976) Latent herpetic infections following experimental viraemia. *Journal of General Virology* **31**, 75–80.

Corey, L., Rubin, R.J. and Thompson, T.R. (1977) Influenza B associated Reye's syndrome incidence in Michigan and potential prevention. *Journal of Infectious Diseases* **135**, 398–407.

Corsellis, J.A.N. (1951) Subacute sclerosing leucoencephalitis: clinical and pathological reports of 2 cases. *Journal of Mental Science* **97**, 570–83.

Craig, C.P. and Nahmias, A.J. (1973) Different patterns of neurological involvement with herpes simplex virus types 1 and 2: isolation of herpes simplex virus type 2 from the buffy coat of two adults with meningitis. *Journal of Infectious Diseases* **127**, 365–72.

Craig, D.E. and Brown, G.C. (1959) The relationship between poliomyelitis antibody and virus excretion from the pharynx and anus of orally infected monkeys. *American Journal of Hygiene* **69**, 1–12.

Cremer, N.E., Oshiro, L.S., Weil, M.L., Lennette, E.H., Itabashi, H.H. and Carnay, L. (1975) Isolation of rubella virus from brain in chronic progressive panencephalitis. *Journal of General Virology* **29**, 143–53.

Cuillé, J. and Chelle, P.-L. (1936) La maladie dite tremblante du mouton est elle inoculable? *Compte Rendu de l'Académie des Sciences (Paris)* **203**, 1552–4.

Davis, L.E. and Johnson, R.T. (1979) An explanation for the localization of herpes simplex encephalitis? *Annals of Neurology* **5**, 2–5.

Davis, L.E., Bodian, D., Price, D., Butler, I.J. and Vickers, J.H. (1977) Chronic progressive poliomyelitis secondary to vaccination in an immunodeficient child. *New England Journal of Medicine* **297**, 241–5.

Dawson, J.R.Jr (1933) Cellular inclusions in cerebral lesions of lethargic encephalitis. *American Journal of Pathology* **9**, 7–15.

Dayan, A.D. and Stokes, M.I. (1973) Rapid diagnosis of encephalitis by immunofluorescent examination of cerebrospinal fluid cells. *Lancet* **1**, 177–9.

Dean, D.J., Evans, W.M. and McClure, R.C. (1963) Pathogenesis of rabies. *Bulletin of the World Health Organization* **29**, 803–11.

De Brito, T., Araujo, M.D. and Tiriba, A. (1973) Ultrastructure of the Negri body in human rabies. *Journal of the Neurological Sciences* **20**, 363–72.

Department of Health and Social Security (1981) *Report of the advisory group on the management of patients with spongiform encephalopathy (Creutzfeldt–Jakob Disease (CJD))*. HMSO, London.

Department of Health and Social Security, Scottish Home and Health Department, Department of Health and Social Services Northern Ireland, and Welsh Office (1978) *Code of Practice for the Prevention of Infection in Clinical Laboratories and Post-mortem Rooms*. HMSO, London.

Dickinson, A.G. (1976) Scrapie in sheep and goats. In *Slow Virus Diseases of Animals and Man* (Ed. Kimberlin, R.H.), pp. 209–41. North-Holland, Amsterdam.

Dinn, J.J. (1979) Distribution of herpes simplex virus in acute necrotising encephalitis. *Journal of Pathology* **129**, 135–8.

Dinn, J.J. (1980) Transolfactory spread of virus in herpes simplex encephalitis. *British Medical Journal* **281**, 1392.

Dowdle, W.R., Nahmias, A.J., Harwell, R.W. and Pauls, F.P. (1967) Association of antigenic type of *Herpesvirus hominis* with site of viral recovery. *Journal of Immunology* **99**, 974–80.

Doyle, P., Gibson, G.M. and Dolman, C.L. (1982) Proved herpes zoster arteritis with cerebral infarct. *Journal of Neuropathology and Experimental Neurology* **41**, 351.

Drysdale, H.C., Jones, L.F., Oppenheimer, D.R. and Tomlinson, A.H. (1976) Measles inclusion-body encephalitis in a child with treated lymphoblastic leukaemia. *Journal of Clinical Pathology* **29**, 865–72.

Dudgeon, J.A. (1961) Virological aspects of Behçet's disease. *Proceedings of Royal Society of Medicine* **54**, 104–6.

Duffy, P., Wolf, J., Collins, G., Devoe, A.G., Streeten, B. and Cowen, D. (1974) Possible person-to-person transmission of Creutzfeldt–Jakob disease. *New England Journal of Medicine* **290**, 692–3.

Dupont, J.R. and Earle, K.M. (1965) Human rabies

encephalitis: a study of forty-nine fatal cases with a review of the literature. *Neurology* **15,** 1023–34.

von Economo, C. (1917) Encephalitis lethargica. *Wiener klinische Wochenschrift* **30,** 581–5.

von Economo, C. (1931) *Encephalitis Lethargica. Its Sequelae and Treatment.* Oxford University Press, London.

Editorial (1982) Reye's syndrome—epidemiological considerations. *Lancet* **1,** 941–3.

Esiri, M.M. (1982a) Herpes simplex encephalitis: an immunohistological study of the distribution of viral antigen within the brain. *Journal of the Neurological Sciences* **54,** 209–26.

Esiri, M.M. (1982b) Viruses and Alzheimer's disease. *Journal of Neurology, Neurosurgery and Psychiatry* **45,** 759.

Esiri, M.M. and Tomlinson, A.H. (1972) Herpes zoster. Demonstration of virus in trigeminal nerve and ganglion by immunofluorescence and electron microscopy. *Journal of the Neurological Sciences* **15,** 35–48.

Esiri, M.M., Oppenheimer, D.R., Brownell, B. and Haire, M. (1981) Distribution of measles antigen and immunoglobulin-containing cells in the CNS in subacute sclerosing panencephalitis (SSPE) and atypical measles encephalitis. *Journal of the Neurological Sciences* **53,** 29–43.

Fekadu, M. (1975) Asymptomatic non-fatal canine rabies. *Lancet* **1,** 569.

Flewett, T.H. (1973) The rapid diagnosis of herpes encephalitis. *Postgraduate Medical Journal* **49,** 398–400.

Fowler, M. and Robertson, E.G. (1959) Observations on kuru III. Pathological features in five cases. *Australasian Annals of Medicine* **8,** 16–26.

Fox, J.P. (1980) Eradication of poliomyelitis in the United States: a commentary in the Salk reviews. *Reviews of Infectious Diseases* **2,** 277–87.

Fraser, N.W., Lawrence, W.C., Wroblewska, Z., Gilden, D.H. and Koprowski, H. (1981) Herpes simplex type I DNA in human brain tissue. *Proceedings of the National Academy of Sciences of the USA* **78,** 6461–5.

Gajdusek, D.C., Gibbs, C.J.Jr and Alpers, M. (1966) Experimental transmission of kuru-like syndrome to chimpanzees. *Nature (London)* **209,** 794–6.

Gajdusek, D.C. and Zigas, V. (1957) Degeneration disease of the central nervous system in New Guinea: the endemic occurrence of kuru in the native population. *New England Journal of Medicine* **257,** 974–8.

Gardner, S.D. (1973) Prevalence in England of antibody to human polyomavirus (BK). *British Medical Journal* **1,** 77–8.

Gardner, S.D., Field, A.M., Coleman, D.V. and Hulme, B. (1971) New human papovirus (BK) isolated from urine after renal transplantation. *Lancet* **1,** 1253–7.

Gibbs, C.J.Jr, Gajdusek, D.C., Asher, D.M., Alpers, M.P., Beck, E., Daniel, P.M. et al. (1968) Creutzfeldt–Jakob disease (spongiform encephalopathy): transmission to the chimpanzee. *Science* **161,** 388–9.

Gibbs, C.J.Jr, Gajdusek, D.C. and Amyx, H. (1979) Strain variation in the viruses of Creutzfeldt–Jakob disease and kuru. In *Slow Transmissible Diseases of the Nervous System*, vol. 2 (Eds. Prusiner, S.B. and Hadlow, W.J.), pp. 87–110. Academic Press, New York.

Goodpasture, E.W. and Teague, O. (1923) The transmission of the virus of herpes febrilis along sensory nerves with resulting unilateral lesions in the central nervous system in the rabbit. *Proceedings of the Society for Experimental Biology and Medicine* **20,** 545–7.

Greenberg, J. (1970) Herpes zoster with motor involvement. *Journal of the American Medical Association* **212,** 322.

Greenfield, J.G. (1950) Encephalitis and encephalomyelitis in England and Wales during the last decade. *Brain* **73,** 141–66.

Griffin, N., Keeling, J.W. and Tomlinson, A.H. (1979) Reye's syndrome associated with respiratory syncytial virus infection. *Archives of Disease in Childhood* **54,** 74–6.

Grose, C., Henle, W., Henle, G. and Feorino, P.M. (1975) Primary Epstein–Barr virus infections in acute neurologic diseases. *New England Journal of Medicine* **292,** 392–5.

Hadlow, W.J. (1959) Scrapie and kuru. *Lancet* **2,** 289–90.

Hall, W.W. and Choppin, P.W. (1979) Evidence for lack of synthesis of the M polypeptide of measles virus in brain cells in subacute sclerosing panencephalitis. *Virology* **99,** 443–7.

Hall, W.W., Lamb, R.A. and Choppin, P.W. (1979) Measles and SSPE virus proteins: lack of antibodies to the M protein in patients with subacute sclerosing panencephalitis. *Proceedings of the National Academy of Sciences of the USA* **76,** 2047–51.

Halsey, N.A., Hurwitz, E.S. and Micklejohn, G. (1980) An epidemic of Reye's syndrome associated with influenza A in Colorado. *Journal of Pediatrics* **97,** 535–9.

Hammon, W.McD., Coriell, L.L., Wehrle, P.F. and Stokes, J.Jr (1953) Evaluation of Red Cross gamma globulin as a prophylactic agent for poliomyelitis 4. Final report of results based on clinical diagnoses. *Journal of the American Medical Association* **151,** 1272–85.

Hart, M.N. and Earle, K.M. (1975) Haemorrhagic and perivenous encephalitis: a clinical-pathological review of 38 cases. *Journal of Neurology, Neurosurgery and Psychiatry* **38,** 585–91.

Haymaker, W. (1961) Mosquito-borne encephalitides. In *Encephalitides* (Eds. van Bogaert, L., Radermecker, J., Hozay, J. and Lowenthal, A.), pp. 38–56. Elsevier, Amsterdam.

Head, H. and Campbell, A.W. (1900) Pathology of herpes zoster and its bearing on sensory localization. *Brain* **23,** 353–523.

Hill, T.J., Field, H.J. and Roome, A.P.C. (1972) Intra-axonal location of herpes simplex virus particles. *Journal of General Virology* **15,** 253–5.

Hogan, E.L. and Krigman, M.R. (1973) Herpes zoster myelitis: evidence for viral invasion of spinal cord. *Archives of Neurology* **29,** 309–13.

Hope-Simpson, R.E. (1965) The nature of herpes zoster: a long-term study and a new hypothesis. *Proceedings of the Royal Society of Medicine* **58,** 9–20.

Hornabrook, R.W. (1979) Kuru and clinical neurology. In *Slow Transmissible Disease of the Nervous System*, vol. 1 (Eds. Prusiner, S.B. and Hadlow, W.J.), pp. 37–66. Academic Press, New York.

Horstmann, D.M. (1982) Control of poliomyelitis: a continuing paradox. *Journal of Infectious Diseases* **146,** 540–51.

Horstmann, D.M., McCollum, R.W. and Mascola, A.D. (1954) Viremia in human poliomyelitis. *Journal of Experimental Medicine* **99,** 355–70.

Horta-Barbosa, L., Fuccillo, D.A., Sever, J.L. and Zeman, W. (1969) Subacute sclerosing panencephalitis: isolation of measles virus from a brain biopsy. *Nature (London)* **221,** 974.

Hughes, J.T. (1969) Pathology of herpes simplex encephalitis. In *Virus Diseases and the Nervous System* (Eds. Whitty, C.W.M., Hughes, J.T. and MacCallum, F.O.), pp. 39–37. Blackwell Scientific, Oxford and Edinburgh.

Hull, R.N. (1973) The simian herpesviruses. In *The Herpesviruses* (Ed. Kaplan, A.S.), pp. 390–426. Academic Press, New York.

Illis, L.S. and Gostling, J.V.T. (1972) *Herpes Simplex Encephalitis*. Scientechnica, Bristol.

Jabbour, J.T., Duenas, D.A., Sever, J.L., Krebs, H.M. and Horta-Barbosa, L. (1972) Epidemiology of subacute sclerosing panencephalitis. *Journal of the American Medical Association* **220,** 959–62.

Jakob, A. (1921) Über eigenartige Erkrankungen des Zentralnervensystems mit bemerkenswerten anatomischen Befunde (Spastische Pseudosklerose-Encephalomyelopathie mit disseminierten Degenerationsherden). *Zeitschrift für die gesamte Neurologie und Psychiatrie* **64,** 147–228.

Johnson, H.N. (1979) Rabies virus. In *Diagnostic Procedures for Viral Rickettsial and Chlamydial Infections*, 5th edn. (Eds. Lennette, E.H. and Schmidt, N.J.), pp. 843–77. American Public Health Association, Washington DC.

Johnson, R.T. (1964) The pathogenesis of herpes virus encephalitis. I. Virus pathways to the nervous system of suckling mice demonstrated by fluorescent antibody staining. *Journal of Experimental Medicine* **119,** 343–56.

Johnson, R.T. (1980) Selective vulnerability of neural cells to viral infection. *Brain* **103,** 447–72.

Johnson, R.T. (1982) *Viral Infections in the Nervous System*. Raven Press, New York.

Johnson, R.T. and Herndon, R.M. (1974) Virologic studies of multiple sclerosis and other chronic and relapsing neurological diseases. *Progress in Medical Virology* **18,** 214–28.

Johnson, R.T. and Mims, C.A. (1968) Pathogenesis of viral infections of the nervous system. *New England Journal of Medicine* **278,** 23–30, 84–92.

Johnson, R.T., Olson, L.C. and Buescher, E.L. (1968) Herpes simplex virus infections of the nervous system. Problems in laboratory diagnosis. *Archives of Neurology* **18,** 260–4.

Juel-Jensen, B.E. and MacCallum, F.O. (1972) *Herpes simplex, Varicella and Zoster*. Heinemann Medical, London.

Kastrukoff, L., Long C., Doherty, P.C., Wroblewska, Z. and Koprowski, H. (1981) Isolation of virus from brain after immunosuppression of mice with latent herpes simplex. *Nature (London)* **291,** 432–3.

Kiessling, W.R., Hall, W.W., Yung, L.L. and ter Meulen, V. (1977) Measles-virus-specific immunoglobulin-M response in subacute sclerosing panencephalitis. *Lancet* **1,** 324–7.

Kimberlin, R.H., Walker, C.A., Millson, G.C., Taylor, D.M., Robertson, P.A., Tomlinson, A.H. et al. (1983) Disinfection studies with two strains of mouse-passaged scrapie agent—guidelines for Creutzfeldt-Jakob and related agents. *Journal of the Neurological Sciences* **59,** 355–69.

Klapper, P.E., Laing, I. and Longson, M. (1981) Rapid non-invasive diagnosis of herpes encephalitis. *Lancet* **2,** 607–9.

Klatzo, I., Gajdusek, D.C. and Zigas, V. (1959) Pathology of kuru. *Laboratory Investigation* **8,** 799–847.

Koschel, K. and Muenzel, P. (1980) Persistent paramyxovirus infections and behaviour of β-adrenergic receptors in C-6 rat glioma cells. *Journal of General Virology* **47,** 513–17.

Kristensson, K., Vahlne, A., Persson, L.A. and Lycke, E. (1978) Neural spread of herpes simplex virus types 1 & 2 in mice after corneal or subcutaneous (foot-pad) inoculation. *Journal of the Neurological Sciences* **35,** 331–40.

Lampert, P.W., Earl, K.M., Gibbs, C.J.Jr and Gajdusek, D.C (1969) Experimental kuru encephalopathy in chimpanzees and spider monkeys.

Journal of Neuropathology and Experimental Neurology **28,** 353–70.

Landrigan, P.J. and Witte, J.J. (1973) Neurologic disorders following live measles virus vaccination. *Journal of the American Medical Association* **223,** 1459–62.

Landsteiner, K. and Popper, E. (1909) Uebertragung der Poliomyelitis acuta auf Affen. *Zeitschrift für Immunitätsforschung* **2,** 377–90.

Latarjet, R. (1979) Inactivation of the agents of scrapie, Creutzfeldt–Jakob disease and kuru by radiations. In *Slow Transmissible Diseases of the Nervous System*, vol. 2 (Eds. Prusiner, S.B. and Hadlow, W.J.), pp. 387–407. Academic Press, New York.

Lebon, P. and Lyon, G. (1974) Non-congenital rubella encephalitis. *Lancet* **2,** 468.

Leech, R.W. and Harris, J.C. (1977) The neuropathology of Western equine and St Louis encephalitis: a review of the 1975 North Dakota epidemic. *Journal of Neuropathology and Experimental Neurology* **36,** 611.

Legrain, M., Graveleau, J., Brion, S., Mikol, J. and Küss, R. (1974) Leuco-éncephalopathie multifocale après transplantation rénale. *Journal of the Neurological Sciences* **23,** 49–62.

Leonard, J.C. and Tobin, J.O'H. (1971) Polyneuritis associated with cytomegalovirus infections. *Quarterly Journal of Medicine* **40,** 435–42.

Lindenberg, R. and Haymaker, W. (1982) Tissue reactions in the gray matter of the central nervous system. In *Histology and Histopathology of the Nervous System* (Eds. Haymaker, W. and Adams, R.D.), pp. 1037–1228. Thomas, Springfield, Illinois.

Linneman, C.C.Jr and Alvira, M.M. (1980) Pathogenesis of varicella-zoster angiitis in the CNS. *Archives of Neurology* **37,** 239–40.

Longson, M. (1979) Herpes encephalitis. In *Virus Diseases.* (Ed. Heath, R.B.), pp. 73–86. Pitman Medical, Tunbridge Wells.

Longson, M. and Bailey, A.S. (1977) Herpes encephalitis. In *Recent Advances in Clinical Virology, 1* (Ed. Waterson, A.P.), pp. 1–19. Churchill Livingstone, Edinburgh.

Luria, S.E., Darnell, J.E., Baltimore, D. and Campbell, A. (1978) *General Virology*, 3rd edn. Wiley, New York.

Lyon, G. (1972) Action des immuno-suppresseurs sur une encéphalitis virale (roueole): inhibition de la réaction inflammatoire. *Compte Rendu de l'Academie des Sciences* (*Paris*) (D) **274,** 1878–9.

MacCallum, F.O., Chinn, I.J. and Gostling, J.V.T. (1974) Antibodies to herpes simplex virus in the cerebrospinal fluid of patients with herpetic encephalitis. *Journal of Medical Microbiology* **7,** 325–31.

MacCallum, F.O., Potter, J.M. and Edwards, D.H. (1964) Early diagnosis of herpes simplex encephalitis by brain biopsy. *Lancet* **2,** 332–4.

McCormick, W.F., Rodnitzky, R.L., Schochet, S.S. and McKee, A.P. (1969) Varicella-zoster encephalomyelitis. *Archives of Neurology* **21,** 559–70.

McLennan, J.L. and Derby, G. (1980) Herpes simplex virus latency: the cellular localization of virus in dorsal root ganglia and the fate of the infected cell following virus activation. *Journal of General Virology* **51,** 233–43.

Madeley, C.R. (1972) *Virus Morphology.* Churchill Livingstone, Edinburgh and London.

Malamud, N., Haymaker, W. and Pinkerton, H. (1950) Inclusion encephalitis with a clinicopathologic report of three cases. *American Journal of Pathology* **26,** 133–53.

Marinesco, G. and Dragonesco, S. (1923) Recherches expérimentales sur le neurotropisme du virus herpetique. *Annales Institut Pasteur* **37,** 753–83.

Masters, C.L., Harris, J.O., Gajdusek, D.C., Gibbs, C.J.Jr, Bernoulli, C. and Asher, D.M. (1979) Creutzfeldt–Jakob disease: patterns of worldwide occurrence and the significance of familial and sporadic clustering. *Annals of Neurology* **5,** 177–88.

Maton, P.N., Pollard, J.D. and Newsom Davis, J. (1976) Human rabies encephalomyelitis. *British Medical Journal* **1,** 1038–40.

Melnick, J.L., Wenner, H.A. and Phillips, C.A. (1979) Enteroviruses. In *Diagnostic Procedures for Viral Rickettsial and Chlamydial Infections*, 5th edn. (Eds. Lennette, E.H. and Schmidt, N.J.), pp. 471–534. American Public Health Association, Washington DC.

ter Meulen, V., Müller, D., Käckell, Y.M., Katz, M. and Meyermann, R. (1972) Isolation of infectious measles virus in measles encephalitis. *Lancet* **2,** 1172–5.

Miller, A.E. (1980) Selective decline in cellular immune response to varicella zoster in the elderly. *Neurology* **30,** 582–7.

Miller, D.L. (1964) Frequency of complications of measles, 1963. *British Medical Journal* **2,** 75–8.

Miller, H.G., Stanton, J.B. and Gibbons, J.L. (1956) Parainfectious encephalomyelitis and related syndromes. *Quarterly Journal of Medicine* **25,** 427–505.

Miller, J.D. and Ross, C.A.C. (1968) Encephalitis: a four-year survey. *Lancet* **1,** 1121–6.

Mims, C.A. (1977) *The Pathogenesis of Infectious Disease.* Academic Press, London and New York.

Modlin, J.F., Jabbour, J.T., Witte, J.J. and Halsey, N.A. (1977) Epidemiologic studies of measles, measles vaccine and subacute sclerosing panencephalitis. *Pediatrics* **59,** 505–12.

Moore, M., Katona, P., Kaplan, J.E., Schonberger, L.B. and Hatch, M.H. (1982) Poliomyelitis in the

United States, 1969–1981. *Journal of Infectious Diseases* **146,** 558–63.

Murphy, F.A., Bauer, S.P., Harrison, A.K. and Winn, W.C. (1973a) Comparative pathogenesis of rabies and rabies-like viruses. Viral infection and transit from inoculation site to central nervous system. *Laboratory Investigation* **28,** 361–76.

Murphy, F.A., Harrison, A.K., Winn, W.C. and Bauer, S.P. (1973b) Comparative pathogenesis of rabies and rabies-like viruses. Infection of the central nervous system and centrifugal spread of virus to peripheral tissues. *Laboratory Investigation* **29,** 1–16.

Nahmias, A.J., Whitley, R.J., Visintine, A.N., Takei, Y., Alford, C.A.Jr and the Collaborative Antiviral Study Group. (1982) Herpes simplex virus encephalitis: laboratory evaluations and their diagnostic significance. *Journal of Infectious Diseases* **145,** 829–36.

Narayan, O., Penney, J.B., Johnson, R.T., Herndon, R.M. and Weiner, L.P. (1973) Etiology of progressive multifocal leukoencephalopathy. Identification of papova virus. *New England Journal of Medicine* **289,** 1278–82.

Nathanson, N. and Martin, J.R. (1979) The epidemiology of poliomyelitis: enigmas surrounding its appearance, epidemicity and disappearance. *American Journal of Epidemiology* **110,** 672–92.

Negri, A. (1903) Beitrag zum Studium der Aetiologie der Tollwuth. *Zeitschrift für Hygiene und Infektionskrankheiten* **43,** 507–28.

Netter, A. and Urbain, A. (1926) Les relations du zona et de la varicelle. Etude sérologique de 100 cas de zona. *Comptes Rendus de la Société de Biologie* **94,** 98–102.

Nicholson, K. (1983) Human rabies. In *Rabies a Growing Threat.* (Ed. Pattison, J.R.), pp. 6–17. Van Nostrand Reinhold, Wokingham.

Ohya, T., Martinez, A.J., Jabbour, J.T., Lemmi, H. and Duenas, D.A. (1974) Subacute sclerosing panencephalitis. *Neurology* **24,** 211–18.

Oldstone, M.B.A., Holmstoen, J. and Welsh, R.M.Jr (1977) Alterations of acetylcholine enzymes in neuroblastoma cells persistently infected with lymphocytic choriomeningitis virus. *Journal of Cellular Physiology* **91,** 459–72.

Olson, L.C., Buescher, E.L., Artenstein, M.S. and Parkman, P.D. (1967) Herpes virus infections of the human central nervous system. *New England Journal of Medicine* **277,** 1271–7.

Padgett, B.L. and Walker, D.L. (1973) Prevalence of antibodies in human sera against JC virus: an isolate from a case of multifocal leukoencephalopathy. *Journal of Infectious Diseases* **127,** 467–70.

Padgett, B.L., Walker, D.L., ZuRhein, G.M., Eckroade, R.J. and Dessel, B.H. (1971) Cultivation of papova-like virus from human brain with progressive multifocal leucoencephalopathy. *Lancet* **1,** 1257–60.

Parsons, A.C. (1922) *Encephalitis Lethargica.* Reports on Public Health and Medical Subjects, no. 11. Ministry of Health, London.

Partin, J.C., Partin, J.S., Schubert, W.K. and McLaurin, R.L. (1975) Brain ultrastructure in Reye's syndrome (encephalopathy and fatty degeneration of the viscera). *Journal of Neuropathology and Experimental Neurology* **34,** 425–44.

Partin, J.S., McAdams, A.J., Partin, J.C., Schubert, W.K. and McLaurin, R.L. (1978) Brain ultrastructure in Reye's disease. II. Acute injury and recovery processes in three children. *Journal of Neuropathology and Experimental Neurology* **37,** 796–819.

Paterson, P.Y. (1960) Transfer of allergic encephalomyelitis in rats by means of lymph node cells. *Journal of Experimental Medicine* **111,** 119–36.

Paul, J.R. (1971) *A History of Poliomyelitis.* Yale University Press, New Haven, Conn.

Payne, F.E., Baublis, J.V. and Habashi, H.H. (1969) Isolation of measles virus from cell cultures of brain from a patient with subacute sclerosing panencephalitis. *New England Journal of Medicine* **281,** 585–9.

Penney, J.B. and Narayan, O. (1973) Studies of the antigenic relationships of the new human papova viruses by electron microscopy agglutination. *Infection and Immunity* **8,** 299–300.

Phillips, C.A., Fanning, W.L., Gump, D.W. and Phillips, C.F. (1977) Cytomegalovirus encephalitis in immunologically normal adults. Successful treatment with vidarabine. *Journal of the American Medical Association* **238,** 2299–300.

Prusiner, S.B. (1982) Novel proteinaceous infectious particles cause scrapie. *Science* **216,** 136–44.

Purdham, D.R. and Batty, P.F. (1974) A case of acute measles meningoencephalitis with virus isolation. *Journal of Clinical Pathology* **27,** 994–6.

Reye, R.D.K., Morgan, G. and Baral, J. (1963) Encephalopathy and fatty degeneration of viscera: a disease entity in childhood. *Lancet* **2,** 749–52.

Reyes, M.G., Gardner, J.J., Poland, J.D. and Monath, T.P. (1981) St Louis encephalitis: quantitative, histologic and immunofluorescent studies. *Archives of Neurology* **38,** 329–34.

Richardson, E.P. Jr (1961) Progressive multifocal leukoencephalopathy. *New England Journal of Medicine* **265,** 815–23.

Rivers, T.M. and Schwentker, F.F. (1935) Encephalomyelitis accompanied by myelin destruction experimentally produced in monkeys. *Journal of Experimental Medicine* **61,** 689–702.

Ross, E. and Armentrout, S.A. (1962) Myocarditis associated with rabies. *New England Journal of Medicine* **266,** 1087–9.

Russell, R.R. and Donald, J.C. (1958) The nervous complications of mumps. *British Medical Journal* **2,** 27–30.

Sabin, A. (1981) Paralytic poliomyelitis: old dogmas and new perspectives. *Reviews of Infectious Diseases* **3,** 543–64.

Sabin, A.B. and Wright, A.M. (1934) Acute ascending myelitis following a monkey bite, with isolation of virus capable of reproducing the disease. *Journal of Experimental Medicine* **59,** 115–35.

Schmitz, H. and Enders, G. (1977) Cytomegalovirus as a frequent cause of Guillain–Barré syndrome. *Journal of Medical Virology* **1,** 21–7.

Schneider, L.G. (1982) Antigenic variants of rabies virus. *Comparative Immunology, Microbiology and Infectious Diseases* **5,** 101–7.

Schneweis, K.E. (1962) Serologische Untersuchungen zur Typendifferenzierung des Herpesvirus hominis. *Zeitschrift für Immunitätsforschungund experimentelle Therapy* **124,** 24–48.

Scott, T.F.McN. (1967) Postinfectious and vaccinial encephalitis. *Medical Clinics of North America* **51,** 701–7.

Sequiera, L.W., Jennings, L.C., Carrasco, L.H., Lord, M.A., Curry, A. and Sutton, R.N.P. (1979) Detection of herpes simplex viral genome in brain tissue. *Lancet* **2,** 609–12.

Shope, R.E. (1982) Rabies related viruses. *Yale Journal of Biology and Medicine* **55,** 271–5.

Shope, R.E. and Sather, G.E. (1979) Arboviruses. In *Diagnostic Procedures for Viral, Rickettsial and Chlamydial Infections* (Eds. Lennette, E.H. and Schmidt, N.J.), pp. 767–814. American Public Health Association, Washington DC.

Silverstein, A., Steinberg, G. and Nathanson, M. (1972) Nervous system involvement in infectious mononucleosis. *Archives of Neurology* **26,** 353–8.

Sköldenberg, B., Jeansson, S. and Wolontis, S. (1973) Herpes simplex virus type 2 in acute aseptic meningitis. *Lancet* **1,** 611.

Smith, M.G., Lennette, E.H. and Reames, H.R. (1941) Isolation of the virus of herpes simplex and the demonstration of intranuclear inclusions in a case of acute encephalitis. *American Journal of Pathology* **17,** 55–68.

Spillane, J.D. and Wells, C.E.C. (1964) The neurology of Jennerian vaccination. A clinical account of the neurological complications which occurred during the smallpox epidemic in South Wales in 1962. *Brain* **87,** 1–44.

Sullivan-Bolyai, J.Z. and Corey, L. (1981) Epidemiology of Reye's syndrome. *Epidemiologic Reviews* **3,** 1–26.

Sullivan-Bolyai, J.Z., Marks, J.S. and Johnston, D. (1980) Reye's syndrome in Ohio, 1973–77. *American Journal of Epidemiology* **112,** 627–38.

Sung, J.H., Hayano, M., Mastri, A.R. and Okagaki, T. (1976) A case of human rabies and ultrastructure of the Negri body. *Journal of Neuropathology and Experimental Neurology* **35,** 541–59.

Takashima, S. and Becker, L.E. (1979) Neuropathology of fatal varicella. *Archives of Pathology and Laboratory Medicine* **103,** 209–13.

Tangchai, P. and Vejjajiva, A. (1971) Pathology of the peripheral nervous system in human rabies. *Brain* **94,** 299–306.

Tomlinson, A.H., Chinn, I.J. and MacCallum, F.O. (1974) Immunofluorescence staining for the diagnosis of herpes encephalitis. *Journal of Clinical Pathology* **27,** 495–9.

Tomlinson, A.H. and Esiri, M.M. (1983) Herpes simplex encephalitis: immunohistological demonstration of spread of virus via olfactory pathways in mice. *Journal of the Neurological Sciences* **60,** 473–84.

Tomlinson, A.H. and MacCallum, F.O. (1970) The incidence of complement-fixing antibody to varicella-zoster virus in hospital patients and blood donors. *Journal of Hygiene* **68,** 411–16.

Townsend, J.J., Baringer, J.R., Wolinsky, J.S., Malamud, N., Mednick, J.P., Panitch, H.S. et al. (1975) Progressive rubella panencephalitis: late onset after congenital rubella. *New England Journal of Medicine* **292,** 990–3.

Townsend, J.J., Stroop, W.G., Baringer, J.R., Wolinsky, J.S., McKerrow, J.H. and Berg, B.O. (1982) Neuropathology of progressive rubella panencephalitis after childhood rubella. *Neurology* **32,** 185–90.

Tsiang, H., Ermine, A. and Marcovistz, R. (1982) Aspects moléculaires et cellulaires de la pathogenie dans la rage. *Comparative Immunology, Microbiology and Infectious Diseases* **5,** 61–5.

de Vries, E. (1960) *Postvaccinial Perivenous Encephalitis.* Elsevier, Amsterdam.

Walker, D.L. (1978) Progressive multifocal leukoencephalopathy: an opportunistic viral infection of the central nervous system. In *Handbook of Clinical Neurology* (Eds. Vinken, P.J. and Bruyn, G.W.), pp. 307–41. Elsevier/North-Holland, Amsterdam.

Watson, K., Stevens, J.G., Cook, M.L. and Subak-Sharpe, J.H. (1980) Latency competence of thirteen HSV-I temperature sensitive mutants. *Journal of General Virology* **49,** 149–59.

Weil, M.L., Itabashi, H.H., Cremer, N.E., Oshiro, L.S., Lennette, E.H. and Carnay, L. (1975) Chronic progressive panencephalitis due to rubella virus simulating subacute sclerosing panencephalitis. *New England Journal of Medicine* **292,** 994–8.

Weiner, L.P., Herndon, R.M., Narayan, O., Johnson, R.T., Shah, K., Rubinstein, L.J. et al. (1972) Isolation of virus related to SV40 from patients with progressive multifocal leukoencephalopathy. *New England Journal of Medicine* **286,** 385–90.

Weller, T.H. and Stoddard, M.B. (1952) Intranuclear inclusion bodies in cultures of human tissue inoculated with varicella vesicle fluid. *Journal of Immunology* **68,** 311–19.

Wickman, I. (1907) quoted by Paul, J. (1971) in *A History of Poliomyelitis*, p. 89. Yale University Press, New Haven and London.

Wildy, P. (1967) The progression of herpes simplex virus to the central nervous system of the mouse. *Journal of Hygiene* **65,** 173–92.

Wilfert, C.M., Buckley, R.H., Mokanakumar, T., Griffith, J.F., Katz, S.L., Whisnaut, J.K. et al. (1977) Persistent and fatal central nervous system echovirus infections in patients with agammaglobulinemia. *New England Journal of Medicine* **296,** 1485–9.

Will, R.G. and Matthews, W.B. (1982) Evidence for case-to-case transmission of Creutzfeldt-Jakob disease. *Journal of Neurology, Neurosurgery and Psychiatry* **45,** 235–8.

Willoughby, E., Price, R.W., Padgett, B.L., Walker, D.L. and Dupont, B. (1980) Progressive multifocal leukoencephalopathy (PML): in vitro cell-mediated immune responses to mitogens and JC virus. *Neurology* **30,** 256–62.

Wolf, S.M., Schotland, D.L. and Phillips, L.L. (1965) Involvement of nervous system in Behçet's syndrome. *Archives of Neurology* **12,** 315–25.

ZuRhein, G.M. and Chou, S.M. (1965) Particles resembling papovaviruses in human cerebral demyelinating disease. *Science* 148, 1477–9.

ZuRhein, G.,M. and Varakis, J. (1974) Progressive multifocal leukoencephalopathy in a renal allograft recipient. *New England Journal of Medicine* **291,** 798.

8

Parasitic and fungal infections of the nervous system

F. Scaravilli

Protozoal infections

Amoebiasis

It is customary to give separate descriptions of the cerebral lesions produced by *Entamoeba histolytica* and of the primary meningoencephalitis caused by free-living amoebae.

Amoebic abscess of the brain

This infection is caused by *Entamoeba histolytica*. The parasite infests man and other primates (Levine, 1961) and is found throughout the world with the highest incidence in Latin America. Amoebiasis is commonest in tropical and subtropical climates and among urban populations where poverty predominates. In man the infection begins in the mucosa of the colon and may remain localized there for years.

The organism exists in two forms: *trophozoites* and *cysts*. Trophozoites are spherical or oval organisms, 15–25 μm in diameter, with vacuolated cytoplasm and a single nucleus (Fig. 8.1); pseudopodia are occasionally seen. In routinely stained sections the nuclei are round and have a small central karyosome and peripheral chromatin; the cytoplasm contains abundant glycogen. Cysts are spherical, 2–25 μm in diameter and contain four to eight nuclei.

Cerebral involvement is a rare and late complication, and is secondary to haematogenous dissemination from a primary intestinal, pulmonary or hepatic focus. Very occasionally, amoebic abscesses of the brain may be found apparently without extraneural infection (Connor, Neafie and Meyers, 1976). Meningoencephalitis occurs in 0.9–8.1 per cent of fatal cases, the latter rate being found in Mexico (Lombardo et al., 1964). Odunjo (1969) found a frequency of 4 per cent in 135 autopsy cases in Nigeria. In the brain the site of predilection is in the richly vascularized cortical grey matter and basal ganglia. The early lesion is a soft red focus surrounded by petechiae. This single abscess usually cavitates. Occasionally multiple abscesses have been found (Odunjo, 1969). The contents of the cavity are yellow-green, the walls surrounding it are irregular and there is no evidence of encapsulation. Superficial lesions may involve the meninges.

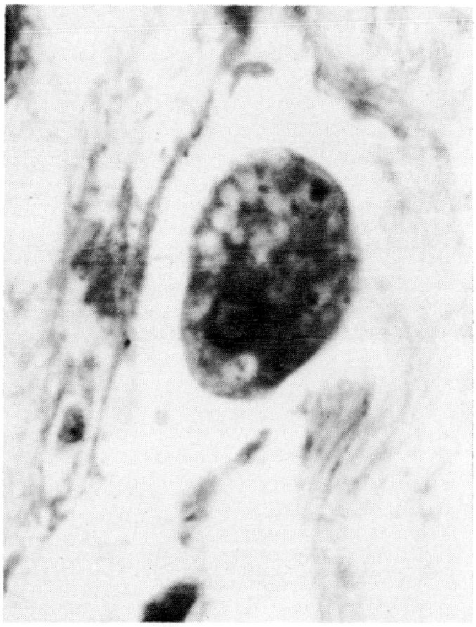

Fig. 8.1 Trophozoite of *Entamoeba histolytica*. The oval cell body contains an easily recognized nucleus and numerous vacuoles. Haematoxylin and eosin × 1725.

Microscopically, the abscess wall has an inner zone of necrotic tissue and a broad outer zone of congestion and vascular proliferation. The surrounding brain undergoes degenerative changes and is infiltrated by lymphocytes, plasma cells and scanty polymorphs around blood vessels. There is also a reactive astrocytosis. Trophozoites can be identified in the necrotic wall of the abscess: they are large with relatively small, eccentric nuclei and can be confused with phagocytes although the latter are smaller.

The prognosis for a patient with an amoebic brain abscess is extremely poor and only seven cases with survival had been recorded in the literature by 1980 (Becker et al., 1980). Although emetine and chloroquine reach therapeutic levels in the liver, there is no evidence that they do so in the brain (Parmer and Cottrill, 1949).

Primary amoebic encephalitis

Following the first report by Fowler and Carter (1965), it became apparent that amoebae, other than *E. histolytica*, were capable of invading the central nervous system in man, producing encephalitis. The term 'primary encephalitis' was introduced by Butt (1966) and Carter (1968) and now includes primary amoebic meningoencephalitis due to *Naegleria fowleri* and granulomatous amoebic encephalitis due to the *Hartmannella-Acanthamoeba* group.

Primary amoebic meningoencephalitis

Naegleria fowleri is a free-living, highly motile organism which can exist also in a flagellate form. According to Culbertson (1976) *Naegleria* has been found in almost every continent and cases have been described in the USA, England, Ireland, Belgium, Czechoslovakia, Zambia, Brazil, Australia and New Zealand.

Previously healthy children and young adults are those mainly affected, in summer and autumn, as isolated cases or in small outbreaks. The infection is acquired by swimming in warm lakes or pools contaminated with the amoebae. The post-mortem finding of severe involvement of the olfactory area and experimental work (Mar-

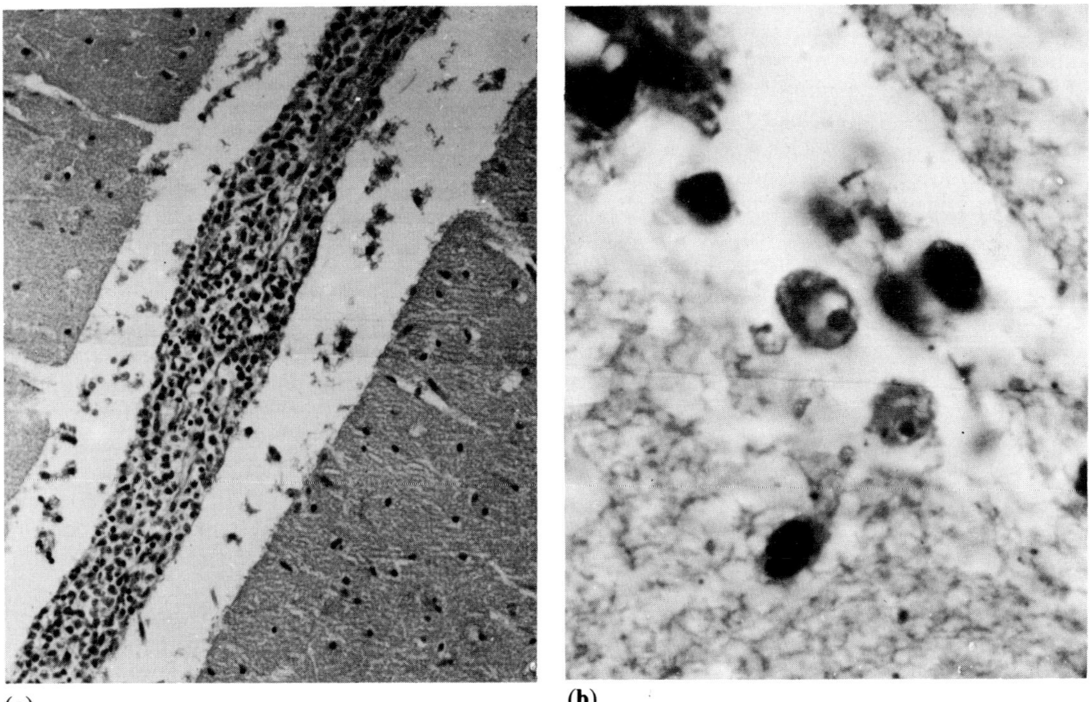

(a) **(b)**

Fig. 8.2 Primary amoebic meningoencephalitis. (**a**) Thin layer of leptomeningeal exudate in the cerebellum. × 175. (**b**) Trophozoite of *Naegleria fowleri* with pale vesicular nucleus and prominent nucleolus. Haematoxylin and eosin × 1300. (Courtesy of Dr M. Nielsen.)

tinez et al., 1973) support the hypothesis that the protozoa enter the CNS through the nasal mucosa and the cribriform plate. Headache, neck stiffness and fever are the usual symptoms, and disturbances of taste and olfaction may be the only localizing signs. The clinical course usually is fatal within 2–7 days. Up to 1981 over 80 rapidly fatal cases from all parts of the world were reported by Cain et al. (1981). Recently, however, a few successfully treated cases have been reported (see Rothrock and Buchsbaum, 1980; Seidel et al., 1982) and amphotericin B may have influenced the long survival of the second patient described by Apley et al. (1970).

Lesions may be found anywhere in the central nervous system, including the posterior fossa and the upper spinal cord. The affected areas are swollen and slightly soft, and take the form of an acute necrotizing and haemorrhagic meningoencephalitis. The layer of purulent leptomeningeal exudate is relatively thin (Fig. 8.2a) and consists of mononuclear cells and lymphocytes; there is massive destruction of brain and blood vessels, some of which are thrombosed. Occasionally the ventricular system and the choroid plexuses are involved. Amoebae are present in the subarachnoid exudate (Fig. 8.2b) but it may be difficult to differentiate them from macrophages.

The parasites are slightly smaller than *Entamoeba histolytica* and measure about 10–20 μm in diameter. Their nuclei have a distinct membrane, are pale and contain a prominent nucleolus. The presence of vacuoles may obscure the nuclear margins. These features are typical of the resting cell; when in motion *Naegleria* becomes elongated and has a single lobose pseudopodium. When amoebae are exposed to distilled water, they change to biflagellate forms. Cysts, 9–10 μm in diameter, have been observed in cultures on agar; they are never present in tissue sections, presumably because of the rapid course of the illness.

Granulomatous amoebic encephalitis

Unlike *Naegleria*, amoebae of the *Hartmannella-Acanthamoeba* group usually produce multifocal chronic illnesses in debilitated patients or in immunodeficient individuals. In this group of diseases, ages range from 5 to 58 years, both sexes are equally affected and a history of swimming has never been reported. In a series of 15 patients reviewed by Martinez (1980) 13 were suffering from an associated disorder such as liver disease, diabetes mellitus or Hodgkin's disease, and all of them had been or were receiving treatment which included antibiotics, radiotherapy or steroids. Two patients were pregnant and three were alcoholics. A few cases with no known pre-existing illness have, however, also been recorded (see Martinez, 1982). The clinical course is longer than in encephalitis due to *Naegleria* and varies from 12 to 120 days. Grunnet, Cannon and Kushner (1981) have, however, reported a case with a rapidly fatal course of 7 days' duration. toms include mental abnormalities, fits, headache, hemiparesis and fever; less frequently there may be visual disturbances, ataxia and aphasia.

The macroscopic findings consist of a diffuse meningitis with exudate in the subarachnoid space. The cerebral hemispheres are slightly swollen and may show areas of softening, haemorrhage and necrosis. Any region may be involved, but lesions are particularly severe in the cerebellum, the brain stem, the thalamus and the anterior parts of the cerebral hemispheres. Occasionally involvement of the brain can present as a mass simulating a tumour or other expanding lesion (Martinez et al., 1980). The spinal cord is spared.

Histologically there is a subacute or chronic meningitis. Within the brain there is a vasculitis involving both arteries and veins, with perivascular cuffing by lymphocytes, macrophages and plasma cells. Many blood vessels may contain thrombi in various stages of organization. Giant cells are present in the walls of the thrombosed vessels as well as outside them and are associated with discrete reactive gliosis and with foci of microglial proliferation. Giant cells are absent, however, in the brains of immunosuppressed patients in whom a slight increase in the number of eosinophils has been described. Trophozoites may be found in vessel walls and in areas free of any inflammatory reaction. In six of the patients reported by Martinez (1980) there were lesions in the liver, lungs, kidney, lymph nodes and skin. He suggests that they were the result of haematogenous dissemination.

Acanthamoebae are 15–45 μm in diameter, have a clear nucleus with a dense central nucleolus and cytoplasm that contains granules and vacuoles. Unlike *Naegleria*, organisms of the *Acanthamoeba* group move slowly. The cystic form is rather irregular in shape and measures 15–20 μm in diameter.

Brain lesions due to *Hartmannella* have also been described: Kernohan, Magath and Schloss (1960) reported a case in a child, and, more recently, Jager and Stamm (1972) described a case presenting as an abscess in a patient suffering from Hodgkin's disease.

Meningoencephalitis due to the *Hartmannella-Acanthamoeba* group is fatal. Although no effective treatment has been found, it seems that sulphadiazine and clotrimazole are effective against at least some strains of *Acanthamoeba* (Martinez, 1982).

Cerebral malaria

Cerebral malaria occurs only in malignant tertian malaria due to *Plasmodium falciparum*. In the UK 56 fatal cases were reported between 1968 and 1977 in patients coming from malarial areas (Janota and Doshi, 1979). Children in hyperendemic areas, pregnant women and non-immune adults who have interrupted prophylactic treatment are particularly susceptible to this complication which has a 33 per cent mortality rate (Marsden and Bruce-Chwatt, 1975).

In 19 fatal cases studied by Toro and Román (1978), the main macroscopic abnormalities in the brain were oedema, vascular congestion, petechial haemorrhages, dark grey discoloration of the grey matter and some opacity of the leptomeninges. Histological examination shows that the oedema is both perivascular and diffuse; in some cases endothelial cells are swollen and prominent, whilst occasional veins have necrotic walls; perivascular oedema and diapedesis of red cells, thrombosis of the vessels by plugs of hyaline material, and demyelination and necrosis of nerve fibres are also observed in such cases. The red blood cells in capillaries in the grey matter contain malaria parasites (Fig. 8.3a). Granules of dark malarial pigment (related to haematin) are also seen in capillaries (Fig. 8.3b). Although haemorrhages are associated with the entire capillary network, they are more abundant in the white matter (Fig. 8.3c). Hypoxic-ischaemic changes are also observed in the brain and are accompanied by glial proliferation. This can be seen as a generalized excess of microglia or as nodular aggregates of astrocytes and microglial cells containing neutral lipids and iron pigment. The nodules, called the malarial granulomas of Dürck (Fig. 8.3d) in spite of the fact that they are not true granulomas, are morphologically similar to those seen after the resolution of fat emboli. They represent the final stage of glial reaction, and were observed by Toro and Román (1978) in six of their 19 cases. An inflammatory infiltrate consisting of lymphocytes and mononuclear cells may spread to the leptomeninges. Occasionally the pituitary gland is affected and may even become infarcted (Janota and Doshi, 1979). These lesions are morphologically similar to those observed in fat embolism, parasitized red cells playing a similar role to fat globules in interfering with capillary circulation. The physiopathology, however, is more complex, and Maegraith (1974) supported the view that the packing of cerebral capillaries by red cells and thrombosis are terminal events, not essential to the pathogenesis of cerebral malaria. Migasena and Maegraith (1967) have shown that there is early alteration of the endothelial wall with breakdown of the blood-brain barrier. Further experimental work by Rest and Wright (1979) confirmed this finding by showing that the damage is initiated by the presence of specific antigen-antibody complexes in the blood stream. The process parallels the involvement of the glomerular basal lamina in the malarial nephrotic syndrome caused by *P. malariae* infection (Houba et al., 1971). Complexes are taken up by endothelial cells through pinocytosis and their presence in the cytoplasm attracts monocytes, leading to damage to endothelial cells and consequent oedema and haemorrhage. These features closely resemble those for which Poser (1969) coined the name 'vasculomyelinopathy'. The term includes forms of hyperergic reaction of the nervous system to various proteins. The natural outcome is a vasculopathy with involvement of the surrounding myelin. Toro and Román (1978) have confirmed all of the observations described by Poser. Moreover, clinical manifestations in malaria suggest an acute hyperergic reaction within the CNS, similar to that following vaccination or the injection of foreign proteins. The onset is usually acute, with convulsions, changes in the level of consciousness leading to coma and few, if any, localizing signs. Despite the extreme severity of the clinical picture, cerebral malaria can be completely reversible (Daroff et al., 1967). The various stages of the vasculomyelinopathy can be halted by the administration of corticosteroids and antimalarial drugs.

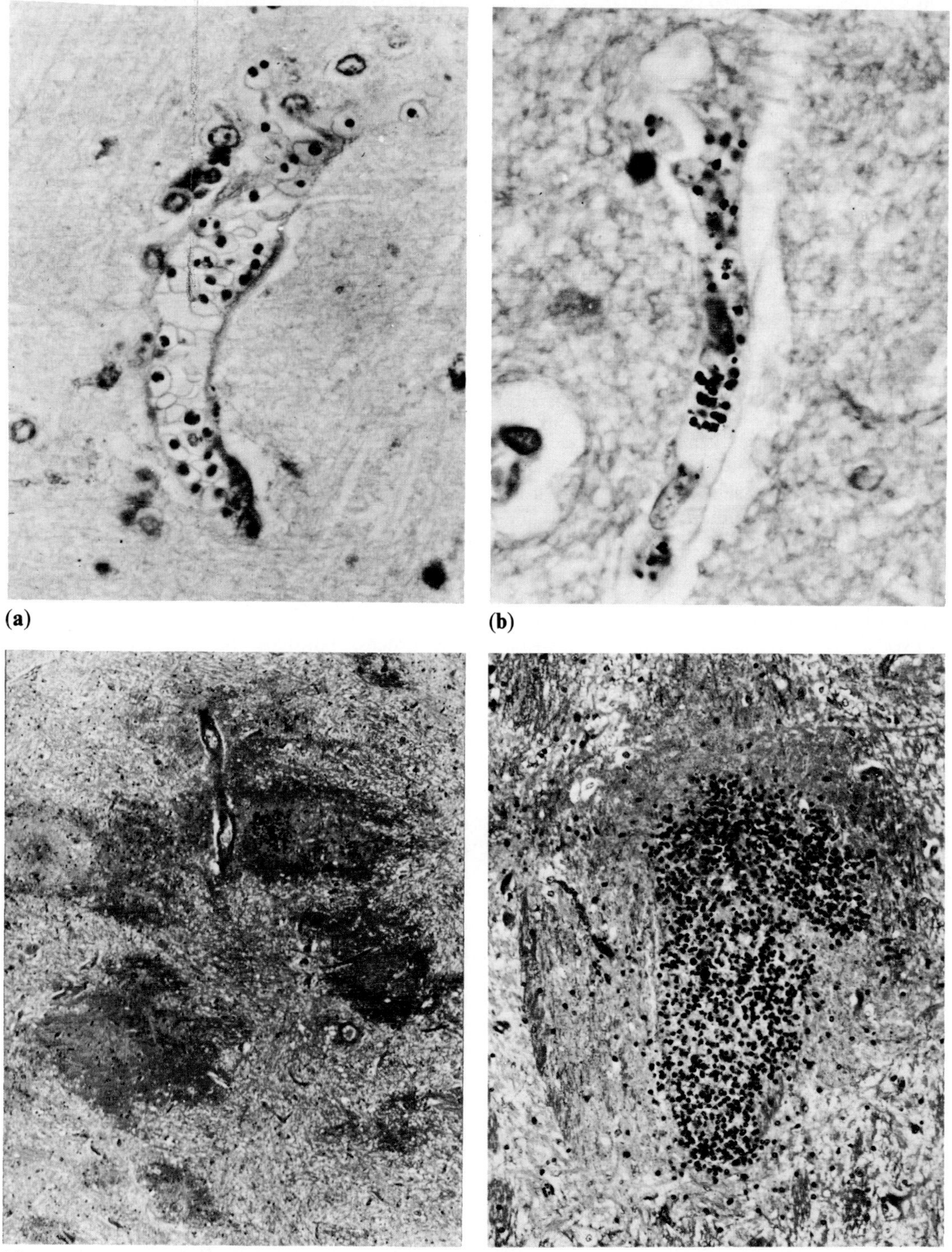

(a) (b) (c) (d)

Fig. 8.3 Cerebral malaria. (**a**) Numerous red cells in a capillary contain parasites. Colophonium-Giemsa × 720 (**b**) A capillary in the grey matter contains malarial pigment. Haematoxylin and eosin × 800. (**c**) Perivascular haemorrhages in the white matter. Haematoxylin and eosin × 50. (**d**) A Dürck's granuloma with reactive gliosis in a small area of infarction. Haematoxylin and eosin × 130. (**a** and **b** courtesy of Dr M. Nielsen; **c** and **d** courtesy of Dr S. Daniel.)

Toxoplasmosis

Toxoplasma, a coccidian organism of the order Sporozoa, is known to infect mammals and birds; its relevance to human pathology was pointed out by Wolf and Cowen (1937) who reported toxoplasmosis in a 1-month-old baby. Since then many cases have been described in infants in North and South America, continental Europe and Great Britain. The frequency of human infection varies in different countries. Remington and Klein (1976) found that the incidence of antibodies to Toxoplasma in women under 35 years was 33 per cent in London and New York whilst it reached 85 per cent in Paris.

The specific name *Toxoplasma gondii* is derived from the animal in which the parasite was first described, the North American rodent, gondi. The organism is an obligatory intracellular parasite, and studies by Krick and Remington (1978) have elucidated its life-cycle. The definitive hosts for toxoplasma are the cat family, where the entire life-cycle can be completed. Both sexual and asexual forms may be found in the intestinal mucosa. The organisms exist as trophozoites, cysts and oöcysts. The oöcysts are found only in cats after they have eaten raw prey previously infected by cysts from another cat. The infective oöcysts contain two sporocysts, each of which harbours eight sporozoites. These are liberated in the intestine and invade the cells of the mucosa; eventually oöcysts are produced and excreted. Animals and man acquire the infection by eating meat from chronically infected animals or by ingesting oöcysts deposited in soil, sand or litterpans of cats. It should be emphasized that although infective forms enter through the intestine, man does not develop enteritis; furthermore, infection and clinical disease do not necessarily correspond: clinical evidence of the disease occurs only in a minority of individuals in whom the parasite has entered, invaded organs and induced a chronic infection.

Toxoplasma cysts may contain several hundred merozoites, active motile organisms with a single glycogen granule, similar in size to the nucleus, whilst trophozoites (the form of the parasite that lives outside the cyst) contain smaller dispersed granules. Cyst walls vary in thickness and stain faintly with the PAS technique. They consist of an outer membrane and an inner layer of variable thickness and are granular or tubular in appearance (Powell et al., 1978). Individual sporozoites in the cysts are 2–3 μm in length, crescent-shaped, with a pointed anterior end opposite the nucleus. Each organism is enveloped by a two-layered membranous structure. Organisms divide by endodyogeny (Jacobs, 1967) and are then called bradyzoites or tachyzoites according to whether they have a low or a high rate of multiplication. Studies by Aikawa et al. (1977) have shown that, although passive entry into macrophages can occur, there is evidence for active penetration of host cells by invagination without disruption of the cell membrane. Electron microscopic studies have revealed that the tachyzoite (Fig. 8.4) is specifically modified for host cell penetration. The conoid is the part of the organism structurally equipped to facilitate entry (Powell et al., 1978). After penetration, the vacuole then formed becomes the site of replication of organisms (cyst). The cysts enlarge and ultimately rupture the host cell—which dies, leaving viable cysts within which replication may continue. These may remain embedded in the tissues of the host without producing further disease (Frenkel, 1972).

The development of toxoplasmosis in man de-

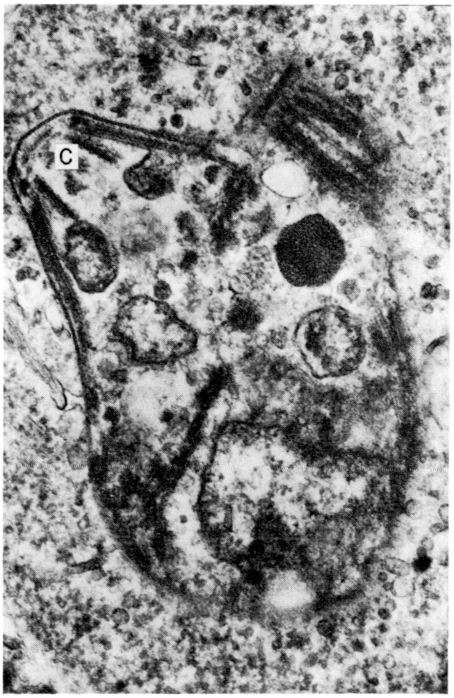

Fig. 8.4 Toxoplasmosis. Tachyzoite (motile form) of *T. gondii*, showing the conoid (C) at the anterior end of the organism. × 40 000. (Courtesy of Dr F. Gray.)

pends very much on the host's susceptibility and immunological status. Of the two types of immunity, that due to circulating antibodies is the first to appear and plays a role in limiting extracellular dissemination of the organism. Hypersensitivity to Toxoplasma is a further complication and can lead to death of non-infected cells. According to whether the disease is acquired in an immunologically mature individual or before the development of immunological competence, there are two different patterns of disease—one occurring in adults and the other in neonates.

Toxoplasmosis in the adult

The most common signs of infection are lymphadenopathy—localized (mostly cervical) or generalized—malaise, fever and lymphocytosis. In the large majority of patients spontaneous resolution follows but, in some, pneumonia, hepatitis, myocarditis or encephalitis may supervene.

Encephalitis due to toxoplasma manifests itself as a febrile illness. Pathological features include lymphocytic infiltration of the leptomeninges and, within the brain, glial nodules composed of astrocytes and microglia (Fig. 8.5a), with or without necrosis, and occasional parasitic cysts that measure 20–100 μm in diameter (Fig. 8.5b). An inflammatory reaction occurs only if there is cell necrosis, and it is known that intracellular organisms do not elicit any inflammatory response. Blood vessels cuffed with lymphocytes can also be seen. Unless the parasite can be clearly identified, the lesions lack specificity. Kass et al. (1952) described a patient with diffuse encephalitis and microglial nodules, whilst Bobowski and Reed (1958) reported an atypical case in whom the disease presented as a space-occupying lesion with numerous cysts, necrosis and multinucleated giant cells.

Foci of asymptomatic toxoplasmosis may occasionally be found in the brains of patients dying from unrelated causes. Persistence of toxoplasma cysts in the brain after the acquisition of immunity is of special interest because it allows relapse to occur if immunity fails.

In the *eye*, toxoplasmosis may attack the choroid, the ciliary body or the retina, producing

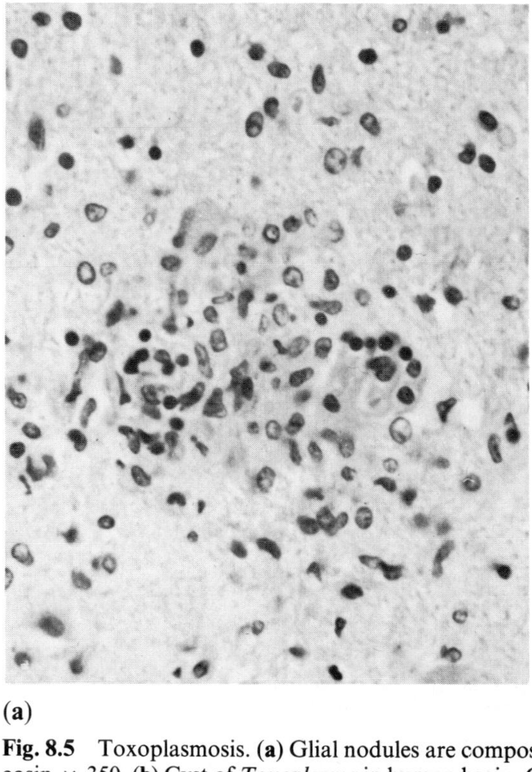

(a)

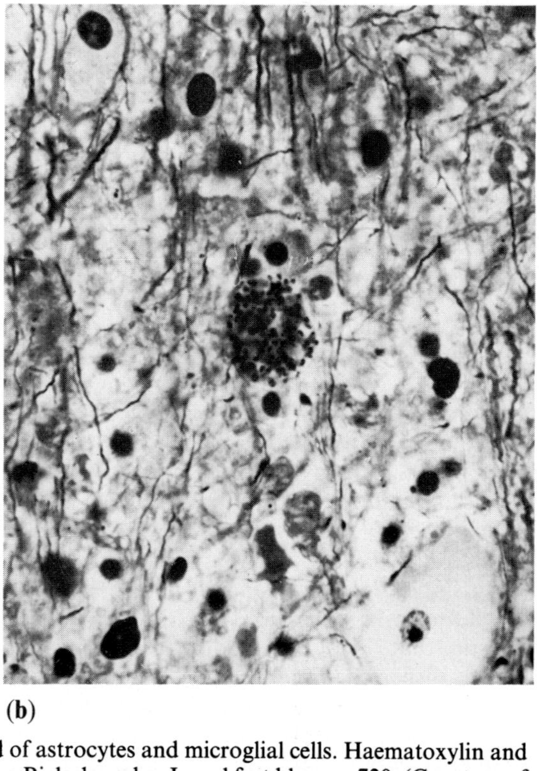

(b)

Fig. 8.5 Toxoplasmosis. (**a**) Glial nodules are composed of astrocytes and microglial cells. Haematoxylin and eosin × 350. (**b**) Cyst of *Toxoplasma* in human brain. Gros Bielschowsky–Luxol fast blue. × 720. (Courtesy of Dr F. Gray.)

small foci of granulomatous inflammation followed by scarring.

Toxoplasmosis, although a relatively benign disease in normal adults, is often fatal in patients being treated with antimitotic or immunosuppressive drugs. Some 50 per cent of such patients show clinical signs of encephalitis and 90 per cent of fatal cases have encephalitis (Krick and Remington, 1978). Impaired cellular immunity is thought to be responsible for this loss of resistance to toxoplasma (Lindberg and Frenkel, 1977). Several authors (Ghatak and Sawyer, 1978; Powell et al., 1978; Best and Finlayson, 1979) have emphasized the morphological similarity between toxoplasma encephalitis in immunosuppressed patients and that occurring in the newborn (see below); in both instances there are large areas of necrosis with variable numbers of inflammatory cells. Cysts packed with organisms are present as well as isolated organisms. Insufficient data are available about the rate of progression of the encephalitis in these patients, but from single case reports it appears that the large necrotic lesions seen at autopsy evolve rapidly (Ghatak and Sawyer, 1978).

Congenital toxoplasmosis

Toxoplasmosis in the newborn is completely different from that seen in the normal adult. The reason is that, of the two factors acting in the adult form—proliferation of the organism with rupture of the cyst and spreading of the antigen in an immune background—only the first occurs in the neonate, whose immune system is still immature. Congenital toxoplasmosis occurs only if maternal infection is acquired during pregnancy. Infection of the fetus is via the placenta and is found in 2-3 per 1000 births (Larroche, 1977). The type of damage produced depends on the time of infection. Fetal infection does not occur during the first 2 months of pregnancy, probably because the placenta has not yet been formed (Robertson, 1962). During the next 3 months the risk of infection is very high (1 in 3) and the damage is severe; during the sixth and seventh months the risk of infection is higher but damage is less and there is a high rate of prematurity. Towards the end of the pregnancy, the fetus is seldom affected. The pathogenesis of the diffuse, highly destructive process typical of neonatal toxoplasmosis is described in detail by Binford and Connor (1976). In the nervous system, toxoplasma proliferates in the ependymal and subependymal tissues and spreads widely because of the absence of circulating antibodies. Contact between circulating antibodies passively transferred from the mother and toxoplasma antigen in the walls of the vessels may account for perivascular inflammation and thrombosis. The relative sparing of the fourth ventricle by the necrotizing process is thought to be due to the lower protein content of the CSF there due to drainage through the foramina.

Morphological features reflect the pathogenesis: they include lymphocytes and occasional polymorphs in the subarachnoid space and foci of complete destruction of both grey and white matter. Focal calcification is present around the ventricles and the aqueduct may be obstructed, leading to internal hydrocephalus. Microcephaly is found in cases in which destruction of the brain has been severe. Congenital toxoplasmosis can also affect the eyes, and chorioretinitis is a common late result of congenital infection.

Trypanosomiasis

This disease is due to protozoa of the family Trypanosomatidae, and has been known for centuries since the first reported human case, that of a Sudanese king who died in 1373. Not all trypanosomes are pathogenic to man: those involved in human disease are *Trypanosoma gambiense* and *T. rhodesiense* in Africa and *T. cruzi* in South America.

African trypanosomiasis

This illness is endemic in areas of tropical forest near rivers. Its cause was demonstrated in 1902, the year in which an epidemic killed two-thirds of the population of 300 000 in Uganda. Flies of the genus *Glossina* are the vectors; *G. palpalis* transmits *T. gambiense* whilst *G. morsitans* carries *T. rhodesiense*. However, this association of trypanosome with a particular genus of fly is only ecological and does not indicate any host–parasite specificity (Hutt and Wilks, 1971). The disease is transmitted via the bite of an infected fly. There is a local reaction in the skin where the patient has been bitten. Invasion of the blood occurs after a few days and is accompanied by fever, erythema, oedema and tachycardia. The disease caused by *T. rhodesiense* usually follows a fairly acute course and structural abnormalities in the brain are often not severe. On the other hand, *T. gambiense* may be associated with a chronic progressive neurological disease—classic West African *sleeping sickness*—and very striking structural abnormalities in the brain.

During the early systemic phase of the disease lesions are found in the reticuloendothelial system, heart and serous membranes. Meningoencephalitis is characteristic of the late phases of the disease; affected patients show increasing disability, slow gait, a mask-like expression, somnolence and restlessness, and, terminally, tremor of the hands, choreic movements, varying degrees of paralysis and convulsions. Cerebral involvement is more severe in infections with *T. gambiense* than with *T. rhodesiense*.

In fatal cases, the brain is often of entirely normal appearance macroscopically but in chronic cases there may be some thickening of leptomeninges, more over the convexity than at the base of the brain. Histological examination shows a diffuse meningoencephalitis consisting of lymphocytes, histiocytes and plasma cells (Fig. 8.6a) in the subarachnoid space and around blood vessels in the brain. Lymphocytes and plasma cells often extend out from these vessels into the adjacent brain tissue, and there is diffuse microglial hyperplasia. There may also be large astrocytes and glial nodules. In some cases capillaries show endothelial proliferation and appear to be surrounded by small haemorrhages or, in later stages, by haemosiderin-laden histiocytes. A characteristic but by no means pathognomonic feature of trypanosomiasis is the morular cell, a modified plasma cell with a small, peripheral nucleus and cytoplasm filled with Russell bodies (Fig. 8.6b). These cells are present in the inflammatory infiltrate in the meninges and brain, but also may be found isolated in otherwise unaffected areas. Damage to neurons and demyelination are rare, although Janssen, van Bogaert and Haymaker (1956) described peripheral nerve lesions in six patients with chronic meningoencephalitis. Trypanosomes have never been described in histological sections; in blood or CSF they may be seen as elongated and flagellated with an undulating

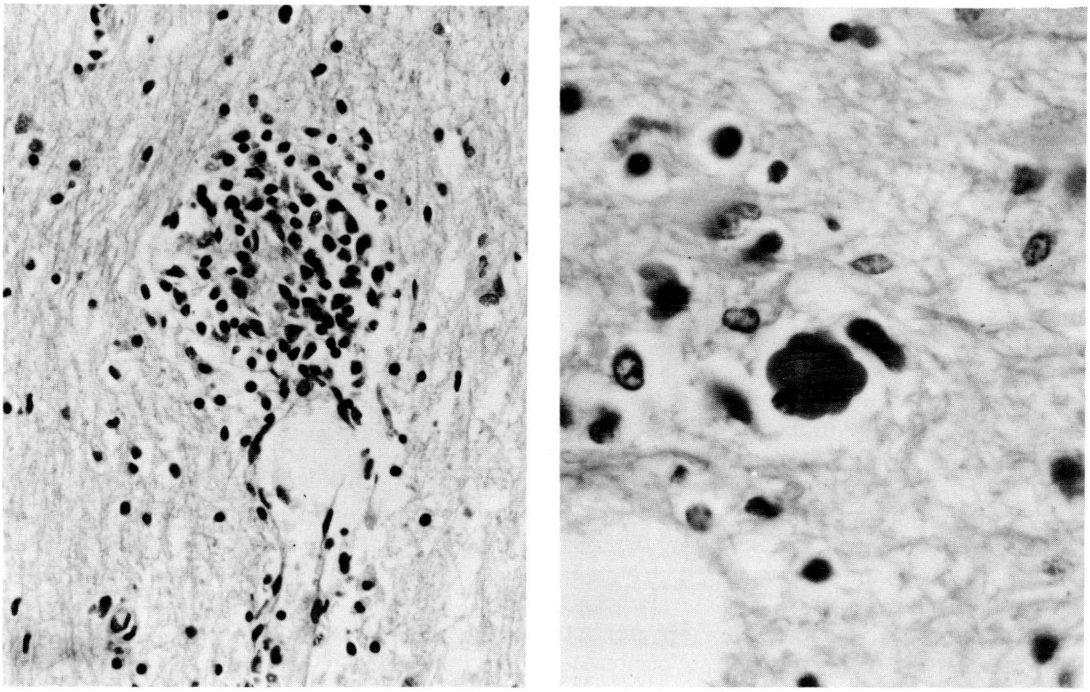

(a) **(b)**

Fig. 8.6 Human African trypanosomiasis. **(a)** Inflammatory nodule composed of lymphocytes and histiocytes around a blood vessel. Haematoxylin and eosin × 520. **(b)** A morular cell in the brain with a peripheral nucleus and numerous globules filling the cytoplasm. Haematoxylin and eosin × 560. (Courtesy of Dr M. Nielsen.)

membrane. Multiplication occurs by binary fission.

Most of the descriptions of the neuropathology of African trypanosomiasis have been based on cases of *T. gambiense* encephalitis. In the two cases of *T. rhodesiense* infection described by Hawkings and Greenfield (1941) meningeal opacity was patchy and limited to the exposed surfaces of gyri and there was no involvement of the brain tissue. On the other hand, Calwell (1937) described pathological changes similar to those seen in treated cases due to *T. gambiense*.

Hutt and Wilks (1971) have suggested that the differences are probably related to the stage at which observations were made. If the patients die early from cardiac involvement, as is common in patients with *T. rhodesiense* infection, lesions in the brain are likely to be less apparent than in those who die later.

Recent experimental studies (Poltera, Lambert and Miescher, 1979; Poltera, 1980) have clarified the mode and tempo of brain involvement. Invasion of the brain takes place simultaneously with cardiac involvement and begins in the choroid plexus where parasites multiply and induce an inflammatory reaction.

American trypanosomiasis (Chagas' disease)

This is a disease of rural districts, and is caused by *T. cruzi*. It was discovered in Brazil by Chagas in 1909 and was described later in almost all the countries of the three Americas, in Java (Malamos, 1935) and in India (Fulton and Harrison, 1946).

Insects of the family Reduviidae carry the parasite in their faeces. As they suck the victim's blood, they defaecate and parasites can enter through the skin wound around which a firm nodule develops. The protozoon has a particular tropism for muscle tissue (Fig. 8.7a) and, according to its environment, it can take a Leishmania-like form (amastigotes).

The disease is usually acquired during childhood and may be acute in children or chronic both in children and in adults. The infection may remain dormant for as long as 10–20 years (Laranja et al., 1956) during which the infected individuals appear normal. Encephalitis is more common in acute than in chronic cases (Manuelidis, 1972).

Macroscopically, changes in the brains of patients who die in the acute stage consist of oedema, and congestion and petechial haemorrhages in the white matter. Microscopically the appearances are those of a generalized nodular encephalitis in which the parasites can be found as leishmaniae in glial cells (Fig. 8.7b). Similar lesions have been reproduced in experimental animals, especially newborn dogs and rats, and have the appearances of a generalized nodular encephalitis. Unencapsulated nodules (Fig. 8.7c) vary in size and are mainly related to small vessels in the cortex and white matter; they consist of aggregates of microglial cells with fewer astrocytes, histiocytes and polymorphs and occasional central necrosis. Perivascular infiltrates of lymphocytes and some polymorphs are common. Two cases that do not conform to this description have been reported by Johnson and DeRivas (1936) and by De Quieroz (1973): these presented respectively as a diffuse granulomatous process, and as an isolated and haemorrhagic tumour-like mass in the left occipital lobe consisting of multiple areas of necrotic tissue with perifocal glial reaction and identifiable parasites.

It is believed that trypanosomes initially invade the endothelium of cerebral vessels and subsequently pass into astrocytes (Alencar, 1972). There is no cellular reaction until pseudocysts rupture, liberating parasites. Unlike acute toxoplasmic encephalopathy, neurons in the CNS are relatively well preserved, although Köberle (1968) reported a decrease in their numbers in man and animals. Demyelination has not been observed, except where the cellular aggregates are present. In contrast with the CNS, autonomic ganglion cells degenerate during the acute phases of Chagas' disease (Tafuri, 1970), before an inflammatory infiltrate appears. The recent finding of common neuronal and trypanosomal antigens (Wood et al., 1982) may contribute to understanding the precise mechanism underlying neuronal degeneration.

About 10 per cent of the acute cases of Chagas' disease are believed to evolve into the chronic phase in which the heart, hollow viscera and autonomic viscera are affected (Brown and Voge, 1982) and show lesions of the autonomic ganglia.

Congenital trypanosomiasis Congenital cases of Chagas' disease are well recognized, whereas those due to the African trypanosomes have only been reported in small numbers (Daveloose,

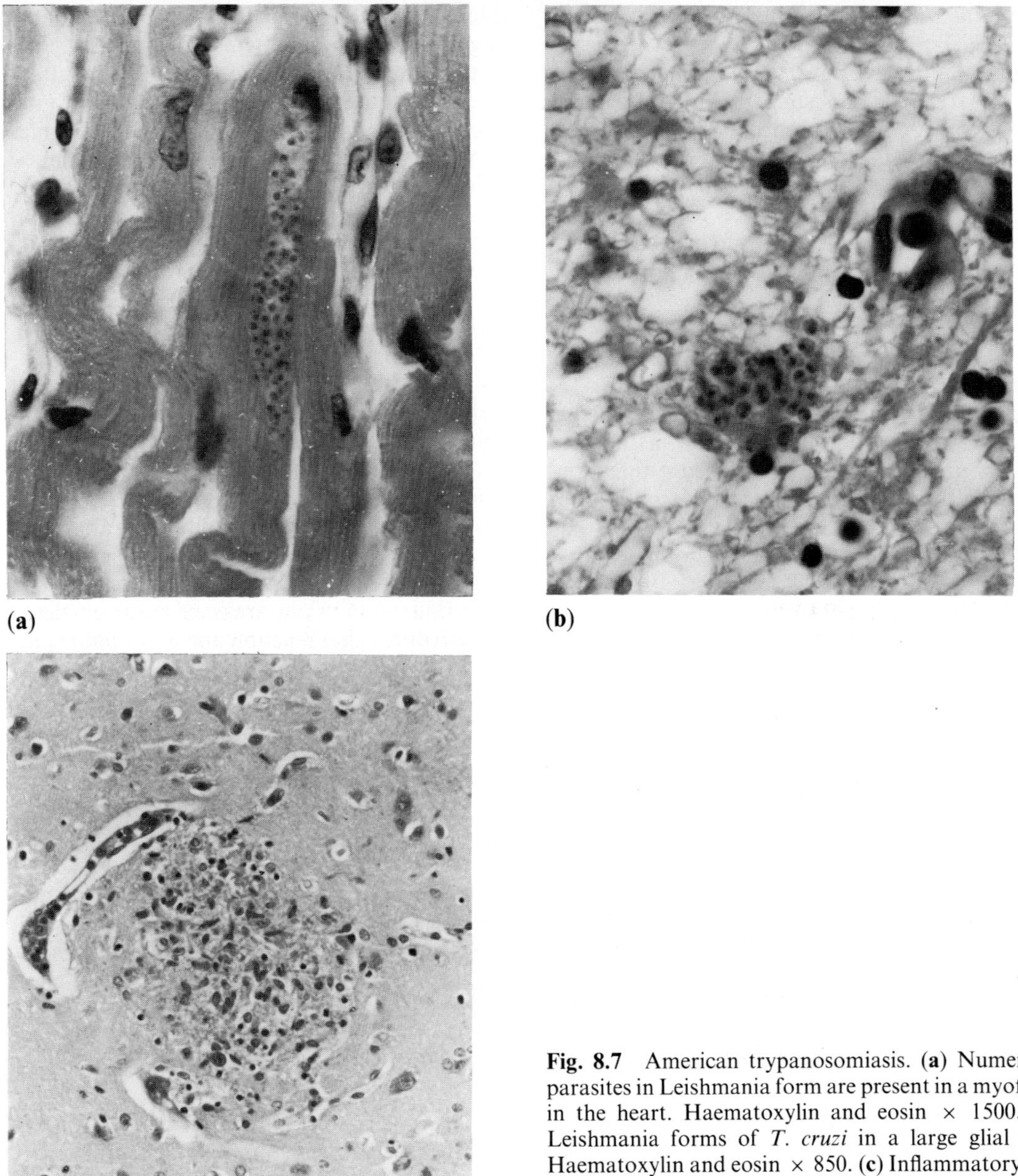

(a) **(b)** (c)

Fig. 8.7 American trypanosomiasis. (**a**) Numerous parasites in Leishmania form are present in a myofibre in the heart. Haematoxylin and eosin × 1500. (**b**) Leishmania forms of *T. cruzi* in a large glial cell. Haematoxylin and eosin × 850. (**c**) Inflammatory nodule in close contact with two capillaries in the cerebral cortex. Haematoxylin and eosin × 200. (**a** and **c** courtesy of Dr E. M. Tani; **b** courtesy of Dr J. E. H. Pittella.)

1972; Burke, Bengoni and Diantete, 1974). The infection can occur during any phase of the maternal disease (Bittencourt, 1976). It is believed that the trophoblast acts as a barrier to *T. cruzi*, and the presence in some cases of a lesion and inflammation of the villi of the placenta and the identification of trypanosomes in the trophoblast support the idea that the infection takes place through a focal break in the barrier. Transplacental infection may lead to abortion, prematurity or small-for-dates babies.

Meningoencephalitis, that may not be clinically apparent, is less severe than in acquired forms of the disease and has the morphological features of a chronic disease with, occasionally, epithelioid and giant cells. It is associated with inflammatory lesions of the heart, skeletal muscle, oesophagus and intestine.

In the case reported by Traub et al. (1978) and due to *T. rhodesiense*, a baby girl had been delivered by caesarian section. She developed the disease 9 days after delivery and the parasite was isolated from the blood and CSF. Traub et al. (1978) are in favour of transplacental transmission. However, transmission through mucous membranes contaminated by maternal blood cannot be ruled out since Zeledón (1974) has demonstrated that *T. cruzi* can invade the normal skin of the mouse.

Metazoal infections

Cestodes

Cysticercosis

Cerebral cysticercosis is world-wide, but is particularly frequent in South America and India. In Mexico it is the cause of death in 2–3 per cent of all post-mortem material and of up to 33 per cent of all brain tumours (Hernandez, 1960; Olivé and Angulo-Rivero, 1962). In the past it was rarely found in the USA, where only 50 cases were reported in about 30 years (Latovitzki et al., 1978); but in the last decade its frequency has considerably increased in that country (McCormick, Zee and Heiden, 1982).

The organism responsible for this disease is *Taenia solium*, a pork tapeworm whose permanent host is man. The adult worm lives in the small intestine to which it is attached by four suckers and two rows of hooklets and where it absorbs food. Eggs excreted in the faeces are ingested by animals that act as intermediate hosts. Man, however, can also become an intermediate host when he eats food contaminated with viable eggs or, in individuals harbouring the adult tapeworm, either when gravid proglottids are regurgitated into the stomach by antiperistalsis or are ingested by the faecal–oral route.

In the duodenum of both man and pig, the shells of the ova are dissolved; embryos penetrate the wall of the intestine and are carried by the circulation to all organs, including brain and muscle. Escobar and Nieto (1972) quoted a case in which congenital infection was suggested.

In the brain, larvae develop a cystic wall in about 2 months and the cysts take several forms. In most cases they remain small, sequestrated and eventually die; less frequently, thin-walled, racemose cysts develop in the basal cisterns causing hydrocephalus or cranial nerve palsies. In children and, occasionally, in adults cysts may behave as space-occupying lesions.

The clinical manifestations are varied. In 17 patients examined by Vijayan et al. (1977) six presented with fits; four showed signs of meningoencephalitis with fever, headaches, blurred vision and papilloedema; two had symptoms of space-occupying lesions; two presented with psychiatric manifestations; two complained of impaired vision; and one had muscular pseudohypertrophy. Cysts in the vertebral bodies are rare but they may lead to compression of the spinal cord with motor and sensory disturbances. In the visual system, blindness may result from a fibrous adhesive arachnoiditis due to compression of the optic nerves and chiasma or from live encysted parasites in the vitreous (Brown and Voge, 1982).

The presence of cysts—*cysticerci*—in the brain and meninges induces changes in the CSF that tend to become less evident or to disappear with time. Cells are increased up to 1000/mm^3 and consist of lymphocytes and eosinophils. The colloidal gold curve may be of meningitic or even paretic type. Complement fixation tests are positive in about three-quarters of the cases. The blood count, ESR and serum protein electrophoresis are usually normal, but serum indirect haemagglutination titres for cysticercosis give positive results in approximately 90 per cent of patients. In chronic cases the diagnosis often rests on the presence in muscle of cysts which may be palpable or appear radiologically as small, oval or elongated opacities. Calcified intracerebral nodules are less easily detected owing to the density of the skull shadow.

Macroscopically the appearances are variable and depend on the number, size and location of cysts as well as on their stage of evolution. Their number can vary from just one to several hundred and they are commonly found in brain tissue, and less frequently in the meninges and ventricles. In the meninges they appear as small, colourless structures, adherent to the pia or ing freely in the subarachnoid space, particularly in the sylvian fissure. They can be single or multiple and in the latter case they may be attached to a central pedicle and resemble a bunch of grapes. The basal meninges become thickened and the cysts within them tend to shrink. In slices of the brain, cysts measuring up to 1 cm may be numerous in the cortex but they can be found also in the deep grey and white matter. They occur rarely in the cerebellum. They can project into the ventricles or appear on the cortical surface. In chronic cases, many of the cysts become calcified. Larger cysts have a tense, grey capsule in which, unless they are sterile, there is a mural nodule in which the embryo lies. When the disease has reached the chronic stage or there are racemose or intraventricular cysts, hydrocephalus may develop.

Whatever the location of a cyst, its wall has three histologically distinct layers: an outer or cuticular layer, about 3 μm thick; a middle cellular layer with a pseudoepithelial structure; and an inner reticular or fibrillary layer (Fig. 8.8a). If present, the parasite (Fig. 8.8b) in the mural nodule has a double row of hooklets; however, most subarachnoid racemose cysts are sterile. Intracerebral cysts are surrounded by a collagenous capsule produced by the host. Larvae elicit a slight inflammatory reaction which becomes more evident after the death of the parasite. The reaction remains circumscribed to the tissue immediately adjacent to the parasite and consists, in the early stages after death of the larva, of an inner layer of polymorphs, mononuclear and foreign body giant cells and eosinophils, and an outer zone of granulation tissue. In

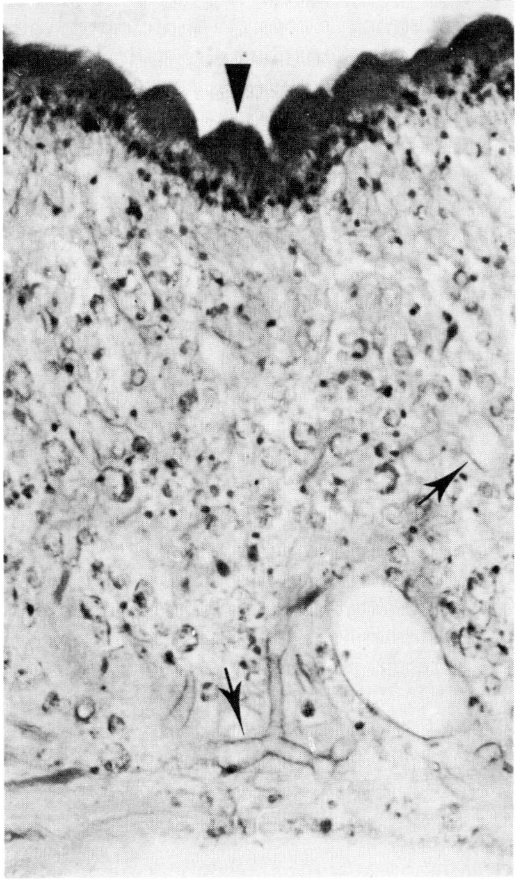

(a)

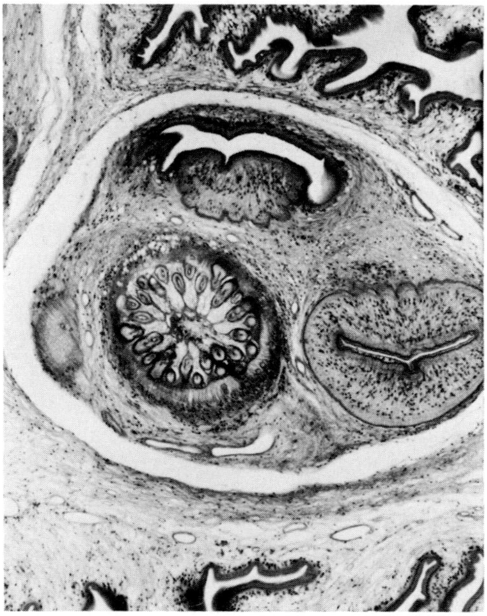

(b)

Fig. 8.8 Cysticercosis. (**a**) Wall of a cyst of cysticercus, showing the three layers. The outer cuticular (arrowhead) and the intermediate layers are thin. The inner is thicker and shows a rich network of small canaliculi (arrows). PAS × 850. (**b**) Scolex of cysticercus, showing the rostellum carrying hooklets and two muscular suckers. Haematoxylin and eosin × 160.

some smaller nodules the fibrous capsule may be lined by a layer of foreign body giant cells and surrounded by a core of necrotic tissue, cholesterol and calcium. Old nodules may be entirely fibrotic. Ventricular cysticerci tend to become attached to the ependyma and elicit a granular ependymitis. Active cysts in the basal meninges induce an intense inflammatory reaction and proliferation of collagen leading to degeneration of the parasite.

Meningeal and small intracerebral arteries in the vicinity of cysts undergo characteristic reactions consisting of concentric or eccentric fibroblastic or collagenous thickening of the intima or local excrescences, sometimes forming bridges across the lumen. The elastica is not duplicated but may be discontinuous in places. There is usually little fibrosis of the media and the adventitia is infiltrated with plasma cells.

Echinococcosis

Hydatid disease of the central nervous system is produced by the larval stage of *Echinococcus granulosus*. The disease is not uncommon in sheep-rearing countries and numerous reports have come from Australia, New Zealand, Uruguay and Argentina. In the British Isles, the majority of the cases occur in Wales and in the Shetland Islands.

The life-cycle of the parasite is similar to that of *Taenia solium*. The dog is the definitive host of the adult worm, and its ova, excreted in faeces, infect herbage and are eaten by sheep. Hatched embryos infiltrate through the wall of the duodenum to the veins of the portal system and thence to the liver, lungs and general circulation. Encysted embryos develop in the liver, lungs and abdominal organs of sheep, the cycle being completed when dogs eat these infected organs, thus introducing the parasite into the intestine where it remains. Man is infected by ingesting food contaminated with ova, or by direct contact with dogs, which is probably the reason why most cases are seen in children.

Hydatidosis can be described as *primary*, when the cyst is caused by the larval development, or *secondary*, when it develops as a result of the rupture of a primary hydatid cyst elsewhere in the body (Arana-Iñiguez, 1973). Primary hydatid cysts of the brain comprise about 5 per cent of all cases in children, but are rarer in adults. In the series of 145 cases observed by Arana-Iñiguez in Uruguay (1973), 76 per cent were intracerebral, 7 per cent cranial and 17 per cent in vertebral bodies. Cerebral hydatid cyst was more frequent in children and the cranial localization slightly higher in the same group, whilst the vertebral form was observed almost exclusively in adults.

Hydatid cysts of the brain are usually solitary, spherical and unilocular. They are almost always found in the cerebral hemispheres, particularly in the region supplied by the middle cerebral artery; according to Escobar and Nieto (1972), they are usually retrorolandic. Because of the large size they attain, they usually lie only a few millimetres below the cortex which is flattened over them and appears bluish. Cysts can develop in the lateral ventricles and their rupture can lead to a secondary hydatidosis. Cysts rarely cause serious symptoms until they reach about 6 cm in diameter, but they can be much larger; in Phillips' series (1948), two had a diameter of 10 cm, two contained 600 ml of fluid, and two were described as being of the size of an orange. Langmaid and Rogers (1940) found two cysts side by side, one 8 cm the other 6 cm in diameter. Cysts may be successfully removed at operation because the capsule is readily detached from surrounding brain tissue. Involvement of the spinal cord is nearly always secondary to vertebral involvement.

The contents of most cysts are a clear, colourless fluid which usually contains small daughter cysts and a granular deposit of scolices. A few cysts are sterile and some contain turbid or, more rarely, yellowish fluid. If cysts are ruptured at operation, new ones are formed in contaminated areas and may grow rapidly. In a case reported by Phillips (1948) numerous new cysts, some of which were 2.5 cm in diameter, were found at autopsy 8 months after an operation to remove one hydatid cyst.

Histologically (Fig. 8.9) the wall of the cyst, which is 2–3 mm thick, consists of three layers; an outer layer of fibrous tissue, derived from the host; an intermediate, laminated, chitinous or cuticular layer; and an inner germinal layer to which oval capsules are usually attached. Apart from mild gliosis and lymphocytic cuffing of vessels in the immediate vicinity, there is little other reaction to the cysts.

The CSF is normal apart from a possible increase in pressure.

Because of the tendency of the parasite to de-

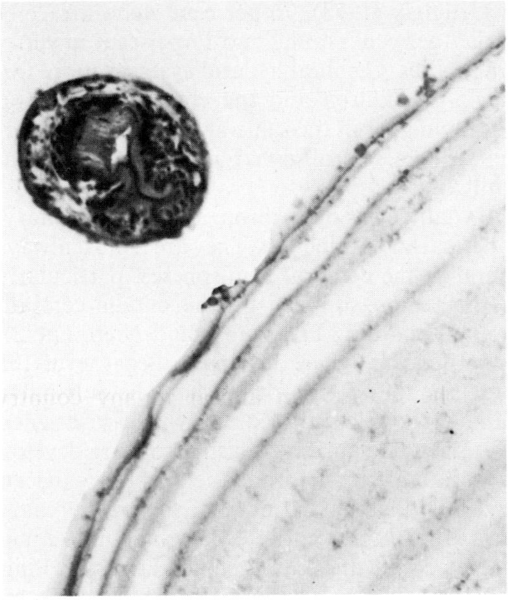

Fig. 8.9 Section of hydatid cyst, showing the intermediate, laminated and germinative layers with one scolex. The outer layer is not included in the picture. Haematoxylin and eosin × 580.

velop in areas of least resistance, cysts in bone arise in the cancellous tissue of epiphyses and in the bodies of vertebrae. Diaphyses are rarely affected, and involvement of the skull is uncommon. According to Arana-Iñiguez (1973) and Samiy and Zadeh (1965), skull involvement accounts for 7.5 per cent and 10 per cent of cases with hydatidosis affecting respectively the CNS and the brain. The cysts are multilocular, and progressively invasive leading to thinning and erosion of cortical bone with involvement of periosteum and spread to neighbouring tissues. The spinal cord may be damaged by compression of cysts growing into the spinal canal and/or by fracture or subluxation of the affected spine.

Coenurosis

Coenurosis, a rare infection of man, is caused by *Coenurus cerebralis*, the larval stage of the dog tapeworm, *Multiceps multiceps* (*Taenia multiceps*), a parasite with a life-cycle similar to that of *Echinococcus granulosus*. Coenurosis is more common in sheep-rearing countries and the intermediate host may be any one of a variety of herbivorous and omnivorous animals, particularly sheep and other ungulates, rabbits and rodents. Man, too, may be the intermediate host by ingesting food contaminated with ova from canine faeces. Despite the fact that most cases of human coenurosis occur in tropical Africa, the only ones reported to have cerebral involvement come from temperate climates and only three cases of coenurosis were reported in the USA up to 1970 (Johnstone and Jones, 1950; Hermos et al., 1970; Orihel, Gonzales and Beaver, 1970). Ingested ova hatch in the intestine and, after migration through the intestinal walls, larvae settle in the organs where they metamorphose into coenurus. This takes the form of a cyst, usually unilocular, measuring up to 5 cm in diameter.

In most cases only one cyst develops in the CNS, but multiple cysts have been described, forming grape-like collections of vesicles that closely resemble the racemose type of cysticercus. They are found in the ventricles, usually the fourth, or in the subarachnoid space. According to Kuper, Mendelow and Proctor (1958) they develop only in regions bathed by the CSF, but they have been found in the cerebral hemispheres; in addition, cases with spinal cord involvement have been described (Templeton, 1968). The arachnoid surrounding the cysts is thickened. Unlike hydatid cysts, the wall of coenurus is thin, opaque and milky-white. It is not surrounded by a fibrous capsule and does not show any laminar structure. Multiple scolices—up to 400—may project from the inner surface into the lumen. Sometimes the cyst is sterile. The head of each scolex carries a rostellum, armed with a double row of hooklets. In the adjacent brain tissue there is astrocytic proliferation, collagen formation and a chronic inflammatory reaction with occasional giant cells. Marked meningeal adhesions and thrombosis of major vessels have been described by Hermos et al. (1970). The serum complement fixation reaction with hydatid antigen is usually positive. In infestations of this type the CSF is often normal or there may be only a slight increase in cells.

Trematodes

Paragonimiasis

The lung fluke *Paragonimus* spp. is found in the Far East, Africa and Latin America. In its life-cycle there is a final host (man and mammals), a first intermediate host (snails) and a second intermediate host (crustacea). Adult worms are found in the lungs, where they lay eggs that are eliminated with the sputum and the faeces. Once eggs reach water they hatch and miracidia invade freshwater snails in which the asexual cycle takes place. Cercariae emerging from snails into water invade crustacea, where they encyst and mature into metacercariae. When metacercariae are swallowed by the final host they undergo excystation into the small intestine and enter the peritoneal cavity. They subsequently migrate to various organs and most of them enter the pleural cavity and invade the lungs (Miyazaki and Nishimura, 1975).

In the brain, *Paragonimus* occurs predominantly in the temporal and occipital lobes (Miyazaki and Nishimura, 1975), although other regions are not exempt. The lesion may have the appearances of a granuloma, an encapsulated abscess or a cyst that seem to represent stages of evolution of the pathological process. Less frequently the lesion may appear as a haemorrhagic focus surrounded by a halo of eosinophils (Brenes Madrigal et al., 1982).

Histological examination discloses a central necrotic zone surrounded by a layer of collagen. The eggs of the parasite can be found in the necrotic tissue, mainly near the collagen, and they are often surrounded by foreign-body giant cells. Mature worms are rarely found in the brain in man. In the adjacent meninges there is a lymphocytic infiltrate and fibrosis.

Individuals suffering from paragonimiasis have a history of residence in or travelling to affected regions. Their blood and CSF leucocytes show an increased percentage of eosinophils, and their sputum is rust-coloured and may contain eggs of the parasite.

Schistosomiasis

The CNS is one of the rarest sites of schistosomal infection. A comprehensive review of the literature by Kane and Most (1948) showed that during the period 1899–1944, 24 cases of schistosomiasis of the CNS had been reported. In the following 19 months during the American campaign of the Leyte Islands in the Philippines, the same authors reported a further 27 cases. Since then other cases have been described, and in 1972 Herskowitz was able to find 104 cases of schistosomiasis of the CNS, 29 of which were restricted to the spinal cord. Budzilovich, Most and Feigin (1964), however, suggested that schistosomiasis of the CNS may be more common than generally reported and that many cases escape diagnosis.

Three species of schistosomes infect man: *Schistosoma mansoni* in South America, Puerto Rico, the West Indies, the Middle East and Africa; *S. haematobium* in Africa and the Middle East; and *S. japonicum* in China, the Philippines, Japan, Thailand, Laos and Kampuchea. Although a geographic factor is of importance (schistosomiasis is unknown in certain parts of the world), the movement of large numbers of people and the scarcity of travel controls is such that the disease can appear in any country. Lesions of the CNS are always secondary to a primary infection elsewhere in the body (Brown and Voge, 1982). They occur in the brain in cases of infections by *S. japonicum* or in the spinal cord in cases due to *S. mansoni* and *S. haematobium* (Marcial-Rojas and Fiol, 1963).

The life-cycle of the parasite requires an intermediate host. Eggs passed in the faeces (*S. mansoni* and *S. japonicum*) or urine (*S. haematobium*) reach fresh water, where they hatch. Miracidia then invade a snail (*Biomphalaria* spp. for *S. mansoni*; *Bulinus* spp. for *S. haematobium*; *Oncomelania* spp. for *S. japonicum*) where they reproduce asexually; cercariae emerging from infected snails enter the water and penetrate the skin of people coming into contact with them. From the site of entry, larvae reach the lungs through the veins, and from there the hepatic portal system. After mating, female worms reach the most peripheral veins where they lay eggs: *S. mansoni* goes to the inferior mesenteric vein; *S. haematobium* to the vesical, prostatic and uterine plexuses; and *S. japonicum* to the superior mesenteric veins. Ova either pass through the mucosa into the lumen of the gut or the urinary bladder, or are carried by the blood stream to the various parts of the body.

The path by which eggs reach the CNS is still not clear (Pittella and Lana-Peixoto, 1981). Embolization through the arterial system necessitates the presence of an abnormal pulmonary arteriovenous shunt, but another possible route is anastomoses between the portal and pulmonary circulation via the azygos veins. On the other hand, the concentration of numerous ova in localized areas of the brain suggests that they might be deposited there by a female worm lying either in a cerebral venous sinus or in a large superficial vein (Greenfield and Pritchard, 1937). Faust (1948) suggested that the parasite could reach the CNS through anastomoses between veins of the CNS and the portal system. Although positive evidence of the occurrence of the worm in the human nervous system is scanty (Raper, 1948; Barros et al., 1956; Chitiyo, 1972), the possible migration of adult worms to the brain is supported by the experimental work by Fujinami (cited by Shimidzu, 1935) who found adult schistosomes in the cerebral veins of monkeys exposed to cercariae.

The interval between exposure to infection and the appearance of symptoms ranges from 4 weeks to 2–4 years. In the former case ova are usually abundant in the patient's faeces or urine and the diagnosis is easily made. In cases with later onset, ova may be difficult to find. In the CSF there is usually an increase of protein with a slight to moderate number of lymphocytes, but there are no eosinophils or ova. Lesions of the nervous system can be disseminated or localized. In the former condition, miliary granulomas may be found in all parts of the brain, most commonly in the cerebral and cerebellar cortex and in the deep grey matter. Bassett and Lowenberg (1949) described the appearance at operation of innumerable, shotty, yellow-orange, glistening nodules ranging from 1–2 mm to 0.5 cm in diameter, scattered over the exposed cortical surface of the parietal, temporal and occipital lobes. Localized lesions can mimic tumours or appear as an agglomeration of smaller nodules up to 3 cm in diameter that can be seen on the surface of the brain occasionally invading the dura. In cases where the spinal cord is involved, Brown and Voge (1982) describe the region as being encased within a bulging and tense dural sac; on opening the dura, copious clear fluid was released and numerous whitish nodules 1–2 mm in diameter were seen along the anterior and posterior surfaces of the congested cord at thoracic and lumbar levels sometimes involving the roots.

Histological examination shows chronic inflammation of the leptomeninges and small granulomas (Fig. 8.10). The meningitis consists of lymphocytes, plasma cells, eosinophils and macrophages. The granulomas contain a variable number of ova; these are oval and measure 60–90 μm in length and 40–60 μm in width. When the ova lie singly they may be surrounded by a zone of radially arranged fibroblasts or may be partly enclosed in a multinucleated foreign-body giant cell. When several lie together there is a central zone of pyknotic nuclei surrounded by fibroblasts, epithelioid cells and occasional giant cells. This zone is surrounded in turn by a wall of varying thickness consisting of collagen infiltrated by inflammatory cells. In early lesions these consist mainly of eosinophils which are later replaced by lymphocytes and plasma cells. This fibrous wall may be thick, forming the greater part of the granuloma and giving the mass a firm, rubbery texture. Degenerated nerve cells and swollen astrocytes are seen in the surrounding nervous tissue which is also oedematous. Some arteries can show severe vasculitis. Cases have been described in which the deposition of ova occurred without there being any clinical manifestation or evidence of granulomas. It is clear that the granuloma is formed by the reaction of the host tissue to an irritant or toxic substance in the ova which is present only when ova are viable, as, after treatment with antimony, neurological symptoms usually clear up rapidly.

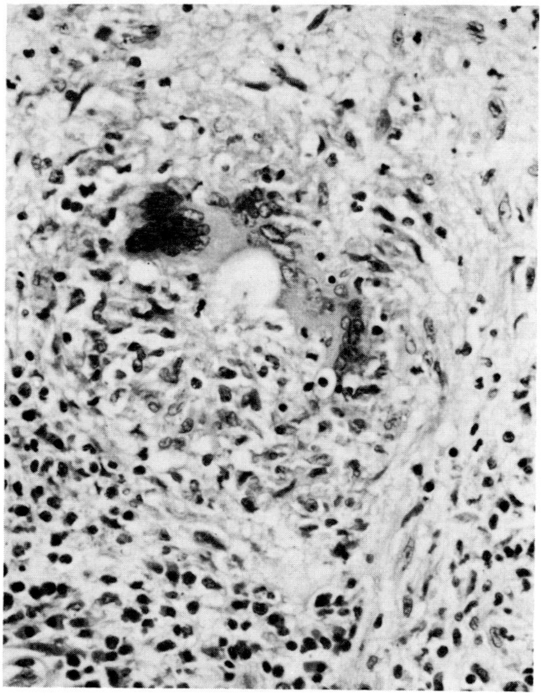

Fig. 8.10 Schistosomiasis (*S. japonicum*). Small granuloma with lymphocytes, epithelioid cells and giant cells. Haematoxylin and eosin × 300. (Courtesy of Dr M. Nielsen.)

Other trematode infections

Trematodes that are normally parasites of animals can accidentally infect man. *Philophthalmus* sp., a parasite of birds, was reported by Dissanaike and Bilimoria (1958) to be responsible for eye involvement in a patient who could have acquired the infection bathing in a stream visited by birds. Another worm, *Alaria americana*, is a parasite of frogs. Shea et al. (1973) reported a case in which the parasite was found in the retina of a patient who became infected by preparing frogs' legs for a meal. A fatal case was reported by Fernandes et al. (1976) in a patient who acquired the infection by eating inadequately cooked frogs' legs: at autopsy there were extensive haemorrhages in almost all viscera; in the CNS there was subarachnoid haemorrhage, petechiae in the cortex and white matter, and thromboses. Mesocercariae of *A. americana* were seen histologically without any cellular reaction around them.

Nematodes

Larva migrans

Under this heading are included three nematodes that have as their definitive hosts mammals other than man. Human infestation is due to ingestion of food contaminated with larvae, the further development of which does not reach the complete maturation. The parasites are *Toxocara*, *Angiostrongylus* and *Gnathostoma*.

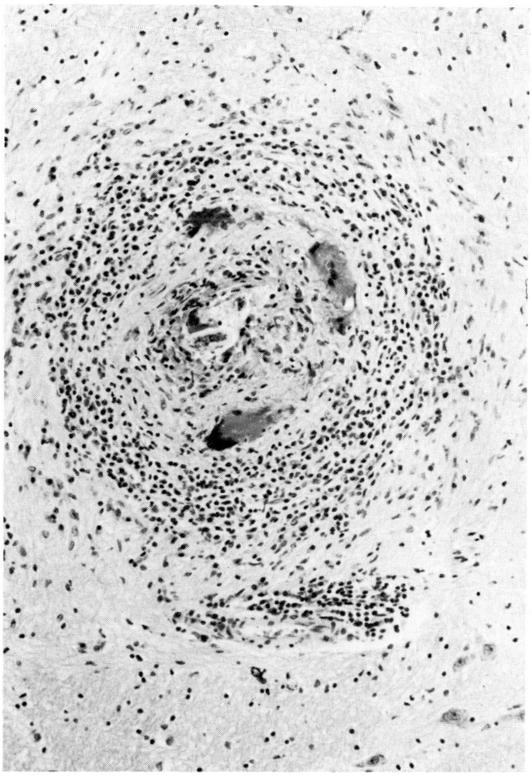

Fig. 8.11 Granulomatous reaction around a larva of *Toxocara canis*. The granuloma was situated in the pons, and shows an outer layer of lymphocytes, plasma cells, eosinophils and fibroblasts, and a central area consisting of epithelioid and multinucleated giant cells. Two segments of the larva are also seen. Haematoxylin and eosin × 400 reduced to 85%. (Courtesy of Dr C. Scholtz.)

Toxocariasis Children acquire this infection by ingesting material contaminated with the ova of *Toxocara canis* or *T. cati*, from dog or cat faeces respectively. The ova may remain viable for months and are frequently mixed with the ova of *Ascaris lumbricoides*, giving rise to mixed infections (Dent et al., 1956). The ova that have been swallowed hatch in the stomach and intestine. Larvae migrate through the intestinal wall to other organs via blood vessels and lymphatics, and although they are unable to complete their life cycle in man they are, nevertheless, capable of a long survival. The resulting clinical syndrome is called 'visceral larva migrans'; before the demonstration of the parasite it was referred to by a variety of terms such as Loeffler's syndrome, tropical eosinophilia and benign eosinophilic leukaemia. It has been proven experimentally in mice (Sprent, 1955) that Toxocara reaches the brain 2 days after infection. The parasite is arrested in a vessel similar in diameter to its size; this then ruptures, with consequent haemorrhage. The death of the parasite is followed by a non-encapsulated granulomatous reaction (Fig. 8.11) consisting of lymphocytes, eosinophils, plasma cells, fibroblasts and epithelioid cells. Such lesions have been found in the leptomeninges, cerebral cortex, brain stem and spinal cord (Dent et al., 1956). The eyes may also be involved, giving rise to a lesion which can be confused with retinoblastoma and leading to unnecessary enucleation of the eye. Pathological investigation of the eye reveals small foci of inflammatory necrosis in the retina, containing lymphocytes and eosinophils with occasional granulomatous areas. Usually the worm or part of it can be recognized.

Angiostrongyliasis The disease is produced by invasion of the CNS by larvae of the rat lung worm *Angiostrongylus cantonensis* that in the adult form lives in the pulmonary arteries of various species of rat and other murine rodents (Jindrak, 1975). The life-cycle consists of ova that, eliminated in the lungs, hatch in 6 days. Larvae infiltrate through the respiratory tract into the digestive system of the rat and are eliminated with the faeces. The first stage larvae are able to survive for long periods and have as intermediate hosts several species of snail or slug in which, through successive stages, they acquire a stage that is infective for mammals. Rats become infected by eating molluscs; larvae penetrate the wall of the stomach and reach the general circulation through the portal vein and liver. The larvae reach the nervous system in two ways: either directly from cerebral blood vessels or by way of a peripheral nerve. They may then enter the subarachnoid spaces.

Man represents an accidental host after the ingestion of infested slugs or snails, and epidemics of the disease have been described among populations in the Pacific Islands and South-East Asia. The migration of larvae has not been observed in man but information about the visceral stage of infection obtained from experimental work may be applicable to man in whom, however, migrating larvae never reach the stomach (Nye et al., 1970).

Lesions in the CNS include: (1) a meningeal reaction with lymphocytes, plasma cells and Charcot–Leyden crystals; (2) tracks made by the worm, some of which may resemble artefacts, but others being surrounded by products of degeneration including fragments of axons, myelin debris and macrophages; (3) a granulomatous reaction with giant cells around dead larvae; and (4) vascular necrosis, thrombosis and infarction. Involvement of the eye was reported by Prommindaroj, Leelawongs and Pradatsundarsar (1962). In cases of involvement of the CNS, the CSF shows pleocytosis with 100–3000 eosinophils/mm^3, and, very occasionally, adult *A. cantonensis* have been recovered from it (Hsieh, 1967).

Gnathostomiasis. *Gnathostoma spinigerum*, the nematode responsible for a form of eosinophilic meningoencephalitis in man, occurs in the adult stage in both wild and domestic dogs and cats and has been reported in Japan, Thailand and the Philippines. The life-cycle of this parasite is similar to that of *A. cantonesis*: eggs eliminated by cats and dogs are ingested by copepods where they reach larval development. Further growth of the larvae occurs in fish, reptiles, amphibians and birds that eat copepods. Man becomes infected by eating raw fish or meat containing larvae that do not mature completely and infiltrate through the subcutaneous tissues from where they can reach the brain, the spinal cord and the eye. They can survive for many years.

The main lesions that are found in the cerebral hemispheres, brain stem and spinal cord are caused by the sexually immature adult, and consist of scattered haemorrhagic foci and areas of necrosis surrounded by oedema and a cellular reaction consisting of eosinophils and macrophages. Granulomas have not been observed. The parasite has occasionally been found in small cystic cavities in the grey matter.

Whilst the definitive diagnosis resides in the recovery of the parasite, eosinophilia is suggestive of the disease. The CSF may contain up to 700 leucocytes/mm^3, with a large proportion of eosinophils.

Onchocerciasis and loiasis

The nematodes responsible for these diseases are, in the adult form, parasites of the subcutaneous tissues of man. Adult forms of *Onchocerca volvulus*, a worm found in Africa and Central and South America, do not cause much damage; females, however, produce microfilariae some of which migrate through the dermis and into the anterior segment of the eye. Others are ingested by flies; after proliferating in the thoracic muscles they move to the proboscis, from where they can return to man where they mature. Onchocerciasis is also known as 'river blindness' because it is spread by flies living near fast-moving water. A detailed description and discussion of the lesions of the eye in onchocerciasis have been given by Buck (1974) and by Brown and Voge (1982). Lesions vary in intensity and in size, ranging from minute corneal opacities with an associated inflammatory reaction to the microfilariae to bullae that result from epithelial detachment from Bowman's membrane and infiltration with neutrophils, eosinophils, plasma cells and lymphocytes. The pupillary opening becomes obscured by exudate, and the cornea becomes vascularized and keratinized. The inflammatory process extends inwards inducing iridocyclitis, and the filtration angle may become occluded with ensuing glaucoma. The melanocytes of the iris can be displaced in the stroma or be extruded into the fluid of the anterior chamber. Pathological changes within the brain and the spinal cord have not been described, yet microfilariae have been found in the CSF (Mazzotti, 1959).

According to Ogumba (1972) 8.9 per cent of the population living on the coasts of West Equatorial Africa suffer from **loiasis**, a condition caused by the larvae of *Loa loa*, a worm with a life-cycle similar to that of *O. volvulus*. Macroscopically the lesions in the CNS consist of mild oedema and small haemorrhages. Histological abnormalities include occlusions of small vessels by microfilariae and perivascular infiltrates and granulomas. Van Bogaert et al. (1955) reported microscopic granulomatous nodules, usually perivascular, scattered throughout the cerebral and cerebellar hemispheres, including the basal ganglia and the brain stem, and containing microfilariae. They consisted of microglial cells, lymphocytes and giant cells, and some of them contained a necrotic area. In addition, the cortical grey matter showed a diffuse microglial proliferation, with rod cells and astrocytic proliferation. Lesions of the other organs include occlusion of the central artery of the retina and multiple small necrotic areas containing microfilariae in the portal spaces of the liver.

Other filarial infections Other filariae are known to infect man. Among these, *Dirofilaria conjunctivae*, *D. repens*, *D. immitis* and *D. tenuis* mainly affect the eye although neurological involvement has also been reported (Dissanaike et al., 1977).

Strongyloidiasis

This infection, caused by *Strongyloides stercoralis*—a nematode with a wide geographical distribution—is most common in the tropics; it is estimated that in some areas of Brazil up to 80 per cent of the population is affected (Meyers, Connor and Neafie, 1976). The worms have a free-living phase in damp, warm soil where they deposit eggs that give rise to rhabditiform larvae. Under adverse conditions rhabditiform larvae become filariform larvae that can infect man by penetrating the skin. In temperate climates, however, infection occurs through contact and ingestion. Larvae reach the lungs from where they are coughed up and swallowed, and they become adult forms in the duodenum. Females produce rhabditiform larvae, some of which are eliminated with the faeces whilst others become filariform larvae which return to the circulation thus completing the endogenous cycle.

In fatal cases the clinical manifestations that include paralytic ileus, malabsorption and meningitis are related by hyperinfection with an altered host–parasite relationship. Rivera et al. (1970) have suggested that this hyperinfectious situation may be produced by drugs that cause paralytic ileus and subsequent reinvasion by larvae.

Pathological findings include the presence of larvae in the subarachnoid space (Owor and Wamukota, 1976) or in microinfarcts produced by obstruction of capillaries by the parasite (Neefe et al. (1973). In a case described by Masdeu et al. (1982) five abscesses were found in the brain in addition to microinfarcts.

Trichinosis

Trichinella spiralis is a nematode of world-wide distribution. Infection in man occurs by eating raw or undercooked pork containing larvae that, after being released from the muscle fibres in the stomach, migrate to the intestine where the male dies after copulation. Females produce embryos that are distributed to various organs via the blood stream. The lethal complications of trichinosis are myocarditis, pneumonitis and involvement of the nervous system, whilst involvement of skeletal muscle is common.

Cerebral involvement is a rare event and only follows infection with a large number of larvae (Brown and Voge, 1982). It can be secondary to embolization from a thrombus in the heart or to an allergic reaction with inflammation of the walls of small vessels. The macroscopic features may be limited to a non-purulent meningitis, mild oedema and occasional small haemorrhages. Histological abnormalities include granulomatous nodules, more numerous in the white than in the grey matter, consisting of lymphocytes, microglia and histiocytes. Larvae may be identifiable in the nodules. Moderate to heavy perivascular lymphocytic infiltrations have been found in the brain and in the meninges. In addition, the subcortical white matter may contain spherical cavities filled with amorphous mucinoid material. Nerve cells can be secondarily involved in the process and show degenerative changes. Larvae can also be found in the brain without there being any surrounding cellular reaction.

Infections by fungi

For practical purposes, fungal infections of the nervous system can be divided into two principal categories: those induced by pathogens, and those produced by saprophytes in patients whose resistance to infection is lowered by conditions such as diabetes, leukaemia, the lymphomas and other disseminated malignant processes, or by the prolonged use of antibiotics, corticosteroids, cytotoxic drugs or immunosuppressive agents. Infections produced by saprophytic fungi are often referred to as *opportunistic* (or opportunist). Lesions in the CNS include meningitis, the formation of abscesses and granulomas, and, because the organisms invade the walls of vessels, the occurrence of thromboses leading to necrosis and infarction of brain tissue.

The types and incidences of mycoses, their evolution and the changes undergone by these diseases in recent years, have been reviewed by Fraser et al (1979). Infection of the brain by a fungus is always secondary to a primary focus elsewhere, usually in the lung or intestine. The site of entry may, however, remain unrecognized and cases are reported in which the only evidence of infection is in the nervous system.

In the identification of fungi in tissue sections, certain staining techniques are of considerable value; for example, the periodic acid–Schiff method and methenamine silver (Fetter, Klintworth and Hendry, 1967). More recently, immunocytological methods have been introduced for the diagnosis of fungal infections. Immunofluorescence has been used more for the identification of microbial (White and McGavran, 1965) than for fungal antigens (Kaplan and Kraft, 1969). Immunoperoxidase, on the other hand, has proved very helpful and relatively easy to perform because it provides permanent material that can be examined with conventional histological methods (Fig. 8.12). Although at present it does not allow one to distinguish between different species of the same fungus (Saeed and Hay, 1981), it can make diagnosis possible in cases where fungi lack some of their characteristic morphological features.

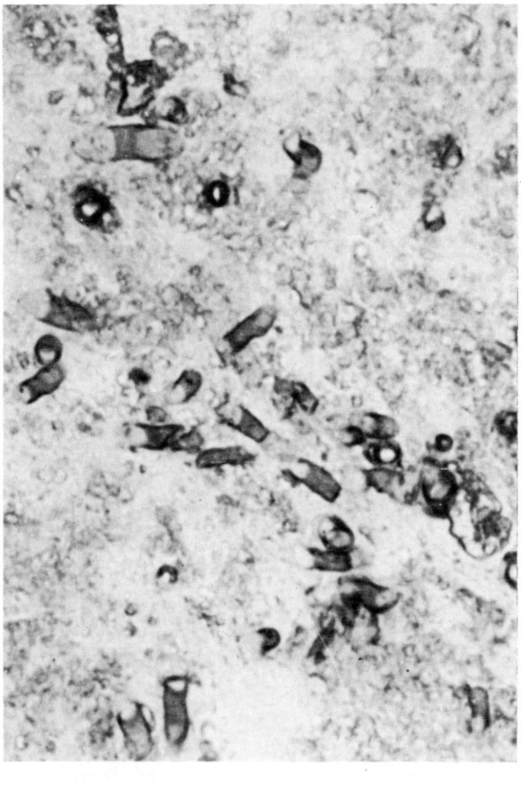

Fig. 8.12 *Aspergillus fumigatus* stained by the immunoperoxidase technique. The walls of the hyphae are shown by the presence of a dark precipitate. × 275. (Courtesy of Dr R.J. Hay.)

Actinomycosis

Actinomyces is a small anaerobic organism of world-wide distribution occurring mainly in rural areas. Infection of the CNS was first reported by Ponfick, in 1882.

The incidence of involvement of the brain is low; Sanford and Voelker (1925) found only eight cases amongst 587 patients with actinomycosis. Lesions in the CNS are usually secondary to a focus elsewhere in the body, spreading to the nervous system either by direct extension (a cervicofacial lesion) or by the blood stream, in the latter case from a thoracic or abdominal focus. Multilocular abscesses are formed with central zones consisting of polymorphs, necrotic debris and colonies of a branching mycelium surrounded by granulation tissue. When the abscess is near the surface, a meningitic reaction may be induced.

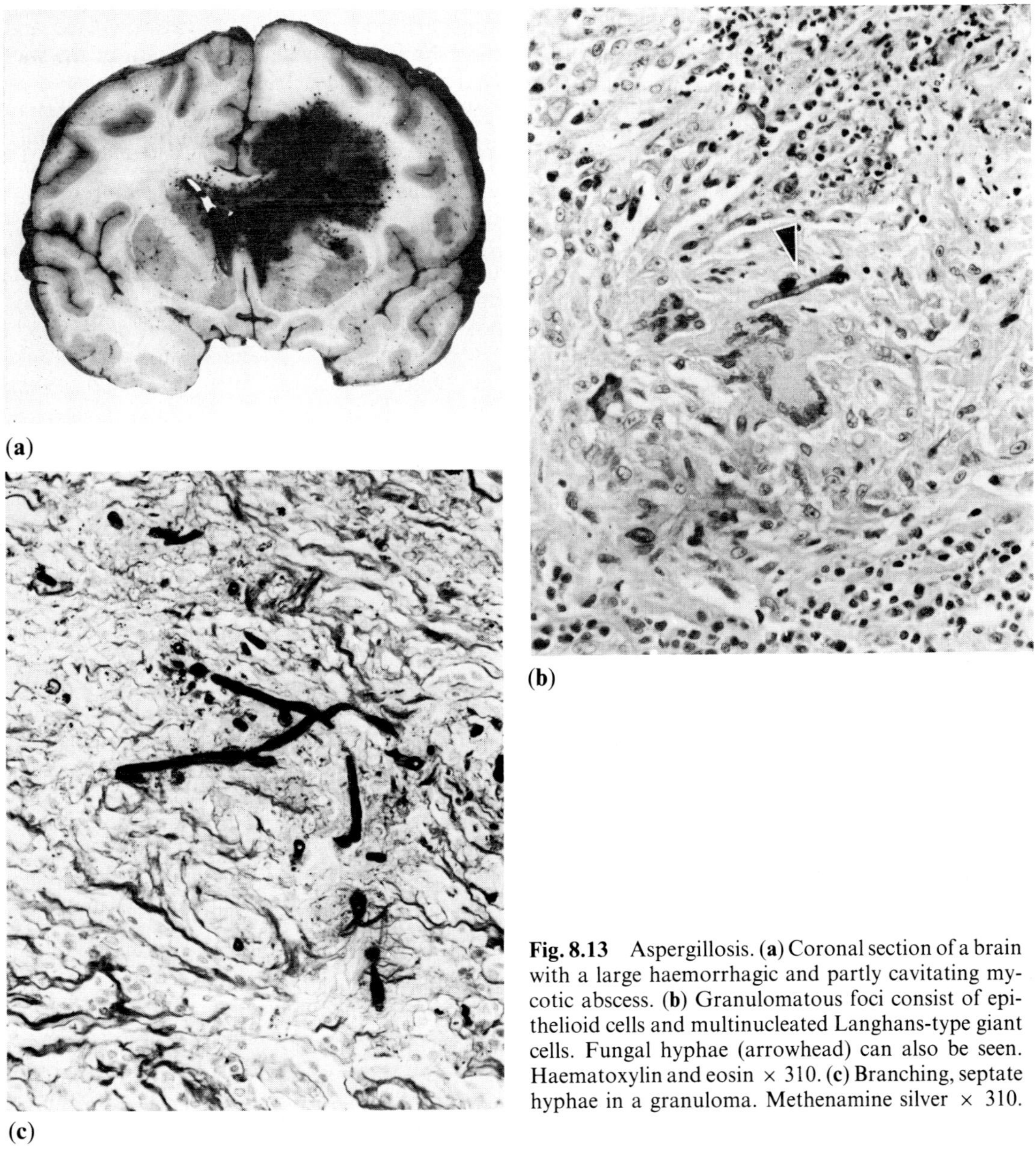

Fig. 8.13 Aspergillosis. (**a**) Coronal section of a brain with a large haemorrhagic and partly cavitating mycotic abscess. (**b**) Granulomatous foci consist of epithelioid cells and multinucleated Langhans-type giant cells. Fungal hyphae (arrowhead) can also be seen. Haematoxylin and eosin × 310. (**c**) Branching, septate hyphae in a granuloma. Methenamine silver × 310.

Aspergillosis

Aspergillus is ubiquitous and over 350 species are known, although only a few are pathogenic in man—amongst them *A. fumigatus*, *A. niger*, *A. flavus* and *A. oryzae*. The organism consists of branching septate hyphae, with a diameter of 3–10 μm.

In man the disease is becoming more common and usually is localized to one site (e.g. the external ear, lungs, or paranasal sinuses). A generalized form with involvement of the CNS is less frequently encountered (MacKenzie, 1979) and usually occurs in patients debilitated by neoplastic or collagen disorders (Pillay et al., 1968; Aisner et al., 1979), drug addiction (Kaufman, Thal and Farmer 1976), alcoholism (Mukoyama, Gimple and Poser, 1969) or immunosuppression (Ingwer et al., 1978).

The true incidence of cerebral involvement is difficult to ascertain. Grčević and Matthews (1959) and Carbone et al. (1964) estimated that 60–70 per cent of cases with disseminated forms of aspergillosis have neurological lesions. More recently, Meyer et al., (1973) found cerebral lesions in nine out of 93 patients suffering from various types of tumour.

The infection may spread to the CNS either directly from the paranasal sinuses (Warder, Chikes and Hudson, 1975) or the orbit (Hedges and Leung, 1976), or blood-borne from the lungs or gastrointestinal tract (Young et al., 1970). perimental intranasal administration of *Aspergillus* spores in mice has shown that direct venous spread may occur from the nasal region to the brain and that this spread is enhanced by concomitant steroid administration (Epstein et al., 1968). In some cases, however, no evident source of infection has been found (Linares, McGarry and Baker, 1971).

Granulomas may develop in the brains of patients with disseminated disease, but commonly abscesses, which may be single or multiple, develop. Meyer et al. (1973) found 50 in a single patient. Their gross appearance is either that of a pale, soft area, sometimes with petechiae, or a necrotic and haemorrhagic lesion with central cavitation (Fig. 8.13a). Histologically, the most striking feature is the intensity of vascular invasion with thrombosis. The amount of inflammation varies according to the stage of the disease and from patient to patient. Polymorphonuclear leucocytes predominate in the early phases whilst treated cases show no inflammatory cells (Young et al., 1970). Granulomas in the brain due to aspergilli occur either in association with a chronic infection (Fetter, Klintworth and Hendry, 1967) or, more rarely, as a solitary lesion (Jackson, Earle and Kuri, 1955; Tveten, 1965). Microscopically, these lesions consist of aggregates of lymphocytes, plasma cells and epithelioid cells with variable amounts of collagen and necrotic tissue. Multinucleated giant cells of Langhans type may also be present as well as fungal hyphae (Fig. 8.13b and c). Blood vessels are always involved and may show thrombosis and invasion of the wall by fungi. In the case reported by Wiles et al. (1981) the lesion was limited to one gasserian ganglion and contained numerous eosinophils. The meninges, overlying both abscesses and granulomas, are involved by a variable amount of exudate.

Treatment of cerebral lesions was ineffective until the recent introduction of combined therapy with amphotericin B and flucytosine, which has been used successfully in four cases (Feely and Steinberg, 1977; Mohandas et al., 1978; Sekhar, Dujouny and Rao, 1980; Wiles et al., 1981).

Blastomycosis

This disease exists predominantly in North American countries and is endemic in the south-eastern regions of the USA, but it has also been reported widely in Africa. The causative agent *Blastomyces dermatitidis*, found in soil and decayed wood, predominantly affects adult males, mainly agricultural workers. The fungus usually gains access to the lungs and spreads to the brain through the blood stream. A primary lesion in the skin has been reported but is rare (Fetter, Klintworth and Hendry, 1967). Although blastomycosis may be a primary disease, it may also occur as an opportunistic infection (Black and Wilson, 1953). The incidence of cerebral involvement in affected cases varies considerably in different pathological studies. Wade and Bel (1916) reported 33 per cent whilst Chick et al. (1956) gave a figure as low as 6 per cent.

In the nervous system, the disease can present as a meningitis or as single or multiple abscesses. The meninges may be involved in the form of an extradural lesion that causes pachymeningitis leading to compression of the underlying brain or spinal cord. When the leptomeninges are involved, the lesion may be diffuse or localized to the base of the brain overlying an abscess. A fibrinopurulent exudate results which may cause an obstructive hydrocephalus and/or become adherent to the dura. This condition can run a subacute or chronic course, and the prognosis is exceedingly poor.

The centre of an abscess contains caseous necrotic material, neutrophils and lymphocytes and is surrounded by epithelioid and multinucleated giant cells of Langhans type, some of which have phagocytosed organisms. Long-standing lesions are enclosed within a thick capsule of hyalinized connective tissue infiltrated with plasma cells.

Blastomyces is usually identifiable in sections stained with haematoxylin and eosin, the fungus appearing as a central basophilic body surrounded by a clear space which presumably corresponds to the lamellar cell wall described in electron micrographs by Mirra, Trombley and Miles (1980). The total size of the yeast varies from 10 to 25 μm. The fungus multiplies by a single bud with a broad base.

The South American form of blastomycosis has also been reported to cause cerebral lesions (Baker, 1972), and is due to *Paracoccidioides brasiliensis*, an organism similar to *B dermatitidis* except for having multiple buds.

Candidosis

Candidosis is a world-wide fungal opportunistic infection due to *Candida* spp. a normal constituent of human flora. It can occur in the oral cavity in infants and as a disseminated disease in individuals suffering from lymphomas, diabetes and other debilitating diseases.

The CNS is only occasionally involved, usually by haematogenous dissemination from a primary focus in the respiratory or gastrointestinal tracts. Yet post-mortem studies have established that candidosis is the most common fungal infection in the CNS, and occurs more frequently than aspergillosis or cryptococcosis (Parker, McCloskey and Lee, 1981). Moreover, Louria, Stiff and Bennett (1962) collected ten cases from the literature in which involvement of the brain occurred in previously healthy persons.

Cerebral lesions occur late in cases with visceral candidosis, and are usually complicated by cardiac and renal lesions (Parker, McCloskey and Lee, 1981). These authors found lesions scattered throughout the brain in 19 cases. In the early stages they resemble haemorrhagic infarcts (Fig. 8.14). Later they consist of abscesses and granulomas without central foci of necrosis. In addition, infarcts may occur as a result of thrombosis of small vessels caused by filaments and budding cells. The cellular reaction around the fungus, which may be minimal, consists of lymphocytes, plasma cells, a few polymorphs and occasional giant cells. Meningitis can also be present.

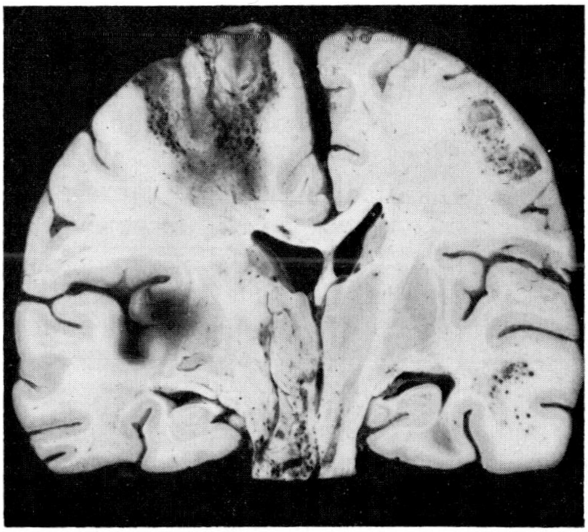

Fig. 8.14 Candidosis. Coronal section of brain showing numerous haemorrhagic areas.

The fungus usually produces pseudohyphae, a chain of elongated cylindrical cells and oval budding cells 2–3 μm long.

Cladosporiosis

The causative agent is a pigmented fungus, *Cladosporium bantianum* (formerly known as *C. trichoides*), a non-opportunistic organism found in temperate regions of all continents. Symmers (1960) reported a personal case and reviewed 14 cases in the literature up to 1960. According to Sandhyamani et al. (1981), who reported two cases, cerebral cladosporiosis is a rare disease.

A primary site for the mycosis is rarely found, although it is assumed (Baker, 1972) to be in the lungs. The paranasal sinuses were involved in the case published by Brown et al. (1976), and an immunological deficiency was present in the case described by Musella and Collins (1974).

The usual manifestation of involvement of the brain is abscess formation (Middleton et al., 1976), with or without meningitis. The characteristic brown colour of the mycelium can be recognized macroscopically. Abscesses can be multiple and may extend into the ventricles. In histological sections, *C. bantianum* appears as hyphae, 2–3 μm in diameter with septa marked by indentations at 5–15 μm intervals. Both hyphae and spores are pigmented. Abscesses, sometimes containing the fungus, consist of lymphocytes, polymorphs, histiocytes and giant cells, and may be surrounded by fibrosis and gliosis. The prognosis is probably good since both patients described by Sandhyamani et al. (1981) survived without specific antimycotic therapy.

Coccidioidomycosis

Coccidioidomycosis is endemic in some southwestern regions of North America (California and Mexico) and in South America, particularly in Argentina and Paraguay. The fungus (*Coccidioides immitis*) is restricted to regions with a semi-arid climate. Fungi and their spores may be carried a considerable distance by wind or by rodents (Baker, 1972). The fungus is not an opportunistic organism. Initially it causes a mild febrile illness, but in a number of cases this is followed by infection of the lungs, leading to the formation of nodules that may calcify. Primary infection of skin occurs more rarely.

The CNS may be involved, usually as a terminal event, as a result of diffuse haematogenous spread. It is estimated that in the USA up to 100 people, mainly black adults, die from this mycosis every year. The majority of patients with involvement of the CNS present as cases of meningitis. At the base of the brain there is commonly thickening, opacity and the formation of small nodules in the meninges. Hydrocephalus or involvement of vessels may follow. Microscopically the lesions consist of granulomas or small abscesses with caseous necrosis and giant cells. Less commonly, there are larger granulomatous lesions within the brain and, occasionally, in the spinal cord.

Fungi occur in tissue as round spherules 20–35 μm in diameter, mature forms containing endospores. They also exist in nature and in culture as hyphae with arthrospores. Budding is rarely observed.

Cryptococcosis

The disease is caused by *Cryptococcus neoformans*, also known as *Torula histolytica*, which usually is harboured in fruit, milk, soil and the manure of some birds. The disease has a worldwide distribution, but most reported cases have occurred in the southern parts of the USA and in Australia. Cryptococcosis affects individuals of all races, predominantly males. The infection sometimes develops spontaneously in previously healthy people, but up to 85 per cent of cases are associated with debilitating diseases (Collins, Gellhorn and Trimble, 1951; Hay et al., 1980). The lungs and the brain are the target organs and involvement of the CNS is thought to be secondary to a focus in the lung, although the latter may not be apparent or can have disappeared several years before manifestation of the cerebral lesion (Palmrose and Losli, 1952).

The majority of cases of cerebral involvement present as a meningitis, in some as a space-occupying lesion. Mortality is high, although remissions have been described (Baker, 1972). The CSF ranges from clear, with only an increase in lymphocytes and protein, to turbid and with a large number of cells, including polymorphs. Cryptococci are often identifiable and may be cultured. The protein also varies greatly, ranging from almost normal to more than 500 mg/dl.

In meningitic forms, the exudate is found mainly at the base, although it may be diffuse and there may be tubercle-like formations, 2–3 mm in diameter, adjacent to blood vessels. Lesions of short duration consist of collections of organisms that distort rather than destroy brain tissue, and there is little or no surrounding inflammatory reaction and gliosis. The absence of inflammatory changes in acute cases is supported by the experimental observations of Bergman (1961) who found a delay between the arrival of organisms and tissue reactions in the brain.

In cases of longer survival there may be hydrocephalus and the formation of cysts in the Virchow–Robin spaces which are distended by organisms, particularly in the superficial layers of the cortex, although more deeply placed cysts of similar appearance have been reported.

The inflammatory response consists of collections of lymphocytes, plasma cells, eosinophils and multinucleated giant cells (Fig. 8.15a). In the latter, nuclei are often more centrally located than in typical Langhans-type cells, and crypto-

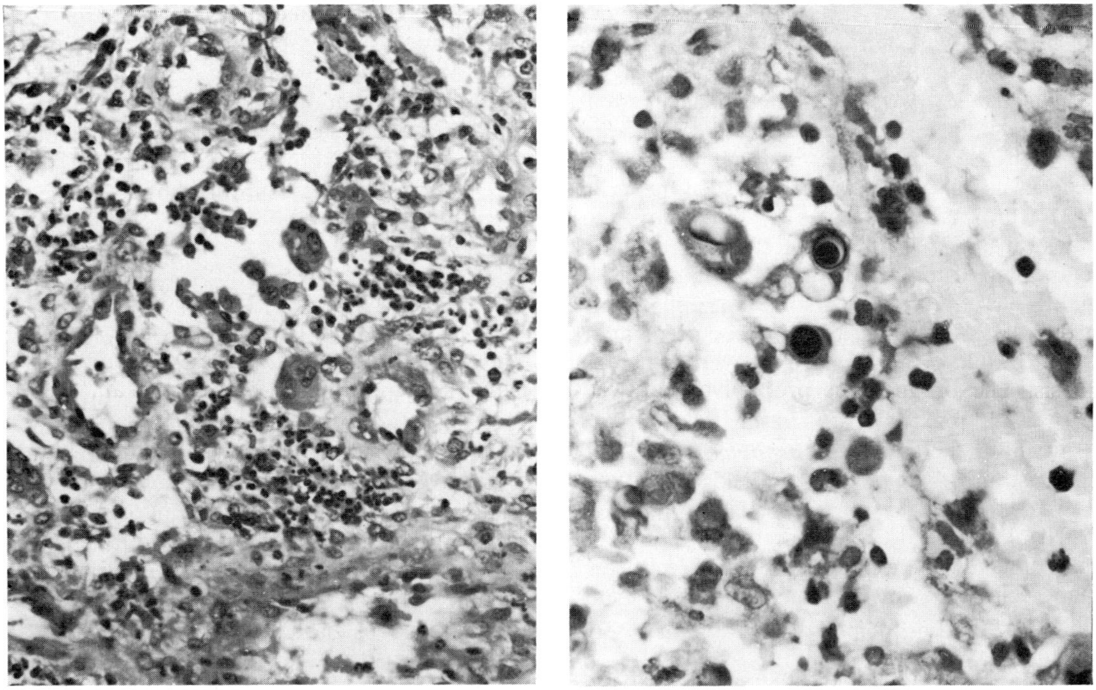

(a) (b)

Fig. 8.15 Cryptococcosis. (**a**) The inflammatory reaction to the fungus includes a few giant cells. Haematoxylin and eosin × 220. (**b**) The fungus appears as a round body surrounded by a capsule. PAS × 500.

cocci (with or without capsules) can frequently be seen within them.

In routinely stained sections (H and E, and PAS) the organism is easily identified (Fig. 8.15b) as a round body, 4–7 μm in diameter, surrounded by a capsule 3–5 μm thick (Binford and Dooley, 1976). Small buds are attached to the main body through a short neck. The classic, simple way of demonstrating the capsule is by adding a few drops of diluted India ink to the fresh preparation. This provides a dark background against which the capsule is clearly seen. The pathologist should be warned, however, that *C. neoformans* has staining reactions similar to corpora amylacea.

Histoplasmosis

The disease is endemic in some regions of the USA (Ohio Valley and Central Mississippi Valley) and cases have also been reported from Brazil, Argentina, Panama, Zimbabwe and Australia. Epidemics have occurred as a result of exposure to chicken, pigeon and starling manure and to bat guano, and have also been observed in the middle-west states of the USA among people working in undergound mines. The fungus, *Histoplasma capsulatum*, can be isolated also from the soil and from domestic and wild animals. The disease originates from the inhalation of air-borne spores. All ages and races and both sexes can be affected but there are two peaks of incidence, one in infancy and childhood, during which the disease involves the reticular system, and the other in the fifth and sixth decades, in which males are predominantly affected.

Histoplasmosis may occur as isolated, benign foci or in a disseminated form which is usually due to reinfection involving the lungs. Despite the freqnency of the disease in endemic zones, involvement of the CNS is uncommon. Baker (1972) has claimed that cerebral infection is invariably secondary to pulmonary infection. Cooper and Goldstein (1963) found involvement of the CNS in 7 per cent of cases of histoplasmosis and suggested that this low frequency is due to the fact that the primary lesions become inactivated and calcified and, unlike tuberculosis, cannot progress. Of 26 cases with lesions in the CNS reported in the English literature and reviewed by them, five had no neurological symptoms or signs, although there was pathological evidence of involvement of the nervous system; six others had clinical and pathological evidence of the disease and in 15 there was meningitis. This last was usually confined to the base of the brain.

In acute cases there are grey and yellow exudates consisting of lymphocytes, plasma cells and macrophages containing organisms but without giant cells. The exudate sometimes surrounds blood vessels and tracks along them for short distances into the brain itself or overlies swollen brain tissue. In chronic cases there is meningeal fibrosis and foci of necrosis in the brain.

A solitary granuloma (*histoplasmoma*) was first described by Cooper and Goldstein (1963). It was localized to the cerebellar vermis and sisted of a central caseous area surrounded by macrophages, lymphocytes, plasma cells and giant cells. The ependyma showed numerous small foci of granuloma with macrophages containing organisms.

The fungus can be identified as small ovoid, PAS positive bodies, 1–5 μm in size. In preparations stained with haematoxylin and eosin they appear much smaller because only the central part of the organism is stained.

An African form of histoplasmosis caused by *H. duboisii* is known to affect man, in whom it produces lesions of skin, subcutaneous tissue and bone. Involvement of CNS has not so far been described.

Nocardiosis

Nocardia asteroides, the causative agent of nocardiosis, is a ubiquitous actinomycete that acts as an opportunistic parasite and is therefore found mainly in patients with debilitating disorders. There is no racial predominance, but men seem to be more susceptible to infection than are women. *Nocardia* has been isolated from water, grass and soil. The CNS is invaded from a primary pulmonary lesion, but there are cases in which no apparent disease was identified outside the brain (Jacobs and Gibson, 1963; King et al., 1966).

Nocardia produces abscesses (Fig. 8.16a) and/or meningitis, but the latter is usually found in

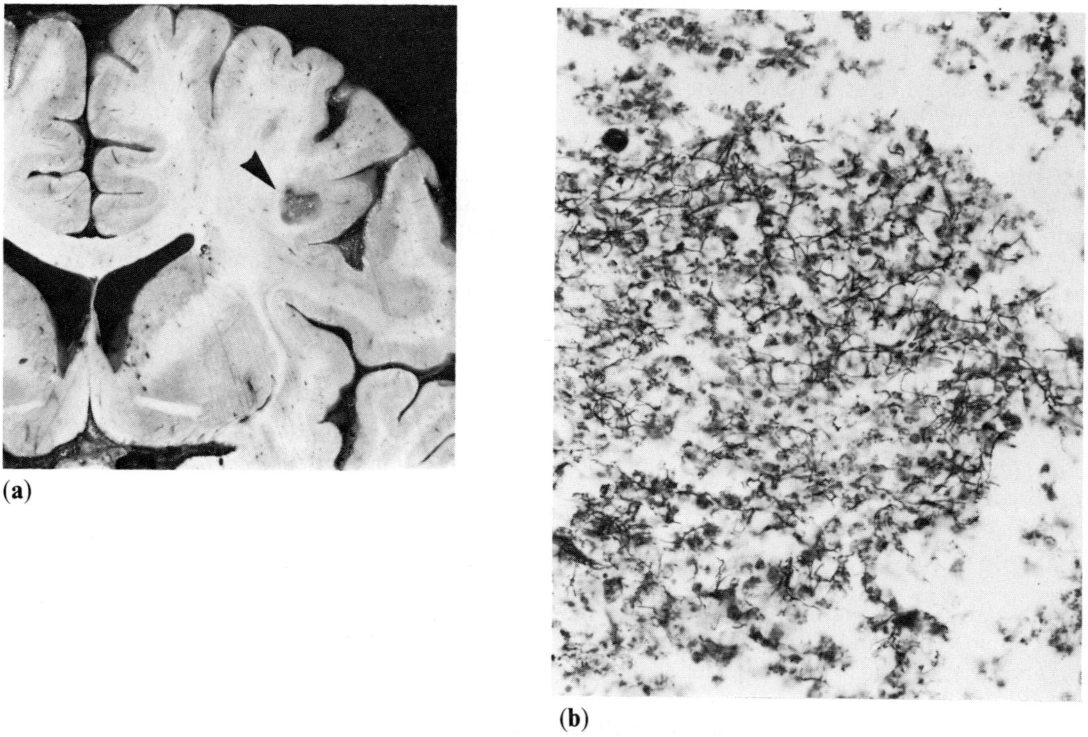

(a) (b)

Fig. 8.16 Nocardiosis. (**a**) Small abscess (arrowhead) in the brain. (**b**) Delicate branching hyphae are seen in the abscess. Methenamine silver × 320. (**b**) Courtesy of Dr M. Nielsen.

contiguity with an underlying abscess. Occasionally the spinal cord also is involved (Welsh, Rhodes and Jacques, 1961). Microscopically the abscesses, which sometimes appear to be produced by the confluence of smaller lesions, have a fibrous wall and consist of neutrophils. Granulomatous reactions are rare (Epstein et al., 1963) and there are no giant cells. The fungi appear as thin branching hyphae, about 1 μm in diameter (Fig. 8.16b). They cannot be recognized in routinely stained preparations but can be identified by using Grocott's methenamine silver stain for a longer time than usual (up to 1 hour).

Zygomycosis (mucormycosis)

The causative agents are opportunistic fungi belonging to the class of *Zygomycetes*. They are ubiquitous and are found in soil, manure and decaying vegetable material. Both sexes and all ages and races are affected. Diabetic patients are particularly susceptible to infection, the predisposing factor, according to Baker (1972), being acidosis rather than hyperglycaemia. Patients being treated with ACTH, steroids, antibiotics and cytostatic drugs as well as drug abusers (Pierce et al., 1982) seem to be more vulnerable than others. The disease usually runs an acute course, death supervening within a few days.

Unlike most other mycoses, in which cerebral involvement is secondary to a primary focus in the lung, cerebral zygomycosis develops most frequently from an infection of the skin of the face or in the mucosa of the nose. In a personal case the infection involved the sphenoidal sinus and the bone of the floor of the sella was necrotic. From the primary sites the infection spreads to surrounding regions and to the arteries of the orbit and the internal carotid arteries with eventual thrombosis. Pathologists should be aware of the possibility of zygomycosis when they are examining a necrotic and inflammatory specimen from the orbital or nasal region of a diabetic

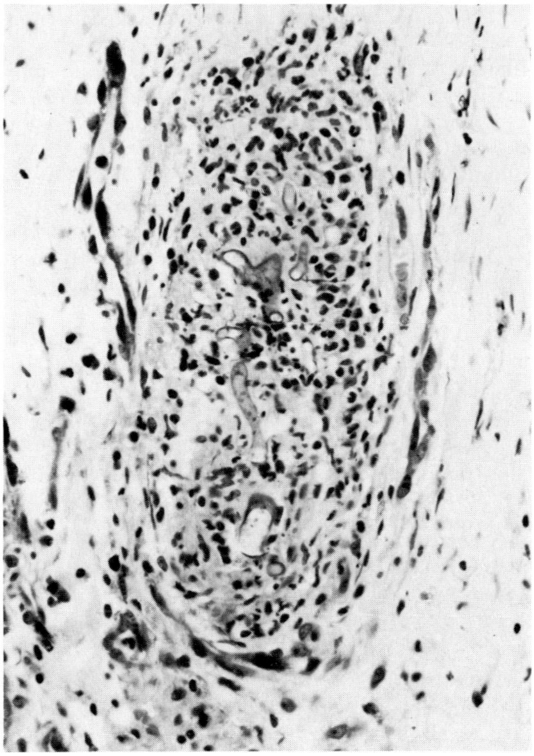

(a)

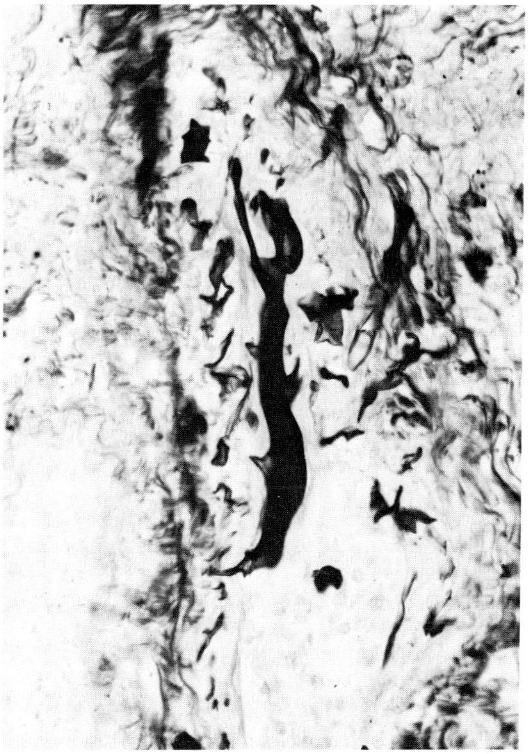

(b)

Fig. 8.17 Zygomycosis. (**a**) The inflammatory reaction is more intense around blood vessels and consists of polymorphs. Hyphae are seen within and throughout the walls of blood vessels. Haematoxylin and eosin × 250. (**b**) The fungal hyphae are broad, irregular and non-septate. Methenamine silver × 310.

patient. The lungs, the gastrointestinal tract or areas of trauma may be alternative, though less frequent, routes of entry.

Microscopically, the inflammatory reaction, which may be absent in areas of infarction, consists of polymorphs and is present mainly around blood vessels; hyphae are also numerous around and within the walls of blood vessels in the meninges and brain (Fig. 8.17a). In only one case (Lie Kian et al., 1956) has a granulomatous reaction with giant cells been observed.

The most characteristic morphological feature of zygomycetes are the broad hyphae (Fig. 8.17b) which range in width from 3 to 12 μm, are non-septate and branch at irregular intervals at right angles.

Other mycoses

In addition to those described above, *Allescheria* (Winston, Jordan and Rhodes, 1977), *Penicillium* (Fetter, Klintworth and Hendry, 1967) and numerous other fungi may be a cause of infection of the CNS. More exhaustive lists with morphological details and biological properties have been reported by Fetter, Klintworth and Hendry (1967), Baker (1972) and Binford and Connor (1976).

References

Aikawa, M., Komata, Y., Asai, T. and Midorikawa, O. (1977) Transmission and scanning electron microscopy of host cell entry by *Toxoplasma gondii. American Journal of Pathology* **87,** 285–96.

Aisner, J., Murillo, J., Schimpff, S.C. and Steere, A.C. (1979) Invasive aspergillosis in acute leukemia: correlation with nose cultures and antibiotic use. *Annals of Internal Medicine* **90,** 4–9.

Alencar, A. (1972) Chagas' disease. In *Pathology of the Nervous System*, vol. 3 (Ed. Minckler, J.), pp. 2559–65. McGraw-Hill, New York.

Apley, J., Clarke, S.K.R., Roome, A.P.C.H., Sandry, S.A., Saygi, G., Silk, B. and Warhurst, D.C. (1970). Primary amoebic meningoencephalitis in Britain. *British Medical Journal* **1,** 596–9.

Arana-Iñiguez, R. (1973) Hydatid echinococcosis of the nervous system. In *Tropical Neurology* (Ed. Spillane, J.D.), pp. 408–17. University Press, London.

Baker, R.D. (1972) Fungus infection of the central nervous system. In *Pathology of the Nervous System*, vol. 3 (Ed. Minckler, J.), pp. 2476–2503. McGraw-Hill, New York.

Barros, O.M., Giannoni, F.G., Marigo, C. and Frizzo, F.J. (1956) Cor pulmonale e miocardite esquistossomóticos. Considerações clínico-patológicas a propósito de dois casos. *Arquivos do Hospital da Santa Casa de São Paulo* **2,** 33–72.

Bassett, R.C. and Lowenberg, K. (1949) Cerebral schistosomiasis. *Journal of Neuropathology and Experimental Neurology* **8,** 220–5.

Becker, G.L., Knep, S., Lance, K.P. and Kaufman, L. (1980) Amebic abscess of the brain. *Neurosurgery* **6,** 192–4.

Bergman, F. (1961) Pathology of experimental cryptococcosis: a study of course and tissue response in subcutaneously induced infection in mice. *Acta Pathologica et Microbiologica Scandinavica* **51,** Suppl. 147, 1–163.

Best, T. and Finlayson, M. (1979) Two forms of encephalitis in opportunistic toxoplasmosis. *Archives of Pathology and Laboratory Medicine* **103,** 693–6.

Binford, C.H. and Connor, D.H. (Eds.) (1976) *Pathology of Tropical and Extraordinary Diseases.* Armed Forces Institute of Pathology, Washington DC.

Binford, C.H. and Dooley, J.R. (1976) Diseases caused by fungi and actinomycetes. Deep mycoses. In *Pathology of Tropical and Extraordinary Diseases*, vol. 2 (Eds. Binford, C.H. and Connor, D.H.), pp. 551–609. Armed Forces Institute of Pathology, Washington DC.

Bittencourt, A.L. (1976) Congenital Chagas' disease. *American Journal of Diseases of Children* **130,** 97–103.

Black, T.C. and Wilson, H.M. (1953) Coexistent pulmonary tuberculosis and systemic blastomycosis: report of case successfully treated with streptomycin, *p*-aminosalicylic acid and stilbamidine. *American Review of Tuberculosis and Pulmonary Diseases* **68,** 615–21.

Bobowski, S.J. and Reed, W.G. (1958) Toxoplasmosis in an adult, presenting as a space-occupying cerebral lesion. *Archives of Pathology* **65,** 460–4.

van Bogaert, L., Dubois, A., Janssens, P.G., Radermecker, J., Tverdy, G. and Wanson, M. (1955) Encephalitis in *Loa-loa* filariasis. *Journal of Neurology, Neurosurgery and Psychiatry* **18,** 103–9.

Brenes Madrigal, R., Rodriguez-Ortiz, B., Vargas Solano, G., Ocampo Obando, E.M. and Ruiz-Sotela, P.J. (1982) Cerebral hemorrhagic lesions produced by *Paragonimus mexicanus.* Report of three cases in Costa Rica. *American Journal of Tropical Medicine and Hygiene* **31,** 522–6.

Brown, J.W. III, Nadell, J., Sanders, C.V. and Sardenga, L. (1976) Brain abscess caused by *Cladosporium trichoides* (*Bantianum*): a case with paranasal sinus involvement. *Southern Medical Journal* **69,** 1519–21.

Brown, W.J. and Voge, M. (1982) *Neuropathology of Parasitic Infections.* Oxford University Press, Oxford.

Buck, A.A. (Ed.) (1974) *Onchocerciasis: symptomatology, pathology, diagnosis.* World Health Organization, Geneva.

Budzilovich, G.N., Most, H. and Feigin, I. (1964) Pathogenesis and latency of spinal cord schistosomiasis. *Archives of Pathology* **77,** 383–8.

Burke, J., Bengoni, K. and Diantete, N.L. (1974) Un cas de trypanosomiase africaine (*T. gambiense*) congénitale. *Annales de la Société Belge de Médecine Tropicale* **54,** 1–4.

Butt, C.G. (1966) Primary amebic meningoencephalitis. *New England Journal of Medicine* **274,** 1473–6.

Cain, A.R., Wiley, P.F., Brownell, B. and Warhurst, D.C. (1981) Primary amoebic meningoencephalitis. *Archives of Disease in Childhood* **56,** 140–3.

Calwell, H.G. (1937) Pathology of brain in Rhodesian trypanosomiasis. *Transactions of the Royal Society of Tropical Medicine and Hygiene* **30,** 611–24.

Carbone, P.P., Sabesin, S.M., Sidranski, H. and Frei, E. III (1964) Secondary aspergillosis. *Annals of Internal Medicine* **60,** 556–67.

Carter, R.F. (1968) Primary amoebic meningo-encephalitis: clinical, pathological and epidemiological features of six fatal cases. *Journal of Pathology and Bacteriology* **96,** 1–25.

Chagas, C. (1909) Nova tripanosomíase humana, *Memórias do Instituto Oswaldo Cruz* **1,** 159–218.

Chick, E.W., Sutliff, W.D., Rakich, J.H. and Furcolow, M.L. (1956) Epidemiological aspects of cases of blastomycosis admitted to Memphis, Tennessee, hospitals during the period 1922–1954: review of 86 cases. *American Journal of the Medical Sciences* **231,** 253–62.

Chitiyo, M.E. (1972) Schistosomal involvement of the choroid plexus. *Central African Journal of Medicine* **18,** 45–7.

Collins, V.P., Gellhorn, A. and Trimble, J.R. (1951) The coincidence of cryptococcosis and disease of the reticulo-endothelial and lymphatic systems. *Cancer* **4,** 883–9.

Connor, D.H., Neafie, R.C. and Meyers, W.M. (1976) Amebiasis. In *Pathology of Tropical and Extraordinary Diseases* (Eds. Binford, C.H. and Connor, D.H.), pp. 379–481. Armed Forces Institute of Pathology, Washington DC.

Cooper, R.A. Jr and Goldstein, E. (1963) Histoplasmosis of the central nervous system. Report of two cases and review of the literature. *American Journal of Medicine* **35,** 45–57.

Culbertson, C.G. (1976) Amebic meningoencephalitis. In *Pathology of Tropical and Extraordinary Diseases* (Eds. Binford, C.H. and Connor, D.H.), pp. 482–545. Armed Forces Institute of Pathology, Washington DC.

Daroff, R.B., Deller, J.J., Kastl, A.J. and Webster-Blocker, W. (1967) Cerebral malaria. *Journal of the American Medical Association* **202,** 679–82.

Daveloose, P. (1972) Un cas de trypanosomiase africaine congénitale. *Annales de la Société Belge de Médicine Tropicale* **52,** 63.

Dent, J.H., Nichols, R.L., Beaver, P.C., Carrera, G.M. and Staggers, R.J. (1956) Visceral larva migrans. With a case report. *American Journal of Pathology* **32,** 777–803.

De Queiroz, A.C. (1973) Tumour-like lesion of the brain caused by *Trypanosoma cruzi. American Journal of Tropical Medicine and Hygiene* **22,** 473–6.

Dissanaike, A.S. and Bilimoria, D.P. (1958) On an infection of the human eye with *Philophthalmus sp.* in Ceylon. *Journal of Helminthology* **32,** 115–18.

Dissanaike, A.S., Ramalingam, S., Fong, A., Pathmayokan, S., Thomas, V. and Kan, S.P. (1977) Filaria in the vitreous of the eye of man in peninsular Malaysia. *American Journal of Tropical Medicine and Hygiene* **26,** 1143–7.

Epstein, S., Holden, M., Feldshun, J. and Singer, J.M. (1963) Unusual cause of spinal cord compression: nocardiosis. *New York Journal of Medicine* **63,** 3422–7.

Epstein, S.M., Miale, T.D., Moossy, J., Verney, E. and Sidransky, H. (1968). Experimental intracranial aspergillosis. *Journal of Neuropathology and Experimental Neurology* **27,** 473–82.

Escobar, A. and Nieto, D. (1972) Parasitic diseases. In *Pathology of the Nervous System*, vol. 3 (Ed. Minckler, J.), pp. 2503–21. McGraw-Hill New York.

Faust, E.C. (1948) An enquiry into the ectopic lesions in schistosomiasis. *American Journal of Tropical Medicine and Hygiene* **28,** 175–99.

Feely, M. and Steinberg, M. (1977) Aspergillus infection complicating transsphenoidal yttrium-90 pituitary implant. Report of two cases. *Journal of Neurosurgery* **46,** 530–2.

Fernandes, B.J., Cooper, J.D., Cullen, J.B., Freeman, R.S., Ritchie, A.C., Scott, A.A. et al. (1976) Systemic infection with *Alaria americana* (*Trematoda*). *Canadian Medical Association Journal* **115,** 1111–14.

Fetter, B.F., Klintworth, G.K. and Hendry, W.S. (1967) *Mycoses of the Central Nervous System.* William and Wilkins, Baltimore.

Fowler, M. and Carter, R.F. (1965) Acute pyogenic meningitis probably due to *Acanthamoeba sp.*: a preliminary report. *British Medical Journal* **2,** 740–2.

Fraser, D.W., Ward, J.I., Ajello, L. and Plikaytis, B.D. (1979) Aspergillosis and other systemic mycoses. The growing problem. *Journal of the American Medical Association* **242,** 1631–5.

Frenkel, J.K. (1972) Toxoplasmosis. In *Pathology of the Nervous System*, vol. 3 (Ed. Minckler, J.), pp. 2521–38. McGraw-Hill New York.

Fulton, J.D. and Harrison, C.V. (1946) Outbreak of *Trypanosoma cruzi* infection in Indian monkeys. *Transactions of the Royal Society of Tropical Medicine and Hygiene* **39,** 513–20.

Ghatak, N.R. and Sawyer, D.R. (1978) A morphologic study of opportunistic cerebral toxoplasmosis. *Acta Neuropathologica* **42,** 217–21.

Grčević, N. and Matthews, W.F. (1959) Pathologic changes in acute disseminated aspergillosis, particularly involvement of the central nervous system. *American Journal of Clinical Pathology* **32,** 536–51.

Greenfield, J.G. and Pritchard, B. (1937) Cerebral infection with *Schistosoma japonicum*. *Brain* **60,** 361–72.

Grunnet, M.L., Cannon, G.H. and Kushner, J.P. (1981) Fulminant amebic meningoencephalitis due to *Acanthamoeba*. *Neurology* **31,** 174–7.

Hawkings, F. and Greenfield, J.G. (1941). Two autopsies on Rhodesiense sleeping sickness: visceral lesions and significance of change in cerebrospinal fluid. *Transactions of the Royal Society of Tropical Medicine and Hygiene* **35,** 155–64.

Hay, R.J., Mackenzie, D.W.R., Campbell, C.K. and Philpot, C.M. (1980) Cryptococcosis in the United Kingdom and the Irish Republic, an analysis of 69 cases. *Journal of Infection* **2,** 13–22.

Hedges, T.R. and Leung, L.E. (1976). Parasellar and orbital apex syndrome caused by aspergillosis. *Neurology* **26,** 117–20.

Hermos, J.A., Healy, G.R., Schultz, M.G., Barlow, J. and Church, W.G. (1970) Fatal human cerebral coenurosis. *Journal of the American Medical Association* **213,** 1461–4.

Hernandez, H.G. (1960) Cerebral cysticercosis. *Arizona Medicine* **17,** 390–3.

Herskowitz, A. (1972) Spinal cord involvement with *Schistosoma mansoni*. *Journal of Neurosurgery* **36,** 494–8.

Houba, V., Allison, A.C., Adeniyi, A. and Houba, J-E. (1971) Immunoglobulin classes and complement in biopsies of Nigerian children with the nephrotic syndrome. *Clinical and Experimental Immunology* **8,** 761–74.

Hsieh, H.C. (1967) *Angiostrongylus cantonensis* and eosinophilic meningitis or meningoencephalitis due to its infection. *Taiwan Clinical Medicine* **3,** 467–71 (in Chinese).

Hutt, M.S.R. and Wilks, N.E. (1971) African trypanosomiasis (sleeping sickness). In *Pathology of Protozoal and Helminthic Diseases with Clinical Correlations* (Ed. Marcial-Rojas, R.A.), pp. 57–68. Williams and Wilkins, Baltimore, Md.

Ingwer, I., McLeish, K.R., Tight, R.R. and White, A.C. (1978) *Aspergillus fumigatus* epidural abscess in a renal transplant recipient. *Archives of Internal Medicine* **138,** 153–4.

Jackson, I.J., Earle, K. and Kuri, J. (1955). Solitary aspergillus ganuloma of the brain. Report of 2 cases. *Journal of Neurosurgery* **12,** 53–61.

Jacobs, L. (1967) Toxoplasma and toxoplasmosis. *Advances in Parasitology* **5,** 1–45.

Jacobs, S.I. and Gibson, R.M. (1963) A fatal case of cerebral abscess due to *Nocardia asteroides*. *Journal of Neurology, Neurosurgery and Psychiatry* **26,** 363–7.

Jager, B.V. and Stamm, W.P. (1972) Brain abscesses caused by free-living amoeba probably of the genus *Hartmannella* in a patient with Hodgkin's disease. *Lancet* **2,** 1343–5.

Janota, I. and Doshi, B. (1979) Cerebral malaria in the United Kingdom. *Journal of Neurology, Neurosurgery and Psychiatry* **32,** 769–72.

Janssen, P., van Bogaert, L. and Haymaker, W. (1956) Pathology of the peripheral nervous system in African trypanosomiasis. A study of seven cases. *Journal of Neuropathology and Experimental Neurology* **15,** 269–87.

Jindrak, K. (1975). Angiostrongyliasis cantonensis (eosinophilic meningitis, Alicata's disease). In *Topics on Tropical Neurology*, vol. 12, pp. 133–64. Contemporary Neurology series (Ed. Hornabrook, R.W.) F.A. Davis, Philadelphia, Pa.

Johnson, C.M. and DeRivas, G.T. (1936) Six new cases of Chagas' disease in Panama, with review of previous cases. *American Journal of Tropical Medicine* **16,** 47–57.

Johnstone, H.G. and Jones, O.W. Jr (1950) Cerebral coenurosis in infant. *American Journal of Tropical Medicine* **30,** 431–41.

Kane, C.A. and Most, H. (1948) Schistosomiasis of the central nervous system. Experiences in World War II and a review of the literature. *Archives of Neurology and Psychiatry* **59,** 141–83.

Kaplan, W. and Kraft, D.E. (1969) Demonstration of pathogenic fungi in formalin-fixed tissues by immunofluorescence. *American Journal of Clinical Pathology* **52,** 420–32.

Kass, E.H., Andrus, S.B., Adams, R.A., Turner, C. and Feldman, H.A. (1952) Toxoplasmosis in the human adult. *Archives of Internal Medicine* **89,** 759–82.

Kaufman, D.M., Thal, L.J. and Farmer, P.M. (1976)

Central nervous system aspergillosis in two young adults. *Neurology* **26,** 484–8.

Kernohan, J.W., Magath, T.B. and Schloss, G.T. (1960) Granuloma of brain probably due to *Endolimax williamsi* (*Iodamoeba bütschlii*). *Archives of Pathology* **70,** 576–80.

King, R.B., Stoops, W.L., Fitzgibbons, J. and Bunn, P. (1966) *Nocardia asteroides* meningitis. A case successfully treated with large doses of sulfadiazine and urea. *Journal of Neurosurgery* **24,** 749–51.

Köberle, F. (1968). Chagas' disease and Chagas' syndromes: the pathology of American trypanosomiasis. In *Advances in Parasitology*, vol. 6 (Ed. Dawes, B.), pp. 63–116. Academic Press, London.

Krick, J.A. and Remington, J.S. (1978) Current concepts in parasitology. Toxoplasmosis in the adult. An overview. *New England Journal of Medicine* **298,** 550–3.

Kuper, S., Mendelow, H. and Proctor, N.S.F. (1958) Internal hydrocephalus caused by parasitic cysts. *Brain* **81,** 235–42.

Langmaid, C. and Rogers, L. (1940) Intracranial hydatids. *Brain* **63,** 184–90.

Laranja, F.S., Dias, E., Nobrega, G. and Miranda, A. (1956) Chagas' disease, a clinical, epidemiologic and pathologic study. *Circulation* **14,** 1035–60.

Larroche, J.C. (1977) *Developmental Pathology of the Neonate*. Excerpta Medica, Amsterdam.

Latovitzki, N., Abrams, G., Clark, C., Mayeux, R., Ascherl, G. Jr and Sciarra, D. (1978) Cerebral cysticercosis. *Neurology* **28,** 838–42.

Levine, N.D. (1961) *Protozoan Parasites of Domestic Animals and of Man*. Burgess Publishing, Minneapolis, Minn.

Lie Kian, J., Njo-Injo Tjoei Eng, Ponan, A. and Van der Muellen, H. (1956) *Basidiobolus ranarum* as a cause of subcutaneous mycosis in Indonesia. *Archives of Dermatology* **74,** 378–83.

Linares, G., McGarry, P.A. and Baker, R.D. (1971) Solid solitary aspergillotic granuloma of the brain. Report of a case due to *Aspergillus candidus* and review of the literature. *Neurology* **21,** 177–84.

Lindberg, R.E. and Frenkel, J.K. (1977) Toxoplasmosis in nude mice. *Journal of Parasitology* **63,** 219–21.

Lombardo, L., Alonso, P., Saénz Arroyo, L., Brandt, H. and Mateos, J.H. (1964) Cerebral amebiasis. Report of 17 cases. *Journal of Neurosurgery* **21,** 704–9.

Louria, D.B., Stiff, D.P. and Bennett, B. (1962) Disseminated moniliasis in the adult. *Medicine* **41,** 307–37.

McCormick, G.F., Zee, C.-S. and Heiden, J. (1982) Cysticercosis cerebri. Review of 127 cases. *Archives of Neurology* **39,** 534–9.

MacKenzie, D.W.R. (1979) Imported fungal infections. *Postgraduate Medical Journal* **55,** 595–7.

Maegraith, B. (1974) Other pathological processes in malaria. *Bulletin of the World Health Organization* **50,** 187–93.

Malamos, B. (1935) Über Vorkommen von Schyzotrypanum cruzi bei Affen in Niederländisch-Indien. *Archiv für Schiffs und Tropenhygiene* **39,** 156–71.

Manuelidis, E.E. (1972). Trypanosomal encephalitides. In *Pathology of the Nervous System*, vol. 3 (Ed. Minckler, J.), pp. 2545–59. McGraw-Hill, New York.

Marcial-Rojas, R.A. and Fiol, R.E. (1963) Neurologic complications of schistosomiasis. Review of the literature and report of two cases of transverse myelitis due to *S. mansoni*. *Annals of Internal Medicine* **59,** 215–30.

Marsden, P.D. and Bruce-Chwatt, L.J. (1975) Cerebral malaria. In *Topics on Tropical Neurology*, vol. 12, pp. 29–44. Contemporary Neurology series (Ed. Hornabrook, R.W.). F.A. Davis, Philadelphia, Pa.

Martinez, A.J. (1980) Is acanthamoebic encephalitis an opportunistic infection? *Neurology* **30,** 567–74.

Martinez, A.J. (1982) Acanthamoebiasis and immunosuppression. *Journal of Neuropathology and Experimental Neurology* **41,** 548–57.

Martinez, A.J., Duma, R.J., Nelson, E.C. and Moretta, F.L. (1973) Experimental Naegleria meningoencephalitis in mice. Penetration of the olfactory mucosal epithelium by *Naegleria* and pathologic changes produced: a light and electron microscope study. *Laboratory Investigation* **29,** 121–33.

Martinez, A.J., Garcia, C.A., Halks-Miller, M. and Arce Vela, R. (1980) Granulomatous amebic encephalitis presenting as a cerebral mass lesion. *Acta Neuropathologica* **51,** 85–91.

Masdeu, J.C., Tantulavanich, S., Gorelick, P.P., Maliwan, N., Heredia, S., Martinez-Lage, J.M. et al. (1982) Brain abscess caused by *Strongyloides stercosalis*. *Archives of Neurology* **39,** 62–3.

Mazzotti, L. (1959) Presencia de microfilarias de *Onchocerca volvulus* en el liquido cefaloraquideo de enfermos tratados con hetrazan. *Revista del Instituto de Salubridad y Enfermedades tropicales* **19,** 1–5.

Meyer, R.D., Young, L.S., Armstrong, D. and Yu, B. (1973) Aspergillosis complicating neoplastic disease. *American Journal of Medicine* **54,** 6–15.

Meyers, W.M., Connor, D.H. and Neafie, R.C. (1976) Strongyloidiasis. In *Pathology of Tropical and Extraordinary Diseases*, vol. 2 (Eds. Binford, C.H. and Connor, D.H.), pp. 428–32. Armed Forces Institute of Pathology, Washington DC.

Middleton, F.G., Jurgenson, P.F., Utz, J.P., Shadomy, S. and Shadomy, H.J. (1976) Brain abscess caused by *Cladosporium trichoides. Archives of Internal Medicine* **136,** 444–8.

Migasena, P. and Maegraith, B. (1967) Pharmacological action of antimalarial drugs. Action of chloroquine and hydrocortisone on blood–brain barrier in *Plasmodiun knowlesi* malaria. *Transactions of the Royal Society of Tropical Medicine and Hygiene* **61,** 6.

Mirra, S.S., Trombley, I.K. and Miles, M.L. (1980) Blastomycoma of the cerebellum. An ultrastructural study. *Acta Neuropathologica* **50,** 109–14.

Miyazaki, I. and Nishimura, K. (1975) Cerebral paragonimiasis. In *Topics on Tropical Neurology*, vol. 12, pp. 109–31. Contemporary Neurology series (Ed. Hornabrook, R.W.), F.A. Davis, Philadelphia, Pa.

Mohandas, S., Ahuja, G.K., Sood, V.P. and Virmani, V. (1978) Aspergillosis of the central nervous system. *Journal of the Neurological Sciences* **38,** 229–33.

Mukoyama, M., Gimple, K. and Poser, C.M. (1969) Aspergillosis of the central nervous system. Report of a brain abscess due to *A. fumigatus* and review of the literature. *Neurology* **19,** 967–74.

Musella, R.A. and Collins, G.H. (1974) Cerebral chromoblastomycosis: case report. *Journal of Neurology* **35,** 219–22.

Neefe, L.I., Pinilla, O., Garagusi, V.F. and Bauer, H. (1973) Disseminated strongyloidiasis with cerebral involvement. A complication of corticosteroid therapy. *American Journal of Medicine* **55,** 832–8.

Nye, S.W., Tangchai, P., Sundarakiti, S. and Panyagupta, S. (1970) Lesions of the brain in eosinophilic meningitis. *Archives of Pathology* **89,** 9–19.

Odunjo, E.O. (1969) Pathological manifestations of amoebiasis in Nigerians. *West African Medical Journal* **18,** 117–20.

Ogumba, E.O. (1972) Ecology of human loiasis in Nigeria. *Transactions of the Royal Society of Tropical Medicine and Hygiene* **66,** 743–8.

Olivé, J.I. and Angulo-Rivero, P. (1962) Panel discussion: Cysticercosis of the nervous system. 1. introduction and general aspects. *Journal of Neurosurgery* **19,** 632–4.

Orihel, T.C., Gonzales, F. and Beaver, P.C. (1970) Coenurus from neck of Texas woman. *American Journal of Tropical Medicine and Hygiene* **19,** 255–7.

Owor, R. and Wamukota, W.N. (1976) A fatal case of strongyloidiasis with *Strongyloides* larvae in the meninges. *Transactions of the Royal Society of Tropical Medicine and Hygiene* **70,** 497–9.

Palmrose, E.C. and Losli, E.J. (1952) Cryptococcus meningitis: report of two cases. *Northwest Medicine* **51,** 121–6.

Parker, J.C. Jr, McCloskey, J.J. and Lee, R.S. (1981) Human cerebral candidosis. A postmortem evaluation of 19 patients. *Human Pathology* **12,** 23–8.

Parmer, L.G. and Cottrill, C.W. (1949) Distribution of emetine in tissues. *Journal of Laboratory and Clinical Medicine* **34,** 818–21.

Phillips, G. (1948) Primary cerebral hydatid cyst. *Journal of Neurology, Neurosurgery and Psychiatry* **11,** 44–52.

Pierce, P.F., Solomon, S.L., Kaufman, L., Garagusi, V.F., Parker, R.H. and Ajello, L. (1982) Zygomycetes brain abscesses in narcotic addicts with serological diagnosis. *Journal of the American Medical Association* **248,** 2881–2.

Pillay, V.K.G., Wilson, D.M., Ing, T.S. and Kark, R.M. (1968) Fungus infection in steroid-treated systemic lupus erythematosus. *Journal of the American Medical Association* **205,** 261–5.

Pittella, J.E. and Lana-Peixoto, M.A. (1981) Brain involvement in hepatosplenic Schistosomiasis mansoni. *Brain* **104,** 621–32.

Poltera, A.A. (1980) Immunopathological and chemotherapeutic studies in experimental trypanosomiasis with special reference to the heart and brain. *Transactions of the Royal Society of Tropical Medicine and Hygiene* **74,** 706–15.

Poltera, A.A., Lambert, P.H. and Miescher, P.A. (1979) Immunopathology of cerebral trypanosomiasis in mice. In *Proceedings of the Menarini Symposium on Immunopathology of the Central and Peripheral Nervous System* (Ed. Miescher, P.A.), pp. 156–64. Schwave, Basle.

Ponfick, E. (1882) *Die Aktinomykose des Menchen.* A. Hirschwald, Berlin.

Poser, C.M. (1969) Disseminated vasculomyelinopathy. A review of the clinical and pathologic reactions of the nervous system in hyperergic diseases. *Acta Neurologica Scandinavica* suppl. 37, 3–44.

Powell, H.C., Gibbs, C.J. Jr, Lorenzo, A.M. Lampert, P.W. and Gajdusek, D.C. (1978) Toxoplasmosis of the central nervous system in the adult. Electron microscopic observations. *Acta Neuropathologica* **41,** 211–16.

Prommindaroj, K., Leelawongs, N. and Pradatsundarsar, A. (1962) Human angiostrongyliasis of the eye of Bangkok. *American Journal of Tropical Medicine and Hygiene* **1,** 759–61.

Raper, A.B. (1948) Cerebral schistosomiasis. *East African Medical Journal* **25,** 262–3.

Remington, J.S. and Klein, J.O. (Eds.) (1976) *Infectious Diseases of the Fetus and Newborn Infant.* W.B. Saunders, Philadelphia, Pa.

Rest, J.R. and Wright, D.H. (1979) Electron microscopy of cerebral malaria in golden hamsters (*Mesocricetus auratus*) infected with *Plasmodium berghei. Journal of Pathology* **127,** 115–20.

Rivera, E., Maldonado, N., Vélez-García, E., Grillo, A.J. and Malaret, G. (1970) Hyperinfection syndrome with *Strongyloides sterconalis*. *Annals of Internal Medicine* **72,** 199–204.

Robertson, J.S. (1962) Toxoplasmosis. *Developmental Medicine and Child Neurology* **4,** 507–18.

Rothrock, J.F. and Buchsbaum, H.W. (1980) Primary amebic meingoencephalitis. *Journal of the American Medical Association* **243,** 2329–30.

Saeed, El.N. and Hay, R.J. (1981) Immunoperoxidase staining in the recognition of Aspergillus infections. *Histopathology* **5,** 437–44.

Samily, E. and Zadeh, F.A. (1965) Cranial and intracranial hydatidosis. With special reference to Roentgen-ray diagnosis. *Journal of Neurosurgery* **22,** 425–33.

Sandhyamani, S., Bhatia, R., Mohapatra, L.N. and Roy, S. (1981) Cerebral cladosporiosis. *Surgical Neurology* **15,** 431–4.

Sanford, A.H. and Voelker, M. (1925) Actinomycosis in the United States. *Archives of Surgery* **11,** 809–41.

Seidel, J.S., Harmatz, P., Visvesvara, G.S., Cohen, A., Edwards, J. and Turner, J. (1982) Successful treatment of primary amebic meningoencephalitis. *New England Journal of Medicine* **306,** 346–8.

Sekhar, L.N., Dujouny, M. and Rao, G.R. (1980) Carotid-cavernous sinus thrombosis caused by *Aspergillus fumigatus*. *Journal of Neurosurgery* **52,** 120–5.

Shea, M., Maberley, A.I., Walters, J., Freeman, R.S. and Fallis, A.M. (1973) Intraretinal larval trematode. *Transactions of the American Academy of Opthalmology and Oto-laringology* **77,** 784–91.

Shimidzu, K. (1935) Ein Operationsfall von Schistosomiasis cerebri. *Archiv für klinische Chirurgie* **182,** 401–7.

Sprent, J.F.A. (1955) On invasion of the central nervous system by nematodes; invasion of the nervous system by ascariasis. *Parasitology* **45,** 41–55.

Symmers, W. St C. (1960) A case of cerebral chromoblastomycosis (cladosporiosis) occurring in Britain as a complication of polyarteritis treated with cortisone. *Brain* **83,** 37–51.

Tafuri, W.L. (1970) Pathogenesis of lesions of the autonomic nervous system of mouse in experimental Chagas' disease. Light and electron microscope studies. *American Journal of Tropical Medicine and Hygiene* **19,** 405–17.

Templeton, A.C. (1968) Human coenurosis infection: a report of 14 cases from Uganda. *Transactions of the Royal Society of Tropical Medicine and Hygiene* **62,** 251–5.

Toro, G. and Román, G. (1978) Cerebral malaria. A disseminated vasculomyelopathy. *Archives of Neurology* **35,** 271–5.

Traub, N., Hira, P.R., Chintu, C. and Mhango, C. (1978) Congenital trypanosomiasis: report of a case due to *Trypanosoma brucei rhodesiense*. *East African Medical Journal* **55,** 477.

Tveten, L. (1965) Cerebral mycosis. A clinicopathological report of four cases. *Acta Neurologica Scandinavica* **41,** 19–33.

Vijayan, G.P., Venkataraman, S., Suri, M.L., Seth, H.N. and Hoon, R.S. (1977) Neurological and related manifestations of cysticercosis. *Tropical and Geographical Medicine* **29,** 271–8.

Wade, H.W. and Bel, G.S. (1916) A critical consideration of systemic blastomycosis with notes of certain special features and report of 5 cases. *Archives of Internal Medicine* **18,** 103–30.

Warder, F.R., Chikes, P.G. and Hudson, W.R. (1975) Aspergillosis of the paranasal sinuses. *Acta Otolaryngologica* **101,** 683–5.

Welsh, J.D., Rhodes, E.R. and Jacques, W. (1961) Disseminated nocardiosis involving spinal cord. Case report. *Archives of Internal Medicine* **108,** 73–9.

White, J.D. and McGavran, M.H. (1965) Identification of *Pasteurella tularensis* by immunofluorescence. *Journal of the American Medical Association* **194,** 294–6.

Wiles, C.M., Kocen, R.S., Symon, L. and Scaravilli, F. (1981) Aspergillus granuloma of the trigeminal ganglion. *Journal of Neurology, Neurosurgery and Psychiatry* **44,** 451–5.

Winston, D.J., Jordan, M.C. and Rhodes, J. (1977) *Allescheria boydii* infections in the immunosuppressed host. *American Journal of Medicine* **63,** 830–5.

Wolf, A. and Cowen, D. (1937) Granulomatous encephalomyelitis due to *Encephalitozoon* (encephalitozoic encephalomyelitis); new protozoan disease of man. *Bulletin of the Neurological Institute of New York* **6,** 306–71.

Wood, J.N., Hudson, L., Jessell, T.M. and Yamamoto, M. (1982) A monoclonal antibody defining antigenic determinants on subpopulations of mammalian neurones and Trypanosoma *cruzi* parasites. *Nature* (*London*) **296,** 34–8.

Young, R.C., Bennett, J.E., Vogel, C.L., Carbone, P.P. and De Vita, T.T. (1970) Aspergillosis. The spectrum of the disease in 98 patients. *Medicine* **49,** 147–73.

Zeledón, R. (1974) Epidemiology, modes of transmission and reservoir hosts of Chagas' disease. In *Trypanosomiasis and Leishmaniasis with Special Reference to Chagas' Disease*, Ciba Foundation Symposium no. 20, pp. 51–77. Elsevier, Amsterdam.

9

Demyelinating diseases

Ingrid V. Allen

The concept and classification of demyelinating disease

The group of disorders known as the *demyelinating diseases* are, with a few rare exceptions, of unknown aetiology and include conditions with differing clinical, epidemiological and pathological features. All, however, have as a cardinal pathological feature *periaxial demyelination*—i.e. myelin destruction with relative axonal preservation—and it is this characteristic which has given rise to the unifying concept of demyelinating disease. These conditions are not to be confused with genetic disorders of myelin formation (i.e. dysmyelination) or with diseases causing myelin breakdown secondary to neuronal destruction (i.e. neuronolytic demyelination or wallerian degeneration). Other conditions of known aetiology, in which periaxial demyelination may occur (e.g. viral infections or intoxications) differ in that demyelination is not the sole or predominant histological abnormality, and these are not therefore included in the category of primary demyelinating diseases even though demyelination may be prominent in them.

The exclusion of genetic disorders of myelin and of disorders associated with axon degeneration and other pathological processes leaves a group of diseases which may be further categorized into those in which the demyelinating disorder is apparently the sole disease process, and a second, much rarer, group in which demyelination occurs in the presence of an associated systemic disease. The former group is by far the more important and includes those conditions commonly referred to as the *primary demyelinating diseases* (Table 9.1). Because the cause of most of these diseases is unknown, classification is based on clinical and pathological description, although recent immunological studies may allow further subclassification. The more uncommon demyelinating disorders associated with systemic diseases are included in the overall classification of demyelinating disease for the sake of completeness. Genetic disorders of myelin, as already stated, are not included in the category of demyelinating disease. These conditions have in the past, however, been confused with Schilder's disease and it is only comparatively recently that this confusion has been resolved. Those genetic disorders associated with known enzyme deficiencies are dealt with in Chapter 12. The X-linked leucodystrophies are documented at the end of this chapter but, for the stated reasons, are not included in the table of demyelinating diseases.

Table 9.1 Classification of demyelinating diseases

Acute disseminated perivenous encephalomyelitis (*acute perivascular myelinoclasis*)
Classic (parainfectious; postimmunization; idiopathic).
Hyperacute (acute haemorrhagic leucoencephalitis)
Multiple sclerosis (*disseminated sclerosis*)
Classic (Charcot type)
Acute (Marburg type)
Diffuse cerebral sclerosis (Schilder type)
Concentric sclerosis (Balò type)
Neuromyelitis optica (Dévic type)
Demyelinating disorders associated with systemic disease
Central pontine myelinolysis
Marchiafava–Bignami disease
Progressive multifocal leucoencephalopathy (see Chapter 7)

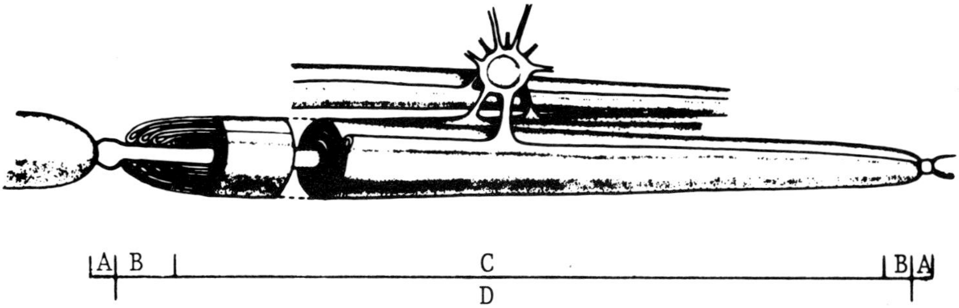

Fig. 9.1 Perspective scale drawing of the interrelationships between the oligodendroglial cell, its processes and the myelin sheath in central nervous tissue. A, node; B, paranodal region; C, perinodal region; D, internode. (Reproduced, with permission from Rumsby, 1978)

Mechanisms and histochemistry of demyelination

In understanding the histological and histochemical changes which occur in the brain and spinal cord secondary to periaxial demyelination, some understanding of the structure and chemistry of myelin is essential (recent reviews include that of Gregson, 1983). Normal myelin has a complicated molecular structure and is formed by modification of the oligodendrocytic cell membrane. The interfascicular oligodendrocyte, unlike the perineuronal satellite oligodendrocyte, has cell processes, each of which forms a segment of the myelin sheath of an axon (Fig. 9.1). It has been calculated that an individual oligodendrocyte may have two or more such processes and may therefore have connection with an equal number of myelin segments, located on one or more axons (Sternberger et al., 1978). Periaxial demyelination occurs through a variety of mechanisms (Table 9.2) which may produce damage to the 'parent' oligodendrocyte, direct damage to the myelin sheath or simultaneous damage to the myelin sheath and the oligodendrocyte cell body.

Much experimental work in recent years has concentrated on immune-mediated demyelination which may be a B-cell effect (Johnson and Bornstein, 1978), a T-cell effect (Lampert, 1983), a T-cell-mediated 'bystander' effect (Wisniewski and Bloom, 1975) or a combined T- and B-cell effect (Raine and Traugott, 1982). Most of the studies of mechanisms of demyelination have been experimental and little is known of mechanisms operating in human disease.

The postulated chemical and known ultrastructural features of myelin are shown in Fig. 9.2. Biochemical and x-ray diffraction studies have contributed to our knowledge of the molecular structure of the myelin sheath which accounts for its histochemical and physical properties. The earliest changes in periaxial demyeli-

Table 9.2 Known causes and mechanisms of primary demyelination in the central nervous system

Primary site of lesion	Cause and mechanism	Human disease	Animal disease
Oligodendrocyte	1 Viral; cytolytic	1 Progressive multifocal leucoencephalopathy	1 JHM mouse hepatitis virus
	2 Chemical; cytolytic	2 Cyanide toxicity	2 Cuprizone toxicity
Myelin sheath	Virus-induced immunological	Herpes simplex	Semliki Forest virus
Myelin sheath	Immunological (various mechanisms)	Acute disseminated perivenous encephalomyelitis	Experimental allergic encephalomyelitis
Myelin sheath	Chemical	Hexachlorophane toxicity	Lysolecithin toxicity
Myelin sheath	Physical	?	Cerebrospinal fluid barbotage

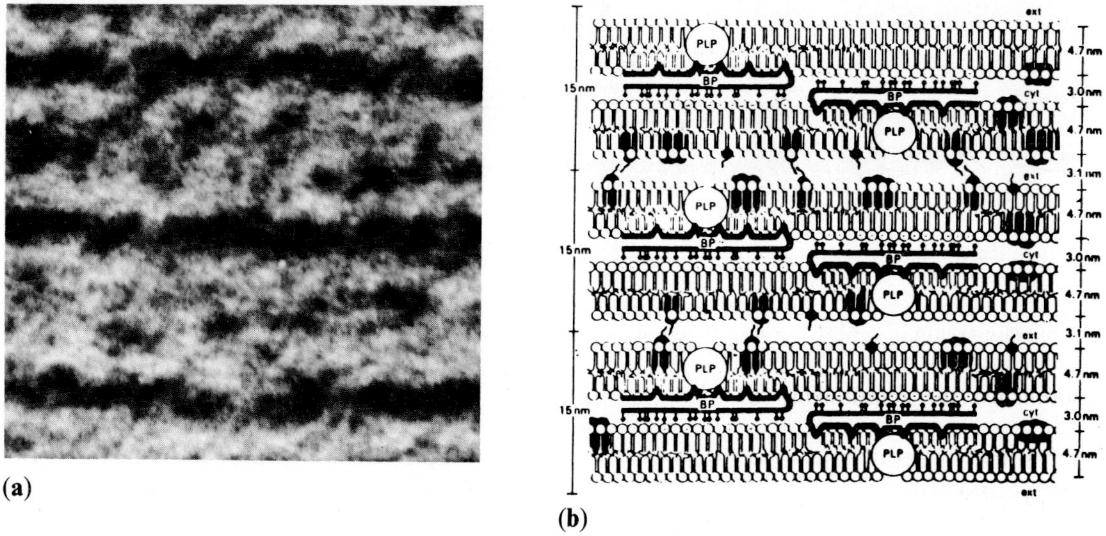

Fig. 9.2 Fine structure and molecular architecture of central nerve myelin. (**a**) Normal human myelin. Electron micrograph ×1 500 000. (**b**) Schematic diagram based on x-ray diffraction and biochemical data. BP, basic protein; PLP, proteolipid protein; cyt, cytoplasmic surfaces of modified oligodendroglial plasma membrane; ext, exterior surfaces of modified oligodendroglial plasma membrane. (**a** courtesy of Dr J. Kirk; **b** reproduced, with permission, from Rumsby, 1978)

nation have possibly not been observed in the human central nervous system, but in experimental animal models various early physical changes have been described, including lamellar separation, fluid accumulation, vesicular transformation and myelinolysis (Lampert, 1983). As the process of disintegration proceeds, whole segments of myelin are destroyed and within the lesion numerous sheaths may be affected. The chemical changes (Fig. 9.3) occurring in the myelin sheath in periaxial demyelination are probably similar to those which occur in wallerian degeneration and result in the liberation of neutral fat which is eventually digested by lysosomal enzymes within macrophages. The formation of neutral fat, however, is a secondary phenomenon and occurs after the early physical changes. Associated chemical changes include an increase in lysosomal enzymes within the lesion and loss of proteins such as the myelin basic protein (Adams, 1981; Ludwin, 1981). It is generally considered that the process of myelinolysis inevitably results in the total disintegration of the myelin sheath within the affected segment. Recently, however, a second effect, known as partial demyelination has been described, in which thinning of the myelin sheath results from sublethal damage to the parent oligodendrocyte (Blakemore, 1982).

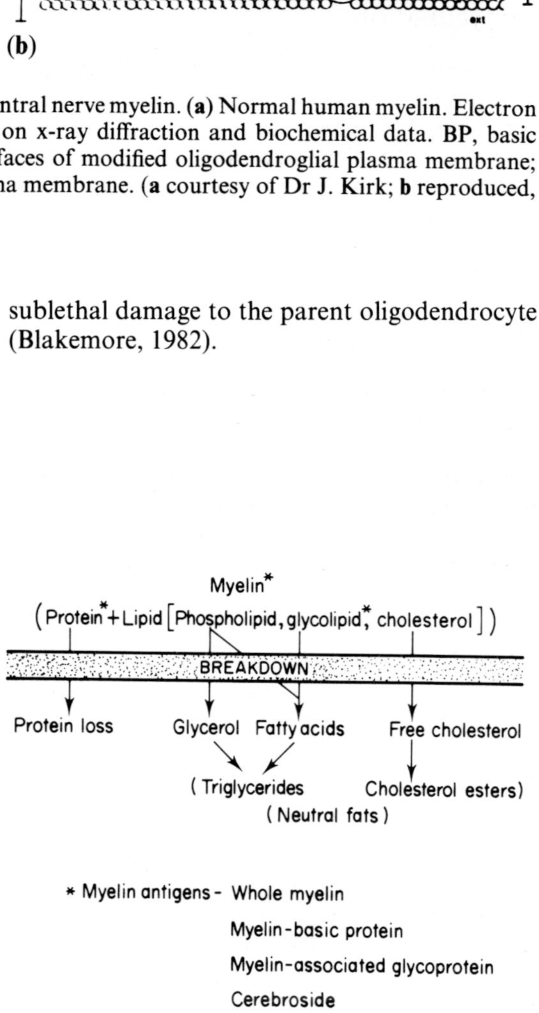

Fig 9.3 Simplified chemical structure of myelin and its breakdown products.

Acute disseminated perivenous encephalomyelitis

Classic type

It has long been recognized that after the acute fevers of childhood or after vaccination (see Chapter 7), the patient occasionally becomes severely ill with diffuse neurological signs indicative of a form of encephalomyelitis usually known, because of the anatomical distribution of the lesions, as acute disseminated perivenous encephalomyelitis. Various clinical studies have established the relationship of this condition with measles, mumps, chickenpox, rubella and whooping cough and with vaccination (Miller, Stanton and Gibbons, 1957; de Vries, 1960; Scott, 1967; Croft, 1969). The relationship with various immunization procedures is more controversial: the effect of Pasteur's rabies vaccine is undisputed but, whilst many authors (e.g. Fenichel, 1982) claim an association with pertussis vaccine, Corsellis, Janota and Marshall (1983) have shown that in cases in which pertussis vaccine has been incriminated, non-specific effects of cerebral anoxia and oedema or pre-existing undiagnosed disease of the central nervous system can explain the neurological signs. Koenig et al. (1979) have described perivenous encephalomyelitis after successfully treated herpes simplex encephalitis, and suggest that it may follow this infection more often than is generally appreciated. A few cases of acute disseminated perivenous encephalomyelitis occur 'spontaneously' or follow non-specific infections. Fisher and Gilmour (1939) suggested that there might be an association with sulphanilamide treatment; one of their patients, however, had systemic lupus erythematosus and, in retrospect, it is possible that this may have caused at least some of the neuropathological abnormalities.

Clinical features The onset of acute disseminated perivenous encephalomyelitis is often sudden, occurring usually 5–14 days after the clinical onset of the initial infection. Unlike classic viral encephalitis, virus has only very rarely been found in brain tissue in this condition and the cerebrospinal fluid may be normal or show a mild, non-specific inflammatory response. The prognosis is good and many patients make a complete recovery; others, however, have some permanent neurological damage, and death occurs in approximately 10 per cent of cases, usually in the acute phase.

Morbid anatomy The early detailed pathological descriptions of this condition were those of Turnbull and McIntosh (1926), Bouman and Bok (1927) and Perdrau (1928); these workers described perivenous demyelination as the pathological hallmark of postvaccinial encephalitis and recognized that this histological abnormality distinguished the condition from classic viral encephalitis. Similar pathological changes were reported in association with measles (Brock, 1926), chickenpox (Glanzmann, 1927), influenza (Greenfield, 1930) and smallpox (Marsden and Hurst, 1932). Turnbull and McIntosh found reactive changes in the spleen in all of their cases and Russell (1955) considered these splenic changes to be an integral part of the disease. The association with childhood illness means that most cases occur in the young, but no post-mortem case under the age of 3 years has been described.

At necropsy, the brain and spinal cord may look normal or merely show congestion and oedema. In a few cases in the sectioned brain, slight grey discoloration of the white matter surrounding small blood vessels may be seen on naked eye examination but it is the histological changes which are characteristic and allow of the diagnosis (Fig. 9.4). Brain and spinal cord are involved in a diffuse inflammatory process in which inflammatory cells are seen around veins and venules, the cerebral hemispheres are usually symmetrically involved and, although the white matter shows more severe changes, the grey matter is also affected. If death occurs very early in the disease, neutrophil polymorphs predominate in the inflammatory reaction; at a later stage, lymphocytes are the predominant cell and a corresponding inflammatory reaction may be seen in the meninges. The most distinctive histological change is *perivascular demyelination:* within these lesions axis cylinders are often relatively unaffected, but myelin sheaths are totally lost and their disintegration is associated with microglial proliferation and lipid phagocytosis. Occasionally the demyelinating lesions are confluent, particularly in the spinal cord (Fig. 9.5), but they do not have the ellipsoid shape of the small perivenous plaques seen in multiple sclerosis. In older lesions there is astrocytic hypertrophy and hyperplasia, and at a very late stage

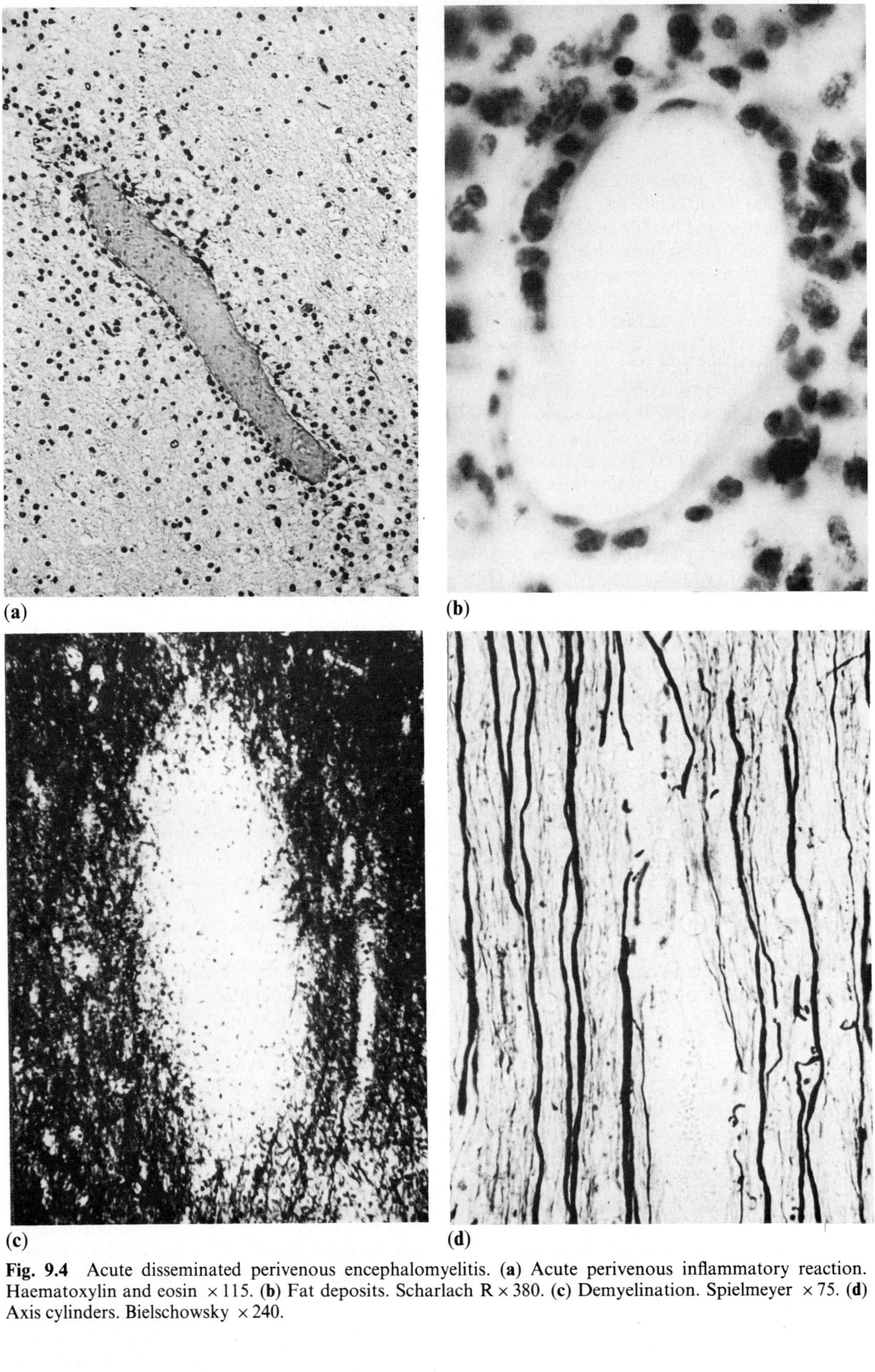

Fig. 9.4 Acute disseminated perivenous encephalomyelitis. (**a**) Acute perivenous inflammatory reaction. Haematoxylin and eosin ×115. (**b**) Fat deposits. Scharlach R × 380. (**c**) Demyelination. Spielmeyer ×75. (**d**) Axis cylinders. Bielschowsky ×240.

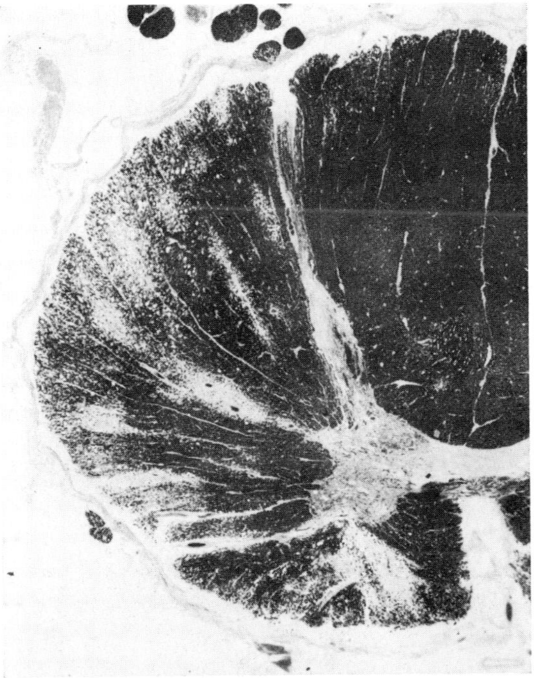

Fig. 9.5 Perivenous encephalomyelitis. Spinal cord in a case of postinfluenzal myelitis (case 2 of Greenfield, 1930). Myelin.

there is gliosis and an increase in perivascular reticulin. Neurons close to lesions often appear normal; some show chromatolysis presumably associated with the destruction of axis cylinders.

Pathology of subacute and late cases Recovery, at least partial, is the usual outcome of acute disseminated perivenous encephalomyelitis and if death occurs it is usually an early event: there have therefore been very few pathological reports of subacute or late cases. Malamud (1939) published a case of post measles encephalitis in which remissions and relapses had occurred, and a further case was described by Bérard-Badier, Gastaut and Payan (1961). The case illustrated in Fig. 9.6 is that published by Oppenheimer (1966); a young man, following vaccination, suffered a subacute relapsing and remitting illness with dementia, blindness and tetraplegia. Pathological features in this type of case include venous adventitial thickening with proliferation of collagen and reticulin, perivenous gliosis with myelin and axis cylinder loss apparently greater than that observed in early cases.

Uchimura and Shiraki (1957) reported nine fatal cases of demyelinating encephalomyelitis following treatment with Pasteur's antirabies vaccine. Death occurred at intervals varying from 10 days to 5 months after the onset of symptoms and in one case the pathology was that of acute disseminated perivenous encephalomyelitis. In the other cases large demyelinated lesions were found adjacent to the ventricular system, in the deep white matter and in the brain stem and spinal cord. The similarity of these lesions to the more acute forms of multiple sclerosis (see below) was striking.

Pathology of recurrent cases It is generally accepted that acute disseminated perivenous encephalomyelitis is a monophasic self-limiting disease. Alcock and Hoffman in 1962, however, reported six clinical cases in which there was recurrence of the syndrome, often related to different antigens. In 1950 van Bogaert reported the case of a girl of 9 who at the age of 6 had encephalitis following measles and 3 years later developed a similar illness from which she died: necropsy revealed widespread demyelination. Chronic, recurrent, demyelinating encephalomyelitis has been described associated with haemophagocytic lymphohistiocytosis, a reticuloendothelial disorder in which it is postulated that there is a 'cross-reactive susceptibility' of erythrocytic, lymphocytic and myelin membranes (Miller, Shulman and Taylor, 1981; Nagashima et al., 1983). Poser, Roman and Emery (1978) have formulated a unifying hypothesis of recurrent disseminated vasculomyelinopathy as the cause of a variety of allergic neurological syndromes, including perivenous demyelination. This is a good working hypothesis with some experimental support (see below) but the pathological and immunological evidence is incomplete.

Pathogenesis Factors which can be cited against a classic infectious aetiology in acute disseminated perivenous encephalomyelitis include the latent interval between the initiating illness and the encephalitis, the failure to recover organisms and the relatively mild inflammatory response. Various hypotheses implicating viruses have, however, been advanced; for example, it is possible that host antigen may become incorporated in the virus envelope, or alternatively viral antigen may become embedded in the host cell membrane: either mechanism could produce cellular destruction by an associated immune re-

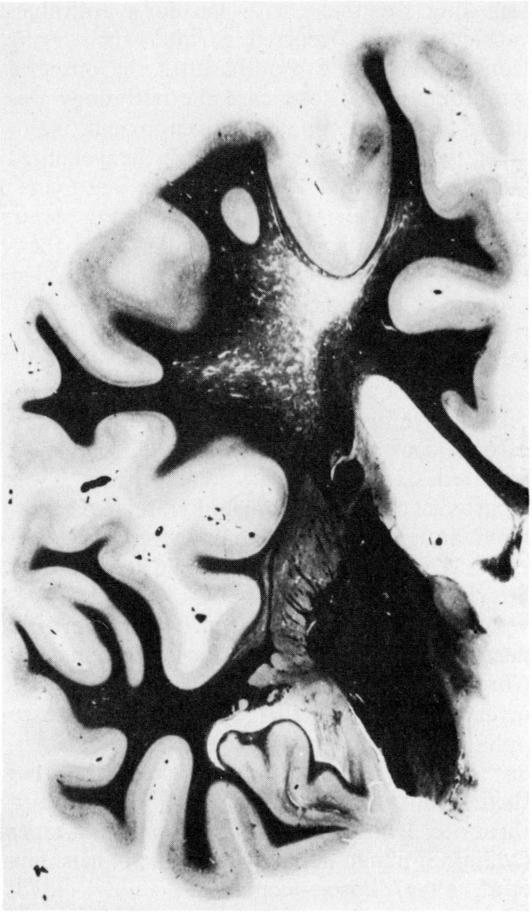

(**a**)

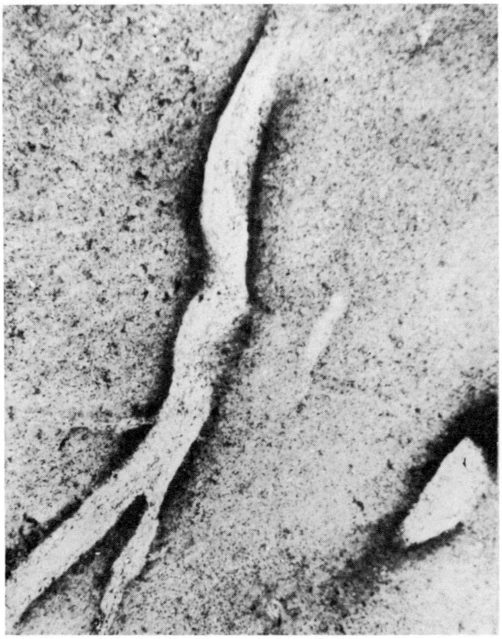

(**b**)

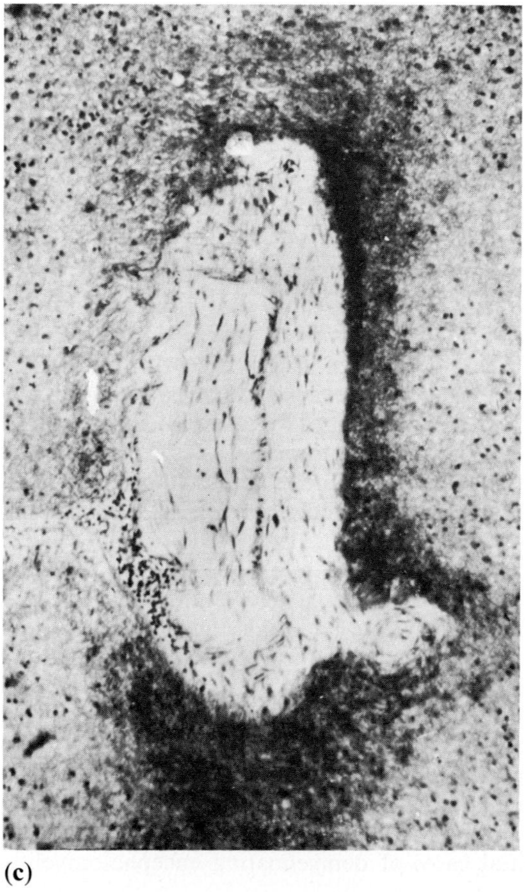

(**c**)

Fig. 9.6 Perivenous encephalitis. Subacute progressive case with remissions and relapses. (**a**) Confluent lesions in centrum semiovale. Myelin ×35. (**b** and **c**) Fibrous scarring of small veins with surrounding gliosis. PTAH × 120.

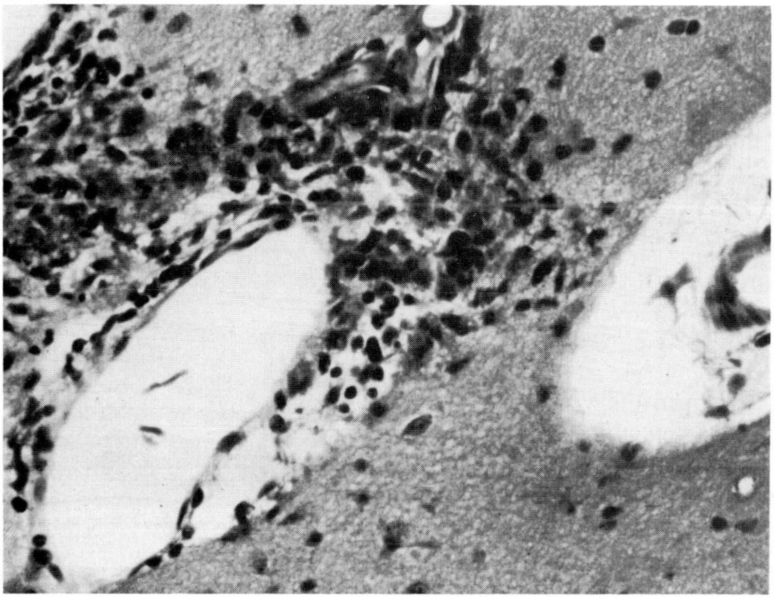

(**a**)

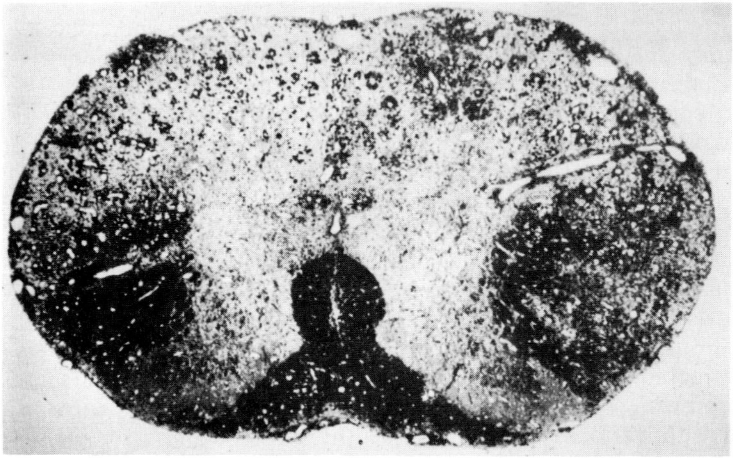

(**b**)

Fig. 9.7 Experimental allergic encephalitis. (**a**) Acute form. Note inflammatory cells. Haematoxylin and eosin ×400. (**b**) Chronic relapsing form. Note demyelination. Myelin ×20.

sponse. Moreover, the oligodendrocyte and its myelin sheath extension do not have to be the primary target; immune damage to surrounding cells may produce 'bystander' demyelination. In support of a viral aetiology Hart and Earle (1975) have described four cases in which typical viral glial nodules (Babès' nodes) were found in addition to perivenous demyelination.

The alternative hypothesis involves an autoallergic response, in which it is postulated that the precipitating illness stimulates host–antibody response against central nervous system antigen. In support of this theory have been cited the fatal cases of encephalitis following antirabies treatment by injection of emulsions of nervous tissues. The lesions following antirabies treatment are generally of the perivascular type and mainly involve the spinal cord, although in some cases the brain or optic nerves are also involved (Bassoe and Grinker, 1930; Lesniowski, 1931; Uchimura and Shiraki, 1957). The production of similar experimental lesions by injection of brain extracts in monkeys (Rivers, Sprunt and Berry, 1933), and later in other species (Fig. 9.7a), supports the idea that autoimmune factors may operate in this form of demyelinating disease (Raine, 1976). This animal model, known as experimental allergic encephalitis, has been further refined by the use of Freund's adjuvant and of various encephalitogenic myelin antigens. The disease can be transferred to a healthy animal by the injection of lymphocytes from an affected animal (Paterson, 1960) and therefore delayed hypersensitivity is at least partly responsible for the pathological reactions. Remyelination in affected animals may occur and it seems possible that, in humans, remyelination may similarly explain the relatively good prognosis in acute disseminated perivenous encephalomyelitis although there is no proof of this. A chronic relapsing model of experimental allergic encephalitis (Fig. 9.7b) has been developed and will be discussed in relation to multiple sclerosis.

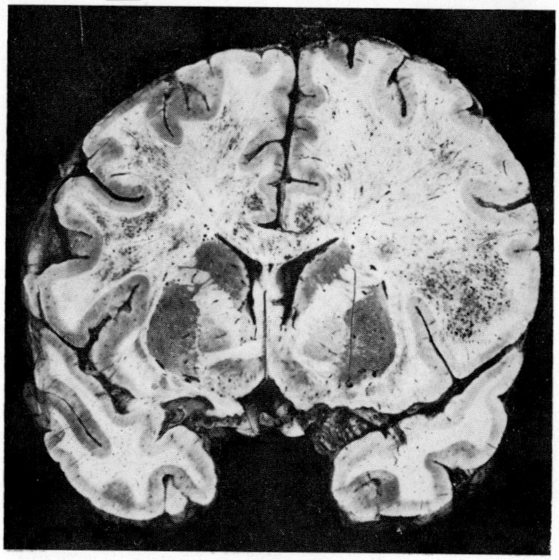

Fig. 9.8 Acute haemorrhagic leucoencephalitis. Case of 3 days' duration following respiratory infection (case 10 of Greenfield, 1950).

Acute haemorrhagic leucoencephalitis

Various forms of haemorrhagic encephalitis or 'brain purpura' are recognized, and toxins, blood dyscrasias, fat embolism and nutritional deficiencies have all been implicated as underlying causes. Within this pathological group there is a residuum of cases, occurring mainly under the age of 30 and characterized by the abrupt onset of encephalitis with pyrexia and coma, death supervening usually within a few days. The cerebrospinal fluid often has a raised protein level and sometimes a high neutrophil polymorph cell count; haemoglobin breakdown products may also be present. Attempts to isolate an infective agent or to demonstrate significant antibody levels have so far failed, and in most cases no cause has been demonstrated. The syndrome may be preceded by an upper respiratory tract infection and has been reported in association with septicaemia, with drug therapy and with various diseases presumed to be allergic: these include ulcerative colitis, acute rheumatism, acute glomerulonephritis and asthma (Graham, Behan and More, 1979).

Morbid anatomy

At necropsy the brain is swollen and soft in consistency, and the meninges are often dull with, occasionally, some subarachnoid exudate. On section (Fig. 9.8), numerous small haemorrhages are seen mainly in white matter: the cerebral cortex and basal ganglia are often spared but there may be involvement of the brain stem, cerebellum and spinal cord. The haemorrhagic lesions are usually symmetrical although in some cases one cerebral hemisphere is more severely affected. Some large haemorrhagic lesions may be seen, giving an appearance of 'confluence'.

Histologically the main abnormalities are related to blood vessels (Fig. 9.9) and consist of necrosis of *vessel walls with fibrinous exudation* (the small veins are most often affected but small necrotic arteries may be seen); *perivascular oedema*, in which swollen astrocytic foot processes may be seen; *neutrophil leucocyte* migration into perivascular spaces and adjacent brain tissue; *perivascular demyelination* with some loss of axis cylinders (these lesions not only surround necrotic venules but may also surround apparently healthy vessels); and *ball and ring haemorrhages* (the ring haemorrhages are usually centred on a thrombosed capillary and are surrounded by a narrow zone of necrotic tissue; some of the haemorrhages are related to necrotic venules). Very acute cases may show only the neutrophil leucocyte infiltration; at a later stage the inflammatory response may be predominantly monocytic and as tissue destruction proceeds, lipophages, siderophages and astrocytes are prominent in the cellular response. Pathological abnormalities in organs outside the central nervous system vary and are either secondary to the encephalitis or related to predisposing diseases.

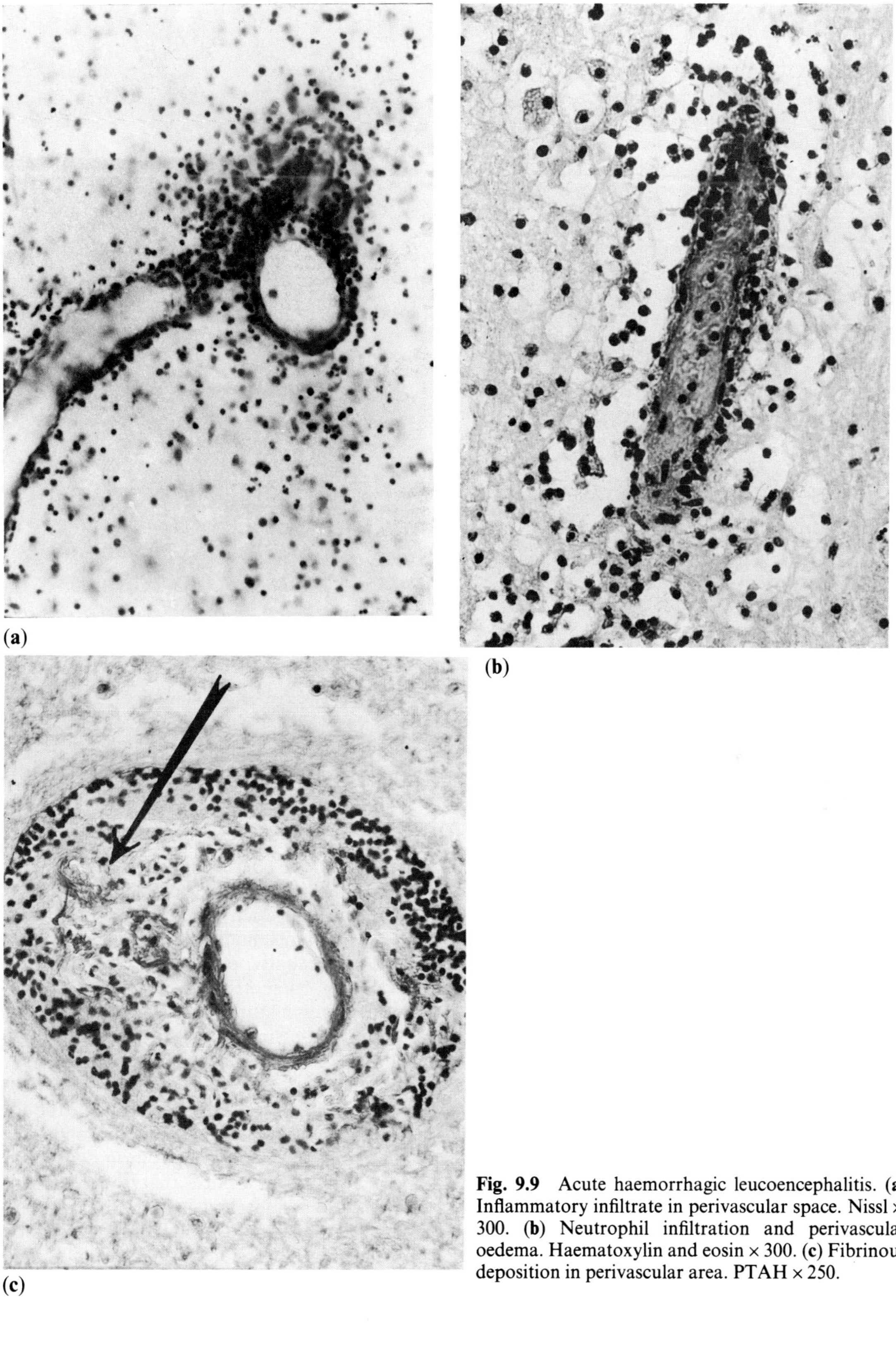

Fig. 9.9 Acute haemorrhagic leucoencephalitis. (**a**) Inflammatory infiltrate in perivascular space. Nissl × 300. (**b**) Neutrophil infiltration and perivascular oedema. Haematoxylin and eosin × 300. (**c**) Fibrinous deposition in perivascular area. PTAH × 250.

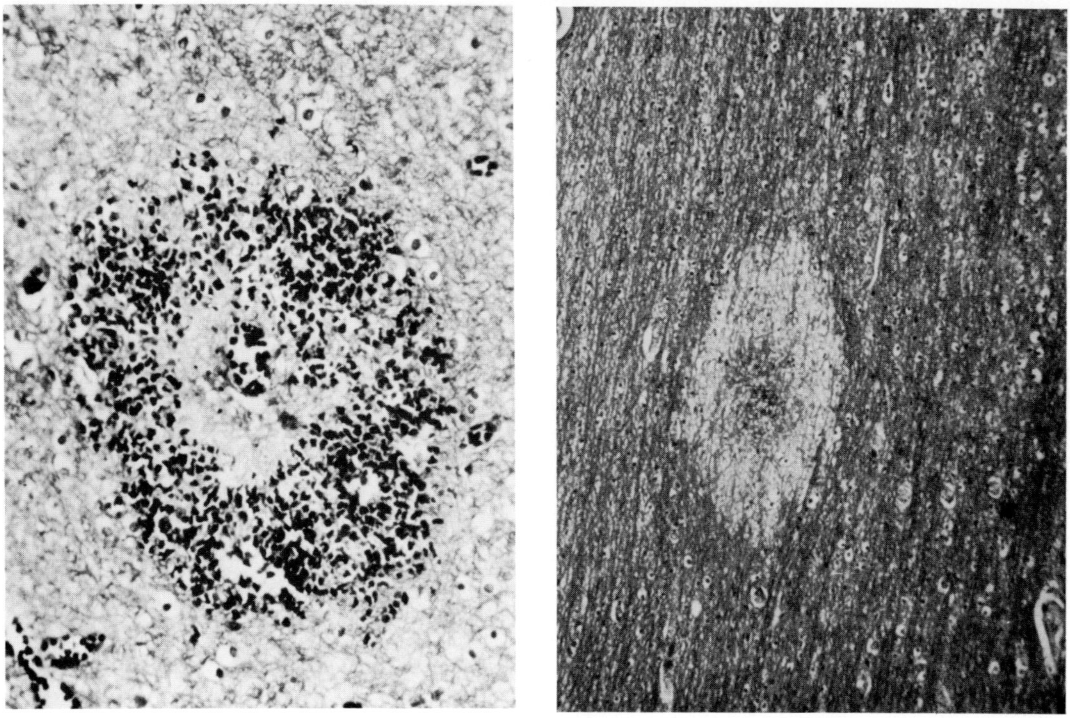

(a) (b)

Fig. 9.10 Cerebral malaria. (**a**) Perivascular inflammatory infiltrate. PTAH × 250. (**b**) Perivascular demyelination. Myelin × 100. (Courtesy of Dr A. Banerjee)

Pathogenesis

Histological comparison of acute haemorrhagic leucoencephalitis and acute perivenous encephalomyelitis would suggest that the two conditions are separate entities. Cases with the features of both conditions have, however, been described (Russell, 1955; Hart and Earle, 1975) and it seems likely that both conditions have an allergic basis and form part of a pathological continuum. This view is supported from the animal model of experimental allergic encephalitis. Levine and Wenk (1965) produced a hyperacute form of this disease in rats by the use of pertussis vaccine as an additional adjuvant, and a similar response has been produced in other species (Paterson, 1976). As a result of these experiments it has been suggested that the classic form of experimental allergic encephalitis is a delayed hypersensitivity response, but that the hyperacute form is caused by the deposition of immune complexes secondary to a circulating antibody response. Clinical and pathological evidence in humans supports this view in that perivascular deposits of immunoglobulins and complement have been demonstrated using immunohistochemistry (Chou, 1982). The pathology of cerebral malaria is strikingly similar to that of acute haemorrhagic leucoencephalitis (Fig. 9.10). Toro and Roman (1978) described 19 fatal cases of malaria and suggested that it is a form of disseminated vasculomyelinopathy with altered endothelial permeability, oedema, perivascular infiltrates, ring haemorrhages and demyelination caused by circulating antigen–antibody complexes. In assessing the pathogenesis of acute haemorrhagic leucoencephalitis it may be significant that Graham, Behan and More (1979) commonly found renal lesions with acute tubular necrosis, evidence of membranoproliferative glomerulonephritis and renal fibrin deposition. These authors concluded that the renal and neurological lesions had a common basis and resembled the endotoxin-induced Shwartzman phenomenon. The lesions probably result, therefore, from activation of complement.

Disseminated or multiple sclerosis

The most common demyelinating disease in temperate climates and one of the more common diseases of the central nervous system generally is that known as disseminated or multiple sclerosis. The disease in its classic form is characterized by relapses and remissions, and about two-thirds of patients ultimately show continuous deterioration (McDonald, 1982). In the majority of patients the disease has this protracted course; a few patients, however, have an acute non-remitting form of the disease, fatal within 5 years; in a further group the course is benign and apparently there is no shortening of life-span. It is apparent, therefore, that multiple sclerosis is a clinical and pathological continuum in which various subcategories are recognized.

The early pathological observations were made by Cruveilhier (1829–42), Carswell (1838), Charcot (1877) and Dawson (1916). It was Charcot, remembered in the eponymous designation of the classic form, who recognized the essential pathological feature of demyelination without axonal destruction, and described the disease as *sclérose en plaques*. Four additional, much rarer, forms are recognized: that of Dévic (1894), in which the optic nerves and spinal cord are mainly affected; Marburg's acute form (1906); Schilder's variety with massive demyelination in the cerebral hemispheres (1913); and the rare type with concentric demyelination, described by Balò (1928).

Classic (Charcot) type

Clinical features

This condition usually presents in adults between the ages of 20 and 40, females having a slightly higher incidence than males (Millar, 1971). The initial symptoms and signs vary, but include paraesthesiae, limb weakness, ataxia, bladder dysfunction, nystagmus, optic neuritis and, very rarely, psychiatric symptoms (Matthews, 1979). The illness usually progresses over many years and most patients die in the chronic stage.

Morbid anatomy

There have been few detailed general pathological studies in multiple sclerosis, but it is widely recognized that most of the pathological abnormalities occurring outside the central nervous system are those commonly associated with chronic neurological illness i.e. infection of the renal and respiratory tracts, limb contractures and pressure sores. Zimmerman and Netsky (1950) suggested that the incidence of malignancy was unduly high in multiple sclerosis, whilst Lumsden (1970) noted a high incidence of mild 'haemosiderosis of the spleen' and of 'thyroid adenomas and involution'. These observations, however, were not confirmed by the study of a controlled series of 120 necropsies (Allen, Millar and Hutchinson, 1978) in which there was no evidence of an increased incidence of vascular disease, endocrine disease or malignancy. The occasional coexistence of multiple sclerosis and cerebral neoplasia is recognized (Anderson et al., 1980; Malmgren, Detels and Verity, 1984; Vieregge et al., 1984), but the significance is debatable and a causal relationship has not been lished although it has been suggested that the two conditions may be related (Russell and Rubinstein, 1977). Peripheral nerve and ocular lesions have not been extensively studied in necropsy cases although there have been reports of an association between multiple sclerosis and polyneuritis (Forrester and Lascelles, 1979) and also hypertrophic neuropathy (Il Ro, Alexander and Oh, 1983).

The brain in chronic cases may appear slightly atrophic, with widening of cerebral sulci and slight ventricular dilatation. Sharply circumscribed, irregular, grey, firm, depressed lesions may be seen on the surface of the pons (Fig. 9.11) and the spinal cord, and on the superior surface of the corpus callosum. Lesions may also be seen in the optic nerves, particularly if the intraorbital portions are examined. Sectioning of the brain often reveals numerous large plaques in the deep white matter of the cerebral hemispheres, usually not extending to the immediate subcortical myelin (Fig. 9.12). Other smaller plaques are scattered, apparently haphazardly, throughout the white and grey matter, although the lesions in the grey matter are usually only detectable microscopically. In the unfixed brain old lesions are grey, often somewhat translucent and feel firm (hence the use of the term 'sclerosis'). In the fixed brain the distinguishing firmness of old

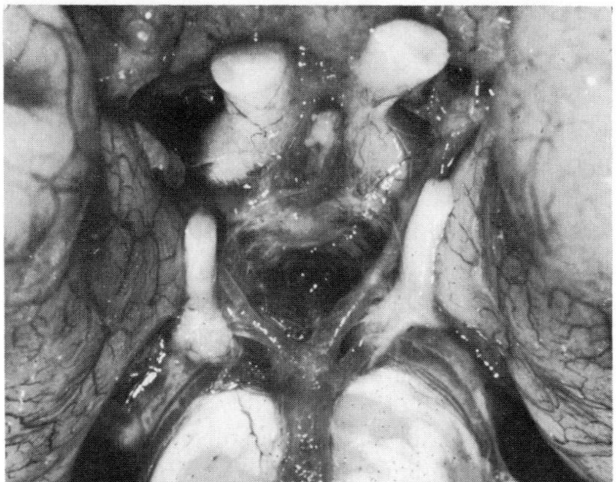

Fig. 9.11 Multiple sclerosis. Male, aged 40; 11-year history. Superficial lesions in pons. The leptomeninges have been removed.

lesions cannot be appreciated and recent lesions, which appear pink in the unfixed brain, may be difficult to see or feel.

Distribution of lesions The pattern of plaque distribution varies considerably from case to case. In severe long-standing cases numerous lesions are found in both cerebral hemispheres and often show a degree of symmetry; predominant involvement of one hemisphere is rare. The relationship of plaques to the ventricular system is a striking feature, in particular to the lateral angles of the lateral ventricles and to the floor of the aqueduct and the fourth ventricle. These periventricular plaques, which look relatively small in the coronal brain section, may in fact extend from the tip of the posterior horn to the tips of the anterior and inferior horns of the lateral ventricle. In this region the relationship with the terminal veins is often striking (Fig. 9.13). The involvement of grey matter is frequently underestimated (Lumsden, 1970), and a significant proportion of plaques occur at the junction of cortex and white matter (Brownell and Hughes, 1962) although often with a rim of subcortical white matter surviving (Fig. 9.14). The optic nerve, brain stem and spinal cord (Fig. 9.15) are often severely involved, and in some patients these sites are selectively affected while the brain may contain only a few plaques. In the spinal cord, lesions in the cervical cord are about twice as common as lesions at lower levels, and Oppenheimer (1978) has shown that there is a striking preponderance of fan-shaped lesions in the lateral columns.

Clinicopathological correlations

The exact basis of the clinical symptomatology in multiple sclerosis is not fully known. Many distinctive clinical signs can be explained in anatomical terms, but the explanation of remission and of a variety of fluctuating symptoms and signs is obscure. Experimental studies in which nerve conduction was studied after diphtheritic demyelination in the spinal cord have established the slowing of conduction following demyelination, and this is probably the major factor in the symptomatology of multiple sclerosis (McDonald, 1974). A careful clinicopathological study based on the optic nerves (Ulrich and Groebke-Lorenz, 1983) supports the importance of demyelination as a cause of clinical symptoms. In this series of 18 cases, 35 of the 36 nerves examined showed demyelination, proportionate in the majority of cases to the deterioration in visual acuity. There was evidence in some cases, however, that nerve conduction can take place in demyelinated fibres, even though the fibres run through relatively large lesions. A further interesting feature emerging from this study was the fact that in only 8 of the 18 patients was there a history of optic neuritis despite the much higher incidence of optic nerve demyelination.

The correlation of anatomically established lesions with clinical signs may not always be easy; for example, it is difficult to understand

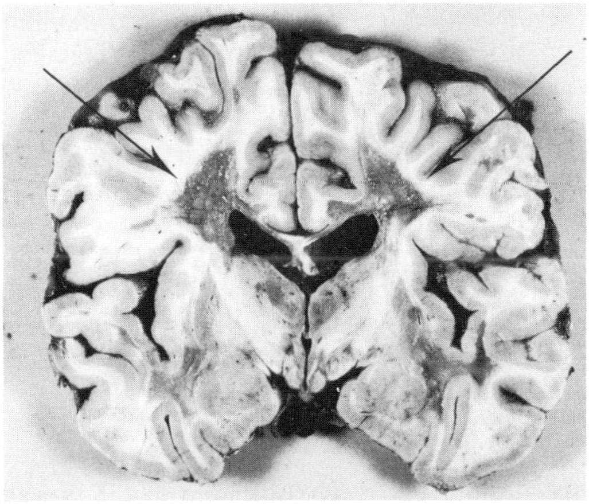

(a)

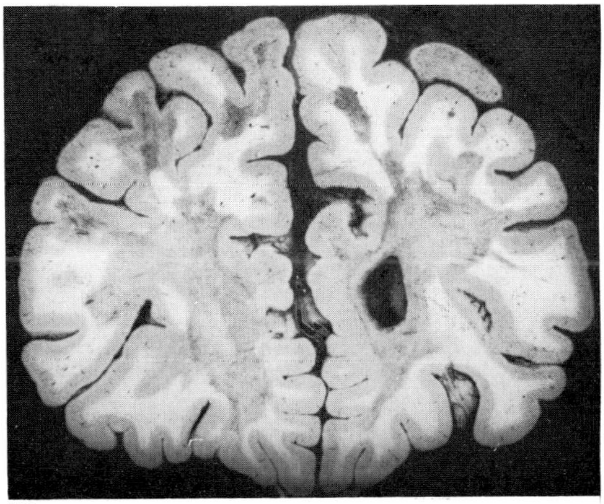

(b)

Fig. 9.12 Multiple sclerosis. (**a**) Periventricular plaques (arrows). (**b**) Symmetrical confluent demyelination and subcortical plaques.

why a plaque in the region of the entry of the sensory root of the Vth cranial nerve to the pons should cause recurrent pain. Equally, it is surprising that the prominent periventricular plaques are not associated with specific clinical symptoms although there is good correlation with the large lesions of deep cerebral white matter and dementia. Occasionally, multiple sclerosis is clinically silent and is discovered unexpectedly at necropsy. A series of such cases has been reported by Phadke and Best (1983), and Ghatak et al. (1974) have reported a case in which a clinically silent plaque was found in the spinal cord at necropsy.

Two other aspects of clinical symptomatology are not fully understood. The recovery from an acute relapse is usually considered to be related to the abatement of plaque oedema and to the disappearance of locally produced substances which may inhibit nerve conduction. There is no doubt that reversible neurological deficit may be caused by secondary phenomena and there is

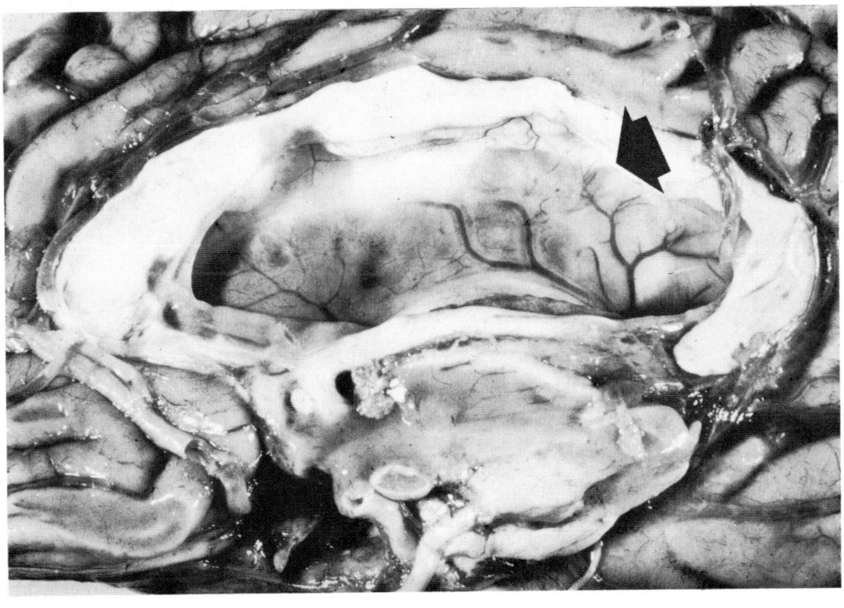

Fig. 9.13 Multiple sclerosis. Plaque formation (arrow) in the wall of the lateral ventricle. Note the close relationship with terminal veins.

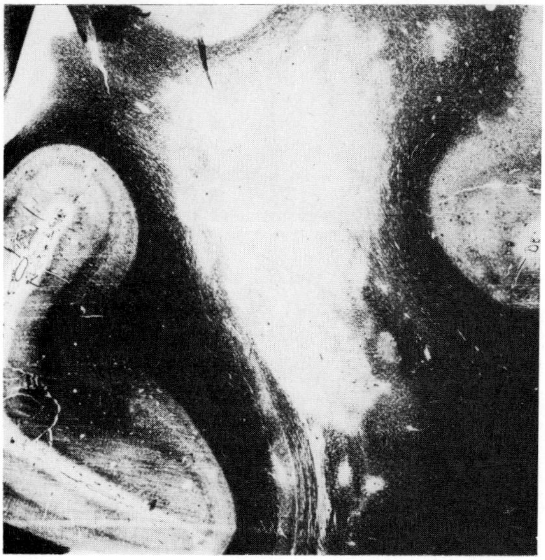

Fig. 9.14 Multiple sclerosis. Subcortical plaque. Myelin × 40.

experimental evidence that astrocytic swelling may produce such an abnormality (Dalakas, Wright and Prineas, 1980). Many patients with multiple sclerosis complain of fluctuating symptoms, including fatigue. The underlying pathology of these symptoms is unknown but factors such as an alteration in the function of the blood–brain barrier (Broman, 1947) and the diffuse astrocytosis characteristic of many cases of multiple sclerosis (Allen and McKeown, 1979) may be significant.

Histology of lesions

Acute lesions are rarely observed in the typical chronic case of multiple sclerosis and it is not therefore surprising that there is controversy as

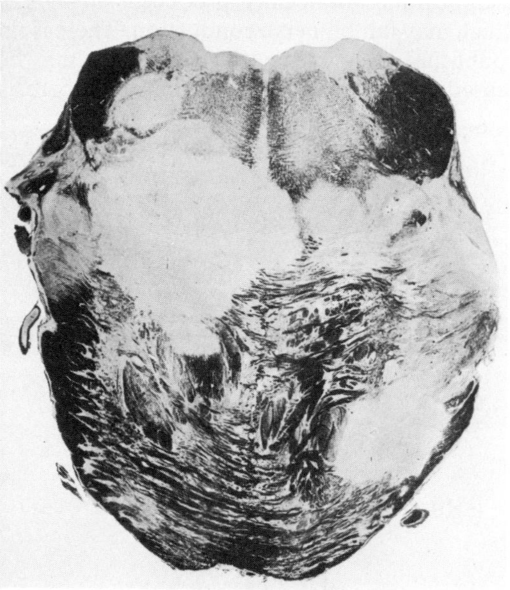

(**a**)

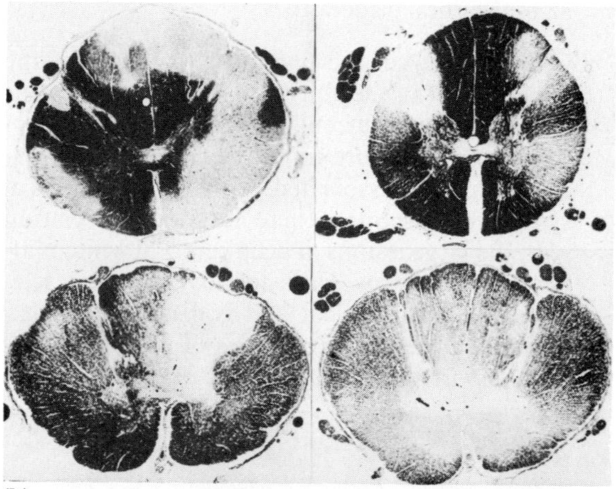

(**b**)

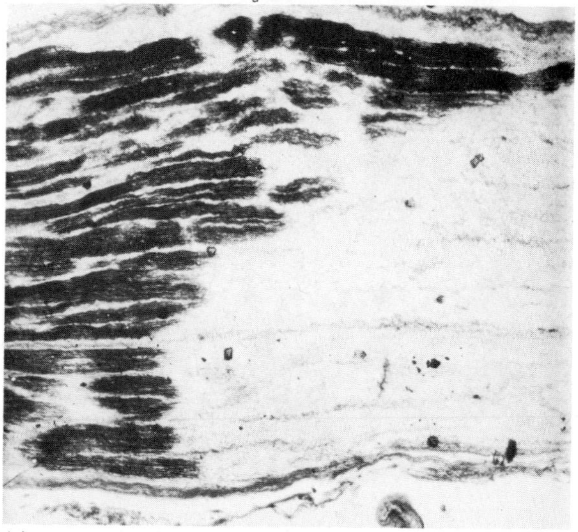

(**c**)

Fig. 9.15 Multiple sclerosis. (**a**) Pontine plaque. Myelin × 4.5. (**b**) Spinal cord plaques. Myelin × 4.5. (**c**) Optic nerve plaque. Myelin × 45.

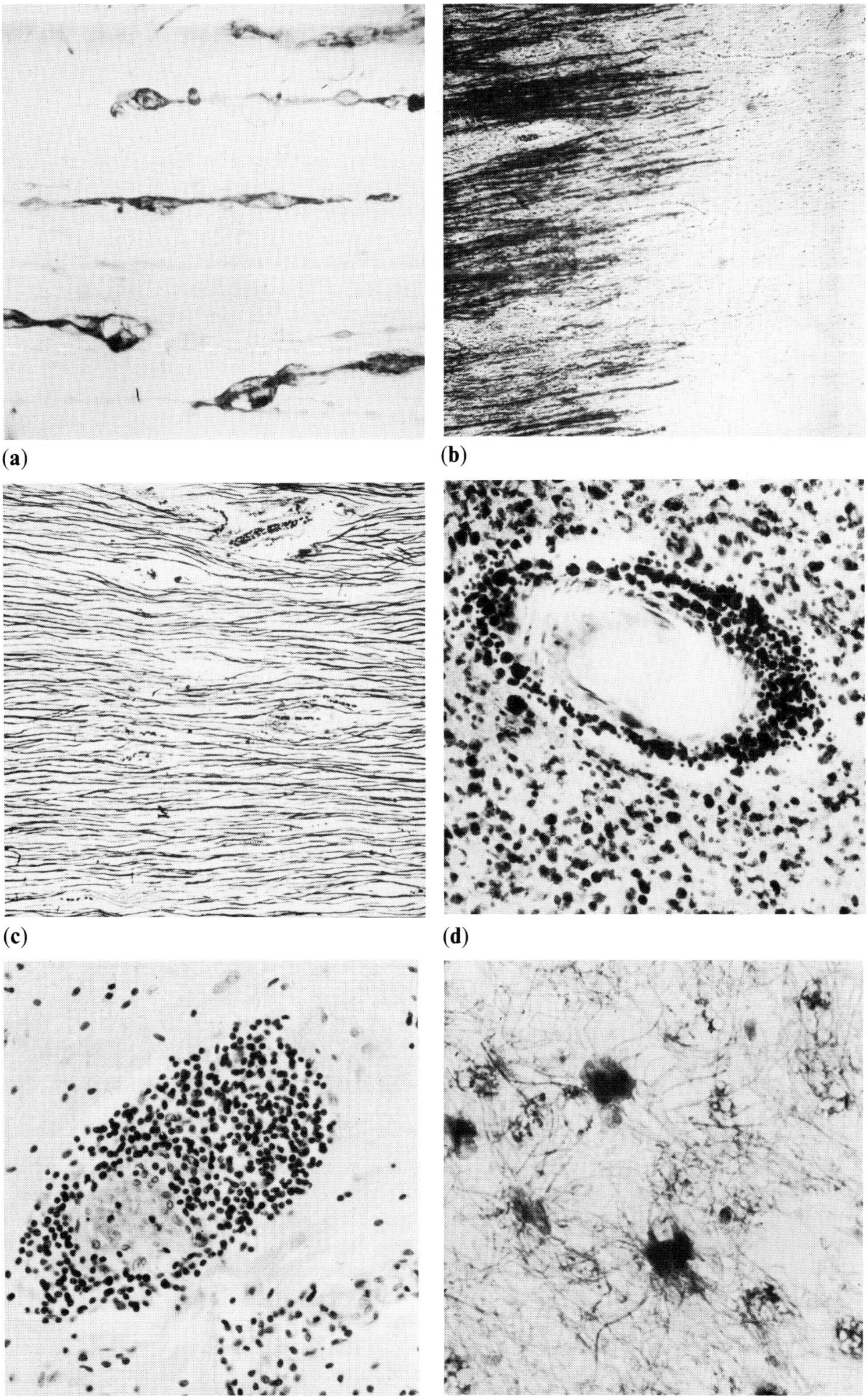

Fig. 9.16 Multiple sclerosis. Acute plaque. (**a**) Myelin beading. Myelin × 425. (**b**) Established lesion. Myelin × 85. (**c**) Axis cylinders. Bielschowsky × 85. (**d**) Fat deposits. Scharlach R × 210. (**e**) Perivascular inflammation. Haematoxylin and eosin × 210. (**f**) Astrocytes. PTAH–acid phosphatase × 425.

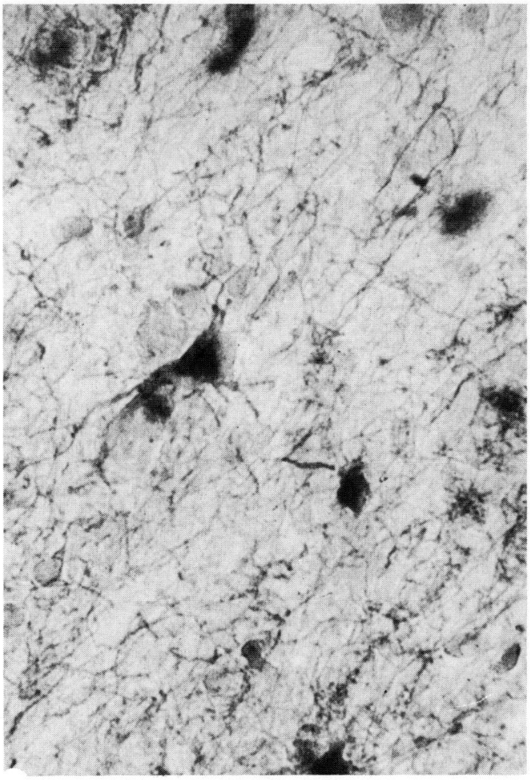

Fig. 9.17 Multiple sclerosis. Old lesion. Astrocytic response. PTAH-acid phosphatase × 465.

to the earliest pathological change (see below). It is generally recognized (Seitelberger, 1960) that the relatively early lesion (Fig. 9.16) is characterized by fragmentation of myelin, relative axonal preservation and microglial proliferation: at this stage oligodendrocytes may still be recognizable. In the ensuing weeks the loss of myelin and oligodendrocytes becomes total, neutral fat can be demonstrated free and within macrophages, and there is marked proliferation of astrocytes with perivascular inflammation (Fig. 9.16). In plaques in grey matter there is a striking preservation of neuronal cell bodies. In lesions of several months' duration inflammation is slight, sudanophilic lipid is less prominent and fibrillary gliosis is established. In the very old plaque the predominant elements are axons and astrocytic processes (Fig. 9.17): the plaque is usually hypocellular, as compared with surrounding tissue, and sudanophilic material is not present. In the chronic stage of the disease some axonal loss occurs and there is evidence of wallerian degeneration, often seen, for example, in the long tracts of the spinal cord. In addition, gliosis, inflammation, perivascular lipofuscin deposition and vascular hyalinization may be seen in the macroscopically normal white matter (Allen and McKeown, 1979) and inflammatory cells may be seen in the meninges. Iron deposition has been demonstrated at the edge of plaques (Craelius et al., 1982) but the amounts are small and the significance is unknown.

Shadow plaques and remyelination In some plaques, loss of myelin is not total, nor do they have the clear-cut outline of the typical plaque: such lesions are known as *shadow plaques* (Fig. 9.18). There are various possible explanations for this appearance (Lumsden, 1970): the lesion may be early and the myelin not totally lost; the demyelination may be selective, involving certain fibres only, or may be partial with sheath thinning rather than total loss; finally, the lesion may be partially or totally remyelinated. Shadow plaques are often severely gliosed and are observed adjacent to a completely demyelinated lesion.

Electron microscopical studies have shown a variety of abnormalities in the structure of myelin at the edge of plaques (Prineas and Connell, 1979), including uniform, thin, short, internodes suggestive of remyelinated segments (Fig. 9.19). Remyelination with peripheral-type myelin in multiple sclerosis is also well documented (Ghatak et al., 1973; Ogata and Feigin, 1975; Schoene et al., 1977; Itoyama et al., 1983) and is associated with Schwann cell proliferation. The evidence, therefore, that some shadow plaques are partially remyelinated lesions is strong.

Other varieties of multiple sclerosis

Acute multiple sclerosis—Marburg type

Marburg in 1906 described three cases in which a relatively acute illness was associated with multiple recently demyelinated lesions in the central nervous system. This variety is probably not as rare as some authors would suggest and occurs most commonly in relatively young patients, often preceded by a feverish illness and characterized by rapid deterioration and death within a few months. Occasionally an acute fulminant phase of the disease may occur as a terminal event in a more chronic case and this observation

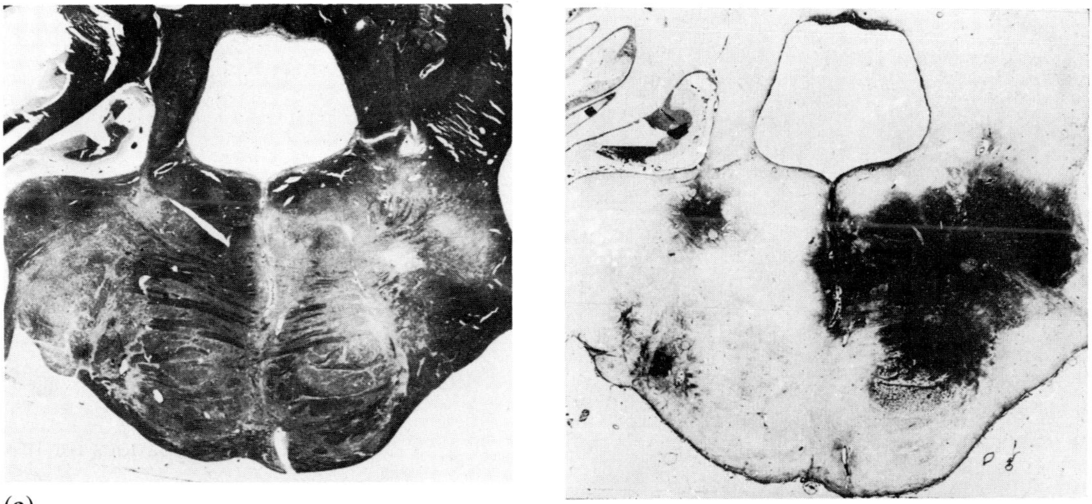

(a) (b)

Fig. 9.18 Multiple sclerosis. Male, aged 56. Shadow plaques in pons. (**a**) Myelin. (**b**) Glial fibres.

strengthens Peters' (1968) argument that the differences between acute and classic multiple sclerosis are merely quantitative. *At necropsy* in these cases, myelin destruction may be very extensive and axonal loss severe. Oedema is a feature of the early phase and the abnormalities observed are probably a combination of the primary disorder, wallerian degeneration and the effects of oedema. Treatment with anti-inflammatory drugs may modify the inflammatory response, which is greater in untreated cases than in classic multiple sclerosis (Fig. 9.20).

Schilder type (Schilder's cerebral sclerosis, Schilder's disease, sudanophilic diffuse sclerosis)

It is generally accepted that a severe and usually fairly acute form of demyelinating disease can occur in previously healthy children. Schilder's original description (1912) describes such a case, but his later publications (1913, 1924) caused confusion in that he classified two further cases as this form of demyelinating disease, although these cases clearly had a different pathology and were probably examples of leucodystrophy and subacute sclerosing panencephalitis respectively (Lumsden, 1951). This confusion, however, has now been resolved and, on exclusion of the leucodystrophies and other forms of diffuse white matter damage, a group of cases can be distinguished with characteristic pathological features. *At necropsy*, widespread demyelination with variable axonal damage is observed in both cerebral hemispheres and often in the brain stem and cerebellum. The hemispheric lesions are not usually symmetrical, they have a sharp edge and do not involve the subcortical rim of white matter (Fig. 9.21). Wallerian degeneration occurs throughout the central nervous system, and is most easily seen in the spinal cord. Transitional forms are seen in which the characteristic large lesions are associated with multiple small plaques. This 'combined' type has a later onset and a more variable clinical course.

Concentric sclerosis—Balò type

This is a rare variety of multiple sclerosis, first recognized by Balò in 1928 although similar cases had already been described by Marburg in 1906 and by Barré et al. in 1926. The onset is acute, occurring usually in the second and third decades of life, and the course is fulminant. *At necropsy*, alternating zones of myelinated and demyelinated tissue are seen (Fig. 9.22), either with a concentric pattern or with a more irregular arrangement. Cases have been described in older patients in whom the illness was more chronic and differed pathologically in that bands of loose tissue alternated with spongy, demyelinated gliosed zones in which axons were preserved. In the case reported by Currie, Roberts and Urich (1970), concentric sclerosis was associated with neuromyelitis optica.

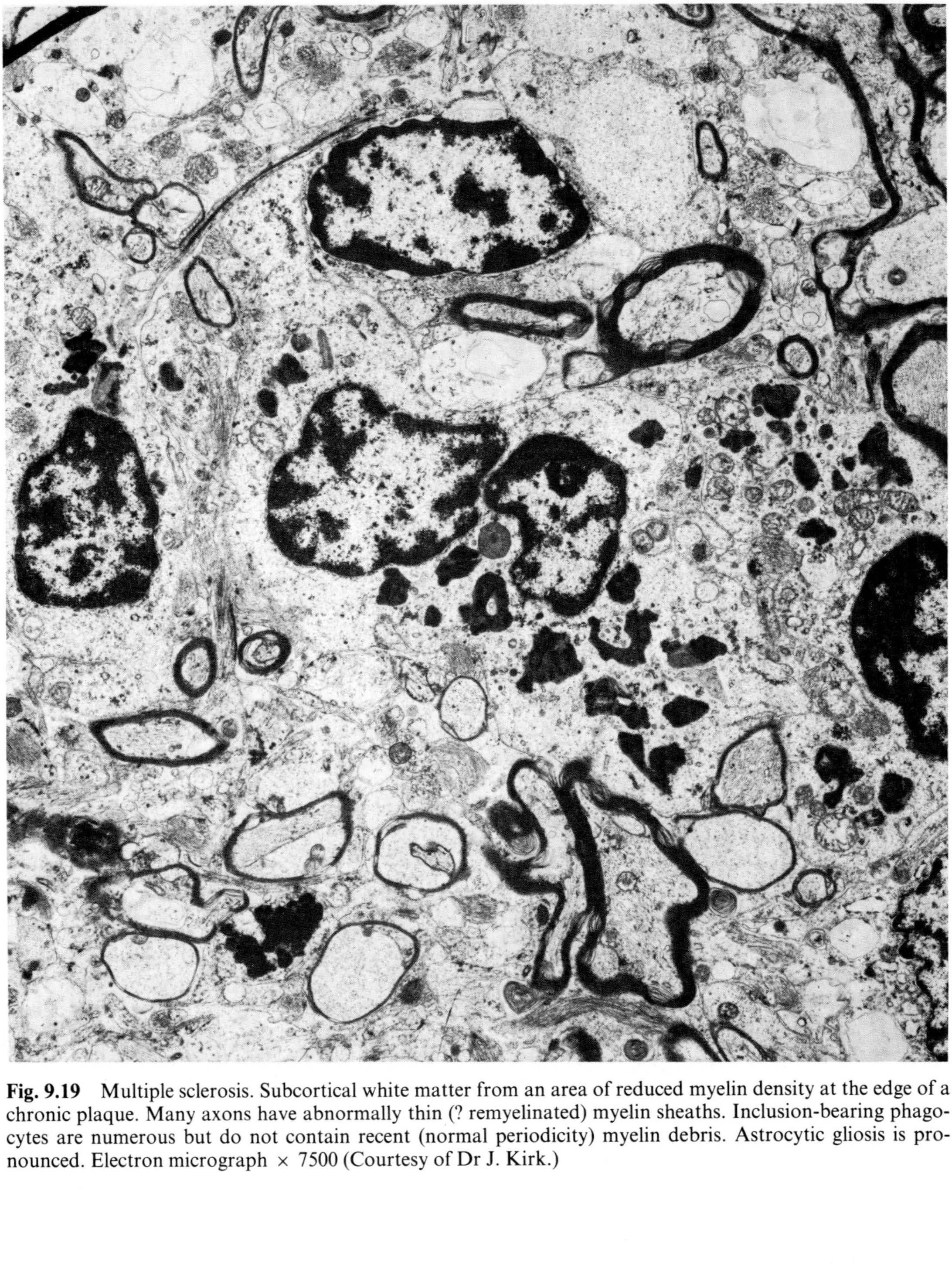

Fig. 9.19 Multiple sclerosis. Subcortical white matter from an area of reduced myelin density at the edge of a chronic plaque. Many axons have abnormally thin (? remyelinated) myelin sheaths. Inclusion-bearing phagocytes are numerous but do not contain recent (normal periodicity) myelin debris. Astrocytic gliosis is pronounced. Electron micrograph × 7500 (Courtesy of Dr J. Kirk.)

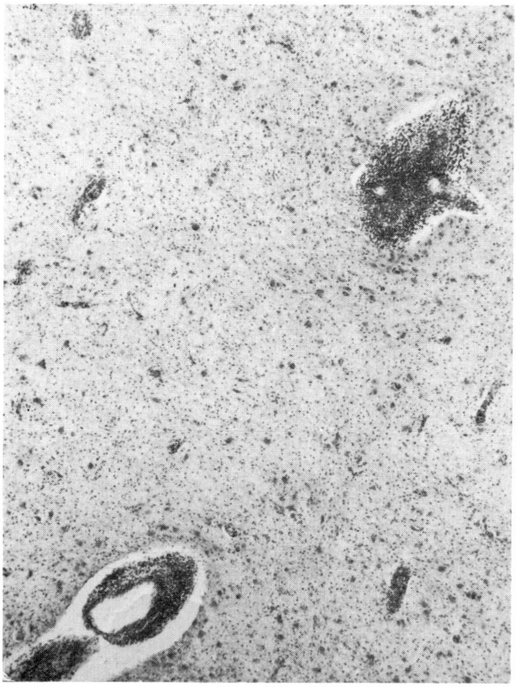

(a)

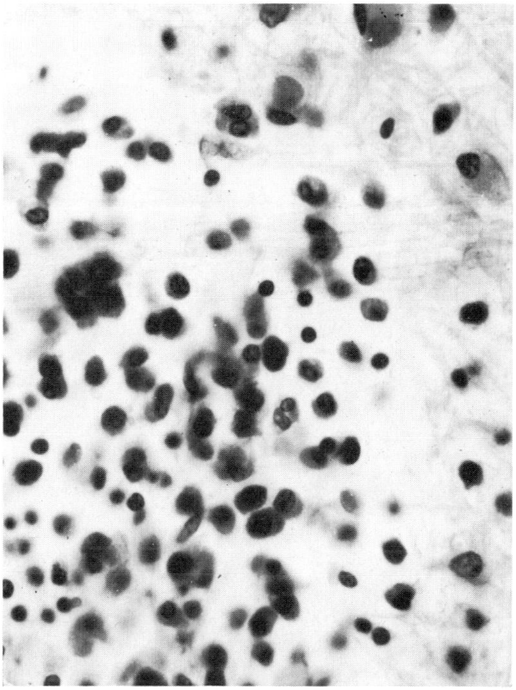

(b)

Fig. 9.20 Acute multiple sclerosis. (**a**) Lesion in white matter with an intense perivascular inflammatory infiltrate, microglial proliferation and astrocytic hypertrophy. Haematoxylin and eosin × 35. (**b**) Detail of perivascular inflammation showing mixed cells, including many plasma cells. Haematoxylin and eosin × 560.

Neuromyelitis optica—Dévic type

In severe chronic cases of multiple sclerosis the combination of partial or complete blindness with paraplegia is not unusual, although often there is evidence of more generalized involvement of the central nervous system. The term 'neuromyelitis optica' is reserved for those cases in which the visual and spinal cord signs occur within an interval of days or weeks. In most of these cases there is an acute onset, death occurring in 50 per cent within months, whilst in the remainder there may be partial or total recovery. Allbutt (1870) described this association between blindness and myelopathy, but it was Gault (1895), stimulated by his teacher Dévic's publication (1894), who reviewed the published cases and coined the term 'neuroptica-myélite'.

Since the original description there has been controversy on two points—first, whether neuromyelitis optica has a single pathological basis and, secondly, the relationship between the condition and multiple sclerosis. The arguments for and against a common pathological basis were well summarized by Cloys and Netsky (1970), and clearly visual and spinal cord abnormalities can be associated with a variety of easily defined diseases. The term 'neuromyelitis optica', however, is not used for conditions such as syphilis or systemic lupus erythematosus which can mimic multiple sclerosis (Allen et al., 1979), but is reserved for cases in which no underlying disease process can be identified. Within this 'idiopathic' group clinical delineation of the syndrome is relatively easy, but the question arises as to whether there is a common aetiology and similar pathology in all cases. Hassin (1937) argued that the pathological findings in his case were distinctive and that neuromyelitis optica was therefore a separate disease entity. Few, however, would agree with this view, and careful clinicopathological studies (Greenfield and Norman, 1963; Cloys and Netsky, 1970) indicate that a variety of demyelinating disorders may produce the syndrome. As the cause of these disorders is unknown (see below), the question of common aetiology remains open and the recent observation that antibody to glial fibrillary

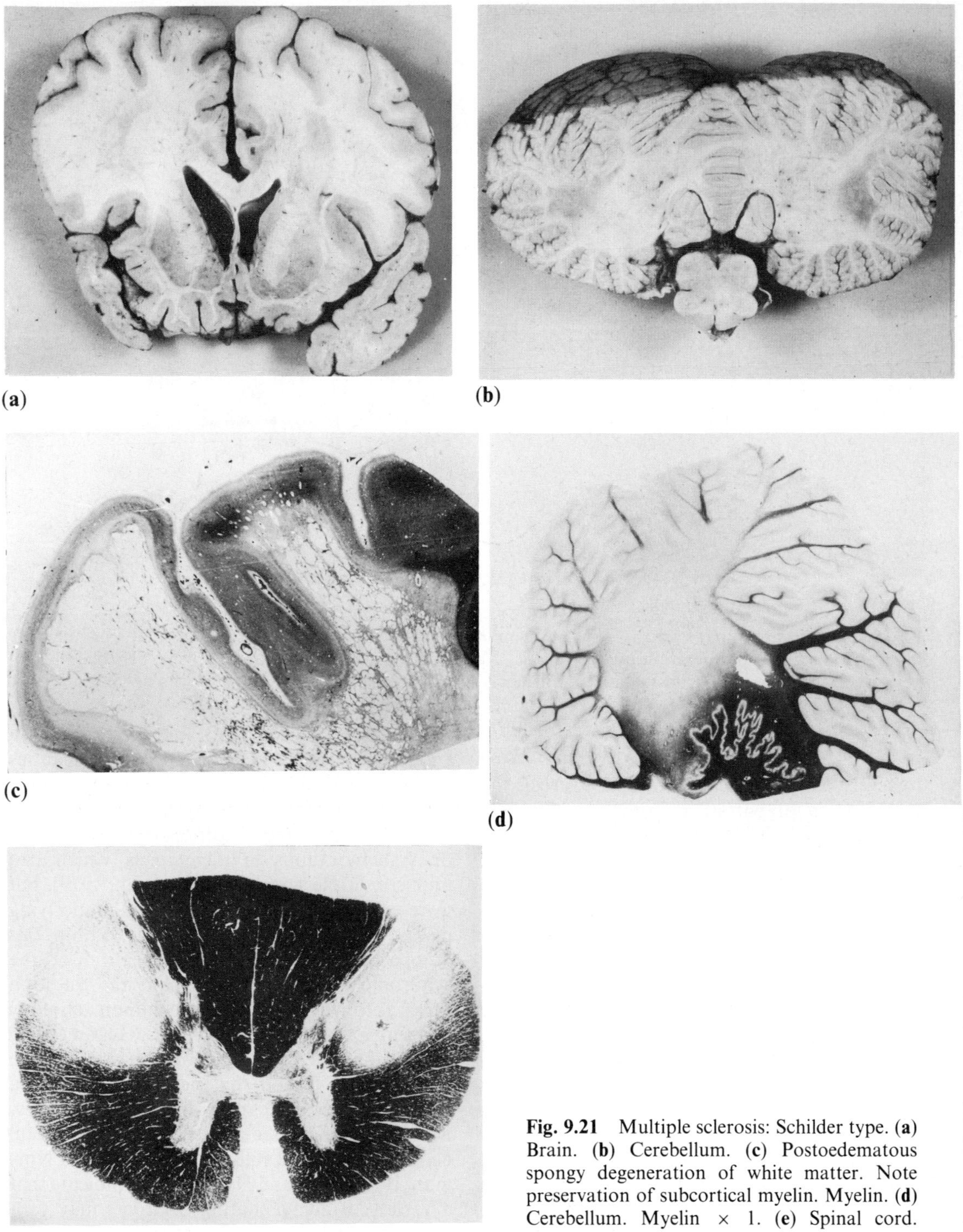

(a) (b) (c) (d) (e)

Fig. 9.21 Multiple sclerosis: Schilder type. (**a**) Brain. (**b**) Cerebellum. (**c**) Postoedematous spongy degeneration of white matter. Note preservation of subcortical myelin. Myelin. (**d**) Cerebellum. Myelin × 1. (**e**) Spinal cord. Myelin × 7.5.

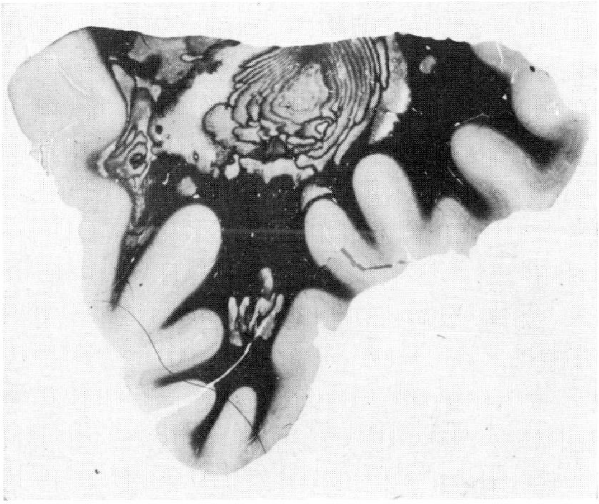

(**a**)

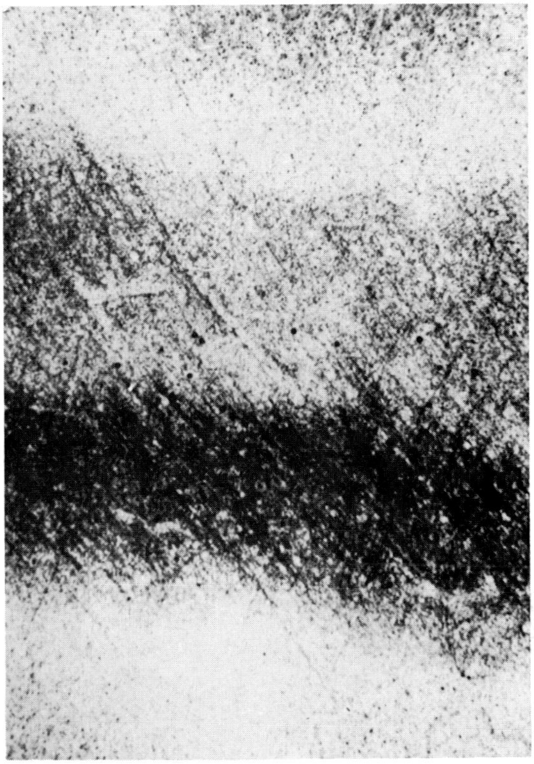

(**b**)

Fig. 9.22 Multiple sclerosis. Balò type. (**a**) Concentric demyelination in subcortical white matter. Myelin. (**b**) Complete demyelination, partial demyelination and preserved myelin in one field. Myelin × 45.

acidic protein could be demonstrated in the cerebrospinal fluid of a case of neuromyelitis optica as opposed to multiple sclerosis is of unknown significance (Chou, et al., 1984). All fatal cases of neuromyelitis optica have in common *at necropsy* partial or total demyelination of the optic nerves as well as demyelination in the spinal cord (Fig. 9.23). If the condition has been chronic the affected segment of the cord (most frequently the upper thoracic) will show a marked gliomesodermal reaction, and peripheral nerve type remyelination is often seen in the posterior root entry zone (Fig. 9.24).

Associated histological abnormalities, not necessarily confined to the optic nerves and spinal cord, allow further subcategorization, although with some overlap. Five groups can be recognized in which the associated lesions may be those of: (1) acute or chronic multiple sclerosis, (2) Schilder's disease (Fig. 9.25), (3) perivenous encephalomyelitis, (4) diffuse encephalomyelitis, or (5) acute multiple sclerosis with tissue necrosis (Fig. 9.26). It has been argued that the term 'demyelinating disease' by definition excludes conditions in which general tissue necrosis is prominent and that therefore cases of neuromyelitis optica exhibiting this feature should be considered a separate entity. It is possible, however, that in the acute phase of the demyelinating process, large lesions may be associated with severe oedema and tissue ischaemia. These secondary effects are likely to be particularly severe in the spinal cord, encircled by pia, and in the optic nerves, similarly encircled and traversing the optic foramina. Hughes (1978) has collected a series of cases of so-called *acute necrotic myelopathy* and has reviewed a further 20 well-documented cases. He tends to place these cases among the demyelinating diseases, and this view is supported by a previous history of optic neuritis in one case and of associated plaque formation in the brain of a second case.

Aetiology and pathogenesis of multiple sclerosis

Numerous hypotheses have been formulated as to the pathogenesis of multiple sclerosis and over the years suggestions as to aetiology have tended to follow scientific fashion. Current hypotheses

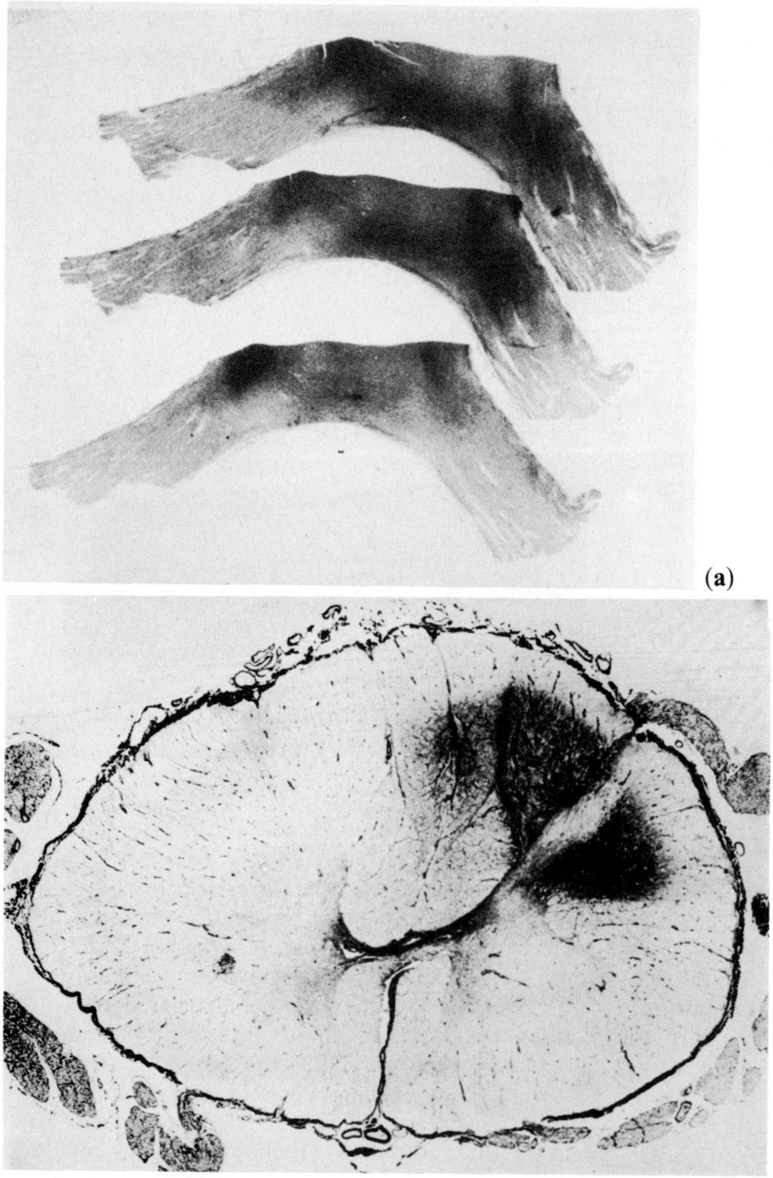

(a)

(b)

Fig. 9.23 Neuromyelitis optica. (**a**) Optic nerve and chiasma. Myelin × 20. (**b**) Spinal cord. Myelin × 10.

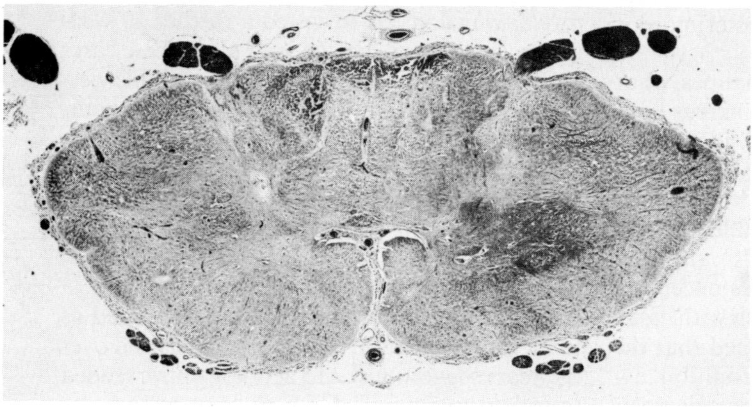

Fig. 9.24 Multiple sclerosis. Dévic type. Woman aged 35, dying after a 15-year illness with remissions and relapses. Necropsy findings. Demyelination of optic nerves and necrosis of thoracic cord. Section from C7 segment, showing mixture of necrosis and wallerian degeneration, and invasion of posterior columns by myelinated nerve fibres from the posterior roots. Myelin.

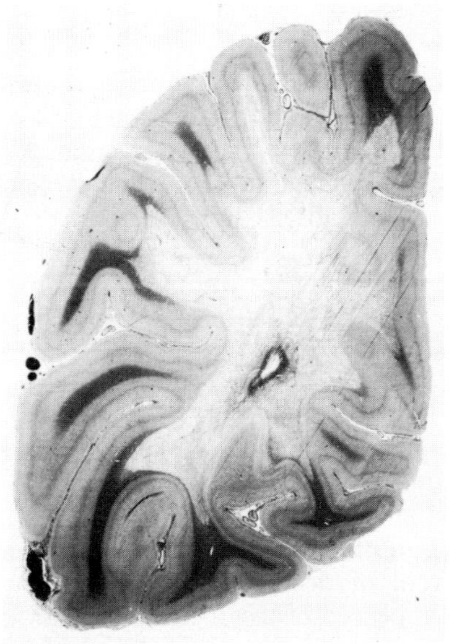

(a)

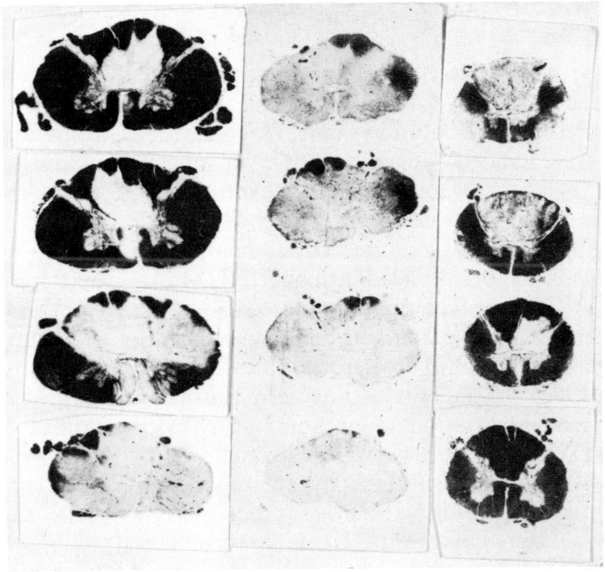

(b)

Fig. 9.25 Multiple sclerosis: mixed Schilder and Dévic type. (Case reported by Greenfield, 1950.) (**a**) Left occipital lobe. PTAH. (**b**) Cord, C6–T5 and T11–L2. The intervening thoracic segments were completely demyelinated. Myelin.

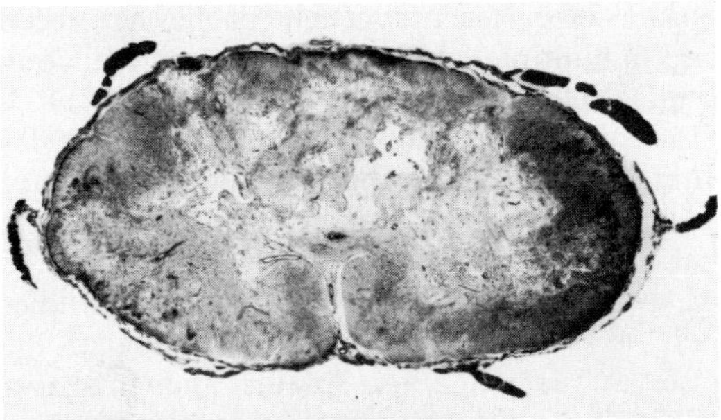

(**a**)

(**b**)

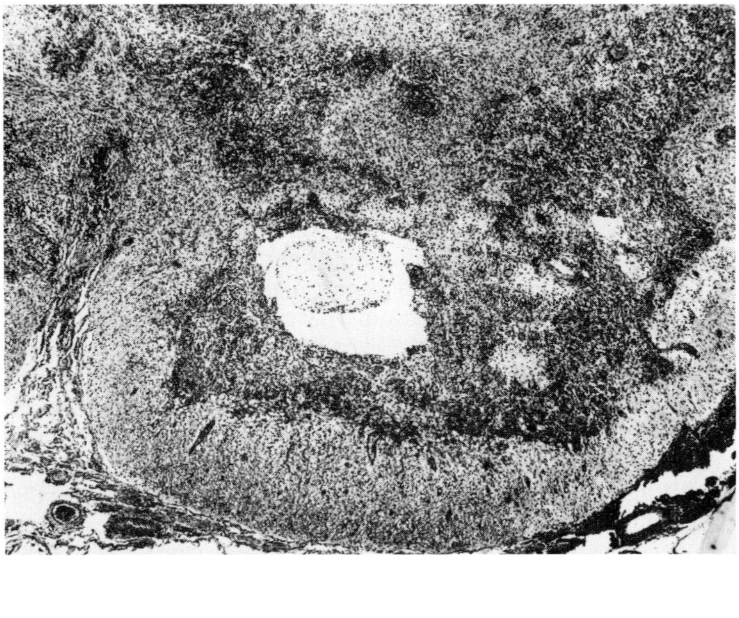

Fig. 9.26 Multiple sclerosis: Dévic type. Woman, aged 56. (**a**) Low power and (**b**) higher power views of a severely destructive lesion in the cervical cord, associated with a previous attack of retrobulbar neuritis with residual demyelination of one optic nerve.

may be categorized as infective, autoallergic, combined infective-allergic, metabolic and toxic. Perhaps the only aetiological factor which has been excluded is classic mendelian inheritance. There is, however, strong evidence of some genetic predisposition in that the incidence of multiple sclerosis among immediate relatives of patients is 15 to 20 times that expected (McAlpine, 1972); moreover, there is a loose correlation between a certain pattern of histocompatibility antigens and multiple sclerosis (Stewart and Kirk, 1983). In patients of northern European origin the association is predominantly with HLA-DW2 and DR2, with a less strong association with B7 and A3. It is likely, therefore, that susceptibility to multiple sclerosis is increased by a gene residing close to the HLA-D locus. This association, however, is far from constant and, even in families with several cases, has not been a consistent finding (Stewart et al., 1981). Twin studies support this view in that the risk of developing multiple sclerosis for a patient's monozygotic twin is 533 times that of the normal population, and for a dizygotic twin 259 times (Kuwert, 1977). These findings are suggestive of a genetic background to the disease, but the fact that 75 per cent of identical twins are discordant for multiple sclerosis indicates that genetic background is not sufficient to produce the disease.

Epidemiological studies have established the geographical distribution of the disease (Kurtzke, 1983) and also support the environmental hypothesis. High, medium and low frequency zones are recognized throughout the world: high frequency zones include northern Europe, southern Canada, northern USA, New Zealand and south-eastern Australia. Migration studies suggest that the multiple sclerosis factor operates during adolescence and that there is then a latent period until the disease develops in early adult life. Migration to a low frequency zone before the age of 15 therefore reduces the risk of developing multiple sclerosis, while migration after that age does not produce any change in risk (Dean, 1970).

The idea that multiple sclerosis is an acquired infection is of long standing and is supported by several observations. For example, Dean (1970) argued that the epidemiological studies are best explained by exposure to an infective agent in childhood. The well-established abnormalities in the cerebrospinal fluid, including elevation of immunoglobulin G, with oligoclonal banding (Roström, 1981) again suggest an infective aetiology. There are many claims of isolation of infectious agents from multiple sclerosis brain, including protozoa, bacteria, spirochaetes and mycoplasma. These observations are now considered to be failures in laboratory technique, and in recent years those favouring an infective aetiology have concentrated on a possible viral infection. Various viruses have been isolated from multiple sclerosis tissue (ter Meulen and Stephenson, 1983) but again no consistent pattern has emerged. Some of the isolates are now considered laboratory contaminants; others are frequently isolated from control tissue and are therefore of doubtful pathological significance. With the advent of electron microscopy many reports have appeared of 'virus-like particles' in multiple sclerosis tissue. Again, however, there has been no consistent pattern, and with more careful study it is apparent that many of these particles are artefacts or normal intracellular organelles (Fig. 9.27) (Kirk and Hutchinson, 1978; Kirk, 1979b). Recently genetic probes have been used in multiple sclerosis tissue, with conflicting results (Stevens et al., 1980; Haase et al., 1981). Pilot studies suggested the presence of measles antigen in a significant number of cases of multiple sclerosis but further evidence suggests that controls may give similar results.

Despite the failure of viral isolation studies there is no doubt as to the accuracy of the observations made by Adams and Imagawa (1962), that patients with multiple sclerosis have high titres of measles antibody in serum and cerebrospinal fluid. Further work has shown that, in addition to measles, other viral antibody levels may be raised (Norrby et al., 1974) and that viral antibody is apparently synthesized locally within the cerebrospinal fluid pathway. The significance of these antibody responses is unknown and their relationship to the elevated cerebrospinal fluid immunoglobulin and oligoclonal bands is not a simple one. Viral antigen will absorb only part of the elevated immunoglobulin and even the oligoclonal bands are not absorbed entirely (Roström, 1981). It may well be that non-specific immunostimulation is responsible for the increased levels of cerebrospinal fluid viral antibodies (Leinikki et al., 1982); nevertheless, the viral hypothesis cannot be dismissed and is supported by many experimental viral models of demyelination (for reviews of this subject, see Lampert (1978) and Martin and

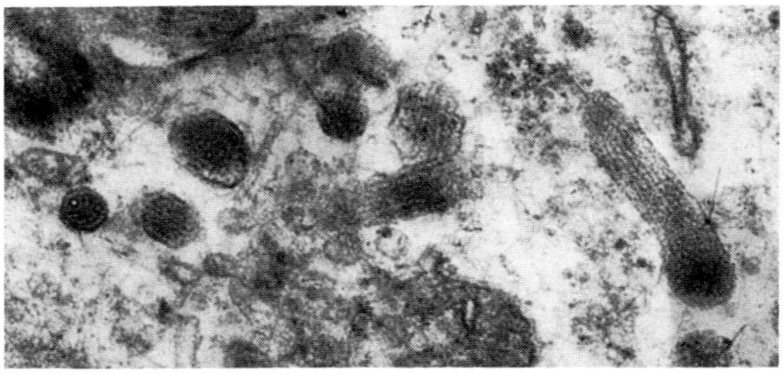

(**a**)

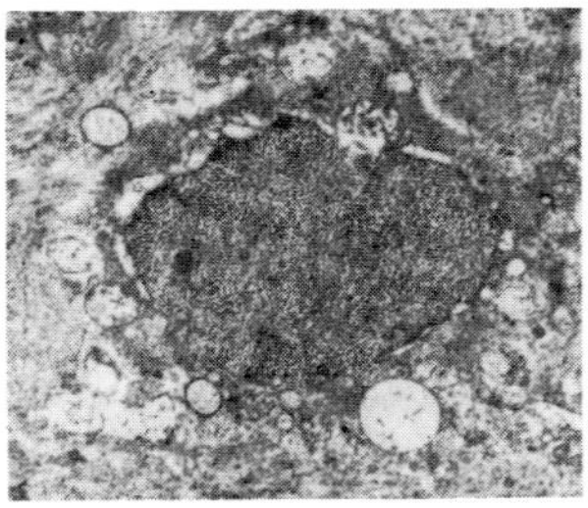

(**b**)

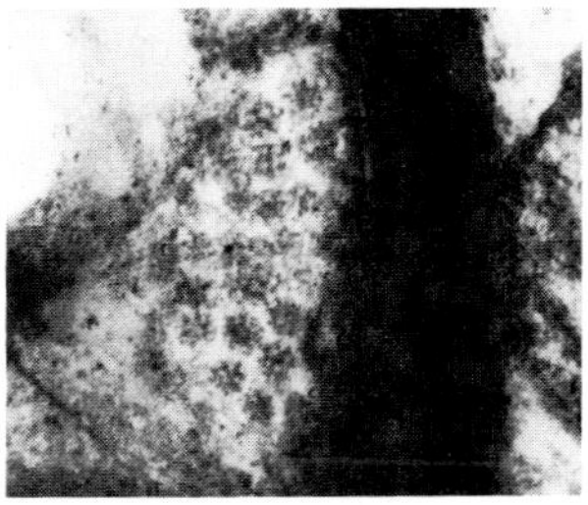

(**c**)

Fig. 9.27 Multiple sclerosis. Structures previously mistaken for paramyxoviruses (**a** and **b**) and papovavirus (**c**). (**a**) Tubule-containing Weibel–Palade bodies; specific granules of endothelial cell. Electron micrograph × 54 500. (**b**) Nucleoprotein filamentous aggregates in perivascular cell nucleus. Electron micrograph × 7000. (**c**) Clathrin-coated vesicles and clathrin coats. Electron micrograph × 40 000. (**a** and **c** reproduced, with permission, from Kirk and Hutchinson, 1978; **b** courtesy of Dr J. Kirk.)

Nathanson (1979)). Many of the viruses used in these experimental models are not common human pathogens; it is therefore of interest that experimental demyelination has been produced using a common human pathogen—i.e. herpes simplex virus type 2 (Martin, 1982). In evaluating the viral hypothesis it must be remembered that virus does not have to be present in the central nervous system to produce an effect. Persistence in the reticuloendothelial system is recognized and persistent virus has been demonstrated in other tissues; for example, in the uvea in canine distemper (Summers, Greison and Appel, 1983). Moreover, immunological theory implies that persistence of virus is not essential for a target effect. Viruses may trigger an autoallergic response against myelin or against an adjacent tissue, producing 'bystander' demyelination.

The idea that multiple sclerosis develops as an autoallergic response to myelin or one of its components has, like the viral theory, received wide attention. Diseases such as rheumatoid arthritis and systemic lupus erythematosus are characterized by high viral antibody levels and disordered immune regulation; similar abnormalities have been found in multiple sclerosis (Arnason and Waksman, 1980; Goust et al., 1980; Goust, Hogan and Arnaud, 1982). These tests of immune function must be interpreted with caution (Leibowitz, 1983). The techniques employed are difficult, little is known of natural variation, and the same effect can be produced by a wide variety of antigens, both autologous and heterologous.

Evidence for autoimmunity in multiple sclerosis is not strong. Despite many studies for antibodies against myelin or its components in serum and cerebrospinal fluid, no consistent pattern has emerged (Ryberg 1981; Chou et al., 1983). The presence of IgG with a constant oligoclonal isofocusing spectrum in cerebrospinal fluid is not specific for multiple sclerosis (Chu et al., 1983) and there is no evidence that serum from patients with multiple sclerosis contains antibodies against human glial cells (Kennedy and Lisak, 1981). Bornstein (1963), however, reported demyelinating factors in serum from patients with multiple sclerosis and there have been several confirmatory reports (Seil et al., 1983). Recently, autoantibodies against pituitary peptides have been demonstrated in sera from patients with multiple sclerosis (Hansen et al., 1983), and these may have a demyelinating effect.

For many years it has been considered possible that multiple sclerosis may be caused by the release of a toxin from cerebrospinal fluid to surrounding brain and spinal cord. No firm evidence for this theory has emerged although Wolfgram (1979) has argued that the toxic hypothesis has been ignored, and suggests that such a toxin might be endogenous and of low molecular weight. In view of Wolfgram's argument it is interesting that Swank in 1950 suggested that dietary lipids may be important in the aetiology of multiple sclerosis, and there have been several claims that modification of lipid in the diet gives a significant improvement in the course of the disease (Millar, 1975; Bates, Fawcett and Weightman, 1978). More recently it has been shown that there are significant differences in essential fatty acids in the serum and cerebrospinal fluids of multiple sclerosis patients as compared with healthy subjects (Neu, 1983). Lipid analysis of the macroscopically normal white matter in multiple sclerosis indicates that there is undoubted abnormality, but it is generally considered that these changes are the result of microscopic lesions and do not indicate an intrinsic abnormality of lipid metabolism (Norton, 1977). Similarly it can be shown that abnormal protein and hydrolytic enzyme values in the macroscopically normal white matter are associated with histological abnormality (Allen and McKeown, 1979; Cuzner, 1980; Allen, 1983). The relationship of abnormal serum and brain levels of various trace elements to neurological disease in farm animals is well known, and it has been postulated that similar abnormalities could cause multiple sclerosis either by a direct toxic effect or by potentiating viral infection. As with other biochemical studies, interpretation of results is difficult because of the possible effects of diffuse histological abnormality; however, abnormalities in trace elements have been reported in serum and in brain from cases of multiple sclerosis (Craelius, Jacobs and Lee Jones, 1980; Hallmans, 1982; Palm and Hallmans, 1982; Warren and Horsky, 1983).

Evolution of the plaque in multiple sclerosis and its pathogenetic significance

Histopathological studies in multiple sclerosis have a limited role in testing fundamental aetiological hypotheses. Nevertheless, many of the histological observations could be of cardinal significance. A constant and well-documented feature in multiple sclerosis is the anatomical distribution of the lesions and several studies have confirmed the peculiar vulnerability of myelin in the optic nerves, in the periventricular region (Brownell and Hughes, 1962) and in the spinal cord (Oppenheimer, 1978), yet the significance of plaque distribution is unknown. As already stated, the vulnerability of the periventricular white matter has been explained on the basis of a toxin circulating in the cerebrospinal fluid. Against this view, however, is the fact that not all of the periventricular white matter is equally vulnerable. A vascular basis for plaque formation was proposed in some of the original descriptions of the disease and, although it is now accepted that there is no evidence of vascular thrombosis as the basis of plaque formation, it has been suggested that local susceptibility may be particularly great in regions situated in the boundary zones between the territories of supply of major cerebral arteries (Brownell and Hughes, 1962). Fog (1965), in a detailed study of the relationship of plaques to cerebral veins, observed that most plaques had a close anatomical relationship with one, two or more cerebral veins and considered this relationship of pathogenetic significance. Oppenheimer (1978), in a study of the spinal cord in 18 cases of multiple sclerosis, has emphasized the presence of fan-shaped lesions in the lateral columns and has suggested that mechanical stress might be a factor in the anatomical siting of some plaques. In summarizing the evidence of pathogenesis accruing from anatomical studies, it may be said that all central nervous system white matter is susceptible in multiple sclerosis, the cause of the increased vulnerability of certain anatomical sites is unknown, a relationship of plaques to veins seems to be significant, and the possibility that these are the site of protein and cellular leakage early in the disease requires investigation.

The known histological and chemical abnormalities in an established plaque are represented diagrammatically in Fig. 9.28, the only controversial observation being the apparent increase in oligodendrocytes in the plaque edge (Ibrahim and Adams, 1965). As yet there is no evidence that oligodendrocytes in the adult human can respond in this way (Cavanagh, 1970). It may, however, occur in other species (Lampert, 1978), and Raine, Scheinberg and Waltz (1981) have described the survival and proliferation of oligodendrocytes in an active established multiple sclerosis lesion. Despite several publications referring to the 'early lesion' in multiple sclerosis, nothing is known of the initial stages of plaque formation (i.e. within a few hours of a clinical relapse). Pathologists using post-mortem material have had to approach this problem either by studying the plaque edge or by random

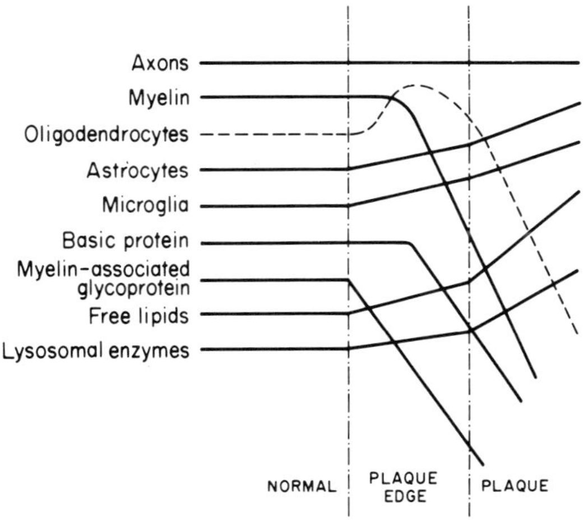

Fig. 9.28 Multiple sclerosis. Schematic view of the plaque and periplaque. The changes in oligodendrocytes are controversial.

sampling of macroscopically normal white matter. Both methods have scientific disadvantages: the plaque edge because it is the site of interaction between diseased and healthy tissue; the macroscopically normal white matter because it may show abnormality of a secondary nature consequent on plaque formation. With this variation in approach, three differing descriptive views of the early lesion are held: that the early lesion is characterized by hypercellularity with microglial proliferation, by physical disintegration of myelin, and by perivascular lymphocytic reaction. The hypercellularity of the relatively early lesion was recognized by Dawson (1916) but this histological picture is characteristic of an established plaque, possibly of several weeks' duration. A series of histopathological studies (Zimmerman and Netsky, 1950; Seitelberger, 1960; Lumsden, 1970) support the view that the earliest morphological feature is disintegration

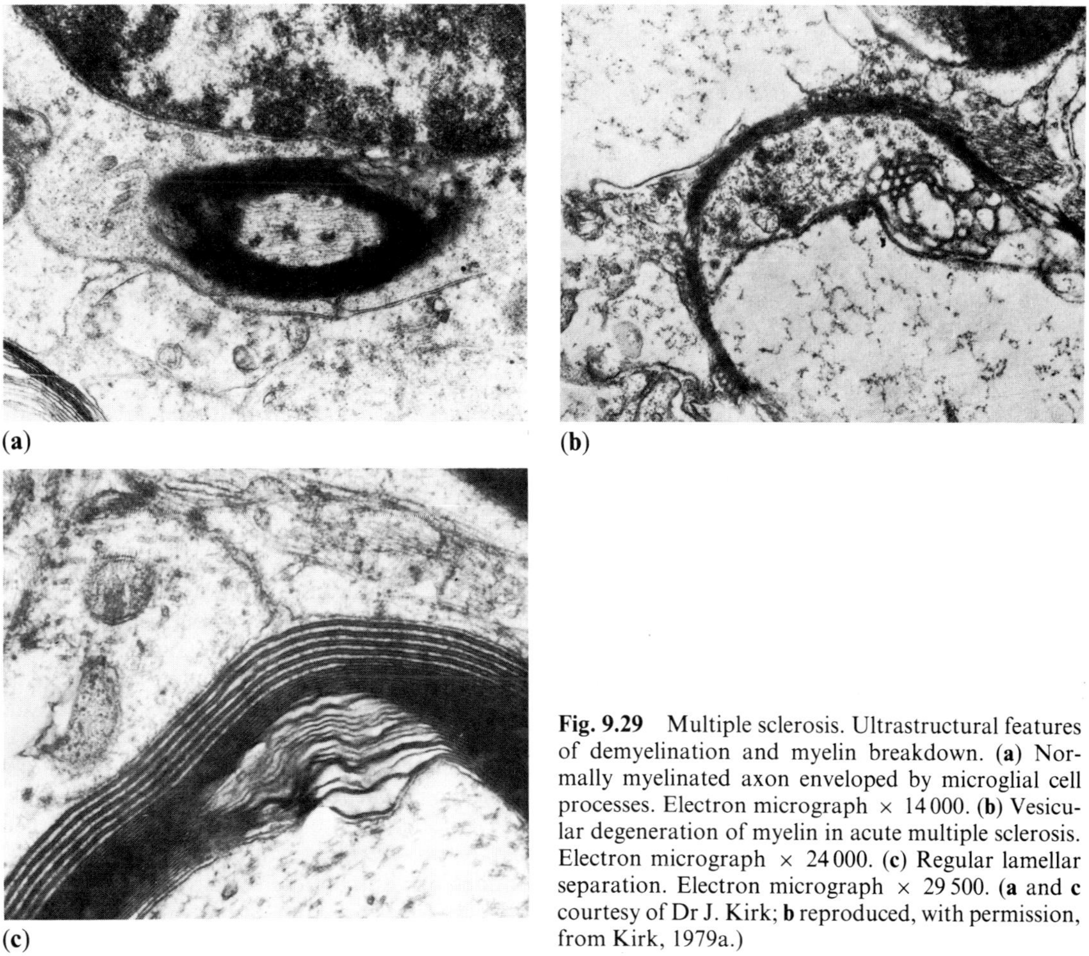

(a) (b) (c)

Fig. 9.29 Multiple sclerosis. Ultrastructural features of demyelination and myelin breakdown. (**a**) Normally myelinated axon enveloped by microglial cell processes. Electron micrograph × 14 000. (**b**) Vesicular degeneration of myelin in acute multiple sclerosis. Electron micrograph × 24 000. (**c**) Regular lamellar separation. Electron micrograph × 29 500. (**a** and **c** courtesy of Dr J. Kirk; **b** reproduced, with permission, from Kirk, 1979a.)

of myelin and that this fragmentation is then followed by chemical breakdown. With the formulation of the autoallergic hypothesis more emphasis has been placed on the inflammatory reaction in multiple sclerosis, and Adams (1977) has suggested that perivascular lymphocytic cuffs in normally myelinated tissue may represent the initial lesion. Electron microscopy has extended our knowledge of the established plaque (Figs. 9.29 and 9.30) and has confirmed the importance of microglial cells in the phagocytosis of myelin debris but no consensus has been reached regarding the actual mechanism of demyelination (Prineas, 1975; Prineas and Connell, 1978; Kirk, 1979a; Lassman, 1983; Raine, 1983).

Support for immune-mediated demyelination has come from many light and electron-microscopical studies (Guseo and Jellinger, 1975; Tanaka, Iwasaki and Koprowski, 1975; Prineas and Wright, 1978) in which lymphocytes and plasma cells have been demonstrated in the perivascular region and in myelinated tissue. These studies have been extended by the use of immunohistochemistry, and immunoglobulin-containing cells have been demonstrated within the central nervous system (Mussini, Hauw and Escourolle, 1977; Esiri, 1980). Recently the lymphocytic response has been studied using T- and B-cell markers (Nyland, Mork and Matre, 1982; Kreth et al., 1982) and T-cell subset markers (Traugott, Reinherz and Raine, 1983; Booss et al., 1983). The results, however, are conflicting and as yet no uniform pattern has been established. Moreover, the relationship of these cells to the elevated immunoglobulin in the cerebrospinal fluid is unknown. In a combined histological and biochemical study (Cuzner et al., 1981), plaque levels of immunoglobulin could not be correlated positively with the inflammatory cell response. The possibility that the astrocytic response may be a cardinal event in early demyelination has been suggested from the time of the earliest observations on multiple sclerosis (Dawson, 1916; Field, 1967). The fact that a diffuse astrocytosis is observed in the white matter in cases in which demyelination is slight or the involvement predominantly spinal (Allen, Glover and Anderson, 1981) could be interpreted as supportive evidence for the primary involvement of astrocytes in the pathological response. It must be remembered, however, that astrocytes respond early and vigorously to many pathogenetic stimuli and that this response cannot be considered to be specific. It would seem that the most fruitful approach to recognition of the early lesion in multiple sclerosis is a combination of histological and histochemical techniques including immunohistochemistry.

Relationship between multiple sclerosis, perivenous encephalomyelitis and experimental allergic encephalitis

The similarity between acute perivenous encephalomyelitis and experimental allergic encephalitis is strong and has already been discussed. Neither of these conditions, however, at least on superficial comparison, has much in common with multiple sclerosis. For example, acute perivenous encephalomyelitis and experimental allergic encephalitis are acute monophasic illnesses with distinctive patterns of inflammation and a variable degree of demyelination. In comparing the two human conditions, however, possible evidence for a common pathogenesis lies in the recognition of cases with structural abnormalities suggestive of both multiple sclerosis and acute perivenous encephalomyelitis. Döring (1941) and Pette (1942) emphasized the similarities between cases of acute multiple sclerosis of the Marburg type and acute perivenous encephalomyelitis, and for these cases used the term 'demyelinating encephalitis'. The pathology of the Japanese cases, described by Uchimura and Shiraki (1957), of demyelinating disease following antirabies vaccine and of Jellinger and Seitelberger's case (1958) following calf's brain extract injections for paralysis agitans, was that of acute perivenous encephalomyelitis with larger 'plaque-like' lesions. In these conditions the antigen was administered repeatedly and there was no evidence of an autonomous, relapsing–remitting condition; similar 'cumulative demyelination' can be produced experimentally by repeated cyanide intoxication (Lumsden, 1950). Despite the dissimilarity of acute experimental allergic encephalitis and multiple sclerosis, the introduction of a chronic relapsing model of experimental allergic encephalitis has shown that immunological and structural abnormalities very similar to those seen in multiple sclerosis can be produced by manipulation of this animal model in susceptible strains (Raine, 1978; Brown, McFarlin and Raine, 1982; Lassmann, 1983). Other similarities between experimental

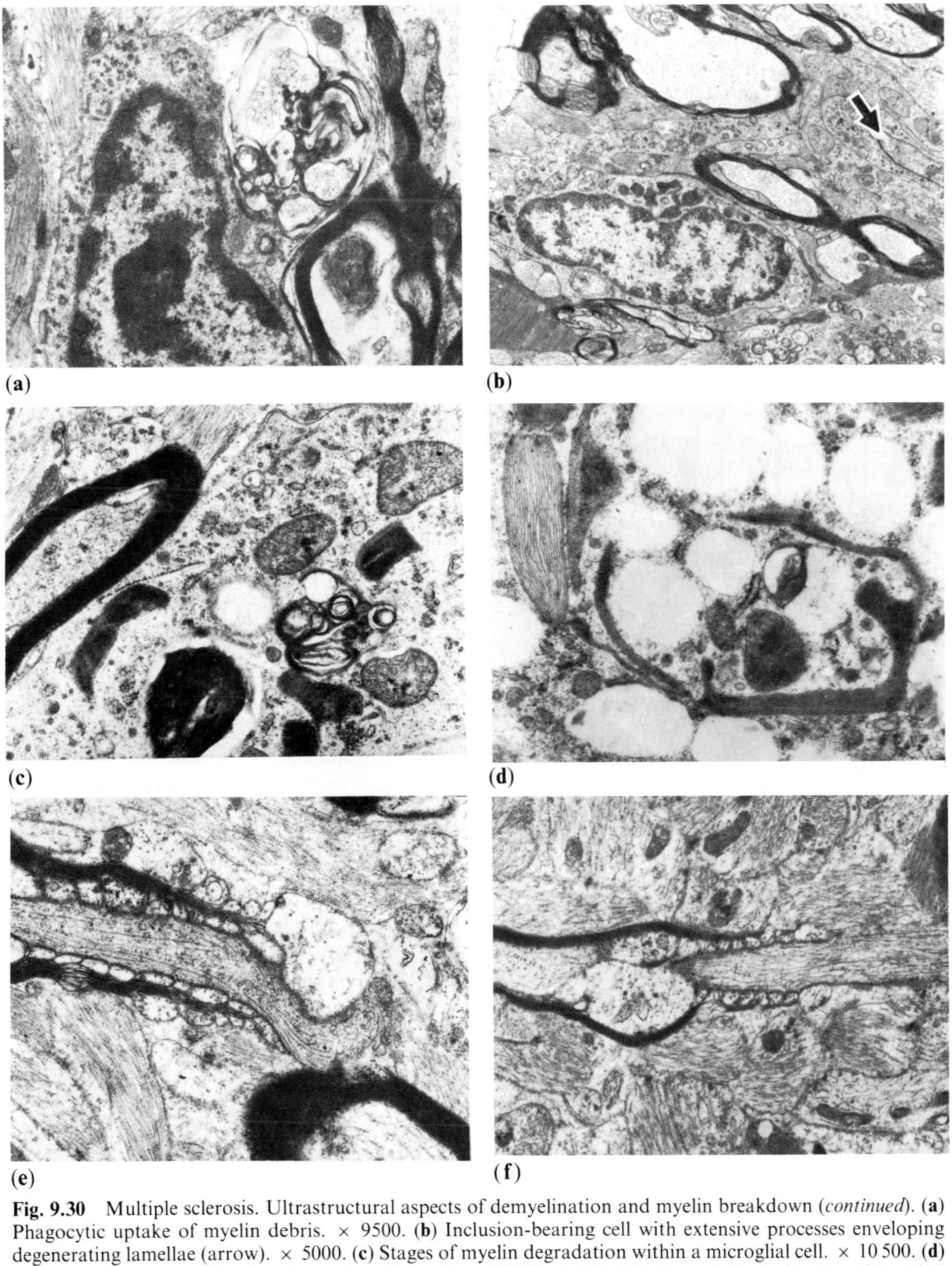

Fig. 9.30 Multiple sclerosis. Ultrastructural aspects of demyelination and myelin breakdown (*continued*). (**a**) Phagocytic uptake of myelin debris. × 9500. (**b**) Inclusion-bearing cell with extensive processes enveloping degenerating lamellae (arrow). × 5000. (**c**) Stages of myelin degradation within a microglial cell. × 10 500. (**d**) Lyre bodies and lipid droplets in a microglial cell. × 20 000. (**e**) Nodal abnormality indicative of 'partial' demyelination; retraction of outer nodal loops of myelin. × 14 500. (**f**) Segmental demyelination and fibrous astrogliosis. × 10 500. (**a, c** and **d** courtesy of Dr M. Hutchinson; **b, e** and **f** courtesy of Dr J. Kirk.)

allergic encephalomyelitis and multiple sclerosis exist; for example, Grundke-Iqbal, Lassmann and Wisniewski (1980) have found the immunohistochemistry to be similar, whilst Mehta, Lassmann and Wisniewski (1981) have found oligoclonal bands in the cerebrospinal fluid in experimental allergic encephalitis and Bornstein and Raine (1977) have demonstrated that both multiple sclerosis serum and experimental allergic encephalitic serum can demyelinate spinal cord organotypic cultures. The development of a chronic relapsing model of experimental allergic encephalitis with a clinical state very similar to that of multiple sclerosis has led to the widely stated view that the pathogenesis might be similar to that of multiple sclerosis. However, doubts have been cast on this view and it has been suggested that a pool of antigen must be present continuously outside the central nervous system to produce the chronic relapsing model of experimental allergic encephalitis. The model is therefore that of cumulative demyelination induced by recurrent acute episodes, dependent on persistent antigen.

Demyelination in other diseases

Periaxial demyelination occurs in a variety of disorders associated with systemic diseases unrelated to multiple sclerosis. Some of these, such as progressive multifocal leucoencephalopathy, are viral in origin (see Chapter 7) while others are toxic or metabolic disorders. Several are of uncertain pathogenesis and these include central pontine myelinolysis and Marchiafava-Bignami disease.

Central pontine myelinolysis

In 1959 Adams, Victor and Mancall described a rare demyelinating condition affecting the pons predominantly although white matter in other parts of the central nervous system may also be affected (Adams, 1962; Wright, Laureno and Victor, 1979; Endo, Oda and Hara, 1981; Goldman and Horoupian, 1981). In the original cases chronic alcoholism and malnutrition were the underlying factors, but since that time central pontine myelinolysis has been associated with many other systemic disorders including viral hepatitis (Ho et al., 1979) chronic pulmonary disease, chronic liver and kidney disease and neoplasia (Endo, Oda and Hara, 1981). In all cases, in addition to the signs of the underlying disease, localizing signs referable to the pontine lesion were observed. At *necropsy* areas of grey softening are seen in the central part of the upper and middle pons, impinging on the tegmentum but not reaching the pial or ventricular surfaces. Histologically (Fig. 9.31) a sharply defined area of myelin breakdown with relative preservation of nerve cell bodies and axis cylinders is seen. Within the lesion, myelin breakdown products are present and there is oligodendrocytic loss and reactive astrocytosis.

Pathogenesis

An increasingly strong association between central pontine myelinolysis and an abnormality of plasma sodium has become apparent. In most

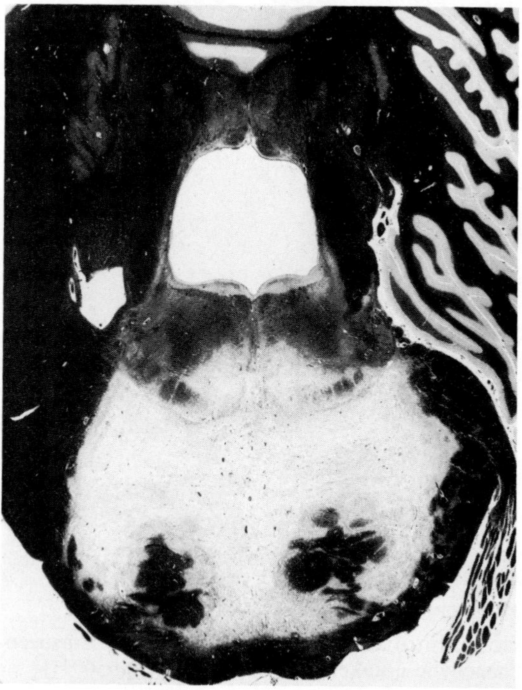

Fig. 9.31 Central pontine myelinolysis. Woman, aged 47, dying after a 2-month illness. Myelin stain showing lesion in pons, with partial sparing of pyramidal bundles.

cases hyponatraemia has been observed and the biochemical abnormality can be correlated with the histological age of the lesion (Wright, Laureno and Victor, 1979). The association with hyponatraemia is not simple, however, and it has been suggested that demyelination may be caused by a rapid, iatrogenic, rise in plasma sodium from hyponatraemic levels (Norenberg, Leslie and Robertson, 1982). This view is supported by experimental evidence in which demyelination was induced in dogs following rapid correction of hyponatraemia (Laureno, 1982).

Marchiafava-Bignami disease

In this exceedingly rare disorder, first described by Marchiafava and Bignami in 1903, demyelination occurs in the corpus callosum. The disease is most common in male drinkers who prefer crude red wine. Ironside, Bosanquet and McMenemey (1961) listed 88 documented cases including one of their own. Italian and French nationalities predominated, and cases from other countries were rare.

At necropsy the sharply demarcated lesion in the corpus callosum is apparent, but in addition degeneration of other symmetrical pathways such as the anterior commissure and the middle cerebellar peduncles is seen (Lumsden 1970). In some cases there is loss of axis cylinders while in others this feature is not seen. Oligodendrocytic loss is total but lipophage and astrocytic responses are often slight. The features of Wernicke's encephalopathy and pellagroid neuronal changes may also be found (Koeppen and Barron, 1978).

Pathogenesis

The pathogenesis of the lesion remains obscure. Chronic alcoholism and malnutrition *per se* cannot be the explanation because Marchiafava-Bignami disease is not associated with all forms of alcoholism. Chronic cyanide intoxication can produce similar lesions, as can chronic methyl alcohol intoxication (Poser, 1973). The association with alcoholism is not invariable: the condition is rare in Asians but in the first Chinese case to be described there was no history of alcoholism or other drug addiction (Kuo-Chun and Kuan-Jung, 1983).

X-linked leucodystrophy

The leucodystrophies may be classified according to clinical, pathological, genetic and biochemical criteria. A genetic classification has much to commend it, as ultimately genetic factors must determine the other features. Various patterns of inheritance are recognized within the broad group of leucodystrophies; those associated with lysosomal enzyme deficiencies are generally inherited on an autosomal recessive basis, but a further group of X-linked leucodystrophies is now recognized. A classification of this group is given in Table 9.3 (Baraitser, 1982).

Table 9.3 X-linked leucodystrophy

Adrenoleucodystrophy:
Classic type
Adrenomyeloneuropathy
Pelizaeus-Merzbacher disease:
Type I—classic
Type II—Seitelberger, connatal or congenital
Type III—transitional
Type IV—adult
Type V—atypical
Type VI—Cockayne

Adrenoleucodystrophy

Classic type For many years the association of a demyelinating disease of the Schilder type with adrenocortical insufficiency has been recognized. The early reports of Siemerling and Creutzfeldt (1923), Pfister (1936) and Hampel (1937) were followed by a series of case reports of 'bronzed Schilder's disease' or 'melanodermic leucodystrophy': more recently the term 'adrenoleucodystrophy' has gained wide acceptance. Schaumburg and his colleagues (1972, 1974, 1975) have collected 50 cases from the literature and published a detailed clinicopathological study of a further 17 cases. The hereditary nature of the disorder was established by the studies of Gagnon and LeBlanc (1959), Hoefnagel, Vanden Noort and Ingbar (1962), Crome and Zapella (1963), Fanconi et al. (1963) and Peiffer and Zerbin-Rudin (1963). It is apparent that males are almost exclusively affected and that in most cases there is an X-linked recessive transmission. The case for this pattern of inheritance is supported not only by male predominance in the disorder but also by the report of an affected heterozygotic female with two affected sons (Morariu et al., 1982). In a recent report, however, Jaffe et al. (1982) have suggested that an autosomal recessive form of the disease exists affecting neonatal males and females equally.

Clinical presentation is usually in the latter half of the first decade but, in addition to this juvenile form, connatal (Ulrich et al., 1978), neonatal (Manz et al., 1980), infantile and adult (Powers and Schaumburg, 1980, 1981) forms are recognized. Early abnormalities are often visual, with motor signs occurring later, and there is usually steady neurological deterioration with death occurring about 5 years after the onset of clinical signs. Occasional patients with the juvenile form have had long survival, and in the adult form the presentation may be of a psychiatric disorder with neurological and endocrine abnormalities occurring later (Bresnan et al., 1979). Variable presentation of the syndrome may be seen within one pedigree (Gagnon and LeBlanc, 1959; Schaumburg et al., 1975) with some members suffering from Addison's disease alone, whereas others have the combined abnormality.

Pathology *Nervous system* The external appearances of the brain and spinal cord are usually normal, but on section the involved white matter is grey in colour and of firm consistency. The occipital, parietal and temporal lobes are most severely affected and show symmetrical diffuse abnormality of the white matter (Blaw et al., 1964; Blaw, 1970; Schaumburg et al., 1975). The frontal lobes often are affected less severely but usually show some demyelination. The subcortical arcuate fibres and band of Gennari show at least partial sparing, whilst the optic nerves and tracts, fornix, hippocampal commissure, posterior cingulum and corpus callosum are usually severely affected. Lesions in the cerebellum are recorded but the brain stem and spinal cord usually show only secondary long tract degeneration.

The lesions are characterized histopathologically by three zones: (1) there is destruction of myelin, axonal sparing and a scattering of PAS-positive and sudanophilic macrophages; (2) myelinated and demyelinated axons are seen with an associated inflammatory and lipophage response; (3) there is dense gliosis with loss of oligodendrocytes, myelin and axons. Neurons are generally well preserved although those in the deeper layer of the cerebral cortex may show an increase in lipofuscin. Degeneration of the medial and lateral geniculate bodies, hippocampal formation and dentate nuclei is usually severe.

Several electron microscopical studies have confirmed and extended the light microscopical findings, and the important observation has been that of distinctive curvilinear inclusions within macrophages (Schaumburg et al., 1974, 1975).

The adrenal glands These glands are atrophic and may be affected so severely that they cannot be identified at necropsy. On histological examination the medulla is normal but the cortex is abnormal (Fig. 9.32) although there may be relative sparing of the zona glomerulosa (Blaw et al., 1964). Lymphocytic infiltration may be seen, and the cortical epithelial cells may show ballooning (Schaumburg et al., 1972) and contain inclusions similar to those seen in cerebral macrophages (Powers and Schaumburg, 1974). These abnormalities have been demonstrated in the fetal adrenal (Powers et al., 1982).

Other organs Electron microscopical examination of testis and peripheral nerve has demonstrated lamellar profiles in the interstitial cells of the testis and in Schwann cells (Schaumburg et al., 1975). Manz et al. (1980) have described similar inclusions in macrophages and in lymph nodes, liver and spleen.

Biochemistry Several studies have demonstrated increases in cholesterol esters within brain tissue; it has been suggested that there is a defect in very-long-chain fatty acid metabolism (Igarashi et al., 1976; Menkes and Corbo, 1977; Manz et al., 1980) and studies on fibroblasts support this view (Rizzo et al., 1984). The biochemical properties of myelin membrane from white matter of affected cases indicate significant enrichment in abnormal cholesterol ester (Brown et al., 1983). It is not known how these biochemical changes relate to the process of demyelination.

Adrenomyeloneuropathy

In 1957 Hewitt described two sisters with Addison's disease, one of whom had spasticity of the legs. Since then, other cases have been reported; Schaumburg et al. (1977) have reported five cases, all male, with a slowly progressive spastic

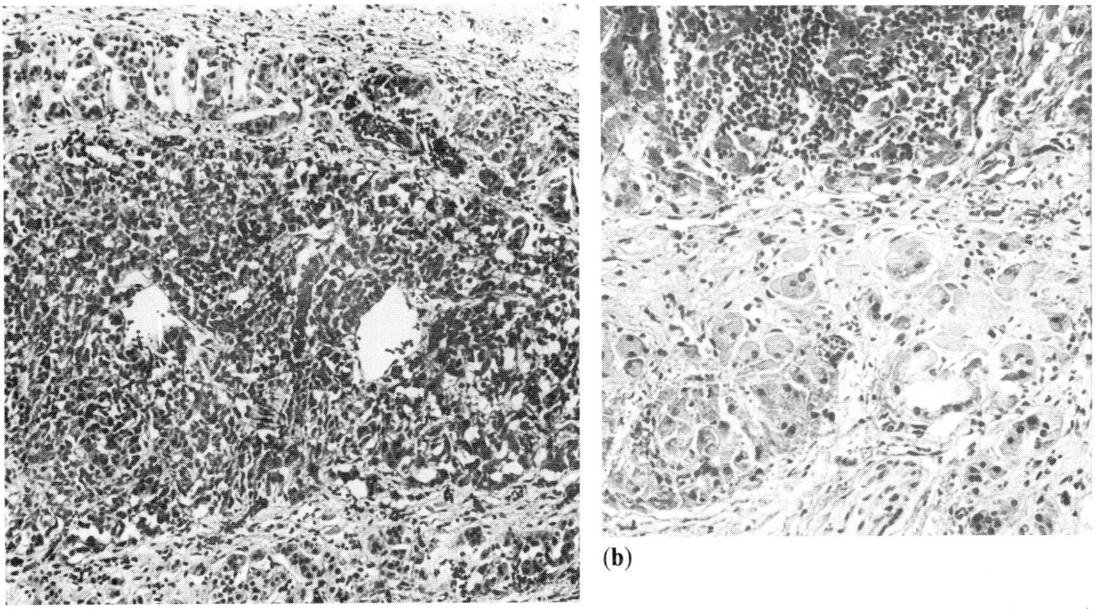

(a) (b)

Fig. 9.32 Adrenoleucodystrophy. (**a**) 'Pseudolaminar' atrophy of the adrenal without marked lymphocytic infiltration. Haematoxylin and eosin × 110. (**b**) Atrophy of the adrenal with lymphocytic infiltration and distension of some cells. Haematoxylin and eosin × 160.

paraparesis, distal symmetrical polyneuropathy, Addison's disease and hypogonadism. Davis et al. (1979) have reported a pedigree in which adrenoleucodystrophy and adrenomyeloneuropathy coexisted; this suggests that the two conditions may be caused by the same mutant gene. In support of this hypothesis, cytoplasmic inclusions similar to those described in adrenoleucodystrophy have been described in the brain, spinal nerve roots, adrenal glands and interstitial cells of the testis in a case of adrenomyeloneuropathy (Probst et al., 1980), and similar biochemical abnormalities have been described in the two conditions (Askanas et al., 1979). Preliminary attempts to treat patients with either adrenoleucodystrophy or adrenomyeloneuropathy by dietary restriction of very-long-chain fatty acids has produced some clinical improvement (Moser et al., 1982).

Pelizaeus-Merzbacher disease

A rare, X-linked, demyelinating disease was described in one family by Pelizaeus (1885) and Merzbacher (1910). Since then similar families have been reported on a world-wide basis, and the diagnosis is based on clinical, genetic and neuropathological grounds. As the result of various detailed studies, particularly those of Seitelberger (1954, 1957, 1963, 1970), Norman and colleagues (Norman, 1962; Norman and Tingey, 1963; Norman et al., 1966; Peiffer and Zerbin-Rudin, 1963), various subtypes are now recognized.

Type I—Classic The classic variety described by Pelizaeus and Merzbacher is characterized by the onset of neurological symptoms in the infantile or late infantile period. Dementia is often a feature, and death occurs approximately 5 years after the onset of symptoms.

At necropsy the brain is generally atrophic and the brain stem and cerebellum are often particularly severely affected. Histologically the pattern of demyelination is 'tigroid'; i.e. there is widespread myelin loss but irregular 'islands' of myelin are preserved, particularly around blood vessels (Fig. 9.33). Microscopical examination of fields in which myelin is apparently well preserved reveals degeneration of individual myelinated fibres. Axis cylinders tend to be preserved and there is a vigorous astrocytic response but the degeneration of myelin is not accompanied by liberation of sudanophilic material.

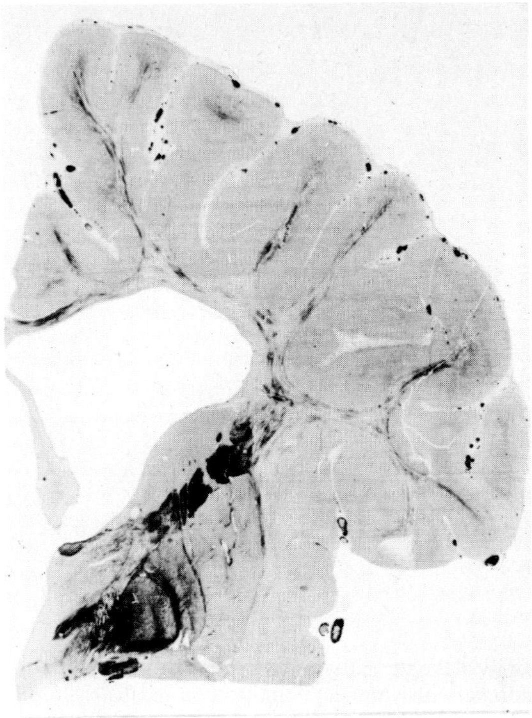

(a)

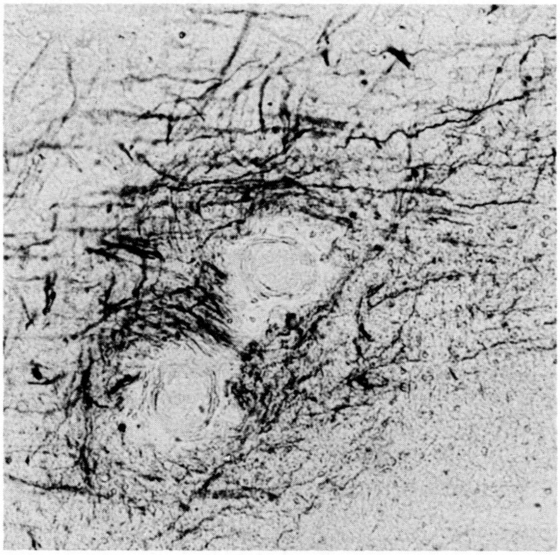

(b)

Fig. 9.33 Pelizaeus–Merzbacher disease. (**a**) Profound demyelination of the white matter, with sparing of islets of myelin. (**b**) A surviving perivascular islet of myelin in the midst of widespread demyelination.

This latter observation has led to the postulation that the intrinsic abnormality is in myelin formation (Blackwood and Cumings, 1954).

Type II—Seitelberger, connatal or congenital type This is a severe variety, characterized by very poor neurological development with nystagmus, involuntary movements and spasticity of the lower limbs. The 13 cases reviewed and described by Seitelberger were all male and the inheritance X-linked, but the syndrome has been described in females (Nisenbaum, Sandbank and Kohn, 1965) and there is confusion as to the exact criteria for diagnosis.

At necropsy the brain shows generalized atrophy, and the white matter of the centrum semiovale and corpus callosum is thin and discoloured. Histologically there is severe demyelination (Fig. 9.34) but a few islands of surviving myelin may be present. Nerve cells and axis cylinders tend to be well preserved and sudanophil products of myelin degradation are scarce. The cerebellum may show loss of nerve cells, demyelination and astrocytosis, and the occurrence of concomitant microgyria has been reported. As in the classic form of the disease, the white matter shows a reduction of total lipids chemically. In a possible case, Adachi et al. (1970) found on electron microscopy only occasional lamellar myelin sheaths; cortical neurons were normal.

Type III—transitional between I and II Seitelberger (1970) has drawn attention to the occurrence of some cases resembling both the congenital and the classic form of Pelizaeus–Merzbacher's disease and he has listed these separately as 'transitional' forms. All cases have been sporadic and both males and females have been affected.

Type IV—adult type Onset is in the fifth decade, with neurological abnormalities and intellectual deterioration. Unlike other forms, the inheritance appears to be autosomal dominant.

Type V Seitelberger (1970) included six atypical cases in this category. Since then further cases have been reported.

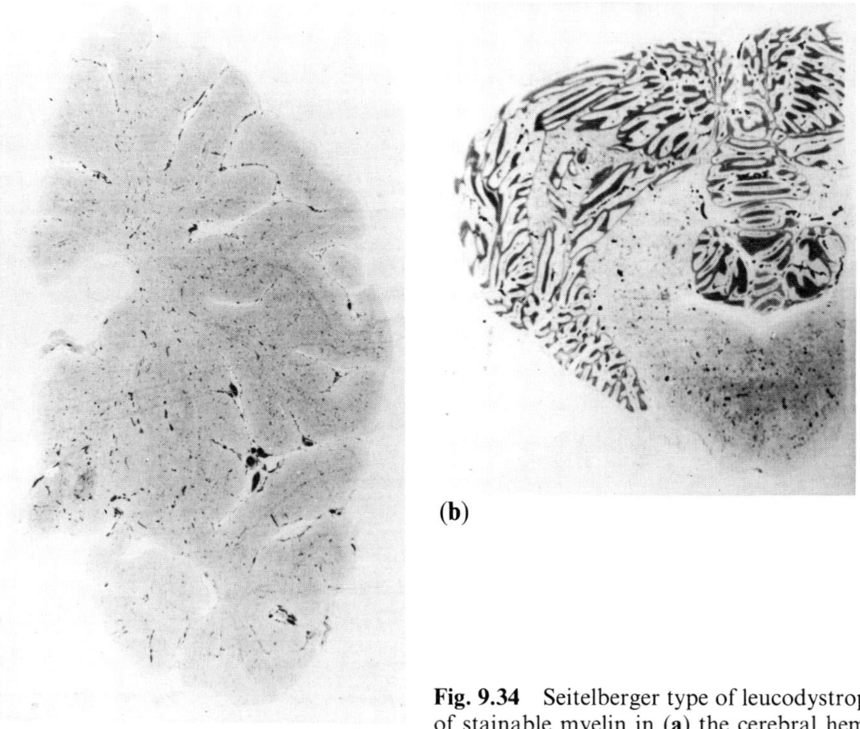

(a) (b)

Fig. 9.34 Seitelberger type of leucodystrophy. Complete absence of stainable myelin in (**a**) the cerebral hemisphere and in (**b**) the cerebellum and brain stem. Heidenhain's method for myelin.

Type VI In this syndrome there is widespread involvement of the white matter with a 'tigroid' pattern of demyelination. In addition, there may be segmental demyelination in peripheral nerves with dwarfism, cataracts, joint contractures, hypersensitivity to sunlight, severe dental caries and intracranial calcification. The disease is probably a leucodystrophy but the exact relationship to other forms of Pelizaeus-Merzbacher disease is unknown. The condition has been reviewed by Soffer et al. (1979).

The Alexander type of leucodystrophy

This condition, first described by Alexander (1949), commences in infancy or later childhood, the clinical picture being of progressive dementia, paralysis and epilepsy. With onset before the union of the cranial sutures the patients become megalencephalic. All reported cases have been sporadic. The large brain shows a somewhat indurated, uniformly white, cortical ribbon. The subjacent white matter is discoloured and may be loosened in texture, soft, jelly-like, collapsed or broken down (Fig. 9.35). Histological examination reveals diffuse demyelination and rarefac-

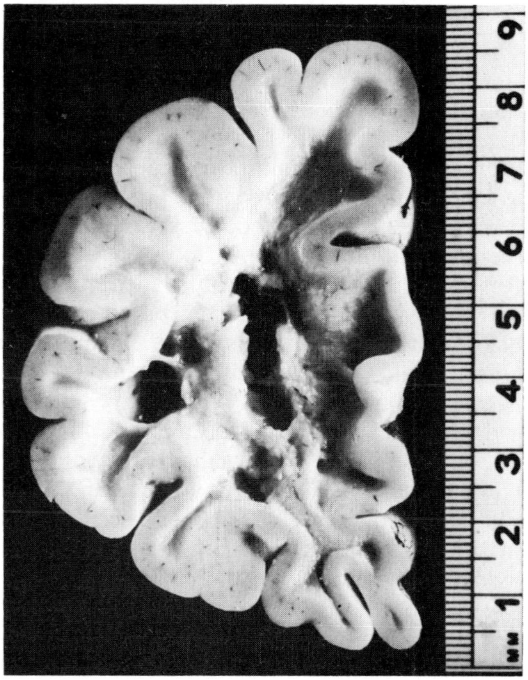

Fig. 9.35 Coronal block of the frontal lobe from a case of Alexander's leucodystrophy.

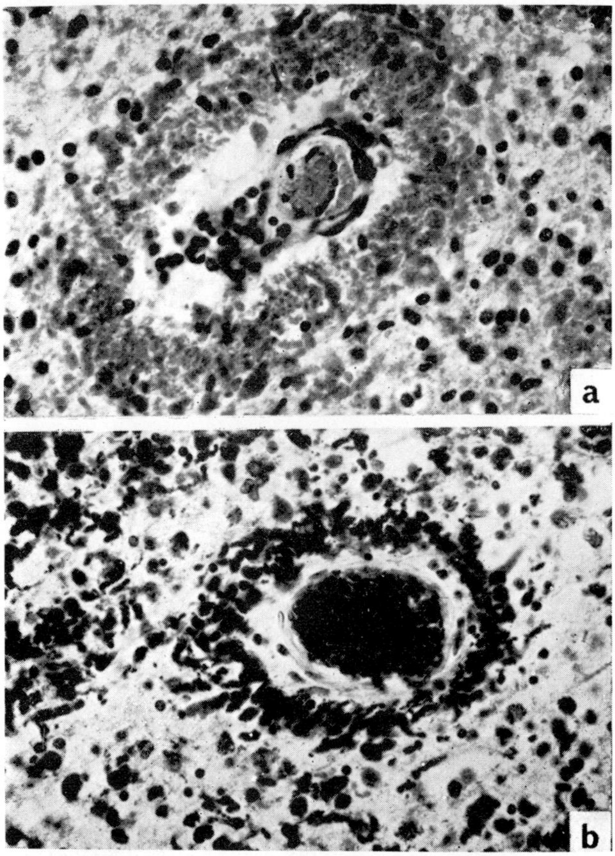

Fig. 9.36 Rosenthal fibres in a case of Alexander's leucodystrophy are particularly dense and numerous around a blood vessel. (**a**) Haematoxylin and eosin × 400. (**b**) Heidenhain–Woelcke × 400.

tion of the white matter, with little or no sparing of the arcuate fibres. The distinctive feature is the presence throughout the central nervous system of innumerable Rosenthal fibres arranged most densely around blood vessels and deep to the external and internal surfaces of the brain. Rosenthal fibres are irregularly shaped elongated or rounded hyaline eosinophil bodies staining black with the myelin stains (Fig. 9.36), and deep purple with Mallory's phosphotungstic acid haematoxylin. They are PAS-negative and not sudanophil. Their precise nature has not been established but it is obvious that they contain or consist mainly of proteins including glial fibrillary acidic protein. They also occur, albeit in smaller numbers, in many other conditions associated with reactive or neoplastic astrocytosis. Some areas of the cerebral cortex in Alexander's disease show fibrous gliosis and there may be diffuse neuronal loss both in the cerebral cortex and in subcortical formations.

On electron microscopy Rosenthal fibres appear as dense round osmiophilic structures merging with thickened glial fibrils.

Further details of the condition will be found in case reports, such as those by Vogel and Hallervorden (1962), Herndon and Rubinstein (1968), Schochet, Lampert and Earle (1968) and Herndon et al. (1970).

Spongiform leucodystrophy

Non-specific spongiform degeneration or rarefaction of neural tissue, the status spongiosus of German authors, is a relatively common neuropathological finding in diverse conditions. It has been regarded by some as a consequence of long-standing widespread or localized brain oedema. On histological examination, tissue sections, especially of the white matter, show rarification, displaying countless vacuoles which coalesce into grosser cavities (Fig. 9.37). Such spongiform degeneration may be associated with lack of myelination, demyelination or gliotic change. In some children spongiform degeneration of the white matter is the sole ascertainable

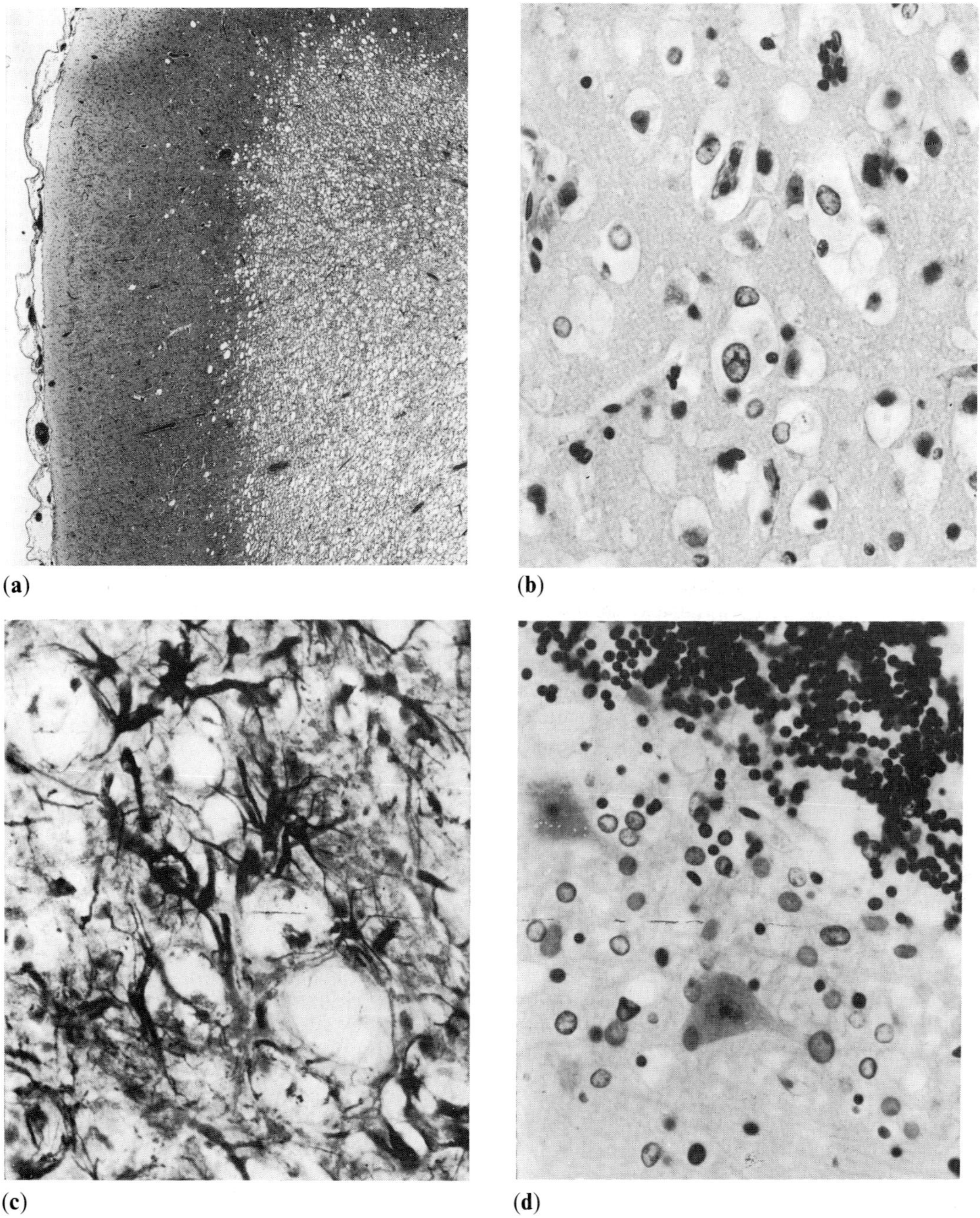

Fig. 9.37 Spongiform leucodystrophy. (**a**) Low power view of the cortex and white matter. (**b**) Deeper layers of the cortex. (**c**) White matter. × 400. (**d**) Cerebellar cortex with large vesicular astrocytic nuclei. × 400.

pathological change. Such cases, especially if familial, have been named *spongiform leucodystrophy* or, less appropriately, *Canavan's type of diffuse sclerosis*. Three forms of the condition have been described: a *congenital*, an *infantile* and a *juvenile*. The infantile cases were often Jewish. They showed severe mental retardation, enlargement of the head and hypotonia followed by spastic paralysis. The CSF protein was sometimes raised. The condition tended to be transmitted as a mendelian recessive trait. In addition to the status spongiosus, the cerebral cortex of these cases (and subcortical grey matter) shows numerous enlarged, bare vesicular astrocytic nuclei resembling Alzheimer II cells. Although there is considerable variation in the extent and position of the demyelination and spongiform change, the part most affected is the centrum semiovale where the white matter may be converted into a loose meshwork of bare glial and axonal fibres. The arcuate fibres are often involved and the degeneration may extend into the deeper layers of the cerebral cortex where Alzheimer II cells are particularly numerous. The basal ganglia may be affected. In the cerebellum there is frequently an oedematous space (lamina dissecans) between the granular and molecular layers, Purkinje cells being displaced outwards. Spongiform leucodystrophy was fully described in a monograph by van Bogaert and Bertrand (1967) and has been reviewed by Adachi et al. (1973). For a detailed description, including characteristic electron microscopical data, readers are referred to the case reports of two siblings by Kolkmann, Rana and Nützenadel (1971). Most of the infantile cases die in infancy but more chronic ones surviving into later childhood are known to occur (Adachi and Volk, 1968). No specific enzyme deficiency has been identified as a cause of the leucodystrophy, and, indeed, the condition is probably not homogeneous. A somewhat similar disorder, sometimes associated with retinitis pigmentosa, has been reported in older children. This was first described by Kearns and Sayre (1958) and about 20 cases have been reviewed by Tridon, *et al.* (1974). None was familial.

Spongiform leucodystrophy, a disease primarily of the white matter, is not to be confused with 'spongy degeneration of the grey matter' which may also occur in children (Janota, 1974).

References

Adachi, M. and Volk, B.W. (1968) Protracted form of spongy degeneration of the central nervous system (van Bogaert and Bertrand type). *Neurology* **18,** 1084–92.

Adachi, M., Schneck, L., Volk, B.W. and Torii, J. (1970) Histochemical, ultrastructural and biochemical studies of a case with leucodystrophy due to congenital deficiency of myelin. *Journal of Neuropathology and Experimental Neurology* **29,** 149–50.

Adachi, M., Schneck, L., Cara, J. and Volk, B.W. (1973) Spongy degeneration of the central nervous system (van Bogaert and Bertrand type, Canavan's disease). A review. *Human Pathology* **4,** 331–47.

Adams, C.W.M. (1977) Pathology of multiple sclerosis: progression of the lesion. *British Medical Bulletin* **33,** 15–20.

Adams, C.W.M. (1981) Histochemical contributions to the study of multiple sclerosis. In *Histochemistry. The Widening Horizons of its Application in the Biomedical Sciences* (Eds. Stoward, P.J. and Polak, J.M.), pp. 163–82. John Wiley, Chichester, New York, Brisbane, Toronto, Singapore.

Adams, J.H. (1962) Central pontine myelinolysis. In *Proceedings of the 4th International Congress of Neuropathology*, vol. 3 (Ed. Jacob, H.), pp. 303–08. Thieme, Stuttgart.

Adams, J.M. and Imagawa, D.T. (1962) Measles antibodies in multiple sclerosis. *Proceedings of the Society for Experimental Biology and Medicine* **111,** 562–6.

Adams, R.D., Victor, M. and Mancall, E.L. (1959) Central pontine myelinolysis. *Archives of Neurology and Psychiatry* **81,** 154–72.

Alcock, N.S. and Hoffman, H.L. (1962) Recurrent encephalomyelitis in childhood. *Archives of Disease in Childhood* **37,** 40–4.

Alexander, W.S. (1949) Progressive fibrinoid degeneration of fibrillary astrocytes. *Brain* **72,** 373–81.

Allbutt, T.C. (1870) On the ophthalmoscopic signs of spinal disease. *Lancet* **1,** 76–8.

Allen, I.V. (1983) Hydrolytic enzymes in multiple sclerosis. In *Progress in Neuropathology*, Vol 5 (Ed. Zimmerman, H.M.), pp. 1–17. Raven Press, New York.

Allen, I.V. and McKeown, S.R. (1979) A histological,

histochemical and biochemical study of the macroscopically normal white matter in multiple sclerosis. *Journal of the Neurological Sciences* **41,** 81–91.

Allen, I.V., Millar, J.H.D. and Hutchinson, M.J. (1978) General disease in 120 necropsy-proven cases of multiple sclerosis. *Neuropathology and Applied Neurobiology* **4,** 279–84.

Allen, I.V., Glover, G. and Anderson, R. (1981) Abnormalities in the macroscopically normal white matter in cases of mild or spinal multiple sclerosis (MS). *Acta Neuropathologica* Suppl 7, 176–8.

Allen, I.V., Millar, J.H.D., Kirk, J. and Shillington, R.K.A. (1979) Systemic lupus erythematosus clinically resembling multiple sclerosis and with unusual pathological and ultrastructural features. *Journal of Neurology, Neurosurgery and Psychiatry* **42,** 392–401.

Anderson, M., Hughes, B., Jefferson, M., Smith, W.T. and Waterhouse, J.A.H. (1980) Gliomatous transformation and demyelinating diseases. *Brain* **103,** 603–22.

Arnason, B.G.W. and Waksman, B.H. (1980) Immunoregulation in multiple sclerosis. *Annals of Neurology* **8,** 237–40.

Askanas, V., McLaughlin, J., Engel, W.K. and Adornato, B.T. (1979) Abnormalities in cultured muscle and peripheral nerve of a patient with adrenomyeloneuropathy. *New England Journal of Medicine* **301,** 588–90.

Balò, J. (1928) Encephalitis periaxialis concentrica. *Archives of Neurology and Psychiatry* **19,** 242–64.

Baraitser, M. (1982) *The Genetics of Neurological Disorders*. Oxford University Press, Oxford.

Barré, J.A., Morin, V., Draganesco, S. and Reys, L. (1926) Encéphalite periaxiale diffuse. *Revue Neurologique* **2,** 541–57.

Bassoe, P. and Grinker, R.R. (1930) Human rabies and rabies vaccine encephalomyelitis. *Archives of Neurology and Psychiatry* **23,** 1138–60.

Bates, D., Fawcett, P.R.W. and Weightman, D. (1978) Polyunsaturated fatty acid in treatment of acute remitting multiple sclerosis. *British Medical Journal* **2,** 1390–1.

Bérard-Badier, M., Gastaut, H. and Payan, H. (1961) Comparative clinico-pathological study of one early and two late cases of measles encephalitis (with an electroencephalographic study of one case). In *Encephalitides: Proceedings of a Symposium on the Neuropathology, Electronencephalography and Biochemistry of Encephalitides*, Antwerp, 1959 (Eds. van Bogaert, L., Radermecker, J., Hozay, J. and Lowenthal, A.), pp. 106–23. Elsevier, Amsterdam, London, New York, Princeton.

Blackwood, W. and Cumings, J.N. (1954) A histological and chemical study of three cases of diffuse cerebral sclerosis. *Journal of Neurology, Neurosurgery and Psychiatry* **17,** 33–49.

Blakemore, W.F. (1982) Myelination, demyelination and remyelination in the CNS. In *Recent Advances in Neuropathology—2* (Eds. Smith, W.T. and Cavanagh, J.B.), pp. 53–81. Churchill Livingstone, London.

Blaw, M.E. (1970) Melanodermic type leukodystrophy (adrenoleukodystrophy). In *Handbook of Clinical Neurology*, vol. 10 (Eds. Vinken, P.J. and Bruyn, G.W.), pp. 128–33. North-Holland, Amsterdam; American Elsevier, New York.

Blaw, M.E., Osterberg, K., Kozak, P. and Nelson, E. (1964) Sudanophilic leukodystrophy and adrenal cortical atrophy. *Archives of Neurology* **11,** 626–31.

van Bogaert, L. (1950) Post-infectious encephalomyelitis and multiple sclerosis. *Journal of Neuropathology and Experimental Neurology* **9,** 219–49.

van Bogaert, L. and Bertrand, I. (1967) *Spongy Degeneration of the Brain in Infancy*. North-Holland, Amsterdam.

Booss, J., Esiri, M.M., Tourtellotte, W.W. and Mason, D.Y. (1983) Immunohistological analysis of T lymphocyte subsets in the central nervous system in chronic progressive multiple sclerosis. *Journal of the Neurological Sciences* **62,** 219–32.

Bornstein, M.B. (1963) A tissue-culture approach to demyelinative disorders. *National Cancer Institute Monographs* **11,** 197–214.

Bornstein, M.B. and Raine, C.S. (1977) Multiple sclerosis and experimental allergic encephalomyelitis: specific demyelination of CNS in culture. *Neuropathology and Applied Neurobiology* **3,** 359–67.

Bouman, L. and Bok, S.T. (1927) Die Histopathologie der Encephalitis post vaccinationem. *Zeitschrift für die gesamte Neurologie und Psychiatrie* **111,** 495–510.

Bresnan, M.J., Davis, K.R., Richardson, E.P., Kliman, B., Dickersin, G.R. and Kolodny, E.H. (1979) Case records of the Massachusetts General Hospital, case 18-1979. *New England Journal of Medicine* **300,** 1037–45.

Brock, J. (1926) Ueber Systematik und Klinik meningoencephaler Krankheitszustände im Kindesalter. *Zeitschrift für Kinderheilkunde* **40,** 552–72.

Broman, T. (1947) Supravital analysis of disorders in the cerebral vascular permeability. II. Two cases of multiple sclerosis. *Acta Psychiatrica et Neurologica Scandinavica* suppl. 46, 58–71.

Brown, A., McFarlin, D.E. and Raine, C.S. (1982) Chronologic neuropathology of relapsing experimental allergic encephalomyelitis in the mouse. *Laboratory Investigation* **46,** 171–85.

Brown, F.R. III, Chen, W.W., Kirschner, D.A., Frayer, K.L., Powers, J.M., Moser, A.B. and Moser, H.W. (1983) Myelin membrane from adrenoleukodystrophy brain white matter—biochemical properties. *Journal of Neurochemistry* **41,** 341–8.

Brownell, B. and Hughes, J.T. (1962) The distribution of plaques in the cerebrum in multiple sclerosis. *Journal of Neurology, Neurosurgery and Psychiatry* **25,** 315–20.

Carswell, R. (1838) Atrophy. In *Pathological Anatomy. Illustration of Elementary Forms of Disease,* Plate IV. Longman, Orme, Brown, Green and Longman, London.

Cavanagh, J.B. (1970) Reactions of neuroglial cells to injury. In *Modern Trends in Neurology—5,* pp. 149–164. Butterworths, London.

Charcot, J.M. (1877) *Lectures on the Diseases of the Nervous System* (Trans. G. Sigerson). The New Sydenham Society, London. 1st series lecture 6 (delivered 1868).

Chou, C.H.J., Chou, F.C.H., Tourtellotte, W.W. and Kibler, R.F. (1983) Search for a multiple sclerosis-specific brain antigen. *Neurology* **33,** 1300–4.

Chou, C.H.J., Chou, F.C.H., Tourtellotte, W.W. and Kibler, R.F. (1984) Dévic's syndrome: antibody to glial fibrillary acidic protein in cerebrospinal fluid. *Neurology* **34,** 86–8.

Chou, S.M. (1982) Acute haemorrhagic leucoencephalitis as a disseminated vasculomyelinopathy: immunoperoxidase study. *Journal of Neuropathology and Experimental Neurology* **41,** 357.

Chu, B., Sever, J.L., Madden, D.L., Iivanainen, M., Leon, M., Wallen, W. et al. (1983) Oligoclonal IgG bands in cerebrospinal fluid in various neurological diseases. *Annals of Neurology* **13,** 434–9.

Cloys, D.E. and Netsky, M.G. (1970) Neuromyelitis optica. In *Handbook of Neurology,* vol. 9 (Eds. Vinken, P.J. and Bruyn, G.W.), pp. 426–35. North-Holland, Amsterdam; American Elsevier, New York.

Corsellis, J.A.N., Janota, I. and Marshall, A.K. (1983) Immunization against whooping cough: a neuropathological review. *Neuropathology and Applied Neurobiology* **9,** 261–70.

Craelius, W., Jacobs, R.M. and Lee Jones, A.O. (1980) Mineral composition of brains of normal and multiple sclerosis victims. *Proceedings of the Society for Experimental Biology and Medicine* **165,** 327–9.

Craelius, W., Migdal, M.W., Luessenhop, C.P., Sugar, A. and Mihalakis, I. (1982) Iron deposits surrounding multiple sclerosis plaques. *Archives of Pathology and Laboratory Medicine* **106,** 397–9.

Croft, P.B. (1969) Para-infectious and post-vaccinial encephalomyelitis. *Postgraduate Medical Journal* **43,** 392–400.

Crome, L. and Zapella, M. (1963) Schilder's disease (sudanophilic leucodystrophy) in five male members of one family. *Journal of Neurology, Neurosurgery and Psychiatry* **26,** 431–8.

Cruveilhier, J. (1829–42) *Anatomie Pathologique du Corps Humain,* vol. 2, livraison 52, Plate 2. Baillière, Paris.

Currie, S., Roberts, A.H. and Urich, H. (1970) The nosological position of concentric lacunar leucoencephalopathy. *Journal of Neurology, Neurosurgery and Psychiatry* **33,** 131–7.

Cuzner, M.L. (1980) Recent biochemical and immunological observations in multiple sclerosis. *Neuropathology and Applied Neurobiology* **6,** 405–14.

Cuzner, M.L., Allen, I.V., Glynn, P. and Newcombe, J. (1981) Antigenic specificity of intrathecally synthesised immunoglobulins in multiple sclerosis. *Neuropathology and Applied Neurobiology* **7,** 503.

Dalakas, M., Wright, R.G. and Prineas, J.W. (1980) Nature of the reversible white matter lesion in multiple sclerosis. Effects of acute inflammation on myelinated tissue studied in the rabbit eye. *Brain* **103,** 515–24.

Davis, L.E., Snyder, R.D., Orth, D.N., Nicholson, W.E., Kornfeld, M. and Seelinger, D.F. (1979) Adrenoleukodystrophy and adrenomyeloneuropathy associated with partial adrenal insufficiency in three generations of a kindred. *American Journal of Medicine* **66,** 342–7.

Dawson, J.W. (1916) The histology of disseminated sclerosis. *Transactions of the Royal Society of Edinburgh* **50,** 517–740.

Dean, G. (1970) The multiple sclerosis problem. *Scientific American* **223,** 40–6.

Dévic, M.E. (1894) Myélite subaiguë compliquée de névrite optique. *Bulletin Médical (Paris)* **8,** 1033.

Döring, G. (1941) Zur Pathologie und Klinik der Entmarkungsencephalomyelitis. *Deutsche Zeitschrift für Nervenheilkunde* **153,** 73–139.

Endo, Y., Oda, M. and Hara, M. (1981) Central pontine myelinolysis. A study of 37 cases in 1,000 consecutive autopsies. *Acta Neuropathologica* **53,** 145–53.

Esiri, M.M. (1980) Multiple sclerosis: a quantitative and qualitative study of immunoglobulin-containing cells in the central nervous system. *Neuropathology and Applied Neurobiology* **6,** 9–21.

Fanconi, A., Prader, A., Isler, W., Lüthy, F. and Siebenmann, R. (1963) Morbus Addison with cerebral sclerosis in childhood. A hereditary syndrome with X chromosomal inheritance? *Helvetica Paediatrica Acta* **18,** 480–501.

Fenichel, G.M. (1982) Neurological complications of immunization. *Annals of Neurology* **12,** 119–28.

Field, E.J. (1967) The significance of astroglial hypertrophy in scrapie, kuru, multiple sclerosis and old age together with a note on the possible nature of the scrapie agent. *Deutsche Zeitschrift für Nervenheilkunde* **192,** 265–74.

Fisher, J.H. and Gilmour, J.R. (1939) Encephalomyelitis following administration of sulphanilamide. *Lancet* **2,** 301–5.

Fog, T. (1965) Multiple sclerosis. *Acta Neurologica Scandinavica* suppl. 15, 5–161.

Forrester, C. and Lascelles, R.G. (1979) Association between polyneuritis and multiple sclerosis. *Journal of Neurology, Neurosurgery and Psychiatry* **42,** 864–6.

Gagnon, J. and LeBlanc, R. (1959) Sclérose cérébrale diffuse avec melanodermie et atrophie surrenale. Maladie d'Addison-Scholz. *Union Médicale de Canada* **88,** 392–412.

Gault, F. (1895) De la Neuromyélite Optique Aiguë. Thesis, University of Lyon.

Ghatak, N.R., Hirano, A., Doron, Y. and Zimmerman, H.M. (1973) Remyelination in multiple sclerosis with peripheral type myelin. *Archives of Neurology* **29,** 262–7.

Ghatak, N.R., Hirano, A., Lijtmaer, H. and Zimmerman, H.M. (1974) Asymptomatic demyelinated plaque in the spinal cord. *Archives of Neurology* **30,** 484–6.

Glanzmann, E. (1927) Die nervösen Komplikationen der Varizellen, Variola und Vakzine. *Schweizerische medizinische Wochenschrift* **57,** 145–54.

Goldman, J.E. and Horoupian, D.S. (1981) Demyelination of the lateral geniculate nucleus in central pontine myelinolysis. *Annals of Neurology* **9,** 185–9.

Goust, J.M., Hoffman, P.M., Pryjma, J., Hogan, E.L. and Fudenberg, H.H. (1980) Defective immunoregulation in multiple sclerosis. *Annals of Neurology* **8,** 526–33.

Goust, J.M., Hogan, E.L. and Arnaud, P. (1982) Abnormal regulation of IgG production in multiple sclerosis. *Neurology* **32,** 228–34.

Graham, D.I., Behan, P.O. and More, I.A.R. (1979) Brain damage complicating septic shock. Acute haemorrhagic leucoencephalitis as a complication of the generalised Shwartzman reaction. *Journal of Neurology, Neurosurgery and Psychiatry* **42,** 19–28.

Greenfield, J.G. (1930) Acute disseminated encephalomyelitis as sequel to 'influenza'. *Journal of Pathology and Bacteriology* **33,** 453–62.

Greenfield, J.G. (1950) Encephalitis and encephalomyelitis in England and Wales during the last decade. *Brain* **73,** 141–66.

Greenfield, J.G. and Norman, R.M. (1963) Demyelinating diseases. In *Greenfield's Neuropathology*, 2nd edn (Eds. Blackwood, W., McMenemey, W.H., Meyer, A., Norman, R.M. and Russell, D.S.), pp. 475–519. Edward Arnold, London.

Gregson, N.A. (1983) The molecular biology of myelin. In *Multiple Sclerosis: pathology, diagnosis and management*. (Eds. Hallpike, J.F., Adams, C.W.M. and Tourtellotte, W.W.), pp. 1–28. Chapman and Hall, London.

Grundke-Iqbal, I., Lassmann, H. and Wisniewski, H.M. (1980) Chronic relapsing experimental allergic encephalomyelitis. *Archives of Neurology* **37,** 651–6.

Guseo, A. and Jellinger, K. (1975) The significance of perivascular infiltrations in multiple sclerosis. *Journal of Neurology* **211,** 51–60.

Haase, A.T., Ventura, P., Gibbs, C.J. and Tourtellotte, W.W. (1981) Measles virus nucleotide sequences: detection by hybridization in situ. *Science* **212,** 672–5.

Hallmans, G. (1982) Zinc and copper in multiple sclerosis. *Journal of Neurology, Neurosurgery and Psychiatry* **45,** 691–8.

Hampel, E. (1937) Morbus Addisonii und sklerosierende Erkrankung des Hemisphärenmarks. *Deutsche Zeitschrift für Nervenheilkunde* **142,** 186.

Hansen, B.L., Hansen, G.N., Hagen, C. and Brodersen, P. (1983) Autoantibodies against pituitary peptides in sera from patients with multiple sclerosis. *Journal of Neuroimmunology* **5,** 171–83.

Hart, M.N. and Earle, K.M. (1975) Haemorrhagic and perivenous encephalitis: a clinical-pathological review of 38 cases. *Journal of Neurology, Neurosurgery and Psychiatry* **38,** 585–91.

Hassin, G.B. (1937) Neuroptic myelitis versus multiple sclerosis. A pathologic study. *Archives of Neurology and Psychiatry* **37,** 1083–99.

Herndon, R.M. and Rubinstein, L.J. (1968) Leukodystrophy with Rosenthal fibers (Alexander's disease): a histochemical and electron microscopic study. *Neurology* **18,** 300.

Herndon, R.M., Rubinstein, L.J., Freeman, J.M. and Mathieson, G. (1970) Light and electron microscopic observations on Rosenthal fibers in Alexander's disease and in multiple sclerosis. *Journal of Neuropathology and Experimental Neurology* **29,** 524–51.

Hewitt, P.H. (1957) Addison's disease occurring in sisters. *British Medical Journal* **2,** 1530–1.

Ho, K.C., Hodach, R., Varman, R., Thorsteinson, V., Hess, T. and Dale, D. (1979) Kernicterus and central pontine myelinolysis in a 14-year-old boy with fulminating viral hepatitis. *Annals of Neurology* **8,** 633–6.

Hoefnagel, D., Vanden Noort, S. and Ingbar, S.H. (1962) Diffuse cerebral sclerosis with endocrine abnormalities in young males. *Brain* **85,** 553–69.

Hughes, J.T. (1978) *Pathology of the Spinal Cord*, pp. 152–6. Lloyd-Luke, London.

Ibrahim, M.Z.M. and Adams, C.W.M. (1965) The relation between enzyme activity and neuroglia in early plaques of multiple sclerosis. *Journal of Pathology and Bacteriology* **90,** 239–43.

Igarashi, M., Schaumburg, H.H., Powers, J., Kishimoto, Y., Kolodny, E. and Suzuki, K. (1976) Fatty acid abnormality in adrenoleukodystrophy. *Journal of Neurochemistry* **26,** 851–60.

Il Ro, Y., Alexander, B. and Oh, S.J. (1983) Multiple sclerosis and hypertrophic demyelinating peripheral neuropathy. *Muscle and Nerve* **6,** 312–16.

Ironside, R., Bosanquet, F.D. and McMenemey, W.H. (1961) Central demyelination of the corpus callosum (Marchiafava–Bignami disease). *Brain* **84,** 212–30.

Itoyama, Y., Webster, H. de F., Richardson, E.P. Jr and Trapp, B.D. (1983) Schwann cell remyelination of demyelinated axons in spinal cord multiple sclerosis lesions. *Annals of Neurology* **14,** 339–46.

Jaffe, R., Crumrine, P., Hashida, Y. and Moser, H.W. (1982) Neonatal adrenoleukodystrophy. Clinical, pathologic, and biochemical delineation of a syndrome affecting both males and females. *American Journal of Pathology* **108,** 100–11.

Janota, I. (1974) Spongy degeneration of grey matter in 3 children. Neuropathological report. *Archives of Disease in Childhood* **49,** 571–5.

Jellinger, K. and Seitelberger, F. (1958) Akute tödliche Entmarkungsencephalitis nach wiederholten Hirntrockenzelleninjektionen. *Klinische Wochenschrift* **36,** 437–41.

Johnson, A.B. and Bornstein, M.B. (1978) Myelin-binding antibodies *in vitro*. Immunoperoxidase studies with experimental allergic encephalomyelitis, anti-galactocerebroside and multiple sclerosis sera. *Brain Reserarch* **159,** 173–82.

Kearns, T.P. and Sayre, G.P. (1958) Retinitis pigmentosa, external ophthalmoplegia and complete heart block. *Archives of Ophthalmology* **60,** 183.

Kennedy, P.G.E. and Lisak, R.P. (1981) Do patients with demyelinating diseases have antibodies against human glial cells in their sera? *Journal of Neurology, Neurosurgery and Psychiatry* **44,** 164–67

Kirk, J. (1979a) The fine structure of the CNS in multiple sclerosis. II. Vesicular demyelination in an acute case. *Neuropathology and Applied Neurobiology* **5,** 289–94.

Kirk, J. (1979b) Pseudoviral hollow-cored vesicles in multiple sclerosis brain. *Acta Neuropathologica* **48,** 63–6.

Kirk, J. and Hutchinson, W.M. (1978) The fine structure of the CNS in multiple sclerosis. I. Interpretation of cytoplasmic papovavirus-like and paramyxovirus-like inclusions. *Neuropathology and Applied Neurobiology* **4,** 343–56.

Koenig, H., Rabinowitz, S.G., Day, E. and Miller, V. (1979) Post-infectious encephalomyelitis after successful treatment of herpes simplex encephalitis with adenine arabinoside. Ultrastructural observations. *New England Journal of Medicine* **300,** 1089–93.

Koeppen, A.H. and Barron, K.D. (1978) Marchiafava–Bignami disease. *Neurology* **28,** 290–4.

Kolkmann, F.-W., Rana, B.N. and Nützenadel, W. (1971) Zur Frage der Beziehungen zwischen Morbus Canavan (infantile spongiöse Neurodystrophie van Bogaert–Bertrand) und Pelizaeus–Merzbachersche Krankheit. Kasuistischer, feinstruktureller und zytochemischer Beitrag. *Neuropädiatrie* **2,** 305–24.

Kreth, H.W., Dunker, R., Rodt, H. and Meyermann, R. (1982) Immunohistochemical identification of T-lymphocytes in the central nervous system of patients with multiple sclerosis and subacute sclerosing panencephalitis. *Journal of Neuroimmunology* **2,** 177–83.

Kuo-Chun, M. and Kuan-Jung, C. (1983) Primary necrosis of corpus callosum with dystrophic astrogliosis and rosenthal-like fiber formation. The first Chinese case of Marchiafava–Bignami's disease (MBD). *Acta Neuropathologica* **60,** 283–90.

Kurtzke, J.F. (1983) Epidemiology of multiple sclerosis. In *Multiple Sclerosis: pathology, diagnosis and management*. (Eds. Hallpike, J.F., Adams, C.W.M. and Tourtellotte, W.W.), pp. 47–95. Chapman and Hall, London.

Kuwert, E.K. (1977) Genetical aspects of multiple sclerosis with special regard to histocompatibility determinants. In *The Histocompatibility System in Multiple Sclerosis*, (Ed. Fog, T.), pp. 23–42. Munksgaard, Copenhagen.

Lampert, P.W. (1978) Autoimmune and virus-induced demyelinating diseases. A review. *American Journal of Pathology* **91,** 175–208.

Lampert, P.W. (1983) Fine structure of the demyelinating process. In *Multiple Sclerosis: pathology, diagnosis and management*. (Eds. Hallpike, J.F., Adams, C.W.M. and Tourtellotte, W.W.), pp. 29–46. Chapman and Hall, London.

Lassmann, H. (1983) *Comparative Neuropathology of Chronic Experimental Allergic Encephalomyelitis and Multiple Sclerosis*. Springer, Berlin, Heidelberg, New York, Tokyo.

Laureno, R. (1982) Central pontine myelinolysis following rapid correction of hyponatremia. *Annals of Neurology* **13,** 232–42.

Leibowitz, S. (1983) The immunology of multiple sclerosis. In *Multiple Sclerosis: pathology, diagnosis and management* (Eds. Hallpike, J.F., Adams, C.W.M. and Tourtellotte, W.W.), pp. 379–412. Chapman and Hall, London.

Leinikki, P., Shekarchi, I., Ilvanainen, M., Taskinen, E., Holmes, K.V., Madden, D. and Sever, J.L. (1982) Virus antibodies in the cerebrospinal fluid of multiple sclerosis patients detected with Elisa tests. *Journal of the Neurological Sciences* **57,** 249–55.

Lesniowski, S. (1931) Inflammation de la substance grise du tronc cérébral (polioencephalitis superior et inférior) après vaccination antirabique. *Journal of Neurology and Psychiatry* **31,** 427–40.

Levine, S. and Wenk, E.J. (1965) A hyperacute form of allergic encephalomyelitis. *American Journal of Pathology* **47,** 61–88.

Ludwin, S.K. (1981) Pathology of demyelination and remyelination. In *Demyelinating Disease: Basic and Clinical Electrophysiology*. (Ed. Waxman, S.G. and Ritchie, J.M.), pp. 123–68. Raven Press, New York.

Lumsden, C.E. (1950) Cyanide leucoencephalopathy in rats and observations on the vascular and ferment hypotheses of demyelinating diseases. *Journal of Neurology, Neurosurgery and Psychiatry* **13,** 1–15.

Lumsden, C.E. (1951) Fundamental problems in the pathology of multiple sclerosis and allied demyelinating diseases. *British Medical Journal* **1,** 1035–43.

Lumsden, C.E. (1970) The neuropathology of multiple sclerosis. In *Handbook of Clinical Neurology*, vol. 9 (Eds. Vinken, P.J. and Bruyn, G.W.), pp. 296–8. North-Holland, Amsterdam.

McAlpine, D. (1972) Some aspects of the natural history. In *Multiple Sclerosis. A Reappraisal* (Eds. McAlpine, D., Lumsden, C.E. and Acheson, E.D.), pp. 83–98. Churchill Livingstone, Edinburgh.

McDonald, W.I. (1974) Pathophysiology in multiple sclerosis. *Brain* **97,** 179–96.

McDonald, W.I. (1982) Clinical problems of multiple sclerosis. In *Neuronal-Glial Cell Interrelationships* (Ed. Sears, T.A.), Dahlem Konferenzen 1982, pp. 11–24. Springer, Berlin, Heidelberg, New York.

Malamud, N. (1939) Sequelae of postmeasles encephalomyelitis. A clinicopathologic study. *Archives of Neurology and Psychiatry* **41,** 943–54.

Malmgren, R.M., Detels, R. and Verity, M.A. (1984) Co-occurrence of multiple sclerosis and glioma—case report and neuropathologic and epidemiologic review. *Clinical Neuropathology* **3,** 1–9.

Manz, H.J., Schuelein, M., McCullough, D.C., Kishimoto, Y. and Eiben, R.M. (1980) New phenotypic variant of adrenoleukodystrophy: pathologic, ultrastructural and biochemical study in two brothers. *Journal of the Neurological Sciences* **45,** 245–60.

Marburg, O. (1906) Die sogenannte 'akute multiple Sklerose'. *Jahrbuch für Psychiatrie und Neurologie* **27,** 211–312.

Marchiafava, E. and Bignami, A. (1903) Sopra un' alterazione del corpo calloso osservata in sogetti alcoolisti. *Rivista di Patologia Nervosa e Mentale* **8,** 544–9.

Marsden, J.P. and Hurst, E.W. (1932) Acute perivascular myelinoclasis ('acute disseminated encephalomyelitis') in smallpox. *Brain* **55,** 181–225.

Martin, J.R. (1982) Spinal cord and optic nerve demyelination in experimental herpes simplex virus type 2 infection. *Journal of Neuropathology and Experimental Neurology* **41,** 253–66.

Martin, J.R. and Nathanson, N. (1979) Animal models of virus-induced demyelination. In *Progress in Neuropathology*, vol. 4 (Ed. Zimmerman, H.M.), pp. 27–46. Raven Press, New York.

Matthews, W.B. (1979) Multiple sclerosis presenting with acute remitting psychiatric symptoms. *Journal of Neurology, Neurosurgery and Psychiatry* **42,** 859–63.

Mehta, P.J., Lassmann, H. and Wisniewski, H.M. (1981) Immunologic studies of chronic relapsing EAE in guinea pigs: similarities to multiple sclerosis. *Journal of Immunology* **12,** 334–8.

Menkes, J.H. and Corbo, L.M. (1977) Adrenoleukodystrophy—accumulation of cholesterol esters with very-long-chain fatty acids. *Neurology* **27,** 928–32.

Merzbacher, L. (1910) Eine eigenartige familiäre Erkrankungsform (Aplasia axialis extracorticalis congenita). *Zeitschrift für die gesamte Neurologie und Psychiatrie* **3,** 1–138.

ter Meulen, V. and Stephenson, J.R. (1983) The possible role of viral infections in multiple sclerosis and other related demyelinating diseases. In *Multiple Sclerosis: pathology, diagnosis and management* (Eds. Hallpike, J.F., Adams, C.W.M. and Tourtellotte, W.W.), pp. 241–75. Chapman and Hall, London.

Millar, J.H.D. (1971) *Multiple Sclerosis. A Disease Acquired in Childhood.* Thomas, Springfield, Illinois.

Millar, J.H.D. (1975) Clinical management: linoleic acid diet. In *Multiple Sclerosis Research* (Eds. Davison, A.N., Humphrey, J.H., Liversedge, A.L., McDonald, W.J. and Porterfield, S.J.), pp. 217–40. HMSO, London; Elsevier Scientific, Amsterdam and New York.

Miller, C.A., Shulman, I. and Taylor, C. (1981) Demyelination with hemophagocytic lymphohistiocytosis of the CNS. *Acta Neuropathologica* **54,** 153–5.

Miller, H.G., Stanton, J.B. and Gibbons, J.L. (1957) Acute disseminated encephalomyelitis and related syndromes. *British Medical Journal* **1,** 668–71.

Morariu, M. A., Chason, J. L., Norum, R. A., Moser, H. W. and Migeon, B. (1982) Adrenoleukodystrophy variant in a heterozygous female. (abstract) *Neurology* **32,** A81.

Moser, H.W., Schulman, J.D., Rizzo, W.B., Brown, F.R. III, Van Duyn, M.A. and Moser, A.B. (1982) Dietary restriction of very-long-chain fatty acids in adrenoleukodystrophy. (abstract) *Neurology* **32,** A81.

Mussini, J.M., Hauw, J.J. and Escourolle, R. (1977) Immunofluorescence studies of intra cytoplasmic immunoglobulin binding lymphoid cells (CILC) in the central nervous system. Report of 32 cases including 19 multiple sclerosis. *Acta Neuropathologica* **40,** 227-32.

Nagashima, T., Yamada, K., Uono, M., Tsubaki, Y., Morimatsu, Y. and Nagashima, K. (1983) Chronic recurrent demyelinating encephalomyelitis associated with hemophagocytic lymphohistiocytosis. *Acta Neuropathologica* **59,** 25-30.

Neu, I.S. (1983) Essential fatty acids in the serum and cerebrospinal fluid of multiple sclerosis patients. *Acta Neurologica Scandinavica* **67,** 151-63.

Nisenbaum, C., Sandbank, U. and Kohn, R. (1965) Pelizaeus-Merzbacher disease 'infantile acute type' Report of a family. *Annales Paediatricia (Basel)* **204,** 365-76.

Norenberg, M.D., Leslie, K.O. and Robertson, A.S. (1982) Association between rise in serum sodium and central pontine myelinolysis. *Annals of Neurology* **11,** 128-35.

Norman, R.M. (1962) Lipid diseases of the brain. In *Modern Trends in Neurology—3* (Ed. Williams, D.), pp. 173-99. Butterworths, London.

Norman, R.M. and Tingey, A.H. (1963) Sudanophil leucodystrophy and Pelizaeus-Merzbacher disease. In *Brain Lipids and Lipoproteins and the Leucodystrophies.* (Eds. Folch-Pi, J. and Bauer, H.), pp. 169-86. Elsevier, Amsterdam.

Norman, R.M., Tingey, A.H., Harvey, P.A. and Gregory, A.M. (1966) Pelizaeus-Merzbacher disease: a form of sudanophil leucodystrophy. *Journal of Neurology, Neurosurgery and Psychiatry* **29,** 521-9.

Norrby, E., Link, H., Olsson, J., Panelius, M., Salmi, A. and Vandvik, B. (1974) Comparison of antibodies against different viruses in cerebrospinal fluid and serum samples from patients with multiple sclerosis. *Infection and Immunity* **10,** 688-94.

Norton, W.T. (1977) Isolation and characterization of myelin. In *Myelin* (Ed. Morell, P.), pp. 161-99. Plenum Press, New York.

Nyland, H., Mork, S. and Matre, R. (1982) In-situ characterization of mononuclear cell infiltrates in lesions of multiple sclerosis. *Neuropathology and Applied Neurobiology* **8,** 403-11.

Ogata, J. and Feigin, I. (1975) Schwann cells and regenerated peripheral myelin in multiple sclerosis: an ultrastructural study. *Neurology* **25,** 713-16.

Oppenheimer, D.R. (1966) A case of so-called demyelination encephalitis. *Neuropatologia Polska* **4,** suppl., pp. 717-21.

Oppenheimer, D.R. (1978) The cervical cord in multiple sclerosis. *Neuropathology and Applied Neurobiology* **4,** 151-62.

Palm, R. and Hallmans, G. (1982) Zinc and copper in multiple sclerosis. *Journal of Neurology, Neurosurgery and Psychiatry* **45,** 691-8.

Paterson, P.Y. (1960) Transfer of allergic encephalomyelitis in rats by means of lymph node cells. *Journal of Experimental Medicine* **111,** 119-35.

Paterson, P.Y. (1976) Experimental allergic encephalomyelitis: role of fibrin deposition in immunopathogenesis of inflammation in rats. *Federation Proceedings* **35,** 2428-34.

Peiffer, J. and Zerbin-Rudin, E. (1963) On the diversity of Pelizaeus-Merzbacher disease (at the same time a contribution on familial multiple sclerosis). *Acta Neuropathologica* **3,** 87-107.

Pelizaeus, F. (1885) Über eine eigentümliche Form spastischer Lähmung mit Zerebralerscheinungen auf hereditärer Grundlage (multiple Sklerose). *Archiv für Psychiatrie und Nervenkrankheiten* **16,** 698-710.

Perdrau, J.R. (1928) The histology of post-vaccinal encephalitis. *Journal of Pathology and Bacteriology* **31,** 17-32.

Peters, G. (1968) Multiple sclerosis. In *Pathology of the Nervous System,* vol. 1 (Ed. Minckler, J.), pp. 821-43. McGraw-Hill, New York.

Pette, H. (1942) *Die akutentzündlichen Erkrankungen des Nervensystems.* Thieme, Leipzig.

Pfister, R. (1936) Beitrag zur Kenntnis der diffusen Hirnsklerose. *Archiv für Psychiatrie und Nervenkrankheiten* **105,** 1-16.

Phadke, J.G. and Best, P.V. (1983) Atypical and clinically silent multiple sclerosis: a report of 12 cases discovered unexpectedly at necropsy. *Journal of Neurology, Neurosurgery and Psychiatry* **46,** 414-20.

Poser, C.M. (1973) Demyelination in the central nervous system in chronic alcoholism: central pontine myelinolysis and Marchiafava-Bignami's disease. *Annals of the New York Academy of Sciences* **215,** 373-81.

Poser, C.M., Roman, G. and Emery, E.S. III (1978) Recurrent disseminated vasculomyelinopathy. *Archives of Neurology* **35,** 166-70.

Powers, J.M. and Schaumburg, H.H. (1974) Adrenoleukodystrophy. Similar ultrastructural changes in adrenal cortical and Schwann cells. *Archives of Neurology* **30,** 406-11.

Powers, J.M. and Schaumburg, H.H. (1980) A fatal cause of sexual inadequacy in the male: adrenoleukodystrophy. *Journal of Urology* **124,** 583.

Powers, J.M. and Schaumburg, H.H. (1981) The testis in adrenoleukodystrophy. *American Journal of Pathology* **102,** 90.

Powers, J.M., Moser, H.W., Moser, A.B. and Schaumburg, H.H. (1982) Fetal adrenoleukodystrophy: the significance of pathologic lesions in adrenal gland and testis. *Human Pathology* **13,** 1013-19.

Prineas, J.W. (1975) Pathology of the early lesion in multiple sclerosis. *Human Pathology* **6,** 531–54.

Prineas, J.W. and Connell, F. (1978) The fine structure of chronically active multiple sclerosis plaques. *Neurology* **28,** 68–75.

Prineas, J.W. and Connell, F. (1979) Remyelination in multiple sclerosis. *Annals of Neurology* **5,** 22–31.

Prineas, J.W. and Wright, R.G. (1978) Macrophages, lymphocytes, and plasma cells in the perivascular compartment in chronic multiple sclerosis. *Laboratory Investigation* **38,** 409–21.

Probst, A., Ulrich, J., Heitz, Ph.U. and Herschkowitz, N. (1980) Adrenomyeloneuropathy. A protracted, pseudosystematic variant of adrenoleukodystrophy. *Acta Neuropathologica* **49,** 105–15.

Raine, C.S. (1976) Experimental allergic encephalomyelitis and related conditions. In *Progress in Neuropathology*, Vol. 3 (Ed. Zimmerman, H.M.), pp. 225–50. Grune & Stratton, New York, San Francisco, London.

Raine, C.S. (1978) Membrane specialisations between demyelinated axons and astroglia in chronic EAE lesions and multiple sclerosis plaques. *Nature (London)* **275,** 326–7.

Raine, C.S. (1983) Multiple sclerosis and chronic relapsing EAE: comparative ultrastructural neuropathology. In *Multiple Sclerosis: pathology, diagnosis and management* (Eds. Hallpike, J.F., Adams, C.W.M. and Tourtellotte, W.W.), pp. 413–60. Chapman and Hall, London.

Raine, C.S., Scheinberg, L. and Waltz, J.M. (1981) Multiple sclerosis. Oligodendrocyte survival and proliferation in an active established lesion. *Laboratory Investigation* **45,** 534–46.

Raine, C.S. and Traugott, U. (1982) The pathogenesis and therapy of multiple sclerosis is based upon the requirement of a combination of myelin antigens for autoimmune demyelination. *Journal of Neuroimmunology* **2,** 83–91.

Rivers, T.M., Sprunt, D.H. and Berry, G.P. (1933) Observations on attempts to produce acute disseminated encephalomyelitis in monkeys. *Journal of Experimental Medicine* **58,** 39–53.

Rizzo, W.B., Avigan, J., Chemke, J. and Schulman, J.D. (1984) Adrenoleukodystrophy: very-long-chain fatty acid metabolism in fibroblasts. *Neurology* **34,** 163–9.

Roström, B. (1981) Specificity of antibodies in oligoclonal bands in patients with multiple sclerosis and cerebrovascular disease. *Acta Neurologica Scandinavica* suppl. 86.

Rumsby, M.G. (1978) Organization and structure in central-nerve myelin. *Biochemical Society Transactions* **6,** 448–62.

Russell, D.S. (1955) The nosological unity of acute haemorrhagic leucoencephalitis and acute disseminated encephalomyelitis. *Brain* **78,** 369–76.

Russell, D.S. and Rubinstein, L.J. (1977) *Pathology of Tumours of the Nervous System*, 4th edn. Edward Arnold, London.

Ryberg, B. (1981) Studies on Complement-fixing Antibrain Antibodies in Multiple Sclerosis. Thesis from the Department of Neurology, University Hospital, Lund, Sweden.

Schaumburg, H.H., Richardson, E.P., Johnson, P.C., Cohen, R.B., Powers, J.M. and Raine, C.S. (1972) Schilder's disease. Sex-linked recessive transmission with specific adrenal changes. *Archives of Neurology* **27,** 458–60.

Schaumburg, H.H., Powers, J.M., Suzuki, K. and Raine, C.S. (1974) Adreno-leukodystrophy (sex-linked Schilder disease). Ultrastructural demonstration of specific cytoplasmic inclusions in the central nervous system. *Archives of Neurology* **31,** 210–13.

Schaumburg, H.H., Powers, J.M., Raine, C.S., Suzuki, K. and Richardson, E.P.Jr (1975) Adrenoleukodystrophy. A clinical and pathological study of 17 cases. *Archives of Neurology* **32,** 577–91.

Schaumburg, H.H., Powers, J.M., Raine, C.S., Spencer, P.S., Griffin, J.W., Prineas, J.W. and Boehme, D.M. (1977) Adrenomyeloneuropathy: a probable variant of adrenoleukodystrophy. II. General pathologic, neuropathologic and biochemical aspects. *Neurology* **27,** 1114–19.

Schilder, P. (1912) Zur Kenntnis der sogenannte diffusen Sklerose. *Zeitschrift für die gesamte Neurologie und Psychiatrie* **10,** 1–60.

Schilder, P. (1913) Zur Frage der Encephalitis diffusa. *Zeitschrift für die gesamte Neurologie und Psychiatrie* **15,** 358–76.

Schilder, P. (1924) Die Encephalitis periaxialis diffusa. *Archiv für Psychiatrie und Nervenkrankheiten* **71,** 327–56.

Schochet, S.S., Lampert, P.W. and Earle, K.M. (1968) Alexander's disease. A case report with electron microscopic observations. *Neurology* **18,** 543–9.

Schoene, W.C., Carpenter, S., Behan, P.O. and Geschwind, N. (1977) 'Onion bulb' formations in the central and peripheral nervous system in association with multiple sclerosis and hypertrophic polyneuropathy. *Brain* **100,** 755–73.

Scott, T.F.McN. (1967) Postinfectious and vaccinial encephalitis. *Medical Clinics of North America* **51,** 701–17.

Seil, F.J., Westall, F.C., Romine, J.S. and Salk, J. (1983) Serum demyelinating factors in multiple sclerosis. *Annals of Neurology* **13,** 664–7.

Seitelberger, F. (1954) Die Pelizaeus-Merzbachersche Krankheit. Klinisch-anatomische Untersuchungen zum Problem ihrer Stellung unter den diffusen Sklerosen. *Wiener Zeitschrift für Nervenheilkunde* **9,** 228–89.

Seitelberger, F. (1957) Histochemistry and classification of the Pelizaeus–Merzbacher disease. In *Cerebral Lipidoses*, pp. 92–7. Blackwell Scientific, Oxford.

Seitelberger, F. (1960) Histochemistry of demyelinating diseases proper, including allergic encephalomyelitis and Pelizaeus–Merzbacher's disease. In *Modern Scientific Aspects of Neurology* (Ed. Cummings, J.N.), pp. 146–87. Edward Arnold, London.

Seitelberger, F. (1963) Contribution to Pelizaeus–Merzbacher's disease. In *Brain Lipids and Lipoproteins, and the Leucodystrophies* (Eds. Folchi-Pi, J. and Baurer, H.), pp. 187–98. Elsevier, Amsterdam.

Seitelberger, F. (1970) Pelizaeus–Merzbacher disease. In *Handbook of Clinical Neurology*, vol. 10 (Eds. Vinken, P.J. and Bruyn, G.W.), pp. 150–202. North-Holland, Amsterdam.

Siemerling, E. and Creutzfeldt, H.G. (1923) Bronzekrankheit und sklerosierende Encephalomyelitis. *Archiv für Psychiatrie und Nervenkrankheit* **68,** 217–44.

Soffer, D., Grotsky, H.W., Rapin, I. and Suzuki, K. (1979) Cockayne syndrome: unusual neuropathological findings and review of the literature. *Annals of Neurology* **6,** 340–8.

Sternberger, N.H., Itoyama, Y., Kies, M.W. and Webster, H. de F. (1978) Immunocytochemical method to identify basic protein in myelin-forming oligodendrocytes of newborn rat CNS. *Journal of Neurocytology* **7,** 251–63.

Stevens, J.G., Bastone, V.B., Ellison, G.W. and Myers, L.W. (1980) No measles virus genetic information detected in multiple sclerosis-derived brains. *Annals of Neurology* **8,** 625–7.

Stewart, G. J. and Kirk, R.L. (1983) The genetics of multiple sclerosis: the HLA system and other genetic markers. In *Multiple Sclerosis: pathology, diagnosis and management* (Ed. Hallpike, J.F., Adams, C.W.M. and Tourtellotte, W.W.), pp. 97–128. Chapman and Hall, London.

Stewart, G.J., McLeod, J.G., Basten, A. and Bashir, H.V. (1981) HLA family studies and susceptibility to multiple sclerosis: a common gene, dominantly expressed. *Human Immunology* **3,** 13–29.

Summers, B.A., Greisen, H.A. and Appel, M.J.G. (1983) Does virus persist in the uvea in multiple sclerosis, as in canine distemper encephalomyelitis? *Lancet* **2,** 372–6.

Swank, R.L. (1950) Multiple sclerosis: a correlation of its incidence with dietary fat. *American Journal of Medical Science* **220,** 421–30.

Tanaka, R., Iwasaki, Y. and Koprowski, H. (1975) Ultrastructural studies of perivascular cuffing cells in multiple sclerosis brain. *American Journal of Pathology* **81,** 467–74.

Toro, G. and Roman, G. (1978) Cerebral malaria. A disseminated vasculomyelinopathy. *Archives of Neurology* **35,** 271–5.

Traugott, U., Reinherz, E.L. and Raine, C.S. (1983) Multiple sclerosis. Distribution of T cells, T cell subsets and Ia-positive macrophages in lesions of different ages. *Journal of Neuroimmunology* **4,** 201–21.

Tridon, P., Martin, J.-J., Vidailhet, M., Floquet, J., Philippart, M. and Neimann, M. (1974) Spongiose cérébrale juvénile. *Pédiatrie* **29,** 235–47.

Turnbull, H.M. and McIntosh, J. (1926) Encephalomyelitis following vaccination. *British Journal of Experimental Pathology* **7,** 181–222.

Uchimura, I. and Shiraki, H. (1957) A contribution to the classification and the pathogenesis of demyelinating encephalomyelitis. With special reference to the central nervous system lesions caused by preventative inoculation against rabies. *Journal of Neuropathology and Experimental Neurology* **16,** 139–208.

Ulrich, J. and Groebke-Lorenz, W. (1983) The optic nerve in multiple sclerosis. A morphological study with retrospective clinicopathological correlations. *Neuro-ophthalmology* **3,** 149–59.

Ulrich, J., Herschkowitz, N., Heitz, P.H., Sigrist, T.H. and Baerlocher, P. (1978) Adrenoleukodystrophy: preliminary report of a connatal case. Light and electron microscopical, immunohistochemical and biochemical findings. *Acta Neuropathologica* **43,** 77–83.

Vieregge, P., Nahser, H.C., Gerhard, L., Reinhardt, V. and Nau, H.E. (1984) Multiple sclerosis and cerebral tumour. *Clinical Neuropathology* **3,**10–21.

Vogel, F.S. and Hallervorden, J. (1962) Leukodystrophy with diffuse Rosenthal fibre formation. *Acta Neuropathologica* **2,** 126–43.

de Vries, E. (1960) *Postvaccinial Perivenous Encephalitis.* Elsevier, Amsterdam.

Warren, H.V. and Horsky, S.J. (1983) Quantitative analysis of zinc, copper, lead, molybdenum, bismuth, mercury and arsenic in brain and other tissues from multiple sclerosis and non-multiple sclerosis cases. *Science of the Total Environment* **29,** 163–9.

Wisniewski, H.M. and Bloom, B.R. (1975) Primary demyelination as a nonspecific consequence of a cell-mediated immune reaction. *Journal of Experimental Medicine* **141,** 346–59.

Wolfgram, F. (1979) What if multiple sclerosis isn't an immunological or a viral disease? The case for a circulating toxin. *Neurochemical Research* **4,** 1–14.

Wright, D.G., Laureno, R. and Victor, M. (1979) Pontine and extrapontine myelinolysis. *Brain* **102,** 361–85.

Zimmerman, H.M. and Netsky, M.G. (1950) The pathology of multiple sclerosis. *Association for Research into Nervous Diseases. Proceedings* **28,** 271–312.

10

Malformations of the nervous system

Jeanne-Claudie Larroche

Congenital malformations continue to be a major cause of infant death in the western world, and of these the malformations involving the nervous system are among the commonest. Warkany (1971) has outlined the problems in obtaining accurate statistics. Incidence figures vary considerably, depending on the accuracy of observation, the population groups under consideration and other factors such as whether abortion and stillbirths are included in assessments. Some general points can be made, however. The incidence of malformations is higher in children with intrauterine growth retardation and in multiple pregnancies, and racial and geographical factors may be of importance as exemplified by the variation in the incidence of anencephaly which has been reported as 20 times higher in Belfast than in Paris (Penrose, 1957).

The development of the human brain continues for years after birth and the term 'malformation' as applied to the nervous system must therefore include anomalies arising postnatally. The immature nervous system does not react to injury in the same way as it does in the adult. Inflammatory responses are not seen before the sixth fetal month (Eicke, 1959) and parts may be absorbed without trace of neuroglial or connective tissue repair. Moreover, it is known from observations on animals that the same anomaly may be produced by both genetic and environmental causes. Monographs by Warkany (1971), Crome and Stern (1972) and Baraitser (1982) give detailed accounts of malformations and their inheritance.

The findings of experimental teratology

Much light has been thrown on the mechanisms of abnormal development by the study of experimentally induced malformations in animals. Since the observations of von Hippel (1907) that irradiation of pregnant rabbits produces malformations of the eye in the offspring, a very large literature has grown up around the subject. Kalter (1968) reviewed in detail both malformations induced experimentally and those occurring spontaneously in a wide range of species. The following brief account of the various teratogenic agents is largely based on Kalter's work.

Vitamin deficiencies A wide range of malformations are induced by feeding pregnant animals with diets deficient in specific vitamins, or by administering counteracting substances such as inactive analogues, antimetabolites and antagonists. *Riboflavin* deficiency, with rare exceptions, produced mainly skeletal malformations. Addition of the riboflavin-antagonist galactoflavin produces a wider range of lesions, including hydrocephalus. In mice the hydrocephalus is associated with an enormous expansion of the fourth ventricle resembling the Dandy–Walker malformation in man. *Folic acid* deficiency produces hydrocephalus in rats, either without an obvious obstruction in the cerebrospinal fluid pathway or with aqueduct stenosis. Combined *vitamin* B_{12} and folic acid deficiency also produces hydrocephalus. Exencephaly and eye anomalies can be caused by *pantothenic acid* deficiency. *Vitamin A* deficiency is known to be teratogenic in pigs and rabbits. Cerebral malformations are also induced occasionally by deficiencies of *vitamin E* and of *nicotinic acid.*

Hypervitaminosis A The teratogenic effect of an excessive intake of vitamin A was discovered by Cohlan (1953). Severe cerebral malformations, of which exencephaly was the most common, were produced with a high degree of consistency in rats (Cohlan, 1954; Giroud and Martinet, 1956) and subsequently in other species.

Trypan blue Gillman et al. (1948) reported that injection of pregnant rats with trypan blue produced a wide range of malformations in the offspring, including those of the central nervous system. The most common lesions are hydrocephalus and spina bifida, whilst exencephaly is relatively uncommon (Gillman et al., 1951). A hindbrain malformation resembling the Arnold–Chiari deformity in man has also been recorded. The mechanism of action of trypan blue remained controversial for many years. Beck, Lloyd and Griffiths (1967) adduced convincing evidence that its action is on the lysosomal enzymes in the epithelium of the yolk sac, blocking its histotrophic activity, particularly the uptake of protein.

Tissue antibodies Malformations can be induced in fetal rats by injections of heterologous antisera against rat kidney, rat placenta and rat yolk sac (Brent and Johnson, 1967). The nephrotoxic serum is concentrated in the basement membrane of the maternal renal glomeruli, in the adrenal glands and in the visceral and parietal layers of the yolk sacs, but not in the embryonic tissues (Slotnick and Brent, 1966). The most common malformation caused by the apparent yolk sac dysfunction is a non-obstructive hydrocephalus, the morphology of which was studied by Duckett, Brent and Jensch (1974).

Ionizing radiation X-rays have long been used as a teratogenic agent which can be timed and dosed with considerable accuracy. The systematic studies of Hicks (1952, 1953a, b, 1954) still retain their validity. Pregnant rats were subjected to a single dose of ionizing radiation on successive days of their 3 weeks' gestation and a timetable of predictable malformations was constructed. Exposure prior to day 9 did not affect the primitive neural tube, but a similar dose given on day 9 led to severe head deformities and anencephaly. Stenosis of the aqueduct followed radiation on day 11, and from day 13 to day 18 various cortical and striatal disturbances and absence of the corpus callosum were brought about. Minor degrees of damage led to micrencephaly without obvious loss of nerve cells, whilst irradiation shortly before birth caused a cerebellar malformation with distortion of the granular layer. The exact mechanism by which radiation induces malformations is still controversial. Hicks' view that the 'stage specificity' of the changes correlates well with phases of enhanced metabolic activity of the neuroblasts, associated with increased formation of nucleic acid and proteins, is probably an oversimplification as it does not explain the relative immunity of the primitive neuroepithelium in the first few days of embryonal life during which mitotic activity is intense. It is probable that the teratogenic activity of x-rays depends on the balance of destruction and repair processes. In the earliest stages of growth, destruction of a few cells can easily be compensated for by the still totipotential remaining cells. With advancing differentiation this is no longer possible and the combination of destruction and partial repair leads to malformations.

Other chemical substances Numerous drugs have now been tested for teratogenic properties and many have been found to induce occasional malformations of the central nervous system. These include alkylating substances, antimetabolites, alkaloids, hypoglycaemic agents, antithyroid drugs, salicylates, antibiotics, antihistamines, thalidomide and many others. Hydrocephalus has been induced in the offspring of pregnant rats by administration of tellurium between day 9 and day 15 of gestation (Duckett, 1971, 1972).

Hypoxia Experiments using diminished oxygen supply as the teratogenic agent are of interest as this factor may be concerned in human malformations. Owing to its ability to utilize anaerobic as well as aerobic sources of energy, the neuroblast is much more resistant to anoxia than is the mature neuron. It is therefore not surprising that these experiments met with only limited success. Anoxia in chick embryos has been shown to lead to anencephaly, cyclopia and forking of the aqueduct. Exencephaly or hydrocephalus appeared in a small number of offspring of hypoxic pregnant mice. Instances of exencephaly and one of cyclopia in the offspring of pregnant hypoxic rabbits have been observed. Rats and hamsters are apparently less susceptible to the teratogenic effects of oxygen deprivation.

Infection This is another subject of great interest in view of the undoubted teratogenic effect of some virus infections in man. It has been critically reviewed by Elizan and Fabiyi (1970). The two well-established human teratogenic viruses, rubella and cytomegalovirus, do not produce malformations in animals. A variety of developmental abnormalities is produced in various species by viruses normally pathogenic to those species. Thus intrauterine infection with bluetongue virus can produce hydranencephaly in sheep. Hydrocephalus and cerebellar hypoplasia can be similarly produced in pigs infected by the hog cholera virus. The rat virus, the HI virus of hamsters and the feline panleucopenia virus can all cause cerebellar hypoplasia in their respective species.

General conclusions It may be concluded from this review of experimental teratology that several factors play a part in teratogenesis. Probably the most important is the time of injury, as widely disparate mechanisms operating at the same stage of development will produce similar end-results. Nevertheless, the nature of the noxa is of importance as some agents produce highly specific disorders. Genetic factors must also be taken into account. The susceptibility to noxious agents varies from species to species and from strain to strain within the same species. The common experience that in an exposed litter only some fetuses are affected whilst others invariably escape damage has also been attributed to genetic differences between littermates. This interplay between genetic and environmental factors may be of importance in human teratology.

Nutrition and brain growth Variations in size of the brain as opposed to specific malformations have received little attention from experimental teratologists, but a considerable amount of evidence has accumulated to indicate that starvation may affect the growth of the brain. The adult brain is remarkably resistant to starvation but nutritional deprivation during the period of growth leads both to a reduction in brain size and to abnormalities of behaviour. An analysis of the factors involved in brain growth reveals the great complexity of the problem (Dobbing, 1970). Impairment of growth may be due to inhibition of cell division or interference with cell maturation. Cell division occurs in two phases, neuronal and glial. Multiplication of neuroblasts occurs early and is completed in fetal life, whilst the peak of proliferation of glial cells occurs much later and extends into postnatal life. Maturation involves development of cell processes, establishment of synaptic connections and myelination. The extent to which all these processes may be affected by nutrition or other exogenous factors offers a wide field for further research.

Aetiology of human malformations

Despite intensive investigations the causation of prenatal malformations in man remains largely undetermined. The problem is complicated by the fact that the same type of structural anomaly may be produced both by genetic and by exogenous causes. Some important factors have come to light in recent years which point the way to further fields of research.

Genetic factors Very few cerebral malformations are caused by simple mendelian inheritance and these are fully listed in McKusick's (1978) catalogue. The following conditions may be cited as examples. Some forms of micrencephaly may be inherited as autosomal recessive traits; for instance, the type which occurs in bird-headed dwarfs. A sex-linked variety of hydrocephalus, associated with stenosis of the aqueduct, is known. Hereditary congenital facial paralysis is an example of dominant inheritance.

Epidemiological studies of common malformations, such as anencephaly, spina bifida and hydrocephalus, have revealed a high risk of recurrence of these conditions in the same families (Record and McKeown, 1950; Carter, David and Laurence, 1968). Detailed analysis of the data suggests the interplay of environmental and genetic factors, the latter probably polygenic in nature.

Finally, malformations have been reported in association with inborn errors of metabolism such as sudanophil leucodystrophy (Norman et al., 1962) and maple syrup urine disease (Martin and Norman, 1967). Whilst these observations are too rare to exclude fortuitous association, the possibility of genetic links must be considered.

Cytogenetic abnormalities The study of disordered chromosome patterns has thrown important light on congenital anomalies of the nervous system (for full reviews, see Källén and

Levan 1970; Crome and Stern, 1972). The most important anomalies are the *trisomies*, in which an additional chromosome is present in one group. Trisomy in the G (21–22) group is commonly found in mongolism. D (13–15) trisomy is associated with multiple congenital abnormalities which include cyclopia and other forms of holoprosencephaly and arhinencephaly. Multiple anomalies also occur in E (17–18) trisomy, in which the CNS malformations are largely confined to the cerebellum. *Translocations*, of either the D/G or the G/G type are found in cases of mongolism with 46 chromosomes. *Deletions* of part of one chromosome are often associated with mental subnormality; the best known is the 'cri du chat' syndrome associated with deletion of the short arm of the no. 5 chromosome. Abnormalities of *sex chromosomes* include Klinefelter's syndrome (XXY) and Turner's syndrome (XO) as well as a variety of more complex chromosomal combinations. Many of them are associated with mental retardation, but little is known of the structural changes in their brains. Most cases of Turner's syndrome who survive to adult life show no cerebral malformations. Cortical dysplasia and grey matter heterotopias were described in a mentally subnormal girl with the syndrome (Brun and Sköld, 1968), and cerebellar malformations were found in a girl dying in infancy (Molland and Purcell, 1975). However, most XO fetuses undergo spontaneous abortion (Carr, 1967) and these often show gross malformation. *Mosaicism* in which an abnormal karyotype is found only in a proportion of cells, the remainder being normal, occurs in several conditions, such as Turner's syndrome or mongolism. These patients tend to be less severely affected than those who present chromosomal abnormalities in pure form.

Maternal age That mongoloid children are often born when their mothers approach the end of their reproductive period has been amply confirmed. This applies only to the common trisomic type of mongolism, the rare translocation type being genetically determined and appearing at any age. A higher average maternal age was also found in a group of miscellaneous malformations (Pitt, 1962) and in a series of mentally subnormal subjects from which mongolism was excluded (Åkesson, 1966).

Maternal infections The demonstration of a relationship between maternal infection during pregnancy and maldevelopment of the offspring has furnished additional evidence of the pathogenetic importance of environmental factors. It is well established that maternal infections other than syphilis may pass the placenta and interfere with development, and Gregg's (1941) original observations on the malign effect of rubella have been amply confirmed. Swan (1949) estimated that no fewer than 93 per cent of the mothers of his 558 collected cases had been infected during the first 4 months of pregnancy. This selected group of patients, however, gives far too high an incidence. In mothers infected with rubella during the first 4 months of pregnancy the incidence of stillbirths, neonatal deaths, immaturity and malformations was 17 per cent compared with 6 per cent in the controls. Transmission to the embryo may occur without overt disease in the mother. It is likely that the teratogenic virulence of the virus varies in different epidemics since there are numerous instances of maternal infection in early pregnancy without untoward consequences to the child. More recent observations on the effects of maternal rubella and other infections have been summarized by Johnson (1982).

In Swan's (1949) large series the commonest abnormalities were microcephaly, cardiac defects, deafness and cataract. Hydrocephalus, absent corpus callosum, mongolism, epilepsy and spastic syndromes were also represented. The deafness is due to defective development of the organ of Corti and is seldom total. The critical stage for the development of the cochlea is about a month later than that for the lens, so cataract and deafness are not often found in the same individual. Swan, however, noted that the time of the clinical onset of the maternal infection did not always coincide with the known stage of active differentiation of the affected organ in the offspring and suggested that these discrepancies might be due to variation in the proliferation of the virus or in the resistance of the cells to infection. Very few adequate examinations have been made of the micrencephalic brains following rubella embryopathy. Friedman and Cohen's (1947) case showed absence of the corpus callosum and anomalies of the cerebral cortex. In the two cases described by Mutrux, Wildi and Bourquin (1949) the gyral pattern was normal. The abnormal features were mild hydrocephalus, a small corpus callosum and perivascular and marginal gliosis. Töndury and Smith (1966) reviewed their experience of 57 fetuses aborted after maternal infections with rubella; 68 per cent showed evidence of damage to various organs. In none was any direct disease found in brain cells, but endothelial damage with focal haemorrhages was seen in some. In 10 affected fetuses the width of the cerebral cortex was reduced in comparison with normal controls.

The effects on the human fetus of other viral infections is summarized by Johnson (1982). Microcephaly, perhaps the result of chronic encephalitis, is the commonest sequel.

Cytomegalovirus can infect the fetal nervous system and lead to hydrocephalus with widespread evidence of inflammation and periventricular calcifications. In Diezel's (1954) case the maternal infection was thought to have occurred in the fourth month of pregnancy, and the infant's brain showed the malformation of micropolygyria in addition to the usual destructive lesions. Several similar cases have been recorded (Haymaker et al., 1954; Crome and France 1959; Bignami and Appicciutoli 1964). All these cases showed micrencephaly with extensive cortical microgyria, occasional cerebellar microgyria, subependymal calcifications and typical giant intranuclear inclusions, mainly in glial cells. Occasionally cases are encountered in older children which display all these features with the exception of inclusion bodies. These may well represent burnt-out cases of intrauterine cytomegalovirus infections though proof may be difficult to obtain.

Granulomatous meningoencephalitis is another group of diseases which may attack the developing nervous system. Of these, *toxoplasmosis* is the best known. A condition also characterized by hydrocephalus, widespread calcifications, thickened leptomeninges and eccentric degenerative changes in the smaller blood vessels was described as a separate disease by Sabin and Feldman (1948) on the grounds of the negative serological tests (Sabin's non-toxoplasmic vascular encephalopathy).

Intrauterine meningitis following *staphylococcal* infection is another very rare cause of congenital hydrocephalus (Crosby, Mosberg and Smith, 1951). A comprehensive account of the prenatal and perinatal infections of the central nervous system has been given by Wolf and Cowen (1959).

Irradiation Deep x-ray therapy to the pelvis during the first 4 months of pregnancy has produced many cases of microcephaly. Anomalies of the eye (optic atrophy, choroidoretinitis, abnormal retinal pigmentation) are much commoner in these cases than in micrencephaly of genetic origin. Four histologically examined cases in which therapeutic irradiation has been carried out during pregnancy were quoted by Cowen and Geller (1960). Various anomalies of the eyes, cerebral hemispheres and thalamus were present in Johnson's (1938) cases. Courville and Edmondson (1958) reported microcephaly with diffuse loss of cortical nerve cells. Cerebellar microgyria with some structural disorientation was the main feature of the cases of Miskolczy (1931) and of van Bogaert and Radermecker (1955). It is interesting to note that at autopsy three of these brains exhibited meningoencephalitis. To these cases may be added that of Uiberrack (1942) which showed pachygyria of the cerebral cortex and defective development of the vermis. Studies on children exposed *in utero* to the atomic explosions at Hiroshima and Nagasaki revealed a relatively high incidence of microcephaly and mental retardation, but no specific malformations (Plummer, 1952; Yamazaki, Wright and Wright, 1954). Follow-up studies confirmed these observations (Wood, Johnson and Omori, 1967; Miller, 1968).

Other environmental factors Children of mothers with *phenylketonuria* are known to be at risk. If the mother is homozygous and untreated the offspring are likely to show microcephaly and severe mental retardation.

Neural tube defects—dysraphic disorders

Two theories have been proposed to explain the morphogenesis of most dysraphic states—reopening of a previously closed neural tube or failure of the neural walls to close. Patten (1952) attributed rupture of the neural tube to overgrowth of parts of the encephalon and Gardner (1961, 1965, 1973), who coined the term *dysraphic states*, suggested that when the roof of the fourth ventricle becomes impermeable (Weed, 1917) reopening or rupture of the neural tube might occur as a result of abnormal distension by CSF. The proponent of the second theory was von Recklinghausen (1886). Today this theory is generally accepted but the precise sequence of events and the tissues involved in the morphogenesis of these defects are still subject to controversy. In the very few human embryos studied by Dekaban (1963) and by Lemire, Shepard and Alvord (1965) the neural groove had never closed, and Padget (1968, 1970) described abnormal neural cleft formations, which she called neuroschisis, and fluid-filled blebs raising the ectoderm and subsequently rupturing.

Most of the information on dysraphic disorders has been derived from experimental studies in which abnormalities similar to those observed in man have been induced repeatedly by hypervitaminosis A or by trypan blue (Giroud, 1960, 1977; Kalter, 1968; Warkany, 1971; among others). Disturbances of the neural tube occur at specific embryonic stages. At 10–11 days in the rat fetus the neural folds separate and display a progressive eversion, the ependymal surface being then exposed. Structures other than the neuroectoderm, such as the mesoderm and notochord, may also be involved. Marin-Padilla (1978, 1980) has stated that the supporting mesodermal tissue is primarily affected, being inadequately developed at the sites of the neural tube defect. Thus the morphological expression of dysraphism ranges from a localized defect in the membranous bone of the cranial vault (*crania lacunosa*) and vertebral anomalies to partial or severe neural tube anomalies.

Craniorrhachischisis

Craniorrhachischisis is the most severe form of dysraphism. Brain and spinal cord are exposed to the surrounding amniotic fluid, resulting in necrosis, degeneration or angioma-like formations.

Exencephaly

Exencephaly and anencephaly are different stages of the same developmental anomaly. Exencephaly has been rarely described in human fetal pathology (Marin-Padilla, 1970), probably because of the rapid necrosis of brain tissue exposed to amniotic fluid, leading to anencephaly.

Anencephaly

Anencephaly was known in Egyptian antiquity, and in 1761 Morgagni compared the human monster to a toad. It was also described by Geoffroy Saint-Hilaire in 1825 (see Giroud, 1977, for a historical review). The calvaria is hypoplastic or absent, the base of the skull is thick and flattened, and there is a constant anomaly of the sphenoid bone resembling 'a bat with folded wings' (Marin-Padilla, 1965). The orbits are shallow, causing protrusion of the eyes. The forebrain is replaced by a reddish irregular mass of vascular tissue with multiple cavities containing CSF. If the occipital bones are formed, disorganized tissue resembling brain stem and cerebellum may be found (Friede, 1975).

Histological examination of the vascular tissue discloses thin-walled veins and capillaries embedded within a dense meshwork of connective tissue described as the *area cerebrovasculosa* (André-Thomas, Laruelle and Reumont, 1955). Communication with the systemic circulation is slight or absent (Vogel, 1961). Glial nodules, ependyma-like epithelium and choroid plexus may be identifiable. Careful dissection discloses trigeminal ganglia and hypoplastic anterior pituitary tissue but the intermediate and posterior lobes are always missing. The absence of these structures and of the hypothalamus is associated with a hypoplastic adrenal cortex (Angevine, 1938; Tuchmann-Duplessis and Larroche, 1958). Various other visceral abnormalities have been reported in cases of anencephaly (Nakado, 1973), a large thymus and hypoplastic lungs being the most frequent. Spina bifida was associated with anencephaly in 17 per cent in the series of Frezal et al. (1964) and in 14 per cent of that of Cassidy (1969). Polyhydramnios is observed in about half of the cases but its pathogenesis is unclear.

Epidemiological studies have shown a high incidence of anencephaly in Ireland and in Wales, 1–6 per 1000 live births compared with about 0.5–2 per 1000 in the USA and 0.5 in France (Nevin, Johnston and Merrett, 1981). Females are affected more frequently than males. Anencephaly is the most common congenital malformation of the brain in human fetuses. Familial cases of anencephaly and/or spina bifida have been observed, but transmission is poorly understood. The role of diet and social class is still debated.

Early prenatal detection of neural tube defects is possible by the estimation of alpha-fetoprotein (AFP) in amniotic fluid, first described by Brock and Sutcliffe (1972). This protein, synthesized by fetal liver and excreted in the urine, is increased in amount in the amniotic fluid in various malformations, mainly those which involve the neural tube. More recently AFP has been determined in maternal serum (Wald et al., 1977; Milunsky et al., 1980). The test is not entirely reliable, however, and is likely to be replaced by measurement of acetylcholinesterase in the amniotic fluid. This enzyme, produced specifically in nervous tissue, is excreted in the CSF and passes into the amniotic fluid only in cases with defects of the neural tube. Specific isoenzymes of amniotic fluid cholinesterase can now be assessed by electrophoresis (Brock, 1981; Guibaud et al., 1982. Anencephaly can also be detected as early as the twelfth week by ultrasonography.

Encephalocele and cranial meningocele

These malformations consist of a protrusion of brain or meninges through a cranial defect. They occur most frequently in the occipital region, 75–80 per cent of cases occurring there, the frontal and lateral parts of the skull being much less often affected.

Occipital encephalocele The herniation occurs through the occipital bone, with or without involvement of the foramen magnum. The mass of tissue is often voluminous (Fig. 10.1), is attached to one of the cerebral hemispheres by a narrow pedicle, and is partially covered with normal skin and hair. Ulceration of the skin and secondary infection are frequent. On section, small convolutions with a normally laminated or microgyric cortex and underlying white matter often surround a cavity which may communicate with one of the cerebral ventricles. Occipital encephalocele may be associated with the Meckel syndrome (microcephaly, microphthalmia, craniofacial clefts and other skeletal and visceral anomalies).

Parietal encephalocele or meningocele occurs only occasionally (McLaurin, 1964). Deformities of the brain are usually present and are not confined to the ipsilateral hemisphere. They include asymmetry, distortion of the ventricular walls, agenesis of the corpus callosum and hydrocephalus.

Anterior encephalocele (Fig. 10.2) is most commonly found at the frontoethmoidal junction. It is usually visible at the bridge of the nose (in 60 per cent of cases) as a bulging subcutaneous nodule and mild hypertelorism or as a mass of brain tissue. The encephalocele may expand into the nasal cavity (30 per cent of cases), ethmoidal or sphenoidal air sinuses, pharynx or orbit (Ziter and Bramwit, 1970). The abnormal mass may contain brain tissue with oligodendrocytes, fibrous or hypertrophic astrocytes and, occa-

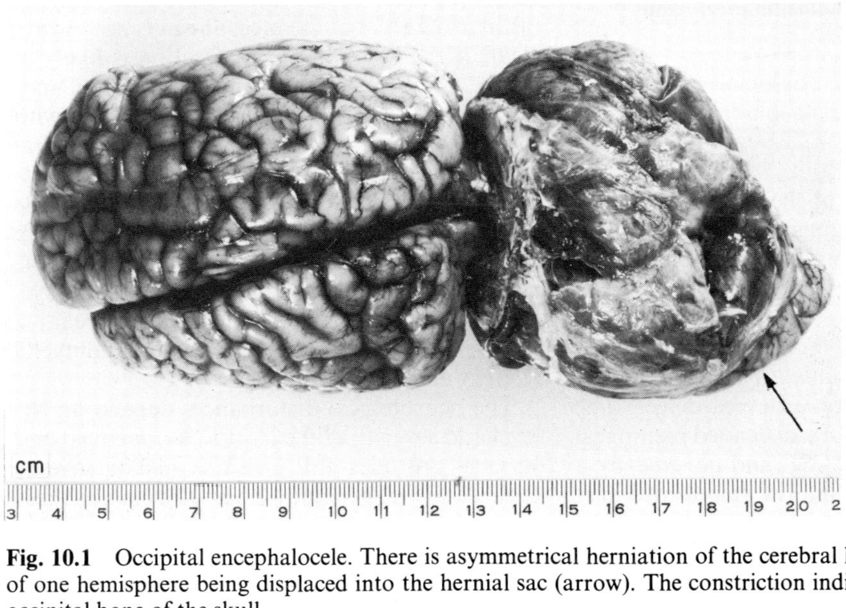

Fig. 10.1 Occipital encephalocele. There is asymmetrical herniation of the cerebral hemispheres, almost half of one hemisphere being displaced into the hernial sac (arrow). The constriction indicates the position of the occipital bone of the skull.

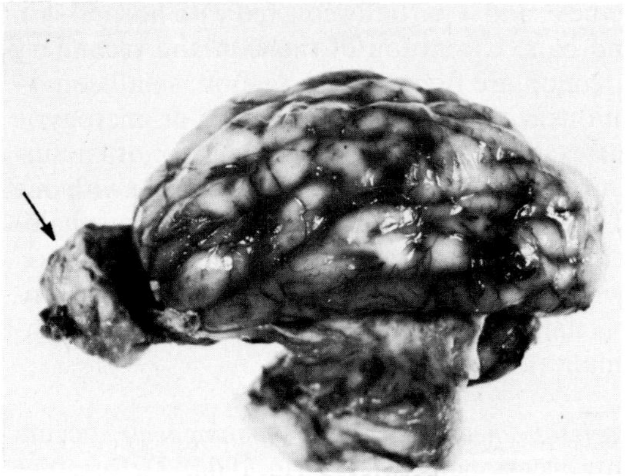

Fig. 10.2 Anterior (frontal) encephalocele (arrow).

sionally, atrophic and pyknotic neurons. The clinical diagnosis may be difficult if only the meninges protrude through the cribriform plate of the ethmoid bone. Cerebrospinal fluid passing into the nasal cavity is indicative of a free communication between the subarachnoid space and the encephalocele.

Since frontoethmoidal meningocele and encephalocele are rare in western Europe but relatively common in south-east Asia, genetic and geographical factors may be of importance in their aetiology (Flatz and Sukthomya, 1970; Suwanwela and Suwanwela, 1972).

Spinal meningocele, myelomeningocele and myelocele

These three anomalies are associated with a defect in the vertebrae (spina bifida), of varying severity (Barson, 1970).

Meningocele consists of herniation of both dura and arachnoid through a vertebral defect, the spinal cord remaining in a normal position in the spinal canal.

Meningomyelocele is a more severe malformation (Fig. 10.3). Both meninges and spinal cord herniate through a large vertebral defect. The fluctuant mass consists of a distended meningeal sac which is filled with CSF and covered by a thin membrane or by skin. The spinal cord may be closed, floating on the posterior surface of the arachnoid cyst. The central canal is often dilated and the posterior part herniates with the meninges. In other cases, often referred to as *myelocele*, the malformation appears as a flat open lesion, CSF leaking on to the exposed area. The spinal cord at the site of the bony defect forms a flat discoidal mass, highly vascular and often covered with granulation tissue. The posterior surface of the spinal cord is open and the central canal blends into the skin.

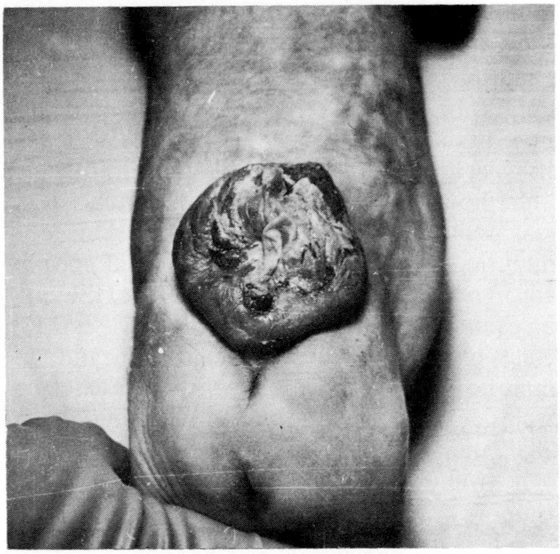

Fig. 10.3 Lumbar meningomyelocele, showing ulceration of the surface, in an infant with hydrocephalus and paraplegia.

Hydrocephalus occurs in many infants with one of these defects but the mechanism is not always clear. If the lesion is open, infection is likely to occur. The Arnold–Chiari malformation (Chiari type II malformation) is usually associated with these dysraphic states. In some cases, lateral compression, dorsal displacement and angulation of the brain stem and aqueduct may be the cause of the hydrocephalus (Emery, 1974). In addition, anomalies in the spinal cord above the meningomyelocele are common and include syringomyelia, hydromyelia, diastematomyelia, a double or multiple central canal and diplomyelia (Emery and Lendon, 1973).

The neurological disturbances depend on the level and severity of the lesions, but medical and surgical attitudes still give rise to controversy because of the generally poor outcome in these cases (Laurence and Tew, 1967; Lorber, 1971; Deonna, 1981).

Environmental factors, geographical and social class distribution and dietary conditions seem to play a role in the pathogenesis. Genetic factors have also been incriminated because of a preponderance in girls and recurrence in siblings.

Arnold-Chiari malformation

This complex deformity of brain stem and cerebellum was first described by Cleland (1883) and subsequently by Chiari (1891, 1895) and Arnold (1894). The deformity has become generally known as the Arnold-Chiari malformation, and Friede (1975) considered that no useful purpose would be served by changing it. The term, however, should be confined to the type II malformation described below.

The individual components of the disorder may be found in various combinations and may vary in severity, and although the eponym may be questionable, Chiari's classification is still appropriate.

Type I (Fig. 10.4) is ectopia of the cerebellar tonsils. This malformation, encountered in adults and a not uncommon cause of late-onset hydrocephalus, is usually an isolated feature or is associated with minor deformity of the medulla.

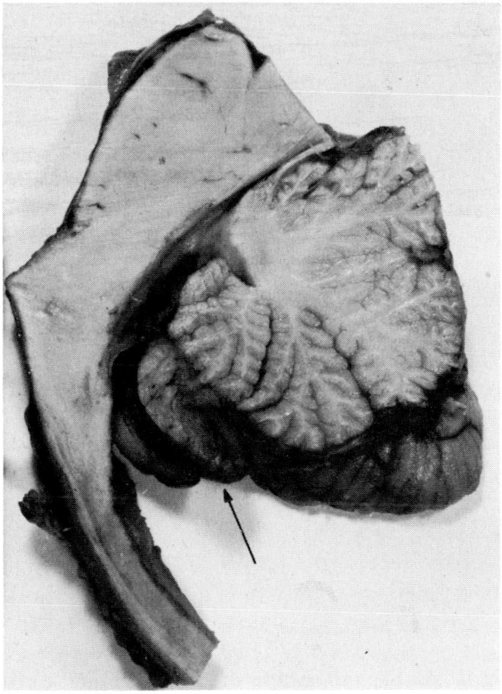

Fig. 10.4 Chiari type I malformation. The ectopic nodule of cerebellar tissue (arrow) has no connection with the normal vermis.

Type II is recognized as the Arnold-Chiari malformation. Is by far the most common type seen in neonates and is almost always associated with a lumbosacral myelomeningocele. It consists of lengthening of the vermis and tonsils of the cerebellum and their downward displacement through the foramen magnum into the spinal canal (Fig. 10.5). The dorsal part of the elongated medulla is shifted caudally and overrides the upper cervical cord, resulting in a characteristic Z-shaped kink at the junction between medulla and cord (Fig. 10.6). The inferior part of the fourth ventricle and everted choroid plexuses form, with the herniated cerebellum, a compact mass of tissue tightly adherent to the foramen magnum and the upper cervical spinal canal. The cerebellar hemispheres are often asymmetrical and flattened. The vermis, although present, is often buried between the hemispheres, which may expand ventrally, surrounding the medulla oblongata.

The posterior fossa is small, broadened and shallow, with a low position of the venous sinuses. The tentorium may be rudimentary and inserted at a low level. The foramen magnum is enlarged. Anomalies of the cranial vault, such as craniolacunia, are common. Hydromyelia, syringomyelia and diastematomyelia are also frequent.

Type III is a cervical spina bifida, the entire cerebellum being herniated through the foramen magnum, forming a myelocerebellomeningocele.

Type IV is cerebellar hypoplasia.

The Arnold-Chiari deformity (type II) is almost always associated with hydrocephalus; ventricular dilatation may be caused by compression (Emery, 1974) or stenosis of the aqueduct of Sylvius or, in cases with an open spinal defect, by secondary meningitis. The hydrocephalus is usually of communicating type. This is clearly shown if meningitis develops as a result of infection of the lumbar myelomeningocele: the infection spreads into the ventricles to produce pyocephalus, but not into the intracranial subarachnoid space. There often appear to be numerous small gyri on the surface of the brain, but on histological examination there is no true micropolygyria. Heterotopias are a constant finding in the cerebellum.

Several hypotheses have been proposed to explain the Arnold-Chiari (type II) malformation.

1. The spinal cord is attached to the mal-

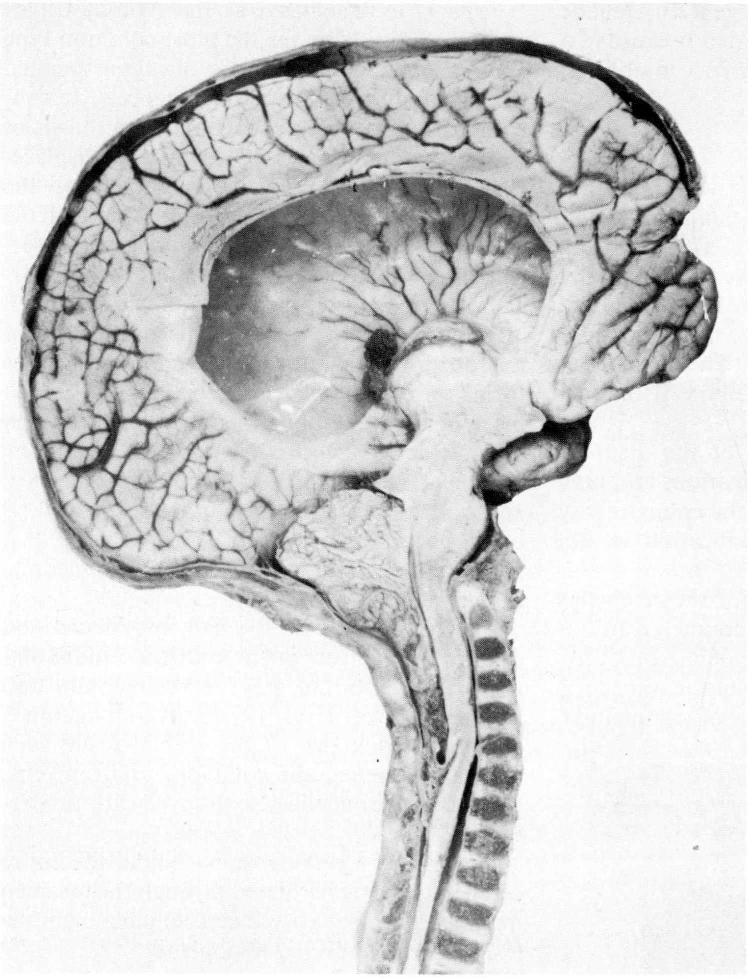

Fig. 10.5 Arnold–Chiari malformation (Chiari type II) and hydrocephalus in a 7-week-old infant. Note the downward displacement of the cerebellar vermis and tonsils through the foramen magnum into the spinal canal and the beak-like deformity of the quadri-geminal plate.

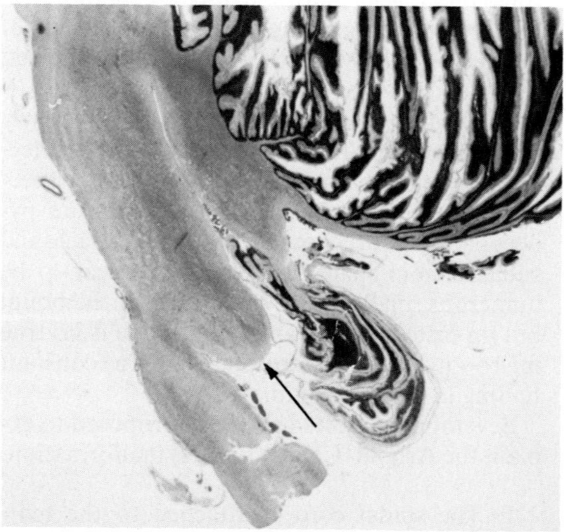

Fig. 10.6 Sagittal section of brain stem and cerebellum in the Arnold–Chiari malformation. The herniated cerebellar tissue lies posterior to the Z-shaped kink (arrow) at the junction of medulla and spinal cord.

formed vertebrae at the level of the myelomeningocele, thus preventing its normal ascent during development and causing a downward displacement of the brain stem and cerebellum (Penfield and Coburn, 1938). Against this hypothesis are the facts that the spinal nerves in the thoracic region are normally orientated (Barry, Patten and Stewart, 1957), and that the Arnold-Chiari malformation can occur, although rarely, without an associated myelomeningocele (Peach, 1965; Duckett, 1966).

2. Hydrocephalus is the initial event (Padget, 1970; Gardner, 1961, 1973); the cerebellum is then displaced caudally through the foramen magnum, with consequent herniation of the vermis and of the elongated medulla which overlaps the upper cervical cord. But hydrocephalus is occasionally absent in individuals with the Arnold-Chiari deformity.

3. The pontine flexure fails to form; this leads in turn to an elongated brain stem and subsequently the medulla forms an acute bend over the upper cervical cord. The outpouching of the choroid plexuses and the 'extraventricular' appearance of part of the cerebellum would therefore be a remnant of the embryonic anlage of the rhombencephalon (Daniel and Strich, 1958). There is, however, no disorganization in the topographical distribution of the nuclei in the affected areas.

None of these hypotheses explains satisfactorily the various types of Arnold-Chiari malformation. Their only common denominator is the abnormal occipital bone with a disproportion between the size of the posterior fossa, which is small and shallow, and the size of the cerebellum and brain stem, which is normal. The deformity develops early in gestation at the age of 10 weeks and may be related to the group of dysraphic disorders (Marin-Padilla, 1978) with localized mesodermal and posterior fossa abnormalities.

Malformations of the spinal cord

In addition to the several gross malformations described above under the heading of dysraphic states and usually obvious in the neonatal period, other less severe abnormalities may not be suspected on gross examination. Histological examination at many levels of the cord may be required for their identification. These anomalies, usually described in the adult, also raise the question as to whether they are primary malformations or acquired lesions.

Hydromyelia is an overdistension of the central canal, either because of incomplete fusion of the posterior columns (Staemmler, 1942) or as a persistence of the primitive large canal of the embryo. The dilatation may be focal and is often more pronounced in the lumbar region. In the neonate, isolated hydromyelia is usually asymptomatic and is an incidental finding at autopsy. It may be found only on serial slices of the spinal cord (Benda, 1959). Hydromyelia may also be one anomaly in a more complex syndrome. It is, for instance, associated with the Arnold-Chiari malformation in approximately 40 per cent of cases (MacKenzie and Emery, 1971). The central canal may be lined by normal ependyma, which becomes replaced by glial tissue (Fig. 10.7).

Diastematomyelia and diplomyelia may be difficult to distinguish from each other without careful study of serial sections. The two anomalies may coexist in different segments of the cord. Diastematomyelia consists of two hemicords either within a single dural sac and separated by a vascular mass of connective tissue or in two separate dural sacs between which there may be a bony septum (James and Lassman, 1972). This condition may be asymptomatic in neonates. It has been described in childhood, when symptoms develop (Matson et al., 1950; Lefevre, Klein and Fauré, 1956), and is often associated with spina bifida.

Diplomyelia consists of a duplicated spinal cord, instead of two facing hemicords as in diastematomyelia. Its embryogenesis is poorly understood (Dryden, 1980). Duplication of the central canal over a short distance may be an incidental finding and is usually associated with other malformations. Many abnormalities of form, size and distribution of grey and white matter in the spinal cord have been described by, among others, Gardner (1973). The filum terminale may be absent with dilatation of the conus medullaris or may be long and folded in an S-shaped fashion. Abnormal fila may contain disorganized cord elements or mesenchymal structures, as in hamartomas (Emery and Lendon, 1969; Talwalker and Dastur, 1974).

Asymmetry (Fig. 10.8) or *absence of the ventral pyramidal tracts* is a not uncommon finding upon systematic examination of the spinal cord

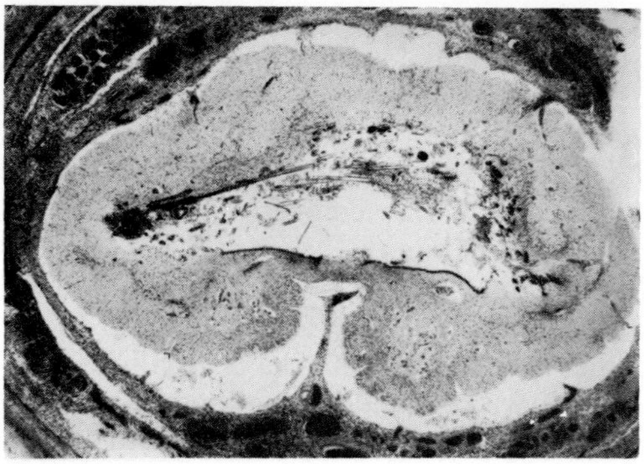

(a)

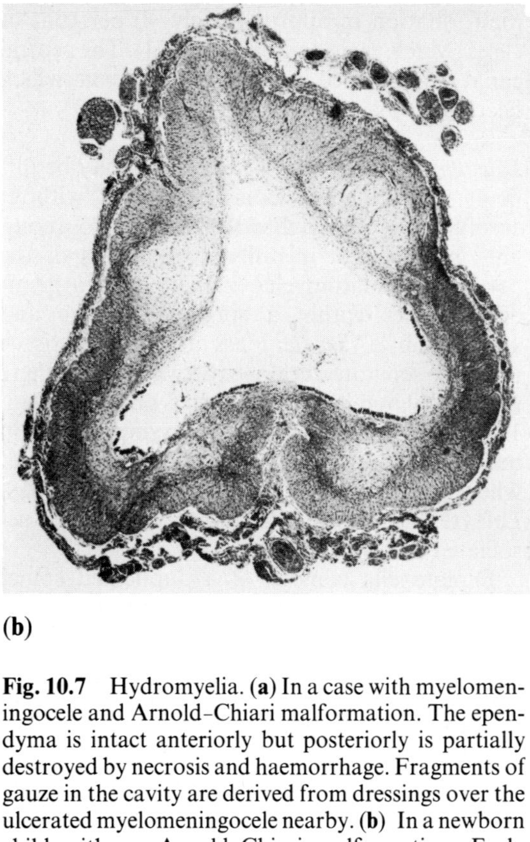

(b)

Fig. 10.7 Hydromyelia. (**a**) In a case with myelomeningocele and Arnold–Chiari malformation. The ependyma is intact anteriorly but posteriorly is partially destroyed by necrosis and haemorrhage. Fragments of gauze in the cavity are derived from dressings over the ulcerated myelomeningocele nearby. (**b**) In a newborn child with an Arnold–Chiari malformation. Early gliosis replaces the ependymal lining in the posterior half of the cavity.

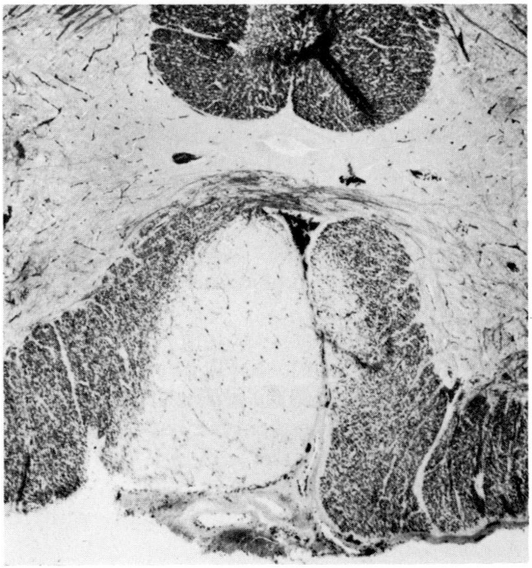

Fig. 10.8 Transverse section of cervical spinal cord. There is marked asymmetry of the direct pyramidal tracts (unmyelinated in the neonate and therefore pale in sections stained for myelin).

of neonates. The classical concept of the decussation of the pyramidal tract and of anterior (direct) and lateral (crossed) fibres has been revised by Yakovlev (1972) who studied fetal and neonatal brains in serial sections stained for myelin. The pyramidal tracts are readily identified in the spinal cord of the very young because they are poorly myelinated and their size and shape can be studied more easily than in adults. Most frequently, the fibres of the left pyramidal tract cross the midline first, and pass anteriorly to those of the right. The tracts are usually symmetrical but six variations have been observed, differing according to the number of crossed fibres, one or both direct pyramidal tracts showing great variability in size.

Syringomyelia and syringobulbia

The name *syringomyelia* is used for a disease in which there is tubular cavitation of the spinal cord extending over many segments. Cavities which involve only two or three segments are not usually considered syringomyelic, although they may be of essentially similar nature. It is not always possible even at necropsy to distinguish syringomyelia from hydromyelia, but the distinction is important as will appear when the aetiology of the two conditions is considered. The name *syringobulbia* is used for a similar condition in which the cavities are situated in the medulla and these syringes are often associated with syringomyelia. The name is rather less appropriate because the cavities are more slit-like than tubular. Rarely, the cavitation extends into the pons and in exceptional cases it may reach the midbrain and even the internal capsule (Spiller, 1906). Clinically the disease usually begins during the second and third decade and is slowly progressive, or the symptoms may increase at first rapidly and then more slowly. They may cease to progress at any time. Unless associated with bulbar symptoms, the disease rarely causes death directly but considerable disability is produced by the weakness of limbs and trunk and by the almost invariable spinal deformity. Syringomyelia is usually encountered in adults but has occasionally occurred in infants, the youngest reported being 5 weeks old (Duffy and Ziter, 1964).

Pathological changes in syringomyelia

When exposed at operation or autopsy the spinal cord appears swollen and tense in the cervical region and may fill the spinal canal. During life the enlargement can be demonstrated radiologically by myelography, an important diagnostic procedure in the disease. Externally, apart from the swelling, the spinal cord appears normal and there is no leptomeningeal thickening. The syrinx is filled with a clear fluid, which in many cases (Gardner, 1973) proves to have a similar composition to that of cerebrospinal fluid. The syrinx fluid may, however, be yellow with a high protein content. When at necropsy the fluid within the syrinx is allowed to escape, the cord becomes flattened, most often in its anteroposterior diameter. The syrinx may best be examined by numerous transverse sections but clearly a thorough examination at every segmental level is a very time-consuming task. A complete examination throughout the cord would require many thousands of sections and is scarcely feasible. In cases carefully examined at necropsy the following features recur. The cavity is usually found to be largest in the cervical region but is often absent from the first cervical segment. In the consideration of some of the theories of aetiology of syringomyelia this complete absence of any trace of the syrinx at this high cervical level is important. The syrinx commonly extends through the upper thoracic segments for a varying distance and usually terminates at a lower thoracic level. The lumbosacral enlargement is rarely involved. In typical cases the cavity in the cervical enlargement extends transversely across the cord, involving the more posterior parts of the ventral horns and passing across the midline behind the central canal. It often extends also into the posterior horns (Fig. 10.9a). When very

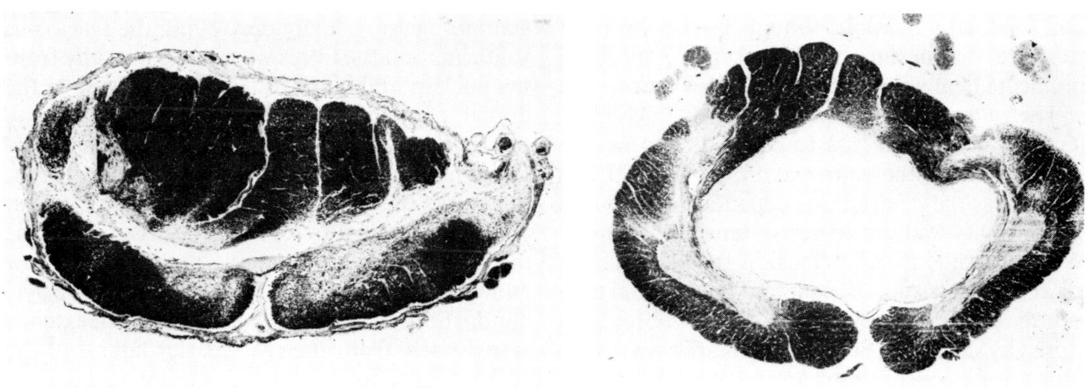

(a) **(b)**

Fig. 10.9 Syringomyelia. Transverse sections of the spinal cord stained to demonstrate myelin. (**a**) Cervical level. The slit-like cavity extends into both posterior horns. (**b**) Thoracic level. The cavity merges with the central canal. Loyez method.

large it occupies most of the cross-sectional area of the cord; the more anterior groups of motor nerve cells lie in front of it but otherwise little grey matter remains, and the lateral and posterior white columns are reduced by compression to a narrow zone of fibres (Fig. 10.9b). Extensions in the midline, or more laterally into the posterior columns, are common and the anterior white commissure is often destroyed either by pressure or by a midline anterior extension of the cavity. A transverse cavity with midline posterior and anterior extensions, such as is sometimes seen at this level, closely resembles the cruciform shape of the central canal during the stage of fetal development before the alar and basal laminae fuse with one another. That this is more than a chance resemblance is shown by the most usual position of the cavity in the medulla which also lies between the nuclei arising respectively from the alar and the basal laminae. In the thoracic cord the cavity commonly lies in the posterior horns and is often unilateral. When bilateral the cavities may be separate or may be joined in the region of the grey commissure and so form a single U-shaped cavity. Serial sections show that cavities which are double at one level usually join into a single cavity at some point above, and it is usual for the cavity on one side to end at a higher level than the other. More rarely two cavities join in the lower thoracic region. Although the grey matter is the common site of cavitation, extensions into the posterior or lateral columns or across the white commissure are not unusual, and the cavity may reach the pial surface at the tips of the dorsal horns at any level. It is possible, though usually difficult to prove, that in some cases the syrinx may communicate here with the subarachnoid space.

The walls of the cavity vary greatly in character, especially from case to case but also in different parts of the same cavity. Greenfield believed that these variations depended on the age of the cavity and the degree of tension within it. Where there is recent extension the wall is irregular and consists of degenerated neuroglial and neural elements. Myelinated nerve fibres enclosed by sheaths of Schwann cells are commonly found in the wall of syrinx and have been thought (Hughes and Brownell, 1963) to arise by regeneration from damaged posterior nerve roots. The myelin around the syrinx stains poorly, as it does in oedematous white matter, and the appearances suggest tearing of the tissues and transudation of serous fluid into them. When the cavity has been established for a longer time there is neuroglial hyperplasia around it with large fibre-forming astrocytes lying chiefly in a tangential direction. These finally form a dense concentric wall of neuroglial sclerosis which may be 1–2 mm in thickness. It is common to find a thin layer of collagen covering some part of the wall. Thicker strands of collagen, or blood vessels with hyalinized walls, may be seen passing across the cavity from one wall to another. Where the cavity communicates with the central canal, as it not uncommonly does especially in the cervical region, part of the central wall of the cavity is lined with ependymal cells, but in most places these take no part in the formation of the wall. This is an obvious but sometimes overlooked feature distinguishing syringomyelia from hydromyelia. When in syringomyelia there is a lining of ependyma the layer of neuroglial tissue which is deep to the ependymal layer is usually thinner than that surrounding the rest of the cavity.

Syringobulbia

Slit-like cavities in the medulla usually lie in one of three positions (Jonesco-Sisesti, 1932).

1. The most common is a slit running out in an anterolateral direction from the floor of the fourth ventricle external to the hypoglossal nucleus. It may communicate with the cavity of the ventricle but sometimes begins anterior to this. It passes outwards and forwards for a variable distance towards the descending tract of the trigeminal nerve, usually destroying the fasciculus solitarius and the fibres which pass dorsally from the nucleus ambiguus to join those arising in the dorsal vagal nucleus (Fig. 10.10c). A cavity in this position is most commonly limited to the lower half or two-thirds of the medulla where it interrupts the fibres passing from the nuclei gracilis and cuneatus to form the decussation of the medial lemniscus. It may also descend low enough to interrupt many of the decussating pyramidal fibres (Fig. 10.10d). At this level it extends transversely from the grey matter lateral to the central canal to a position anterior to the substantia gelatinosa and descending tract of the trigeminal nerve. Cavities in this position usually have thin walls of neuroglial tissue. Occasionally the slit is replaced by a neuroglial scar which interrupts the fibre system as completely as a slit

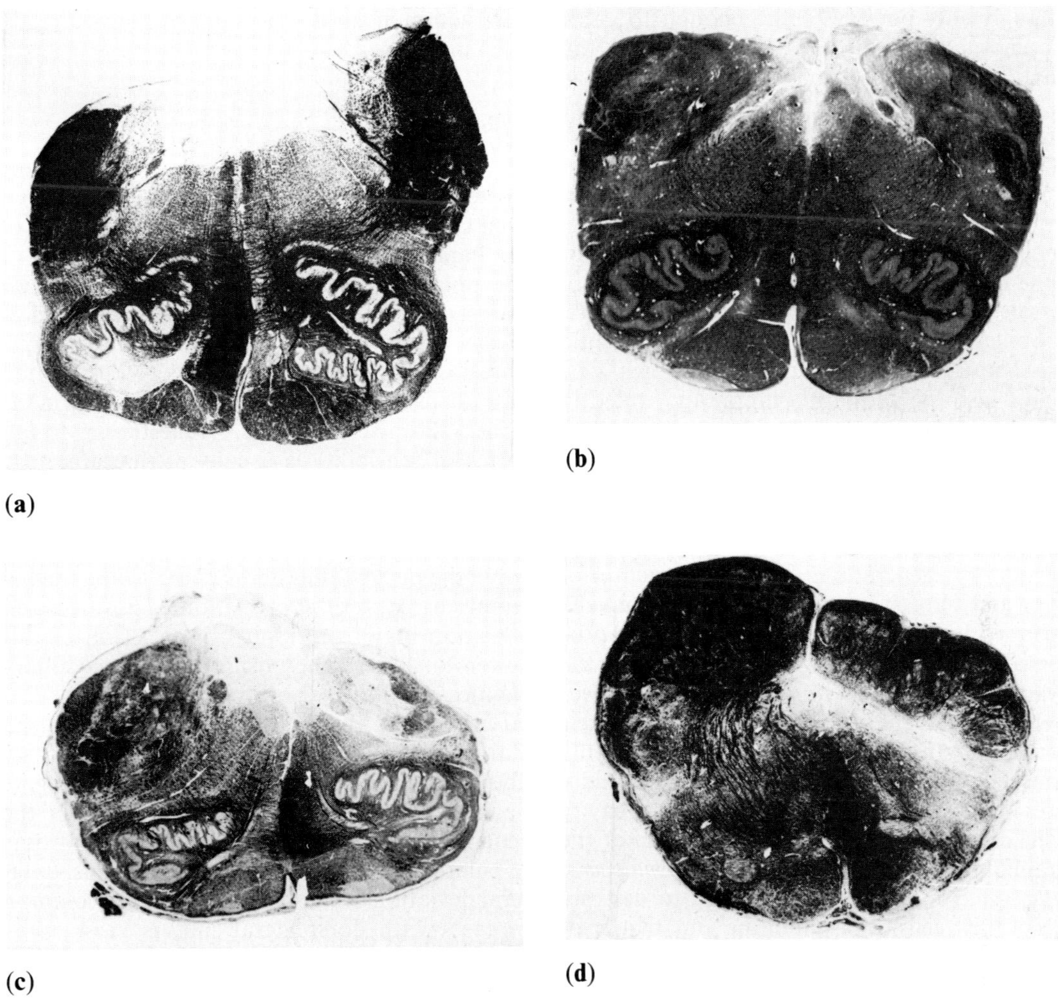

Fig. 10.10 Syringobulbia. Transverse sections of medulla. (**a**) Case with ventral slit between olive and pyramid and dorsolateral slit at a lower level which has produced degeneration of the contralateral medial lemniscus. (**b**) Case with bilateral dorsolateral and dorsomedial slits. (**c**) Case with dorsolateral slit producing degeneration of the medial lemniscus. (**d**) Section at the level of the pyramidal decussation. The lateral extension of the cavity has destroyed the crossed pyramidal fibres. Loyez method for myelin.

or cavity. Such appearances are not uncommon at the upper and lower ends of a cavity, and may arise from secondary fusion of its walls. These cavities are usually unilateral but may be bilateral and roughly symmetrical (Fig. 10.10b). In such a case one cavity extends to a higher or lower level than the other.

2. Almost equally common is an extension of the fourth ventricle along the median raphe for a shorter or longer distance. This is usually lined by ependyma, but occasionally is replaced by a neuroglial scar containing ependymal cells or small ependyma-lined tubules, like those seen in forking of the aqueduct (Fig. 10.10b). By interrupting the decussation of fibres passing from the descending vestibular nucleus to the median longitudinal fasciculus these slits may cause nystagmus, but are otherwise asymptomatic. When this median extension is small and is not associated with other cavitation in the medulla it scarcely merits the name of syringobulbia

3. A rarer position for a cavity is between the pyramid and the inferior olive where it interrupts the emerging fibres of the hypoglossal nerve (Fig. 10.10a). These cavities are usually unilateral; in Spiller's (1906) case they were bilateral,

although only one was large enough to cause atrophic palsy of the tongue. A cavity in this situation may also damage the anteromedian part of the olive or the posterior part of the pyramid.

Cavities in the pons usually lie in the tegmentum where they may destroy the fibres of the sixth or seventh cranial nerves, or the central tegmental tract. They may pass down posterior to the olive for a short distance. Extensions of the cavity to a higher level are extremely rare. In Spiller's case the cavity in one pyramid passed up among the corticospinal fibres, destroying also the substantia nigra, and ended in the internal capsule and caudate and lenticular nuclei.

Secondary degenerations

Secondary degenerations follow destruction of tracts and fibre systems both in syringomyelia and in syringobulbia. The pyramidal tracts may be pressed on by an anterior cavity between the pyramid and medullary olive, or a slit at a lower level may interrupt pyramidal fibres during their decussation. In the latter case there is commonly some retrograde degeneration of the pyramidal fibres in the medulla. Alternatively, a large cavity in the cervical region may destroy much of the pyramidal tract by compression. The *spinocerebellar tracts* may degenerate owing to destruction of their cells of origin in the grey matter of the cord or of the fibres leaving these. The fibres passing in the posterior columns may be compressed or destroyed by extensions of the cavity in the cord. In cases of syringobulbia the fibres relayed to the thalamus from the nuclei gracilis and cuneatus are commonly destroyed as they pass towards the decussation of the medial lemniscus, so there is more or less complete absence of the medial lemniscus on the side opposite to the lesion (Fig. 10.10a and c); retrograde degeneration occurs in the nerve cells of the nuclei gracilis and cuneatus. Fibres passing to the spinothalamic tracts are very commonly involved either at or near their cells of origin in the posterior horns or as they cross the midline in the central commissure. The dorsolateral cavities in the medulla commonly interrupt some of the fibres passing inwards from the descending trigeminal nucleus to the medial lemniscus. The destruction of the motor fibres arising in the nucleus ambiguus and hypoglossal nuclei and destruction of the tractus solitarius have already been mentioned.

Symptomatology

The symptomatology of syringomyelia is closely related to the extent of the destruction of individual cells and fibres. Wasting of the muscles of the hands and forearms is related to lesions of the posterolateral cell groups in the anterior horns of the cervical cord. Dissociated anaesthesia results from damage to spinothalamic fibres and autonomic symptoms to destruction of the cells of the intermediolateral column in the upper thoracic segments. Anaesthesia to all forms of sensibility is usually attributable to a combination of a spinothalamic lesion either with a lesion in the posterior columns or, more often, with a cavity in the medulla which interrupts the decussating fibres going to the medial lemniscus. Loss of appreciation of position and vibration may also result from a lesion of this system of fibres. The position of the medullary cavities explains the paralyses of the lower cranial nerves and the facial and corneal analgesia. Rarely, extensions into the pons may cause paralysis of one abducens nerve or of conjugate deviation to one side, or by destruction of the central tegmental tract may lead to the syndrome of palatolaryngeal nystagmus. Nystagmus, or lateral deviation of the eyes, which is very common in cases with dorsolateral slits, is most easily explained by the destruction of fibres which pass from the descending vestibular nucleus to the medial longitudinal fasciculus.

Secondary syringomyelia

This term should be reserved for longitudinal cysts secondary to clearly evident causes. Tumours, trauma, adhesive arachnoiditis, haematomyelia and vascular softenings account for most cases. Most of the cysts are small but in tumours the associated cystic lesion may be extensive and progressive.

Poser (1956) reviewed 254 necropsied cases of syringomyelia and found that 40 (about 16 per cent) had an associated intramedullary tumour. Out of 209 cases of intramedullary tumours there was an incidence of 31 per cent of syringomyelia. Extrinsic tumours can cause syringomyelia, as in the case reported by Kosary et al., (1969) who found an occipital meningioma. Post-traumatic syringomyelia is dealt with in Chapter 17. Syringomyelia has occasionally been described following adhesive arachnoiditis (Schwartz, 1897) and a case was described by Appleby et al. (1969) following tuberculous meningitis. Carroll (1967) described syringomyelia following an attack of acute anterior poliomyelitis and reviewed other case reports of this association.

The cavitation associated with spinal tumours presents a more difficult problem. In some cases there is only a small cavity which extends for one or two segments above and below the tumour. Such cavities may arise as a result of transudation from the tumour. In other cases the cavities may be very extensive and may involve most of the spinal cord above and below the tumour. Such cavities are most often associated either with tumours of ependymal character or with haemangioblastomas. In the former case it is possible that the cavitation was a true syringomyelia and preceded the growth of the tumour. In two cases examined at the National Hospital, Queen Square, an ependymal tumour at the mid-thoracic level was associated with cavitation which extended from the C2 segment to the conus terminalis. This had all the characters of a syringomyelic cavity but had not caused any anaesthesia or other symptoms above the level of the tumour. The cavitation associated with haemangioblastomas of the spinal cord may, like the cerebellar cysts, be caused by transudation from the tumour acting over many years. Such cavities also are often very extensive. Brain, Greenfield and Northfield (1943) reported a case with a tumour at the T9 level, and cavitation extending from the medulla to the conus terminalis, and in the cases of Craig, Wagener and Kernohan (1941) the cavity was almost equally extensive. It would appear that cavities associated with tumours extend into the lumbosacral enlargement more often than do those of simple syringomyelia. The venous congestion which is often found below the level of a spinal tumour may be a contributory factor to this lumbosacral extension. The linkage of syringomyelia to cerebral tumours on which Langhans based his theory of pathogenesis is probably a chance association since asymptomatic cavitation of the cervical cord is not rare.

Aetiology and pathogenesis

The inclusion of syringomyelia in the large group of spinal cord malformations appears justified at first sight on anatomical grounds, but this may not be correct and in any case brings us little nearer to an understanding of its cause. One difficulty is the distinction of syringomyelia from hydromyelia. Gardner (1973) has summarized his conclusions in the statement that 'syringomyelia is symptomatic hydromyelia'. This view was derived from the finding of a malformation of the hindbrain obstructing the foramen of Magendie in a high proportion of cases. Gardner's view is that this obstruction causes distension initially of the central canal which may then rupture allowing CSF to escape into the substance of the spinal cord. In hydromyelia there is an undoubted association with neural tube malformations. It is also possible in some cases to trace the development of a syringomyelic cavity from hydromyelia, for example in cases of the Arnold-Chiari malformation in the adult. But this is true for only a minority of cases. Syringomyelia is rarely familial. The so-called 'hereditary lumbosacral syringomyelia' has been shown to be an affection of the dorsal root ganglia and primary sensory neurons (Denny-Brown, 1951).

Several different factors may be combined in the pathogenesis of cavitation in syringomyelia: (1) instability in the lines of junction of the alar and basal laminae with each other; (2) the constant movements of flexion and torsion to which the cervical cord and lower medulla are exposed; (3) the tendency for cysts within nervous tissue to undergo alterations of tension and so to enlarge.

1. As has been seen, the cavitation, both in the spinal cord and especially in the medulla, tends to occur along lines of fusion which take place comparatively late in fetal life. The ventral cavity in the medulla may thus be related to the migration of the olivary cells from the rhomboid lip across the median raphe to their final position behind the pyramids. Many of the earlier writers described the cells in the walls of a syringomyelic cavity as of embryonal character (Gowers and Taylor, 1899). There is little evidence of this in many cases which have been expertly examined. Ependymal cells are often seen in the tissue in front of the cavity; in those that result from a hydromyelia they may also be found under its

lateral walls; but these cells do not differ from those seen in the grey commissure in normal cords. The theory that cavitation takes place by the breakdown of abnormal neuroglial tissue appears to have no firm histological basis since this is a feature of no other pathological condition either in the medulla or in the spinal cord.

2. The reason why syringomyelic cavities tend to begin in the cervical region of the cord, and attain their greatest size there, may well be related to the great mobility of the cervical spine. Bending of the neck in all directions and torsion when the head is turned (Schaltenbrandt, 1951) must impose stresses and strains on the cervical cord to which it is less subject at lower levels, and which may well cause small tears of the tissue in the centre of the cord. Movements of the head on the atlanto-occipital joint must affect the lower medulla in a similar way.

3. Once cavitation in the spinal cord has begun it may be enlarged by transudation of fluid into it under pressure. This expansion is more likely to occur in the grey matter than in the firmer columns of white matter and, owing to the restricting investment of pia mater, must take place chiefly upwards and downwards. It is favoured by anything which increases venous congestion in the body cavity, such as muscular effort, since there are no valves on the veins draining the spinal cord, but it may also depend to some extent on the electrolyte content of the blood. In this connection the fact that a syringomyelic cavity usually ceases at the C2 level and has no communications with the fourth ventricle may be of considerable importance (see also Barnett, Foster and Hudgson, 1973).

Malformations of the cerebellum

The classification of cerebellar abnormalities is somewhat unsatisfactory because of the diversity of the phylogenetic status of the affected regions, the heterogeneity of associated malformations and the various possible pathogenetic mechanisms for a given abnormality. In addition, most abnormalities have been described after the neonatal period, when the pathological picture may be complicated by degenerative changes or by the sequelae of birth injury or perinatal vascular disturbance.

Agenesis of the cerebellum is a very uncommon anomaly that has been described in a heterogeneous group of patients. In the literature total agenesis has been reported in children aged 11 years (Combette, 1831), 15 years (Ferrier, 1876) and 4 months, the last with spina bifida and a lumbar meningocele (Priestley, 1920). There was no histological study in these cases. Riccardi and Marcus (1978) reported two male siblings born with congenital hydrocephalus who died, respectively, 4 days and a few minutes after birth. Autopsy, of one child only, revealed no cerebellar tissue. The authors suggested that cerebellar agenesis was the primary pathology, the non-communicating hydrocephalus being secondary to absence of the foramina of Magendie and Luschka, and that the anomaly was transmitted on an X-linked recessive basis.

The author's only personally studied instance of total absence of the cerebellum (Fig. 10.11) was in a male stillborn premature infant with hydrocephalus. A large arachnoid cyst filled the interhemispheric fissure, the ventricles were enlarged, and the corpus callosum and septum pellucidum absent. Macchi and Bentivoglio (1977)

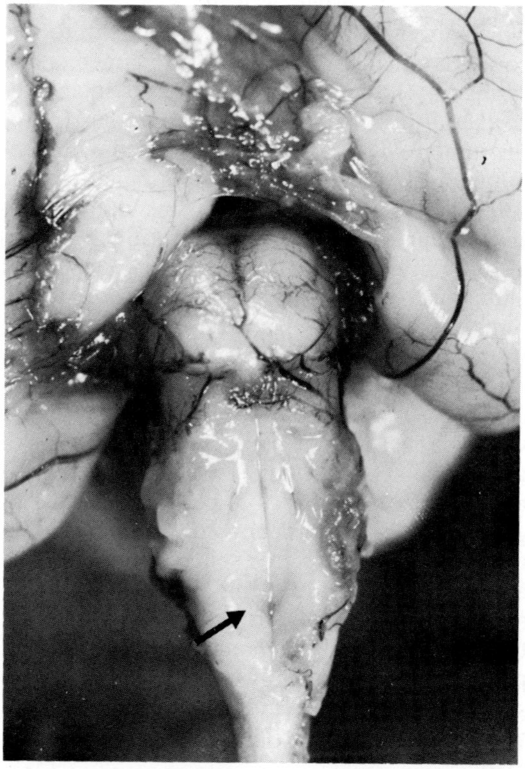

Fig. 10.11 Agenesis of the cerebellum in a premature infant. The floor of the fourth ventricle (arrow) is exposed by the total absence of cerebellar tissue.

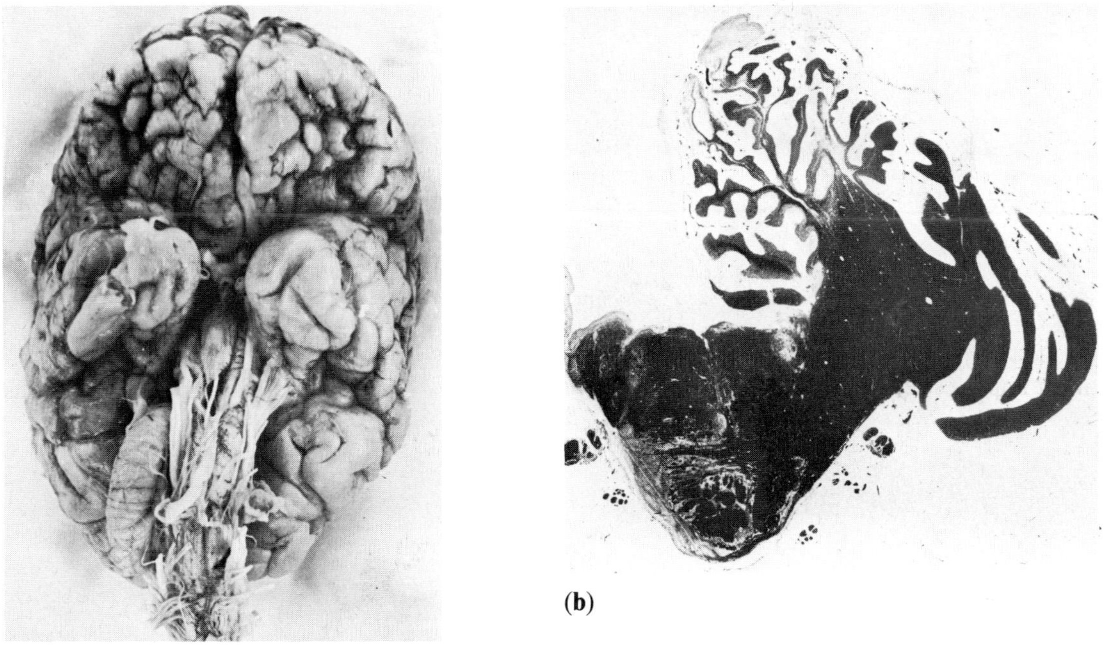

(a) (b)

Fig. 10.12 Absence of the left cerebellar hemisphere and middle cerebellar peduncle and marked reduction in the size of the contralateral pontine nuclei.

surveyed the literature and collected a dozen cases of 'agenesis of the cerebellum' although in some, as in Baker and Graves' two cases (1931), remnants of cerebellar tissue could be demonstrated. In total or nearly total absence of the cerebellum, related structures such as the pontine nuclei, inferior olives and cerebellar peduncles are either hypoplastic or malformed. Usually, both mental and physical handicaps are described in these patients. The cerebellar defect, however, may not be suspected during life (Rubinstein and Freeman, 1940). Absence of one hemisphere is much less rare (Fig. 10.12) and is associated with anomalies of the contralateral inferior olive and pons which may take the form of atrophy rather than maldevelopment.

Hypoplasia of the cerebellum

This anomaly forms a large and heterogeneous group. It has been found in cases of amaurotic familial idiocy (Bielschowsky, 1920; Norman, 1940; Jervis, 1950; Ule, 1952; Friede, 1964; Urich, 1977) associated with a paucity or absence of granule cells. The molecular layer was wide, usually gliosed, and myelination poor. Friede (1964) suggested that there was arrest of development of the external granular layer during early fetal life. Subsequently the condition was reproduced experimentally by the injection of cycasin to newborn mice (Hirano, Dembitzer and Jones, 1972), and an analogous disorder is seen in *Weaver* mutant mice (Hirano et al., 1973; Rakic and Sidman, 1973). The aetiology of this granule cell type of cerebellar hypoplasia is still controversial, but it may be that a disorder of the Bergmann glia precedes the failure of migration of granule cells which, in turn, leads to the death of granule cells. Purkinje cells are only mildly affected but their dendrites grow abnormally and dendritic spines are present in excess (Fig. 10.13).

Another form of cerebellar hypoplasia with communicating hydrocephalus and mental retardation was described in two brothers and a maternal uncle in a family in which five members had a branchial fistula (Renier et al., 1983).

R. Brun (1917, 1918a, b) described, under the title of pontoneocerebellar hypoplasia, cerebellum with hypoplastic, flattened, lateral lobes and well-developed vermis and flocculi (Fig. 10.14). In the cerebellar hemispheres the mossy and climbing fibres are largely absent. The ventral

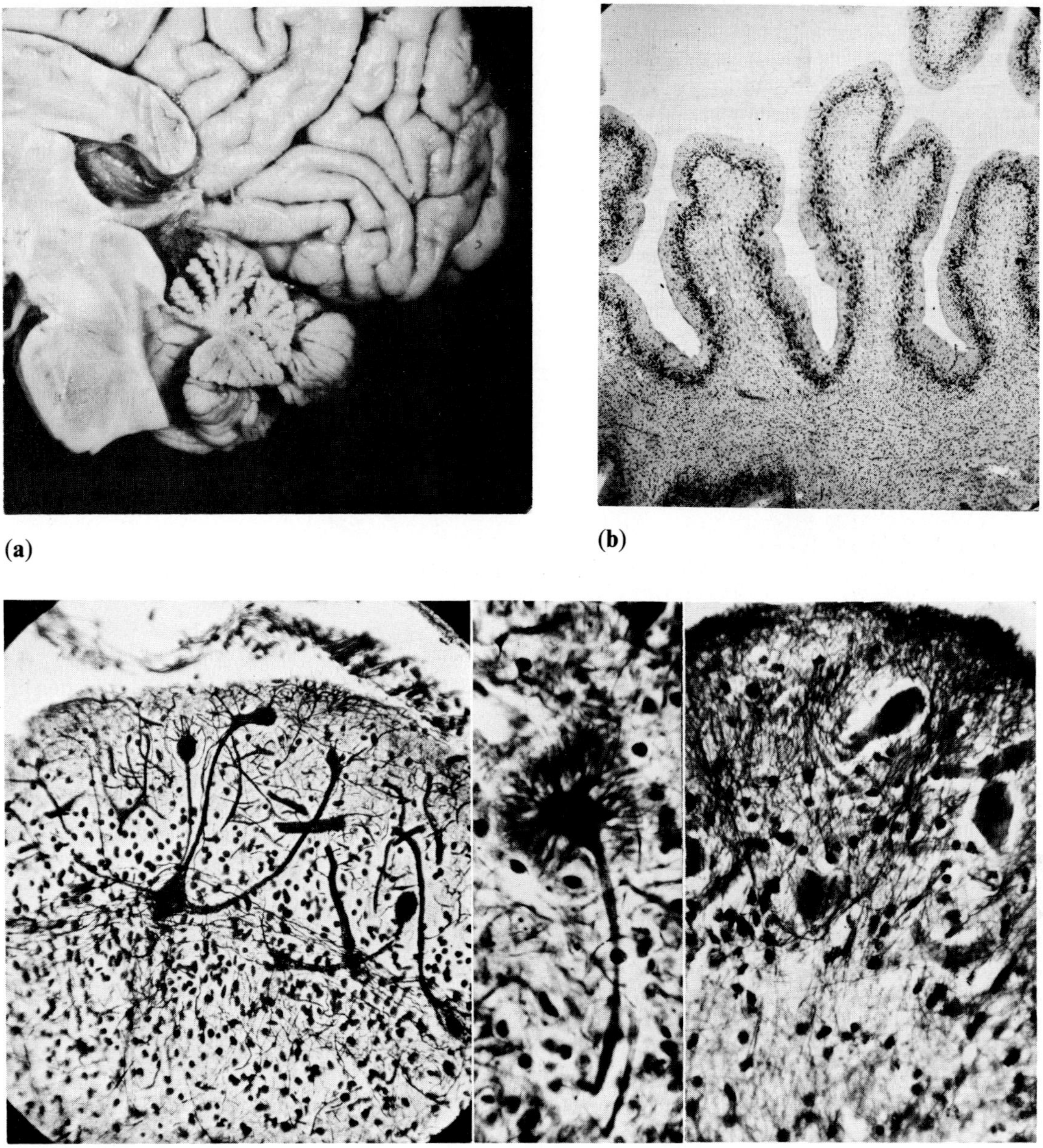

(a) (b) (c) (d) (e)

Fig. 10.13 Cerebellar hypoplasia of granule cell type. (**a**) Mid-sagittal section showing small cerebellum and shrinkage of the superior vermis. (**b**) Atrophy of the granule cell layer and preservation of the Purkinje cells, many of which are present in the molecular layer. Cresyl violet. (**c**) Cactus-like expansion of the dendrites of the Purkinje cells. Note the tangential fibres lying low in the molecular layer. Cajal's silver nitrate pyridine method. (**d**) Dendritic expansion with fine terminal brushwork of fibres. Bielschowsky's silver method. (**e**) Fibrillary gliosis is mainly in the molecular layer. Heterotopic Purkinje cells are shown. Holzer's method.

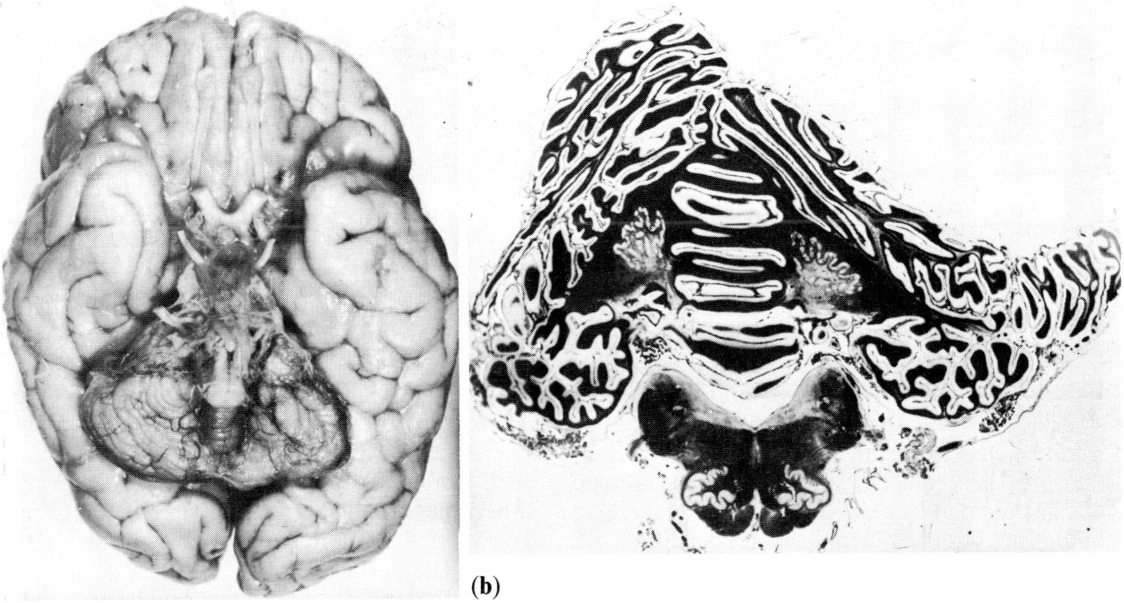

(b)

(a)

Fig. 10.14 Pontoneocerebellar hypoplasia. (**a**) The cerebellum is small and flattened—like a pressed fig. (**b**) Section of medulla and cerebellum. Note the relatively large vermis and flocculi compared with the lateral lobes. Loyez method for myelin.

part of the pons is unduly small and its transverse fibres and the nuclei pontis are markedly reduced in numbers. The dentate nuclei are composed of isolated clumps, a malformation also present in the cases of Brouwer (1924) and Biemond (1955). Biemond suggested that this malformation of the dentate nucleus may be the primary event, the other cerebellar changes being of a secondary character.

In this condition the small volume of the neocerebellum must be attributed to hypoplasia. The minor losses of Purkinje cells and patchy thinning of the granular layer in Biemond's case would not account for the great reduction in the size of the hemispheres. In other parts of the nervous system, however, signs of a degenerative process may sometimes be found. Thus in an example of pontoneocerebellar hypoplasia occurring in an infant of 3 months both dentate nuclei were almost completely degenerated and gliosed, except for the most dorsal convolutions (i.e. the part connected with the vermis) where groups of cells had survived. The original crenated outline of the nerve cell bands was, however, clearly distinguishable. This lesion was evidently related to the atrophy of the nucleus ventralis of each thalamus. A severe loss of nerve cells was also found in the inferior olives, particularly in the dorsal convolutions, and this was accompanied by marked fibrillary gliosis. The ventral pons was about half as thick as in the newborn and showed a great numerical reduction in its transverse fibres and in the nerve cells in the nuclei pontis. The remaining cells were often of small size, suggesting a retardation in development, but a heavy gliosis of the region was nevertheless seen. On the other hand, the small lateral lobes of the cerebellum showed no evidence of degeneration. In the brain stem certain nuclei with cerebellar connections were either absent or very poorly developed, their sites showing no traces of a destructive process (Norman and Urich, 1958). Gross and Kaltenback (1959) also noted the combination of malformation and system degenerations in their case.

Pontoneocerebellar hypoplasia has been found assocated with cerebral pachygyria (Kramer, 1956).

Hypoplasia and atrophy of the cerebellum were reported in children with Werdnig-Hoffmann disease (Norman, 1961; Weinberg and Kirkpatrick 1975; Gouttières, Aicardi and

Farkas, 1977) and in infants with Down's syndrome (Norman, 1963). In two patients, aged 4 and 5 months, reported by Norman and Urich (1958) there was a small but normally lobulated cerebellum with an underdeveloped pons and peduncles. Severe neuronal necrosis, fibrillary gliosis and poor myelination were found mainly in the dentate and pontine nuclei, the inferior olives and in the preposital and other nuclei of the medulla. In addition, the nucleus ventralis of both thalami, mamillary bodies and corpora luysi showed signs of degeneration. In the light of these observations, the authors raised the question of whether degenerative changes affected several structures simultaneously, the brain stem lesions not necessarily being secondary to the cerebellar anomaly. Acute anoxic-ischaemic necrosis, predominantly in these regions, is frequent in the neonatal period, and cerebellar hypoplasia, in the broadest sense, would be expected to occur more often as a sequel of these episodes. Friede (1975) suggested that cases of neocerebellar hypoplasia with atrophy of the pons might result from neonatal neuronal necrosis.

In the neonate, hypoplasia of the cerebellum involving the neo- and palaeocerebellum may be an incidental finding at autopsy. Neurological abnormalities are often obscured by respiratory distress, or are not specific. In one of the author's cases there were broad cerebral convolutions and a focally sparsely cellular layer III. The cerebellum consisted of a small mass with only a few lamellae. Microscopically the dentate nucleus was only poorly defined and contained few large neurons. The molecular layer was ill-defined and only occasional Purkinje cells were identified. For the most part the tissue was undifferentiated and uniformly highly cellular.

Partial defects of the cerebellum are often associated with malformation in the cerebrum such as anencephaly, total rachischisis and the Arnold-Chiari malformation. Cerebellar hypoplasia with atresia of the fourth ventricle and massive heterotopias were found by Friede (1975) in a case of arhinencephaly. Occipital encephaloceles may also be associated with severe cerebellar defects (Evrard and Caviness, 1974; Friede, 1975).

Total or partial absence of the vermis (i.e. rhombencephaloschisis) is not uncommon and has been described either as an isolated malformation or as part of a syndrome. In the Dandy-Walker malformation the vermis is absent in approximately one-fourth of the cases. The posterior lobes may be missing or attenuated and merge into the cyst wall. When the defect is isolated the posterior part of the vermis is usually absent or hypoplastic. Total absence of, or a rudimentary, vermis have also been described in association with complex deformities of the cerebral hemispheres, such as encephalocele, polymicrogyria, fusion of thalamic nuclei and hypoplastic corpus callosum (Karch and Urich, 1972; Padget and Lindenberg, 1972; Smith and Huntington, 1977).

Less frequently the vermis is absent and there is fusion of both cerebellar hemispheres and dentate nuclei. The defect is associated with absence or hypoplasia of the commissural system and other brain anomalies (De Morsier, 1955; Gross and Hoff, 1959; Michaud, Mizrahi and Urich, 1982). The pathogenesis is not known. Teratogenic agents, if any, must operate early in embryonic life, affecting both the commissural plate and the cerebellar primordium.

An uncommon familial syndrome of aplasia of the vermis was described by Joubert et al. (1969) and was associated with episodic hyperpnoea, abnormal eye movements, ataxia and mental retardation. Another case, well documented anatomically, has been reported by Friede and Boltshauser (1978). Almost total absence of the vermis was associated with atresia of both lateral cerebellar foramina, heterotopias, dysplasia of the inferior olives, fasciculated anterior corticospinal tracts, and definite hypoplasia or abnormal distribution of the solitary tract and gracile nucleus.

Cysts within the posterior fossa may occur in the von Hippel-Lindau syndrome. Cystic lesions secondary to intracerebellar infarction or haemorrhage are usually encountered in adults, and may be secondary to the acute lesions that can be observed in the neonatal period. Lemire et al. (1975) have suggested that intrauterine viral infection might be the cause of cerebellar and subependymal cysts observed in a 10-month-old boy who died of congenital heart disease.

Dandy-Walker malformation

This malformation, first recognized by Dandy and Blackfan (1914), was further described by Taggart and Walker (1942). Later, Benda (1954) proposed the eponym Dandy-Walker syndrome,

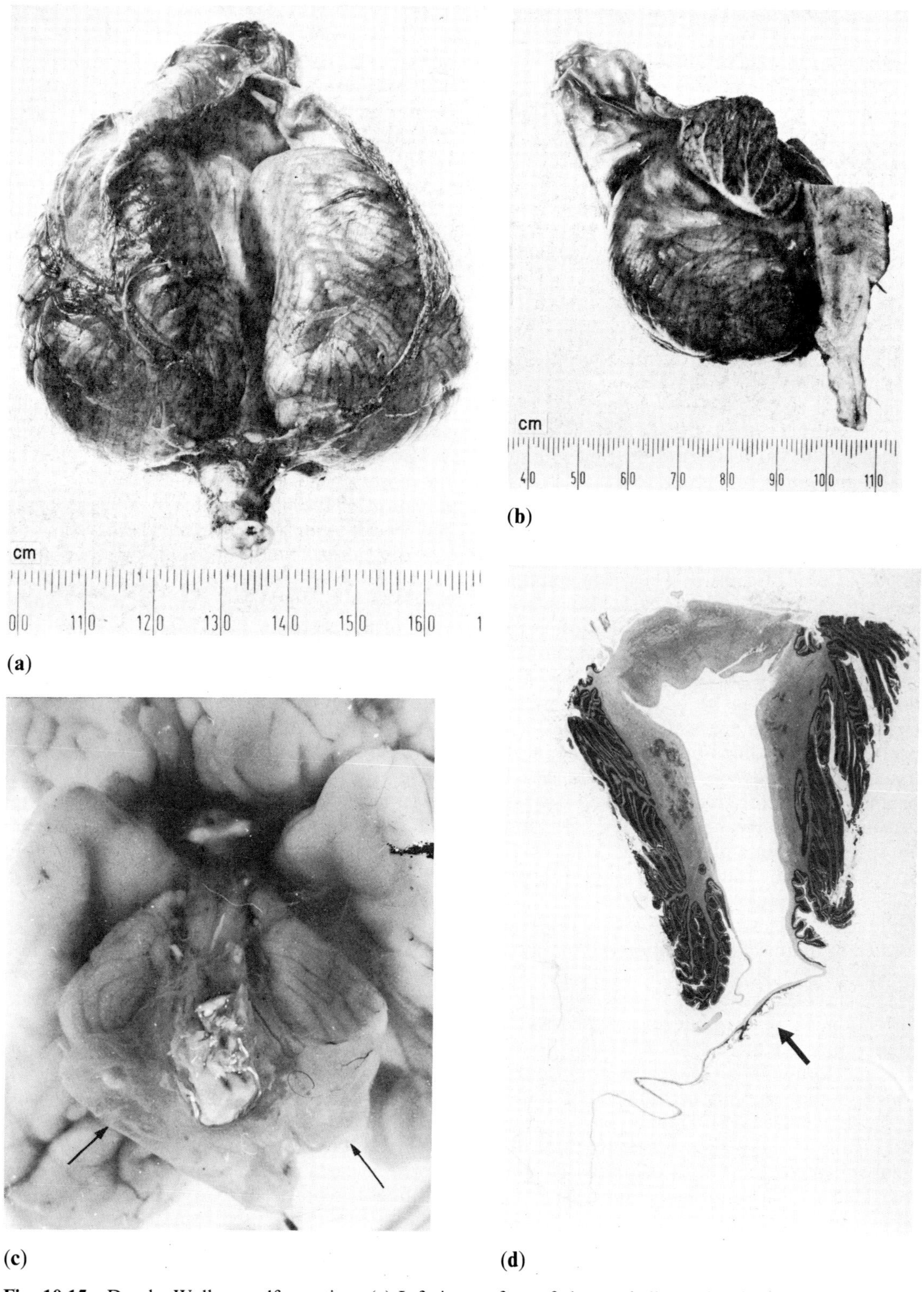

Fig. 10.15 Dandy–Walker malformation. (**a**) Inferior surface of the cerebellum, showing the defect in the vermis and the line of attachment of the tent-like cyst. (**b**) Sagittal section of brain stem and cerebellum showing preservation of the superior vermis and incorporation of the rudimentary inferior vermis into the cyst wall. (**c**) Base of neonatal brain, photographed under water. The delicate membrane (arrows) forming the cyst wall is shown floating in the water. (**d**) Horizontal section of brain stem and cerebellum. There is complete absence of the vermis and remnants of cerebellar tissue (arrow) are incorporated into the cyst wall.

by which it is now generally known. Large series of cases and general reviews include those by D'Agostino, Kernohan and Brown (1963), Hart, Malamud and Ellis (1972), Brown (1977) and Tal et al. (1980). Neonates with the Dandy-Walker malformation have a large head with signs of raised intracranial pressure and noticeable bulging of the occipital region. Pathological examination discloses distended hemispheres due to dilatation of the ventricular system and a large posterior fossa with high insertion of the sinuses and tentorium. The cerebellar hemispheres are normal in size but are often flattened. The vermis is either absent or hypoplastic (Fig. 10.15a and b). The distended roof of the fourth ventricle forms a large cyst (Fig. 10.15c and d) with blood vessels meandering within the membrane which is often thicker than a normal ventricular roof and splits easily.

Total or partial absence of the corpus callosum is a common association, and was found in 60 per cent of cases by Hart, Malamud and Ellis (1972). The third ventricle is also enlarged, and at autopsy its distended roof is often torn, or mistaken for a cyst. Other cerebral anomalies such as a bizarre gyral pattern, heterotopias and polymicrogyria may be observed. On microscopic examination the wall of the cyst in the posterior fossa is lined by a layer of connective tissue which blends into the leptomeninges. The patency of the foramina is difficult to assess because the membranes are often torn during autopsy. Remnants of cerebellar cortex or ectopic cells may be found in the wall of the cyst. Heterotopic nodules are usually scattered in the white matter. The inferior olives are often malformed or in an ectopic position (Hanaway and Netsky, 1971).

The pathogenesis of the Dandy-Walker malformation is unknown but several theories have been proposed. One, accepted for many years, is that the foramina of Magendie and Luschka, which should normally become patent at about 8-10 weeks (Weed, 1917) remain sealed (Dandy, 1921; Taggart and Walker, 1942), resulting in the enlargement of the fourth ventricle. However, the patency of these foramina has been demonstrated in some cases (Lemire et al., 1975). In another hypothesis Friede (1975) has suggested that an anomaly of the rostral part of the fourth ventricle (i.e. a developmental arrest in the hindbrain with persistence of the embryonic anterior part of the roof of the fourth ventricle) caused non-opening of the pia-arachnoid foramina. The malpositioned tentorium and torcular may also be interpreted as an arrest in development. Lemire et al. (1975) considered that the malformation results from an anomaly of the posterior medullary velum and impaired cell migration, the rostral part of the roof of the fourth ventricle being involved in the development of the vermis, hence the combined anomaly. Remnants of cerebellar cells in the walls of the cyst may be related to this process. Gardner, O'Rahilly and Prolo (1975) observed that the Dandy-Walker syndrome has certain features in common with the Arnold-Chiari malformation, but a review of numerous pertinent embryological studies failed to elucidate the primary cause and pathogenesis.

The clinical diagnosis, based on the shape of the infant's head, can be confirmed by transillumination of the posterior fossa. Ultrasonography or CT scan may give satisfactory images. The diagnosis *in utero* is possible by ultrasonography (Hatjis, Horber and Anderson, 1981; Newman et al., 1982). Differentiation from other cysts of the posterior fossa can be made radiologically. In the Dandy-Walker malformation the posterior venous sinuses are inserted higher than normally (Fauré, Lepintre and Lyon, 1963) and the cerebellar arteries are either displaced downwards or are absent or hypoplastic (La Torre, Fortuna and Occhipinti, 1973). With longer survival, neurological signs are related to increasing intracranial pressure. Papilloedema, optic atrophy and blindness, mental retardation and spasticity have been described.

Lhermitte-Duclos disease

It seems appropriate to include in the category of cerebellar malformations this condition known variously as *diffuse ganglioneuroma* (Lhermitte and Duclos, 1920), *diffuse hypertrophy of the cerebellar cortex* (Oppenheimer, 1955) and *granule cell hypertrophy* (Ambler, Pogacar and Sidman, 1969). This is not a common condition. Ambler, Pogacar and Sidman (1969) reviewed 36 cases in all, and since then only a few additional reports have appeared. Although some of the names used to describe the lesion suggest that it is neoplastic, and it is considered by Russell and Rubinstein (1977) to be hamartomatous in nature, there are features which indicate that it is malformative in origin with a strangely progressive course. The clinical presen-

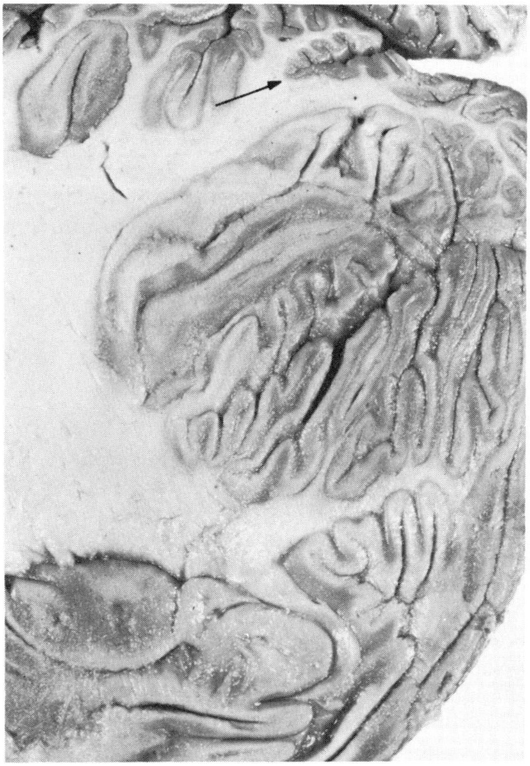

Fig. 10.16 Lhermitte–Duclos disease. Cut surface of cerebellum after fixation. Note the broad pale folia merging with normal folia (arrow). The underlying white matter shows slit-like cavities beneath the widened cortex. (Courtesy of Dr D.G.F. Harriman.)

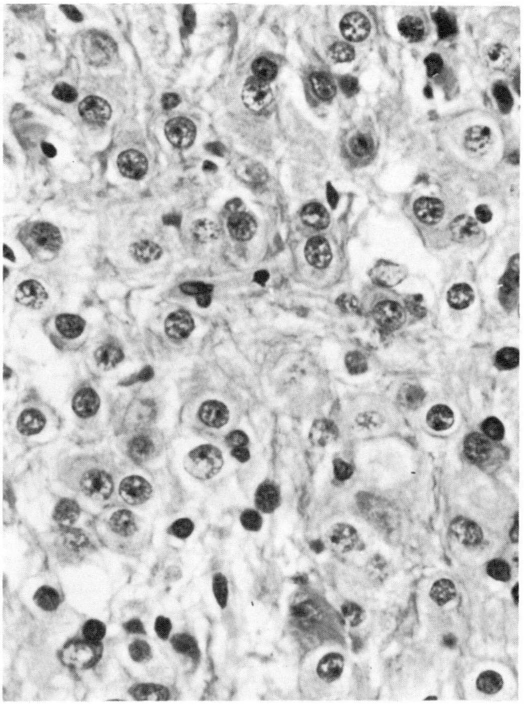

Fig. 10.17 Lhermitte–Duclos disease. Section of abnormal cortex from a biopsy of the cerebellum. The granule cells in the affected region are replaced by large abnormal neurons. Haematoxylin and eosin × 400.

tation is usually of raised intracranial pressure developing in adult life but many of the reported cases had megalencephaly, some cases were familial and some had other neural malformations. In some instances the finding was made incidentally at autopsy.

The structural abnormality consists of broadening of folia in regions of the cerebellum (Fig. 10.16), these regions varying greatly in size from case to case. Macroscopically the folia appear whitened whilst the cores of the folia lack white matter which is replaced by a slit-like cavity. Histologically the thick outer ('molecular') layer contains myelinated axons but no Purkinje dendrites. The inner layer adjoining the cavity consists of large neurons (Fig. 10.17) with rounded nuclei and peripheral Nissl bodies. No Purkinje cells are present in this layer.

The prognosis seems to be good in cases presenting as cerebellar tumours which are subsequently surgically resected, but why raised intracranial pressure develops is not clear. Ambler, Pogacar and Sidman (1969) considered the disease to be a developmental disorder of cell growth.

Holoprosencephaly (arhinencephaly)

This complex malformation covers a large spectrum of anomalies ranging from cyclopia to agenesis of one olfactory bulb.

Cyclopia, known in antiquity, was fully described with other facial anomalies by Geoffroy Saint-Hilaire (1832). A detailed description of the brain was given by Kundrat in 1882 (cited by Yakovlev and Wadsworth, 1946b), who coined the term *arhinencephaly* because of the absence of the olfactory bulbs and tracts which he considered were the cardinal feature of the malformation. Yakovlev (1959a) introduced the term *holotelencephaly* because of failure of evagination of the secondary telencephalic vesicles. His

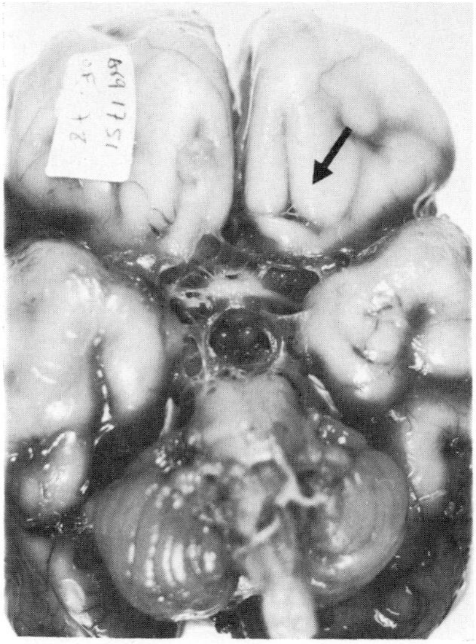

Fig. 10.18 Holoprosencephaly. Base of brain showing absence of left olfactory bulb and tract (arrow).

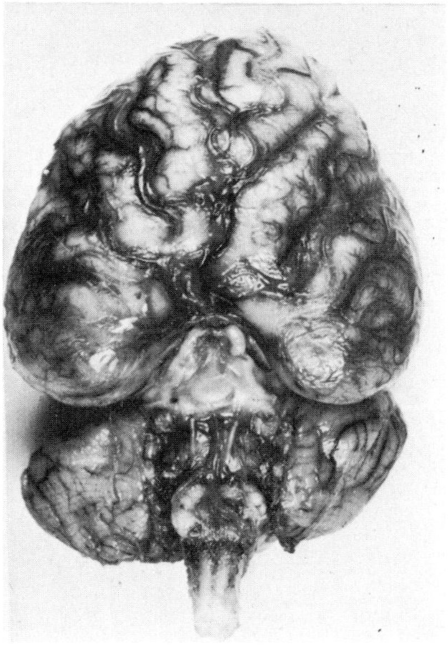

Fig. 10.19 Holoprosencephaly. An example of the most severe form of this malformation associated with cyclopia. There is no interhemispheric fissure, the hemispheres are fused, olfactory and optic nerves are absent and gyri are broad and have an abnormal pattern.

study was based on several brains, cut in serial sections, in which the entire cytoarchitecture was reconstructed.

The term *holoprosencephaly*, coined by De Myer, Zeman and Palmer (1963), emphasizes the failure of cleavage of the prosencephalon. The holoprosencephalies comprise a large spectrum of anomalies of the embryonic forebrain, ranging from the absence of the olfactory bulbs and tracts (Fig. 10.18), the 'lobar holoprosencephaly' of De Myer, Zeman and Palmer (1964) which should be correctly named 'olfactory aplasia', to the most severe form, an anterior holosphere, with no interhemispheric fissure and a single ventricle or 'alobar' holoprosencephaly (Fig. 10.19). Another form, with fusion of the frontal lobes or frontal and parietal lobes across the midline and posterior interhemispheric fissure, is called 'semi-lobar'.

In severe forms, the brain is often smaller than normal. Neither the sagittal sinus nor the falx cerebri is identifiable. Olfactory bulbs and tracts are absent and the broad convolutions have a bizarre pattern. Optic tracts are absent in the form associated with cyclopia. Brain stem and cranial nerves may be normal, although the pes pedunculi and the bulbar pyramids are often hypoplastic. Viewed from above, the horseshoe-shaped mass of brain represents the uncleaved telencephalic vesicles. The medial part of the brain consists of a thin membrane which often ruptures during autopsy, as it is usually distended by hydrocephalus. Although microcephaly is a common feature, the size of the head may be normal because of the distended ventricles. When the pia-arachnoid membrane is removed, the basal ganglia and thalami are exposed and the meatus of the aqueduct is readily visible.

In other cases the forebrain may be spherical, with broad and bizarre gyri and without an interhemispheric fissure. On coronal section, there is no corpus callosum and no septum pellucidum. The single ventricle is large and the deep grey nuclei are fused, the claustrum lying ventrally.

From the cytoarchitectonic study and mapping of Yakovlev (1959a) it became clear that although the posterior half of the brain is absent in most cases, the only missing architectonic fields are those characteristic of the frontal lobes, anterior to the motor area. Lamination, however, is often abnormal, with ectopic cells or sparsely cellular layers. The cerebellum may be hypoplastic and there are always dysplastic nodules of granular, spindle or ganglionic cells dispersed in the white matter and in the dentate and roof nuclei.

The association of certain facial malformations with holoprosencephaly is so frequent that De Myer, Zeman and Palmer (1964) could write 'The face predicts the brain'. During the third embryonic week, the prechordal mesoderm normally migrates forwards into the area anterior to the notochord, induces the morphogenesis of the forebrain, and initiates the formation of various buds. These structures are therefore linked in their morphogenesis. Depending on the time of its occurrence, there will be failure of formation or of fusion of these facial buds. Cyclopia and agnathia are the major forms. Frontonasal dysplasia is considered by Roubicek, Spranger and Wende (1981) to be an expression of holoprosencephaly. Fissures or clefts may be uni- or bilateral, isolated or multiple, and include hare lip with or without a cleft palate. Chromosomal aberrations are often associated with these features. The most common is trisomy 13-15 (Patau et al., 1960) followed by trisomy 18 (Butler et al., 1965; Robain and Gorce, 1972), deletion of 18, and ring 18 and triploidy. Holoprosencephaly has also been described with significant frequency in infants of diabetic mothers (Dekaban, 1959). Since, however, there is a large spectrum of malformations in this group, it would be hazardous to ascribe them to a single cause.

Various anomalies of other organs are common in this setting, but their severity does not necessarily correlate with the severity of the cerebral malformations. Hydramnios and intrauterine growth retardation are frequent.

The diagnosis of holotelencephaly can be made *in utero* by ultrasonography (Blackwell et al., 1982). Postnatally either CT scan or ultrasound gives a well-defined image of the malformation. In all cases the prognosis is poor.

Anomalies of cell migration

Anomalies or defects of neuronal migration are manifest in a variety of ways, depending on whether there is complete failure of migration, arrest of migration leading to an ectopic position of neurons, or a simple malorientation of neurons.

Mechanisms and pathogenesis are poorly understood but an important role may be played by the glia in the regulation of neuronal migration.

Ectopias and heterotopias

Arrest or curtailment is much more common than complete failure of migration and affects both cerebrum and cerebellum. The localization of ectopias varies from case to case according to when the failure of migration occurs.

In the cerebrum cases of ectopia or heterotopia with total absence of the cortical ribbon are not known. It may therefore be assumed that the first wave of migration at 8-10 weeks takes place normally, whereas the second wave between weeks 10 and 16 is probably disturbed. In the cerebrum, ectopic neurons form irregular nodules (Fig 10.20) at varying distances from the ventricles, or concentric striae in the white matter, or radial columns which mimic normal neuronal migration. The nature of the cells in these periventricular nodules may be difficult to identify in the neonate and the distinction from

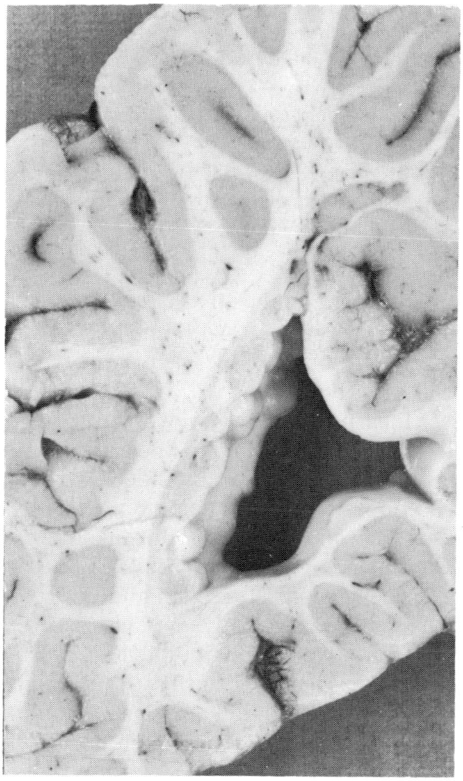

Fig. 10.20 Subependymal nodules of ectopic grey matter lie deep to the central white matter, having remained in the position of the original matrix layer. Note the characteristic bossed appearance of the ventricular wall.

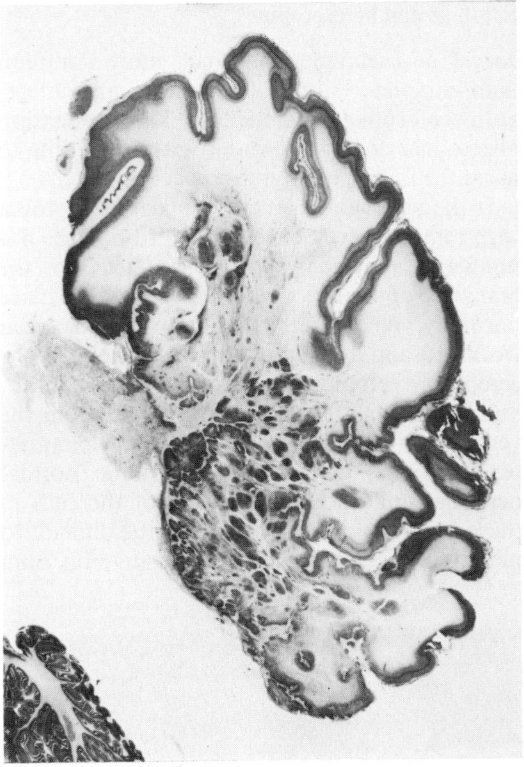

Fig. 10.21 Irregularly shaped masses of neurons lie in the white matter. The gyral pattern of the overlying cortex is also abnormal. Cresyl violet.

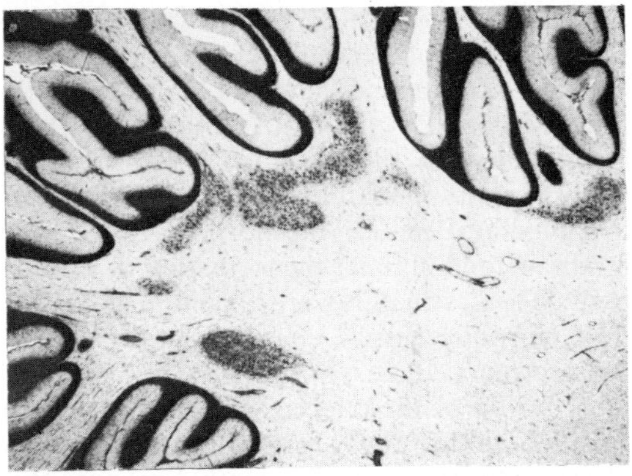

Fig. 10.22 Heterotopic islands of nerve cells in the cerebellar white matter in a case of cerebral pachygyria. Carbol azure.

tuberous sclerosis is difficult. In older patients pneumoencephalography has been used to demonstrate heterotopic nodules deforming the lateral ventricles (Bergeron 1969; Mueller, 1970). Whatever their position or number, ectopic cells (Fig 10.21) are usually found in association with other anomalies of cerebral organogenesis such as microcephaly, microgyria, agyria and pachygyria, the cerebrohepatorenal syndrome of Zellweger or other complex malformations. In an unusual and unclassified case with multiple cerebral clefts, there was a totally anarchic distribution of neurons associated with polymicrogyria.

Isolated ectopic mature neurons, in either subcortical or deep white matter, are fairly common features in the neonatal brain. They should probably not be considered as malformations, although it is not known if these cells are only temporarily arrested or what their ultimate fate would be.

Another minor abnormality consists of malposition or malorientation of neurons in the cortex or subcortical white matter. This subtle anomaly is not easily seen with routine neurohistological stains but is more readily demonstrable in Golgi preparations. Their significance is not known.

Heterotopias and ectopic neurons occur more frequently in the cerebellum (Fig. 10.22) than in the cerebrum, and have been recognized for many years (Pfleger, 1880). Medulloblastoma (a midline cerebellar tumour in children) has been thought to originate in heterotopias in the posterior medullary velum (Stevenson and Echlin, 1934). Brzustowicz and Kernohan (1952) correlated the sites of cerebellar gliomas with the sites of ectopic neurons (cell rests). More recently, cerebellar heterotopias have been described in various chromosomal aberrations such as trisomy D (13–15) (Atkins and Rosenthal, 1961; Miller et al, 1963; Snodgrass et al., 1966) and trisomy 17–18 (Norman, 1966; Terplan, Sandberg and Aceto, 1966; Sumi, 1970).

Three types of neurons are found in cerebellar ectopias—small granule cells, spindle cells and mature neurons. They usually occur in clusters of homogeneous or heterogeneous (mixed cell type) components. Each type of ectopic neuron tends to occur with a predilection for a specific site. The small granule cells are found mainly in the axes of the folia in the form of long striae of cells, or in groups often around vessels. The spindle cells are found almost anywhere, often around vessels, in the dentate and roof nuclei, in the nodulus and flocculus and in the cochlear nuclei and often coexistent with granule cells. It is difficult to decide whether or not they represent the same type of cell but in different planes. Their shape may be like that of the external granular layer cells which become elongated when migrating. The large mature neurons are usually located in the deep white mater where they form compact masses surrounded by a ring of granule cells. Foci of mixed cells are found mainly in the flocculus and nodulus.

Studies of large series of cerebellar heterotopias (Rorke, Fogelson and Riggs, 1968; Larroche, 1969, 1977a) have demonstrated the frequency of cerebellar dysplasia in otherwise normal fetuses and neonates. Small clusters of mature neurons, granule or spindle cells may be seen scattered in the folia or in the white matter. However, large nodules of mixed cells are always associated with other brain malformations and, to a lesser degree, with visceral malformations.

Teratogenic agents such as x-irradiation (Altman, Anderson and Wright, 1969; Phemister, Shively and Young, 1969a,b) viral infections (Kilham and Margolis, 1964) and drugs (Nathanson, Cole and Van der Loos, 1969) can induce cerebellar ectopias in laboratory animals. In the human fetus abnormal neuronal migration was recently reported in maternal methylmercury poisoning (Choi et al., 1978).

Cerebellar cortical dysplasia is often associated with polymicrogyria. The normal sequence of fetal cerebellar cortical development is well established (Larroche, 1962). In the full-term newborn, the cerebellar cortex is still composed of four layers—external granular, molecular, Purkinje cell and internal granular layers. The postmitotic neurons of the external granular layer migrate inwards to form the internal granular layer, along the radially disposed Bergmann glial fibres (Rakic, 1971). This process is protracted over a long period of time *in utero* and after birth. It is not known when the disturbances of migration occur. The disordered distribution of granule and Purkinje cells observed in young fetuses suggests an early disorganization of cell migration but focal vascular impairment occurring later cannot be ruled out. A minor anomaly of the cerebellum consists of a proliferation of the external granule cells which tend to form a bridge between adjacent folia (Fig. 10.23).

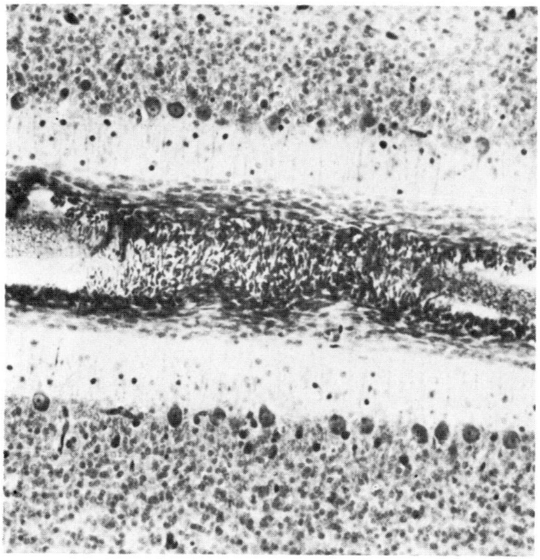

Fig. 10.23 Section of neonatal cerebellar cortex showing cells of the external granular layer forming a bridge between adjacent folia.

Other structures, in particular the inferior olivary nuclei, may be found in an ectopic position, an anomaly usually associated with agyria.

Agyria (lissencephaly) and pachygyria

These terms are used to describe an abnormal surface configuration of the brain, either a total absence of gyri (agyria or lissencephaly) (Fig. 10.24) or, more frequently, a few broad malformed gyri (pachygyria) varying in site and number (Fig. 10.25). Since the classic description by Bielschowsky (1923) many cases have been reported in the literature, among them the well-documented cases of Greenfield and Wolfsohn

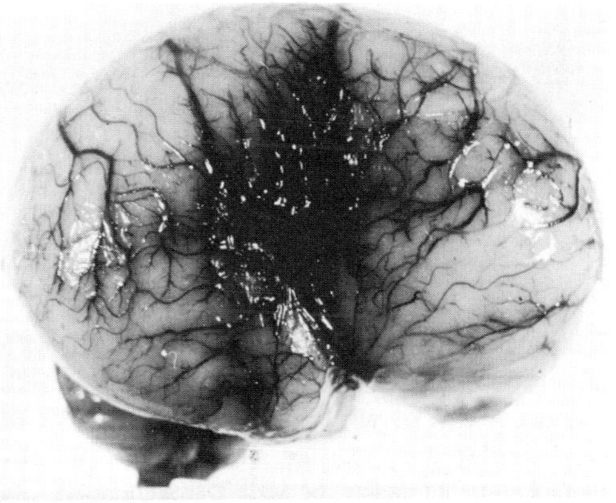

Fig. 10.24 Lateral surface of a neonatal brain showing a smooth surface in which there is a complete absence of gyri. There is a shallow sylvian fissure and a small temporal lobe.

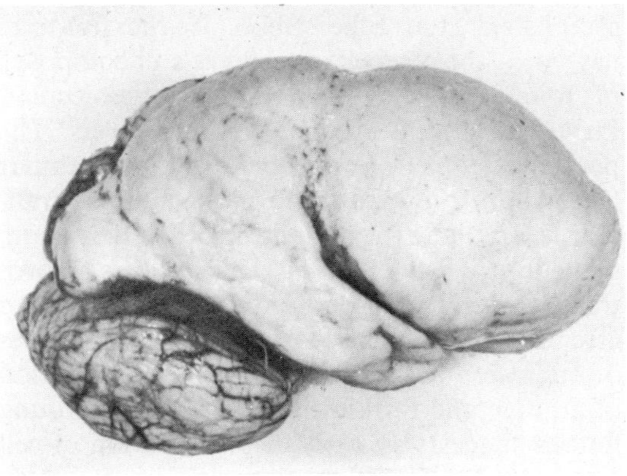

Fig. 10.25 Agyria and pachygyria.

(1935), de Lange (1939) Walker (1942) and Crome (1956). The brain is usually smaller than normal, the primary rolandic and sylvian fissures are poorly defined, whilst temporal and hippocampal gyri are often well preserved (Daube and Chou, 1966). The falx cerebri is either short or absent. The ventricles may be enlarged, and nodules of heterotopic grey matter bulge beneath the ependyma (Fig. 10.26).

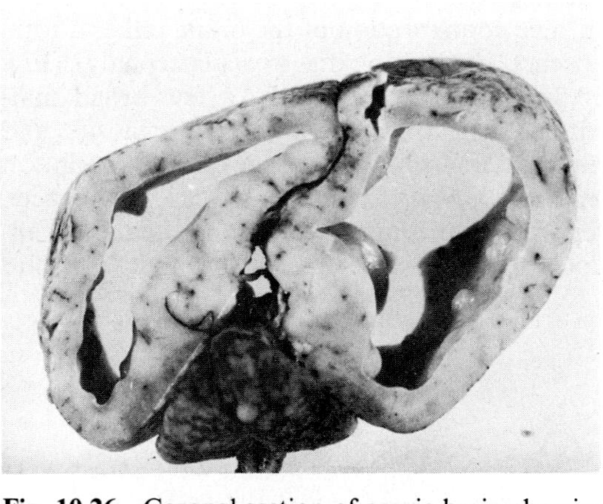

Fig. 10.26 Coronal section of agyric brain showing enlarged ventricles and nodules of heterotopic grey matter beneath the ependyma.

Histologically (Fig. 10.27), four layers are seen in the cerebral mantle—a molecular layer, a thick grey zone, a rim of white matter and a layer of periventricular grey matter. In the neonate the subpial granular layer is still present and the molecular layer may be very cellular. There is no identifiable horizontal stratification, and a clear unmyelinated zone separates the 'cortical plate' from the deeper concentric layers or columns of neurons which have not accomplished their migration. Jellinger and Rett (1976) attempted to identify the classic cortical layers by the size and shape of the cells. The deep periventricular white matter is much reduced with interspersed heterotopic nodules (Fig. 10.28). The claustrum and

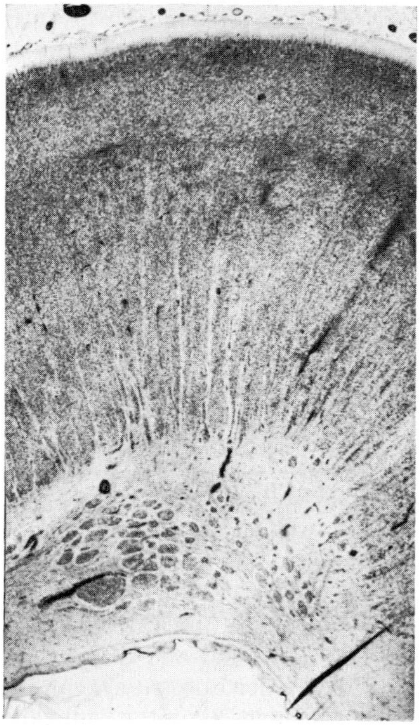

Fig. 10.27 Section through the wall of the hemisphere of an agyric brain, showing the great depth of grey matter. There are numerous heterotopias near the ventricular wall. Carbol azure.

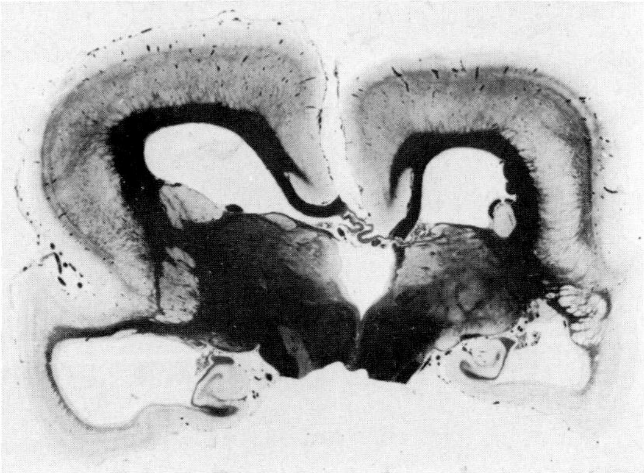

Fig. 10.28 Section through both hemispheres of an agyric brain to show the relative proportions of grey and white matter and the well-developed thalami and Ammon's horns. Heidenhain's myelin method.

capsula extrema are absent but the striatum and thalamus show only minor changes.

The corticobulbar and corticospinal tracts are hypoplastic, and the inferior olives incomplete or malformed. In the cerebellum there are often numerous heterotopic foci. Defective formation of the corpus callosum, a structure which is developing by week 12 of gestation may be of some interest in dating the onset of the cortical malformation (Josephy, 1944; Jellinger and Rett, 1976). Turricephaly and spina bifida have also been described in familial cases of lissencephaly (Alberca-Serrano and Reznik, 1964).

Visceral abnormalities, such as heart malformation, renal agenesis or polycystic kidneys, and minor skeletal deformities have been observed with agyria or pachygyria.

The *pathogenesis* is not known. In one group (walker's type), arrested or abnormal neuronal migration seems to be the end-result of some pathological process that may begin as early as the eighth gestational week, when the first young neurons start migrating, and may continue for many weeks since cells are arrested at various distances from their proper destination. Agyria coexisting with pachygyria in the same brain suggests a different timing or a gradient of severity of the pathogenesis in different regions of the brain within the limit of the programmed cell migration—i.e. between 8 and 16 weeks. In one of the writer's cases, calcifications were found in the midline structures, suggesting some pathology during early fetal life. A hypothesis proposed by Stewart, Richman and Caviness (1975) is that the late migrating neurons destined to become the superficial cortical layer (II and IV) are arrested by a deep cortical and subcortical laminar necrosis at about the fourth fetal month. Neurons destined for layer II and IV either do not migrate or degenerate. In certain cases the topography of the abnormal cortex suggests a hypoxic-ischaemic aetiology with a proximodistal vascular pattern of pathology.

In a second group (Miller-Dieker type) the extent and the severity of the lesions and the massive periventricular nodular heterotopias can hardly be explained by vascular impairment during the late migratory period. Norman et al. (1962) reported a case of pachygyria occurring in the setting of sudanophil leucodystrophy, and a familial occurrence (Miller 1963; Dieker et al., 1969; Garcia, Dunn and Trevor, 1978; Barth et al., 1982) and parental consanguinity (Norman et al., 1976) suggest an autosomal recessive inheritance. The malformation was classified as such by McKusick (1971). Clinical features consist of microcephaly with frequent minor facial anomalies, hypotonia with seizures or a decerebrate state and arrest of psychomotor development (Druckman, Chao and Alvord, 1959).

Polymicrogyria

The term 'microgyria' was introduced by Bielschowsky in 1916 to describe certain gross and microscopical abnormalities of the cerebral cortex. Bresler (1899) had already differentiated this malformation from ulegyria, a sequela of perinatal hypoxic-ischaemic damage. There is, in polymicrogyria, an increased number of gyri (Fig. 10.29), some of which may be very small,

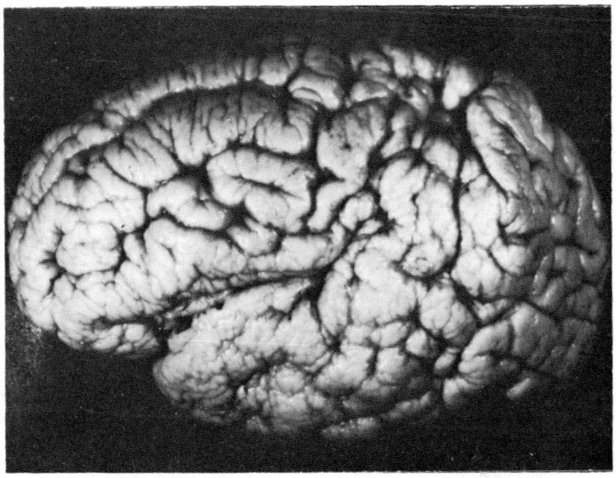

Fig. 10.29 Polymicrogyria affecting most of the cortex but particularly marked in the temporal lobe. The surface of the broad gyri is finely and irregularly bossed or wrinkled, giving it a 'chestnut' appearance.

separated by shallow sulci, and without the normal spatial arrangement, an appearance which was compared to a cauliflower by Bielschowsky (1916). However, polymicrogyria is most often a histological finding (internal microgyria), the abnormal cortical plate being covered by a normal or even a pachygyric surface (Fig. 10.30).

The *cerebral polymicrogyric cortex* is composed of four layers (Fig. 10.31) (Ranke, 1910; Bielschowsky, 1916; Crome, 1952). The first or superficial molecular layer is sparsely cellular and may contain randomly distributed neurons. The boundary between the first and second layer is often ill-defined. The second or outer dense

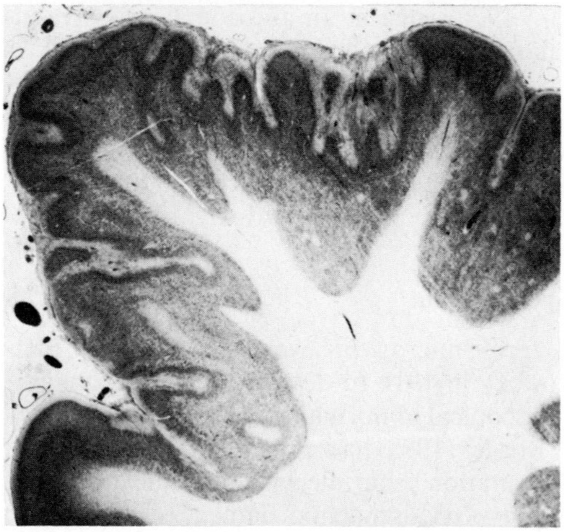

(a)

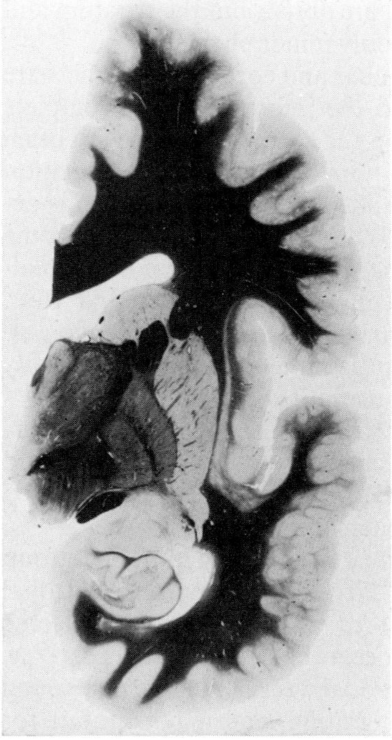

(b)

Fig. 10.30 (**a**) Section of polymicrogyric cortex. Miniature convolutions are found below the surface but are not demarcated externally by sulci. Carbol azure. (**b**) Coronal section of hemisphere shown in (**a**) stained to demonstrate myelin. Note the polymicrogyria in the temporal lobe which has an unfissured pachygyric surface. Kultschitsky–Pal method.

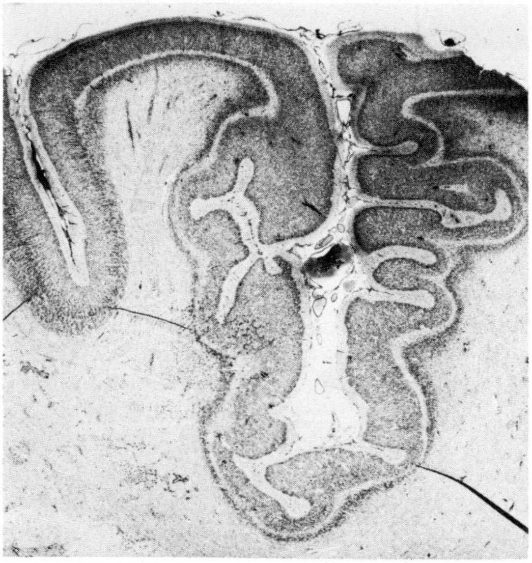

Fig. 10.31 The four-layered type of polymicrogyric cortex. Carbol azure.

layer is irregular, forming a garland-like structure with projections into the molecular layer. Neurons are small, fusiform or pyramidal, and are sometimes orientated tangentially to the surface. The third or sparsely cellular layer of Ranke (1910) is irregular and follows the convoluted pattern of the second layer. In older infants it contains a horizontal plexus of myelinated fibres. The fourth layer consists of round or fusiform cells with an even or patchy distribution, which Bielschowsky (1916) considered to correspond to ectopic neurons, arrested in their migration. This four-layered pattern may, however, not be clearly visible, and the chaotic arrangement of the cells prevents any attempt at classification. The cortex may be deeply indented so that two molecular layers become juxtaposed with a vessel forming the axis of each abnormal sulcus. Distinction between nodules of ectopic cells and infolding of layer II is therefore difficult. Abnormal tangential or fan-like myelinated fibres may be seen in the molecular layer. The polymicrogyric cortex may cover the entire surface of the hemispheres or may occur in limited areas. The transition from normal to malformed cortex is usually abrupt. However, as the malformed cortex is approached, layer II may become irregular though still within a normal six-layered cortex. Over the microgyric cortex, the meninges are thickened and in places interrupted by bundles of fibroblasts (Bertrand and Gruner, 1955). Arteries are numerous and often penetrate the cortex obliquely. The veins are dilated, forming an angiomatous meshwork within the leptomeninges.

The pathogenesis and time of occurrence of polymicrogyria are still debated. A disturbance of cell migration in terms of timing and spatial arrangement or a postmigratory selective destruction of specific layers are possible mechanisms. The authoritative studies of Bielschowsky were based on the old concept of development of the cortical plate in which it was thought that the superficial layers were formed by neurons which migrated first, the deeper layers being formed by late-migrating neurons. Thus Bielschowsky (1916) considered the fourth layer, which failed to reach the cortex, as an ectopic deep cortical layer, with the sparsely cellular third layer containing a myelinated fibre plexus corresponding to the subcortical U-fibres. It is now known, from experimental work, that the sequence of normal migration is the reverse—i.e. the deep layers are formed first, the superficial ones later. Nevertheless, the association of large heterotopic nodules in both cerebrum and cerebellum with polymicrogyria and the presence of polymicrogyria in the lips of the clefts in schizencephaly suggest an early impairment of cell migration. In Norman's case (1980) of bilateral symmetrical encephaloclastic lesions with polymicrogyria the history and morphology suggest that there was a defect of cell migration before the third and fourth fetal month. Furthermore, polymicrogyria and pachygyria, which have been described in Zellweger's cerebrohepatorenal syndrome (Volpe and Adams, 1972), might be a primary disorder of neuronal migration.

The second hypothesis, suggesting a postmigratory deleterious effect on the cortical lamination, probably of hypoxic-ischaemic origin (Jakob, 1940; Smith and Linell, 1959; Dekaban, 1965; De León, 1972), was developed and extended by Richman, Stewart and Caviness (1974) who mapped the cortex in cases of agyria and pachygyria and demonstrated a homology between layers in abnormal and normal cortices. Layers II and IV are missing in agyria and sparsely cellular in pachygyria. The poorly cellular layer may represent a laminar necrosis, secondary to hypoxia or ischaemia. In their case the developmental disturbance was dated at about 20–24 weeks—i.e. at a postmigratory period. Animal experiments give some support to this hypothesis. Partial necrosis of layers IV and VI by contact-freezing in newborn rats (Dvorak and Feit, 1977) stops neuroblasts destined for layers I, II and III and reproduces the four-layered cortex observed in human pathology. The presence of calcium deposits and gliosis in some malformed brains also suggests an ischaemic pathogenesis. In addition, polymicrogyria is almost always present in porencephaly. In this connection it is worth noting that polymicrogyria has been described in cases of maternal carbon monoxide exposure (Hallervorden, 1949; Bankl and Jellinger, 1967). Furthermore, micropolygyria has been reported in a great variety of intrauterine infections such as cytomegalovirus (Diezel, 1954; Marie et al., 1957; Crome and France, 1959; Bignami and Appicciutoli, 1964; Friede and Mikolasek, 1978), toxoplasmosis (De León, 1972) and syphilis (Lyon, 1972, personal communication). The mechanism is not known but probably involves neuronal necrosis as in the case of vascular impairment. The time of maternofetal infection is not known and it is still undecided as to whether damage to the matrix cells and/or glial fibres impairs cortical plate formation, or whether there is damage to the already formed cortical plate so that late migrating neurons are unable to pass through to reach their superficial destination.

In *cerebellar polymicrogyria* (Figs. 10.32 and 10.33), also called cerebellar cortical dysplasia (Larroche, 1977b), the folia fail to develop normally but this is rarely recognizable on gross examination (Urich, 1977). Microscopical studies reveal a disordered distribution of granule cells and Purkinje cells within an ill-defined molecular layer. In the neonate, the external granular layer which normally still forms the outermost limit of the folia is often disrupted or irregular (Fig. 10.33). The term 'polymicrogyria' is not really appropriate unless folium is equated with gyrus. Cerebellar microgyria is often

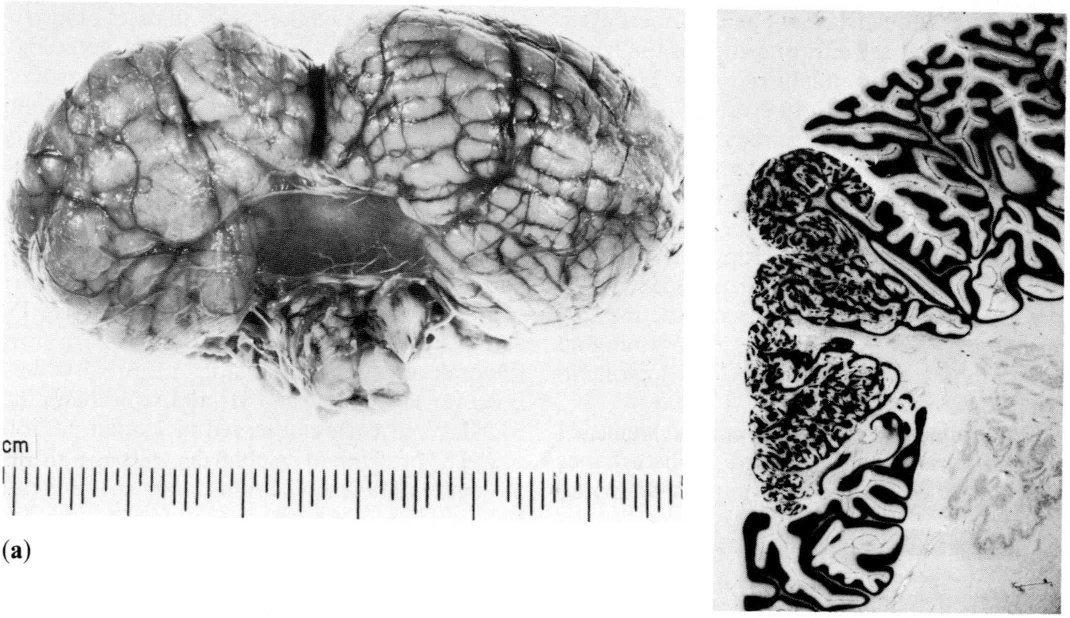

(a)

(b)

Fig. 10.32 (**a**) Cerebellar pachygyria ('microgyria'). The gyri of one hemisphere appear broad and irregularly flat, replacing the normal pattern of lobules and folia. (**b**) Section of cerebellum showing microgyria. In the cortex the granule and Purkinje cells are irregularly distributed in the molecular layer.

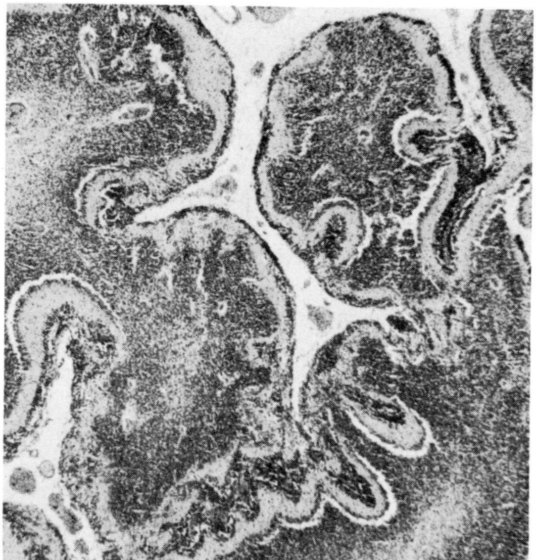

Fig. 10.33 Section of neonatal microgyric cerebellum. The external granular layer is irregularly thickened or interrupted.

associated with foci of ectopic neurons in the white matter of folia and central nuclei. The cause and mechanism of the impairment in cell migration are poorly understood.

Cerebellar polymicrogyria is a rare anomaly. It is associated with cerebral malformations such as holoprosencephaly in 6.6 per cent of cases, and with severe visceral malformations in 10 per cent of cases. It has also been described with cerebral polymicrogyria in a case of cytomegalovirus infection (Bignami and Appicciutoli, 1964).

Status verrucosus This anomaly is extremely rare and has never been described in the neonate. Successively called 'status corticis verrucosus deformis' by Ranke (1905), 'status verrucosus' by Bertrand and Gruner (1955), 'état verruqueux' by van Bogaert and Ley (1929), 'warts' by Jakob (1940), 'dysgénésie nodulaire' by Morel and Wildi (1952) and 'verrucose dysplasia' by Grčević and Robert (1961), the deformity consists of superficial cortical nodules 1–5 mm in diameter, scattered over the surface of the hemispheres with a predilection for the frontal lobe. The overlying pia mater is often adherent to the nodule.

Histological examination shows that the second and third layers herniate through the molecular layer, which is often thin or absent. The nodule consists of neurons of varying size, grouped in a homogeneous fashion or disposed around an axis composed of radial myelinated fibres. At times a blood vessel lies in the centre of the bundle. The nodules may be found in an otherwise normal cortex, but are more often associated with polymicrogyria, for which they may be mistaken, or with other malformations (Bertrand and Gruner, 1955; Crome, 1969).

The pathogenesis of the deformity is not clear, but the associated vascular pattern suggests a close relationship between vascular and tissue dysplasia.

Status pseudoverrucosus or status verrucosus simplex (Retzius, 1895) may be either a transient stage of development or, more likely, an artefact (Streeter, 1912) caused by fixing fetal brains in a gauze bag which leaves its imprint on the surface of the brain. Another artefact is caused by leptomeninges being focally peeled off fetal brains before fixation, and appears as a fine shrinkage of the surface of the brain, mimicking status verrucosus or polymicrogyria. The underlying cortex is normal. Another type of anomaly is found, on microscopic examination only, in the brains of some fetuses of about 20 weeks. The second layer of the cortex forms irregular protrusions into the molecular layer, the external surface remaining smooth. It might be a transient stage of migration or a true malformation or precursor of polymicrogyria.

Schizencephalies

Yakovlev and Wadsworth (1946a, b) and Yakovlev (1959b) made the distinction between encephaloclastic porencephalies and schizencephalies. The former result from destruction of cerebral tissue, the latter from 'failure of development of the cerebral mantle in the zones of cleavage of the primary cerebral fissures'. The schizencephalies are usually bilateral and symmetrical. These abnormalities are rare, the most used nomenclature being that of Yakovlev and Wadsworth (1946a, b), who described several forms of congenital cleft. The first consists of a cleft with fused lips involving the entire thickness of the cerebral wall (Fig. 10.34) without com-

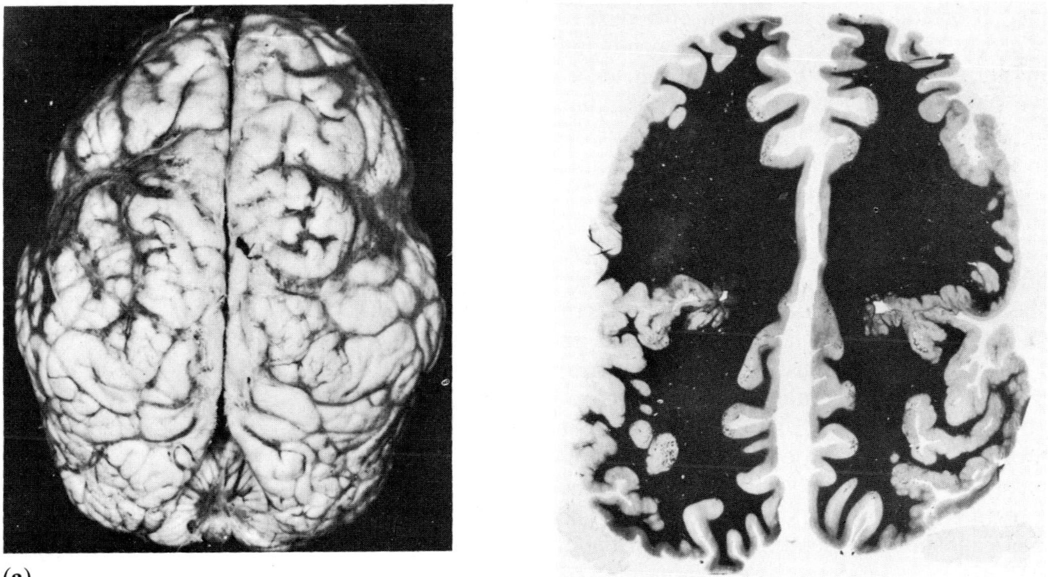

(a)

(b)

Fig. 10.34 Schizencephaly. (**a**) Bilateral symmetrical clefts with fused lips indenting the region of the central fissures are visible on the surfaces of the hemispheres. (**b**) Section stained for myelin. The clefts extend deeply into the brain and are bordered by small malformed gyri. Loyez method. (From Yakovlev and Wadsworth, 1946a. Reproduced by permission of the Editor, *Journal of Neuropathology and Experimental Neurology*.)

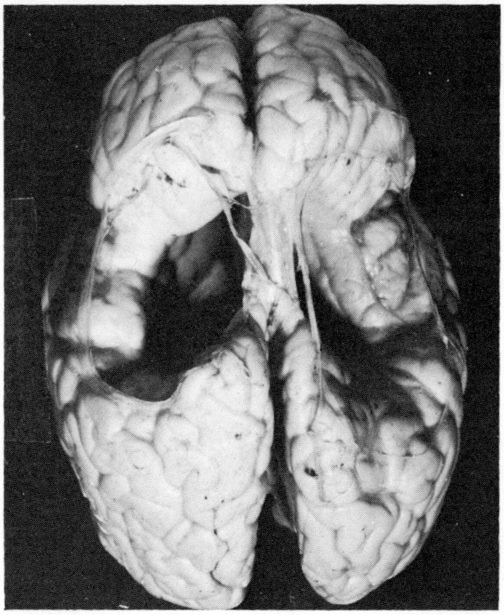

Fig. 10.35 Schizencephaly with separated lips. Symmetrical clefts extend down to the lateral ventricles (From Yakovlev, 1959a. Reproduced by permission of the Editor, *Journal of Neuropathology and Experimental Neurology*.)

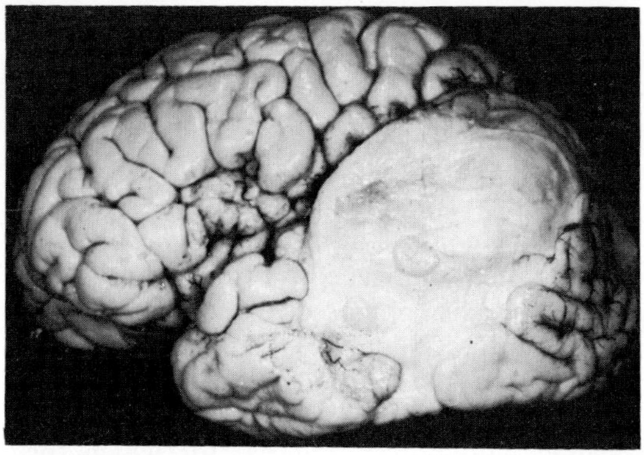

Fig. 10.36 Prenatal 'porencephaly'. A thin membrane, in which there are islands of neural tissue, forms the wall of the enlarged lateral ventricle. There is an area of microgyria in the upper bank of the sylvian fissure. The condition was bilateral.

munication between the subarachnoid space and ventricle. The cleft lies in the region of the central or medial orbital fissures. In the deeper part of the furrow the presence of a 'pia-ependymal seam' appears to be the hallmark of schizencephaly. In this group there is no hydrocephalus. The convolutions bordering the clefts are malformed and microgyric. Elsewhere, areas of normal cortex alternate with microgyria or pachygyria and heterotopias are present in the centrum semiovale. The other structures of the brain are normal.

The second form of schizencephaly consists of clefts with hydrocephalus and lips separated. In one case there was extensive and symmetrical agenesis of the entire mantle, anterior and dorsal to the sylvian fissure, a thin transparent membrane forming the roof of the symmetrical hemispheric defects. The sagittal sinus and the falx cerebri were present only posteriorly. The corpus callosum and septum pellucidum were absent and the lateral ventricles communicated widely. Descending cortical fibres were absent at all levels. In other cases there were symmetrical defects in the region of the central fissure (Fig. 10.35), roofed by a transparent membrane, and severe hydrocephalus. Convolutions bordering the defects showed microgyria (Fig. 10.36), and heterotopias were found elsewhere. The characteristic fusion between the cystic defect and the lateral ventricle was also found and there was no trace of the bulbar pyramids. Similar cases have been described under different names such as 'basket-brain' (Cohn and Neumann, 1946), porencephaly (Feld and Gruner, 1957; Friede, 1975), hydranencephaly or hydrenencephaly (Norman, Urich and Woods, 1958) or cerebral defects (Dekaban, 1965) and porencephaly with microgyria (Levine, Fisher and Caviness, 1974). Norman (1980) has suggested that the features

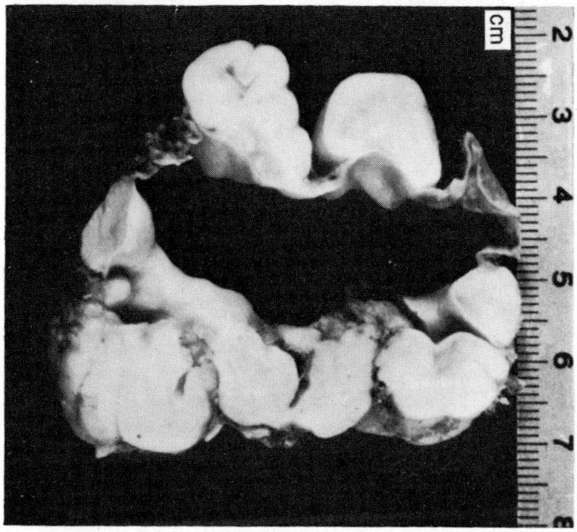

Fig. 10.37 Coronal section of a neonatal brain, showing bilateral symmetrical defects covered by thin membranes. (Courtesy of Dr. D. Gaillard.)

described as bilateral encephaloclastic lesions in a young fetus could have resulted in the appearance of schizencephaly had survival been longer. In one of the writer's cases with bilateral symmetrical defects and hydrocephalus (Fig. 10.37), numerous calcium deposits were scattered in the malformed cortex around the cleft.

The origin of these malformations is not clear. Yakovlev and Wadsworth (1946a, b) considered schizencephalies to be anomalies of the 'fundamental plan of structural organization of the brain'. The tendency now is to implicate a failure of blood supply to the cerebral mantle during early fetal development at a critical period of neuronal migration.

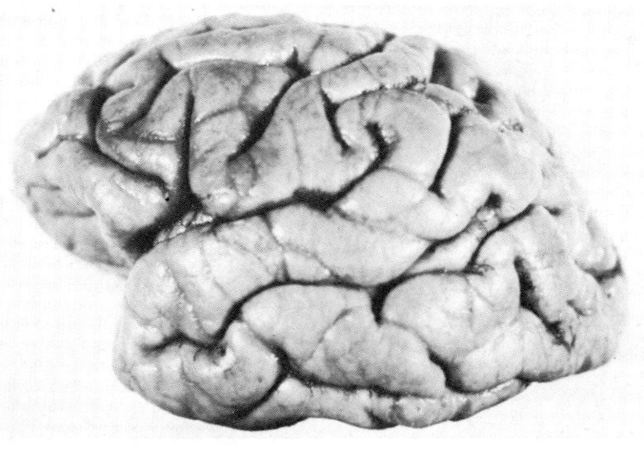

Fig. 10.38 Familial microcephaly. Note the simple convolutional pattern formed by the relatively broad gyri.

Microcephaly

Etymologically, 'microcephaly' means a small head. To describe a small brain, the term 'micrencephaly' would be more appropriate. However, because brain and skull usually grow in parallel the term 'microcephaly' is generally used to indicate smallness of the brain occurring usually as a malformation. Data on the normal range of head circumference from birth to adulthood were published by Eichorn and Bayley (1962) and Nellhaus (1968), and intrauterine growth curves were established by Lubchenco et al. (1963). The weight of the fresh brain can be used as a measure of fetal development (Potter, 1953; Gruenwald and Minh, 1960; Larroche and Maunoury, 1973). With ultrasonography the size of the fetal head can be assessed accurately *in utero* from the biparietal diameter. Figures of 2 or more standard deviations below the mean are abnormal.

'Microcephaly' is a descriptive term and does not refer to a particular aetiology; classification is therefore difficult. Böök, Schut and Reed (1953) proposed two types, one due to non-genetic disease and the other inherited. Warkany and Dignan (1973) proposed three types, one due to gene mutation, the second to chromosomal changes and the third to environmental influences. Ross and Frias (1977) proposed two large groups—with or without associated malformations. Microcephaly with associated malformations includes genetic disorders (chromosomal aberrations and single gene defects), environmental causes and cases of unknown aetiology. Familial cases (Robain and Lyon, 1972) show severe cortical anomalies (Fig. 10.38). Microcephaly without associated malformations includes primary microcephaly of proven or doubtful genetic transmission due to inborn errors of metabolism or due to environmental factors, and those of unknown aetiology. In the neonatal period, microcephaly without associated malformations should arouse the suspicion of intrauterine infection (Remington and Klein, 1976). The central nervous system of the fetus is particularly vulnerable to rubella virus, cytomegalovirus and herpesvirus. The mechanism of action of the viruses is poorly understood but the destruction of immature neurons and glial cells during mitosis or migration might explain the underdevelopment of the brain. Toxoplasmosis is known to be commonly associated with hydrocephalus due to occlusion of the aqueduct of Sylvius. However, some infants with inapparent congenital toxoplasmosis at birth may later develop microcephaly. Herpesvirus contamination occurs usually during birth, and microcephaly may develop after birth if the infection is not rapidly fatal.

Microcephaly may be associated with intrauterine growth retardation (Larroche and Maunoury, 1973; Larroche, 1977a), a condition which occurs in heterogeneous pathological conditions such as malformation (visceral and/or cerebral) and infections, multiple pregnancy, and placental insufficiency with maternal toxaemia or renal diseases. Hypotrophic infants usually have a large brain in relation to body weight and within normal limits for gestational age. However, in only very few cases of a large series of infants showing retarded intrauterine growth was the brain weight 2 s.d. below the mean—i.e. microcephalic by definition. The external configuration of the brain corresponds to gestational age, and cytoarchitecture and myelination are not significantly modified in the neonatal period. Placental deficiency, which develops usually during the second half of pregnancy, probably does not affect the number of neurons but may possibly damage glial cells and impair subsequent myelination, which could play a part in pathogenesis of so-called minimal brain damage. Dobbing and Sands (1971) have emphasized the vulnerability of the fetal brain at certain periods of its development, and it is possible that microcephaly may be induced by undernutrition.

In multiple pregnancies fetal brain growth may be more retarded than body weight (Hofman, 1983). This may be very pronounced in cases of monochorionic placenta with the so-called transfusion syndrome.

Megalencephaly

Fletcher (1900) defined megalencephaly as a 'proportionate enlargement of the whole brain, associated with the presence of a variable mental or nervous aberration'. Today the accepted definition is a brain weight 2.5 standard deviations above the mean for the age and sex. Various descriptive terms have been used, such as cerebral gigantism and macrocephaly. Megalencephaly includes a variety of clinical and pathological conditions and no classification is entirely satisfactory (Dennis, Rosenberg and Alvord, 1961; Norman, 1963; Fontan and Battin, 1965).

Dekaban and Sakuragawa (1977) subdivided the megalencephalies into three main categories and various subgroups, based on their own and previously reported cases. *Primary megalencephaly* may be an isolated finding or associated with achondroplasia and endocrine disorders, or it may be familial. Males are affected twice as often as females, and in the majority of patients the large head is noticed within the first year of life. In about 25 per cent of the cases reviewed by Dekaban and Sakuragawa there was no obvious abnormality of the brain other than its size. In the remaining cases half showed some cytoarchitectonic or neuronal abnormalities, and half severe macroscopically visible malformations (Fig. 10.39). Mental retardation and neurological disorders of some sort were present in the majority of patients. *Secondary megalencephaly* is associated with genetic disorders, such as the sphingolipidoses, mucopolysaccharidoses and amaurotic idiocy, and with various leucodystrophies (including Alexander's disease) and neurocutaneous syndromes. Megalencephaly may be present at birth or may become manifest during the early postnatal years. The *third group* includes unilateral megalencephaly which may

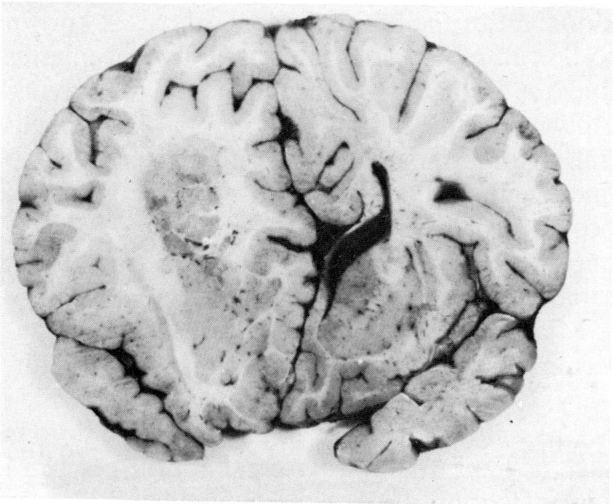

(a)

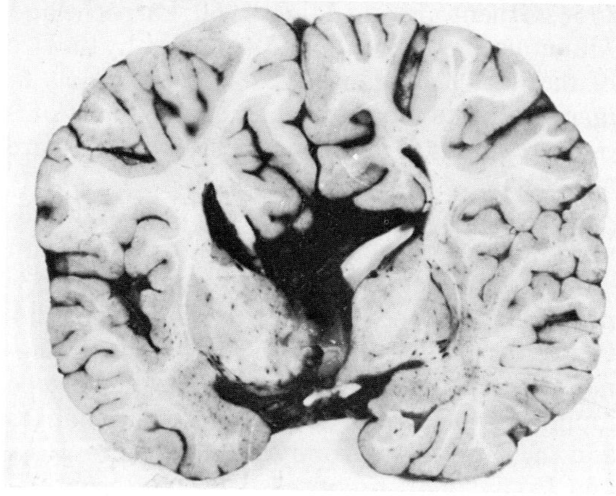

(b)

Fig. 10.39 Megalencephaly with multiple cerebral anomalies, including absence of the corpus callosum and an abnormal gyral pattern. From a child aged 3 years with total brain weight of 1554 g (cerebellum 186 g). **(a)** Coronal section showing large heterotopias in the white matter on the left and a longitudinal callosal bundle on the right. **(b)** At a more posterior level a malformed left thalamus and polygyria in the right temporal lobe are shown.

be associated with hypertrophy of one side of the body. Seizures and mental retardation have been reported. The brain shows both gross and microscopical abnormalities. A particular form of megalencephaly described as cerebral gigantism was reported by Sotos et al. (1964) and has been known since then as Sotos' syndrome. Evident at birth are large hands, feet and cranium with moderate prognathism, and advanced osseous maturation for the age. There have been sporadic as well as familial cases (Hansen and Friis, 1976).

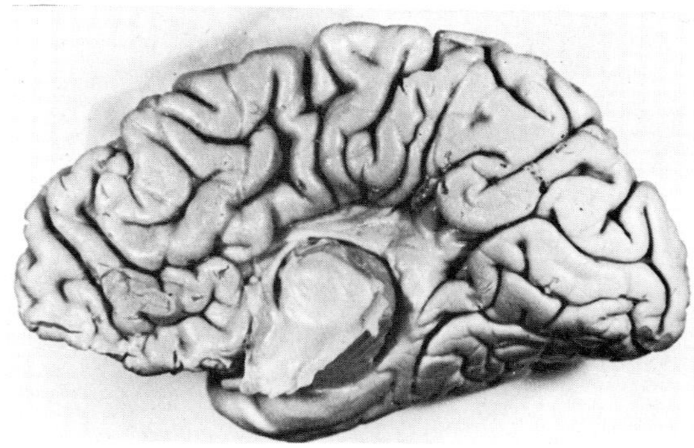

Fig. 10.40 Agenesis of the corpus callosum. Note the radiate pattern of gyri and sulci.

Commissures and midline structures

The corpus callosum develops within the commissural plate, a thickening of the lamina terminalis, which is a midline structure forming the most rostral part of the neural tube or future prosencephalon (Johnston, 1913; Hochstetter, 1929; Rakic and Yakovlev, 1968). In embryos of 6–8 weeks the commissural plate or lamina reuniens consists of a cellular area within which, a few weeks later, fibres will pass from one hemisphere to the other. By 13–14 weeks the rostral part of the corpus callosum is forming and this is progressively separated from the anterior commissure (which develops in the same commissural plate) by a midline cavity, the cavum septi pellucidi. The fornix and hippocampal commissures, which also originate in the commissural plate, follow the backward growth of the corpus callosum.

Agenesis of the corpus callosum

Agenesis of the corpus callosum may be part of complex malformations, such as holoprosencephaly with absence of the anterior commissure, or the Dandy–Walker syndrome. It may also be totally or partially absent or hypoplastic in an otherwise normal brain. Extensive descriptions of the defect have been made by de Morsier and Mozer (1935), Marburg (1949), Loeser and Alvord (1968a, b), Jellinger and Gross (1973), Field, Ashton and White (1978) among others. In partial agenesis, the posterior portion is generally missing. In total absence of the corpus callosum the medial hemispheric surface has an abnormal gyral pattern. The cingulum is poorly outlined and most of the gyri extend perpendicularly to the roof of the third ventricle (Fig. 10.40). The psalterium, normally beneath the splenium, is absent. A prominent bundle of fibres, myelinated at the time when the corpus callosum should be myelinated, the so-called Probst's bundle (1901), runs in the apex of the lateral ventricles or in the roof, near the interhemispheric fissure (Fig. 10.41). On coronal sections of the brain no structure seems to separate the lateral ventricles in the midline. The roof of the third ventricle is a membrane composed of pia-arachnoid and ependyma. It is often distended, bulging into the interhemispheric fissure and displacing the fornices laterally. The septum pellucidum is said to be absent. However, Loeser and Alvord (1968b) have demonstrated an analogous structure between Probst's bundle and the fornix.

Familial cases have been reported (Naiman and Frazer, 1955; Menkes, Philippart and Clark, 1964), as well as sporadic. No overt neurological signs were detected in one case of Field, Ashton and White (1978) whilst epilepsy, hydrocephalus or mental retardation were described by Grogono (1968). A syndrome, including agenesis of the corpus callosum, chorioretinopathy and infantile spasms, has occasionally been reported (Aicardi and Chevrie, 1969; Renier et al., 1973). In neonates total or partial agenesis may be an incidental finding.

The malformation was recognized on pneumoencephalograms by Davidoff and Dyke (1934) and by Penfield and Hyndman (1934), and the characteristic 'butterfly wing' shape of the ventricles was described (see Fig. 10.41a). Large series were subsequently published by Carpenter and Druckemiller (1953), Grogono (1968) and Probst (1973). The diagnosis is readily made in the neonate by ultrasound or CT scan.

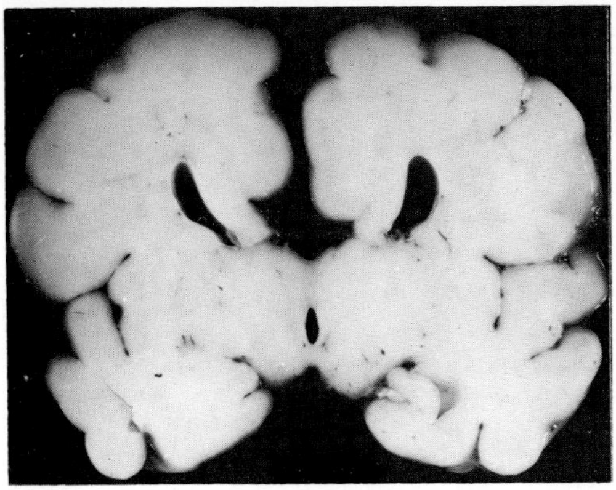

(a)

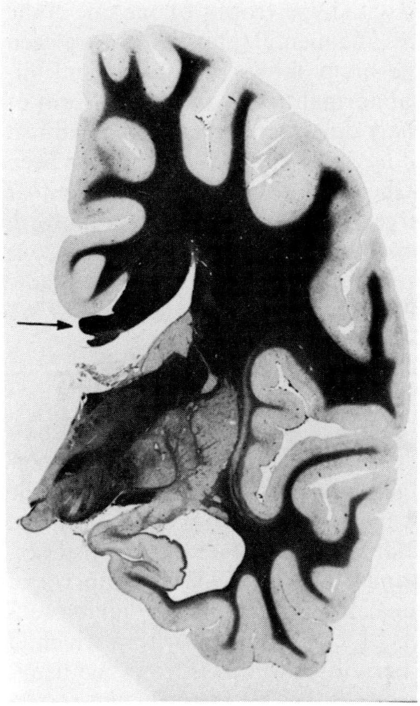

(b)

Fig. 10.41 (**a**) Coronal section of a neonatal brain, showing agenesis of the corpus callosum, bilateral prominent callosal bundles and the characteristic 'butterfly wing' shape of the lateral ventricles. (**b**) Coronal section of a hemisphere, showing the myelinated callosal bundle ('Probst's bundle'—arrow). Heidenhain's method for myelin.

Anomalies of the septum pellucidum

One leaf of the septum may be missing or the septum may be totally absent, with a normal corpus callosum indicating a relative independence of these two structures. Absence of the septum pellucidum may be the only abnormality in the brain (Dolgopol, 1938) or it may be part of a complex syndrome. Absence of the septum may be associated with uni- or bilateral porencephaly, microgyria and heterotopias (de Morsier, 1956; Gross and Hoff, 1959). Similar features were found in pneumoencephalograms by Zellweger and von Muralt (1952) and more recently in CT scan by Harwood-Nash and Fitz (1976) and Aicardi and Goutières (1981). The pathogenesis of this complex syndrome is still debated but it does not seem to be genetically determined. The clinical picture is usually very severe, and may include moderate or severe mental retardation, hemiplegia or tetraplegia, and defective vision or blindness.

Cavum septi pellucidi and cavum vergae Sometimes misnamed fifth and sixth ventricles (Dandy, 1931), these midline cavities are bounded above by the corpus callosum, and laterally by the two leaves of the septum pellucidum and the fornices. Anteriorly, the cavum septi pellucidi (Fig. 10.42) lies between the transverse fibres of the genu of the corpus callosum and the anterior commissure. As the corpus cal-

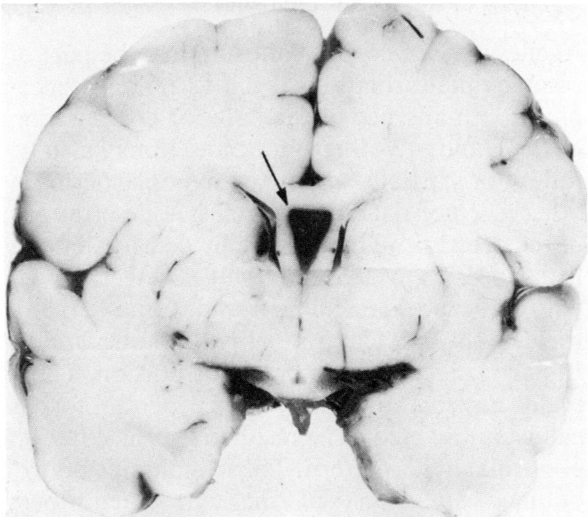

Fig. 10.42 Cavum septi pellucidi (arrow) in a coronal section of a neonatal brain.

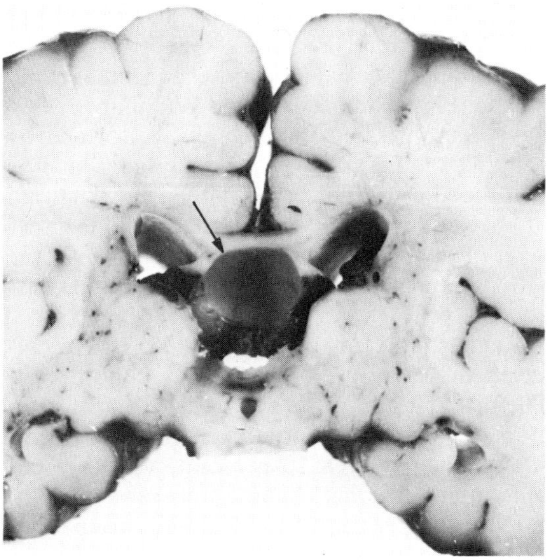

Fig. 10.43 Cavum vergae (arrow) in a neonatal brain.

losum develops caudally, the cavity stretches backward. Its posterior limit is ill-defined and there is considerable individual variation. At times it is prolonged posteriorly by another cavity, the cavum vergae (Fig. 10.43). In the neonate this often bulges below the splenium of the corpus callosum. Cavum septi pellucidi and the less common cavum vergae usually communicate freely but at times they may be separated by a bridge of cerebral tissue. The cavum septi pellucidi is constantly present in the human fetus but tends to become obliterated toward term (Larroche and Baudey, 1961; Shaw and Alvord, 1969). In adults the cavity is found in about 20 per cent of brains studied at autopsy (Schwidde, 1952). The cavum vergae has never been described alone.

The walls of the cavities are lined by neuroglial tissue without a definite epithelial structure. At times, large undifferentiated cells or macrophages are found in the walls or within the lumen. Under normal conditions, the cavity does not communicate with the lateral ventricles. In premature infants presenting with germinal layer and intraventricular haemorrhage, the veins of the septum are often overdistended and blood may be found in the cavum.

Cavum septi pellucidi and cavum vergae have been demonstrated *in utero* by ultrasound as early as 16 weeks (Plaix, 1983). In premature and full-term infants the midline cavities are readily detectable in CT scan and echography (Mack, Rumack and Johnson, 1980).

Cavum veli interpositi Although this structure is not a commissural formation but a leptomeningeal cistern of minor importance, it seems appropriate to describe it here because of its relationship with the cavum vergae. This cistern, well known when pneumoencephalograms were commonly utilized, is normally patent in premature infants and progressively seals off. Sandwiched between the floor of the cavum vergae above and the roof of the third ventricle below, it communicates posteriorly with the cistern of the great vein of Galen. On X-ray it is difficult to distinguish it from a cavum vergae (Larroche and Baudey, 1961). Occasionally, haemorrhage has been described in this area, collecting over the roof of the third ventricle and leading to obstructive hydrocephalus (Lourie and Berne, 1961).

Anomalies of the wall of the lateral ventricles

Adhesions between two facing ventricular walls have been described under various names such as coarctation (Davidoff, 1946) or coaptation (Bates and Netsky, 1955) of the walls, goniosynapses (Costoulas, 1958) or transventricular adhesions (Norman and McMenemey, 1955). The sites of adhesion are between caudate nucleus and corpus callosum or between opposing walls of the anterior horn of the lateral ventricle or, less often, of the occipital and temporal horns. The affected ventricle may be reduced in size and the contralateral cavity enlarged. Ventricular adhesions have been described in a large series of brains of demented patients by Morel and Wildi (1954) and by Costoulas (1958), and the diagnosis was made during life on pneumoencephalograms by Davidoff (1946). On microscopical examination the surface of the cavities may be lined with ependymal cells (Davidoff, 1946) and, in neonates, by a dense feltwork of glial fibres with tufts of germinal cells (Larroche, 1977a). The pathogenesis is obscure. In two children aged 9 months and 13 years respectively, presenting with transventricular adhesions, Norman and McMenemey (1955) described haemosiderin-laden macrophages on the ependymal wall and in the caudate nucleus, suggestive of birth injury with residual haemorrhage and scarring. Davidoff (1946) and Epstein (1953) considered that these anomalies probably represent developmental impairment, taking place between weeks 9 and 15 of gestation. The hypothesis of Bates and Netsky (1955) that overgrowth of the caudate nucleus leads to its adherence to the opposite ventricular wall is improbable, since other sites of adhesion have been described. The association of these apparently minor abnormalities with other brain malformations such as heterotopias, status verrucosus and micropolygyria and with neurological disorders suggests an early lesion possibly vascular in origin (Dambska et al., 1968).

Arachnoid cysts

Arachnoid cysts have been the subject of an abundant literature, summarized recently by Shaw and Alvord (1977). However, there seems to be some confusion concerning the definition itself as well as the pathogenesis of the lesions. Under the term 'congenital arachnoid cyst' anomalies as diverse as dilated cisterns, ependymal cysts of the cavum vergae, diverticula of the ventricles and cysts of neural origin have been described. Strictly speaking, the so-called primary arachnoid cyst should be regarded as a developmental abnormality of the arachnoid (Oliver, 1958; Starkman, Brown and Linell, 1958; Grollmus, Wilson and Newton, 1976). Ultrastructural studies (Choux et al., 1978; Schachenmayr and Friede, 1979; Rengachary and Watanabe, 1982) have demonstrated that the cyst is formed by splitting of the arachnoid membrane, which is reinforced by a thick layer of collagen. The wall of the cyst is totally independent of the inner layer of the dura mater. The fine structure of the cells is similar to that of normal trabecular arachnoid cells.

Rengachary and Watanabe (1982) have collected more than 200 cases of arachnoid cyst. The distribution of the cysts was sylvian fissure 49 per cent, cerebellopontine angle 11 per cent, supracollicular area 10 per cent, vermis 9 per cent, interhemispheric fissure 5 per cent, cerebral convexity 4 per cent, the clival and interpeduncular area 3 per cent.

Arachnoid cysts are rare in neonates. In about 3000 consecutive fetal and neonatal autopsies, performed by the author, only five were found. Two extended over the convexity of the hemispheres (Fig. 10.44a) or filled the interhemispheric fissure (Fig. 10.44b) (in one there was an associated absence of the septum pellucidum); one occurred over the temporal pole; and two in the posterior fossa over a cerebellar hemisphere clearly differing from a Dandy–Walker mal-

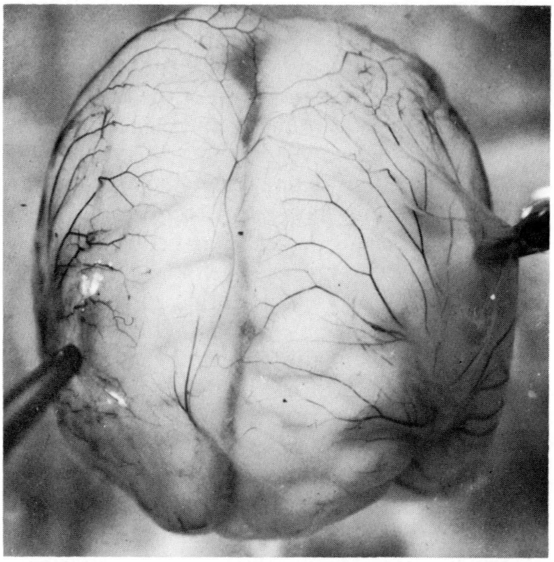

(a)

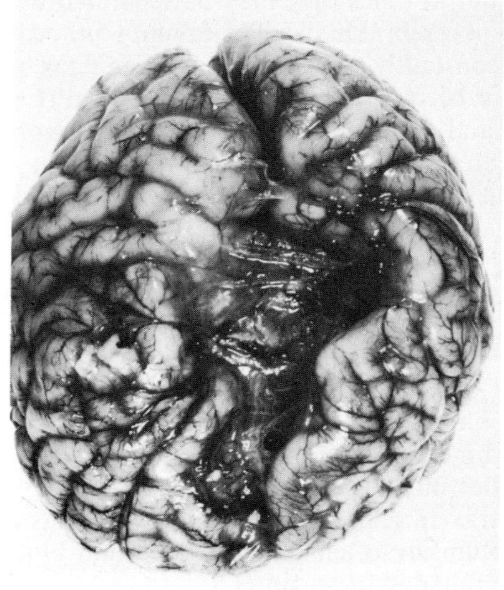

(b)

Fig. 10.44 (**a**) Cystic distension of subarachnoid space extending over the convexities of both hemispheres in a neonatal brain. (**b**) Arachnoid cyst in the interhemispheric fissure.

formation. This incidence is surprisingly low. Other types of cyst have been reported in the neonatal period. Loeser and Alvord (1968a) described a cluster of interhemispheric cysts attached to the falx, with absence of the corpus callosum. These were lined by ependyma and contained choroid plexus, features which might be found in diverticula of the third ventricle. A dilated cavum veli interpositi may be mistaken for a cyst or a posterior fossa tumour (Taveras and Poser, 1959). Haemorrhage in this area with secondary hydrocephalus due to compression of the aqueduct of Sylvius was reported by Lourie and Berne (1961), and a paracollicular plate cyst described in a baby born after a difficult labour and containing stigmata of old haemorrhage (Kruyff, 1965) may represent a link between primary and secondary arachnoid cysts. One may then wonder whether the anomalies are overlooked at autopsy in fetuses and neonates, or whether certain cysts develop and become symptomatic only after birth. Recently, isolated cases have been diagnosed in neonates by CT scan (Harwood-Nash and Fitz, 1976) and by ultrasound (Mack, Rumack and Johnson, 1980).

Cysts of the choroid plexus are extremely rare. This minor abnormality may be an incidental finding in systematic examination of fetal brains.

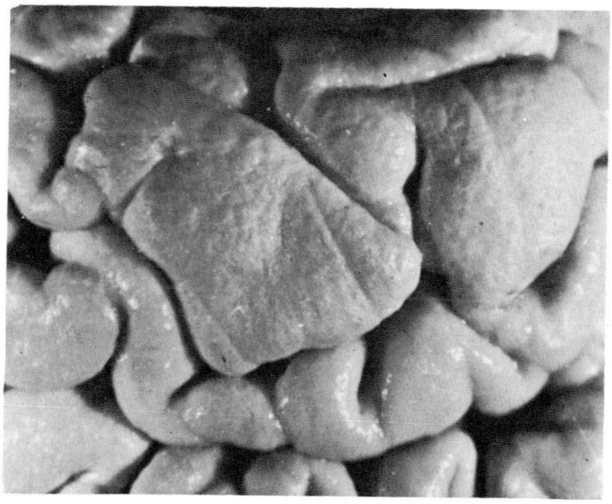

Fig. 10.45 Tuberous sclerosis. A cortical tuber (Pellizzi type 1) is shown as a widened and flattened region of a gyrus. The surface is slightly granular and the tuber is pale and firm to the touch. The leptomeninges have been stripped off.

Tuberous sclerosis complex (Bourneville's disease)

The lesions of tuberous sclerosis, a name first used by Bourneville (1880), were described by von Recklinghausen (1862) in a neonate with cardiac rhabdomyomata. An extensive review of the literature was made by Borberg (1951). The syndrome includes multiple anomalies of the brain, skin, retina and viscera.

When the leptomeninges are removed, hard nodules (the tubers) may project slightly above the surface of the gyri (Figs 10.45 and 10.46). But

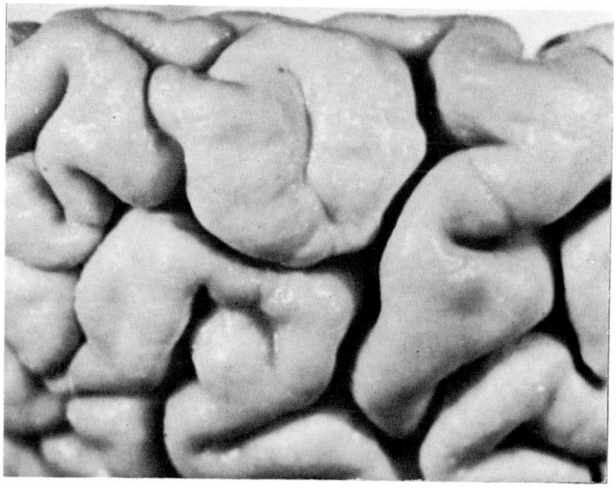

Fig. 10.46 Tuberous sclerosis. A cortical tuber (Pellizzi type 2) appears as a rounded flattened nodule with a rough and dimpled surface. The tuber is elevated above the surrounding brain from which it is demarcated by a sulcus.

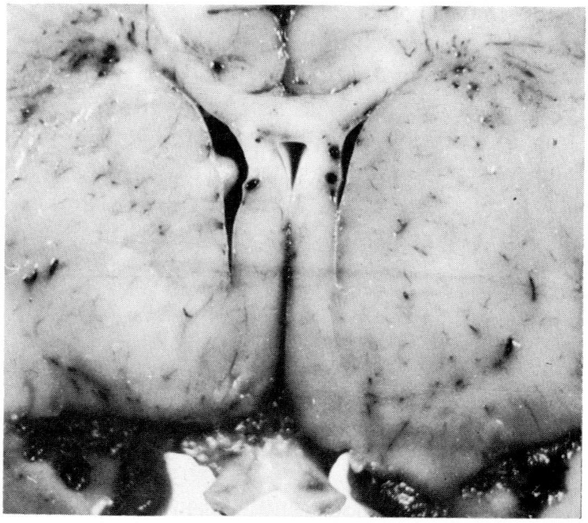

Fig. 10.47 Tuberous sclerosis. A subependymal nodule bulges into the lateral ventricle.

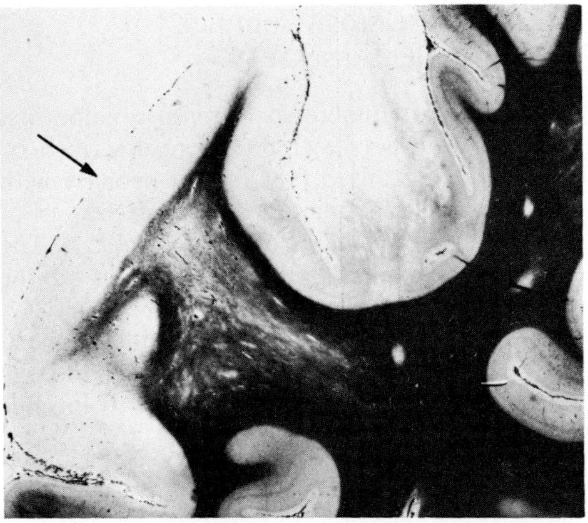

Fig. 10.48 A cortical tuber (arrow) overlies the flat margin of the central core of white matter which shows a poverty of myelin and is also gliosed. Heidenhain's method for myelin.

it is on coronal sections that the subependymal nodules are best seen, even in the newborn (Fig. 10.47). (Simopoulos and Breslow, 1966; A. Probst and Ohnacker, 1977; Larroche, 1977a). Ranging in size from a few millimeters to 1–2 cm, they bulge under the ependyma into the ventricles and may cause obstructive hydrocephalus or lie in the subjacent white matter. They are occasionally found in the brain stem and cerebellum. In older patients the cortical nodules are often associated with underlying patches of gliosed white matter (Fig. 10.48).

On microscopic examination (Figs. 10.49 to 10.53) the tubers contain large, elongated or oval cells resembling astrocytes with thick processes. The nucleus is clear with a prominent nucleolus, and sometimes the cytoplasm contains vacuoles. The subependymal nodules are composed of large cells which have abundant cytoplasm, irregularly shaped, sometimes multiple nuclei and processes which contribute to a fibrillary stroma (Fig. 10.54). Electron microscopic studies of subependymal nodules have demonstrated that these large cells have features of differentiated astrocytes with abundant glycogen, vesicles and filaments, large mitochondria and characteristic processes filled with glial filaments (Ribadeau-Dumas, Poirier and Escourolle, 1973; De Chadarevian and Hollenberg, 1979). In the cortical tubers, puncta adhaerentia or short desmosome-like junctions have been observed between glial cells (Trombley and Mirra, 1981) and were considered by the authors to be embryonic features, supporting the hypothesis of a dysplastic type of tumour.

The tuberous lesions may undergo calcification visible on skull x-rays, and are described in the adult brain as 'brain stones' by Yakovlev and Guthrie (1931) and in the cerebellum by Schafer, Berg and Norman (1975). CT scanning (Harwood-Nash and Breckbill, 1976; Kuhlendahl et al., 1977) and ultrasound (Couture and Cadier, 1983) are of particular value for early diagnosis. Associated dysplasia of the corpus callosum has been described in the newborn by Barth, Stam and Harten (1978).

Slow enlargement of the subependymal nodules in childhood may be followed by malignant transformation into diffusely infiltrating astrocytomas or glioblastomas (Fig. 10.55).

Neurological signs may be misinterpreted in neonates and seizures underestimated. In most cases, generalized convulsions and electroencephalographic abnormalities such as hypsarrhythmia develop within a few months. Later, mental retardation and characteristic retinal phakomas are common (Debré et al., 1952; Ponsot and Lyon, 1977; Monaghan et al., 1981).

Skin lesions are usually absent at birth. They develop during the first year of life or later and consist of areas of vitiligo or 'café au lait' spots,

Fig. 10.49 Section of a cortical tuber showing giant cells. Hortega's silver carbonate method for astrocytes.

Fig. 10.50 A group of large abnormal cells in a cortical tuber. They are stained by Bielschowsky's silver method and so could be neuronal in type.

Fig. 10.51 Giant cells of astrocytic type in a cortical tuber: (**a**) Hortega's method; (**b**) Cajal's gold sublimate method.

Fig. 10.52 Anomalous cells in a cortical tuber: (**a**) multinucleated cell; (**b**) large cells showing cytoplasmic vacuolation. Carbol azure.

Fig. 10.53 Sheaf-like bundles of neuroglial fibres lie in the superficial part of a cortical tuber. Holzer's method.

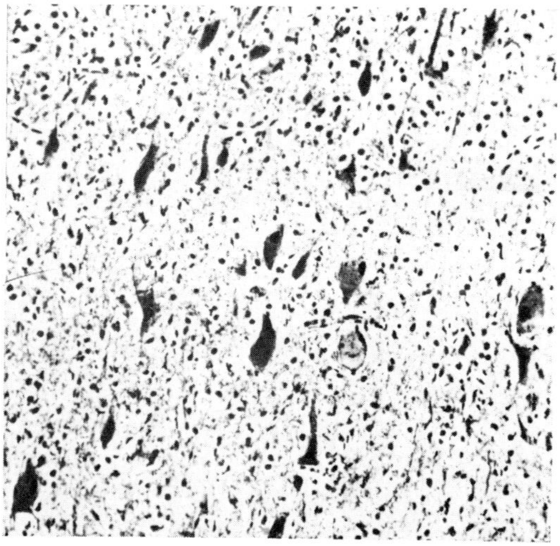

Fig. 10.49

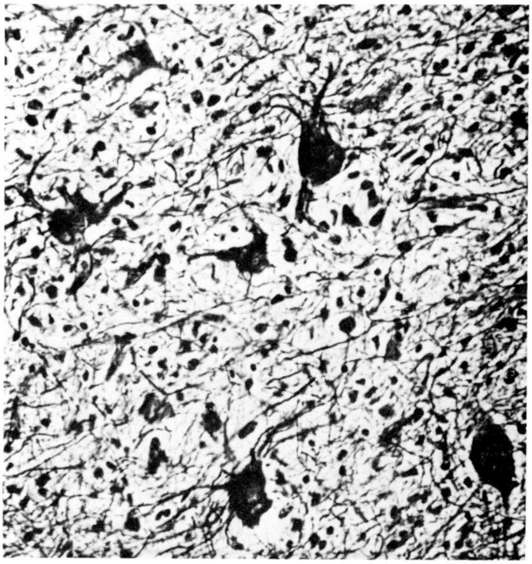

Fig. 10.50

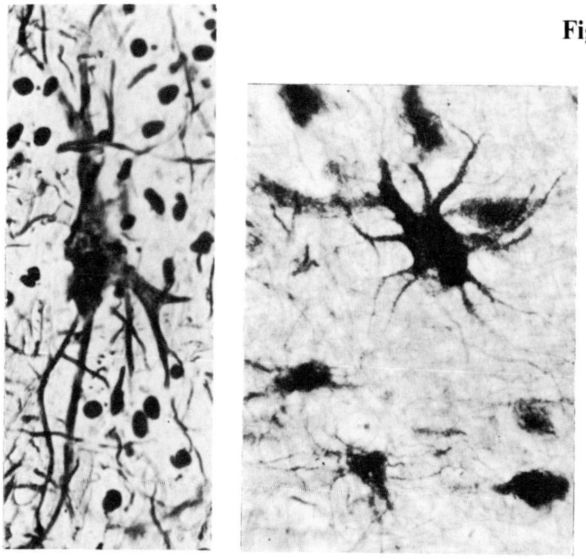

Fig. 10.51 (a) (b)

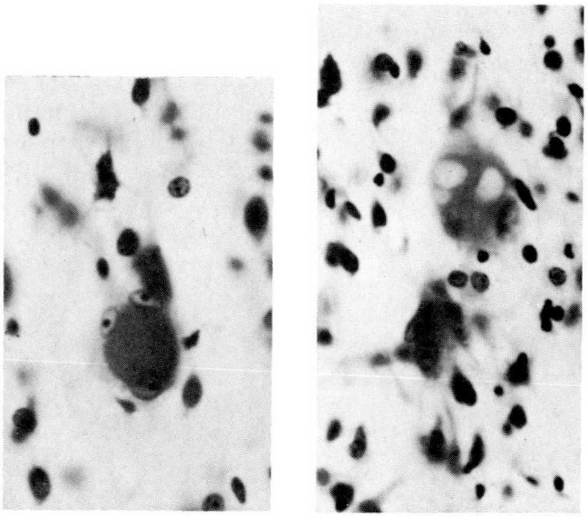

Fig. 10.52 (a) (b)

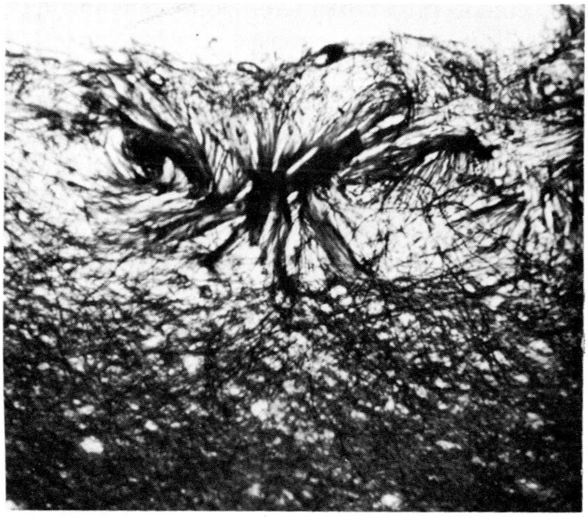

Fig. 10.53

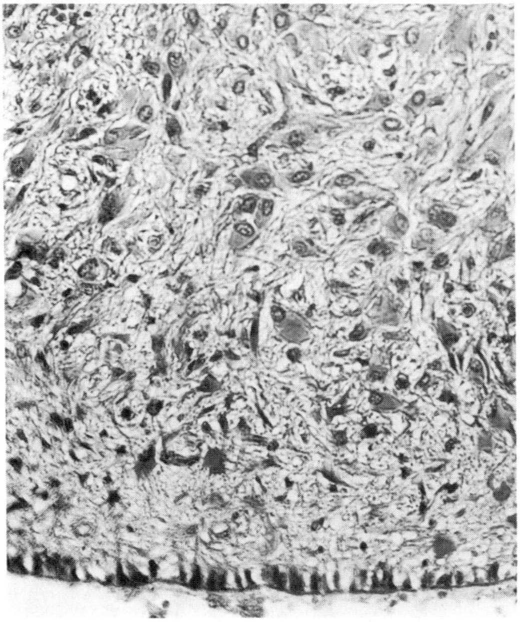

Fig. 10.54 Subependymal nodule in a neonatal case of tuberous sclerosis. The cells are large with a single rounded nucleus and abundant eosinophilic cytoplasm and are intermingled with leashes or whorls of glial fibres.

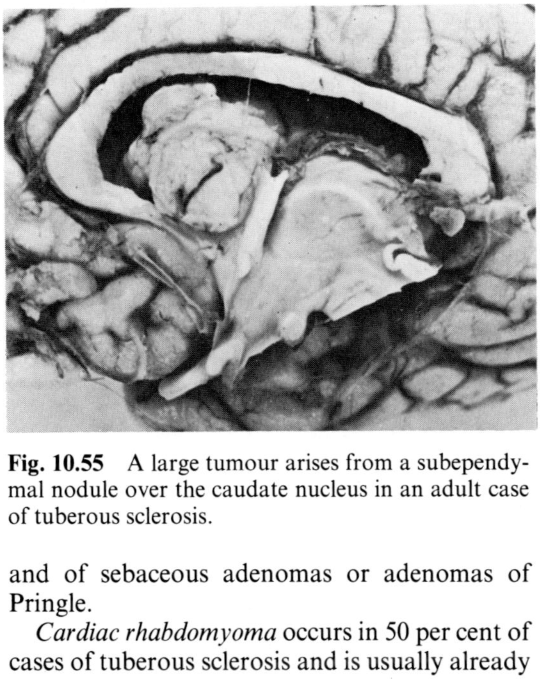

Fig. 10.55 A large tumour arises from a subependymal nodule over the caudate nucleus in an adult case of tuberous sclerosis.

and of sebaceous adenomas or adenomas of Pringle.

Cardiac rhabdomyoma occurs in 50 per cent of cases of tuberous sclerosis and is usually already present in the neonatal period. It was first described by von Recklinghausen (1862) in an infant with tuberous sclerosis. It is a slowly grow-

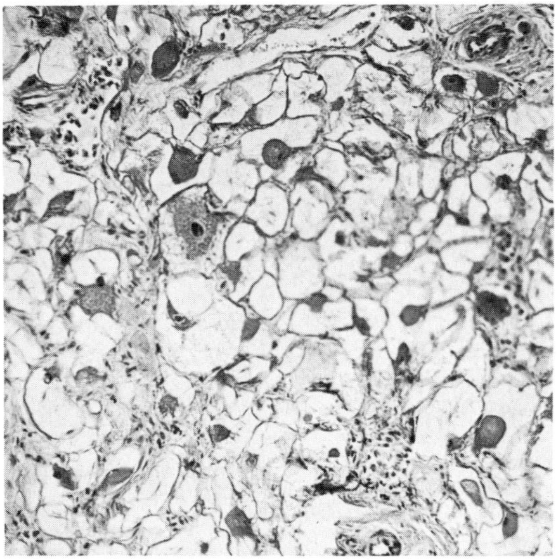

Fig. 10.56 Typical microscopic appearance of one of the multiple rhabdomyomatous nodules found in the tuberous sclerosis complex. Haematoxylin and eosin.

ing tumour, but it may become large enough to cause severe haemodynamic disturbances and death (Pratt-Thomas, 1947; Pernot, Worms and Merlin, 1972; Tsarkraklides et al., 1974). The tumour lies essentially within the ventricular wall and may consist of a single or, more usually, multiple nodules composed histologically (Fig. 10.56) of large cells up to 20 μm in diameter with one or several nuclei and abundant eosinophilic granular cytoplasm, glycogen-rich vacuoles and interweaving processes which may have striations of skeletal muscle fibres. In older patients tumour nodules may be found in kidneys and lungs as well. In 80 per cent of cases renal involvement consists of angiomyolipomas and, less frequently, of cystic lesions.

Tuberous sclerosis has an irregular autosomal dominant inheritance although sporadic cases have been described. Genetic counselling is recommended. It occurs in about 1 per 150 000 births, girls being affected more often than boys.

Von Hippel–Lindau's angiomatosis

Von Hippel-Lindau's angiomatosis is a syndrome comprising disseminated capillary angiomas in the skin and viscera with, at times, cyst formation. Von Hippel (1904) described angiomatosis retinae, and Lindau (1926) established the association between angiomas and cysts of the cerebellum, cysts of the pancreas, kidneys, liver and lung, and tumours of kidney and adrenal. The tumours in the CNS are better known as capillary haemangioblastomas and may be found in cerebellum, brain stem or spinal cord, rarely in cerebral hemispheres. In the case of Bernard, Payan and Toga (1962) angiomas were found in the conjunctiva, retina and brain. In another case (Larroche, 1977a) which represents the most diffuse and complete form, the infant was born at term and died at 6 weeks with angiomas widely disseminated in the skin of the extremities, trunk and head. Their size ranged from a few millimetres to several centimetres in diameter. Angiomas were also present in almost all viscera, in some autonomic ganglia, in the umbilical cord and in bones. Several tumours were found in the cerebrum and cerebellum, and on the inferior surface of the cerebellum a cyst blocked the foramina of the fourth ventricle, causing hydrocephalus.

Both sexes are affected. Sporadic cases have been reported, but in familial cases transmission is by an autosomal dominant gene (Shokeir, 1970). The occurrence in identical twins has been reported by Wesolowski et al. (1981). Most commonly the neurological picture becomes manifest during adolescence, dominated by progressive signs of raised intracranial pressure and cerebellar dysfunction.

Sturge–Weber syndrome (encephalofacial angiomatosis)

This syndrome is characterized by naevus formation in the skin in the territories of the sensory branches of the fifth cranial nerve, and by ocular abnormalities such as glaucoma and choroidal angioma. This neurocutaneous syndrome was first described clinically by Sturge in 1879. In 1897 Kalischer demonstrated the meningeal angiomatosis, and Dimitri (1923) described in x-rays of the skull calcification which was later shown to be intracerebral (Weber, 1929; Krabbe, 1934). There is excessive vascularity of the meninges, the small veins being tortuous and increased in number, giving a dark purple colour to the cerebral surface. On sectioning the brain, calcification may be readily visible beneath the hypervascularized meninges in the outer cortical layers. On microscopic examination (Fig. 10.57), the vessel walls are encrusted with deposits of iron and calcium, and calcific granular deposits of varying size lie freely in the parenchyma. Micropolygyria and heterotopias may also be found in the cerebrum and cerebellum.

The port wine stain of the face is present at birth, as is buphthalmos in 70 per cent of the cases (Nellhaus, Haberland and Hill, 1967). Intracranial calcification has exceptionally been reported in neonates (Fanconi, 1962; Kitahara and Maki, 1978) and diagnosed on CT scan (Alonso et al., 1979).

Focal neurological signs and cerebral atrophy may be evident at birth, but most of the symptoms such as hemiparesis, hemiplegia, epilepsy and mental retardation begin within the first year of life (Blum and Mutrux, 1949) and in early childhood (Wohlwill and Yakovlev, 1957; Roizin et al., 1959). The pathogenesis of the disease is not known, but incomplete involution of the embryonal vasculature has been proposed (Roizin et al., 1959). Although familial cases have been reported, there is no clear evidence for hereditary transmission.

Von Recklinghausen's disease

Neurofibromatosis of von Recklinghausen (1882) (neuroectodermosis of Yakovlev and Guthrie (1931), congenital neuroectodermal dysplasia of van Bogaert (1935)) is a syndrome outside the scope of this chapter. However, it was diagnosed by Hsi-Chih-Chao (1959) in a neonate who presented with convulsions and café au lait spots. The lesion consists essentially of proliferation and hyperplasia of Schwann cells in peripheral nerves and nerve roots including cranial nerves, the most commonly affected being the acoustic. Ocular lesions, usually present at birth, include glaucoma and neurofibroma of the eyelids and may be associated with hemihypertrophy of the face, orbital enlargement and exophthalmos. Visceral lesions and elephantiasis may be present. Inheritance of the disease is by autosomal dominant transmission. Neurinoma of the eighth nerve was observed once as an incidental finding in the author's series of autopsies of neonates.

Arteriovenous malformation

Aneurysmal malformation of the vein of Galen is the most frequent form observed in the neonate. The first recognition of the abnormality is attributed to Wohak (1923). More than 100 cases

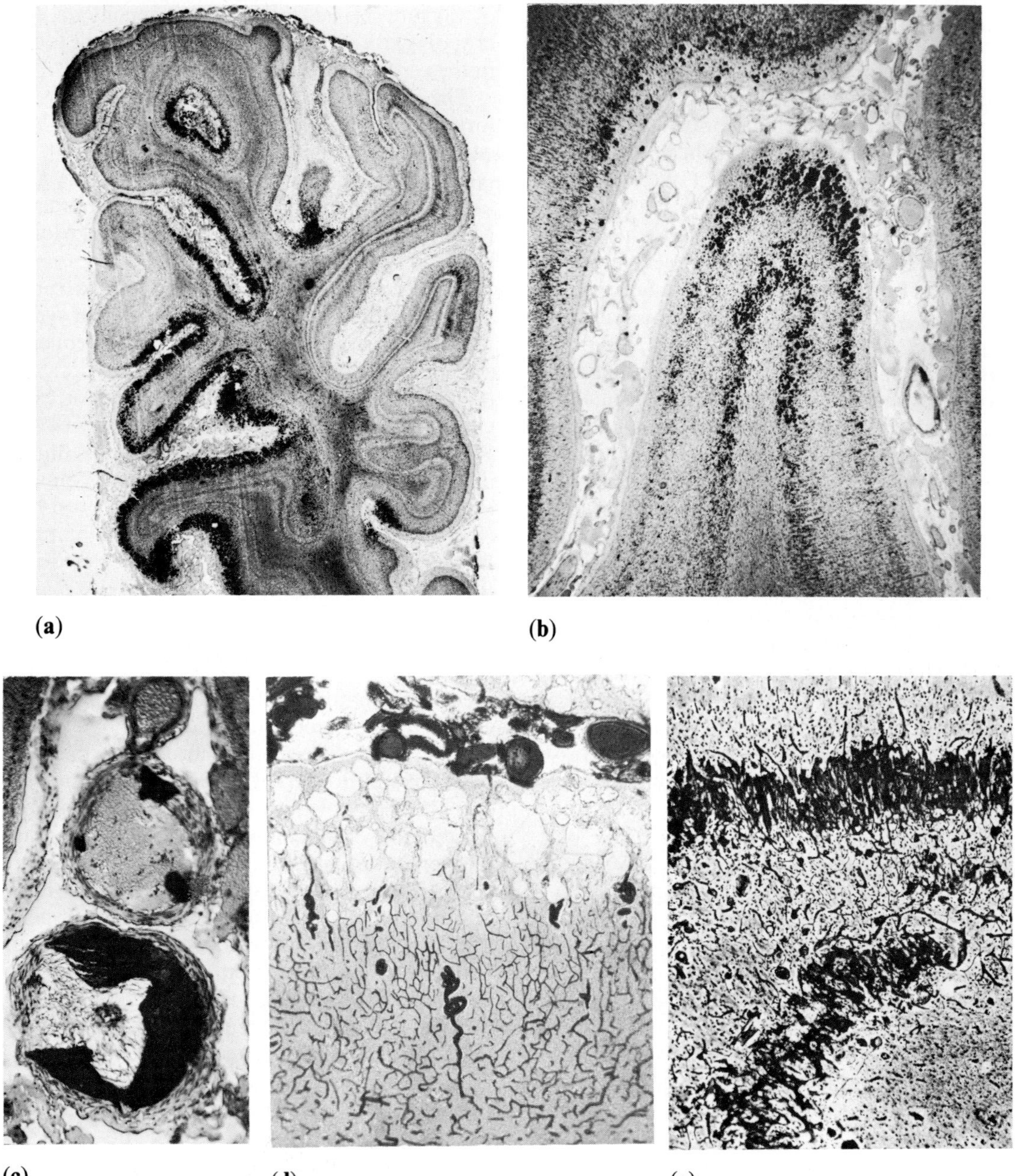

(a) (b) (c) (d) (e)

Fig. 10.57 Sturge–Weber's disease. (**a**) Low power view of section through the occipital pole showing the meningeal venous angioma and the darkly stained dense calcification mainly in the outer layers of the cortex. Carbol azure. (**b**) A higher power view of the meninges and cortex of the occipital pole. The calcification affects deeper as well as superficial layers of the cortex. Carbol azure. (**c**) Calcified meningeal arteries. Carbol azure. (**d**) Abnormal convoluted blood vessels in the non-calcified layers of the cerebral cortex. Masson's trichrome. (**e**) Adventitial fibrosis occasionally found in areas of laminar calcification. The calcium deposits are peculiarly dense and powdery in these areas. Gomori's reticulin.

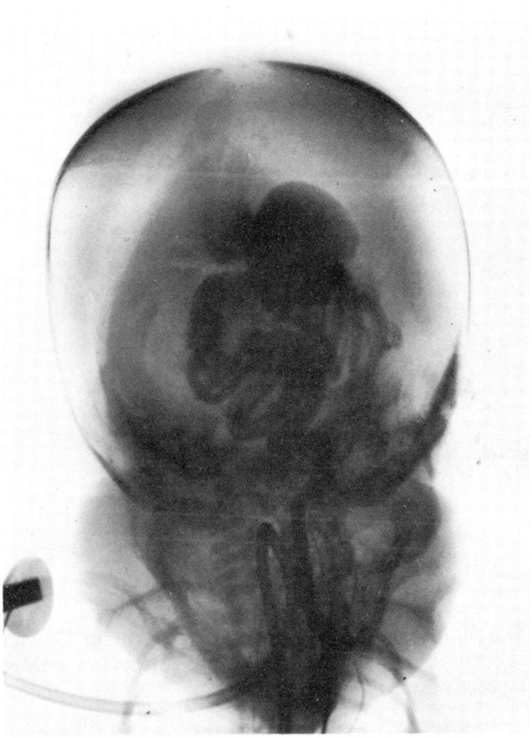

Fig. 10.58 Vertebral arteriogram in an infant. The aneurysmal dilatation of the vein of Galen is shown. (Courtesy of Dr J.C. Gabilan and Dr M. Dehan.)

have been reviewed by Lagos (1977). The malformation is not a true aneurysm but an arteriovenous fistula, the vein of Galen undergoing aneurysmal dilatation (Hirano and Solomon, 1960; O'Brien and Schechter, 1970). The dilated vein of Galen (Fig. 10.58) is generally fed by blood from one or both posterior cerebral arteries or one of their branches, less frequently from small posterior branches of the middle cerebral arteries. The aneurysm may also be fed by anomalous branches of the carotid and/or basilar circulation (Litvak, Yahr and Ransohoff, 1960). The vessels may have a normal architecture, but more often a lace-like network of tortuous vessels empties into the saccular vein of Galen which may be up to several centimetres in diameter. The entire venous system, including transverse and straight sinuses, is dilated. If the shunt is large, clinical signs may develop soon after birth or within a few weeks. Silverman et al. (1955) and Pollock and Laslett (1958) were the first to point out that cerebral arteriovenous fistula can lead to cardiomegaly and congestive cardiac failure in the newborn, and many cases have since been recognized (Gomez et al., 1963; Holden et al., 1972; Loth, Casasoprana and Thibert, 1972).

The differential diagnosis from congenital heart defect is important. In arteriovenous fistula, auscultation over the surface of the skull may reveal a continuous murmur, indicating the flow of blood through the fistula (Levine et al., 1962 and Loth, Casasoprana and Thibert, 1972). In the series of Holden et al. (1972) this sign was found in 80 per cent of cases. In addition, twitching or generalized tonic convulsions (Claireaux and Newman, 1960) and hydrocephalus may occur as a result of compression of the aqueduct (Russell and Nevin, 1940; Clément et al., 1954; Montoya, Dohn and Mercer, 1971).

Various cerebral lesions, either in the territory of the corresponding arteries or elsewhere, have been described in association with this vascular malformation. Periventricular infarction and intraventricular haemorrhage due to compression by the tumour-like vascular mass (Norman and Becker, 1974; Schum et al., 1979) and periventricular calcification (Perez-Fontan et al., 1982) have been described. In addition, the aneurysm itself may become calcified (Siqueira and Murray, 1972) or thrombosed (Lazar, 1974).

Other arteriovenous malformations may be located elsewhere. In the neonate, communication between the anterior or middle cerebral arteries and the sagittal sinus (Stern, Ramos and Wigglesworth, 1968) or between a branch of the middle cerebral artery and the lateral sinus (Carrea and Girado, 1968) have been described. An arteriovenous malformation involving cerebellar veins and arteries in a complicated network of vessels over the vermis was found in a premature infant (Baird and Stitt, 1959). These vascular malformations probably result from failure of the primitive capillary plexus to differentiate into mature arterial and venous channels.

Down's syndrome

The external appearance of the 'mongoloid' brain is much more diagnostic than are the microscopic findings. The weight of the fully grown brain seldom exceeds 1200 g and is usually nearer 1000 g. The brain is abnormally rounded and short with a steeply rising, almost vertical, occipital contour. The convolutional pattern usually shows no gross departure from normality, but there may be asymmetries on the two sides and

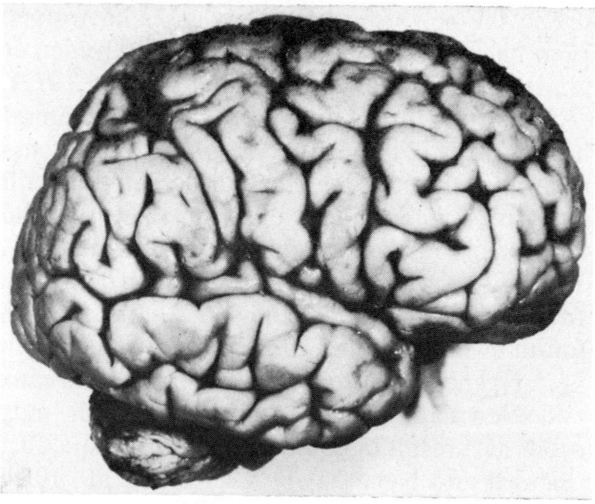

Fig. 10.59 The right hemisphere of the brain in Down's syndrome. The cerebellum is small and the occipital contour flatter than normal. The frontal lobe is reduced in its anteroposterior diameter and the superior temporal gyrus poorly developed.

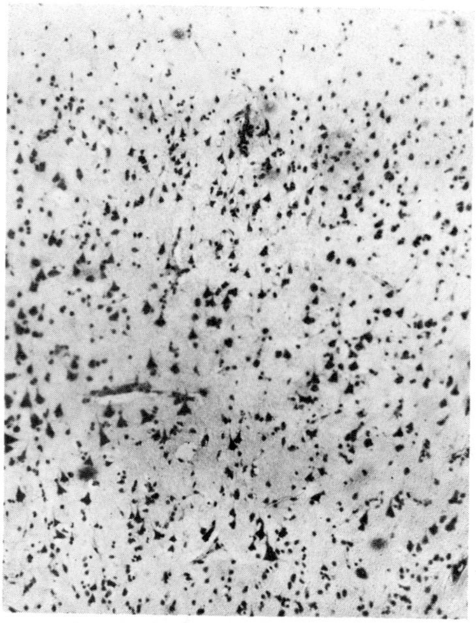

Fig. 10.60 Section of the angular gyrus in Down's syndrome showing diffuse loss of neurons in the third layer. Cresyl violet.

the insula is often exposed on account of the poor development of the third frontal gyrus. Compared with the brain of a normal adult there is a poverty of secondary sulci, but the ape-like simplification of genetic micrencephaly is never found. Very characteristic of the 'mongol' brain, though not peculiar to it, is narrowness of the superior temporal gyrus (Fig. 10.59). The anomaly is often bilateral and is present in about half the cases. Conspicuous smallness of the cerebellum and brain stem in comparison with the cerebrum as a whole is also a common feature (Crome, Cowie and Slater, 1966).

Benda (1947) proposed that most of these abnormalities of shape have been impressed on the developing brain by the retarded growth of the mongol skull and pointed out that the crowns of gyri may be flattened, that the sagittally arranged sulci may show S-shaped distortion and that fibrous union may bind contiguous parts of the convolutions together.

Many microscopic anomalies have been described in the syndrome but they are all shared by other forms of severe oligophrenia. Davidoff (1928) reported patchy cerebral calcifications and a poverty of nerve cells in the third cortical layer of his cases (Fig 10.60). This finding is not very common, but irregularities of grouping certainly occur so that relatively acellular areas adjoin those which display an increased density due to the presence of clusters of small nerve cells. Systematic cell counts in random sections indicate that the nerve cells are, in fact, often increased on the average per unit area. This seeming paradox may be related to the small size of the brain as a whole, since, as a general rule, the more underdeveloped the state of the brain, the closer together are the cortical neurons. Benda (1947), however, considered that an active destruction of the nerve cells associated with anoxia and oedema takes place in mongols dying in infancy. The same author lay stress upon the poor myelination of the grey and white matter and demonstrated a striking poverty of myelin in the U-fibres. Meyer and Jones (1939) were the first to demonstrate a conspicuous fibrillary gliosis of the central white matter in many, but by no means all, cases. There was often no corresponding pallor in myelin preparations, although patchy areas of demyelination were sometimes seen, as they were in Davidoff's cases. Benda reported frequent minor malformations in the spinal cords and drew attention to a finding which he considered peculiar to the condition, namely the fusion of the columns of Clarke, so that the nerve cells occupy a strip of grey matter lying behind the central canal. Except for undoubted signs of retarded or mildly perverted development, the brain thus shows few pathological changes which cannot be explained on the basis of intercurrent disease. Whether such fortuitous lesions are in some way related to abnormal constitutional factors, such as general circulatory asthenia or endocrine anomalies, have not been precisely determined. Certainly the frequent association of congenital heart disease is an important factor. Arterial and venous thromboses are well-known complications of Fallot's tetralogy, as are embolism and cerebral abscess due to detachment of vegetations from congenitally malformed or infected valves.

Middle-aged mongols often show clinical signs of premature senility and this may be reflected in the brain by the presence of senile plaques and Alzheimer's neurofibrillary change (Jervis, 1948; Solitare and Lamarche, 1966; Olson and Shaw, 1969). In Malamud's (1972) series the brains of all mongoloids dying over the age of 40 showed lesions of this type in various degrees of severity. Ultrastructurally the neurofibrillary tangles are identical with those seen in typical cases of Alzheimer's disease (Schochet, Lampert and McCormick, 1973) (See also Chapter 20).

Aetiology Most, if not all, cases of Down's syndrome display various chromosomal abnormalities, such as trisomy G, D/G or G/G translocations or mosaicism. The additional chromosome in trisomy G is no. 21. The relative incidence of different chromosomal types has been remarkably constant in recorded series. Trisomy G occurs in over 90 per cent of cases, translocations in 2–4 per cent and mosaicism in 2–3 per cent. The incidence of trisomy increases with advancing maternal age; a relatively higher proportion of translocations occurs in children of younger mothers. Most familial cases are associated with translocations. The risk of a mother carrying a translocation chromosome producing another mongoloid child is somewhat less than the theoretical one in three in a D/G or G21/G22 translocation. In the rare G21/G21 translocation all children are invariably affected. For a full discussion on the cytogenetics of Down's syndrome the reader is referred to a series of articles by Polani and his collaborators, (Giannelli, Hamerton and Carter, 1965; Hamerton, Giannelli and Polani, 1965; Polani et al., 1965). The *pathogenesis* of the condition, or the mechanism by which an additional chromosome can cause a wide range of abnormalities with variable expressivity, has been the subject of abundant speculation, yet remains obscure.

Hydrocephalus

This subject is dealt with in general in Chapter 2, and only congenital hydrocephalus will be described here. Its main cause is obstruction to the flow of CSF. Thus in the Dandy–Walker syndrome (see p. 406) the exit foramina in the fourth ventricle are malformed or sealed, leading to great distension of the fourth ventricle as well as the lateral ventricles. In the Chiari type II malformation, elongation of the fourth ventricle and possibly arachnoiditis prevent the flow of CSF into the intracranial subarachnoid space.

The importance of malformations of the aqueduct, such as stenosis and forking, have been emphasized (Russell, 1949). Histological examination shows slit-like lumina with irregular contours (de Lange, 1929). Emery (1974), however, did not find complete obliteration of the aqueduct in a study of serial sections of the midbrain in cases of hydrocephalus and myelocele. The 'occlusion' of the aqueduct is probably contributed to by compression and angulation of the brain stem. Stenosis and forking of the aqueduct are usually associated with other malformations of the brain. A special form of familial congenital hydrocephalus due to stenosis of the aqueduct of Sylvius was described by Bickers and Adams (1949). In the report by Edwards, Norman and Roberts (1961), seven male infants were affected in two generations of the same family. These children showed, in addition, deformity of the hands with the thumb flexed over the palm and a short first metacarpal. Other cases have been published and have confirmed the recessive X-linked inheritance (Gilly et al., 1971; Holmes et al., 1973). Membranous occlusion of the aqueduct was also described by Russell (1949). Gliosis around the aqueduct tends to narrow the lumen or to obliterate it completely. There is no associated developmental abnormality of the brain and the presence of ependymitis in other parts of the ventricular system suggests an ante- or perinatal infection.

In full-term infants who suffer severe perinatal hypoxic-ischaemic brain damage, *ex vacuo* hydrocephalus may develop. The enlarged ventricles are usually symmetrical. In premature infants when leucomalacia evolves to sclerosis or to cavitation of the white matter, lesions may be asymmetrical with unilateral ventricular dilation.

There remain cases of hydrocephalus for which the cause is still unknown. Unclassifiable, bizarre and complex malformations of the brain, fluid-filled cysts over the hemispheres, cerebellar agenesis and abnormal meninges and vessels (Norman, Thurber and Woolley, 1981) have been observed but no clear relationship between these anomalies and the hydrocephalus has been established.

The distended hemispheres are fragile and easily torn *post mortem*, and collapse when CSF escapes. In many cases, however, even after complete draining of CSF, the brain is heavier than that of an infant of the same age. This may be due to infiltration of fluid into the brain tissue. In addition, the external surface of the brain may show small gyri and shallow sulci without any underlying cytoarchitectonic abnormality. Postnatal growth of the cortical surface seems to proceed normally in spite of the expanding hydrocephalus, and Friede (1975) has suggested that with the abnormal distension of the hemisphere 'a great portion of intrasulcal cortex is exposed resulting in redundant gyration'.

Sections of the brain show the enlarged cavities, a grossly distended infundibulum reduced to a thin transparent membrane, and a fenestrated or absent septum pellucidum. The corpus callosum becomes extremely thin. The anterior horns of the ventricles are usually less dilated than the temporal and occipital horns, where the cerebral mantle may be reduced in thickness to a few millimetres. Whilst the cortex is relatively well preserved, the white matter is severely reduced in amount. Degenerative changes may be due to the stretching and tearing of nerve fibres, diffusion of CSF into the periventricular white matter causing interstitial oedema, or chronic compression. Remarkable re-expansion of the cerebral mantle may occur after shunting, this suggesting that a mechanical cause is at least partly responsible for the thinning of the white matter. On microscopic examination the ventricular walls are denuded and the ependyma is replaced by a layer of glial tissue.

References

Aicardi, J. and Chevrie, J. J. (1969) Le syndrome agénésie calleuse, spasmes en flexion, lacunes choriorétiniennes. *Archives Françaises de Pédiatrie* **26,** 7–12.

Aicardi, J. and Goutières, F. (1981) The syndrome of absence of the septum pellucidum with porencephalies and other developmental defects. *Neuropediatrics* **12,** 319–29.

Åkesson, H. O. (1966) Condition at birth and mental deficiency. *Acta Genetica et Statistica Medica* **16,** 283–304.

Alberca-Serrano, R. and Reznik, M. (1964) Turricéphalie héréditaire, microcéphalie familiale avec lissencéphalie. Rapport de ce syndrome malformatif avec les dystrophies cérébro-médullaires. *Journal of the Neurological Sciences* **1,** 555–77.

Alonso, A., Taboada, D., Ceres, L., Beltran, J., Olague, R. and Nogues, A. (1979) Intracranial calcification in a neonate with the Sturge–Weber syndrome and additional problems. *Pediatric Radiology* **8,** 39–41.

Altman, J., Anderson, W. J. and Wright, K. A. (1969) Reconstitution of the external granular layer of the cerebellar cortex in infant rats after low-level X-irradiation. *Anatomical Record* **163,** 453–72.

Ambler, M., Pogacar, S. and Sidman, R. (1969) Lhermitte–Duclos disease (granule cell hypertrophy of the cerebellum). Pathological analysis of the first familial case. *Journal of Neuropathology and Experimental Neurology* **28,** 622–47.

André-Thomas, T., Laruelle, L. and Reumont, J. (1955) Anencéphalie et collagène. *Annales de Médecine* **56,** 325–51

Angevine, D. M. (1938) Pathologic anatomy of hypophysis and adrenals in anencephaly. *Archives of Pathology* **26,** 507–18.

Appleby, A., Bradley, W. G., Foster, J. B., Hankinson, J. and Hudgson, P. (1969) Syringomyelia due to chronic arachnoiditis at the foramen magnum. *Journal of the Neurological Sciences* **8,** 451–64.

Arnold, J. (1894) Myelocyste, Transposition von Gewebskeimen und Sympodie. *Beiträge zur Pathologischen Anatomie und zur allgemeinen Pathologie* **16,** 1–28.

Atkins, S. and Rosenthal, M. K. (1961) Multiple congenital abnormalities associated with chromosomal trisomy. *New England Journal of Medicine* **265,** 314–18.

Baird, W. F. and Stitt, D. G. (1959) Arteriovenous

aneurysm of the cerebellum in a premature infant. *Pediatrics* **24,** 455–7.

Baker, R. C. and Graves, G. O. (1931) Cerebellar agenesis. *Archives of Neurology and Psychiatry* **25,** 547–55.

Bankl, H. and Jellinger, J. (1967) Zentralnervöse Schäden nach fötaler Kohlenoxydvergiftung. *Beiträge zur Pathologischen Anatomie und Allgemeinen Pathologie* **135,** 350–76.

Baraitser, M. (1982) *The Genetics of Neurological Disorders.* Oxford University Press, Oxford.

Barnett, H. J. M., Foster, J. B. and Hudgson, P. (1973) *Syringomyelia.* Saunders, London.

Barry, A., Patten, B. M. and Stewart, B. H. (1957) Possible factors in the development of the Arnold–Chiari malformation. *Journal of Neurosurgery* **14,** 285–301.

Barson, A. J. (1970) Spina bifida: the significance of the level and extent of the defect to the morphogenesis. *Developmental Medicine and Child Neurology* **12,** 129–44.

Barth, P. G., Stam, F. C. and van den Harten, J. J. (1978) Tuberous sclerosis and dysplasia of the corpus callosum. Case report of their combined occurrence in a newborn. *Acta Neuropathologica* **42,** 63–4.

Barth, P. G., Mullaart, R., Stam, F. C. and Slooff, J. L. (1982) Familial lissencephaly with extreme neopallial hypoplasia. *Brain and Development* **4,** 145–51.

Bates, J. I. and Netsky, M. G. (1955) Developmental anomalies of the horns of the lateral ventricles. *Journal of Neuropathology and Experimental Neurology* **14,** 316–25.

Beck, F., Lloyd, J. B. and Griffiths, A. (1967) Lysosomal enzyme inhibition by trypan blue: a theory of teratogenesis. *Science* **157,** 1180–2.

Benda, C. E. (1947) *Mongolism and Cretinism.* Grune and Stratton, New York.

Benda, C. E. (1954) The Dandy–Walker syndrome or the so-called atresia of the foramen of Magendie. *Journal of Neuropathology and Experimental Neurology* **13,** 14–29.

Benda, C. E. (1959) Dysraphic states. *Journal of Neuropathology and Experimental Neurology* **18,** 56–74.

Bergeron, T. (1969) Radiographic demonstration of cortical heterotopia. *Acta Radiologica* **9,** 135–9.

Bernard, R., Payan, H. and Toga, M. (1962) Angiomatose neuro-ectodermique évolutive et mortelle à brève échéance chez un nouveau-né. *Archives d'Anatomie Pathologique* **10,** 298–301.

Bertrand, I. and Gruner, J. (1955) The status verrucosus of the cerebral cortex. *Journal of Neuropathology and Experimental Neurology* **14,** 331–47.

Bickers, D. S. and Adams, R. D. (1949) Hereditary stenosis of the aqueduct of Sylvius as a cause of congenital hydrocephalus. *Brain* **72,** 246–62.

Bielschowsky, M. (1916) Uber Mikrogyrie. *Journal für Psychologie und Neurologie* **22,** 1–47.

Bielschowsky, M. (1920) Zur Histopathologie und Pathogenese der amaurotischen Idiotie mit besonderer Berücksichtigung der zerebellären Veränderungen. *Journal für Psychologie und Neurologie* **26,** 123–244.

Bielschowsky, M. (1923) Über die Oberflächengestaltung des Grosshirnmantels bei Pachygyrie, Mikrogyrie und bei normaler Entwicklung. *Journal für Psychologie und Neurologie* **30,** 29–76.

Biemond, A. (1955) Hypoplasia ponto-neocerebellaris, with malformation of the dentate nucleus. *Folia Psychiatrica, Neurologica et Neurochirurgica Neerlandica* **58,** 2–7.

Bignami, A. and Appicciutoli, L. (1964) Micropolygyria and cerebral calcification in cytomegalic inclusion disease. *Acta Neuropathologica* **4,** 127–37.

Blackwell, D. E., Spinnato, J. A., Hirsch, G., Giles, H. R. and Sackler, J. (1982) Antenatal ultrasound diagnosis of holoprosencephaly: a case report. *American Journal of Obstetrics and Gynecology* **143,** 848–9.

Blum, J. D. and Mutrux, S (1949) La maladie de Sturge–Weber–Krabbe. *Ophthalmologica* **118,** 781–95.

van Bogaert, L. and Ley, R. (1929) L'état verruqueux de la corticalité cérébrale et cérébelleuse dans un cas d'idiotie avec rigidité et amaurose. *Archives Suisse de Neurologie* **24,** 194–230.

van Bogaert, L. (1935) Les dysplasies neuroectodermiques congenitales. *Revue Neurologique* **63,** 354–98.

van Bogaert, L. and Radermecker, M. A. (1955) Une dysgénésie cérébelleuse chez un enfant du radium. *Revue Neurologique* **93,** 65–82.

Böök, J. A., Schut, J. W. and Reed, S. C. (1953) A clinical and genetical study of microcephaly. *American Journal of Mental Deficiency* **57,** 637–60.

Borberg, A. (1951) Clinical and genetic investigations into tuberous sclerosis and Recklinghausen's neurofibromatosis. *Acta Psychologica et Neurologica Scandinavica* Suppl. 71, pp. 239.

Bourneville, D. M. (1880) Sclérose tubéreuse des circonvolutions cérébrales: idiotie et épilepsie hémiplégique. *Archives de Neurologie* **1,** 81–91.

Brain, W. R., Greenfield, J. G. and Northfield, D. W. C. (1943) A case of atypical Lindau's disease. *Journal of Neurology and Psychiatry* **6,** 32–7.

Brent, R. L. and Johnson, A. (1967). The production of congenital malformations using tissue antisera. VII. Yolk sac. *Federation Proceedings* **26,** 701.

Bresler, N. C. (1899) Klinische und pathologisch-anatomische Beiträge zur Mikrogyrie. *Archiv für Psychiatrie und Nervenkrankeiten* **31,** 566–73.

Brock, D. J. H. (1981) Amniotic fluid acetylcholinesterase. *Lancet* **i,** 95.

Brock, D. J. H. and Sutcliffe, R. G. (1972) Alpha-fetoprotein in the antenatal diagnosis of anencephaly and spina bifida. *Lancet* **2,** 197–8.

Brouwer, B. (1924) Hypoplasia ponto-neocerebellaris. *Psychiatrische en Neurologische Bladen* **6,** 461–9.

Brown, J. R. (1977) The Dandy–Walker syndrome. In *Handbook of Clinical Neurology* vol 30 (Eds. Vinken, P. J. and Bruyn, G. W.), pp. 623–46. North-Holland, Amsterdam.

Brun, A. and Sköld, G. (1968) CNS malformations in Turner's syndrome. An integral part of the syndrome? *Acta Neuropathologica* **10,** 159–61.

Brun, R. (1917, 1918a, b) Zur Kenntnis der Bildungsfehler des Kleinhirns. *Schweizer Archiv für Neurologie und Psychiatrie* **1,** 61–123; **2,** 48–105; **3,** 13–88.

Brzustowicz, R. J. and Kernohan, J. W. (1952) Cell rests in region of fourth ventricle, histologic and embryologic consideration. *Archives of Neurology and Psychiatry* **67,** 585–91, 592–601, 602–11.

Butler, L. J., Snodgrass, G. J., France, N., Sinclaire, C. and Russel, A. (1965) Trisomy syndrome. Analysis of 13 cases. *Archives of Disease in Childhood* **40,** 600–11.

Carpenter, M. B. and Druckemiller, W. H. (1953) Agenesis of the corpus callosum diagnosed during life. *Archives of Neurology and Psychiatry* **69,** 305–22.

Carr, D. H. (1967) Chromosome anomalies as a cause of spontaneous abortion. *American Journal of Obstetrics and Gynecology* **97,** 283–93.

Carrea, R. and Girado, J. M. (1968) Angiomatous and fistulous arteriovenous aneurysm in children. In *Progress in Brain Research*, Vol. 30, Cerebral circulation. (Ed. Luyendijk, W.), pp. 433–9. Elsevier, Amsterdam.

Carroll, J. D. (1967) Syringomyelia as a possible complication of poliomyelitis. *Neurology* **17,** 213–15.

Carter, C. O., David, P. A. and Laurence, K. M. (1968) A family study of major central nervous system malformations in South Wales. *Journal of Medical Genetics* **5,** 81–106.

Cassady, G. (1969) Anencephaly: a 6 year study of 367 cases. *American Journal of Obstetrics and Gynecology* **103,** 1154–9.

Chiari, H. (1891) Über Veränderungen des Kleinhirns, des Pons und der Medulla oblongata infolge von congenitaler Hydrocephalie des Grosshirns. *Deutsche Medizinische Wochenschrift* **27,** 1172–5.

Chiari, H. (1895) Über die Veränderungen des Kleinhirns, des Pons, und der Medulla oblongata infolge von congenitaler Hydrocephalie des Grosshirns. *Denkschriften der Akademie der Wissenschaften, Wien* **63,** 71–116.

Choi, B. H., Lapham, L. W., Amin-Zaki, L. and Saleem, T. (1978) Abnormal neuronal migration, deranged cerebral cortical organization, and diffuse white matter astrocytosis of human fetal brain: a major effect of methylmercury poisoning in utero. *Journal of Neuropathology and Experimental Neurology* **37,** 719–33.

Choux, M., Raybaud, C., Puisard, N., Hassoun, J. and Gambarelli, D. (1978) Intracranial supratentorial cysts in children excluding tumour and parasitic cysts. *Child's Brain* **4,** 15–32.

Claireaux, E. R. and Newman, C. G. H. (1960) Arterio-venous fistula (aneurysm) of the great vein of Galen with heart failure in the neonatal period. *Archives of Disease in Childhood* **35,** 605–12.

Cleland, J. (1883) Contribution to the study of spina bifida, encephalocele and anencephalus. *Journal of Anatomy and Physiology* **17,** 257–92.

Clément, R., Gerbeaux, J., Combes-Hamelle, A., Pertuiset, B. and Petranca, C. (1954) Anévrysmes arterio-veineux de l'ampoule de Galien chez le nourrisson. Leur rôle dans l'hydrocéphalie communicante. *Presse Médicale* **62,** 658–61.

Cohlan, S. Q. (1953) Excessive intake of vitamin A during pregnancy as a cause of congenital anomalies in the rat. *Science* **117,** 535–6.

Cohlan, S. Q. (1954) Congenital anomalies in the rat produced by the excessive intake of vitamin A during pregnancy. *Pediatrics* **13,** 556–67.

Cohn, R. and Neumann, M. A. (1946) Porencephaly. A clinicopathologic study. *Journal of Neuropathology and Experimental Neurology* **5,** 257–70.

Combette, M. (1831) Absence complète du cervelet, des pédoncules postérieurs et de la protubérance cérébrale chez une jeune fille morte dans sa onzième année. *Bulletin de la Société des Anatomistes, Paris* **5,** 148–53.

Costoulas, G. (1958) Un type peu connu d'anomalies des ventricules cérébraux: les goniosynapses (étude anatomo-clinique et statistique). *Annales d'Anatomie Pathologique* **3,** 268–83.

Courville, C. B. and Edmonson, H. A. (1958) Mental deficiency from intrauterine exposure to radiation. *Bulletin of the Los Angeles Neurological Society* **23,** 11–20.

Couture, A. and Cadier, L. (1983) *Echographie Cérébrale par Voie Transfontanellaire.* Vigot, Paris.

Cowen, D. and Geller, L. M. (1960) Long-term pathological effects of prenatal X-irradiation on the central nervous system of the rat. *Journal of Neuropathology and Experimental Neurology* **19,** 488–527.

Craig, W. M., Wagener, H. P. and Kernohan, J. W. (1941) Lindau–von Hippel disease. *Archives of Neurology and Psychiatry* **46,** 36–58.

Crome, L. (1952) Microgyria. *Journal of Pathology and Bacteriology* **64,** 479–95.

Crome, L. (1956) Pachygyria. *Journal of Pathology and Bacteriology* **71,** 335–52.

Crome, L. (1969) Brain warts. *Journal of Mental Deficiency Research* **13,** 60–5.

Crome, L., Cowie, V. and Slater, R. E. (1966) A statistical note on cerebellar and brain-stem weight in mongolism. *Journal of Mental Deficiency Research* **10,** 69–72.

Crome, L. and France, N. (1959) Microgyria and cytomegalic inclusion disease in infancy. *Journal of Clinical Pathology* **12,** 427–34.

Crome, L. and Stern, J. (1972) *Pathology of Mental Retardation,* 2nd edn. Churchill Livingstone, Edinburgh and London.

Crosby, R. M. N., Mosberg, W. H. Jr and Smith, G. W. (1951). Intrauterine meningitis as cause of hydrocephalus. *Journal of Pediatrics* **39,** 94–101.

D'Agostino, A. N., Kernohan, J. N. and Brown, J. R. (1963) The Dandy–Walker Syndrome. *Journal of Neuropathology and Experimental Neurology* **22,** 450–70.

Dambska, M., Berard-Badier, M., Toga, M. and Pinsard, N. (1968) A propos des malformations complexes du cortex, des ventricules et du noyau caudé dans un cas d'une fratrie de microcéphales. *Neuropathologia Polska* **6,** 319–24.

Dandy, W. E. (1921) The diagnosis and treatment of hydrocephalus due to occlusion of the foramina of Magendie and Luschka. *Surgery, Gynecology and Obstetrics* **32,** 112–24.

Dandy, W. E. (1931) Congenital cerebral cysts of the cavum septi pellucidi (fifth ventricle) and cavum vergae (sixth ventricle) *Archives of Neurology and Psychiatry* **25,** 44–66.

Dandy, W. E. and Blackfan, K. D. (1914) Internal hydrocephalus, an experimental clinical and pathological study. *American Journal of Diseases of Children* **8,** 406–82.

Daniel, P. M. and Strich, S. J. (1958) Some observations on the congenital deformity of the central nervous system known as the Arnold–Chiari malformation. *Journal of Neuropathology and Experimental Neurology* **17,** 255–66.

Daube, J. R. and Chou, S. M. (1966) Lissencephaly. Two cases. *Neurology* **16,** 179–91.

Davidoff, L. M. (1928) Brain in mongolian idiocy; report of 10 cases. *Archives of Neurology and Psychiatry* **20,** 1229–57.

Davidoff, L., and Dyke, G. (1934) Agenesis of the corpus callosum. Diagnosis by encephalography; report of 3 cases. *American Journal of Roentgenology* **32,** 1–10.

Davidoff, L. M. (1946) coarctation of the walls of the lateral angles of the lateral cerebral ventricles. *Journal of Neurosurgery* **3,** 250–6.

Debré, R., Thieffy, S., Mozziconacci, S., Bargeton, E. and Ramade, J. (1952) La sclérose tubéreuse de Bourneville chez le nourrisson et le petit enfant. *Archives Françaises de Pédiatrie* **9,** 342–82.

De Chadarevian, J. P. and Hollenberg, R. D. (1979) Subependymal giant cell tumor of tuberose sclerosis: a light and ultrastructural study. *Journal of Neuropathology and Experimental Neurology* **38,** 419–33.

Dekaban, A. (1959) Arhinencephaly in an infant born to a diabetic mother. *Journal of Neuropathology and Experimental Neurology* **18,** 620–6.

Dekaban, A. S. (1963) Anencephaly in early human embryos. *Journal of Neuropathology and Experimental Neurology* **22,** 533–48.

Dekaban, A. (1965) Large defects in cerebral hemispheres associated with cortical dysgenesis. *Journal of Neuropathology and Experimental Neurology* **24,** 512–30.

Dekaban, A. S. and Sakuragawa, N. (1977) Megalencephaly. In *Handbook of Clinical Neurology* vol 30 (Eds. Vinken, P. J. and Bruyn, G. W.), pp 647–60. North-Holland, Amsterdam.

De León, G. (1972) Observations on cerebral and cerebellar microgyria. *Acta Neuropathologica* **20,** 278–87.

De Morsier, G. (1955) Etudes sur les dysraphies cranio-encéphaliques. II. Agénésie du vermis cérébelleux—dysraphie rhombocéphalique médiane (rhomboschisis). *Monatsschrift für Psychiatrie und Neurologie* **129,** 321–44.

De Morsier, G. (1956) Agénésie du septum lucidum avec malformations du tractus optique—la dysplasie septo-optique. *Schweizer Archiv für Neurologie und Psychiatrie* **77,** 267–92.

De Morsier, G. and Mozer, J.J. (1935) Agénésie complète de la commissure calleuse et troubles du développement de l'hémisphère gauche avec hémiparesie droite et intégrité mentale. (Le syndrome embryonnaire précoce de l'artère cérébrale antérieure.) *Schweizer Archiv für Neurologie und Psychiatrie* **35,** 64–95.

De Myer, W., Zeman, W. and Palmer, C. (1963) Familial alobar holoprosencephaly (arhinencephaly with median cleft lips and palate. Report of patient with 46 chromosomes. *Neurology* **13,** 913–18.

De Myer, W., Zeman, W. and Palmer, C. (1964) The face predicts the brain: diagnostic significance of median facial anomalies for holoprosencephaly (arhinencephaly). *Pediatrics* **34,** 256–63.

Dennis, J. P., Rosenberg, H. S. and Alvord, E. C. Jr (1961) Megalencephaly, internal hydrocephalus and other neurological aspects of achondroplasia. *Brain* **84,** 427–45.

Denny-Brown, D. (1951) Hereditary sensory radicular neuropathy. *Journal of Neurology, Neurosurgery and Psychiatry* **14,** 237–52.

Deonna, T. (1981) Prognostic des myeloméningocèles.

Journal de Gynécologie Obstétrique et Biologie de la Reproduction **10,** 181–4.

Dieker, H., Edwards, R.H., ZuRhein, G., Chou, S.M., Hartman, H.A. and Opitz, J.M. (1969) The lissencephaly syndrome. *Birth Defects Original Articles Series* **5,** 53–64.

Diezel, P. (1954) Mikrogyrie infolge cerebraler Speicheldrüsenvirusinfektion im Rahmen einer generalisierten Cytomegalie bei einem Säugling zugleich ein Beitrag zur Theorie der Windungsbildung. *Virchows Archiv für Pathologie und Anatomie* **325,** 109–30.

Dimitri, V. (1923) Tumor cerebral congénito (angioma cavernoso) *Revista del Asociacion Medica Argentina* **36,** 1029.

Dobbing, J. (1970) Undernutrition and the developing brain. *American Journal of Diseases of Children* **120,** 411–15.

Dobbing, J. and Sands, J. (1971) Vulnerability of developing brain. IX. The effect of nutritional growth retardation on the timing of the brain growth spurt. *Biology of the Neonate* **19,** 363–78.

Dolgopol, V. B. (1938) Absence of the septum pellucidum as the only anomaly in the brain. *Archives of Neurology and Psychiatry* **40,** 1244–8.

Druckman, R., Chao, D. and Alvord E. C. Jr (1959) A case of atonic cerebral diplegia with lissencephaly. *Neurology* **9,** 806–14.

Dryden, R. J. (1980) Duplication of the spinal cord: a discussion of the possible embryogenesis of diplomyelia. *Developmental Medicine and Child Neurology* **22,** 234–43.

Duckett, S. (1966) Foetal Arnold–Chiari malformation. *Acta Neuropathologica* **7,** 175–9.

Duckett, S. (1971) The morphology of tellurium-induced hydrocephalus. *Experimental Neurology* **31,** 1–16.

Duckett, S. (1972) Teratogenesis of tellurium. *Annals of the New York Academy of Sciences* **192,** 220–6.

Duckett, S., Brent, R. L. and Jensch, R. P. (1974) The morphology of immunologically induced hydrocephalus in the newborn rat. *Journal of Neuropathology and Experimental Neurology* **33,** 365–73.

Duffy, P. E. and Ziter, F. A. (1964) Infantile syringobulbia: a study of its pathology and a proposed relationship to neurogenic stridor in infancy. *Neurology* **14,** 500–9.

Dvorak, K. and Feit, J. (1977) Migration of neuroblasts through partial necrosis of the cerebral cortex in newborn rats. Contribution to the problems of morphological development and developmental period of cerebral microgyria. *Acta Neuropathologica* **38,** 203–12.

Edwards, J.H., Norman, R.M. and Roberts, J.M. (1961) Sex-linked hydrocephalus. Report of a family with 15 affected members. *Archives of Disease in Childhood* **36,** 481–85.

Eichorn, D.H. and Bayley, N. (1962) Growth in head circumference from birth through young adulthood. *Child Development* **33,** 257–71.

Eicke, W.J. (1959) Les maladies inflammatoires de l'encéphale chez le foetus. In *Malformations Congénitales du Cerveau* (Eds. Heuyer, G., Feld, M. and Gruner, J.), pp. 81–92. Masson, Paris.

Elizan, T.S. and Fabiyi, A. (1970) Congenital and neonatal anomalies linked with viral infections in experimental animals. *American Journal of Obstetrics and Gynecology* **106,** 147–65.

Emery, J.L. (1974) Deformity of the aqueduct of Sylvius in children with hydrocephalus and myelomeningocele. *Developmental Medicine and Child Neurology* **16,** suppl. 32, 40–48.

Emery, J.L. and Lendon, R.G. (1969) Lipomas of the cauda equina and other fatty tumours related to neurospinal dysraphism. *Developmental Medicine and Child Neurology* suppl. 20, 62–70.

Emery, J.L. and Lendon, R.G. (1973) The local cord lesion in neurospinal dysraphism (meningomyelocele). *Journal of Pathology* **110,** 83–96.

Epstein, J.A. (1953) Coarctation of the walls of the lateral angles of the lateral cerebral ventricles; a comparative anatomical study. *Journal of Neuropathology and Experimental Neurology* **12,** 302–9.

Evrard, P. and Caviness, V.S. (1974) Extensive developmental defect of the cerebellum associated with posterior fossa ventriculocele. *Journal of Neuropathology and Experimental Neurology* **33,** 385–99.

Fanconi, G. (1962) Sturge–Weber Syndrom beim Neugeborenen. *Helvetica Paediatrica Acta* **17,** 486.

Fauré, C., Lepintre, J. and Lyon, G. (1963) Etude radiologique du syndrome de Dandy–Walker. *Acta Radiologica* **1,** 843–56.

Feld, M. and Gruner, J. (1957) Sur deux cas de porencéphalie hemisphérique malformative associée à une agénésie septale. *Presse Médicale* **15,** 329–82.

Ferrier, D. (1876) *Functions of the Brain.* Smith and Elder, London.

Field, M., Ashton, R. and White, K. (1978) Agenesis of the corpus callosum; report of two preschool children and review of the literature. *Developmental Medicine and Child Neurology* **20,** 47–61.

Flatz, G. and Sukthomya, C. (1970) Fronto-ethmoidal encephalomeningoceles in the population of Northern Thailand. *Humangenetik* **11,** 1–9.

Fletcher, H.M. (1900) A case of megalencephaly. *Transactions of the Pathological Society of London* **51,** 230–2.

Fontan, A. and Battin, J.J. (1965) La mégalencéphalie primitive. *Archives Françaises de Pédiatrie* **22,** 521–9.

Frezal, J., Kelley, J., Guillemot, M.L. and Lamy, M. (1964) Anencephaly in France. *American Journal of Human Genetics* **16,** 336–50.

Friede, R.L. (1964) Arrested cerebellar development. A type of cerebellar degeneration in amaurotic idiocy. *Journal of Neurology, Neurosurgery and Psychiatry* **27,** 41–5.

Friede, R.L. (1975) *Developmental Neuropathology.* Springer, Vienna.

Friede, R.L. and Boltshauser, E. (1978) Uncommon syndromes of cerebellar vermis aplasia. I. Joubert syndrome. *Developmental Medicine and Child Neurology* **20,** 758–63.

Friede, R.L. and Mikolasek, J. (1978) Postencephalitic porencephaly hydranencephaly or polymicrogyria. A review. *Acta Neuropathologica* **43,** 161–8.

Friedman, M. and Cohen, P. (1947) Agenesis of corpus callosum as a possible sequel to maternal rubella during pregnancy. *American Journal of Diseases of Children* **73,** 178–85.

Garcia, C.A., Dunn, D. and Trevor, R. (1978) The lissencephaly (agyria) syndrome in siblings, computerized tomographic and neuropathologic findings. *Archives of Neurology* **35,** 608–11.

Gardner, E., O'Rahilly, R. and Prolo, D. (1975) The Dandy-Walker and Arnold-Chiari malformations: clinical developmental and teratological considerations. *Archives of Neurology* **32,** 393–407.

Gardner, W.J. (1961) Rupture of the neural tube. The cause of myelomeningocele. *Archives of Neurology* **4,** 1–7.

Gardner, W.J. (1965) Hydrodynamic mechanism of syringomyelia: its relationship to myelocele. *Journal of Neurology, Neurosurgery and Psychiatry* **28,** 247–59.

Gardner, W.J. (1973). *The Dysraphic States.* Excerpta Medica, Amsterdam.

Geoffroy Saint-Hilaire, I. (1825) Sur de nouveaux anencéphales humains confirmant par leur fait d'organisation la derniée théorie sur les monstres. *Mémoires du Muséum d'histoire Naturelle* (*Paris*) **12,** 233–56.

Geoffroy Saint-Hilaire, I. (1832) *Histoire générale et particulière des Anomalies de l'organisation chez l'homme et les animaux.* J.B. Baillère, Paris.

Giannelli, F., Hamerton, J.L. and Carter, C.O. (1965) Cytogenetics of Down's syndrome (mongolism). II. The frequency of interchange trisomy in patients born at a maternal age of less than 30 years. *Cytogenetics* **4,** 186–92.

Gillman, J., Gilbert, C., Gillman, T. and Spence, I. (1948) A preliminary report on hydrocephalus, spina bifida, and other congenital anomalies in the rat produced by trypan blue. *South African Journal of Medical Sciences* **13,** 47–90.

Gillman, J., Gilbert, C., Spence, I. and Gillman, T. (1951) A further report on congenital anomalies in the rat produced by trypan blue. *South African Journal of Medical Sciences* **16,** 125–35.

Gilly, R., Cotton, J., Farouz, S., Noiret, A. and Maclet, M. (1971) Hydrocéphalie congénitale et anomalie bilatérale des pouces: syndrome malformatif lié au chromosome 'X'. *Pédiatrie* **26,** 365–78.

Giroud, A. (1960) Causes and morphogenesis of anencephaly. In *Congenital Malformations*, Ciba Foundation Symposium, pp. 199–212. Churchill, London.

Giroud, A. (1977) Anencephaly. In *Handbook of Clinical Neurology*, vol. 30 (Eds. Vinken, P.J. and Bruyn, G.W.), pp. 173–208. North-Holland, Amsterdam.

Giroud, A. and Martinet, M. (1956) Tératogénèse par hautes doses de vitamine A en fonction des stades du développement. *Archives d'Anatomie Microscopique et de Morphologie Expérimentale* **46,** 77–99.

Gomez, M.R., Whitten, C.F., Nolke, A., Berstein, J. and Meyer, J.S. (1963) Aneurysmal malformation of the great vein of Galen causing heart failure in early infancy: report of 5 cases. *Pediatrics* **31,** 400–11.

Gouttières, F., Aicardi, J. and Farkas, E. (1977) Anterior horn cell disease associated with pontocerebellar hypoplasia in infants. *Journal of Neurology, Neurosurgery and Psychiatry* **40,** 370–8.

Gowers, W.R. and Taylor, J. (1899) *A Manual of Diseases of the Nervous System*, 3rd edn. Churchill, London.

Grčević N. and Robert, F. (1961) Verrucose dysplasia of the cerebral cortex (dysgénésie nodulaire disséminée de Morel et Wildi). *Journal of Neuropathology and Experimental Neurology* **20,** 399–411.

Greenfield, G. and Wolfsohn, J. (1935) Microcephalia vera. A study of two brains illustrating the agyric form and the complex microgyric form. *Archives of Neurology and Psychiatry* **33,** 1296–316.

Gregg, N. McA. (1941) Congenital cataract following German measles in the mother. *Transactions of the Ophthalmological Society of Australia* **3,** 35–46.

Grogono, J.L. (1968) Children with agenesis of the corpus callosum. *Developmental Medicine and Child Neurology* **10,** 613–16.

Grollmus, J.M., Wilson, C.B. and Newton, T.H. (1976) Paramesencephalic arachnoid cysts. *Neurology* **26,** 128–34.

Gross, H. and Hoff, H. (1959) Sur les dysraphies cranio-encéphaliques. In *Malformations congénitales du Cerveau* (Eds. Heuyer, G., Feld, M. and Gruner, J.), pp. 287–96. Masson, Paris.

Gross, H. and Kaltenback, E. (1959) Uber eine kombinierte progressive pontocerebelläre Systematrophie bei einem Kleinkind. *Deutsche Zeitschrift für Nervenheilkunde* **179,** 388–400.

Gruenwald, P. and Minh, H. (1960) Evaluation of body and organ weights in perinatal pathology. I. Normal standard derived from autopsies. *American Journal of Clinical Pathology* **39,** 247–53.

Guibaud, S., Simplot, A., Bonnet, M., Thoulon, J.M., Guibaud, P. and Robert, J.M. (1982) Acétylcholinestérase du liquide amniotique. Application au diagnostic prénatal des défauts de fermeture du tube neural. II. Test qualitatif. *Journal de Génétique Humaine* **30,** 119–34.

Hallervorden, J. (1949) Ueber eine Kohlenoxydvergiftung im Fötalleben mit Entwicklungsstörung der Hirnrinde. *Allgemeine Zeitschrift für Psychiatrie* **124,** 289–98.

Hamerton, J.L., Giannelli, F. and Polani, P.E. (1965) Cytogenetics of Down's syndrome (mongolism). I. Data on a consecutive series of patients referred for genetic counselling and diagnosis. *Cytogenetics* **4,** 171–85.

Hanaway, J. and Netsky, M. (1971) Heterotopias of the inferior olive: relation to Dandy–Walker malformation and correlation with experimental data. *Journal of Neuropathology and Experimental Neurology* **30,** 380–389.

Hansen, F.J. and Friis, B. (1976) Familial occurrence of cerebral gigantism. Sotos' syndrome. *Acta Paediatrica Scandinavica* **65,** 387–9.

Hart, M.N., Malamud, N. and Ellis, W.G. (1972) The Dandy–Walker syndrome. A clinicopathological study based on 28 cases. *Neurology* **22,** 771–80.

Harwood-Nash, D.C. and Breckbill, D. (1976) Computed tomography in children: a new diagnostic technique. *Journal of Pediatrics* **89,** 343–57.

Harwood-Nash, D.C. and Fitz, C.R. (1976) *Neuroradiology in Infants and Children*, vol. III, pp. 1026–33. Mosby, St Louis, Mo.

Hatjis, C.G., Horber, J.D. and Anderson, G.G. (1981) The *in utero* diagnosis of a posterior fossa intracranial cyst (Dandy–Walker cyst). *American Journal of Obstetrics and Gynecology* **140,** 473–4.

Haymaker, W., Girdany, B.R., Stephens, J., Lillie, R.D. and Fetterman, G.H. (1954) Cerebral involvement with advanced periventricular calcification in generalized cytomegalic inclusion disease of the newborn. *Journal of Neuropathology and Experimental Neurology* **13,** 562–86.

Hicks, S.P. (1952) Symposium on cerebral palsy: some effects of ionizing radiation and metabolic inhibition on developing mammalian nervous system. *Journal of Pediatrics* **40,** 489–513.

Hicks, S.P. (1953a) Developmental brain metabolism—effects of cortisone, anoxia, fluoroacetate, radiation, insulin and other inhibitors on the embryo, newborn and adult. *Archives of Pathology* **55,** 302–27.

Hicks, S.P. (1953b) Developmental malformations produced by radiation. *American Journal of Roentgenology* **69,** 272–93.

Hicks, S.P. (1954) Mechanism of radiation anencephaly, anophthalmia and pituitary anomalies repair in the mammalian embryo. *Archives of Pathology* **57,** 363–78.

von Hippel, E.V. (1904) Ueber eine sehr seltene Erkrankung der Netzhaut. *Albrecht von Graefes Archiv für Ophthalmologie* **59,** 83–106.

von Hippel, E. (1907) Über experimentelle Erzeugung von angeborenen Star bei Kaninchen nebst Bemerkungen über gleichzeitig beobachteten Mikrophthalmus und Lidcolobom. *Albrecht von Graefes Archiv für Ophthalmologie* **65,** 326–60.

Hirano, A., Dembitzer, H.M. and Jones, M. (1972) An electron microscopic study of cycasin-induced cerebellar alterations. *Journal of Neuropathology and Experimental Neurology* **31,** 113–25.

Hirano, A. and Solomon, S. (1960) Arteriovenous aneurysm of the vein of Galen. *Archives of Neurology* **3,** 589–93.

Hirano, A., Dembitzer, H.M., Ghatak, N.R., Fan, K.J. and Zimmerman, H.M. (1973) On the relationship between human and experimental granule cell type cerebellar degeneration. *Journal of Neuropathology and Experimental Neurology* **32,** 493–502.

Hochstetter, F. (1929) *Beiträge zur Entwicklungsgeschichte des menschlichen Gehirns.* Deuticke, Vienna and Leipzig.

Hofman, M.A. (1984) Energy metabolism and relative brain size in human neonates from single and multiple gestations: an allometric study. *Biology of the Neonate* **45,** 157–64.

Holden, A.M., Fyler, D.C., Shillito, J. Jr and Nadas, A. S. (1972) Congestive heart failure from intracranial arteriovenous fistula in infancy. *Pediatrics* **49,** 30–9.

Holmes, L., Nash, A., Zurhein, G., Levin, M. and Opitz, J. (1973) X-linked aqueductal stenosis: clinical and morphological finding in two families. *Pediatrics* **51,** 697–704.

Hsi-Chih-Chao, D. (1959) Congenital neurocutaneous syndrome in children. I. Neurofibromatosis; II. Tuberous sclerosis; III. Sturge–Weber disease. *Journal of Pediatrics* **55,** 189–99; 447–59; 635–49.

Hughes, J.T. and Brownell, B. (1963) Aberrant nerve fibres within the spinal cord. *Journal of Neurology, Neurosurgery and Psychiatry* **26,** 528–34.

Jakob, H. (1940) Die feinere Oberflächengestaltung der Hirnwindungen; die Hirnwarzenbildung und die Mikropolygyrie. *Zeitschrift für die gesamte Neurologie und Psychiatrie* **170,** 64–84.

James, C.C.M. and Lassman, L.P. (1972) *Spinal Dysraphism; spina bifida occulta.* Butterworths, London.

Jellinger, K. and Gross, H. (1973) Congenital telencephalic midline defects. *Neuropädiatrie* **4**, 446–52.

Jellinger, K. and Rett, A. (1976) Agyria-pachygyria (lissencephaly syndrome). *Neuropädiatrie* **7**, 66–91.

Jervis, G.A. (1948) Early senile dementia in mongoloid idiocy. *American Journal of Psychiatry* **105**, 102–6.

Jervis, G.A. (1950) Early familial cerebellar degeneration: report of 3 cases in one family. *Journal of Nervous and Mental Disease* **111**, 398–407.

Johnson, F.E. (1938) Injury of the child by Roentgen ray during pregnancy. Report of a case. *Journal of Pediatrics* **13**, 894–901.

Johnson, R.T. (1982) *Viral Infections of the Nervous System*. Raven Press, New York.

Johnston, J.B. (1913) The morphology of the septum, hippocampus and pallial commissure in reptiles and mammals. *Journal of Comparative Neurology* **23**, 371–478.

Jonesco-Sisesti, N. (1932) *La Syringobulbie*. Masson, Paris.

Josephy, H. (1944) Congenital agyria and defect of the corpus callosum. *Journal of Neuropathology and Experimental Neurology* **3**, 69–72.

Joubert, M., Eisenring, J.J., Robb, J.P. and Andermann, F. (1969) Familial agenesis of the cerebellar vermis. A syndrome of episodic hyperpnea, abnormal eye movements, ataxia and retardation. *Neurology* **19**, 813–25.

Kalischer, S. (1897) Demonstration des Gehirns eines Kindes mit Telangectasie der links-seitigen Gesicht und Kopfhaut und der Hirnoberfläche. *Klinische Wochenschrift* **34**, 1059.

Källén, B. and Levan, A. (1970) Chromosomes in man, with special reference to neuropathological disorders in *Neuropathology: Methods and Diagnosis* (Ed. Tedeschi, C.G.), pp. 547–82. Little, Brown, Boston, Mass.

Kalter, H. (1968) *Teratology of the central nervous system* (induced and spontaneous malformations of laboratory, agricultural and domestic mammals). University of Chicago Press, Chicago and London.

Karch, S.B. and Urich, H. (1972) Occipital encephalocele: a morphological study. *Journal of Neurological Sciences* **15**, 89–112.

Kilham, L. and Margolis, G. (1964) Cerebellar ataxia in hamsters inoculated with rat virus. *Science* **143**, 1047–8.

Kitahara, T. and Maki, U. (1978) A case of Sturge-Weber disease with epilepsy and intracranial calcification at the neonatal period. *European Neurology* **17**, 8–12.

Kosary, I.Z., Braham, J., Shaked, I. and Tadmor, R. (1969) Cervical syringomyelia associated with occipital meningioma. *Neurology* **19**, 1127–30.

Krabbe, K.B. (1934) Facial and meningeal anomalies associated with calcifications of brain cortex; clinical and anatomopathologic contribution. *Archives of Neurology and Psychiatry* **32**, 737–55.

Kramer, W. (1956) Dysgenetic gliosis of the brain—a case of macrogyria. *Journal of Neuropathology and Experimental Neurology* **15**, 471–84.

Kruyff, E. (1965) Paracollicular plate cysts. *American Journal of Roentgenology* **95**, 899–916.

Kuhlendahl, H.D., Gross-Selbeck, G., Doose, H., Klinge, H. and Jensen, H.P. (1977) Cranial computer tomography in children with tuberous sclerosis. *Neuropädiatrie* **8**, 325–32.

Lagos, J.C. (1977) Congenital aneurysms and arteriovenous malformations. In *Handbook of Clinical Neurology*, vol. 31 (Eds. Vinken, P.J. and Bruyn, G.N.), pp. 137–209. North-Holland, Amsterdam.

de Lange, C. (1929) Klinische und pathologisch anatomische Mitteilungen über Hydrocephalus chronicus congenitus und acquisitus. *Zeitschrift für die gesamte Neurologie und Psychiatrie* **120**, 433.

de Lange, C. (1939) Lissenzephalie beim Menschen. *Monatschrift für Psychiatrie und Neurologie* **101**, 350–81.

Larroche, J.Cl. (1962) Quelques aspects anatomiques du développement cérébral. *Biology of the Neonate* **4**, 126–53.

Larroche, J.Cl. (1969) Histologic anomalies in the cerebellum (incidence and interpretation). In *Third International Conference on Congenital Malformations, The Hague*. Excerpta Medica, Amsterdam.

Larroche, J.Cl. (1977a) *Developmental Pathology of the Neonate*. Excerpta Medica, Amsterdam.

Larroche, J.Cl. (1977b) Cytoarchitectonic abnormalities (abnormalities of cell migration). In *Handbook of Clinical Neurology*, vol. 30 (Eds. Vinken, P.J. and Bruyn, G.W.), pp. 479–506. North-Holland, Amsterdam.

Larroche, J.Cl. and Baudey, J. (1961) Cavum septi lucidi, cavum vergae, cavum veli interpositi: cavités de la ligne médiane (étude anatomique et pneumoencephalographique dans la période néonatale). *Biologia Neonatorum* **3**, 193–236.

Larroche, J.Cl. and Maunoury, T. (1973) Analyse statistique de la croissance pondérale des foetus et des viscères pendant la vie intrautérine. *Archives Françaises de Pédiatrie* **30**, 927–49.

La Torre, E., Fortuna, A. and Occhipinti, E. (1973) Angiographic differentiation between Dandy-Walker cyst and arachnoid cyst of the posterior fossa in newborn infants and children. *Journal of Neurosurgery* **38**, 298–308.

Laurence, K.M. and Tew, B.J. (1967) Follow-up of 65 survivors from the 425 cases of spina bifida born in South Wales between 1956 and 1962. *Developmental Medicine and Child Neurology* suppl. 13, 1–13.

Lazar, M.L. (1974) Vein of Galen aneurysm: successful excision of a completely thrombosed aneurysm in an infant. *Surgical Neurology* **2,** 22-4.

Lefevre, J., Klein, M.R. and Fauré, C. (1956) La diastématomyélie. *Revue Neurologique* **94,** 357-62.

Lemire, R.J., Loeser, J.D., Leech, R.W. and Alvord, E.C. (1975) *Normal and Abnormal Development of the Human Nervous System.* Harper and Row, Hagerstown, Md.

Levine, D.N., Fisher, M.A. and Caviness, V.S. (1974) Porencephaly with microgyria: a pathological study. *Acta Neuropathologica* **29,** 99-113.

Levine, O.R., Jameson, A., Nellhaus, G. and Gold, A.P. (1962) Cardiac complications of cerebral arterio-venous fistula in infancy. *Pediatrics* **30,** 563-75.

Lhermitte, J. and Duclos, P. (1920) Sur un ganglioneurome diffus du cortex du cervelet. *Bulletin de l'Association Francaise pour l'étude du Cancer* **9,** 99-107.

Lindau, A. (1926) Studien über Kleinhirncysten. Bau, Pathogenese und Beziehungen zur Angiomatosis retinae. *Acta Pathologica et Microbiologica Scandinavica* suppl. 1, 1-128.

Litvak, J., Yahr, M.D. and Ransohoff, J. (1960) Aneurysms of great vein of Galen and midline cerebral arteriovenous anomalies. *Journal of Neurosurgery* **17,** 945-54.

Loeser, J.D. and Alvord, E.C. (1968a) Clinicopathological correlation in agenesis of the corpus callosum. *Neurology* **18,** 745-56.

Loeser, J.D. and Alvord, E.C. (1968b) Agenesis of the corpus callosum. *Brain* **91,** 553-70.

Lorber, J. (1971) Results of treatment of myelomeningocele. An analysis of 524 unselected cases, with special reference to possible selection for treatment. *Developmental Medicine and Child Neurology* suppl. **13,** 279.

Loth, P., Casasoprana, A. and Thibert, M. (1972) Une cause rare de défaillance cardiaque néonatale: l'anévrysme arterio-veineux intracranien. *Archives Française de Pédiatrie* **24,** 255-68.

Lourie, H. and Berne, A. (1961) A contribution on the etiology and pathogenesis of congenital communicating hydrocephalus. *Biologia Neonatorum* **15,** 815-22.

Lubchenco, L.O., Hansman, C., Dresseler, M. and Boyd, E. (1963) Intrauterine growth as estimated from live born birth weight data at 24 and 42 weeks of gestation. *Pediatrics* **32,** 793-800.

Macchi, G. and Bentivoglio, M. (1977) Agenesis or hypoplasia of cerebellar structures. In *Handbook of Clinical Neurology*, vol. 30 (Eds. Vinken, P.J. and Bruyn, G.N.), pp. 367-93. Elsevier/North-Holland, Amsterdam.

Mack, L.D., Rumack, C.M. and Johnson, M.L. (1980) Ultrasound evaluation of cystic intracranial lesions in the neonate. *Radiology* **137,** 451-5.

MacKenzie, N.G. and Emery, J.L. (1971) Deformities of the cervical cord in children with neurospinal dysraphism. *Developmental Medicine and Child Neurology* **13,** suppl. 25, 58-61.

McKusick, V.A. (1971) *Mendelian Inheritance in Man: catalogue of autosomal dominant, autosomal recessive, and X-linked phenotypes*, 3rd edn, pp. 440-1. Johns Hopkins Press, Baltimore, Md.

McKusick, V.A. (1978) *Mendelian inheritance in Man: catalogs of autosomal dominant, autosomal recessive and X-linked phenotypes*, 5th edn. Johns Hopkins Press, Baltimore, Md.

McLaurin, R.L. (1964) Parietal cephaloceles. *Neurology* **14,** 764-74.

Malamud, N. (1972) Neuropathology of organic brain syndromes associated with aging. In *Aging and the Brain* (Ed. Gaitz, C.M.), pp. 63-87. Plenum, New York.

Marburg, O. (1949) So-called agenesis of the corpus callosum (callosal defect). *Archives of Neurology and Psychiatry* **61,** 297-312.

Marie, J., See, G., Gruner, J., Hebert, S., de Gennes, J.L. and de Fouquet, J. (1957) Manifestations cérébrales de la maladie des inclusions cytomégaliques. *Annales de Pédiatrie* **25,** 248-56.

Marin-Padilla, M. (1965) Study of the skull in human cranioschisis. *Acta Anatomica* **62,** 1-20.

Marin-Padilla, M. (1970) Morphogenesis of anencephaly and related malformations. *Current Topics in Pathology* **51,** 145-74.

Marin-Padilla, M. (1978) Clinical and experimental rachischisis. In *Handbook of Clinical Neurology*, vol. 32 (Eds. Vinken, P.J. and Bruyn, G.W.), pp.159-91. Elsevier/North-Holland, Amsterdam.

Marin-Padilla, M. (1980) Morphogenesis of experimental encephalocele (cranioschisis occulta). *Journal of the Neurological Sciences* **46,** 83-99.

Martin, J.K. and Norman, R.M. (1967) Maple syrup urine disease in an infant with microgyria. *Developmental Medicine and Child Neurology* **9,** 152-9.

Matson, D., Woods, R., Campbell, J. and Ingraham, F. (1950) Diastematomyelia: diagnosis and surgical treatment. *Pediatrics* **6,** 98-112.

Menkes, J.H., Philippart, M. and Clark, D.E. (1964) Hereditary partial agenesis of the corpus callosum. *Archives of Neurology* **11,** 198-208.

Meyer, A. and Jones, T.B. (1939) Histological changes in brain in mongolism. *Journal of Mental Science* **85,** 206-21.

Michaud, J., Mizrahi, E.M. and Urich, H. (1982) Agenesis of the vermis with fusion of the cerebellar hemispheres. septo-optic dysplasia and associated anomalies. Report of a case. *Acta Neuropathologica* **56,** 161-6.

Miller, J. (1963) Lissencephaly in two siblings. *Neurology* **13,** 841–50.

Miller, L.Q., Picard, E., Elkan, M., Warner, B. and Gerald, P. (1963) A specific congenital brain defect (arhinencephaly) in 13–15 trisomy. *New England Journal of Medicine* **268,** 120–4.

Miller, R.W. (1968) Effects of ionizing radiation from the atomic bomb on Japanese children. *Pediatrics* **41,** 257–63.

Milunsky, A., Ellcott, A., Neff, R.K. and Frigoletto, F.D. Jr (1980) Prenatal diagnosis of neural tube defects. IV. Maternal serum alpha-fetoprotein screening. *Obstetrics and Gynecology* **55,** 60.

Miskolczy, D. (1931) Ein Fall von Kleinhirnmissbildung. *Archiv für Psychiatrie und Nervenkrankheiten* **93,** 596–615.

Molland, E.A. and Purcell, M. (1975) Biliary atresia and the Dandy–Walker anomaly, in a neonate with 45X Turner's syndrome. *Journal of Pathology* **115,** 227–30.

Monaghan, H.P., Krafchik, B.R., Macgregor, D.L. and Fitz, C.R. (1981) Tuberous sclerosis complex in children. *American Journal of Diseases of Children* **135,** 912–17.

Montoya, G., Dohn, D.F. and Mercer, R.D. (1971) Arteriovenous malformation of the vein of Galen as a cause of heart failure and hydrocephalus in infants. *Neurology* **21,** 1054–8.

Morel, F. and Wildi, E. (1952) Dysgénésie nodulaire disséminée de l'écorce frontale. *Revue Neurologique* **87,** 251–70.

Morel, F. and Wildi, E. (1954) Les ventricules cérébraux dans la démence précoce. *Monatsschrift für Psychiatrie und Neurologie* **127,** 1–10.

Morgagni, J.B. (1761) *De Sedibus et Causis Morborum.* Trans. by B. Alexander (1769) *The Seats and Causes of Diseases Investigated by Anatomy,* vols. I, II and III.

Mueller, C. (1970) Heterotopic gray matter. *Radiology* **94,** 357–8.

Mutrux, S., Wildi, E. and Bourquin, J. (1949) Contribution à l'étude clinique et anatomo-pathologique des troubles cérébraux de l'embryopathie rubéoleuse. *Schweizer Archiv für Neurologie und Psychiatrie* **64,** 369–83.

Naiman, J. and Frazer, F.C. (1955) Agenesis of the corpus callosum. *Archives of Neurology and Psychiatry* **74,** 182–5.

Nakado, K.K. (1973) Anencephaly: a review. *Developmental Medicine and Child Neurology* **15,** 383–400.

Nathanson, N., Cole, G. and Van der Loos, H. (1969) Heterotopic cerebellar granule cells following administration of cyclophosphamide to suckling rats. *Brain Research* **15,** 532–6.

Nellhaus, G. (1968) Head circumference from birth to eighteen years. Practical composite international and interracial graphs. *Pediatrics* **41,** 106–19.

Nellhaus, G., Haberland, C. and Hill, B. (1967) Sturge–Weber disease with bilateral intracranial calcifications at birth and unusual pathologic findings. *Acta Neurologica Scandinavica* **43,** 314–27.

Nevin, N.C., Johnston, W.P. and Merrett, J.D. (1981) Influence of social class on the risk of recurrence of anencephalus and spina bifida. *Developmental Medicine and Child Neurology* **23,** 155–9.

Newman, G.C., Buschi, A.I., Sugg, N.K., Kelly, T.E. and Miller, J.Q. (1982) Dandy–Walker syndrome diagnosed in utero by ultrasonography. *Neurology* **32,** 180–4.

Norman, M.G. (1980) Bilateral encephaloclastic lesions in a 26 week gestation fetus: effect on neuroblast migration. *Journal Canadien des Sciences Neurologiques* **7,** 191–4.

Norman, M.G. and Becker, L.E. (1974) Cerebral damage in neonates resulting from arterio-venous malformations in the vein of Galen. *Journal of Neurology, Neurosurgery and Psychiatry* **37,** 252–8.

Norman, M.G., Thurber, L.A. and Woolley, H.E. (1981) Abnormal leptomeninges and vessels causing fetal hydrocephalus. Diagnosis of hydrocephalus at 19 weeks' gestation by ultrasound. *Acta Neuropathologica* **54,** 283–6.

Norman, M.G., Roberts, J., Siroid, J. and Tremblay, L.J.M. (1976) Lissencephaly. *Journal Canadien des Sciences Neurologiques* **3,** 39–46.

Norman, R.M. (1940) Primary degeneration of the granular layer of the cerebellum; an unusual form of familial cerebellar atrophy occurring in early life. *Brain* **63,** 365–79.

Norman, R.M. (1961) Cerebellar hypoplasia in Werdnig–Hoffmann disease. *Archives of Disease in Childhood* **36,** 96–101.

Norman, R.M. (1963) Malformations of the nervous system. In *Neuropathology* (Ed. Greenfield, J.G.), pp. 363–69. Edward Arnold, London.

Norman, R.M. (1966) Neuropathological findings in trisomies 13–15 and 17–18 with special reference to the cerebellum. *Developmental Medicine and Child Neurology* **8,** 170–7.

Norman, R.M. and McMenemey, W.H. (1955) Transventricular adhesion in association with birth injury of the caudate nucleus. *Journal of Neuropathology and Experimental Neurology* **14,** 85–91.

Norman, R.M. and Urich, H. (1958) Cerebellar hypoplasia associated with systemic degeneration in early life. *Journal of Neurology, Neurosurgery and Psychiatry* **21,** 159–66.

Norman, R.M. and Urich, H. (1962) Birth injury due to compression of cerebral arteries. In *London Conference on the Scientific Study of Mental Deficiency*, pp. 299–313. May and Baker, London.

Norman, R.M., Urich, H. and Woods, G.E. (1958) The relationship between prenatal porencephaly and the encephalomalacias of early life. *Journal of Mental Science* **104,** 758–71.

Norman, R.M., Tingey, A.H., Valentine, J.C. and Danby, T.A. (1962) Sudanophil leucodystrophy in a pachygyric brain *Journal of Neurology, Neurosurgery and Psychiatry* **25,** 363–9.

O'Brien, M.S. and Schechter, M.M. (1970) Arteriovenous malformations involving the Galenic system. *American Journal of Roentgenology* **110,** 50–5.

Oliver, L.C. (1958) Primary arachnoid cysts. Report of two cases. *British Medical Journal* **1,** 1147–9.

Olson, M.I. and Shaw, C.M. (1969) Presenile dementia and Alzheimer's disease in mongolism. *Brain* **92,** 147–56.

Oppenheimer, D.R. (1955) A benign 'tumour' of the cerebellum. *Journal of Neurology, Neurosurgery and Psychiatry* **18,** 199–213.

Padget, D.H. (1968) Spina bifida and embryonic neuroschisis: a causal relationship. *Johns Hopkins Medical Journal* **123,** 233–52.

Padget, D. (1970) Neuroschisis and human embryonic maldevelopment: new evidence on anencephaly, spina bifida and diverse mammalian defects. *Journal of Neuropathology and Experimental Neurology* **29,** 192–216.

Padget, D.H. and Lindenberg, R. (1972) Inverse cerebellum morphogenetically related to Dandy–Walker and Arnold–Chiari syndromes: bizarre malformed brain with occipital encephalocele. *Johns Hopkins Medical journal* **131,** 228–46.

Patau, K., Smith, D.W., Therman, E., Inhorn, S.L. and Wagner, H.P. (1960) Multiple congenital anomaly caused by an extra autosome. *Lancet* **1,** 790–3.

Patten, B.M. (1952) Overgrowth of the neural tube in young human embryos. *Anatomical Record* **113,** 381–93.

Peach, B. (1965) Arnold–Chiari malformation: Morphogenesis. *Archives of Neurology* **12,** 527–35.

Penfield, W. and Coburn, D.F. (1938) Arnold–Chiari malformation and its operative treatment. *Archives of Neurology and Psychiatry* **40,** 328–36.

Penfield, W. and Hyndman, O. (1934) Agenesis of the corpus callosum with discussion of ventriculograms in two living cases. *Transactions of the American Neurological Association* **60,** 182–4.

Penrose, L.S. (1957) Genetics of anencephaly. *Journal of Mental Deficiency Research* **1,** 4–15.

Perez-Fontan, J.J., Herrera, M., Fina, A. and Peguero, G. (1982) Periventricular calcifications in a newborn associated with aneurysm of the great vein of Galen. *Pediatric Radiology* **12,** 249–51.

Pernot, C., Worms, A.M. and Merlin, J.P. (1972) Le rhabdomyome congénital du coeur chez l'enfant. *Pédiatrie* **27,** 5–17.

Pfleger, L. (1880) Beobachtungen über Heterotopie grauer Substanz im Marke des Kleinhirns. *Zentralblatt für die Medizinischen Wissenschaften* **18,** 468–70.

Phemister, R., Shively, J. and Young, S. (1969a) The effects of gamma-irradiation on the postnatally developing canine cerebellar cortex. I. Effects of single sublethal exposures. *Journal of Neuropathology and Experimental Neurology* **28,** 119–27.

Phemister, R., Shively, J. and Young, S. (1969b) The effects of gamma-irradiation on the postnatally developing canine cerebellar cortex. II. Sequential histogenesis of radiation-induced changes. *Journal of Neuropathology and Experimental Neurology* **28,** 128–38.

Pitt, D.B. (1962) A study of congenital malformations. Parts I and II. *Australian and New Zealand Journal of Obstetrics and Gynaecology* **2,** 23–30; 82–90.

Plaix, M.H. (1984) Aspect échographique et évolution des cavités de la ligne médiane chez le foetus. *Journal d'Echographie et de Mèdecine Ultrasonore,* **4,** 239–44.

Plummer, C. (1952) Anomalies occurring in children exposed *in utero* to atomic bomb in Hiroshima. *Pediatrics* **10,** 687–93.

Polani, P.E., Hamerton, J.L., Giannelli, F. and Carter, C.O. (1965) Cytogenetics of Down's syndrome (mongolism). III. Frequency of interchange trisomies and mutation rate of chromosome interchanges. *Cytogenetics* **4,** 193–206.

Pollock, A.Q. and Laslett, P.A. (1958) Cerebral arteriovenous fistula producing cardiac failure in the newborn infant. *Journal of Pediatrics* **53,** 731–6.

Ponsot, G. and Lyon, G. (1977) La sclérose tubéreuse de Bourneville (étude clinique et génétique de 59 observations chez l'enfant). *Archives Françaises de Pédiatrie* **34,** 9–22.

Poser, C.M. (1956) *The Relationship between Syringomyelia and Neoplasm.* Thomas, Springfield, Ill.

Potter, E. (1953) Sturge–Kalischer–Weber syndrome. In *Pathology of the Fetus and the Newborn.* Year Book, Chicago.

Pratt-Thomas, H.R. (1947) Tuberous sclerosis with congenital tumors of heart and kidney. *American Journal of Pathology* **23,** 189–99.

Priestley, D.B. (1920) Complete absence of the cerebellum *Lancet* **2,** 1302–17.

Probst, A. and Ohnacker, H. (1977) Sclérose tubéreuse de Bourneville chez un prématuré. *Acta Neuropathologica* **40,** 157–61.

Probst, F. (1973) Congenital defects of the corpus callosum. Morphology and encephalographic appearances. *Acta Radiologica* suppl. 331, 1–152.

Probst, M. (1901) Über den Bau des vollständig balkenlosen Grosshirns sowie über Mikrogyrie und Heterotopie der grauen Substanz. *Archiv für Psychiatrie und Nervenkrankheiten* **34,** 709–86.

Rakic, P. (1971) Neuron-glia relationship during granule cell migration in developing cerebellar cortex. A Golgi and electron microscopic study in *Macacus rhesus*. *Journal of Comparative Neurology* **141,** 283-312.

Rakic, P. and Sidman, R.L. (1973) Sequence of developmental abnormalities leading to granule cell deficit in cerebellar cortex of weaver mutant mice. *Journal of Comparative Neurology* **152,** 103-32.

Rakic, P. and Yakovlev, P.I. (1968) Development of the corpus callosum and cavum septi in man. *Journal of Comparative Neurology* **132,** 45-72.

Ranke, O. (1905) Status corticis verrucosus deformis. *Zeitschrift für die gesamte Neurologie und Psychiatrie* **28,** 635-750.

Ranke, O. (1910) Beiträge zur Kenntnis der normalen und pathologischen Hirnrindenbildung. *Beiträge zur pathologischen Anatomie und Allgemeinen Pathologie* **47,** 51-125.

von Recklinghausen, F. (1862) Ein Herz von einem Neugeborenen, welches mehrere, theils nach aussen, theils nach den Höhlen prominierende Tumoren (Myome) trug. *Monatsschrift für Geburtshilfe und Gynäkologie* **20,** 1-2.

von Recklinghausen, F. (1882) *Über die multiplen Fibrome der Haut und ihre Beziehung zu den multiplen Neuromen.* Hirschwald, Berlin.

von Recklinghausen, F. (1886) Untersuchungen über die Spina bifida. II.Ueber die Art und die Entstehung der spina bifida, ihre Beziehung zur Rückenmarks- und Darmspalte. *Virchows Archiv für Pathologie und Anatomie* **105,** 296-330.

Record, R.G. and McKeown, T. (1950) Congenital malformations of central nervous system; maternal reproductive history and familial incidence. *British Journal of Social Medicine* **4,** 26-50.

Remington, J.S. and Klein, J.O. (1976) *Infectious Disease of the Fetus and Newborn Infant.* Saunders, Philadelphia, Pa.

Rengachary, S.S. and Watanabe, I. (1982) Ultrastructure and pathogenesis of intracranial arachnoid cysts. *Journal of Neuropathology and Experimental Neurology* **40,** 61-83.

Renier, W., Gabreëls, F., Mol. L. and Korten, J. (1973) Agenesis of the corpus callosum, chorioretinopathy and infantile spasms (Aicardi syndrome). *Psychiatria, Neurologia, Neurochirurgia* **76,** 39-45.

Renier, W.O., Gabreëls, F.J.M., Hustinx, T.W.J., Thyssen, H.O.M. Ter Haar, B.G.A., Kroll, E.W. and Beckers, H. (1983) Cerebellar hypoplasia, communicating hydrocephalus and mental retardation in two brothers and a maternal uncle. *Brain and Development* **5,** 41-5.

Renwick, J.H. (1972) Hypothesis: anencephaly and spina bifida are usually preventable by avoidance of a specific but unidentified substance present in certain potato tubers. *British Journal of Preventive and Social Medicine* **26,** 67-88.

Retzius, G. (1895) In *Das Menschenhirn.* Stockholm (quoted by Streeter, 1912).

Ribadeau-Dumas, J.L., Poirier, J. and Escourolle, R. (1973) Etude ultrastructurale des lésions cérébrales de la sclérose tubéreuse de Bourneville. *Acta Neuropathologica* **25,** 259-70.

Riccardi, V.M. and Marcus, E.S. (1978) Congenital hydrocephalus and cerebellar agenesis. *Clinical Genetics* **13,** 443-7.

Richman, D.P., Stewart, R.M. and Caviness, V.S. (1974) Cerebellar microgyria in a 27 week fetus: an architectonic and topographic analysis. *Journal of Neuropathology and Experimental Neurology* **33,** 374-84.

Robain, O. and Gorce, F. (1972) Arhinencéphalie. *Archives Françaises de Pédiatrie* **29,** 861-79.

Robain, O. and Lyon, G. (1972) Les micrencéphalies familiales par malformations cérébrales. *Acta Neuropathologica* **20,** 96-109.

Roizin, L., Gold, G., Berman, H.H. and Bonafede, V.I. (1959) Congenital vascular anomalies and their histopathology in Sturge-Weber-Dimitri syndrome (naevus flammeus with angiomatosis and encephalosis calcificans). *Journal of Neuropathology and Experimental Neurology* **18,** 75-97.

Rorke, L.B., Fogelson, M.H. and Riggs, H. (1968) Cerebellar heterotopia in infancy. *Developmental Medicine and Child Neurology* **10,** 644-50.

Ross, J.J. and Frias, J.L. (1977) Microcephaly. In *Handbook of Clinical Neurology*, vol. 30, Part I Congenital malformations of the brain and skull. (Eds. Vinken, P.J., Bruyn, G.W.), pp. 507-24. North-Holland, Amsterdam.

Roubicek, M., Spranger, J. and Wende, S. (1981) Frontonasal dysplasia as an expression of holoprosencephaly. *European Journal of Pediatrics* **137,** 229-31.

Rubinstein, H.S. and Freeman, W. (1940) Cerebellar agenesis. *Journal of Nervous and Mental Disease* **92,** 489-502.

Russell, D.S. (1949) Observations on the pathology of hydrocephalus. *Medical Research Council Special Report Series* no 265. HMSO, London.

Russell, D.S. and Nevin, S. (1940) Aneurysm of the great vein of Galen causing internal hydrocephalus: report of two cases. *Journal of Pathology and Bacteriology* **51,** 375-83.

Russell, D.S. and Rubinstein, L.J. (1977) *Pathology of Tumours of the Nervous System*, 4th edn, p. 269. Edward Arnold, London.

Sabin, A.B. and Feldman, H.A. (1948) Chorioretinopathy associated with other evidence of cerebral damage in childhood. A syndrome of unknown aetiology separable from congenital toxoplasmosis. *Journal of Pediatrics* **35,** 296-309.

Schachenmayr, W. and Friede, L.R. (1979) Fine structure of arachnoid cysts. *Journal of Neuropathology and Experimental Neurology* **38,** 434–46.

Schafer, J.A., Berg, B.O. and Norman, D. (1975) Cerebellar calcification in tuberous sclerosis. *Archives of Neurology* **32,** 642–3.

Schaltenbrandt, G. (1951) *Die Nervenkrankheiten.* Thieme, Stuttgart.

Schochet, S.S., Lampert, P.W. and McCormick, W.F. (1973) Neurofibrillary tangles in patients with Down's syndrome: a light and electron microscopic study. *Acta Neuropathologica* **23,** 342–6.

Schum, T.R., Meyer, G.A., Gransz, J.P. and Glaspey, J.C. (1979) Neonatal intraventricular hemorrhage due to an intracranial arteriovenous malformation: a case report. *Pediatrics* **64,** 242–4.

Schwartz, E. (1897) Präparate von einem Falle syphilitischer Meningomyelitis mit Höhlenbildung im Rückenmarke und besonderen degenerativen Veränderungen der Neuroglia. *Wiener Klinische Wochenschrift* **110,** 177.

Schwidde, J.T. (1952) Incidence of cavum septi pellucidi and cavum vergae in 1032 human brains. *Archives of Neurology and Psychiatry* **67,** 625–32.

Shaw, C.M. and Alvord, E.C. (1969) Cava septi pellucidi et vergae: their normal and pathological states. *Brain* **92,** 213–24.

Shaw, C.M. and Alvord, E.C. (1977) 'Congenital arachnoid' cysts and their differential diagnosis. In *Handbook of Clinical Neurology*, vol. 31 (Eds. Vinken, P.J. and Bruyn, G.W.), pp. 75–135. North-Holland, Amsterdam.

Shokeir, M. (1970) Von Hippel–Lindau syndrome. A report on three kindreds. *Journal of Medical Genetics* **7,** 155–7.

Silverman, B.K., Brechx, T., Craig, J. and Nadas, A. (1955) Congestive failure in the newborn, caused by cerebral arterio-venous fistula. *American Journal of Diseases of Children* **89,** 539–43.

Simopoulos, A.P. and Breslow, A. (1966) Tuberous sclerosis in the newborn. *American Journal of Diseases of Children* **111,** 313–16.

Siqueira, E.B. and Murray, K.J. (1972) Calcified aneurysms of the vein of Galen: report of a presumed case and review of the literature. *Neurochirurgia* **15,** 106–12.

Slotnick, V. and Brent, R.L. (1966) The production of congenital malformations using tissue antisera. V. Fluorescent localization of teratogenic antisera in the maternal and fetal tissue of the rat. *Journal of Immunology* **96,** 606–9.

Smith, C. and Linell, E. (1959) Microgyria: a case report. *Neurology* **9,** 689–93.

Smith, M.T. and Huntington, H.W. (1977) Inverse cerebellum and occipital encephalocele: a dorsal fusion defect uniting the Arnold–Chiari and Dandy–Walker spectrum. *Neurology* **27,** 246–51.

Snodgrass, G., Butler, J., France, N., Crome, L. and Russell, A. (1966) The 'D' (13–15) trisomy syndrome: an analysis of 7 examples. *Archives of Disease in Childhood* **41,** 250–61.

Solitare, G.B. and Lamarche, J.B. (1966) Alzheimer's disease and senile dementia as seen in mongoloids: Neuropathological observations. *American Journal of Mental Deficiency* **70,** 840–8.

Sotos, J.F., Dodge, P.R., Muirhead, D., Crawford, J.D. and Talbot, N.B. (1964) Cerebral gigantism in childhood. *New England Journal of Medicine* **271,** 109–16.

Spiller, W.G. (1906) Syringomyelia, extending from the sacral region of the spinal cord through the medulla oblongata, right side of the pons and right cerebral peduncle to the upper part of the right internal capsule (syringobulbia). *British Medical Journal* **2,** 1017–21.

Staemmler, M. (1942) *Hydromyelie, Syringomyelie und Gliose.* Monographien aus dem Gesamtgebiete der Neurologie und Psychiatrie, no. 72 Springer, Berlin.

Starkman, S.P., Brown, T.C. and Linell, E.A. (1958) Cerebral arachnoid cysts. *Journal of Neuropathology and Experimental Neurology* **17,** 484–500.

Stern, L., Ramos, A.D. and Wigglesworth, F.W. (1968) Congenital heart failure secondary to cerebral arteriovenous aneurysm in the newborn infant. *American Journal of Diseases of Children* **115,** 581–7.

Stevenson, L. and Echlin, F. (1934) Nature and origin of some tumors of the cerebellum. *Archives of Neurology* **31,** 93–109.

Stewart, R.M., Richman, D.P. and Caviness, V.S. Jr (1975) Lissencephaly and pachygyria, an architectonic and topographical analysis. *Acta Neuropathologica* **31,** 1–12.

Streeter, G. (1912) The cortex of the brain in the human embryo during the fourth month with special reference to the so-called 'papillae of Retzius'. *American Journal of Anatomy* **7,** 337–44.

Sturge, W.A. (1879) A case of partial epilepsy, apparently due to a lesion of one of the vasomotor centres of the brain. *Transactions of the Clinical Society of London* **12,** 162–7.

Sumi, S.M. (1970) Brain malformations in the trisomy 18 syndrome. *Brain* **93,** 821–30.

Suwanwela, C. and Suwanwela, N. (1972) A morphological classification of sincipital encephalomeningoceles. *Journal of Neurosurgery* **36,** 201–11.

Swan, C. (1949) Rubella in pregnancy as an aetiological factor in congenital malformation, stillbirth, miscarriage and abortion. *Journal of Obstetrics and Gynaecology of the British Empire* **56,** 341–63; 591–605.

Taggart, J.K. and Walker, A.E. (1942) Congenital atresia of the foramina of Luschka and Magendie. *Archives of Neurology and Psychiatry* **48,** 583–612.

Tal, Y., Freigung, B., Dunn, H.G., Durity, F.A. and

Moyes, P.D. (1980) Dandy-Walker syndrome: analysis of 2 cases. *Developmental Medicine and Child Neurology* **22,** 184–201.

Talwalker, V.C. and Dastur, D.K. (1974) Ectopic spinal cord (myelomeningocele) with tethering: a clinico-pathological entity. *Developmental Medicine and Child Neurology* **16** suppl. 32, 159–60.

Taveras, J.M. and Poser, C.M. (1959) Roentgenologic aspects of cerebral angiography in children. *American Journal of Roentgenology* **82,** 371–91.

Terplan, K., Sandberg, A. and Aceto, T. (1966) Structural anomalies in the cerebellum in association with trisomy. *Journal of American Medical Association* **197,** 129–40.

Töndury, G. and Smith, D.W. (1966) Fetal rubella pathology. *Journal of Pediatrics* **68,** 867–79.

Trombley, I.K. and Mirra, S.S. (1981) Ultrastructure of tuberous sclerosis: cortical tuber and subependymal tumor. *Annals of Neurology* **9,** 174–81.

Tsarkraklides, V., Burke, B., Mastri, A., Runge, W., Roe, E. and Anderson, R. (1974) Rhabdomyomas of the heart. *American Journal of Diseases of Children* **128,** 639–46.

Tuchmann-Duplessis, H. and Larroche, J.Cl. (1958) Anencéphalieetatrophiecortico-surrénale. *Comptes rendus de la Société de Biologie* **152,** 300–2.

Uiberrack, F. (1942) Demonstration eines Falles von Ganglienzellerkrankung bei einem Fötus nach Röntgenbestrahlung der Mutter. *Zentralblatt für Allgemeine Pathologie und Pathologische Anatomie* **80,** 187.

Ule, G. (1952) Kleinhirnrindenatrophie vom Körnertyp. *Deutsche Zeitschrift für Nervenheilkunde* **168,** 195–226.

Urich, H. (1977) Malformations of the nervous system. In *Greenfield's Neuropathology,* 3rd edn. (Eds. Blackwood, W. and Corsellis, J.A.N.), pp. 361–469. Edward Arnold, London.

Vogel, S. (1961) The anatomic character of the vascular anomalies associated with anencephaly with consideration of the role of abnormal angiogenesis in the pathogenesis of the cerebral malformation. *American Journal of Pathology* **39,** 163–74.

Volpe, J.J. and Adams, R.D. (1972) Cerebro-hepato-renal syndrome of Zellweger: an inherited disorder of neuronal migration. *Acta Neuropathologica* **20,** 175–98.

Wald, N.J., Cuckle, H., Brock, D.J.H., Peto, R., Polani, P.E. and Woodford, F.P. (1977) Maternal serum alpha-fetoprotein measurement in antenatal screening for anencephaly and spina bifida in early pregnancy. *Lancet* **1,** 1323–32.

Walker, A.E. (1942) Lissencephaly. *Archives of Neurology and Psychiatry,* **48,** 13–29.

Warkany, J. (1971) *Congenital Malformations.* Year Book Medical, Chicago.

Warkany, J. and Dignan, P. StJ. (1973) Congenital malformations and mental retardation: microcephaly. *Mental Retardation* **5,** 113–35.

Weber, F.P. (1929) A note on the association of extensive haemangiomatous naevus of the skin with cerebral (meningeal) haemangioma especially cases of facial vascular naevus with contralateral hemiplegia. *Proceedings of the Royal Society of Medicine* **22,** 431–42.

Weed, L.H. (1917) Development of cerebro-spinal spaces in pig and in man. *Contributions to Embryology* **5,** 1–116.

Weinberg, A.G. and Kirkpatrick, J.B. (1975) Cerebellar hypoplasia in Werdnig–Hoffmann disease. *Developmental Medicine and Child Neurology* **17,** 511–16.

Wesolowski, D.P., Ellwood, R.A., Schwab, R.E. and Farah, J. (1981) Hippel–Lindau syndrome in identical twins. *British Journal of Radiology* **54,** 982–7.

Wohak, H. (1923) Ein Fall von Varix der Vena magna Galeni bei einem Neugeborenen. *Virchows Archiv für Pathologie und Anatomie* **242,** 58–68.

Wohlwill, F.S. and Yakovlev, P.I. (1957) Histopathology of meningo-facial angiomatosis (Sturge–Weber's disease) *Journal of Neuropathology and Experimental Neurology* **16,** 341–64.

Wolf, A. and Cowen, D. (1959) Perinatal infections of the central nervous system. *Journal of Neuropathology and Experimental Neurology* **18,** 191–243.

Wood, J.W., Johnson, K.G. and Omori, Y. (1967) *In utero* exposure to the Hiroshima atomic bomb. An evaluation of head size and mental retardation. Twenty years later. *Pediatrics* **39,** 385–92.

Yakovlev, P.I. (1959a) Pathoarchitectonic studies of the cerebral malformations. III. Arhinencephalies (holotelencephalies). *Journal of Neuropathology and Experimental Neurology* **18,** 22–55.

Yakovlev, P.I. (1959b) Anatomy of the human brain and the problem of mental retardation. In *Mental Retardation* (Eds. Bowman, P.W. and Mautner, H.V.), pp. 1–43. Grune and Stratton, New York.

Yakovlev, P.I. (1972) A proposed definition of the limbic system. In *Limbic System Mechanisms and Autonomic Function* (Ed. Hockman C.H.) pp. 241–83. Thomas, Springfield.

Yakovlev, P.I. and Guthrie, R.H. (1931) Congenital ectodermoses (neurocutaneous syndromes) in epileptic patients. *Archives of Neurology and Psychiatry* **26,** 1145–94.

Yakovlev, P.I. and Wadsworth, R.C. (1946a) Schizencephalies. A study of the congenital clefts in the cerebral mantle. I. Clefts with fused lips. *Journal of Neuropathology ad Experimental Neurology* **5,** 116–30.

Yakovlev, P.I. and Wadsworth, R.C. (1946b) Schizencephalies. A study of the congenital clefts in the cerebral mantle. II. Clefts with hydrocephalus and lips separated. *Journal of Neuropathology and Experimental Neurology* **5,** 169–206.

Yamazaki, J.N., Wright, S.W. and Wright, P.M. (1954) Outcome of pregnancy in women exposed to atomic bomb in Nagasaki. *American Journal of Diseases of Children* **87,** 448–63.

Zellweger, H. and von Muralt, G. (1952). Zur Pathologie des septum pellucidum in Pneumoencephalogram. *Helvetica Paediatrica Acta* **7,** 229–52.

Ziter, F. and Bramwit, D. (1970) Nasal encephaloceles and gliomas. *British Journal of Radiology* **43,** 136.

11

Perinatal brain damage

Jeanne-Claudie Larroche

Intracranial and intracerebral haemorrhage

This term covers a wide spectrum of haemorrhages regardless of the exact localization. Pathologists have tried to be more precise and there has been some attempt to understand the pathogenesis. With the use of new techniques such as CT scan and ultrasonography, clinicians no longer rely exclusively on the clinical history, examination and lumbar puncture to establish the diagnosis, and intracerebral haemorrhages can now be accurately located and their size estimated in living infants.

Intracranial-intracerebral haemorrhages are described in this chapter according to site; known at-risk situations and/or causes are discussed, keeping in mind that the same cause can produce different effects at different gestational ages as the brain matures, and that various causes can produce similar lesions.

In the neonatal period, conditions such as immune thrombocytopenia, haemolytic disease, haemophilia, vitamin K deficiency or meningoencephalitis with coagulation defects may be responsible for intracranial bleeding. These subjects are beyond the scope of this chapter and are not discussed in detail.

Falx and tentorial laceration

Tears of the falx cerebri and of the tentorium in full-term infants are probably traumatic, associated with rupture of the bridging veins and subdural haemorrhage. Isolated tears of the falx (Fig. 11.1), moderate bleeding within the layers of the falx and even true haematomas (Fig. 11.2) are not uncommon, and there is not always a clinical history of trauma. Tears of the great

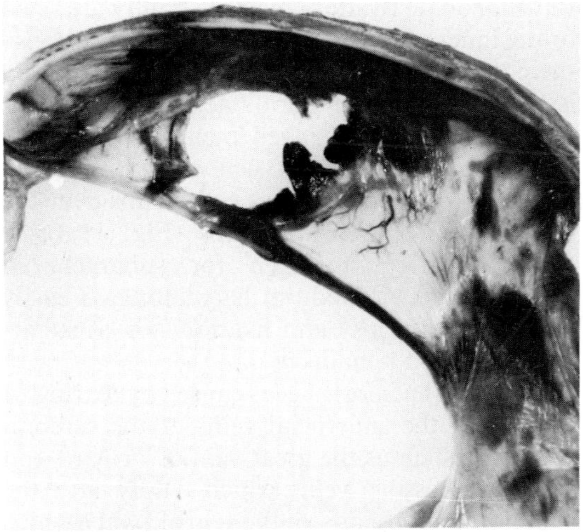

Fig. 11.1 Tear of the falx cerebri which was associated with subdural haemorrhage.

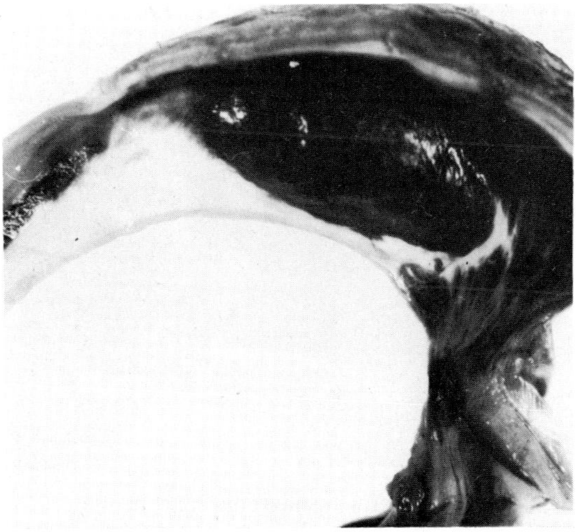

Fig. 11.2 Haematoma in the falx.

cerebral vein (of Galen) or ampulla are extremely rare. Laceration of the superior sheet of the tentorium does not necessarily cause bleeding, and may be overlooked at autopsy. In addition, it may sometimes be difficult to determine whether blood collected over the tentorium originates from small subdural bridging veins or from a lacerated tentorium. Rupture of infratentorial veins resulting in haematomas in the posterior fossa is even more difficult to identify (Blank et al, 1978)

Subdural haemorrhage

In the neonate the dura mater is tightly attached to the inner surface of the skull, and at autopsy the potential space between dura and arachnoid is easily exposed. Subdural haemorrhage ranges from slightly blood-tinged meninges to a clot several millimetres thick which may either be adherent to the skull bones or remains over the convexity of the hemispheres (Fig. 11.3). It should not be mistaken for subarachnoid haemorrhage. A subdural haematoma is easily lost during autopsy and fixation, whilst subarachnoid blood remains *in situ.*

Subdural haemorrhage is caused by tearing or rupture of the superficial veins of the cerebral convexity such as the great vein of Trolard and smaller accessory veins which empty into the superior sagittal sinus, or the vein of Labbé which empties into the transverse sinus. After running in the subarachnoid space, these veins often enter the dura mater and corresponding sinus at right angles. Detailed descriptions were given by Holland (1922), Rydberg (1932), Schipke, Riege and Scoville (1954), Haller, Nesbitt and Anderson (1956) and Schwartz (1961). This lesion is not as common a finding now as it once was.

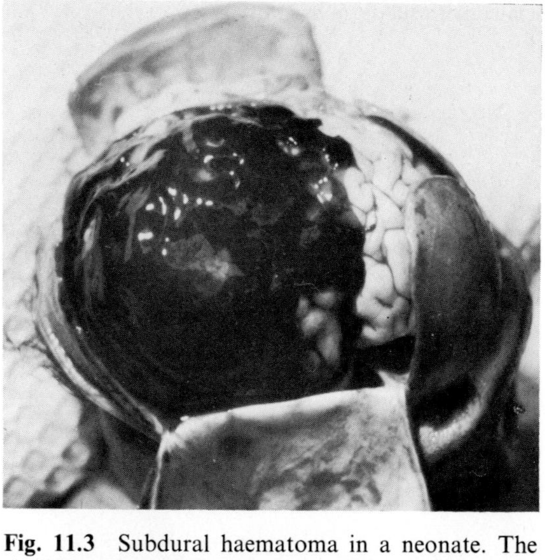

Fig. 11.3 Subdural haematoma in a neonate. The skull bones have been reflected to show the blood clot covering the right parieto-occipital region.

The tears in the veins are the result of opposing forces applied to the fetal head during its passage through the birth canal. They are particularly liable to occur in the full-term infant when the skull is well ossified and in association with cephalopelvic disproportion, a high forceps delivery or breech presentation in a primipara.

In premature infants, subdural haemorrhage may be attributable to the marked malleability of the cranial bones, particularly the parietal bones which readily become distorted and overlapped. Until recently, calculation of the incidence of subdural haematoma was based only on autopsy reports and varied greatly—in 50 per cent of the series reported by Craig (1938) and in 20 per cent in that described by Gröntoft (1953a, b). In 700 consecutive autopsies in 1967–1973, the incidence in the author's department was 18 per cent in full-term infants and 11 per cent in premature infants. In the British Perinatal Survey, Claireaux (1970) gave a figure of 4 per 1000 live births. The incidence in full-term infants has recently significantly decreased because caesarean section is readily undertaken when dystocia is recognized early in labour.

In full-term infants, mechanical difficulties resulting in subdural haemorrhage are often associated with asphyxia and neuronal necrosis, with important clinical implications (Allemand, Monod and Larroche, 1977; Larroche, Amiel-Tison and Dreyfus-Brisac, 1980). In cases of isolated subdural haemorrhage there may be focal or unilateral convulsions, ocular signs or a hemisyndrome with homolateral EEG anomalies. The mixed form is unfortunately more frequent and the clinical picture is that described in hypoxic-ischaemic encephalopathy.

Subdural haematomas without previous trauma may be observed in haemophilic newborn infants (Fig. 11.4) (Volpe et al, 1976).

Thrombosis of sinuses and cerebral veins

Thrombosis of sinuses and large cerebral veins is uncommon in the first few days of life (Larroche, 1977; Rorke, 1982). According to Friede (1975),

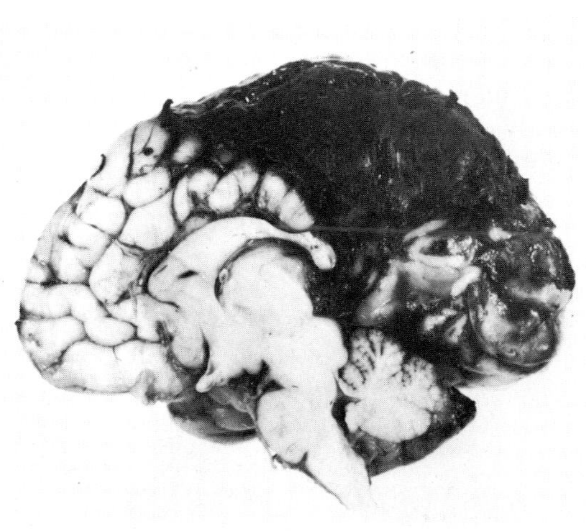

Fig. 11.4 Mid-sagittal cut showing the right hemisphere extensively covered by a thick layer of subdural blood clot.

who reviewed the literature, the many cases described in the nineteenth and early twentieth centuries were secondary to sepsis, dehydration and congenital heart disease—conditions which are better controlled today. Bacterial meningitis or meningoencephalitis may, however, still be complicated by thrombosis of the superficial veins on the convexity (Fig. 11.5) or by microthrombi leading to haemorrhagic encephalopathy. This is particularly so in sepsis due to Gram-negative organisms such as *Pseudomonas* and *Serratia.* Bacteria pass across the vascular wall, which becomes necrotic, and form a cuff or halo around the vessels; disseminated intravascular coagulopathy is a severe complication sometimes observed in these infants. Leucomalacia may be associated with septic haemorrhagic encephalopathies.

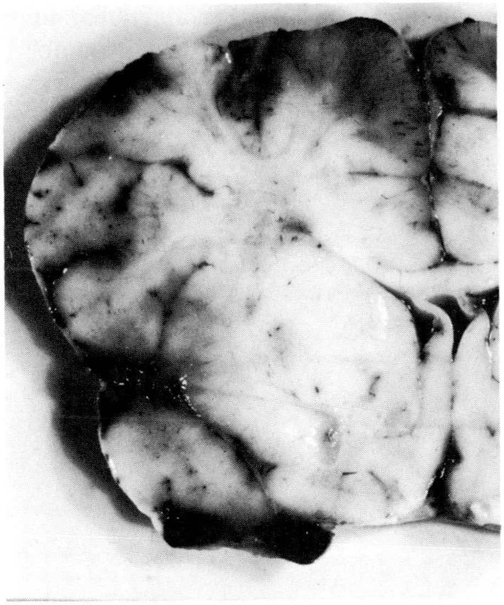

Fig. 11.5 Coronal slice of infant brain, showing extensive thrombosis of superficial veins and haemorrhagic cortical infarction. This was a case with meningitis due to *Pseudomonas aeruginosa.*

Thrombosis in tributaries of the deep venous system of Galen has been described and implicated in the genesis of haemorrhages in subependymal germinal matrix and choroid plexus. In full-term infants, intraventricular haemorrhage has been observed in association with thrombosis of the vein of Galen and haemorrhagic infarcts in the basal ganglia and thalamus.

Classically, when the superior sagittal sinus is thrombosed, haemorrhagic infarcts occur symmetrically in both hemispheres and involve cortex and white matter (Fig. 11.6). Residual lesions (Friede, 1972c) vary from small scars to distinct cavities. The lesions are grossly similar to multicystic encephalomalacia but contain haemosiderin and mineral deposits.

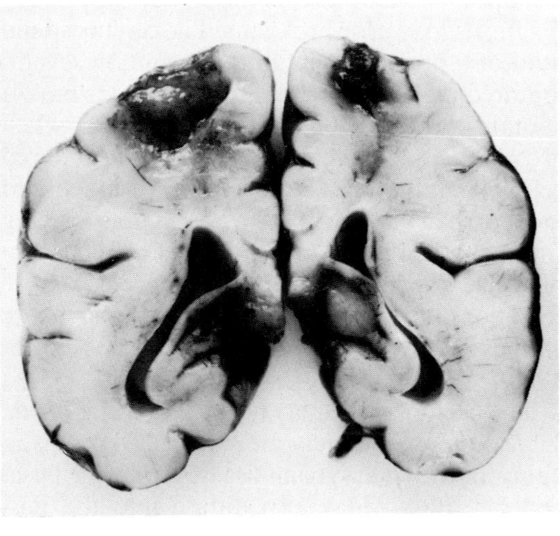

Fig. 11.6 Coronal slice of infant brain, showing bilateral haemorrhagic necrosis of cortex and white matter resulting from sagittal sinus thrombosis.

Subarachnoid haemorrhage

Extravasations of blood in the subarachnoid space are common in both premature and full-term infants. When an isolated phenomenon, they are usually clinically silent. They may be of

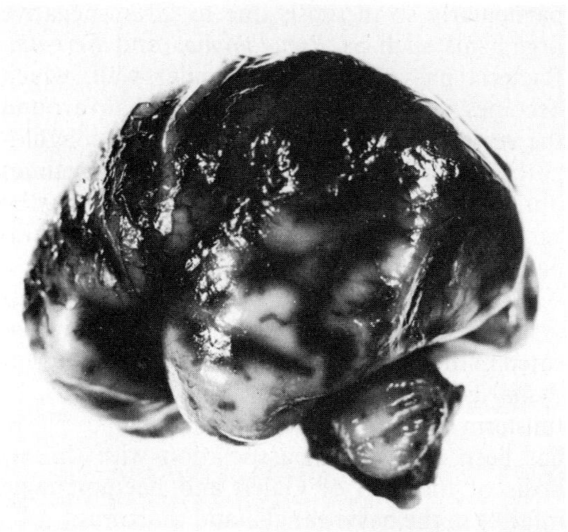

Fig. 11.7 Left hemisphere of a premature infant. There is extensive diffuse subarachnoid haemorrhage.

traumatic origin in cases of forceps or vacuum extraction or may result from asphyxia. Hyperexcitability, an abnormal cry, vasomotor instability, cyanosis and alteration of muscle tone are the typical signs which, in the majority of cases, disappear within several days, but laboratory diagnosis may pose problems. The cerebrospinal fluid of a premature infant may contain several hundred red cells per millilitre. When it is pink it contains 8000–10000 red cells/ml, and when grossly bloody several hundred thousand red cells per millilitre. The incidence of arachnoid haemorrhage is not known, the figures varying from one neonatal unit to another. Subarachnoid haemorrhage is not readily detected on CT scan nor on ultrasonography, and no systematic studies have yet been published (Davis et al., 1980).

The haemorrhage may be focal or diffuse (Fig. 11.7). The blood may be particularly conspicuous in the wide sylvian fissures or in the basal cisterns. Blood may also diffuse into the posterior fossa and must then be differentiated from an extension of intraventricular haemorrhage. Occasionally, hydrocephalus may develop secondary to arachnoid thickening and occlusion of the foramina of Luschka and Magendie (Larroche, 1972a).

A *subarachnoid haematoma* is a well-circumscribed collection of blood over a single or several lobes (Fig. 11.8). Its thickness may vary from several millimetres to 1 cm (Fig. 11.9). The underlying brain may be normal, but haemorrhagic necrosis may occur. In the writer's series (Larroche, 1977) subarachnoid haematoma was found more often over the left hemisphere, particularly over the temporal lobe. Its pathogenesis is not known, but exchange tranfusion had been performed in 80 per cent of cases and arterial thrombo-embolism cannot be ruled out.

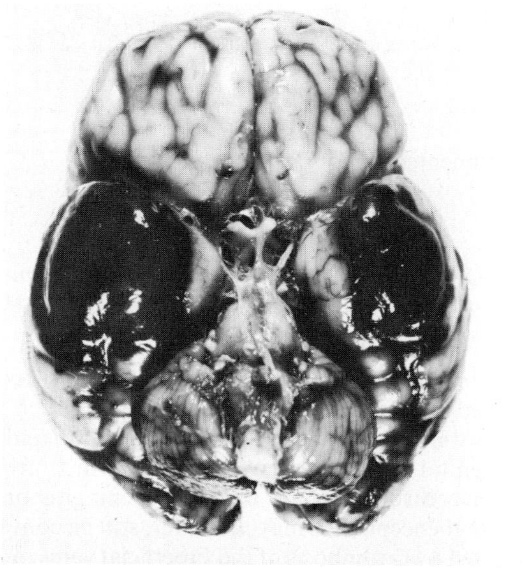

Fig. 11.8 Full-term baby's brain, showing bilateral subarachnoid haematomas over the temporal lobes.

Subpial haemorrhage can be diagnosed only on histological examination. Varying numbers of red blood cells are found between the pia and the molecular layer. In the fetus this layer is

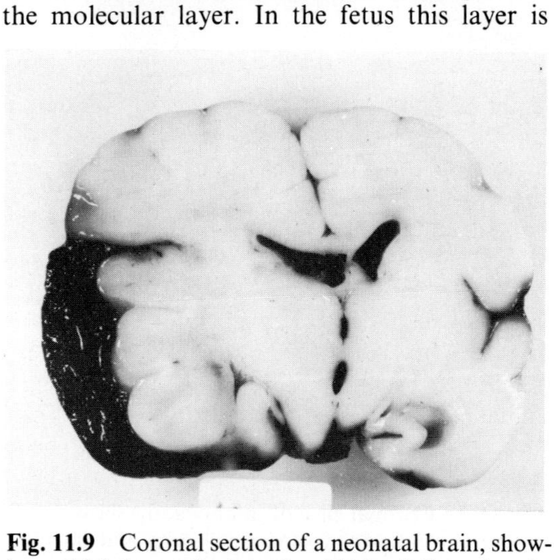

Fig. 11.9 Coronal section of a neonatal brain, showing a thick layer of subarachnoid blood distorting the underlying hemisphere.

highly cellular and red blood cells are often present there. According to Friede (1972a), subpial haemorrhages occur in 15 per cent of cases of perinatal intracranial haemorrhage.

Subependymal and intraventricular haemorrhage in the premature infant

Intraventricular haemorrhage (IVH) is today the most common finding at autopsy in premature infants, and probably the main cause of death. It was first described in 1903 by Couvelaire, and then by Ylppö (1919). Although several well-documented monographs (Rydberg 1932; Gröntoft, 1954; Schwartz, 1961; Larroche, 1964) drew attention to this characteristic cerebral bleeding in premature neonates, it was the introduction of computerized tomography and ultrasonography that led to renewed interest and general recognition of this lesion. Despite the wealth of data on frequency, localization, size and evolution of the haemorrhage, there is still uncertainty as to its pathogenesis, and treatment is unsatisfactory.

Pathological anatomy Intraventricular haemorrhage is usually secondary to bleeding in the subependymal germinal matrix accompanied by rupture of the ependyma, the site of predilection being at the level of the foramen of Monro (Fig. 11.10 and 11.11). The periventricular matrix, which has almost disappeared by 24 weeks, still persists until 35–36 weeks as a conspicuous mass of cells in three major sites—over the head of the caudate nucleus and in the groove between the caudate nucleus and the thalamus, in the roof of the temporal horn, and in the external wall of the occipital horn. The matrix consists of compactly arranged cells with scant cytoplasm and short processes. At 28 weeks, electron microscopy has shown that these cells are immature neurons and mature glial cells. Capillaries cannot be differentiated from small veins but endothelial cells, basal lamina and glial perivascular end-feet are mature by 20 weeks. Endothelial cells, however, show certain outstanding features e.g. large number of organelles, intraluminal microvilli and rod-shaped bodies (Povlishock, Martinez and Moossy, 1977; Larroche, 1982c)—which may be linked to thromboplastic and clotting activity. It has long been said that under normal circumstances this region is highly vascularized; recent work, however, tends to demonstrate the opposite. In microangiographs,

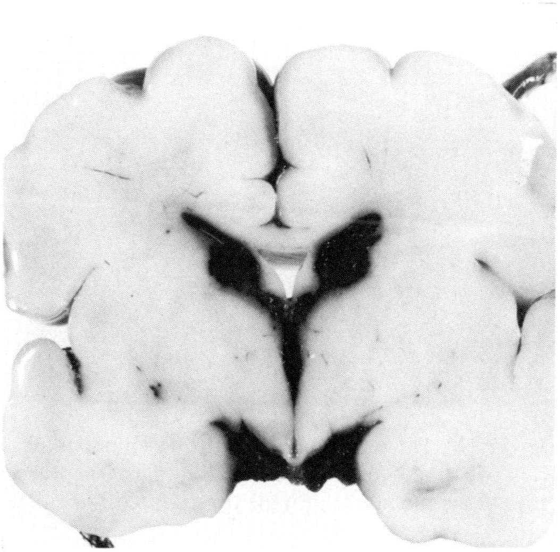

Fig. 11.10 Coronal section of a premature baby's brain, showing bilateral haemorrhage into the subependymal matrix layer, blood clot in the lateral ventricles, the foramina of Monro and the third ventricle. There is also blood in the subarachnoid space over the base of the brain.

Takashima and Tanaka (1978a) showed that the matrix had a rather poor arterial supply, and Pasternak et al. (1982) found a low arterial blood flow in the matrix of the beagle pup. Studies of semithin and ultrathin sections of the matrix in the external wall of the lateral ventricle of human embryos and fetuses have shown a high density of vascular lumina during the active mitotic period until 18–20 weeks; thereafter, there is a significant decrease in the density of vessels in the matrix whereas spectacular proliferation takes place in the cortex. After 26 weeks, the deep venous system of Galen becomes more apparent, draining blood from the expanding hemispheres. The peculiar pattern of these veins renders them vulnerable to haemodynamic disturbances. Veins which drain almost the entire hemisphere (the anterior, septal, choroidal and thalamostriate veins) unite at about the level of the foramen of Monro to form the internal cerebral veins. These flow backwards in the roof of the third ventricle to form the great vein of Galen.

Another source of haemorrhage—in about 15 per cent of cases of IVH—is the choroid plexuses where it may be associated with haemorrhage in the matrix or be isolated; in addition, haemorrhage frequently occurs in the tela choroidea.

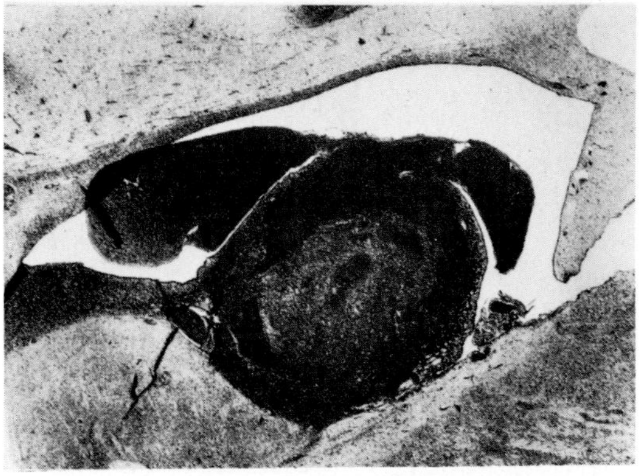

Fig. 11.11 Haemorrhage into the germinal matrix layer over the caudate nucleus. Blood has ruptured through the ependyma into the ventricle. Cresyl violet.

Subependymal haemorrhage may occur at one or several sites and may be unilateral or bilateral. It is remarkable how the haemorrhage can destroy the entire matrix whilst the surrounding structures are spared (Fig. 11.12). Small amounts of blood in the ventricles collect in the occipital horns if the infant lies on its back; more often, however, blood fills the entire ventricular system (Fig. 11.13) and collects in the subarachnoid spaces of the posterior fossa where it compresses the brain stem like a tumour mass. Blood may extend anteriorly to the basal cisterns and downwards to the spinal cord. When the ventricles are very distended, blood may dissect into the parenchyma (Fig. 11.14). This event is not always simply mechanical; often the ependyma is damaged and the overlying white matter is the site of an ischaemic infarct; alternatively, an associated

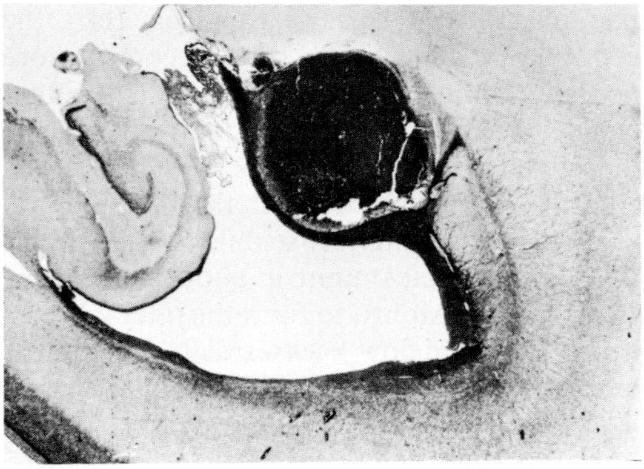

Fig. 11.12 Section showing the temporal horn of the lateral ventricle. Haemorrhage has occurred into the matrix in the region of the tail of the caudate nucleus Cresyl violet.

leucomalacia may secondarily become haemorrhagic and rupture into the ventricle.

These brains are difficult to process in paraffin wax. Celloidin embedding is more appropriate,

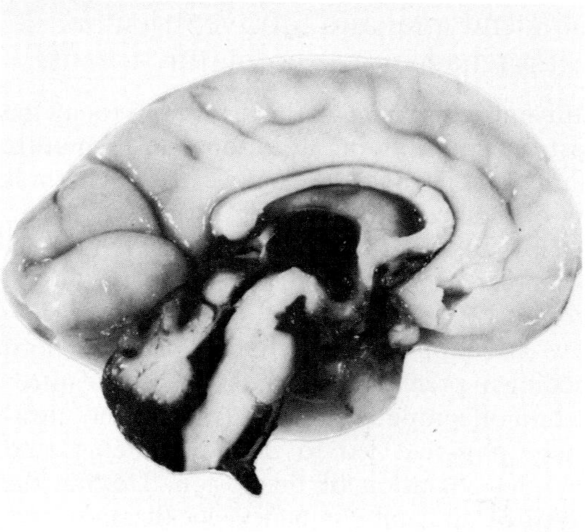

Fig. 11.13 Premature brain cut mid-sagittally. The third ventricle, aqueduct, fourth ventricle and subarachnoid cisterns are filled with blood clot.

allowing serial sections to be prepared without loss of blood clot and without damage to fragile vascular structures.

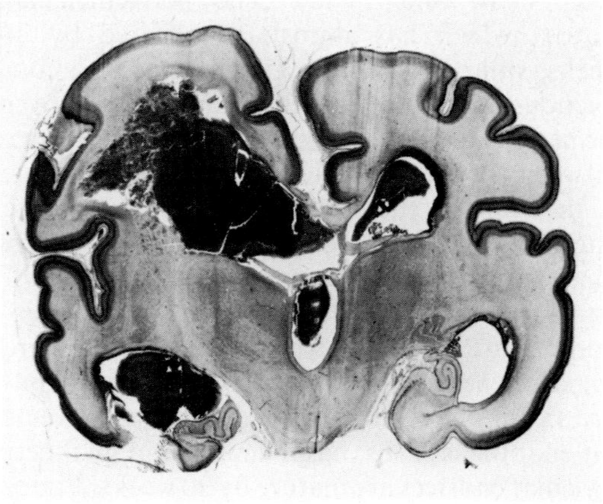

Fig. 11.14 Section of both hemispheres shows enlargement of the ventricular system which is almost filled with blood. The blood has also extended into the white matter of one hemisphere. Cresyl violet.

Microscopic examination discloses congested thin-walled veins (Gruenwald, 1951) and perivascular haemorrhages not only in the matrix but also around the ventricles, in the layers of the septum pellucidum and in the tela choroidea (Rydberg, 1932; Friede, 1975). On serial sections, small thrombi or mural fibrinoid deposits are observed in about 15 per cent of cases of matrix haemorrhage with or without IVH. Ruptured veins are more difficult to identify and their frequency is unknown. According to Friede (1975) there is no microscopic evidence of necrosis antedating the haemorrhage. Rorke (1982), however, has shown partial infarction of the matrix without bleeding whilst Goldstein (1979) has shown that isolated brain capillaries are normally very resistant but, if previously damaged, may rupture under conditions of increased blood flow. Electron microscopic studies of the subependymal layer show that among the first structures to be damaged are the perivascular glial end-feet which become swollen and detached from the basal lamina. This in turn becomes cloudy and ill-defined, whereupon endothelial cells are dislocated and haemorrhage occurs. There seem to exist two sites of bleeding: one around capillaries or small veins, and the other around larger distended veins. Although it has been shown that intraventricular haemorrhage may occur in young fetuses *in utero*, matrix haemorrhages usually develop a few hours after birth. This was demonstrated by Tsiantos et al. (1974), who injected chromium-50-labelled red blood cells in newborns and established a curve of elimination. The time of onset of haemorrhage could be calculated from the concentration of chromium in the ventricular blood clot. Repeated CT scans and ultrasonography have recently confirmed that bleeding occurs most frequently on the first day of life.

Diagnosis Intraventricular haemorrhage in the premature infant is very commonly associated with the respiratory distress syndrome and with hyaline membrane disease (Amiel, 1964; Fedricks and Butler, 1970; Leech and Kohnen, 1974; Thorburn et al., 1982), and it also occurs in small-for-dates infants born prematurely. Acute deterioration in the infant's clinical state occurs, usually after a latent period which corresponds to the time between bleeding into the matrix and rupture of the ependyma leading to intraventricular haemorrhage. Neurological signs range from isolated clonic seizures to a decerebrate state and coma (Amiel, 1964; Volpe, 1981). Abnormal eye movements and mouthing are seizure equivalents. A fall in the haematocrit (Blanc, Rapmund and Silverman, 1957) is a reliable sign of intraventricular haemorrhage and reflects the amount of blood trapped in the brain. At lumbar puncture the CSF is uniformly blood-stained and has a high protein (Cole et al, 1974) and a low glucose content (Deonna et al., 1975). CT scans give accurate information on the time of occurrence, sites of bleeding, and extent and evolution of the lesions (Pevsner et al., 1976; Krishnamoorthy et al., 1977; among others). Papile et al. (1978) have proposed a classification of intraventricular haemorrhage into four grades: I, haemorrhage in the matrix; II, intraventricular haemorrhage without dilatation; III, intraventricular haemorrhage plus dilatation; IV, intraventricular plus intraparenchymal haemorrhage. This classification is useful, although it refers only to the extent of the bleeding, and is valid for ultrasound scannings which are tending to replace CT scans (Pape et al., 1979; Johnson et al., 1979; Allan et al., 1981; Mack et al., 1981; Shankaran et al., 1982).

Epidemiology Until recently, accurate data on the frequency of intraventricular haemorrhage were based on autopsy material only. In premature infants it was found in about 20 per cent of cases as opposed to 2 per cent in infants after 36 weeks of gestation. Fedricks and Butler (1970), using data from the well-documented British Perinatal Mortality Survey in 1958, established an incidence of 25 per 1000 live births under 36 weeks with a maximum of 50 per 1000 under 29 weeks and less than 1 per 1000 after 36 weeks. With improved intensive care techniques, the mortality rate has significantly decreased. Currently, at autopsy, 40–50 per cent of infants of less than 32 weeks' gestation show IVH (Larroche, 1979). Its frequency in mature infants, at autopsy, is still about 2 per cent. CT scan and ultrasound have shown that 40–60 per cent of infants weighing less than 1500 g or at less than 35 weeks' gestation have matrix haemorrhage, either isolated or in association with IVH. The only discordant figure of 90 per cent (Bejar et al., 1980) is unexplained. Boys are affected slightly more frequently than girls.

The *pathogenesis of intraventricular haemorrhage* is complex. Various pathological conditions are associated with it, and their responsibility for the genesis of the bleeding has been variously interpreted. Respiratory distress (hyaline membrane disease) is usually the dominant clinical picture, and at autopsy hyaline membranes in the lungs were found in 80 per cent of the author's cases and in 95 per cent of Leech and Kohnen's cases (1974). Asphyxia, hypercapnia and heart failure increase intracranial venous pressure (Cole et al., 1974; Vert, Nomin and Sibout, 1975), and severe stasis in the right atrium, vena cava and brain (mainly in the deep system of Galen) is commonly found at autopsy. Rupture of a thin-walled vessel may occur and the high fibrinolytic activity of the matrix (Gilles et al., 1971) might explain the rapid and massive spread of an initially minimal haemorrhage. In addition to stasis, altered capillary endothelium and impairment of coagulation factors (Hathaway and Bonnar, 1978) may lead to thrombus formation. On studying serial sections of brains, thrombosis of large veins or minute vessels was found in 10–12 per cent of cases with germinal matrix haemorrhage. Hypernatremia following infusion of bicarbonate has been incriminated by Simmons et al. (1974) and by Papile et al. (1978). However, these observations have not been confirmed (Finberg, 1977; Dykes et al., 1980). Another mechanism, proposed by Hambleton and Wigglesworth (1976) and Pape and Wigglesworth (1979), is that subependymal haemorrhage is due to rupture of the capillary–venous junction secondary to increased pressure in the territory of Heubner's artery. This mechanism does not, however, account for haemorrhages in the temporal and occipital germinal matrix. A few studies necessitating the use of xenon (Lou, Lassen and Friis-Hansen, 1979b) have shown that in the asphyxiated newborn autoregulation of cerebral flow is impaired. Consequently, variations in systemic blood pressure are transmitted to the brain, possibly resulting in ischaemic or haemorrhagic infarcts in vulnerable regions of the brain. Episodes of hypotension or blood pressure instability associated with hypothermia occur frequently on the first day of life in infants who die with intraventricular haemorrhage (Moriette, Relier and Larroche, 1977; Fujimura et al., 1979). In addition, significant variations of blood pressure have been observed during intubation, tracheal aspiration and blood sampling, common nursing manoeuvres in every intensive care unit. This suggests iatrogenic causes of IVH and that sedative drugs might be useful (Wimberley et al., 1982). Recently, pneumothorax with increased intracerebral blood flow has been incriminated in the pathogenesis (Hill, Perlman and Volpe, 1982).

Experimental studies have been few. Asphyxia combined with raised arterial and/or venous pressure increases the frequency of haemorrhages, mostly in the tela choroidea, in fetal sheep (Reynolds et al., 1979). In beagle pups, pathological conditions such as hypercapnia and hypotension followed by hypertension, or injection of drugs such as prostaglandin E, have been associated with IVH (Goddard et al., 1980; Goddard-Finegold, Armstrong and Zeller, 1982).

Small haemorrhages in the matrix are clinically silent. If the infant dies of an intercurrent cause, haemolysed blood, pseudocysts or macrophages loaded with haemosiderin may be found in the surviving matrix. Systematic ultrasonography will permit evaluation of the frequency of such limited haematomas and subsequent scarring in survivors. Unfortunately, it is impossible to appreciate to what extent partial or total destruction of these matrices might interfere with the development of the brain. At risk are immature neurons of the matrix capping the caudate nucleus, which contribute to the late-forming population of the pulvinar, as well as glial cells. Intraventricular haemorrhage is a more serious event and used to be fatal within a few days. Improved general care and assisted ventilation have significantly reduced the mortality rate. As a result, the number of infants coming to autopsy after a long survival has increased. In the author's experience, from 1956 to 1966 only 8 per cent of neonates coming to autopsy had survived for more than 10 days. From 1967 to 1981 this figure increased to 20 per cent and is now 30 per cent (Larroche, 1982b). Consequently, we are now finding the sequelae of lesions that were formerly observed in the acute stage.

Posthaemorrhagic hydrocephalus is one of the major complications of intraventricular haemorrhage. During the period 1956–1966 posthaemorrhagic hydrocephalus occurred in 2 per cent of cases in which intraventricular haemorrhage was found at autopsy. With prolonged survival this complication develops in 20 per cent of cases. However, these autopsy figures do not reflect its true frequency since this depends upon many other factors, including the severity of the haemorrhage. Accurate data based on ultrasonography are still fragmentary.

Blood clot in the posterior fossa is haemolysed and resorbed within about a week but a cell reaction and haemosiderin-laden macrophages thicken the leptomeninges, impeding the normal circulation of CSF. At autopsy, a rusty discoloration of the meninges over the brain stem and the basal part of the cerebellum indicates the previous haemorrhage. The entire ventricular system is usually dilated, the occipital horns more severely than the frontal and temporal horns. The third and fourth ventricles enlarge later than the lateral ventricles. Less frequently, when necrotic haemorrhagic debris occludes the aqueduct the fourth ventricle may be normal. The ependyma is covered with a fine granular rusty deposit containing macrophages laden with haemosiderin. At times, the primary site of bleeding may be identified in the surviving matrix where clusters of germinal cells, cystic cavities, haemolysed blood and macrophages can be identified (Larroche, 1972a, 1977; Takashima, Armstrong and Becker, 1979; Rorke, 1982). The choroid plexuses may be pale, floating in the enlarged ventricles, but in cases of primary haemorrhage they may be brown with a firm consistency. In the first few weeks after haemorrhage there may be no abnormal increase in head circumference in spite of a significant enlargement of the ventricles (Larroche, 1972a; Korobkin, 1975; Volpe, Pasternak and Allan, 1977). This may be due to several factors. The arachnoid spaces over the the convexity and the basal cisterns are wide in premature infants and easily accommodate the enlarging brain. In addition, the unmyelinated hemispheres can be compressed and thinned as the ventricles expand. The ependyma is destroyed not only at the site of haemorrhage but also elsewhere, or it becomes buried beneath proliferating glial cells, forming rosette-like structures. In infants with severe intraventricular haemorrhage who survive under mechanical ventilation, the ventricles may enlarge before the blood clot is entirely resorbed— a condition known as *haemohydrocephalus* (Fig. 11.15). Progressive cystic destruction of the white matter, with formation of diverticula, may occur (Pasternak, Mantovani and Volpe, 1980; Donn and Bowerman, 1982; Grant et al., 1982). The neurological sequelae are not always predictable. They are in part related to the severity of the haemorrhage but especially to the extent of the underlying brain damage, be it haemorrhagic or ischaemic (Fitzhardinge, Flodmark and Ashby, 1982).

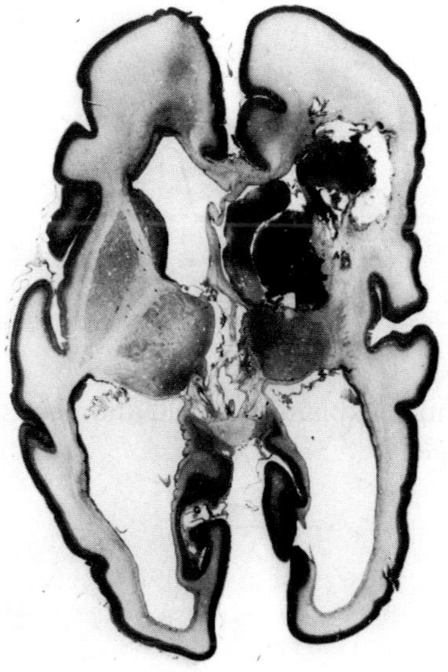

Fig. 11.15 Haemohydrocephalus in the brain of a premature baby. Horizontal section shows grossly dilated ventricles, and one anterior horn filled with blood which has extended into frontal white matter.

Intraventricular haemorrhage in the full-term neonate

Intraventricular haemorrhage occurs infrequently in the mature newborn but the true incidence is not known. Published figures are based only on autopsy cases (Dekaban, 1962; Terplan, 1967). In the writer's experience it occurs in about 2.5 per cent of autopsies on full-term infants. Fedricks and Butler (1970) estimated the incidence to be 0.3–0.6 per 1000 livebirths. With the introduction of CT scan and ultrasound the condition has been diagnosed in infants who survive. Since the germinal matrix has virtually disappeared by 35–36 weeks it is rarely the source of bleeding although Guekos-Thöni et al. (1980), by the use of CT scan, thought that the matrix was the origin in four of their nine cases.

Thrombosis of the deep venous system (Flodmark et al, 1980) and arteriovenous malformations (Schum et al., 1979) have been found in some cases, associated with intracerebral haemorrhage involving the basal ganglia and

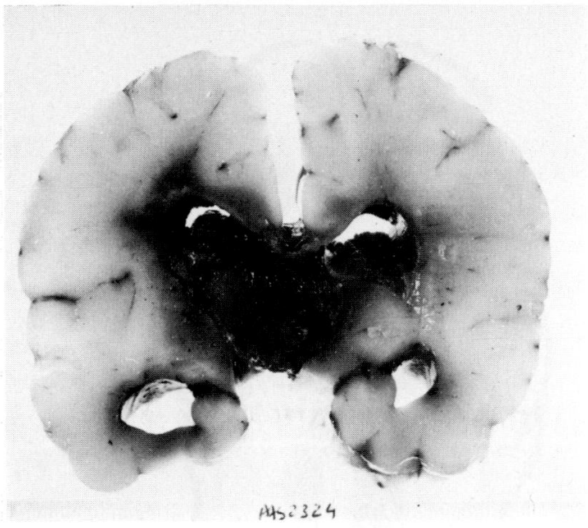

Fig. 11.16 Coronal section of a full-term neonatal brain, showing haemorrhagic necrosis of the thalami and haemorrhage into the ventricles.

thalamus (Fig. 11.16). In the cases of Palma et al. (1979), Cartwright et al. (1979), Scher et al. (1980) and Blanc et al. (1982) the exact origin of the bleeding was not clear and intracerebral haematomas were often present in addition.

In a series of more than 500 consecutive autopsies of infants born at or after 36 weeks of gestation the writer has observed 15 cases of intraventricular haemorrhage. The source was thought to be a vascular malformation in five cases, thrombosis of the vein of Galen in two cases, primary choroid plexus haemorrhage in three cases and matrix haemorrhage in one case. In four others the site of bleeding remained undetermined. Bleeding in the choroid plexus has also been recognized by Donat et al. (1978) and Lacey and Terplan (1982). The prognosis is somewhat better than in premature infants.

Cerebellar haemorrhage

Subarachnoid haemorrhage over the cerebellum, fairly common in premature infants, may occur alone or in association with supratentorial subarachnoid haemorrhage. Blood may collect over the surface of the cerebellum and compress the underlying folia (Fig. 11.17). Primary intracerebellar haemorrhage has recently become a problem in premature baby units, its frequent occurrence in low birth weight infants (Pape, Armstrong and Fitzhardinge, 1976) being attributed to pressure on the infants' occipital bone by facemask attachments. Despite the use of the same techniques, these lesions had not been observed by Helmrath, Hodson and Oliver (1970), and this mechanical cause was not confirmed by Grunnet and Shields (1976) nor by Martin, Roessmann and Fanaroff (1976) who found massive intracerebellar haemorrhage in 21 per cent of neonates born at 26–34 weeks of gestation. The writer found haematomas of the cerebellum in 21 out of 324 premature infants (6.5 per cent from a neonatal unit (1961–1966) and in 77 of 538 infants (14.3 per cent) from an intensive care unit (1967–1980). In neither group was a facemask attached by occipital straps. With decreasing overall mortality, infants who die tend to be younger and smaller, a group especially at risk for haemorrhagic brain lesions.

Haematomas in the cerebellum may be single or multiple. They may bulge above the surface and be readily visible at autopsy or they may be seen only on section. Extension of the haematomas into the vermis with necrosis of the wall of the dilated fourth ventricle may be found in cases of severe intraventricular haemorrhage.

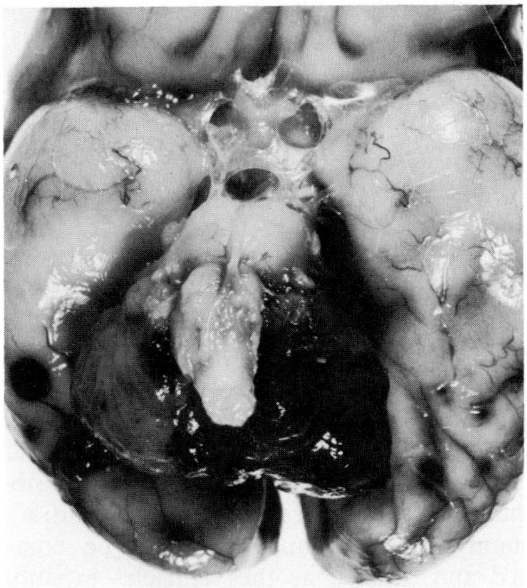

Fig. 11.17 Subarachnoid haematoma over the cerebellum of a premature (30-week) brain.

Microscopic examination discloses petechial haemorrhages in a large number of low birth weight infants presenting with respiratory distress with or without macroscopic haemorrhage. Bacterial sepsis and, in the past, blood incom-

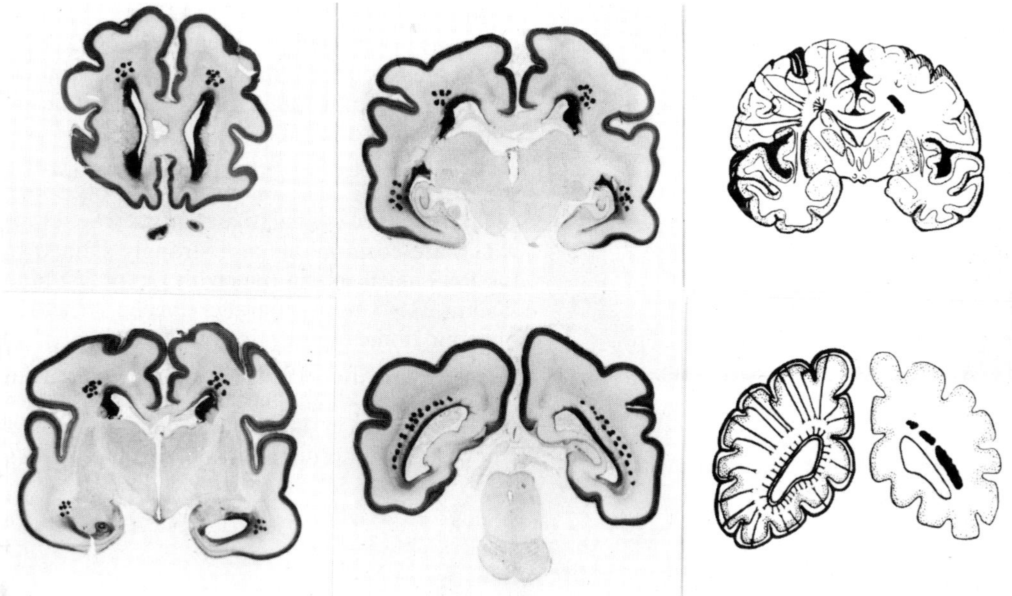

(a) **(b)**

Fig. 11.18 Periventricular leucomalacia. **a**) Sites of predilection of the white matter lesions are superimposed on photographs of coronal sections stained with cresyl violet. **b**) In these diagrams the arterial blood supply is indicated in the left hemisphere whilst the sites of leucomalacia are shown on the right side. These sites correspond to boundary zones between arterial territories in the white matter. (**b**) is reproduced, with permission, from van den Bergh, 1961.)

patibility were often associated with microscopic haemorrhages in the brain, including the cerebellum.

In infants who survive for a few weeks, old haemorrhages appear as golden or olive green staining of the meninges, which may resemble pus. Cystic degeneration and asymmetry of the hemispheres are seen in severe forms. After minor haemorrhage, haemosiderin-laden macrophages and associated neuronal necrosis of varying extent are found on microscopic examination.

The pathogenesis of cerebellar haematomas is really not known. They may be found in the cerebellum, as in other parts of the CNS, in asphyxial states. Vascular malformations are an uncommon cause (Baird and Stitt, 1959). In full-term infants, birth trauma causing skull fractures and tears of the tentorium is a rare cause of posterior fossa haemorrhage and cerebellar damage (Vallée et al., 1981). CT scanning has recently revealed a number of such cases (Rom, Serfontein and Humphreys, 1978; DuBose-Ravenel, 1979; Fishman et al., 1981). The outcome was poor whether management was surgical or conservative.

Intracerebellar haemorrhage was recently detected by ultrasound (Reeder, Setzer and Kaude, 1982) in a small-for-dates infant who weighed 860 g at birth and who presented also with severe intraventricular haemorrhage.

Periventricular leucomalacia

Periventricular leucomalacia was described a century ago and variously interpreted at that time. Virchow (1867) ascribed the lesions to smallpox encephalopathy, and Parrot (1873, 1877) observed them in brains of small debilitated infants. Later, Rydberg (1932) related the lesions to circulatory insufficiency, and Schwartz (1961) incriminated venous stasis during delivery. In 1962, Banker and Larroche emphasized the ischaemic nature of the lesions, their topography in terminal arterial territories (Fig. 11.18) and their frequency in premature infants. They considered leucomalacia to be the structural basis for the spastic mono- and diplegia, described by Little in 1861. More recently, Leech and Alvord (1974), Pape and Wigglesworth (1979), Shuman and Selednik (1980) and Rorke (1982), among others, have described similar morphological features.

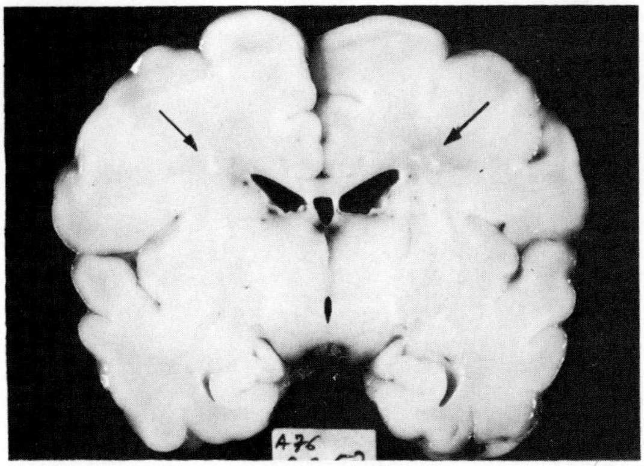

Fig. 11.19 Periventricular leucomalacia. Coronal section of the brain of a premature infant. White spots, each several millimetres in diameter are shown (arrows) close to the lateral ventricles.

On sections of the fixed brain, ill-defined white spots one to several millimetres in diameter are seen in a pale, watery, unmyelinated white matter (Fig. 11.19). The lesions are located in the deep periventricular white matter, especially in the corona radiata near the external angle of the lateral ventricle at the level of the foramen of Monro, in the temporal acoustic radiations, and posteriorly around the trigone in the tapetum and optic radiations. The lesions may be single or multiple, unilateral or bilateral. At first homogeneous, they become outlined by a chalky-white ring and often become centrally cavitated. In the presence of hyperbilirubinaemia, with or without kernicterus, the spots are stained yellow. At times, secondary haemorrhagic foci develop within the ischaemic necrotic zone.

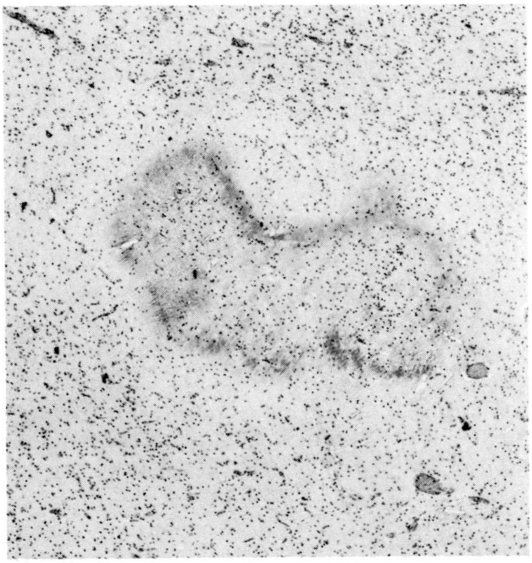

Fig. 11.20 Periventricular leucomalacia. Section shows an irregularly shaped area of necrosis in the white matter. PAS–haematoxylin.

Microscopically the lesions consist of poorly cellular areas of coagulative necrosis (Fig. 11.20) which are eosinophilic and strongly stained by the PAS reaction and blue with Luxol fast blue. Within 24–48 hours, parallel fibrillar structures or round bodies aggregate at the periphery of the necrosis. Silver impregnation reveals swollen, fragmented, club-shaped axis cylinders and retraction balls (Fig. 11.21). Microglia, swollen astrocytes and macrophages soon proliferate. Associated neuronal necrosis may be found in the globus pallidus, dentate nucleus and brain stem nuclei. The ependyma near the necrotic white matter may be destroyed, particularly if the external walls of the occipital horns are affected.

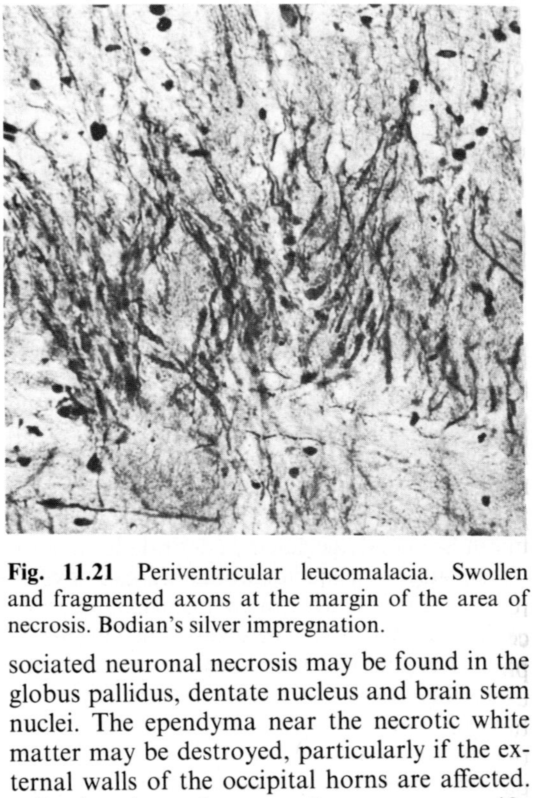

Fig. 11.21 Periventricular leucomalacia. Swollen and fragmented axons at the margin of the area of necrosis. Bodian's silver impregnation.

During the early stages there are no specific clinical signs. The diagnosis is presumptive in a premature infant who is asphyxiated at birth, has prolonged periods of apnoea and hypotension, and has abnormal neurological signs, provided that intraventricular haemorrhage has been excluded. Primary respiratory distress with hyaline membrane disease is less common than in cases of intraventricular haemorrhage. Electroencephalograms, CT scan and ultrasound are not informative (Fitzhardinge, Flodmark and Ashby, 1982).

In full-term infants, areas of hypodensity may correspond to ischaemic lesions but in a different context (Flodmark et al., 1980). The incidence of leucomalacia can therefore be established only on autopsy data. The figures vary from one centre to another, mainly because of the difficulty of recognizing the lesions in the first few days of life and because of the differences in the population under study. Twenty years ago, leucomalacia was described in about 20 per cent of the brains of premature infants. The lesions often occurred alone, without other significant gross pathology. Today, with prolonged survival in intensive care units, the population has changed and leucomalacia is found in about 35 per cent of brains of low birth weight infants (Larroche, 1982a). Similar observations have been made by Shuman and Selednik (1980). In addition, leucomalacia may be associated with intrauterine growth retardation, with hypoglycaemia, congenital heart malformations (Banker and Larroche, 1962; DeReuk, Chattha and Richardson, 1972; Robain and Rosenberg, 1974) and bacterial meningoencephalitis. In these groups there is usually also diffuse neuronal necrosis.

In its pure form, leucomalacia has the morphological attributes of a hypoxic-ischaemic lesion. Its localization at the boundary between ventriculofugal and ventriculopetal cerebral arteries (van den Bergh, 1961; van den Bergh and Vander Eecken, 1968; DeReuk, Chattha and Richardson, 1972), a poorly vascularized area in premature infants (Takashima and Tanaka, 1978a, b), suggests inadequate cerebral perfusion during episodes of apnoea and hypotension commonly found in the history of these premature infants. White matter in the process of myelination is likely to be vulnerable to oxygen lack and circulatory failure. The cortex, by contrast, is relatively spared, perhaps because of the numerous leptomeningeal arterial anastomoses in the fetal brain (Vander Eecken, 1959). Moreover, the oxygen requirement of the cortex is relatively low because of immaturity of the cells, poor development of the neuropil and the absence of oxidative enzymatic activity (Farkas-Bargeton and Diebler, 1978). The high frequency of leucomalacia in cases of meningoencephalitis may be explained by the association with cardiovascular collapse, damage to capillary walls and various metabolic disturbances. In 1969, Gilles and Murphy, suggested that bacterial endotoxin had a role in the genesis of leucomalacia. By intra-abdominal injection of *Escherichia coli* in pregnant animals, the authors produced, in newborn rabbits, lesions similar to those in the early stages described in human neonates.

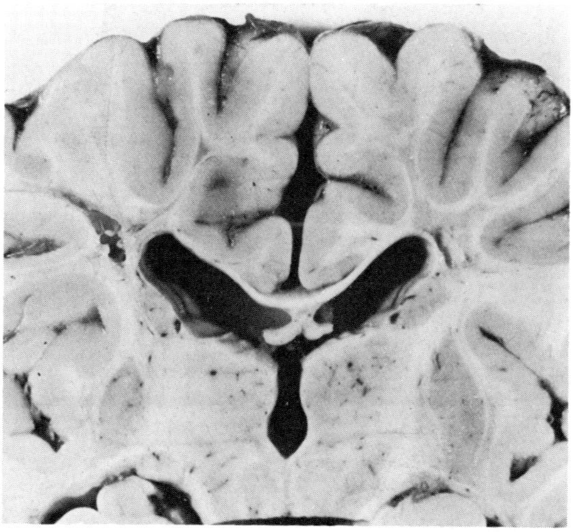

Fig. 11.22 Coronal section of the brain of a 4½-year-old child who was severely retarded. Bilateral cystic softenings are present in the white matter close to the angles of the lateral ventricles which are dilated. The thalami show état marbré.

With improved general care the mortality and morbidity and especially neurological disabilities in low birth weight infants have significantly decreased (Hagberg, Hagberg and Olow, 1975, 1977). Concomitantly, the number of infants who die after surviving more than 10 days has increased. As with intraventricular haemorrhage, lesions are now being observed at a later stage. The morphological sequelae which can be distinguished include a deficiency of myelin in the centrum semiovale (Foix et al., 1926; Marie, Lyon and Bargeton, 1959), which is the end-result of coagulative necrosis and is associated with a glial reaction (Figs. 11.22 and 11.23) the accumulation of macrophages and calcium deposits or mummified cells. Disrupted axons do not myelinate and are unstained with Sudan black or myelin stains (Larroche, 1977). Sclerotic atrophy of the centrum semiovale is compensated for by ex vacuo hydrocephalus.

Multicystic encephalopathy (polyporencephaly) results from the disintegration of brain

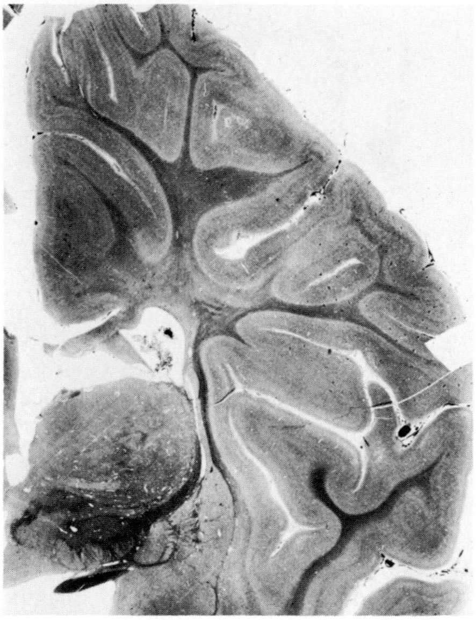

(a)

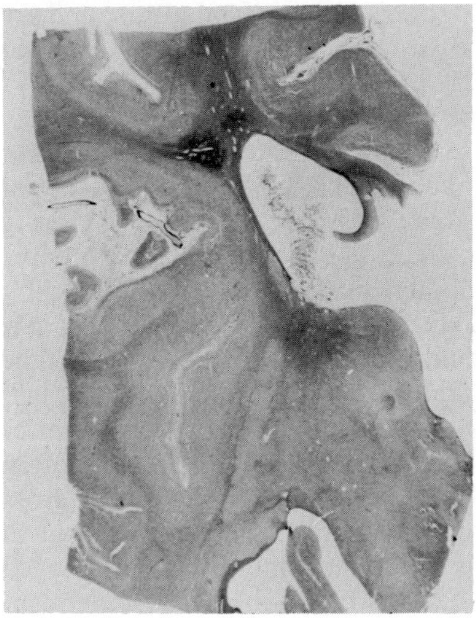

(b)

Fig. 11.23 (**a**) Brain of a 6-year-old child. Section of the parietal lobe stained to demonstrate myelin shows marked pallor in the white matter of the centrum semiovale. Loyez method. (**b**) Section of the same brain, stained by Holzer's method for astrocytes. There is marked astrocytic gliosis of the periventricular white matter (**a** and **b** by courtesy of Dr E. Farkas.)

tissue, the extent of which varies from case to case. When the primary lesion is severe and the unmyelinated white matter oedematous, the lesions become cystic instead of sclerotic (Figs. 11.24 to 11.26). Ex vacuo hydrocephalus will accompany the severe loss of brain tissue. Large astrocytes and macrophages, calcium deposits and damaged axons are commonly found in the walls of the cavities.

Infants who survive with moderate lesions may develop motor deficits, such as spastic mono- or diplegia or auditory and visual impairments, but CT scan may show no significant changes apart from the enlarged ventricles. Multicystic encephalopathy, by contrast, can be detected with CT scan. In the later stages the EEG shows various non-specific abnormal patterns and the absence of bioelectric maturation. The infant may deteriorate and lapse into a state of lethargy, or convulsions and a decerebrate posture may develop.

Hypoxic-ischaemic encephalopathies in full-term neonates

The term 'hypoxic-ischaemic encephalopathy' covers a large part of neonatal neuropathology. Intraventricular haemorrhage in the premature infant and necrosis of white matter or leucomalacia represent particular entities observed either alone or in association with other lesions.

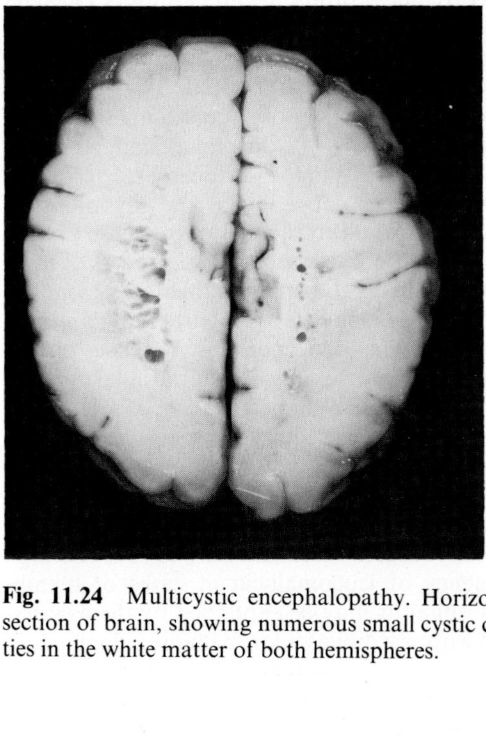

Fig. 11.24 Multicystic encephalopathy. Horizontal section of brain, showing numerous small cystic cavities in the white matter of both hemispheres.

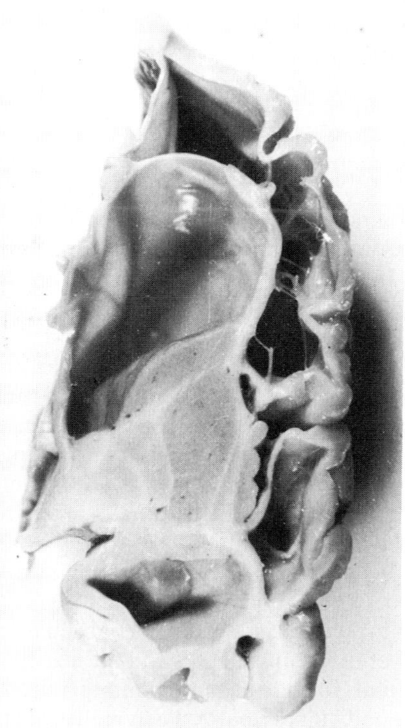

Fig. 11.25 Extensive cavitation of white matter ('central porencephaly'). The condition was bilateral in an 8-month-old retarded child.

In this chapter the term is confined to neuronal necrosis, be it diffuse or focal, which occurs usually in full-term infants in the course of difficult labour and/or delivery, less frequently after birth (Terplan, 1967; Larroche, 1968a). Certain obstetrical situations are known to lead frequently to cerebral damage—for example: occipitoposterior and occipitotransverse position; breech presentation; antepartum haemorrhage due to placenta praevia or abruptio placentae; prolapsed umbilical cord or tight cord around the neck; labour of less than 3 hours in a primipara or of more than 15 hours in a multi- or primipara; a prolonged second stage of labour (more than 2 hours); or a difficult forceps delivery. The risk of serious accidents has been much reduced by better antenatal care and the general use of monitoring of the fetal heart rate (Hon, 1977; Amiel-Tison, Dalisson and Henrion, 1980). In some centres fetal scalp electrodes are used to monitor blood pH and Po_2 as well.

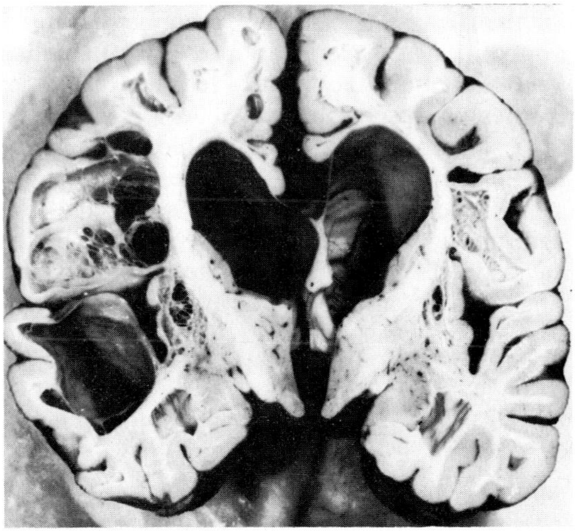

Fig. 11.26 Multicystic encephalopathy (cystic encephalomalacia) of subcortical white matter. There is also bilateral softening of the putamina.

Neurological disorders of varying severity are, however, still observed in neonates who have suffered hypoxic-ischaemic damage before or during birth (Amiel-Tison, 1969; Brown et al., 1974; Volpe, 1981). Amiel-Tison (1979) has defined mild, moderate and severe forms. In mild and moderate forms, there are abnormalities of muscle tone, primary reflexes are temporarily depressed or absent and isolated seizures may occur, but the long-term prognosis is usually good. In large maternity hospitals the incidence of mild and moderate forms has decreased from 1 per 100 live births to 1 per 1000 over the last 15 years. The severe form described below has decreased from 1.6 per 1000 to less than 1 per 1000 during the same period.

In the severe form of hypoxic-ischaemic encephalopathy, the infant is hypotonic at birth, with an Apgar score of less than 3, and requires resuscitation and mechanical ventilation. Abnormal neurological signs develop within a few hours. In the initial period the infant is stuporous or in deep coma and seizures occur in about 50 per cent of cases. Status epilepticus is defined as seizures separated by short intervals without recovery of consciousness. Seizures are often not apparent clinically but the EEG shows bursts of paroxysmal activity or an inactive trace (Dreyfus-Brisac and Monod, 1964). In these cases, the prognosis is very poor. Abnormal eye movements, dilated pupils, inappropriate sucking or subtle movements of the chin are seizure equivalents. In addition, the cry is weak or absent. In many cases it is impossible to obtain CSF at lumbar puncture, probably because of

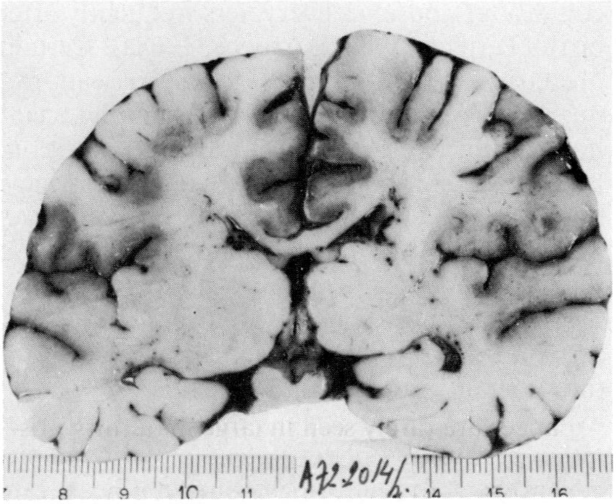

Fig. 11.27 Coronal section of brain of full-term infant. There is extensive dusky discoloration of the cortex with some accentuation in depths of sulci. The temporal cortex on both sides is relatively spared.

oedema. CT scan and ultrasonography show narrow ventricles and sometimes hypodense areas which may represent transient oedema in unmyelinated white matter or severe malacia.

Brain swelling is almost always present. The fontanelles are tense and the sutures separated. There is an absence of CSF in the subarachnoid space, the gyri are flattened and sulci narrowed. Grooving of the uncus and herniation of the cerebellar tonsils through the foramen magnum may be found. The more swollen the brain, the greater its gain in weight during formalin fixation.

On section the brain is pale, sometimes dry but more often watery and tending to disintegrate. The ventricles are compressed with protrusion of the infundibulum into the interpeduncular cistern and there may be a grey-brown discoloration of the cortex (Fig. 11.27), deep grey matter and brain stem structures. The subcortical white matter is often liquefied. The first and second temporal gyri are usually preserved.

Cortical necrosis may be focal or diffuse, patchy or columnar in distribution. It is often more pronounced in the depths of sulci than on the crests of gyri. This topography may be related to the peculiar vascular pattern in the neonate, the depth of the sulcus presenting a relatively avascular triangle (Takashima, Armstrong and Becker, 1978). Necrosis may be laminar (Courville, 1958) involving preferentially layers III and V. Layer II is usually well preserved. It has been suggested (Hopkins, Farkas-Bargeton and Laroche, 1980) that laminar necrosis might correspond to the sites where oxidative enzyme activity first develops in the full-term infant and after birth (Farkas-Bargeton and Diebler, 1978). The hippocampus as a whole, not only Sommer's sector, is vulnerable, cytoplasmic vacuolation, pyknotic nuclei, spindle-shaped neurons and cell loss being found in the pyramidal layer, karyorrhexic forms mostly in the subiculum and presubiculum. In the basal ganglia, large neurons of the globus pallidus are often spindle-shaped, but it may be difficult to identify neuronal damage and loss in the neostriatum. Thalamic nuclei are variably damaged, posterolateral nuclei and centrum medianum being particularly vulnerable. At times, neurons become basophilic with deeply stained processes. Neuronophagia is not a common finding. Damage to the external geniculate body is noteworthy; this necrosis may be global, or somewhat laminar like the underlying structure.

In the brain stem, necrosis occurs particularly in the nuclei of the cranial nerves and the neurons of the reticular formation and pontine nuclei. The inferior colliculi are particularly vulnerable. These lesions are very similar to those demonstrated by Ranck and Windle (1959) in asphyxiated monkeys. The necrosis is rarely visible on gross examination. Histological preparations, show pyknotic neurons, prominent capillaries and, at times, actual infarction.

In the cerebellum, karyorrhexis of the internal granular layer, necrosis of Purkinje cells and cells of the dentate nucleus are prominent features found in nearly every case. Because of swelling and herniation, the tonsils are often the site of both anoxic-ischaemic and haemorrhagic necrosis. Neurons of the medulla oblongata, mainly the inferior olives, and the large anterior horn cells of the spinal cord may also be affected. The few myelinated fibres that are present in the hemispheres of infants at term are poorly stained, swollen, vacuolated and irregular, looking like a string of beads. Later they become fragmented.

Unlike the nearly constant lesions produced in newborn monkeys (Myers, 1972, 1977), where parameters such as duration and severity of anoxic-ischaemic insults can be well controlled, cerebral damage in human neonates is unpredictable in terms of topography and intensity. In most cases, diffuse hypoxic lesions predominate, and there is damage of varying severity in vulnerable areas listed above. Lesions may predominate in the cortex as opposed to the deep grey nuclei, or vice versa. MacAdams (1967) described neuronal necrosis limited to the ventral pons in neonates with pulmonary haemorrhage, and Friede (1972b) observed neuronal necrosis limited to the ventral pons and subicular segment of Ammon's horn in a group of neonates with a history of respiratory distress. A similar distribution of necrosis has been described in severely asphyxiated neonates who sustained an episode of hyperoxaemia (Ahdab-Barmada, Moossy and Painter, 1980).

In other cases, ischaemic lesions predominate in a particular arterial territory or in the boundary zones between two arterial territories. These lesions may be secondary to episodes of hypotension and cerebral hypoperfusion. Volpe and Pasternak (1977) have described three cases of parasagittal cerebral ischaemic injury diagnosed on the basis of technetium brain scan. The areas of probable necrosis were in the terminal fields of the anterior, middle and posterior cerebral arteries. These lesions, however, are rarely pure, and neuronal necrosis is usually observed in other areas as well—mainly in brain stem and dentate nuclei.

Mechanisms by which hypoxic-ischaemic states act upon the brain are complex and have been studied extensively in experimental animals. The changes observed by Myers and colleagues (Myers, 1977, 1979) in fetal rhesus monkeys closely mimic the structural abnormalities in human neonates. Other experiments have been conducted by Brierley and Meldrum (1971), Vannucci and Plum (1975), Duffy and Vannucci (1977) and Vannucci, Nardis and Vannucci (1980), among others. Cerebral hypoxia is discussed in Chapter 4.

Sequelae of hypoxic-ischaemic encephalopathy

In the past, more than 50 per cent of those infants who sustained this type of encephalopathy died within a few days or weeks from diffuse, severe brain dysfunction and/or associated pulmonary complications (Larroche, 1968a). In survivors, lethargy, hypotonia and poor activity persist for weeks. The sucking reflex may reappear and the infant can be bottle-fed. This period of apparent clinical improvement is often misleading, and microcephaly and severe neurological disorders such as spastic paraplegia or quadriplegia, with or without choreo-athetosis, seizures and severe mental retardation may develop in the following months.

CT scans show cerebral atrophy of varying degree, but enlargement of the ventricles is usually less pronounced in infants born at term than in prematurely born infants who develop other forms of cerebral palsy (Kulakowski and Larroche, 1980). Necrosis of the white matter seems to lead to a greater loss of brain substance than does neuronal necrosis of the deep grey nuclei. Nowadays, these severe neurological disturbances are rarely seen in large maternity hospitals, but occasionally an infant who has suffered such brain damage may survive under mechanical ventilation and the neonatal death rate depends to some extent on local ethical decisions.

The structural sequelae are varied and unpredictable. The brain may undergo extensive disintegration and liquefaction, cortex and subcortical white matter presenting a honeycomb appearance, the shape of the gyri being maintained by the molecular layer and leptomeninges. The whole brain may become a multicystic structure. Severe oedema and the high water content of the neonatal brain may explain such evolution. In other cases, because of neuronal loss and poor myelination, the convolutions are thinned and the sulci widened, a sequel known as ulegyria (Fig. 11.28) or gyral scarring (Bresler, 1899; Norman, 1944). Because the initial lesions are usually more severe in the depths of the sulci, the shrinkage is more marked in the deeper parts of the convolution than on the crests, giving them a mushroom shape (Courville, 1960). When shrunken convolutions (ulegyria) are widespread, one may get the impression of polygyria. Laminar atrophy is best seen on sections stained for myelin or by Holzer's method for astrocytes (Fig. 11.29). The ventricle may be enlarged and the corpus callosum thin. Nodular atrophy gives an irregular configuration to the surface of the brain (Courville, 1959, 1960) and glial scars alternate with 'plaques fibromyéliniques'. In the basal ganglia there is the classic *état marbré* or *status marmoratus* first reported by Anton (1893) in a boy with choreo-athetosis who died at 9 years of age, and subsequently by Vogt (1911). Extensively described in the early twentieth century, these lesions are definitively related to birth injury by Norman (1938, 1947) and Malamud (1950), and were said to be often asso-

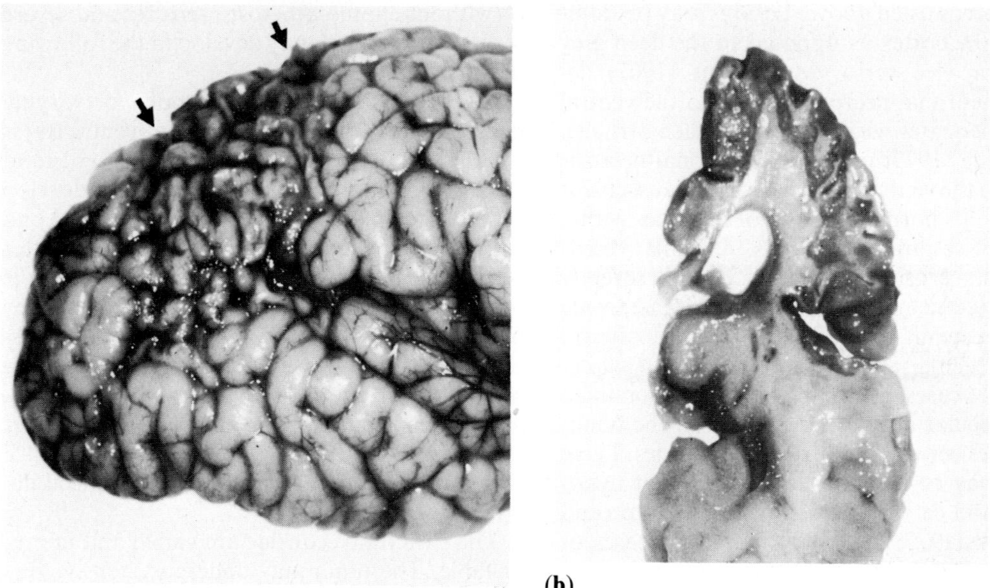

(a) (b)

Fig. 11.28 (**a**) Ulegyria of posterior parietal lobule. Note the small shrunken gyri in the region between the arrows. (**b**) Section of the same brain. The shrunken parietal gyri are contrasted with the temporal which appear normal. (**a** and **b** by courtesy of Dr R.A. Osborne and Dr L. Gupta.)

ciated with cortical lesions. Status marmoratus consists of whitish spots or streaks, resembling the pattern of marble, in the lateral part of the corpus striatum and, less often, in the head of the caudate nucleus and thalamus. The lesions are usually bilateral. Microscopic examination shows bundles of myelinated fibres (once thought to be in excess) focal loss of neurons and glial scarring (Fig. 11.30). The apparent increase in myelin staining is now interpreted as an abnormal distribution of myelinated fibres, a residual lesion due to deviation of myelin formation by astrocytes (Borit and Herndon, 1970). Friede and Schiedmayr (1977), who studied the early stages of status marmoratus in three brains have described maloriented myelinated fibres crossing the scarred tissues but no derangement of the process of myelin formation.

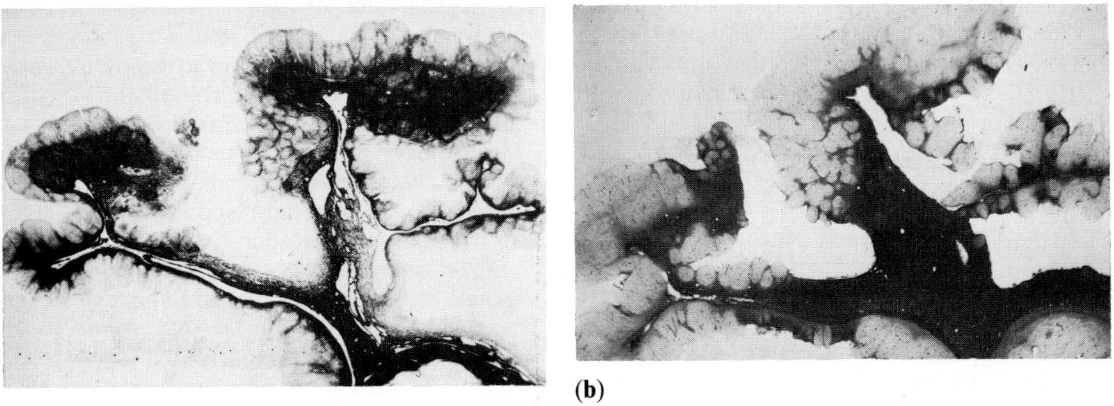

(a) (b)

Fig. 11.29 Ulegyria. Sections of shrunken sclerotic gyri. (**a**) Section stained by Loyez method for myelin. Note the irregular hypermyelination of the cortex and linear cavitation in the underlying white matter. (**b**) Section of the same area stained by Holzer's method for astrocytes. Note dense gliosis in white matter and patchy staining in cortex.

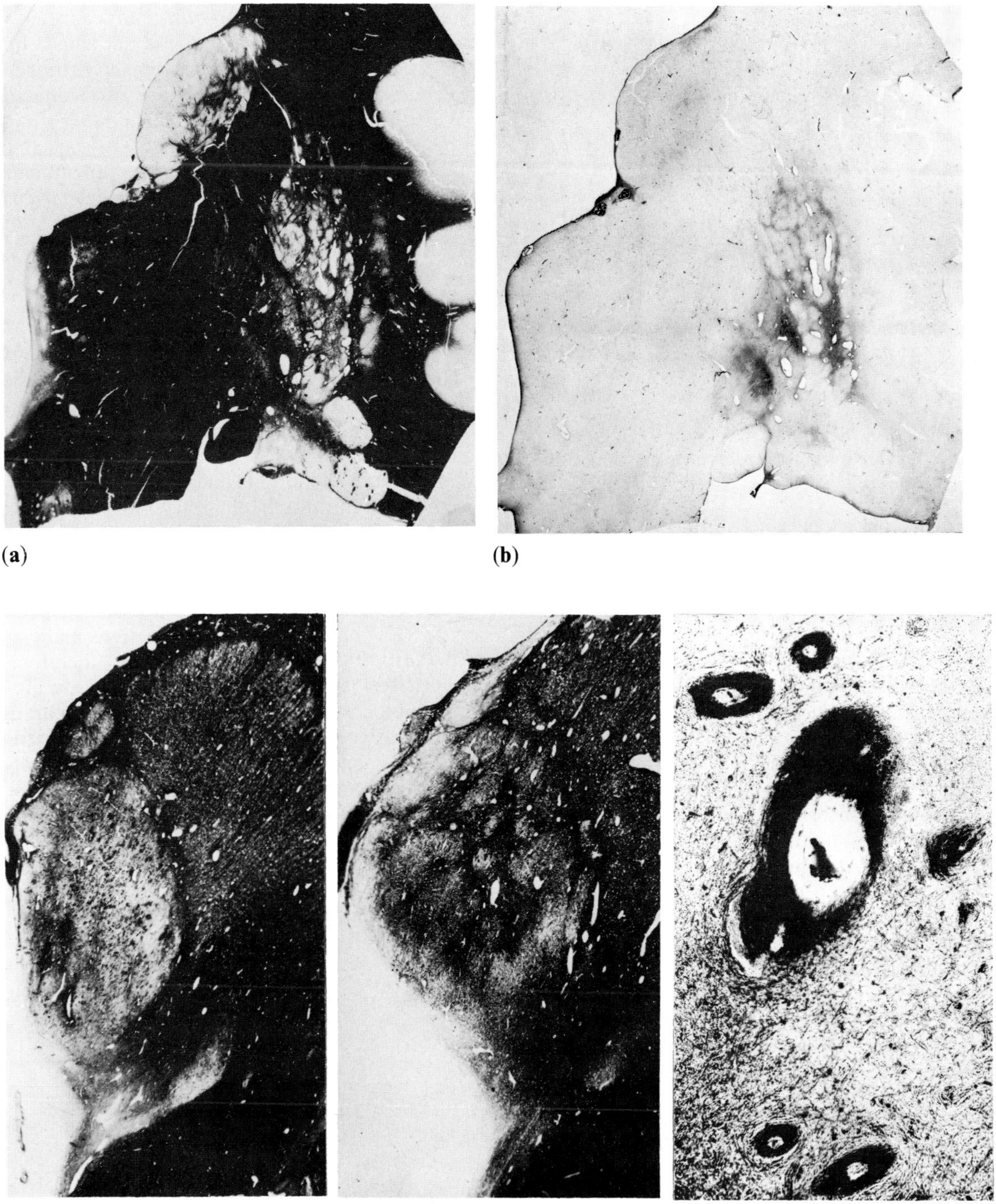

(a) (b)

(c) (d) (e)

Fig. 11.30 Status marmoratus (*état marbré*). Sections stained to demonstrate myelin by the Kultschitsky–Pal method show the irregular pattern of hypermyelination in the caudate nucleus and putamen (**a**) and dorsomedial nucleus of thalamus (**d**) compared with a normal dorsomedial nucleus (**c**). Perivascular hypermyelination in the thalamus (**e**) is an unusual form of *état marbré*. Staining by Holzer's method for astrocytes (**b**) shows marked astrocytic gliosis in putamen and globus pallidus.

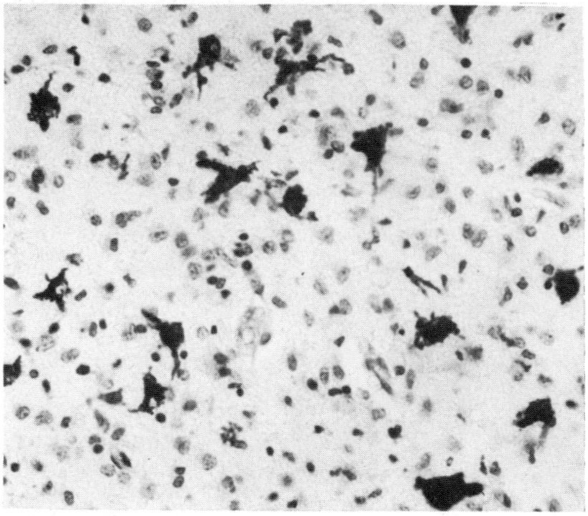

Fig. 11.31 Section of thalamus shows darkly stained ferruginated (mineralized) neurons and astrocytic gliosis.

In addition to neuronal devastation, encrusted or ferruginated neurons (Fig. 11.31) or cystic softening have also been described (Rosales and Riggs, 1962) without marbling. When the cortex has been severely damaged, there may be retrograde degeneration in the thalamus although more usually the lesions in the cortex and deep grey nuclei occur at the same time in the neonate.

Brain damage and congenital heart disease

A variety of brain lesions may occur in infants with congenital heart disease, such as leucomalacia and softening due to thrombosis or emboli, mainly when heart surgery has been performed.

Neuronal necrosis has been observed in some infants with cardiac malformations who die within a few days of birth in a state of severe anoxia and hypotension (Courville, 1955; Ober and Moore, 1955; Cohen, 1960; Terplan, 1973; Robain and Rosenberg, 1974) but the lesions are non-specific. However, the frequency of occurrence and extent of necrotic lesions are noteworthy and explain why neurological signs such as hypertonia and seizures are often observed and may be misleading in neonates with congenital heart disease.

Brain damage and hypoglycaemia

Neuronal necrosis has been attributed to hypoglycaemia in the neonatal period (Anderson, Milner and Strich, 1967). It used to occur frequently in intra-uterine growth-retarded infants, at a time when early feeding was not usual and the blood glucose level was not regularly checked (Brown and Wallis, 1963; Neligan, Robson and Watson, 1963; Haworth and McRae, 1965).

The pathology resembles hypoxic-ischaemic damage to neurons. In experimental animals Myers (1977) found a paradoxical deleterious effect of hyperglycaemia, the mechanism of which is not understood.

Arterial occlusion and cerebral infarction

The frequency of this vascular accident in the neonatal period is not known and, until recently, the diagnosis was rarely made during life because neurological signs are often subtle and overshadowed by hypotonia and respiratory distress. Similarly, during the first few weeks of life, neurological signs are rarely diagnostic. Even at autopsy, if the infarct is small and/or haemorrhagic, it can be missed. The search for vascular occlusion entails minute dissection of the vessels before the brain is cut or serial sections made of the suspected area. Very few cases, therefore, have been reported in neonates. When a major artery is occluded, gross examination of the brain at autopsy or after fixation discloses asymmetrical softening (Fig. 11.32). In neonates, infarcts are often not pale. The presence of secondary or concomitant haemorrhage may be misleading (Larroche and Amiel, 1966; Friede, 1975) and

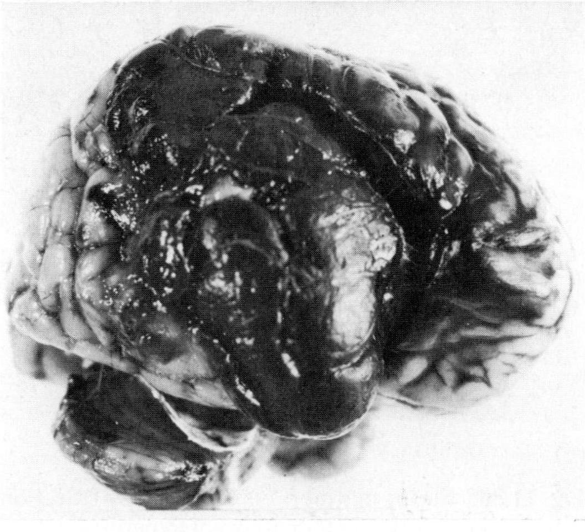

Fig. 11.32 Recent haemorrhagic infarction in the territory of the right middle cerebral artery in a neonate. Note sparing of the occipital and frontal poles.

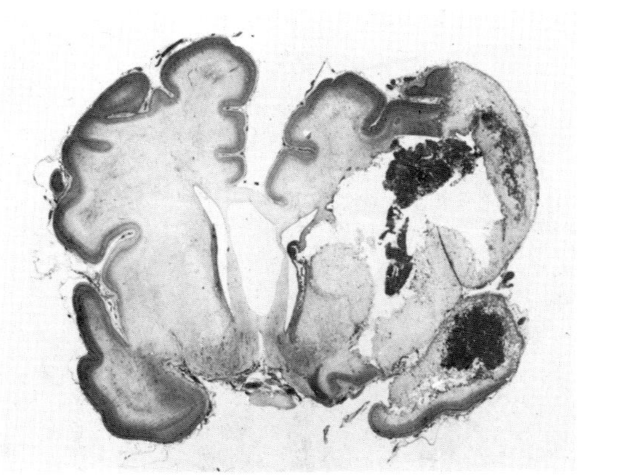

Fig. 11.33 Coronal section showing infarction in the territory of the right middle cerebral artery. The necrotic cortex is sharply demarcated from the unaffected cortex and there has been haemorrhage into the necrotic white matter. Cresyl violet.

may be more prominent in the white matter than in the cortex (Fig. 11.33). The high water content and the absence of myelin probably account for the rapid disintegration of the tissue and the multiple cavities.

Microscopic examination of a recent infarct shows pyknotic neurons or poorly stained cortical areas. A glial reaction with lipid phagocytes and prominent endothelial cells is recognizable within a few days. The affected cortex is disorganized through its full thickness and is sharply demarcated from surrounding normal areas. In recent infarcts it may be difficult to identify fresh thromboemboli. There is no inflammatory reaction and the walls of the vessels may not be damaged. When a large vessel is involved it is usually the middle cerebral artery, more often the left.

Cerebral infarcts occur in premature as well as in full-term infants. Various clinical states are associated with these lesions and may be implicated in their formation, such as respiratory distress, sepsis, congenital heart disease and surgery. Umbilical venous catheters introduced for blood sampling, fluid administration or exchange transfusion have been the source of emboli that may reach the brain as long as the foramen ovale is patent (Larroche, 1977).

Barmada, Moossy and Shuman (1979) found cerebral infarcts in 5.4 per cent of neonates at autopsy, in boys more often than in girls; 18 of the 29 cases reported showed disseminated intravascular coagulation, but the frequency of sepsis and surgery was particularly high in this series. In Friede's cases (1973), cerebral infarcts were thought to be a complication of neonatal leptomeningitis.

In infants who have survived for a time, the morphological features of old infarcts are very similar to those in adults; they have been extensively described (Eicke, 1947; Courville, 1953a; Bertrand and Bargeton, 1955; Norman, Urich and McMenemey, 1957; Urich, 1977). Asymmetrical hemispheres with atrophy, multicystic degeneration and an enlarged ventricle on the side of the lesion are characteristic findings (Fig. 11.34). The lesions may extend to the basal ganglia and thalamus and asymmetrical atrophy of the brain stem is also observed. It is noteworthy that infarcts which occur *in utero* and are described in stillborn infants have a similar appearance. The clinical lesions associated with the infarct become manifest a few months after birth, asymmetrical muscular tone preceding overt hemiplegia. There may be other motor deficits such as choreo-athetosis or, in some cases, recurrent seizures and mental retardation (Aicardi, Amsili and Chevrie, 1969; Kulakowski and Larroche, 1980).

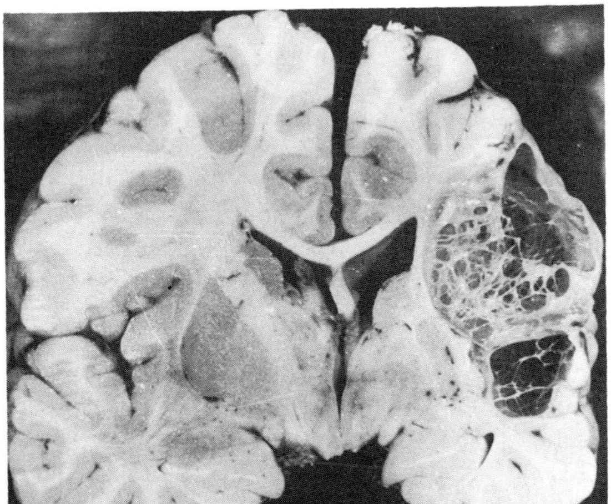

Fig. 11.34 Unilateral old cystic softening in the territory of the middle cerebral artery. Note the small size of the affected hemisphere and the enlarged lateral ventricle.

Multicystic encephalopathy, porencephaly and hydranencephaly

Destructive lesions may involve most of the white matter, with extensive cavitation, or may be limited to the territory of one or more major cerebral arteries. The most severe form, showing almost total destruction of the cerebrum, is hydranencephaly. The differences between multicystic encephalopathy, porencephaly and hydranencephaly are ill-defined, their development depending on the time of occurrence, the extent of the brain damage and survival time. The first parameter—time of occurrence of the lesions in relation to the stage of brain development—is of major importance. Morphogenetic and cytogenetic cortical abnormalities or 'malformations' may develop in association with such clastic lesions, suggesting that the damage occurred *in utero* before neuronal migration was completed. When the injury occurs later in pregnancy, the pathological picture is very similar to that following a comparable lesion after birth. Moreover, congenital porencephaly may progress after birth, evolving into a nearly total loss of parenchyma as in hydranencephaly.

Vascular occlusions or vascular maldevelopment, hypotension, severe anoxia and fetal encephalitis have been incriminated in the pathogenesis of these lesions (Kundrat, 1882; Crome, 1958; Norman, Urich and Woods, 1958; Friede, 1975; Lemire et al, 1975; Smith and Rodeck, 1975; Rorke, 1982; among others). The introduction of CT scan and ultrasonography has brought a new dimension to this problem, confirming some assertions based on autopsy findings and providing irrefutable proof of the intrauterine onset of the lesions in some cases.

Hydranencephaly

This deserves particular attention because of its extensive literature. Cruveilhier (1862) was probably the first to describe hydro-anencephaly. Kluge (1902) coined the term 'hydranencephaly'. Many classic descriptions since published are still valuable, despite variations in terminology (Lange-Cosack, 1944; Crome and Sylvester, 1958; Muir, 1959; Dekaban, 1965; Lyon and Robain, 1967). Post-mortem examination discloses a balloon-like structure which fills the cavity of the skull, and is easily ruptured during dissection. The wall consists of leptomeninges and a gliotic molecular layer, often adherent to the dura. The only remnants of the brain are the lower part of the brain stem and the cerebellum. Exceptionally, however, the lesion may involve structures in the distribution of the vertebral and basilar arteries (Roesmann and Parks, 1978). In certain cases the falx separates two cystic hemispheres. There is no distinct separation between the ventricles and the cavities which are filled with clear colourless or yellow CSF. Basal ganglia and thalamus are often prominent. Parts of the frontal and temporal lobes may also be preserved (Figs. 11.35 and 11.36). In other cases the cingular gyri and parasagittal medial structures are relatively spared. The term 'basket brain' is sometimes used, the preserved medial structures forming the 'handle' of the basket (Norman, Urich and Woods, 1958). Similar anomalies were described by Yakovlev (1959) in his study on schizencephalies.

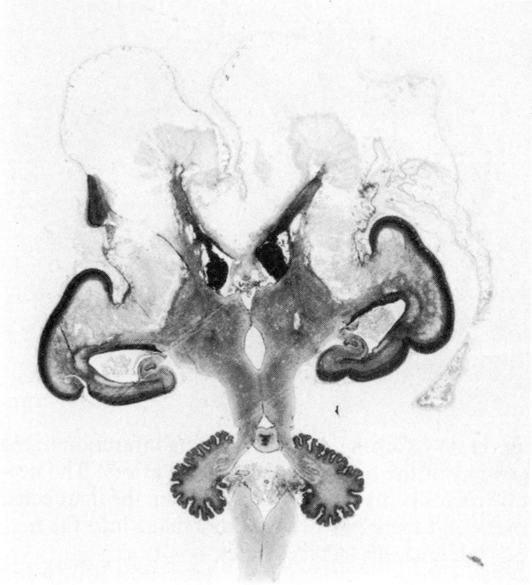

Fig. 11.35 Hydranencephaly. Section of brain showing extensive cavitation of frontal lobes, the wall of the hemispheres consisting of a thin membrane. Temporal lobes, hippocampi, thalami and brain stem and cerebellum are relatively preserved. Cresyl violet.

On histological examination, the wall of the hemisphere consists of a thin membrane of connective tissue and leptomeninges containing vessels. The outer layer of the cortex may persist, as may a residual pattern of convolutions. Where multiple cavities are present, the trabeculae contain lipid macrophages and glial cells. The choroid plexus is usually attached to the floor of the ventricles. The extent of damage to the deep grey nuclei varies but the structures are usually disorganized with focal scarring and mineralization.

Why the clinical signs should sometimes be

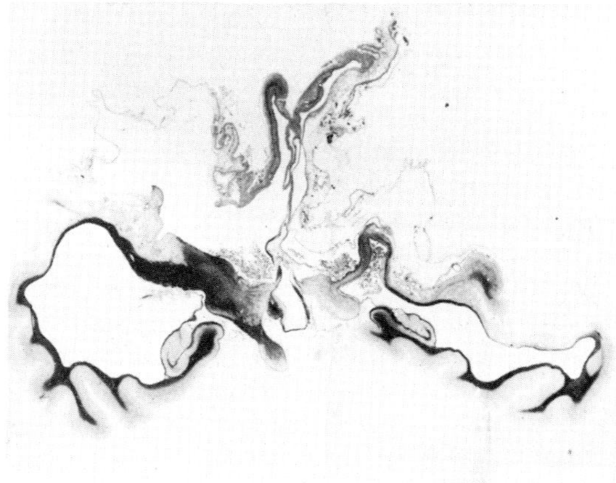

Fig. 11.36 Coronal section of the brain after survival for many years following neonatal meningitis complicated by thrombosis of the middle and anterior cerebral arteries. The preserved areas of brain were in the distribution of the posterior cerebral arteries. The parietal lobes are replaced by cavities bounded by a thin membrane consisting of leptomeninges and neuroglial tissue. Heidenhain method for myelin.

minimal in the neonatal period (Halsey, Allen and Chamberlain, 1971; André et al., 1975) is not well understood. The infant's head may not be enlarged at birth although it may increase rapidly afterwards; whether this is due to obstruction of CSF flow at the aqueduct or overproduction of CSF with defective reabsorption, is not clear.

Spastic quadriplegia and failure of development are the rule in survivors, and it is conceivable that a continuum comprising multicystic encephalopathy, porencephaly and hydranencephaly will be established.

The pathogenesis is probably complex, and various mechanisms have been invoked. Lindenberg and Swanson (1967) believed that hydranencephaly results from cerebral infarction caused by impaired blood flow through the carotid arteries, and, indeed, arteriography has demonstrated hypoplasia of the internal carotid arteries (La Torre and Occhipinti, 1970; André et al., 1975), or bilateral occlusion (Harwood-Nash and Fitz, 1976), or absence of the middle cerebral arteries (Boedecker, Sty and Young, 1981). Polycythaemia, hyperviscosity and decreased tissue perfusion with cerebral ischaemia is the mechanism suggested by Koffler, Keenan and Sutherland (1974). Hydranencephaly has been described in twins. A few cases of familial hydranencephaly have been reported (Fowler et al., 1972; Martin et al., 1977) but the mode of transmission is not clear.

Hydranencephaly has been produced experimentally in monkeys (Myers, 1969) by ligation of the carotid arteries and the jugular veins and, in newborn puppies, by occlusion of the carotid arteries with paraffin. Whilst circulatory impairment is recognized as the main cause, hydranencephaly associated with toxoplasmosis has been described by Altshuler (1973) and by Friede and Mikolasek (1978).

Subependymal pseudocysts

These formations may be related in some way to the anomalies of the walls of the ventricles mentioned in Chapter 10. Until recently, pathologists have paid little attention to them. Schwartz in his monograph (1961) mentioned them briefly. The writer identified 22 examples in 1000 consecutive autopsies (Larroche, 1972b). Isolated or multiple, and not communicating with the ventricles, these cavities can be found at varying depths, but most often are close to the ependyma and anywhere around the ventricular system. The site of predilection, however, is the precaudate germinal matrix. The cavity may be empty and well circumscribed, or irregular and multilocular. Histological examination reveals in some cases remnants of germinal cells and macrophages loaded with iron pigments.

The causes of these cysts are probably diverse. In the writer's series of neonates, various pathological conditions were associated with the cavities, such as respiratory distress with subependymal haemorrhage, hydrops fetalis, cytomegalic inclusion body disease and toxoplasmosis. Subependymal cysts have also been described in the rubella syndrome (Rorke and Spiro, 1967), in various severe congenital malformations and genetic disorders such as lactic acid encephalopathy (Farkas-Bargeton et al., 1971) and in Zellweger's syndrome (Sommer, Bradel and Hamoudi, 1974). The subependymal matrix is probably most vulnerable in early fetal life, and various insults or pathogenetic agents, such as viruses, may destroy some or all of its cells. In intensive care units, premature infants on prolonged mechanical ventilation may survive germinal matrix haemorrhage, and recently, these subependymal cavities have been more widely recognized as a sequel of subependymal haemorrhage (Volpe, 1981; Rorke, 1982).

Fetal encephalopathies of circulatory origin

This is a heterogeneous group of lesions which may be related either to fetal or maternal conditions or to anomalies of the placenta and umbilical cord.

Fetal conditions

Fetal conditions include twinning, arterial occlusions and blood dyscrasias.

Cerebral damage in multiple pregnancies Until recently, the relationship between brain damage and multiple pregnancy was not fully appreciated. Brocher (1932), in an account of five cases of porencephaly, was probably the first to mention that one infant was a twin, the other twin having been macerated and stillborn. A similar situation was reported by Stevenson and McGowan (1942) in one of seven cases of encephalomalacia. Urich (1977) illustrated extensive cavitation of the central white matter in an 8-month-old idiot whose co-twin had been dead *in utero* for several days. Manterola, Towbin and Yakovlev (1966) described cerebral infarction in a non-macerated and underweight stillborn whose co-twin survived. These authors were the first to stress two points: namely, that the infarct had occurred *in utero*, before the onset of labour, and that it was probably due to the so-called transfusion syndrome. Cerebral damage related to pathological conditions in twins with monochorionic placentation has since been described under various terms such as multicystic encephalomalacia (Aicardi, Goutières and Hodebourg de Verbois, 1972; Smith and Rodeck, 1975), cavitated cerebral lesions (Friede, 1975) and encephaloclastic lesions (Norman, 1980). Encephalomalacia has also been described in cases with visceral necroses or ischaemic infarcts occurring in twins (Benirschke, 1961; Reisman and Pathak, 1966; Moore, McAdams and Sutherland, 1969; Dimmick, Hardwick and Ho-Yuen, 1971; Stark and Geiger, 1973).

Yoshioka et al. (1979) and Choulot, Leclerc and Saint-Martin (1982) described cerebral anomalies on CT scan and stressed the relationship between the lesions and multiple pregnancy. Others (Koch et al., 1980) described CT scan images of multicystic spaces in the cerebral hemispheres in similar circumstances.

The lesions vary from recent focal softening with small cavities to extensive destruction and hydranencephaly. At autopsy the brain is soft, usually small but sometimes of normal size for the age of the infant, and the gyri have a normal pattern. Softening may be readily visible on gross examination and the hemispheres may collapse during manipulation. The lesions are often symmetrical and the brain substance largely replaced by a multitude of cavities of varying size, traversed by lace-like trabeculae. Much of the cortex may be reduced to a thin membrane, parts of the frontal and temporal lobes, basal ganglia and thalamus being relatively spared. The brain stem and the cerebellum are grossly preserved, suggesting sparing in the territories of the vertebral and posterior cerebral arteries (see Fig. 11.35).

On histological examination, the affected cortex is totally devoid of neurons, whilst the molecular layer is preserved and highly cellular. The meninges are often hypervascularized. The extent of the lesion with the accumulation of lipid phagocytes and fine calcification varies from one case to another. There is no inflammatory reaction. In the white matter, macrophages and proliferating glial cells are found within a honeycomb-like matrix. There may be areas of necrosis and cavitation in the brain stem. In most cases there is little or no evidence of haemorrhage.

The cause of these severe destructive lesions is not clear. Their distribution is not consistent with venous infarction nor with occlusion of any one major artery although the regions supplied by the vertebral arteries tend to be spared.

Circulatory impairment in twins could arise in several ways. In monochorionic placentas anastomoses between the two fetal placental circulations frequently exist (Benirschke, 1961; Galea, Scott and Goel, 1982) and differences in blood pressure between the two circulations can lead to disparate growth of the fetuses. This is the so-called *transfusion syndrome*. If blood flow is severely impaired in one circulation, the corresponding fetus may die and become macerated. Subsequently, necrotic or thromboplastic material may pass from the macerated placenta to the surviving fetus (Benirschke, 1961), causing multiple emboli (Gosseye, Golaire and Larroche, 1982) or disseminated intravascular coagulation (Moore, McAdams and Sutherland, 1969). Recently, cases with multicystic encephalomalacia in the live twin with a stillborn macerated co-twin were described by Yoshioka et al. (1979), who demonstrated occlusion in large arteries.

Manterola, Towbin and Yakovlev (1966) described a case in which infarction occurred in an underweight stillborn non-macerated twin, the surviving twin being neurologically abnormal. The authors ascribed haemorrhagic infarction to venous stasis but the lesions could have resulted from primary ischaemic infarction with secondary haemorrhage.

Whatever the mechanism, the similarity of cerebral and visceral lesions in sets of twins is not fortuitous. The most severe form of brain damage (i.e. hydranencephaly) is usually observed when one fetus is already macerated at birth, implying a considerable time lapse between brain damage and delivery. The case reported by Norman (1980) illustrates the importance of the time factor in the morphogenesis of brain lesions. Besides the fact that the infant was a twin, the brain showed cortical disorganization with polymicrogyria and schizencephaly.

Neurological signs may be obvious at birth, but they are non-specific and are often overshadowed by respiratory distress. Cases with an interval between birth and the onset of neurological dysfunction have been reported with no satisfactory explanation.

In infants who survive, Aicardi, Goutières and Hodebourg de Verbois (1972) have shown, in pneumoencephalograms, multiple cavities of varying size and progressive enlargement of the ventricles which extend almost to the inner table of the skull, suggesting hydranencephaly. A wide range of psychomotor handicaps develops (Ferrer and Navarro, 1978; Yoshioka et al., 1979; Kulakowski and Larroche, 1980; Choulot, Leclerc and Saint-Martin, 1982), depending on the extent of the lesions and on their localization. Microcephaly is the rule although exceptionally the head circumference may be normal or increased because of raised intracranial pressure. Cerebrospinal fluid is usually clear and colourless but has a high protein content. The EEG is flat or shows paroxysmal spikes.

In multiple pregnancies, growth and vitality of the fetuses can be closely followed by ultrasonography. Unfortunately, this technique is not helpful in detecting a possibly compromised fetal circulation, and damage is likely to occur before appropriate obstetric action can be taken.

Arterial occlusion *in utero*. Intrauterine ischaemic lesions in a defined arterial territory are probably more frequent than was once thought.

A recent infarct of no more than a few days' duration was described by Clark and Linell (1954) in an infant who died 1.5 hours after birth. On serial sections of the middle cerebral artery an occlusion was demonstrated and there were early reactive inflammatory changes in the vessel wall. Banker (1961) found an infarct and old thrombus in a newborn infant who lived 36 hours. Cocker, George and Yates (1965) described infarcts in the territories of the middle cerebral arteries in two infants who presented with neurological signs soon after birth and died at 4 and 11 weeks respectively. The pathogenesis of these occlusions is not clear. It has been suggested that emboli arising from fetal veins or the placenta might reach the cerebral arteries because of the large right-to-left circulatory shunt in the fetus. Old infarcts were identified in a series of systematic autopsies of stillborn infants by Larroche and Amiel (1966) and Larroche (1977). One hemisphere was smaller than the other and was extensively softened and showed cavities of varying size crossed by trabeculae in the territory of the occluded middle cerebral artery (Fig. 11.37).

The cortex was an irregular ribbon-like structure with a relatively preserved and cellular

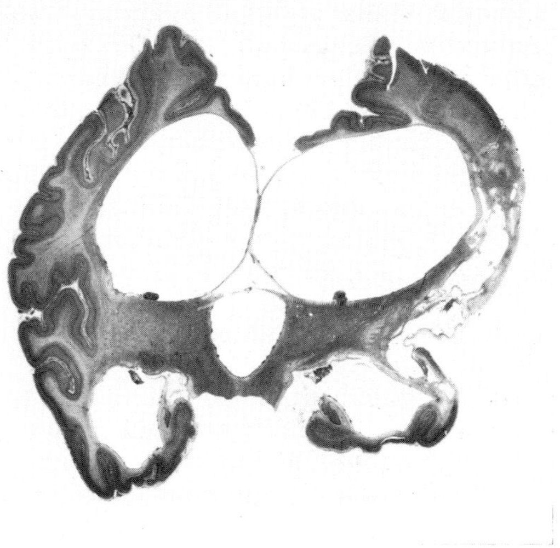

Fig. 11.37 Coronal section of the brain of a stillborn infant. There is old cystic infarction in the territory of the right middle cerebral artery and marked enlargement of the ventricular system (Courtesy of Dr C. Nessmann).

molecular layer. The underlying tissue was cavitated, the walls of these cavities containing glial cells, macrophages and encrusted neurons. The thalamus and basal ganglia of the damaged hemisphere were also partially cavitated. In one case the cerebral peduncles, pons and medulla oblongata were asymmetrical with marked atrophy of the pyramidal tract, suggesting that the vascular accident had occurred long before birth. The middle cerebral artery was occluded by old well-organized thrombus. In another case, the infarct was located in the posterior temporal and occipital lobes and was associated with severe hydrocephalus. In none of these cases could the cause of the occlusion be demonstrated.

In one case, in addition to the softening, there were heavily myelinated glial plaques in the cortex, similar to those described by Borit and Herndon (1970), as well as areas of polymicrogyria. Norman (1980) also described polymicrogyria and cerebral clefts, suggestive of a very early vascular impairment, probably during neuronal migration.

Porencephaly and microgyria were also observed by Stewart et al. (1978) in an infant with an anomalous configuration of the circle of Willis. Examination of the cerebral arteries at autopsy or by *post mortem* angiography would probably provide information on the pathogenesis of both malformations and obviously destructive lesions.

Blood dyscrasias of various origin may lead to fetal cerebral haemorrhage. Bose (1978) has described intracerebral haemorrhage in a case of hydrops fetalis due to haemolytic disease. Similarly, bleeding occurred *in utero* in an infant with isoimmune thrombocytopenia (Zalneraitis, Young and Krishnamoorthy, 1979).

Maternal conditions

These include trauma, systemic diseases and intoxications.

Various maternal conditions have long been incriminated in the pathogenesis of fetal cerebral damage. Anaemia (Norman, 1952; Scharpe and Hale, 1953), toxaemia with hypertension (Courville, 1959), renal disease with oliguria and repeated seizures during the second trimester of pregnancy (Rizzuto and Martin, 1967) and acute circulatory collapse or a persistent low blood pressure have all been incriminated. Multicystic encephalopathy has nearly always been described in older infants, but because of the maternal history and a normal labour and delivery, there was no doubt that the lesions had their onset *in utero*.

A rare case of maternal bee sting anaphylaxis during pregnancy (Erasmus, Blackwood and Wilson, 1982) was followed by delivery 5 weeks later of an infant who died at 9 weeks. At autopsy the brain was atrophic and there were numerous germinal layer cavities and old haemorrhages.

Lesions have been described in the fetus after direct trauma or severe stress to the mother. Direct trauma to the abdominal wall of the mother was reported by Grylack (1982) to have caused cephalhaematoma and hydrocephalus, and multicystic leucomalacia may follow haemorrhage due to trauma.

Severe multicystic encephalomalacia was reported by Ferrer and Navarro (1978) in a 2-day-old full-term infant whose mother suffered abdominal trauma 4 weeks before delivery. Multiple cavitation involved most of the white matter. Bilateral infarcts and atrophy in the territories of the middle cerebral arteries were diagnosed on CT scan (Coignet et al., 1979) in a 3-week-old infant, born prematurely, 1 week after the mother had been injured in a car accident. The extreme form of brain damage—hydranencephaly—was found in a fetus after the mother was involved in an aircraft accident (Fowler, Brown and Cabrera, 1971).

Diffuse ischaemic lesions may result from temporary impairment of placental blood flow due to maternal stress. Myers (1975) has shown, in the pregnant rhesus monkey, that maternal psychological stress may produce episodes of fetal asphyxia and ischaemic brain damage similar to that described in humans. Catecholamine discharge leads to uterine vasoconstriction causing impaired intervillous space perfusion.

Maternal inhalation of toxic gases The toxicity of carbon monoxide (CO) is well known. Fetal brain damage following accidental or deliberate inhalation of CO gas during pregnancy has been described. Microgyria was reported after an accident early in pregnancy (Hallervorden, 1949; Bankl and Jellinger, 1967) whilst softening of white matter and basal ganglia was described when the inhalation had occurred later in pregnancy (Maresch, 1929). The consequences to the fetus of inhalation of butane gas by the mother

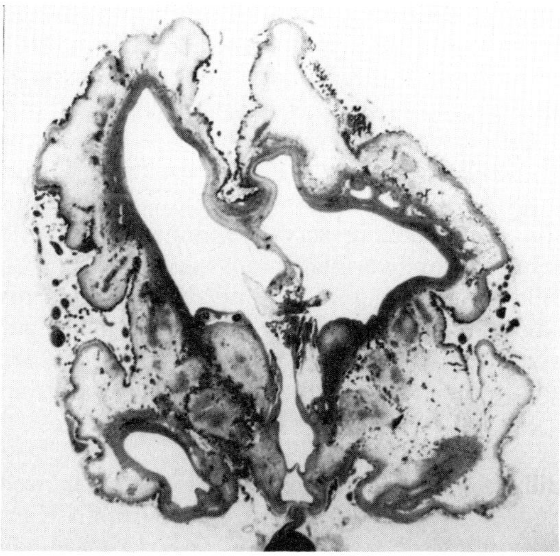

Fig. 11.38 Section of the brain of a newborn 34-week infant whose mother had inhaled butane gas at 30th week of pregnancy. There is extensive destruction of the cortex and deep grey matter, cystic cavitation of the white matter and enlargement of the ventricles.

in a suicide attempt at 30 weeks of pregnancy was reported by Gosseye, Golaire and Larroche (1982). Four weeks after the inhalation of butane, which had resulted in coma of the mother, the infant was delivered and died soon afterwards. The brain was shrunken (weighing only 88 g instead of the expected 220 g) and showed extensive encephalopathy characteristic of hypoxic-ischaemic damage with 4 weeks' survival (Fig. 11.38). The remnants of the cortex consisted of a thin layer of meninges and neurologlial tissue. Multicystic structures were separated by trabeculae containing mineralized neurons, calcium deposits, haemosiderin-laden macrophages and neuroglial cells. The brain stem and cerebellum were also severely damaged, although cells of the external granular layer of the cerebellum were relatively spared. The ventricles were greatly enlarged.

Anomalies of the placenta and cord These may interfere with the fetal circulation and lead to brain damage. Chronic fetal distress due to *placental insufficiency* causing intrauterine growth retardation was commonly observed at a time when maternal renal disease and hypertension during pregnancy were less well controlled than today, and led to much fetal and perinatal mortality. In these cases there was no specific pathology in the brain. If the infant was born alive and survived for a few days, neuronal necrosis was found, but usually only in cases of neonatal asphyxia and hypotension or hypoglycaemia. It was suggested that these lesions developed after birth in association with problems of adaptation, and were not directly related to the chronic fetal distress (Larroche, 1977).

Unusually severe *calcification* of the maternal surface of the placenta may also impair the fetal circulation. Progressive impairment of maternal placental perfusion may result in severe fetal asphyxia. *Abruptio placentae* is a classic cause of fetal death or of severe brain damage. Other conditions such as true knots of the umbilical cord or a tight cord round the neck are potential hazards to fetal cerebral circulation, especially during labour and/or delivery.

Alpers' disease

In 1931 and 1960, Alpers described cases of 'diffuse progressive degeneration of the gray matter of the cerebrum' with severe neurological dysfunction. Similar cases were reported by Blackwood et al. (1963), who proposed the eponym Alpers' disease. The illness starts in early infancy after a normal birth, with convulsions, and thereafter consists of progressive neurological deterioration with spasticity, myoclonus, status epilepticus and dementia. At autopsy, the brain is atrophic and there is generalized shrinkage of the cortex as shown by widened sulci and narrow, firm gyri. The basal ganglia, brain stem and cerebellum may be normal (Laurence and Cavanagh, 1968).

Histologically there is pseudolaminar destruction of neurons in the cerebral cortex, the second, third and fourth layers showing status spongiosus. 'Immature' ganglion cells in the cortex were considered by Alpers to be of pathological significance. There is marked astrocytic gliosis involving both cortex and white matter. The progressive nature of the process was demonstrated by Blackwood et al. (1963), who compared biopsies taken early in the course of the disease with post-mortem findings.

Other terms such as poliodystrophia cerebri progressiva infantilis (Christensen and Krabbe, 1949), walnut brain (Courville, 1953a), hemiatrophy (Norman, 1969) and spongy glioneural dystrophy (Jellinger and Seitelberger, 1970;

Hopkins and Turner, 1973) have been used as synonyms for Alpers' disease. In these cases, however, both the clinical and the morphological findings are too varied to constitute a nosological entity. Several aetiological possibilities have been proposed, such as perinatal asphyxic episodes (Courville, 1953a, b, 1958; Alberca-Serrano et al., 1965) or hypoglycaemia (Laurence and Cavanagh, 1968). Others were familial cases (Blackwood et al., 1963; Liu and Sylvester, 1960) but the underlying aetiology is not known. Focal ulegyria, encephalomalacia of various types and hemiatrophy, with or without contralateral hypertrophy, should not be included in the syndrome of Alpers' disease.

Kernicterus (bilirubin encephalopathy)

More than a century ago Hervieux (1847) described yellow pigmentation of the basal ganglia, and Orth (1875) identified crystals of bile pigment in these same sites. The term 'kernicterus' was coined only in 1903, by Schmorl. This entity has been extensively described by Dereymacker (1949), Claireaux (1950), Bertrand, Bessis and Segarra-Obiol (1952), Gerrard (1952), Haymaker et al. (1961) and Boreau et al. (1964). Other studies which have shed some light on bilirubin metabolism and on the pathophysiology of kernicterus include those of Arias (1960), Hsia (1965) and Maisels (1972).

In the newborn 75 per cent of bilirubin is derived from the normal destruction of circulating erythrocytes in the liver and spleen. Bilirubin, bound to albumin, is conjugated with glucuronic acid by the enzyme uridine diphosphoglucuronyl transferase. In this form, bilirubin passes in the bile to the intestine and is eliminated. Some conjugated bilirubin is hydrolysed by intestinal enzymes and retransported to the liver. Jaundice results mainly from insufficient capacity of the liver to conjugate an overload of bilirubin after abnormal haemolysis in blood group incompatibility (Rh and, less often, ABO), severe septicaemia, resorption of large haematomas, administration of certain drugs or a deficiency of glucose-6-phosphate dehydrogenase. Increased intestinal reabsorption of bilirubin may also lead to bilirubin overload.

Exceptionally, there may exist a primary hepatic enzyme insufficiency such as in Crigler-Najjar disease, an autosomal recessive defect, whilst an inherited deficiency of the enzyme glucuronyl transferase has also been demonstrated in the Gunn rat, a mutant which may develop kernicterus in the neonatal period (Johnson et al, 1959).

In severely asphyxiated neonates, necrosis of liver cells may decrease liver function. Drugs such as sulphonamides, hormones, sodium benzoate (used as a preservative in many injectable solutions) and various anions may compete with bilirubin for albumin-binding sites and thus impair transport (Stern, 1972). A low blood albumin level in premature infants and acidosis are additional factors adversely affecting bilirubin transport.

Bilirubin and brain damage Since it is well established that albumin-bound bilirubin is innocuous (Zuelzer and Mudgett, 1950; Odell, 1959; Diamond and Schmid, 1966), the assessment of albumin concentration, reserve albumin-binding capacity and free bilirubin levels in the blood is of considerable importance (Odell, Storey and Rosenberg, 1970; Odièvre et al., 1970; Zamet et al., 1975; Cashore and Stern, 1982; Pledger, Scott and Belfield, 1982). Less than 340 μmol of indirect serum bilirubin per litre (20 mg/100 ml) is considered a safe threshold, not requiring an exchange transfusion. In premature infants, however, a low serum albumin concentration, respiratory distress and acidosis decrease this safety margin, and kernicterus has been observed with levels as low as 170–205 μmol/l (10–12 mg/100 ml) (Stern and Denton, 1965; Gartner et al., 1970; Lucey, 1972; Zamet et al., 1975).

The mechanism by which bilirubin penetrates the brain and damages certain groups of neurons is not yet well understood. It has been suggested that asphyxia might injure vascular and endothelial cells and alter the blood–brain barrier, thus allowing bilirubin molecules access to neurons. Indeed, Lucey et al. (1964) found that infusion of unconjugated bilirubin in newborn rhesus monkeys produced kernicterus only when the animals were first rendered hypoxic, whilst in infants with septicaemia and meningoencephalitis kernicterus may be due not only to increased haemolysis but also to damage to vessel walls and to the blood–brain barrier.

Biochemical studies on experimental animals (Mustafa, Cowger and King, 1969) and electron microscopic observations (Mustapha, Cowger and King, 1969; Schutta, Johnson and Neville,

1970; Jew and Sandquist, 1979) have shown severe abnormalities of mitochondria in neurons of icteric nuclei and impairment particularly in oxidative phosphorylation processes.

The gross and microscopic features of kernicterus have been extensively described in several monographs (Dereymacker, 1949; Bertrand, Bessis and Segarra-Obiol, 1952; Haymaker et al., 1961; Larroche, 1968b, 1977). The most intense coloration was observed in infants with blood group incompatibility, although it is tending to disappear as a result of anti-D prophylaxis. In premature infants the colour is less intense and restricted to a smaller number of structures.

At autopsy, the CSF and meninges, vermis, flocculus and parahippocampal gyrus may have a yellow tinge. On sections of the brain most of the deep grey nuclei are stained yellow symmetrically (Plate 11.1, *facing* p. 490), including the corpus Luysi, globus pallidus and the lateral nuclei of the thalamus. The lateral geniculate bodies and the putamen are less frequently affected. In the brain stem all the cranial nerve nuclei, especially the oculomotor, vestibular and cochlear and hypoglossal nuclei, as well as the inferior olives, dentate and roof nuclei, nucleus gracilis and cuneatus may be affected, as are the anterior horn cells of the spinal cord. Rarely, the pigment diffuses to other structures such as the hippocampus, fornix, mamillary bodies and habenula. The ependyma and choroid plexuses may also be pigmented. In a few cases the sensorimotor, insular and visual cortices were also yellow but no specific lesions were detected on microscopic study (Martin and Larroche, 1964).

In premature infants, the corpus Luysi, lateral thalamic nuclei, and the oculomotor nerve nuclei are preferentially stained. At times, besides the grey nuclei, the entire brain shows a yellowish tinge where the bilirubin concentration in the plasma is high. The frequency of the association of kernicterus with yellow hyaline membranes (Larroche, 1977) reflects this high concentration in blood. In the fixed brain, the yellow discoloration of the nuclei may fade with time although it may still be bright in sliced brains stored in formalin for more than 10 years. Whilst bile pigments in the liver become green in formalin, bilirubin in the brain remains yellow.

Contrary to common assertion, only part of the pigment is dissolved during the course of processing into paraffin wax or celloidin. Many neurons are (Plate 11.1, *facing* p. 490) yellow, pyknotic and fusiform, with a loss of Nissl bodies. Extracellular pigment remains at the site of neuronal loss.

In mature infants with severe alloimmunization, kernicterus may be the only grossly apparent brain damage and, microscopically, neuronal necrosis is restricted to those nuclei that were bilirubin-stained. Conversely, in premature infants kernicterus is often associated with intraventricular haemorrhage and leucomalacia. In these cases necrotic white matter is often stained yellow because bilirubin is present in fat-laden macrophages. Hypoxic-ischaemic neuronal damage is often superimposed on the bilirubin encephalopathy. This is particularly true of neurons in the subiculum, the pontine nuclei and dentate nuclei which may show necrosis without bilirubin staining.

Kernicterus corresponds to the acute phase of bilirubin encephalopathy and disappears by the end of the first postnatal week. With longer survival, vulnerable structures may not be stained but histological study may show a wide spectrum of lesions. Initially there is neuronal damage with varying degrees of cell loss and a glial reaction followed by fibrillary gliosis and poor myelination. Most of the descriptions of sequelae date back to a time when blood group incompatibility was not yet preventable and when kernicterus developed in spite of repeated exchange transfusions (Fitzgerald, Greenfield and Kounine, 1939; van Bogaert, 1949; Malamud, 1961).

Since the introduction of anti-D prophylactic measures (Scott, 1968), the incidence of kernicterus has significantly changed. Today the main problem is kernicterus in low birth weight infants. Prevention, diagnosis and treatment remain unsatisfactory. In low-birth-weight infants the incidence varies from 32 per cent (Harris, Lucey and Maclean, 1958) to 64 per cent (Gartner et al., 1970) and to zero in the last series of Pearlman et al. (1978). The figure given recently by Pledger, Scott and Belfield (1982) is also very low—2 per cent—but derives from a total autopsy population. Since 1962, the writer has observed at autopsy 64 cases; i.e. about 6 per cent of infants of less than 2000 g.

Bilirubin encephalopathy in the course of haemolytic disease has virtually disappeared in most medical centres. The classic picture consists of restlessness, an abnormal cry, poor sucking and hypertonia, particularly of the neck and extensor muscles of the back. Handling may provoke attacks of opisthotonos with extension and adduction of the lower limbs, flexion of the elbows or slow athetoid movements of the upper extremities. Abnormalities of gaze with the eyes looking downwards are known as the sign of the setting sun.

In infants who survive the acute phase, posticteric encephalopathy with varying degrees of severity develops. The major clinical sign consists of extrapyramidal motor disability. Decerebrate rigidity, affecting particularly the neck and arm muscles, may follow a transient period of hypotonia. Walking may be delayed, impaired by athetoid movements, rigidity of the legs and contortions of the arms and trunk varying widely in amplitude and frequency. If muscle tone is not increased, the distal extremities may show choreiform movements. Speech may be impaired and there may be hearing deficits particularly in the high frequency range. The intellectual level may be relatively little affected. Whilst this form of the disease has practically disappeared, there remains 'the unsolved problem of kernicterus in the susceptible low-birth-weight infants' (Lucey, 1972; Cashore and Stern, 1982). The significance of motor and sensory impairments is difficult to establish, as mild bilirubin encephalopathy may be masked by hypoxic-ischaemic neuronal damage. Hearing and visual deficits may be the only clinical sequelae.

References

Ahdab-Barmada, M., Moossy, J. and Painter, M. (1980) Pontosubicular necrosis and hyperoxemia. *Pediatrics* **66,** 840–7.

Aicardi, J., Amsili, J. and Chevrie, J.J. (1969) Acute hemiplegia in infancy and childhood. *Developmental Medicine and Child Neurology* **11,** 162–73.

Aicardi, J., Goutières, F. and Hodebourg de Verbois, A. (1972) Multicystic encephalomalacia of infants and its relation to abnormal gestation and hydranencephaly. *Journal of the Neurological Sciences* **15,** 357–73.

Alberca-Serrano, R., Fabiani, F., Deneve, V. and Mecken, J. (1965) Familial spastic diplegia due to anoxic encephalopathy (Alpers). *Journal of the Neurological Sciences* **2,** 419–33.

Allan, W.C., Roseto, C.A., Sawyer, L.R. and Courtney, S.E. (1981) Sector scan ultrasound imaging through the anterior fontanelle: its use in diagnosing neonatal periventricular–intraventricular hemorrhage. *American Journal of Diseases of Children* **134,** 1028–31.

Allemand, F., Monod, N. and Larroche, J.Cl. (1977) L'electroencéphalogramme dans les hémorragies sous-durales du nouveau-né. *Revue d'EEG et de Neurophysiologie* **7,** 365.

Alpers, B.J. (1931) Diffuse progressive degeneration of the gray matter of the cerebrum. *Archives of Neurology and Psychiatry* **25,** 469–505.

Alpers, B.J. (1960) Progressive cerebral degeneration of infancy. *Journal of Nervous and Mental Diseases* **130,** 442–8.

Altshuler, G. (1973) Toxoplasmosis as a cause of hydranencephaly. *American Journal of Diseases of Children* **125,** 251–2.

Amiel, C. (1964) Hémorragies cérébrales intra-ventriculaires chez le prématuré. 2. Les éléments du diagnostic clinique. *Biologia Neonatorum* **7,** 57–75.

Amiel-Tison, C. (1969) Cerebral damage in fullterm newborn; aetiological factors, neonatal status and long term followup. *Biologia. Neonatorum* **14,** 234–50.

Amiel-Tison, C. (1979) A method for neurological evaluation within the first year of life. In *Major Mental Handicaps*, Ciba Symposium no. 59, pp. 107–26. Excerpta Medica, Amsterdam.

Amiel-Tison, C., Dalisson, C. and Henrion, R. (1980) Evolution de la pathologie cérébrale du nouveau-né à terme au cours des cinq dernières années dans la maternité de Port-Royal. *Archives Françaises de Pédiatrie* **37,** 87–92.

Anderson, J.M., Milner, R.D. and Strich, S.J. (1967) Effects of neonatal hypoglycaemia on the nervous system: a pathological study. *Journal of Neurology, Neurosurgery and Psychiatry* **30,** 295–310.

André, M., Plenat, E., Floquet, J. and Picard, L. (1975) Hydranencephalie; lésions cérébrales majeures avec comportement neurologique néonatal normal. *Archives Françaises de Pédiatrie* **32,** 915–24.

Anton, G. (1893) Über die Betheiligung der basalen Gehirnganglien bei Bewegungsstörungen und insbesondere bei der Chorea; mit Demonstrationen von Gehirnschnitten. *Wiener Klinische Wochenschrift* **6,** 859–61.

Arias, I.M. (1960) The chemical basis of kernicterus. *Advances in Clinical Chemistry* **3,** 35–82.

Baird, W.F. and Stitt, D.G. (1959) Arteriovenous aneurysm of the cerebellum in a premature infant. *Pediatrics* **24,** 455–7.

Banker, B.Q. (1961) Cerebral vascular disease in infancy and childhood. *Journal of Neuropathology and Experimental Neurology* **20,** 127–40.

Banker, B.Q. and Larroche, J.Cl. (1962) Periventricular leukomalacia of infancy: a form of neonatal anoxic encephalopathy. *Archives of Neurology* **7,** 386–410.

Bankl, H. and Jellinger, K. (1967) Zentralnervöse Schäden nach fötaler Kohlenoxydvergiftung. *Beiträge zur Pathologischen Anatomie* **135,** 350–76.

Barmada, M.A., Moossy, J. and Shuman, R.M. (1979) Cerebral infarcts with arterial occlusion in neonates. *Annals of Neurology* **6,** 495–502.

Bejar, B., Curbelo, V., Coen, R.W., Leopold, G., James, H. and Gluck, L. (1980) Diagnosis and follow-up of intraventricular and intracerebral hemorrhages by ultrasound studies of infants through the fontanelles and sutures. *Pediatrics* **66,** 661–73.

Benirschke, K. (1961) Twin placenta in perinatal mortality. *New York Medical Journal* **61,** 1499–508.

van den Bergh, R. (1961) La vascularisation artérielle intracérébrale. *Acta Neurologica et Psychiatrica Belgica* **61,** 1013–23.

van den Bergh, R. and Vander Eecken, H. (1968) Anatomy and embryology of cerebral circulation. *Progress in Brain Research* **30,** 1–25.

Bertrand, I. and Bargeton, E. (1955) Lésions vasculaires dans l'hémiplégie cérébrale infantile. *Proceedings of 2nd International Congress of Neuropathology*, part II, pp. 519–22. Excerpta Medica Foundation, Amsterdam.

Bertrand, I., Bessis, M. and Segarra-Obiol, J.M. (1952) *L'ictère Nucléaire. Séquelle de la maladie hémolytique du nouveau-né.* Masson, Paris.

Blackwood, W., Buxton, P.H., Cumings, J.N., Robertson, D.J. and Tucker, S.M. (1963) Diffuse cerebral degeneration in infancy (Alpers' disease). *Archives of Disease in Childhood* **38,** 193–204.

Blanc, J.F., Langue, J., Bochu, M., Dutruge, J. and Salle, B. (1982) Les hémorrhagies intra-cérébrales chez le nouveau-né à terme. *Archives Françaises de Pédiatrie* **39,** 251–3.

Blanc, W.A., Rapmund, G. and Silverman, W.A. (1957) Falling hematocrit value in the premature infant as a sign of intraventricular hemorrhage. *American Journal of Diseases of Children* **94,** 430.

Blank, N.K., Strand, R., Gilles, F.H. and Palakshappa, A. (1978) Posterior fossa subdural hematomas in neonates. *Archives of Neurology* **35,** 108–11.

Boedecker, R.A., Sty, J.R. and Young, L.W. (1981) Radiological case of the month. *American Journal of Diseases of Children* **135,** 1135–6.

van Bogaert, L. (1949) Aspects cliniques et pathologiques des séquelles tardives de l'ictére nucléaire. *Acta Neurologica Belgica* **49,** 961–4.

Boreau, Th., Martin, L., Larroche, J.Cl. and Sautriot, G. (1964) Etude clinique et anatomique de quelques cas d'ictère nucléaire du nouveau-né par maladie hémolytique à évolution rapidement mortelle. *Gynécologie et Obstétrique* **63,** 289–336.

Borit, A. and Herndon, R.M. (1970) The fine structure of *plaques fibromyéliniques* in ulegyria and in status marmoratus. *Acta Neuropathologica* **14,** 304–11.

Bose, C. (1978) Hydrops fetalis and in utero intracranial hemorrhage. *Journal of Pediatrics* **93,** 1023–4.

Bresler, J. (1899) Klinische und pathologisch-anatomische Beiträge zur Mikrogyrie. *Archiv für Psychiatrie* **31,** 566–73.

Brierley, J.B. and Meldrum, B.S. (1971) *Brain Hypoxia.* Heinemann Medical, London.

Brocher, J.E.W. (1932) Polyporencephalie. *Zeitschrift für die gesamte Neurologie und Psychiatrie* **142,** 107–19.

Brown, J.K., Purvis, R.J., Forfar, J.O. and Cockburn, F. (1974) Neurological aspects of perinatal asphyxia. *Developmental Medicine and Child Neurology* **16,** 567–80.

Brown, R. and Wallis, P. (1963) Hypoglycaemia in the newborn. *Lancet* **i,** 1278.

Cartwright, G.W., Culbertson, K., Schreiner, R.L. and Garg, B.P. (1979) Changes in clinical presentation of term infants with intracranial haemorrhage. *Developmental Medicine and Child Neurology* **21,** 730–7.

Cashore, W.J. and Stern, L. (1982) Neonatal hyperbilirubinemia. *Pediatric Clinics of North America* **29,** 1191–203.

Choulot, J.J., Leclerc, M.A. and Saint-Martin, J. (1982) Malformation cérébrale et jumeau survivant. *Archives Françaises de Pédiatrie* **39,** 105–7.

Christensen, A. and Krabbe, K.H. (1949) Poliodystrophia cerebri progressiva (infantilis). *Archives of Neurology and Psychiatry* **61,** 28–43.

Claireaux, A. (1950) Haemolytic disease of the newborn. II. Nuclear jaundice (kernicterus). *Archives of Disease in Childhood* **25,** 61–81.

Claireaux, A. (1970) Stillbirth and first-week deaths. In *British Births*, vol. 1: *The first week of life*, Heinemann Medical, London.

Clark, R.M. and Linell, E.A. (1954) Case report: premature occlusion of the internal carotid artery. *Journal of Neurology, Neurosurgery and Psychiatry* **17,** 295–7.

Cocker, J., George, S.W. and Yates, P.O. (1965) Perinatal occlusion of the middle cerebral artery. *Developmental Medicine and Child Neurology* **7,** 235–43.

Cohen, M.M. (1960) The central nervous system in congenital heart disease. *Neurology* **10,** 452–6.

Coignet, J., Palix, C., Tommassi, C. and Raybaud, Ch. (1979) Rapport de la scanographie dans la souffrance cérébrale du nouveau-né. *Pédiatrie* **34,** 787–97.

Cole, V.A., Durbin, G.M., Olaffson, A., Reynolds, E.O.R., Rivers, R.P.A. and Smith, J.F. (1974) Pathogenesis of intraventricular haemorrhage in newborn infants. *Archives of Disease in Childhood* **49,** 722–8.

Courville, C.B. (1953a) *Contributions to the Study of Cerebral Anoxia.* San Lucas Press, Los Angeles.

Courville, C. (1953b) Long survival with hemiplegia incident to paranatal anoxia. *Bulletin of the Los Angeles Neurological Society* **18,** 110–15.

Courville, C.B. (1955) Case studies in cerebral anoxia; focal cortical necrosis superimposed upon a malformed brain in a case of congenital heart disease. *Bulletins of the Los Angeles Neurological Society* **20,** 69–73

Courville, C.B. (1958) Etiology and pathogenesis of laminar cortical necrosis. *Archives of Neurology and Psychiatry* **79,** 17–30.

Courville, C.B. (1959) Antenatal and paranatal circulatory disorders as a cause of cerebral damage in early life. *Journal of Neuropathology and Experimental Neurology* **18,** 115–39.

Courville, C.B. (1960) Pathogenesis of nodular atrophy of the cerebral cortex. A common cortical change found in cases of cerebral palsy. *Archives of Pediatrics* **77,** 101–29.

Couvelaire, A. (1903) Hémorrhagies du système nerveux central des nouveaux-nés. *Annales de Gynécologie et Obstétrique* **59,** 253–68.

Craig, W.S. (1938) Intracranial haemorrhage in the newborn. *Archives of Disease in Childhood* **13,** 89–124.

Crome, L. (1958) Multilocular cystic encephalopathy of infants. *Journal of Neurosurgery and Psychiatry* **21,** 146–52.

Crome, L. and Sylvester, P.E. (1958) Hydranencephaly (hydrencephaly). *Archives of Disease in Childhood* **35,** 235–45.

Cruveilhier, J. (1862) *Traité d'Anatomie Pathologique Générale*, vol. 3. J.B. Baillière, Paris.

Davis, J.M., Ploetz, J., Davis, K.R., Black, P.M. and Zervas, N.T. (1980) Cranial computed tomography in subarachnoid hemorrhage. Relationship between blood detected by CT and lumbar puncture. *Journal of Computer Assisted Tomography* **4,** 794–6.

Dekaban, A. (1962) Cerebral birth injury. Pathology of hemorrhagic lesions. *Mental Retardation* **39,** 196–227.

Dekaban, A. (1965) Large defects in cerebral hemispheres associated with cortical dysgenesis. *Journal of Neuropathology and Experimental Neurology* **24,** 512–30.

Deonna, T., Payot, M., Probst, A. and Prod'hom, L.S. (1975) Neonatal intracranial hemorrhage in premature infants. *Pediatrics* **56,** 1056–64.

DeReuk, J., Chattha, A.S. and Richardson, E.P. (1972) Pathogenesis and evolution of periventricular leukomalacia in infancy. *Archives of Neurology* **27,** 229–36.

Dereymacker, A. (1949) *Contribution à l'Étude Clinique, Anatomique et Expérimentale de l'Ictère Nucléaire du Nouveau-né.* Masson, Paris.

Diamond, I. and Schmid, R. (1966) Experimental bilirubin encephalopathy. The mode of entry of bilirubin ^{14}C into the C.N.S. *Journal of Clinical Investigation* **45,** 678–89.

Dimmick, J.E., Hardwick, D.F. and Ho-Yuen, B. (1971) A case of renal necrosis and fibrosis in the immediate newborn period. *American Journal of Diseases of Children* **122,** 345–7.

Donat, J.F., Okazaki, H., Kleinberg, F. and Reagan, R. (1978) Intraventricular hemorrhages in full-term and premature infants. *Mayo Clinic Proceedings* **53,** 437–41.

Donn, S.M. and Bowerman, R.A. (1982) Neonatal posthemorrhagic porencephaly Ultrasonographic features. *American Journal of Diseases of Children* **136,** 707–9.

Dreyfus-Brisac, C. and Monod, N. (1964) Electroclinical studies of status epilepticus and convulsions in the newborn. In *Neurologic and Electroencephalographic Correlative Studies in Infancy* (Eds. Kellaway, P. and Peterson, I.), Grune and Stratton, New York.

DuBose-Ravenel, S. (1979) Posterior fossa hemorrhage in the term newborn: report of two cases. *Pediatrics* **64,** 39–42.

Duffy, T.E. and Vannucci, R.C. (1977) Metabolic aspects of cerebral anoxia-asphyxia in the fetus and newborn. In *Brain: Fetal and Infant* (Ed. Berenberg, S.R.), pp. 316–23. Martinus Nijhoff, The Hague.

Dykes, F.D., Lazzara, A., Ahmann, P., Blumenstein, B., Schartz, J. and Braun, A.W. (1980) Intraventricular hemorrhage: a prospective evaluation of etiopathogenesis. *Pediatrics* **66,** 42–9.

Eicke, W.J. (1947) Gefässveränderungen bei Meningitis und ihre Bedeutung für die Pathogenese frühkindlicher Hirnschäden. *Virchows Archiv* **314,** 88–124.

Erasmus, C., Blackwood, W. and Wilson, J. (1982) Infantile multicystic encephalomalacia after maternal bee sting anaphylaxis during pregnancy. *Archives of Disease in Childhood* **57,** 785–7.

Farkas-Bargeton, E. and Diebler, M.F. (1978) A topographical study of enzyme maturation in human cerebral neocortex: a histochemical and biochemical study. In *Architectonics of the Cerebral Cortex* (Eds. Brazier, M.A.B. and Petsche, H.), Raven Press, New York. pp. 175–90.

Farkas-Bargeton, E., Goutières, F., Richardet, J.M., Thieffry, S. and Brissaud, H.E. (1971) Leucoencephalopathie familiale associée à une acidose lactique congénitale. *Acta Neuropathologica* **17,** 156–68.

Fedricks, J. and Butler, N.R. (1970) Certain causes of

neonatal death. II. Intraventricular haemorrhage. *Biology of the Neonate* **15,** 257–90.

Ferrer, I. and Navarro, C. (1978) Multicystic encephalomalacia of infancy. *Journal of the Neurological Sciences* **38,** 179–89.

Finberg, L. (1977) The relationship of intravenous infusions and intracranial hemorrhage. A commentary. *Journal of Pediatrics* **91,** 777–8.

Fishman, M.A., Percy, A.K., Cheek, W.R. and Speer, M.E. (1981) Successful conservative management of cerebellar hematomas in term neonates. *Journal of Pediatrics* **98,** 466–8.

Fitzgerald, G.M., Greenfield, J.G. and Kounine, B. (1939) Neurological sequelae of 'kernicterus'. *Brain* **62,** 292–310.

Fitzhardinge, P.M., Flodmark, O. and Ashby, S. (1982) The prognostic value of computed tomography of the brain in asphyxiated premature infants. *Journal of Pediatrics* **100,** 476–81.

Flodmark, O., Becker, L.E., Harwood-Nash, D.C., Fitzhardinge, P.M., Fitz, C.R. and Chuang, S.H. (1980) Correlation between computed tomography and autopsy in premature and fullterm neonates that have suffered perinatal asphyxia. *Radiology* **137,** 93–103.

Foix, Ch., Bariety, M., Baruch, H. and Marie, J. (1926) A propos d'un nouveau cas de sclérose intracérébrale centro-lobaire et symmétrique. *Revue Neurologique* **33,** 930–42.

Fowler, M., Brown, C. and Cabrera, K.F. (1971) Hydranencephaly in a baby after an aircraft accident to the mother. Case report and autopsy. *Pathology* **3,** 21–30.

Fowler, M., Dow, R., White, T.A. and Greer, C.H. (1972) Congenital hydrocephalus. Hydrencephaly in five siblings, with autopsy studies: a new disease. *Developmental Medicine and Child Neurology* **14,** 173–88.

Friede, R. (1972a) Subpial hemorrhage in the newborn. *Journal of Neuropathology and Experimental Neurology* **31,** 548–56.

Friede, R.L. (1972b) Ponto-subicular lesions in perinatal anoxia. *Archives of Pathology* **94,** 343–54.

Friede, R.L. (1972c) Residual lesions of infantile cerebral phlebothrombosis. *Acta Neuropathologica* **22,** 319–32.

Friede, R.L. (1973) Cerebral infarcts complicating neonatal leptomeningitis. Acute and residual lesions. *Acta Neuropathologica* **23,** 245–53.

Friede, R.L. (1975) *Developmental Neuropathology.* Springer, Vienna.

Friede, R.L. and Mikolasek, J. (1978) Postencephalitic porencephaly, hydranencephaly or polymicrogyria. A review. *Acta Neuropathologica* **43,** 161–8.

Friede, R.L. and Schiedmayr, W. (1977) Early stages of status marmoratus. *Acta Neuropathologica* **38,** 123–7.

Fujimura, M., Salisbury, D.M., Robinson, R.O., Howat, P., Emerson, P.M., Keeling, J.N. et al. (1979) Clinical events relating to intraventricular haemorrhage in the newborn. *Archives of Disease in Childhood* **54,** 409–14.

Galea, P., Scott, J.M. and Goel, K.M. (1982) Feto-fetal transfusion syndrome. *Archives of Disease in Childhood* **57,** 781–94.

Gartner, L.M., Snyder, R.N., Chabon, R.S. and Bernstein, J. (1970) Kernicterus: high incidence in premature infants with low serum bilirubin concentrations. *Pediatrics* **45,** 906–17.

Gerrard, J. (1952) Kernicterus. *Brain* **75,** 526–71.

Gilles, F.H. and Murphy, S.F. (1969) Perinatal telencephalic leucoencephalopathy. *Journal of Neurology, Neurosurgery and Psychiatry* **32,** 404–13.

Gilles, F., Price, R., Kevy, S. and Berenberg, W. (1971) Fibrinolytic activity in the ganglionic eminence of the premature human brain. *Biology of the Neonate* **18,** 426–32.

Goddard, J., Lewis, R.M., Alcala, H. and Zeller, R.S. (1980) Intraventricular hemorrhage. An animal model. *Biology of the Neonate* **37,** 39–52.

Goddard-Finegold, J., Armstrong, D. and Zeller, R.S. (1982) Intraventricular hemorrhage following volume expansion after hypovolemic hypotension in the newborn beagle. *Journal of Pediatrics* **100,** 798–802.

Goldstein, G.W. (1979) Pathogenesis of brain edema and hemorrhage: role of the brain capillary. *Pediatrics* **64,** 357–60.

Gosseye, S., Golaire, M.C. and Larroche, J.Cl. (1982) Cerebral, renal and splenic lesions due to fetal anoxia and their relationship to malformations. *Developmental Medicine and Child Neurology* **24,** 510–18.

Grant, E.G., Kerner, M., Schellinger, D., Borts, F.T., McCullough, D.C., Smith, Y. et al. (1982) Evolution of porencephalic cysts from intraparenchymal hemorrhage in neonates. Sonographic evidence. *American Journal of Neuroradiology* **3,** 467–70.

Gröntoft, O. (1953a) Intracerebral and meningeal haemorrhages in perinatally deceased infants. I. Intracerebral haemorrhages. *Acta Obstetrica et Gynecologica Scandinavica* **32,** 308–34.

Gröntoft, O. (1953b) Intracerebral and meningeal haemorrhages in perinatally deceased infants. II. Meningeal haemorrhages. *Acta Obstetrica et Gynecologica Scandinavica* **32,** 458–97.

Gröntoft, O. (1954) Intracranial hemorrhage and blood brain barrier problems in the newborn. *Acta Pathologica and Microbiologica Scandinavica* suppl. C, 30, 109.

Gruenwald, P. (1951) Subependymal cerebral hemorrhage in premature infants and its relation to various injurious influences at birth. *American*

Journal of Obstetrics and Gynecology **61,** 1285–92.

Grunnet, M.L. and Shields, W.D. (1976) Cerebellar hemorrhage in the premature infant. *Journal of Pediatrics* **88,** 605–8.

Grylack, L. (1982) Prenatal sonographic diagnosis of cephalohematoma due to pre-labor trauma. *Pediatric Radiology* **12,** 145–7.

Guekos-Thöni, U., Boltshauser, E., Mieth, D. and Isler, N. (1980) Intracranial haemorrhage in the term infant confirmed by computed tomography. *Helvetica Paediatrica Acta* **35,** 531–44.

Hagberg, B., Hagberg, G. and Olow, I. (1975) The changing panorama of cerebral palsy in Sweden 1954–1970. I. Analysis of the general changes. II. Analysis of the various syndromes. *Acta Paediatrica Scandinavica* **64,** 187–200.

Hagberg, B., Hagberg, G. and Olow, I. (1977) The panorama of cerebral palsy in Swedish children born 1954–1974. *Neuropädiatrie* **8,** suppl., 516–21.

Haller, E., Nesbitt, R. and Anderson, G. (1956) Clinical and pathological concepts of gross intracranial hemorrhage in perinatal mortality. *Journal of Obstetrics and Gynecology* **11,** 179–204.

Hallervorden, J. (1949) Uber eine Kohlenoxydvergiftung im Fötalleben mit Entwicklungsstörung der Hirnrinde. *Allgemeine Zeitschrift für Psychiatrie* **124,** 289–98.

Halsey, J.H., Allen, N. and Chamberlain, H.R. (1971) The morphogenesis of hydranencephaly. *Journal of the Neurological Sciences* **12,** 187–218.

Hambleton, G. and Wigglesworth, J.S. (1976) Origin of intraventricular haemorrhage in the preterm infant. *Archives of Diseases in Childhood* **51,** 651–9.

Harris, R.C., Lucey, J.F. and Maclean, J.R. (1958) Kernicterus in premature infants associated with low concentrations of bilirubin in plasma. *Pediatrics* **21,** 875–83.

Harwood-Nash, D.C. and Fitz, C.R. (1976) *Neuroradiology in Infants and Children.* Mosby, St Louis, Mo.

Hathaway, N.H. and Bonnar, J. (1978). Perinatal coagulation. In *Monographs in Neonatology* (Ed. Oliver, T.K. Jr) Grune and Stratton, New York.

Haworth, J.C. and McRae, K.N. (1965) The neurological and developmental effects of neonatal hypoglycemia. A follow-up of 22 cases. *Canadian Medical Association Journal* **92,** 861–5.

Haymaker, W., Margoles, C., Pentschew, A., Jacob, H., Lindenberg, R., Arroyo, L. et al. (1961) Pathology of kernicterus and posticteric encephalopathy. Presentation of 87 cases, with a consideration of pathogenesis and etiology. In *Kernicterus and its Importance in Cerebral Palsy*, pp. 21–228. Charles Thomas, Springfield, Ill.

Helmrath, R.A., Hodson, W.A. and Oliver, T.K. (1970) Positive pressure ventilation in the newborn infant: the use of a face mask. *Journal of Pediatrics* **76,** 202–7.

Hervieux, J. (1847) *De l'ictère des nouveaux-nés.* MD thesis, Paris.

Hill, A., Perlman, J.M. and Volpe, J.J. (1982) Relationship of pneumothorax to occurrence of intraventricular hemorrhage in the premature newborn *Pediatrics* **69,** 144.

Holland, E. (1922) Cranial stress in the foetus during labour. *Journal of Obstetrics and Gynaecology of the British Empire* **29,** 549–71.

Hon, E.H. (1977) Detection of asphyxia *in utero*—fetal heart rate. In *Intrauterine Asphyxia and the Developing Fetal Brain* (Ed. Gluck, L.), pp. 167–77. Year Book, Chicago.

Hopkins, I., Farkas-Bargeton, E. and Larroche, J.Cl. (1980) Neonatal neuronal necrosis: its relationship to the distribution and maturation of oxidative enzymes of newborn cerebral and cerebellar cortex. *Early Human Development* **4,** 51–60.

Hopkins, I.J. and Turner, B. (1973) Spongy glioneuronal dystrophy: a degenerative disease of the nervous system. *Journal of Neurology, Neurosurgery and Psychiatry* **36,** 50–6.

Hsia, D.Y.Y. (1965) Bilirubin metabolism. *Pediatric Clinics of North America* **12,** 713–22.

Jellinger, K. and Seitelberger, F. (1970) Spongy glioneural dystrophy in infancy and childhood. *Acta Neuropathologica* **16,** 125–40.

Jew, J.Y. and Sandquist, D. (1979) CNS changes in hyperbilirubinemia. *Archives of Neurology* **36,** 149–54.

Johnson, L., Sarmiento, F., Blanc, N.A. and Day, R. (1959) Kernicterus in rats with an inherited deficiency of glucuronyl transferase. *American Journal of Diseases of Children* **97,** 591–608.

Johnson, M.L., Mack, L.A., Rumack, C.M., Frost, M. and Rashbaum, C. (1979) B mode echoencephalography in the normal and high risk infant. *American Journal of Roentgenology* **133,** 375–81.

Kluge, H. (1902) Untersuchungen über Hydranencephalie (Cruveilhier) quoted by Friede (1975).

Koch, B., Braillier, D., Eng, G. and Binder, H. (1980) Computerized tomography in cerebral-palsied children. *Developmental Medicine and Child Neurology* **22,** 595–607.

Koffler, H., Keenan, W. and Sutherland, J. (1974) Hydranencephaly following elevated hematocrit values in a newly born infant. *Pediatrics* **54,** 770–2.

Korobkin, R. (1975) The relationship between, head circumference and the development of communicating hydrocephalus in infants following intraventricular hemorrhage. *Pediatrics* **56,** 74–7.

Krishnamoorthy, K.S., Fernandez, R.A., Momose, K.J., Delong, G.R., Moylan, F.M.B., Todres, I.D. and Shannon, D.C. (1977) Evaluation of neonatal intracranial hemorrhage by computerized tomography. *Pediatrics* **59,** 165–72.

Kulakowski, S. and Larroche, J.Cl. (1980) Cranial computerized tomography in cerebral palsy. An attempt at anatomoclinical and radiological correlations. *Neuropediatrics* **11,** 339–53.

Kundrat, H. (1882) Die Porencephalie. Eine anatomische Studie. quoted by Yakovlev (1959).

Lacey, D.J. and Terplan, K. (1982) Intraventricular hemorrhage in the fullterm neonate. *Annals of Neurology* **8,** 227.

Lange-Cosack, H. (1944) Die Hydranencephalie als Sonderform der Grosshirnlosigkeit. *Archiv für Psychiatrie und Nervenkrankheiten* **117,** 1–51, 595–640.

Larroche, J.Cl. (1964) Les hémorrhagies cérébrales intraventriculaires chez les prématurés. 1. Anatomie et physiopathologie. *Biologia Neonatorum* **7,** 26–56.

Larroche, J.Cl. (1968a) Nécrose cérébrale massive chez le nouveau-né. Ses rapports avec la maturation, son expression clinique et bioélectrique. *Biology of the Neonate* **13,** 340–60.

Larroche, J.Cl. (1968b) Kernicterus. In *Handbook of Clinical Neurology*, vol. 6 (Eds. Vinken, P. and Bruyn, G.W.), pp. 491–515. North-Holland, Amsterdam.

Larroche, J.Cl. (1972a) Post haemorrhagic hydrocephalus in infancy. Anatomical study. *Biology of the Neonate* **20,** 287–99.

Larroche, J.Cl. (1972b) Subependymal pseudocysts in the newborn. *Biology of the Neonate* **21,** 170–83.

Larroche, J.Cl. (1977) *Developmental Pathology of the Neonate*, Exerpta Medica, Amsterdam.

Larroche, J.Cl. (1979) Intraventricular hemorrhage in the premature neonate: anatomy, pathogenesis and diagnosis. In *Advances in Perinatal Neurology* (Eds Korobkin, R. and Guilleminault, C.) pp. 115–40. SP Medical and Scientific, New York.

Larroche, J.Cl. (1982a) Hypoxic brain damage in fetus and newborn. Morphological characters. Pathogenesis. Prevention. *Journal of Perinatal Medicine* **10,** suppl. 2, 29–31.

Larroche, J.Cl. (1982b) *Intraventrikuläre Blutung. Neue morphologische und epidemiologische Aspekte seit der Intensivpflege*, pp. 165–8. Thieme, Stuttgart.

Larroche, J.Cl. (1982c) The fine structure of matrix capillaries in human embryos and young fetuses. The Second Ross Conference on Intraventricular Hemorrhage, Washington DC.

Larroche, J.Cl. and Amiel, Cl. (1966) Thrombose de l'artère sylvienne à la période néonatale. Etude anatomique et discussion pathogénique des hémiplégies dites congénitales. *Archives Françaises de Pédiatrie* **23,** 257–74.

Larroche, J.Cl., Amiel-Tison, Cl. and Dreyfus-Brisac, C. (1980) Fetal and neonatal brains. In *Clinical Perinatology* (Eds Aladjem, S., Brown, A.K. and Sureau, C.) pp. 116–59. Mosby, St Louis, Mo.

Larroche, J.Cl., Amiel, Cl., Relier, J.P. and Korn, G. (1975) Leucomalacie et avenir cérébral en relation avec les soins intensifs néonataux. *Annales de l'Anesthésiologie Française* **16,** 171–5.

La Torre, E. and Occhipinti, E. (1970) Angiographic findings in some malformations of the brain. *European Neurology* **4,** 210–25.

Laurence, K.M. and Cavanagh, J.B. (1968) Progressive degeneration of the cerebral cortex in infancy. *Brain* **91,** 261–80.

Leech, R.W. and Alvord, E.C. Jr (1974) Morphologic variations in periventricular leukomalacia. *American Journal of Pathology* **74,** 591–602.

Leech, R.W. and Kohnen, P. (1974) Subependymal and intraventricular hemorrhage in the newborn. *American Journal of Pathology* **77,** 465–76.

Lemire, R.J., Loeser, J.D., Leech, R.W. and Alvord, E.C. (1975) *Normal and Abnormal Development of the Human Nervous System.* Harper and Row, Hagerstown, Md.

Lemire, R.J., Shepard, T.H. and Alvord, E.C. Jr. (1965). Caudal myeloschisis (lumbo sacral spina bifida cystica) in a five millimeter (Horizon XIV) human embryo. *Anatomical Record* **152,** 9–16.

Lindenberg, R. and Swanson, P.D. (1967) Infantile hydranencephaly: a report of 5 cases of infarction of both cerebral hemispheres in infancy. *Brain* **90,** 839–41.

Little, W. (1861) The influence of abnormal parturition, difficult labour, premature birth and asphyxia neonatorum, on the mental and physical condition of the child, especially in relation to deformities. *Transactions of the Obstetrical Society of London* **3,** 293–344.

Liu, M.C. and Sylvester, P. (1960) Familial diffuse progressive encephalopathy. *Archives of Disease in Childhood* **35,** 345–51.

Lou, H.C., Lassen, N.A. and Friis-Hansen, B. (1979a) Impaired autoregulation of cerebral blood flow in the distressed newborn infant. *Journal of Pediatrics* **94,** 118–21.

Lou, H.C., Lassen, N.A. and Friis-Hansen, B. (1979b) Is arterial hypertension crucial for the development of cerebral haemorrhage in premature infants? *Lancet* **1,** 1215–17.

Lucey, J. (1972) The unsolved problem of kernicterus in the susceptible low birth weight infant. *Pediatrics* **48,** 646–7.

Lucey, J.F., Hibbard, E., Behrman, R.E., Esquivel (de Gallardo), F.O. and Windle, W.F. (1964) Kernicterus in asphyxiated newborn Rhesus monkeys. *Experimental Neurology* **9,** 43–58.

Lyon, G. and Robain, O. (1967) Etude comparative des encéphalopathies circulatoires prénatales et paranatales (hydranencéphalies et encéphalomalacies kystiques de la substance blanche). *Acta Neuropathologica* **9,** 79–98.

MacAdams, J. (1967) Pulmonary hemorrhage in the newborn. *American Journal of Diseases of Children* **113,** 255–62.

Mack, L.A., Wright, K., Hirch, J.H., Alvord, E.C., Guthrie, R.D., Shuman, W.P. et al. (1981) Intracranial hemorrhage in premature infants: accuracy of sonographic evaluation. *American Journal of Roentgenology* **137,** 245–50.

Maisels, J. (1972) Bilirubin. On understanding and influencing its metabolism in the newborn infant. Symposium on recent clinical advances. *Pediatric Clinics of North America* **19,** 447–501.

Malamud, N. (1950) Status marmoratus: a form of cerebral palsy following either birth injury or inflammation of the central nervous system. *Journal of Pediatrics* **37,** 610–19.

Malamud, N. (1961) Pathogenesis of kernicterus in the light of its sequelae. In *Kernicterus and its Importance in Cerebral Palsy*, pp. 230–46. Thomas, Springfield, Ill.

Manterola, A., Towbin, A. and Yakovlev, P.I. (1966) Cerebral infarction in the human fetus near term. *Journal of Neuropathology and Experimental Neurology* **25,** 479–88.

Maresch, R. (1929) Ueber einen Fall von Kohlenoxydgasschädigung der Kinder in der Gebärmutter. *Wiener Klinische Wochenschrift* **79,** 454–6.

Marie, J., Lyon, G. and Bargeton, E. (1959) La sclérose cérébrale centro-lobaire. A propos de l'étude anatomo-clinique d'un cas de diplégie spasmodique congénitale (syndrome de Little). *Presse Médicale* **60,** 2286–9.

Martin, Cl., Allain, D., Vital, C., Babin, J.P., Demarquez, J.L. and San Juan, B. (1977) Hydranencéphalie familiale. *Annales de Pédiatrie* **24,** 673–8.

Martin, L. and Larroche, J.Cl. (1964) Incidence et interprétation actuelle des lésions corticales dans l'ictère nucléaire. *Revue Neurologique* **6,** 545–55.

Martin, R., Roessmann, U. and Fanaroff, A. (1976) Massive intracerebellar hemorrhage in low-birth-weight infants. *Journal of Pediatrics* **89,** 290–3.

Moore, C.M., McAdams, A.J. and Sutherland, J. (1969) Intrauterine disseminated intravascular coagulation. A syndrome of multiple pregnancy with a dead twin fetus. *Journal of Pediatrics* **74,** 523–8.

Moriette, G., Relier, J.P. and Larroche, J.Cl. (1977) Les hémorhagies intraventriculaires au cours de la maladie des membranes hyalines. *Archives Françaises de Pédiatrie* **34,** 492–504.

Muir, C.S. (1959) Hydrencephaly and allied disorders: a study of cerebral defects in Chinese children. *Archives of Disease in Childhood* **34,** 231–46.

Mustafa, M.G., Cowger, M.L. and King, T.E. (1969) Effects of bilirubin on mitochondrial reactions. *Journal of Biological Chemistry* **244,** 6403–14.

Myers, R.E. (1969) Brain pathology following fetal vascular occlusion: an experimental study. *Investigations in Ophthalmology* **8,** 41–50.

Myers, R.E. (1972) Two patterns of perinatal brain damage and their conditions of occurrence. *American Journal of Obstetrics and Gynecology* **112,** 246–76.

Myers, R.E. (1975) Maternal psychological stress and fetal asphyxia. A study in the monkey. *American Journal of Obstetrics and Gynecology* **122,** 47–59.

Myers, R.E. (1977) Experimental models of perinatal brain damage: relevance to human pathology. In *Intrauterine Asphyxia and the Developing Fetal Brain* (Ed. Gluck, L.), pp. 37–97. Year Book, Chicago.

Myers, R.E. (1979) Lactic acid accumulation as a cause of brain oedema and cerebral necrosis resulting from oxygen deprivation. In *Advances in Perinatal Neurology* (Eds Korobkin, R. and Guilleminault, C.), pp. 85–114. S.P. Medical and Scientific, New York.

Neligan, G.A., Robson, E. and Watson, J. (1963) Hypoglycaemia in the newborn; a sequel of intrauterine malnutrition. *Lancet* **1,** 1282–4.

Norman, M.G. (1980) Bilateral encephaloclastic lesions in a 26 weeks gestation fetus; effect on neuroblastic migration. *Journal Canadien des Sciences Neurologiques* **7,** 191–4.

Norman, R.M. (1938) An example of status marmoratus of the cerebral cortex. *Journal of Neurology and Psychiatry* **1,** 1–10.

Norman, R.M. (1944) Atrophic sclerosis of the cerebral cortex associated with birth injury. *Archives of Disease in Childhood* **19,** 111–21.

Norman, R.M. (1947) Etat marbré of the corpus striatum following birth injury. *Journal of Neurology, Neurosurgery and Psychiatry* **10,** 12–25.

Norman, R.M. (1952) Mental deficiencies. In *Proceedings of the 1st International Congress of Neuropathology (Rome)*, vol. 2, pp. 276–82. Rosenberg and Sellier, Torino.

Norman, R.M. (1969) Malformations of the nervous system. In *Greenfield's Neuropathology*, 2nd edn (Eds Norman, R.M., Blackwood, W., Meyer, A., McMenemey, W.H. and Russell, Dorothy S.) pp. 324–441. Edward Arnold, London.

Norman, R.M., Urich, H. and McMenemey, W.H. (1957) Vascular mechanisms of birth injury. *Brain* **80,** 49–58.

Norman, R.M., Urich, H. and Woods, G.E. (1958) The relationship between prenatal porencephaly and the encephalomalacias of early life. *Journal of Mental Science* **104,** 758–71.

Ober, W.B. and Moore, T.E. (1955) Congenital cardiac malformations in neonatal period;

autopsy study. *New England Journal of Medicine* **253,** 271–5.

Odell, G.B. (1959) Studies in kernicterus. I. The protein binding of bilirubin. *Journal of Clinical Investigation* **38,** 823–33.

Odell, G.B., Storey, G.N. and Rosenberg, L.A. (1970) Studies in kernicterus. III. The saturation of serum proteins with bilirubin during neonatal life and its relationship to brain damage at five years. *Journal of Pediatrics* **76,** 12–21.

Odièvre, M., Pinon, F., Schirar, M., Luzeau, R. and Sauvageot, M. (1970) La fraction de bilirubine non conjuguée et non liée à l'albumine au cours des hyperbilirubinémies néonatales. *Archives Françaises de Pédiatrie* **27,** 225–35.

Orth, T. (1875) Über das Vorkommen von Bilirubinkrystallen bei neugeborenen Kindern. *Virchows Archiv* **63,** 447–62.

Palma, P.A., Miner, M.E., Morriss, F.H., Adcock, E.W. and Denson, S.E. (1979) Intraventricular hemorrhage in the neonate born at term. *American Journal of Diseases of Children* **133,** 941–4.

Pape, K.E., Armstrong, D.L. and Fitzhardinge, P.M. (1976) Central nervous system pathology associated with mask ventilation in the very low birth weight infant: a new etiology for intracerebellar hemorrhages. *Pediatrics* **58,** 473–83.

Pape, K.E. and Wigglesworth, J.S. (1979) *Haemorrhage, Ischaemia and Perinatal Brain,* Heinemann Medical, London.

Pape, K.E., Blackwell, R.J., Cusick, G., Sherwood, A., Houang, M.T.W., Thorburn, R.J. et al. (1979) Ultrasound detection of brain damage in preterm infants. *Lancet* **1,** 1261–4.

Papile, L.A., Burstein, J., Burstein, R. and Koffler, H. (1978) Incidence and evolution of subependymal and intraventricular hemorrhage: a study of infants with birth weights less than 1500 g. *Journal of Pediatrics* **92,** 529–34.

Parrot, J. (1873) Etude sur le ramollissement de l'encéphale chez le nouveau-né. *Archives de Physiologie Normale et Pathologique (Paris)* **5,** 59–73, 176–95, 283–303.

Parrot, J. (1877) *Cliniques des Nouveau-nés: l'Athrepsie,* pp. 281–345. Masson, Paris.

Pasternak, J.F., Mantovani, J.F. and Volpe, J.J. (1980) Porencephaly from periventricular intracerebral hemorrhage in a premature infant. *American Journal of Diseases of Children* **134,** 673–5.

Pasternak, J.F., Groothuis, D.R., Fischer, J.M. and Fischer, D.P. (1982) Regional cerebral blood flow in the newborn beagle pup: the germinal matrix is a 'low-flow' structure. *Pediatric Research* **16,** 499–503.

Pearlman, M.A., Gartner, L.M., Lee, K.S., Morecki, R. and Horoupian, D.S. (1978) Absence of kernicterus in low birth weight infants from 1971 through 1976: comparison with findings in 1966 and 1967. *Pediatrics* **62,** 460–4.

Pevsner, P.H., Garcia-Bunel, R., Leeds, N. and Finkelstein, M. (1976) Subependymal and intraventricular hemorrhage in neonates. *Radiology* **119,** 111–14.

Pledger, D.R., Scott, J.M. and Belfield, A. (1982) Kernicterus at low levels of serum bilirubin: the impact of bilirubin albumin-binding capacity. *Biology of the Neonate* **41,** 38–44.

Povlishock, J.T., Martinez, A.J. and Moossy, J. (1977) The fine structure of blood vessels of the telencephalic germinal matrix in the human fetus. *American Journal of Anatomy* **149,** 439–52.

Ranck, J.B. and Windle, W.F. (1959) Brain damage in the monkey *Macaca mulatta* by asphyxia neonatorum. *Experimental Neurology* **1,** 130–54.

Reeder, J.D., Setzer, E.S. and Kaude, J.V. (1982) Ultrasonic detection of perinatal intracerebellar hemorrhage. *Pediatrics* **70,** 385–6.

Reisman, L.E. and Pathak, A. (1966) Bilateral renal cortical necrosis in the newborn. *American Journal of Diseases of Children* **111,** 541–3.

Reynolds, M.L., Evans, C.A.N., Reynolds, E.D., Saunders, R., Durbin, N.R. and Wigglesworth, J.S. (1979) Intracranial haemorrhage in the preterm sheep fetus. *Early Human Development* **3,** 163–86.

Rizzuto, N. and Martin, L. (1967) Le problème de l'encéphalopathie foetale kystique survenant au cours du deuxième tiers de la grossesse. *Biology of the Neonate* **11,** 115–27.

Robain, O. and Rosenberg, S. (1974) Ramollissement cérébraux localisés à la substance blanche paraventriculaire au cours des cardiopathies congénitales de l'enfant. *Annales d'Anatomie Pathologique* **19,** 311–20.

Roesmann, U. and Parks, P.J. Jr (1978) Hydranencephaly in vertebral-basilar territory. *Acta Neuropathologica* **44,** 141–3.

Rom, S., Serfontein, G.L. and Humphreys, R.P. (1978) Intracerebellar hematoma in the neonate. *Journal of Pediatrics* **93,** 486–8.

Rorke, L.B. (1982) *Pathology of Perinatal Brain Injury,* Raven Press, New York.

Rorke, L.B. and Spiro, A.J. (1967) Cerebral lesions in congenital rubella syndrome. *Journal of Pediatrics* **70,** 243–55.

Rosales, R.K. and Riggs, H.E. (1962) Symmetrical thalamic degeneration in infants. *Journal of Neuropathology and Experimental Neurology* **21,** 372–6.

Rydberg, E. (1932) Cerebral injury of the newborn children consequent on birth trauma with an inquiry into the normal and pathological anatomy of the neuroglia. *Acta Pathologica et Microbiologica Scandinavica* suppl. 10, 1–247.

Scharpe, O. and Hale, E.G. (1953) Renal impairment, hypertension and encephalomalacia in infant surviving severe intrauterine anoxia. *Proceedings of the Royal Society of Medicine* **46,** 1063–5.

Scher, M.S., Wright, F.S., Cockman, L.A. and Thompson, T.R. (1980) Intraventricular hemorrhage in the fullterm neonate. *Archives of Neurology* **39,** 769–72.

Schipke, R., Riege, D. and Scoville, W.B. (1954) Acute subdural hemorrhage at birth. *Pediatrics* **14,** 468–74.

Schmorl, G. (1903) Zur Kenntnis des Ikterus neonatorum. *Verhandlungen der Deutschen Pathologischen Gesellschaft* **6,** 109–15.

Schneider, H., Ballowitz, L., Schachinger, H., Hanefeld, F. and Dröszus, J.V. (1975) Anoxic encephalopathy with predominant involvement of basal ganglia, brainstem and spinal cord in the perinatal period. *Acta Neuropathologica* **33,** 287–98.

Schum, T.R., Meyer, G.A., Grausz, J.P. and Glaspay, J.C. (1979) Neonatal intraventricular hemorrhage due to an intracranial arteriovenous malformation: a case report. *Pediatrics* **64,** 242–4.

Schutta, H.S., Johnson, L. and Neville, H.E. (1970) Mitochondrial abnormalities in bilirubin encephalopathy. *Journal of Neuropathology and Experimental Neurology* **29,** 296–305.

Schwartz, P. (1961) *Birth Injuries of the Newborn.* Karger, Basel.

Scott, J.M. (1968) Preventing rhesus haemolytic disease. *British Medical Journal* **2,** 827–8.

Shankaran, S., Slovis, T.L., Bedard, M.P. and Poland, R.L. (1982) Sonographic classification of intracranial hemorrhage. A prognostic indication of mortality, morbidity and short term neurologic outcome. *Journal of Pediatrics* **100,** 469–75.

Shuman, R.M. and Selednik, L.J. (1980) Periventricular leukomalacia. A one-year autopsy study. *Archives of Neurology* **37,** 231–5.

Simmons, M.A., Adcock, E.W., Bard, H. and Battaglia, F.C. (1974) Hypernatremia and intracranial hemorrhage in neonates. *New England Journal of Medicine* **291,** 6–10.

Smith, J.F. and Rodeck, C. (1975) Multiple cystic and focal encephalomalacia in infancy and childhood with brain stem damage. *Journal of the Neurological Sciences* **25,** 377–88.

Sommer, A., Bradel, E.J. and Hamoudi, A. (1974) The cerebrohepatorenal syndrome (Zellweger's syndrome). *Biology of the Neonate* **25,** 219–29.

Stark, H. and Geiger, R. (1973) Renal tubular dysfunction following vascular accidents of the kidneys in the newborn period. *Journal of Pediatrics* **83,** 933–40.

Stern, L. (1972) Drug interactions. II. Drugs, the newborn infant, and the binding of bilirubin to albumin. *Pediatrics* **49,** 916–18.

Stern, L. and Denton, R. (1965) Kernicterus in small premature infants. *Pediatrics* **35,** 483–5.

Stevenson, L.D. and McGowan, L.E. (1942) Encephalomalacia with cavity formation in infants. *Archives of Pathology* **34,** 286–300.

Stewart, R.M., Williams, R.S., Kukl, P. and Schoenen, J. (1978) Ventral porencephaly: a cerebral defect associated with multiple congenital anomalies. *Acta Neuropathologica* **42,** 231–5.

Takashima, S., Armstrong, D.L. and Becker, L.E. (1978) Subcortical leukomalacia; relationship to development of the cerebral sulcus and its vascular supply. *Archives of Neurology* **35,** 470–2.

Takashima, S., Armstrong, D. and Becker, L.E. (1979) Old subependymal necrosis and hemorrhage in the prematurely born infants. *Brain and Development* **1,** 299–304.

Takashima, S. and Tanaka, K. (1978a) Microangiography and vascular permeability of the subependymal matrix in the premature infant. *Canadian Journal of Neurological Sciences* **5,** 45–50.

Takashima, S. and Tanaka, K. (1978b) Development of cerebrovascular architecture and its relationship to periventricular leukomalacia. *Archives of Neurology* **35,** 11–16.

Terplan, K.L. (1967) Histopathologic brain changes in 1152 cases of the perinatal and early infancy period. *Biology of the Neonate* **11,** 348–66.

Terplan, K.L. (1973) Patterns of brain damage in infants and children with congenital heart disease. *American Journal of Diseases of Children* **125,** 175–85.

Thorburn, R.J., Lipscomb, A.P., Stewart, A.L., Reynolds, E.O.R. and Hope, P.L. (1982) Timing and antecedents of periventricular haemorrhage and cerebral atrophy in very preterm infants. *Early Human Development* **7,** 221–38.

Tsiantos, A., Victorin, L., Relier, J.P., Dyer, N., Sundell, H., Brill, A.B. et al. (1974) Intracranial hemorrhage in the prematurely born infant: timing of clots and evaluation of clinical signs and symptoms. *Journal of Pediatrics* **85,** 854–9.

Urich, H. (1977) Malformations of the nervous system, perinatal damage and related conditions in early life. In *Greenfield's Neuropathology* 3rd edn (Eds Blackwood, W. and Corsellis, J.A.N.), pp. 361–469. Edward Arnold, London.

Vallée, B., Besson, G., Alix, D., Monnerie, J.L., Bellet, M. and Castel, Y. (1981) Hématome intracérébelleux chez un nouveau-né à terme. *Annales de Pédiatrie* **28,** 679–83.

Vander Eecken, H. (1959) *Anastomoses between the Leptomeningeal Arteries of the Brain: their morphological, pathological and clinical significance.* Thomas, Springfield, Ill.

Vannucci, R.C. and Plum, F. (1975) Pathophysiology of perinatal hypoxic-ischemic brain damage. In

Biology of Brain Dysfunction, vol. 3 (Ed. Gaull, G.E.), pp. 1-45. Plenum Press, New York.

Vannucci, R.C., Nardis, E.E. and Vannucci, S.J. (1980) Cerebral metabolism during hypoglycemia and asphyxia in newborn dogs. *Biology of the Neonate* **38,** 276-86.

Vert, P., Nomin, P. and Sibout, M. (1975) Intracranial venous pressure in newborn: variations in physiological state and in neurologic and respiratory disorders. In *Intensive Care in the Newborn* (Ed. Stern, L.), pp. 185-96. Masson, New York.

Virchow, R. (1867) Zur pathologischen Anatomie des Gehirns. I. Congenitale Encephalitis und Myelitis. *Virchows Archiv für Pathologie und Anatomie* **38,** 129-42.

Vogt, C. (1911) Ein neuer Fall von état marbré des Corpus striatum. *Journal für Psychologie und Neurologie* **18,** 489.

Volpe, J.J. (1981) *Neurology of the Newborn*. Saunders, Philadelphia, Pa.

Volpe, J.J. and Pasternak, J.F. (1977) Parasagittal cerebral injury in neonatal hypoxic-ischemic encephalopathy: clinical and neuroradiologic features. *Journal of Pediatrics* **91,** 472-6.

Volpe, J.J., Pasternak, J.F. and Allan, W.C. (1977) Ventricular dilation preceding rapid head growth following neonatal intracranial hemorrhage. *American Journal of Diseases of Children* **131,** 1212-15.

Volpe, J.J., Manica, J.P., Land, V.J. and Coxe, W.S. (1976) Neonatal subdural hematoma associated with severe hemophilia A. *Journal of Pediatrics* **88,** 1023-5.

Wimberley, P.D., Lou, H.C., Pedersen, H., Hejl, M., Lassen, N.A. and Friis-Hansen, B. (1982) Hypertensive peaks in the pathogenesis of intraventricular hemorrhage in the newborn. Abolition by phenobarbitone sedation. *Acta Paediatrica Scandinavica* **71,** 537-42.

Yakovlev, P.I. (1959) Anatomy of the human brain and the problem of mental retardation. In *Mental Retardation* (Eds Bowman, P.W. and Mautner, H.V.), pp. 1-43,. Grune and Stratton, New York.

Ylppö, A. (1919) Pathologisch-anatomische Studien bei Frühgeborenen. *Zeitschrift für Kinderheilkunde* **20,** 212-431.

Yoshioka, H., Kadomoto, Y., Mino, M., Morikawa, Y., Kasabuchi, Y. and Kusonoki, T. (1979) Multicystic encephalomacia in liveborn twin with a stillborn macerated co-twin. *Journal of Pediatrics* **95,** 798-800.

Zalneraitis, E.L., Young, R.S.K. and Krishnamoorthy, K.S. (1979) Intracranial hemorrhage in utero as a complication of isoimmune thrombocytopenia. *Journal of Pediatrics* **95,** 611-14.

Zamet, P., Nakamura, H., Perez-Robles, S., Larroche, J.Cl. and Minkowski, A. (1975) The use of critical levels of birth weight and 'free bilirubin' as an approach for prevention of kernicterus. *Biology of the Neonate* **26,** 274-82.

Zuelzer, W.W. and Mudgett, R.T. (1950) Kernicterus: etiologic study based on an analysis of 55 cases. *Pediatrics* **6,** 452-74.

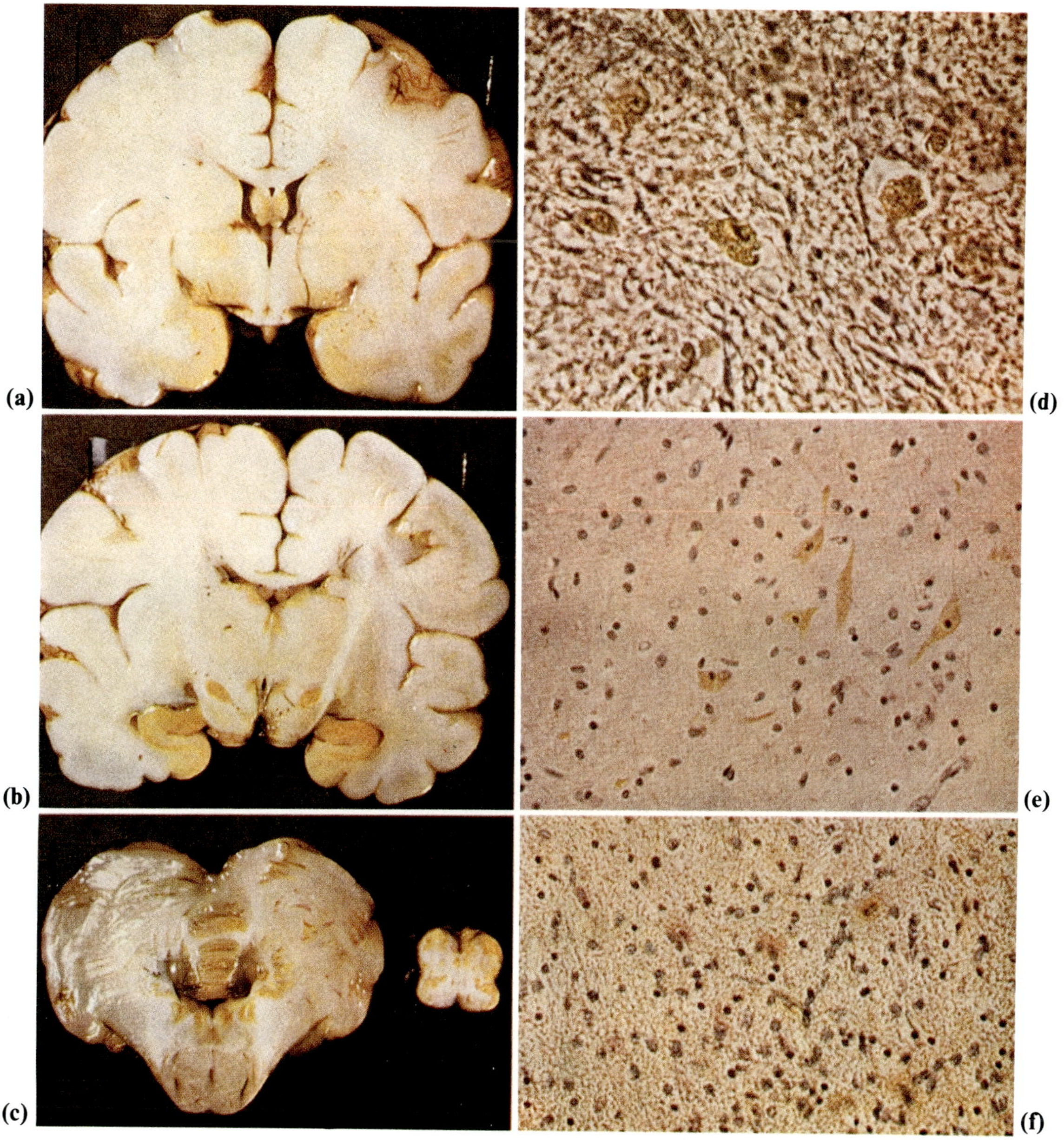

Plate 11.1 Kernicterus. On the left sections of the formalin-fixed brain show staining by bilirubin of (**a**) fornices and temporal cortex, (**b**) hippocampi and subthalamic nuclei, (**c**) dentate and olivary nuclei. On the right damaged pigmented neurons are seen in (**d**) frozen section of abducens nucleus, (**e**) paraffin section of globus pallidus and (**f**) paraffin section of subthalamic nucleus.

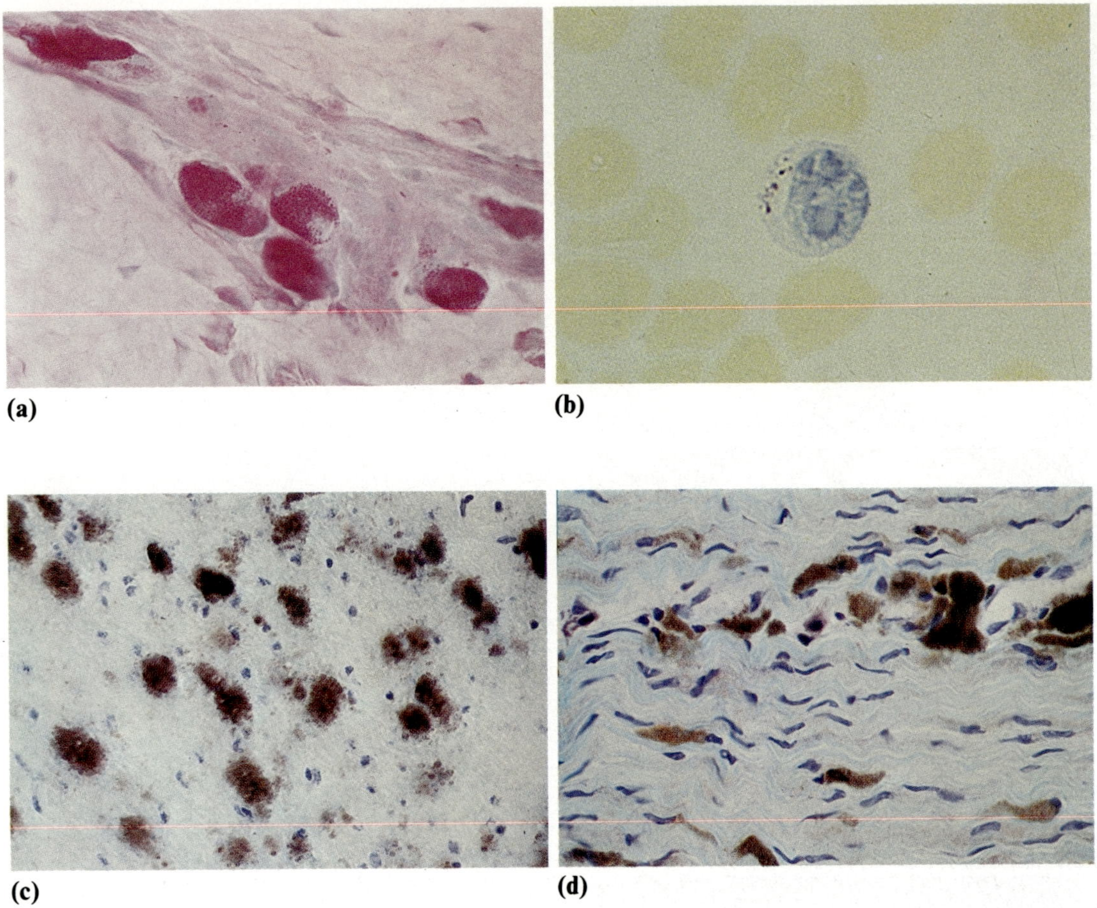

Plate 12.1

(**a**) Sialidosis. Cryostat section of rectal biopsy. Neurons in the submucosal plexus are packed with granules stained strongly by PAS. Similar changes occur in G_{M1} and G_{M2} gangliosidosis. × 320

(**b**) Mucopolysaccharidosis. Peripheral blood film from a patient with MPS III (Sanfilippo). Red metachromatic granules lie in the cytoplasm of a lymphocyte. Toluidine blue method (Filipe and Lake, 1983). × 1600

(**c**) Metachromatic leucodystrophy. Cryostat section of cerebral biopsy stained as a permanent preparation by the toluidine blue method of Bodian and Lake (1963). Note brown metachromasia in macrophages in the white matter. × 200

(**d**) Metachromatic leucodystrophy. Cryostat section of a sural nerve biopsy stained by toluidine blue (Bodian and Lake, 1963) as a permanent preparation. Brown metachromatic deposits are present in Schwann cells and macrophages. A mast cell contains red granules. × 320

12

Lysosomal enzyme deficiencies

Brian D. Lake

The storage diseases have always attracted attention because of their dramatic clinical presentations and striking pathology. The microscopic appearance of the enlarged neurons in patients with 'amaurotic familial idiocy' appeared similar in all cases before special stains and electron microscopy were available. Consequently there was confusion in the terminology and classification of the storage diseases. Chemical studies on extracted tissues were often crude by today's standards, but by the mid-1920s cerebroside had been established as the stored product in Gaucher's disease, and sphingomyelin was isolated from the liver and spleen in Niemann-Pick disease. Work by Klenk in the 1930s led to the isolation of gangliosides from the brain and the recognition that Tay-Sachs disease was characterized by excess ganglioside. Chromatography, particularly thin-layer chromatography with silica gel on glass plates, was introduced in the early 1960s and has allowed the separation and identification of lipid components in milligram quantities of tissue.

Early theories to account for the accumulation of large amounts of lipid in the storage disorders centred about altered metabolism and suggestions of increased synthesis and imbalance of enzymes within reticulum cells and histiocytes. Interest in intracellular digestion has its origins in the eighteenth century, and, through the experiments of Metchnikoff and others in the nineteenth century and DeDuve and his colleagues in 1955, the lysosomal theory was introduced. The development of the lysosomal concept was reviewed by Aterman (1979) and the wider aspects of the theory have been covered by Hers and Van Hoof (1973).

Following the discovery of a lysosomal enzyme deficiency as a cause for Pompe's disease in 1963, Hers (1965) suggested a set of criteria by which a disorder could be included in the group of lysosomal storage disorders. Because the metabolic block is in intralysosomal digestion the storage should be intravacuolar, and enlarged and altered lysosomes should be seen by electron microscopic examination. The vacuoles should be associated with acid phosphatase activity, as this is an activity readily localizable by electron histochemistry. Although acid phosphatase is not entirely a lysosomal enzyme, its association with the stored product is sufficient proof of the lysosomal nature of the storage. Enzymes are not usually specific for a single substance but rather they have a specificity for a group; as a consequence Hers (1965) predicted that the stored material could be heterogeneous, and several of the storage disorders have now been shown to accumulate more than one storage product. It was also part of the criteria that there should be a primary defect in one lysosomal protein.

Most of the lysosomal storage disorders have these criteria but, with increasing clinical and pathological awareness, defects which did not appear to conform have been described. In at least two instances—in metachromatic leucodystrophy and one form of G_{M2}-gangliosidosis—no *enzyme* defect has been found, but there is a deficiency of a protein cofactor which facilitates the binding of the enzyme to the substrate. These protein cofactors are part of the lysosomal system and still fall within the original criteria of a defect in one lysosomal protein. There is also recent evidence that in cases where a dual enzyme deficiency is apparent, the defect may lie in a protector protein which normally prevents intralysosomal digestion of the lysosomal enzyme proteins. The addition of leupeptin to the culture medium restores the activity of β-galactosidase in an otherwise dual deficiency of β-galactosidase and neuraminidase expressed in cultured fibroblasts (Sakuraba, Aoyagi and Suzuki, 1982). Secondary defects are found where the stored product inhibits enzyme activity. In the mucopolysaccharidoses, reduced activity of β-galactosidase and hyaluronidase have been ascribed to the complexing of mucopolysaccharide to the enzyme protein, resulting in abnormal kinetics and the apparent production of abnormal isoenzymes.

A greater understanding of the mechanisms of secretion has led to the recognition of the defect in mucolipidosis II and mucolipidosis III where, because of faulty recognition signals on the synthesized enzyme protein, the enzyme is exported rather than being diverted to the lysosome. This results in a high activity of some lysosomal enzymes in serum and the virtual absence of the same enzyme in tissue samples. Here the defect is not primarily in a lysosomal protein. With deeper understanding of the synthesis of lysosomal enzyme proteins, their protection from digestion within the lysosome and the nature of their cofactors, it should be possible in time to identify the defect in the few remaining lysosomal enzyme disorders in which the defect is not yet known.

Investigation of the lysosomal storage disorders involves detailed clinical descriptions, gross pathology, histology, histochemistry, electron microscopy, chemistry and enzymology. The studies must be thorough and wherever possible conclusive, because in most of them prenatal diagnosis is possible, and detailed study may allow the mechanisms of mental retardation to be revealed. In this respect the various animal models with well defined enzyme defects may prove useful and may also be of use in monitoring the effect of various treatments, including bone marrow transplantation.

The chemistry and enzymology of the lysosomal storage disorders are reviewed in Stanbury et al. (1983) and by Brady and Barranger (1981), and the reader is referred to these sources for more detailed information regarding the individual disorders. For details of histochemical methods and their application in this group of disorders the reader is referred to Filipe and Lake (1983).

The gangliosidoses

The gangliosidoses are a group of disorders in which increased amounts of gangliosides of normal structure are present in the brain and sometimes in other organs. There are two main groups:

G_{M2}-gangliosidoses and G_{M1}-gangliosidoses.

G_{M2}-gangliosidosis

At one time (in the early 1960s) G_{M2}-gangliosidosis was synonymous with Tay–Sachs disease, but with the recognition of the enzyme deficiency characteristic of most of the patients with Tay–Sachs disease, clinical variants with the same or similar deficiencies have become common. 'Tay–Sachs disease' is best used as a clinical term for the infantile form of G_{M2}-gangliosidosis because, although the enzyme deficiencies are different in each of the three infantile forms (Table 12.1), the clinical presentations, symptoms and course are identical. Late-infantile, juvenile and adult forms of G_{M2}-gangliosidosis have also been described.

Table 12.1 G_{M2}-gangliosidosis

Clinical type	Enzyme defect
Infantile (Tay–Sachs disease):	
Type 1 (or type B)	Hexosaminidase A
Type 2 (or type O) (Sandhoff's disease)	Hexosaminidase A and B
Type 3 (or type AB)	Hexosaminidase A activator protein
Late-infantile	Hexosaminidase A (partial or profound)
Juvenile	Hexosaminidase A (partial or profound)
Adult	Hexosaminidase A (partial or profound)

Each disorder is inherited as an autosomal recessive trait. Tay–Sachs disease is relatively common in Ashkenazi Jews, who have a carrier frequency of about 1 in 30, and although it was thought at one time to be an almost exclusively Jewish disease it has been found in other races but with a lower carrier frequency of about 1 in 300. The initial descriptions by Tay (1881) and Sachs (1887) were of the clinical Tay–Sachs type and it is impossible to guess which enzyme deficiency their patients had.

Clinical features

The clinical features of the *three infantile* types of G_{M2}-gangliosidosis are essentially identical. The children appear normal at birth and develop normally for up to 4 or 5 months, when psychomotor retardation becomes apparent. In retrospect, an abnormal startle response to sounds, usually consisting of brisk extension of the arms, may be recalled by the parents. Increasing psychomotor retardation with hypotonia and spasticity of the limbs leads to a cachectic, decerebrate state by the age of 3 years. Megalencephaly will have been noted during the second year, and fits of a generalized tonic–clonic nature or minor motor seizures occur from about 12–15 months. The children are blind before the end of the first year and bilateral cherry red spots are seen at the macula. Hepatomegaly, splenomegaly or skeletal abnormalities do not occur. Death usually occurs before the age of 5 years, often from bronchopneumonia. In the Sandhoff variant some patients show mild splenomegaly.

The onset of the *late-infantile* form of G_{M2}-gangliosidosis (Brett et al., 1973) is after 18 months of age with progressive dementia and fits. An abnormal startle response may be found and bilateral cherry red spots at the macula are present in some patients. The *juvenile* form begins at between 4 and 6 years with dementia, and progresses slowly. Spasticity increases and fits occur. The cherry red spots, so common in the infantile form, are uncommon and less well defined when they are present. Death occurs up to 10 years from the onset of clinical symptoms.

The much rarer *adult* form (Rapin et al., 1976) presents with slowly progressive deterioration from early childhood. There is evidence of neurogenic muscular atrophy (Johnston et al., 1982), ataxia, dystonia and dysarthria. Fits and ocular abnormalities do not occur. Mental retardation may only be slight.

Chemistry The ganglioside isolated by Klenk was identified by chromatography as ganglioside G_{M2} by Svennerholm (1964), and its structure is shown in Fig. 12.1. In the brain, G_{M2}-ganglioside

ceramide – glucose – galactose – *N*-acetylgalactosamine
(galactose attached to:) *N*-acetylneuraminic acid

G_{M2}- ganglioside

ceramide - glucose - galactose - *N*-acetylgalactosamine

Asialo - G_{M2} (G_{A2})

ceramide - glucose - galactose - *N*-acetylgalactosamine - galactose
(galactose attached to:) *N*-acetylneuraminic acid

G_{M1} - ganglioside

ceramide - glucose - galactose - *N*-acetylgalactosamine - galactose

Asialo - G_{M1} (G_{A1})

ceramide - glucose - galactose - galactose - *N*-acetylgalactosamine

Globoside

Fig. 12.1 Structures of gangliosides and asialoderivatives.

is increased more than 100-fold in all types, although the increase is less marked in the juvenile type. Small increases are also noted in the liver and spleen. Because the enzyme involved does not have absolute specificity and recognizes the terminal group, the asialoderivative (G_{A2}) also accumulates but not to the same degree as G_{M2}-ganglioside. Minor increases are also to be expected in other compounds containing a terminal *N*-acetylhexosamine.

In the variant known as Sandhoff's disease there is also significant storage of the glycolipid globoside, normally degraded by hexosaminidase B. Globoside is increased to a minor extent in the brain but greater concentrations are found in liver, spleen and, particularly, kidney. No such increases are found in hexosaminidase A deficiency. Other evidence for involvement of disturbed glycolipid and glycoprotein catabolism in Sandhoff's disease is provided by the occurrence in the urine of oligosaccharides containing mannose and *N*-acetylglucosamine (Strecker and Montreuil, 1971). Urine from patients with hexosaminidase A deficiency does not contain these oligosaccharides.

Enzyme defect The chemical analysis of the isolated G_{M2}-ganglioside showed a terminal *N*-acetylgalactosamine residue (Fig. 12.1), which led to the conclusion that a deficiency of β-galactosaminidase (hexosaminidase) was responsible for the disorder. However, apart from Sandhoff, Andreae and Jatzkewitz (1968) who showed a deficiency of this activity in one case, they and others found slightly increased hexosaminidase activity in other cases of Tay–Sachs disease. Robinson and Stirling (1968) showed that hexosaminidase in human spleen had two components which they labelled A and B. The A form was heat labile and could also be separated from the B component by gel electrophoresis. Okada and O'Brien (1969) showed that most cases of Tay–Sachs disease were deficient in the A component. Both components are deficient in Sandhoff's disease. Occasional cases were described in which there was clearly neuronal storage with excess ganglioside G_{M2} but in which both hexosaminidase A and hexosaminidase B were present and active against artificial and natural substrates. Conzelmann and Sandhoff (1978) have shown that the activator protein necessary for the degradation of G_{M2}-ganglioside by hexosaminidase A (Hechtman and LeBlanc, 1977) was deficient in such cases, and this has been confirmed in other similar cases (Hechtman et al., 1982).

Enzyme assay can be conveniently carried out on separated white blood cells, serum, cultured fibroblasts, tears or tissue samples. The heterozygous state of the most common form (hexosaminidase A deficiency) can be readily detected, and screening programmes have been established among populations which are particularly at risk (Kaback, 1977). In the normal individual, of the total hexosaminidase activity in serum, 50–65 per cent is hexosaminidase A. The figure for fibroblasts is similar, and in separated white blood cells is 60–70 per cent as hexosaminidase A. Heterozygotes show approximately half this level, whilst affected patients show less than 5 per cent as hexosaminidase A. Screening has also disclosed several clinically normal adult individuals with hexosaminidase A deficiency (Thomas et al., 1982; Vidgoff, Buist and O'Brien 1973).

Prenatal detection of an affected or normal fetus can be achieved through amniocentesis at 16–18 weeks of pregnancy. The amniotic fluid cells are cultured and the cultured cells assayed for hexosaminidases A and B. Amniotic fluid (cell free) can also be used. It is of course necessary to know the exact defect being sought, either through assay of cells from a previously affected sibling or through the screening programme, bearing in mind the caveat in the paragraph above.

Neuropathology

The brain is, depending on the duration of the disease, normal in size, micrencephalic or megalencephalic. The enlargement is thought to be due to neuronal swelling and astrocytic hyperplasia. It is usually firm, even indurated at times. There may be ulegyria with narrowing of the cortex together with discoloration and loss of a clear distinction between grey and white matter. Myelin loss is evident in the infantile cases but not in the late-infantile or juvenile cases.

The microscopical changes and histochemical reactions are the same for all types of G_{M2}-gangliosidosis (de Baecque et al., 1975) and will be described together.

Neurons, wherever they occur, are enlarged, the cytoplasm is ballooned and the nucleus pushed to one pole of the cell (Fig. 12.2). Thus neurons throughout the central nervous system, in the myenteric and submucosal plexuses of the whole of the gastrointestinal tract, in the adrenal

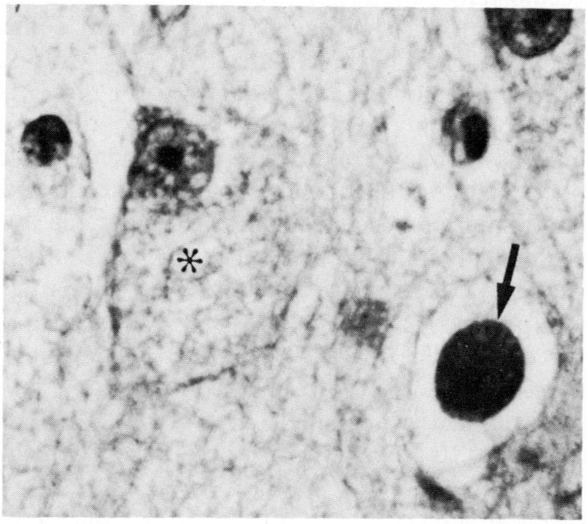

Fig. 12.2 G_{M2}-gangliosidosis. The distended cortical neurons (*) are PAS negative in this section of paraffin-embedded tissue, whilst a glial cell (arrow) retains PAS positivity. PAS × 830.

medulla, and in the various ganglia show the same changes.

In paraffin sections, stained with haematoxylin and eosin the neuronal cytoplasm appears foamy, and microglial cells in the cortex also show evidence of storage. The stored ganglioside is extracted from neurons during processing and the periodic acid–Schiff (PAS) reaction is negative. The glial cells, however, remain strongly positive, indicating that the stored material may not be ganglioside or that it is more strongly bound in the storage complex. The granular material in neurons and glial cells stains strongly with Luxol fast blue and with Sudan black. In formalin-fixed frozen sections and cryostat sections neurons are strongly PAS positive (Figs. 12.3 and 12.4) and show strong metachromasia

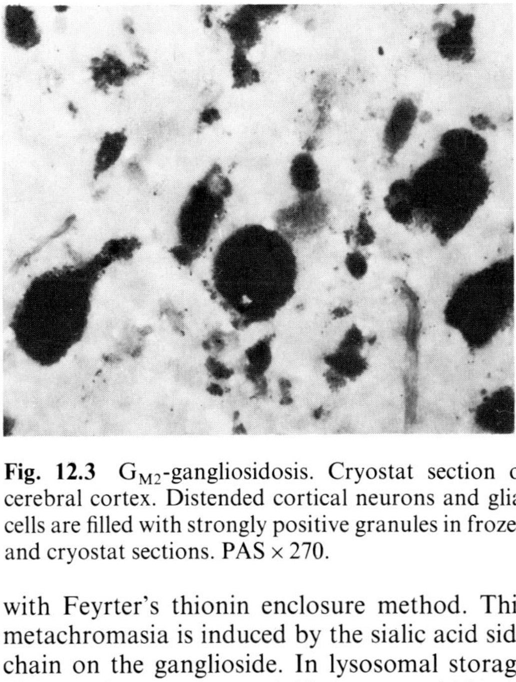

Fig. 12.3 G_{M2}-gangliosidosis. Cryostat section of cerebral cortex. Distended cortical neurons and glial cells are filled with strongly positive granules in frozen and cryostat sections. PAS × 270.

with Feyrter's thionin enclosure method. This metachromasia is induced by the sialic acid side chain on the ganglioside. In lysosomal storage diseases the stored material is present within enlarged lysosomes which are increased in number; consequently reactions for the demonstration of lysosomal enzyme activity (acid phosphatase, β-glucuronidase, β-galactosidase) show greatly enhanced activity with larger and more numerous granules of reaction product. The histochemical method for the demonstration of hexosaminidase activity is reliable for the diagnosis of the Sandhoff variant of Tay–Sachs disease (total hexosaminidase deficiency). The heat inactivation methods for discrimination between hexo-

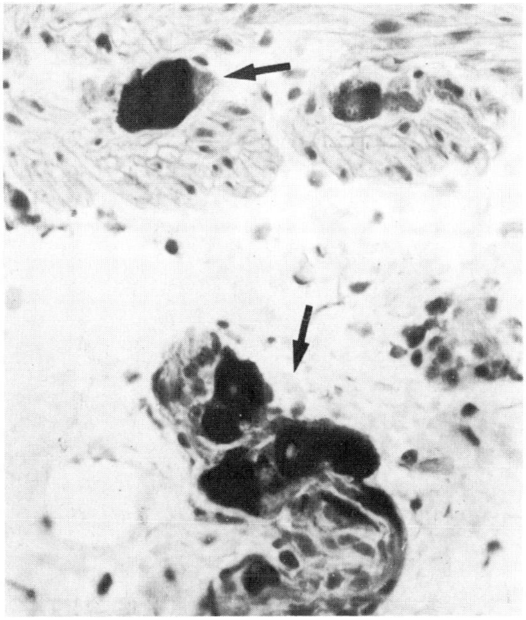

Fig. 12.4 Juvenile G_{M2}-gangliosidosis. Neurons (arrows) in Meissner's plexus of the gut contain PAS positive granules. × 300.

saminidases A and B are, however, not suitable for tissue sections and an absence of hexosaminidase A cannot be detected in the presence of hexosaminidase B by histochemical staining methods.

The staining reactions of the neurons and glial cells are identical to those in G_{M1}-gangliosidosis. This is to be expected because the two gangliosides differ only by a terminal galactose unit.

Electron microscopy of the stored material, as first shown by Terry and Weiss (1963), demonstrates membranous cytoplasmic bodies (MCBs). These are membrane-bound structures which may have parallel or concentric lamellae and are present in neurons and glial cells alike (Fig. 12.5). The MCBs have been isolated by differential gradient centrifugation and shown to contain G_{M2}-ganglioside, cholesterol and phospholipid. A protein component may also be present.

Visceral organs generally show no evidence of storage although in the occasional case storage cells can be detected in the sinusoids of the liver. These cells are strongly PAS positive in frozen or cryostat sections and contain either ganglioside G_{M2} or its asialoderivative G_{A2}. There is no vacuolation in lymphocytes and no storage can be

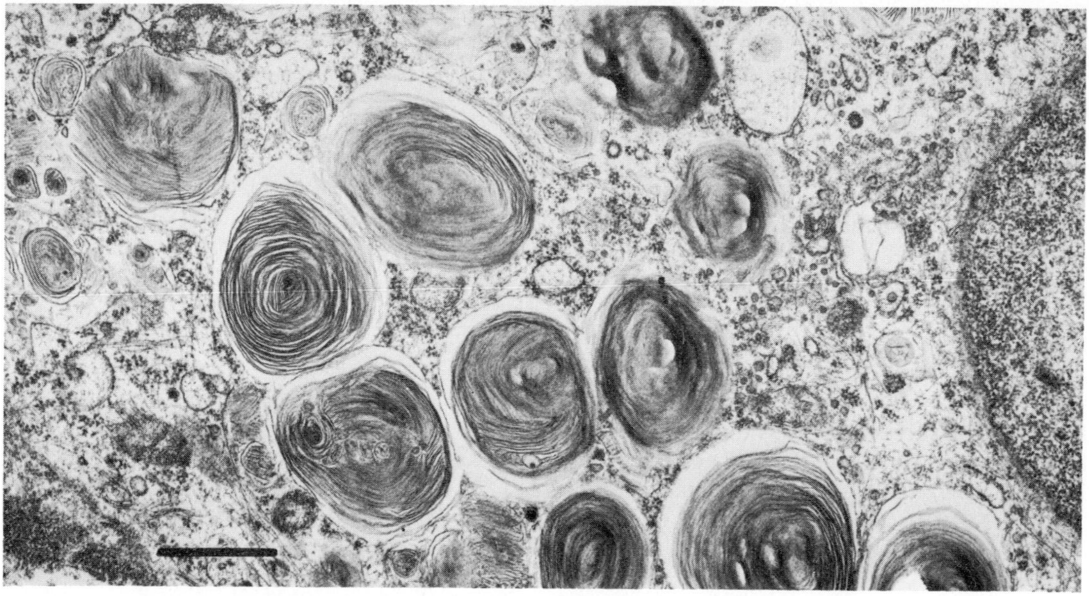

Fig. 12.5 G_{M2}-gangliosidosis. Membranous cytoplasmic bodies in a neuron. Bar = 1 μm × 16000.

reliably detected by electron microscopy. The bone marrow contains no storage cells although occasional foamy cells may be found in the Sandhoff variant. In skin and conjunctival biopsies studied by electron microscopy Schwann cells may show membranous cytoplasmic bodies, but these are not completely characteristic of G_{M2}-gangliosidosis and can be found in many other disorders. Their discovery in a skin or conjunctival biopsy, therefore, does not necessarily establish the diagnosis.

In affected fetuses light microscopy is not very helpful, and no convincing storage can be demonstrated in neurons of the cortex or brain stem. This applies to gestational ages up to about 20 weeks. Electron microscopy, however, shows evidence of storage in the form of early, loosely packed MCBs (Fig. 12.6) and this is found readily in the brain stem (Adachi, Schneck and Volk, 1974) even as early as 12 weeks. In lipid extracts subjected to thin layer chromatography there is an excess of ganglioside G_{M2} when compared with extracts from fetal brain tissue of a similar age. In the placenta there is no evidence of storage, except in Sandhoff's disease in which a few large foamy storage cells may be found in the stroma of the villi. The cells contain membrane-bound vacuoles. No hexosaminidase activity can be demonstrated within the trophoblast in Sandhoff's disease.

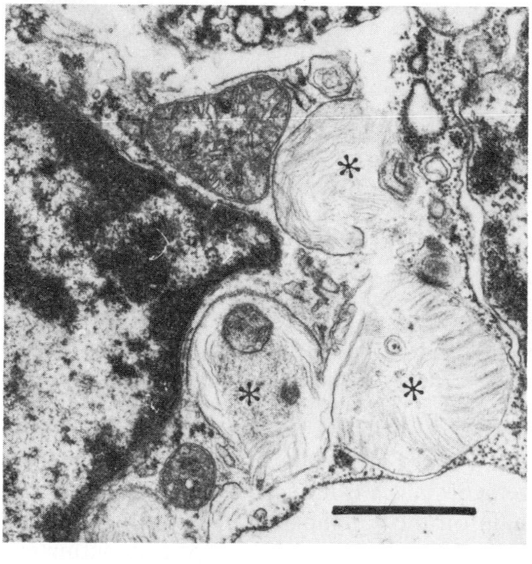

Fig. 12.6 G_{M2}-gangliosidosis. Neurons in the brain stem of a 17-week fetus show early MCBs(*). Bar = 1 μm. × 19000.

Diagnosis The diagnosis of Tay–Sachs disease and its variants must be made by enzyme assay of a suitable sample (serum, white blood cells, fibroblasts). The microscopical diagnosis can be made by examination of neurons obtained in a biopsy of intestine. A suction rectal biopsy, of the type performed for the investigation of

Hirschsprung's disease, is adequate although some pathologists prefer a full-thickness biopsy or an appendix. Cryostat sections or, less satisfactory, frozen sections are necessary. The changes are similar to those of G_{M1}-gangliosidosis and to exclude this possibility the demonstration of β-galactosidase activity is necessary. Thin layer chromatography of a solvent extract will show excess G_{M2}-ganglioside, and electron microscopy will show the presence of neuronal membranous cytoplasmic bodies.

Animal models Cats with a deficiency of hexosaminidase A and B and a gross excess of ganglioside G_{M2} have been described (Cork et al., 1977). Globoside was increased in the liver and the ultrastructural changes in the brain were the same as those seen in the human disorder. These cats have the equivalent of Sandhoff's disease. Bernheimer and Karbe (1970) described the morphology and neurochemistry in German shorthair pointer dogs affected with G_{M2}-gangliosidosis. The ultrastructural changes and chemistry appear identical to the human counterpart. Visceral changes were not recorded. A similar disorder has also been described in Yorkshire swine (Pierce et al., 1976).

G_{M1}-gangliosidosis

There are two forms of G_{M1}-gangliosidosis presenting in childhood. The *infantile* form (type 1) presents at or soon after birth with failure to thrive, hepatosplenomegaly, accompanied by x-ray changes and facial dysmorphism similar to those found in the mucopolysaccharidoses (Landing et al., 1964). The patients may show peripheral oedema. Sometimes the onset is milder occurring later, about the end of the first year. The dysmorphic features and hepatosplenomegaly gave rise to the early descriptions of 'pseudo-Hurler disease', and the presence of bilateral cherry red spots at the macula led to the description 'Tay-Sachs disease with visceral involvement' (Norman et al., 1959). Other terms that have been used are familial neurovisceral lipidosis (Landing et al., 1964), Landing's disease (Sacrez et al., 1967) and generalized gangliosidosis (O'Brien et al., 1965). Later symptoms of psychomotor retardation and fits in some patients occur and death, usually as a result of pneumonia, supervenes before the second birthday.

The rarer *late-infantile/juvenile* form (type 2) (Derry et al., 1968; L.S. Wolfe et al., 1970) begins with progressive mental and motor retardation at between 1 and 5 years of age. Fits are common, and spastic tetraplegia develops with cerebellar and extrapyramidal signs. Decerebrate rigidity follows and death occurs at between 3 and 10 years. There are no visceral signs and x-ray changes are minor, being restricted to the vertebral bodies.

Both forms are inherited as autosomal recessive traits.

The occurrence of an *adult* form of G_{M1}-gangliosidosis has been complicated by enzymology. Many older patients appear to have the same enzyme defect as that in the infantile and juvenile forms, but on closer inspection the primary deficiency is in neuraminidase activity with secondary β-galactosidase deficiency. Similar secondary β-galactosidase deficiencies have been reported in the mucopolysaccharidoses (Patel, Tappel and O'Brien, 1970). A rare patient presenting with dystonia had G_{M1}-ganglioside storage in the brain, deficient β-galactosidase activity but normal neuraminidase activity, and may represent the adult form (T. Kobayashi and Suzuki, 1981).

Chemistry The lipid that accumulates in the brain has been identified (O'Brien et al., 1965) as ganglioside G_{M1} (see Fig. 12.1), and this accounts for 70–80 per cent of the total ganglioside as compared with about 20 per cent in the normal brain. The asialo-G_{A1} also is increased. Cholesterol and phospholipid have also been found in the isolated membranous bodies.

Although G_{M1}-ganglioside also accumulates in the viscera to a small extent, there is extensive visceral storage in the infantile form of oligosaccharides, often referred to as keratan-sulphate-like mucopolysaccharide even though the sulphate content is almost non-existent. Some fractions contain sialic acid. The constant feature of the oligosaccharides is a terminal galactose residue with a β-link, and with this linkage occurring in blood group substances, immunoglobulins and glycolipids and glycopeptides of membranes a wide variety of oligosaccharides can be expected to accumulate or be excreted. Wolfe and his colleagues (1974) have identified an octasaccharide as a major component in the liver of the infantile form.

Enzymology A deficiency of β-galactosidase activity in the infantile form was first reported by Sacrez et al. in 1967 and this was later confirmed by other workers (Dacremont and Kint, 1968; Okada and O'Brien, 1968). A similar deficiency in the late-infantile/juvenile form was shown by Kint, Dacremont and Vlietinck (1969), Wolfe et al. (1970) and others. Studies by Ho and O'Brien (1969) suggested that the acid β-galactosidase activity of human liver could be separated into three isoenzymes (A, B and C) on starch gel electrophoresis, and O'Brien (1969) reported that all three isoenzyme bands showed no activity in the infantile form of G_{M1}-gangliosidosis. The fast-moving A isoenzyme, however, was preserved in the late-infantile/juvenile form whilst the B and C isoenzymes were deficient. These findings were not confirmed by Y. Suzuki, Crocker and Suzuki (1971) or by Lowden et al. (1974).

The enzyme assay can be performed on fresh (or frozen) liver or brain tissue, and the defect has been demonstrated in all organs with some differences in characteristics between the residual activity and the normal enzyme (Pinsky, Powell and Callahan, 1970; Chou, Kaye and Nadler, 1974). It is more convenient to perform the assay on a leucocyte preparation, as white cells can readily be prepared for assay, or whole blood sent with appropriate anticoagulant on ice to a laboratory proficient in the assay of lysosomal enzymes and their defects. Less than 10 per cent of normal activity is found in affected patients whilst parental levels are in the heterozygote (approximately 50 per cent) range. In all cases of suspected G_{M1}-gangliosidosis the β-galactosidase activity in the leucocytes of the parents is an important diagnostic test because in at least one form of sialidosis (mucolipidosis I, MLI) the patient is deficient in β-galactosidase as well as sialidase. Parental leucocyte β-galactosidase activity is normal in these cases.

The assay is performed using the sensitive 4-methylumbelliferyl-β-galactoside as substrate measuring the fluorescence of released 4-methylumbelliferone. The enzyme β-galactosidase also appears to exhibit α-arabinosidase activity (Van Hoof and Hers, 1968) and β-fucosidase activity (Wiederschain, 1980), and deficiencies have been recorded in patients with G_{M1}-gangliosidosis by using α-arabinoside and β-fucoside substrates.

Pathology

In both forms the brain may appear grossly normal and the megalencephaly sometimes seen in Tay–Sachs disease is not found. Some cortical atrophy and increased consistency of the white matter is sometimes noted. Enlargement of the liver and spleen (both up to two to three times the normal weight), with kidneys of normal size—although enlarged kidneys are occasionally recorded—are the usual findings at post-mortem in the infantile form. In the late-infantile/juvenile form organ weights are normal.

In both forms neuronal storage with ballooning of neuronal cytoplasm occurs throughout the cortex, brain stem and spinal cord and is also evident in the submucosal and myenteric plexuses of the gut. The neurons have a foamy appearance in routine sections and are indistinguishable from those seen in G_{M2}-gangliosidosis. Because the structure of gangliosides G_{M1} and G_{M2} differs only in the terminal *N*-acetylgalactosamine, and they are stored together with cholesterol and phospholipid, the neuronal staining reactions and ultrastructure (Fig. 12.7) are identical. In routinely processed tissue the ganglioside has been extracted and the neurons are thus mostly PAS negative, in contrast with glial cells which are strongly positive. In sections stained with Luxol fast blue or Sudan black granular

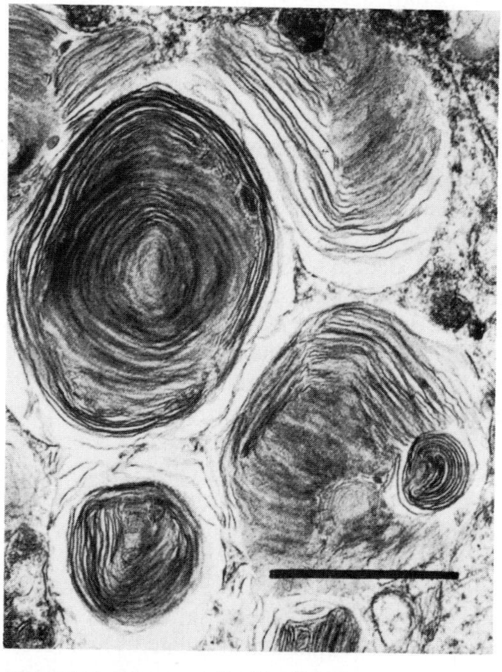

Fig. 12.7 G_{M1}-gangliosidosis. Neuronal membranous cytoplasmic bodies are identical to those in G_{M2}-gangliosidosis. Bar = 1 μm. × 25000.

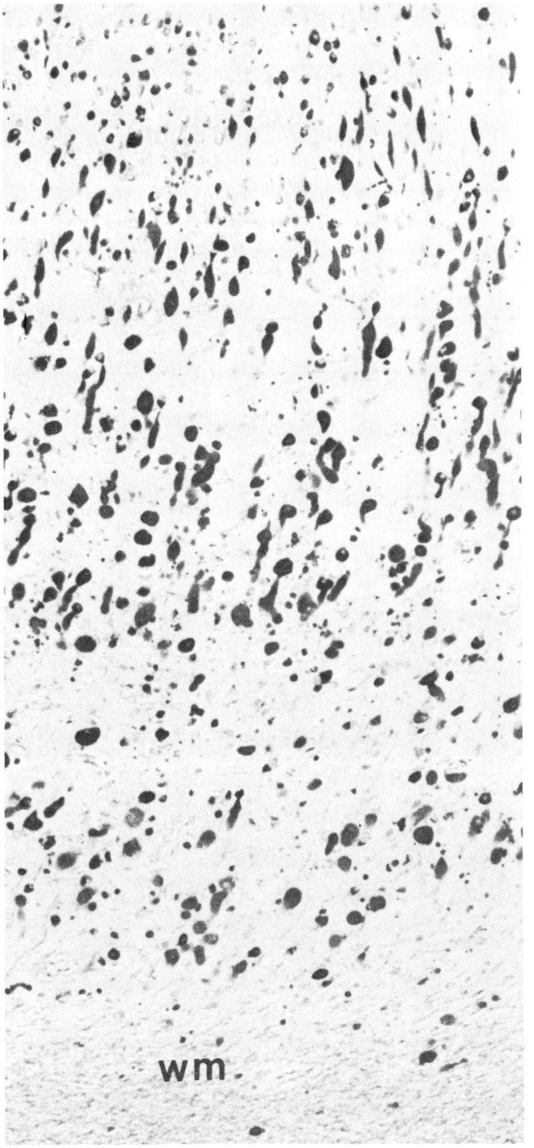

Fig. 12.8 G_{M1}-gangliosidosis type 2 (late-infantile/juvenile). Section of cerebral cortex. Neuronal, axonal and glial storage is evident in all layers. There is some loss of myelin in the white matter (wm). Luxol fast blue × 120.

neuronal, axonal and glial storage bodies (Fig. 12.8) are demonstrable. The white matter is gliotic and there is loss of myelin in the infantile form, but not in the late-infantile/juvenile form.

In frozen or cryostat sections the stored ganglioside in neurons and glia is brightly PAS positive, is mildly sudanophilic with Sudan black

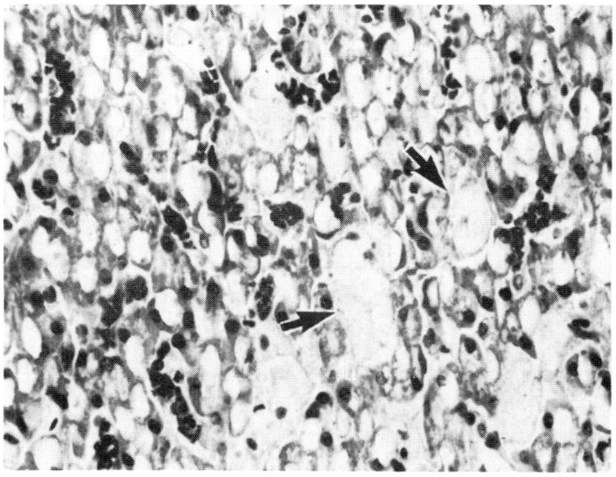

Fig. 12.9 G_{M1}-gangliosidosis type 1 (infantile). Section of liver. The hepatocytes show prominent vacuolation and storage cells (arrows) are evident in the sinusoids. Haematoxylin and eosin × 240.

and gives a rose metachromasia with Feyrter's thionin enclosure staining. The Bial reaction for sialic acid is a little capricious but should be positive. The presence of the cholesterol associated with the ganglioside can be shown by either the Schultz or the perchloric acid–naphthoquinone reaction.

The stored oligosaccharide in visceral organs of patients with the infantile form is extremely water soluble and is lost on fixation; even with protective measures using cryostat sections of

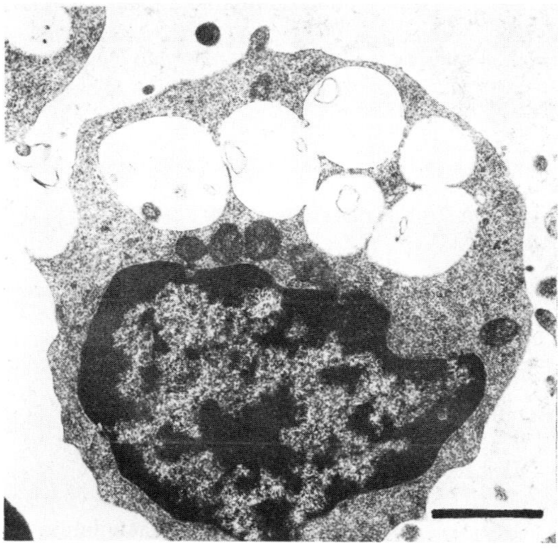

Fig. 12.10 G_{M1}-gangliosidosis type 1. Electron micrograph of a lymphocyte showing prominent membrane-bound empty vacuoles. A large proportion of lymphocytes show this change. Bar = 1 μm. × 14500.

snap-frozen tissue the low molecular weight of the oligosaccharides conspires with their solubility to prevent microscopic detection. As a consequence affected cells appear empty. Marked storage in the hepatocytes gives the appearance at first glance of a very fatty liver (Fig. 12.9) but no lipid can be demonstrated. Foamy storage cells of the mononuclear phagocyte system are present in the liver sinusoids (Fig. 12.9) and these contain deposits of ganglioside which stain with the PAS reaction and are Alcian blue positive. The renal glomerular epithelium shows marked cytoplasmic vacuolization and appears to contain a water soluble oligosaccharide similar to that in the liver cells. The spleen contains numerous foamy histocytes in the red pulp and in the follicles. Lymph nodes are similarly affected. Skin biopsies prepared for 1 μm plastic

Table 12.2 Light miscroscopy of routinely stained blood films in lysosomal storage diseases

Disorder	Feature
G_{M1}-gangliosidosis:	
Infantile	Numerous large cytoplasmic vacuoles in many lymphocytes
Late-infantile/juvenile	No vacuolated lymphocytes
G_{M2}-gangliosidosis (all types)	No vacuolated lymphocytes
Batten:	
Infantile	No change at light microscopy
Late-infantile	No change at light microscopy
Early-juvenile	No change at light microscopy
Juvenile	Several large cytoplasmic vacuoles in a large proportion of lymphocytes
Adult	No change at light microscopy
Gaucher (all types)	No vacuolated lymphocytes
Niemann–Pick type A	A few (1–6) small discrete vacuoles in a variable proportion of lymphocytes
Niemann–Pick type B	No vacuolated lymphocytes
Niemann–Pick type C	Occasional cases show a few vacuoles in some lymphocytes
Fabry's disease	No vacuolated lymphocytes
Metachromatic leucodystrophy	No changes
Austin's disease (mucosulphatidosis)	Alder granulation of neutrophils; Gasser cells; absent eosinophils
Krabbe's leucodystrophy	No changes
Aspartylglucosaminuria	Large bold vacuoles present in some lymphocytes
Salla disease	Large bold vacuoles present in up to 30% of lymphocytes
Fucosidosis	Numerous small vacuoles in some lymphocytes—inconstant
Mannosidosis	Numerous large and small vacuoles present in many lymphocytes
Glycogen storage disease type 2 (all forms)	A few (1–6) small vacuoles in most lymphocytes
Mucopolysaccharidosis:	
Types 1–3	Occasional vacuoles in some lymphocytes; occasional Gasser cells
Type 6	Alder granulation in all neutrophils
Type 7	Alder granulation in all neutrophils
Mucolipidosis:	
ML I type 1	No consistent change
ML I type 2	Large cytoplasmic vacuoles in a variable proportion of lymphocytes
ML II	Large cytoplasmic vacuoles in ” ” ”
ML III	Vacuolation of lymphocytes is variable
ML IV	No change at light microscopy
Farber's disease	No vacuolation of lymphocytes
Wolman's disease (and cholesteryl ester storage disease)	A few (1–6) small vacuoles in many lymphocytes

sections are useful for the demonstration of foamy vacuolation of sweat gland epithelium, foamy histiocytes and vacuolated fibroblasts. Endothelial cells of blood vessels are also heavily vacuolated throughout and are seen in skin, brain and gut. Numerous PAS-positive histiocytes are present in the lamina propria of the gut in both forms of G_{M1}-gangliosidosis. Lymphocytes contain numerous bold cytoplasmic vacuoles (Fig. 12.10), readily seen in peripheral blood films stained with Giemsa, Leishman or other routine haematological method (Table 12.2). Large foamy histiocytes of the 'Niemann–Pick' type are present in bone marrow aspirates.

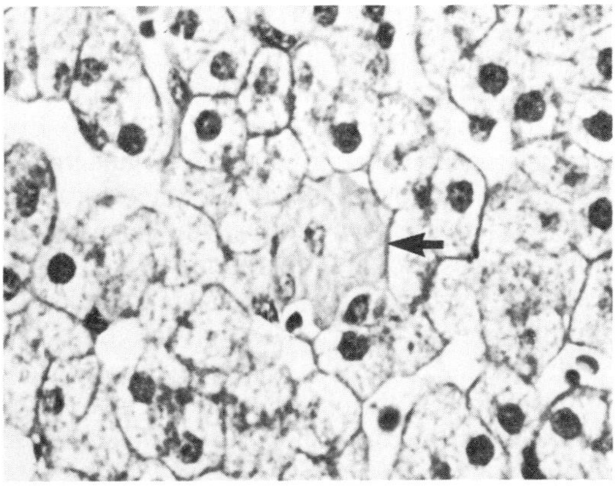

Fig. 12.11 G_{M1}-gangliosidosis type 2. Section of liver. The hepatocytes appear normal. Storage cell (arrow) with a faintly striated cytoplasm is shown in a sinusoid. Haematoxylin and eosin ×500.

The lymphocytic vacuoles and the bone marrow histiocytes appear empty and are unstained by PAS or Sudan black methods.

In the late-infantile/juvenile form there are some differences in the visceral organs. The liver may appear relatively normal in routine sections with no involvement of the hepatocytes although scattered histiocytes are found in the sinusoids (Fig. 12.11). They contain a gangliosidic-like substance which has the same characteristics as that in the liver histiocytes of the infantile type. Few storage cells are found in the spleen but ballooning of the renal glomerular epithelium is found as in the infantile type. No vacuolated lymphocytes are seen and the bone marrow aspirates show storage cells which are few in number and bear a superficial resemblance to Gaucher cells. In May–Grünwald–Giemsa-stained marrow films the cells stain a sky-blue colour and have a finely striated appearance. They are PAS positive.

Enzyme histochemistry As with most lysosomal disorders, there is an alteration in the state of affected cells and consequently it is possible to show enhanced acid phosphatase activity in those cells affected by storage (Fig. 12.12). This is a useful screening procedure and will detect storage cells and the involved endothelial cells as well as confirming the storage in other cell types such as heart muscle. The method for the detection of β-galactosidase activity using a substituted indoxyl-β-galactoside substrate is reliable

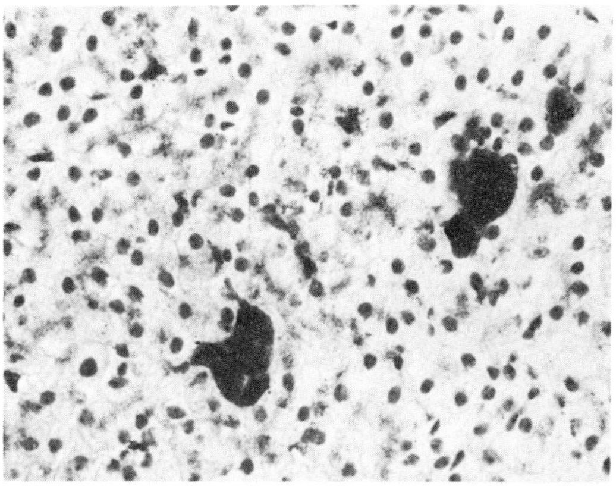

Fig. 12.12 G_{M1}-gangliosidosis type 2. Liver, stained to demonstrate acid phosphatase activity. The hepatocytes show normal activity but the storage cells are strongly stained. ×280.

(Lake, 1974) and can be used on leucocytes, cultured fibroblasts and sections of snap-frozen tissue. In normal white cells activity is present diffusely in neutrophils and discrete droplet form in lymphocytes. Platelets show activity and eosinophils show weak granular activity. In both forms of G_{M1}-gangliosidosis no activity can be demonstrated in neutrophils, lymphocytes or platelets. Eosinophils retain their activity. Normal neurons have strong β-galactosidase activity but no activity is present in the distended neurons of G_{M1}-gangliosidosis. Reactive astrocytes, however, show some enzyme activity, perhaps of a different isoenzyme. In the liver of patients with the late-infantile/juvenile form where the liver appears superficially normal no β-galactosidase activity is seen and it is thus surprising that there is no demonstrable storage in the hepatocytes. The β-galactosidase in the brush border of enterocytes, also shown by the indoxyl method, is normal in the small intestine but β-galactosidase within the enterocytes is decreased.

Fetal pathology Studies on 17- to 22-week-old fetuses aborted after deficient β-galactosidase activity had been detected in cultured amniotic fluid cells obtained at amniocentesis at about 16 weeks gestation show that there are no macroscopic features of the disease. In particular there are no dysmorphic features, organ weights are within normal limits and no radiological changes can be found. Routine microscopy of the brain and spinal cord shows no convincing storage, but foamy storage cells can be detected in the liver and spleen and ballooning of the glomerular epithelium is evident (Kaback et al., 1973; Lowden et al., 1973). Foamy cells are present in the bone marrow and vacuolated lymphocytes may be found in the peripheral blood. There are numerous large foamy histiocytes in the stroma of the placental villi and fine vacuoles in endothelial cells in the fetal vessels (Fig. 12.13). Electron microscopy shows, in addition, the beginnings of neuronal storage (Yamano et al., 1983), particularly in the brain stem and dorsal root ganglia, and vacuolation of endothelial cells of capillaries in the cerebral cortex (Fig. 12.14). Enzyme histochemistry shows absent β-galactosidase activity in most organs, but in the liver there is some activity in the periportal hepatocytes only, and this probably represents either a non-lysosomal enzyme or an isoenzyme similar to that observed in the brain or even activity of the residual altered enzyme. The vacuolated trophoblast layer of the placenta and the histiocytes of the villous stroma have no β-galactosidase activity.

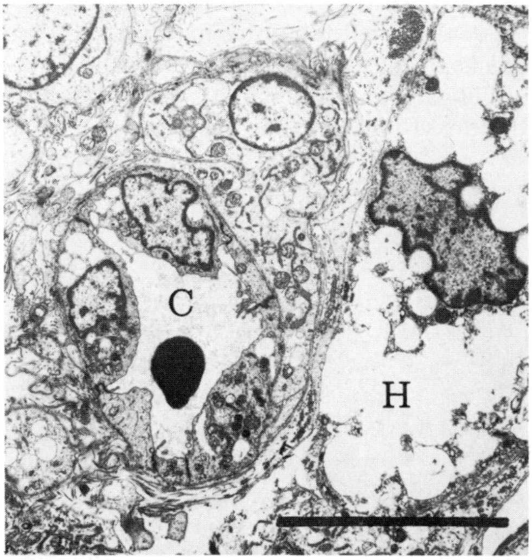

Fig. 12.13 G_{M1}-gangliosidosis type 1. Placenta. Large membrane-bound vacuoles are present in a histiocyte (H) and small vacuoles are seen in endothelial cells of a capillary (C). Bar = 10 μm. × 2900.

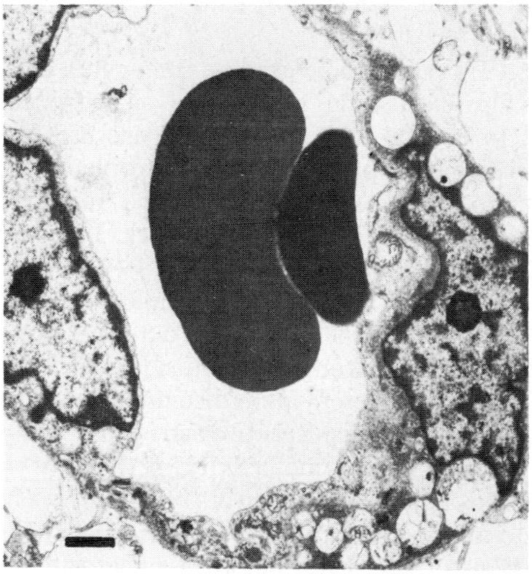

Fig. 12.14 G_{M1}-gangliosidosis type 1. Fetal cerebral cortex. Membrane-bound vacuoles are present in the endothelial cells of a capillary. Bar = 1 μm. × 5300.

Diagnosis Assay of leucocytes for β-galactosidase activity affords the simplest and most effective means of diagnosis, bearing in mind the secondary deficiencies seen in some of the mucopolysaccharidoses and in sialidosis. The β-galactosidase activity of parental leucocytes should also be determined. Where enzyme assay is not available, or it may take some time to realize a result, microscopy of blood films showing marked vacuolation of lymphocytic cytoplasm is a helpful guide for the infantile form. Vacuolation is not present in the late-infantile/juvenile form. Cryostat sections of a rectal biopsy (suction type, full-thickness or even appendix) will show in infantile and juvenile forms neuronal storage of a ganglioside-like material and the presence of numerous PAS-positive histiocytes in the lamina propria. Large foamy histiocytes are present in the bone marrow of the infantile form, whilst in the late-infantile/juvenform the bone marrow storage cells are fewer in number and are reminiscent of Gaucher cells. Electron microscopy of rectum showing neuronal MCBs may be helpful, but examination of conjunctiva or skin favoured by some, although showing storage, does not provide a precise enough diagnosis for routine use. Brain biopsy should never be necessary.

Animal models G_{M1}-gangliosidosis has been described in cats and the neuronal storage appears to be identical to that in man (Baker et al., 1971; Farrell et al., 1973). The ganglioside concentration in the brain is up to eight times the normal and β-galactosidase activity is grossly decreased. There is minor evidence of storage in visceral organs (Barnes et al., 1981) but in two cases seen personally no vacuolated lymphocytes were apparent. The disorder has also been reported in cattle (Donelly, Sheahan and Rogers, 1973) and in dogs (Rodriguez et al., 1982). In contrast with the human disease, no storage in the renal glomerulus has been noted in the animal models. No sensible comparison can be made in relation to infantile or juvenile forms in the animal model because the presentation might be regarded as infantile yet the pathology more closely resembles the human juvenile form.

G_{M3}-gangliosidosis

Several patients considered to represent G_{M3}-gangliosidosis have been reported (Jørgensen et al., 1964; Pilz, Sandhoff and Jatzkewitz, 1966), but since these also showed a storage of other gangliosides and storage disorders of the brain are well known to show non-specific increases in gangliosides these cases cannot be regarded as examples of G_{M3}-gangliosidosis. Chemical analysis was performed on tissues stored in formalin which is known to induce changes in ganglioside structure. It may well be that both the described cases are part of the Niemann–Pick type C disorder.

Max and his colleagues (Max et al., 1974; Tanaka et al., 1975; Maclaren et al., 1976) have described a unique case in which in the brain G_{M3}-ganglioside accounted for 67 per cent of the total ganglioside, the remainder being G_{D3}. Gangliosides G_{M1}, G_{M2} and G_{D1A} were absent.

A defect of ganglioside synthesis was suggested by this finding and an absence of G_{M3}-uridine diphosphate: *N*-acetylgalactosaminyl transferase was demonstrated.

The patient resembled a case of infantile G_{M1}-gangliosidosis with coarse facies, macroglossia and gingival hypertrophy. The skin was thickened and hirsute and there were flexion contractures of the fingers. He had hepatosplenomegaly but no cataract or corneal opacity was seen. The patient was unresponsive, hypotonic, had frequent seizures and died aged 14 weeks after recurrent attacks of bronchopneumonia.

The brain showed slight increase in weight and on section there was widespread spongy degeneration particularly severe in the brain stem. No inflammatory cells or lipid macrophages were present but some degree of gliosis with Alzheimer type II astrocytes was shown. An increase in the total amount of G_{M3}-ganglioside was found in the liver but no microscopical evidence of visceral storage was found. The exact status of this patient is unclear.

Batten's disease (neuronal ceroid lipofuscinosis)

This group of disorders still has one of the most confusing set of eponyms. In 1903 F. E. Batten, then pathologist to the National Hospital, Queen Square, described two sisters whose initial symptoms were failing vision at about the age of 6 years followed by dementia. He described the characteristic visual sign of 'looking out of the corners of her eyes to see an object' which has been commented on recently (Spalton, Taylor and Sanders, 1980). In the next year Mayou (1904) reported three siblings with cerebral degeneration and similar macular changes. This early situation was complicated by F. E. Batten's elder brother, R. D. Batten, who in 1897 presented to the Ophthalmological Society of the United Kingdom 'two brothers with symmetrical disease of the macula, commencing at the age of fourteen'. These two patients, however, showed no evidence of mental defect and probably represent examples of retinitis pigmentosa. F. E. Batten, as physician to the Hospital for Sick Children, Great Ormond Street, later published details of another two families whose children's illness began with fits at about 3 years of age (Batten,

1914). During this time Spielmeyer (1905), Vogt (1905), Jansky (1908), Bielschowsky (1913) and others had described similar disorders. Although at first Batten considered that the pathological changes in his and other cases were distinct from those of amaurotic family idiocy (Sachs, 1896), or 'Waren Tay–Sachs disease' as he called it, he later (Batten and Mayou, 1915) changed his view and felt that there was one large group of maculocerebral degeneration of which there were three types beginning at different ages. He believed that the name Waren Tay–Sachs family amaurotic idiocy should be maintained. A large series of cases of juvenile amaurotic idiocy was described by Sjögren (1931) and an adult form was reported by Kufs (1925). In these and others the term 'amaurotic idiocy' was used. The term persisted for many years until Zeman and Dyken (1969) coined the term 'neuronal ceroid lipofuscinoses' to describe those disorders in which neuronal deposition of an autofluorescent lipopigment was present, in contrast to the ganglioside accumulation in Tay-Sachs disease and generalized gangliosidosis. Other groups have preferred 'Batten's disease', a term which is widely used although 'Bielschowsky–Jansky' and 'Spielmeyer–Vogt–Sjögren' have also been used, depending on national preference. Recent descriptions of other variants (Santavuori et al., 1973; Lake and Cavanagh, 1978) have led to these eponyms also being used. Researches in recent years have uncovered what is probably the earliest description of the juvenile type in a family of four children in Norway (Stengel, 1826). Some might therefore argue that Stengel's disease would be appropriate. With such a plethora of eponyms and terms (Tables 12.3 and 12.4) it is not surprising that some of the literature is confusing and even misleading. It has even been claimed (Menkes, Andrews and Cancilla, 1971) that Freud (1893) first described juvenile amaurotic idiocy in a paper on familial cerebral diplegia. Freud's cases were not demented and were examples of one of the spinocerebellar syndromes.

Table 12.3 Eponyms for Batten's disease and its subgroups

Batten	Santavuori
Bielschowsky	Sjögren
Hagberg	Spielmeyer
Jansky	Stengel
Kufs	Stock
Mayou	Vogt

Table 12.4 Other terms used for Batten's disease

Amaurotic family idiocy
Cerebral lipidosis with onset past infancy
Cerebromacular degeneration
Diffuse lipofuscinosis
Generalized ceroid lipofuscinosis
Heredofamilial lipidosis
Maculocerebral degeneration
Neuronal ceroid lipofuscinosis
Neurovisceral storage disease with curvilinear bodies
Polyunsaturated fatty acid lipidosis

The term 'neuronal ceroid lipofuscinosis' is not perfect, as Zeman and Dyken (1969) acknowledged, but, since the storage is in all tissues and the substance, though having staining characteristics of ceroid or lipofuscin, is probably neither of these substances, it is preferable to use the more common term 'Batten's disease'. This acknowledges the clinical and pathological contributions of F. E. Batten in describing two forms of the disease. Other much more cumbersome terms (cerebral lipidosis with onset past infancy, etc.) are clearly open to confusion with the later onset forms of the gangliosidoses and with Niemann–Pick type C disease.

Table 12.5 Batten's disease: present classification

Infantile	(Hagberg–Santavuori)
Late-infantile	(Bielschowsky–Jansky)
Early-juvenile	(Lake–Cavanagh)
Juvenile	(Batten–Mayou; Spielmeyer–Vogt)
Adult	(Kufs)

In this chapter a classification based on clinical presentation, age of onset, pathology and electrophysiology will be used. It has been found over many years of study of a large series of patients at the Hospital for Sick Children, Great Ormond Street, that the combined diagnostic approach has provided the most useful classification (Table 12.5).

Clinical features

Infantile Batten's disease The patients develop normally for up to about 8 months, reaching their milestones at the expected times, and then present with rapidly progressive psychomotor retardation. This begins between the ages of 8 and 18 months and is accompanied by hypotonia and ataxia. Myoclonic jerking and visual loss follow but fits are not a prominent feature. All patients show microcephaly and reach a 'burnt out' state by 3 years of age. The EEG by this time has become isoelectric. Death occurs at between 3 and 10 years.

Late-infantile Batten's disease Early development is normal and patients learn to walk and talk at the normal time. The first symptom which brings the child to the attention of a physician is often the sudden onset of fits which are difficult to control. This occurs at between 18 months and 4 years. Retrospectively some disturbance of gait and slurring of speech may have been noticed before the onset of fits. Regression, with insidious impairment of vision, spastic tetraplegia and bulbar paralysis, leads to death at between 4 and 10 years.

Juvenile Batten's disease The first sign is deterioration of vision with a pigmentary retinopathy occurring between the ages of 4 and 9 years. Although the children may not be quite as bright as their peers the dementia is often not noticed until several years later. The onset of fits some 2–4 years after visual failure, gait disturbances, slurred speech and anxiety follow. Spastic tetraplegia leads to death in the late teens to early twenties.

Adult Batten's disease (Kufs' disease) The adult form of Batten's disease differs from the other forms in that there are no ocular symptoms. The early signs, occurring at any time from childhood to adult life, are of behavioural disturbances with progressive dementia, ataxia and grand mal fits. Extrapyramidal signs and cerebellar symptoms follow. Slowness of speech leading to dysarthria is a feature.

Early-juvenile Batten's disease Several patients with the early presentation similar to late-infantile Batten's disease but whose course and pathological changes have similarities to the juvenile form have been described (Lake and Cavanagh, 1978; Libert, Martin and Ceuterick, 1982).

Protracted juvenile form of Batten's disease The onset and symptoms are the same as for the juvenile form but occur later and are spread over a longer time (Libert, Martin and Ceuterick, 1982). The presence of visual failure serves to differentiate this form from Kufs' disease.

Other forms The literature abounds with 'atypical' cases, but close inspection of the clinical history and pathology usually allows precise identification of a typical form. Occasional rare patients have been described whose symptoms and clinical course are in keeping with the juvenile form but whose pathology (see below) is entirely consistent with the infantile form (Carpenter et al., 1973; Crome and Lake, 1974, unpublished observation). The status of these truly atypical cases will be revealed only when the defect has been identified.

Inheritance

An autosomal recessive mode of inheritance is evident for most of the forms of Batten's disease. An exception is a possible dominantly inherited form of Kufs' disease in five generations of a family (Boehme et al., 1971; Leonberg, Armstrong and Boehme, 1982). Scattered reports of two forms of Batten's disease in one family can be discounted. Zeman and Hoffman (1962) described two siblings with juvenile Batten's disease and a distant relative with a neuronal storage disease who died at the age of 53 with optic atrophy, retinitis pigmentosa and dementia. Some degree of consanguinity was evident and a variety of other disorders (fits, eye defects, intellectual deficits) were scattered in the family. The mother of two children with juvenile Batten's disease was diagnosed by rectal biopsy as having the adult form (Kamijyo et al., 1974). Because neurons in the intestinal tract of the adult contain much lipofuscin the diagnosis cannot be upheld. More recently, Badurska, Fidzianska and Jedrzejowska (1981) claim that the father of a child with the late-infantile form showed inclusions in lymphocytes which resembled fingerprint bodies (also in the child) and others which resembled curvilinear bodies. The latter were prolific in the child and were found in 4 per cent of the father's lymphocytes. They concluded that the father had Kufs' disease and that this was evidence of nosological unity of all forms of Batten's disease. However, the fingerprint inclusions in the lymphocytes represent the parallel tubular arrays normally present in variable proportions in the normal population; the curvilinear inclusions in the father's lymphocytes are more difficult to explain but probably represent collections of vesicles sometimes found in lymphocytes of normal individuals.

Chemistry Extraction and isolation techniques applied to tissues of patients with Batten's disease have revealed no consistent abnormalities. In the infantile form a disturbance of polyunsaturated lipids led to the term 'polyunsaturated fatty acid lipidosis' (Hagberg et al., 1974), but there is no real storage and similar changes have been found in other demyelinated brains. The fluorescent component of age pigment (lipofuscin) seems to contain a polymer of malonaldehyde (Siakotos and Munkres, 1982) and is unrelated to the stored material in Batten's disease which has a different autofluorescence emission spectrum (Dowson et al., 1982). Wolfe et al. (1977) identified retinoyl complexes as the autofluorescent component of the neuronal storage material in Batten's disease, but there is some dispute regarding interpretation of proton NMR spectra and an accumulation of a polyprenol (dolichol) is now favoured (Wolfe and Ng Ying Kin, 1982). Dolichols are involved in glycoprotein synthesis but no evidence for accumulation of glycoproteins or glycolipids has yet been found. The nature of the stored material(s) in the various types of Batten's disease is unknown but a series of compounds similar to the gangliosides can be envisaged with defects at various points leading to a family of disorders not dissimilar to the gangliosidoses.

Enzymology Because the stored substance has not been identified, apart from the dolichol mentioned in the preceding section, no enzyme defect relating to the storage has been found. Armstrong, Dimmitt and van Wormer (1974) described a partial deficiency of *p*-phenylenediamine-mediated peroxidase activity in granulocytes, but considerable controversy exists over the preparation of the sample and not all laboratories confirm the deficiency. A difference in the ratio of the bound and soluble forms of peroxidase was shown, with the later suggestion that one of the isoenzymes might also be low (Armstrong, 1982). Treatment with vitamins and antioxidants removed the deficiency after 7 weeks in one case, but low levels were again recorded after 28 weeks' treatment (Srivastava et al., 1982). It has been further shown that *p*-phenylenediamine cannot be reliably used as an electron acceptor in the reaction medium (Tsan et al., 1978) and that there is no peroxidase deficiency in brain or liver of patients with Batten's disease (Srivastava et al., 1982) although Armstrong et al. (1975) have shown decreased levels in the thyroid. It seems clear that the decreased peroxidatic activity observed by some is a secondary phenomenon influenced by a variety of factors.

Pathology In all forms of Batten's disease the brain is greatly atrophic. The most severe atrophy is in the *infantile form* where the brain may weigh only 200–400 g in a child of 10 years. There is cerebral gyral atrophy and the cerebellum is also atrophic (Fig. 12.15) but the brain stem appears relatively spared. The dura is thick and there is usually a conspicuous subdural gelatin-

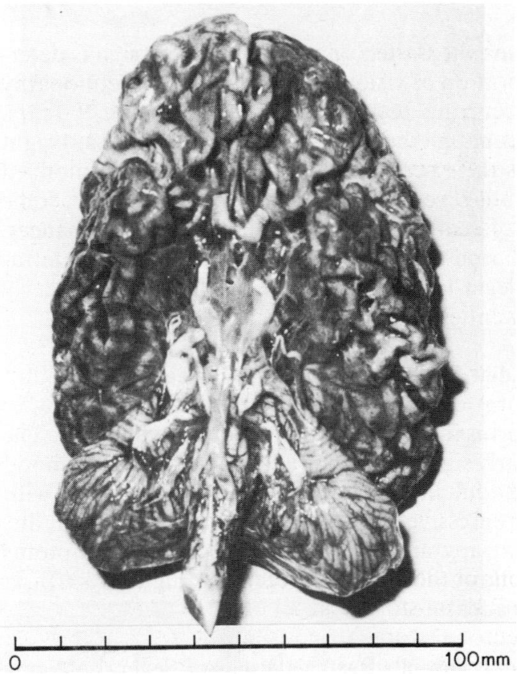

Fig. 12.15 Infantile Batten's disease. Grossly atrophic brain weighing 300 g from a 9-year-old boy. Both cerebral and cerebellar atrophy are severe.

ous layer. The skull is thickened and may be up to 1.5 cm thick. On slicing, the cortex may be a mere 1–2 mm layer over a tough rubbery white matter.

In the *late-infantile form* the brain may weigh 600–900 g at the age of 6–10 years, with varying degrees of atrophy sometimes more pronounced in the cerebellum. The cortex may be thin and the white matter firm. In younger patients the degree of atrophy may be minimal. The brain in the *juvenile form* is usually grossly atrophic and in patients of up to 17 years may weigh only 600–700 g, the degree of atrophy being directly proportional to the duration of the disease. A less severe degree of atrophy is seen in the *adult type* in which frontal lobes show the greatest changes. Widening of the sulci, a thinned cerebral cortex and greyness of centrum semiovale are features.

As in any generalized neuronal storage disease, neurons wherever they occur contain the stored material. In contrast with the gangliosidoses, the neurons in Batten's disease are not ballooned, but the existing cytoplasm is filled with a finely granular material having the histochemical characteristics of lipofuscin or ceroid.

The changes seen in the brain of the *infantile type* vary considerably with age, and the following sequence is usually observed (Haltia, Rapola and Santavuori, 1973). Up to about $2\frac{1}{2}$ years neuronal storage is observed with some degree of neuronal loss, an astrocytosis and the presence of macrophages. From the age of $2\frac{1}{2}$ years the neurons are grossly depleted in number, astrocytes contain stored material and there are numerous macrophages. Loss of myelin is evident. By 4 years of age, cortical neurons have disappeared, resulting in an isoelectric EEG (Santavuori, Haltia and Rapola, 1974), and there is a complete loss of myelin including the subcortical U-fibres. The brain has been largely replaced by hypertrophic astrocytes storing the lipopigment (Fig. 12.16). Neurons in the basal ganglia, brain stem and spinal cord are still present. In the peripheral nervous system, neurons of the gastrointestinal tract are also present and show storage at all ages. In addition to the neuronal storage, deposition is found in macrophages in groups in the spleen, and in lymph nodes and lamina propria of the gut. Smooth muscle cells of the intestinal wall, of arterioles and arteries, skeletal and cardiac muscle, renal

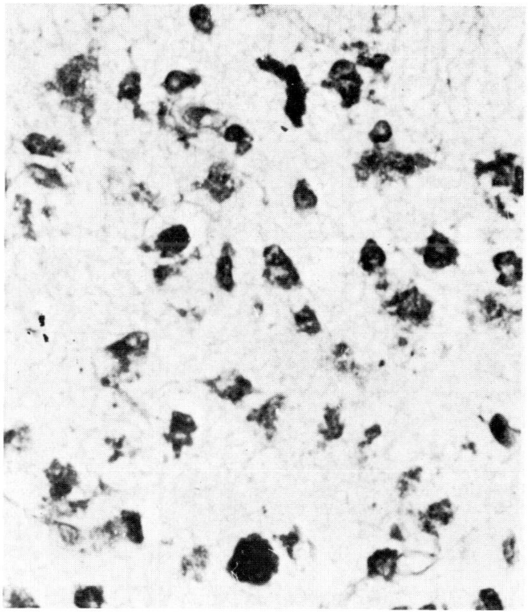

Fig. 12.16 Infantile Batten's disease. Section of cerebral cortex in the later stages of the disease. Neurons are replaced by hypertrophic astrocytes and a few macrophages. The cells contain stored material which is stained strongly by the PAS reaction. PAS ×390.

glomerular endothelium, distal tubular epithelium of the kidney, germinal epithelium of the testis, thyroid follicles and cells of the exocrine and endocrine pancreas also show deposition. Endothelial cells of capillaries and other blood vessels also show deposits of the lipopigment. The neuronal and other deposits are readily shown in routinely fixed, paraffin-wax-embedded sections stained with Sudan black. In paraffin sections, and particularly in frozen sections, the substance stains strongly with PAS and shows strong autofluorescence. In contrast with other forms of Batten's disease the substance does not stain with Luxol fast blue. An acid phosphatase reaction shows the increased activity in affected cells and will detect deposition shown otherwise only by an autofluorescence examination. Hepatocytes appear to be uninvolved but Kupffer cells show storage. By light microscopy no evidence of storage is seen in lymphocytes in a peripheral blood film.

The ultrastructural appearance of the stored or deposited material is very similar in all organs. The substance is osmiophilic and consists of globules with a granular matrix either single and measuring up to 0.5 μm or as aggregates of glob-

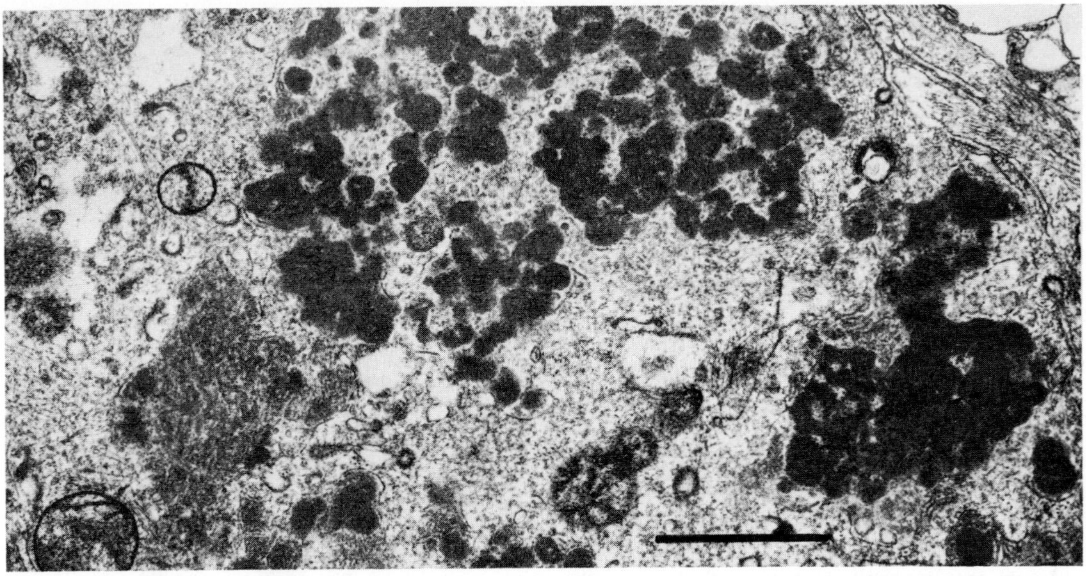

Fig. 12.17 Infantile Batten's disease. Electron micrograph of a neuron containing granular osmiophilic deposits. Bar = 1 μm. ×23000.

ules measuring up to 3 μm in diameter (Fig. 12.17). The single globules and the aggregates are surrounded by a unit membrane and show a strong reaction for acid phosphatase activity. The deposits have been described as granular osmiophilic deposits (GROD) and are also known as 'Finnish snowballs'. In skin biopsies the deposits are best seen in endothelial cells, though some may be found in Schwann cells, smooth muscle cells, epithelial cells in sweat glands, basal epithelial cells and in fibroblasts (Ceuterick et al., 1976). Similar deposits are found in about 10 per cent of lymphocytes (Haynes et al., 1979). In the renal glomerular epithelium the deposits are larger, less well defined and often do not possess a limiting membrane. Although the deposits wherever they are found have a superficial resemblance to lipofuscin (wear and tear) pigment, they differ in not being associated with the characteristic electron-lucent vacuoles found with most lipofuscin deposits.

In the *late-infantile form* the changes are less severe and although some neuronal loss is seen with a mild to moderate astrocytosis, neurons are present in the cortex even in older patients. The granular deposition in the neuronal cytoplasm (Fig. 12.18), displacing the Nissl substance, has a pale yellowish colour in haematoxylin and eosin preparations. The substance resists processing and stains positively with PAS, Sudan black and Luxol fast blue in paraffin, frozen and cryostat sections. Examination with

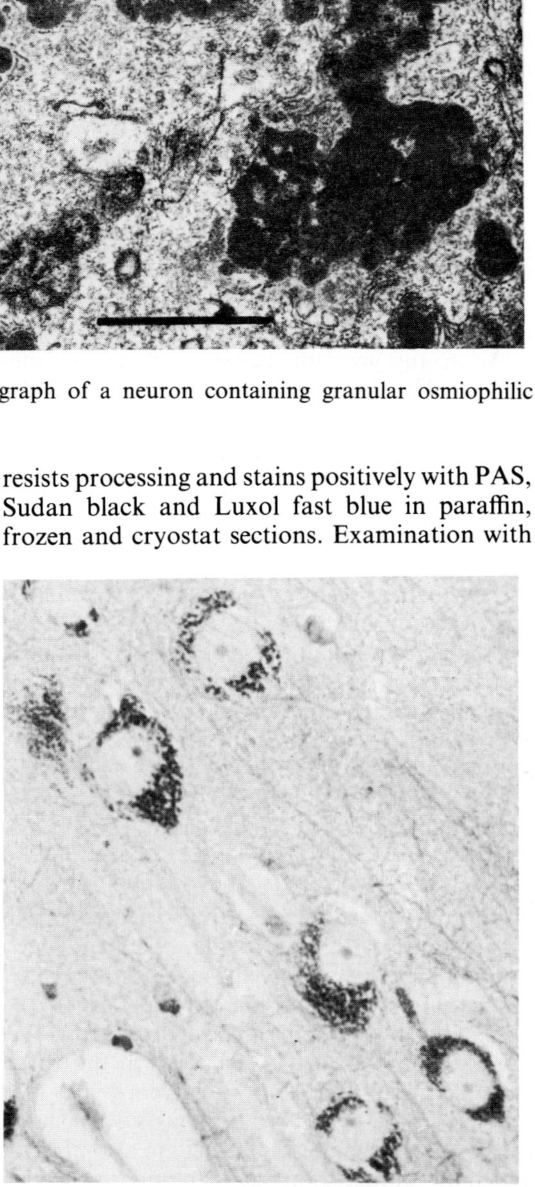

Fig. 12.18 Late-infantile Batten's disease. Neurons in a cortical biopsy contain storage granules which stain strongly with Luxol fast blue. The cell body does not show the distension found in the gangliosidoses. ×580.

ultraviolet light reveals bright yellow autofluorescence contrasting with the orange autofluorescence of normal lipofuscin. Neuronal deposition of this material is observed throughout the central nervous system. There may be some loss of myelin in the white matter but this is not marked. In the peripheral nervous system the deposits in the neurons of the gastrointestinal tract show some slight differences in staining properties, and in the ganglia of Auerbach and Meissner the granules are not PAS positive. The deposits in frozen or cryostat sections show sudanophilia with Sudan black (staining greyish rather than the blue-black of neutral fat), are positive with Luxol fast blue and show an autofluorescence which is paler than that observed in infantile or juvenile Batten's disease. In cryostat sections of rectal biopsies, or from the appendix, similar deposits are present in smooth muscle cells and endothelial cells of capillaries and arterioles. The deposits are readily shown by an acid phosphatase reaction which is usually negative in these sites. Widespread deposition of the substance is also observed in sweat gland epithelium, thyroid, pancreas, skeletal muscle, adrenal and kidney tubules.

Electron microscopy in late-infantile Batten's disease is relatively uniform with the characteristic curvilinear body present in all sites where deposition is shown by light microscopy (Figs.

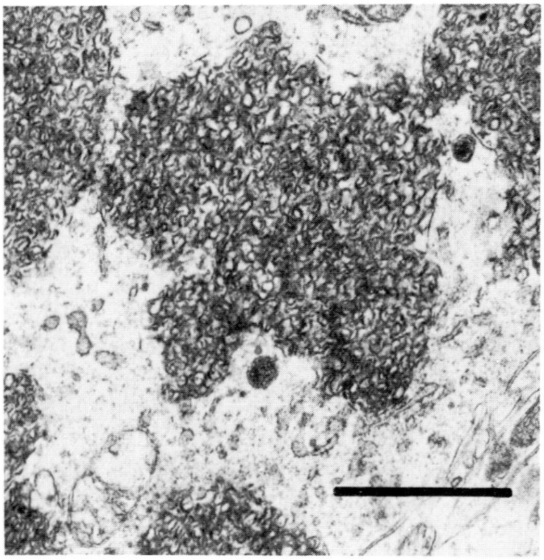

Fig. 12.19 Late-infantile Batten's disease. Curvilinear bodies are present in a cortical neuron. Bar = 1 μm. × 23000.

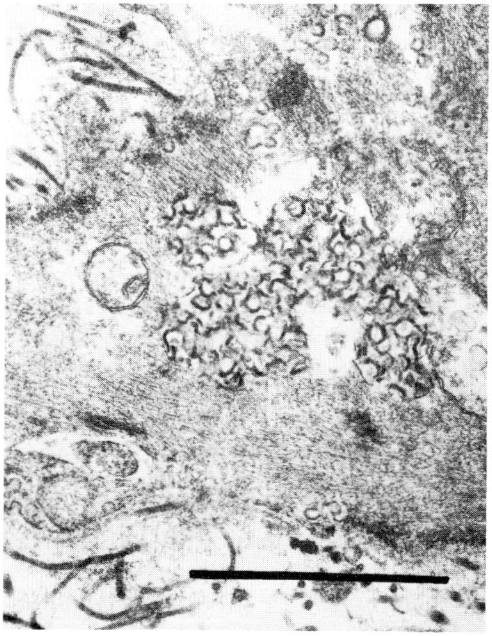

Fig. 12.20 Late-infantile Batten's disease. Curvilinear profiles are present within a smooth muscle cell. Bar = 1 μm. × 35000.

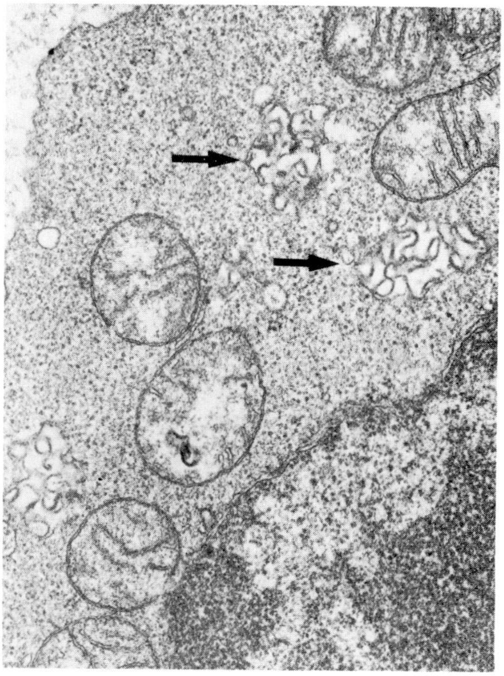

Fig. 12.21 Late-infantile Batten's disease. Several collections of curvilinear profiles (arrows) are present in a peripheral lymphocyte. × 26000.

12.19 and 12.20), as well as in other cells (e.g. cells of the diffuse neuroendocrine system, astrocytes and oligodendroglia). Lymphocytes, while without evidence of storage by light microscopy, contain collections of cytoplasmic curvilinear bodies (Fig. 12.21). The term 'curvilinear body' was introduced by Duffy, Kornfeld and Suzuki (1968) and it is now used in preference to the terms proposed by Gonatas, Gambetti and Baird (1968) and Zeman and Donahue (1963). Urinary sediment also contains curvilinear bodies present within renal tubular cells and lying free (de Baecque, 1975).

In *juvenile Batten's disease* the cortical neurons show a similar degree of accumulation to those in the late-infantile form. There is a varying degree of gliosis, usually mild, and little evidence of myelin loss. The granular deposits in neurons are stained by PAS, Sudan black and Luxol fast blue, and show strong autofluorescence. These reactions are seen both in routine paraffin sections and in sections of frozen tissue.

In the gastrointestinal tract the stored material in neurons stains as that in the brain, in contrast to late-infantile Batten's disease. In addition to the neuronal storage, deposits can be detected in smooth muscle cells (Fig. 12.22), endothelial cells and macrophages. The deposits are best detected by autofluorescent studies on cryostat sections and by acid phosphatase staining procedures, both of which are negative in these sites in normal tissue. The neurons show a strong coarse reaction for acid phosphatase, whilst normal neurons show only a few fine granules of activity.

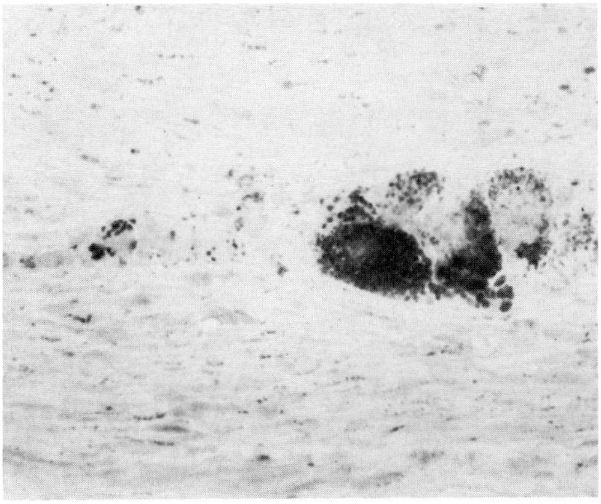

Fig. 12.22 Juvenile Batten's disease. Granular sudanophilic deposits within neurons and smooth muscle cells in a rectal biopsy. Sudan black ×390.

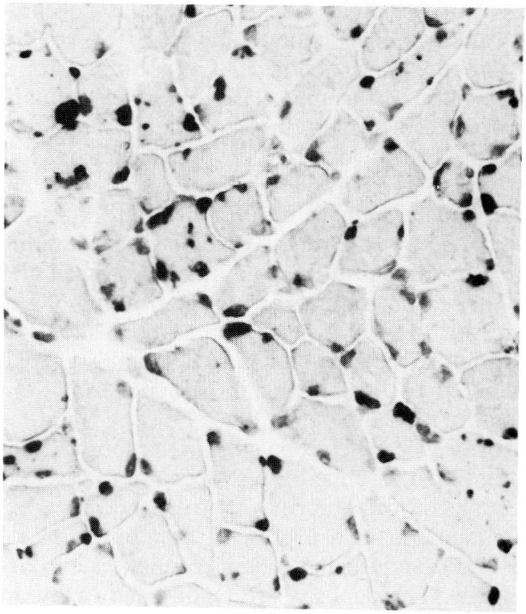

Fig. 12.23 Juvenile Batten's disease. Cryostat section of skeletal muscle. Fibres show strong acid phosphatase activity at sites of storage. Normal muscle would be negative. ×520.

In distinction from other forms of Batten's disease, small numbers of intensely acid-phosphatase-positive histiocytes are found between the smooth muscle cells in rectal biopsies (Lake, 1976, 1981, 1983a). Deposits can be detected on most organs, including skeletal muscle (Fig. 12.23), pancreas, kidney and sural nerve (Nakano et al., 1978).

Electron microscopically, the situation in juvenile Batten's disease is not as straightforward as in the infantile or late-infantile types. In general the deposits in neurons have a fingerprint appearance and this pattern predominates (Fig. 12.24). Inclusions, mostly fingerprint, are found in endothelial cells and smooth muscle but they may be admixed with curvilinear profiles (Schwendemann et al., 1978), a pattern also seen in pancreas (Fig. 12.25). In sweat glands it is sometimes impossible to find inclusions (O'Brien et al., 1975) or they may have fingerprint or rectilinear profiles (Carpenter, Karpati and Andermann, 1972; Carpenter et al., 1977). Skeletal muscle cells do not contain fingerprint bodies; rather, rectilinear profiles are found. These somewhat resemble curvilinear bodies with stacks of lamellae which are straight as often as curved (Carpenter et al., 1977).

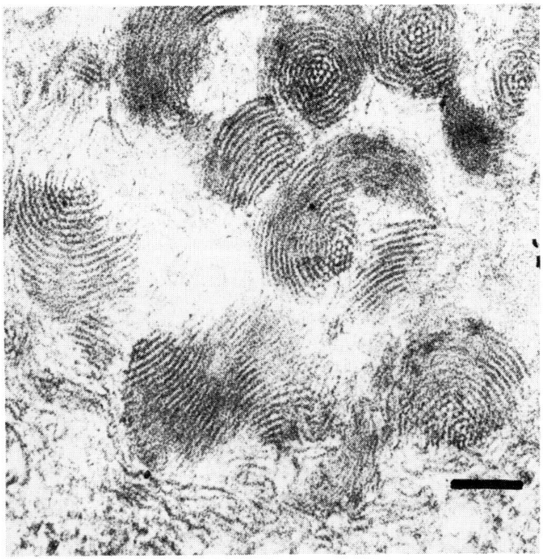

Fig. 12.24 Juvenile Batten's disease. 'Fingerprint' bodies in a neuron from the gastrointestinal tract. Bar = 0.1 μm. × 86000.

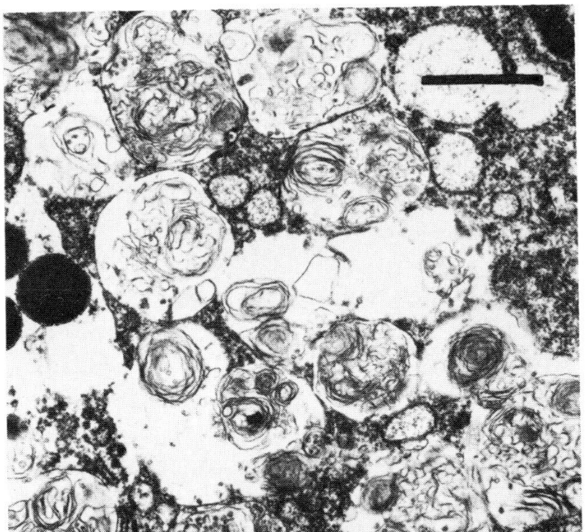

Fig. 12.25 Juvenile Batten's disease. Pancreas. A mixture of curvilinear and lamellar profiles lie in the cytoplasm of an exocrine cell. Bar = 1 μm. × 13800.

All cases of juvenile Batten's disease show vacuolated lymphocytes, the proportion varying from a few per cent up to 50 per cent. The vacuoles are bold and well delineated, and are readily seen in routine blood films stained with the May-Grünwald-Giemsa method (or other routine haematological stain). The cells with vacuoles tend to be found in greater numbers towards the tail of the film. Vacuoles are present in the presymptomatic state and are not found in heterozygotes (Bürrig, Schwendemann and Löhler, 1982). Attention was first drawn to the presence of lymphocytic vacuoles in the juvenile form by Bagh and Hortling (1948) and its uses as a screening procedure were described by Rayner and Böök (1958) and Melchior, Terslev and Friis-Hansen (1962). The vacuoles are empty and have no staining characteristics. By electron microscopy the vacuoles are membrane bound and a small proportion contain fragments of fingerprint inclusions (Schwendemann, 1976). Fingerprint inclusions should not be confused with the normally occurring parallel tubular arrays once thought to be characteristic (Schwendemann, 1982).

The pathology of *adult Batten's disease* (Kufs' disease) is not clear because it is difficult to define clinically, and different workers have described different conditions under the label of Kufs' disease. No consensus of opinion has emerged. It is clear that there is excessive deposition of a lipofuscin-like substance in neurons in the brain (Fig. 12.26) and gastrointestinal tract (Kornfeld, 1972; Dom et al., 1979; Goebel et al., 1982) which has staining characteristics very similar to that in the juvenile form. In older brains normal lipofuscin often appears excessive and it has staining characteristics not dissimilar to the abnormal pigment in Kufs' disease. Goebel and his colleagues (1982) have commented that in Kufs'

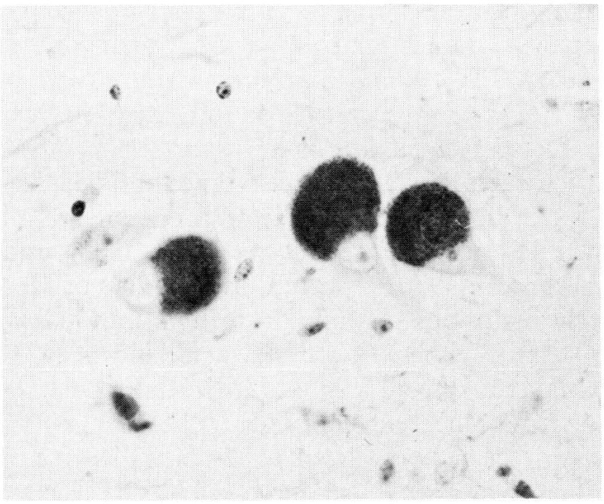

Fig. 12.26 Adult Batten's (Kufs') disease. Stored material in distended neurons in the end-plate of the hippocampus is strongly stained by Luxol fast blue. × 450.

disease the pigment occurs not only in the neuronal perikarya but also within axonal hillocks (Fig. 12.27). Dowson (1983) has shown differences in the autofluorescence emission spectra between normal, Kufs' and other forms of Batten's disease. Visceral storage, in Kupffer cells, hepatocytes, macrophages in spleen, muscle and kidney, is present in some cases yet is reported as being absent in others (Fine, Barron and Hirano, 1960; Kornfeld, 1972; Libert, Martin and Ceuterick, 1982). No vacuolated lymphocytes are present, and no storage was detected in skin or conjunctival biopsies by Dom et al. (1979) although Carpenter et al. (1977)

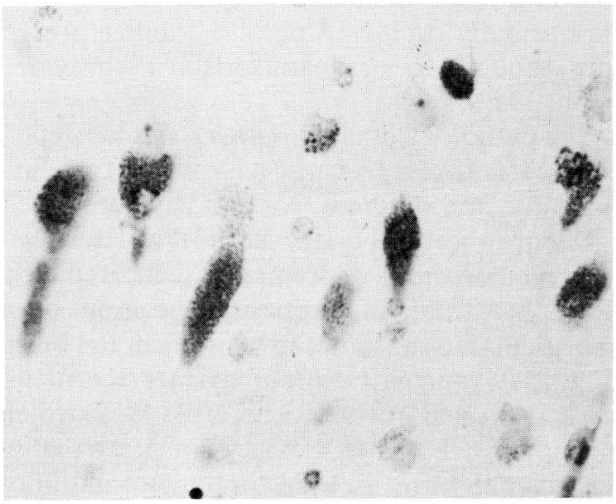

Fig. 12.27 Adult Batten's (Kufs') disease. Cerebral cortex. Neuronal and axonal storage is prominent and readily demonstrated by Luxol fast blue staining. ×470.

found inclusions in eccrine sweat glands in two patients. The last-named authors found no evidence of skeletal muscle storage whilst Dom et al. (1979) showed muscle involvement in two brothers. The inclusions show no clear ultrastructural uniformity but curvilinear bodies, fingerprint bodies and rectilinear profiles have all been described (Goebel et al., 1982). Chou and Thompson (1970) reported on granular osmiophilic inclusions and 'miniature membranous cytoplasmic bodies' (more characteristic of Niemann–Pick type C) in a rather dubious case which has more in common with the unusual type described by Carpenter et al. (1973) than with the more 'typical' cases of Kufs' disease. Others also have described granular deposits (Goebel et al., 1982) sometimes associated with prominent lipid droplets (Zeman and Siakotos, 1973) which are difficult to separate from the normal wear and tear pigment present in relatively large amounts in the normal brain at this age.

Similar changes have been reported in the dominantly inherited form of Kufs' disease (Boehme et al., 1971).

In some of the *unusual forms* the staining reactions, distribution of changes and ultrastructure are very similar to those seen in patients who present with a typical history of a clearly defined type. The juvenile case reported by Carpenter et al. (1973) has the staining reactions and ultrastructure typical of the infantile form and a similar case has been seen by Crome and Lake (1974, unpublished observations). In other patients, whose presentation has similarities to the late-infantile type, the pathology is that of the juvenile type but without changes in lymphocytes. These patients are referred to as the early-juvenile type (Lake and Cavanagh, 1978; Libert, Martin and Ceuterick, 1982).

Lipofuscin-like deposits also occur in the mucolipidoses, and although in mucolipidoses types I, II and III there should be no confusion because the clinical picture is quite different, mucolipidosis type IV presenting with psychomotor retardation in the first year may appear as an unusual type of Batten's disease in a rectal biopsy. The staining reactions are very similar but the ultrastructure is different (see later section, 'Mucolipidoses').

Diagnosis The diagnosis will be suspected in many of the cases from the clinical history and electrophysiology (Pampiglione and Harden, 1977) and a confirmatory biopsy is usually all that is necessary. Brain biopsy is not justified when neurons in the rectal submucosa show the changes which mirror those in the brain. Cryostat sections of a suction rectal biopsy, taken about 5 cm from the anal verge, stained as described by Lake (1976, 1981, 1983a) are adequate for the diagnosis and subtyping of the disorder. A second suction rectal biopsy should be processed for electron microscopy, and neurons, smooth muscle and endothelial cells examined. The ultrastructural changes in the rectum are often more definitive than those in brain or muscle. Although skin, conjunctival or muscle biopsies are preferred by some, there can be no substitute for the examination of neurons in a neurodegenerative condition, particularly when the dementia is hardly apparent or where a clinically unaffected younger sibling is being investigated. Screening of blood films for vacuoles in lymphocytes in the juvenile form, electron microscopy of lymphocytes in the late-infantile form and skin biopsies in the infantile form are useful in the initial work-up. Urinary dolichols are increased and may, in the future, provide another diagnostic route.

Animal models Several species of animal have been reported with a condition analogous to Batten's disease. It is difficult to assign the disorders to a particular group but it would seem that the late-infantile and juvenile types are represented. English setter dogs (Hagen, 1953; Koppang, 1982), chihuahuas (Rač and Giesecke, 1975) and dachshunds (Cummings and deLahunta, 1977) have been reported to have a disorder similar to the juvenile form whilst sheep (Jolly et al., 1980; Jolly et al., 1982) and a Siamese cat (Green and Little, 1974) appear to have the late-infantile counterpart.

Congenital amaurotic idiocy

This term has been used to describe a condition which has been only rarely reported. Two of the cases (Norman and Wood, 1941; Brown, Corner and Dodgson, 1954) were in the same family. The third was reported from Sweden by Hagberg et al. (1965). A fourth case with great similarities to the earlier reported cases has been described by Humphreys, Lake and Scholtz (1985, in preparation). In each case the brain was extremely small, weighing from 65 g in a 7-day-old girl to 139 g in a 19-month-old boy. There was pachygyria affecting the frontal lobes and gross loss of myelin with neutral fat accumulation. There was severe neuronal loss in the cortex and proliferated astrocytes and numerous macrophages, particularly in the deeper layers of the cortex, contained deposits which were PAS positive, sudanophilic and autofluorescent. Neurons in the brain stem and spinal cord showed storage, and storage in macrophages was also evident in liver, spleen, thymus, adrenal and kidney.

Chemical analysis of the brain of Hagberg's case showed a marked decrease of myelin lipids and the presence of a small amount of a ganglioside not found in normal brain. This ganglioside (G_{D3}) migrated between G_{M1} and G_{D1A}; the total ganglioside concentration was not increased. The stored substance has many of the characteristics of lipofuscin, and by electron microscopy consists of granular deposits with some membranous profiles within a limiting membrane. The disorder may represent a form of Batten's disease.

Niemann-Pick disease

The early description of a disorder showing hepatosplenomegaly and progressive deterioration, leading to death before the age of 2 years showed some similarities to Gaucher's disease but Niemann (1914) considered it to be different. Further similar cases were reported (see Thannhauser, 1940), and Pick (1927) studied the pathology of Niemann's case and others. The disorder was known as Niemann-Pick disease by 1927 although many other terms were, and have been, used. The importance of phospholipid accumulation was recognized but it was Klenk (1934) who discovered that sphingomyelin was the major storage substance. Crocker and Farber (1958) published a review of the clinical, pathological and chemical findings in 18 patients with Niemann-Pick disease, based especially on the increase of sphingomyelin in the spleen and the presence of foam cells in tissues. Crocker and Farber noted that not all their patients showed increased liver sphingomyelin and that others showed no evidence of neurological involvement. They speculated that Niemann-Pick disease was a disorder with a broad range of biological behaviour. Crocker later (1961) classified the disorder into four tentative groups which he called A, B, C and D;

Group A 'Classic' Niemann-Pick disease with severe early CNS deterioration and chest x-ray changes.

Group B Heavy visceral involvement, normal CNS function, chest x-ray changes.

Group C Moderate course with moderate CNS problems.

Group D Nova Scotian group. Late, eventually severe CNS defect.

A deficiency of sphingomyelinase activity was later reported (Brady et al., 1966) in the infantile (group A) form. Groups A, B, C and D were investigated by P. B. Schneider and Kennedy (1967) and they showed that groups A and B had deficient sphingomyelinase activity whilst groups C and D had activities in the normal range. Because of the clinical and chemical variability noted by Crocker and Farber and the lack of deficient sphingomyelinase activity in groups C and D, numerous reports of atypical storage orders have appeared, causing confusion to the uninitiated. Many terms have been used (Table 12.6) and some of the cases of juvenile Gaucher's disease undoubtedly belong to groups C and D. The 'groups' were designated 'types' by Fredrickson and Sloan (1972b).

Table 12.6 Terms associated with Niemann–Pick disease types C and D

Juvenile dystonic lipidosis
Juvenile dystonic idiocy without amaurosis
Atypical cerebral lipidosis
Atypical juvenile lipidosis
Subacute Niemann–Pick disease
Juvenile Niemann–Pick disease
Ophthalmoplegic lipidosis
Neurovisceral storage disease with vertical supranuclear ophthalmoplegia
Neville–Lake syndrome
Neville's disease
Subacute neurovisceral lipidosis
Lactosylceramidosis
Sea-blue histiocyte disease
Chronic reticuloendothelial cell storage disease
Nova Scotian variant of Niemann–Pick disease

At a recent international symposium the classification of Niemann-Pick disease was refined (Elleder and Jirásek, 1983). Two major groups are now recognized—*group I* in which there is sphingomyelinase deficiency, and *group II* in which sphingomyelinase activity is essentially normal (Table 12.7). Group I includes types A and B and some of the atypical cases with long survival, neurological involvement and deficient sphingomyelinase activity (Elleder et al., 1980).

Table 12.7 Current classification of Niemann–Pick disease

Group I Sphingomyelinase deficient
1. Type A: Neurovisceral (infantile, juvenile and adult)
2. Type B: Visceral only (infantile, juvenile and adult)
Group II Not sphingomyelinase deficient
1. Type C: Neurovisceral
2. Possible pure visceral form
This group includes type D, which is in most respects identical to type C.

Group II includes types C and D, the latter being regarded as a pure strain of type C disease originating from a single family from south-west Nova Scotia in the seventeenth century. It was acknowledged that group II may have no relationship with group I, but rather than change the name again when the defect is defined it was decided to retain the original label of Niemann–Pick disease.

Clinical features

In group I, the neurovisceral form presents early with hepatosplenomegaly and failure to thrive. By the age of 1 year the mental retardation is usually evident although in some patients the onset of dementia is a little later. Cherry red spots at the macula are common in this form, and a diffuse reticular infiltration is usually found in both lungs. Death occurs before the age of 4 years. The chronic non-neuropathic visceral form may present with hepatosplenomegaly within the first year or, more usually, later in childhood. Adult cases without CNS involvement and formerly classified by Fredrickson and Sloan (1972b) as type E, are also recognized. They often present with hepatosplenomegaly and haematological problems (Long et al., 1977). Radiological evidence of lung infiltration is common.

Group II (type C) presents with a wide-ranging variety of symptoms and signs, which tend to be similar in any one family. Early presentation of failure to thrive with marked hepatosplenomegaly from, or soon after, birth may be complicated by severe prolonged neonatal obstructive jaundice which is often considered as neonatal giant cell hepatitis, and may lead to death. The jaundice may fade after several months and the spleen becomes smaller. Signs of dementia and ataxia are insidious in onset and, together with fits, can occur from any age but are more usual between the ages of 2 and 10 years. Other patients present with unexplained splenomegaly without any initial neurological symptoms. Mild splenomegaly may be found in juveniles or adults presenting with dementia and ataxia. Dystonia has been noted in about one-quarter of patients. One of the later characteristic signs is the loss of vertical eye movements (Neville et al., 1973), which may not have developed in all patients before death. A similar wide range of symptoms and signs is present in those patients of Nova Scotian ancestry (M. W. Spence, 1982, personal communication). Occasional families with group II disease show differing presenting features in siblings (Wenger, Barth and Githens, 1977).

The symptoms and signs are similar to those in the syndrome described by Rosenblum et al. (1981) in which prolonged jaundice associated with vitamin E deficiency leads to a peripheral neuropathy, posterior column dysfunction and a vertical supranuclear ophthalmoplegia. There is, however, no splenomegaly and no dementia. Some patients with group II disease presenting with jaundice also show vitamin E deficiency (Lake and Muller, 1981, unpublished observations) and the possible relationship between the symptoms in the two conditions remains to be clarified.

An autosomal recessive mode of inheritance is found in all forms of Niemann–Pick disease. The infantile sphingomyelinase-deficient type A is more common among patients of Ashkenazi Jewish ancestry.

Chemistry In group I Niemann–Pick disease (types A and B) the phospholipid content of liver and spleen is increased three to five times, and sphingomyelin accounts for about 50 per cent of the phospholipid compared with less than 10 per cent in the normal. In type A there is an increase of sphingomyelin in both grey and white matter of the brain whilst normal amounts are recorded in type B (Pilz, 1970). In most organs there is a striking increase in sphingomyelin content.

Kamoshita et al. (1969) isolated the storage bodies and showed that they contain high concentrations of sphingomyelin and cholesterol, and a small amount of glucocerebroside. The brain in type A shows a mild increase in gangliosides G_{M3} and G_{M2}. *Bis*-(monoacylglycero)-phosphate (or lysobisphosphatidic acid), although a minor component, is regularly detected in tissue from patients with Niemann–Pick disease type A (Elleder et al., 1980). Normally this compound is undetectable.

In group II patients (types C and D) the chemistry is variable. In many there is a marked accumulation of sphingomyelin in the spleen, reaching levels found in group I patients. However, liver sphingomyelin is usually only slightly raised, and no excess of sphingomyelin is found in the brain. *Bis*-(monoacylglycero)-phosphate is present (Seng et al., 1971) and an increase in several ceramide hexosides and monosialogangliosides is found but the increases are insufficient to account for the microscopical evidence of marked storage within neurons and hepatocytes. The increased ceramide lactoside content led to the label 'lactosyl ceramidosis' in one patient (G. Dawson, Matalon and Stein, 1971), whilst Hagberg et al. (1978) isolated lactose and other oligosaccharides from the spleen of another.

Enzymology In group I patients there is a profound deficiency of lysosomal sphingomyelinase activity (Brady et al., 1966; P. B. Schneider and Kennedy, 1967) which can be assayed using radio-labelled sphingomyelin as substrate. Magnesium-dependent neutral sphingomyelinase activity is normal. Prenatal diagnosis is possible by analysis of cultured amniotic fluid cells obtained at amniocentesis (E. L. Schneider et al., 1972a; Patrick et al., 1977). A radio-labelled substrate or a chromogenic substrate (2-hexadecanoylamino-4-nitrophenyl phosphorylcholine) may be used in the assay on white blood cells, cultured fibroblasts or tissue samples. Lysosomal sphingomyelinase can also be estimated with thin layer chromatography by the detection of released ceramide (Harzer and Benz, 1973).

The enzymological basis of group II patients is not clear. Claims that the sphingomyelinase activity in cultured fibroblasts is decreased are not consistent, and absences of components of sphingomyelinase on electrofocusing, which might account for the decreased activity in some, are found to be non-specific (Vanier, Rousson and Louisot, 1983). Indeed it would be surprising if sphingomyelinase were involved, except perhaps secondarily, since no sphingomyelin is stored in the brain, an organ in which there is marked neuronal deposition of an as yet unidentified substance.

Baraton and Revol (1977) and Christomanou (1980) have suggested that an activator protein deficiency was responsible for the decreased sphingomyelinase and β-glucosidase activities observed in some cases of group II patients. This suggestion has not been confirmed by other workers (Harzer et al., 1978).

Pathology. *Niemann–Pick disease group I.* The most striking abnormality is the gross enlargement of the liver and spleen in patients with and without CNS involvement. In type A patients the brain may show slight atrophy and the white matter is usually firm. No gross changes are found in the brain of the few type B patients who have come to autopsy. There may be hepatic cirrhosis

Sections of brain from type A patients show generalized neuronal and glial ballooning (Fig. 12.28) similar to that found in Tay–Sachs disease, and marked demyelination with gliosis and numerous storage cells in the white matter. Neurons in the plexuses of Auerbach and Meissner in the gastrointestinal tract are also ballooned (Pick, 1927).

The foamy storage cell (Niemann–Pick cell) which is present throughout the mononuclear phagocyte system is large (20–90 μm in diameter) and has a 'mulberry-like' appearance with the cytoplasm filled with relatively uniform vacuoles (Fig. 12.29). The cells are usually mononucleate and rarely multinucleate, and only occasional ingested red blood cells or other blood cell debris is present. Niemann–Pick cells are found filling the red pulp of the spleen, in the sinusoids of the liver (Fig. 12.30) and may replace the structure of lymph nodes. In the lungs the alveolar spaces and septa are filled with Niemann–Pick cells. The thymus is replaced by foam cells which are also numerous in the adrenal medulla (Fig. 12.31). Niemann–Pick cells are found in most organs

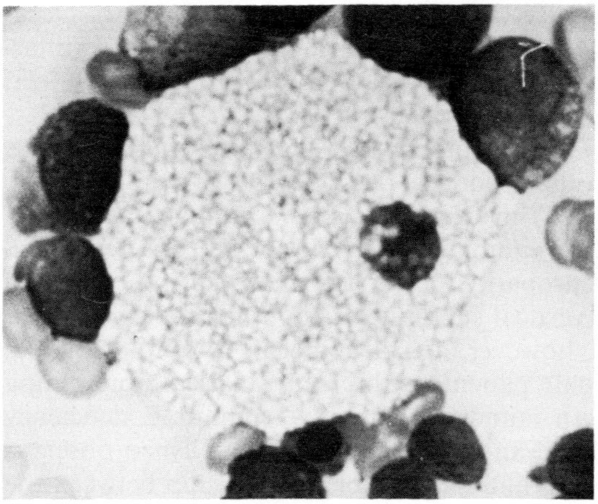

Fig. 12.29 Niemann–Pick disease type A. Bone marrow film. The large foamy cell is filled with small vacuoles of uniform size. May–Grünwald–Giemsa × 980.

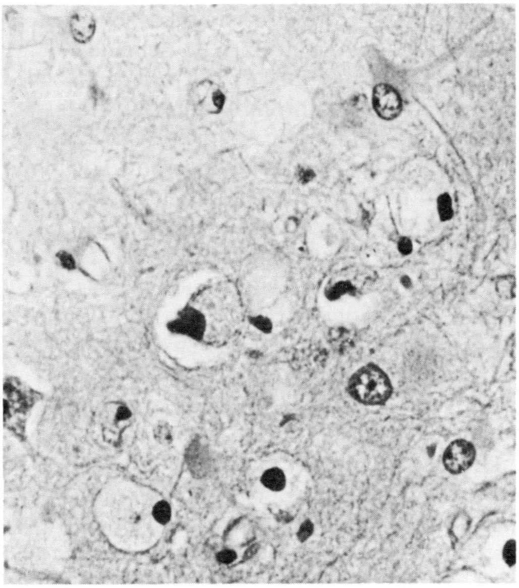

Fig. 12.28 Niemann–Pick disease type A. Cerebral cortex. Neurons and microglial cells are greatly distended by stored material. Reactive astrocytes are not affected. Haematoxylin and eosin ×470.

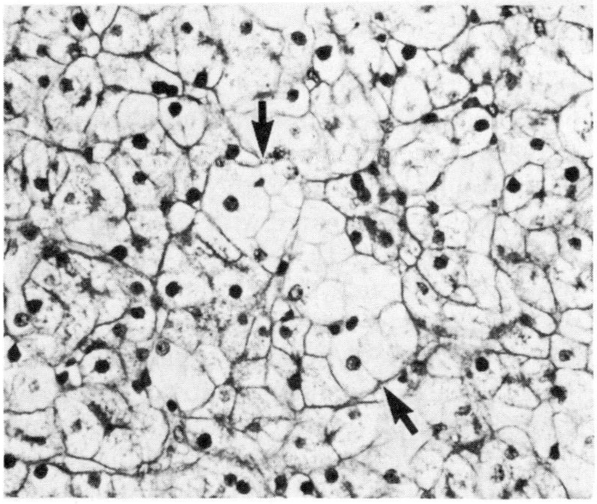

Fig. 12.30 Niemann–Pick disease type A. Liver. Large foamy storage cells (arrows) in the sinusoids. The hepatocytes are also foamy. Type B disease presents an essentially similar picture. Haematoxylin and eosin ×250.

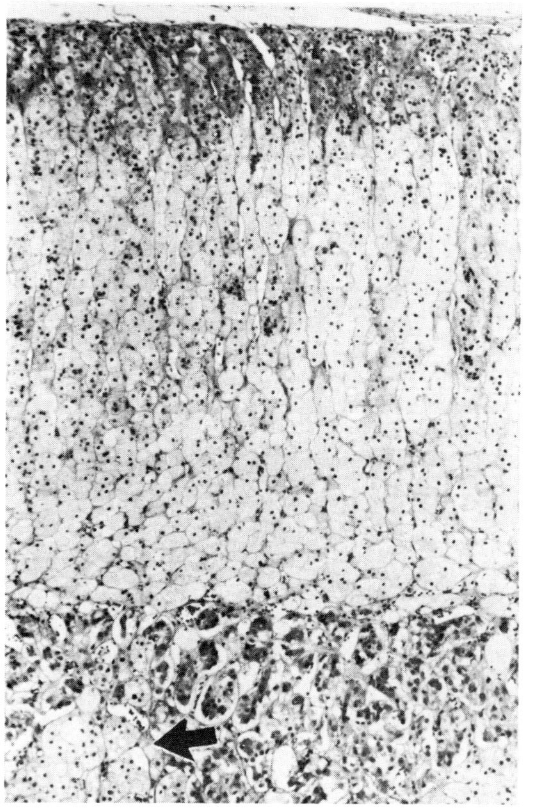

Fig. 12.31 Niemann–Pick disease type A. Adrenal gland. The cortical cells are foamy and the medulla contains nests of Niemann–Pick cells (arrow). (In type C disease there is no adrenal involvement.) Haematoxylin and eosin ×80.

and are common in bone marrow preparations which are used for the initial diagnosis. Deposits of sphingomyelin are also present in smooth muscle cells, in the endothelial cells of capillaries and other blood vessels and in hepatocytes. Schwann cells and unmyelinated nerve fibres also show inclusions. The lymphocytes of patients with type A Niemann–Pick disease show cytoplasmic vacuoles which are small and discrete (Baty, 1930) in contrast with the patients with type B in whom there is minimal or no lymphocytic vacuolation (Crocker and Farber, 1958).

Bone marrow aspirates, best examined as films rather than as fixed embedded blocks, show collections of Niemann–Pick cells (see Fig. 12.29) in type A and in the younger patients with type B. However, in the older patients with type B disease the numbers of foamy Niemann–Pick cells are fewer and the most prominent cell is one in which the cytoplasm is filled with small granules staining intensely blue with the Giemsa or Wright stain. The granules have the staining characteristics of ceroid/lipofuscin and their distinctive appearance has attracted the picturesque term 'sea-blue histiocytes' which in turn has led to the 'syndrome of the sea-blue histiocyte' becoming applied to a hotch-potch of patients (Silverstein, Ellefson and Ahern, 1970). Although sea-blue histiocytes can occur in a variety of conditions including lecithin: cholesterol acyl transferase deficiency, when the cells are numerous and their cytoplasm is filled with granules, type B Niemann–Pick disease is the most probable diagnosis (Bayer and Wewalka, 1973; Long et al., 1977, Dewhurst et al., 1979).

The lipid deposition is best detected in frozen or cryostat sections because the sphingomyelin and cholesterol are extracted during routine processing. The usual acid haematein reaction (Lake, 1966) does not always give reliable evidence of sphingomyelin deposition, possibly because of variability of the fatty acid side chain. The results are consistent but not always reliable, and the more recently introduced ferric-haematoxylin method (Elleder and Lojda, 1973) is preferred. Sudan black stains the cells and deposits, which in polarized light show as a red birefringence due to the molecular organization of the lipids within the cell. Cholesterol, shown by the Schultz or PAN methods, is constantly present in association with the sphingomyelin. The occurrence of ceramide hexosides and gangliosides is shown by a positive PAS reaction. Niemann–Pick cells and the deposits of sphingomyelin within lysosomes of other cell types all show strong acid phosphatase activity outlining the vacuoles, and this is often the simplest way to demonstrate involvement of a particular cell type. Alkaline phosphatase activity is present in the sinusoids of the red pulp of the spleen in patients with Niemann–Pick disease and some other storage diseases but not in the normal or in haematological disorders (Elleder, 1979).

By electron microscopy the neuronal inclusions consist of loosely packed lipid lamellae within membrane-bound vacuoles measuring 1–2 μm. The appearance is somewhat similar to that of the gangliosidoses but the lamellae are less ordered and there is more electron-lucent space (Wallace et al., 1965). The hepatocytic inclusions (Fig. 12.32) are less regularly shaped (Volk and Wallace, 1966) whilst the lymphocytes

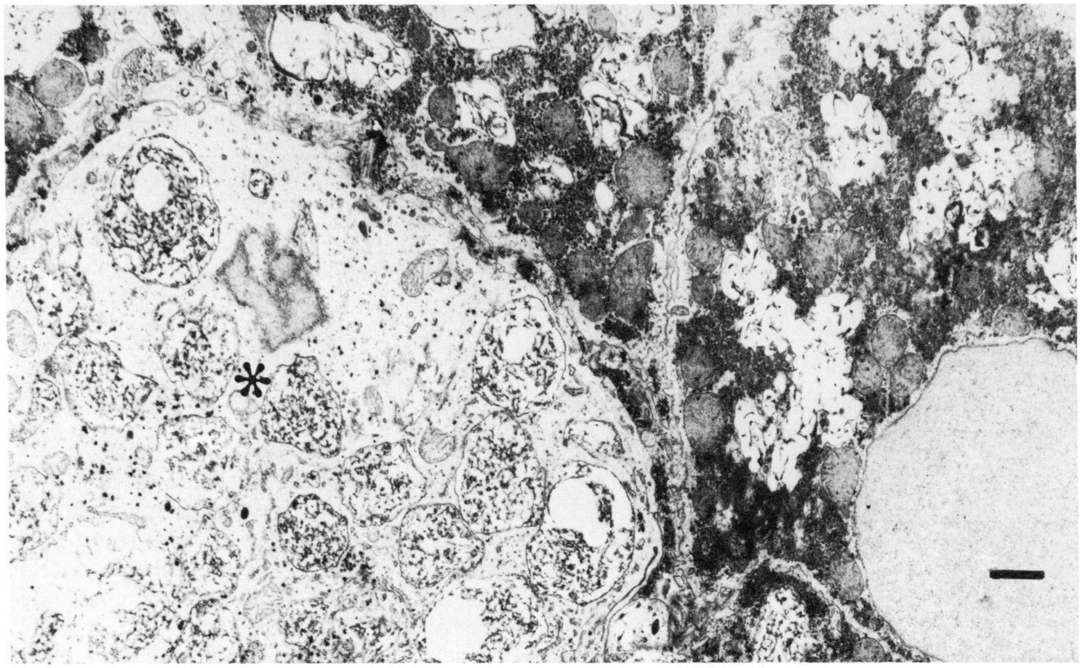

Fig. 12.32 Niemann–Pick disease type A. Liver. Electron micrograph showing a Niemann–Pick cell (*) and portions of two hepatocytes containing membrane-bound collections of less tightly packed lamellae. Bar = 1 μm. × 7000.

show more tightly packed lipid lamellae (Lazarus et al., 1967). Similar inclusions are observed in other tissues (Fig. 12.33) and in the Niemann–Pick cells (Lynn and Terry, 1964). The granules of the sea-blue histiocytes and the deposits in the sinusoidal lining cells of the spleen show well-ordered tightly packed concentric lamellae (Golde et al., 1975; Long et al., 1977) which are different from the inclusions elsewhere accounting for the differing staining reactions.

A study of the ultrastructure of the eye showed inclusions within most of the cell types, including retinal ganglion cells, retinal pigment epithelium, corneal stromal cells, lens epithelium, corneal endothelium and sphincter muscle of the iris (Robb and Kuwabara, 1973). The authors concluded that the changes account for the slight corneal haze seen in some patients with type A disease.

Fetal pathology In affected fetuses no increase in sphingomyelin is found in brain but a tenfold increase is found in the liver and there is also excess within the placenta (E.L. Schneider et al., 1972a; Klibansky et al., 1979). Histochemical studies of the liver showed an increase in sudanophil, acid-haematein-positive staining material in hepatocytes, and an increase in acid phosphatase activity. Electron microscopy showed lam-

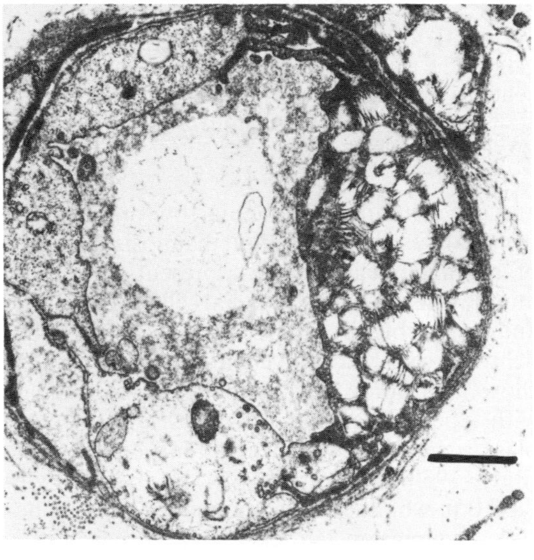

Fig. 12.33 Niemann–Pick disease type A. Capillary. Electron micrograph showing angular inclusions in one of the endothelial cells. Bar = 1 μm. × 11500.

ellated lipid cytosomes in hepatocytes and Kupffer cells and within neurons of the basal ganglia. In the brain and spinal cord, storage bodies were present in endothelial cells and pericytes of most vessels examined.

Pathology. *Niemann-Pick disease group II* Although the clinical features are diverse in this group the unifying feature is the pathology, which is almost identical in all cases. There may be some degree of cerebral atrophy and the white matter is firm, showing an astrocytosis without demyelination. The neuronal ballooning seen in all regions is particularly prominent in the basal ganglia, brain stem (Fig. 12.34) and spinal cord (Norman, Forrester and Tingey, 1967; Hagberg et al., 1978) and is accompanied by axonal swellings also containing the finely granular storage material (Fig. 12.35). A neuroaxonal dystrophy is found in the brain stem and spinal cord (Harzer and Peiffer, 1981; Elleder, Jirásek and Vlk, 1983), and in others neurofibrillary tangles are observed (Horoupian and Yang, 1978). Neurons, including those of the gastrointestinal tract, store a substance which is not sphingomyelin. In frozen and cryostat sections the substance is only weakly sudanophilic and does not give a positive acid haematein reaction. The ferric-haematoxylin method, controlled with alkaline hydrolysis, indicates the presence of phospholipid whilst a water-soluble sugar-containing compound can be demonstrated by the PAS reaction. In processed embedded tissue no storage material can be shown.

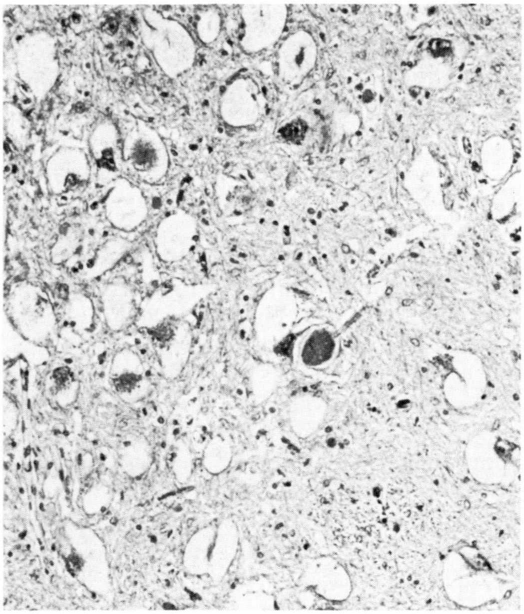

Fig. 12.34 Niemann-Pick disease type C. Marked neuronal storage in the substantia nigra. Haematoxylin and eosin × 145.

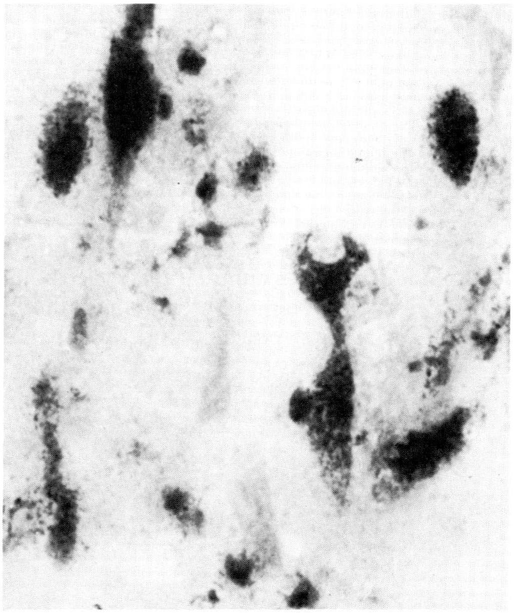

Fig. 12.35 Niemann-Pick disease type C. Cortex. Cryostat section stained with the protected (celloidinized) PAS method showing strongly positive storage granules in neurons and in distended axonal processes. This substance is extracted by aqueous fixatives × 570.

The numerous foam cells present in the spleen usually contain sphingomyelin and cholesterol, and are sudanophilic and positive with ferric haematoxylin. They have a positive PAS reaction in frozen and cryostat sections. Differentiation of group I patients from group II patients is not possible by chemical analysis of spleen because both are essentially identical with regard to sphingomyelin content. In group II, sinusoidal cells, show little or no storage in contrast with group I. Occasional patients have no splenic sphingomyelin accumulation. Their storage cells give staining characteristics similar to those of neurons and are PAS positive. The increase in hexosides has led to patients with this disorder being erroneously labelled juvenile Gaucher's disease (Maloney and Cumings, 1960).

The cell which has led to much of the confusion is the foam cell present in bone marrow aspirates taken for the investigation of hepatosplenomegaly. In contrast with group I Niemann–Pick disease, the foamy cells in the bone marrow of patients with group II have non-uniform vacuoles and an occasional ingested erythrocyte, and often contain densely staining nuclear fragments (Fig. 12.36). These differences were noted by Crocker and Farber (1958) in those patients who did not fit the 'classic' Niemann–Pick disease and who showed no gross liver sphingomyelin accumulation. The bone marrow cells are not sudanophilic, stain diffusely with PAS and show strong acid phosphatase activity. In older patients occasional pale sea-blue histiocytes containing lipofuscin and showing autofluorescence may be found.

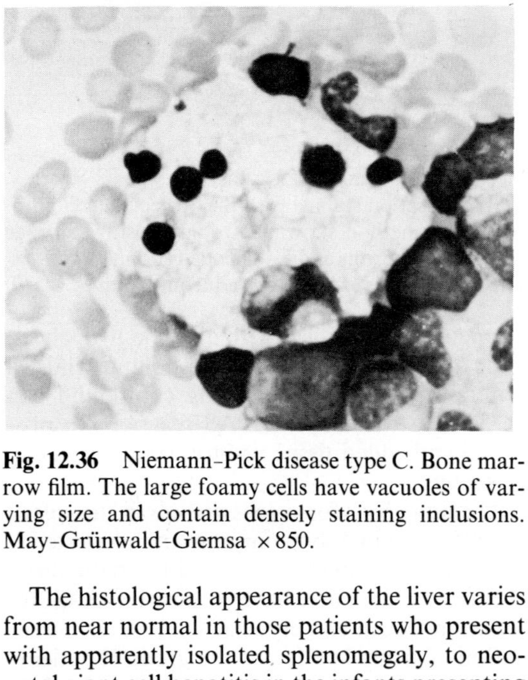

Fig. 12.36 Niemann–Pick disease type C. Bone marrow film. The large foamy cells have vacuoles of varying size and contain densely staining inclusions. May-Grünwald-Giemsa ×850.

The histological appearance of the liver varies from near normal in those patients who present with apparently isolated splenomegaly, to neonatal giant cell hepatitis in the infants presenting with hepatosplenomegaly and severe prolonged obstructive jaundice. In routine sections in the former cases the acinar architecture is undisturbed, the hepatocytes do not appear to be involved in storage, and the enlarged Kupffer cells and storage cells in the sinusoids can only be identified by the PAS reaction after digestion of glycogen (Neville et al., 1973; Hagberg et al., 1978). In frozen or cryostat sections the storage cells are weakly sudanophilic and may show some evidence of sphingomyelin deposition. Acid phosphatase preparations show very strong activity in hepatocytes and storage cells, indicating involvement of both cell types in storage (Lake, 1983b) which can be confirmed by electron microscopy. The storage disease in the patients presenting with severe jaundice is often masked by marked bile pigment deposition, a giant cell hepatitic change and fibrosis leading to cirrhosis in some patients (Ivemark et al., 1963; Guibaud et al., 1979). The storage cells can be masked by the PAS-positive histiocytes present normally in giant cell hepatitis of other causes. The Kupffer cells show storage and there can be collections of storage cells in the portal areas. Lipofuscin pigment in hepatocytes is more abundant than normal. Storage cells are abundant in lymph nodes and may be present in thymus and lung. Smooth muscle cells, heart, skeletal muscle and adrenals are not involved. Usually there is no storage in endothelial cells although in some cases acid phosphatase activity is present in them. The majority of patients do not exhibit vacuolation of lymphocytes but some show a small percentage with a few vacuoles.

The ultrastructure of the neuronal storage material has a distinctive appearance. The membrane-bound polymorphous cytoplasmic bodies (Elfenbein, 1968) measure up to 3 μm and contain loosely packed lamellae which are concentric in some planes of section (Fig. 12.37). Sometimes the limiting membrane contains two or three collections of lamellae and some have fused to produce more complex bodies (Neville et al., 1973); Pellissier et al., 1975). Dense osmiophilic inclusions are often found. Lipid lamellae, similar to those in group I patients, are found in the spleen (Anzil et al., 1973). The involvement of hepatocytes is variable, sometimes showing marked accumulation of mainly empty membrane-bound vacuoles (Fig. 12.38). A few lipid lamellae may be present. In other areas the inclusions are sparse, and may be indistinguishable from those of neonatal hepatitis. The Kupffer cells and storage cells are filled by coalescing membrane-bound vacuoles and electron-dense deposits with occasional lipid lamellae (Wiedemann et al., 1972).

Because the enzymatic basis for the disease is unknown, and the depression of sphingomyelinase activity is probably secondary, prenatal detection is not reliable. In one fetus, of 20 weeks in whom the diagnosis was probable, lipid changes were present (Harzer et al., 1978).

Diagnosis Bone marrow films, stained appro-

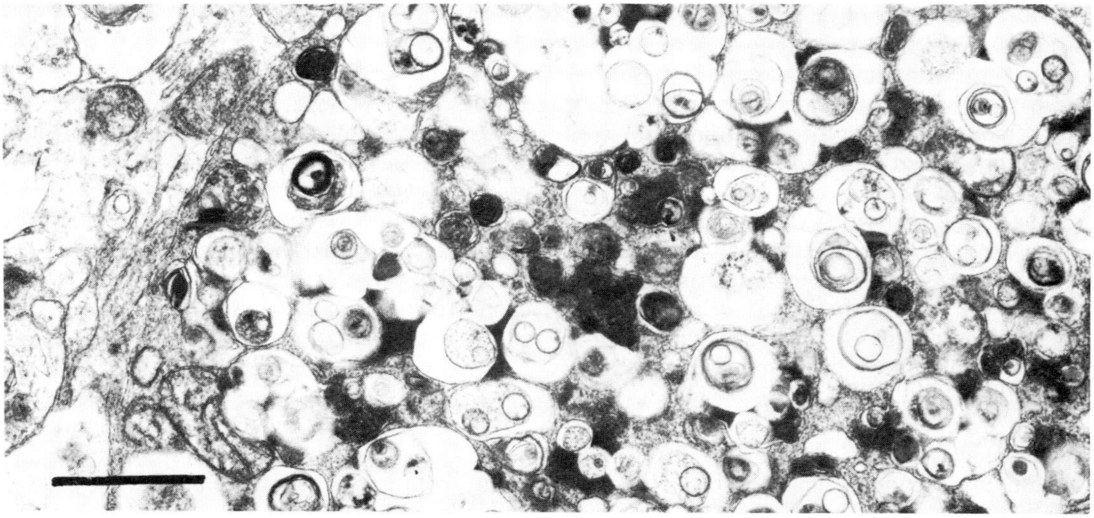

Fig. 12.37 Niemann–Pick disease type C. Electron micrograph of cortical biopsy showing polymorphous cytoplasmic bodies packed in a neuron. Bar = 1 μm. × 20000.

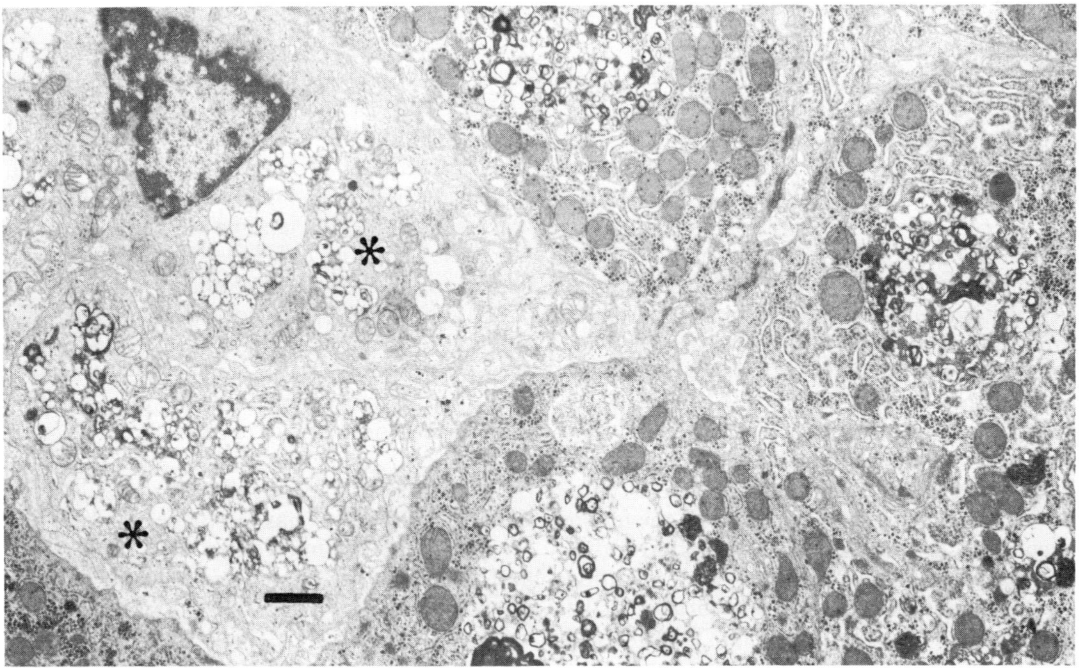

Fig. 12.38 Niemann–Pick disease type C. Electron micrograph of liver showing two storage cells (*) and hepatocytes (right) containing numerous lipid lamellae and membrane-bound vacuoles. Bar = 1 μm. × 7300.

priately and examined carefully, will differentiate between group I and group II patients. Many vacuolated lymphocytes are consistently present in the infantile form of group I. Sphingomyelinase activity may be measured in leucocytes, cultured fibroblasts or tissue samples. To confirm the neuronal storage in the infantile form of group I (and its absence in type B), a suction rectal biopsy will also show smooth muscle cell and endothelial cell involvement, in addition to the numerous foamy cells in the lamina propria. In group II patients there is no smooth muscle storage, endothelial cells are rarely involved, and scattered small foamy histiocytes not containing sudanophilic lipid are present in the submucosa. Neuronal storage is best demonstrated in cryostat sections, protected with a thin film of celloidin, stained by the PAS method (Lake, 1983a).

It has been reported (Vethamany, Welch and Vethamany, 1972) that heterozygote carriers of group II disease show the characteristic storage cells in bone marrow. In the author's experience, the number of cells is small, and heterozygote detection would be difficult and probably unreliable.

Animal models The drug AY9944 causes a reduction in sphingomyelinase activity without gross increase in sphingomyelin content. AY9944 is an inhibitor of cholesterol metabolism and an increase of 7-dehydrocholesterol is found.

Niemann–Pick disease has been reported in a poodle dog (Bundza, Lowden and Charlton, 1979) and in Siamese cats (Snyder, Kingston and Wenger, 1982). In the cats the disorder is analogous to type A.

Feline lipidosis (Percy and Jortner, 1971), though often quoted as an animal model of Niemann–Pick type A, has the morphology and chemistry most closely resembling type C disease. Mice with a disorder similar to type C disease have recently been reported (Morris et al., 1982).

The morphology and chemistry of the FM mice (Lyon, Hulse and Rowe, 1965) is quite different from any form of Niemann–Pick disease and their inclusion in this group is unjustified.

Gaucher's disease

Three main types of Gaucher's disease are recognized, affecting adults, infants and juveniles respectively. *Type 1, chronic non-neuronopathic Gaucher's disease*, is generally regarded as the adult form but its onset can be at any age from birth onwards. Those with early onset show massive splenomegaly with a lesser degree of hepatomegaly. Hypersplenism may necessitate removal of the spleen, which can weigh up to 8 kg. Episodes of bone pain caused by vascular changes in the metaphysis of long bones brought about by the massive deposits of Gaucher cells are a feature in older children and adolescents, and fractures at the head and neck of the femur are common. Destruction of the vertebral bodies may occur. In older patients the presenting symptoms may be a tendency to bruise easily; their course is usually mild. No neurological symptoms occur. *Type 2, acute neuronopathic Gaucher's disease*, presents usually within 6 months of birth, the neonatal period often being normal. The first signs of hepatosplenomegaly, failure to thrive, or difficulty in feeding can occur singly or in combination. Motor delay is evident by 6 months and this progresses to cranial nerve and extrapyramidal tract involvement. Fits are not common. Death, usually from pulmonary infection, occurs before the second birthday.

Type 3, subacute or juvenile neuronopathic Gaucher's disease has been studied extensively in two large kindreds in Sweden (Dreborg, Erikson and Hagberg, 1980) and in a family in West Cameroon (Tripp et al., 1977). The essential features are of early asymptomatic splenomegaly which progresses to symptoms of hypersplenism. Intellectual deterioration is usually evident by about 5 years. Myoclonic epilepsy and spasticity are found in many patients and a large proportion have a horizontal gaze palsy. Bone necrosis and fractures as in the adult (type 1) patients occur later. Neurological disease in adults with Gaucher's disease has also been described (Miller, McCleuer and Kanfer, 1973; King, 1975) and this may be regarded as a chronic form of type 3. Several other scattered reports seem to show a wider variety of symptoms but most of these cases are probably not examples of Gaucher's disease.

All forms of Gaucher's disease are inherited in an autosomal recessive mode. Type 1 is more common among patients with Ashkenazi Jewish ancestors (Groen, 1964).

Chemistry A marked increase in glucocerebroside is present in spleen (100 × normal) and liver (up to 10 × normal). No increase is found in brain. In visceral organs there is also a mild increase in ganglioside G_{M3}. Cholesterol is not increased and no increase is found in lactosylceramide in true Gaucher's disease.

Enzymology Brady, Kanfer and Shapiro (1965) showed a deficiency of glucocerebrosidase in the soluble fraction of a spleen extract acting at neutral pH. However, Patrick (1965) demonstrated that, using artificial and natural substrates under acidic conditions, there was no activity of glucocerebrosidase and a marked reduction of β-glucosidase present in homogenates of tissue from patients with Gaucher's disease. He speculated that Gaucher's disease was a defect of the lysosomal system. Further work has shown that only one of the isoenzymes of β-glucosidase is deficient and that the enzyme protein is present but inactive. Problems of solubilization of the enzyme and cerebroside have given rise to difficulties in assay and suggestions of a two-component system. The enzymology has recently been reviewed by Patrick (1982). The defect is similar in all types, although some differences between the neuronopathic and non-neuronopathic forms are reported (Glew et al., 1982; Ginns et al., 1982).

The enzyme assay can be performed on leucocytes, cultured fibroblasts and cultured amniotic fluid cells allowing prenatal diagnosis.

Tartrate-stable serum acid phosphatase is usually elevated in patients with all forms of Gaucher's disease, although similar increases are found in several other conditions but usually not in other lipid storage diseases.

Pathology The gross appearance of the brain is not abnormal in type 2 Gaucher's disease, and in the few reports of neuropathology in type 1 brains no macroscopic changes were noted. The most striking features are the massive splenomegaly, hepatomegaly and enlargement of lymph nodes. The spleen shows white areas of infarction on its surface and the cut surface is almost uniform, with the malpighian bodies widely separated and barely visible to the naked eye.

The characteristic Gaucher cell, present in almost all organs and tissues, is large, measuring 20–100 μm and containing one or more nuclei. The cytoplasm is filled with finely or coarsely fibrillar material (Fig. 12.39) which gives an appearance of crumpled tissue paper. Sections of

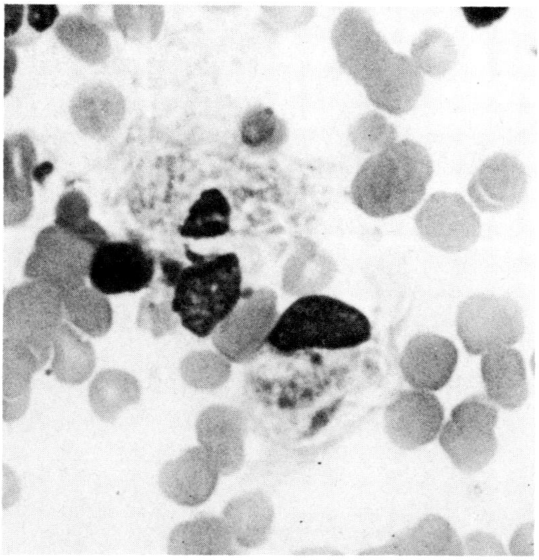

Fig. 12.39 Gaucher's disease. Bone marrow film. Two Gaucher cells are present, their cytoplasm having a striated appearance. May-Grünwald-Giemsa. × 850.

the cell usually show the fibrillar nature although in some planes of section the cell may have a vacuolar appearance. The cerebroside content of the cell gives rise to positive PAS staining, and because cerebroside is essentially the only substance stored, Gaucher cells are negative with fat stains, do not stain for cholesterol and show no reaction with the acid haematein or ferric-haematoxylin methods. Acid phosphatase activity is strong in Gaucher cells, as in all storage cells of lysosomal origin. Iron pigment is sometimes present in Gaucher cells, reflecting the haematological origin of the cerebroside. By electron microscopy the fibrillar inclusions (Fig. 12.40) appear as membrane-bound elongated bodies containing a tubular arrangement of the glucocerebroside (Fredrickson and Sloan, 1972a). Negative staining shows that the walls of the tubules consist of fibrils 60–80Å in diameter in a right-handed twisted arrangement (Lee and Ellis, 1971). Cells similar to Gaucher cells are occasionally found in chronic myeloid leukaemia and, light microscopically, are indistinguishable from Gaucher cells. However, by electron microscopy the 'storage' bodies contain filamentous inclusions rather than the tubules found in Gaucher cells (Lee and Ellis, 1971).

Detailed studies of the brain in acute neuronopathic Gaucher's disease are those reported by Norman, Urich and Lloyd (1956) and by Banker,

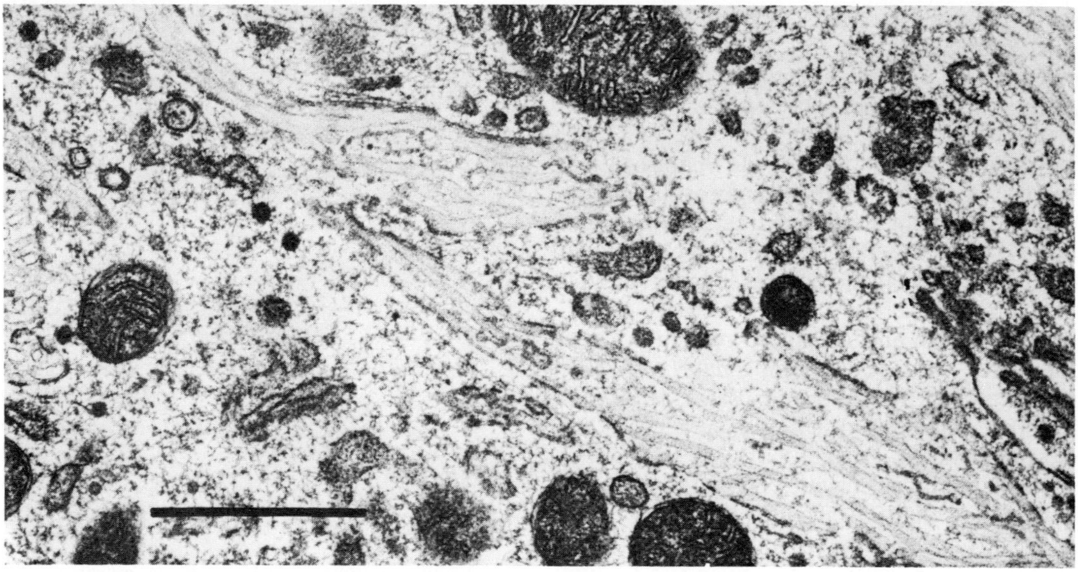

Fig. 12.40 Gaucher's disease. Electron micrograph of a Gaucher cell showing the striated inclusions which consist of a tubular arrangement of the cerebroside. Bar = 1 μm. × 29000.

Miller and Crocker (1962). In the cerebral cortex there is no evidence of neuronal storage and only a mild loss of neurons is seen in layers 3 and 5. Myelination appears normal for age. Gaucher cells are found lying free in the cortex and perivascularly (Figs. 12.41, 12.42). In the basal ganglia and brain stem marked to moderate neuronophagia and gliosis is evident, while in other neurons there is mild cytoplasmic swelling suggesting storage. By electron microscopy the typical tubular inclusions are not seen in the swollen neurons and there is no evidence of generalized neuronal storage (Adachi et al., 1972). These authors did find occasional neuronal Gaucher bodies and some evidence of membranous cytosomes. Although these are not characteristic of Gaucher's disease, similar cytosomes have been found in the foamy cells present in a 17-week fetus with Gaucher's disease, in addition to the typical tubular inclusions (E. L. Schneider et al., 1972b).

Few reports of CNS pathology in the non-

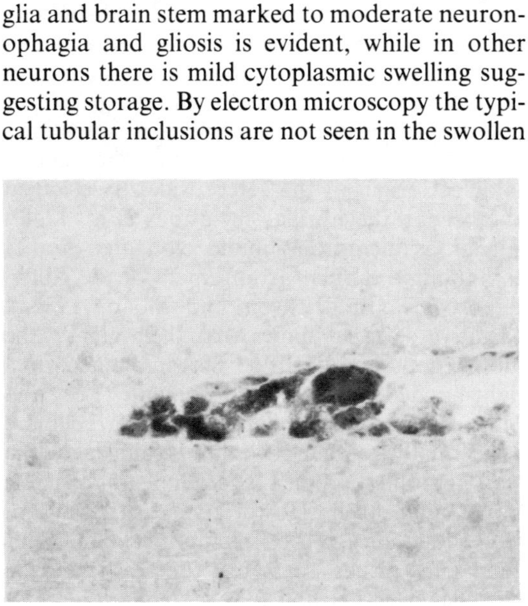

Fig. 12.41 Gaucher's disease type 2. Frontal cortex. Perivascular Gaucher cells showing strong acid phosphatase activity in cryostat section. × 280.

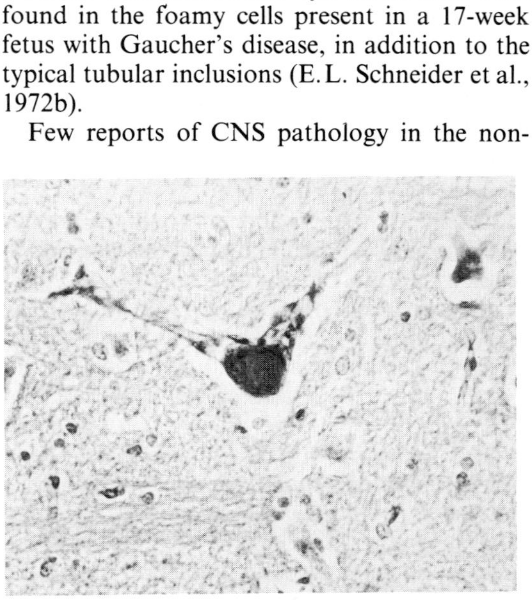

Fig. 12.42 Gaucher's disease, type 2. Basal ganglia. A Gaucher cell lies adjacent to a capillary. PAS × 280.

neuronopathic form (type 1) are available, but Gaucher cells are seen in periadventitial tissue (Brady and Barranger, 1983).

Gaucher cells are present in large numbers in the spleen (Fig. 12.43), where they form characteristic nests, the centres of which may be necrotic. Lymph nodes and bone marrow contain numerous Gaucher cells which are also present in liver portal areas and sinusoids (Fig. 12.44). Hepatocytes are not involved in storage of glucocerebroside. Gaucher cells are found in pancreas, thyroid, lung and adrenal and occasionally

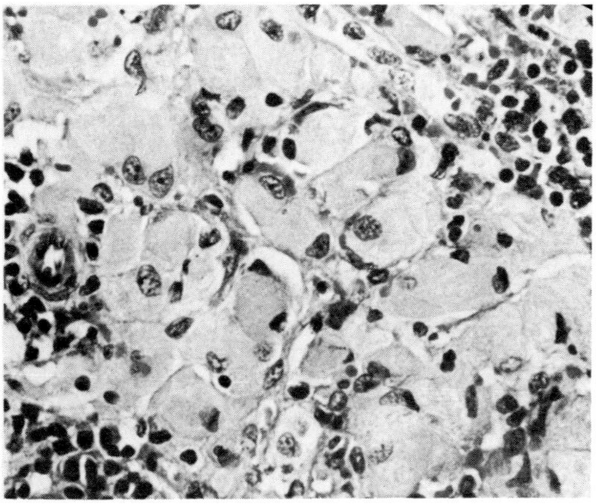

Fig. 12.43 Gaucher's disease. Spleen. Gaucher cells in tissue sections do not all show the striped appearance of those in marrow films. Haematoxylin and eosin × 300.

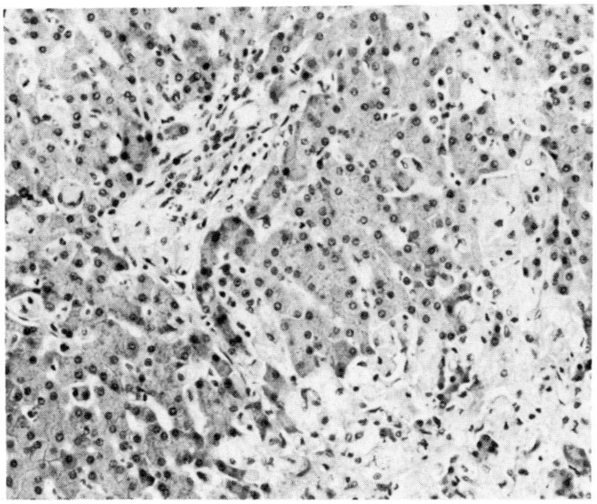

Fig. 12.44 Gaucher's disease. Liver. Numerous Gaucher cells are present in portal areas and in sinusoids. In contrast with Niemann–Pick disease, the hepatocytes are not involved. Haematoxylin and eosin × 120.

in the renal glomerulus. W. Collier noted (1895) that the adenoids contained the large 'epithelioid' cells in a 6-year-old child whose spleen weighed one-sixth of her body weight at death.

No evidence of neuronal storage disease is present in neurons of the gastrointestinal tract and the lymphoreticular aggregates do not contain Gaucher cells. Bone marrow aspirates contain numerous Gaucher cells but lymphocytes are not vacuolated.

Several unusual cases of Gaucher's disease have been reported. In one family both the neuronopathic and the non-neuronopathic forms occurred (Wenger, Roth and Sattler, 1982) in enzymatically proven cases. The authors suggested that the father was a carrier for the non-neuronopathic type and that the mother was a carrier for the neuronopathic form. In an even more bizarre case, no evidence of microscopical or chemical storage was found in a 12½-year-old girl who presented with myoclonic epilepsy, spasticity and mild mental retardation. There was no hepatosplenomegaly. The activity of β-glucocerebrosidase was deficient using natural and artificial substrates and there was no complementation of fibroblast cultures with other forms of Gaucher's disease (Wenger et al., 1983). Her second cousin, however, showed microscop-

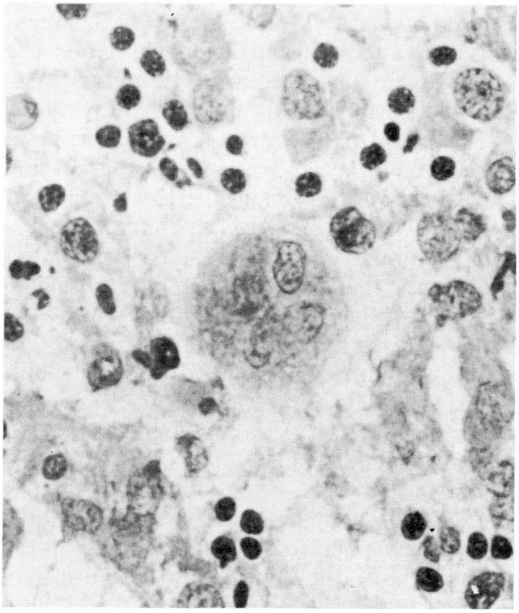

Fig. 12.45 Gaucher's disease. Fetal liver (19 weeks' gestation) showing a pale but positively stained Gaucher cell in a sinusoid. PAS × 700.

ical evidence of storage and had deficient enzyme activity.

A significant proportion of patients with type 1 (non-neuronopathic) Gaucher's disease develop malignancy of some type. Hodgkin's disease (Sharer et al., 1974), glioblastoma multiforme (Lyons, Scheithauer and Ginsburg, 1982) and myeloma, myeloid leukaemia and lymphoma (Lee, 1981) have been reported. Shoenfeld et al. (1982) found that immunoglobulins were significantly increased and suggest that there is a chronic stimulation of the immune system which can lead to the development of malignancy.

Fetal pathology A 17-week fetus with infantile (type II) Gaucher's disease showed a three- to fourfold increase in liver glucocerebroside. (Schneider et al., 1972b). By light microscopy scattered multinucleate Gaucher cells are present in liver (Fig. 12.45), spleen, thymus and bone marrow. There was no abnormality in the brain. Ultrastructural studies show characteristic tubular inclusions, membranous cytosomes and finely filamentous inclusions in the storage cells.

Animal models Gaucher's disease has been reported in silky haired terriers (Van der Water, Jolly and Farrow, 1979) and sheep (Laws and Saal, 1968). The disease has been induced in mice by injection of conduritol-β-epoxide, which is a potent inhibitor of glucocerebrosidase (Adachi and Volk, 1977). However, although electron microscopically and chemically there is evidence of glucocerebroside storage, no Gaucher cells are seen.

Metachromatic leucodystrophy

Leucodystrophy, Scholz type or Greenfield's disease, is now known as metachromatic leucodystrophy and derives its name from the staining properties of the stored sulphatides. The disorder was first described by Alzheimer (1910) and later reported by Witte (1921), Scholz (1925), Greenfield (1933) and Brain and Greenfield (1950). The clinical details have been reviewed by Lyon, Arthuis and Thieffry (1961) and, more recently, by MacFaul et al. (1982) for the cases occurring in children. Three types are recognized according to the age of onset and clinical presentation. Gait disorders with progressive loss of abilities are the main features of the late-infantile type (onset before 2 years) and intermediate type (onset 4–6 years), whilst the juvenile type (onset 6–10 years) is characterized by educational and behavioural problems followed by gait disorder. An adult form is also described (Witte, 1921; Kraus-Ruppert et al., 1972) characterized by psychosis and dementia with motor signs appearing later.

Studies of peripheral nerve function show slowing of the nerve conduction velocity in the late-infantile and intermediate cases but it may not be found in all of the juvenile cases, and conduction is usually normal in the adult form (Fullerton, 1964; MacFaul et al., 1982).

Inheritance is by autosomal recessive transmission in most cases (Schutta et al., 1966). Occasional families show dominant inheritance.

The similar condition, mucosulphatidosis or Austin variant of metachromatic leucodystrophy, is considered later under the heading 'Mucosulphatidosis'.

Chemistry In 1958 three independent reports (Austin; Jatzkewitz; Hagberg et al. (published 1959)) showed that the metachromatic lipids accumulating in the white matter and kidney consist mainly of cerebroside sulphate. Mårtensson reported that kidney contains cerebroside dihexose sulphate in addition (Mårtensson, Percy and Svennerholm, 1966). Myelin lipids are decreased. The sulphatide in the white matter can be up to ten times the normal level in the late-infantile type, and lesser increases are present in the adult type (Jatzkewitz, Pilz and Holländer, 1964). Kidney sulphatides are increased up to seventy times the normal.

Enzymology The deficiency of arylsulphatase A reported by Austin et al. (1964) was shown by Mehl and Jatzkewitz (1965) to be due to deficiency of the heat-labile component of cerebroside sulphatase. The heat-stable component which co-purifies with cerebroside sulphatase has no effect on arylsulphatase A activity. The deficiency can be demonstrated in urine, leucocytes and fibroblasts as well as in tissue samples. Other arylsulphatases (B and C) are normal, and steroid sulphatase activity is normal. Values of arylsulphatase A in heterozygotes are not always as high as expected and may fall almost in the homozygous range (MacFaul et al., 1982).

Prenatal diagnosis is possible by assay of cultured amniotic fluid cells obtained by amniocentesis at about 16 weeks. Because some parents show very low activities this should be taken into account before prenatal diagnosis is attempted.

The arylsulphatase A protein is present but inactive and the defect is similar in all forms of metachromatic leucodystrophy because complementation does not occur in cell lines from patients with the late-infantile and adult forms (Kolodny and Moser, 1983). The defect in mucosulphatidosis is different in that complementation does occur in cell lines fused with those from patients with metachromatic leucodystrophy.

More recently, the activator of cerebroside sulphatase has been characterized (Fischer and Jatzkewitz, 1978), and several patients with confirmed (microscopical and chemical) metachromatic leucodystrophy *without* arylsulphatase A deficiency have presumed or proven activator protein deficiency (Shapiro et al., 1979; Stevens et al., 1981; Hahn et al., 1981, 1982).

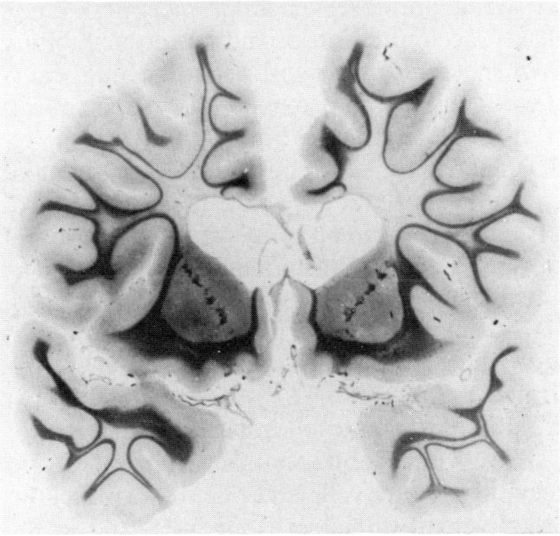

Fig. 12.46 Metachromatic leucodystrophy. Coronal celloidin section through both hemispheres stained by Heidenhain's method for myelin. There is symmetrical and extensive loss of myelin in the white matter. Note preservation of U-fibres.

Pathology The brain at post-mortem is usually externally normal in appearance although some cases show slight atrophy. The white matter has a firm feel. On slicing, the white matter may have a dull chalky white appearance with a clear demarcation from the cortex. Viscera show no gross abnormality except for the gall bladder which may exhibit papillomatous changes.

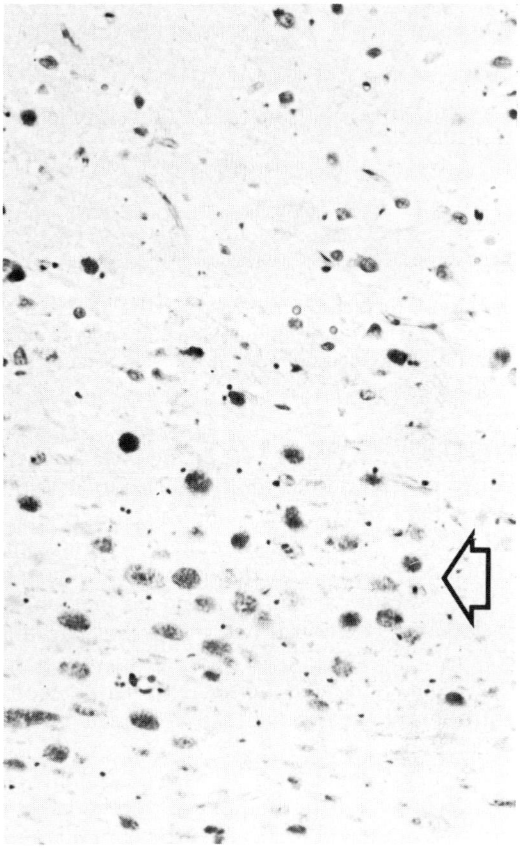

Fig. 12.47 Metachromatic leucodystrophy. PAS-positive macrophages present in the white matter (arrow). Cortical neurons are normal. Paraffin section. PAS ×200.

On microscopy, the white matter of the brain shows marked loss of myelin (Fig. 12.46) and replacement by numerous macrophages which in paraffin sections are PAS positive (Fig. 12.47). In contrast with Krabbe's leucodystrophy the storage cells do not form clusters and are rarely multinucleate.

The macrophages contain cerebroside sulphate (sulphatide) which is responsible for the metachromasia in frozen or cryostat sections

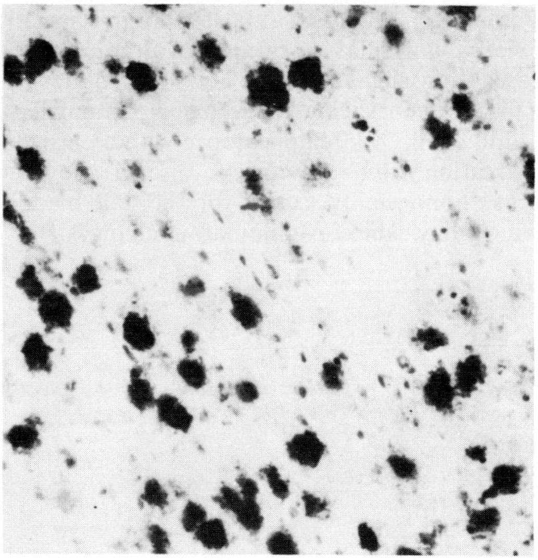

Fig. 12.48 Metachromatic leucodystrophy. Cryostat section stained with toluidine blue showing strongly metachromatic macrophages in the white matter. × 180.

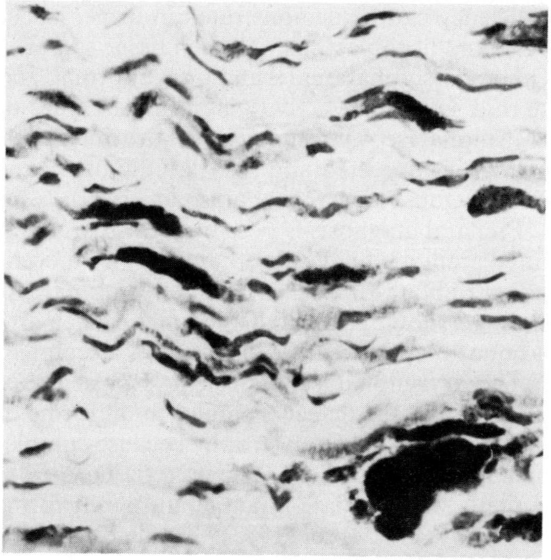

Fig. 12.49 Metachromatic leucodystrophy. Cryostat section of a sural nerve biopsy. Macrophages and Schwann cells are stained metachromatically. Toluidine blue ×430.

(Fig. 12.48; and Plate 12.1c, *facing* p. 491) when stained with acidified cresyl fast violet (von Hirsch and Peiffer, 1955), toluidine blue (Bodian and Lake, 1963) or thionin or acriflavine (Holländer, 1963). The lipid is extracted during processing into paraffin wax and no metachromasia can be demonstrated in routine paraffin sections. The sulphatides stain positively with Alcian blue and have a critical electrolyte concentration of greater than 0.8 M $MgCl_2$ (Lampert and Lewis, 1975). Cholesterol is present with the sulphatide and is positive with the Schultz or perchloric acid naphthoquinone methods. No storage is present in cortical neurons but marked storage is present in nuclei of the basal ganglia, brain stem and cerebellum. The distribution of affected nuclei has been described (Peiffer, 1959; Norman, Urich and Tingey, 1960; Abraham and Lampert, 1963). Neurons of the gastrointestinal tract generally do not store sulphatides although occasional reports mention metachromatic deposits in neurons of the myenteric and submucosal plexuses (Kamoshita et al., 1963). In mucosulphatidosis (see below) there is marked neuronal storage of a gangliosidic nature in cortical and gastrointestinal neurons in addition to the sulphatide deposition in white matter and elsewhere.

Sulphatides accumulate in macrophages and Schwann cells of peripheral nerves (Olsson and Sourander, 1969) and with toluidine blue staining (Fig. 12.49; and Plate 12.1d, *facing* p. 491) exhibit a range of colours from yellow to brown to purple, in contrast to the reddish purple in the brain. In other conditions where there is breakdown of myelin, metachromatic reactions are very weak and are generally pale pink only. Marked accumulation of sulphatides exhibiting brown metachromasia with toluidine blue occurs in the kidney within proximal, distal and collecting tubular epithelium (Fig. 12.50), with the result of increased sulphatides in urinary sediment (Austin, 1957; MacFaul et al., 1982). Metachromatic deposits *within* cells are diagnostic, but casts and granular clusters may also occur. The stained deposits have a green birefringence in polarized light, reflecting the structural organization of the stored sulphatide (Guseo, Deák and Szirmai, 1975).

Sulphatides are stored in peripheral nerves of all sizes, in macrophages of lymph nodes and spleen, in Kupffer cells and bile duct epithelium of the liver, in the adrenal medulla, and in the islets of Langerhans of the pancreas (Wolfe and Pietra, 1964) and are also seen in most other organs (Thieffry, 1962; Hagberg, Sourander and Svennerholm, 1962). The gall bladder may be small and fibrotic or show papillomatous

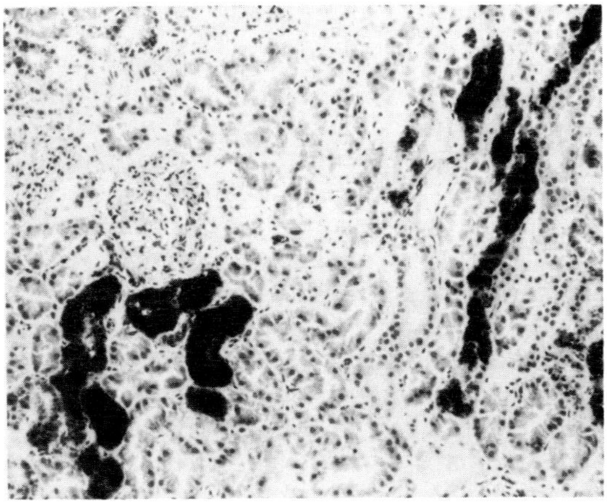

Fig. 12.50 Metachromatic leucodystrophy. Cryostat section of kidney stained with toluidine blue. Metachromatic deposits are shown in tubular epithelium. × 100.

change, and contains deposited sulphatides in the epithelium and in macrophages in the stroma. The white blood cells are not abnormal in contrast with mucosulphatidosis, and no storage cells are present in bone marrow aspirates. Cerebrospinal fluid may show no evidence of sulphatide accumulation (Hagberg, Sourander and Svennerholm, 1961) or may contain metachromatic bodies in some cases (Canelas et al., 1964). These latter authors also demonstrated metachromatic deposits in saliva and in parotid gland biopsies.

Fetal tissues (Leroy et al., 1973) show a mild biochemical increase in brain sulphatides but no metachromatic deposits are present in brain, liver or gall bladder. In the kidney, however, metachromasia is found in Henle's loop and in distal tubular epithelium.

Electron microscopy Three main types of inclusion are recognized. The most typical is the prismatic inclusion consisting of stacked discs giving a herringbone appearance in one plane and a hexagonal honeycomb in another (Fig. 12.51). Tuffstone inclusions, named after their resemblance to volcanic limestone, consist of concentric and radial lamellae in a granular matrix (Bischoff and Ulrich, 1967; Guseo, Deák and Szirmai, 1975). Laminated structures consisting of pairs of membranes and zebra-like bodies can also be found. The less structured bodies show acid phosphatase activity which is not so marked in the more organized prismatic inclusions

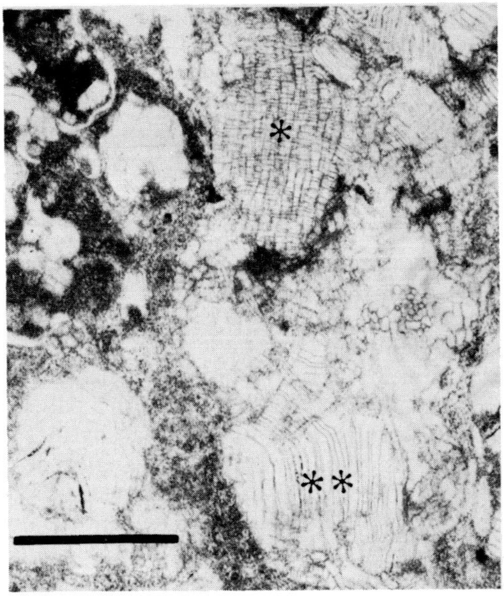

Fig. 12.51 Metachromatic leucodystrophy. Electron micrograph of macrophage in the white matter showing prismatic (*) and lamellar (**) inclusions in a granular matrix. Bar = 1 μm. × 22000.

(Résibois, 1969). Similar deposits are noted in peripheral nerves (Brion, Mikol and Graveleau, 1970) and can be induced in sulphatase-deficient fibroblasts grown in the presence of sulphatide (Rutsaert, Menu and Résibois, 1973). Peripheral nerve myelin shows a variety of changes with concentric zones of loose lamellae with loss of the intraperiod line alternating with apparently normal myelin. The outer myelin lamellae only may be involved. Occasional linear densities may be present in otherwise normal myelin sheaths. Sulphatide deposits also occur in the Schwann cells of unmyelinated fibres.

Diagnosis Initial screening for metachromatic leucodystrophy can be reliably done by the examination of urinary sediment for metachromatic deposits. Assay of arylsulphatase A activity in leucocytes, cultured fibroblasts or urine is necessary for confirmation of the diagnosis (MacFaul et al., 1982). Neutrophils should be examined to ensure that no Alder granulation is present (see below, 'Mucosulphatidosis').

If a biopsy is considered necessary (e.g. where enzyme assay is not available or in the presumed activator protein deficiency) then frozen sections of a sural nerve biopsy will provide the diagnosis.

Biopsies of other tissues are either too invasive or may not provide consistent results.

Animal model Sulphatide deposits have been described in white matter, Schwann cells and kidney of a Hawaiian goose (Wight, 1976) but no enzyme studies were reported.

Mucosulphatidosis

Mucosulphatidosis (Rampini et al., 1970) is a condition in which the pathological changes of metachromatic leucodystrophy exist in a patient who shows evidence of mucopolysaccharidosis and gross neuronal storage of gangliosides. Patients present with pyschomotor retardation at about 1 year, progressing to dementia with death occurring at between 3 and 10 years. Mild skeletal changes may be seen on x-ray and some of the patients have ichthyosis. Corneal clouding occurs in some and there is increased urinary excretion of glycosaminoglycans as in the mucopolysaccharidoses.

The defect affects many different sulphatases (Basner et al., 1979) which degrade a variety of sulphate esters within lysosomes and in the cell cytoplasm. The deficiency of many sulphatases has led to the name 'multiple sulphatase' deficiency (Austin, 1973) and the condition is also known as the Austin variant of metachromatic leucodystrophy. Chemically an increase in sulphatides, gangliosides and ceramide lactoside as well as an increase in mucopolysaccharides is shown in the brain (Pilz and Jatzkewitz, 1968; Austin, 1973).

The early cases described (Mossakowski, Mathieson and Cumings, 1961; Bischoff and Ulrich, 1967; Thieffry, Lyon and Maroteaux, 1967) showed the pathological changes of two disorders. In the white matter of the brain and peripheral nerves abundant deposits of metachromatic sulphatides are demonstrated while the neurons are ballooned by storage of gangliosidic-like substances giving the appearance of those in Tay–Sachs disease. Visceral organs have evidence of water-soluble acid mucopolysaccharide deposition in addition to sulphatide deposition in liver, spleen and kidney. Metachromatic granules are present in urinary sediment and are indistinguishable from those in metachromatic leucodystrophy. In contrast with metachromatic leucodystrophy, the neutrophils contain Alder granules (see Fig. 12.59), and eosinophil granules are usually absent. Alder granulation is also present in the granulocytic series of cells in bone marrow aspirates. Gasser cells and Buhot cells are seen in peripheral blood and bone marrow.

Electron microscopy reveals zebra bodies and lamellated inclusions within neurons, membrane bound vacuoles in capillary endothelial cells and typical sulphatide inclusions within macrophages (Raynaud et al., 1975).

Diagnosis The presence of urinary sulphatides in the absence of arylsulphatases A and B in leucocytes or cultured fibroblasts is diagnostic. Peripheral blood films should be examined and the diagnosis should not be entertained in the absence of Alder granulation. Urinary mucopolysaccharides may be slightly increased.

Krabbe's leucodystrophy

The first generally accepted descriptions of infantile cerebral sclerosis was by Krabbe in 1916, although there may have been earlier reports. It was not until 1924 that Collier and Greenfield used the term 'globoid cells' in a late-onset form, to describe the cells that are characteristic of the disorder now known as Krabbe's leucodystrophy or Krabbe's globoid cell leucodystrophy.

Most cases are of the infantile form, but some of later onset are described. The clinical course of the infantile form was described in Krabbe's (1916) five cases and more recently by Hagberg et al. (1969) in a large series from Sweden. After a normal neonatal development in which they learn to follow with their eyes, to laugh and smile and to have some head control, the patients become irritable and have episodes of intensive crying. The mean age of onset is 4 months. Their development ceases and violent tonic spasms occur in response to noises or bright lights. Deterioration of motor function leads to a permanent opisthotonic posture with hypertonic flexion in the arms and extension in the legs. Hyperpyrexial episodes are common. Myoclonic jerking, optic atrophy and blindness follow and the patients become decerebrate and die, from an intercurrent respiratory infection or bulbar paralysis usually by 15 months of age.

Cases of later onset present at about 2 years with gait problems followed by blindness and spasticity (Christensen, Melchior and Andersen, 1960) or with failing vision, ataxia and spastic paraparesis from 2 to 6 years (Collier and Greenfield, 1924; Crome et al., 1973). A patient reported by Crome et al. (1973) presented in status epilepticus at $6\frac{1}{2}$ years and began losing vision 18 months later.

The oldest verified case (Kolodny et al., 1980) diagnosed at the age of 18 years, presented with difficulty in walking at 2 years. He was mentally subnormal and had pale optic discs and slow dysarthric speech. The adult case described by Guillain, Bertrand and Gruner (1941) presented with a tearful right eye and difficulty in chewing and swallowing. He had an unsteady gait but vision was normal. The pathological description of the brain lesions appears to fit that for Krabbe's leucodystrophy but there are some differences and without enzyme analysis this case should be regarded with interest rather than as a clear-cut example of the adult form.

Krabbe's leucodystrophy is transmitted by autosomal recessive inheritance.

Chemistry Lipid analysis of the brain shows severe loss of myelin lipids, with a high concentration of galactocerebroside in enriched globoid cell fractions (Austin, 1963a). Extracts of the devastated white matter have no absolute increase in galactocerebroside but a change in the ratio of galactocerebroside to sulphatide (Austin, 1963b). Normal myelin has a ratio of about 3:1 for galactocerebroside:sulphatide but in Krabbe's leucodystrophy the ratio rises to between 5:1 and 10:1 with an overall *decrease* in galactocerebroside content. In cases where the myelin appears normal the chemical composition is normal. Psychosine (galactosylsphingosine) is normally present in white matter in very small amounts but up to 100-fold increases are found in Krabbe's leucodystrophy (Svennerholm, Vanier and Mansson, 1980). Although Krabbe's leucodystrophy is a demyelinating disease there is no increase in white matter cholesteryl esters even in the more recently demyelinated areas.

In a series of experiments Austin and his colleagues (Austin, 1962a; Austin and Lehfeldt, 1965) showed that of over 30 different compounds only galactocerebroside caused a globoid cell reaction when injected into the white matter of rat brains. Suzuki and Suzuki (1983) noted that if the galactocerebroside contains as little as 3 per cent psychosine the response is far greater than for galactocerebroside alone. This supports the hypothesis that psychosine is a highly toxic compound which poisons the oligodendroglial cells, preventing further myelin production, and consequently there is no great accumulation of globoid cells or galactocerebroside.

Enzymology Early studies suggested a deficient synthesis of myelin, and a defect of cerebroside sulphotransferase was reported (Bachhawat, Austin and Armstrong, 1967). Further studies proved that deficient activity of lysosomal galactocerebroside-β-galactosidase is the primary defect and that the activity of this enzyme is profoundly reduced in grey and white matter, liver and spleen (Suzuki and Suzuki, 1970), and in serum, leucocytes and fibroblasts (Suzuki and Suzuki, 1971). The defect in sulphotransferase is not consistent in all tissues (Austin et al., 1970) and is probably secondary to the loss of oligodendroglia. The enzyme is substrate specific and artificial substrates do not reveal the defect.

The enzyme deficiency is found also in the late-onset form of the disease (Young et al., 1972; Kolodny et al., 1980). Because it is expressed in fibroblasts and cultured amniotic fluid cells, prenatal diagnosis is now possible (Suzuki, Schneider and Epstein, 1971; Harzer, 1982).

The enzyme is also active when psychosine is used as substrate, and deficient activity would account for the increased concentration of psychosine and its toxic effects.

Pathology The brain is generally small and weighs about 600–800 g with a normal external apperance. The gyri, however, may be shrunken and the sulci widened and the cerebellar folia may be prominent. The white matter is firm under a cortex of normal consistency, giving the feel of an 'iron fist in a velvet glove'. On cut section the white matter has a greyish appearance but the subcortical arcuate fibres are preserved and form a distinct white line some 1–2 mm thick (Krabbe, 1916). The appearance is similar in the infantile and later onset forms. Visceral organs are normal.

Microscopically the main features are of relatively normal cortex with no evidence of storage. The white matter shows gross loss of myelin (Fig. 12.52), a marked astrocytic gliosis and the pres-

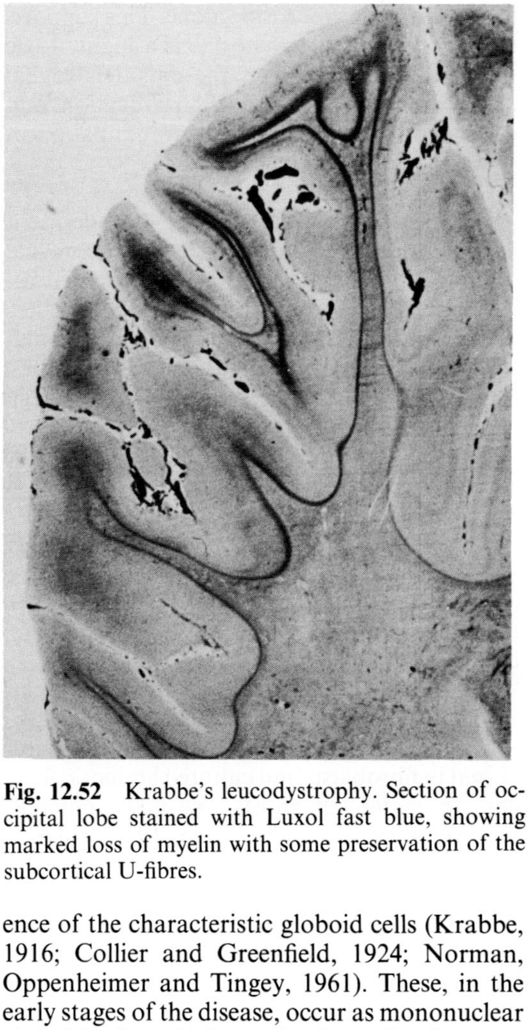

Fig. 12.52 Krabbe's leucodystrophy. Section of occipital lobe stained with Luxol fast blue, showing marked loss of myelin with some preservation of the subcortical U-fibres.

ence of the characteristic globoid cells (Krabbe, 1916; Collier and Greenfield, 1924; Norman, Oppenheimer and Tingey, 1961). These, in the early stages of the disease, occur as mononuclear globoid cells, which, as the demyelination proceeds, form clusters of globoid cells (Fig. 12.53) each up to 50 μm in diameter and containing up to 20 peripherally located nuclei. The clusters generally occur around blood vessels. As the demyelination becomes more severe, with loss of oligodendroglia due to psychosine toxicity, the numbers of globoid cells first increase and then

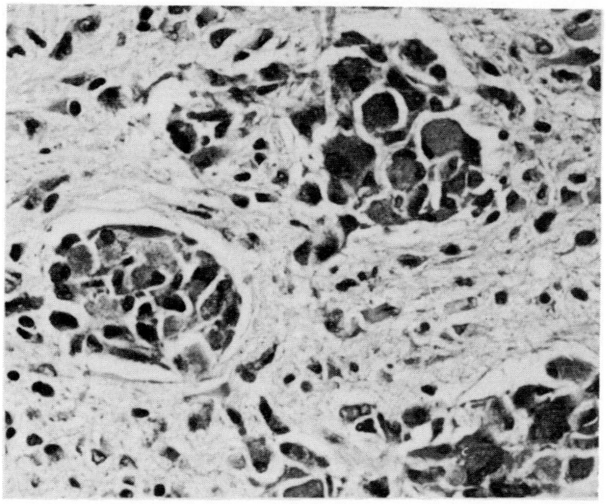

Fig. 12.53 Krabbe's leucodystrophy. Clusters of globoid cells in the white matter. PAS ×280.

decrease. A point is reached in areas of longstanding myelin loss where all that may be left is a few scattered single or clusters of globoid cells, an intense astrocytic gliosis and almost total loss of axons (D'Agostino, Sayre and Hayles, 1963). In some cases there may be no globoid cells at this stage (Dunn et al., 1976). In the late-onset cases the appearance of globoid cells may be delayed and a brain biopsy can appear entirely normal histologically and chemically (Crome et al., 1973).

There has been controversy over the identity and origin of globoid cells and it has been suggested that they arise from microglia, oligodendroglia, astrocytes or adventitial cells. Christensen, Melchior and Andersen (1960) referred to them as gemistocytic astrocytes but no processes have ever been seen. It is now clear that they are macrophages arising from non-neural mesodermal cells and previous distinctions between 'epithelioid' and 'globoid' are not valid.

The globoid cells are PAS positive (Blackwood and Cumings, 1954) and stain only faintly with Sudan dyes (Diezel, 1955). Lipid laden macrophages are not usually present, unlike most other demyelinating conditions, and cholesteryl esters are not increased. The globoid cells do not exhibit metachromasia but show strong activity of acid phosphatase and other lysosomal enzymes.

Although the cerebral cortex shows only minor changes there is almost total loss of neurons in the dentate nucleus and in the inferior olives (Norman, Oppenheimer and Tingey, 1961; Shaw and Carlson, 1970; Crome et al., 1973),

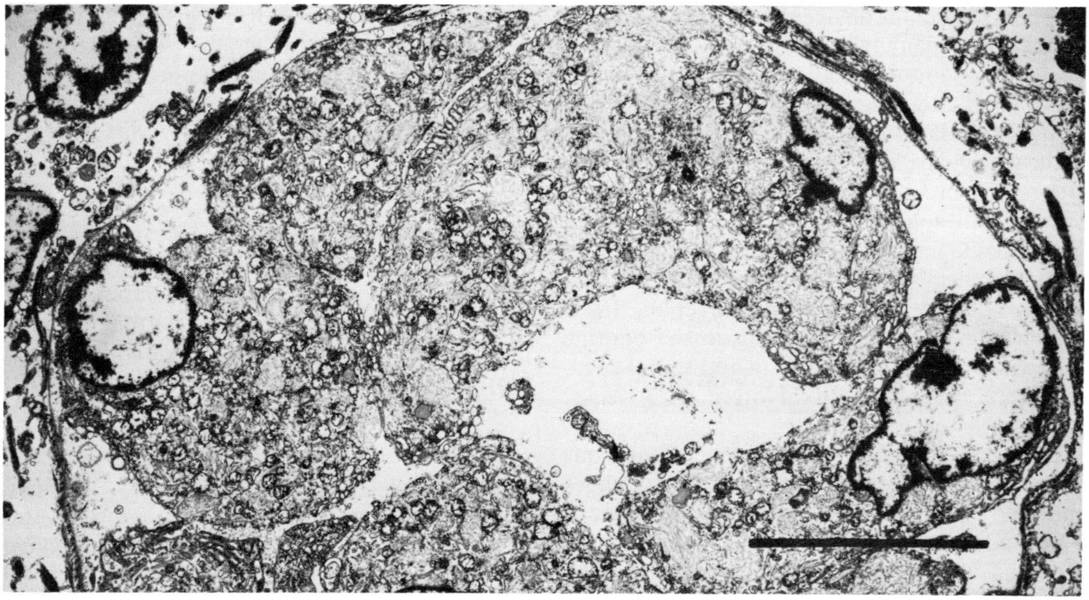

Fig. 12.54 Krabbe's leucodystrophy. Electron micrograph of brain biopsy shows a cluster of globoid cells. Bar = 10 μm. × 3200.

whilst other nuclei in the brain stem and Purkinje cells in the cerebellum are less severely affected.

By electron microscopy (Fig. 12.54) abnormal inclusions are found within the globoid cells only. Apart from the usual characteristics of busy macrophages, straight or curved tubular profiles (Fig. 12.55) which appear irregularly crystalloid in cross-section are present scattered in the cell or sometimes aggregated in an electron-dense matrix (Nelson et al., 1963; Shaw and Carlson, 1970; Suzuki and Grover, 1970; Schochet, McCormick and Powell, 1976). A second type of twisted tubular inclusion is also present (Yunis and Lee, 1969) which has some similarities to the cerebroside storage in Gaucher's disease.

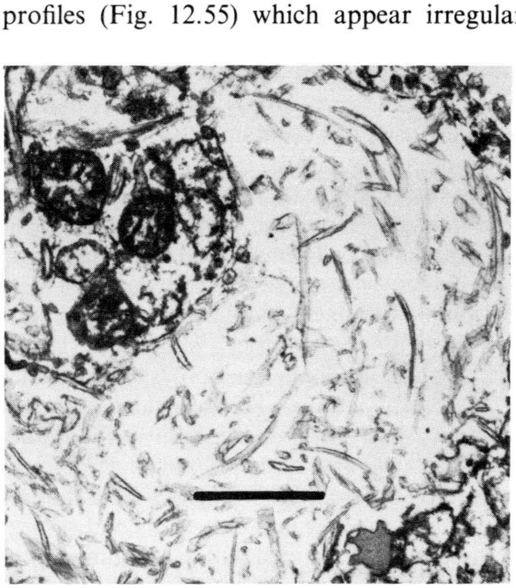

Fig. 12.55 Krabbe's leucodystrophy. Electron micrograph showing the curved tubular inclusions in cytoplasm of a globoid cell. Bar = 1 μm. × 17000.

Early reports suggested that peripheral nerves were normal in Krabbe's disease but Austin (1962b) noted that there were segmental areas of myelin breakdown in one sural nerve biopsy, and Matsuyama, Minoshima and Watamabe (1963) reported on changes in cranial and spinal nerve roots. Allen and de Veyra (1967) and Sourander and Olsson (1968) demonstrated degenerative changes in peripheral nerves, and Lake (1968) showed that segmental demyelination with increased acid phosphatase activity was a feature. An extensive study of seven cases confirmed the peripheral neuropathy (Dunn et al., 1969) which could be detected at 6 weeks of age before any clinical signs were evident. The degenerative changes found in the clinically affected patients consisted of demyelination with prominent Elzholz bodies, presence of macrophages and increased endoneurial fibrosis. Schwann cells with strong acid phosphatase activity, teased fibres showing segmental demyelination and an occasional lipid laden macrophage, were all demonstrated. No globoid cells are found in peripheral nerves. By electron microscopy the curved or straight tubular profiles (splinter shaped) found in the globoid cells in the central nervous system are rarely present in Schwann cells but are present in the macrophages (Bischoff and Ulrich, 1969; Suzuki and Grover, 1970).

Pathological changes are present in affected fetuses (Ellis et al., 1973; Martin et al., 1981; Harzer, 1982) with globoid cells in the pontine tegmentum, medulla oblongata and spinal cord. Peripheral nerves are also involved at 23 weeks' gestation.

Outside the central and peripheral nervous system most authors have not noted any changes although Austin (1962a) reported minor inconstant sudanophilic degenerative change in the proximal and collecting tubules of the kidney and was able to see similar cells in urinary sediment. Giant cells, similar to globoid cells, have been reported in lung, lymph nodes and spleen in one patient (Hager and Oehlert, 1957). No changes are seen in peripheral blood cells (Suzuki and Grover, 1970). Skeletal muscle can show the changes of congenital fibre type disproportion (Martin et al., 1976; Dehkharghani et al., 1981) but this appearance is not specific and is seen in a variety of muscle disorders (Cavanagh, Lake and McMeniman, 1979).

Diagnosis The diagnosis of Krabbe's leucodystrophy is best made by enzyme assay of leucocytes or cultured fibroblasts. Indications of the disorder can be obtained from a peripheral nerve biopsy; if these facilities are not available, a brain biopsy should establish the diagnosis in most cases.

Animal models A morphologically identical disorder has been reported in cats, sheep, several species of dogs (West Highland terriers, cairn terriers, blue-tick hounds and beagles) and in the mutant mouse *twitcher* (Duchen et al., 1980). The defect in the terriers (Suzuki et al., 1970) and the mice is identical to that in the human disease, with deficient activity of galactocerebroside-β-galactosidase (Suzuki and Suzuki, 1983).

The mucopolysaccharidoses

The current classification of the mucopolysaccharidoses (Table 12.8) is based on a mixture of historical eponyms, specific enzyme defects and analysis of urinary mucopolysaccharides (also known as glycosaminoglycans or GAGs). Although Thomson in Edinburgh recognized some of the earliest cases at the turn of the century he did not publish the observations but referred to the condition as 'Johnny McLeod's disease' (Henderson, 1940), Johnny McLeod being the first of three siblings who are now recognized as having had Hurler's syndrome. Hunter (1917) and Hurler (1919) published the first definitive descriptions of the disorder which now bear their names, and later Morquio, Sanfilippo, Maroteaux and Lamy, and Scheie described other conditions which are now included in the general classification. McKusick (1972) has reviewed the early history and clinical manifestations, and McKusick and Neufeld (1983) describe the more recent findings.

Of the many names applied to this group of conditions, the term 'gargoylism' is fortunately only rarely used now, and apart from its unnecessarily offensive nature, its derivation was erroneous since 'gargoyle' refers to the rainspout rather than the grotesque carvings with which they are associated. The term 'mucopolysaccharidosis' (MPS) was suggested by Brante (1952) who isolated dermatan sulphate from the livers of two patients with Hurler's syndrome. Later workers showed that mucopolysacchariduria was a constant feature. The general pattern of excretion is shown in Table 12.8 but it should be noted that urinary mucopolysaccharides are examined by different laboratories with different methods, and the way in which each condition is diagnosed and subdivided will vary from centre to centre. Chondroitin sulphate is always present and is a component of normal urine but its amount is not generally increased in the mucopolysaccharidoses. Although MPS I and MPS II

Table 12.8 Classification of the mucopolysaccharidoses

Type	Eponym	Subtype	Urinary GAGS	Enzyme defect
MPS I	Hurler Scheie Hurler/Scheie	IH IS IH/S	Dermatan sulphate and heparan sulphates	α-L-Iduronidase
MPS II	Hunter	A Severe B Mild C Autosomal recessive	Dermatan sulphate and heparan sulphates	Sulpho-iduronate sulphatase
MPS III	Sanfilippo	A	Heparan sulphates	2-Deoxyglucose-2-sulphamate sulphatase (sulphamidase)
		B	Heparan sulphates	α-*N*-Acetylglucosaminidase
		C	Heparan sulphates	Acetyl CoA: α-glucosaminide: *N*-acetyl transferase
		D	Heparan sulphates	*N*-Acetylglucosamine-6-sulphate sulphatase
MPS IV	Morquio	A Severe	Keratan sulphate	*N*-Acetylgalactosamine-6-sulphate sulphatase
		B Mild	—	β-Galactosidase
MPS VI	Maroteaux-Lamy	A Severe	Dermatan sulphate	*N*-Acetylgalactosamine-4-sulphate sulphatase (aryl sulphatase B)
		B Mild	—	
		C Intermediate	—	
MPS VII	—		Dermatan sulphate	β-Glucuronidase

are both shown with dermatan sulphate and heparan sulphate as the main components, the proportions are different and differences in two heparan sulphate components may be evident. The Sanfilippo syndrome (MPS III) was characterized by heparan sulphate excretion, and now four types of MPS III have been described (Coppa et al., 1983) each with a different enzyme defect but each excreting heparan sulphates. Similarly, MPS IV (Morquio) is recognized by keratan sulphate excretion but the two forms have different enzyme defects and the mild form (type B) sometimes shows only minimal or no keratan sulphaturia. On the other hand, MPS I (Hurler) and the former MPS V (Scheie) have been brought together on the basis of their common defect of α-L-iduronidase activity, leaving MPS V now unfilled. A number of 'atypical' mucopolysaccharidoses have been described and these may eventually be fitted into the classification which will no doubt undergo revisions and expansion in the future.

The mucopolysaccharidoses are generally inherited in an autosomal recessive fashion with the exception of MPS II (Hunter) which is an X-linked recessive condition although a few cases of MPS II in females are recorded (Mossman et al., 1983).

Prenatal diagnosis by assay of cultured amniotic fluid cells (von Figura, van de Kamp and Niermeijer, 1982), by analysis of amniotic fluid mucopolysaccharides derived from fetal urine (Mossman et al., 1981) or combination of the two (Harper et al., 1974) is possible from 14 weeks of pregnancy.

The **pathology** of all types of mucopolysaccharidosis is dominated by the storage of mucopolysaccharides within lysosomes of cells of most tissues and organs. In addition there may be neuronal storage of several gangliosides which may also occur within macrophages in the liver.

The mucopolysaccharides are not protein bound and are extremely water-soluble, a factor which resulted in failure to detect them in sections of fixed tissue and the preoccupation with neuronal lipid storage as the major pathological change in the early cases examined.

The gross appearance of the brain is usually normal although the skull is sometimes grossly thickened and the dura and leptomeninges are opaque and thickened. Slicing of the fixed brain will usually show perivascular pits in the white matter (Norman, Urich and France, 1959) in cases where there is mental retardation as well as in those cases where no mental retardation is evident. Figure 12.56 shows the appearance in Maroteaux–Lamy syndrome but in MPS IVA no such changes are seen (Koto et al., 1978). The myelin is often normal but the perivascular areas contain collections of foamy cells in which water-soluble acid mucopolysaccharides can be detected in cryostat sections of snap-frozen tissue stained by a suitable metachromatic method (Lake, 1983a). Cystic changes may also be seen in these areas. Wallace et al. (1966) reported diffuse demyelination in two cases of MPS III.

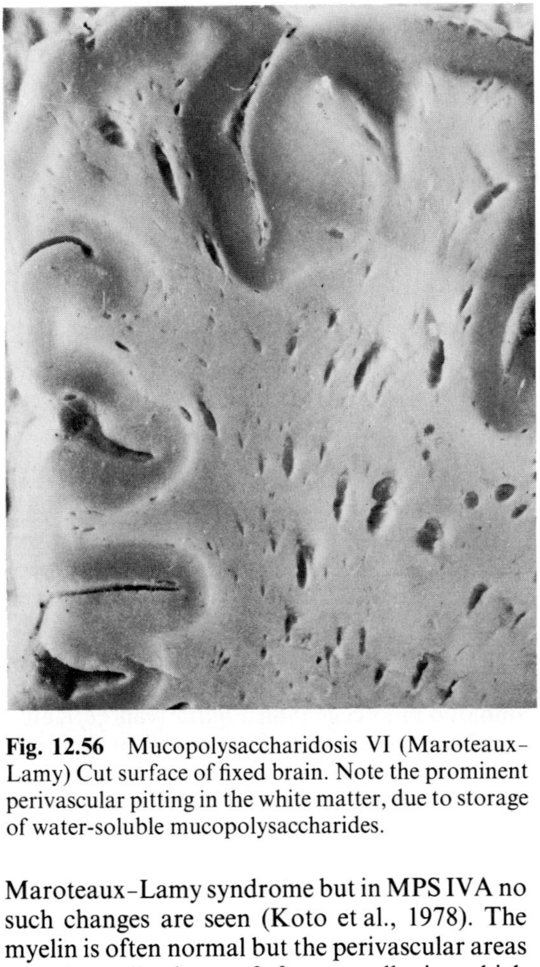

Fig. 12.56 Mucopolysaccharidosis VI (Maroteaux–Lamy) Cut surface of fixed brain. Note the prominent perivascular pitting in the white matter, due to storage of water-soluble mucopolysaccharides.

Chemical analysis of the brain shows increases in dermatan sulphate in MPS I and MPS II, with a large excess of heparan sulphate in MPS III (Dekaban and Constantopoulos, 1977). Separation of gangliosides shows a normal pattern in MPS IS (Dekaban et al., 1976), with non-specific increases in gangliosides G_{M3} and G_{M2} in MPS IH, similar to that seen in Niemann–Pick disease type A and Krabbe's leucodystrophy.

Neuronal storage may be gross and resemble that seen in the gangliosidoses, or may be less evident. Where no mental retardation is present (e.g. in MPS IS and MPS VI), no neuronal storage is seen (Dekaban et al., 1976; Lake, 1978, personal observation). However, in cases of MPS IV (Gilles and Deuel, 1971; Koto et al., 1978) neuronal storage of PAS-positive globules was observed in the cerebral cortex, Ammon's horn, basal ganglia and the thalamic nuclei. None was seen in the anterior horn cells or neurons of the gastrointestinal tract or retina. In MPS IH, MPS IH/S, MPS II and MPS III the neuronal storage is present throughout the brain, spinal cord and ganglia of the gastrointestinal tract. The stored gangliosides are PAS positive, sudanophilic and are stained strongly with Luxol fast blue. In frozen sections cholesterol can be demonstrated as part of the stored material (Schnabel, 1961). No neuronal storage of mucopolysaccharide can be demonstrated.

In visceral organs routine microscopy may reveal a mild degree of cellular vacuolation but this is not gross and no mucopolysaccharide can be demonstrated in tissues fixed in aqueous media. Alcohol or picric-acid/dioxan mixtures have been used to preserve the soluble mucopolysaccharide but even then preservation is poor. Cryostat sections of snap-frozen tissue retain much more of the mucopolysaccharide, which even under optimal conditions will diffuse during staining giving an area of metachromasia in and around the storing cells. Hepatocytes and Kupffer cells store acid mucopolysaccharides in all forms of mucopolysaccharidosis, the degree of storage being marked in hepatocytes in MPS I, II and III while lesser amounts are present in MPS IV and VI. Kupffer cells may in addition accumulate gangliosides which are PAS positive and show a positivity with colloidal iron staining which can be abolished by treatment with sialidase. Mucopolysaccharide storage is found in lymph nodes, spleen, kidney (Kobayashi, 1959) and heart (Dawson, 1954). Mitral incompetence is a common complication of the mucopolysaccharidoses and is caused by infiltration of the mitral valves by large foamy cells and connective

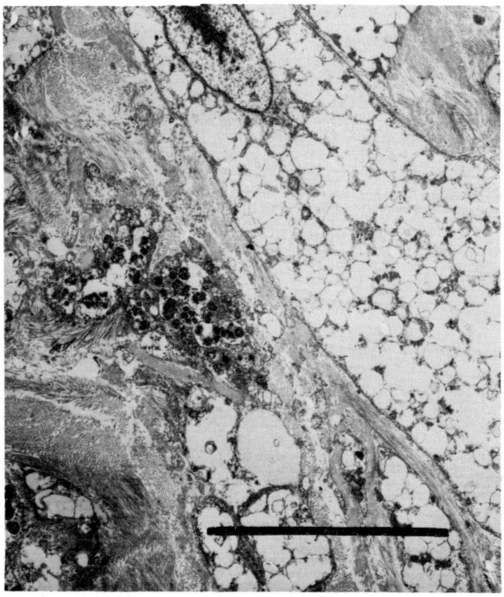

Fig. 12.57 Mucopolysaccharidosis VI (Maroteaux-Lamy). Electron micrograph showing large foamy cells in the mitral valve together with electron-dense lipofuscin-like deposits. Similar changes are present in the other mucopolysaccharidoses. Bar = 10 μm. × 3200.

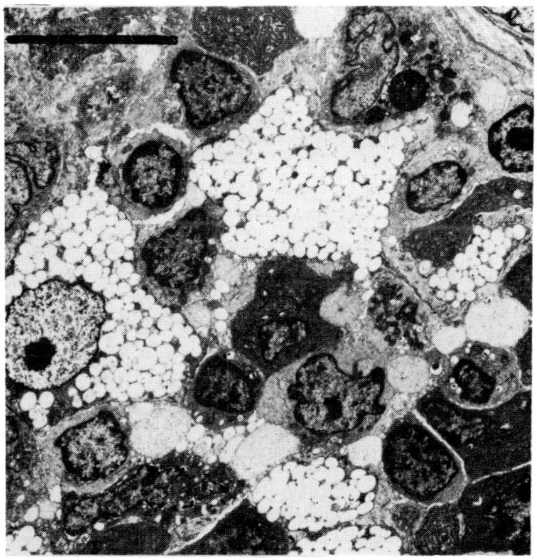

Fig. 12.58 Mucopolysaccharidosis IV (Morquio). Electron micrograph of tonsil shows histiocytes distended by membrane-bound vacuoles. Bar = 10 μm. × 2100.

tissue. Figure 12.57 shows the infiltration in the biopsy of the mitral valve of a young woman with Maroteaux-Lamy disease who had mitral insufficiency. Fibroblasts in skin, conjunctiva, cornea and endothelial cells of the vascular system also store mucopolysaccharides. Kenyon (1976) has reviewed the ocular pathology of the systemic mucopolysaccharides. Deposition of mucopolysaccharide in tonsils may not be gross but is present in fibroblasts and in histiocytes in the subcapsular regions (Fig. 12.58).

Peripheral blood cells show changes which, in very broad terms, relate to the specific type of mucopolysaccharidosis (Lake, 1981). Alder granulation, a coarse reddish violet granulation present in neutrophils in blood films stained with May-Grünwald-Giemsa or Wright stain (Fig. 12.59) is found in MPS VI and MPS VII and is also seen in mucosulphatidosis. All neutrophils are affected and the appearance is similar to an exaggerated toxic granulation. All granulocytes are affected and Alder granulation is also striking in bone marrow cells. Vacuolated lymphocytes are not usually prominent, except in MPS IVB, but occasional Gasser cells—vacuolated lymphocytes with basophilic inclusions—may be seen in any of the mucopolysaccharidoses. Metachromatic inclusions in the cytoplasm of lymphocytes (Fig. 12.60; Plate 12.1b, *facing* p. 491) are generally seen in a greater proportion of lymphocytes in MPS III than in MPS I and MPS II.

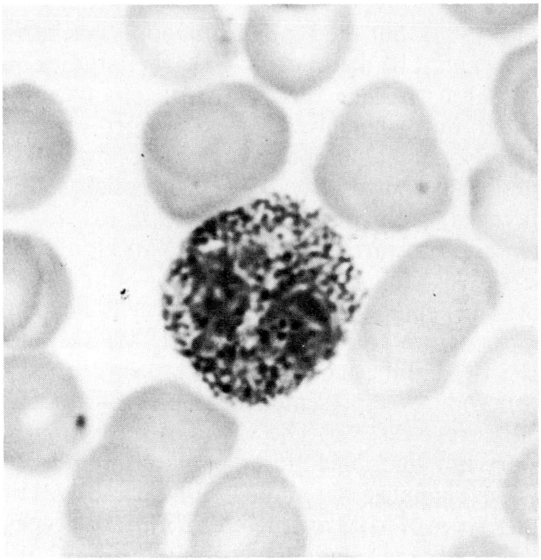

Fig. 12.59 Mucopolysaccharidosis VI (Maroteaux-Lamy). Alder granulation in a neutrophil stained with May-Grünwald-Giemsa × 2000.

Bone marrow aspirates will show storage cells containing acid mucopolysaccharide (Hann

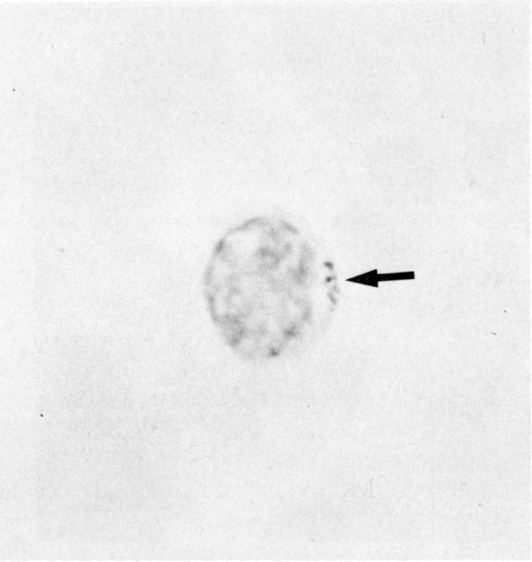

Fig. 12.60 Mucopolysaccharidosis III (Sanfilippo). Metachromatic granular inclusions (arrow) in the cytoplasm of a circulating lymphocyte. Toluidine blue ×1370.

et al., 1983), but the type of mucopolysaccharidosis cannot be determined. In earlier studies of bone and cartilage there were no changes recorded but later investigators report on the foamy vacuolated appearance of chondrocytes, osteoblasts and periosteal cells (McKusick, 1972; Maynard, Cooper and Ponseti, 1973).

In *electron microscopic* studies Van Hoof and Hers (1964) found large membrane-bound vacuoles in hepatocytes and Kupffer cells in liver biopsies from patients with MPS I, MPS II and MPS III, and they concluded that the mucopolysaccharidoses represented examples of lysosomal storage disease. The vacuoles were mainly empty but some fine granular material and occasional lamellae were noted. Similar changes in other types of MPS are present in most cell types and membrane-bound vacuoles (see Fig. 12.58) are observed in fibroblasts, endothelial cells, smooth muscle cells, skeletal muscle, macrophages and epithelium of distal and collecting tubules of kidney, conjunctiva and cornea (Van Hoof, 1973a; Kenyon, 1976). Where corneal clouding is not evident by slit-lamp examination, ultrastructural changes are minimal and confined to the stromal keratinocytes. The neuronal storage is present in various forms. Some of the storage bodies are very similar to those of the primary gangliosidoses and can be described as MCBs. In others the lamellae are more loosely arranged and are often parallel rather than concentric. The parallel arrays may aggregate, leaving spaces between aggregates and giving rise to the zebra body. The changes are not consistent for any particular type of MPS but reflect the secondary storage of ganglioside (Dekaban et al., 1976; Winters et al., 1976; Hadfield et al., 1980; Murphy et al., 1983). Pericytes and perivascular macrophages may contain clear vacuoles or membranous fragments. Neuronal storage in MPS IV (Koto et al., 1978) consists of loosė lamellae which are stacked, straight or tangled in the form of conglomerates up to 7 μm in diameter. Zebra bodies or MCBs were rarely present. Endothelial and perithelial cells showed membrane-bound empty vacuoles (Gilles and Deuel, 1971) with absence of perivascular lacunae by light microscopy. Tubulovesicular inclusions, similar to those found in neuroaxonal dyştrophy, were observed in MPS IIIB (Hadfield et al., 1980).

Prenatal diagnosis by examination of amniotic fluid glycoaminoglycans (Whiteman and Henderson, 1977) and assay of cultured amniotic fluid cells for the particular enzyme has been confirmed by study of the affected fetus in MPS I, MPS II, MPS III, MPS IV and MPS VI. Histochemical examination of liver and placenta shows evidence of acid mucopolysaccharide accumulation within hepatocytes and macrophages respectively. Electron microscopically, membrane-bound vacuoles within hepatocytes (Harper et al., 1974; Ceuterick et al., 1980) and macrophages and fibroblasts in the placenta have been found (Lake, 1981, unpublished observations). Neuronal storage, not visible by light microscopy, is present in the brain stem and spinal cord where zebra bodies (Fig. 12.61) are seen as early as 15 weeks in MPS II (Lake, 1983, unpublished observation). Storage cells are present in the bone marrow at this time (Fig. 12.62), and in MPS VI Alder granulation can be seen in circulating neutrophils by 19 weeks (Lake, 1982, unpublished observations). Radiological changes are not present in any type by 20 weeks (Hall and Lake, 1982, unpublished observations).

Diagnosis of the mucopolysaccharidoses is best accomplished by a combined clinical and radiological approach with studies of urinary GAGs, microscopy of leucocytes and enzyme assay of leucocytes or cultured fibroblasts. Ultra-

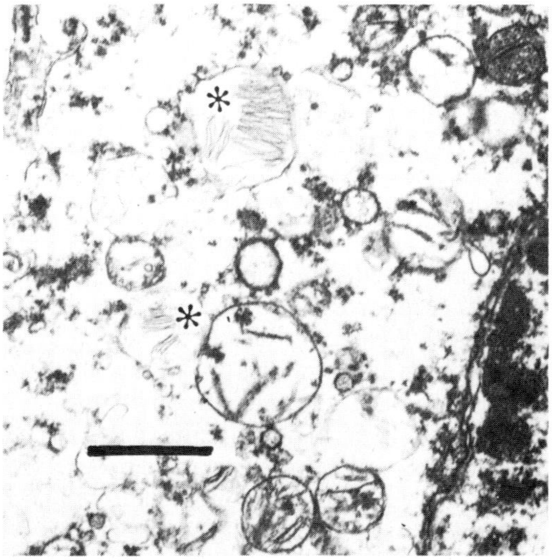

Fig. 12.61 Mucopolysaccharidosis II. Fetal (15 weeks) spinal cord. Membrane-bound stacks of lamellae (*) are seen in neuronal perikaryon. Bar = 1 μm. × 15000.

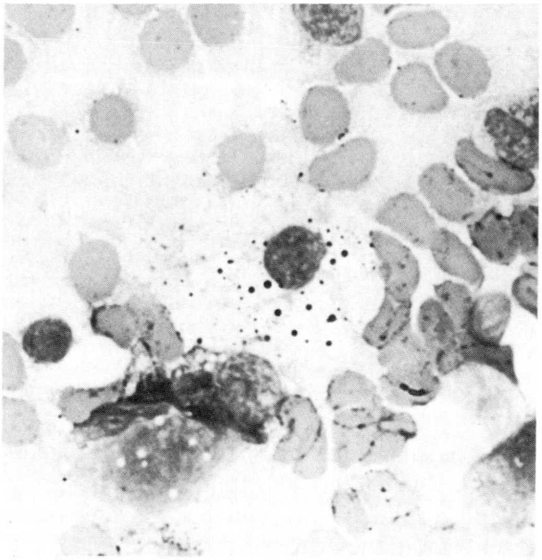

Fig. 12.62 Mucopolysaccharidosis II. Fetal (15 weeks) bone marrow contains storage cells with basophilic, metachromatic inclusions. May-Grünwald-Giemsa × 800.

structural studies of skin or conjunctival biopsies, although providing morphological evidence of a storage disorder of the mucopolysaccharidosis/mucolipidosis type, do not allow its precise identification.

Treatment of patients with transplants of HLA-compatible fibroblasts does not appear to be an effective means of enzyme replacement (Munnich et al., 1982; Crow et al., 1983) but bone marrow transplantation does seem to reverse the clinical features. Leucocyte α-L-iduronidase activity returned in a patient with MPS IH who was given maternal bone marrow cells (Hobbs et al., 1981) and the urinary GAGs changed towards a normal pattern. Although the visceral and skeletal changes appear to be corrected by this form of treatment it is not known whether the neuronal component is similarly reversed.

α-L-iduronidase deficiency has been described in the short-haired cat (Haskins et al., 1979) and in the Plott hound (Schull et al., 1982). The pathology is similar to MPS I in man. Maroteaux-Lamy disease (MPS VI) appears in Siamese cats (Haskins et al., 1981) with neutrophil Alder granulation and arylsulphatase B deficiency. Visceral storage is present but storage in the brain is confined to the perithelium of the brain and cord and connective tissue cells of the meninges and choroid plexus. Spinal cord compression due to atlantoaxial subluxation consequent upon hypoplasia of the odontoid process occurs in the cats as in the severe form in man. Mice of the C3H strain have a partial deficiency of β-glucuronidase activity, and a mucopolysaccharidosis can be induced in rats by suramin which inhibits iduronate sulphatase, β-glucuronidase and hyaluronidase (Constantopoulos et al., 1980). The animal models, particularly those with MPS I, should provide useful information on the effect of bone marrow transplants on the pathology of the brain.

Mucolipidosis I

A deficiency of lysosomal sialidase activity in the various types of mucolipidosis I (ML I) is complicated by varying deficiencies of β-galactosidase and a very wide clinical spectrum. As further biochemical pathways are discovered and the specificity of sialidases become defined it is possible that many of the patients, now considered within this group, will fit into other categories. In broad terms, ML I consists of two main groups, which have been classified as: sialidosis type 1—normosomatic group; and sialidosis type 2—dysmorphic group. The dysmorphic group can be divided into infantile and juvenile forms (Lowden and O'Brien, 1979).

Sialidosis type 1 is also known as the cherry-red spot myoclonus syndrome (Rapin et al., 1978) and presents in the first decade with bilateral cherry red spots at the macula. An alternating periodic nystagmus is seen in some and cataracts may be present in others. Severe myoclonus develops and in most patients there is no intellectual impairment. In the earliest reported patient (Glasgow, 1957) there was thinning and scalloping of cortical bone with cystic changes. No hepatosplenomegaly is found. Vacuolated lymphocytes may be present, and foamy cells in

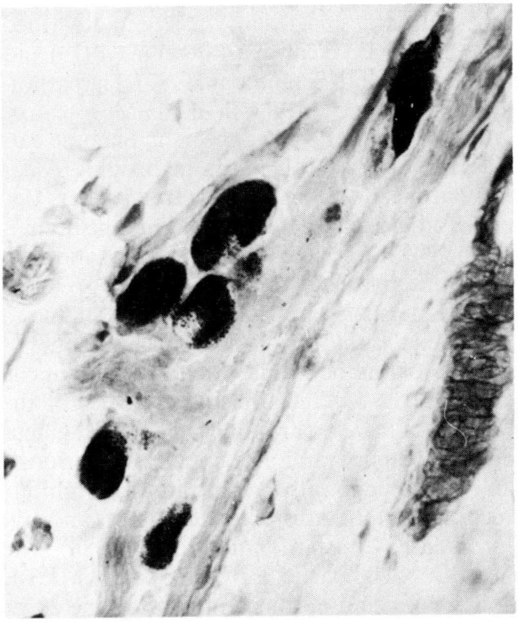

Fig. 12.63 Sialidosis type 1 (cherry red spot–myoclonus syndrome). Section of rectal biopsy from an 11-year-old girl without dementia. There is marked storage in neurons of Meissner's plexus. Cryostat section; PAS ×350.

the bone marrow staining strongly with PAS are found in some patients. Neuronal storage in the brain cortex and neurons of the gastrointestinal tract (Fig. 12.63; Plate 12.1a, *facing* p. 491), very similar to and indistinguishable from that of the gangliosidoses, is present in spite of the absence of neurological deficit. Kupffer cells show marked vacuolation, and some evidence of hepatocytic storage is also visible on electron microscopy. The stored substance has sialic acid residues and stains with Alcian blue and PAS reactions if care is taken to prevent its loss. A defect of lysosomal neuraminidase activity is present, with normal β-galactosidase activity. The urinary excretion of sialyloligosaccharides is increased.

Sialidosis type 2 has a variety of names attached, reflecting the early and continuing uncertainty of the nature of the disorder. Spranger et al. (1968) described 'lipomucopolysaccharidosis', Goldberg et al. (1971) reported on cases with cherry red spots at the macula, corneal clouding and β-galactosidase deficiency, and Orii et al. (1972) reported on a new type of mucolipidosis with β-galactosidase deficiency. Earlier the disorder was known as mucopolysaccharidosis Gal +, reflecting the hyperactivity of β-galactosidase in liver. The patients have coarse facial features, skeletal dysplasia and progressive loss of vision with corneal clouding and bilateral cherry red spots at the macula. Most patients are deaf and show mild to moderate mental retardation. Mucopolysaccharide excretion is normal but sialyloligosaccharides are increased. Neuronal storage of a ganglioside-like substance is present in the brain and gastrointestinal tract. The liver shows foamy Kupffer cells and vacuoles in hepatocytes. By electron microscopy the vacuoles contain a delicate protein-like precipitate with numerous dense granules and many unstructured osmiophilic round inclusions (Loeb et al., 1969b). This appearance serves to differentiate ML I from mucopolysaccharidosis type I (Hurler) where the vacuoles are essentially empty. The cytoplasm of renal glomerular epithelial cells is vacuolated. Large foamy cells are found in the bone marrow and a high proportion of cases have had vacuolated lymphocytes. Metachromatic deposits in the urinary sediment reported by Spranger et al. (1968) indicate the sialyloligosaccharide excretion and are different from the deposits in metachromatic leucodystrophy which resist acetone dehydration.

Nephrosialidosis is a further variant which presents in infancy with features of a mucopolysaccharidosis and a glomerulopathy with an increasing proteinuria (Maroteaux et al., 1978). In the few cases recorded, death has occurred before the age of 5 years. Widespread neuronal storage, storage in cells of the mononuclear phagocyte system in the liver, spleen and lungs, with ballooning of the renal glomerular epithelium and proximal tubules are the major features (Le Sec, Stanescu and Lyon, 1978). Numerous bone marrow foam cells and prominent vacuolated lymphocytes are present. Deficient activity of lysosomal neuraminidase directed towards the

$\alpha(2 \rightarrow 6)$ linkage was found, with normal activity against $\alpha(2 \rightarrow 3)$ substrates.

Severe cases of mucolipidosis I have also been described with congenital ascites and hepatomegaly (Riches and Smuckler, 1983). The placenta showed a markedly vacuolated trophoblast layer and many vacuolated foamy cells in the stroma of the villi. Vacuoles were not noted in the vascular endothelial cells or smooth muscle cells. Prenatal diagnosis has been successful in a severe form of ML I in which absent sialidase activity with normal β-galactosidase was found (Johnson et al., 1980).

In an adult type of mucolipidosis with deficiency of sialidase and β-galactosidase (Kobayashi et al., 1979), angiokeratomata were present in a patient with corneal clouding and ataxia. Appendiceal neurons showed marked storage of a ganglioside-like material which was PAS positive and was composed of membranous cytoplasmic bodies at electron microscopy. Smooth muscle cells were also affected. Vacuolated lymphocytes and PAS-positive foamy bone marrow cells were found and urinary sialyloligosaccharide excretion was up to ten times more than normal.

Mucolipidoses II and III

Although these were originally considered to be different disorders, both have the same enzyme defect and can be considered as the severe and mild forms respectively. A defect in uridine-5′-diphosphate-*N*-acetylglucosamine: glycoprotein-*N*-acetylglucosaminylphosphotransferase is described in both, and there is no complementation in cell fusion studies (Neufeld and McKusick, 1983). Some workers find that mucolipidosis III is genetically heterogeneous (Honey et al., 1982), reflecting the rapidly changing state of biochemical knowledge in the mucolipidoses.

Mucolipidosis II (also known as I-cell disease) presents very similarly to Hurler's syndrome (MPS IH) with marked skull and skeletal deformities, short stature and psychomotor retardation but without mucopolysacchariduria. Onset is in the first year, and later joint contractures and cardiac problems develop. The label I-cell disease originates from the appearance of cultured fibroblasts by phase microscopy. The cytoplasm of the cells is filled with *Inclusions*, and although this seemed relatively specific at the time, similar appearances are seen in many other disorders. Mucolipidosis III (or pseudo-Hurler polydystrophy) is milder, presenting in early childhood with gradually increasing restriction of joint mobility, mild skeletal dysplasia, corneal clouding and mild mental retardation (Kelly et al., 1975). In both ML II and ML III there are grossly elevated levels of serum lysosomal enzymes—particularly β-glucuronidase and arylsulphatase A—with decreased or even absent activities in cultured fibroblasts.

Vacuolated lymphocytes in peripheral blood films (Fig. 12.64) and foam cells in bone marrow aspirates are present in both types. Little tissue evidence of storage by light microscopy is present but the renal glomerular epithelium is grossly ballooned in ML II (Fig. 12.65) even in the affected fetus. By electron microscopy clear vacuoles are found in fibroblasts, Schwann cells and astrocytes, and to a minor extent in hepatocytes (Van Hoof, 1973a). In the heart, the myofibres show some degree of vacuolation with increased lipofuscin deposits even in the early cases, and acid phosphatase activity is grossly increased (Lake, 1983a). This increase is evident even in the affected fetus. Placenta shows endothelial cell and smooth muscle storage, and histiocytes with vacuoles containing partially degraded collagen fibres are also present (Lake, 1982, unpublished observations).

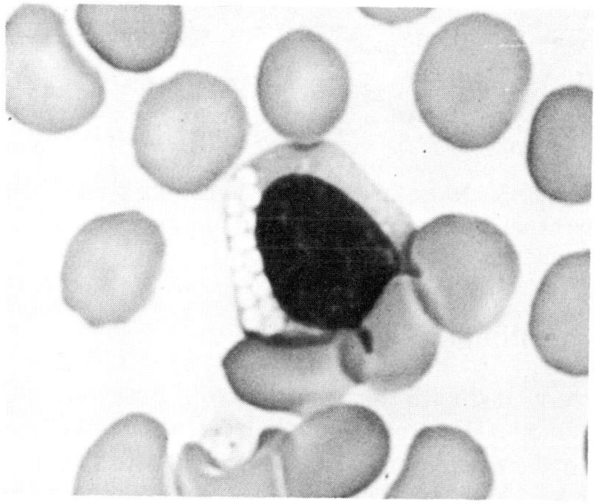

Fig. 12.64 Mucolipidosis II. Numerous prominent vacuoles in a lymphocyte in peripheral blood. May-Grünwald-Giemsa × 1800.

Urinary excretion of sialyloligosaccharides of a wide variety of structure is increased (Farriaux and Strecker, 1979) and can be demonstrated by thin layer chromatography.

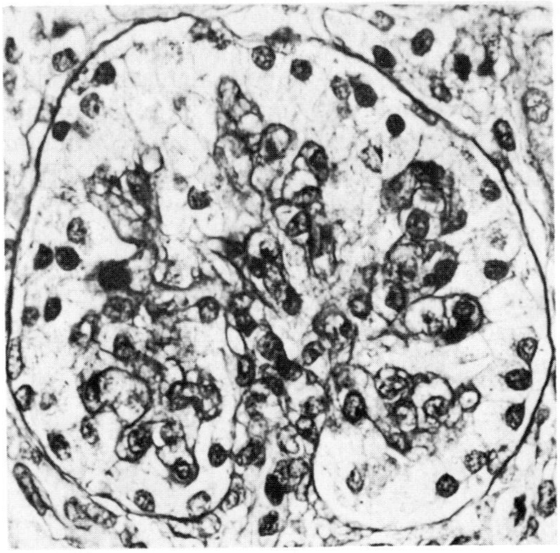

Fig. 12.65 Mucolipidosis II. Kidney. The glomerular epithelial cells are foamy and contain empty vacuoles. Haematoxylin and eosin ×475.

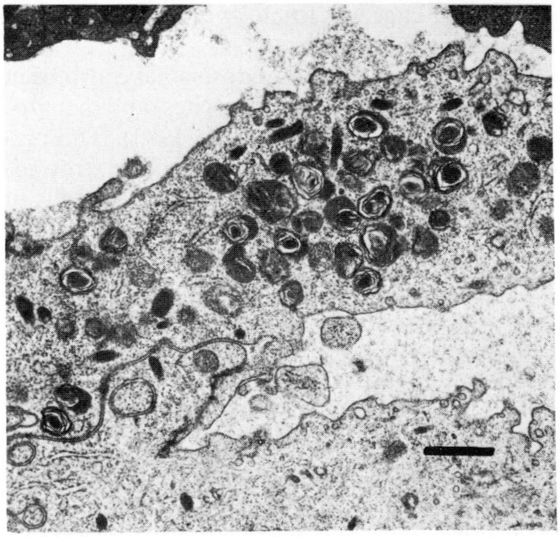

Fig. 12.66 Mucolipidosis IV. Electron micrograph showing membranous cytoplasmic bodies in the endothelial cells of a blood vessel. Bar = 1 μm. ×8800.

Mucolipidosis IV

In contrast with the other mucolipidoses, mucolipidosis IV shows no skeletal abnormalities. Early corneal clouding and progressive psychomotor retardation evident by 1 year are the main features (Goutières, Arsenio-Nunes and Aicardi, 1979). Hepatosplenomegaly may be present. Milder cases have been described with corneal clouding and ataxia as the main problems (Lake et al., 1982). Many described patients have had Ashkenazi Jewish origins.

Urinary mucopolysaccharides are normal but some degree of sialyloligosacchariduria is present. A defect of ganglioside sialidase has been described (Bach et al., 1979).

Neuronal storage in the central (Tellez-Nagel et al., 1976) and peripheral nervous system (Goebel, Kohlschütter and Lenard, 1982) demonstrated by PAS, Sudan black and Luxol fast blue stains is in the form of a few granules. An excess of autofluorescent lipofuscin is also present. The storage bodies are membrane bound and are packed with lamellae similar to the MCBs of the gangliosidoses. Similar inclusions are present in endothelial cells of capillaries (Fig. 12.66), the epithelium of the conjunctiva and skin, and in Schwann cells and fibroblasts. Skeletal muscle cells show numerous inclusions which are red with the modified Gomori trichrome and show acid phosphatase activity (Goebel, Kohlschütter

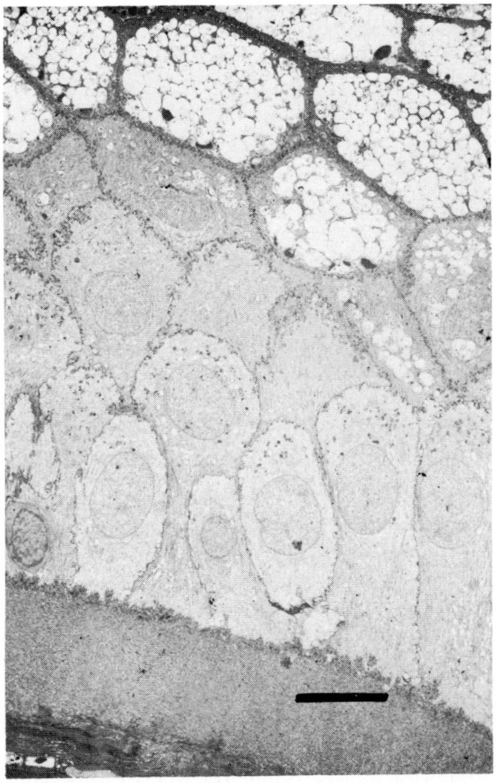

Fig. 12.67 Mucolipidosis IV. Electron micrograph of the corneal epithelium showing marked vacuolation of the surface layers. Bar = 10 μm. ×1200.

and Lenard, 1982). The inclusions are composed of membrane-bound collections of lamellae. Smooth muscle cells and hepatocytes (Livni and Merin, 1978) are similarly affected. Clear vacuoles are present in Kupffer cells, sweat gland epithelium and the superficial epithelial cells of the cornea (Fig. 12.67).

Cultured fibroblasts (Fig. 12.68) and cultured amniotic fluid cells of affected fetuses contain numerous membrane-bound multilamellated inclusions (Livni and Merin, 1978), allowing reliable prenatal diagnosis (Kohn et al., 1982).

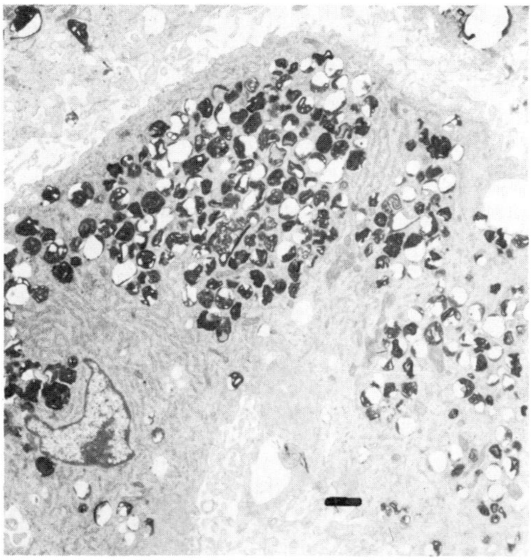

Fig. 12.68 Mucolipidosis IV. Fibroblasts in tissue culture contain numerous membrane-bound multilamellar inclusions. Bar = 1 μm. ×4200.

Mannosidosis

Since the description by Öckerman (1967) of a generalized storage disorder resembling Hurler's syndrome, two main types have emerged (Beaudet, 1983). Cases generally fall into a severe infantile type I or a milder juvenile-adult type II. They all show, to a greater or lesser extent, psychomotor retardation, coarse facies, dysostosis multiplex and recurrent bacterial infections. Deafness, hepatosplenomegaly and corneal or lenticular opacities are also common findings. Although the patients show physical resemblances to patients with mucopolysaccharidosis, the urinary mucopolysaccharide excretion is normal. The disorder is inherited in an autosomal recessive manner.

A defect in lysosomal α-mannosidase activity affecting the isoenzymes A and B, with normal activity of the neutral isoenzyme C, leads to the intralysosomal accumulation of mannose-rich oligosaccharides. The urinary excretion of tri- and tetramannosides is grossly elevated and these can be detected by thin layer chromatography (Humbel and Collart, 1975).

Routine microscopy reveals widespread vacuolation of nerve cells in the cerebral cortex, brain stem and spinal cord with little evidence of storage in the basal ganglia. In the cerebellum there is loss of the granular layer and only a few Purkinje cells remain (Kjellman et al., 1969). Neurons in the peripheral nervous system show marked storage. Apart from neurons, vacuoles are observed in astrocytes, endothelial cells and pericytes (Sung, Hayano and Desnick, 1977). A diffuse gliosis and some loss of myelin may also be seen.

The liver may appear normal in routine sections, but close examination, using plastic sections, will reveal occasional vacuoles in hepatocytes, foamy Kupffer cells and a mild degree of vacuolation in bile duct epithelium. Storage cells similarly may not be evident in the spleen or lymph nodes in routine sections. Fibroblasts, endothelial cells, histiocytes and some epithelial cells are also vacuolated, seen especially clearly in plastic sections.

Marked cytoplasmic vacuolation is present in peripheral blood lymphocytes with some showing a few large discrete vacuoles and others being filled with numerous small discrete vacuoles. In bone marrow aspirate large foamy storage cells are evident in addition to the vacuolated lymphocytes. Characteristically, plasma cells contain several large vacuoles (Fig. 12.69).

The stored oligosaccharides are extremely water-soluble and are lost to routine staining methods. Cryostat sections of snap-frozen tissue, stained by the PAS reaction with reagents made up in 70–90% alcohol (Kjellman et al., 1969), or protected with celloidin before staining by the PAS reaction (Lake, 1983b), will demonstrate the mannose-rich oligosaccharides. Blood films can be stained similarly and the lymphocytes in the thicker parts of the film are positive, in contrast with those in the tail of the film whose vacuoles have probably been ruptured during spreading. No lipid inclusions are present in the brain or visceral organs. An acid phosphatase reaction will show enhanced activity in affected cells and indicate involvement where none may

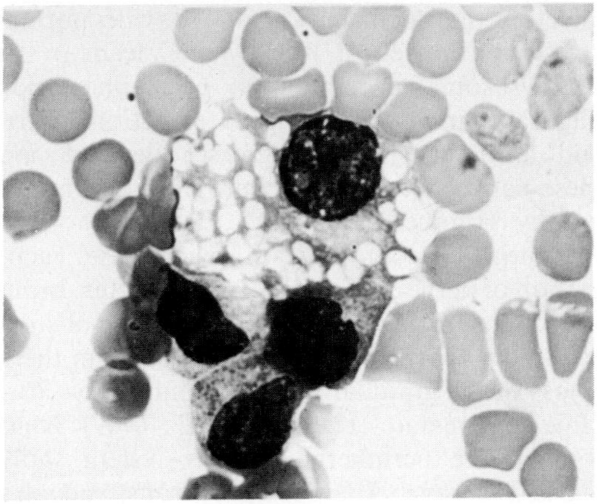

Fig. 12.69 Mannosidosis. Bone marrow film. A plasma cell contains clearly defined vacuoles. May-Grünwald-Giemsa ×950.

be apparent by routine methods. The histochemical method for demonstration of α-mannosidase activity cannot be used for diagnosis because of the presence of isoenzyme C in mannosidosis.

Electron microscopy shows that the membrane-bound vacuoles contain a reticulogranular material without specific features. The vacuoles in plasma cells contain in addition a few lamellar structures.

Diagnosis is made from the clinical presentation, absence of mucopolysacchariduria, presence of vacuolated lymphocytes and assay of α-mannosidase in leucocytes.

Mannosidosis occurs in Angus cattle (Jolly, 1971; Hocking, Jolly and Batt, 1972) and in Persian cats (Vandeville et al., 1982). The disorder can be induced by the α-mannosidase inhibitor swainsonine (an indolizidine alkaloid) which occurs naturally in legumes of the genus *Swainsona* and has been responsible for outbreaks of Swainsona toxicosis in sheep, horses and cattle (Huxtable, Dorling and Walkley, 1982). The animal model shows similar pathology to the human disorder, but axonal spheroids appear more frequently.

Jones et al. (1983) have described the clinical and pathological features of mannosidosis in Nubian goats caused by a deficiency of β-mannosidase activity. Membrane-bound vacuoles were present in most cell types. This disorder has so far not been described in man.

Fucosidosis

Fucosidosis exists in two main forms (Beaudet, 1983). Type I, first described by Durand, Borrone and Della Cella (1969), presents before the age of 1 year with respiratory infections followed at about 1 year by mental and motor regression. Hepatomegaly may be present, and mild to moderate dysostosis multiplex resembling mucopolysaccharidosis type I is found. A high ionic concentration of sweat electrolytes is common. Death occurs in the first decade. Type II has a milder more prolonged course with mental retardation becoming evident at between 1 and 2 years (Patel, Watanabe and Zeman, 1972). Facial appearance and skeletal x-rays are very similar to mucopolysaccharidosis type I, and angiokeratomata, identical to those in Fabry's disease, are found in all cases. Sweat electrolytes are normal. Clear-cut distinction between the two types is complicated by the occurrence of both types within one family (Romeo et al., 1977).

A defect in α-fucosidase activity was first recognized and it was later shown that α-fucosidase isoenzymes separated by electrophoresis show no activity in patients with the disease (MacPhee and Logan, 1977). The enzyme can be assayed in tissues, leucocytes and cultured fibroblasts. Prenatal detection is possible. Fucose-rich compounds have been isolated in large amounts from urine, liver and serum. The structure of these glycolipids and oligosaccharides shows a terminal fucose group and has similarities to the H and Lewis blood group substances.

The brain may be enlarged (Durand, Borrone and Della Cella, 1969) or small (Dahms et al., 1979), and shows marked neuronal ballooning with some neuronal loss particularly in the thalamus and dentate nucleus. Purkinje cells are severely depleted. There is loss of myelin with advanced gliosis, and in one case numerous Rosenthal fibres were present giving an appearance of Alexander's leucodystrophy (Garcia, McGarry and Duncan, 1980). Marked vacuolar storage is present in hepatocytes, Kupffer cells and bile duct epithelium, and the gall bladder has been described as 'strawberry-like' and nonfunctioning in two cases (Durand, Borrone and Della Cella, 1969). The adrenals in these cases were small and atrophic. Granulovacuolar storage is seen in almost all organs, including kidney (where the glomerular epithelium shows ballooning), spleen, lymph nodes, lungs, heart and endocrine glands. Vascular endothelial cells, fibroblasts and sweat glands all show marked vacuolation. Foam cells are present (variably) in bone marrow and vacuolated lymphocytes are common in type I but less frequent in type II. Extensive granuloma-like nodules composed of storage cells were present in the lungs of one case (Dahms et al., 1979). The stored material is extremely soluble and eludes most attempts to demonstrate the contents of the vacuoles. By electron microscopy the vacuoles are membrane-bound and are generally empty although some contain parallel lamellae around the periphery of the vacuole (Freitag et al., 1971). Lamellar inclusions and empty inclusions are present in neurons and astrocytes whilst clear inclusions only are observed in oligodendroglia (Loeb et al., 1969a). Cultured fibroblasts contain numerous vacuoles with parallel lamellae occupying part of the vacuole (Van Hoof, 1973b). Vascular tortuosities can be observed in the conjunctival capillaries and retinal veins late and inconstantly, and electron microscopy of conjunctival biopsies can provide useful diagnostic information (Libert and Toussaint, 1982).

Aspartylglycosaminuria

Aspartylglycosaminuria is a slowly progressive condition which presents in the first year of life with recurrent infections, diarrhoea and umbilical or inguinal hernia (Beaudet, 1983). Coarse facies and sagging coarse skin are evident in the first decade, and by this time mental retardation is apparent. Joint laxity, macroglossia, short stature, a systolic murmur and mild dysostosis multiplex are also described. Hepatosplenomegaly is not frequently observed, but where present regresses with age. Excitable, psychotic behaviour may develop in adult patients. One patient with angiokeratomata has been described (Gehler et al., 1981).

There is marked urinary excretion of aspartylglycosylamine and other glycoasparagines, and a mild increase in tissue levels of aspartylglycosylamine (Palo and Savolainen, 1972). The activity of the lysosomal enzyme aspartylglycosylamine amidohydrolase is very low in plasma, reduced to less than 25 per cent of normal in liver, somewhat reduced in brain but is normal in kidney in spite of ample evidence of storage (Arstila et al., 1972; Palo et al., 1972). Leucocytes show no activity (Isenberg and Sharp, 1975).

The mode of inheritance is autosomal recessive. The disorder is common in Finland but has also been described in England, Italy, the United States and Norway.

In the few cases which have come to autopsy, no consistent macroscopic change is seen in the brain. One Finnish patient showed cranial hyperostosis and cerebral atrophy, whilst in one of the English patients the brain was grossly normal and the patient died of bronchial carcinoma with secondaries in the liver. Her heart showed thickened and crenated mitral valves, a feature also noted in the Finnish patient (Haltia, Palo and Autio, 1975).

By light microscopy the neuronal cytoplasm is seen to be filled with poorly defined vacuoles, the changes being noticeable in the cerebral cortex and basal ganglia but less evident in the brain stem. No storage material can be detected in the neuronal vacuoles. Neurons and glial cells also contain excess lipofuscin, which may also be present in the liver. Marked vacuolation is found in hepatocytes, with the vacuoles often being larger than the nucleus. Kupffer cells are packed with vacuoles and the bile duct epithelium is also vacuolated (Haltia, Palo and Autio, 1975). The vacuoles appear empty, and no lipid, carbohydrate or mucopolysaccharide can be detected. Acid phosphatase activity is strong in the hepatocytes, Kupffer cells and bile duct epithelium. In the kidney, abnormally large lysosomes are present in the glomerular epithelial cells and in the proximal tubules. Minor vacuolar changes may be seen in other visceral organs.

Electron microscopy shows that the vacuoles are membrane bound and essentially empty. A few wispy lamellae may be present. The lipofuscin in enlarged lysosomes is present in neurons, glial cells and the kidney.

Peripheral blood films contain vacuolated lymphocytes and although they may be difficult to find in some patients the vacuoles are large, bold and membrane bound.

The marked vacuolation in the liver and brain is surprising in view of the relatively small amount of storage material present and it is possible that osmotic effects or detergent action may be responsible for the changes.

Salla disease

A group of patients from the Salla area of north-eastern Finland have severe mental retardation, coarse facial features and clumsiness (Aula et al., 1979). Onset is in the first year with psychomotor retardation. No corneal clouding is seen, and fits occur in only about one-third of patients. No enzyme defect is known, and apart from a raised urinary free sialic acid no biochemical abnormality has been found. Urinary mucopolysaccharides and aspartylglycosylamine are normal.

Vacuolated lymphocytes are present in peripheral blood, and by electron microscopy dermal fibroblasts, sweat gland epithelium and Schwann cells show membrane-bound vacuoles. Occasional vacuolation is also found in endothelial and smooth muscle cell cytoplasm. Cultured fibroblasts are filled with membrane-bound vacuoles.

Fabry's disease

Fabry's disease (Desnick and Sweeley, 1983) often presents first with the skin lesion which occurs as clusters of punctate red-black telangiectases in the bathing trunk area and mucous membranes, and it is this lesion which led to the early label of angiokeratoma corporis diffusum. The lesions are not specific for Fabry's disease and occur in fucosidosis, sialidosis (ML I) and aspartylglucosaminuria. However, although they are present in the majority of patients with Fabry's disease, absence of angiokeratomata does not exclude the diagnosis (Clarke et al., 1971; Flynn et al., 1972). Proteinuria is often found early in the disease and the renal problems progress to total renal insufficiency. Retinal, conjunctival and corneal abnormalities are present in most if not all patients from an early age (Franceschetti, 1976). Attacks of burning pain in the extremities and paraesthesiae are present often associated with fever in many patients. Impairment of autonomic function, with diminished sweating, reduced tear and saliva formation and disordered intestinal mobility, is well recognized (Cable, Kolodny and Adams, 1982). The disorder is X-linked and nearly all patients have the Xg^a blood group antigen. Minor manifestations can occur in the female heterozygote.

The defect of ceramide trihexosidase activity described by Brady et al. (1967) was later shown by Kint (1970) to be an α-galactosidase deficiency. Further studies have shown that, of the two forms of α-galactosidase, the heat-labile A form is deficient in Fabry's disease. The defect results in the accumulation of ceramide trihexoside and ceramide dihexoside, both with terminal α-galactosyl residues, arising from degradation of blood group antigens and globoside. Prenatal diagnosis is possible.

Biopsies of the skin lesions show dilated vessels in the upper dermis with flattening of the overlying basal keratinocytes. Occasionally thrombosed vessels may be observed, and slight to moderate keratosis is seen in some cases. Endothelial cells of all vessels contain, in frozen sections, PAS-positive deposits which mostly stain with Sudan black and show birefringence in polarized light. In the smaller vessels the endothelial cells bulge into the lumen. The smooth muscle cells of arterial and arteriolar walls and pericytes, as well as the arrector pili muscles, contain similar deposits. Sweat gland epithelium is also involved. Although inclusions can be demonstrated in cultural fibroblasts, they are not usually observed in skin biopsy specimens.

In renal biopsies the glomerular epithelium shows marked ballooning and vacuolation, a feature also found in the mucolipidoses, some forms of chronic glomerulonephritis, in the nephrotic syndrome and in hyperlipidaemia (McKenzie and Kincaid-Smith, 1969). Interstitial foam cells and vacuolation of the cells in the loop of Henle and distal tubular epithelium are observed. The staining reactions of these are similar to those observed in the endothelial and smooth muscle cells. The cells of the distal tubules desquamate and the lipid deposits are found in urinary sediment (Frost, Tanaka and Spaeth, 1966) where they occur as large mulberry-like cells and casts which are intensely PAS positive, birefringent and non-metachromatic. Urinary sediment can be extracted with lipid solvents and the lipids characterized by thin layer chromatography. Marked excesses of ceramide trihexoside and ceramide dihexoside are present in all cases and can be detected in asymptomatic individuals even in the neonatal period (Philippart, Sarlieve and Manacorda, 1969). Heterozygotes show mild increases. In the later stages of the disease the renal changes are severe, with glomerular sclerosis and other findings being the sequelae of non-specific end-stage renal disease.

Cardiac muscle fibres also accumulate the deposited lipids, and in some patients mitral insufficiency has been noted in addition to the cardiac hypertrophy and vascular deposition leading to infarction. Foam cells and cells resembling sea-blue histiocytes are present in bone marrow aspirates, but peripheral blood cells show no abnormalities. The cells of the mononuclear-phagocyte system in lymph nodes, spleen and liver and elsewhere exhibit storage, as do the ganglion cells of the peripheral nervous system (Rahman and Lindenberg, 1963; Frost, Tanaka and Spaeth, 1966). Storage is demonstrable in certain neurons in the central nervous system (Kahn, 1973), particularly those in the amygdala, hypothalamus and brain stem. Anterior horn cells and dorsal root ganglia similarly contain deposits of the ceramide trihexoside. The pathology of the brain is mostly related to the vascular changes with small infarcts and ischaemic episodes leading to seizures, hemiplegia and dementia even in the absence of any of the usual symptoms or signs (Morgan-Hughes and Lake, 1982, unpublished observations). Peripheral nerves are only slightly involved, with minor reductions in the numbers of small myelinated fibres (Kocen and Thomas, 1970; Tomé, Fardeau and Lenoir, 1977) and evidence of storage in perineurial cells and in the vascular endothelium.

Histochemical studies of the deposits (Lehner and Adams, 1968) in all sites show that they are generally removed during processing, but in frozen or cryostat sections the deposits stain strongly with PAS (Fig. 12.70), are positive with Sudan black and show birefringence. The deposits also contain cholesterol. In routine paraffin sections some sudanophilia and birefringence are retained and the deposits also stain with Luxol fast blue. Acid phosphatase activity is demonstrable within the affected endothelial, epithelial, muscle and phagocytic cells. The presence of α-galactose-linked residues in the deposits can be shown using peroxidase-labelled lectin from *Bandeiraea simplicifolia* which binds specifically to α-galactosyl residues. Electron

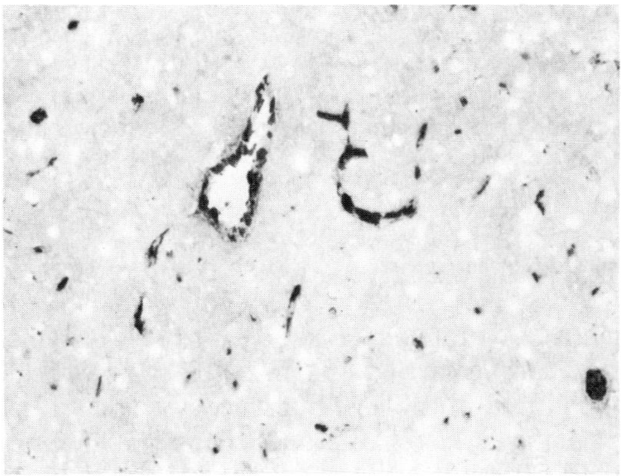

Fig. 12.70 Fabry's disease. Cortical biopsy. Cryostat section. Strongly PAS-positive deposits are seen in endothelial cells of capillaries and larger vessels. × 120.

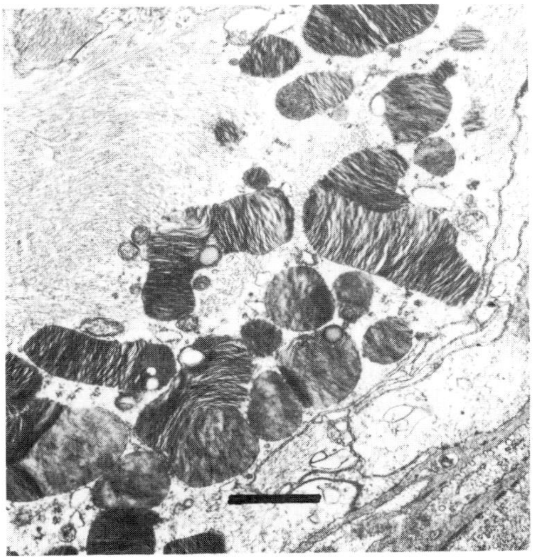

Fig. 12.71 Fabry's disease. Electron micrograph of cortical biopsy. Membrane-bound collections of lipid lamellae are present in the cytoplasm of an astrocyte. Bar = 1 μm. × 11500.

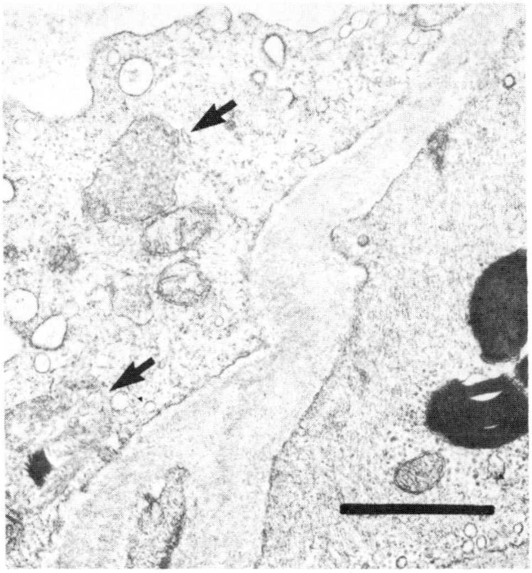

Fig. 12.72 Fabry's disease. Electron micrograph showing tubular inclusions (arrows) in an endothelial cell, and lipid lamellae in a smooth muscle cell. Bar = 1 μm. × 18600.

microscopic examination of affected cells and tissues (Frost, Tanaka and Spaeth, 1966; Malmqvist et al., 1971; Kint and Carton, 1973) shows collections of inclusions measuring 0.1–10 μm which are composed of tightly packed lipid lamellae with a periodicity of 40–100 Å depending on the site, the age of the patient and/or the processing schedule used. The lamellae may be concentric or parallel and can appear as stacks or as interwoven curved segments (Tomé, Fardeau and Lenoir, 1977). Although, by light microscopy, skeletal muscle cells do not appear to be involved, rare inclusions may be found at ultrastructural study. In the brain, astrocytes may show marked storage (Fig. 12.71) in addition to the vascular accumulation. Most inclusions appear as lamellae but occasionally tubular inclusions (Fig. 12.72) not dissimilar to those in Gaucher's disease may be found in endothelial cells (Frost, Tanaka and Spaeth, 1966), hepatocytes and skeletal muscle. These tubular inclusions correspond to the brightly PAS-positive, non-sudanophilic and non-birefringent deposits.

Prenatal diagnosis, achieved by assay of α-galactosidase A in cultured amniotic fluid cells, has been successful in detecting affected and normal fetuses (Brady, Uhlendorf and Jacobson, 1971; Galjaard et al., 1974; Malouf, Kirkman and Buchanan, 1976). Light microscopic examination of affected terminated fetuses is unremarkable but by electron microscopy involvement of the renal glomerulus and tubules is apparent. Increased ceramide trihexoside levels are present in all tissues except brain.

Type II glycogenosis

Type II glycogenosis (Pompe's disease, generalized glycogenosis, acid maltase deficiency) was the first of the lysosomal enzyme deficiencies to be recognized (Hers, 1963) and it was soon found that there was a wide spectrum of clinical presentation with juveniles and adults being affected (Hers and de Barsy, 1973).

Infants present at or soon after birth with marked hypotonia, cardiomegaly and sometimes hepatomegaly. Occasionally, macroglossia is seen and respiratory problems related to cardiac dysfunction lead to death from pulmonary infection or cardiorespiratory insufficiency before the age of 2 years. Juveniles present similarly to patients with muscular dystrophy. Limb girdle and trunk weakness, a positive Gowers' manoeuvre and respiratory problems may be found. Adults with respiratory muscle weakness and weakness of other skeletal muscles present in the second or third decade (Engel et al., 1973). The disorder is inherited as an autosomal recessive trait.

The gross deposition of glycogen is caused by deficient activity of acid maltase (acid α-1,4-glucosidase), the enzyme protein being present but

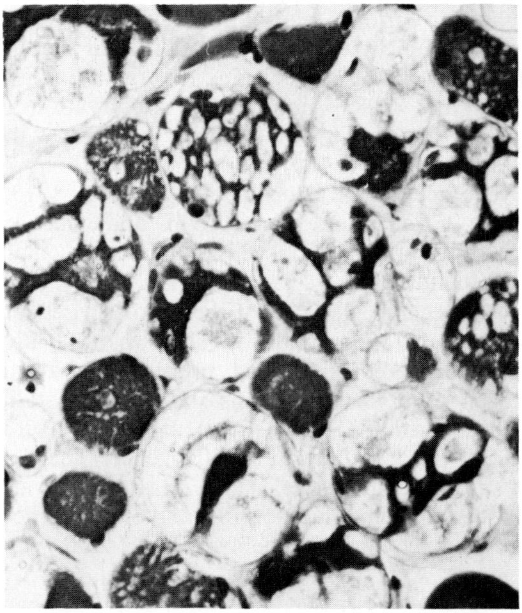

Fig. 12.73 Juvenile type II glycogenosis. Transverse cryostat section of muscle biopsy. There is marked vacuolar change within the myofibres. Gomori trichrome ×330.

inactive (Ninomiya et al., 1983). The enzyme assay can be carried out on tissue samples and on cultured fibroblasts but leucocyte assays are not sufficiently reliable due to the presence of other α-1,4-glucosidases. Prenatal detection is possible by assay of cultured amniotic fluid cells obtained by amniocentesis.

Skeletal muscle is affected in all forms of the disease. A vacuolar myopathy (Fig. 12.73), which is extreme in infants and moderate in juveniles and most adults, may be mild or nonexistent in some adults. The vacuoles are filled with glycogen and have strong acid phosphatase activity. In the infant the glycogen content can be up to ten times the normal with almost complete distortion of the architecture. Type 2 muscle fibres are often more affected than type 1 fibres in the adult. The presence of a metachromatic substance, putatively identified as an acid mucosubstance, has been noted in most of the infantile and juvenile cases but is rare in the adult patient (Wolfe and Cohen, 1968; Engel et al., 1973). Areas where the excess glycogen is deposited show strong acid phosphatase activity, and even fibres which appear normal have discrete foci of acid phosphatase activity. Capillary endothelium and smooth muscle cells of large and small arteries and arterioles contain excess glycogen and show acid phosphatase activity. In the infantile form, the heart is grossly enlarged and all fibres are vacuolated and contain excess glycogen. Although the acid maltase activity of the heart in the juvenile and adult forms is deficient, excess glycogen is not seen (Engel et al., 1973). Kupffer cells in the liver and hepatocytes both store an excess of glycogen and show strong acid phosphatase activity. As in the heart, the juvenile and adult forms have little evidence of storage despite deficient hepatic acid maltase activity. Cells of the mononuclear-phagocyte system in the spleen contain excess glycogen, and smooth muscle cells of the circular and longitudinal muscle coats of the gastrointestinal tract are similarly involved. Neuronal glycogen storage is evident in the myenteric and submucosal plexuses of the gut in the anterior horn cells of the spinal cord (Fig. 12.74), motor cranial nerve nuclei and parts of the basal ganglia and brain stem in the infantile (Mancall, Aponte and Berry,

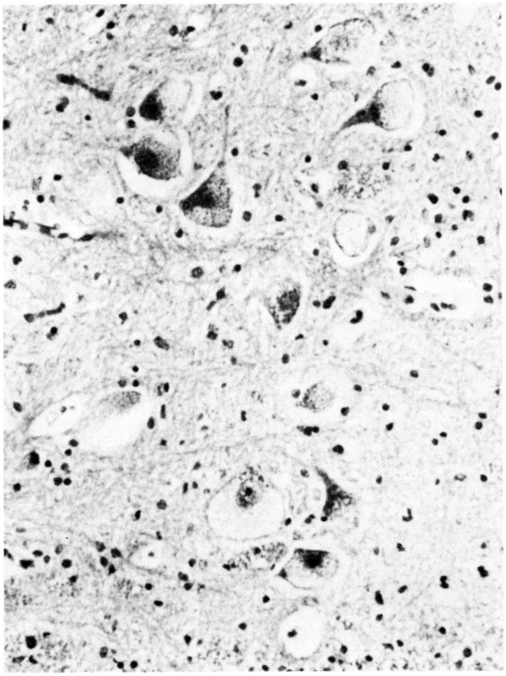

Fig. 12.74 Infantile type II glycogenosis. Anterior horn cells of the spinal cord are markedly ballooned by storage of glycogen. Haematoxylin and eosin × 200.

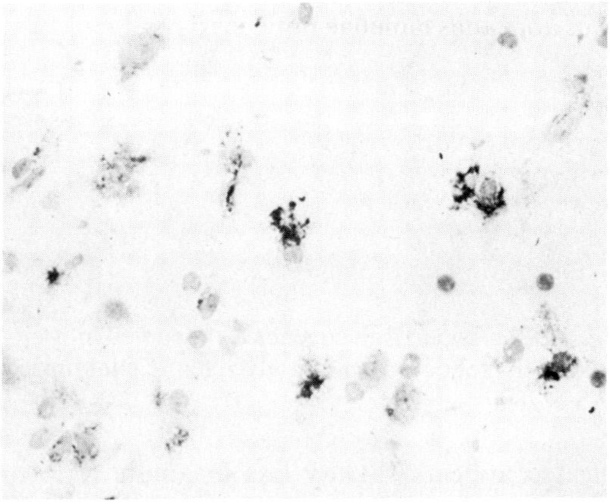

Fig. 12.75 Infantile type II glycogenosis. Cerebral cortex. Glycogen storage is marked in astrocytes but not in neurons. Cryostat section. Celloidinized PAS × 270.

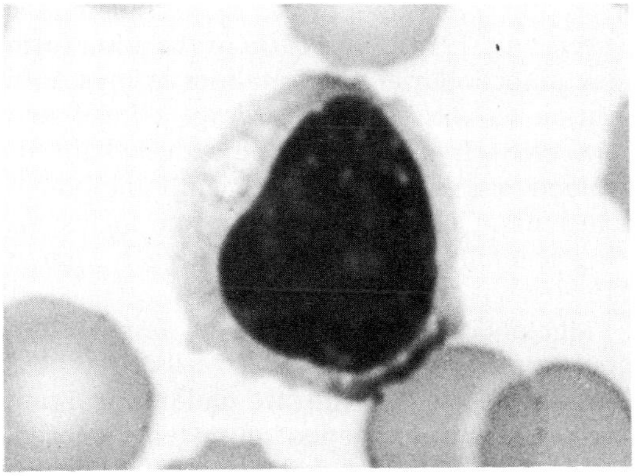

Fig. 12.76 Type II glycogenosis. A lymphocyte from peripheral blood contains several small discrete vacuoles. May-Grünwald-Giemsa × 2800.

1965) and childhood forms (Matsuishi et al., 1982). Glycogen deposition is prominent in astrocytes (Fig. 12.75) in the cerebral cortex and white matter. Some degree of gliosis may be evident but myelination appears normal.

In all forms of the disease, peripheral blood lymphocytes show small discrete cytoplasmic vacuoles which contain glycogen (Figs. 12.76 and 12.77). The proportion of lymphocytes

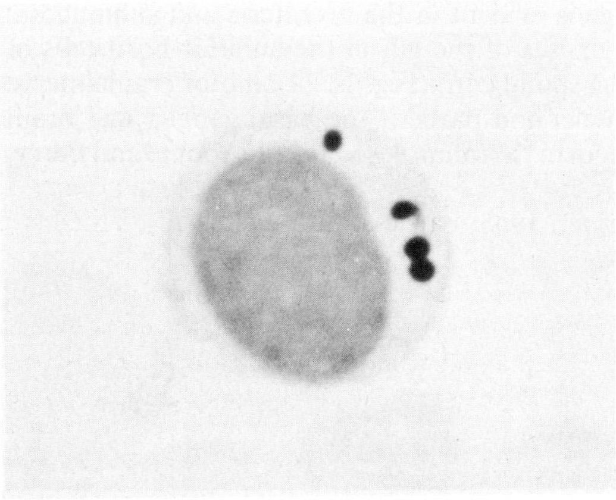

Fig. 12.77 Type II glycogenosis. Vacuoles in a circulating lymphocyte contain glycogen. Celloidinized PAS ×2800.

affected appears slightly less in adults than in infants where most lymphocytes are involved. Screening of peripheral blood films is reliable and affords the simplest diagnostic procedure without resort to biopsy.

Electron microscopy reveals the glycogen within membrane-bound vacuoles in the liver (Baudhuin, Hers and Loeb, 1964) and muscle (Engel et al., 1973). Rare cases of the adult form show mitochondrial abnormalities in muscle in addition to the glycogen storage (Engel and Dale, 1968). Lymphocytes and endothelial cells of blood vessels also contain membrane-bound inclusions of glycogen particles, the inclusions being generally round and measuring 1–2 μm in diameter.

Prenatal detection is possible by assay of cultured amniotic fluid cells. These cells, and those from skin biopsies of affected children, contain discrete membrane-bound glycogen deposits, and diagnosis by electron microscopy may be made even on uncultured amniotic fluid cells (Hug, 1974). Affected fetuses show excess glycogen in Kupffer cells and hepatocytes, but heart and skeletal muscle do not appear abnormal by light microscopy. The placenta affords good evidence of lysosomal storage within endothelial cells and smooth muscle cells of vessel walls (Fig. 12.78). Generalized glycogenosis has been described in cats, dogs, sheep and Japanese quails (Desnick, Patterson and Scarpelli, 1982) and in cattle (Howell et al., 1981).

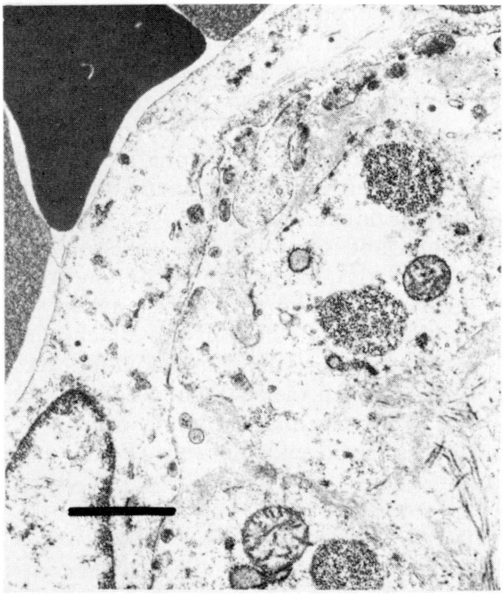

Fig. 12.78 Type II glycogenosis. Placenta. Membrane-bound glycogen deposits are seen within a smooth muscle cell adjacent to a capillary endothelial cell in a villus. Bar = 1 μm. × 14000.

Farber's disease

Farber's disease (Farber's lipogranulomatosis) is characterized by onset in the early months of life with painful swelling of joints and subcutaneous nodules over the affected joints, a hoarse cry and respiratory and feeding difficulties. Psychomotor retardation is usually evident. Death usually occurs within the first or second year of life although a number of patients with milder involvement and long survival have now been reported (Moser and Chen, 1983).

Chemical studies show a marked increase in the concentration of free ceramide. Liver, brain and kidney ceramides contain mainly hydroxylated fatty acids, whilst those isolated from the subcutaneous nodules contain exclusively non-hydroxylated fatty acids. Increases in glycolipids and mucopolysaccharides have been reported but the increases probably represent the high concentrations of ganglioside G_{M3} described by Moser et al. (1969). The ceramide excess is a result of a deficiency of lysosomal ceramidase. Neutral and alkaline ceramidase activity is normal (Sugita, Dulaney and Moser, 1972).

Neuronal storage is present and is particularly marked in the brain stem, basal ganglia and anterior horn cells of the spinal cord. Cortical neurons and neurons in the gastrointestinal tract also show storage but to a lesser extent. Nerve cell loss, neuronophagia and gliosis may also be present. Routine microscopy of the liver is essentially normal but numerous foamy cells are present in the red pulp of the spleen, in the lungs and in lymph nodes where the architecture may be grossly distorted. Collections of storage cells may also be found in the endocardium, and endothelial cells of blood vessels and the epithelial cells of bile ducts also display storage. The subcutaneous nodules consist of collections of foam cells, which in some areas occur as granulomata with macrophages lymphocytes and multinucleate giant cells. Similar granulomata occur in the lungs. Scattered foam cells are present in the bone marrow.

The stored material in neurons shows strong PAS positivity and weak sudanophila and is birefringent in polarized light. The substance also is positive with Alcian blue. Similar staining reactions are also present among the foam cells. It is probable that the PAS and Alcian blue reactions indicate the increased ganglioside content, and the weak sudanophilia and birefringence relate to the ceramide deposition. An acid phosphatase reaction shows marked involvement of the hepatocytes and identifies the affected endothelial cells and foamy cells.

Electron microscopy of neurons shows zebra bodies which may also be present in endothelial cells. Membrane-bound collections of lipid lamellae are found in hepatocytes together with large empty membrane-bound vacuoles. The vacuoles in other organs are usually empty except in the dermal foamy cells where small curvilinear tubular structures fill the vacuoles. Curvilinear inclusions, which occasionally may be found elsewhere, are considered an indication of ceramides containing non-hydroxylated fatty acids (Rutsaert et al., 1977).

Prenatal diagnosis by assay of acid ceramidase activity in cultured amniotic fluid cells is possible; an affected fetus showed increased ceramide levels in liver and kidney with ultrastructural evidence of zebra bodies in the brain stem (Fensom et al., 1979).

Wolman's disease and cholesteryl ester storage disease

These disorders represent both ends of the spectrum of acid lipase (acid esterase) deficiency. Wolman's disease presents in early infancy with diarrhoea, vomiting and failure to thrive. There is hepatosplenomegaly, and adrenal calcification in most; a rapid course with anaemia and fevers leads to death usually before the age of 6 months (Abramov, Schorr and Wolman, 1956; Crocker et al., 1965; Patrick and Lake, 1973). There is a slightly milder variant in infants who present with abdominal distension and mild attacks of diarrhoea and vomiting. Their course is variable but most survive to enjoy reasonable health and suffer only mild hepatomegaly (Yamaguchi, Tsuchiyama and Tabata, 1971; Patrick and Lake, 1973). In the early 1960s Fredrickson described at a meeting of the American College of Physicians in Denver a single case of cholesteryl ester storage disease in an adult, and later Lageron et al. (1967) and Schiff et al. (1968) described further cases in which asymptomatic hepatomegaly was associated with excessive deposition of cholesteryl esters. Since that time further cases of cholesteryl ester storage disease have been described (Gautier, Lapons and Raulin, 1978), some with a hepatitis-like illness leading to death (Beaudet et al., 1977) and others with radiological evidence of adrenal calcification and pulmonary vascular obstruction (Beaudet et al., 1977; Michels et al., 1979).

An autosomal recessive mode of inheritance is evident in each type and no racial predilection is found.

The lipids deposited in visceral organs consist of a mixture of triglycerides and cholesteryl esters which can be increased up to the order of 100 times the normal level (Assmann and Fredrickson, 1983). The increases in the milder clinical forms are not as marked as in the severe infantile form. In addition to the cholesteryl esters and triglycerides, increases in diglycerides, monoglycerides and free fatty acids are seen, and Lin, Tie and Ho (1976) have reported an increased amount of glyceryl ethers in adrenal, liver and spleen in Wolman's disease. Analysis of lipids in the central nervous system of patients with Wolman's disease has shown a slight increase in cholesteryl esters, with normal gangliosides and variable myelin-lipid decreases. These decreases, or lower levels than normal for age, are probably related to the poor nutritional state of the patients.

Deficient activity of the lysosomal enzyme acid lipase, reported by Patrick and Lake (1969) accounts for the extensive deposition of glycerol esters (triglycerides) and cholesteryl esters. The enzyme also has characteristics as an acid esterase (Lake and Patrick, 1970; Young and Patrick, 1970) and can be assayed using labelled natural substrates, *p*-nitrophenyl esters or long chain esters of 4-methylumbelliferone (Schaub et al., 1980). The defect is the same in all variants and can be assayed in tissues (Patrick and Lake, 1969), leucocytes (Young and Patrick, 1970) or cultured fibroblasts (Beaudet et al., 1974). Acid esterase is present in normal cultured amniotic fluid cells, allowing prenatal detection of a fetus affected with Wolman's disease (Patrick et al., 1976). Fetal tissues from the abortus showed increased cholesteryl esters and a severe deficiency of acid esterase.

In Wolman's disease the liver and spleen are enlarged and may weigh between two and five times the normal weight for age. The cut surface of these organs appears yellow/orange and has a greasy homogeneous appearance. Lymph nodes, thymus and tonsils are enlarged and yellowish. The adrenals are, in most cases, symmetrically enlarged with a normal configuration and are yellow and gritty on cutting. Diffuse calcification, evident by radiology during life, is more pronounced in the deeper layers of the cortex. Rare cases show no radiological evidence of calcification (Guazzi et al., 1968; Kyriakides et al., 1970) whilst others may show no adrenal enlargement at autopsy (Schaub et al., 1980). The surface of the small intestine has a yellowish velvet-like appearance, more noticeable proximally. The colon is often grossly normal although yellow patches may be seen. Kidney, heart, lungs and muscles appear normal. The brain shows no gross changes and the cut surface reveals normal demarcation between cortex and white matter (Byrd and Powers, 1979).

In cholesteryl ester storage disease, few gross pathological studies have been made (Assmann and Fredrickson, 1983) but those that have report on the brilliant orange-yellow colour of the liver, which Lageron et al. (1967) referred to as the colour of fresh butter. The spleen may or may not be enlarged; adrenal enlargement was seen in two cases (Beaudet et al., 1977) and in one case adrenal calcification was visible on radiological examination. Atheromatous plaques present in the coronary artery were not thought to be significant in one patient (Assmann and Fredrickson, 1983). Death was due to aortic valvular stenosis in that case. In none of the patients has there been clinical evidence of coronary or systemic atherosclerosis.

Microscopically the main feature of Wolman's disease is the abundant nature of lipid-laden foamy cells of the mononuclear-phagocyte system which are present in the liver, spleen, lymph nodes, bone marrow, lungs, testes, ovaries, thyroid, thymus and adrenals. The hepatocytes also have a foamy appearance and there may be pronounced portal fibrosis or even cirrhosis. Occasional foamy cells may be seen in the renal glomerulus whilst the lamina propria of the small intestine is filled with foamy cells which also occur to a lesser degree in the large intestine. Some of the foam cells, particularly those of the liver and adrenal show acicular crystalline inclusions of cholesteryl esters (Fig. 12.79). In the

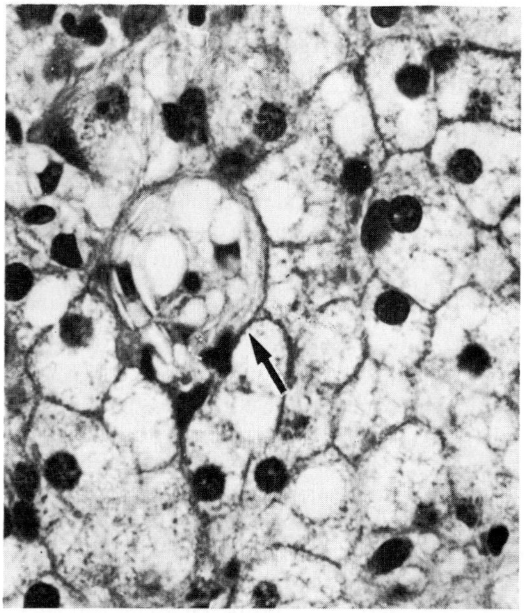

Fig. 12.79 Wolman's disease. Liver biopsy. Lipid vacuoles are present within hepatocytes, and a storage cell (arrow) contains crystalline shapes of cholesteryl esters. Haematoxylin and eosin ×720.

adrenal the zona glomerulosa is preserved and the outer zona fasciculata is less severely affected. Most change occurs in the inner portion of the zona fasciculata and the zona reticularis where large foamy cells (Fig. 12.80), some containing large 'cholesterol clefts', fill the space. Focal areas of necrosis are common, and calcification in fine granular deposits or larger aggregates accounts for the gritty feel. The medulla is generally unaffected.

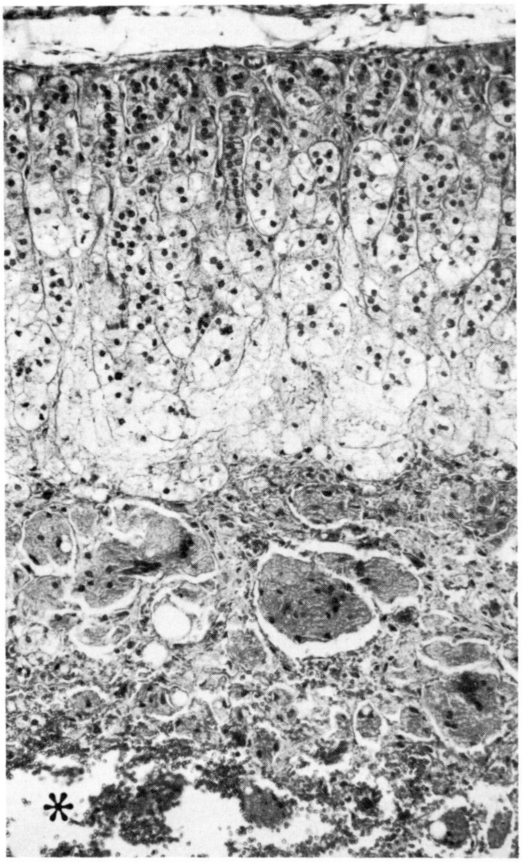

Fig. 12.80 Wolman's disease. Adrenal. The zona fasciculata and zona reticularis contain many large multinucleated histiocytes. Necrosis and calcification are evident (*). Haematoxylin and eosin × 140.

In the central nervous system, light microscopy reveals only minor changes (Byrd and Powers, 1979) but there may be a diffuse fibrillary gliosis throughout the white matter (Guazzi et al., 1968), with foamy cells present in the leptomeninges and choroid plexus.

The foamy storage cells contain vacuoles which 'whether large or small have clear cut margins' (Abramov, Schorr and Wolman, 1956) and stain intensely with the Sudan dyes. The Schultz reaction, or the perchloric acid-naphthoquinone method for cholesterol and its esters (Filipe and Lake, 1983) is strongly positive in the foamy cells and hepatocytes. With Nile blue the hepatocytes stain red, whilst the portal macrophages and Kupffer cells are purple—indicating the presence of free fatty acids in addition to cholesteryl esters. The Sudan dyes demonstrate lipid deposition in endothelial cells and there may be marked lipid accumulation in smooth, skeletal and cardiac muscle. Neurons of the central nervous system do not contain lipid but those in the myenteric and submucosal plexuses of the gut may show marked storage which is particularly evident in the small intestine (Kamoshita and Landing, 1968). Occasional lipid deposition may be noted in astrocytes and oligodendroglial cells. Lipid deposits are markedly birefringent when examined mounted in aqueous media. Maltese crosses may be apparent but most of the lipid is present in the form of acicular crystals (Marshall et al., 1969).

In all organs the foamy storage cells possess strong acid phosphatase activity with the reaction product outlining the lipid droplets or crystals. Acid esterase activity is deficient in appropriately prepared tissue sections (Lake and Patrick, 1970; Patrick and Lake, 1973), and in peripheral lymphocytes (Lake, 1971) which also show lipid deposits in cytoplasmic vacuoles.

Electron microscopy reveals that the lipid droplets and crystals are membrane bound (Fig. 12.81) and that the membranes are associated with acid phosphatase activity, indicating their derivation from lysosomes (Lake and Patrick, 1970). In the central nervous system (Byrd and Powers, 1979) lipid deposition occurs in oligodendrocytes and astrocytes but not in neurons. In peripheral nerve, perineurial, endoneurial and Schwann cells lipid inclusions were mostly membrane bound.

In the fetus affected by Wolman's disease (Patrick et al., 1976) increased triglyceride and cholesteryl esters were present in liver and adrenal. The deposits stained strongly with Sudan dyes, and macrophages staining purple with Nile blue were present in the liver (Lake, 1977). Calcification was already apparent in the adrenals at 19 weeks' gestation. No lipid deposits were seen in the small bowel.

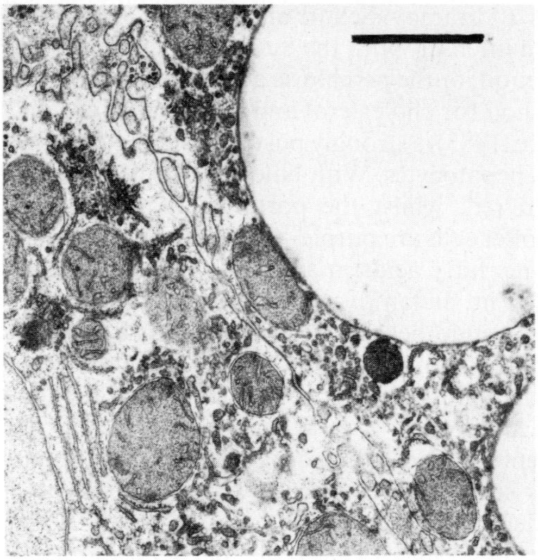

Fig. 12.81 Wolman's disease. Electron micrograph of liver biopsy. Lipid deposits in the hepatocytes are membrane-bound. Bar = 1 μm. × 16000.

Initial screening of peripheral blood films reveals a few small discrete vacuoles in the cytoplasm of many lymphocytes, and these vacuoles stain with the Sudan dyes. The number of affected lymphocytes is greater in Wolman's disease, but a significant number can also be found in cholesteryl ester storage disease. Bone marrow samples, prepared as films rather than embedded tissue blocks, contain large foamy lipid-laden macrophages which are more prominent in Wolman's disease. A combination of vacuolated lymphocytes and bone marrow histiocytes in which neutral fat can be demonstrated is almost diagnostic. The activity of acid esterase can be assayed in leucocytes or cultured fibroblasts, or by histochemical staining. Where enzyme assay is not available a liver biopsy will establish the diagnosis, particularly if frozen tissue is examined and electron microscopy is carried out on an appropriately fixed sample.

Leav et al. (1968) described budgerigars with a lipidosis resembling Wolman's disease, but although lipid analyses were done no enzymic studies are available. The distribution of lesions, with hepatocytes apparently uninvolved and with no distinction being made between ester cholesterol and free cholesterol, no conclusions can be drawn.

Cystinosis

Three forms of cystinosis occur (Seegmiller, 1973). The severe nephropathic form presents in infants with failure to thrive and a Fanconi syndrome with progressive renal failure leading to death in the first decade. Deposition of cystine crystals within the conjunctiva and a mass of needle-shaped crystals in the cornea with depigmentation of the retina give rise to symptoms of photophobia (Wong, 1976). The patients are generally of fair complexion and have fair hair. An intermediate form, with the onset of renal disease later and survival to the second or third decade, is also known. A benign form of cystinosis without apparent renal involvement, but with the corneal and retinal changes, is also described.

Deposition of cystine is widespread and the crystals are mainly present within cells of the mononuclear-phagocyte system of liver, spleen and lymph nodes. Abundant crystals are present in the lamina propria of the gastrointestinal tract. Smooth muscle cells are also affected, and some cells containing cystine are present in the renal medulla and occasionally in the glomerulus. Diagnosis is usually made with unfixed films of bone marrow aspirates examined by polarized light (Fig. 12.82). The crystals of cystine are relatively soluble and are lost from tissues and

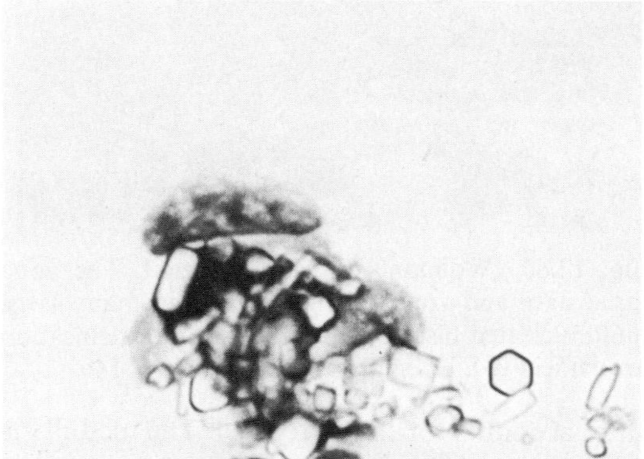

Fig. 12.82 Cystinosis. Bone marrow film in partially polarized light. Note the hexagonal and rectangular crystals. × 1000.

touch preparations during fixation in aqueous agents and in the floating out and staining of sections. Cryostat sections of snap-frozen tissue, bone marrow films or touch preparations can be stained with 1% basic fuchsin in 70% alcohol to show nuclei without loss of crystals. No neuronal storage is seen but in occasional cases cystine crystals are found in the brain. Levine and Paparo (1982) found demyelination of the internal capsule and bilateral necrosis of the internal capsule and brachium pontis with abundant cystine deposition in the choroid plexus.

By electron microscopy the crystals are present within lysosomes, are membrane bound and associated with acid phosphatase activity (Patrick and Lake, 1968). Although leucocytes and cultured cells have a high cystine content, crystals are not observed.

Prenatal diagnosis by estimation of ^{35}S-cystine incorporation in cultured amniotic fluid cells (Willcox and Patrick, 1974) is successful in detecting affected fetuses. In fetuses of less than 20 weeks' gestation the only microscopical abnormality is vacuolation of the retinal epithelium. No evidence of cystine crystal deposition is present. However, Haynes et al., (1980) have shown by light and electron microscopy that cystine crystals were present in Kupffer cells of the liver of a 22-week-old fetus.

Renal transplantation initially corrects the renal failure but has no effect on the leucocyte cystine concentration and eventually cystine crystals appear within the transplanted kidney.

References

Abraham, K. and Lampert, P. (1963) Intraneuronal lipid deposits in metachromatic leukodystrophy. *Neurology* **13,** 686–92.

Abramov, A., Schorr, S. and Wolman, M. (1956) Generalized xanthomatosis with calcified adrenals. *American Journal of Diseases of Children* **91,** 282–6.

Adachi, M., Schneck, L. and Volk, B. W. (1974) Ultrastructural studies of eight cases of fetal Tay-Sachs disease. *Laboratory Investigation* **30,** 102–12.

Adachi, M. and Volk, B. W. (1977) Gaucher disease in mice induced by conduritol-β-epoxide. Morphologic features. *Archives of Pathology and Laboratory Medicine* **101,** 255–9.

Adachi, M., Wallace, B.J., Schneck, L. and Volk, B.W. (1972) Fine structure of central nervous system in early infantile Gaucher's disease. *Archives of Pathology* **83,** 513–26.

Allen, N. and de Veyra, E. (1967) Microchemical and histochemical observations in a case of Krabbe's leukodystrophy. *Journal of Neuropathology and Experimental Neurology* **26,** 456–74.

Alzheimer, A. (1910) Beiträge zur Kenntis der pathologischen Neuroglia und ihrer Beziehungen zu den Abbauvorgängen im Nervengewebe. *Histologische und histopathologische Arbeiten über die Grosshirnrinde* **3,** 401–562.

Anzil, A. P., Blinzinger, K., Mehraein, P. and Dozic, S. (1973) Niemann-Pick disease type C: case report with ultrastructural findings. *Neuropädiatrie* **4,** 207–25.

Armstrong, D. (1982) Peroxidase activity in human and canine ceroid-lipofuscinosis, with special emphasis on the eye. In *Ceroid-lipofuscinosis (Batten's disease)* (Eds. Armstrong, D., Koppang, N. and Rider, J.A.), pp. 247–70. Elsevier Biomedical, Amsterdam.

Armstrong, D., Dimmitt, S. and van Wormer, D. (1974) Studies in Batten's disease. I. Peroxidase deficiency in granulocytes. *Archives of Neurology* **30,** 144–52.

Armstrong, D., van Wormer, D., Neville, H., Dimmitt, S. and Clingan, F. (1975) Thyroid peroxidase deficiency in Batten-Spielmeyer-Vogt disease. *Archives of Pathology and Laboratory Medicine* **99,** 430–5.

Arstila, A. U., Palo, J., Haltia, M., Riekkinen, P. and Autio, S. (1972) Aspartylglucosaminuria, I. Fine structural studies on liver, kidney and brain. *Acta Neuropathologica* **20,** 207–16.

Assmann, G. and Fredrickson, D. S. (1983) Acid lipase deficiency: Wolman's disease and cholesteryl ester storage disease. In *The Metabolic Basis of Inherited Disease.* (Eds. Stanbury, J. B., Wyngaarden, J. B., Fredrickson, D. S., Goldstein, J. L. and Brown, M. S.) 5th edn, pp. 803–19. McGraw-Hill, New York.

Aterman, K. (1979) The development of the concept of lysosomes. A historical survey, with particular reference to liver. *Histochemical Journal* **11,** 503–41.

Aula, P., Autio, S., Raivio, K. O., Rapola, J., Thodén, C.-J., Koskela, S.-L. and Yamashina, I. (1979) Salla disease. A new lysosomal storage disorder. *Archives of Neurology* **36,** 88–94.

Austin, J. H. (1957) Metachromatic form of diffuse sclerosis. I. Diagnosis during life by urine sediment examination. *Neurology* **7,** 415–26.

Austin, J. H. (1958) Observations in metachromatic leukoencephalopathy. *Transactions of the American Neurological Association* **83,** 149–52.

Austin, J.H. (1962a) Recent studies in the metachromatic and globoid forms of diffuse sclerosis. *Ultrastructure and Metabolism of the Nervous System* **40,** 189–221.

Austin, J. H. (1962b) Some newer findings in Krabbe (globoid) leukodystrophy. *Transactions of the American Neurological Association* **87,** 66–71.

Austin, J. H. (1963a) Studies in globoid (Krabbe) leukodystrophy. II. Controlled thin-layer chromatographic studies of globoid body fractions in seven patients. *Journal of Neurochemistry* **10,** 921–30.

Austin, J.H. (1963b) Studies in globoid (Krabbe) leukodystrophy. *Archives of Neurology* **9,** 207–31.

Austin, J. H. (1973) Studies in metachromatic leukodystrophy. XII. Multiple sulfatase deficiency. *Archives of Neurology* **28,** 258–64.

Austin, J.H. and Lehfeldt, D. (1965) Studies in globoid (Krabbe) leucodystrophy. III. Significance of experimentally produced globoid-like elements in rat white matter and spleen. *Journal of Neuropathology and Experimental Neurology* **24,** 265–89.

Austin, J., McAfee, D., Armstrong, D., O'Rourke, M., Shearer, L. and Bachhawat, B. (1964) Abnormal sulphatase activities in two human diseases. *Biochemical Journal* **93,** 15c.

Austin, J., Suzuki, K., Armstrong, D., Brady, R., Bachhawat, B.K., Schlenker, J. and Stumpf, D. (1970) Studies in globoid (Krabbe) leukodystrophy (GLD). V. Controlled enzymic studies in ten human cases. *Archives of Neurology* **23,** 502–12.

Bach, G., Zeigler, M., Schaap, T. and Kohn, G. (1979) Mucolipidosis type IV. Ganglioside sialidase deficiency. *Biochemical and Biophysical Research Communications* **90,** 1341–7.

Bachhawat, B. K., Austin, J. H. and Armstrong, D. (1967) A cerebroside sulphotransferase deficiency in a human disorder of myelin. *Biochemical Journal* **104,** 15c–17c.

Badurska, B., Fidzianska, A. and Jedrzejowska, H. (1981) A dominant form of neuronal ceroid-lipofuscinosis. An ultrastructural study of sural nerve and peripheral lymphocytes. *Journal of Neurology* **226,** 205–12.

de Baecque, C. (1975) Diagnosis of neuronal ceroid-lipofuscinosis by electron microscopy of urinary sediment. *New England Journal of Medicine* **292,** 1408.

de Baecque, C. M., Suzuki, K., Rapin, I., Johnson, A. B., Whethers, D. L. and Suzuki, K. (1975) G_{M2}-gangliosidosis AB variant. Clinicopathological study of a case. *Acta Neuropathologica* **33,** 207–26.

Bagh, Kv. and Hortling, H. (1948) Blodfynd vid juvenil amaurotisk idioti. *Nordisk Medicin* **38,** 1072–6.

Baker, H. J., Lindsey, J. R., McKhann, G. M. and Farrell, D. F. (1971) Neuronal G_{MI}-gangliosidosis in a Siamese cat with β-galactosidase deficiency. *Science* **174,** 838–9.

Banker, B. Q., Miller, J. Q. and Crocker, A. C. (1962) The cerebral pathology of infantile Gaucher's disease. In *Cerebral Sphingolipidoses* (Eds. Aronson, S. M. and Volk, B. W.), pp. 73–99. Academic Press, New York.

Baraton, G. and Revol, A. (1977) Activateur des sphingohydrolases et nature du déficit en sphingomyelinase dans la maladie de Niemann–Pick type A, B et C. *Clinica Chimica Acta* **76,** 339–43.

Barnes, I. C., Kelly, D. F., Pennock, C. A. and Randell, J. A. J. (1981) Hepatic beta-galactosidase and feline G_{MI}-gangliosidosis. *Neuropathology and Applied Neurobiology* **7,** 463–76.

Basner, R., von Figura, K., Glossl, J., Klein, U., Kresse, H. and Mlenkush, U. (1979) Multiple deficiency of mucopolysaccharide sulphatases in mucosulphatidosis. *Pediatric Research* **13,** 1316–19.

Batten, F. E. (1903) Cerebral degeneration with symmetrical changes in the maculae in two members of a family. *Transactions of the Ophthalmological Society of the United Kingdom* **23,** 386–90.

Batten, F. E. (1914) Family cerebral degeneration with macular change (so-called juvenile form of family amaurotic idiocy). *Quarterly Journal of Medicine* **7,** 444–54.

Batten, F. E. and Mayou, M. S. (1915) Family cerebral degeneration with macular changes. *Proceedings of the Royal Society of Medicine* **8,** 70–90.

Batten, R. D. (1897) Two brothers with symmetrical disease of the macula, commencing at the age of fourteen. *Transactions of the Ophthalmological Society of the United Kingdom* **17,** 48–9.

Baty, J. M. (1930) Lipoid histiocytosis (Niemann's disease). *American Journal of Diseases of Children* **39,** 573–85.

Baudhuin, P., Hers, H. G. and Loeb, H. (1964) An electron microscopic and biochemical study of type II glycogenosis. *Laboratory Investigation* **13,** 1140–52.

Bayer, P. M. and Wewalka, F. (1973) Syndrom der 'Sea-blue histiocytes' bzw. der sogenannten 'Blauen Pigmentmakrophagen'. Lipidchemische Untersuchungen bei der Erstbeobachtung. *Wiener klinische Wochenschrift* **85,** 514–17.

Beaudet, A. L. (1983) Disorders of glycoprotein degradation. Mannosidosis, fucosidosis, sialidosis and aspartylglucosaminuria. In *The Metabolic Basis of Inherited Disease* (Eds. Stanbury, J. B., Wyngarden, J. B., Fredrickson, D. S., Goldstein, J. L. and Brown, M. S.), 5th edn, pp. 788-802. McGraw-Hill, New York.

Beaudet, A. L., Lipson, M. H., Ferry, G. D. and Nichols, B. L. (1974) Acid lipase in cultured fibroblasts: cholesterol ester storage disease. *Journal of Laboratory and Clinical Medicine* **84,** 54-61.

Beaudet, A. L., Ferry, G. D., Nichols, B. L. and Rosenberg, H. S. (1977) Cholesterol ester storage disease: clinical, biochemical and pathological studies. *Journal of Pediatrics* **90,** 910-14.

Bernheimer, H. and Karbe, E. (1970) Morphologische und neurochemische Untersuchungen von 2 Formen der amaurotischen Idiotie des Hundes: Nachweis einer G_{M2}-Gangliosidose. *Acta Neuropathologica* **16,** 243-61.

Bielschowsky, M. (1913) Über spät-infantile familiäre amaurotische Idiotie mit Kleinhirnsymptomen. *Deutsche Zeitschrift für Nervenheilkunde* **50,** 7-29.

Bischoff, A. and Ulrich, J. (1967) Amaurotische Idiote in Verbindung mit metachromatishcher Leukodystrophie: Übergangsform oder Kombination? *Acta Neuropathologica* **8,** 292-308.

Bischoff, A. and Ulrich, J. (1969) Peripheral neuropathy in globoid cell leukodystrophy (Krabbe's disease). Ultrastructural and histochemical findings. *Brain* **92,** 861-70.

Blackwood, W. and Cumings, J. N. (1954) A histological and chemical study of three cases of diffuse cerebral sclerosis. *Journal of Neurology, Neurosurgery and Psychiatry* **17,** 33-49.

Bodian, M. and Lake, B. D. (1963) The rectal approach to neuropathology. *British Journal of Surgery* **50,** 702-14.

Boehme, D., Cottrell, J., Leonberg, S. and Zeman, W. (1971) A dominant form of neuronal ceroid-lipofuscinosis. *Brain* **94,** 745-60.

Brady, R. O. and Barranger, J. A. (1981) Inborn lysosomal enzyme deficiencies. In *The Molecular Basis of Neuropathology* (Eds. Davison, A. N. and Thompson, R. H. S.), pp. 188-220. Edward Arnold, London.

Brady, R. O. and Barranger, J. A. (1983) Glucosylceramide lipidosis. Gaucher's disease. In *The Metabolic Basis of Inherited Disease* (Eds. Stanbury, J. B., Wyngaarden, J. B., Fredrickson, D. S., Goldstein, J. L. and Brown, M. S.), 5th edn, pp. 842-56. McGraw-Hill, New York.

Brady, R. O., Kanfer, J. N. and Shapiro, D. (1965) Metabolism of glucocerebrosides. II. Evidence of an enzymatic deficiency in Gaucher's disease. *Biochemical and Biophysical Research Communications* **18,** 221-5.

Brady, R. O., Uhlendorf, B. W. and Jacobson, C. B. (1971) Fabry's disease: antenatal detection. *Science* **172,** 174-5.

Brady, R. O., Kanfer, J. N., Mock, M. B. and rickson, D. S. (1966) The metabolism of sphingomyelin. II. Evidence of an enzymatic deficiency in Niemann-Pick disease. *Proceedings of the National Academy of Sciences of the USA* **55,** 366-9.

Brady, R. O., Gal, A. E., Bradley, R. M., Martensson, E., Warshaw, A. L. and Lester, L. (1967) Enzymatic defect in Fabry's disease: ceramide trihexosidase deficiency. *New England Journal of Medicine* **276,** 1163-7.

Brain, W. R. and Greenfield, J.G. (1950) Late infantile metachromatic leucoencephalopathy with primary degeneration of the interfascicular oligodendroglia. *Brain,* **73,** 291-317.

Brante, G. (1952) Gargoylism: a mucopolysaccharidosis. *Scandinavian Journal of Clinical and Laboratory Investigation* **4,** 43-8.

Brett, E. M., Ellis, R. B., Haas, L., Ikonne, J. U., Lake, B. D., Patrick, A. D. and Stephens, R. (1973) Late onset G_{M2} gangliosidosis. Clinical, pathological and biochemical studies on eight patients. *Archives of Disease in Childhood* **48,** 775-85.

Brion, S., Mikol, J. and Graveleau, J. (1970) Leucodystrophie métachromatique de l'adulte jeune. Étude clinique, biologique et ultrastructurale. *Révue Neurologique* **122,** 161-76.

Brown, N. J., Corner, B. D. and Dodgson, M. H. C. (1954) A second case in the same family of congenital familial cerebral lipoidosis resembling amaurotic family idocy. *Archives of Disease in Childhood* **29,** 48-54.

Bundza, A., Lowden, J. A. and Charlton, K. M. (1979) Niemann-Pick disease in a poodle dog. *Veterinary Pathology* **16,** 530-8.

Bürrig, K.-F., Schwendemann, G. and Löhler, J. (1982) Lack of structural abnormalities in lymphocytes from heterozygotes of juvenile type of generalized ceroid-lipofuscinosis. A light and electron microscopic study. *Neuropediatrics* **13,** 216-18.

Byrd, J. C. and Powers, J. M. (1979) Wolman's disease: ultrastructural evidence of lipid accumulation in central and peripheral nervous systems. *Acta Neuropathologica* **45,** 37-42.

Cable, W. J. L., Kolodny, E. H. and Adams, R. D. (1982) Fabry disease: impaired autonomic function. *Neurology* **32,** 498-502.

Canelas, H. M., Escalante, O. D., Iriya, K. and de Jorge, F. B. (1964) The diagnosis of metachromatic leucodystrophy during life. Metachromatic lipids in saliva and cerebrospinal fluid sediments and in the parotid glands. *Arquivos de Neuro-Psiquiatria* **22,** 122-8.

Carpenter, S., Karpati, G. and Andermann, F. (1972) Specific involvement of muscle nerve and skin in late infantile and juvenile amaurotic idiocy. *Neurology* **22,** 170-86.

Carpenter, S., Karpati, G., Wolfe, L. S. and Andermann, F. (1973) A type of juvenile cerebromacular degeneration characterized by granular osmiophilic deposits. *Journal of the Neurological Sciences* **18,** 67–87.

Carpenter, S., Karpati, G., Andermann, F., Jacob, J. C. and Andermann, E. (1977) The ultrastructural characteristics of the abnormal cytosomes in Batten–Kufs' disease. *Brain* **100,** 137–56.

Cavanagh, N. P. C., Lake, B. D. and McMeniman, P. (1979) Congenital fibre type disproportion myopathy: a histological diagnosis with an uncertain clinical outlook. *Archives of Disease in Childhood* **54,** 735–43.

Ceuterick, C. H., Martin, J. J., Casaer, P. and Edgar, G. W. F. (1976) The diagnosis of infantile generalized ceroid-lipofuscinosis (type Hagberg-Santavuori) using skin biopsy. *Neuropädiatrie* **7,** 250–60.

Ceuterick, C., Martin, J. J., Libert, J. and Farriaux, J.-P. (1980) Sanfilippo A disease in the fetus. Comparison with pre- and postnatal cases. *Neuropädiatrie* **11,** 176–85.

Chou, L., Kaye, C. I. and Nadler, H. L. (1974) Brain β-galactosidase and G_{M1}-gangliosidosis. *Pediatric Research* **8,** 120–5.

Chou, S. M. and Thompson, H. G. (1970) Electron microscopy of storage cytosomes in Kufs' disease. *Archives of Neurology* **23,** 489–501.

Christensen, E., Melchior, J. C. and Andersen, H. (1960) Diffuse infantile familial sclerosis (Krabbe type). *Acta Psychiatrica et Neurologica Scandinavica* **35,** 431–9.

Christomanou, H. (1980) Niemann–Pick disease type C: evidence for the deficiency of an activating factor stimulating sphingomyelin and glucocerebroside degradation. *Hoppe-Seyler's Zeitschrift für physiologische Chemie* **361,** 1489–1502.

Clarke, J. T. R., Knaack, J., Crawhall, J. C. and Wolfe, L. S. (1971) Ceramide trihexosidosis (Fabry's disease) without skin lesions. *New England Journal of Medicine* **284,** 233–5.

Collier, J. and Greenfield, J. G. (1924) The encephalitis periaxialis of Schilder: a clinical and pathological study, with an account of two cases, one of which was diagnosed during life. *Brain* **47,** 489–519.

Collier, W. (1895) A case of enlarged spleen in a child aged six. *Transactions of the Pathological Society of London* **46,** 148–50.

Constantopoulos, G., Rees, S., Cragg, B. G., Barranger, J. A. and Brady, R. O. (1980) Experimental animal model for mucopolysaccharidosis. Suramin-induced glycosaminoglycan and sphingolipid accumulation in the rat. *Proceedings of the National Academy of Sciences of the USA* **77,** 3700–4.

Conzelmann, E. and Sandhoff, K. (1978) AB variant of infantile G_{M2}-gangliosidosis: deficiency of a factor necessary for stimulation of hexosaminidase A-catalyzed degradation of ganglioside G_{M2} and glycolipid G_{A2}. *Proceedings of the National Academy of Sciences of the USA* **75,** 3979.

Coppa, G. V., Giorgi, P. L., Felici, L., Gabrielli, O., Donti, E., Bernasconi, S. et al. (1983) Clinical heterogeneity in Sanfilippo disease (mucopolysaccharidosis III) type D: presentation of two new cases. *European Journal of Pediatrics* **140,** 130–3.

Cork, L. C., Munnell, J. F., Lorenz, M. D., Murphy, J. V., Baker, H. J. and Rattazzi, M. C. (1977) G_{M2}-ganglioside lysosomal storage disease in cats with β-hexosaminidase deficiency. *Science* **196,** 1014–17.

Crocker, A. C. (1961) The cerebral defect in Tay–Sachs disease and Niemann–Pick disease. *Journal of Neurochemistry* **7,** 69–80.

Crocker, A. C. and Farber, S. (1958) Niemann–Pick disease: a review of eighteen patients. *Medicine* **37,** 1–95.

Crocker, A. C., Vawter, G. F., Neuhauser, E. B. D. and Rosowsky, A. (1965). Wolman's disease: three new patients with a recently described lipidosis. *Pediatrics* **35,** 627–40.

Crome, L., Hanefeld, F., Patrick, D. and Wilson, J. (1973) Late onset globoid cell leucodystrophy. *Brain* **96,** 841–8.

Crow, J., Gibbs, D. A., Cozens, W., Spellacy, E. and Watts, R. W. E. (1983) Biochemical and histopathological studies on patients with mucopolysaccharidoses, two of whom had been treated by fibroblast transplantation. *Journal of Clinical Pathology* **36,** 415–30.

Cummings, J. F. and deLahunta, A. (1977) An adult case of canine neuronal ceroid-lipofuscinosis. *Acta Neuropathologica* **39,** 43–51.

Dacremont, G. and Kint, J. A. (1968) G_{M1}-ganglioside accumulation and β-galactosidase deficiency in a case of G_{M1}-gangliosidosis (Landing disease). *Clinica Chimica Acta* **21,** 421–5.

D'Agostino, A. N., Sayre, G. P. and Hayles, A. B. (1963) Krabbe's disease. *Archives of Neurology* **8,** 82–96.

Dahms, B. B., Davis, R. L., Neustein, H. B. and Landing, B. H. (1979) Fucosidosis—light, histochemical and ultrastructural findings. *Laboratory Investigation* **40,** 302–3 (abstract).

Dawson, G., Matalon, R. and Stein, A. O. (1971) Lactosylceramidosis: lactosylceramide galactosyl hydrolase deficiency and accumulation of lactosylceramide in cultured skin fibroblasts. *Journal of Pediatrics* **79,** 423–9.

Dawson, I. M. P. (1954) The histology and histochemistry of gargoylism. *Journal of Pathology and Bacteriology* **67,** 587–604.

Dehkharghani, F., Sarnat, H. B., Brewster, M. A. and Roth, S. I. (1981) Congenital muscle fibre type disproportion in Krabbe's leukodystrophy. *Archives of Neurology* **38,** 585–7.

Dekaban, A. S. and Constantopoulos, G. (1977) Mucopolysaccharidosis types I, II, IIIa and V. Pathological and biochemical abnormalities in the neuronal and mesenchymal elements of the brain. *Acta Neuropathologica* **39,** 1–7.

Dekaban, A. S., Constantopoulos, G., Herman, M. M. and Steusing, J. K. (1976) Mucopolysaccharidosis type V (Scheie syndrome). A post-mortem study by multidisciplinary techniques with emphasis on the brain. *Archives of Pathology and Laboratory Medicine* **100,** 237–45.

Derry, D. M., Fawcett, J. S., Andermann, F. and Wolfe, L. S. (1968) Late infantile systemic lipidosis: major monosialogangliosidosis, delineation of two types. *Neurology* **18,** 340–8.

Desnick, R. J., Patterson, D. F. and Scarpelli, D. G. (Eds.) (1982) In *Animal Models of Inherited Metabolic Diseases*, p. 475. Alan R. Liss, New York.

Desnick, R. J. and Sweeley, C. C. (1983) Fabry's disease: α-galactosidase A deficiency. In *The Metabolic Basis of Inherited Disease* (Eds. Stanbury, J. B., Wyngaarden, J. B., Fredrickson, D. S., Goldstein, J. L. and Brown, M. S.), 5th edn, pp. 906–44. McGraw-Hill, New York.

Dewhurst, N., Besley, G. T. N., Finlayson, N. D. C. and Parker, A. C. (1979) Sea-blue histiocytosis in a patient with chronic non-neuropathic Niemann–Pick disease. *Journal of Clinical Pathology* **32,** 1121–7.

Diezel, P. B. (1955) Histochemische Untersuchungen an den Globoidzellen der familiären infantilen diffusen Sklerose vom Typus Krabbe. *Virchows Archiv für pathologische Anatomie und Physiologie und für klinische Medizin* **327,** 206–28.

Dom, R., Brucher, J. M., Ceuterick, C., Carton, H. and Mattin, J. J. (1979) Adult ceroid-lipofuscinosis (Kufs' disease) in two brothers. Retinal and visceral storage in one; diagnostic muscle biopsy in the other. *Acta Neuropathologica* **45,** 67–72.

Donelly, W. J., Sheahan, B. J. and Rogers, T. A. (1973) G_{M1}-gangliosidosis in Friesian calves. *Journal of Pathology* **111,** 173–9.

Dowson, J. H. (1983) Autofluorescence emission spectra of neuronal lipopigment in a case of adult-onset ceroidosis (Kufs' disease). *Acta Neuropathologica* **59,** 241–5.

Dowson, J. H., Armstrong, D., Koppang, N., Lake, B. D. and Jolly, R. D. (1982) Autofluorescence emission spectra of neuronal lipopigment in animal and human ceroidoses (ceroid lipofuscinosis). *Acta Neuropathologica* **58,** 152–6.

Dreborg, S., Erikson, A. and Hagberg, B. (1980) Gaucher's disease Norrbottnian type I. General clinical description. *European Journal of Pediatrics* **133,** 107–18.

Duchen, L. W., Eicher, E. M., Jacobs, J. M., Scaravilli, F. and Teixeira, F. (1980) Hereditary leucodystrophy in the mouse: the new mutant twitcher. *Brain* **103,** 695–710.

Duffy, P. E., Kornfeld, M. and Suzuki, K. (1968) Neurovisceral storage disease with curvilinear bodies. *Journal of Neuropathology and Experimental Neurology* **27,** 351–70.

Dunn, H. G., Lake, B. D., Dolman, C. L. and Wilson, J. (1969) The neuropathy of Krabbe's infantile cerebral sclerosis (globoid cell leucodystrophy). *Brain* **92,** 329–44.

Dunn, H. G., Dolman, C. L., Farrell, D. F., Tischler, B., Hasinoff, C. and Woolf, L. I. (1976) Krabbe's leukodystrophy without globoid cells. *Neurology* **26,** 1035–41.

Durand, P., Borrone, C. and Della Cella, G. (1969) Fucosidosis. *Journal of Pediatrics* **75,** 665–74.

Elfenbein, I. B. (1968) Dystonic juvenile idiocy without amaurosis. A new syndrome. Light and electron microscopic observations of cerebrum. *Johns Hopkins Medical Journal* **123,** 205–21.

Elleder, M. (1979) Alkaline phosphatase activity induction in human spleen sinuses in storage disorders. *Virchows Archiv. Abteilung B. Zellpathologie* **32,** 89–92.

Elleder, M. and Jirásek, A. (1983) International symposium on Niemann–Pick disease. *European Journal of Pediatrics* **140,** 90–1.

Elleder, M., Jirásek, A. and Vlk, J. (1983) Adult neurovisceral lipidosis compatible with Niemann–Pick disease type C. *Virchows Archiv. Abteilung A. Pathologische Anatomie* **401,** 35–43.

Elleder, M. and Lojda, Z. (1973) Studies in lipid histochemistry. XI. New rapid simple and selective method for the demonstration of phospholipids. *Histochemie* **36,** 149–66.

Elleder, M., Šmid, F., Harzer, K. and Čihula, J. (1980) Niemann–Pick disease. Analysis of liver tissue in sphingomyelinase-deficient patients. *Virchows Archiv. Abteilung A. Pathologische Anatomie* **385,** 215–31.

Ellis, W. G., Schneider, E. L., McCulloch, J. R., Suzuki, K. and Epstein, C. J. (1973) Fetal globoid cell leukodystrophy (Krabbe disease). *Archives of Neurology* **29,** 253–7.

Engel, A. G. and Dale, A. J. D. (1968) Autophagic glycogenosis of late onset with mitochondrial abnormalities: light and electron microscopic observations. *Mayo Clinic Proceedings* **43,** 233–79.

Engel, A. G., Gomez, M. R., Seybold, M. E. and Lambert, E. H. (1973) The spectrum and diagnosis of acid maltase deficiency. *Neurology* **23,** 95–106.

Farrell, D. F., Baker, H. J., Herndon, R. M., Lindsey, J. R. and McKhann, G. M. (1973) Feline G_{M1}-gangliosidosis: biochemical and ultrastructural comparison with the disease in man. *Journal of Neuropathology and Experimental Neurology* **32,** 1–18.

Farriaux, J.-P. and Strecker, G. (1979) La mucolipidose II (I cell disease): une sialidose? *Archives Françaises de Pédiatrie* **36,** 225–34.

Fensom, A. H., Benson, P. F., Neville, B. R. G., Moser, H. W., Moser, A. B. and Dulaney, J. T. (1979) Prenatal diagnosis of Farber's disease. *Lancet* **2,** 990–2.

von Figura, K., van de Kamp, J. J. and Niermeijer, M. F. (1982) Prenatal diagnosis of Morquio's disease type A (*N*-acetylgalactosamine-6-sulphate sulphatase deficiency). *Prenatal Diagnosis* **2,** 67–9.

Filipe, M. I. and Lake, B. D. (1983) *Histochemistry in Pathology*. Churchill Livingstone, Edinburgh.

Fine, D. I. M., Barron, K. D. and Hirano, A. (1960) Central nervous system lipidosis in an adult with atrophy of the cerebellar granular layer. *Journal of Neuropathology and Experimental Neurology* **19,** 355–69.

Fischer, G. and Jatzkewitz, H. (1978) The activator of cerebroside sulphatase. A model of the activation. *Biochimica Biophysica Acta* **528,** 69–76.

Flynn, D. M., Lake, B. D., Boothby, C. B. and Young, E. P. (1972) Gut lesions in Fabry's disease without a rash. *Archives of Disease in Childhood* **47,** 26–33.

Franceschetti, A. T. L. (1976) Fabry's disease: ocular manifestations. *Birth Defects. Original Article Series* **12,** 195–208.

Fredrickson, D. S. and Sloan, H. R. (1972a) Glucosyl ceramide lipidosis. Gaucher's disease. In *The Metabolic Basis of Inherited Disease* (Eds. Stanbury, J. B., Wyngaarden, J. B. and Fredrickson, D. S.) 3rd edn, pp. 730–59. McGraw-Hill, New York.

Fredrickson, D. S. and Sloan, H. R. (1972b) Sphingomyelin lipidoses: Niemann–Pick disease. In *The Metabolic Basis of Inherited Disease* (Eds. Stanbury, J. B., Wyngaarden, J. B. and Fredrickson, D. S.), 3rd edn, pp. 783–807. McGraw-Hill, New York.

Freitag, E., Küchemann, K., Blümke, S. and Spranger, J. (1971) Hepatic ultrastructure in fucosidosis. *Virchows Archiv. Abteilung B. Zellpathologie* **7,** 99–113.

Freud, S. (1893) Ueber familiäre Formen von cerebralen Diplegien. *Neurologisches Zentralblatt* **12,** 512–15 and 542–7.

Frost, P., Tanaka, Y. and Spaeth, G. L. (1966) Fabry's disease—glycolipid lipidosis. Histochemical and electron microscopic studies of two cases. *American Journal of Medicine* **40,** 618–27.

Fullerton, P. M. (1964) Peripheral nerve conduction in metachromatic leucodystrophy (sulphatide lipidosis). *Journal of Neurology, Neurosurgery and Psychiatry* **27,** 100–5.

Galjaard, H., Niermeijer, M. F., Hahnemann, N., Mohr, J. and Sørensen, S. A. (1974) An example of rapid prenatal diagnosis of Fabry's disease using microtechniques. *International Journal of Clinical Genetics* **5,** 368–77.

Garcia, C. P., McGarry, P. A. and Duncan, C. M. (1980) Fucosidosis and Alexander's leucodystrophy. *Journal of Neuropathology and Experimental Neurology* **39,** 353 (abstract).

Gautier, M., Lapons, D. and Raulin, J. (1978) Maladie de surcharge à esters du cholesterol chez l'enfant. *Archives françaises de Pédiatrie* **35,** suppl. 11, 38–49.

Gehler, J., Sewell, A. C., Becker, C., Spranger, J. and Hartmann, J. (1981) Aspartylglucosaminuria in an Italian family. Clinical and biochemical characteristics. *Journal of Inherited Metabolic Diseases* **4,** 229–30.

Gilles, F. H. and Deuel, R. K. (1971) Neuronal cytoplasmic globules in the brain in Morquio's syndrome. *Archives of Neurology* **25,** 393–403.

Ginns, E. I., Brady, R. O., Pirruccello, S., Moore, C., Sorrell, S., Furbish, F. S. et al. (1982) Mutations of glucocerebrosidase: discrimination of neurologic and non-neurological phenotypes of Gaucher disease. *Proceedings of the National Academy of Sciences of the USA* **79,** 5607–10.

Glasgow, G. L. (1957) A case of amaurotic family idiocy with lipid storage disease of bone. *Australasian Annals of Medicine* **6,** 295–9.

Glew, R. H., Daniels, L. B., Clark, L. S. and Hoyer, S. W. (1982) Enzymic differentiation of neurologic and non-neurologic forms of Gaucher's disease. *Journal of Neuropathology and Experimental Neurology* **41,** 630–41.

Goebel, H. H., Kohlschütter, A. and Lenard, H. G. (1982) Morphologic and chemical biopsy findings in mucolipidosis IV. *Clinical Neuropathology* **1,** 73–82.

Goebel, H. H., Braak, H., Seidel, D., Doshi, R., Marsden, C. D. and Gullotta, F. (1982) Morphologic studies on adult neuronal-ceroid lipofuscinosis (NCL). *Clinical Neuropathology* **1,** 151–62.

Goldberg, M. F., Cotlier, E., Fichenscher, L. G., Kenyon, K., Enat, R. and Borowsky, S. A. (1971) Macular cherry red spot, corneal clouding and β-galactosidase deficiency. *Archives of Internal Medicine* **128,** 387–9.

Golde, D. W., Schneider, E. L., Bainton, D. F., Pentchev, P. G., Brady, R. O., Epstein, C. J. and Cline, M. J. (1975) Pathogenesis of one variant of sea-blue histiocytosis. *Laboratory Investigation* **33,** 371–8.

Gonatas, N. K., Gambetti, P. and Baird, H. (1968) A second type of late infantile amaurotic idiocy with multilamellar cytosomes. *Journal of Neuropathology and Experimental Neurology* **27,** 371–89.

Goutières, F., Arsenio-Nunes, M. L. and Aicardi, J. (1979) Mucolipidosis IV. *Neuropädiatrie* **10,** 321–31.

Green, P. D. and Little, P. B. (1974) Neuronal ceroid

lipofuscin storage in Siamese cats. *Canadian Journal of Comparative Medicine* **38,** 207–12.

Greenfield, J. G. (1933) A form of progressive cerebral sclerosis in infants associated with primary degeneration of the interfascicular glia. *Journal of Neurology and Psychopathology* **13,** 289–302.

Groen, J. J. (1964) Gaucher's disease. Hereditary transmission and racial distribution. *Archives of Internal Medicine* **113,** 543–9.

Guazzi, G. C., Martin, J. J., Philippart, M., Roels, H., van der Eecken, H., Vrints, L. et al. (1968) Wolman's disease. *European Neurology* 1, 334–62.

Guibaud, P., Vanier, M.-T., Malpuech, G., Gaulme, J., Houllemare, L., Goddon, R. and Rousson, R. (1979) Forme infantile précoce, cholestatique, rapidement mortelle de la sphingomyelinase type C. *Pédiatrie* **34,** 103–14.

Guillain, G., Bertrand, I. and Gruner, J. (1941) Sur une type anatomo-clinique spéciale de leucoencéphalite à nodules morulés gliogènes. *Revue Neurologique* **73,** 401–14.

Guseo, A., Deák, G. and Szirmai, I. (1975) An adult case of metachromatic leucodystrophy. A light polarization and electron microscopic study. *Acta Neuropathologica* **32,** 333–9.

Hadfield, M. G., Ghatak, N. R., Nakoneczna, I., Lippman, H. R., Myer, E. E., Constantopoulos, G. and Bradley, R. M. (1980) Pathologic findings in mucopolysaccharidosis type III B (Sanfilippo's syndrome B). *Archives of Neurology* **37,** 645–50.

Hagberg, B., Sourander, P. and Svennerholm, L. (1961) Clinical and laboratory diagnosis of metachromatic leucodystrophy. *Cerebral Palsy Bulletin* **3,** 438–43.

Hagberg, B., Sourander, P. and Svennerholm, L. (1962) Sulphatide lipidosis in childhood. *American Journal of Diseases of Children* **104,** 644–56.

Hagberg, B., Sourander, P., Svennerholm, L. and Voss, H. (1959) Late infantile metachromatic leucodystrophy of genetic type. *Acta Paediatrica* **48,** 200.

Hagberg, B., Hultquist, G., Ohman, R. and Svennerholm, L. (1965) Congenital amaurotic idiocy. *Acta Paediatrica Scandinavica* **54,** 116–30.

Hagberg, B., Kollberg, H., Sourander, P. and Åkesson, H. O. (1969) Infantile globoid cell leucodystrophy (Krabbe's disease). *Neuropädiatrie* **1,** 74–88.

Hagberg, B., Haltia, M., Sourander, P., Svennerholm, L. and Eeg-Olofsson, O. (1974) Polyunsaturated fatty acid lipidosis—infantile form of so-called neuronal ceroid-lipofuscinosis. *Acta Paediatrica Scandinavica* **63,** 753–63.

Hagberg, B., Haltia, M., Sourander, P., Svennerholm, L., Vanier, M.-T. and Ljunggren, C.-G. (1978) Neurovisceral storage disorder simulating Niemann–Pick disease. A new form of oligosaccharidosis? *Neuropädiatrie* **9,** 59–73.

Hagen, L. (1953) Lipid dystrophic changes in the central nervous system in dogs. *Acta Pathologica et Microbiologica Scandinavica* **33,** 22–35.

Hager, H. and Oehlert, W. (1957) Ist die diffuse Hirnsklerose des Typ Krabbe eine entzündliche Allgemeinerkrankung? *Zeitschrift für Kinderheilkunde* **80,** 82–6.

Hahn, A. F., Gordon, B. A., Gilbert, J. J. and Hinton, G. G. (1981) The AB-variant of metachromatic leukodystrophy (postulated activator protein deficiency). Light and electron microscopic findings in a sural nerve biopsy. *Acta Neuropathologica* **55,** 281–7.

Hahn, A. F., Gordon, B. A., Feleki, V., Hinton, G. G. and Gilbert, J. J. (1982) A variant form of metachromatic leukodystrophy without arylsulphatase deficiency. *Annals of Neurology* **12,** 33–6.

Haltia, M., Palo, J. and Autio, S. (1975) Aspartylglycosaminuria. A generalized storage disease. Morphological and histochemical studies. *Acta Neuropathologica* **31,** 243–55.

Haltia, M., Rapola, J. and Santavuori, P. (1973) Infantile type of so-called neuronal ceroid-lipofuscinosis. *Acta Neuropathologica* **26,** 157–70.

Hann, I., Rankin, A., Pritchard, J. and Lake, B. D. (1983) *Atlas of Paediatric Haematology*. Oxford University Press, Oxford.

Harper, P. S., Laurence, K. M., Parkes, A., Wusteman, F. S., Kresse, H., von Figura, K., et al. (1974) Sanfilippo A disease in the fetus. *Journal of Medical Genetics* 11, 123–32.

Harzer, K. (1982) Prenatal enzymic diagnosis in 24 pregnancies with risk of Krabbe disease. *Clinica Chimica Acta* **122,** 21–8.

Harzer, K. and Benz, H. U. (1973) A simple sphingomyelinase determination for Niemann–Pick disease: differential diagnosis of types A, B and C. *Journal of Neurochemistry* **21,** 999–1001.

Harzer, K. and Peiffer, J. (1981) Morbus Niemann–Pick type C (subakute neuroviscerale Lipidosis). *Archiv für Psychiatrie und Nervenkrankheiten* **230,** 71–9.

Harzer, K., Schlote, W., Peiffer, J., Benz, H. U. and Anzil, A. P. (1978) Neurovisceral lipidosis compatible with Niemann–Pick disease type C. Morphological and biochemical studies of a late infantile case and enzyme and lipid assays in a prenatal case of the same family. *Acta Neuropathologica* **43,** 97–104.

Haskins, M. E., Jezyk, P. F., Desnick, R. J., McDonough, S. K. and Patterson, D. F. (1979) Alpha-L-iduronidase deficiency in a cat: a model of mucopolysaccharidosis I. *Pediatric Research* **13,** 1294–7.

Haskins, M. E., Jezyk, P. F., Desnick, R. J. and Patterson, D. F. (1981) Mucopolysaccharidosis VI, Maroteaux-Lamy syndrome. Arylsulphatase B-deficient mucopolysaccharidosis in the Siamese cat. *American Journal of Pathology* **105,** 191–3.

Haynes, M. E., Manson, J. I., Carter, R. F. and Robertson, E. (1979) Electron microscopy of skin and peripheral blood lymphocytes in infantile (Santavuori) neuronal ceroid lipofuscinosis. *Neuropädiatrie* **10,** 245–63.

Haynes, M. E., Carter, R. F., Pollard, A. C. and Carey, W. F. (1980) Light and electron microscopy of infantile and fetal tissues in cystinosis. *Micron* **11,** 443–4.

Hechtman, P. and LeBlanc, D. (1977) Purification and properties of the hexosaminidase A activity protein from human liver. *Biochemical Journal* **167,** 693–701.

Hechtman, P., Gordon, B. A. and Ng Ying Kin, N. M. K. (1982) Deficiency of hexosaminidase A activator protein in a case of G_{M2} gangliosidosis: variant AB. *Pediatric Research* **16,** 217–22.

Henderson, J. L. (1940) Gargoylism. A review of the principal features with a report of five cases. *Archives of Disease in Childhood* **15,** 201–14.

Hers, H. G. (1963) α-Glucosidase deficiency in generalized glycogen storage disease (Pompe's disease). *Biochemical Journal* **86,** 11–16.

Hers, H. G. (1965) Inborn lysosomal disorders. *Gastroenterology* **48,** 625–33.

Hers, H. G. and de Barsy, T. (1973) Type II glycogenosis (acid maltase deficiency). In *Lysosomes and Storage Diseases* (Eds. Hers, H. G. and Van Hoof, F.), pp. 197–216. Academic Press, New York.

Hers, H. G. and Van Hoof, F. (Eds.) (1973). *Lysosomes and Storage Diseases.* Academic Press, New York.

von Hirsch, T. and Peiffer, J. (1955) Über histologische Methoden in der Differentialdiagnose von Leukodystrophien und Lipoidosen. *Archiv für Psychiatrie und Nervenkrankheiten* **194,** 88–104.

Ho, M. W. and O'Brien, J. S. (1969) Hurler's syndrome: deficiency of a specific beta-galactosidase isoenzyme. *Science* **165,** 611–13.

Hobbs, J. R., Barrett, A. J., Chambers, D., James, D. C. O., Hugh-Jones, K., Byrom, N. et al. (1981) Reversal of clinical features of Hurler's disease and biochemical improvement after treatment by bone-marrow transplantation. *Lancet* **2,** 709–12.

Hocking, J. D., Jolly, R. D. and Batt, R. D. (1972) Deficiency of α-mannosidase in Angus cattle. An inherited lysosomal storage disease. *Biochemical Journal* **128,** 69–78.

Holländer, H. (1963) A staining method for cerebroside sulfuric acid-esters in brain tissue. *Journal of Histochemistry and Cytochemistry* **11,** 118–19.

Honey, N. K., Mueller, O. T., Little, L. E., Miller, A. L. and Shows, T. B. (1982) Mucolipidosis III is genetically heterogeneous. *Proceedings of the National Academy of Sciences of the USA* **79,** 7420–4.

Horoupian, D. S. and Yang, S. S. (1978) Paired helical filaments in neurovisceral lipidosis (juvenile dystonic lipidosis). *Annals of Neurology* **4,** 404–11.

Howell, J. McC., Dorling, P. R., Cork, R. D., Robinson, W. F., Bradley, S. and Gawthorne, J. M. (1981) Infantile and late infantile onset form of generalized glycogenosis type II in cattle. *Journal of Pathology* **134,** 266–77.

Hug, G. (1974) Enzyme therapy and prenatal diagnosis in glycogenosis type II. *American Journal of Diseases of Children* **128,** 607–9.

Humbel, R. and Collart, M. (1975) Oligosaccharides in urine of patients with glycoprotein storage diseases. 1. Rapid detection by thin layer chromatography. *Clinica Chimica Acta* **60,** 143–5.

Hunter, C. (1917) A rare disease in two brothers. *Proceedings of the Royal Society of Medicine* **10,** 104–16.

Hurler, G. (1919). Über einen Typ multipler Abartungen, vorwiegend am Skelettsystem. *Zeitschrift für Kinderheilkunde* **24,** 220–34.

Huxtable, C. R., Dorling, P. R. and Walkley, S. U. (1982) Onset and regression of neuroaxonal lesions in sheep with mannosidosis induced experimentally with swainsonine. *Acta Neuropathologica* **58,** 27–33.

Isenberg, J. N. and Sharp, H. L. (1975) Aspartylglucosaminuria: psychomotor retardation masquerading as a mucopolysaccharidosis. *Journal of Pediatrics* **86,** 713–17.

Ivemark, B. I., Svennerholm, L., Thorén, C. and Tunell, R. (1963) Niemann–Pick disease in infancy. Report of two siblings with clinical, histologic and chemical studies. *Acta Paediatrica* **52,** 391–404.

Jansky, J. (1908) Dosud nepopsany pripad familiarni amauroticke idiotie komplikovane hypoplasii mozeckovou. *Sborník Lékařský v Praze* **13,** 165.

Jatzkewitz, H. (1958) Zwei Typen von Cerebrosidschwefelsäureestern als sog. 'Prälipoide' und Speichersubstanzen bei der Leukodystrophie. Typ Scholz (metachromatische Form der diffusen Sklerose). *Hoppe-Seyler's Zeitschrift für physiologische Chemie* **311,** 279–90.

Jatzkewitz, H., Pilz, H. and Holländer, H. (1964) Biochemische und vergleichende histochemische Untersuchungen in umschriebenen Gebieten des Gehirns bei Fällen von adulter and infantiler metachromatischer Leukodystrophie. *Acta Neuropathologica* **4,** 75–89.

Johnson, W. G., Thomas, G. H., Miranda, A. F., Driscoll, J. M., Wigger, J. H., Yeh, M.-Y. et al. (1980) Prenatal diagnosis in two pregnancies at risk for congenital sialidosis. *Annals of Neurology* **8,** 216 (abstract).

Johnston, W. G., Wigger, J., Karp, H. R., Glaubiger, L. M. and Rowland, L. P. (1982) Juvenile spinal muscular atrophy: a new hexosaminidase deficiency phenotype. *Annals of Neurology* **11,** 11–16.

Jolly, R. D. (1971) The pathology of the central nervous system in pseudolipidosis of Angus cattle. *Journal of Pathology* **103,** 113–21.

Jolly, R. D., Janmaat, A., West, D. M. and Morrison, I. (1980) Ovine ceroid-lipofuscinosis: a model of Batten's disease. *Neuropathology and Applied Neurobiology* **6,** 195–209.

Jolly, R. D., Janmaat, A., Graydon, R. J. and Clemett, R. S. (1982) Ceroid-lipofuscinosis the ovine model. In *Ceroid-Lipofuscinosis (Batten's disease)* (Eds. Armstrong, D., Koppang, N. and Rider, J. A.), pp. 219–28. Elsevier Biomedical, Amsterdam.

Jones, M. Z., Cunningham, J. G., Dade, A. W., Alessi, D. M., Mostosky, U. V. Vorro, J. R. et al. (1983) Caprine β-mannosidosis: clinical and pathological features. *Journal of Neuropathology and Experimental Neurology* **42,** 268–85.

Jørgensen, L., Blackstad, Th. W., Harkmark, W. and Steen, J. A. (1964) Niemann–Pick's disease. Report of a case with histochemical evidence of neuronal storage of acid glycolipids. *Acta Neuropathologica* **4,** 90–106.

Kaback, M. M. (1977). *Tay-Sachs Disease: screening and prevention.* Alan R. Liss, New York.

Kaback, M. M., Sloan, H. R., Sonneborn, M., Herndon, R. M. and Percy, A. K. (1973) G_{M1}-gangliosidosis type I: in utero detection and fetal manifestations. *Journal of Pediatrics* **82,** 1037–41.

Kahn, P. (1973) Anderson–Fabry disease: a histopathological study of three cases with observations on the mechanism of production of pain. *Journal of Neurology, Neurosurgery and Psychiatry* **36,** 1053–62.

Kamijyo, Y., Kawamura, J., Garcia, J. H. and Lindenberg, R. (1974) Ultrastructural observations of cerebral ceroid-lipofuscinosis; juvenile and adult types in the same family. *Journal of Neuropathology and Experimental Neurology* **33,** 181 (abstract).

Kamoshita, S. (1981) Fetal pathology of lipidoses. *Acta Paediatrica Japonica* **23,** 16–23.

Kamoshita, S. and Landing, B. H. (1968) Distribution of lesions in myenteric plexus and gastrointestinal mucosa in lipidoses and other neurologic disorders of children. *American Journal of Clinical Pathology* **49,** 312–18.

Kamoshita, S., Matsubayashi, A., Suzuki, M. and Arima, M. (1963) An autopsied case of metachromatic leucodystrophy. *Paediatria Universitatis Tokyo* **8,** 43–8.

Kamoshita, S., Aron, A. M., Suzuki, K. and Suzuki, K. (1969) Infantile Niemann–Pick disease. A chemical study with isolation and characterization of membranous cytoplasmic bodies and myelin. *American Journal of Diseases in Children* 117, 379–94.

Kelly, T. E., Thomas, G. H., Taylor, H. A., McKusick, V. A., Sly, W. S., Glaser, J. H. et al. (1975) Mucolipidosis III (pseudo Hurler polydystrophy). Clinical and laboratory studies in a series of 12 patients. *Johns Hopkins Medical Journal* **137,** 156–75.

Kenyon, K. R. (1976) Ocular manifestations and pathology of systemic mucopolysaccharidoses. *Birth Defects. Original Article Series* **12,** *133–53.*

King, J. O. (1975) Progressive myoclonic epilepsy due to Gaucher's disease in an adult. *Journal of Neurology, Neurosurgery and Psychiatry* **38,** 849–54.

Kint, J. A. (1970) Fabry's disease: α-galactosidase deficiency. *Science* **167,** 1268–9.

Kint, J. A. and Carton, D. (1973) Fabry's disease. In *Lysosomes and Storage Diseases* (Eds. Hers, H. G. and Van Hoof, F.), pp. 357–80. Academic Press, New York.

Kint, J. A., Dacremont, G. and Vlietinck, R. (1969) Type II G_{M1} gangliosidosis? *Lancet* **2,** 108–9.

Kjellman, B., Gamstorp, I., Brun, A., Öckerman, P.-A. and Palmgren, B. (1969) Mannosidosis: a clinical and histopathological study. *Journal of Pediatrics* **75,** 366–73.

Klenk, E. (1934) Über die Natur der Phosphatide in der Milz bei Niemann–Pickscher Krankheit. *Hoppe-Seyler's Zeitschrift für physiologische Chemie* **222,** 151–6.

Klibansky, C., Chazan, S., Schoenfeld, A. and Abramovici, A. (1979) Chemical and biochemical studies in human fetuses affected with Niemann–Pick disease type A. *Clinica Chimica Acta* **91,** 243–50.

Kobayashi, N. (1959) Acid mucopolysaccharide granules in the glomerular epithelium in gargoylism. *American Journal of Pathology* **35,** 591–605.

Kobayashi, T. and Suzuki, K. (1981) Chronic G_{M1}-gangliosidosis presenting as dystonia. II. Biochemical studies. *Annals of Neurology* **9,** 476–83.

Kobayashi, T., Ohta, M., Goto, I., Tanaka, Y. and Kuroiwa, Y. (1979) Adult type mucolipidosis with β-galactosidase and sialidase deficiency. *Journal of Neurology* **221,** 137–49.

Kocen, R. S. and Thomas, P. K. (1970) Peripheral nerve involvement in Fabry's disease. *Archives of Neurology* **22,** 81–8.

Kohn, G., Sekeles, E., Arron, J. and Ornoy, A. (1982) Mucolipidosis IV. Prenatal diagnosis by electron microscopy. *Prenatal Diagnosis* **2,** 301–7.

Kolodny, E. H. and Moser, H. W. (1983) Sulphatide lipidosis: metachromatic leukodystrophy. In *The Metabolic Basis of Inherited Disease* (Eds. Stanbury, J. B., Wyngaarden, J. B., Fredrickson, D. S., Goldstein, J. L. and Brown, M. S), 5th edn, pp. 881–905. McGraw-Hill, New York.

Kolodny, E. H., Adams, R. D., Haller, J. S., Joseph, J., Crumrine, P. K. and Raghavan, S. S. (1980) Late onset globoid cell leucodystrophy. *Annals of Neurology* **8,** 219 (abstract).

Koppang, N. (1982) Ceroid-lipofuscinosis in the English setter. A review. In *Ceroid-Lipofuscinosis (Batten's disease)* (Eds. Armstrong, D., Koppang, N. and Rider, J. A.), pp. 201–17. Elsevier Biomedical, Amsterdam.

Kornfeld, M. (1972) Generalized lipofuscinosis (generalized Kufs' disease). *Journal of Neuropathology and Experimental Neurology* **31,** 668–82.

Koto, A., Horwitz, A. L., Suzuki, K., Tiffany, C. W. and Suzuki, K. (1978) The Morquio syndrome. Neuropathology and biochemistry. *Annals of Neurology* **4,** 26–36.

Krabbe, K. (1916) A new familial, infantile form of diffuse brain-sclerosis. *Brain* **39,** 74–114.

Kraus-Ruppert, R., Wildbolz, A., Matthieu, J. M. and Herschkowitz, N. (1972) The late form of metachromatic leukodystrophy. *Journal of the Neurological Sciences* **17,** 373–81.

Kufs, H. (1925) Über eine Spätform der amaurotischem Idiotie und ihre heredofamiliären Grundlagen. *Zentralblatt für die gesamte Neurologie und Psychiatrie* **95,** 169–88.

Kyriakides, E. C., Filippone, N., Paul, B., Grattan, W. and Balint, J. A. (1970) Lipid studies in Wolman's disease. *Pediatrics* **46,** 431–6.

Lageron, A., Caroli, J., Stralin, H. and Barbier, P. (1967) Polycorie cholestérolique de l'adulte. I. Etude clinique, électronique, histochimique. *Presse Médicale* **75,** 2785–98.

Lake, B. D. (1966) A histochemical study of Gaucher's disease and Niemann–Pick's disease. *Journal of the Royal Microscopical Society* **86,** 417–25.

Lake, B. D. (1968) Segmental demyelination of peripheral nerves in Krabbe's disease. *Nature (London)* **217,** 171–2.

Lake, B. D. (1971) Histochemical detection of the enzyme deficiency in blood films in Wolman's disease. *Journal of Clinical Pathology* **24,** 617–20.

Lake, B. D. (1974) An improved method for the detection of β-galactosidase activity and its application to G_{M1}-gangliosidosis and mucopolysaccharidoses. *Histochemical Journal* **6,** 211–18.

Lake, B. D. (1976) The differential diagnosis of the various forms of Batten disease by rectal biopsy. *Birth Defects. Original Article Series* **12,** 455–62.

Lake, B. D. (1977) Histochemical and ultrastructural studies in the diagnosis of inborn errors of metabolism. *Records of Adelaide Children's Hospital* **1,** 337–45.

Lake, B. D. (1981) Metabolic disorders—general considerations. In *Pediatric Pathology* (Ed. Berry, C. L.), pp. 617–39. Springer, Berlin.

Lake, B. D. (1983a) Metabolic disorders of the central and peripheral nervous system. In *Histochemistry in Pathology* (Eds. Filipe, M. I. and Lake, B. D.), pp. 53–69. Churchill-Livingstone, Edinburgh.

Lake, B. D. (1983b) Metabolic disorders of the liver. In *Histochemistry in Pathology* (Eds. Filipe, M. I. and Lake, B. D.), pp. 160–72. Churchill-Livingstone, Edinburgh.

Lake, B. D. and Cavanagh, N. P. C. (1978) Early juvenile Batten's disease. A recognizable subgroup distinct from other forms of Batten's disease. *Journal of the Neurological Sciences* **36,** 265–71.

Lake, B. D. and Patrick, A. D. (1970) Wolman's disease: deficiency of E-600 resistant acid esterase activity with storage of lipids in lysosomes. *Journal of Pediatrics* **76,** 262–6.

Lake, B. D., Milla, P. J., Taylor, D. S. I. and Young, E. P. (1982) A mild variant of mucolipidosis type 4 (ML4). *Birth Defects. Original Article Series* **18,** 391–404.

Lampert, I. A. and Lewis, P. D. (1975) Staining of sulphatides in metachromatic leukodystrophy with alcian blue at high salt concentrations. *Histochemistry* **43,** 269–74.

Landing, B. H., Silverman, F. N., Craig, J. M., Jacoby, M. D., Lahey, M. E. and Chadwick, D. L. (1964) Familial neurovisceral lipidosis. *American Journal of Diseases of Children* **108,** 503–22.

Laws, L. and Saal, J. R. (1968) Lipidosis of the hepatic reticulo-endothelial cells in a sheep. *Australian Veterinary Journal* **44,** 416.

Lazarus, S., Vethamany, V., Schneck, L. and Volk, B. W. (1967) Fine structure and histochemistry of peripheral blood cells in Niemann–Pick disease. *Laboratory Investigation* **17,** 155–70.

Leav, I., Crocker, A. A., Petrak, M. and Jones, T. C. (1968) A naturally occurring lipidosis in shell parakeets. *Laboratory Investigation* **18,** 433–7.

Lee, R. E. (1981) The high incidence of malignant tumours in adults with Gaucher's disease. *Laboratory Investigation* **44,** 37A.

Lee, R. E. and Ellis, L. D. (1971) The storage cells of chronic myelogenous leukaemia. *Laboratory Investigation* **24,** 261–4.

Lehner, T. and Adams, C. W. M. (1968) Lipid histochemistry of Fabry's disease. *Journal of Pathology and Bacteriology* **95,** 411–15.

Leonberg, S. C., Armstrong, D. and Boehme, D. (1982) A century of Kufs disease in an American family. In *Ceroid-lipofuscinosis (Batten's disease)* (Eds. Armstrong, D., Koppang, N. and Rider, J. A.), pp. 87–94. Elsevier Biomedical, Amsterdam.

Leroy, J. G., van Elsen, A. F., Martin, J.-J., Dumon, J. E., Hulet, A. E., Okada, S. and Navarro, C. (1973) Infantile metachromatic leukodystrophy. Confirmation of a prenatal diagnosis. *New England Journal of Medicine* **288,** 1365–9.

Le Sec, G., Stanescu, R. and Lyon, G. (1978) Un nouveau type de sialidase avec atteinte renale: la nephrosialidase. II. Etude anatomique. *Archives Françaises de Pédiatrie* **35,** 830–44.

Levine, S. and Paparo, G. (1982) Brain lesions in a case of cystinosis. *Acta Neuropathologica* **57,** 217–20.

Libert, J., Martin, J.-J. and Ceuterick, C. (1982) Protracted and atypical forms of ceroid-lipofuscinosis. In *Ceroid-lipofuscinosis* (*Batten's disease*) (Eds. Armstrong, D., Koppang, N. and Rider, J. A.), pp. 45–59. Elsevier Biomedical, Amsterdam.

Libert, J. and Toussaint, D. (1982) Tortuosities of retinal and conjunctival vessels in lysosomal storage disorders. *Birth Defects. Original Article Series* **18,** 347–58.

Lin, H. J., Tie, M. S. F. and Ho, F. (1976) Accumulation of glycerylether lipids in Wolman's disease. *Journal of Lipid Research* **17,** 53–6.

Livni, N. and Merin, S. (1978) Mucolipidosis IV. Ultrastructural diagnosis of recently defined genetic disorder. *Archives of Pathology and Laboratory Medicine* **102,** 600–4.

Loeb, H., Tondeur, M., Jonniaux, G., Mockel-Pohl, S. and Vamos-Hurwitz, E. (1969a) Biochemical and ultrastructural studies in a case of mucopolysaccharidosis 'F' (fucosidosis). *Helvetica Paediatrica Acta* **24,** 519–37.

Loeb, H., Tondeur, M., Toppet, M. and Cremer, N. (1969b) Clinical, biochemical and ultrastructural studies of an atypical form of mucopolysaccharidosis. *Acta Paediatrica Scandinavica* **58,** 220–8.

Long, R. G., Lake, B. D., Pettit, J. E., Scheuer, P. J. and Sherlock, S. (1977) Adult Niemann–Pick disease: its relationship to the syndrome of the sea-blue histiocyte. *American Journal of Medicine* **62,** 627–35.

Lowden, J. A. and O'Brien, J. S. (1979) Sialidosis: a review of human neuraminidase deficiency. *American Journal of Human Genetics* **31,** 1–18.

Lowden, J. A., Cutz, E., Conen, P. E., Rudd, N. and Doran, T. A. (1973) Prenatal diagnosis of G_{M1}-gangliosidosis. *New England Journal of Medicine* **288,** 225–8.

Lowden, J. A., Callahan, J. W., Norman, M. G., Thain, M. and Prichard, J. S. (1974) Juvenile G_{M1}-gangliosidosis. *Archives of Neurology* **31,** 200–3.

Lynn, R. and Terry, R. D. (1964) Lipid histochemistry and electron microscopy in adult Niemann–Pick disease. *American Journal of Medicine* **37,** 987–94.

Lyon, G., Arthuis, M. and Thieffry, S. (1961) Leucodystrophie métachromatique infantile familiale. *Revue Neurologique* **104,** 508–32.

Lyon, M. F., Hulse, E. V. and Rowe, C. E. (1965) Foam-cell reticulosis of mice, an inherited condition resembling Gaucher's and Niemann–Pick disease. *Journal of Medical Genetics* **2,** 99–106.

Lyons, J. C., Scheithauer, B. W. and Ginsburg, W. W. (1982) Gaucher disease and glioblastoma multiforme in two siblings. A clinicopathological study. *Journal of Neuropathology and Experimental Neurology* **41,** 45–53.

MacFaul, R., Cavanagh, N., Lake, B. D., Stephens, R. and Whitfield, A. E. (1982) Metachromatic leucodystrophy: review of 38 cases. *Archives of Disease in Childhood* **57,** 168–75.

McKenzie, I. F. C. and Kincaid-Smith, P. (1969) Foam cells in the renal glomerulus. *Journal of Pathology* **97,** 151–4.

McKusick, V. A. (1972) The mucopolysaccharidosis. In *Heritable Disorders of Connective Tissue* 4th edition, C. V. Mosby, Saint Louis, pp. 521–686.

McKusick, V. A. and Neufeld, E. F. (1983) The mucopolysaccharide storage diseases. In *The Metabolic Basis of Inherited Disease* (Eds. Stanbury, J. B., Wyngaarden, J. B., Fredrickson, D. S., Goldstein, J. L. and Brown, M. S.), 5th edn, pp. 751–77. McGraw-Hill, New York.

Maclaren, W. K., Max, N. K., Cornblath, M., Brady, R. O., Ozand, P., Campbell, R. et al. (1976) G_{M3}-gangliosidosis: a novel sphingolipodystrophy. *Pediatrics* **57,** 106–10.

MacPhee, G. B. and Logan, R. W. (1977) Fucosidosis in a native-born Briton. *Journal of Clinical Pathology* **30,** 278–83.

Malmqvist, E., Ivemark, B. I., Lindsten, J., Mannsbach, A. B. and Mårtensson, E. (1971) Pathologic lysosomes and increased urinary glycosylceramide excretion in Fabry's disease. Studies on a family with evidence of linkage with the sex-linked blood group Xg. *Laboratory Investigation* **25,** 1–14.

Maloney, A. F. J. and Cumings, J. N. (1960) A case of juvenile Gaucher's disease with intraneuronal lipid storage. *Journal of Neurology, Neurosurgery and Psychiatry* **23,** 207–13.

Malouf, M., Kirkman, H. N. and Buchanan, P. D. (1976) Ultrastructural changes in antenatal Fabry's disease. *American Journal of Pathology* **82,** 13a.

Mancall, E. L., Aponte, G. E. and Berry, R. G. (1965) Pompe's disease (diffuse glycogenosis) with neuronal storage. *Journal of Neuropathology and Experimental Neurology* **24,** 85–96.

Maroteaux, P., Humbel, R., Strecker, G., Michalski, J.-C. and Mande, R. (1978) Un nouveau type de sialidose avec atteinte renale. La nephrosialidose. I. Etude clinique, radiologique et nosologique. *Archives Françaises de Pédiatrie* **35,** 812–29.

Marshall, W. C., Ockenden, B. G., Fosbrooke, A. S. and Cumings, J. N. (1969) Wolman's disease: a rare lipidosis with adrenal calcification. *Archives of Disease in Childhood* **44,** 331–41.

Mårtensson, E., Percy, A. and Svennerholm, L. (1966) Kidney glycolipids in late infantile metachromatic leucodystrophy. *Acta Paediatrica Scandinavica* **55,** 1–9.

Martin, J. J., Clara, R., Ceuterick, C. and Joris, C. (1976) Is congenital fibre type disproportion a true myopathy? *Acta Neurologica et Psychiatrica Belgica* **76,** 335–44.

Martin, J. J., Leroy, J. G., Ceuterick, C., Libert, J., Dodinval, P. and Martin, L. (1981) Fetal Krabbe leukodystrophy. A morphological study of two cases. *Acta Neuropathologica* **53,** 87–91.

Matsuishi, T., Terasawa, K., Yoshida, I., Yano, E., Yamashita, F., Hidaka, T. et al. (1982) Vacuolar myopathy with type 2A fiber strophy and type 2B fiber deficiency. A case of childhood form acid α-1,4-glucosidase deficiency. *Neuropediatrics* **13,** 173–6.

Matsuyama, H., Minoshima, I. and Watamabe, I. (1963) An autopsy case of leucodystrophy of Krabbe type. *Acta Pathologica Japonica* **13,** 195–9.

Max, S. R., Maclaren, N. K., Brady, R. O., Bradley, R. M., Rennels, M. B., Tanaka, J. et al. (1974) G_{M3} (haematoside) sphingolipodystrophy. *New England Journal of Medicine* **291,** 929–31.

Maynard, J. A., Cooper, R. R. and Ponseti, I. V. (1973) Morquio's disease (mucopolysaccharidosis type IV). Ultrastructure of epiphyseal plates. *Laboratory Investigation* **28,** 194–205.

Mayou, M. S. (1904) Cerebral degeneration with symmetrical changes at the maculae in three members of a family. *Transactions of the Ophthalmological Society of the United Kingdom* **24,** 142.

Mehl, E. and Jatzkewitz, H. (1965) Evidence for the genetic block in metachromatic leucodystrophy (ML). *Biochemical and Biophysical Research Communications* **19,** 407–11.

Melchior, J. C., Terslev, E. and Friis-Hansen, B. (1962) Vacuolized lymphocytes in peripheral blood as a screening test in progressive neurological diseases. *Danish Medical Bulletin* **9,** 83–6.

Menkes, J. H., Andrews, J. M. and Cancilla, P. A. (1971) The cerebroretinal degenerations. *Journal of Pediatrics* **79,** 183–96.

Michels, V. V., Driscoll, D. J., Ferry, G. D., Duff, D. F. and Beaudet, A. L. (1979) Pulmonary vascular obstruction associated with cholesteryl ester storage disease. *Journal of Pediatrics* **94,** 621–3.

Miller, J. D., McCleuer, R. and Kanfer, J. N. (1973) Gaucher's disease: neurologic disorder in adult siblings. *Annals of Internal Medicine* **78,** 883–7.

Morris, M. D., Bhuvaneswaran, C., Shio, H. and Fowler, S. (1982) Lysosome lipid storage disorder in NCTR-BALB/c mice. *American Journal of Pathology* **108,** 140–70.

Moser, H. W. and Chen, W. W. (1983) Ceramidase deficiency: Farber's lipogranulomatosis. In *The Metabolic Basis of Inherited Disease* (Eds. Stanbury, J. B., Wyngaarden, J. B., Fredrickson, D. S., Goldstein, J. L. and Brown, M. S.), 5th edn, pp. 820–30. McGraw-Hill, New York.

Moser, H. W., Prensky, A. L., Wolfe, H. J. and Rosman, N. P., with the technical assistance of Carr, S. and Ferriera, G. (1969) Farber's lipogranulomatosis. Report of a case and demonstration of an excess of free ceramide and ganglioside. *American Journal of Medicine* **47,** 869–90.

Mossakowski, M., Mathieson, G. and Cumings, J. N. (1961) On the relationship of metachromatic leucodystrophy and amaurotic idiocy. *Brain* **84,** 585–604.

Mossman, J., Patrick, A. D., Fensom, A. H., Tansley, L. R., Benson, P. F., Der Kaloustian, V. M. and Dudin, G. (1981) Correct prenatal diagnosis of a Hurler fetus whose amniotic fluid cell cultures were of maternal origin. *Prenatal Diagnosis* **1,** 121–4.

Mossman, J., Blunt, S., Stephens, R., Jones, E. E. and Pembrey, M. (1983) Hunter's disease in a girl: association with X:5 chromosomal translocation disrupting the Hunter gene. *Archives of Disease in Childhood* **58,** 511–15.

Munnich, A., Saudubray, J. M., Hors-Cayla, M. C., Poenaru, L., Ogier, H., Strecker, G. et al. (1982) Enzyme replacement therapy by transplantation of HLA-compatible fibroblasts in Sanfilippo syndrome: another trial. *Pediatric Research* **16,** 259–61.

Murphy, J. V., Hodach, A. E., Gilbert, E. F., Deanching, M. and Matalon, R. (1983) Hunter's syndrome. Ultrastructural features in young children. *Archives of Pathology and Laboratory Medicine* **107,** 495–9.

Nakano, T., Sakai, H., Kinoshita, J., Yagishita, S. and Ito, Y. (1978) Spielmeyer–Vogt disease (generalized juvenile ceroid-lipofuscinosis). Distribution and morphology of inclusions. *Advances in Neurological Sciences* **22,** 1376–91.

Nelson, E., Aurebeck, G., Osterberg, K., Berry, J., Jabbour, J. T. and Bornhoffen, J. (1963) Ultrastructural and chemical studies on Krabbe's disease. *Journal of Neuropathology and Experimental Neurology* **22,** 414–34.

Neufeld, E. and McKusick, V. A. (1983) Disorders of lysosomal enzyme synthesis and localization. I-cell disease and pseudo-Hurler polydystrophy. In *The Metabolic Basis of Inherited Disease* (Eds. Stanbury, J. B., Wyngaarden, J. B., Fredrickson, D. S., Goldstein, J. L. and Brown, M. S.), 5th edn, pp. 778–87. McGraw-Hill, New York.

Neville, B. G. R., Lake, B. D., Stephens, R. and Sanders, M. D. (1973) A neurovisceral storage disease with vertical supranuclear ophthalmoplegia and its relationship to Niemann–Pick disease. A report of nine patients. *Brain* **96,** 97–120.

Niemann, A. (1914). Ein unbekanntes Krankheitsbild. *Jahrbuch für Kinderheilkunde* **79,** 1–10.

Ninomiya, N., Matsuda, I., Fukuda, S., Iwamasa, T. and Osame, T. (1983) Immunohistochemical demonstration of acid α-glucosidase in Pompe's disease. *Histochemical Journal* **15,** 601–604.

Norman, R. M., Forrester, R. M. and Tingey, A. H.

(1967) The juvenile form of Niemann–Pick disease. *Archives of Disease in Childhood* **42,** 91–6.

Norman, R. M., Oppenheimer, D. R. and Tingey, A. H. (1961) Histological and chemical findings in Krabbe's leucodystrophy. *Journal of Neurology, Neurosurgery and Psychiatry* **24,** 223–32.

Norman, R. M., Urich, H. and France, N. E. (1959) Perivascular cavitation of the basal ganglia in gargoylism. *Journal of Mental Science* **105,** 1070–7.

Norman, R. M., Urich, H. and Lloyd, O. C. (1956) The neuropathology of infantile Gaucher's disease. *Journal of Pathology and Bacteriology* **72,** 121–31.

Norman, R. M., Urich, H. and Tingey, A. H. (1960) Metachromatic leuco-encephalopathy. A form of lipidosis. *Brain* **83,** 369–80.

Norman, R. M. and Wood, N. (1941) A congenital form of amaurotic family idiocy. *Journal of Neurology and Psychiatry* **4,** 175–90.

Norman, R. M., Urich, H., Tingey, A. H. and Goodbody, R. A. (1959) Tay–Sachs disease with visceral involvement and its relationship to Niemann–Pick disease. *Journal of Pathology and Bacteriology* **78,** 409–21.

O'Brien, J. S. (1969). Five gangliosidoses. *Lancet* **2,** 805.

O'Brien, J. S., Stern, M. B., Landing, B. H., O'Brien, J. K. and Donnell, G. N. (1965) Generalized gangliosidosis. *American Journal of Diseases of Children* **109,** 338.

O'Brien, J. S., Bernett, J., Veath, L. and Paa, D. (1975) Lysosomal storage disorders. Diagnosis by ultrastructural examination of skin biopsy specimens. *Archives of Neurology* **33,** 592–9.

Öckerman, P. A. (1967) A generalized storage disorder resembling Hurler's syndrome. *Lancet* **2,** 239–41.

Okada, S. and O'Brien, J. S. (1968) Generalized gangliosidosis; beta-galactosidase deficiency. *Science* **160,** 1002–4.

Okada, S. and O'Brien, J. S. (1969) Tay–Sachs disease: generalized absence of a β-D-*N*-acetylhexosaminidase component. *Science* **165,** 698–700.

Olsson, Y. and Sourander, P. (1969) The reliability of the diagnosis of metachromatic leucodystrophy by peripheral nerve biopsy. *Acta Paediatrica Scandinavica* **58,** 15–24.

Orii, T., Minami, R., Sukagawa, K., Sato, S., Tsugawa, S., Horino, K. et al. (1972) A new type of mucolipidosis with β-galactosidase deficiency and glycopeptiduria. *Tohoku Journal of Experimental Medicine* **107,** 303–15.

Palo, J. and Savolainen, H. (1972) Thin-layer chromatographic demonstration of aspartylglycosylamine and a novel acidic carbohydrate in human tissues. *Journal of Chromatography* **65,** 447–50.

Palo, J., Riekkinen, P., Arstila, A. U., Autio, S. and Kivimäki, T. (1972) Aspartylglucosaminuria II. Biochemical studies on brain, liver, kidney and spleen. *Acta Neuropathologica* **20,** 217–24.

Pampiglione, G. and Harden A. (1977) So-called neuronal ceroid lipofuscinosis. Neurophysiological studies in 60 children. *Journal of Neurology, Neurosurgery and Psychiatry* **40,** 323–30.

Patel, V., Tappel, A. L. and O'Brien, J. S. (1970) Hyaluronidase and sulphatase deficiency in Hurler's syndrome. *Biochemical Medicine* **3,** 447–57.

Patel, V., Watanabe, I. and Zeman, W. (1972) Deficiency of α-L-fucosidase. *Science* **176,** 426–7.

Patrick, A. D. (1965) A deficiency of glucocerebrosidase in Gaucher's disease. *Biochemical Journal* **97,** 17c–18c.

Patrick, A. D. (1982) The β-glucosidase isoenzymes and the enzymatic defect in Gaucher's disease. In *Gaucher's Disease: a century of delineation and research* (Eds. Desnick, R. J., Gatt, S. and Grabowski, G. A.), pp. 287–308. Alan R. Liss, New York.

Patrick, A. D. and Lake, B. D. (1968) Cystinosis. Electron microscopic evidence of lysosomal storage of cystine in lymph node. *Journal of Clinical Pathology* **21,** 571–5.

Patrick, A. D. and Lake, B. D. (1969) Deficiency of an acid lipase in Wolman's disease. *Nature (London)* **222,** 1067–8.

Patrick, A. D. and Lake, B. D. (1973) Wolman's disease. In *Lysosomes and Storage Diseases* (Eds. Hers, H. G. and van Hoof, F.), pp. 453–73. Academic Press, New York.

Patrick, A. D., Willcox, P., Stephens, R. and Kenyon, V. G. (1976) Prenatal diagnosis of Wolman's disease. *Journal of Medical Genetics* **13,** 49–51.

Patrick, A. D., Young, E., Kleijer, W. T. and Niermeijer, M. F. (1977) Prenatal diagnosis of Niemann–Pick disease type A using chromogenic substrate. *Lancet* **2,** 144.

Peiffer, J. (1959) Über die metachromatischen Leukodystrophien (typ Scholz). *Archiv für Psychiatrie und Zeitschrift für die gesamte Neurologie* **199,** 386–416.

Pellissier, J. F., Gambarelli, D., Hassoun, J., Roger, J., Suzuki, K. and Toga, M. (1975) Neurolipidose juvénile atypique. Étude ultrastructurelle d'une biopsie cérébrale. *Journal of the Neurological Sciences* **25,** 183–96.

Percy, D. H. and Jortner, B. S. (1971) Feline lipidosis. Light and electron microscopic studies. *Archives of Pathology* **92,** 136–44.

Philippart, M., Sarlieve, L. and Manacorda, A. (1969) Urinary glycolipids in Fabry's disease. Their examination in the detection of atypical variants and the pre-symptomatic state. *Pediatrics* **43,** 201–6.

Pick, L. (1927) Über die lipoidzelligen Splenohepatomegalie Typus Niemann–Pick als Stoffwechselerkrankung. *Medizinische Klinik* **23,** 1483–8.

Pierce, K.R., Kosanke, S.D., Bay, W.W. and Bridges, C.H. (1976) G_{M2}-gangliosidosis. Porcine cerebrospinal lipodystrophy. *American Journal of Pathology* **83,** 419–21.

Pilz, H. (1970) Niemann–Picksche Krankheit im Erwachsenenalter. *Deutsche medizinische Wochenschrift* **95,** 1–15.

Pilz, H. and Jatzkewitz, H. (1968) Biochemical evaluation of a combined sulfatidosis and gangliosidosis (glycolipidosis) of the brain. *Pathologia Europaea* **3,** 409–15.

Pilz, H., Sandhoff, K. and Jatzkewitz, H. (1966) Eine Gangliosidstoffwechsel-störung mit Anhäufung von Ceramid-lactosid, Monosialo-ceramid-lactosid und Tay–Sachs-Gangliosid im Gehirn. *Journal of Neurochemistry* **13,** 1273–82.

Pilz, H., Muller, D., Sandhoff, K. and Menlen, V. (1968) Tay–Sachssche Krankheit mit Hexosaminidase-Defekt. *Deutsche medizinische Wochenschrift* **98,** 1833.

Pinsky, L., Powell, E. and Callahan, J. (1970) G_{M1}-gangliosidosis types 1 and 2: enzymatic differences in cultured fibroblasts. *Nature (London)* **228,** 1093–5.

Rac, R. and Giesecke, P. R. (1975) Lysosomal storage disease in chihuahuas. *Australian Veterinary Journal* **51,** 403–4.

Rahman, A. N. and Lindenberg, R. (1963) The neuropathology of hereditary dystopic lipidosis. *Archives of Neurology* **9,** 373–85.

Rampini, S., Isler, W., Baerlocher, K., Bischoff, A., Ulrich, J. and Plüss, H. J. (1970) Die Kombination von metachromatischer Leukodystrophie und Mukopolysaccharidose als selbständiges Krankheitsbild (Mukosulfatidose). *Helvetica Paediatrica Acta* **25,** 436–61.

Rapin, I., Suzuki, K., Suzuki, K. and Valsamin, M. P. (1976) Adult (chronic) G_{M2}-gangliosidosis. Atypical spinocerebellar degeneration in a Jewish sibship. *Archives of Neurology* **33,** 120–30.

Rapin, I., Goldfischer, S., Katzman, R., Engel, J. and O'Brien, J. S. (1978) The cherry-red spot myoclonus syndrome. *Annals of Neurology* **3,** 234–42.

Raynaud, E.-J., Escourolle, R., Baumann, N., Turpin, J.-C., Dubois, G., Malpuech, G. and Lagarde, R. (1975) Metachromatic leukodystrophy. Ultrastructural and enzymatic study of a case of variant O form. *Archives of Neurology* **32,** 834–8.

Rayner, S. and Böök, J. A. (1958) Genetics and blood morphology in amaurotic idiocy. *Lancet* **1,** 1077–8.

Résibois, A. (1969) Electron microscopic study of metachromatic leucodystrophy. III. Lysosomal nature of the inclusions. *Acta Neuropathologica* **13,** 149–56.

Riches, W. G. and Smuckler, E. A. (1983) A severe infantile mucolipidosis. Clinical biochemical and pathologic features. *Archives of Pathology and Laboratory Medicine* **107,** 147–52.

Robb, R. M. and Kuwabara, T. (1973) The ocular pathology of type A Niemann–Pick disease. *Investigative Ophthalmology* **12,** 366–77.

Robinson, D. and Stirling, J. L. (1968) *N*-acetyl-β-glucosaminidases in human spleen. *Biochemical Journal* **107,** 321–327.

Rodriguez, M., O'Brien, J. S., Garrett, R. S. and Powell, H. C. (1982) Canine G_{M1}-gangliosidosis. An ultrastructural and biochemical study. *Journal of Neuropathology and Experimental Neurology* **41,** 618–629.

Romeo, G., Borrone, C., Gatti, R. and Durand, P. (1977) Fucosidosis in Calabria: founder effect or high gene frequency? *Lancet* **1,** 368–9.

Rosenblum, J. L., Keating, J. P., Prensky, A. A. and Nelson, J. S. (1981) A progressive neurologic syndrome in children with chronic liver disease. *New England Journal of Medicine* **304,** 503–8.

Rutsaert, J., Menu, R. and Résibois, A. (1973) Ultrastructure of sulfatide storage in normal and sulfatase-deficient fibroblasts in vitro. *Laboratory Investigation* **29,** 527–35.

Rutsaert, J., Tondeur, M., Vamos-Hurwitz, E. and Dustin, P. (1977) The cellular lesions of Farber's disease and their experimental reproduction in tissue culture. *Laboratory Investigation* **36,** 474–80.

Sachs, B. (1887) On arrested cerebral development with special reference to its cortical pathology. *Journal of Nervous and Mental Disease* **14,** 541.

Sachs, B. (1896) A family form of idiocy, generally fatal associated with early blindness. *Journal of Nervous and Mental Disease* **21,** 475–9.

Sacrez, R., Juif, J. G., Gigonnet, J. M. and Gruner, J. E. (1967) La maladie de Landing, ou idiote amaurotique infantile précoce avec gangliosidose généralisée. *Pédiatrie* **22,** 143–62.

Sakuraba, H., Aoyagi, T. and Suzuki, Y. (1982) Galactosialidosis (β-galactosidase-neuraminidase deficiency): a possible role of serine-thiol proteases in the degradation of β-galactosidase molecules. *Clinica Chimica Acta* **125,** 275–82.

Sandhoff, K., Andreae, U. and Jatzkewitz, H. (1968) Deficient hexosaminidase activity in an exceptional case of Tay–Sachs disease with additional storage of kidney globoside in visceral organs. *Pathologia Europaea* **3,** 278.

Santavuori, P., Haltia, M. and Rapola, J. (1974) Infantile type of so-called neuronal ceroid-lipofuscinosis. *Developmental Medicine and Child Neurology* **16,** 644–53.

Santavuori, P., Haltia, M., Rapola, J. and Raitta, C. (1973) Infantile type of so-called neuronal ceroid-lipofuscinosis I. A clinical study of 15 cases. *Journal of the Neurological Sciences* **18,** 257–67.

Schaub, J., Janka, G. E., Christomanou, H., Sandhoff, K., Permanetter, W., Hübner, G. and Meister, P. (1980) Wolman's disease: clinical biochemical and ultrastructural studies in an unusual case without striking adrenal calcification. *European Journal of Pediatrics* **135,** 45–53.

Schiff, L., Schubert, W. K., McAdams, A. J., Spiegel, E. L. and O'Donnell, J. F. (1968) Hepatic cholesterol ester storage disease. A familial disorder. I. Clinical aspects. *American Journal of Medicine* **44,** 538–46.

Schnabel, R. (1961) Histochemische und biochemische Untersuchungen beim Gargoylismus (Pfaundler–Hurler Syndrom). *Virchows Archiv für pathologische Anatomie und Physiologie und für klinische Medizin* **334,** 379–98.

Schneider, E. L., Ellis, W. G., Brady, R. O., McCulloch, J. R. and Epstein, C. J. (1972a) Prenatal Niemann–Pick disease: biochemical and histologic examination of a 19-gestational week fetus. *Pediatric Research* **6,** 720–9.

Schneider, E. L., Ellis, W. G., Brady, R. O., McCulloch, J. R. and Epstein, C. J. (1972b) Infantile (type 2) Gaucher's disease: *in utero* diagnosis and fetal pathology. *Journal of Pediatrics* **81,** 1134–9.

Schneider, P. B. and Kennedy, E. P. (1967) Sphingomyelinase in normal human spleens and in spleens from subjects with Niemann–Pick disease. *Journal of Lipid Research* **8,** 202–9.

Schochet, S. S., McCormick, W. F. and Powell, G. F. (1976) Krabbe's disease: a light and electron microscopical study. *Acta Neuropathologica* **36,** 153–60.

Scholz, W. (1925) Klinische, pathologisch-anatomische, und erbbiologische Untersuchungen bei familiärer diffuser Hirnsklerose im Kindesalter. *Zeitschrift für die gesamte Neurologie und Psychiatrie* **99,** 651–85.

Schull, R. M., Munger, R. J., Spellacy, E., Hall, C. W., Constantopoulos, G. and Neufeld, E. F. (1982) Canine α-L-iduronidase deficiency. A model of mucopolysaccharidosis I. *American Journal of Pathology* **109,** 244–8.

Schutta, H. S., Pratt, R. T. C., Metz, H., Evans, K. A. and Carter, C. O. (1966) A family study of the late infantile and juvenile forms of metachromatic leucodystrophy. *Journal of Medical Genetics* **3,** 86–91.

Schwendemann, G. (1976) Lymphocytic inclusions in the juvenile type of generalized ceroid-lipofuscinosis. An electron microscopic study. *Acta Neuropathologica* **36,** 327–38.

Schwendemann, G. (1982) Diagnosis of juvenile ceroid-lipofuscinosis by electron microscopy of lymphocytes and of rectal, skin and sural nerve biopsy tissues. In *Ceroid-lipofuscinosis* (*Batten's disease*) (Eds. Armstrong, D., Koppang, N. and Rider, J. A.), pp. 117–40. Elsevier Biomedical, Amsterdam.

Schwendemann, G., Colmant, H. J.; Elze, K.-L., Koepp, P., Lagenstein, I. and Steinhausen, H.-C. (1978) Juvenile type of generalized ceroid-lipofuscinosis (Spielmeyer–Sjogren syndrome). II. Biopsy findings. *Neuropädiatrie* **9,** 28–48.

Seegmiller, J. E. (1973). Cytinosis. In *Lysosomes and Storage Diseases* (Eds. Hers, H. G. and Van Hoof, F.), pp. 485–518. Academic Press, New York.

Seng, P. N., Debuch, H., Witter, B. and Wiedemann, H.-R. (1971) *Bis*(monoacylglycerin) phosphorsäure-Vermehrung bei sphingomyelinose (M. Niemann–Pick?). *Hoppe-Seyler's Zeitschrift für physiologische Chemie* **352,** 280–8.

Shapiro, L. T., Aleck, K. A., Kaback, M. M., Itabashi, H., Desnick, R. J., Brand, N. et al. (1979) Metachromatic leukodystrophy without arylsulfatase A deficiency. *Pediatric Research* **13,** 1179–81.

Sharer, L. R., Barondess, J. A., Silver, R. T. and Gray, G. F. (1974) Association of Hodgkin's disease and Gaucher's disease. *Archives of Pathology* **98,** 376–8.

Shaw, C. M. and Carlson, C. B. (1970) Crystalline structures in globoid-epitheloid cells: an electron microscopic study of globoid leukodystrophy (Krabbe's disease). *Journal of Neuropathology and Experimental Neurology* **29,** 306–19.

Shoenfeld, Y., Gallant, L. A., Shaklai, M., Livini, E., Djaldetti, M. and Pinkhas, J. (1982) Gaucher's disease. A disease with chronic stimulation of the immune system. *Archives of Pathology and Laboratory Medicine* **106,** 388–91.

Siakotos, A. N. and Munkres, K. D. (1982) Recent developments in the isolation and properties of autofluorescent lipopigments. In *Ceroid-lipofuscinosis* (*Batten's disease*) (Eds. Armstrong, D., Koppang, N. and Rider, J. A.), pp. 167–83. Elsevier Biomedical, Amsterdam.

Silverstein, M. N., Ellefson, R. D. and Ahern, E. J. (1970) The syndrome of the sea-blue histiocyte. *New England Journal of Medicine* **282,** 1–4.

Sjögren, T. (1931) Die juvenile amaurotische Idiotie. Klinische und erblichkeitsmedizinische Untersuchungen. *Hereditas* **14,** 197–426.

Snyder, S. P., Kingston, R. S. and Wenger, D. A. (1982) Niemann–Pick disease: sphingomyelinosis of Siamese cats. *American Journal of Pathology* **108,** 252–4.

Sourander, P. and Olsson, Y. (1968) Peripheral neuropathy in globoid cell leucodystrophy (morbus Krabbe). *Acta Neuropathologica* **11,** 69–81.

Spalton, D. J., Taylor, D. S. I. and Sanders, M. D. (1980) Juvenile Batten's disease: an ophthalmological assessment of 26 patients. *British Journal of Ophthalmology* **64,** 726–32.

Spielmeyer, W. (1905) Über familiäre amaurotische

Idioten. *Neurologisches Zentralblatt* **24,** 620–1.

Spranger, J., Wiedemann, H.-R., Tolksdorf, M., Graucob, E. and Caesar, R. (1968) Lipomucopolysaccharidose. Eine neue Speicherkrankheit. *Zeitschrift für Kinderheilkunde* **103,** 285–306.

Srivastava, S. K., Garg, H. S., Neff, W. A. and Awasthi, Y. C. (1982) Peroxidase isoenzymes in the tissues of normal and a Batten's disease patient. In *Ceroid-lipofuscinosis* (*Batten's disease*) (Eds. Armstrong, D., Koppang, N. and Rider, J. A.), pp. 291–9. Elsevier Biomedical, Amsterdam.

Stanbury, J. B., Wyngaarden, J. B., Fredrickson, D. S., Goldstein, J. L. and Brown, M. S. (Eds.) (1983) *The Metabolic Basis of Inherited Disease*, 5th edn. McGraw-Hill, New York.

Stevens, R. L., Fluharty, A. L., Kihara, H., Kaback, M. M., Shapiro, L. J., Marsh et al. (1981) Cerebroside sulfatase activator deficiency induced metachromatic leukodystrophy. *American Journal of Human Genetics* **33,** 900–6.

Stengel, C. (1826) Beretning om et maerkeligt Sygdomstilfoelde hos fire Sodskende i Naerheden af Roraas. *Eyr* (*Christiania*) **1,** 347–52.

Strecker, G. and Montreuil, J. (1971) Description d'une oligosaccharidosurie accompagnant une gangliosidose G_{M2} a deficit total en *N*-acetyl hexosaminidases. *Clinica Chimica Acta* **33,** 395–401.

Sugita, M., Dulaney, J. T. and Moser, H. W. (1972) Ceramidase deficiency in Farber's disease (lipogranulomatosis). *Science* **178,** 1100–2.

Sung, J. H., Hayano, M. and Desnick, R. J. (1977) Mannosidosis: pathology of the nervous system. *Journal of Neuropathology and Experimental Neurology* **36,** 807–20.

Suzuki, K. and Grover, W. D. (1970) Krabbe's leukodystrophy (globoid cell leukodystrophy): an ultrastructural study. *Archives of Neurology* **22,** 385–96.

Suzuki, K., Schneider, E. L. and Epstein, C. J. (1971) *In utero* diagnosis of globoid cell leukodystrophy (Krabbe's disease). *Biochemical and Biophysical Research Communications* **45,** 1363–6.

Suzuki, K. and Suzuki, Y. (1970) Globoid cell leukodystrophy (Krabbe's disease): deficiency of galactocerebroside β-galactosidase. *Proceedings of the National Academy of Sciences of the USA* **66,** 302–9.

Suzuki, K. and Suzuki, Y. (1983) Galactosylceramide lipidosis: globoid cell leukodystrophy (Krabbe's disease). In *The Metabolic Basis of Inherited Disease* (Eds. Stanbury, J. B., Wyngaarden, J. B., Fredrickson, D. S., Goldstein, J. L. and Brown, M. S.), 5th edn, pp. 857–80. McGraw-Hill, New York.

Suzuki, Y., Crocker, A. C. and Suzuki, K. (1971) G_{M1}-gangliosidosis. Correlation of clinical and biochemical data. *Archives of Neurology* **24,** 58–64.

Suzuki, Y. and Suzuki, K. (1971) Krabbe's globoid cell leukodystrophy: deficiency of galactocerebrosidase in serum, leukocytes and fibroblasts. *Science* **171,** 73–5.

Suzuki, Y., Austin, J., Armstrong, D., Suzuki, K., Schlenker, J. and Fletcher, T. (1970) Studies in globoid leukodystrophy: enzymatic and lipid findings in the canine form. *Experimental Neurology* **29,** 65–75.

Svennerholm, L. (1964) The gangliosides. *Journal of Lipid Research* **5,** 145.

Svennerholm, L., Vanier, M.-T. and Mansson, J. E. (1980) Krabbe's disease. A galactosyl-sphingosine (psychosine) lipidosis. *Journal of Lipid Research* **21,** 53–64.

Tanaka, J., Garcia, J. H., Max, S. R., Viloria, J. E., Karaijyo, Y., Maclaren, N. K. et al. (1975) Cerebral sponginess and G_{M3} gangliosidosis: ultrastructure and probable pathogenesis. *Journal of Neuropathology and Experimental Neurology* **34,** 249–62.

Tay, W. (1881) Symmetrical changes in the region of the yellow spot in each eye of an infant. *Transactions of the Ophthalmological Society of the United Kingdom* **1,** 55–7.

Tellez-Nagel, I., Rapin, I., Iwamoto, T., Johnson, A. B., Norton, W. T. and Nitowsky, H. (1976) Mucolipidosis IV. Clinical, ultrastructural, histochemical and chemical studies of a case including brain biopsy. *Archives of Neurology* **33,** 828–35.

Terry, R. D. and Weiss, M. (1963) Studies in Tay-Sachs disease. II. Ultrastructure of the cerebrum. *Journal of Neuropathology and Experimental Neurology* **22,** 18–55.

Thannhauser, S. J. (1940) In *Lipidoses: Diseases of the Cellular Lipid Metabolism.* Oxford University Press, London.

Thieffry, S. (1962) La leucodystrophie métachromatique infantile familiale; maladie de Scholz-Greenfield. *Pédiatrie* **17,** 593–606.

Thieffry, S., Lyon, G. and Maroteaux, P. (1967) Encephalopathie metabolique associant une mucopolysaccharidose et une sulphatidose. *Archives françaises de pédiatrie* **24,** 425–32.

Thomas, G. H., Raghavan, S., Kolodny, E. H., Frisch, A., Neufeld, E. F., O'Brien, J. S. et al. (1982) Nonuniform deficiency of hexosaminidase A in tissues and fluids of two unrelated individuals. *Pediatric Research* **16,** 232–7.

Tomé, F. M. S., Fardeau, M. and Lenoir, G. (1977) Ultrastructure of muscle and sensory nerve in Fabry's disease. *Acta Neuropathologica* **38,** 187–94.

Tripp, J. H., Lake, B. D., Young, E., Ngu, J. and Brett, E. M. (1977) Juvenile Gaucher's disease with horizontal gaze palsy in three siblings. *Journal of Neurology, Neurosurgery and Psychiatry* **40,** 470–8.

Tsan, M. F., Gale, A. N., Murphy, E. A. and McIntyre, P. A. (1978) Neuronal ceroid-lipofuscinosis. Studies of granulocyte enzyme activities. *Journal of the Neurological Sciences* **36,** 13–24.

Van der Water, N. S., Jolly, R. D. and Farrow, B. R. H. (1979) Canine Gaucher disease—the enzymic defect. *Australian Journal of Experimental Biology and Medical Science* **57,** 551.

Vandeville, M., Fankhauser, R., Bichsel, P., Wiesmann, U. and Herschkowitz, N. (1982) Hereditary neurovisceral mannosidosis associated with α-mannosidase deficiency in a family of Persian cats. *Acta Neuropathologica* **58,** 64–8.

Van Hoof, F. (1973a) Mucopolysaccharidoses. In *Lysosomes and Storage Diseases* (Eds. Hers, H. G. and Van Hoof, F.), pp. 217–59. Academic Press, New York.

Van Hoof, F. (1973b) Fucosidosis. In *Lysosomes and Storage Diseases* (Eds. Hers, H. G. and Van Hoof, F.), pp. 277–90. Academic Press, New York.

Van Hoof, F. and Hers, H. G. (1964) L'ultrastructure des cellules hépatiques dans la maladie de Hurler (gargoylisme). *Comptes Rendus de l'Academie des Sciences, Paris* **259,** 1281–3.

Van Hoof, F. and Hers, H. G. (1968) The abnormalities of lysosomal enzymes in mucopolysaccharidoses. *European Journal of Biochemistry* **7,** 34–44.

Vanier, M. T., Rousson, R. and Louisot, P. (1983) Chromatofocussing of skin fibroblast sphingomyelinase: alterations in Niemann–Pick disease type C shared by G_{M1}-gangliosidosis. *Clinica Chimica Acta* **130,** 155–61.

Vethamany, V. G., Welch, J. P. and Vethamany, S. K. (1972) Type D Niemann–Pick disease (Nova Scotia variant). Ultrastructure of blood, skin fibroblasts and bone marrow. *Archives of Pathology* **93,** 537–43.

Vidgoff, J., Buist, N. R. M. and O'Brien, J. S. (1973) Absence of *β-N*-acetyl-D-hexosaminidase A activity in a healthy woman. *American Journal of Human Genetics* **25,** 372.

Vogt, H. (1905) Über familiäre amaurotische Idiotie und verwandte Krankheitsbilder. *Monatsschrift für Psychiatrie und Neurologie* **18,** 161–71; 310–57.

Volk, B. W. and Wallace, B. J. (1966) The liver in lipidosis. An electron microscopic and histochemical study. *American Journal of Pathology* **49,** 203–25.

Wallace, B. J., Schneck, L., Kaplan, H. and Volk, B. W. (1965) Fine structure of the cerebellum of children with lipidoses. *Archives of Pathology* **80,** 466–86.

Wallace, B. J., Kaplan, D., Adachi, M., Schneck, L. and Volk, B. W. (1966) Mucopolysaccharidosis type III. Morphologic and biochemical studies of two siblings with Sanfilippo syndrome. *Archives of Pathology* **82,** 462–73.

Wenger, D. A., Barth, G. and Githens, J. H. (1977) Nine cases of sphingomyelin lipidosis, a new variant in Spanish-American children. Juvenile variant of Niemann–Pick disease with foamy and sea-blue histiocytes. *American Journal of Diseases of Children* **131,** 955–61.

Wenger, D. A., Roth, S. and Sattler, M. (1982) Acute neuronopathic (infantile) and chronic non-neuropathic (adult) Gaucher disease in full siblings. *Journal of Pediatrics* **100,** 252–4.

Wenger, D. A., Roth, S., Kudoh, T., Grover, W. R., Tucker, S. H., Kaye, E. M. and Ullman, M. D. (1983) Biochemical studies in a patient with subacute neuropathic Gaucher disease without visceral glucosylceramide storage. *Pediatric Research* **17,** 3448.

Whiteman, P. and Henderson, H. (1977) A method for the determination of amniotic fluid glycosaminoglycans and its application to the prenatal diagnosis of Hurler and Sanfilippo diseases. *Clinica Chimica Acta* **79,** 99–105.

Wiedemann, H.-R., Debuch, H., Lennert, K., Caesar, R., Blümke, S., Harms, D., Tolksdorf, M. et al. (1972) Über eine infantil-juvenile, subchronisch verlaufende, den Sphingomyelinosen (Niemann–Pick) anzureihende Form der Lipidosen ein neuer Typ? *Zeitschrift für Kinderheilkunde* **112,** 187–225.

Wiederschain, G. (1980) Detection of generalized G_{M1}-gangliosidosis. *Lancet* **1,** 881–2.

Wight, P. A. L. (1976) The histopathology of a cerebral lipidosis in the Hawaiian goose *Branta sandvicensis*. *Neuropathology and Applied Neurobiology* **2,** 335–47.

Willcox, P. and Patrick, A. D. (1974) Biochemical diagnosis of cystinosis using cultured cells. *Archives of Disease in Childhood* **49,** 209–12.

Winters, P. R., Harrod, M. J., Molenich-Eleetred, S. A., Kirkpatrick, J. and Rosenberg, R. N. (1976) α-L-Iduronidase deficiency and possible Hurler–Scheie genetic compound. Clinical, pathologic and biochemical findings. *Neurology* **26,** 1003–7.

Witte, F. (1921) Ueber pathologische Abbauvorgänge im Zentralnervensystem. *Münchener medizinische Wochenschrift* **68,** 69–72.

Wolfe, H. J. and Cohen, R. B. (1968) Nonglycogen polysaccharide storage in glycogenosis type 2 (Pompe's disease). *Archives of Pathology* **86,** 579–84.

Wolfe, H. J. and Pietra, G. G. (1964) The visceral lesions of metachromatic leukodystrophy. *American Journal of Pathology* **44,** 921–30.

Wolfe, L. S. and Ng Ying Kin, N. M. K. (1982) Batten's disease: new research findings on the biochemical defect. *Birth Defects. Original Article Series* **18,** 233–9.

Wolfe, L. S., Senior, R. G. and Ng Ying Kin, N. M. K. (1974) The structures of oligosaccharides accumulating in the liver of G_{M1}-gangliosidosis type I. *Journal of Biological Chemistry* **249,** 1828–38.

Wolfe, L. S., Callahan, J., Fawcett, J. S., Andermann, F. and Scriver, C. (1970) G_{M1}-gangliosidosis without chondrodystrophy or visceromegaly: β-galactosidase deficiency with gangliosidosis and the excessive excretion of a keratan sulphate. *Neurology* **20,** 23–44.

Wolfe, L. S., Ng Ying Kin, N. M. K., Baker, R. R., Carpenter, S. and Andermann, F. (1977) Identification of retinoyl complexes as the autofluorescent component of the neuronal storage material in Batten's disease. *Science* **195,** 1360–2.

Wong, V. G. (1976) Ocular manifestations in cystinosis. *Birth Defects. Original Article Series* **12,** 181–6.

Yamaguchi, K., Tsuchiyama, H. and Tabata, K. (1971) Two male siblings' cases of specific lipidosis found by electron microscopy. *Acta Pathologica Japonica* **21,** 445–58.

Yamano, T., Shimada, M., Okada, S., Yutaka, T., Kato, T., Inui, K. et al. (1983) Ultrastructural study on nervous system of fetus with G_{M1}-gangliosidosis type 1. *Acta Neuropathologica* **61,** 15–20.

Young, E. P. and Patrick, A. D. (1970) Deficiency of acid esterase activity in Wolman's disease. *Archives of Disease in Childhood* **45,** 664–8.

Young, E., Wilson, J., Patrick, A. D. and Crome, L. (1972) Galactocerebrosidase deficiency in globoid cell leucodystrophy of late onset. *Archives of Disease in Childhood* **47,** 449–50.

Yunis, E. J. and Lee, R. E. (1969) The ultrastructure of globoid (Krabbe) leukodystrophy. *Laboratory Investigation* **21,** 415–19.

Zeman, W. and Donahue, S. (1963) Fine structure of the lipid bodies in juvenile amaurotic idiocy. *Acta Neuropathologica* **3,** 144–9.

Zeman, W. and Dyken, P. (1969) Neuronal ceroid-lipofuscinosis (Batten's disease). Relationship to amaurotic familial idocy. *Pediatrics* **44,** 570–83.

Zeman, W. and Hoffman, J. (1962) Juvenile and late forms of amaurotic idiocy in one family. *Journal of Neurology, Neurosurgery and Psychiatry* **25,** 352–62.

Zeman, W. and Siakotos, A. N. (1973) The neuronal ceroid-lipofuscinoses. In *Lysosomes and Storage Diseases* (Eds. Hers, H. G. and Van Hoof, F.), pp. 519–51. Academic Press, New York.

13

Nutritional deficiencies and metabolic disorders

L.W. Duchen and Jean M. Jacobs

Vitamin deficiencies

The biochemical role of vitamins in the metabolism of the nervous system has been reviewed by McIlwain and Bachelard (1984). The B group is of greater importance than the other vitamins. Deficiency, whether of thiamine (B_1), nicotinic acid, riboflavin and pantothenic acid (B_2 group), pyridoxine (B_6) or cyanocobalamin (B_{12}), produces a well-known clinical syndrome. The significance of other B vitamins such as choline, biotin, inositol and para-aminobenzoic acid is not so well understood.

Thiamine

Thiamine is not synthesized in the central nervous system and must be transported from the blood. The entry of thiamine into brain and cerebrospinal fluid is via a saturable transport mechanism at blood-brain and blood-CSF barriers where its concentration in the extracellular space of the CNS is regulated. Cells within the brain also have saturable uptake and release systems, whilst gut and kidneys regulate total thiamine levels by a group of saturable transport systems and metabolism. Thiamine's importance in the nervous system, and in particular the role of its deficiency in the production of neurological syndromes associated with alcoholism, is shown by the continued abundance of research on clinical and experimental aspects of thiamine deficiency (see Sable and Gubler, 1982). Decreased blood thiamine levels are associated with impaired oxidation of pyruvic acid, raised pyruvate and lactate levels, and reduced levels of erythrocyte transketolase. Thiamine deficiency syndromes are particularly associated with chronic alcoholism although they may complicate nutritional deficiency occurring in patients with carcinoma of the intestinal tract (especially of the stomach), chronic gastritis, gastric ulcer, persistent vomiting as in hyperemesis gravidarum, and pernicious anaemia.

Thiamine deficiency associated with alcoholism

The Wernicke and Korsakoff syndromes

First described by Wernicke (1881), this syndrome, which may be acute or subacute, is characterized by: mental disturbance; impairment of memory and disorientation; ataxia and nystagmus; extraocular palsies, miotic pupils and sluggish pupillary reflexes; peripheral neuropathy and reduced tendon reflexes. Recent reviews of the clinical and pathological features of Wernicke's encephalopathy have been those of Victor, Adams and Collins (1971); Victor (1976); Harper (1979) and Leevy (1982). Clearly this syndrome is not rare, an overall incidence of 1.7 per cent being found by Harper (1979) in 2891 consecutive autopsies over the years 1973–76. Victor, Adams and Collins (1971) and Lishman (1981) have reviewed the historical aspects of Wernicke's encephalopathy and its relationship to the Korsakoff syndrome which is often its sequel.

Pathological changes The main lesions occur in the periventricular regions around the third and fourth ventricles and aqueduct. The mamillary bodies are most consistently involved (Fig. 13.1b–d) and may contain petechial haemor-

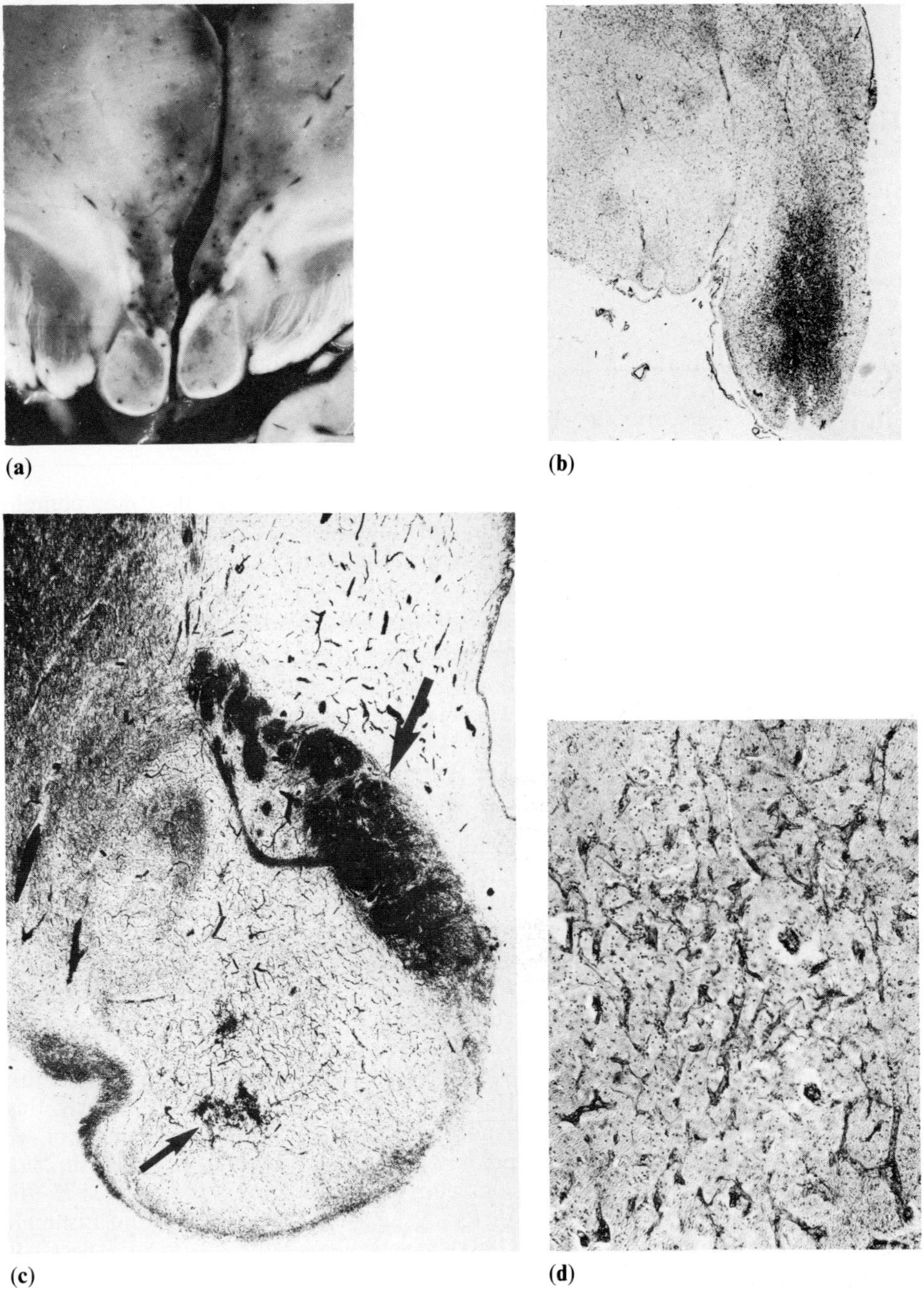

Fig. 13.1 Wernicke's encephalopathy. (**a**) Coronal section through mamillary bodies and third ventricle. Numerous haemorrhages in the wall of the third ventricle are shown. (**b**) Section through mamillary body showing recent haemorrhage. Cresyl violet ×7. (**c**) Haemorrhages (arrows) in the mamillary body shown in a section stained for myelin. Heidenhain ×10. (**d**) Section of mamillary body shows prominence of capillaries and increased pericapillary cellularity. Holzer ×60.

rhages visible macroscopically. Macroscopic haemorrhages may also be found in grey matter around ventricles and aqueduct, and in the colliculi, fornices, thalamus and inferior olives (Wernicke's original name for the pathology was acute superior haemorrhagic polioencephalitis). Non-haemorrhagic necrosis or foci of softening may also be present in these areas, and are probably older lesions.

Microscopically the *acute* stage of Wernicke's encephalopathy is characterized by prominence and dilatation of capillaries with a marked increase in cellularity due to the increased size and numbers of endothelial and adventitial cells (Fig. 13.1d). Capillary dilatation is particularly prominent in the mamillary bodies and pericapillary haemorrhages may be present. The adventitial thickening is due to the presence of large numbers of histiocytes. Neurons may show degenerative changes but myelinated fibres seem to be more vulnerable than nerve cells, many of which tend to be preserved.

Rarely, the lesions may not centre on the mamillary bodies but on the anterior hypothalamus, and the optic chiasm may be involved and become severely gliosed (Meyer, 1944). Campbell and Russell (1941) noted involvement of optic nerves. The acute lesions tend to be similar in whatever structure is affected.

In the *later* stages (Figs. 13.2 and 13.3) the pathological changes depend on the severity and on the duration of survival. The most severe lesions include complete tissue necrosis, the formation of cysts, neuronal loss of varying degree, usually severe loss of myelinated fibres (particularly around the mamillary bodies) and reactive changes. Microglial, histiocytic and macrophage cells are increased in number, fibrous gliosis being prominent in older lesions. Haemosiderin-laden macrophages indicate previous haemorrhages. In the cerebellum there may be loss of Purkinje cells, patchy loss of granule cells, an increase in Bergmann astrocytes and thinning of the molecular layer. These changes tend to occur only in the anterior (superior) vermis, rarely elsewhere in the cerebellum.

The *pathogenesis* of the acute lesions of Wernicke's encephalopathy is not clearly understood but the localization of lesions may be related to the effects of thiamine deficiency on serotoninergic neurons (Chan-Palay, 1977; Plaitakis et al., 1982). Various hypotheses have been put forward, including a postulated toxic effect of pyruvic acid on grey matter around the walls and floor of the third and fourth ventricles and aqueduct, or, alternatively, an increased requirement for thiamine in these areas. Thiamine deficiency in alcoholics may be due to decreased intake, reduced absorption, malutilization or increased excretion. The lesions of Wernicke's

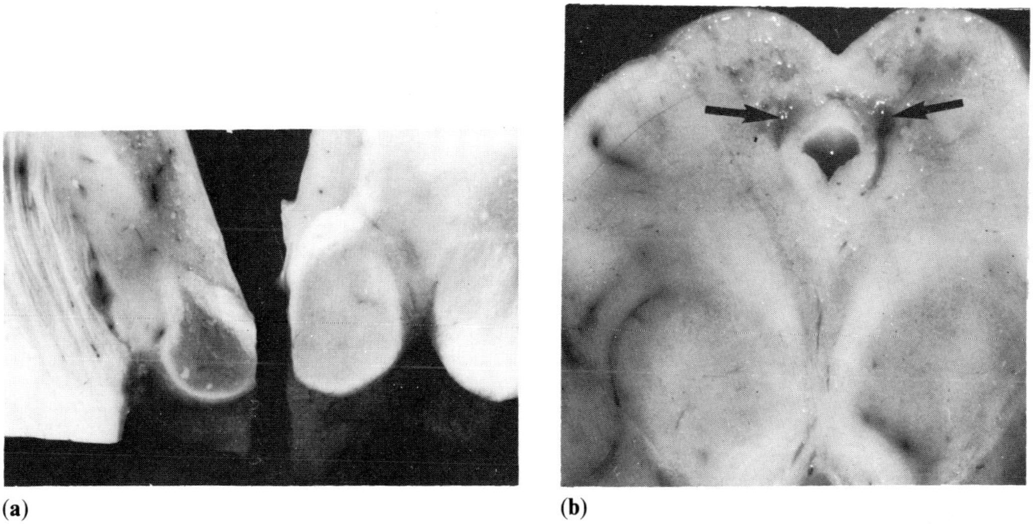

(a) (b)

Fig. 13.2 Chronic lesions in Wernicke–Korsakoff syndrome. (**a**) Coronal sections showing shrinkage and discolouration of mamillary bodies (left) compared with mamillary body from a normal brain (right). (**b**) Midbrain. Small cystic cavities (arrows) are shown in periaqueductal grey matter. (Courtesy of Prof. J.A.N. Corsellis.)

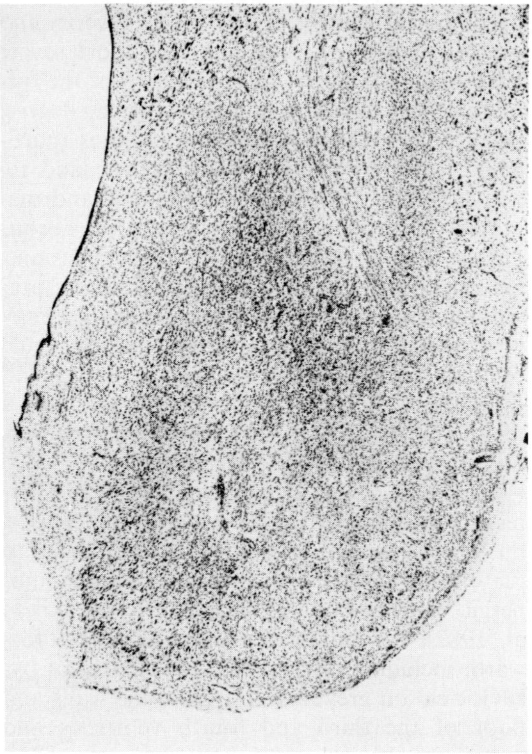

(a)

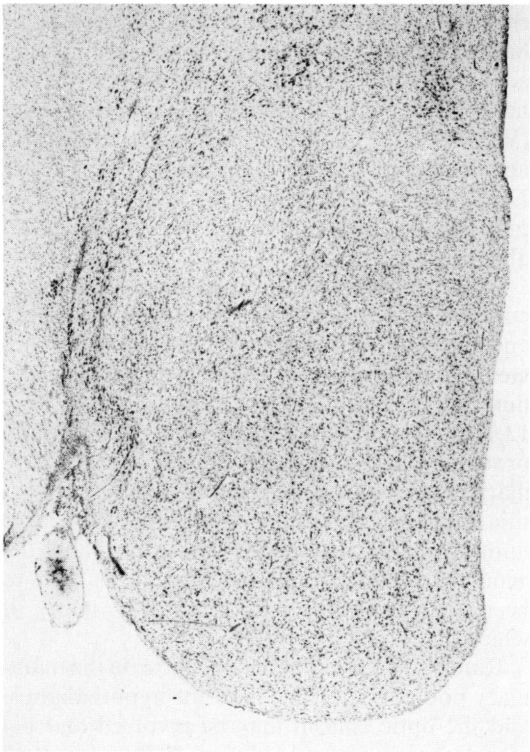

(b)

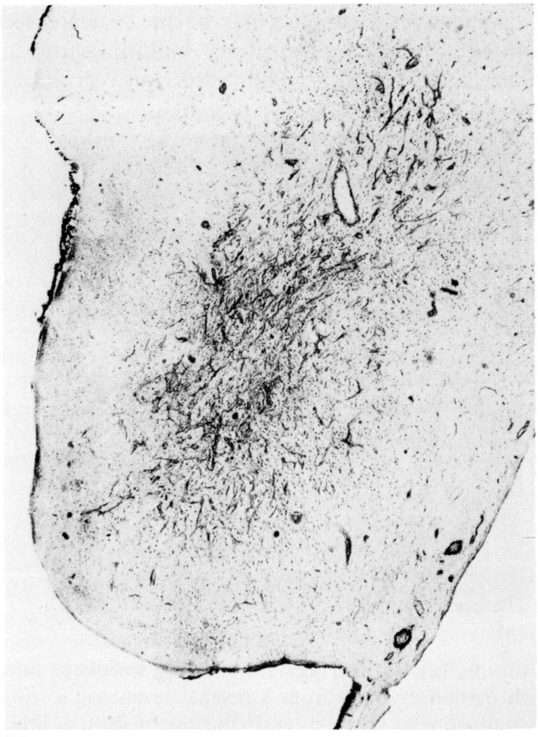

(c)

Fig. 13.3 Chronic lesions in Wernicke–Korsakoff syndrome. (**a**) Section of mamillary body. Increased cellularity is due to marked gliosis. (**b**) Section of mamillary body of a normal brain for comparison with (a). Cresyl violet ×20. (**c**) In the same mamillary body as shown in (**a**), Holzer's stain shows a marked increase in glial fibres and prominence of capillaries. ×20.

encephalopathy develop only after prolonged alcohol abuse and not all alcoholics are necessarily equally at risk. Blass and Gibson (1977) have suggested that the Wernicke-Korsakoff syndrome may develop because of an inherited abnormality of the thiamine-dependent enzyme transketolase.

The transition between the acute syndrome and the chronic amnesic syndrome of Korsakoff (also dealt with in Chapter 20) is now well established. In fully developed Korsakoff psychosis the mamillary bodies are macroscopically shrunken and microscopically there is severe neuronal loss and gliosis. Lesions are found at other sites, and considerable interest attaches to the aetiology of the striking impairment of memory. Victor, Adams and Collins (1971) found that only if there was no pathology in the dorsomedial nucleus of the thalamus was there definitely no defect of memory. Mair, Warrington and Weiskrantz (1979) observed, in addition to shrinkage and gliosis of the mamillary bodies, a thin band of severe gliosis between the third ventricle and the dorsomedial thalamic nuclei. Lishman (1981) has pointed out that not all patients with Korsakoff's psychosis have a previous history of acute Wernicke's encephalopathy, and supposes that the lesions caused by thiamine deficiency may develop insidiously.

Multiple vitamin deficiencies may occur concomitantly with thiamine deficiency and may contribute to the pathological changes, particularly in the spinal cord. Associated peripheral neuropathy and sensory ganglion cell loss may lead to loss of myelinated fibres in ascending sensory pathways in the spinal cord.

Alcoholic peripheral neuropathy The pathological changes in the *peripheral nerves* and *autonomic ganglia* in alcoholism are described in Chapter 18.

Acute alcoholic intoxication seldom leads to death and necropsy reports are rare. Cerebral congestion, oedema and diffuse petechial haemorrhages have been described (Courville and Myers, 1954) and when cardiovascular degeneration is present, in particular cerebral arteriosclerosis with hypertension, a toxic dose of alcohol may lead to massive haemorrhage or infarction (Meyer, 1963; *Lancet*, 1982).

According to McIlwain (1966), severe intoxication is accompanied by decreased cerebral blood flow and decreased respiration. The oxidation of ethanol proceeds through acetaldehyde, the blood level of which is normally low but is elevated following ingestion of alcohol. The depressant action of alcohol is, however, due not to these oxidation products but to the presence of the actual compound in cerebral tissue, as also occurs with drugs such as anaesthetics and hypnotics. Acetaldehyde, like other toxic substances such as the heavy metals, probably combines with lipoic acid which is then no longer available for the oxidation of pyruvates.

Other cerebral disorders in alcoholism

Amblyopia occurring in association with chronic alcohol abuse has been reviewed by Dreyfus (1976). In this disorder (also known as tobacco-alcohol or nutritional amblyopia, or retrobulbar neuropathy) there is blurring of vision, diminished visual acuity and scotomas. Other deficiency syndromes are also usually present. The few cases which have been examined pathologically show bilateral symmetrical loss of myelinated fibres in the central parts of the optic nerves and loss of ganglion cells in the retina, particularly in the region of the fovea. In severe cases where there is advanced disease, fibres of the optic nerves are replaced by collagenous connective tissue. The disorder is probably the result of a deficiency of several vitamins.

Disturbances of cerebral function other than Wernicke's encephalopathy have long been recognized as associated with chronic alcoholism. Dreyfus (1976) used the term 'alcoholic dementia' in association with cerebral degeneration and pointed out that it should not be used synonymously with Korsakoff's psychosis, and must be distinguished from delirium tremens, pellagra psychosis and hepatic encephalopathy occurring as a consequence of cirrhosis.

A moderate degree of atrophy of frontal and parietal lobes, with meningeal thickening and ventricular enlargement, was described by Mott (1910), Courville (1955) and Lynch (1960). Astrocytic proliferation and neuronal loss in the third layer of the frontal cortex was described by Morel (1939). Cerebellar degeneration in alcoholics was noted by Jakob (1912), Stender and Lüthy (1931) and Lhermitte (1935), whilst Neuburger (1957) found that degeneration of the cerebellar granular layer was relatively common in his investigation of 42 cases of alcoholism.

Cerebellar degeneration in alcoholism was reviewed by Victor, Adams and Mancall (1959) and Allsop and Turner (1966). Lesions are predominant in the anterior (superior) vermis and, to a lesser degree, in the anterior lobe of the cerebellar hemispheres. The earliest changes affect the granule cell layer, followed by Purkinje cell degeneration and astrocytic proliferation. Degeneration of the inferior olives appears to be secondary.

Cerebral abnormalities in chronic alcoholics have been identified by the use of the CT scan (see Ideström, 1980; Ron et al., 1982). Although there may be no overt signs of brain damage, ventricular enlargement and cortical atrophy were noted. The pathological basis for these changes is not known. Abstinence from alcohol seemed to be followed by a reversal of the abnormalities. Leevy (1982) uses the term 'thiamine dementia' to describe reversible non-specific mental abnormalities in alcoholics and subdivides the progression of abnormalities into successive grades: I is a trivial defect of awareness with euphoria or depression; II comprises apathy, personality changes and uncontrollable alcohol intake; III includes confusion, disorientation and encephalopathy. These cases have reduced blood thiamine levels, electroencephalographic abnormalities and evidence of cerebral atrophy on CT scan, and may respond to the administration of thiamine.

Nicotinic acid deficiency is found amongst alcoholics and may cause obvious pellagra with stomatitis, dermatitis, cogwheel rigidity and delirium or stupor. In such cases there may be little response to treatment until nicotinic acid is added. The mortality rate is, however, high and, characteristically, chromatolysis is present in neurons particularly of the brain stem and spinal cord.

Marchiafava–Bignami syndrome

Degeneration of the corpus callosum in chronic alcoholics was described by Marchiafava and Bignami (1903) and has subsequently been reported from other European and American countries. Reviews of the literature include those by Ironside, Bosanquet and McMenemey (1961) and Brion (1976) (see also Chapter 9). Although a high proportion of reported cases were Italians drinking Italian wine, the condition has been described in many non-Italians drinking non-Italian wine. Most of those affected have been middle-aged males who have been drinking 2 litres or more of red wine a day for many years. There may be associated nutritional deficiencies, including Wernicke's encephalopathy.

The principal pathological change is necrosis of the corpus callosum (Fig. 13.4a). This may involve the whole anteroposterior extent of the corpus callosum or only part, and the central fibres are mainly affected with preservation usually of an upper and lower rim. The lesion extends to the lateral edges of the corpus callosum. Macroscopically the lesion appears as a greyish softened band which histologically shows glial and vascular remnants. Glial proliferation is not usually very marked and axons may be relatively preserved in some cases. A striking feature usually is the proliferation and fibrous sclerosis of blood vessels.

Other regions of white matter which are sometimes involved include the cerebellar peduncles (Fig. 13.4b) and the centrum semiovale in frontal and parietal regions in the lateral extensions of the corpus callosum. The anterior commissures and optic chiasma are less often affected (Victor and Adams, 1961) whilst the fornix is said never to be involved. There is occasionally cortical laminar necrosis affecting the third layer and necrosis in the basal ganglia is another inconstant finding.

Clinically the illness may be of acute onset with convulsions rapidly progressing to coma and death. A subacute form is more common in which there is longer survival after a fairly acute onset of dementia. Rarely is there a chronic progressive disease lasting several years.

The pathogenesis is still unknown and a toxic factor in cheap red wine has seemed the closest constant association. The lesions most closely resemble those of hypoxic-ischaemic origin and it may be relevant that similar lesions of the white matter, affecting the corpus callosum and anterior commissure, have been described following experimental cyanide and, less often, carbon monoxide intoxication.

Central pontine myelinolysis

This syndrome, a considerable number of the reported cases of which have been in chronic alcoholics, is characterized by a usually sym-

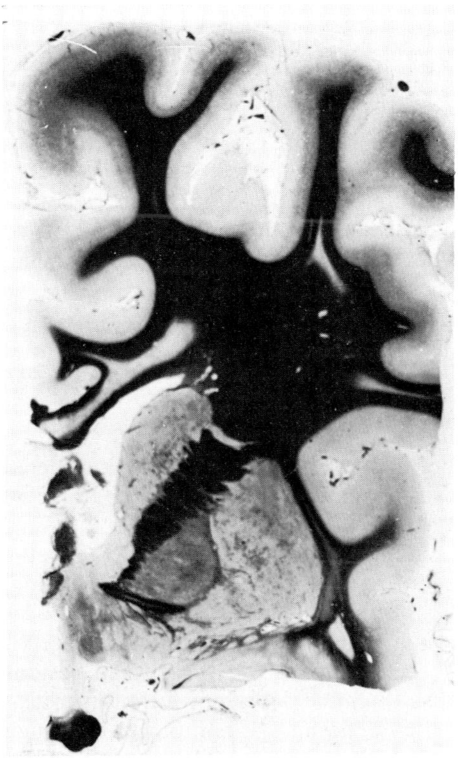

(a)

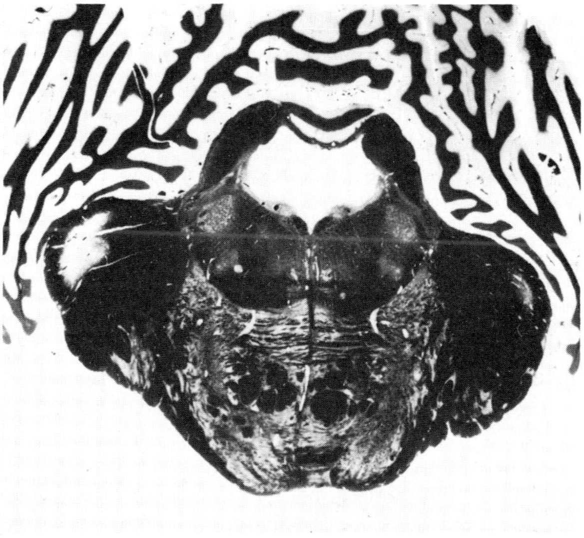

(b)

Fig. 13.4 Marchiafava–Bignami disease. Sections stained to demonstrate myelin show degeneration of (**a**) the central fibres in the corpus callosum, anterior commissure and white matter at the base of gyri, and (**b**) of the middle cerebellar peduncle. Heidenhain.

metrical area of myelin breakdown in the pons. Axons and nerve cells tend to be preserved. The condition is discussed in Chapter 9.

Beriberi

Beriberi occurs mainly in the Far East, and in tropical climates, but was prevalent in both World Wars in other localities, particularly during periods of famine which occurred in prisoner-of-war camps and in some occupied countries in Europe. Acute, subacute and chronic forms are described; furthermore, wet and dry beriberi are also recognized, according to whether or not oedema is present. Peripheral neuropathies more frequently occur in the chronic form, and may be complicated by the characteristic heart condition and oedema. In the infant, beriberi is usually acute and the underlying abnormality is likely to be the sequel of combined protein and thiamine deficiency (Platt, 1958a); such cases tend to be very oedematous.

The heart lesion consists of acute dilatation, particularly on the right side. Symmetrical oedema, starting usually at the ankles, spreads upwards, and the scrotum may be involved early. Polyneuritis begins distally in the lower extremities, and may become widespread and involve cranial nerves, laryngeal nerves, posterior roots and autonomic nerves.

Mental disturbances are said to be rare; when persistent, it is difficult to exclude the Wernicke syndrome.

The pathology of the peripheral neuropathy is discussed in Chapter 18. With regard to the other pathological manifestations, Buzzard and Greenfield's (1921) description still stands; in the wet form anasarca and hydropericardium are present together with congestion of the spleen and with nutmeg liver. In all fatal cases great dilatation of the right side of the heart has been noted and histologically its muscle shows hydropic swelling of fibres, loss of striations and replacement by granulation and fibrous tissue.

Some of the findings described in the spinal cord are, if not due to other concomitant vitamin deficiency, likely to be secondary to the peripheral neuropathy.

Experimental thiamine deficiency

The early literature on the experimental induction of thiamine deficiency states has been reviewed by Smith (1976). Lesions similar to those of the human Wernicke syndrome have been found in many species of animal with either naturally occurring or experimentally induced deficiency. Symmetrical haemorrhages and focal necrosis have been observed in periventricular grey matter, brain stem nuclei and thalamus in the rat, mouse, pigeon and dog (Dreyfus and Victor, 1961). Animals eating a raw fish diet may develop lesions because of its high content of thiaminase, an enzyme which destroys thiamine (Chastek paralysis in foxes—Evans, Carlson and Green, 1942; a similar disease in cats—Jubb, Saunders and Coates, 1956). Thiamine deficiency may be induced experimentally either by its complete absence from the diet or by the administration of an antimetabolite pyrithiamine (Watanabe et al., 1981). A dietary deficiency alone causes symptoms of neurological impairment in the rat in 3–4 weeks. The combination of dietary deficiency with pyrithiamine leads to ataxia, opisthotonos and convulsions within 11–12 days (Plaitakis et al., 1982).

In electron microscopic studies Robertson, Wasan and Skinner (1968) and Watanabe et al. (1981) found swelling of glial cytoplasm in the early stages of thiamine deficiency. Later, swelling of the inner loop of the myelin sheath developed and there was ballooning of the periaxonal space. Robertson, Wasan and Skinner (1968) postulated a breakdown of energy-dependent electrolyte transport by perivascular glia leading to the influx of fluid across the blood-brain barrier, the failure of transport being due to a lack of thiamine-dependent enzymes.

Chan-Palay (1977) has shown that serotoninergic neurons are particularly numerous in the raphe and reticular formation of pons and medulla, in hypothalamic, mamillary, trabecular and interpeduncular nuclei in the rat, regions in which acute lesions develop in thiamine deficiency. These neurons as well as their axonal plexuses in many areas, especially in spinal cord and medulla, normally take up tritium labelled 5-hydroxytryptamine (5HT). Thiamine deficiency causes a failure of these neurons to take up 5HT. Plaitakis et al. (1982) has shown that the high affinity uptake of 5HT by synaptosomes, particularly from cerebellum and less so from hypothalamus, is greatly reduced by thiamine deficiency.

Vitamins of the B_2 group

Pantothenic acid

Deficiency of pantothenic acid will be considered first because it is more closely related to thiamine deficiency than are the other B_2 vitamins. Like thiamine, pantothenic acid is concerned with the oxidation of pyruvate, its absence or 'blocking' likewise resulting in hyperpyruvaemia. As coenzyme A, it is an important catalyst of the acetylation of acetylcholine. For this reason, lesions ascribed to thiamine deficiency were thought to be caused by deficiency of pantothenate though this has not been confirmed (North and Sinclair, 1956).

It has been suggested (Gopalan, 1946) that the 'burning feet' syndrome may be due, at least in part, to pantothenic acid deficiency. Human volunteers in whom deficiency was induced by Bean, Hodges and Daum (1955), either by a diet devoid of the vitamin or by administration of its antagonist comethyl pantothenic acid, showed signs of fatigue and paraesthesiae of the 'burning feet' type which improved on large doses of the vitamin. Davidson and Passmore (1969), however, considered that the syndrome results from prolonged lack of protein and the B group of vitamins.

The deficiency of pantothenic acid in rats results in alopecia, generalized dermatitis and ulceration of the gastrointestinal tract, particularly of the colon. Haemorrhagic necrosis of the adrenal has been reported in rats but not in other animals. In monkeys with pantothenic acid deficiency, ataxia was the main clinical sign (McCall et al., 1946). Follis and Wintrobe (1945) and Swank and Adams (1948) observed degeneration of peripheral nerves, the posterior roots and their ganglia and the posterior columns of the spinal cord in pigs; the earliest lesion was central chromatolysis in neurons of the posterior root ganglia, followed by degeneration of myelin and axons in nerves, spinal roots or spinal cord; central chromatolysis of some anterior horn neurons and occasional degeneration in the pyramidal tracts were also found.

Nicotinic acid: pellagra

Pellagra is the commonest complication of nicotinic acid deficiency. The disease was known in eighteenth century Spain and received its present name (*pelle*, skin; and *agra*, rough) from peasants in northern Italy.

A toxic or infective cause had been suspected until the clinical studies of Goldberger and Wheeler (1915, 1920) indicated its relationship to dietary deficiency in human patients, and also in dogs with 'black tongue' disease, which has similar features. (Terris (1963) edited a selection of Goldberger's papers written between 1913 and 1928.) *Clinically* pellagra is characterized by lesions of the skin and mucous membranes, and by neurological and psychiatric disturbances. The typical skin lesions begin as erythema and are followed by atrophy. Diarrhoea, glossitis, gastric achylia and anaemia are frequent. Changes in the nervous system develop later, and polyneuritis, spastic paralysis and ataxia, tremor and rigidity, visual disturbances (particularly retrobulbar neuritis) and deafness have all been described. Mental changes may occur early and are of 'psychoneurotic' type, which later develop into depressive or manic states, followed in severe cases by progressive dementia (Leigh, 1952). Epileptic convulsions are not uncommon.

Usually pellagra takes a chronic intermittent course over several years, and morphological lesions of the central nervous system appear only in the later stages.

An acute syndrome was reported by various authors (Hardwick, 1943; Spillane, 1947) and has been termed 'nicotinic acid deficiency encephalopathy'. Clinically there is clouding of consciousness, cogwheel rigidity, and grasping and sucking reflexes. The patients are usually elderly with chronic organic illness and have often been living on an obviously inadequate diet. Signs of other vitamin B complex deficiency states are frequently present. Patients with this encephalopathy may respond dramatically to nicotinic acid therapy.

Pellagra was diagnosed on neuropathological evidence in 20 post-mortem cases of chronic alcoholism (Ishii and Nishihara, 1981). The patients presented with various mental, neurological and gastrointestinal symptoms, but with no skin lesions. The neuropathological changes closely resembled those described in 1952 by Leigh (see 'Pathological studies', below).

A syndrome exhibiting pellagra-like symptoms (light-sensitive dermatitis, cerebellar ataxia and psychotic manifestations) has been described by Baron et al. (1956). Cases examined by Hersov (1955), Rodnight and McIlwain (1955), and Hersov and Rodnight (1960), though originally interpreted differently, have been identified as having the same condition, which has been named *Hartnup disease* after one of the affected families. Biochemically, it is characterized by a pronounced and persistent aminoaciduria of a special pattern and an abnormally large output of indolic compounds. The basic metabolic defect results from a genetically induced disorder of cell membranes which involves the transport mechanisms of certain neutral amino acids; this defect in the proximal convoluted tubule results in aminoaciduria. Malabsorption in the jejunum leads to an intraluminal increase in tryptophan, which is broken down to indolic compounds by the colonic flora and subsequently excreted in the urine. The abnormal metabolism of tryptophan probably prevents its conversion to nicotinamide, and thus increases the threshold at which the diet becomes inadequate to provide enough nicotinamide for bodily requirements (Milne, 1969). Post-mortem investigations have not been traced.

Patients with the carcinoid syndrome due to a malignant argentaffinoma occasionally develop tryptophan deficiency and a pellagra-like state, because of circulating serotonin.

Pathological studies on pellagra include those made by Wilson (1914), Greenfield and Holmes (1939), Hsü (1942) and Leigh (1952).

The change found most consistently in the brain is central chromatolysis (Fig. 13.5a and b), first described as 'central neuritis' by Meyer (1901), although there has been controversy about its distribution. Leigh examined 14 cases and found the highest incidence in Betz cells, followed by pontine nuclei (Fig. 13.5b), dorsal vagal nucleus, gracile and cuneate nuclei, nucleus ambiguus, descending trigeminal nucleus, oculomotor nucleus, basal ganglia, vestibular nucleus and reticular and arcuate nuclei in that

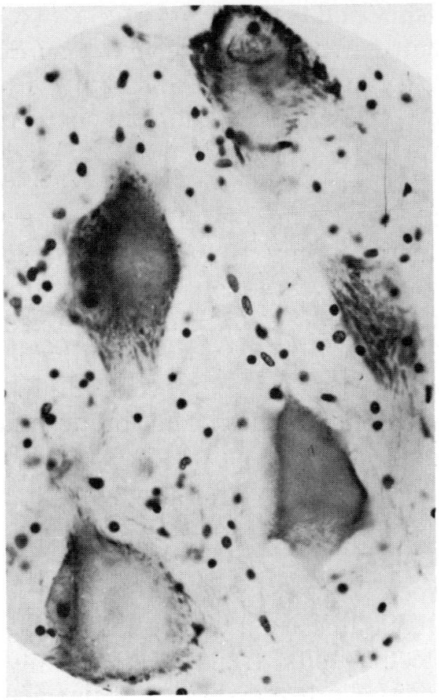

(a)

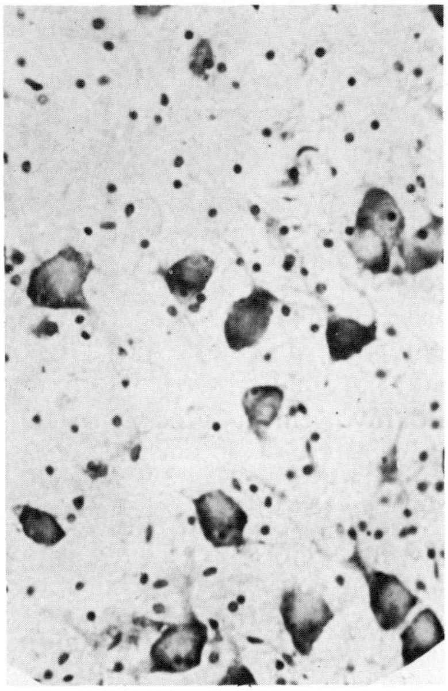

(b)

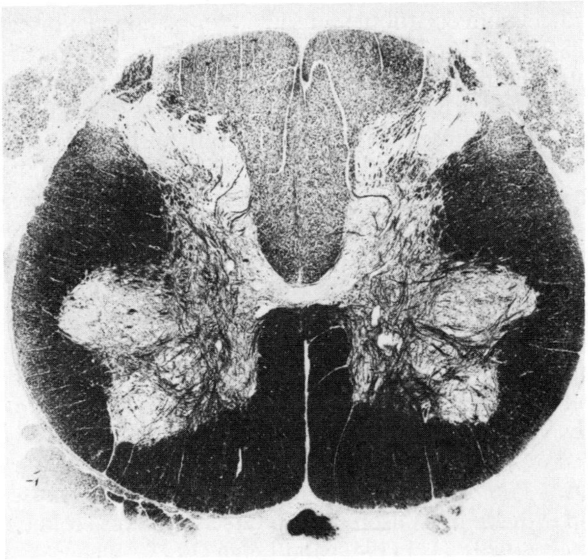

(c)

Fig. 13.5 Pellagra. Central chromatolysis in (**a**) anterior horn cells and (**b**) pontine cells. Cresyl violet ×250. (**c**) Lumbar spinal cord. Note loss of myelinated fibres in the posterior columns. Heidenhain's method for myelin. (b courtesy of Dr D. Leigh.)

order. Of the six spinal cords studied, central chromatolysis of anterior horn neurons was seen in four. Axonal damage is too inconsistent in the central nervous system to account for the widespread chromatolysis, which is more likely to be related to the effects of a metabolic defect on neuronal perikarya.

Proliferation of the neuroglia is not a feature. The fibrosis and hyaline change of the blood vessels emphasized by Hsü (1942) were infrequent in Leigh's (1952) material; increase of lipofuscin is, according to Hsü, often seen in pellagra, but this also was not a prominent feature in Leigh's cases.

Degeneration of the posterior and lateral tracts of the cord has been described (Fig. 13.5c). In Greenfield and Holmes' (1939) case, degeneration was most severe in the fasciculus gracilis, with lesions of lesser severity in the spinocerebellar and crossed and uncrossed pyramidal tracts. In the study by Hsü (1942) of 13 Chinese soldiers who died from inanition, most showed degeneration of the posterior columns. Pellagrinous degeneration of posterior and lateral tracts differs histologically from that seen in the same tracts in vitamin B_{12} deficiency. The characteristic honeycomb appearance caused by the discontinuous degeneration of myelin sheaths is absent in pellagra, which more closely resembles wallerian-type degeneration. Greenfield and Holmes found that both posterior and anterior roots are affected. Involvement of the peripheral nerves has also been noted by many workers including Aring et al. (1941) and Greenfield and Carmichael (1935). The latter authors counted fibres in the cutaneous nerves of the toe and found reduced fibre densities in pellagrous compared to normal nerves. In severe cases both myelin and axons showed evidence of degeneration, but in milder cases only the myelin was affected.

Both central and peripheral lesions may occur together, though experience in World War II made it clear that certain components of the syndrome of pellagra can also occur independently. Polyneuritis, for example, is likely to be an admixture rather than an integral part of pellagra and is probably due to deficiency of other vitamins, especially thiamine or other components of the B_2 complex. Combined degeneration of posterior and lateral columns identical to that found in pellagra has been described as an isolated deficiency syndrome, sometimes combined with retrobulbar neuritis and deafness (Spillane, 1947).

Experimental and biochemical studies Elvehjem et al. (1937) showed that nicotinic acid cured black tongue in dogs. Denton (1928), who studied Goldberger's dogs, described histological lesions of the skin and mucous membranes that were indistinguishable from those in human pellagra. Histological changes in the central nervous system were not mentioned.

In rats fed on a diet poor in vitamin B_2, there was degeneration of anterior horn cells, rather than the central chromatolysis of human pellagra (Stern and Findlay, 1929). Antagonistic analogues of nicotinic acid (antinicotinamides) have also failed to produce pellagra-like lesions. Hicks (1955) found that 3-acetylpyridine caused neuronal changes in spinal and sympathetic ganglia, the supraoptic nucleus and the pyramidal layer of Ammon's horn, in mice and rats, although Coggeshall and MacLean (1958) described lesions that were confined almost exclusively to Lorente de No's fields CA3 and CA4 of Ammon's horn. Another antimetabolite, 6-aminonicotinamide, produces lesions in anterior horns and nuclei of the medulla; these are described more fully in Chapter 14.

Although nicotinic acid is important in the diet, most of the requirement is provided by biosynthesis in the intestines. Destruction of intestinal flora by sulphonamides or antibiotics may cause pellagrous changes. Nicotinic acid is synthesized from tryptophan, and the absence of this amino acid from maize probably explains why a wholly maize diet often results in pellagra. Blood tryptophan levels are relatively low in pellagra. Woolley (1946) isolated a pellagra-inducing factor from maize, which may be chemically related to one of the acetylpyridine antinicotinamides.

The complex nature of the deficiency in experimental pellagra was demonstrated by Wintrobe et al. (1943) in pigs, and by Krehl et al. (1945) in dogs and rats. A diet poor in nicotinamide but adequate in thiamine, riboflavin, pantothenic acid and choline, and with optimal protein, had few ill-effects; but when the protein was reduced, signs of deficiency developed. In affected animals there was chromatolysis of the small nerve cells of the posterior root ganglia, but no myelin degeneration in peripheral nerves.

Madhaven, Belavady and Gopalan (1968) concluded that pellagra occurring in the Hyderabad region of India is related to consumption of the millet jowar, and that its high leucine content is a factor. Black tongue was induced in dogs fed with maize or jowar or casein-plus-leucine. The animals showed extensive ulceration of the gastrointestinal mucosa. Changes in the spinal cord included focal haemorrhages and chromatolysis, satellitosis and neuronal phagocytosis. Excess leucine interferes with tryptophan and nicotinic acid metabolism, causing pellagra. Gopalan (1969) proposed this to be the first evidence that an important deficiency can arise because of particular proportions of different dietary amino acids.

Riboflavin

Riboflavin was the first constituent of an enzyme

system to be isolated and synthesized. As riboflavin phosphate it is part of several 'yellow' flavoprotein enzymes, and in combination with adenylic acid it functions as coenzyme in the dehydrogenase group.

In experimental animals of various species the most prominent changes resulting from deficiency occur in the skin, eyes and nervous system. The skin lesions vary in extent and type according to the species; usually there is dermatitis followed by atrophy of sebaceous glands and hair follicles. Lesions tend to occur in the angle of the mouth and in the nasolabial folds. Bessey and Wolbach (1939) drew attention to abnormal capillary growth in the cornea. Cataracts have been noted in rats and pigs.

Myelin degeneration in peripheral nerves and in the fibre tracts of the spinal cord, especially in the posterior columns, has been described in rats (Shaw and Phillips, 1941), dogs (Street, Cowgill and Zimmerman, 1941), mice (Lippincott and Morris, 1942) and young pigs (Wintrobe et al., 1944).

Norton et al. (1976) have produced riboflavin deficiency in rats by diet and treatment with galactoflavin (10-D-dulcityl-7, 8-dimethylisoalloxazine), a riboflavin antagonist. In their ultrastructural study they described demyelination of sciatic nerve fibres, although their illustrations appear to show some axonal degeneration.

In man the main change, induced experimentally by Sebrell and Butler (1939), is a dermatitis about the mouth resulting in fissure formation (cheilosis) and reddening of the lips. Vascularization of the cornea, occasionally resulting in ulceration has been reported. Lane, Smith and Alfrey (1975) have described peripheral neuropathy in man after a prolonged riboflavin-deficient diet and treatment with the riboflavin antagonist, galactoflavin. Perception of pain, temperature, vibration, touch and spatial orientation was reduced, and there was a reduction in sensory conduction velocity. Riboflavin has occasionally been suggested as a cause of 'burning feet' syndrome (Peraita, 1946; Lai and Ransome, 1970). Stannus (1944) suggested that Strachan's syndrome of amblyopia, painful neuropathy and orogenital dermatitis (Jamaican neuritis) may be caused by riboflavin deficiency because treatment with the vitamin has beneficial effects, particularly on the mucocutaneous lesion. Strachan's syndrome and other similar disorders have been discussed by Victor (1975).

In one of the few neuropathological studies of Strachan's syndrome, Scott (1918) showed Marchi-positive staining in posterior columns which was most severe in the cervical region. There was little damage in the anterolateral funiculi and none in the corticospinal tracts. Some peripheral nerves and spinal roots showed marked degenerative changes; optic nerves and auditory nerves were also affected to varying degrees. Fisher (1955) examined men who had been prisoners of war in the Far East, had developed Strachan's syndrome and nutritional deficiency and who had died several years later from unrelated causes. He found selective degeneration in the gracile tract, severely affecting the cervical regions of the cord and speculated that both central and peripheral fibres of sensory ganglion cells were affected by a 'dying-back' neuropathy.

Pyridoxine

Goldberger and Lillie (1926) described a pellagra-like condition in rats fed on a maize diet extracted by alcohol. György (1934) and his collaborators excluded nicotinic acid and riboflavin deficiency as causes and showed that another factor, pyridoxine, was involved. Pyridoxine, together with pyridoxal and pyridoxamine comprise the vitamin B_6 group, but these are active physiologically only in their phosphorylated forms. More than 50 pyridoxine phosphate-dependent enzyme reactions have been identified and many of these occur in the nervous system. Of particular importance in CNS metabolism is their role as coenzymes for the decarboxylation of amino acids and also for the formation of the amines noradrenaline, adrenaline, tyramine, dopamine and serotonin. Pyridoxine phosphate is a cofactor in a rate-limiting stage of the production of the inhibitory amine γ-aminobutyric acid (GABA).

Experimental lesions have been described in several species fed on a pyridoxine-deficient diet. These are most prominent in skin, erythropoietic tissue and the nervous system. The skin lesions consist of pellagra-like symmetrical dermatitis which is not influenced by sunlight. Anaemia (usually normocytic) develops, the liver may show fatty infiltration and there may be extensive deposits of iron pigment in liver, spleen and bone marrow. Rinehart and Greenberg (1956) found intimal proliferation (which closely resembles human atherosclerosis) in many arteries of monkeys completely deprived of pyridoxine for 5–6 months.

Epileptiform fits (grand mal and petit mal) lasting several minutes have been described in pyridoxine deficient rats and pigs (Chick, El Sadr and Worden, 1940; Wintrobe et al., 1943). The fits, which may be related to the known biochemical effects on GABA synthesis, responded to replacement therapy. Demyelination of peripheral nerves, posterior root fibres and fibres in the posterior columns has also been described in experimental studies, but significant chromatolysis in posterior root ganglia was not noted (Follis and Wintrobe, 1945, Swank and Adams, 1948), even though the neurons later atrophy and disappear.

Purpura and Gonzales-Monteagudo (1960) described necrosis in the end-folium of the hippocampus (fields CA2 and CA4 of Lorente de Nó) of cats which developed within 2 hours of a single injection of methoxypyridoxine, a pyridoxine antagonist. In Nissl preparations the nerve cells were shrunken, deeply basophilic and showed loss of intracellular architecture. In view of the incidence of convulsions, the authors stressed that they failed to produce similar changes in so short a time either by hypoxia or by metrazol *or* pentylene tetrazol and strychnine. The animals had been paralysed with succinylcholine chloride. Similarly localized lesions were also found in rats treated with analogues of nicotinic acid.

Monkeys fed on a pyridoxine-deficient diet, or given deoxypyridine, a pyridoxine antagonist, showed swelling of Betz cells in the motor cortex and, to a lesser degree, of small pyramidal cells, with eccentric displacement of the nucleus and loss of Nissl substance. Myelin degeneration was noted in peripheral nerves (Victor and Adams, 1956).

Morre and Kirksey (1980) examined the dendritic trees of Purkinje cells in the developing cerebellum of progeny of mother rats kept on a vitamin B_6-deficient diet. By the fifteenth day there was a decrease in Purkinje cell dendritic arborization which persisted for more than 50 days.

Formation of the physiologically active phosphorylated form of pyridoxine is affected by the drug isoniazid, resulting in peripheral neuropathy and other neurological disturbances in man and experimental animals (see Chapter 14). Pyridoxine deficiency has also been noted as a complication of therapy with the antihypertensive drug hydralazine. The hydrazine (—$NHNH_2$) group in the structure of hydralazine relates the drug to the family of compounds the hydrazines and hydrazides (—$CONHNH_2$) which have been shown to induce pyridoxine-responsive convulsions in laboratory animals (Raskin and Fishman, 1965). Penicillamine may act as a pyridoxine antagonist (Jaffe, Altman and Merryman, 1964).

Cavanagh and Ridley (1967) suggested that the neuropathy associated with acute intermittent porphyria may be due to consumptive tissue deficiency of pyridoxal phosphate resulting from its overuse by the active conjugating enzyme amino-laevulinic acid synthetase, the enzyme whose overactivity is an important metabolic lesion in this disease.

In 1952–53 there was an epidemic of vitamin B_6-deficiency symptoms in babies, caused by excessive use of a milk preparation which was deficient in the vitamin (Molony and Parmelee, 1954). The most prominent clinical feature was epileptiform convulsions which were promptly relieved by administration of pyridoxine. Convulsions in breast-fed babies fed with milk low in vitamin B_6 have also been described (Bessey, Adam and Hansen, 1957). The convulsions disappear after pyridoxine treatment.

In a review on the regulation and function of pyridoxal phosphate, Ebadi (1981) refers to a number of reports of convulsions in children caused by vitamin B_6 deficiency. He states that vitamin B_6-related seizures continue to occur in parts of the world where there is widespread undernutrition.

The pyridoxine antagonist deoxypyridoxine has been reported to cause human peripheral neuropathy which is relieved by treatment with the vitamin (Vilter et al., 1953).

Vitamin B_{12}

Synthesis of crystalline vitamin B_{12} by Lester-Smith (1948) and Rickes et al. (1948) marked the culminating point of a great scientific achievement which evolved through the empirical discovery of the value of liver in the treatment of pernicious anaemia by Minot and Murphy (1926), the distinction between intrinsic (gastric) and extrinsic (dietary) factors by Castle (1929), and the identification and eventual synthesis of folic acid in 1946. Vitamin B_{12} has reduced mortality from neurological effects of deficiency by prevention, by cure of early disease and by arrest of the fully developed disease. Folic acid, however, although it has an effect on macrocytic anaemia, is of no value in the treatment or prevention of the neurological complication. Although vitamin B_{12} is now known to be Castle's extrinsic factor, the intrinsic factor is still unidentified. The latter is a glycoprotein which chelates with and serves as a carrier for vitamin B_{12}, the resultant complex being absorbed in the terminal ileum.

Deficiency of vitamin B_{12} affects particularly haemopoietic tissue, epithelial surfaces and the nervous system. The vitamin is found in several forms which all belong to a class of compounds called cobalamins. At present, two vitamin B_{12}-dependent enzymes are known to occur in man: methylmalonyl CoA mutase, which uses the deoxyadenyl form for the degradation of propionate through methylmalonyl CoA to succinate; and folate-dependent methionine synthetase, which utilizes the methyl form to synthesize methionine.

In 1973, Gandy, Jacobson and Sidman discovered by chance that a single injection of 1-aminocyclopentane carboxylic acid (cycloleucine) caused a neurological disorder in mice. The animals became ataxic, and proprioception and muscle strength were decreased. Histologically there was a myelopathy with resemblances to that seen in vitamin B_{12} deficiency. It was suggested that cycloleucine acts by blocking the formation of methionine which is required for the biosynthesis of choline, an important constituent of myelin. Its action might therefore reproduce the effects of B_{12} deficiency on methionine synthesis. Small, Carnegie and Anderson (1981) produced a myelin abnormality in chicks by the intraperitoneal injection of cycloleucine. Electron microscopy showed myelin vacuolation with splitting at the intraperiod lines similar to that produced by triethyltin and hexachlorophane (see Chapter 14). Small, Carnegie and Anderson found decreased incorporation of methyl groups into methylarginine in myelin basic protein.

Experimental studies in monkeys (Dinn et al., 1980) have shown that exposure to nitrous oxide for 1.5–8 weeks caused spinal cord lesions similar to those found in human B_{12} deficiency. Degeneration of sensory nerves was also found. Nitrous oxide is thought to inactivate methionine synthetase (one of the vitamin B_{12}-dependent enzymes), causing a depletion of methionine and consequent methyl group deficiency. This hypothesis might explain the neurological lesions associated with B_{12} deficiency.

Cox and White (1962) suggested that accumulation of methylmalonic acid may cause lesions in the nervous system, and Vivacqua et al. (1966) found increased amounts of methylmalonic acid in the urine of B_{12}-deficient patients with neurological symptoms. However, infants with methylmalonic aciduria may show no evidence of neurological disease (Rosenberg, 1972).

The possibility of a link between B_{12} deficiency and cyanide poisoning originated from the observation that treatment with this vitamin led to an improvement in tobacco amblyopia (Heaton, McCormick and Freeman, 1958). Also, a visual disturbance similar to tobacco amblyopia develops occasionally in patients with pernicious anaemia (Hamilton, Ellis and Sheets, 1959); this occurs more frequently in smokers who inhale cyanide from tobacco.

Hypotheses implicating cobalamin in the normal detoxification of cyanide and the consequent increased toxic hazard from cyanide in patients with B_{12} deficiency have been reviewed by Victor (1970) and Potts (1973) who found no evidence to support these theories.

Causes of neurological disorders in vitamin B_{12} deficiency Addisonian pernicious anaemia, which results from a failure of production of intrinsic factor due to autoimmune gastritis is the commonest cause of B_{12} deficiency associated with neurological disease. Other conditions such as total or subtotal gastrectomy, and organic diseases of the intestine, including strictures, fistulae, diverticula, tuberculous ulceration, tumour, regional ileitis and idiopathic and tropical sprue, may also be causative factors.

Vitamin B_{12} is synthesized by micro-organisms which occur in water, soils, sewage and the intestines of man and animals. However, man is dependent upon food for the vitamin, because bacterial synthesis occurs too far distally in the intestine for the vitamin to be absorbed.

Vitamin B_{12} deficiency of dietary origin is rare. It can occur in vegans—strict vegetarians who eat no egg or milk products. Low serum B_{12} levels were found in British vegans (Wokes, Badenoch and Sinclair, 1955). A vegetarian diet is common in India for religious and economic reasons and is associated with low serum B_{12} levels (Mehta, Rege and Satoskar, 1964; Dastur et al., 1972). Conditions such as intestinal disease, folate deficiency of nutritional origin, and iron deficiency can also affect absorption of B_{12}.

Neurological sequelae of dietary deficiency are also rare. A syndrome of pallor of mucous membranes, hyperpigmentation of the skin, developmental regression and involuntary movements of the head, trunk and limbs was reported in breast-fed infants of vitamin B_{12}-deficient mothers (Jadhar et al., 1962; Baker et al., 1962). The six affected infants were all well nourished but had megaloblastic marrows and low serum B_{12} levels. All responded well to oral B_{12}.

Badenoch (1954) recorded definite clinical signs of neuropathy in a boy of 15, a strict vegetarian, who improved dramatically after treatment with B_{12}. Pallis and Lewis (1974) have pointed out, however, that the association of a low serum B_{12} and a neurological disorder may not imply a causal relationship.

Neurological effects of vitamin B_{12} deficiency Leichtenstern (1884) reported the association of pernicious anaemia with disease of the spinal cord but he considered that the anaemia came on in the course of tabes dorsalis, to which he attributed the cord lesion. Lichtheim (1887) appears to have been the first to recognize that the spinal lesions of pernicious anaemia differed in several respects from those of tabes. The lesions, which were subacute, as shown both by the short history and by the abundant lipophages in the degenerate tracts of the cord, involved both the dorsal and the anterolateral columns; there was no thickening of the leptomeninges and only slight atrophy of the dorsal nerve roots in the lumbar region. Lichtheim's pupil, Minnich (1892), supplemented these observations when he found slight degeneration in the posterior and lateral columns in five fatal cases of pernicious anaemia with no neurological symptoms or signs.

The first full clinical and pathological description of the disease was given by Russell, Batten and Collier (1900) who named it subacute combined degeneration of the spinal cord; they were not satisfied with this term but were unable to suggest a better one. The name gives no indication of the association of the spinal cord lesions with macrocytic anaemia, neither does it suggest involvement of peripheral nerves or the brain. Richmond and Davidson (1958) proposed the term 'vitamin B_{12} neuropathy', although, again, this fails to encompass all aspects of the disease.

Clinical features The term 'subacute' describes the course of most untreated cases in which functional disturbances increase fairly rapidly and cause severe disability in a few weeks or months. The course may be so rapid that the patient is unable to stand after 2–3 weeks or it may be more gradual and allow the patient to continue at work for a year or more. Russell, Batten and Collier (1900) distinguished three stages in the disease. (1) A stage of spastic paraparesis and slight ataxia, with marked paraesthesiae including numbness, stiffness or tingling, which may precede the onset of motor disability by several months. The upper limbs are usually affected after the lower limbs, although clumsiness in writing is often an early feature of the disease. (2) A stage of severe ataxic paraplegia which may develop very rapidly, with marked anaesthesia of the legs and trunk. (3) The final stage of complete paraplegia with total anaesthesia is seldom seen in treated patients. The main danger to patients is in the first stage, when the anaemia is slight and the significance of the early, largely subjective, symptoms is not recognized. Recovery from the first stage is usually remarkably complete with adequate treatment, but in untreated patients the transition to the second stage may be so rapid that it cannot be arrested before grave and irremediable damage to the spinal cord has taken place.

Various mental changes have been observed and range from neurasthenia and depression to confusional states, amnesic syndromes and dementia ('megaloblastic madness'). Several workers (Ferraro, Arieti and English, 1945; Mayer-Gross, Slater and Roth, 1954) stressed the frequency of paranoid psychoses. The overall incidence of mental disorder was estimated by Woltmann (1924) to be 4 per cent of nearly 1500 cases of pernicious anaemia seen at the Mayo Clinic, but it is not clear whether this estimate includes minor affective aberrations. Epileptic seizures occur occasionally.

Pallis and Lewis (1974) have stressed the importance of peripheral neuropathy in B_{12} deficiency. They emphasized the difficulties in identifying neurological symptoms and signs as being of either central (myelopathic) or peripheral origin and concluded that peripheral neuropathy is the commonest neurological complication of vitamin B_{12} deficiency, recognition of its prevalence having been long delayed as a result of faulty interpretation of physical signs. Victor (1975) considers that spinal cord lesions are mainly responsible for the neurological complications of pernicious anaemia, peripheral neuropathy being less frequent and of less clinical significance.

Certainly there are variable reports of the incidence of peripheral neuropathy in pernicious anaemia. Woltmann (1919) carried out careful neurological examinations of 150 patients with pernicious anaemia and found 4.9 per cent to have symptoms and signs of a peripheral neuropathy; 80 per cent of these patients also showed evidence of spinal cord disease. Dynes and Norcross (1943) found signs of peripheral neuropathy in 23 per cent of their patients, whilst a higher incidence still was reported by Hamilton and Nixon (1921) and van der Scheer and Koek (1938).

Evidence from electrophysiological studies suggests that peripheral neuropathy is a common feature of pernicious anaemia. Gilliatt, Goodman and Willison (1961) found abnormalities of the nerve action potential from the lateral popliteal nerve in three patients who had impairment of superficial sensation in a 'stocking' distribution. Mayer (1965) studied 32 patients with pernicious anaemia or low serum B_{12} levels who had symptoms or signs secondary to central or peripheral nerve dysfunction. He found a reduced mean conduction velocity in distal sensory fibres in the median and ulnar nerves, although velocities in the proximal motor and sensory nerves were normal. A study by Lockner et al. (1969) showed that electrophysiological evidence of peripheral neuropathy was many times more common than symptoms. Cox-Klazinga and Endtz (1980) found that 65 per cent of untreated patients had reduced nerve conduction velocities; they suggest that peripheral nerve involvement in pernicious anaemia is more frequent than might be expected from the literature.

Pathology of subacute combined degeneration of the cord Early descriptions of spinal cord lesions were generally based on examination of preparations stained for myelin, and the terms 'demyelination' and 'degeneration' were used interchangeably.

Russell, Batten and Collier (1900) noted that the disease mainly involved the mid-thoracic segments of the cord, where a zone of destruction of white matter might extend all round the cord, affecting not only the long tracts but endogenous and exogenous fibres alike. In severe cases only fibres adjacent to the grey horns were spared (Fig. 13.6a). Degeneration diminished towards cervical levels of the cord, particularly in the anterolateral columns. In the upper cervical segments only the posterior columns, especially the funiculus gracilis, and the spinocerebellar tracts were demyelinated. At lower lumbar levels, lesions affected only the pyramidal tracts (Fig. 13.6a). This descending tract was usually unaffected in the region of the medullary pyramids, although some degeneration was occasionally seen at this level.

The early lesions consist of swelling of myelin sheaths with little change in the axons. Later, axonal degeneration is seen at the primary site of the lesion (usually the mid-thoracic segments), leading to subsequent wallerian-type degeneration of the long tracts in cervical and lumbar segments. Loss of fibres results in the formation of spaces, giving the tissue a loose, vacuolated appearance.

The distribution of the lesions is remarkably constant. The earliest changes occur in the centre of the posterior columns, producing irregular oval-shaped areas of pallor (Clarke, 1904) (Fig. 13.6b). At the same time, or slightly later, lateral column lesions appear at the surface of the cord immediately anterior to the posterior horns (Fig. 13.6c). More often, small distinct foci of degeneration appear on the surface of the cord or in the lips of the anteromedian fissure. Early lesions in posterior and anterolateral columns do not have the distribution of tract degeneration, but they may eventually involve much of the posterior columns and the pyramidal and spinocerebellar tracts.

The question of demyelination without axonal damage has been raised with reference to the lesions caused by B_{12} deficiency. There is evidence that in early lesions only myelin sheaths are affected and this seems to be confirmed in experimental studies (see below). However, axonal degeneration follows soon after the myelin changes. The remission and apparent complete cure of early cases by suitable treatment may indicate that the disease has been arrested at a stage when only a small proportion of axons has been damaged in any tract. Whether remyelina-

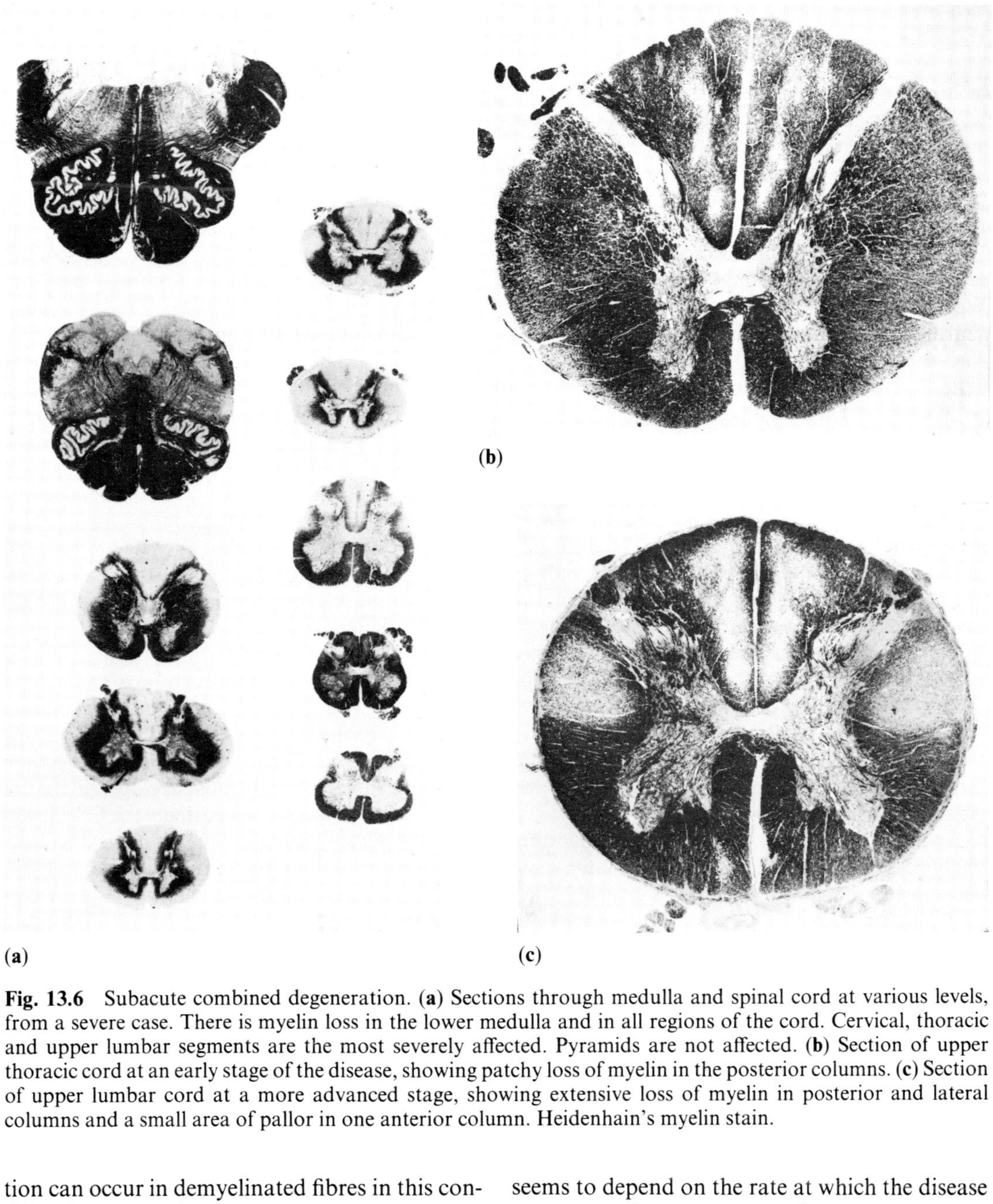

Fig. 13.6 Subacute combined degeneration. (**a**) Sections through medulla and spinal cord at various levels, from a severe case. There is myelin loss in the lower medulla and in all regions of the cord. Cervical, thoracic and upper lumbar segments are the most severely affected. Pyramids are not affected. (**b**) Section of upper thoracic cord at an early stage of the disease, showing patchy loss of myelin in the posterior columns. (**c**) Section of upper lumbar cord at a more advanced stage, showing extensive loss of myelin in posterior and lateral columns and a small area of pallor in one anterior column. Heidenhain's myelin stain.

tion can occur in demyelinated fibres in this condition is not certain.

It has been said that neuroglial scarring occurs only during remissions and especially as a result of treatment. However, Russell, Batten and Collier (1900) observed fibrous gliosis in some of their cases, and it has been seen by others in untreated cases which had progressed steadily but not very rapidly. The astrocytic reaction seems to depend on the rate at which the disease progresses. In acute cases the astrocytes may appear inactive or undergo regressive changes. In less acute cases the cell bodies of the astrocytes swell slightly and their processes become thicker and more numerous. In the more slowly progressive cases there is often considerable fibrous gliosis in the areas first affected although none may be seen in areas of recent degeneration.

There are insignificant changes in the meninges, nerve roots or the grey matter of the cord. The anterior horn cells often contain some excess of lipofuscin but otherwise appear normal. In severe cases there may be chromatolysis of the neurons of Clarke's column and in the Betz cells of the precentral gyrus. Posterior roots have occasionally shown loss of fibres (Putnam, 1891; Zimmerman, 1943).

More extensive changes in the brain have been reported in a relatively small number of cases by Woltmann (1918), Adams and Kubik (1944), Ferraro, Arieti and English (1945) and others. The most characteristic lesions are small, ill-defined, often perivascular foci of demyelination within the cerebral white matter. They may be scanty, detectable only on careful search, or they may be disseminated over wide areas of the corona radiata. The large ascending and descending tracts in the internal capsule, cerebral peduncles and pons are relatively spared. The histology of these foci is similar to that of the focal changes in the spinal cord, with fusiform swelling of myelin sheaths and axons in recent foci, followed by fibre degeneration and proliferation of lipophages in older foci. In some cases there may be perivascular and diffuse fibrous gliosis of greater severity than is usually seen in the spinal cord. Degeneration of the optic nerves (papillomacular bundle) was described by Bickel (1914) and Adams and Kubik (1944).

Apart from these foci of demyelination, haemorrhages and fibrosis of capillaries and small arterioles may be found. Ferraro, Arieti and English (1945) described widespread degeneration of cortical neurons.

Pernicious anaemia is one of the conditions associated with the Wernicke syndrome (p. 572).

The pathology of peripheral nerve changes has been reviewed by Pant, Asbury and Richardson (1968) and Victor (1975). Despite its importance in vitamin B_{12} deficiency, the peripheral nerve changes are poorly understood, and no single detailed study of the peripheral nervous system is available.

Russell, Batten and Collier (1900) found peripheral nerves to be normal or only slightly degenerated in most of their cases, although in chronic cases there was considerable degeneration in the larger nerves and in their small intramuscular branches. Peripheral nerve degeneration was also found by van der Scheer and Koek (1938), Foster (1945) and Coërs and Woolf (1959).

Greenfield and Carmichael (1935) made a quantitative study of biopsies of a small cutaneous branch of the anterior tibial nerve from patients with pernicious anaemia. There were reduced numbers of fibres, particularly those of large size, in preparations stained for myelin with osmic acid. However, when the nerves were examined by the Gros–Bielschowsky method, there was no reduction in numbers nor any change in appearance of the axons. Although this finding suggests the presence of a demyelinating neuropathy, other descriptions are more consistent with an axonal type of neuropathy. Foster (1945) described reduced numbers of myelin sheaths and axons, and increased numbers of Schwann cells, with axon reaction changes in posterior root ganglion cells and degenerative changes in the centrally directed posterior root fibres. Coërs and Woolf (1959) found abnormalities in preterminal axons and end-plates in muscle biopsies of patients with vitamin B_{12} deficiency.

Clinical pathology The cerebrospinal fluid usually shows a slight excess of protein. Vitamin B_{12} levels in the CSF have been studied by various authors (see Girdwood, 1968) and, though there are discrepancies, most are agreed that in both normal and affected patients the CSF levels are considerably less than the serum levels. Estimations of the blood serum show reduction, but rarely complete absence of vitamin B_{12}. In pernicious anaemia, vitamin B_{12} absorption using radioactive B_{12} (Berlyne, Liversedge and Emery, 1957) is almost nil, although with the addition of intrinsic factor it becomes normal. The Schilling test (measurement of urinary excretion of radio-labelled vitamin B_{12} after oral administration) can also be used to distinguish addisonian from non-addisonian cases.

Vitamin B_{12} deficiency in animals Demyelinating lesions associated with vitamin B_{12} deficiency states have been described in chicks, rats and calves (Alexander, 1957). In 1963, Krohn, Oxnard and Chalmers showed that primates in captivity kept on a vegetarian diet spontaneously developed a disease called cage paralysis. In a study of 15 rhesus monkeys maintained on a strict vegetarian diet for many years (Oxnard and Smith, 1966), five developed paralysis. The spinal cords showed spongiform demyelination of posterior and lateral columns without significant gliosis; severe demyelination of peripheral nerves, more marked distally, was found in three of the animals. Neuropathological changes were also found in animals which did not become paralysed. Four paralysed monkeys given cyanocobalamin showed clinical improvement. Further studies (Torres, Smith and Oxnard, 1971) have confirmed the peripheral nerve pathology, and shown additionally that segmental demyelination was the main lesion

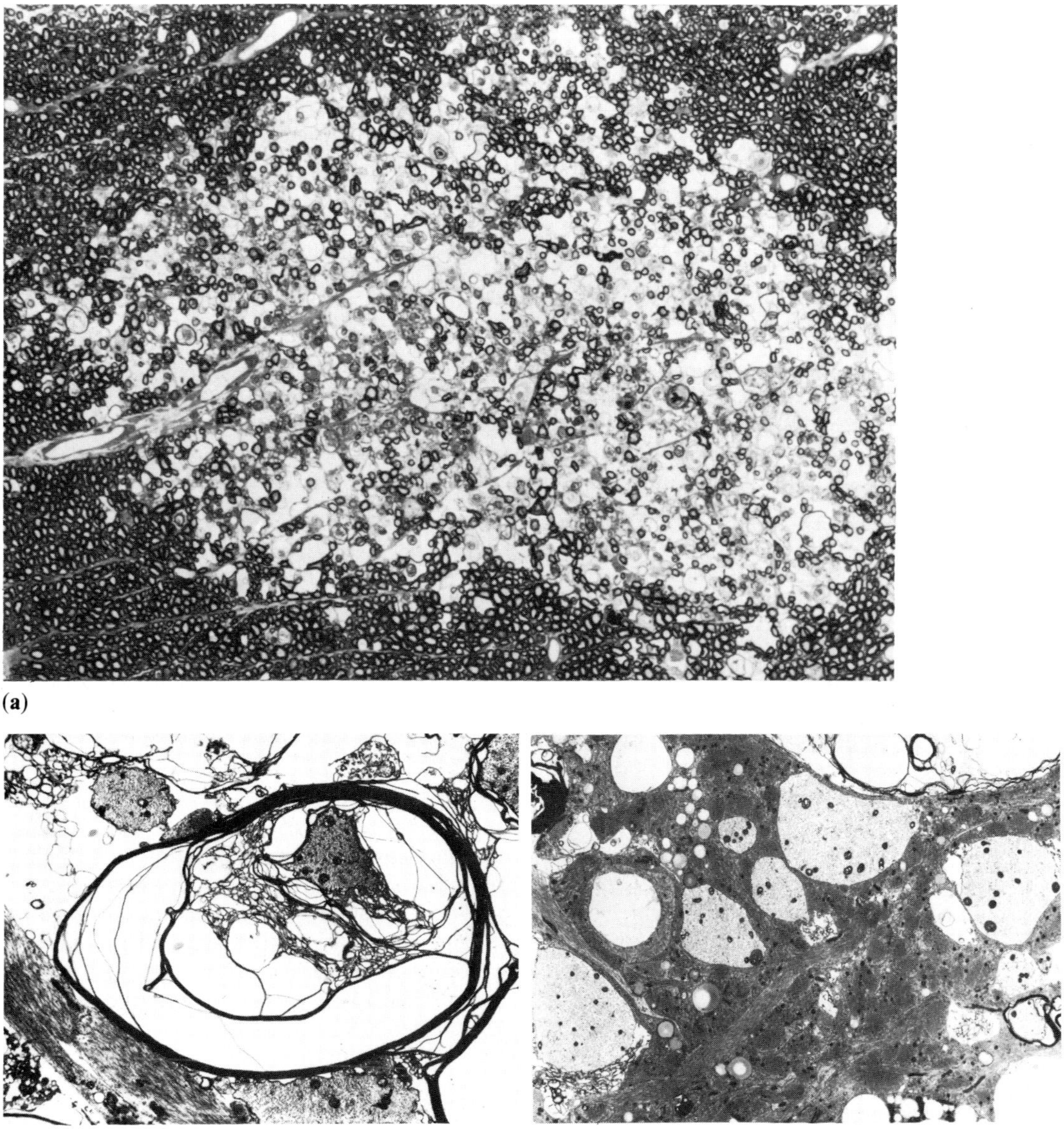

(a) (b) (c)

Fig. 13.7 Spinal cord from monkeys with vitamin B_{12} deficiency. (**a**) Section from posterior column showing a focal area of spongy change. 1 μm epon section. Crystal violet ×100. (**b**) Electron micrograph from area of spongiosus showing breakdown of myelin sheath with honeycomb-like appearance. ×5000. (**c**) Electron micrograph from area of spongiosus at a later stage. Several demyelinated axons are seen embedded in a dense network of astrocytic processes. ×2700. (From Agamanolis et al., 1978. Reproduced by courtesy of the Editor, *Journal of Neuropathology and Experimental Neurology*.)

with axonal degeneration in the most severe cases.

Agamanolis et al. (1978) have reported an electron microscope study of central nervous system changes in monkeys kept on a diet deficient in B_{12}, but supplemented with other vitamins. The lesions were indistinguishable topographically and histologically from those of human subacute combined degeneration of the cord. Affected posterior and lateral columns were studied in detail. The mildest changes were of a focal spongy nature (Fig. 13.7a), caused by distension of the myelin sheaths, wide separation of myelin lamellae forming extensive vacuoles or the formation of periaxonal spaces. The extracellular space was also increased. At later stages, myelin sheaths showed honeycomb-like breakdown and other types of degenerative change (Fig. 13.7b). Axons disappeared from some fibres with abnormalities, but a great many remained intact, although denuded of myelin, embedded in a dense network of astrocyte processes (Fig. 13.7c). A substantial number of axons contained accumulations of dense bodies and mitochondria, often causing axonal swelling.

Folic acid

Folic acid was first identified as an antianaemic factor in 1935. It is present in high concentration in all green-leaved vegetables, yeast and liver.

Folic acid deficiency in man causes haematological changes similar to those of pernicious anaemia. Deficiency can result from poor diet conditions such as steatorrhoea and tropical sprue, leading to malabsorption and from treatment with anticonvulsive drugs such as phenytoin and primidone.

Although there are several reports which suggest that folic acid deficiency can cause neurological disorders, the evidence of a direct causal relationship is not very persuasive.

Pallis and Lewis (1974) have reviewed a number of cases of neuropathy and encephalopathy in which folate deficiency was present and possibly a causative factor. The most convincing are cases of 'congenital specific folate malabsorption' in which defective transport of folic acid across the intestinal mucosa is attributed to a new inborn error of metabolism. The neurological disorder was characterized by moderate mental and physical retardation, ataxia and seizures (Luhby and Cooperman, 1967). A similar case was reported by Lanzkowsky, Erlandson and Bezan (1969), in which there was profound mental retardation, dysarthria and athetotic movements. Folate administration decreased the frequency of seizures in the cases described by Luhby and Cooperman but caused an increase in numbers of seizures in the patient described by Lanzkowsky, Erlandson and Bezan.

Pallis and Lewis (1974) have referred to three other separate cases of inborn errors of folate metabolism associated with mental retardation and abnormally *high* levels of folate activity in the serum. In these patients there seems to be a defect of folate metabolism rather than of absorption.

Low serum folate levels are often found in conditions which themselves may be the cause of neurological disorders. Psychiatric disturbances, particularly in the elderly, have been associated with folate depletion (Girdwood, 1968). However, as Pallis and Lewis have emphasized, a low serum folate is not uncommon in elderly patients in whom neurological signs are present which are sometimes unrelated to recognized clinical entities.

Martinez Figueroa et al. (1980) have found some improvement in electrophysiological abnormalities in the peripheral nerves of patients on long-term anticonvulsant therapy who were treated with folate for a month.

There are no reports of neuropathological lesions resulting from folic acid deficiency.

Vitamin A

This substance, a carotene, is the precursor of the light-sensitive pigment rhodopsin, which is present in the rods of the retina. Deficiency of the vitamin leads to nyctalopia and also to keratinizing metaplasia of the conjunctival and corneal epithelium (xerosis). Vitamin A is also necessary in the synthesis of active sulphate (Sundaresen, 1966) which is transferred to galactoceramide, thus forming sulphatide. Melchior and Clausen (1968) attempted to reduce sulphatide synthesis in human metachromatic leucodystrophy: they fed a diet poor in vitamin A but failed to induce significant clinical improvement.

Experimental deficiency in animals has been associated with degeneration of the cranial and peripheral nerves and grey and white matter of the spinal cord (Wolbach and Bessey, 1941; Mellanby, 1944) but this is the result of selective cessation of growth of bone and subsequent increase of pressure and not to a direct effect on the neural tissue. Hayes, Nielsen and Eaton (1968) found that optic nerve lesions in vitamin A-deficient calves resulted from raised CSF pressure due to an increased resistance to bulk absorption of the CSF, and an abnormal development of the sphenoid bone. Howell and Thompson (1967a, b) found cerebral herniation, thinning of cerebellar flocculi and ridging of the lumbosacral spine in chicks. Fluorescence microscopy detects very little of this enzyme in the normal central nervous system (Popper, 1941).

Hydrocephalus in young rabbits whose mothers had suffered from vitamin A deficiency was described by Millen and Woollam (1956); the hydrocephalus was not caused by stenosis of the aqueduct, and its pathogenesis is obscure.

A case of benign intracranial hypertension induced by deficiency of vitamin A during infancy has been reported by Karsakis and Bass (1982); CSF pressure became normal after parenteral therapy with vitamin A. Excessive vitamin A also causes raised intracranial pressure.

Vitamin C (ascorbic acid)

Gross vitamin C deficiency causes scurvy, a disease characterized by multiple haemorrhages. These may occur anywhere in the body, most frequently under the periosteum of the long bones, but also in the nervous system, including the retina and cerebrum.

Vitamin K

Similar diapedetic haemorrhages in numerous sites were reported by Ferraro and Roizin (1943) in the brains of fowls and cats deprived of vitamin K. The haemorrhages are related to the reduction of prothrombin levels which follow deficiency of the vitamin. Hypoprothrombinaemia with similar haemorrhagic manifestations is occasionally seen in patients suffering from obstructive jaundice, diarrhoea or sprue, and in such cases therapy with vitamin K has been successful.

Vitamin E

Vitamin E deficiency was found to cause reproductive abnormalties in rats, and Evans and Bishop (1922) demonstrated that these abnormalities could be prevented by a factor present in lettuce and wheat germ oil, later identified as α-tocopherol (vitamin E).

Vitamin E is a highly non-polar lipid. Its intestinal absorption is linked to fat absorption and facilitated by the presence of bile salts.

Neurological disease has been reported in a number of conditions in which there is defective fat absorption or which lead to reduced concentrations of bile salts in the small intestine. These include biliary atresia (Rosenblum et al., 1981), cystic fibrosis (Geller, Gilles and Schwachman, 1977), childhood chronic liver disease (Tomasi, 1979), steatorrhoea (Binder, Solitaire and Spiro, 1967) intrahepatic cholestasis (Saito et al., 1982) and abetalipoproteinaemia (Bassen–Kornzweig syndrome) (Guggenheim et al., 1982).

A number of these conditions are associated with deficiency of vitamin E. Indeed, in abetalipoproteinaemia there are undetectable levels of the vitamin in the serum from birth. In some cases oral administration of vitamin E has led to an improvement in neurological symptoms. The association between vitamin E and neurological function has recently been reviewed by Muller, Lloyd and Wolff (1983).

The neuropathology of progressive neuromuscular disease in a girl with fatal familial intrahepatic cholestasis has been described by Saito et al. (1982). The serum vitamin E level was very low. A distal axonopathy was found affecting both central and peripheral axons of sensory ganglion cells. There was also neuronal loss in sensory and oculomotor nuclei of the brain stem, basal ganglia, Clarke's column, posterior horn and dorsal root ganglia. Neuronal lipofuscinosis was reported, and swollen dystrophic axons (spheroids) were seen in gracile and cuneate nuclei, many other brain stem nuclei, basal ganglia, spinal cord grey matter and dorsal root ganglia. Harding et al. (1982) have reported the cases of two adults who developed progressive neurological disorders more than 20 years after the onset of fat malabsorption. The neurological syndrome was suggestive of spinocerebellar degeneration with an associated peripheral neuropathy. Vitamin E was undetectable in the serum of both cases. One patient showed improvement clinically and electrophysiologically after treatment with vitamin E. Harding et al. discuss the role of vitamin deficiency in neurological disorders associated with chronic fat malabsorption. They also point out the similarity between the neuropathological findings in man (Geller, Gilles and Schwachman, 1977; Rosenblum et al., 1981; Saito et al., 1982), rats (Towfighi, 1981), and monkeys (Nelson et al., 1981), which suggest that vitamin E deficiency produces a 'dying-back' neuropathy in both central and peripherally directed fibres of the sensory neurons, the central fibre degeneration being more marked than that in the peripheral fibres.

Vitamin E deficiency in animals Vitamin E deficiency has been studied in a number of species. It causes degeneration of testicular epithelium, fetal resorption, myopathy and nervous system defects. Ringsted (1935) described a nervous system disorder in adult rats. These neuropathological changes were reviewed by Einarson and Ringsted (1938) and confirmed by Lutrell and Mason (1949) and Malamud, Nelson and Evans (1949). The earliest central nervous system lesions are seen as degeneration of posterior columns and associated spinal roots, and gliosis. Anterior horn cells first show chromatolysis; they then accumulate lipid-containing material which later forms ceroid pigment; the cells eventually degenerate. There may be some pyramidal tract degeneration. Alongside these nervous system changes there is hyaline degeneration and necrosis of muscle associated with the accumulation of pigment. The pigment is also found in neurons, glial cells and blood vessels in the brain. It has been suggested that the accumulated pigment is an end-product of excessive lipid peroxidation in the absence of the protective antioxidant effect of vitamin E. In an electron microscope study of vitamin E-deficient rats Miyagishi, Takahata and Iizuka (1967) concluded that the pigment was similar to that seen in aged rats.

Verma and Wei King (1967) described narrowing of the aqueduct of Sylvius leading to hydrocephalus in the developing brain of vitamin E-deficient rats. There was also a reduction in numbers of neurons, gliosis and abnormalities of the choroid plexus.

Pentschew and Schwarz (1962) found eosinophilic bodies in the gracile and cuneate nuclei of rats fed a vitamin E-deficient diet for many months. By electron microscopy these were identified as axons which contained large numbers of neurofilaments, dense bodies, mitochondria and vesicular profiles. Similar axonal swellings (spheroids) were described in infantile neuraxonal dystrophy (Cowen and Olmstead, 1963; Seitelberger, 1971) and rats poisoned with parabromophenylacetylurea (Blakemore and Cavanagh, 1969). Lampert, Blumberg and Pentschew (1964) discussed their resemblance to regenerated axons, and Blakemore and Cavanagh (1969) suggested that they represent attempted axonal regeneration.

In a more recent study, Nelson et al. (1981) kept rhesus monkeys on a vitamin E-deficient diet for 30–33 months. Distal axonal degeneration was found in central (posterior column) fibres and peripheral nerves, the central fibres being the more severely affected. Some dorsal root ganglion cells had degenerated.

Swollen, dystrophic axons (spheroids) were seen less frequently in these monkeys than in vitamin E-deficient rats. Accumulations of lipoprotein were evident in neuronal perikarya and in endothelial cells within the central nervous system.

Hunger oedema

Hunger oedema has been a prominent feature of many famines and occurred as a consequence of impoverished diets in Europe during and immediately after the two World Wars. Reduction in plasma protein has been held to be its main cause, but according to McCance (1951) this may not be as important a factor as the replacement of fat and of tissue volume by fluid; posture, renal function, salt intake and perhaps hormonal imbalance all play their part. The central nervous system is the last region to lose weight and tissue volume and there are no specific neuropathological changes. The central and peripheral neuropathies of vitamin B deficiencies are uncommon.

Kwashiorkor

Clinicopathological descriptions were given by Trowell, Davies and Dean (1954), Follis (1958) and Platt (1958b). Although a diet deficient mainly in protein has been considered the principal causative factor, Golden (1982), who re-evaluated its role, found that in children with oedematous malnutrition the oedema disappeared rapidly on diets low in protein but producing energy. A 'dietary energy intake' below 245–270 KJ/kg per day led to oedema.

Kwashiorkor has been reported from poverty-stricken areas in Africa, India, Jamaica and elsewhere, and usually affects children between the ages of 6 months and 4 years; an adult form has also been recognized. Clinically kwashiorkor is characterized by retardation in growth, muscular wasting, oedema, diarrhoea, a dermatosis resembling pellagra (though not sensitive to sunlight), enlargement of the liver, and a mental apathy and behaviour disturbance which may be profound. If left untreated, the condition is fatal, but severe manifestations of the syndrome may respond favourably to an adequate diet.

Neurological signs are not prominent, and although a rhythmic and coarse tremor, hypotonia and areflexia have been described during the recovery period, these signs usually disappear. Balmer, Howells and Wharton (1968) described acute encephalopathy with drowsiness deepening into coma. In fatal cases the brain showed no macroscopic changes. Garrow (1967) suggested that mental signs in kwashiorkor may be related to deficiency in brain potassium.

Pathological changes in kwashiorkor These include fatty liver and atrophy of the pancreas and mucosal glands of the intestine. The brain has usually shown only non-specific oedema and congestion or no identifiable changes at all.

van Bogaert et al. (1962) investigated the muscles of Congolese infants with kwashiorkor and found changes which they considered to be characteristic; the muscle fibres showed foamy and eosinophilic degeneration, accompanied by an intermysial oedema which was followed by fibrosis.

The salient signs of kwashiorkor have been reproduced in experimental animals, and with particular ease in young pigs fed on a 'Gambia diet'. Platt and his associates were able to study many of the features of this syndrome in strictly controlled conditions. The central nervous system was only slightly (though consistently) affected (Meyer, Stewart and Platt, 1961); there was chromatolysis, especially in the neurons of the anterior horns in the spinal cord, and slight activation of astrocytes and oligodendrocytes. These changes were interpreted as a reversible adaptation to deficient nutrition, rather than as evidence of progressive degeneration and glial replacement. Similar though more severe changes were found in the pups of bitches fed on a low protein diet. Stewart and Platt (1968) noted neurological disorders (tremors, abnormal gait, ataxia, convulsions) in protein-calorie deficient pups. Platt and Stewart (1969) subsequently reviewed the whole question of experimental protein-calorie deficiency: as well as the chromatolysis and neuroglial hyperplasia in the cord mentioned above, they noted thinning of myelin sheaths and similar though less pronounced brain involvement; the peripheral nerves showed widening of the nodes of Ranvier a change which Oldfors and Nordberg (1977) were unable to confirm in rats. It was suggested that malnutrition during intrauterine or early postnatal life may lead to irreversible neurological changes.

Neuropathological changes associated with liver disease

Encephalopathy is a common and serious complication of various forms of liver disease. Three different clinical syndromes can be recognised: (1) chronic, familial type of cerebral hepatolenticular degeneration (Wilson's disease); (2) acquired (non-wilsonian) chronic hepatocerebral degeneration; and (3) a relatively acute neurological disease often progressing to hepatic coma, which may accompany liver failure.

Familial hepatolenticular degeneration (Wilson's disease)

The term 'hepatolenticular degeneration' was applied to a familial metabolic disease, transmitted as an autosomal recessive, in which cirrhosis of the liver is associated with degeneration of the corpus striatum. Onset of the disease is from the first to the fourth decade, but it most usually appears towards the end of the second decade. In untreated cases the duration of the illness is usually between 3 and 10 years but it may be considerably longer. The onset usually follows, at an interval of months or years, an attack of febrile jaundice which may be transient. In many instances the hepatic cirrhosis remains occult throughout the course of the disease but there may be variable ascites, swelling of the ankles and/or splenomegaly. A heavy urinary excretion of amino acids, including types that are not usually found in hepatic cirrhosis, has been noted in the majority of cases.

Clinically there is progressive rigidity and coarse tremor of the limbs, a spastic condition of the face, mouth and pharynx causing dysarthria and dysphagia, and, in the terminal stages of the disease, some degree of dementia.

Historical Wilson (1912) reported six cases with three necropsies and added eight more from the literature. Two or three members of some families were affected. Hoesslin and Alzheimer (1912) reported a case with full postmortem examination and termed the condition *pseudosclerosis*. In addition to cirrhosis of the liver they found widespread degenerative changes in the brain, especially in the striatum; they emphasized the presence in all the degenerated areas of large astrocytes with swollen, vesicular and sometimes multiple nuclei which are now named after Alzheimer (see below). Kayser (1902) and Fleischer (1903) described a ring of brown pigmentation in the cornea (Fig. 13.8a) in cases of pseudosclerosis associated with cirrhosis of the liver. These observations were collated by Hall (1921), who added 53 further cases from the literature and four cases of his own. In some of these the lesions were widespread in the brain, involving the cerebral cortex, the basal ganglia and brain stem nuclei and the dentate nucleus and cerebellar peduncle; but lesions were always most severe in the striatum. Opalski (1930) subsequently described the large phagocytic cells which bear his name (Fig. 13.8b), and Haurowitz (1930) and Lüthy (1931) found an excess of copper in both corpus striatum and liver. By 1948 Denny-Brown had found over 150 case reports in the literature and, with Uzman, described the aminoaciduria which so often occurs in the disease (Uzman and Denny-Brown, 1948). Cumings (1948) showed that patients dying of Wilson's disease had excess copper in the brain, liver and kidneys. This discovery led to the development of therapy involving the continuous administration of β,β-dimethylcysteine (D-penicillamine), which is effective in most cases (Walshe, 1976). Further details have been given by Cumings (1959), Bergsma (1968), Bearn (1972) and Scheinberg and Sternlieb (1974).

Pathological changes The brain usually shows no external abnormality except some shrinking of the insular cortex. On section the corpus striatum appears shrunken, especially in its middle third, so that on horizontal section the outline of its external border is sinuous, resembling a Cupid's bow. This is less obvious in coronal sections in which the outline is flatter than normal and at some levels may even be concave. The corpus striatum, and sometimes the thalamus, has a brownish or brick-red colour according to the duration of formalin fixation. Cavitation is often found in the putamen. In milder forms cavitation is chiefly perivascular, but when severe

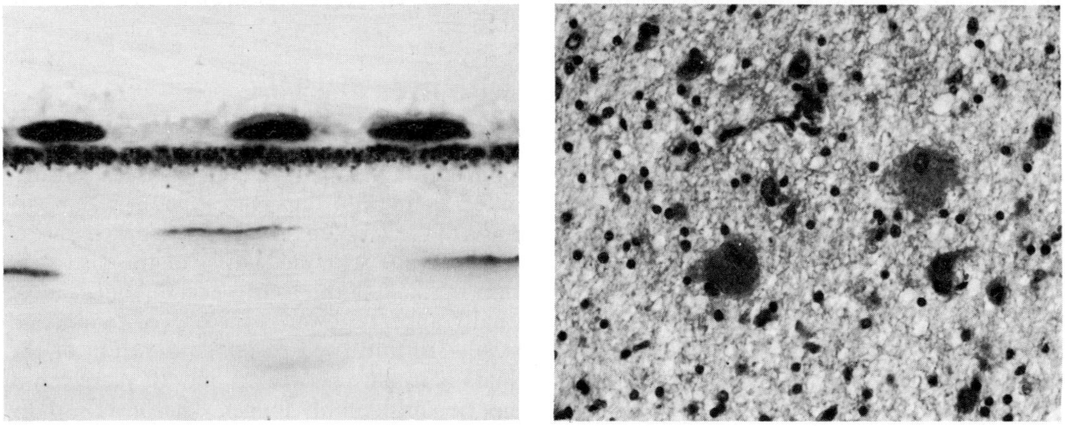

(a) **(b)**

Fig. 13.8 Wilson's disease. (**a**) Section of cornea showing the Kayser–Fleischer zone of pigment granules in Descemet's membrane. ×1200. (**b**) Opalski cells in the subthalamic nucleus. The cells are large with finely granular cytoplasm and have no processes. The nuclei are relatively small. Haematoxylin and van Gieson × 250.

may involve most of the central and anterior parts of the putamen and spread into the caudate nucleus. Very rarely it has been found in other nuclei such as the thalamus and red nucleus (Howard and Royce, 1919). The central white matter of the cerebral and cerebellar hemispheres may also show spongy softening or cavitation, and the overlying cortex may then be atrophic (Schulman, 1968).

Histology The putamen shows, in most cases, increased cellularity due chiefly to proliferation of astrocytes. Many astrocytic nuclei are larger and more vesicular than normal with one or more basophilic nucleoli (Fig. 13.9), and so they

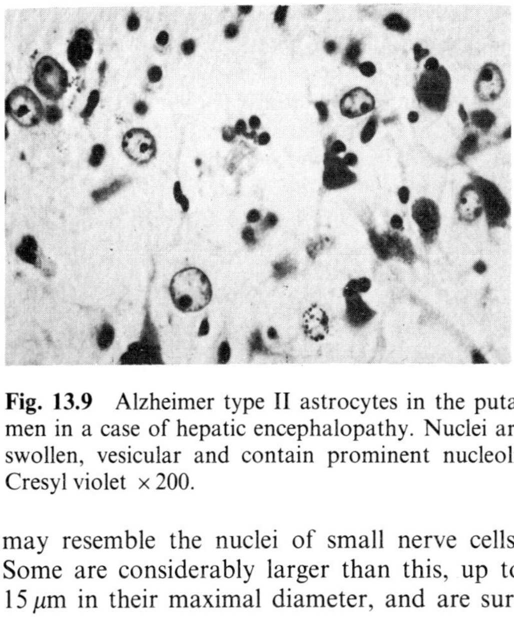

Fig. 13.9 Alzheimer type II astrocytes in the putamen in a case of hepatic encephalopathy. Nuclei are swollen, vesicular and contain prominent nucleoli. Cresyl violet ×200.

may resemble the nuclei of small nerve cells. Some are considerably larger than this, up to 15 μm in their maximal diameter, and are surrounded by fine yellow granules which appear to be enclosed in tenuous processes. It is not clear whether the granules correspond to the copper-containing cytoplasmic material demonstrated histochemically by Uzman (1956). These nuclei belong to cells of Alzheimer type II, which do not form neuroglial fibres. Large multinucleated cells of Alzheimer type I are much rarer and are not present in every case; Lapham (1962) demonstrated that such cells had double the normal amount of nuclear DNA. Scharenberg and Drew (1954) studied Alzheimer-type astrocytes by metallic impregnation methods and showed that their cytoplasm and processes are more prominent than routine stains suggest.

Both in the putamen and caudate nucleus there is a general reduction in the number of neurons. In some cases the loss is mainly of large neurons; in others small neurons are most affected.

When cavities are present they have ragged edges which show little evidence of reactive scarring by either neuroglial or collagen fibres. Lipophages and siderophages in variable numbers are seen in relation to cavities; old or recent haemorrhages (occasionally extensive) have been described. Lüthy (1931) and Lichtenstein and Gore (1955) found pericapillary concentrations which stained heavily for copper in the putamen.

The globus pallidus consistently shows less change, though there is a reduction in the number of its myelinated fibres, and Alzheimer type II nuclei and Opalski cells are usually seen; cystic transformation is rare. In the subthalamic nucleus also, Alzheimer-type astrocytes and Opalski cells may be present and there is often degeneration and loss of neurons. Focal degeneration of the cerebral cortex is not uncommon, especially in the frontal lobes. There may be areas of hypermyelination, status spongiosus or diffuse loss of nerve cells and fibres, both in the cortex and in the white matter of the convolutions (Barnes and Hurst, 1926). In the thalamus and the nuclei of the brain stem, Alzheimer and Opalski cells may be found. Phagocytes containing iron pigment are commonly found in the globus pallidus and substantia nigra. In the latter nucleus, Lichtenstein and Gore (1955) found unilateral scarring, but this is unusual. Degeneration of the dentate nucleus, often associated with Marchi or sudanophilic degeneration of the superior cerebellar peduncle, has been found in a number of cases (Greenfield, Poynton and Walshe, 1924).

Careful examination will usually reveal a variable degree of involvement of the cerebral and cerebellar cortices and white matter, similar to that in the lentiform nucleus but usually less severe, cystic changes being uncommon. The brain stem and cord are rarely affected and then only to a limited extent. Victor, Adams and Cole (1965) showed that lesions identical to those found in Wilson's disease can occur with other varieties of cirrhosis in which copper metabolism is not affected; they therefore questioned the causative effect of copper accumulation, though Popoff et al. (1965) came to the opposite conclusion.

Opalski cells Opalski (1930) described an unusual cell type which he found only in cases of hepatolenticular degeneration. These are large cells the nuclei of which are small when compared to the size of the perikarya (in contrast to Alzheimer's glial cells) (see Fig. 13.8b). Opalski cells are oval or rounded, without processes, and have a finely granular or slightly foamy cytoplasm, staining a light-rose colour by Nissl's method. The small nucleus is usually oval and central and more darkly stained than that of Alzheimer type II cells. Very rarely a larger nucleus is present or the cells are multinucleated. Regressive changes in which the nucleus lies peripherally and the cytoplasm is vacuolated are frequently seen. These cells are very much less frequent than Alzheimer type II cells, and Opalski found them mainly in the thalamus, globus pallidus and zona reticularis of substantia nigra but very rarely in the striatum; their presence in hepatolenticular degeneration has been confirmed by numerous subsequent writers. Such cells measure up to 35 μm and stand out prominently when stained with van Gieson's counterstain by the bright orange-brown colour and rounded outline of the cell body. In the lentiform nuclei they are usually found in relation to foci of degeneration and in association with Alzheimer glia; they are less common in the cerebral cortex and elsewhere in the basal ganglia, though they have been seen in the subthalamus (see Fig. 13.8b). Their origin is uncertain and they have been regarded as degenerate neurons (Victor, Adams and Cole, 1965) or derivatives of either astrocytes (Opalski) or phagocytes (Greenfield, 1963).

Kayser–Fleischer ring Sections of the cornea show granules of brown pigment in Descemet's membrane near the limbus of the cornea, and this is pathognomonic of Wilson's disease (see Fig. 13.8a). The granules do not give a Prussian blue reaction for iron, and, unlike melanin, do not bleach with oxidizing agents. They react for copper with rubeanic acid and rhodanine, and have been shown to contain copper by spectroscopic analysis.

Johnson and Campbell (1982) have studied the cornea by electron microscopy. Dense granules were found in the posterior non-banded portion of Descemet's membrane, and very occasionally in endothelial cells. X-ray energy spectroscopy showed the granules to contain copper and sulphur. Deposition of copper in the lens produces a sunflower cataract.

Liver In the early stages of the disease hepatomegaly may occur, though there is usually atrophy terminally, when the liver is coarsely cirrhotic with nodules which may vary in size from 1 mm to 2 cm or more. The colour varies in different cases and the individual lobules may also vary, some being yellow, others brick-red, greenish or brown. This appears to be due to differences in the amount of copper storage, fatty degeneration or bile staining. Microscopically the characteristic appearances of macronodular cirrhosis are seen, but the fibrous septa are less heavily collagenous than in most cirrhotic livers, and may contain perivascular collections of lymphocytes and numerous small bile ducts. In some early cases the appearances have been those of subacute hepatitis. Granules giving staining reactions for copper have been described in liver cells. Iron-containing pigment and bile pigment may also be present. Anderson and Popper (1960) studied 19 cases in detail and noted that marked glycogen infiltration of nuclei was an early and typical feature and that the cirrhosis was postnecrotic in type.

Changes in other organs The spleen is often enlarged, congested and firmer than normal, with fibrosis of the pulp and trabeculae secondary to portal hypertension; when hepatic cirrhosis has been clinically silent, it shows no abnormality. Böttiger and Möllerberg (1959) described cardiomegaly in this disease; histology showed coarse dark intracellular pigment, which failed to give the staining reactions for iron, around the nuclei of the cardiac muscle cells. Various forms of skeletal disease may occur in association with Wilson's disease, including osteoporosis (Rosenoer and Mitchell, 1959).

Biochemistry The chief metabolic abnormality in hepatolenticular degeneration is failure to use the copper absorbed in excess from the intestines to synthesize the serum copper-carrying protein caeruloplasmin. Normally copper is taken up from the intestine in loose combination with albumin and after about 24 hours is transferred to globulin, to which it is more firmly bound (Bearn and Kunkel, 1954). In the blood serum copper is attached to the alpha-, beta- and gamma-globulins in proportions of about 25, 50 and 20 per cent; only 2–5 per cent remains attached to albumin. In hepatolenticular degeneration, on the other hand, only 40–60 per cent of the total serum copper is bound to globulin, chiefly to the beta and gamma fractions; in four out of five cases Cumings, Goodman and Earl (1955) found only traces of copper in combination with alpha-globulin. The remainder is loosely attached to albumin from which it more easily becomes detached and is either taken up by the proteins of the brain and liver or excreted by the kidneys. The urinary excretion therefore rises from the normal 10 to 100 μg Cu per day to amounts of 400–600 μg or even higher. Under treatment with BAL or the chelating agent penicillamine these figures may be greatly exceeded. Holmberg and Laurell (1948) isolated from human serum a blue protein substance in which copper was combined with alpha-globulin. They called this substance caeruloplasmin and found that, using *p*-phenylenediamine as a substrate, it could act as an oxidase. In hepatolenticular degeneration, caeruloplasmin is normally absent or present in very small amounts and has no oxidase activity (Bearn and Kunkel, 1954). In two out of 40 cases, however, Cumings (1962) found it present in normal quantity, and there appears to be poor correlation between caeruloplasmin concentration and the duration and severity of the clinical course of the illness (Cartwright et al., 1960). The serum copper level was normal in four out of the 40 cases. The amount of caeruloplasmin may also be diminished in a patient's siblings who themselves show no sign of the disease (Turpin, Jerome and Schmidt, 1953). The physiology of copper in man and its relation to Wilson's disease has been reviewed by Walshe (1957) and Cumings (1972).

It has been suggested that the caeruloplasmin present in some patients with Wilson's disease is structurally and therefore functionally abnormal. Thus there may be two different alleles mediating the disease—one leading to failure of protein synthesis and one to abnormalities of protein structure; either could result in the same derangement of copper transport (British Medical Journal, 1967). However, Holtzmann et al. (1967) studied the caeruloplasmin from a patient in whom the levels of the protein were near normal and found that the tryptic peptide map, electrophoretic analysis, amino acid and sugar composition, copper content and oxidase activity were all normal and not consistent with the theory that there is a structural abnormality of caeruloplasmin in Wilson's disease; they suggested that there was a reduced rate of caeruloplasmin synthesis in their patient, because treatment with penicillamine caused the protein to disappear from the plasma. Penicillamine lowers body copper stores, and caeruloplasmin synthesis in the normal individual may be stimulated by a fall in body copper. Although caeruloplasmin appears to prevent hepatolenticular degeneration, the precise way in which it does this remains obscure.

The increase of amino acids in the urine, which may reach 300–800 mg of amino acid nitrogen per day (about four to six times normal), affects all those normally present, and the abnormal amino acids, proline and citrulline have occasionally been found. There is no alteration in the amino acids of the blood serum and it is probable that the increased excretion is related to defective reabsorption in the convoluted tubules of the kidneys. The relation of aminoaciduria to the abnormal copper metabolism is not clear. Excess of amino acids appears in the urine in other diseases of the liver, but only when its function is gravely disturbed as in acute yellow atrophy; it is rarely seen in cases of hepatic cirrhosis without jaundice. In hepatolenticular degeneration the aminoaciduria is therefore out of proportion to the disturbance of liver function, which is usually slight and in many cases is not evident on routine testing. Plasma inorganic phosphate and urate concentrations are reduced and there may be proteinuria, glycosuria, hypercalciuria and hyperphosphaturia (Eastham and Jancar, 1968). In untreated cases the blood pyruvate concentrations are increased and pyruvate tolerence is abnormal after glucose ingestion; treatment with penicillamine reverses these features.

Acquired (non-wilsonian) hepatocerebral degeneration

Victor (1974) has pointed out that the acute encephalopathy progressing to hepatic coma and chronic hepatocerebral (largely irreversible) disease are two ends of a spectrum of forms of disease which may blend imperceptibly. Permanent neurological changes may ensue in patients who survive an episode of hepatic coma, or in others with chronic liver disease who deteriorate over a period of years without reaching a state of coma. Such patients may show tremor of the head and limbs, grimacing, dysarthria, cerebellar ataxia, choreoathetosis and dementia. There are diffuse electroencephalographic abnormalities which resemble those found in patients with hepatic coma except that they are irreversible, whilst those in hepatic coma are either evanescent or terminal. Either type may be associated with all varieties of chronic liver disease, but the chronic encephalopathy may be based more on the portal-systemic shunting of blood than on hepatocellular disease.

Neuropathological changes Macroscopically, patchy but diffuse laminar necrosis is found with microcavitation at the junction of cortex and white matter, in the striatum (especially in the superior pole of the putamen) and in cerebellar white matter (Victor, 1974; Finlayson and Superville, 1981).

Victor, Adams and Cole (1965) described three main histological findings: diffuse increase in the size and number of protoplasmic astrocytes; intranuclear inclusions (mainly glycogen) in astrocytes; and diffuse but patchy degeneration of neurons and myelin especially in the deeper cortex and subcortex, basal ganglia and cerebellum. Abnormal astrocytes were Alzheimer type II (see Fig. 13.9) with large, pale, occasionally lobulated or irregular nuclei, one or two nucleoli and a distinct nuclear membrane, along the surface of which lipofuscin-like granules could be seen. Cell cytoplasm was very scanty in sections stained by routine methods. These astrocytes were most numerous in the deeper cerebral cortex but were also found in variable numbers throughout the basal ganglia, hypothalamus, brain stem, cerebellum and even spinal grey matter. Immunohistochemical staining of basal ganglia and other brain regions from ten patients with hepatic encephalopathy, including some with acquired hepatocerebral degeneration, gave negative results for glial fibrillary astrocyte (GFA) protein in Alzheimer type II cells (Sobel et al., 1981). GFA protein is normally present in all types of astrocytes. Giant Alzheimer type I astrocytes were rarely seen.

In some cases, degeneration and loss of neurons and myelin in the deeper cortex was associated with pronounced microcavitation which had a pseudolaminar or laminar distribution, sometimes extending into the subcortical white matter. In places, loss of neurons involved the whole cortex and then microcavitation was not a feature. A variable degree of neuronal loss was usually present in the basal ganglia, together with microcavitation (mainly in the putamen) when cortical cavitation was present. Victor, Adams and Cole (1965) also found many Opalski cells in the cerebral cortex and basal ganglia and noted a transition from obvious neurons to Opalski forms.

Shiraki (1968) found central pontine myelinolysis in cases of acquired hepatocerebral degeneration and in Wilson's disease, which supports the suggestion of Adams, Victor and Mancall (1959) that the pontine disease may result from liver damage. Shiraki also noted that cerebral damage suggestive of 'circulatory inadequacy' and ischaemia were commonly found in all forms of hepatocerebral disease.

Peripheral nerve lesions Hepatic neuropathy has been reviewed by Asbury (1975). Dayan and Williams (1967) found evidence of segmental demyelination in teased single peripheral nerve fibres from ten patients with hepatic failure due to various causes. Clinical evidence of neuropathy was not always present. Patients with clinical signs (sensory impairment, diminished tendon jerks) included all patients with alcoholic cirrhosis and one with haemochromatosis; in these instances multiple factors had to be considered, though alcohol is an unlikely cause of segmental demyelination. It was concluded that the metabolic effects of hepatic failure, perhaps related to disturbed carbohydrate metabolism, were the most likely basis for the neuropathy.

Knill-Jones et al. (1972) studied 14 similar patients with various forms of liver disease, and confirmed the presence of indolent demyelination and remyelination; wallerian-type degeneration was less frequently seen. The occurrence of the neuropathy could not be correlated with either the duration of the liver disease or the results of liver function tests, although affected patients showed high immunoglobulin (IgA and IgM) levels. It was concluded that causal factors other than diabetes or excessive alcohol intake were responsible and that collateral shunting of portal blood was important because of the interference with hepatic detoxification which ensues.

Hepatic coma The acute disorder associated with liver failure, leading to hepatic coma, has been fully described by Victor (1974). The association between liver disease and derangement of mental functions has long been recognized. The term 'hepatic coma' came into use in the 1940s when a number of papers appeared drawing attention to coma as a complication of chronic liver disease (Murphy et al., 1948). Coma was not invariably terminal; it could occur as a transient abnormality and could recur. It was generally thought that coma or change in mentation was the only neurological abnormality in these patients.

Although nitrogen metabolism had been studied in patients with liver disease, abnormalities had not been related to the development of coma. However, in 1934, Monguio and Krause suggested an association between blood ammonia content and a neurological syndrome of stupor, convulsions and coma in dogs with a portacaval anastomosis (an Eck fistula).

Adams and Foley (1949) described the clinical findings in neurological disorder associated with liver disease. Before coma developed, there was an intervening stage of deranged consciousness with mental confusion causing either increased or decreased psychomotor activity, progressive drowsiness and stupor. In the confused state, there were frequently intermittent but sustained contractions of outstretched arms and legs causing a 'flapping' movement or asterixis. The electroencephalogram became abnormal during the early stages.

In a survey of the neuropathology of more than 150 cases of severe liver disease (Adams and Foley, 1953), gross examination of the brain revealed little of importance. Microscopically there was diffuse hyperplasia of protoplasmic astrocytes in lenticular and dentate nuclei, cerebral cortex, diencephalic and other brain stem nuclei. There was little or no visible alteration in nerve cells or other parenchymal elements.

McDermott and Adams in 1954 reported their observations on a patient in whom removal of a carcinoma of the head of the pancreas had necessitated the creation of an Eck fistula; the liver only showed fatty change at autopsy. Administration of nitrogenous substances such as ammonium chloride and urea caused episodes of stupor which corresponded to increased blood ammonia levels.

At the time of Adams and Foley's (1953) observations, the diuretic properties of ammonia-cation exchange resins were being investigated. Oral administration of the resins in patients with hepatic cirrhosis often induced early manifestations of hepatic coma.

The association between abnormal nitrogen metabolism and hepatic coma was now established and was further confirmed and amplified by Sherlock and her colleagues (Sherlock et al., 1954).

The astrocyte changes which are frequently the only histopathological alteration in patients dying of hepatic encephalopathy have been reviewed by Norenberg (1981); both Alzheimer type I and II changes were described.

Experimental portacaval anastomosis Hahn et al. (1893) performed Eck fistula operations in dogs and noted that they developed neurological symptoms provided that they were fed with raw meat. 'Meat intoxication' was associated with increased arterial blood ammonia levels. Although it was suggested that the cerebral changes were the result of carbamic acid absorbed from the gut, no structural changes were described in the brain.

More recently, Kline et al. (1966) and Doyle (1967) described astrocyte changes in dogs with a portacaval anastomosis. Doyle measured plasma ammonia and related increased levels to the appearance of swelling and lobulation of astrocyte nuclei.

Cavanagh and Kyu (1971) described astrocyte changes in rats with portacaval shunts. Although astrocytes were not increased in number and showed no 'nuclear' glycogen, other changes were considered to resemble those found in human encephalopathy associated with chronic liver disease. Cavanagh (1974) has reviewed the value of portacaval anastomosis as a model for studying astrocyte (Alzheimer type II) changes, which, he points out, are central both morphologically and metabolically to the problem of hepatic encephalopathy.

Alzheimer type II changes in astrocytes appear 4 weeks after operation. With perfusion-fixation, the nuclear changes are limited to a tortuosity in outline and an increase in nucleolar size; swelling is found only after delayed fixation and is not seen after adequate perfusion-fixation. Ultrastructural studies (Zamora, Cavanagh and Kyu, 1973) showed generalized swelling of astrocyte cytoplasm within a week of operation in all of the brain regions sampled, with early swelling of end-feet. Vacuoles formed from distended sacs of rough endoplasmic reticulum, and the basement membrane around blood vessels became folded, increasing the surface relationship between end-feet and capillary endothelial cells. Astrocyte filaments appeared to be reduced, and glycogen was diminished in quantity or lost. With the appearance of degenerative changes in myelinated fibres in the neuropil, reactive changes were seen including increases of glycogen and filaments.

Cavanagh et al. (1972) also described changes in the cerebellar cortex in rats with portacaval anastomosis. Focal vacuolations were seen in the molecular layer in the depths of sulci. Electron microscopy showed that these represented swellings of glial cell processes which in the early stages are related to Purkinje dendrites but do not affect the end-feet. Vacuolar changes tended to be related to the plasma ammonia nitrogen levels. Homogenizing cell change or loss of Purkinje cells was also reported.

Norenberg (1981) studied portacaval shunted rats given ammoniacal cation exchange resins to cause encephalopathy. Electron microscopy of astrocytes at an early stage of the encephalopathy showed an increase in the cytoplasmic compartment with proliferation of mitochondria and rough endoplasmic reticulum; the end-feet were often prominently affected. During the period of coma, the cytoplasm became electron-lucent, and empty vacuoles and degenerated mitochondria were seen. This degenerative appearance was thought to represent the electron microscopic correlate of Alzheimer type II changes seen by light microscopy. The astrocytic appearances were reversible provided that feeding of the resin was discontinued before the onset of coma.

The pathology seen in hepatic encephalopathy can be interpreted as an ammonia-induced gliopathy. The role of other agents and conditions which have been associated with hepatic encephalopathy, such as short chain fatty acids, hypokalaemia, hyponatraemia, hypercapnia, sedatives and amino acids are reviewed and discussed by Norenberg (1981) in his comprehensive survey of the astrocyte in liver disease.

Reye's syndrome

First reported in 1929 by Brain, Hunter and Turnbull, the clinical and pathological features were defined by Reye, Morgan and Baral (1963) and Mowat (1973). The onset is acute, with vomiting, convulsions, disturbance of consciousness and coma. Children of 2 months to 15 years have been affected and about 50 per cent show clinical hepatomegaly. Mortality estimates have varied from 20 to 80 per cent, and many survivors show CNS sequelae such as mental impairment, fits or hemiplegia.

Neuropathological findings in five acute cases of Reye's disease have been summarized by Manz and Colon (1982). Marked cerebral oedema was evident in all cases, with brain stem herniation in three. Acute, multifocal or diffuse ischaemic change or necrosis, often with a laminar distribution, affected the cortex, basal ganglia, diencephalon and brain stem. Small foci of haemorrhagic infarction and microhaemorrhages were found in two brains. There was no acute inflammatory cell infiltration. Two subacute cases of Reye's disease showed multifocal resolving microinfarcts of the cortex, with either astrocytosis or complete necrosis of all cortical layers. A single chronic case showed small foci of old microinfarcts with associated gliosis in the cerebral cortex, basal ganglia and diencephalon. Diffuse depopulation of Purkinje and granule cells and Bergmann astrocytosis was found in the cerebellum.

The *liver* in Reye's disease is swollen, greasy, shows severe periportal fatty infiltration and in fatal cases (as opposed to biopsy material) is often necrotic.

Partin et al. (1978) took brain biopsies of three patients at the acute stage of the disease, during decompressive craniotomy, and again after recovery and examined them by electron microscopy. Pleomorphic changes were described in neuronal mitochondria in the acute stage biopsies, although interpretation of these appearances is made difficult because of concurrent hypoxic and/or ischaemic changes. Mitochondria were normal in the recovery specimens. Astrocyte swelling was present in all of the acute biopsies; the cells appeared watery with vacuolation of endoplasmic cisternae but the mitochondria were normal. In recovery specimens, fibrous astrocytes were seen in the one case in which there was considerable neuronal loss. Myelin vacuolation was widespread in all acute biopsies; accounting for much of the brain swelling. Myelin lamellae were split at the intraperiod line. Many non-specific changes, including crystalloid and fibrillar nuclear inclusions, and residual bodies (lipofuscin) in neurons and astrocytes, were noted.

The *pathogenesis* of Reye's syndrome has been reviewed by DeLong and Glick (1982) and several hypotheses were considered. The most convincing evidence points to hyperammonaemia as a cause, and this is used as the criterion for case assessment by the Center for Disease Control. The time-course of hyperammonaemia generally correlates closely with the progression of the disease and is consistently elevated early in the course of the disease. The association of myelin vacuole formation with hyperammonaemia is not clear, but the observed swelling of astrocytes might be expected.

Other hypotheses implicating hyperfatty acidaemia, generalized mitochondrial dysfunction and lactic acidosis were also considered.

The cause of the disease is not certain, although an association with previous viral disease has been observed. Serological data have demonstrated an epidemiological association of Reye's syndrome with at least 23 different antecedent virus infections (De Vivo and Keating, 1976). In a national surveillance study over a 5-year period (1973–74, 1976–80) in the USA, the highest reported incidence of the disease occurred during influenza B and A(H1N1) outbreaks (Hurwitz et al., 1982). Salicylate treatment during the antecedent illness is also suggested as a causative factor (Halpin et al., 1982; Hurwitz et al., 1982).

Leigh's disease (infantile subacute necrotizing encephalopathy)

Leigh (1951) first described this disease of infancy and more than 100 cases have since been reported. David, Mamunes and Rosenblum (1976) have comprehensively reviewed these cases. The disease is generally inherited as a mendelian recessive, with males being affected rather more frequently than females (Pincus, 1972). In many cases the disease becomes evident before the age of 1 year and in most by the age of 2 years; its progress is inexorable. Adolescent and adult forms have been described (Sipe, 1973; Whetsell and Plaitakis, 1978) and also a chronic type (Christensen, Melchior and Plum, 1963). Clinical signs frequently begin with arrest of psychomotor development, although the clinical course may be very variable, making diagnosis difficult. Feeding problems, difficulties in swallowing, weakness, ataxia, loss of vision and external ophthalmoplegia are all described in various combinations. Respiratory problems include periods of hyperventilation of central neurogenic origin. Hypotonia is also an important sign; the deep tendon reflexes may be either decreased or increased. In three cases, reduced conduction velocity and sural nerve biopsy findings suggest a peripheral neuropathy. However, hypotonia may also be of central origin. CSF proteins may be increased.

The lesions as described in Leigh's original paper (1951) were of vascular or endothelial proliferation with far less prominent neuronal changes. Astrocytosis was present and sometimes severe, and there was microglial proliferation.

Studies of 50 cases reviewed by Montpetit et al. (1971) emphasized the capillary proliferation. Neuronal perikarya were relatively spared, the early appearance of 'loosening of the neuropil' possibly being due to degenerative changes in neuronal processes and myelin sheaths.

Lesions predominantly affect grey matter and are usually symmetrical (Fig. 13.10). They occur particularly in the basal ganglia and diencephalon, whilst the spinal cord and cerebellum, are also often affected. Many symptoms are due to brain stem lesions, particularly of the nuclei, which were found in almost every case examined by Montpetit et al. (1971). Egger et al. (1984) reported two cases with involvement of the centrum semiovale, and refers to several others in the literature.

The lesions of Leigh's disease closely resemble

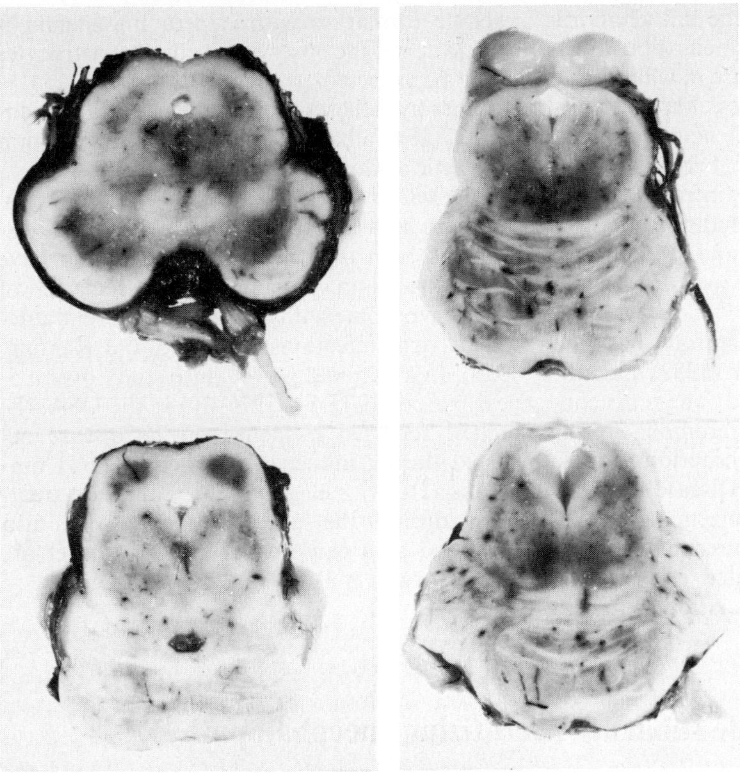

Fig. 13.10 Leigh's disease. Transverse sections of midbrain and pons from an 8-month-old child. Grey matter is symmetrically dark and discoloured. Substantia nigra, colliculi and pontine tegmentum are most severely affected. (Courtesy of Dr B.N. Harding.)

those found in Wernicke's encephalopathy but differ in showing a much smaller incidence of involvement of the mamillary bodies. On the other hand, lesions were found in the substantia nigra in 31 out of 50 cases reviewed by Montpetit et al. but in only 3 out of 57 cases of Wernicke's disease.

The similarity of lesions to those of Wernicke's disease suggested an abnormality of thiamine, but no deficiency has been found. In 1969, Cooper, Itokawa and Pincus found an inhibitor of the mitochondrial enzyme thiamine pyrophosphate-adenosine triphosphate phosphoryl transferase (TTP) in the urine, CSF and blood of a patient with Leigh's disease. This enzyme converts thiamine pyrophosphate to thiamine triphosphate. Further studies (Pincus, 1972; Murphy, 1973) showed that the inhibitor was present in all autopsy-proven cases of Leigh's disease and in obligate carriers. The inhibitor was also demonstrated in the fibroblasts of homozygotes, if the cells were grown in low thiamine media. This provides a possible technique for prenatal diagnosis (Murphy, Diven and Craig, 1974). It is not known whether lack of cerebral TTP resulting from the action of the inhibitor is the primary cause of necrotizing encephalopathy. Another biochemical defect, a deficiency of liver pyruvate carboxylase, has been identified (Hommes, Polman and Reerink, 1968) which causes accumulation of pyruvic and lactic acids and a deficient Krebs cycle, but again it is not known how this abnormality is related to formation of the lesions. Further enzyme abnormalities described include deficiency of pyruvate decarboxylase and pyruvate dehydrogenase. Abnormalities of the endorphin system have also been shown (Brandt, Terenius and Jacobson, 1980).

Leigh's disease has been associated with mitochondrial dysfunction. Egger, Wynne Williams and Erdohazi (1982) described 'ragged red' fibres and abnormal mitochondria in a muscle biopsy from a case having all the features of Leigh's disease. A further two cases of Leigh's disease with mitochondrial abnormalities suggestive of mitochondrial cytopathy are described by Egger et al. (1984) who also review a number of other cases with a similar association.

In addition to the the CNS changes, cardiomyopathy, renal tubular dysfunction, growth hormone deficiency and disturbed haemopoiesis have been described in Leigh's disease (see Egger,

Wynne Williams and Erdohazi, 1982). These are all symptoms occurring in mitochondrial cytopathy, a multisystem disease in which abnormal mitochondria are found in many organs. It is not known whether, or in what way, the mitochondrial changes and the resulting energy deficit might be responsible for the morphological lesions in the CNS.

Hall and Gardner-Medwin (1978) have reported CT scan appearances in four cases of Leigh's disease, of which two were confirmed at autopsy. Further cases have since been reported. Symmetrical areas of low density are seen in the lenticular nucleus which, together with the presence of the enzyme inhibitor in urine, blood or fibroblasts, provides the possibility of an early diagnosis allowing genetic counselling.

Menkes' kinky hair disease

This X-linked recessive disorder, first observed by Menkes et al. (1962), is characterized by mental retardation as well as retardation of growth associated with a curious abnormality of hair. This is erect, undulating and colourless (*pili torti*, *monilethrix* and *trichorrhexis nodosa*). Danks et al. (1972) showed that the severe hypocuprinaemia in these patients is due to impaired absorption of copper from the intestine, the concentration of copper being elevated in the intestinal wall but decreased in the liver and brain. There is decreased activity of copper-dependent enzymes, including cytochrome oxidase. Willemse et al. (1982) found biochemical differences among otherwise typical cases and suggests that more than one allele for the mutation may occur.

The *pathological changes* in the brain have been reviewed by Troost et al. (1982) who also describe three cases. In some cases the brain is severely atrophied. Patchy necrosis, nerve cell loss in the cortex and heterotopic neurons in the molecular layer as well as in the white matter are common findings. There may be widespread fibrillary gliosis. Dilated meningeal vessels have been observed but the earlier suggestion that cerebral lesions are secondary to vascular abnormalities seems not to have been substantiated.

In the cerebellum, which may be hypoplastic, there are usually abnormalities of the dendritic arborizations of Purkinje cells. Dendrites may be swollen and have cactus-like projections, and doubling-back of dendritic branches from beneath the pia, forming a 'weeping-willow' pattern. Branches may arise directly from the Purkinje cell soma.

Electron microscopy of muscle biopsies (Troost et al., 1982) and of cerebral neurons *post mortem* (Yoshimura and Kudo, 1983) suggests that there may be generalized enlargement of mitochondria which tend to have irregularly arranged tubulovesicular cristae.

Mutations in the mouse are known which affect coat colour and are, like human Menkes' disease, X-linked. A number of these mutations, probably alleles, have occurred around the *Mottled* locus and are known as brindled, blotchy, dappled or mosaic. They have varying degrees of abnormality of copper absorption (Hunt, 1974). In the brindled mouse, neuronal degeneration and loss from cerebral and cerebellar cortex were observed. The most consistent finding on electron microscopy was enlargement of neuronal perikaryal mitochondria (Yajima and Suzuki, 1979). These changes could be modified by the parenteral administration of copper, but only if given at critical times of development, viz. 7–10 days postnatally (Nagara, Yajima and Suzuki, 1981).

Disorders of amino acid metabolism

Pathological changes in the nervous system in the aminoacidurias have been reviewed by Crome and Stern (1972) and by Martin and Schlote (1972). Classification of this group of metabolic disorders differentiates the primary aminoacidurias from the so-called secondary form. Martin and Schlote (1972) have emphasized that lesions in the nervous system are generally non-specific, that glial changes in the very young must be distinguished from normal myelination gliosis which is maximal at 6 months and that sudanophil lipid is a normal finding in white matter during myelination in infancy. Fibrillary gliosis in the brain stem in infants is a normal finding, decreasing after the second year. Some pathological changes, such as the presence of Alzheimer type II astrocytes, may be secondary to liver damage.

In *phenylketonuria* cerebral pathology depends on the length of survival and age at death. In untreated cases there tends to be microcephaly, brain weight often being two-thirds normal. Below the age of 5 years there will be gliosis and spongiosus of the white matter, and a delay in myelination. Older patients will show foci of sponginess, myelin pallor, areas of myelin breakdown and gliosis of the white matter (Martin and Schlote, 1972). Bauman and Kemper (1982) have studied profoundly retarded adult male phenylketonurics and observed evidence of impairment of postnatal neuronal development. There was a higher density of the packing of cortical neurons which were smaller than normal and had few Nissl granules. Studied in Golgi preparations the neuronal dendritic arborization was poorly developed and there was a paucity of dendritic spines. Children born of phenylketonuric mothers are at risk and there is the likelihood of their being microcephalic.

Delay in the onset of myelination is also found in *maple syrup urine disease*, *tyrosinaemia* and *arginosuccinic aciduria*. Sponginess in the white matter is a characteristic of several metabolic disorders in which there is hyperammonaemia, and in these cases the spongiosus may begin as intramyelinic vacuolation. A deficiency of *ornithine carbamoyl transferase* is one of the more common inherited disorders of the urea cycle causing hyperammonaemia, and in these cases there may be severe cerebral atrophy, loss of neurons and cystic degeneration, and gliosis of the white matter if the child has survived long enough. More usually, with short survival there may be only spongiosus in white matter and basal ganglia and abnormal (Alzheimer type II) astrocytes (Bruton, Corsellis and Russell, 1970; Harding, Leonard and Erdohazi, 1984). Status spongiosus of white matter ('spongy myelinopathy') was the main neuropathological change in infants dying of hyperglycinaemia studied by Agamanolis et al. (1982). Electron microscopic examination of white matter showed that the vacuoles in this condition also lie within the myelin sheath. The degree of myelination and the severity of vacuolation did not always correspond. In *cystinuria* the brain usually shows no pathological changes, and death was, until recent developments in treatment, due to renal failure. In a case surviving until 19 years of age, deposits of birefringent cystine crystals were present in the choroid plexus in which there were macrophages with foamy cytoplasm and fibrosis as well as symmetrical foci of necrosis in the internal capsules and middle cerebellar peduncles (Levine and Paparo, 1982). The lesions in *homocystinuria* are usually ischaemic in type, infarction developing secondarily to structural abnormalities of cerebral vessels.

Porphyria

Porphyrias are genetic disorders in which there is overproduction and excretion of porphyrins and porphyrin precursors. Two subgroups, hepatic and erythropoietic, can be recognized, based on the site of porphyrin production. Neuropathy occurs only in the acute intermittent, variegate and coproporphyria forms. These are all dominantly inherited disorders. The variegate form is most common in people of European stock in South Africa in whom the incidence is 3:1000 (Dean, 1971).

The metabolic abnormality is now generally accepted to be a breakdown in the mechanism controlling the rate of haem synthesis in liver cells, a role ascribed to amino-laevulinic acid (ALA) synthetase. The control mechanism is probably a negative feedback involving repression of ALA synthetase. The metabolic abnormality is more fully described by Thomas (1981) in the companion volume to this book, and the neuropathy has been reviewed by Ridley (1975).

Similar neurological manifestations occur in the three types of porphyria, suggesting a common mode of action. Ridley (1975) and Thomas

(1981) have discussed hypotheses attempting to relate the metabolic defects to the occurrence of neuropathy. Cavanagh and Ridley (1967) suggested that, in addition to haem synthesis abnormalities, there may be pyridoxine deficiency resulting from consumptive tissue depletion of the vitamin by ALA synthetase which uses pyridoxal phosphate as a cofactor. The similarity in pattern of axonal degeneration in porphyria (see below) and in the neuropathy produced by isoniazid which inhibits formation of this cofactor (see Chapter 14) lends support to this suggestion.

The acute clinical pattern usually occurs in early adult life and is frequently precipitated by the administration of drugs. As Ridley (1975) points out, 'the neuropathy can be regarded as a twentieth century disease whose advent stems from the growth of the modern pharmaceutical industry'. Acute abdominal pain may be the earliest symptom, with nausea, vomiting and constipation. If these symptoms are treated with drugs, particularly barbiturates, a 'psychological stage' with restlessness, crying, insomnia and nightmares can be precipitated. Further treatment with barbiturates leads to a 'neurological stage', with a neuropathy which may prove fatal. Clinically, the neuropathy usually begins with motor symptoms, often affecting the upper limbs first, and involving proximal rather than distal muscles. Weakness is, however, variable in its symmetry, and in the pattern of its progression, which eventually may involve all four limbs. Cranial nerves are often involved, particularly the Xth and VIIth.

Erbsloh (1903) was the first to record neuropathy in a patient with porphyria. No definite changes were found in the cord or roots, but variable degeneration of myelin and axons was noted in peripheral parts of the nerves.

Cavanagh and Mellick (1965) showed, by sampling of various nerves from patients dying with porphyria, that the neuropathy was a dying-back axonal type of degeneration. However, the process was not necessarily confined to the longest fibres, a point also noted by Sweeney, Pathak and Asbury (1970), and in keeping with the clinical signs of proximal weakness. Motor fibres were affected more severely than sensory fibres, the motor axons often degenerating back to the anterior roots, whilst degeneration along sensory fibres was less extensive. In severe cases there was almost total loss of motor nerve fibres in distal muscles, but with sparing of large fibres from muscle spindles.

In the spinal cord, Cavanagh (1973) found degeneration in the posterior columns, more marked in the gracile tract than the cuneate, suggesting that here the longer fibres were preferentially affected. Central chromatolysis of motor neurons was found, and there was evidence of axonal regeneration and collateral sprouting in the muscles in chronic cases.

In a quantitative study of a fatal case, Thorner et al. (1981) showed reduced fibre density in more distal nerves. There was axonal atrophy in a ventral root and tibial nerve, demonstrated by reduced ratios of axon area/myelin lamellar number. Ultrastructural changes were those associated with axonal degeneration. Regenerating clusters were a prominent feature in the ventral root.

Lesions in the cerebrum have been minimal or absent, even when there has been a history of severe mental disturbances. Hierons (1957) described small areas of degeneration or loss of cortical neurons in cerebral or cerebellar cortex, basal ganglia and in the white matter of the hemispheres, and these appeared to be of an ischaemic nature.

No clear evidence of the neurotoxicity of ALA or porphobilinogen has been found in many experimental studies (see Sima et al., 1981). Sima et al. gave ALA to mice and found no morphological changes in the nerves, although motor nerve conduction velocities were decreased, but then returned to normal. Injection of tetraphenyl porphinesulphonate into mice caused some axonal changes with a distal distribution in peripheral nerves.

Steatorrhoea and other gastrointestinal disorders

Adult coeliac disease

Coeliac disease was defined by Booth (1970) as 'a condition in which there is abnormal jejunal mucosa that responds morphologically to treatment with a gluten-free diet'.

Neuropathy developed as a complication in 7 per cent of a series of 302 patients with coeliac disease studied for about 10 years (Cooke, 1976). Clinical and laboratory findings were described by Cooke and Smith (1966) in 16 patients in whom diagnosis was confirmed by jejunal biopsy. Weakness and sensory loss were more marked in the legs than in the arms, and ataxia, mostly of the postural type, became the most prominent feature in nearly all of the patients. Three cases showed signs of cerebellar dysfunction and five had unexplained attacks of unconsciousness.

Kinney et al. (1982) have given a detailed description of post-mortem findings in a case of fatal neuropathy in coeliac disease, comparing it with eight cases of Cooke and Smith (1966) and another case of Finelli et al. (1980). The most consistent pathological findings were depopulation of Purkinje cells with associated gliosis and loss of granule cells. Neuronal loss and gliosis in the dentate nuclei and the olives were features which distinguished the disorder from nutritional cerebellar degenerations (in which the cerebellum is characteristically spared).

Focal loss and/or gliosis in deep grey masses and brain stem nuclei were seen in five of ten cases. Affected structures included the thalamus, caudate nucleus, globus pallidus, putamen, amygdala, anterior hypothalamic nuclei, periaqueductal grey, corpora quadrigemina, substantia nigra, red nuclei and various motor and sensory cranial nerve nuclei.

The spinal cord changes are variable but a common pattern of symmetrical demyelination of posterior columns was found (Fig. 13.11). The fasciculus gracilis and lateral columns were particularly affected.

Cerebral cortex changes include focal neuronal atrophy and/or loss, chromatolysis and, rarely, gliosis.

Terminal branches of peripheral nerve axons were studied in muscle biopsies by Cooke, Johnson and Woolf (1966). They found collateral branching and diffuse swelling of terminal axons.

Aetiological factors in the neuropathy of coeliac disease have been discussed by Cooke (1976) and Kinney et al. (1982). Certain clinical and pathological similarities have been noted between the cases of Cooke and Smith (1966) and a group with carcinomatous neuropathy. Farmer and Richards (1964) and Binder, Solitaire and Spiro (1967) discussed the psychiatric manifestations of adult and childhood coeliac disease, although such features do not usually have a morphological counterpart.

Postgastrectomy states

Operations for peptic ulcer which cause disturbance to the upper small intestine may affect absorption, leading to such complications as osteomalacia, anaemia and, sometimes, neuropathy (Cooke, 1976).

Williams et al. (1969) reported on 14 patients with neuropathy which appeared many years after gastrectomy. The lower limbs were mainly affected, with weakness, wasting, paraesthesiae, difficulty in walking and posterior column deficit. Most of the patients had vitamin B_{12} deficiency. Smith (1976) examined a case which showed demyelination of posterior columns and posterior roots, and atrophy of posterior root ganglia and anterior horn cells; the spongiform degeneration of myelin and the lateral column involvement seen in typical B_{12} deficiency were not present in this case.

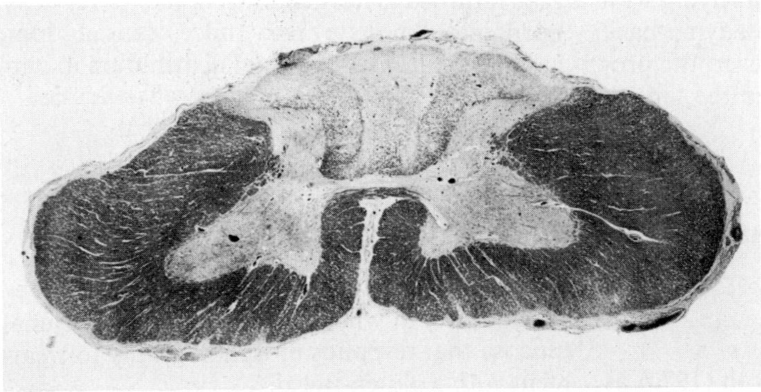

Fig. 13.11 Adult coeliac disease. Degeneration of the posterior columns of the cervical spinal cord from a patient with a long history of coeliac disease and neuropathy, dying of malignant lymphoma. Luxol fast blue–cresyl violet ×8. (Reproduced, with permission, from Cooke and Smith, 1966.)

Whipple's disease

Whipple's disease is a multisystem disorder involving brain and spinal cord; steatorrhoea is a characteristic symptom.

Pallis and Lewis (1974) have summarized features of this disease, including neurological aspects. Clinical findings were reviewed by Maizel, Ruffin and Dobbins (1970). Intellectual impairment, coma, ophthalmoplegia and visual impairment were the most common neurological manifestations.

The specific diagnosis depends on the demonstration of characteristic PAS-staining material in macrophages, particularly in the small intestine. Focal collections of PAS-positive histiocytes have been shown in the brain and spinal cord; these contain organisms which remain unidentified because it has not been possible to culture them.

Ergotism

The common 'fungus of rye' (*Claviceps purpurea*) produces a toxin which in the past has given rise to epidemics of ergotism, particularly in Europe. The toxic components seem to be cornutine, which causes convulsions, and sphacelinic acid, which has a contractile action on smooth muscle fibres, particularly those of vessel walls, causing gangrene.

Poisoning was formerly caused by consumption of bread made with contaminated flour. Now it occurs occasionally from excessive use of ergotamine tartrate in the treatment of migraine (Hudgson and Hart, 1964).

A consistent finding is degeneration of the long tracts, particularly the posterior columns, of the spinal cord (Buzzard and Greenfield, 1921). Thickening of the media and hyaline degeneration of the intima of arteries, sometimes associated with thrombosis, may occur in the gangrenous form. Severe burning pain, known as St Anthony's fire, may precede the onset of gangrene.

Miscellaneous diseases

The Hallervorden–Spatz syndrome

This disorder was originally described in 1922 by Hallervorden and Spatz. Reviews include those of Kalinowsky (1936), Peters (1951), Eicke (1957), Dreese and Netsky (1968) and Jellinger (1973).

Clinically the condition is characterized by progressive rigidity, often preceded or accompanied by choreic or athetoid movements, more rarely by torsion dystonia. Both rigidity and involuntary movements may extend to the muscles of the face, tongue and palate. Progressive mental deterioration and epileptic convulsions have been reported. In most cases the onset is in the first or second decade, and death usually supervenes before the thirtieth year. Later onset has been recorded. Jellinger (1975) recognized three types according to the age of onset: *late infantile* (3 months to 6 years), *classic* (7 to 15 years) and *adult* or *late* (22 to 64 years).

Hallervorden and Spatz (1922) described a clinically identical condition in five of nine siblings; three more siblings had died early from unknown causes. Onset was at between 7 and 9 years, with death occurring at the ages of 16 to 27. Of these, one brain was fully investigated, whilst sections from a second brain revealed identical pathology.

Pathological changes Macroscopically, a rust-brown discoloration of the globus pallidus and the reticular zone of the substantia nigra is a striking finding in most cases. This discoloration is caused by a great increase of pigment in these areas. The pigment has a yellowish-brown colour and, with thionin or cresyl violet, stains in shades of yellow, green and blue. It may be intracellular, in nerve cells, hyperplastic astrocytes and microglia, or may lie free in the tissue, usually around blood vessels. A strong Perl's reaction for iron and positive PAS reaction and sudanophilia are found; reactions for neuraminic acid and acid fastness are negative. This striking picture is in almost all cases enhanced by the presence, in the same areas, of strongly *siderophilic* incrustations of the medium-sized blood vessels and capillaries and of free-lying mulberry concretions (so-called pseudocalcium).

Apart from the consistent pigmentary increase, the other changes within the pallidoreticular zone are more variable. Severe degeneration and loss of nerve cells has been reported in some cases; in others, particularly in familial cases, this may be slight or negligible. Demyelination, particularly of the fine fibres, is usually present, but may be absent in some cases. Proliferation of astrocytes and fibrous gliosis are found in most cases, though to a variable degree.

The finding of large oval or round bodies (spheroids) staining faintly with thionin and lying between the extracellular pigment granules has aroused discussion: the spheroids are now known, as was originally suggested by Hallervorden and Spatz, to be derived from swollen axons. Their occurrence may be widespread. The pallidum, reticular portion of the substantia nigra, subthalamic nucleus, tegmentum of the medulla, cortex and spinal cord are all affected. Neither the axonal changes nor the pigment deposits alone are regarded as specific. In combination, however, they have considerable diagnostic value.

In many cases histological changes in other parts of the brain and in the spinal cord have been reported, but again they vary greatly in intensity and were slight in some of the familial cases. Hallervorden and Spatz described loss of nerve cells in the cerebral cortex and the Purkinje cell layer of the cerebellum; this finding has been confirmed in other cases. The striatum may be involved. The corpus luysii may be considerably demyelinated and gliosed, and gliosis in the dentate nucleus and inferior olives has been recorded. Retinitis pigmentosa accounted for visual disturbances in the cases of Winkelman (1932), Kalinowsky (1927) and Helfand (1935). Degeneration of the pyramidal tracts and of the posterior tracts of the spinal cord was also seen.

Neuroaxonal dystrophy

Jellinger (1973) has summarized convincing evidence that the spheroids in Hallervorden–Spatz disease are dystrophic axons and identical histologically to those seen in normal ageing human and animal brains; in infantile and late infantile neuroaxonal dystrophy (NAD); and in various experimental situations (e.g. vitamin E deficiency; triorthocresyl phosphate or iminodipropionitrile poisoning).

Electron microscopy shows that the spheroids are granular and surrounded by a single unit membrane. They contain cytoplasmic organelles, including normal and enlarged mitochondria, dense bodies, vesicles, neurofilaments, accumulations of smooth membranes, tubules and cisternae. Many spheroids show a whorled arrangement of layered smooth membranes and vesiculotubular structures, 28–40 nm in diameter. The arrangement of the tubulomembranous systems varies from tightly packed, whorled lamellae to loose aggregates of hollow cisternae and longitudinal clefts surrounded by neurofilaments. The spheroids probably arise mainly in preterminal axons of ascending fibres, presynaptic areas participating in axodendritic and axoaxonic synaptic complexes, and even in neuromuscular junctions, according to the underlying cause. Tubulomembranous material and abnormal mitochondria may also be found in neuronal perikarya and dendrites.

The diagnosis of neuroaxonal dystrophy can be made by electron microscopic examination of biopsies which include sensory or autonomic peripheral nerves. Sural nerve, skin, conjunctiva or rectal biopsies (Goebel, Kohlschütter and Schulte, 1980) as well as muscle biopsy have shown the axonal swellings enveloped by Schwann cell processes. In the intestinal autonomic ganglia the axonal enlargements lie close to neuronal perikarya.

As random findings in normal ageing human and animal brains, dystrophic axons occur in the grey matter of the brain stem and spinal cord. In infantile and late-infantile NAD the spheroids are generalized throughout the central, peripheral and autonomic nervous systems.

Seitelberger (1971) distinguished the following types of neuroaxonal dystrophy:

1. Infantile NAD (Seitelberger's disease).
2. Late-infantile NAD (also described as late-infantile type of Hallervorden–Spatz disease).
3. Juvenile form of generalized NAD.
4. Neuroaxonal leucoencephalopathy.
5. Hallervorden–Spatz disease (juvenile and adult types).
6. Presenile NAD and Hallervorden–Spatz disease in other disorders.

NAD seems to represent a non-specific response of axons to injury, either genetically induced or exogenous. The tubulomembranous structures which accumulate in affected axons closely resemble smooth endoplasmic reticulum.

There is at present no satisfactory general explanation of the basic pathogenetic process which determines the appearances of spheroids and it is not unlikely that several different mechanisms may determine this type of axonal pathology. Metabolic or enzymatic axoplasmic deficiencies, axonal injury with redistribution of axoplasm, stasis of axonal flow, altered metabolic activity at axonal terminals with overproduction of smooth endoplasmic reticulum, axoplasmic regeneration, or alterations of synaptic end-complexes have all been proposed as pathogenetic explanations.

Alpers' disease (progressive cerebral degeneration in infancy)

A number of cases have been described which have certain clinical and pathological features in common but which still are sufficiently different to cast doubt on whether they form a nosological entity. The name *Alpers' disease* had been applied to the group by some, because of the original description by Alpers (1931) of a case. The characteristic clinical presentation is of fits beginning in infancy or early childhood and subsequent development of dementia, hypotonia or spasticity and myoclonus. Death usually occurs before the third year.

Histological changes include extensive neuronal loss and status spongiosus in all areas of the cerebral cortex and similar degenerative changes in the deep grey nuclei. The hemispheres may be asymmetrically affected, as in Alpers' (1931) case. Familial cases have been described (Alpers, 1960).

Many more cases have been described in recent years, and reviews include those by Blackwood et al. (1963) and Jellinger and Seitelberger (1977) who divided an obviously heterogeneous collection of cases into three groups: (1) symptomatic, (2) idiopathic, and (3) atypical and unclassified. The first group includes cases with extensive cortical damage resulting from perinatal hypoxia or epilepsy. The second group includes cases with a normal birth history and progressive neurological disease characterized by generalized convulsions, myoclonus, blindness, deafness and profound mental deterioration. Crompton (1968) and Janota (1974) likened the status spongiosus to that of Creutzfeldt–Jakob disease.

The familial nature of a progressive degenerative disease of childhood and its association with hepatic disease has been emphasized by Huttenlocher, Solitaire and Adams (1976). They described pathological changes in the brain indistinguishable from those of so-called Alpers' disease, and also found cirrhosis or hepatitis with superimposed fatty infiltration of the liver. The cases described by Huttenlocher, Solitaire and Adams (1976) were from two sibships, and hereditary recessive transmission was emphasized. In reviewing the literature, Huttenlocher and colleagues found that several of the cases reported (e.g. Blackwood et al. 1963; Wefring and Lamvik, 1967) had been familial and had evidence of liver disease, but those described by Sandbank and Lerman (1972) and Janota (1974) had been sporadic and without liver pathology. Clearly the syndrome of progressive cortical degeneration in infancy includes a number of disparate conditions, and further observations and identification of their aetiology are needed for their adequate definition.

West Indian, Indian and African neuromyelopathy

A variety of neuromyelopathy which closely resembles the rare form of neurosyphilis, in which degeneration of the lateral and posterior tracts of the spinal cord is accompanied by variable degrees of periarteritis and arachnoiditis (so-called 'spastic paraplegia of Erb'), has been recognized in the Caribbean region (Montgomery et al., 1964). Its cause is uncertain but a resemblance to neurolathyrism has supported the possibility that ingested toxins may be responsible; other suggested causes include dietary deficiency, an obscure inflammatory process or a multifactorial background. The process may not be a single entity because a comparable syndrome has been recognized in India (Main, Main and Montgomery, 1969); in West Africa neuromyelopathy also occurs but sensory neuropathy is commoner than paraplegia (Money, 1959; Haddock, Ebrahim and Kapur, 1962). Thus, although there are certain resemblances, the view that West Indian, Indian and African neuromyelopathies are variants of the same disorder is not fully justified. It has been observed that in parts of Nigeria a cassava-containing diet is related to the incidence of ataxic sensory neuropathy, and because cassava has a relatively high cyanide content it may be that the disorder has some connection with cyanide intoxication (Osuntokun, Monekosso and Wilson 1969; Osuntokun et al., 1970).

The clinical features include weakness and unsteadiness of gait, numbness and burning of the feet and legs and, less commonly, formication or pain in the limbs. Deafness and poor vision are also common. In older patients, spasticity and other upper motor neuron lesions are more common than ataxia and posterior column defects.

Histologically, most cases show inflammatory changes of varying severity, mainly perivascular cuffing with lymphocytes, plasma cells and histiocytes. There is reactive fibroblastic proliferation around blood vessels and in the piaarachnoid. Nerve roots and ganglia and the appropriate cranial nerves usually show inflammatory changes in patients with visual or hearing loss. Loss of myelin is found in the lateral pyramidal tracts, the posterior columns and the spinocerebellar tracts. The spinal grey matter usually shows inflammatory changes and neuronal degeneration. Similar but less severe lesions are often present in the cerebral hemispheres, brain stem and cerebellum. In longstanding cases evidence of active inflammation may be less pronounced, although adventitial and leptomeningeal fibrosis may be prominent and has been attributed to previous burnt-out inflammation. Thickening and opacity of the leptomeninges is often recognizable macroscopically, particularly in the basal cisterns.

Although the disease often shows a histological resemblance to meningovascular neurosyphilis, it is not associated with appropriate CSF and serological changes. Furthermore, Argyll Robertson pupils are not present and there is resistance to penicillin therapy.

Syndromes associated with carcinoma

The concurrence of neurological syndromes and malignant disease has given rise to the acceptance that some forms of neoplasm may induce remote pathological changes in the nervous system. Reviews include those by Brain and Norris (1965) and Henson and Urich (1982). The direct effects of metastatic infiltrations, the opportunistic infection of the nervous system by organisms in immunocompromised patients with malignant disease (such as progressive multifocal leucoencephalopathy—dealt with in Chapter 7) and the untoward complications of therapy (see Chapter 14) are excluded from this discussion. Several syndromes have been recognized as associated with carcinoma since Greenfield (1934) and subsequently Brain, Daniel and Greenfield (1951) noted the coincidence of cerebellar degeneration with carcinoma of bronchus and ovary. The others include encephalomyelitis, peripheral neuropathy, myopathy and the myasthenic (Eaton–Lambert) syndrome.

Cerebellar cortical degeneration

The incidence of this form of paraneoplastic disease is probably lower than that of the others. Most reported cases have been associated with carcinoma of the bronchus, the next most common malignancy being of the ovary or breast. The clinical picture is that of acute or subacute cerebellar dysfunction and mental disturbances may be prominent. The cerebrospinal fluid may contain an excess of cells and protein. The histological changes in the cerebellum are those of neuronal degeneration affecting mainly Purkinje cells (Figs. 13.12 and 13.13) and, to a lesser degree, granule cells. Degeneration and loss of Purkinje cells with 'torpedoes' on their degenerating axons is widespread (Fig. 13.13b), the molecular layer is thinner than usual and hyperplasia of Bergmann astrocytes and laying down of glial fibres in an isomorphous fashion are present. The deep cerebellar nuclei are usually preserved but in some cases the dentate nuclei, inferior olives and spinocerebellar pathways have been affected. Lymphocytic infiltrates in the meninges and perivascular cuffing point to some overlap with the encephalomyelitic syndrome (Fig. 13.12a).

Encephalomyelitic syndromes

Although the severity and distribution of lesions varies from case to case the characteristics of the pathology point to a common pathogenesis. The main pathological feature in these cases is inflammatory, consisting of perivascular cuffing and meningeal infiltrations by lymphocytes, and fewer plasma cells, with associated degeneration and loss of neurons. The brunt of the lesions is borne by grey matter, the white matter of the temporal lobes and of the spinal cord being less

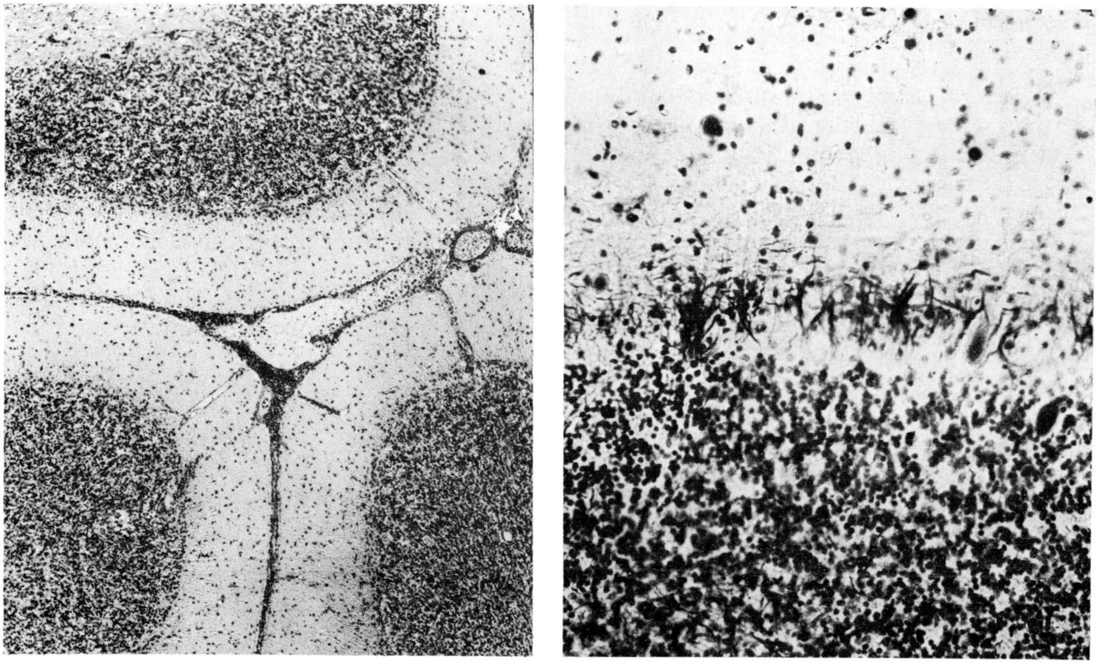

(a) **(b)**

Fig. 13.12 Subacute spinocerebellar degeneration; 3.5 months' history (case 1 of Brain, Daniel and Greenfield, 1951). (**a**) Cerebellum showing widespread loss of Purkinje cells and lymphocytic exudate in the meninges. (**b**) Higher power showing loss of Purkinje cells with persistence of axons of basket cells. Bielschowsky's silver method.

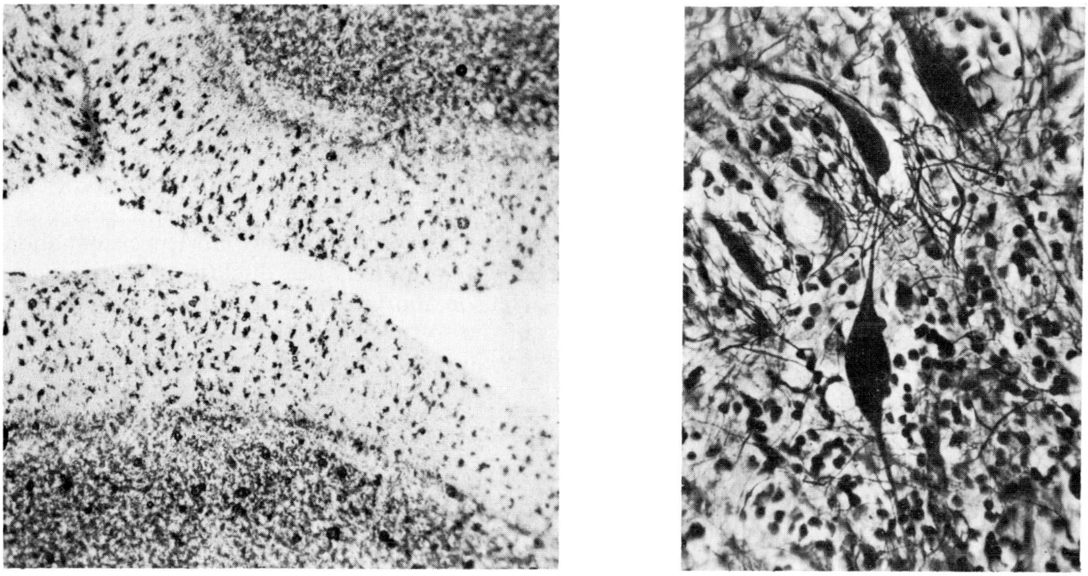

(a) **(b)**

Fig. 13.13 Subacute spinocerebellar degeneration; 6 months' history (case 2 of Brain, Daniel and Greenfield, 1951). (**a**) Cerebellum showing loss of Purkinje cells and phagocytosis of lipid in molecular and granular layers. Scharlach R. and haemalum. (**b**) Degenerated Purkinje cell with torpedo-like swelling on its axon.

involved. The distribution of lesions can be summarized as:

1. *Cerebral hemispheres* predominantly in the medial temporal lobe structures ('limbic encephalitis') affecting the hippocampal formation, amygdaloid complex, cingulate and orbital cortex (Brierley et al., 1960; Corsellis, Goldberg and Norton, 1968). In these cases the principal clinical feature is one of a selective impairment of recent memory combined with other evidence of disturbed temporal lobe function. The duration of the illness has been 5–20 months, very rarely longer than 2 years.
2. *Brain stem* encephalitis, especially involving the medulla.
3. The *cerebellum*, resembling cerebellar cortical degeneration.
4. The *spinal cord*, affecting mainly the grey matter. Lesions may be limited to a few segments or may be very extensive. Loss of anterior horn cells will produce an amyotrophy, and clearly one of the problems is to differentiate coincident amyotrophic lateral sclerosis from the syndrome linked to malignant disease. Another problem is that impairment of the vulnerable blood supply to the spinal cord by masses of carcinomatous para-aortic lymph nodes may cause hypoxic-ischaemic damage to spinal grey matter.
5. *Sensory ganglion cells.* Denny-Brown (1948) described a ganglioradiculitis associated with carcinoma. Neurons of posterior root ganglia may be almost totally degenerated and there is proliferation of satellite cells, leading to the formation of residual nodules of Nageotte. Secondary wallerian degeneration results in loss of myelinated nerve fibres in the sensory roots, posterior columns of the spinal cord and peripheral nerves.

Carcinomatous peripheral neuropathy and neuromuscular syndromes

These are discussed in Chapters 18 and 21 respectively.

Pathogenesis The aetiology of the carcinomatous neuromyopathies is not known with any certainty. Nutritional deficiencies have been postulated but not proved, and therapy with vitamins has been unsuccessful. The inflammatory changes found in encephalomyelitis point to an infective or autoimmune phenomenon. Henson and Urich (1982) summarize the evidence for the various possible aetiologies. They point out the need to take into account the high percentage of oat cell carcinoma and that, although virus-like particles have been reported, no real evidence for a viral infection exists. Bell, Seetharam and McDaniel (1976) have identified antigens which oat cell carcinomas share with Schwann cells and dorsal root ganglion cells. Oat cell carcinoma may be said to be derived from neuroendocrine-programmed cells of the bronchial epithelium and may share hormone or transmitter-secretory functions with neurons.

Other factors which must be taken into account include the occasional very small size of a primary carcinoma which may indeed be so inconspicuous that only the incidental discovery of an infiltrated lymph node points to its presence. Furthermore, the neurological syndrome may precede the discovery of malignancy and clearly in any case with a limbic type of encephalopathy or of cerebellar degeneration, peripheral neuropathy or inflammatory muscle disorder, an associated carcinoma must be suspected and excluded. Even a careful post-mortem examination may, however, fail to disclose any carcinoma. Henson and Urich (1982) emphasize that none of the so-called paraneoplastic disorders has a specific pathology nor are they confined to an association with cancer. All have been found without underlying systemic disease.

References

Adams, R.D. and Foley, J.M. (1949) The neurological changes in the more common types of severe liver disease. *Transactions of the American Neurological Association* **74,** 217–19.

Adams, R.D. and Foley, J.M. (1953) The neurological disorder associated with liver disease. *Research Publications Association for Research in Nervous and Mental Disease* **32,** 198–237.

Adams, R.D. and Kubik, C.S. (1944) Subacute degeneration of the brain in pernicious anemia. *New England Journal of Medicine* **231,** 1–9.

Adams, R.D., Victor, M. and Mancall, E.L. (1959) Central pontine myelinosis. *Archives of Neurology and Psychiatry* **81,** 154–72.

Agamanolis, D.P., Victor, M., Harris, J.W., Hines, J.D., Chester, E.M. and Kark, J.A. (1978) An ultrastructural study of subacute combined degeneration of the spinal cord in vitamin B_{12}-deficient rhesus monkeys. *Journal of Neuropathology and Experimental Neurology* **37,** 273–99.

Agamanolis, D.P., Potter, J.L., Herrick, M.K. and Sternberger, N.H. (1982) The neuropathology of glycine encephalopathy: a report of five cases with immunohistochemical and ultrastructural observations. *Neurology* **32,** 975–85.

Alexander, W.F. (1957) In *Vitamin B_{12} and Intrinsic Factor* (Ed. Heinrich, H.C.) p. 372, Thieme, Stuttgart.

Allsop, J. and Turner, B. (1966) Cerebellar degeneration associated with chronic alcoholism. *Journal of the Neurological Sciences* **3,** 238–58.

Alpers, B.J. (1931) Diffuse progressive degeneration of grey matter of cerebrum. *Archives of Neurology and Psychiatry* **25,** 469–505.

Alpers, B.J. (1960) Progressive cerebral degeneration in infancy. *Journal of Nervous and Mental Diseases* **130,** 442–8.

Anderson, P.J. and Popper, H. (1960) Changes in hepatic structure in Wilson's disease. *American Journal of Pathology* **36,** 483–97.

Aring, C.D., Bean, W.B., Roseman, E., Rosenbaum, M. and Spies, T.D. (1941) Peripheral nerves in cases of nutritional deficiency. *Archives of Neurology and Psychiatry* **45,** 772–87.

Asbury, A.K. (1975) Hepatic neuropathy. In *Peripheral Neuropathy* (Eds. Dyck, P.J., Thomas, P.K. and Lambert, E.H.), pp. 993–8. W.B. Saunders, Philadelphia.

Badenoch, J. (1954) The use of labelled vitamin B_{12} and gastric biopsy in the investigation of anaemia. *Proceedings of the Royal Society of Medicine* **47,** 426–7.

Baker, S.J., Jacob, E., Rajan, K.T. and Swaminathan, S.P. (1962) Vitamin B_{12} deficiency in pregnancy and the puerperium. *British Medical Journal* **1,** 1658–61.

Balmer, S., Howells, G. and Wharton, B.I. (1968) The acute encephalopathy of kwashiorkor. *Developmental Medicine and Child Neurology* **10,** 766–71.

Barnes, S. and Hurst, E.W. (1926) A further note on hepatolenticular degeneration. *Brain* **49,** 36–60.

Baron, D.N., Dent, C.E., Harris, H., Hart, E.W. and Jepson, J.B. (1956) Hereditary pellagra-like skin rash with temporary cerebellar ataxia, constant renal aminoaciduria and other bizarre biochemical features. *Lancet* **2,** 421–8.

Bauman, M.L. and Kemper, T.L. (1982) Morphologic and histoanatomic observations of the brain in untreated human phenylketonuria. *Acta Neuropathologica* **58,** 55–63.

Bean, W.B., Hodges, R.E. and Daum, K. (1955) Pantothenic acid deficiency induced in human subjects. *Journal of Clinical Investigation* **34,** 1073–84.

Bearn, A.G. (1972) Wilson's disease. In *The Metabolic Basis of Inherited Disease* (Eds. Stanbury, J.B., Wyngaarden, J.B. and Fredrickson, D.S.), pp. 1033–50. McGraw-Hill, New York.

Bearn, A.G. and Kunkel, H.G. (1954) Localization of Cu64 in serum following oral administration: alteration in Wilson's disease. *Proceedings for the Society for Experimental Biology and Medicine* **85,** 44–8.

Bell, C.E., Seetharam, S. and McDaniel, R.C. (1976) Endodermally-derived and neural-crest derived differentiation antigens expressed by a human lung tumour. *Journal of Immunology* **116,** 1236–43.

Bergsma, D. (1968) Wilson's disease. *Birth Defects. Original Article Series* **4,** no. 2.

Berlyne, G.M., Liversedge, L.A. and Emery, E.W. (1957) Radioactive vitamin B_{12} in the diagnosis of neurological disorders. *Lancet* **1,** 294.

Bessey, O.A., Adams, D.J.D. and Hansen, A.E. (1957) Intake of vitamin B_6 and infantile convulsions: a first approximation of requirements of pyridoxin in infants. *Pediatrics* **20,** 33–44.

Bessey, O.A. and Wolbach, S.B. (1939) Vascularization of the cornea of the rat in riboflavin deficiency with a note on corneal vascularization in vitamin A deficiency. *Journal of Experimental Medicine* **69,** 1–12.

Bickel, H. (1914) Funikuläre Myelitis mit bulbären und polyneuritischen Symptomen. *Archiv für Psychiatrie und Nervenkrankheiten* **53,** 1106–17.

Binder, H.J., Solitaire, G.B. and Spiro, H.M. (1967) Neuromuscular disease in patients with steatorrhoea. *Gut* **8,** 605–11.

Blackwood, W., Buxton, P.H., Cumings, J.N., Robertson, J. and Tucker, S.M. (1963) Diffuse cerebral degeneration in infancy (Alpers' disease). *Archives of Disease in Childhood* **38,** 193–204.

Blakemore, W.F. and Cavanagh, J.B. (1969) 'Neuroaxonal dystrophy' occurring in an experimental 'dying back' process in the rat. *Brain* **92,** 789–804.

Blass, J.P. and Gibson, G.E. (1977) Abnormality of a thiamine-requiring enzyme in patients with Wernicke–Korsakoff syndrome. *New England Journal of Medicine* **297,** 1367–70.

van Bogaert, L., Radermecker, M.A., Janssen, P. and

Gatera, F. (1962) The muscular lesions of kwashiorkor compared with those of other oedematous conditions and malnutrition in the Congolese infant. *Acta Neuropathologica* **1,** 363-83.

van der Scheer, W.M. and Koek, H.C. (1938) Peripheral nerve lesions in cases of pernicious anaemia. *Acta Psychiatrica and Neurologica* **13,** 61-92.

Booth, C.C. (1970) Enterocyte in coeliac disease. *British Medical Journal* **3,** 725-31.

Böttiger, L.E. and Möllerberg, H. (1959) Increased copper content of hypertrophic myocardium. *Acta Medica Scandinavica* **165,** 413-16.

Brain, W.R., Daniel, P.M. and Greenfield, J.G. (1951) Subacute cortical cerebellar degeneration and its relation to carcinoma. *Journal of Neurology, Neurosurgery and Psychiatry* **14,** 59-75.

Brain, W.R., Hunter, D. and Turnbull, H.M. (1929) Acute meningo-encephalomyelitis of childhood: report of six cases. *Lancet* **1,** 221-7.

Brain, W.R. and Norris, F.H. (1965) *The Remote Effects of Cancer on the Nervous System.* Grune & Stratton, New York.

Brandt, N.J., Terenius, L. and Jacobson, B.B. (1980) Hyperendorphic syndrome in a child with necrotizing encephalomyelopathy. *New England Journal of Medicine* **303,** 914-16.

Brierley, J.B., Corsellis, J.A.N., Hierons, R. and Nevin, S. (1960) Subacute encephalitis of later adult life mainly affecting the limbic areas. *Brain* **83,** 357-68.

Brion, S. (1976) Marchiafava-Bignami syndrome. In *Handbook of Clinical Neurology*, vol. 28 (Eds. Vinken, P.J. and Bruyn, G.W.), pp. 317-29. North-Holland, Amsterdam.

British Medical Journal (1967) Blue blood. (Leading Article) **4,** 435-6.

Bruton, C.J., Corsellis, J.A.N. and Russell, A. (1970) Hereditary hyperammonaemia. *Brain* **93,** 423-34.

Buzzard, E.F. and Greenfield, J.G. (1921) *Pathology of the Nervous System.* Constable, London.

Campbell, A.C.P. and Russell, W.R. (1941) Wernicke's encephalopathy: clinical features and their probable relationship to vitamin B deficiency. *Quarterly Journal of Medicine* **34,** 41-64.

Cartwright, G.E., Markowitz, H., Shields, G.S. and Wintrobe, M.M. (1960) Studies on copper metabolism. XXIX. A critical analysis in normal patients and patients with Wilson's disease and their relatives. *American Journal of Medicine* **28,** 555-63.

Castle, W.B. (1929) Extrinsic factor in pernicious anaemia. *American Journal of the Medical Sciences* **178,** 148.

Cavanagh, J.B. (1973) Peripheral neuropathy caused by chemical agents. *CRC Critical Reviews in Toxicology* **2,** 365-417.

Cavanagh, J.B. (1974) Liver bypass and the glia. *Research Publications Association for Research in Nervous and Mental Disease* **53,** 14-35.

Cavanagh, J.B. and Kyu, M.H. (1971) Type II Alzheimer change experimentally produced in astrocytes in the rat. *Journal of the Neurological Sciences* **12,** 63-75.

Cavanagh, J.B. and Mellick, R.S. (1965) On the nature of the peripheral nerve lesions associated with acute intermittent porphyria. *Journal of Neurology, Neurosurgery and Psychiatry* **28,** 320-7.

Cavanagh, J.B. and Ridley, A. (1967) The nature of the neuropathy complicating acute intermittent porphyria. *Lancet* **2,** 1023-4.

Cavanagh, J.B., Lewis, P.D., Blakemore, W.F. and Kyu, M.H. (1972) Changes in the cerebellar cortex in rats after portocaval anastomosis. *Journal of the Neurological Sciences* **15,** 13-26.

Chan-Palay, V. (1977) Indoleamine neurons and their processes in the normal rat brain and in chronic diet-induced thiamine deficiency demonstrated by uptake of ^{3}H-serotonin. *Journal of Comparative Neurology* **176,** 467-94.

Chick, H., El Sadr, M.M. and Worden, A.N. (1940) Occurrence of fits of an epileptiform nature in rats maintained for a long period on diets deprived of vitamin B_6. *Biochemical Journal* **34,** 595-600.

Christensen, E., Melchior, V.C. and Plum, P. (1963) Combined lesions of basal ganglia, medulla oblongata and spinal cord in a 10-year-old boy. *Acta Paediatrica (Uppsala)* **52,** 304-12.

Clarke, J.M. (1904) On the spinal cord degeneration in anaemia. *Brain* **27,** 441-59.

Coërs, C. and Woolf, A.L. (1959) *The Innervation of Muscle*, p. 91. Blackwell Scientific, Oxford.

Coggeshall, R.E. and MacLean, P.D. (1958) Hippocampal lesions following administration of 3-acetylpyridine. *Proceedings of the Society for Experimental Biology and Medicine* **98,** 687-9.

Cooke, W.T. (1976) Neurological manifestations of malabsorption. In *Handbook of Clinical Neurology*, vol. 28 (Eds. Vinken, P.J. and Bruyn, G.W.), pp. 225-41. North-Holland, Amsterdam.

Cooke, W.T., Johnson, A.G. and Woolf, A.L. (1966) Vital staining and electron microscopy of the intramuscular nerve endings in the neuropathy of adult coeliac disease. *Brain* **89,** 663-82.

Cooke, W.T. and Smith, W.T. (1966) Neurological disorders associated with adult coeliac disease. *Brain* **89,** 683-722.

Cooper, J.R., Itokawa, Y. and Pincus, J.H. (1969) Thiamine triphosphate deficiency in subacute necrotizing encephalomyelopathy. *Science* **164,** 74-5.

Corsellis, J.A.N., Goldberg, G.J. and Norton, A.R.

(1968) Limbic encephalitis and its association with carcinoma. *Brain* **91,** 481–96.

Courville, C.B. (1955) *Effects of Alcohol on the Nervous System of Man*. San Lucas Press, Los Angeles.

Courville, C.B. and Myers, R.O. (1954) Effects of extraneous poisons on the nervous system: alcohols. *Bulletin of the Los Angeles Neurological Society* **19,** 66–95.

Cowen, D. and Olmstead, E.V. (1963) Infantile neuroaxonal dystrophy. *Journal of Neuropathology and Experimental Neurology* **22,** 175–236.

Cox, E.V. and White, A.M. (1962) Methylmalonic acid excretion: an index of vitamin B_{12} deficiency. *Lancet* **2,** 853–6.

Cox-Klazinga, M. and Endtz, L.J. (1980) Peripheral nerve involvement in pernicious anaemia. *Journal of the Neurological Sciences* **45, 367**–71.

Crome, L. and Stern, J. (1972) *The Pathology of Mental Retardation*, 2nd edn, p. 432. Churchill Livingstone, Edinburgh and London.

Crompton, R. (1968) Alpers' disease. A variant of Creutzfeldt–Jakob disease and subacute spongiform encephalopathy. *Acta Neuropathologica* **10,** 99–104.

Cumings, J.N. (1948) The copper and iron content of brain and liver in the normal and in hepatolenticular degeneration. *Brain* **71,** 410–15.

Cumings, J.N. (1959) *Heavy Metals and the Brain*. Blackwell Scientific, Oxford.

Cumings, J.N. (1962) The metabolism of copper and Wilson's disease. *Proceedings of the Nutrition Society* **21,** 29–34.

Cumings, J.N. (1972) Neurochemistry. In *Scientific Foundations of Neurology* (Eds. Critchley, M., O'Leary, J.L. and Jennett, B.), pp. 433–9. Heinemann Medical, London.

Cumings, J.N., Goodman, H.J. and Earl, C.J. (1955) Blood copper and its relationship to globulins. *Journal of Clinical Pathology* **8,** 69–72.

Danks, D.M., Campbell, P.E., Stevens, B.J., Mayne, V. and Cartwright, E. (1972) Menkes' kinky hair syndrome. An inherited defect in copper absorption with widespread effects. *Pediatrics* **50,** 188–201.

Dastur, D.K., Quadros, E.V., Wadia, N.H., Desai, M.M. and Bharucha, E.P. (1972) Effect of vegetarianism and smoking on vitamin B_{12}, thiocyanate and folate levels in the blood of normal subjects. *British Medical Journal* **3,** 260–3.

David, R.B., Mamunes, P. and Rosenblum, W.I. (1976) Necrotizing encephalomyelopathy (Leigh). In *Handbook of Clinical Neurology*, vol. 28 (Eds. Vinken, P.J. and Bruyn, G.W.), pp. 349–63. North-Holland, Amsterdam.

Davidson, L. S. P. and Passmore, R. (1969) *Human Nutrition and Dietetics*, 4th edn. Livingstone, Edinburgh and London.

Dayan, A.D. and Williams, R. (1967) Demyelinating peripheral neuropathy and liver disease. *Lancet* **2,** 133–4.

Dean, G. (1971) *The Porphyrias. A story of inheritance and environment*. Pitman Medical, London.

De Long, G.R. and Glick, T.H. (1982) Encephalopathy of Reye's syndrome: a review of pathogenetic hypotheses. *Pediatrics* **69,** 53–63.

Denny-Brown, D. (1948) Primary sensory neuropathy with muscular changes associated with carcinoma. *Journal of Neurology, Neurosurgery and Psychiatry* **11,** 73–87.

Denton, J. (1928) A study of tissue changes in experimental black tongue in dogs compared with similar changes in pellagra. *American Journal of Pathology* **4,** 341–52.

De Vivo, D.C. and Keating, J.P. (1976) Reye's syndrome. *Advances in Pediatrics* **22,** 175–229.

Dinn, J.J., Weir, D.G., McConn, S., Reed, B., Wilson, P. and Scott, J.M. (1980) Methyl group deficiency in nerve tissues: a hypothesis to explain the lesion of subacute combined degeneration. *Irish Journal of Medical Science* **149,** 1–4.

Doyle, D. (1967) Portocaval Anastomosis in Rats. MD thesis, University of Edinburgh.

Dreese, M.J. and Netsky, M.G. (1968) Degenerative disorders of the basal ganglia. In *Pathology of the Nervous System* vol. 1 (Ed. Minckler, J.), pp. 1185–204. McGraw-Hill, New York.

Dreyfus, P.M. (1976) Amblyopia and other neurological disorders associated with chronic alcoholism. In *Handbook of Clinical Neurology*, vol. 28 (Eds. Vinken, P.J. and Bruyn, G.W.), pp. 331–47. North-Holland, Amsterdam.

Dreyfus, P.M. and Victor, M. (1961) Effects of thiamine deficiency on the central nervous system. *American Journal of Clinical Nutrition* **9,** 414–25.

Dynes, J.B. and Norcross, J.W. (1943) Peripheral neuritis as a complication of pernicious anemia. *Journal of the American Medical Association* **122,** 586–8.

Eastham, R.D. and Jancar, J. (1968) *Clinical Pathology and Retardation*. Wright, Bristol.

Ebadi, M. (1981) Regulation and function of pyridoxal phosphate in CNS. *Neurochemistry International* **3,** 181–206.

Egger, J., Wynne Williams, C.J.E. and Erdohazi, M. (1982) Mitochondrial cytopathy in Leigh's syndrome: mitochondrial abnormalities in spongiform encephalopathies. *Neuropediatrics* **13,** 219–24.

Egger, J., Pincott, J.R., Wilson, J. and Erdohazi, M. (1984) Cortical subacute necrotizing encephalitis. A study of two patients with mitochondrial dysfunction. *Neuropediatrics* In press.

Eicke, W.J. (1957) Die Hallervorden–Spatzsche Krankheit. In *Handbuch der speziellen pathologischen Anatomie und Histologie*, vol. XIII (i).

(Eds. Lubarsch, O., Henke, F. and Rössle, R.), pp. 836–50. Springer, Berlin.

Einarson, L. and Ringsted, A. (1938) *Effect of Chronic Vitamin E Deficiency on the Nervous System and the Skeletal Musculature in Adult Rats*. Levin and Munksgaard, London and Oxford.

Elvehjem, C.A., Madden, R.J., Strong, F.M. and Woolley, D.W. (1937) Relation of nicotinic acid and nicotinic acid amide to canine black tongue. *Journal of the American Chemical Society* **59,** 1767–8.

Erbsloh, W. (1903) Zur Pathologie und pathologischen Anatomie der toxischen Polyneuritis nach Sulfonalgebrauch. *Deutsche Zeitschrift für Nervenheilkunde* **23,** 197–204.

Evans, C.A., Carlson, W.E. and Green, R.G. (1942) The pathology of Chastek paralysis in foxes. A counterpart of Wernicke's hemorrhagic polioencephalitis in man. *American Journal of Pathology* **18,** 79–91.

Evans, H.M. and Bishop, K.S. (1922) On the existence of a hitherto unrecognized dietary factor essential for reproduction. *Science* **56,** 650.

Farmer, R.G. and Richards, H.G. (1964) Malabsorption syndrome and peripheral neuropathy: report of two cases. *Cleveland Clinic Quarterly* **31,** 163–8.

Ferraro, A., Arieti, S. and English, W.H. (1945) Cerebral changes in the course of pernicious anaemia and their relationship to psychic symptoms. *Journal of Neuropathology and Experimental Neurology* **4,** 217–39.

Ferraro, A. and Roizin, L. (1943) Histopathology of central nervous tissue in experimental vitamin K deficiency (vitamin K deficiency haemorrhagic diathesis). *Journal of Neuropathology and Experimental Neurology* **2,** 392–410.

Finelli, P.F., McEntee, W.J., Ambler, M. and Kostenbaum, D. (1980) Adult celiac disease presenting as cerebellar syndrome. *Neurology* **30,** 245–9.

Finlayson, M.H. and Superville, B. (1981) Distribution of cerebral lesions in acquired hepatocerebral degeneration. *Brain* **104,** 79–95.

Fisher, C.M. (1955) Residual neuropathological changes in Canadians held prisoner of war by the Japanese. *Canadian Services Medical Journal* **11,** 157–99.

Fleischer, B. (1903) Quoted by Greenfield, J.G. and McMenemey, W.H. In *Neuropathology*, 2nd edn, p. 580. Edward Arnold, London.

Follis, R.H. Jr (1958) *Deficiency Disease*. Thomas, Springfield, Ill.

Follis, R.H. Jr and Wintrobe, M.M. (1945) A comparison of the effects of pyridoxine and pantothenic acid deficiencies on the nervous system of swine. *Journal of Experimental Medicine* **81,** 539–52.

Foster, D.B. (1945) Degeneration of peripheral nerves in pernicious anemia. *Archives of Neurology and Psychiatry* **54,** 102–9.

Gandy, G., Jacobson, W. and Sidman, R. (1973) Inhibition of a transmethylation reaction in the nervous system—an experimental model for subacute combined degeneration of the cord. *Journal of Physiology* **233,** 1–3.

Garrow, J.S. (1967) Loss of brain potassium in kwashiorkor. *Lancet* **2,** 643–4.

Geller, A., Gilles, F. and Schwachman, H. (1977) Degeneration of fasciculus gracilis in cystic fibrosis. *Neurology* **27,** 185–7.

Gilliatt, R.W., Goodman, H.V. and Willison, R.E. (1961) The recording of lateral popliteal nerve action potentials in man. *Journal of Neurology, Neurosurgery and Psychiatry* **24,** 305–18.

Girdwood, R.H. (1968) Abnormalities of vitamin B_{12} and folic acid metabolism—their influence on the nervous system. *Proceedings of the Nutrition Society* **27,** 101–7.

Goebel, H.H., Kohlschütter, A. and Schulte, F.J. (1980) Rectal biopsy findings in infantile neuroaxonal dystrophy. *Neuropediatrics* **1,** 388–92.

Goldberger, J. and Lillie, R.D. (1926) A note on an experimental pellagra-like condition in the albino rat. *Public Health Reports (Washington DC)* **41,** 1025–9.

Goldberger, J. and Wheeler, G.A. (1915) Experimental pellagra in the human subject brought about by a restricted diet. *Public Health Reports (Washington DC)* **30,** 3336–9.

Goldberger, J. and Wheeler, G.A. (1920) Experimental pellagra in white male convicts. *Archives of Internal Medicine* **25,** 451–71.

Golden, M.H.N. (1982) Protein deficiency, energy deficiency and the oedema of malnutrition. *Lancet* **1,** 1261–5.

Gopalan, C. (1946) The 'burning feet' syndrome. *Indian Medical Gazette* **81,** 22–6.

Gopalan, C. (1969) Possible role for dietary leucine in the pathogenesis of pellagra. *Lancet* **1,** 197–9.

Greenfield, J.G. (1934) Subacute spinocerebellar degeneration occurring in elderly patients. *Brain* **57,** 161–76.

Greenfield, J.G. (1963) *Neuropathology*, 2nd edn. Edward Arnold, London.

Greenfield, J.G. and Carmichael, E.A. (1935) Peripheral nerves in cases of subacute combined degeneration of the cord. *Brain* **58,** 483–91.

Greenfield, J.G. and Holmes, J.M. (1939) A case of pellagra. Pathological changes in the spinal cord. *British Medical Journal* **1,** 815–19.

Greenfield, J.G., Poynton, F.J. and Walshe, F.M.R. (1924) On progressive lenticular degeneration (hepatolenticular degeneration). *Quarterly Journal of Medicine* **17,** 385–403.

Guggenheim, M.A., Ringel, S.P., Silverman, A. and Grabert, B.E. (1982) Progressive neuromuscular disease in children with chronic cholestasis and vitamin E deficiency: diagnosis and treatment with alpha tocopherol. *Journal of Pediatrics* **100,** 51–8.

György, P. (1934) Vitamin B_2 and pellagra-like dermatitis in rats. *Nature* (*London*) 133, 498–9.

Haddock, D.R.W., Ebrahim, G.J. and Kapur, B.B. (1962) Ataxic neurological syndrome found in Tanganyika. *British Medical Journal* **2,** 1442–3.

Hahn, M., Massen, O., Nencki, M. and Pawlow, J.B. (1893) Die Eck'sche Fistel zwischen der unteren Hohlvene und der Pfortader und ihre Folgen für den Organismus. *Archiv für experimentelle Pathologie und Pharmakologie* **32,** 161–210.

Hall, H.C. (1921) *La Dégénérescence Hépato-lenticulaire*. Masson, Paris.

Hall, K. and Gardner-Medwin, D. (1978) CT scan appearances in Leigh's disease. *Neuroradiology* **16,** 48–50.

Hallervorden, J. and Spatz, H. (1922) Eigenartige Erkrankung im extrapyramidalen System mit besonderer Beteiligung des Globus pallidus und der Substantia nigra. *Zentralblatt für die gesamte Neurologie* **79,** 254–302.

Halpin, T.J., Holtzhauer, F.J., Campbell, R.J., Hall, L.J., Correa-Villaseñor, A., Lanese, R. et al. (1982) Reye's syndrome and medication use. *Journal of the American Medical Association* **248,** 687–91.

Hamilton, A.S. and Nixon, C.E. (1921) Sensory changes in the subacute combined degeneration of pernicious anaemia. *Archives of Neurology and Psychiatry* **6,** 1–31.

Hamilton, H.E., Ellis, P.P. and Sheets, R.F. (1959) Visual impairment due to optic neuropathy in pernicious anaemia: report of a case and review of the literature. *Blood* **14,** 378–85.

Harding, A.E., Muller, D.P.R., Thomas, P.K. and Willison, H.J. (1982) Spinocerebellar degeneration secondary to chronic intestinal malabsorption: a vitamin E deficiency syndrome. *Annals of Neurology* **12,** 419–24.

Harding, B.N., Leonard, J.V. and Erdohazi, M. (1984) Ornithine carbamoyl transferase deficiency: a neuropathological study. *European Journal of Pediatrics* **141,** 215–20.

Hardwick, S.W. (1943) Pellagra in psychiatric patients. Twelve recent cases. *Lancet* **2,** 43–5.

Harper, C. (1979) Wernicke's encephalopathy: a more common disease than realised. *Journal of Neurology, Neurosurgery and Psychiatry* **42,** 226–31.

Haurowitz, F. (1930) Über eine Anomalie des Kupferstoffwechsels. *Zeitschrift für physiologische Chemie* **190,** 72–4.

Hayes, K.C., Nielsen, S.W. and Eaton, H.D. (1968) Pathogenesis of the optic nerve lesions in vitamin A deficient calves. *Archives of Ophthalmology* **80,** 777–87.

Heaton, J.M., McCormick, A.J.A. and Freeman, A.G. (1958) Tobacco amblyopia: a clinical manifestation of vitamin B_{12} deficiency. *Lancet* **2,** 286–90.

Helfand, M. (1935) Status pigmentosus, its pathology and its relation to Hallervorden–Spatz disease. *Journal of Nervous and Mental Disease* **81,** 662–75.

Henson, R.A. and Urich, H. (1982) *Cancer and the Nervous System*. Blackwell Scientific, Oxford.

Hersov, L.A. (1955) A case of childhood pellagra with psychosis. *Journal of Mental Science* **101,** 878–83.

Hersov, L.A. and Rodnight, R. (1960) Hartnup disease in psychiatric practice: clinical and biochemical features of three cases. *Journal of Neurology, Neurosurgery and Psychiatry* **23,** 40–5.

Hicks, S.P. (1955) Pathologic effects of antimetabolites; acute lesions in hypothalamus, peripheral ganglia and adrenal medulla caused by 3-acetyl pyridine and prevented by nicotinamide. *American Journal of Pathology* **31,** 189–97.

Hierons, R. (1957) Changes in the nervous system in acute porphyria. *Brain* **80,** 176–92.

Hoesslin, C. von and Alzheimer, A. (1912) Ein Beitrag zur Klinik und pathologischen Anatomie der Westphal–Strümpellschen Pseudosclerose. *Zeitschrift für die gesamte Neurologie und Psychiatrie* **8,** 183–209.

Holmberg, C.G. and Laurell, C.B. (1948) Investigation in serum copper. II. Isolation of the copper-containing protein and a description of some of its properties. *Acta Chemica Scandinavica* **2,** 550–6.

Holtzman, N.A., Naughton, M.A., Iber, F.L. and Gaumnitz, B.M. (1967) Caeruloplasmin in Wilson's disease. *Journal of Clinical Investigation* **46,** 993–1002.

Hommes, F.A., Polman, H.A. and Reerink, J.D. (1968) Leigh's encephalomyelopathy: an inborn error of gluconeogenesis. *Archives of Disease in Childhood* **43,** 423–4.

Howard, C.P. and Royce, C.E. (1919) Progressive lenticular degeneration associated with cirrhosis of the liver (Wilson's disease). *Archives of Internal Medicine* **24,** 497–508.

Howell, J.McC. and Thompson, J.N. (1967a) Lesions associated with the development of ataxia in vitamin A deficient chicks. *British Journal of Nutrition* **21,** 741–50.

Howell, J.McC. and Thompson, J.N. (1967b) Observations on the lesions of vitamin A deficient fowls with particular reference to changes in bone and central nervous system. *British Journal of Experimental Pathology* **48,** 450–4.

Hsü, Y.K. (1942) Pathologic anatomy of the human nervous system in avitaminosis. *Archives of Neurology and Psychiatry* **48,** 271–319.

Hudgson, P. and Hart, J.A.L. (1964) Acute ergotism:

report of a case and a review of the literature. *Medical Journal of Australia* **2,** 589–91.

Hunt, D.M. (1974) Primary defect in copper transport underlies mottled mutants in the mouse. *Nature* (*London*) **248,** 852–3.

Hurwitz, E.S., Nelson, D.B., Davis, C., Morens, D. and Schonberger, L.B. (1982) National surveillance for Reye syndrome: a five year review. *Pediatrics* **70,** 895–900.

Huttenlocher, P., Solitaire, G.B. and Adams, G. (1976) Infantile diffuse cerebral degeneration with hepatic cirrhosis. *Archives of Neurology* **33,** 186–92.

Ideström, C.-M. (Ed.) (1980) Alcohol and brain research. *Acta Psychiatrica Scandinavica* suppl. 286, 62.

Ironside, R., Bosanquet, F.D. and McMenemey, W.H. (1961) Central demyelination of the corpus callosum (Marchiafava–Bignami disease). *Brain* 84, 212–30.

Ishii, N. and Nishihara, Y. (1981) Pellagra among chronic alcoholics: clinical and pathological study of 20 necropsy cases. *Journal of Neurology, Neurosurgery and Psychiatry* **44,** 209–15.

Jadhar, M., Webb, J.K.G., Vaishnava, S. and Baker, S.J. (1962) Vitamin B_{12} deficiency in Indian infants. A clinical syndrome. *Lancet* **2,** 903–7.

Jaffe, I.A., Altman, K. and Merryman, P. (1964) Antipyridoxine effect of penicillamine in man. *Journal of Clinical Investigation* **43,** 1869–73.

Jakob, A. (1912) Zur Klinik und pathologischen Anatomie des chronischen Alkoholismus, zugleich ein Beitrag zu den Erkrankungen des Kleinhirns. *Zeitschrift für die gesamte Neurologie und Psychiatrie* **13,** 132–52.

Janota, I. (1974) Spongy degeneration of grey matter in 3 children. *Archives of Disease in Childhood* **49,** 571–5.

Jellinger, K. (1973) Neuroaxonal dystrophy: its natural history and related disorders. *Progress in Neuropathology* (Ed. Zimmerman, H.M.), vol. 2, 129–80. Grune & Stratton, New York.

Jellinger, K. and Seitelberger, F. (1977) Spongy encephalopathies in infancy: spongy degeneration of CNS and progressive infantile poliodystrophy. In *Scientific Approaches to Clinical Neurology* vol. 1 (Eds. Goldensohn, E.S. and Appel, S.H.), pp. 363–86. Lea & Febiger, Philadelphia.

Johnson, R.E. and Campbell, R.J. (1982) Wilson's disease: electron microscopic, x-ray energy, spectroscopic, and atomic absorption spectroscopic studies of corneal copper deposition and distribution. *Laboratory Investigation* **46,** 564–9.

Jubb, K.V., Saunders, L.Z. and Coates, H.V. (1956) Thiamine deficiency encephalopathy in cats. *Journal of Comparative Pathology and Therapeutics* **66,** 217–27.

Kalinowsky, L. (1927) Familiäre Erkrankungen mit besonderer Beteiligung der Stammganglien. *Monatsschrift für Psychiatrie und Neurologie* **66,** 168–90.

Kalinowsky, L. (1936) Hallervordensche Krankheit. In *Handbuch der Neurologie*, vol. XVI (Eds. Bumke, O. and Foerster, O.), pp. 84–96. Springer, Berlin.

Karsakis, E.J. and Bass, N.H. (1982) Benign intracranial hypertension induced by deficiency of vitamin A during infancy. *Neurology* **32,** 1292–5.

Kayser, B. (1902) Quoted by Greenfield, J.G. and McMenemey, W.H. In *Neuropathology*, 2nd edn, p. 580. Edward Arnold, London.

Kinney, H.C., Burger, P.C., Hurwitz, B.J., Hijmans, J.C. and Grant, J.P. (1982) Degeneration of the central nervous system associated with celiac disease. *Journal of the Neurological Sciences* **53,** 9–22.

Kline, D.G., Doberneck, R.C., Chun, B.K. and Rutherford, R.B. (1966) Encephalopathy in graded portocaval shunts. *Annals of Surgery* **164,** 1003–12.

Knill-Jones, R.P., Goodwill, C.J., Dayan, A.D. and Williams, R. (1972) Peripheral neuropathy in chronic liver disease: clinical, electrodiagnostic and nerve biopsy findings. *Journal of Neurology, Neurosurgery and Psychiatry* **35,** 22–30.

Krehl, W.A., Tepley, L.J., Sarma, P.S. and Elvehjem, C.A. (1945) Growth retarding effect of corn in nicotinic acid low rations and its counteractions by tryptophane. *Science* **101,** 489–90.

Krohn, P.L., Oxnard, C.E. and Chalmers, J.N.M. (1963) Vitamin B_{12} in the serum of the rhesus monkey. *Nature* (*London*) **197,** 186.

Lai, C.S. and Ransome, G.A. (1970) Burning feet syndrome. Case due to malabsorption and responding to riboflavine. *British Medical Journal* **1,** 151–2.

Lampert, P., Blumberg, J.M. and Pentschew, A. (1964) An electronmicroscopic study of dystrophic axons in the gracile and cuneate nuclei of vitamin E deficient rats. *Journal of Neuropathology and Experimental Neurology* **23,** 60–77.

Lancet (1983) 'Binge' drinking and stroke. **2,** 660–1.

Lane, M., Smith, F.E. and Alfrey, C.P. (1975) Experimental dietary and antagonist-induced human riboflavin deficiency. In *Riboflavin* (Ed. Rivlin, R.), pp. 245–77. Plenum Press, New York.

Lanzkowsky, P., Erlandson, M.E. and Bezan, A.I. (1969) Isolated defect of folic acid absorption associated with neural retardation and cerebral calcification. *Blood* **34,** 452–65.

Lapham, L.W. (1962) Cytologic and cytochemical studies of neuroglia. 1. A study of the problem of amitosis in reactive astrocytes. *American Journal of Pathology* **41,** 1–21.

Leevy, C.M. (1982) Thiamine deficiency and alcoholism. *Annals of the New York Academy of Sciences* **378,** 316–26.

Leichtenstern, O. (1884) Über progressive perniciöse Anämie bei Tabeskranken. *Deutsche medizinische Wochenschrift* **10,** 849.

Leigh, D. (1951) Subacute necrotizing encephalomyelopathy in an infant. *Journal of Neurology, Neurosurgery and Psychiatry* **14,** 216–21.

Leigh, D. (1952) Pellagra and the nutritional neuropathies: a neuropathological review. *Journal of Mental Science* **98,** 130–42.

Lester-Smith, E. (1948) Purification of antipernicious anaemia factors from liver. *Nature (London)* **161,** 638–9.

Levine, S. and Paparo, G. (1982) Brain lesions in a case of cystinosis. *Acta Neuropathologica* **57,** 217–20.

Lhermitte, J. (1935) Cortical cerebellar degeneration. *Proceedings of the Royal Society of Medicine* **28,** 379–90.

Lichtenstein, B.W. and Gore, I. (1955) Wilson's disease—chronic form. *Archives of Neurology and Psychiatry* **73,** 13–21.

Lichtheim, H. (1887) Zur Kenntnis der perniciösen Anämie. *Verhandlungen der deutschen Gesellschaft für innere Medizin* **6,** 84–96.

Lippincott, S.W. and Morris, H.P. (1942) Pathologic changes associated with riboflavin deficiency in the mouse. *Journal of the National Cancer Institute* **2,** 601–10.

Lishman, W.A. (1981) Cerebral disorders in alcoholism: syndrome of impairment. *Brain* **104,** 1–20.

Lockner, D., Reizenstein, P., Wennberg, P. and Widen, L. (1969) Peripheral nerve function in pernicious anaemia before and after treatment. *Acta Haematologica* **41,** 257–63.

Luhby, A.L. and Cooperman, J.M. (1967) Congenital megaloblastic anemia and progressive central nervous system degeneration. Further clinical and physiological characterization and therapy of syndrome due to inborn error of folate transport. In *American Pediatric Society Incorporated Annual Meeting*, Atlantic City.

Lüthy, F. (1931) Über Die hepato-lentikuläre Degeneration (Wilson, Westphal, Strumpell). *Deutsche Zeitschrift für Nervenheilkunde* **123,** 101–81.

Lutrell, C.N. and Mason, K.E. (1949) Vitamin E deficiency, dietary fat and spinal cord lesions in the rat. *Annals of the New York Academy of Sciences* **52,** 113–20.

Lynch, M.J. (1960) Brain lesions in chronic alcoholism. *Archives of Pathology* **69,** 342–53.

McCall, K.B., Waisman, H.A., Elvehjem, C.A. and Jones, E.S. (1946) Study of pyridoxine and pantothenic acid deficiencies in the monkey (*Macaca mulatta*). *Journal of Nutrition* **31,** 685–97.

McCance, R.A. (1951) The history, significance and aetiology of hunger oedema. *Medical Research Council Special Report Series* **275,** 21–82.

McDermott, W.V. and Adams, R.D. (1954) Episodic stupor associated with an Eck fistula in the human with particular reference to the metabolism of ammonia. *Journal of Clinical Investigation* **33,** 1–9.

McIlwain, H. (1966) *Biochemistry and the Nervous System*, 3rd edn. Churchill, London.

McIlwain, H. and Bachelard, H.S. (1984) In *Biochemistry and the Central Nervous System*, 5th edn, Churchill Livingstone, Edinburgh and London. (In press.)

Madhaven, T.V., Belavady, B. and Gopalan, C. (1968) Pathology of canine black tongue. *Journal of Pathology and Bacteriology* **95,** 259–63.

Main, K.S., Main, A.J. and Montgomery, R.D. (1969) A spastic paraplegia syndrome in South India. *Journal of the Neurological Sciences* **9,** 179–99.

Mair, W.G.P., Warrington, E.K. and Weiskrantz, L. (1979) Memory disorder in Korsakoff's psychosis. *Brain* **102,** 749–83.

Maizel, H., Ruffin, J.M. and Dobbins, W.O. III (1970) Whipples disease: a review of 19 patients from one hospital and a review of the literature since 1950. *Medicine* **49,** 175–205.

Malamud, N., Nelson, M.M. and Evans, H.M. (1949) The effect of chronic vitamin E deficiency on the nervous system in the rat. *Annals of the New York Academy of Sciences* **52,** 135–8.

Manz, H.J. and Colon, A.R. (1982) Neuropathology, pathogenesis and neuropsychiatric sequelae of Reye syndrome. *Journal of the Neurological Sciences* **53,** 377–95.

Marchiafava, E. and Bignami, A. (1903) Sopra un alterazione del corpo calloso osservata in sogetti alcoolista. *Rivista di Patologia Nervosa e Mentale* **8,** 544–9.

Martin, J.J. and Schlote, W. (1972) Central nervous system lesions in disorders of amino-acid metabolism. *Journal of the Neurological Sciences* **15,** 49–76.

Martinez Figueroa, A., Johnson, R.H., Lambie, D.G. and Shakir, R.A. (1980) The role of folate deficiency in the development of peripheral neuropathy caused by anticonvulsants. *Journal of the Neurological Sciences* **48,** 315–23.

Mayer, R.F. (1965) Peripheral nerve function in vitamin B_{12} deficiency. *Archives of Neurology* **13,** 355–62.

Mayer-Gross, W., Slater, E. and Roth, M. (1954) *Clinical Psychiatry*. Cassell, London.

Mehta, B.M., Rege, D.V. and Satoskar, R.S. (1964) Serum vitamin B_{12} and folic acid activity in lactovegetarian and non-vegetarian healthy adult Indians. *American Journal of Clinical Nutrition* **15,** 77–84.

Melchior, J.C. and Clausen, J. (1968) Metachromatic leucodystrophy in early childhood. Treatment with a diet deficient in vitamin A. *Acta Paediatrica Scandinavica* **57,** 2–8.

Mellanby, E. (1944) Croonian Lecture: Nutrition in relation to bone growth and the nervous system. *Proceedings of the Royal Society, B* **132,** 28–46.

Menkes, J.H., Alter, M., Steigleder, G.K., Weakley, D.R. and Sung, J.H. (1962) A sex-linked recessive disorder with retardation of growth, peculiar hair, and focal cerebral and cerebellar degeneration. *Pediatrics* **29,** 764–79.

Meyer, A. (1901) On parenchymatous systemic degenerations mainly in the central nervous system. *Brain* **24,** 47.

Meyer, A. (1944) The Wernicke syndrome: with special reference to manic syndromes associated with hypothalamic lesions. *Journal of Neurology and Psychiatry* **7,** 66–75.

Meyer, A. (1963) Intoxications. In *Neuropathology* (Eds. Blackwood, W., McMenemey, W.H., Meyer, A., Norman, R.M. and Russell, D.S.), 2nd edn, pp. 233–87. Edward Arnold, London.

Meyer, A., Stewart, R.J.C. and Platt, B.S. (1961) The spinal cord of pigs on low-protein diets. *Proceedings of the Nutrition Society* **20,** xviii.

Millen, J.W. and Woollam, D.H.M. (1956) The effect of the duration of vitamin A deficiency in female rabbits upon the incidence of hydrocephalus in their young. *Journal of Neurology, Neurosurgery and Psychiatry* **19,** 17–20.

Milne, M.D. (1969) Hartnup disease. *Biochemical Journal* **111,** 3–4P.

Minnich, W. (1892) Kenntnis der im Verlaufe der perniciösen Anämie beobachteten Spinalerkrankungen. *Zeitschrift für klinische Medizin* **21,** 264–314.

Minot, G.R. and Murphy, W.P. (1926) Treatment of pernicious anaemia by a special diet. *Journal of the American Medical Association* **87,** 470–6.

Miyagishi, T., Takahata, N. and Iizuka, R. (1967) Electronmicroscope studies on the lipopigments in the cerebral cortex nerve cells of senile and vitamin E deficient rats. *Acta Neuropathologica* **9,** 7–17.

Molony, C.J. and Parmelee, A.H. (1954) Convulsions in young infants as a result of pyridoxine (vitamin B_6) deficiency. *Journal of the American Medical Association* **154,** 405–6.

Money, G.L. (1959) Clinical aspects of tropical ataxic neuropathies related to malnutrition. *West African Medical Journal* **8,** 3–17.

Monguio, J. and Krause, F. (1934) Über die Bedeutung des NH_3-Gehaltes des Blutes für Beurteilung der Leberfunktion: Studien am normalen, lebergeschädigten und Eckschen Fistelhund. *Klinische Wochenschrift* **13,** 1142–7.

Montgomery, R.D., Cruickshank, E.K., Robertson, W.B. and McMenemey, W.H. (1964) Clinical and pathological observations in Jamaican neuropathy. A report on 206 cases. *Brain* **87,** 425–62.

Montpetit, V.J.A., Anderman, F., Carpenter, S., Fawcett, J.S., Zborowska-Sluis, D. and Giberson, H. (1971) Subacute necrotizing encephalomyelopathy—a review and study of two families. *Brain* **94,** 1–30.

Morel, F. (1939) Une forme anatomo-clinique particulaire de l'alcoolisme chronique: sclérose corticale laminaire alcoolique. *Revue Neurologique* **71,** 280–8.

Morre, D.M. and Kirksey, A. (1980) The effect of a deficiency of vitamin B_6 on selected neurons of the developing rat brain. *Nutrition Reports International* **21,** 301–12.

Mott, F.W. (1910) The nervous system in chronic alcoholism. *British Medical Journal* **2,** 1403–8.

Mowat, A.P. (1973) Encephalopathy and fatty degeneration of the viscera: Reye's syndrome. *Archives of Disease in Childhood* **48,** 411–13.

Muller, D.P.R., Lloyd, J.K. and Wolff, O.H. (1983) Vitamin E and neurological function. *Lancet* **1,** 225–8.

Murphy, J.V. (1973) Subacute necrotizing encephalomyelopathy (Leigh's disease): detection of the heterozygous carrier state. *Pediatrics* **51,** 710–15.

Murphy, J.V., Diven, W.F. and Craig, L. (1974) Detection of Leigh's disease in fibroblasts. *Pediatric Research* **8,** 393.

Murphy, T.L., Chalmers, T.C., Eckhardt, R.D. and Davidson, C.S. (1948) Hepatic coma: clinical and laboratory observations on forty patients. *New England Journal of Medicine* **239,** 605–12.

Nagara, H., Yajima, K. and Suzuki, K. (1979) The effect of copper supplementation on the brindled mouse. *Acta Neuropathologica* **40,** 428–46.

Nelson, J.S., Fitch, C.D., Fischer, V.W., Broun, G.O. and Chou, A.C. (1981) Progressive neuropathologic lesions in vitamin E-deficient rhesus monkeys. *Journal of Neuropathology and Experimental Neurology* **40,** 166–86.

Neuburger, K.T. (1957) The changing neuropathologic picture of chronic alcoholism. *Archives of Pathology* **63,** 1–6.

Norenberg, M.D. (1981) The astrocyte in liver disease. In *Advances in Cellular Neurobiology*, vol. 2 (Eds. Federoff, S. and Hertz, L.), pp. 304–52. Academic Press, London.

North, J.D. and Sinclair, H.M. (1956) Nutritional neuropathy: chronic thiamine deficiency in the rat. *Archives of Pathology* **62,** 341–53.

Norton, W.N., Daskal, I., Savage, H.E., Seibert, R.A. and Lane, M. (1976) Effects of riboflavin deficiency on the ultrastructure of rat sciatic nerve fibers. *American Journal of Pathology* **85,** 651–60.

Oldfors, A. and Nordborg, C. (1977). Paranodal

myelin retraction in protein deficient and normal rats. *Acta Neuropathologica*, **40,** 249–252.

Opalski, A. (1930) Über eine besondere Art von Gliazellen bei der Wilson-Pseudosklerosegruppe. *Zeitschrift für die gesamte Neurologie und Psychiatrie* **124,** 420–5.

Osuntokun, B.O., Monekosso, G.L. and Wilson, J. (1969) Relationship of a degenerative tropical neuropathy to diet. Report of a field survey. *British Medical Journal* **1,** 547–50.

Osuntokun, B.O., Langman, M.J.S., Wilson, J. and Aladetoyinbo, A. (1970) Controlled trial of hydroxocobalamin and riboflavine in Nigerian ataxic neuropathy. *Journal of Neurology, Neurosurgery and Psychiatry* **33,** 663–6.

Oxnard, C.E. and Smith, W.T. (1966) Neurological degeneration and reduced serum vitamin B_{12} levels in captive monkeys. *Nature (London)* **210,** 507–9.

Pallis, C.A. and Lewis, P.D. (1974) *The Neurology of Gastrointestinal Disease.* W.B. Saunders, London.

Pant, S.S., Asbury, A.K. and Richardson, E.P. Jr (1968) The myelopathy of pernicious anemia. A neuropathological reappraisal. *Acta Neurologica Scandinavica* **44,** suppl. 35, 1–36.

Partin, J.S., McAdams, A.J., Partin, J.C., Schubert, W.K. and McLaurin, R.L. (1978) Brain ultrastructure in Reye's disease. II. Acute injury and recovery processes in three children. *Journal of Neuropathology and Experimental Neurology* **37,** 796–819.

Pentschew, A. and Schwarz, K. (1962) Systemic axonal dystrophy in vitamin E deficient adult rats. *Acta Neuropathologica* **1,** 303–34.

Peraita, M. (1946) Deficiency neuropathies observed in Madrid during the Civil War (1936–1939). *British Medical Journal* **2,** 784.

Peters, G. (1951) *Spezielle Pathologie der Krankheiten des zentralen und peripheren Nervensystems.* Thieme, Stuttgart.

Pincus, J.H. (1972) Subacute necrotising encephalomyelopathy (Leigh's disease): a consideration of clinical features and aetiology. *Developmental Medicine and Child Neurology* **14,** 87–101.

Plaitakis, A., Hwang, E.C., Van Woert, M.H., Szilagyi, P.I.A. and Berl, S. (1982) Effect of thiamin deficiency on brain transmitter systems. *Annals of the New York Academy of Sciences* **378,** 367–80.

Platt, B.S. (1958a) Clinical features of endemic beriberi. *Federation Proceedings* **17,** suppl. 2, part 2, 8–20.

Platt, B.S. (1958b) Malnutrition and the pathogenesis of disease. *Transactions of the Royal Society of Tropical Medicine and Hygiene* **52,** 189–216.

Platt, B.S. and Stewart, R.J.C. (1969) Effects of protein calorie deficiency on dogs. 2. Morphological changes in the nervous system. *Developmental Medicine and Child Neurology* **11,** 174–92.

Popoff, N., Budzilovich, G., Goodgold, A. and Feigin, I. (1965) Hepatocerebral degeneration. Its occurrence in the presence and in the absence of abnormal copper metabolism. *Neurology* **15,** 919–30.

Popper, H. (1941) Histologic distribution of vitamin A in human organs under normal and under pathologic conditions. *Archives of Pathology* **31,** 766–802.

Potts, A.M. (1973) Tobacco amblyopia. *Survey of Ophthalmology* **17,** 313–39.

Purpura, D.P. and Gonzales-Monteagudo, O. (1960) Acute effects of methoxypyridoxine on hippocampal end-blade neurons: an experimental study of 'special pathoclisis' in the cerebral cortex. *Journal of Neuropathology and Experimental Neurology* **19,** 421–32.

Putnam, J.J. (1891) A group of cases of system scleroses of the spinal cord associated with diffuse collateral degeneration. *Journal of Nervous and Mental Disease* **22,** 51.

Raskin, N.H. and Fishman, R.A. (1965) Pyridoxine deficiency neuropathy due to hydralazine. *New England Journal of Medicine* **273,** 1182–5.

Reye, R.D.K., Morgan, G. and Baral, J. (1963) Encephalopathy and fatty degeneration of the viscera. A disease entity in childhood. *Lancet* **2,** 749–52.

Richmond, J. and Davidson, S. (1958) Subacute combined degeneration of the spinal cord in non-Addisonian megaloblastic anaemia. *Quarterly Journal of Medicine* **27,** 517–31.

Rickes, E.L., Brink, N.G., Konuisky, F.R., Wood, T.R. and Folkers, K. (1948) Vitamin B_{12}, a cobalt complex. *Science* **108,** 134.

Ridley, A. (1975) Porphyric neuropathy. In *Peripheral Neuropathy* (Eds. Dyck, P.J., Thomas, P.K. and Lambert, E.H), pp. 942–55. W.B. Saunders, Philadelphia.

Rinehart, J.F. and Greenberg, L.D. (1956) Arteriosclerotic lesions in pyridoxine deficient monkeys. *American Journal of Pathology* **25,** 481–9.

Ringsted, A. (1935) A preliminary note on the appearance of paresis in adult rats suffering from chronic avitaminosis E. *Biochemical Journal* **29,** 788–95.

Robertson, D.M., Wasan, S.M. and Skinner, D.B. (1968) Ultrastructural features of early brainstem lesions of thiamine deficient rats. *American Journal of Pathology* **52,** 1081–97.

Rodnight, R. and McIlwain, H. (1955) Indicanuria and psychosis of pellagra. *Journal of Mental Science* **101,** 884–9.

Ron, M.A., Acker, W., Shaw, G.K. and Lishman, W.A. (1982) Computerized tomography of the brain in chronic alcoholism. *Brain* **105,** 497–514.

Rosenberg, L.E. (1972) Disorders of propionate, methylmalonate and vitamin B_{12} metabolism. In *The Metabolic Basis of Inherited Disease*, 3rd edn

(Eds. Stanbury, J.B., Wyngaarden, J.B. and Fredrickson, D.S.). McGraw-Hill, New York.

Rosenblum, J.L., Keating, J.P., Prensky, A.L. and Nelson, J.S. (1981) A progressive neurological syndrome in children with chronic liver disease. *New England Journal of Medicine* **304,** 503–8.

Rosenoer, V.M. and Mitchell, R.C. (1959) Skeletal changes in Wilson's disease (hepatolenticular degeneration). *British Journal of Radiology* **32,** 805–9.

Russell, J.S.R., Batten, F.E. and Collier, J. (1900) Subacute combined degeneration of the spinal cord. *Brain* **23,** 39–110.

Sable, H.Z. and Gubler, C.J. (Eds.) (1982) Thiamin: twenty years of progress. *Annals of the New York Academy of Sciences* **378,** 1–468.

Saito, K., Yokoyama, T., Okaniwa, M. and Kamoshita, S. (1982) Neuropathology of chronic vitamin E deficiency in fatal familial intrahepatic cirrhosis. *Acta Neuropathologica* **58,** 187–92.

Sandbank, U. and Lerman, P. (1972) Progressive cerebral poliodystrophy—Alpers' disease. *Journal of Neurology, Neurosurgery and Psychiatry* **35,** 749–55.

Scharenberg, K. and Drew, A.L. (1954) The histopathology of Wilson's disease. *Journal of Neuropathology and Experimental Neurology* **13,** 181–90.

Scheinberg, I.H. and Sternlieb, I. (1974) Wilson's disease. In *Biology of Brain Dysfunction*, vol. 3 (Ed. Gaull, G.E.), pp. 247–64. Plenum Press, New York.

Schulman, S. (1968) Wilson's disease. In *Pathology of the Nervous System*, vol. 1 (Ed. Minckler, J.), pp. 1139–52. McGraw-Hill, New York.

Scott, H.H. (1918) An investigation into an outbreak of 'central neuritis'. *Annals of Tropical Medicine and Parasitology* **12,** 109–89.

Sebrell, W.H. and Butler, R.E. (1939) Riboflavin deficiency in man (ariboflavinosis). *Public Health Reports* (*Washington DC*) **54,** 2121–31.

Seitelberger, F. (1971) Neuropathological conditions related to neuroaxonal dystrophy. *Acta Neuropathologica* suppl. V, 17–29.

Shaw, J.H. and Phillips, P.H. (1941) The pathology of riboflavin deficiency in the rat. *Journal of Nutrition* **22,** 345–58.

Sherlock, S., Summerskill, W.H.J., White, L.P. and Phear, E.A. (1954) Portal-systemic encephalopathy: neurological complications of liver disease. *Lancet* **2,** 453–7.

Shiraki, H. (1968) The comparative study of various types of hepatocerebral diseases in the Japanese. In *The Central Nervous System*, International Academy of Pathology Monograph 9 (Eds. Bailey, O.T. and Smith, D.E.), pp. 252–72. Williams & Wilkins, Baltimore.

Sima, A.A.F., Kennedy, J.C., Blakeslee, D. and Robertson, D.M. (1981) Experimental porphyric neuropathy: a preliminary report. *Canadian Journal of Neurological Sciences* **8,** 105–14.

Sipe, J.C. (1973) Leigh's syndrome: the adult form of subacute necrotizing encephalomyelopathy with predilection for the brain stem. *Neurology* **10,** 1030–8.

Small, D.H., Carnegie, P.R. and Anderson, R. McD. (1981) Cycloleucine-induced vacuolation of myelin is associated with inhibition of protein methylation. *Neuroscience Letters* **21,** 287–92.

Smith, W.T. (1976) Nutritional deficiencies and disorders. In *Greenfield's Neuropathology*, 3rd edn (Eds. Blackwood, W. and Corsellis, J.A.N.), p. 224. Edward Arnold, London.

Sobel, R.A., De Armond, S.J., Forno, L.S. and Eng, L.F. (1981) Glial fibrillary acidic protein in hepatic encephalopathy. An immunohistochemical study. *Journal of Neuropathology and Experimental Neurology* **40,** 625–32.

Spillane, J.D. (1947) *Nutritional Disorders of the Nervous System.* Livingstone, Edinburgh.

Stannus, H.S. (1944) Some problems in riboflavin and allied deficiencies. *British Medical Journal* **2,** 103–5, 140–4.

Stender, A. and Lüthy, F. (1931) Über Spätatrophie der Kleinhirnrinde bei chronischem Alkoholismus. *Deutsche Zeitschrift für Nervenheilkunde* **119,** 604–22.

Stern, R.O. and Findlay, G.M. (1929) Nervous system in rats fed on diets deficient in vitamins B_1 and B_2. *Journal of Pathology and Bacteriology* **32,** 63–9.

Stewart, R.J. and Platt, B.S. (1968) The influence of protein calorie deficiency on the nervous system. *Proceedings of the Nutrition Society* **27,** 95–101.

Street, H.R., Cowgill, G.R. and Zimmerman, H.M. (1941) Further observations on riboflavin deficiency in the dog. *Journal of Nutrition* **22,** 7–24.

Sundaresen, P.S. (1966) Vitamin A and sulphate activating enzymes. *Biochimica et Biophysica Acta* **113,** 95–109.

Swank, R.L. and Adams, R.D. (1948) Pyridoxine and pantothenic acid deficiency in swine. *Journal of Neuropathology and Experimental Neurology* **7,** 274–86.

Sweeney, V.P., Pathak, M.H. and Asbury, A.K. (1970) Acute intermittent porphyria. Increased ALA-synthetase activity during an acute attack. *Brain* **93,** 369–80.

Terris, M. (1963) *Goldberger on Pellagra.* Louisiana State University Press, Baton Rouge.

Thomas, P.K. (1981) Peripheral neuropathy. In *The Molecular Basis of Neuropathology* (Eds. Davison, A.N. and Thompson, R.H.S), pp. 420–1. Edward Arnold, London.

Thorner, P.S., Bilbao, J.M., Sima, A.A.F. and Briggs, S. (1981) Porphyric neuropathy: an ultrastructural and quantitative case study. *Canadian Journal of Neurological Science* **8,** 281–7.

Tomasi, L.G. (1979) Reversibility of human myopathy caused by vitamin E deficiency. *Neurology* **29,** 1182–6.

Torres, I., Smith, W.T. and Oxnard, C.E. (1971) Peripheral neuropathy associated with vitamin B_{12} deficiency in captive monkeys. *Journal of Pathology* **105,** 125–46.

Towfighi, J. (1981) Effects of chronic vitamin E deficiency on the nervous system of the rat. *Acta Neuropathologica* **54,** 261–7.

Troost, D., van Rossum, A., Straks, W. and Willemse, J. (1982) Menkes' kinky hair disease. II. A clinico-pathological report of three cases. *Brain and Development* **4,** 115–26.

Trowell, H.C., Davies, J.N.P. and Dean, R.F.A. (1954) *Kwashiorkor*. Edward Arnold, London.

Turpin, R., Jerome, H. and Schmidt, H.H. (1953) Study of the variations of the caeruloplasmin by an easy technique. *Proceedings of the Royal Society of Medicine* **46,** 1061–2.

Uzman, L.L. (1956) Histochemical localization of copper with rubeanic acid. *Laboratory Investigation* **5,** 299–305.

Uzman, L.L. and Denny-Brown, D. (1948) Aminoaciduria in hepatolenticular degeneration (Wilson's disease). *American Journal of the Medical Sciences* **215,** 599–611.

Verma, K. and Wei King D. (1967) Disorders of the developing nervous system of vitamin E deficient rats. *Acta Anatomica* **67,** 623–5.

Victor, M. (1970) Tobacco amblyopia, cyanide poisoning and vitamin B_{12} deficiency: a critique of current concepts. In *Miami Neuro-Ophthalmology Symposium*, vol. 5 (Ed. Smith, J.L.), pp. 33–48. Huffman, Hallandale, Florida.

Victor, M. (1974) Neurologic changes in liver disease. In Brain Dysfunction in Metabolic disorders. *Research Publications of the Association for Research in Nervous and Mental Disease* **53,** 1–11.

Victor, M. (1975) Polyneuropathy due to nutritional deficiency and alcoholism. In *Peripheral Neuropathy* (Eds. Dyck, P.J., Thomas, P.K. and Lambert, E.H.), pp. 1030–66. W.B. Saunders, Philadelphia.

Victor, M. (1976) The Wernicke-Korsakoff syndrome. In *Handbook of Clinical Neurology*, vol. 28 (Eds. Vinken, P.J. and Bruyn, G.W.), pp. 243–70. North-Holland, Amsterdam.

Victor, M. and Adams, R.D. (1956) Neuropathology of experimental B_6 deficiency in monkeys. *American Journal of Clinical Nutrition* **4,** 346–53.

Victor, M. and Adams, R.D. (1961) On the etiology of the alcoholic neurologic diseases with special reference to the role of nutrition. *American Journal of Clinical Nutrition* **9,** 379–97.

Victor, M., Adams, R.D. and Cole, M. (1965) The acquired (non-Wilsonian) type of chronic hepatocerebral degeneration. *Medicine* **44,** 345–96.

Victor, M., Adams, R.D. and Collins, G.H. (1971). *The Wernicke-Korsakoff Syndrome*. Blackwell Scientific, Oxford.

Victor, M., Adams, R.D. and Mancall, E.L. (1959) A restricted form of cerebellar cortical degeneration occurring in alcoholic patients. *Archives of Neurology* **1,** 579–688.

Vilter, R.W., Mueller, J.F., Glazer, H.S., Jarrold, T., Abraham, J., Thompson, C. and Hawkins, V.R. (1953) The effect of vitamin B_6 deficiency induced by desoxypyridoxine in human beings. *Journal of Laboratory and Clinical Medicine* **42,** 335–57.

Vivacqua, R.J., Myerson, R.M., Prescott, D.J. and Rabinowitz, J.L. (1966) Abnormal propionic-methylmalonic-succinic acid metabolism in vitamin B_{12} deficiency and its possible relationship to the neurologic syndrome of pernicious anemia. *American Journal of the Medical Sciences* **251,** 507–15.

Walshe, J.M. (1967) The physiology of copper in man and its relation to Wilson's disease. *Brain* **90,** 149–76.

Walshe, J.M. (1976) Wilson's disease (hepatolenticular degeneration). In *Handbook of Clinical Neurology*, vol. 27 (Eds. Vinken, P.J., Bruyn, G.W. and Klawans, H.L.), pp. 379–414. North-Holland, Amsterdam.

Watanabe, I., Tomita, T., Hung, K.-S. and Iwasaki, Y. (1981) Edematous necrosis in thiamine-deficient encephalopathy of the mouse. *Journal of Neuropathology and Experimental Neurology* **40,** 454–71.

Wefring, K.W. and Lamvik, J.O. (1967) Familial progressive poliodystrophy with cirrhosis of the liver. *Acta Paediatrica (Uppsala)* **56,** 295–300.

Wernicke, C. (1881–83) *Lehrbuch der Gehirnkrankheiten*, vol. 2. Fischer, Kassel and Berlin.

Whetsell, W.O. and Plaitakis, A. (1978) Leigh's disease in an adult with evidence of 'inhibitor factor' in family members. *Annals of Neurology* **3,** 519–24.

Willemse, J., Van den Hamer, C.J.A., Prins, H.W. and Jonker, P.L. (1982) Menkes' kinky hair disease. I. Comparison of classical and unusual clinical and biochemical features in two patients. *Brain and Development* **4,** 105–14.

Williams, J.A., Hall, G.S., Thompson, A.G. and Cooke, W.T. (1969) Neurological disease after partial gastrectomy. *British Medical Journal* **3,** 210–12.

Wilson, S.A.K. (1912) Progressive lenticular degeneration: a familial nervous disease associated with cirrhosis of the liver. *Brain* **34,** 295–509.

Wilson, S.A.K. (1914) The pathology of pellagra. *Proceedings of the Royal Society of Medicine* **7,** 91.

Winkelman, N.W. (1932) Progressive pallidal degeneration. A new clinico-pathologic syndrome. *Archives of Neurology and Psychiatry* **27,** 1–21.

Wintrobe, M.M., Follis, R.H. Jr, Miller, M.H., Stein, H.J., Alcayaga, R., Humphreys, S. et al. (1943) Pyridoxine deficiency in swine with particular reference to anemia, epileptiform convulsions and fatty liver. *Bulletin of the Johns Hopkins Hospital* **72,** 1–25.

Wintrobe, M.M., Buschke, W., Follis, R.H. Jr and Humphreys, S. (1944) Riboflavin deficiency in the swine with special reference to the occurrence of cataracts. *Bulletin of the Johns Hopkins Hospital* **75,** 102–14.

Wokes, F., Badenoch, J. and Sinclair, H.M. (1955) Human dietary deficiency of vitamin B_{12}. *American Journal of Clinical Nutrition* **3,** 375–82.

Wolbach, S.B. and Bessey, O.A. (1941) Vitamin deficiency and the nervous system. *Archives of Pathology* **32,** 689–722.

Woltmann, H.W. (1918) Brain changes associated with pernicious anemia. *Archives of Internal Medicine* **21,** 791–843.

Woltmann, H.W. (1919) The nervous symptoms in pernicious anemia: an analysis of one hundred and fifty cases. *American Journal of the Medical Sciences* **173,** 400–9.

Woltmann, H.W. (1924) The mental changes with pernicious anemia. *American Journal of Psychiatry* **3,** 435–49.

Woolley, D.W. (1946) Occurrence of 'pellagragenic' agent in corn. *Journal of Biological Chemistry* **163,** 773–4.

Yajima, K. and Suzuki, K. (1979) Neuronal degeneration in the brain of the brindled mouse. *Acta Neuropathologica* **45,** 17–25.

Yoshimura, N. and Kudo, H. (1983) Mitochondrial abnormalities in Menkes' kinky hair disease. *Acta Neuropathologica* **59,** 295–303.

Zamora, A.J., Cavanagh, J.B. and Kyu, M.H. (1973) Ultrastructural response of the astrocytes to portocaval anastomosis in the rat. *Journal of the Neurological Sciences* **18,** 25–45.

Zimmerman, H.M. (1943) Pathology of vitamin B group deficiencies. *Research Publications. Association for Research in Nervous and Mental Disease* **22,** 51–79.

14

Toxic Disorders of the nervous system

Jean M. Jacobs and Pamela M. Le Quesne

Metals

Aluminium

Exposure. Although aluminium is widely distributed and has many industrial uses, toxicity from occupational exposure is extremely rare (McLaughlin et al., 1962). However, it now seems certain that progressive encephalopathy occurring in some patients undergoing chronic dialysis for renal failure (dialysis encephalopathy) is due to aluminium intoxication.

In the early 1970s in some renal dialysis units progressive encephalopathy became one of the commonest causes of death. Alfrey, LeGendre and Kaehny (1976) found that brain aluminium levels were elevated in patients with encephalopathy compared with levels in dialysis patients dying of other causes and with control subjects. This was confirmed by McDermott et al. (1978). The patchy geographical distribution of the disease led to the recognition that the aluminium content of the water used for dialysis was the most important factor (Elliott et al., 1978; Parkinson et al., 1979). Following these reports the aluminium content of water used for dialysis has been kept low by reverse osmosis and the disease has disappeared (Davison et al., 1982).

Clinical features. Dialysis encephalopathy is characterized by progressive dementia with particular speech difficulty, myoclonus, epilepsy which is often focal, and focal neurological signs.

Human pathology. No specific pathological features were found in the brain of the patient with occupational aluminium intoxication described by McLaughlin et al. (1962). In particular it was noted that there were no features of Alzheimer's disease.

Histological changes in the cerebral cortex were demonstrated by Burks et al. (1976) in six patients dying of dialysis encephalopathy. Although no neuronal loss was found in the cortex, many neurons were shrunken with hyperchromatic nuclei and loss of Nissl substance, particularly in the outer granular layer. Enlarged microglial cells were a conspicuous feature and some astroglial proliferation was noted. A spongiform laminar change was present in the second and third cortical layers. Although these histological changes are non-specific, they were not found in uraemic patients of similar clinical severity who had been dialysed for the same length of time but had not developed encephalopathy.

Experimental studies. There have been no reports of experimental studies of clear relevance to dialysis encephalopathy. There has been interest, however, in other aspects of aluminium neurotoxicity since Klatzo, Wiśniewski and Streicher (1965) first reported that neurofibrillary tangles develop following the injection of aluminium into the brains of rabbits, cats and dogs. Because neurofibrillary tangles are a prominent pathological feature of Alzheimer's disease the role of aluminium in the pathogenesis of this disease has frequently been discussed. Raised aluminium levels have been found in some brain regions in patients with Alzheimer's disease. Although there have been some discrepancies in the findings from different laboratories, it seems that these can be attributed to different techniques of sampling (Crapper McLachlan et al., 1980). Perl and Brody (1980), using scanning electron microscopy with x-ray spectrometry, found that aluminium was present in the nuclear region only of tangle-bearing neurons. There is, however, a difference in the structure of the neurofibrillary tangles in the human disease and in the experimental condition. In Alzheimer's disease the tangles are composed of paired helical filaments (M. Kidd, 1964), whereas those following aluminium injection into experimental animals consist of unpaired 100-Å filaments (Wiśniewski, Terry and Hirano, 1970). The similarities and differences in Alzheimer's disease and experimental aluminium encephalopathy have been discussed in detail by Crapper McLachlan and De Boni (1980). Aluminium is unlikely to play a direct causal role in Alzheimer's disease.

Recently it has been reported that the brains of Guamanian Chamorros may contain many neurofibrillary tangles whether or not there had been clinical evidence of the amyotrophic lateral sclerosis - parkinsonism - dementia syndrome which is common in these people (F.H. Anderson et al., 1979). Raised aluminium levels have also been found in these tangle-bearing neurons (Perl et al., 1982). It has been suggested that the aluminium accumulation may be related to high environmental aluminium which has been found in soil and water in certain parts of Guam.

Arsenic

Exposure Intoxication usually occurs accidentally or as a result of criminal action. Arsenic is an important constituent of some weed killers and pesticides, a common source for accidental or deliberate poisoning. Occupational exposure was common in the early part of this century but is now rare, although some exposure may still occur in the smelting industry. A lesser degree of exposure has followed the medicinal use of arsenic for many centuries, particularly during the early part of the present century when organic arsenicals were widely used in the treatment of syphilis and trypanosomiasis.

Although arsenic was used medicinally by the ancient Greeks and Romans, its toxicity was not recognized until the Middle Ages (Buchanan, 1962). Accidental contamination of alcoholic drinks has caused several large outbreaks of poisoning, one of the most famous occurring in 1900 in the Manchester area when contaminated sugar was used in preparing beer (*Lancet*, 1900). Neurological complications associated with the therapeutic use of organic arsenicals were common from about 1920 to 1950. The basis of organic arsenical toxicity may differ from that due to inorganic arsenic.

Clinical features Inorganic arsenic poisoning may occur acutely following a single exposure or chronically following multiple small exposures. After a single toxic exposure, systemic symptoms occur immediately, with gastrointestinal disturbance and shock. If the subject survives there is a latent interval of 2–3 weeks before peripheral neuropathy develops. Sensory symptoms usually occur first and pain is a prominent early feature. Weakness then develops and there may be rapid deterioration for several days or weeks, the severity depending on the degree of exposure. Recovery is slow, continuing for over a year in some instances, and is often incomplete (Le Quesne and McLeod, 1977). Mees' lines (white bands across the nails) develop and gradually move distally.

In chronic poisoning, peripheral neuropathy develops slowly, usually without gastrointestinal symptoms. Hyperkeratosis of the hands and feet is common. Raindrop pigmentation may be seen, particularly on the skin of the trunk.

Toxic complications of organic arsenicals include encephalopathy and exfoliative dermatitis as well as peripheral neuropathy. Treatment with British anti-Lewisite (BAL) is particularly effective for the acute complications produced by organic arsenicals (Peters et al., 1947). It has been suggested that these complications, unlike those due to inorganic arsenic salts, are due to an allergic rather than to a direct toxic effect (Tellenbach, 1949). There is less evidence that chelation has an influence on acute or chronic peripheral neuropathy produced by inorganic arsenic.

Human pathology Little detailed pathological information is available. Nerve biopsies from subjects with arsenic neuropathy have mainly shown axonal degeneration (Heyman et al., 1956; Ota, 1970). Biopsies from four patients following acute intoxication revealed axonal degeneration with more severe involvement of large than small fibres (Le Quesne and McLeod, 1977). There was evidence of continuing degeneration as long as 2–3 months after exposure. In another study, however, prominent segmental demyelination in addition to axonal degeneration was described in nerves from some patients with arsenic neuropathy (Chhuttani and Chopra, 1979). Unfortunately, it is not stated whether these nerves were from patients with acute or chronic intoxication, and this may be an important factor in explaining the different findings. In an ultrastructural study of a nerve from one case of chronic poisoning, Ota (1970) described changes of axonal degeneration only, with occasional 'onion bulb' formation.

Studies of toxic encephalopathy resulting from treatment with organic arsenicals during the 1920s and 1930s revealed pericapillary haemorrhages as a striking feature (Globus and Ginsburg, 1933). The findings were summarized by Hurst (1959). The pons and midbrain were often most severely involved. Small vessel thrombosis and perivascular demyelination were often symmetrically distributed, as were areas of haemorrhagic necrosis.

Experimental studies There have been no successful experimental studies of peripheral neuropathy due to arsenic. It is not clear why this should be so.

Haemorrhagic encephalopathy has been produced in rabbits (Grzycki and Kobusowna, 1951) and monkeys (Hurst, 1959) by administration of various arsenic compounds. The changes were similar to those reported in encephalopathy produced by organic arsenic medication in man. Hurst (1959) found acute haemorrhagic necrosis in grey matter of the brain stem and external geniculate bodies, thalamus and Ammon's horn after high doses of organic arsenic to monkeys.

Lead

Inorganic lead

Exposure. *Children.* The commonest cause of lead poisoning in children during the past 30 years has been ingestion of lead-containing paints, particularly by small children with pica. There are now strict controls concerning the lead content of paint, but some old houses, particularly in inner cities in USA are still covered with lead-based paints.

There is currently much concern about possible deleterious effects of environmental contamination by lead, particularly in relation to its effect on children's intelligence. Exhaust fumes from vehicles using petrol with added lead are blamed for increasing environmental exposure. The scientific evidence is at present under review.

Adults Adult exposure to lead occurs predominantly in relation to occupation. The main industries concerned are lead smelting and electric accumulator manufacture. Plumbosolvent domestic water is a source of lead which has attracted attention. Lead glaze on pottery is still used in some primitive communities, because it can be fired at a lower temperature than other glazes. This can result in dangerous exposure.

Although lead has been used by man throughout the history of civilization, the Romans were the first to use it on a large scale for practical as well as decorative purposes and were the first to recognize lead poisoning as a disease. From the time of the industrial revolution until the need for adequate industrial hygiene became recognized, occupational exposure to lead caused much disease. This is now rare.

Clinical features *Childhood lead poisoning.* The usual manifestation is encephalopathy. There may be a prodromal period of irritability and anorexia for a few weeks, followed by ataxia and vomiting, progressing to fits and coma. There is evidence of raised intracranial pressure with papilloedema. The child is usually anaemic, and x-rays show lead lines at the end of the long bones and increased density of the metacarpals, phalanges and ribs. Control of fits and rapid removal of lead by chelation therapy reduces the mortality.

Adult lead poisoning The onset is usually much more insidious than in children. Ill health due to anaemia may be present for some time. Colic is usually the next manifestation, and if the condition is not recognized and treated at this stage peripheral neuropathy may ensue. Neuropathy is entirely motor, and predominantly affects the muscles exercised most. This led to the typical picture of wrist drop in painters applying leaded paints, because of the frequent use of the forearm extensors.

Peripheral neuropathy due to lead poisoning is rare today because the exposure necessary to produce this condition is rarely found in modern industry.

Human pathology *Acute encephalopathy*. Comprehensive descriptions of acute lead encephalopathy have been made by Blackman (1937), Akelaitis (1941), J.F. Smith et al. (1960), Okazaki et al. (1963), Pentschew (1965) and Osetowska (1971). Macroscopically, brain swelling is a common feature; the cerebral gyri are flattened and sulci narrowed or obliterated. Uncal and tonsillar herniations and a pressure coné are often found. The ventricles are usually compressed although hydrocephalus may result from obliteration of the foramina of Magendie and Luschka, or from impairment of the absorption of CSF. There is vascular engorgement of the leptomeninges, so external surfaces appear hyperaemic and inflamed. The white matter, particularly in the cerebellum, may have a yellowish tint and there may be petechial haemorrhages.

Microscopically there is a wide variety of changes but vascular damage is the predominant and probably the primary lesion. Capillaries may be dilated, narrowed, necrotic or thrombosed, and capillary endothelial cell swelling or 'capillary activation' (Pentschew, 1965) is seen frequently. A perivascular protein-rich transudate, both within the brain and in the meninges, is associated with globules or droplets which are PAS-positive. The normal architecture of the brain may be considerably disrupted by these focal outpourings of fluid; fibres are separated and areas in both grey and white matter have a spongy appearance. Within these foci there are damaged and proliferating glia, degenerating neurons and lipid-laden phagocytes. This spectrum of changes is found throughout the CNS, particularly in the grey matter, but the cerebellum is most severely affected. Lesions are found in the molecular and Purkinje cell layers and there may be severe atrophy of folia.

Chronic encephalopathy Chronic exposure to lead, when it produces an encephalopathy, causes similar changes to those seen in the acute state (Osetowska, 1971), with primary damage to vascular endothelium. There may be a mixture of atrophy and acute swelling—the latter due to a sudden exacerbation of symptoms, possibly as a reaction to previous sensitization.

The presence of toxic levels of lead in the brain is certain evidence of lead-induced encephalopathy. A characteristic feature which may help in the diagnosis of lead intoxication is the presence of intranuclear inclusions in kidney tubule cells.

Neuropathy Before the end of the nineteenth century, lead was widely thought to produce a myopathy; however, in several studies (Gombault, 1873; Zunker, 1880) evidence of nerve fibre degeneration was found in radial nerves. It is not clear from these early records which type of degeneration was seen but it is of interest that endoneurial oedema was noted. Reports of anterior horn cell degeneration in the cervical spinal cord (Zunker, 1880) suggest an axonal degeneration. These early studies have been reviewed by Goldstein, McCall and Dyck (1975).

There are few recent reports of pathological changes in human lead neuropathy, probably because of the decreasing number of cases. Buchthal and Behse (1979) examined the sural nerve of a man exposed to lead for 13 years and who had clinical evidence of neuropathy. They found loss of large ($>7\ \mu m$ diameter) fibres, but no demyelination. Biopsied nerves from lead-exposed men without clinical evidence of neuropathy showed no loss of fibres. In teased fibre preparations there was a rather higher incidence than normal of paranodal demyelination; some individual fibres had multiple internodes of normal length but inappropriately thin diameter. It is not clear whether these internodes were in the process of primary demyelination or if the myelin change is secondary to axonal atrophy.

Experimental studies Animal studies generally confirm clinical experience in man that exposure to high doses of lead causes an encephalopathy in the young and a neuropathy in the adult.

Encephalopathy Suckling rats receiving lead through milk from mothers fed with 4% lead carbonate (Pentschew and Garro, 1966; Thomas, Dallenbach and Thomas 1971; Clasen et al., 1974; Goldstein, Asbury and Diamond, 1974) or by direct administration of lead through an oesophageal catheter (Press, 1977a) develop paraplegia 3–4 weeks after birth; most of the animals die at this stage. The brains of these rats show macroscopic discoloration of the cerebellum due to haemorrhages. Histological examination shows, in addition to haemorrhages, marked oedema with the formation of fluid-filled cavities within the white matter (Fig. 14.1). In general, neurons are preserved; there is glial proliferation and capillaries are conspicuous with endothelial cell proliferation. The cerebellar nuclei, particularly the dentate, show status spongiosus and scattered haemorrhages. The cerebrum is less severely affected but certain areas, for example the striatum, show changes similar to those found in the cerebellum. Michaelson and Sauerhoff (1974) examined the Pentschew and Garro model of poisoning via maternal milk and noticed that by 18 days the suckling rats could gain access to the 4% lead-carbonate-containing (27 000 p.p.m. Pb) food given to the mother. If, at that time, the maternal diet was adjusted to one containing 25 p.p.m. Pb (comparable to the content of lead in maternal milk) a less severe encephalopathy developed; no paraplegia or gross pathological change was evident but the animals showed hyperactivity, aggressiveness and other behavioural abnormalities.

Studies on the pathogenesis of lead encephalopathy point to the developing blood vessels as the primary target of this metal (Thomas, Dallenbach and Thomas, 1971; Goldstein, Asbury and Diamond, 1974). Press (1977a) examined the temporal sequence of the pathological changes in the brain and particularly the cerebellum of poisoned suckling rats long before the onset of clinical signs. Petechial haemorrhages were found in 3-day-old rats and by 5 days extensive haemorrhagic lesions were present throughout molecular and Purkinje cell layers; oedema fluid accumulated later. Regions of haemorrhage correspond to layers undergoing the most active morphogenesis; these regions might also be expected to have a rapidly developing vasculature. Press used Golgi preparations to show developmental vascular abnormalities and found the endothelial buds to be particularly sensitive to lead. Electron microscopy revealed changes in interendothelial junctions of cerebellar capillaries and necrotic endothelial cells (Fig. 14.2) which could affect the integrity of the vessel walls. Toews et al. (1978) found lead to be concentrated in cellular fractions containing brain capillaries from 5-day-old rats dosed acutely with lead and there were morphological abnormalities in the vessels. After a long dosing schedule the vascular changes were reversed and normal vessels were found despite continued dosing. Pentschew and Garro (1966) had also noticed that if rats survived the initial period of acute encephalopathy they often appeared to recover completely.

Pentschew and Garro (1966) demonstrated increased permeability of blood vessels to trypan blue in the brain, particularly the cerebellum of lead-poisoned suckling rats. Stumpf, Sar and Grant (1980) used a single tracer dose of ^{210}Pb in 10-day-old rats in an autoradiographic study of its localization. Radioactivity was concentrated in blood vessels and 'lining' cells of the brain. Activity was also high in circumventricular organs which lack a blood–brain barrier; these findings suggest a basis for neuroendocrine effects in lead intoxication—e.g. retarded growth and decreased serum FSH levels in experimental animals, retarded growth and delayed vaginal opening.

No change in blood–brain barrier permeability was found in adult lead-poisoned rats; neither was there any alteration in the enzymatic transfer of phenylalanine or tyrosine across the barrier (Hertz et al., 1981). Vascular permeability was also unchanged in adult guinea-pigs in which there was no histological evidence of an encephalopathy although the animals showed behavioural disturbances, including seizures, during dosing (Bouldin and Krigman, 1975).

Suckling mice poisoned with maternal milk show less severe changes than rats, possibly because the mother mice could tolerate only a 1% lead carbonate diet. A striking feature in the brains of mice was the presence of large numbers of intervascular strands, and, unlike in rats, the blood–brain barrier remained relatively intact (Rosenblum and Johnson, 1968).

Hirano and Kochen (1976) injected lead into the yolk sac of chick embryos. Brain haemorrhages and cyst formation was seen in embryos younger than 10 days, before the formation of the blood–brain barrier; at later stages no changes were produced.

Newly weaned monkeys dosed orally with lead subacetate and vitamin D (Clasen et al., 1974) developed an encephalopathy with oedematous changes in cerebellar and subcortical white matter, where there was also diffuse astrocytosis and glial nodules. Perivascular PAS-positive granules were considered to be a characteristic feature of lead encephalopathy. Monkeys poisoned by ingestion of lead-containing paint from the bars of their cages developed brain oedema, status spongiosus and endothelial changes (Sauer, Zook and Garner, 1970). Similar changes were

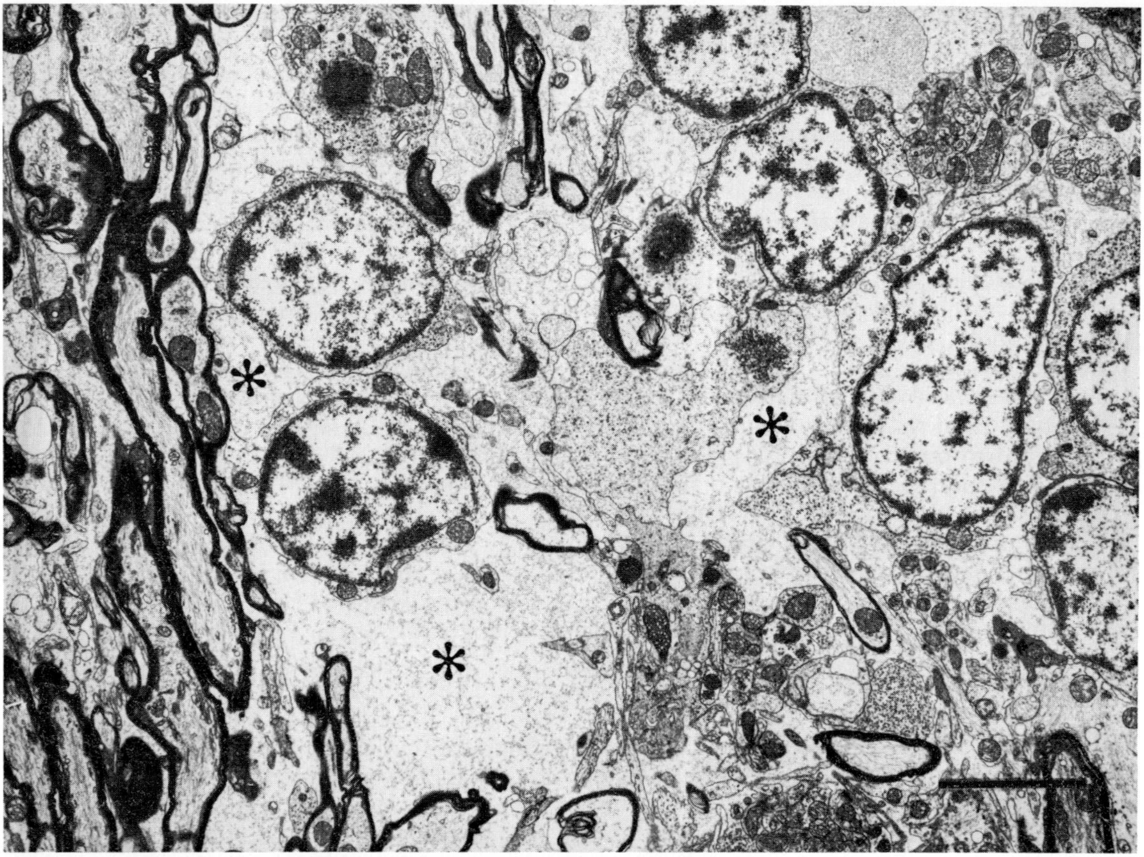

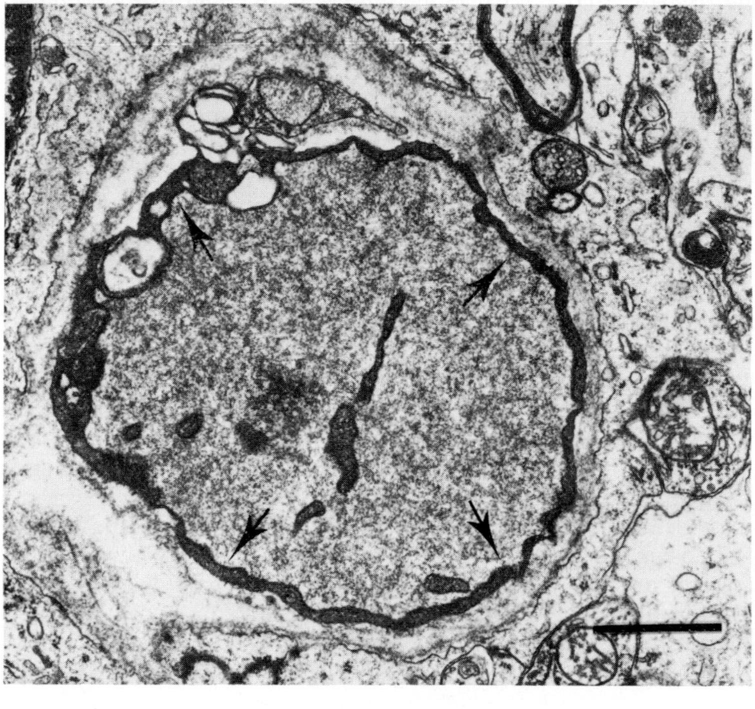

Fig. 14.1 Electron micrograph of cerebellum from a 26-day-old lead-intoxicated rat, showing extensive areas of oedema (*) separating granule cells. Bar = 5 μm.

Fig. 14.2 Electron micrograph showing a capillary with an electron-dense necrotic endothelium (arrows) in the cerebellum of the same rat as in Fig. 14.1. The lumen is filled with granular proteinaceous material. Bar = 1 μm.

found in accidentally poisoned cattle (Christian and Tryphonas, 1971). The suckling rat model of lead encephalopathy has been used to study some parameters of brain development. Press (1977b) gave rats lead by oral gavage; he found decreased numbers of mitotic figures in the external granular layer of the cerebellum, with increased numbers of pyknotic cells leading to a reduction in the thickness of the molecular layer. Purkinje cell development was retarded and the dendritic arborization was less well developed than that of control rats. Krigman and Hogan (1974) found retardation of brain growth with reduced neuronal size, resulting in limited proliferation of processes in the neuropil and a reduction in the number of synapses per neuron. In another study, Krigman et al. (1974) found that axons were reduced in size but the myelin sheath thickness was appropriate for axon diameter.

Lead poisoning by the methods described above involves dosing with large amounts of lead, producing blood lead levels of over 240 μmol/l (500 μg/100 ml); it causes marked weight loss, and this introduces the problem of suitable controls. In many experimental studies no pair-fed controls were used despite the fact that when food contains lead, mother rats consume less and produce less milk. The interpretation of some of these results may therefore be open to question.

Whilst the suckling rat has been a useful model for the study of acute and often fatal encephalopathy, the issue of greatest concern now is the effect of chronic low level lead toxicity, particularly in children. Experimental models producing blood levels of about 17 μmol/l (36 μg/100 ml)—and therefore relevant to human exposure—have shown that synapses in the cerebral cortex are less mature ultrastructurally than are controls (McCauley, Bull and Lutkenhoff, 1979). Winder, Garten and Lewis (1983) have reviewed the effects of lead on the developing nervous system.

Peripheral neuropathy Guinea-pigs fed for several months on a diet containing lead develop peripheral neuropathy, usually without clinical signs (Gombault, 1880; Fullerton, 1966). Examination of teased fibres from these animals shows a predominantly segmental demyelinating lesion with occasional fibres undergoing axonal degeneration. It is of historical interest that Gombault's observations on teased fibres from lead-poisoned guinea-pigs led to the first description of what we now recognize as segmental demyelination. He also noticed that segmental loss of myelin was followed by remyelination with short internodes (Fig. 14.3).

Fullerton (1966) made electrophysiological studies on lead-poisoned guinea-pigs and found motor conduction velocity to be reduced below the control range; a direct correlation was found between the degree of reduction of conduction velocity and the severity of demyelination.

Some species differences have been shown, rabbits developing an axonal type of neuropathy and cats rapidly becoming paralysed due to CNS toxicity (Ferraro and Hernandez, 1932). Although more resistant than other species, rats have been widely used in more recent studies on lead neuropathy. Schlaepfer (1969) dosed rats for 3–18 months with lead; no signs of functional disturbance developed, but demyelination and axonal degeneration were seen in peripheral nerves and roots. In an ultrastructural study, Lampert and Schochet (1968) described myelin vacuolation with splitting of lamellae at major and minor dense lines; Schwann cells were seen in mitosis and remyelination occurred rapidly in the presence of continuing dosing with lead.

In attempting to explain the presence of both demyelination and axonal degeneration, Ohnishi et al. (1977) made a morphometric study of rats with lead neuropathy. They found no change in size and number of dorsal root ganglion cells or of myelinated fibres in proximal and distal parts of the peroneal and sural nerve, results which do not suggest the primary involvement of the nerve cell or axon. Segmental demyelination was equally frequent in proximal and distal parts of these nerves, and the random distribution of demyelinated internodes (Dyck, O'Brien and Ohnishi, 1977) suggested that demyelination was more likely to be a primary event than a secondary change associated with axonal degeneration.

Endoneurial oedema is a conspicuous feature of this model of lead neuropathy; however, no evidence was found of increased permeability of endoneurial blood vessels (Dyck et al., 1980). Lead levels in these nerves were significantly raised at an early stage of the neuropathy, before segmental demyelination or nerve oedema was apparent (Windebank et al., 1980). Presumably lead can pass through intact endoneurial blood vessels. There is no evidence that the pathogenesis of this neuropathy is related to toxic effects

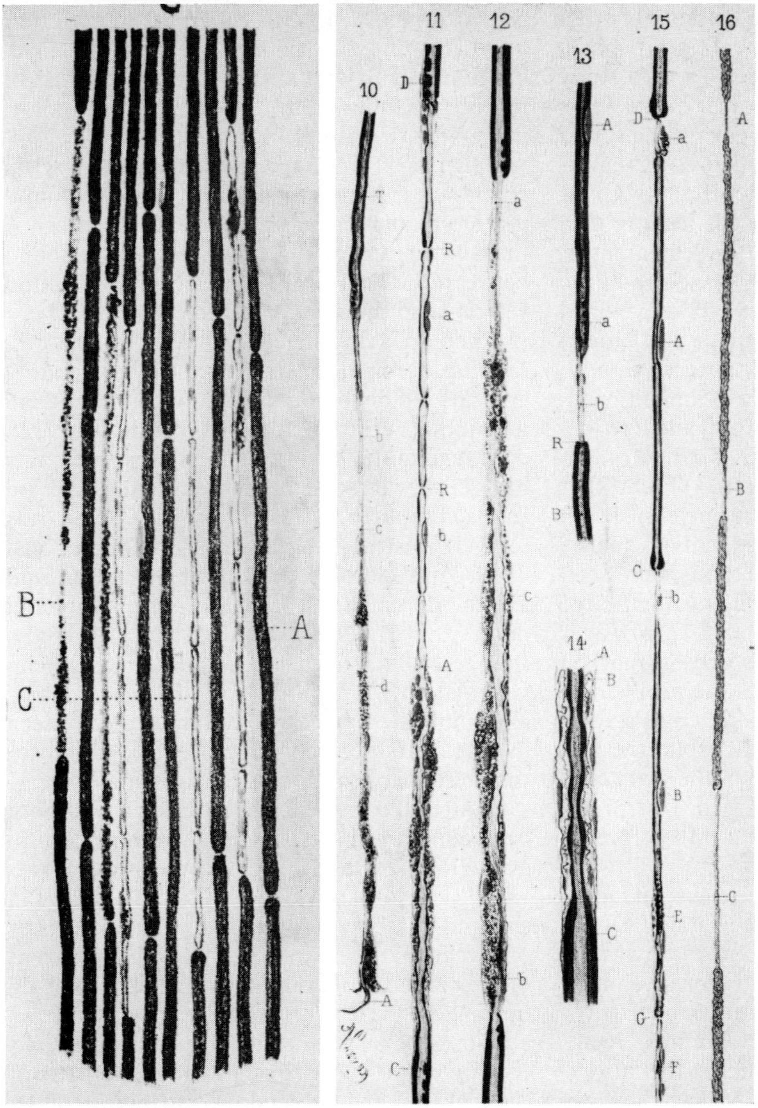

Fig. 14.3 Illustrations from Gombault's (1880) paper on experimental lead neuropathy in guinea-pigs, showing segmental demyelination. Fibres treated with osmium tetroxide and counterstained with picrocarmine.

upon neural blood vessels, as seems to be the case in lead encephalopathy.

Organic lead

Exposure The toxicologically important form of organic lead is tetraethyl lead, which has been added to petrol as an antiknock agent since 1923. Dangerous exposure has occurred only in workers wearing inadequate protective clothing when cleaning out petrol storage tanks. Between 1923 and 1964, 88 workers in the USA and Canada were affected in this way and 16 of them died. In the UK, Cassells and Dodds (1946) described 25 affected subjects and a further 15 cases were reported in five separate incidents over the next 25 years.

Clinical features Sleep disturbances associated with nightmares are recognized early symptoms. Following severe exposure, a constant state of excitement can develop into a manic psychosis. Delusions, hallucinations and intense fear can result in attempted suicide. Sedation is the most effective treatment and no sequelae are recognized in those who survive the acute episode.

Human pathology A case of severe, chronic

petrol (gasoline)-sniffing encephalopathy probably caused by tetraethyl lead in the gasoline has been described by Valpey et al. (1978). The patient died after being admitted with acute encephalopathy four times in as many years. The serum lead was increased and urinary lead acetate was high. The lead content of the brain was at least 5000–6000 p.p.m. The brain showed mild cerebral cortical atrophy with slightly dilated ventricles and patchy cerebellar atrophy. Microscopically there was pyramidal cell loss in the hippocampus, particularly in Roses' fields h3–5 of Ammon's horn. In the cerebellum there was marked but irregular loss of Purkinje cells, and neuronal loss and gliosis in the dentate nucleus. Mild, diffuse astrocyte gliosis was also seen in the pons, striatum, pallidum and thalamus.

Experimental studies Tetraethyl lead is converted to triethyl lead in the liver, and it is the latter form which is neurotoxic. In a study on rats and dogs, R. K. Davis et al. (1963) showed that both triethyl and trimethyl lead produced signs and symptoms of CNS toxicity. In this and another study on rats (Schepers, 1964), histological examination showed widespread neuronal damage.

Seawright et al. (1980) studied the effects of trimethyl or triethyl lead acetate in the rat; a single dose caused hyperexcitability, loss of weight and fine tremor within 2 days. Very aggressive behaviour developed on the third day, leading in some cases to convulsions, paralysis and coma. Some animals died, but surviving rats appeared to behave normally by the tenth day and began to gain weight.

Significant pathological changes were found in the brain. Neuronal necrosis was present 1 day after dosing, affecting the pyriform cortex. By the second day necrotic neurons were seen in the retrohippocampus and entorhinal cortex, the

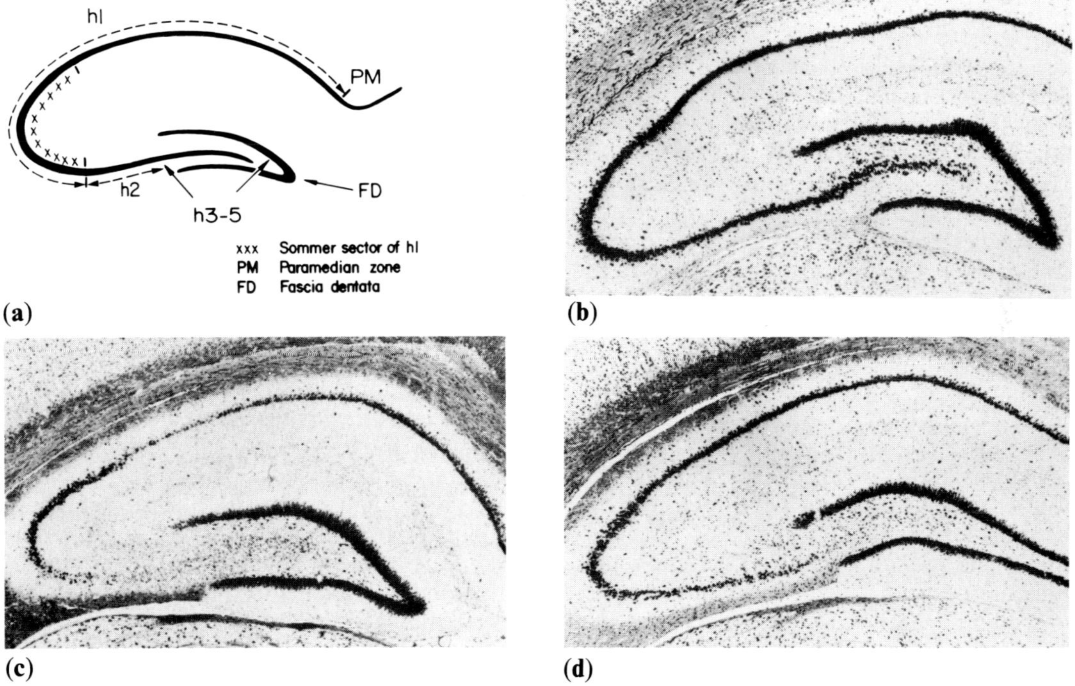

Fig. 14.4 (**a**) Schematic diagram of the rat hippocampus in the coronal plane. (**b**) Hippocampus of control rat, showing well stained neurons of the fascia dentata and pyramidal cell band of regions h1–5. (**c**) Trimethyl tin chloride intoxication: 21 days after a single oral dose of 10 mg/kg. The hippocampus shows extensive loss of neurons in h1 (except dorsolateral portion of Sommer sector), h2 and h3–5. (**d**) Triethyl lead acetate intoxication, following three sublethal weekly oral doses of 10 mg/kg. Rat hippocampus showing marked pyramidal cell loss in h3–5 and to a lesser extent in h2. Luxol fast blue–cresyl violet × 27. (Reproduced from Le Quesne, 1981, by permission of the Editor of the *Journal of Neurology, Neurosurgery and Psychiatry*. Preparations and photographs by A.W. Brown.)

fascia dentata and regions h3–5 of the anterodorsal hippocampus. On the third day there was extensive necrosis in the posteroventral region of the fascia dentata and chromatolysis of most hippocampal neurons. Sporadic neuronal death was found later in the neocortex, with chromatolysis in septal nuclei, amygdaloid complex, caudate nuclei and thalamus, and in the brain stem including vestibular and red nuclei, and the reticular formation.

Multiple dosing caused moderate or extensive loss of neurons in h3–5 of the hippocampus and in the pyriform cortex (Fig. 14.4), with some neuronal necrosis in nuclei of the medulla.

The behavioural changes and limbic system lesions produced by triethyl and trimethyl lead were similar to those casued by trimethyl tin. Organic lead, however, produced more extensive damage although minimal levels of triethyl lead required to produce neuronal damage were higher than those for trimethyl tin.

Manganese

Exposure Intoxication has most commonly occurred in workers in manganese mines, which are to be found in Chile, Morocco and Cuba. Manganese is an essential ingredient of steel, and with the expansion in steel production during the past 30 years industrial exposure has increased in manganese foundries and factories processing manganese ores. Exposure also occurs in electric battery factories, occasionally resulting in intoxication (Lutier, 1963). Environmental pollution may become an increasing problem as manganese replaces lead in petrol as an anti-knock agent (Mena, 1979).

The disease was first described in 1837 by Couper but was not widely recognized until this century. A high incidence of neurological disease was reported from mines in Morocco (Rodier, 1955), Chile and other countries. Several reports of disease occurring in the USA in manganese ore crushing plants and foundries have been reviewed by Mena (1979).

Clinical features Emotional disturbances are the first manifestation, with irritability, nocturnal insomnia and somnolence by day. More severe psychiatric abnormalities may follow with violent or compulsive behaviour and hallucinations (manganese madness). After some months extrapyramidal disorders appear. These have often been described as similar to parkinsonism. Akinesia and rigidity are prominent and most patients have expressionless facies. However, detailed study of a number of patients indicates that variable degrees of dystonia are usually also present. These cause a characteristic gait, differing from that of parkinsonism particularly in the posture of the legs. Repetitive movements are blocked by stiffness (Barbeau, Inoue and Cloutier, 1976; Mena, 1979).

The disease does not progress when exposure ceases, and indeed considerable improvement occurs if neurological abnormalities have been present for only 1 or 2 years.

Biochemistry In Parkinson's disease degeneration of the dopaminergic nigrostriatal pathway results in decreased dopamine within the striatum. Dopamine and homovanillic acid levels are decreased in the striatum in animals given excess manganese (Bonilla and Diez-Ewald, 1974), but noradrenaline (norepinephrine) is reduced to an even greater extent (Barbeau, Inoue and Cloutier, 1976).

L-Dopa treatment has been successful in some patients with manganese encephalopathy both when hypokinetic and when dystonic features predominate (Mena et al., 1970). Mena et al. (1970) have commented that no choreo-athetotic movements occurred in the hypokinetic patients on a drug regimen which would be expected to produce such movements in some parkinsonian patients.

Human pathology Barbeau, Inoue and Cloutier (1976) have discussed the similarities to and differences from the changes found in classic parkinsonism. In chronic manganese intoxication, in contrast to parkinsonism, the main destructive lesions are found in the striatum and pallidum with little change in the substantia nigra. Thus, in contrast to the main involvement of dopaminergic nigrostriatal pathways in parkinsonism, the pallidum–subthalamic nucleus system is preferentially damaged in chronic manganese intoxication.

Experimental studies Extrapyramidal disorders have been produced in rabbits and monkeys by manganese administration (Barbeau, Inoue and Cloutier, 1976). Pentschew, Ebner and Kovatch (1963) carried out the most detailed pathological study in monkeys after intramuscular injection of manganese dioxide suspended in olive oil. Severe selective damage was found in the subthalamic nucleus and pallidum with neuronal loss and gliosis, many astrocytes having abnormal nuclei. Diffuse abnormal astroglial proliferation was seen throughout the cerebrum, brain stem and cerebellum. The structures involved are the same as those in human manganese encephalopathy.

Mercury

Inorganic mercury

Exposure Exposure to inorganic mercury occurs as an occupational hazard in the manufacture of mirrors and scientific instruments. The potential danger from the mixing of amalgams for dental fillings has been questioned.

As with many other occupational diseases of industrial origin, poisoning was common in the early years of this century. The use of mercury in the felt hat trade gave rise to the phrases 'as mad as a hatter' and 'the hatter's shakes'. There should be little danger of serious mercury intoxication in modern industrial environments.

Clinical features Psychological disturbances are the earliest manifestation of mercury poisoning, consisting of emotional lability, depression, outbursts of anger and insomnia. This syndrome is known as erethism. A coarse tremor develops if exposure continues.

Chelating agents (such as BAL and penicillamine) are effective in removing mercury, and clinical improvement follows.

Human pathology No neuropathological studies have been reported to account for the syndrome of 'hatter's shakes', caused by industrial exposure to mercuric salts. Pink disease of infants, probably caused by mercury sublimate, and now only of historical interest, was known to produce motor and sensory nerve degeneration but no changes in spinal tracts (see Cavanagh, 1973).

Two patients developed dementia and erethism following long-term consumption of laxatives containing mercurous chloride (calomel). Loss of cerebellar granule cells was found in both brains (L. E. Davis et al., 1974).

Experimental studies Noetzel (1955) studied the effects of mercuric chloride in the rat. After 3 months of oral administration, focal necrosis of granule cells was found in the cerebellum. Chang and Hartmann (1972) reported finding axonal degeneration in dorsal roots and the sciatic nerve after giving very small doses of mercuric chloride to rats. Jacobs, Cavanagh and Carmichael (1975) gave similar doses to rats; only very occasional axonal degeneration was found. However, ultrastructural studies of dorsal root ganglion cells showed focal areas of disruption of rough endoplasmic reticulum and, later, a more generalized loss of ribosomes from rough endoplasmic reticulum which was confirmed by quantitative methods. The similarities between the ultrastructural findings in inorganic mercury poisoning and those produced by organic mercury possibly indicate a common mechanism of neurotoxicity at a cellular level.

Organic mercury

Exposure Two different sources of exposure have been responsible for poisoning of many subjects with methyl mercury. Inorganic mercury is a waste product of some industrial processes, most notably in the manufacture of paper and in the chlor-alkali industry. Factory effluent is sometimes discharged into nearby rivers or into the sea. Some micro-organisms in the water have the capacity to convert inorganic mercury salts into methyl mercury. This compound then accumulates in fish to an extent that they become toxic to man or animals if eaten.

Methyl mercury is a cheap and effective fungicide. It is particularly useful for treating wheat seed to produce a healthy crop. When used correctly there is no danger in eating the crop which grows from the treated seed. Eating the seed itself, however, is hazardous.

Serious human disease has resulted from both sources of exposure described above. The first recognized outbreak of disease due to methyl mercury resulting from industrial effluent occurred in Minamata in Japan from 1953 to 1956 (Kurland, Faro and Siedler, 1960). Fifty-six people were affected, of whom one-third died (McAlpine and Araki, 1959). A further similar episode occurred in Niigata, also in Japan.

Larger numbers have been affected by mistakenly eating treated wheat seed, as in the episode in Iraq in 1971 (Bakir et al., 1973). In this episode over 6000 people were affected and at least 500 died. In the USA several members of one family developed organic mercury poisoning after eating a pig which had been fed on treated grain (Pierce et al., 1972).

Clinical features Paraesthesiae develop in and around the mouth and in the extremities. Ataxia is marked and affects particularly gait and whole body movements. Concentric constriction of the visual fields with preservation of a small field of normal central vision is characteristic. This triad of clinical signs is unique to adults with methyl mercury poisoning.

In utero intoxication results in more diffuse CNS involvement with psychomotor retardation rather than the specific focal abnormalities that occur in adults (Marsh et al., 1980).

Human pathology The first description of neuropathological changes in organic mercury poisoning was of a man exposed to methylmercury-containing dust for 4 months; he survived, severely disabled, for 15 years (Hunter and Russell, 1954). The findings in this case, in two other accidentally poisoned men and in ten cases of Minamata disease have been assembled by Shiraki (1979a).

The neuropathological changes are consistent whatever the route of administration. Certain areas of the brain are selectively affected. Most severe are the focal, atrophic changes in the calcarine cortex, a region almost invariably involved from the initial stages of the disease. The precentral and cerebellar cortex are also affected, with less severe atrophy in the postcentral and temporal cortex. The calcarine cortical lesions predominantly involve the depths of the sulci; nerve cell degeneration is seen in the second and upper third layers, with associated astrocytosis, glial cell proliferation around capillaries and the presence of macrophages. In chronic cases all layers may be affected, and in Hunter and Russell's (1954) case in the striate region the thickness of brain tissue between the dilated occipital horn and meninges was reduced to 4 mm in places.

In acute cases (Shiraki, 1979a) and in children (Takeuchi, Eto and Eto, 1979) cerebral cortical lesions may be very extensive, almost the entire cortex showing coarse, spongy disruption. This is also the case in infants affected by prenatal exposure to methyl mercury (Reuhl and Chang, 1979).

The cerebellar cortex is always affected, with

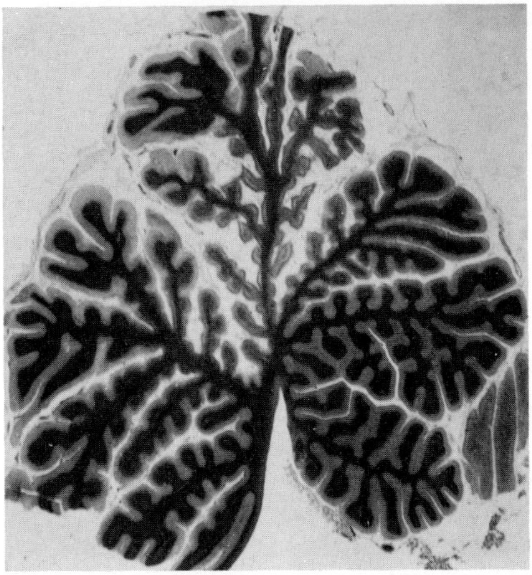

Fig. 14.5 Section of cerebellar vermis from a human case of methyl mercury poisoning. There is lobular atrophy in the declive, extending to adjacent lobules. Loyez' haematoxylin × 2 approx. (Preparation by Professor D. Russell.)

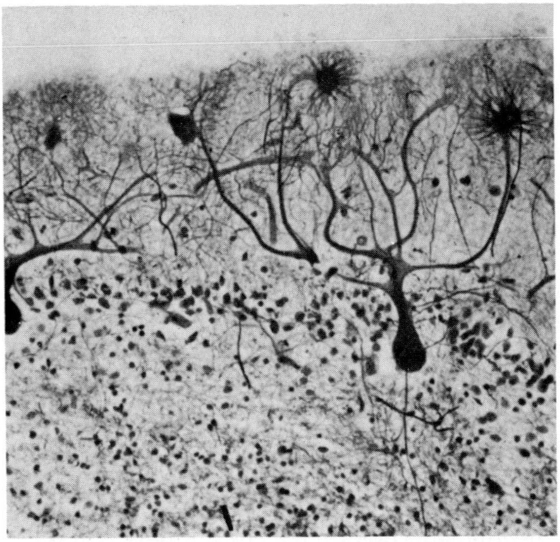

Fig. 14.6 Purkinje cells from a human case of methyl mercury poisoning: the dendrites have radiating spiky processes. Basket fibres are absent from around the cell body. Note loss of granule cells. Hortega's silver impregnation. × 180. (Preparation by Professor D. Russell.)

selective loss of granule cells, particularly in the depths of the sulci (Fig. 14.5); Golgi cell loss was noted by Hunter and Russell (1954). Purkinje cells are usually spared, although curious, radiating, spiny formations at the terminals of the dendrites have been described by Hunter and Russell (Fig. 14.6) and in another chronic case of Minamata disease (Shiraki, 1979a). There were numerous 'torpedoes' on axons of Purkinje cells and also loss of climbing and parallel fibres. Degeneration in the pyramidal tracts was attributed to severe bilateral damage in the precentral cortex in two protracted infant cases. Other regions of the central nervous system were not significantly affected.

There is some uncertainty about changes in the peripheral nervous system. Hunter and Russell (1954) found no abnormalities. Shiraki (1979a) remarked that peripheral nerves have rarely been examined in autopsies of Minamata disease. Eto, Katsuragi and Takeuchi (1976), unpublished data cited by Shiraki, 1979a) and Takeuchi (1977) have described degeneration of posterior columns associated with changes in the dorsal root ganglion cells. Takeuchi noted 'intense involvement of posterior roots and sensory nerve fibres'. In an acute case of poisoning by the intravenous injection of a solution containing ethyl mercury, Shiraki and Nagashima (1977) found degenerative changes in dorsal root ganglion cells, dorsal root and posterior column fibres, although anterior roots were unaffected. The findings in sural nerve biopsies from eight Minamata patients are inconclusive; no degenerative changes were observed although increased numbers of unmyelinated and small myelinated fibres were interpreted as evidence of regeneration (Takeuchi and Eto, 1975, unpublished data cited by Shiraki 1979a). In an electrophysiological study of Iraqi subjects with typical clinical evidence of methyl mercury intoxication, Le Quesne, Damluji and Rustam (1974) found no abnormality of sensory nerves, and suggested that clinical sensory abnormalities in these patients were probably due to lesions in the sensory cortex. It is possible that the degree of sensory nerve involvement may vary according to whether intoxication is acute or chronic.

Experimental studies Different species show variation in the sites of maximal involvement, although the pattern is generally similar to that found in man. Rats were used in the first experimental studies on organic mercury poisoning (Hunter, Bomford and Russell, 1940). A selective involvement of primary sensory neurons was found, which has since been confirmed a number of times (Cavanagh and Chen, 1971). Changes in the CNS are also found in rats (Herman et al., 1973). These include granule cell degeneration and neuronal necrosis in the visual cortex and putamen.

In rabbits, extensive degeneration affected primary sensory neurons, but cerebellar granule and Purkinje cells and neurons in several regions of the forebrain were more severely affected than in rats (Carmichael, Cavanagh and Rodda, 1975). Sensory neurons were particularly affected in the pig (Charlton, 1974). In the cat, lesions predominantly affected the cerebellum, with loss of granule cells (Carbonneau et al., 1974).

In primates, cortical damage is the main feature, and, as in man, the calcarine region is particularly involved (Garman, Weiss and Evans, 1975). Also as in man, peripheral nerves seem to be less affected at an early stage. One monkey exposed to methyl mercury vapour (Hunter, Bomford and Russell, 1940) developed changes in dorsal root ganglion cells, with some peripheral nerve degeneration. Two monkeys acutely intoxicated (Murai et al., 1982) developed abnormal somatosensory evoked potentials but peripheral nerves were normal electrophysiologically and pathologically. These authors suggest that peripheral nerves of primates are less susceptible than those of other species, being affected at a later stage or in chronic poisoning but not in severe acute poisoning.

Ultrastructural studies of the early stages of methyl mercury intoxication in rats showed disorganization of rough endoplasmic reticulum in dorsal root ganglion cells (Herman et al., 1973), which Jacobs, Carmichael and Cavanagh (1975) found to occur focally and particularly at the periphery of cells. The changes observed included degranulation of rough endoplasmic reticulum and, sometimes, complete absence of these protein-synthesizing organelles (Fig. 14.7). Neuronal changes precede axonal degeneration which affects the whole length of nerve fibres with no evidence of a distal pattern. Methyl mercury is thus unusual among neurotoxic substances in causing a neuronopathy rather than distal axonopathy.

In a further ultrastructural study in rabbits,

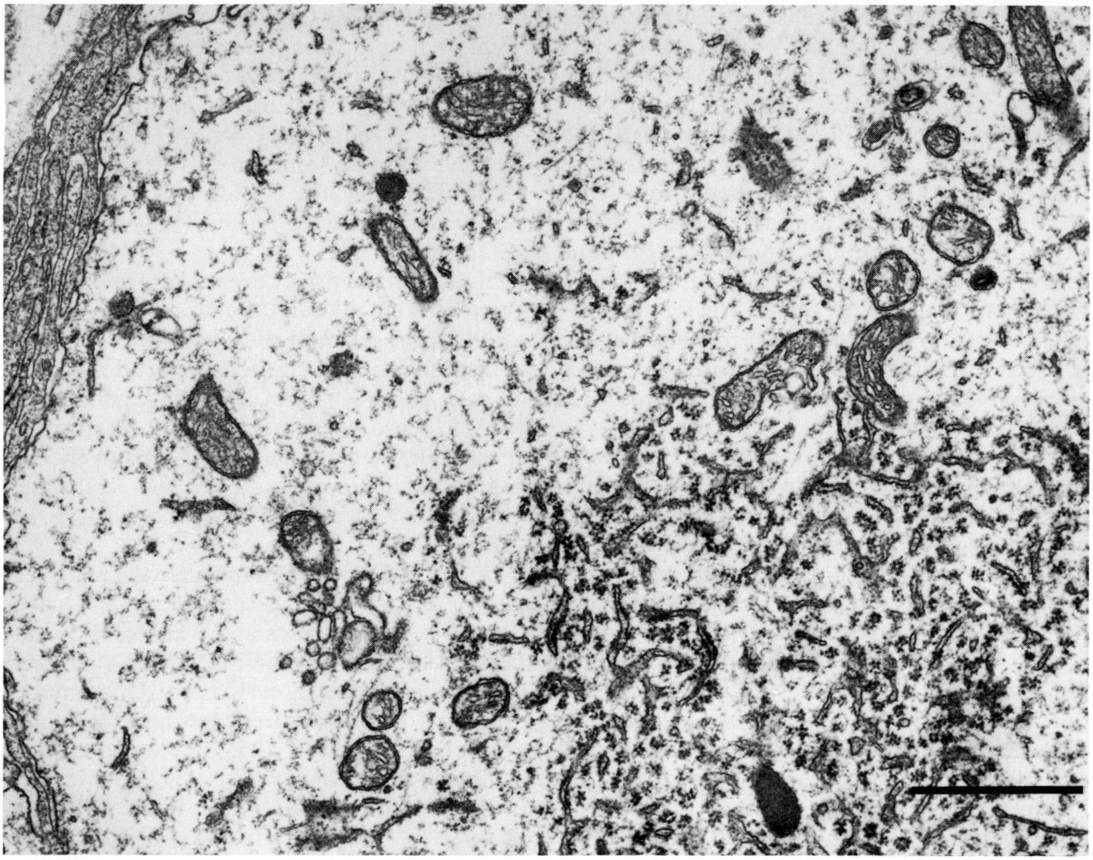

Fig. 14.7 Electron micrograph of part of a dorsal root ganglion cell of a rabbit, showing the changes caused by methyl mercury. There is loss and degranulation of rough endoplasmic reticulum from the peripheral part of the cell. Bar = 1 μm.

Jacobs, Carmichael and Cavanagh (1977) showed that all of the susceptible cell types in the central nervous system (i.e. granule, stellate and basket cells in the cerebellum and neurons of the cerebral cortex) were of small size with a high nuclear/cytoplasmic volume ratio. They suggest that mercury could easily bind to all the rough endoplasmic reticulum in the thin rim of cytoplasm found in these cells, accounting for their selective involvement. The susceptibility of cells in dorsal root ganglia and also in autonomic ganglia may result from the lack of a vascular barrier in these regions, so exposing them to mercury carried in the plasma filtrate (Jacobs, 1980).

Experimental fetal methyl mercury poisoning is known to cause congenital malformations—e.g. exencephaly, encephalocele and hydrocephalus (Reuhl and Chang, 1979). Neuronal loss, cortical cystic change and small haemorrhagic lesions, as well as delayed migration of external granule cells, have been reported.

Biochemistry Short chain alkyl mercury compounds are very neurotoxic. They easily cross the blood–brain barrier, and because of their long biological half-life—about 70 days in man (Magos, 1975)—are rapidly cumulative. Mercurials react with sulphydryl groups that are 'highly unspecific in terms of protein' (Rothstein, 1973). Early *in vitro* studies which had shown that methyl mercury affects protein synthesis were confirmed by Cavanagh and Chen (1971), who found reduced incorporation of amino acids into protein of sensory ganglion cells and peripheral nerves. The ultrastructural finding of ribosomal abnormalities as an early feature of methyl mercury intoxication further corroborated these findings. Methyl mercury probably causes a direct disturbance to ribosomal structure rather than to RNA synthesis (Carmichael and Cavanagh, 1976).

Thallium

Exposure Thallium, one of the heavy metals, was discovered by Sir William Crookes in 1861. Towards the end of that century thallium was found to reduce night sweating in tuberculosis; its depilatory effects were noticed and it came to be used in the treatment of ringworm and also for the removal of hair for cosmetic purposes. Therapeutic usage of thallium was eventually abandoned because of its toxicity.

Thallium is odourless and tasteless; it is employed in a number of industrial processes, but the use of thallium sulphate as a rodenticide and ant-killer presents the most serious hazard for accidental, suicidal and homicidal poisonings. Thallium sulphate is reported to be still widely used in South America and Asia, and is obtainable in the free markets of Italy, France and Germany; it is also used in the southern parts of the USA (Moeschlin, 1980). Kennedy and Cavanagh (1976) described a fatal case of poisoning with Talpinol, a sodium thallate preparation used in Great Britain for killing moles.

One year after Crookes' discovery of thallium, Lamy, a French chemist, also discovered it independently. His suspicions were aroused as to its toxicity when he began to feel pain and weakness in his legs. He fed thallium to various animal species which soon died.

A review of available data by Munch (1934) recorded 778 cases of thallium poisoning, mostly following therapeutic use, with a mortality rate of about 6 per cent. One outbreak of thallium toxicity in California was caused by the consumption of grain treated with thallium to control ground squirrel infestations (Munch, Ginsburg and Nixon, 1933). Moeschlin's review (1980) is based on observations of 70 cases of poisoning since 1939; he points out that thallium has replaced arsenic as a method of homicidal poisoning, and that industrial poisoning is very rare.

Clinical features Clinical effects are dose-dependent. Thallium remains in the tissues for a considerable time, having a half-life of 35 days (Lund, 1956) and so repeated doses are cumulative. A single dose of about 1.5 g thallium sulphate in an adult may cause death due to gastroenteritis, shock and dehydration within a few days (Cavanagh, 1973). Children are apparently less sensitive than adults (Arena, Watson and Sakhadeo, 1965). Following smaller doses the first symptoms are of gastrointestinal disturbance with nausea, vomiting and diarrhoea. One or two weeks later peripheral neuropathy develops, associated with severe pains, particularly in the soles of the feet and the legs but also affecting the joints and sometimes the torso. Disturbed cerebral function results in extreme restlessness, sleep disturbances and theatrical behaviour suggesting a diagnosis of hysteria.

An early sign characteristic of thallium poisoning is dark pigmentation at the root of the hair (Widy, 1959); scalp hairs are more likely to be thus affected than hairs on the chest and legs. Eyebrow and eyelid hairs are least affected because they grow less rapidly. At first, hairs are easily plucked but later they fall out spontaneously; after about 3 weeks there may be total or almost complete alopecia. Body hair and the inner third of the eyebrow hairs are characteristically spared. In the skin there is damage to sweat and sebaceous glands, giving the skin a dry and scaly appearance. Impairment of nail growth results in lunular stripes (Mees' stripes) across the finger nails.

Tachycardia and hypertension may develop during the second week whilst the polyneuropathy becomes increasingly severe. There is numbness of fingers and toes and impaired sensation to pinprick, touch and proprioception. Motor weakness begins distally, later extending to more proximal parts. In severe and fatal cases cranial nerves may be markedly affected. Evidence of central nervous system involvement includes optic neuropathy, psychosis, choreo-athetosis and coma. Ataxia is common and may be of central or peripheral origin.

Biochemistry Thallium has a number of physical properties in common with potassium. These include similarities in the size of their crystal radii and their charges, and also the ability to form complex salts with one another. Thallium ions can compete with potassium ions in biological systems; the affinity of thallium for the potassium site of the enzyme Na^+/K^+-activated adenosine triphosphatase is many times higher than that of potassium. This enzyme is present in membranes of many cell types and particularly in neural tissue, involved as it is in the maintenance of intracellular potassium ion concentration. By becoming part of this enzyme thallium can cross membranes and enter cells. This property provides the rationale for the treatment of thallium poisoning with potassium chloride. Whilst thallium excretion is increased there is also a release of intracellular stores of thallium which exacerbates symptoms often so severely as to limit treatment (Bank et al., 1972).

How thallium acts inside the cell is uncertain; it appears to have an affinity for mitochondria and has been used as a vital stain for their demonstration. Mitochondrial abnormalities have been described in many cell types in thallium-treated rats (Herman and Bensch, 1967), and in sural nerve biopsies from cases of thallium poisoning (Spencer and Schaumburg, 1976a; L.E. Davis et al., 1980). *In vitro* studies have shown striking mitochondrial changes (Spencer et al., 1973).

Thallium probably behaves like other metals in combining with sulphydryl compounds, perhaps affecting the structural proteins, particularly those of the tegmentum, such as keratin, which contain large numbers of cysteine residues. Cavanagh and Gregson (1978) were of the opinion that such changes were unlikely to lead to hair loss, and their studies on mitosis in hair follicles in rats showed a decline in mitotic rate, possibly associated with a disturbance of energy metabolism.

Distal fibre degeneration affecting both central and peripheral nerves is now recognized as a characteristic feature of thallium intoxication (see the sections below on 'Human pathology' and 'Experimental studies'). The biochemical defects underlying this pattern of degeneration have been the subject of much speculation, particularly since similar patterns of nerve fibre damage are found in a wide variety of toxic conditions and enzyme deficiency states as well as in diseases such as motor neuron disease and Friedreich's ataxia. In seeking a common denominator to explain these neuropathies, Cavanagh (1979) has drawn attention to similarities between vitamin deficiencies and toxic neuropathies; he suggests that defects in energy metabolism, and in particular coenzymes, may be common to many of them. Thallium is known to interact with riboflavin, and might therefore cause a depletion of flavin coenzymes. Cavanagh (1979) has postulated that loss of such enzymes from multiple sites along the fibre may lead to axonal degeneration; proximal parts of the axon would be spared because of replacement of the depleted enzymes from their site of synthesis in the perikaryon.

Diagnostic tests Conclusive evidence of thallium intoxication rests on the demonstration of thallium in tissues, excreta and body fluids. A simple screening test using rhodamine B to form a red fluorescent colour (Bank et al., 1972) is sensitive to 0.03 μg/ml. Microgram quantities can be detected using flame spectrophotometry (Amore, 1974), and neutron activation methods will give the thallium content of a single hair (Specht and Rohner, 1960). Thallium can be detected in cremation ash despite the high temperatures used (1000°C). Black pigmentation in the root of the hair is an early diagnostic sign; repeated doses produce zones of pigmentation.

There is no evidence that BAL or EDTA are beneficial in the treatment of thallium poisoning. Prussian blue (potassium ferric cyanoferrate II) appears to be the most effective therapy, binding thallium which is excreted in bile in an unabsorbable form. Kamerback et al. (1971) reported increased faecal excretion and clinical improvement following its use.

Human pathology Except for evidence of hepatotoxicity, the principal pathological changes are found in the nervous system (Cavanagh et al., 1974). The brain may appear swollen and oedematous with scattered haemorrhages. Microscopical examination shows variable degrees of oedema in the white matter of cerebral and cerebellar hemispheres (Prick, 1979). Cavanagh et al. (1974) noticed extensive and recent areas of oedema and necrosis in the subthalamic regions, substantia nigra and across corticospinal pathways but found no neuronal changes. Prick (1979) describes degenerative changes in nerve cells in the cerebral and cerebellar cortex, hypothalamic nuclei, olivary nuclei and corpus striatum without a glial reaction.

Degeneration of peripheral nerves and chromatolysis of motor neurons has long been a recognized feature of thallium intoxication (Munch, Ginsburg and Nixon, 1933; Gettler and Weiss, 1943). An extensive study of these changes was made by Cavanagh et al. (1974) in three victims of a poisoner, and by Kennedy and Cavanagh

(1976) in another fatal case. Careful sampling showed a distal pattern of nerve degeneration, large intramuscular nerve bundles, the sural nerve and the vagus nerve in the chest showing widespread fibre degeneration whilst the more proximal nerves such as the upper sciatic, the spinal roots, and the cranial nerves at their origins showed minimal changes. Shorter nerves such as the oculomotor were affected and they also showed a distal pattern of fibre degeneration.

The spinal changes in the case described by Kennedy and Cavanagh (1976) confirm that the central axons of sensory ganglion cells also show a distal or 'dying-back' type of degeneration. In spinal ganglia, Nageotte nodules were seen in addition to chromatolytic ganglion cells. Apart from occasional degenerating fibres in the corticospinal tracts, the posterior columns contained the only tracts in the spinal cord showing pathological change.

Experimental studies No entirely satisfactory animal model of human thallotoxicosis has yet been found, although a few species are known to be susceptible and to display signs of nervous system involvement. Kaeser (1962) described electrophysiological abnormalities and degeneration of peripheral nerve fibres in guinea-pigs following thallium administration. Although rats injected with thallium show no clinical evidence of neuropathy, ultrastructural changes were found in their peripheral nerves (Spencer and Schaumburg, 1976a). The axons contained swollen mitochondria similar to those found in a sural nerve biopsy in human thallium poisoning. These mitochondrial abnormalities were felt to be non-specific but more numerous than in other toxic axonopathies. *In vitro* studies of cord–ganglia–muscle cultures exposed to thallium salts showed axonal swellings (Peterson and Murray, 1965) later found to be caused by swelling of mitochondria in axons but not in other cell types; these changes were reversible on withdrawal of thallium from the cultures (Spencer at al., 1973).

Kennedy and Cavanagh (1977) studied the effects of thallium on the nervous system in the cat. After careful dosing, the cats developed functional neurological disturbances such as ataxia and hypotonia. Pathological changes were confined to the axons of primary sensory neurons, motor nerves being unaffected. Evidence of fibre degeneration was found in posterior columns of the cord, particularly in the cervical region where the longer gracile tracts were more severely affected than the cuneate tracts, a pattern suggesting distal degeneration of the longest fibres. In peripheral nerves, sensory fibre degeneration caused denervation changes in the skin, particularly of the hindfeet. Chromatolytic cells were found in spinal and trigeminal ganglia. The sparing of motor fibres may be explained by the presence, within muscle, of a large reservoir of potassium ions which could 'dilute' the thallium ions, reducing their damaging effects.

Tin

Exposure Inorganic tin is not neurotoxic. Of the 200–300 organic tin compounds synthesized, only two are known to be neurotoxic. Each produces a completely different type of lesion in the CNS.

Triethyl tin, present as an impurity in a preparation used to treat boils, was the cause of an outbreak of poisoning in France in 1953–54. The preparation, called Stalinon, was supposed to consist of diethyltin diiodide, but triethyltin diiodide was found in concentrations of up to 10 per cent. Neurological symptoms due to raised intracranial pressure appeared suddenly within a few days of taking the drug; 110 patients died and at least 100 others were permanently affected.

Trimethyl tin poisoning has been reported in two chemists who were synthesizing an organotin compound. Both developed mental confusion and generalized epileptic seizures after an acute exposure; they appeared to recover completely after removal from exposure (Fortemps et al., 1978).

Triethyl tin

Clinical features The clinical course of triethyl tin intoxication in the patients treated with Stalinon was described by Alajouanine, Derobert and Thieffry (1958). Severe and persistent headache, photophobia, vomiting and drowsiness developed within about 4 days of starting treatment. In addition to symptoms and signs of raised intracranial pressure, some patients developed a flaccid paraparesis, sensory loss with a distinct upper limit and loss of sphincter control. Death occurred in almost half of the cases within 4–10 days. Patients with cerebral symptoms recovered slowly, but paraplegia was irreversible.

Human pathology Cossa et al. (1958) and Gruner (1958) each examined 4 fatal cases of poisoning following Stalinon treatment. Macroscopic brain swelling was seen in all cases, with compression of the ventricles. There was generalized oedema of the white matter, particularly striking in the centrum semiovale. The oedema seemed to be caused by large numbers of microvacuoles affecting, or related to, the myelin sheaths. Axons were relatively unaffected. Grey matter showed only slight oedema and there was no evidence of neuronal degeneration.

Experimental studies It has been known for over a century that triethyl tin causes paralysis, convulsions and coma in experimental animals (see Foncin and Gruner, 1979). In 1957, Magee, Stoner and Barnes (1957) fed rats with the compound in their diet for 7–9 days. The animals developed paralysis, first affecting the hindlimbs but later involving all limbs. Two-thirds of the rats died during the third week; the others, still receiving tin but at a lower dose, appeared to recover for about 2 weeks and then developed tremors and convulsions. Watanabe (1980) refers to a number of other experimental studies; weakness or paralysis was a common finding, with functional recovery when triethyl tin administration was discontinued. Young mice were more sensitive to triethyl tin than were mature animals (Watanabe, 1977).

Acute intoxication of suckling rats caused diffuse haemorrhagic lesions throughout the brain but particularly in the cerebellum (Suzuki, 1971).

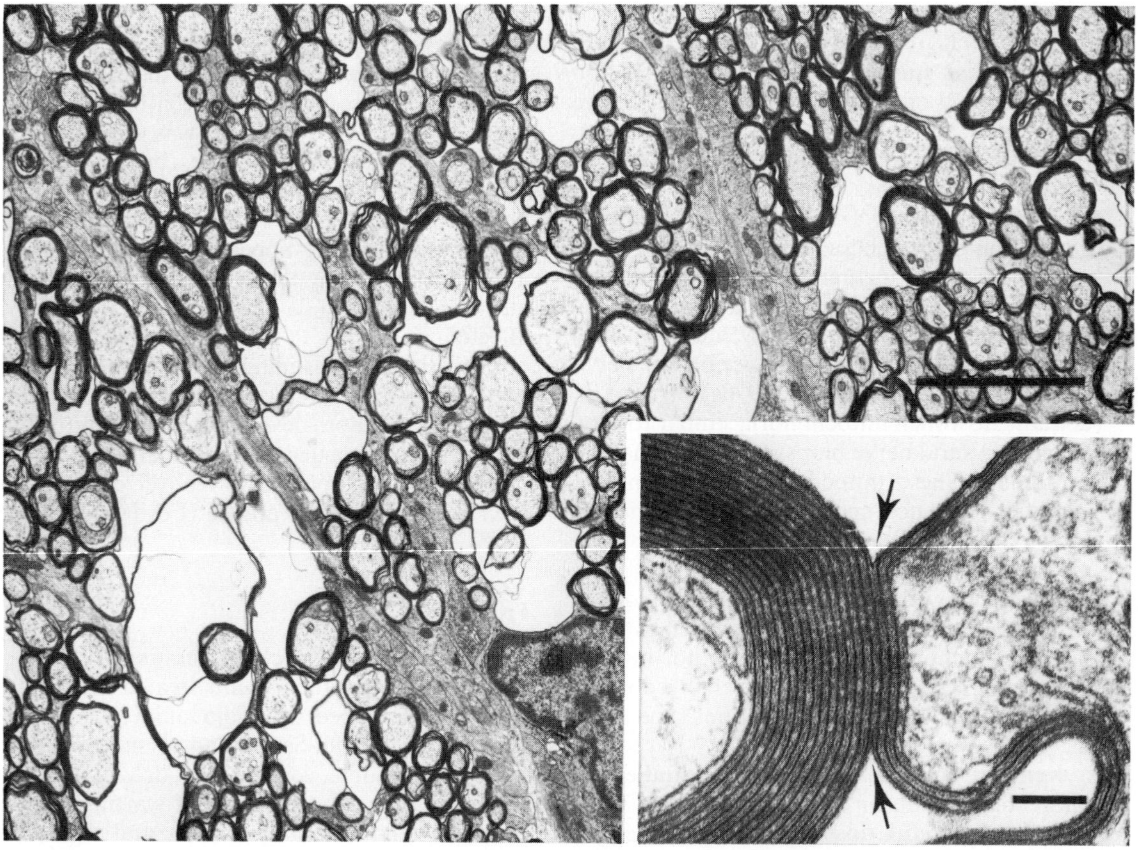

Fig. 14.8 Electron micrograph of optic nerve from a rat given intravenous triethyl tin (10 mg/kg) 4 hours previously. Numerous intramyelinic vacuoles are shown; there is no swelling of astrocyte or glial processes. Bar = 5 μm. *Inset*. Electron micrograph at higher magnification from the same optic nerve, showing separation of myelin at the intraperiod line (arrows). Bar = 0.1 μm.

Similar haemorrhagic lesions were found in suckling rats poisoned with lead, indium, terbium, thallium and mercury (Gabbiani, Baic and Deziel, 1967).

Magee, Stoner and Barnes (1957) found the brain and spinal cord of rats treated with triethyl tin to be grossly enlarged; there was bulging of the white matter at the cut surface. The diffuse sponginess of white matter was due to vacuolations which, by light microscopy, appeared to be closely associated with myelin sheaths. Later electron microscope studies showed that the vacuoles formed within the myelin sheath by splitting of lamellae at the intraperiod line (Aleu, Katzman and Terry, 1963). Myelin vacuolation appears to be the sole pathological change induced by triethyl tin. Astrocyte swelling has been described by Torack, Gordon and Prokop (1970) who felt this was an intermediate step in the movement of fluid into the myelin sheath. Jacobs, Cremer and Cavanagh (1977) examined the brains of rats within 1–2 hours of intravenous triethyl tin; they found that intramyelin vacuoles appeared directly in the sheaths with no accompanying or preceding changes in astrocytes or oligodendrocytes (Fig. 14.8). Triethyl tin is known to have a high affinity binding constant for myelin (Lock and Aldridge, 1975) and this property may explain the extremely selective localization of the vacuoles. Kirschner and Sapirstein (1982) used x-ray diffraction to detect myelin swelling, producing a periodicity of 200Å (normally 150–165 Å), which preceded movement of fluid into the sheath. In these studies of triethyl-tin-treated rats, changes were seen in the myelin of the central but not of the peripheral nervous system. Graham and Gonatas (1973) described myelin changes in the peripheral nerves of rats fed with triethyl tin; however, few fibres were affected and there is clearly a difference in susceptibility between central and peripheral myelin.

Trimethyl tin

Experimental studies The neurotoxicity of trimethyl tin was investigated following suggestions that it could be used in dentures to make them radio-opaque (see Le Quesne, 1981). Brown et al. (1979) dosed rats with trimethyl tin; the animals developed tremors, hyperexcitability and aggressive behaviour. Histological studies showed significant pathology only in the nervous system; bilateral and symmetrical loss of neurons was found, first affecting the hippocampus (h2 and h3–5) with later involvement of h1 (see Fig. 14.4), the pyriform cortex and the amygdaloid nucleus. In affected regions the neurons showed condensation and clumping of nuclear chromatin, with shrunken and eosinophilic cytoplasm. Dissolution of Nissl substance appeared to be an early change, eventually leading to cell death and removal by phagocytosis. Another type of neuronal change described as 'selective chromatolysis' was seen in some animals.

Bouldin et al. (1981) studied the ultrastructural changes in the hippocampal formation and pyriform cortex of rats after acute and chronic dosing with trimethyl tin. Earliest changes were the appearance of dense-cored vesicles and tubules which showed acid phosphatase activity and resembled Golgi-associated endoplasmic reticulum. Later, autophagic vacuoles and polymorphic dense bodies accumulated in affected neurons. These changes appear to be unique to trimethyl tin intoxication. The 'selective chromatolysis' in some neurons was found to be associated with collections of dense-cored vesicles; the cells did not show the typical changes of chromatolysis which particularly involve the rough endoplasmic reticulum.

Bismuth

Exposure Bismuth salts are used medicinally in the management of chronic gastrointestinal disorders and for colostomy control. They are used infrequently in the UK but, until recently, on a wider scale in some other countries (e.g. France).

Neurological disease ascribable to bismuth occurred as an epidemic in France between 1974 and 1978, when approximately 1000 patients were affected (Martin-Bouyer, 1978). A few patients were affected in Australia, from where the disease was first reported (Burns, Thomas and Barron, 1974).

Clinical features Bismuth encephalopathy becomes manifest gradually with anxiety, depression and irritability followed by rapid deterioration associated with confusion, dysarthria and myclonus. Gait disturbance is prominent. Coma and death may supervene. On stopping the drug recovery is often complete, or there may be some residual memory loss.

Biochemistry Raised blood bismuth levels have been found in all those with bismuth encephalopathy. Values ranging from 100 to 3000 $\mu g/l$ were recorded in 58 affected subjects (Hillemand et al., 1977) compared with levels less than 50 $\mu g/l$ in asymptomatic patients on comparable doses. Raised levels in cerebral tissue have also been detected at post-mortem, the highest values being found in frontal cortex, basal ganglia and cerebellar cortex (Escourolle et al., 1977). The reasons why some patients become ill and others on a similar dose regimen do not is unknown, as are the reasons why this hitherto unknown disease should suddenly appear in epidemic proportions in a circumscribed part of the world.

Human pathology Marked loss of cerebellar Purkinje cells has been described with necrotic lesions in h1, h2 and h3 fields of Ammon's horn (Liessens et al., 1978). Neuronal loss with microglial proliferation was also described in the basal ganglia. The patient described by Liessens et al. (1978) died of septicaemia, and some cerebral lesions were attributed to infection and anoxia. No specific diagnostic pathological features were identified.

Cadmium

Exposure Cadmium is found in low concentrations as a natural constituent of some soils and waters. More important sources of contamination are industrial processes such as smelting and refining of zinc and lead ores, combustion of coal and oil, and the disposal of waste products. Non-occupational exposure to cadmium is mainly through contaminated food; cigarette smoking also causes an increase in the body burden of cadmium (Webb, 1975).

Cadmium is not known to be neurotoxic to man. In Japan, severe and prolonged exposure to cadmium from industrially polluted waters produced a syndrome of osteomalacia, multiple fractures and renal tubular dysfunction, predominantly affecting postmenopausal women and called itai-itai disease (Friberg et al., 1974). Continuous low level exposure to cadmium may cause kidney damage and is possibly a causative factor in producing hypertension (Schroeder and Vinton, 1969).

Experimental studies Cadmium-induced damage to the CNS has been produced only in neonatal animals. Rats and rabbits (Gabbiani, Baic and Deziel, 1967) and mice (Webster and Valois, 1981) given cadmium chloride subcutaneously during the first 3 weeks of life developed haemorrhages with neuronal destruction in the cerebrum and cerebellum. The youngest animals were the most vulnerable; the localization of damage was apparently to regions with only partially differentiated capillaries (Webster and Valois, 1981). Electron microscopy showed abnormalities of capillaries, vacuolation and thinning of endothelial cells, widening of interendothelial gaps and eventual degeneration. Damage to neural elements appeared to be secondary to these endothelial changes. No CNS changes were produced after giving cadmium to animals more than 3 weeks old.

In older animals, subcutaneous administration of cadmium produced haemorrhagic lesions in dorsal root and gasserian ganglia, with necrosis of some ganglion cells; guinea-pigs, golden hamsters, rats and mice were all affected (Gabbiani, Gregory and Baic, 1967). Vascular changes similar to those found in the CNS were described by Schlaepfer (1971a) and Gabbiani et al. (1974). These lesions were thought to be selective for sensory ganglion cells, but in a more recent study in mice, Arvidson (1980) described similar vascular changes in the sciatic nerve and superior cervical ganglion but not in the coeliac ganglion. Neuronal changes were limited to sensory ganglion cells.

It is not clear why only certain parts of the nervous system vasculature should be affected. Although ganglionic blood vessels are fenestrated this feature appears not to be essential for cadmium-induced damage.

Long-term exposure to cadmium in drinking water produced a peripheral neuropathy in rats, demyelination being found in nerves and roots (Sato et al., 1978). A characteristic feature was the presence of glycogenosomes in peripheral nerve axons, possibly related to the inhibition of alpha-glucosidase by cadmium (Hamada et al., 1981).

Gold

Exposure Exposure to gold occurs through the use of sodium aurothiomalate in the treatment of rheumatoid arthritis. It was widely used for many years following its introduction in 1927. Since the advent of other potent drugs (e.g. steroids) it has become less used, but still has a place in therapy.

Clinical features Neurological complications of gold therapy are rare compared with skin lesions, which are common (Hartfall, Garland and Goldie, 1937). In addition to peripheral neuropathy, cranial nerve disorders and psychiatric symptoms have been described (Endtz, 1958). Neuropathy may be symmetrical and distal but in some instances rapid onset of asymmetrical weakness and sensory symptoms has been described (Lescher, 1936). The sudden onset of asymmetrical neurological abnormalities, sometimes associated with fever and rash, suggests that there may be an immune basis to the condition in such instances.

Human pathology Some data are available from nerve biopsy studies by Walsh (1970) and Katrak et al. (1980): findings have varied. Walsh (1970) described acute axonal degeneration affecting fibres of all sizes in the sural nerve of one patient. Amongst the three nerves studied by Katrak et al (1980), one showed predominant segmental demyelination. Thus, full pathological details about this type of neuropathy remain to be elucidated.

Experimental studies A mixture of axonal degeneration and segmental demyelination which was dose-related in severity has been produced in peripheral nerves of rats treated with sodium aurothiomalate (Katrak et al., 1980). This observation makes it likely that a direct toxic rather than an immune mechanism is responsible for the development of this experimental neuropathy. However, the rarity of the complication in clinical practice suggests that there might be some predisposing factor necessary for the development of clinical neuropathy.

Platinum

Cis-platinum (*cis*-diamminedichloroplatinum, *cis*-platin) was introduced as a chemotherapeutic agent during the 1970s. The dose that can be given is limited mainly by renal toxicity. Ototoxicity, with tinnitus and high frequency hearing loss, is also a complication. Sensory peripheral neuropathy has occurred in a number of patients on high doses (several courses of 75–100 mg/m^2 body surface area).

Biopsy of a sural nerve from one patient showed loss of axons; loss of axons with gliosis in the posterior columns were found in a *post mortem* study of a child who had been treated with high doses of platinum (Hemphill et al., 1980).

Weakness of the hindlimbs and unsteadiness developed in rats given high doses of *cis*-platinum (Clark et al., 1980). Pathological examination showed axonal degeneration in peripheral nerves and also abnormal axons in the optic disc, retrolaminar optic nerve and long tracts of the spinal cord. Affected axons were filled with malorientated neurofilaments and some were degenerating.

Tellurium

Exposure Tellurium is an uncommon metal, widely distributed and found mostly as the telluride of other metals. Its industrial uses are varied, particularly because it has both metallic and non-metallic properties. Tellurium-containing fumes are the most common source of industrial exposure. Tellurium-132 is one of the fission products released in atomic reactor accidents.

Tellurium compounds were formerly used in the treatment of leprosy, syphilis, trypanosomiasis, seborrhoeic dermatitis, and in pulmonary tuberculosis to relieve night sweating.

Clinical features Reports of cases of acute and chronic exposure to tellurium-containing fumes describe symptoms and signs which include epigastric tenderness, headache, dizziness, nausea, somnolence, a skin rash and suppression of sweating. Black discoloration of exposed skin can persist for many weeks. The lethal dose is approximately 2 g.

Biochemistry Tellurium fumes are readily absorbed in the lungs. After oral administration tellurium compounds are reduced to elemental tellurium in the gut and most is excreted in the faeces. De Meio and Henriques (1947) showed the brain to contain less of an injected dose than did other organs.

Experimental studies Tellurium is neurotoxic to experimental animals, and three different effects have been described depending on the age at which the substance is administered; hydrocephalus, peripheral neuropathy and lipofuscinosis.

Hydrocephalus Pregnant rats fed on a diet containing 3500 p.p.m. elemental tellurium produce offspring with hydrocephalus; most die within 1 month (Garro and Pentschew, 1964). Duckett, Sandler and Scott (1971) found that the tenth to fifteenth day of gestation was the critical period for development of hydrocephalus. Agnew, Fauvre and Pudenz (1968) had shown that radioactive tellurium crosses the placental barrier and rapidly reaches the fetal brain, where uptake is higher than in the maternal brain. Initially, the hydrocephalus is of a communicating (non-obstructive) type which appears to develop at birth. Later, obstructions, such as closure of the foramina of the fourth ventricle or of the cerebral aqueduct, may develop. The cause of the hydrocephalus is not known. Ultrastructural studies show flattening of ventricular ependymal cells and subependymal oedema, but these are probably secondary changes (Duckett, 1971). Possible mechanisms in the formation of hydrocephalus include overproduction of CSF or failure of its absorption. In man, CSF is absorbed by arachnoidal granulations, but many animals (including the rat) have no arachnoidal granulations. The hydrocephalus produced by tellurium is an interesting experimental model which is both selective and reproducible.

Peripheral neuropathy Weanling rats about 18 days of age, fed on a diet containing elemental tellurium, develop peripheral neuropathy mainly involving sciatic nerves and lumbar spinal roots (Lampert, Garro and Pentschew, 1970). The rats show hindlimb paralysis from about the fourth day of feeding; by the tenth day they begin to recover despite continued intake of tellurium.

Electron microscopy shows the earliest changes to take place in Schwann cells after 2 days of feeding. Endoplasmic reticulum becomes dilated and appears to engulf small quantities of cytoplasm, with eventual formation of membranous whorls surrounding altered cytoplasm; other organelles are relatively unaffected. The Schwann cell cytoplasm retracts, leaving myelin lamellae in direct contact with basal lamina. Myelin sheaths then degenerate, beginning at Schmidt–Lanterman clefts and nodes of Ranvier. Lamellae split at the intraperiod line, separate and form vesicular debris. By 1 week macrophages have penetrated the basal lamina and removed the myelin. Schwann cells associated with unmyelinated fibres are not affected (Lampert and Garrett, 1971).

Teased sciatic nerves show myelin irregularities in most fibres by the second day of feeding with tellurium; a day later paranodal and segmental demyelination is widespread. Some fibres also show axonal degeneration (Duckett et al., 1979). Marked endoneurial oedema develops subsequent to the myelin degeneration (Lampert and Garrett, 1971). Remyelination begins from the tenth day by a normal process of myelinogenesis, coinciding with functional recovery.

Recent studies by Said and Duckett (1981) describe changes in the peripheral nerves and roots of adult rats fed with tellurium for 3 months; these changes are similar to, but less severe than, those found in young rats.

Lipofuscinosis Chronic administration of tellurium causes a gross blackening of the brain (and other organs) in a number of experimental animals. Duckett and White (1974) found electron-dense needle-shaped crystals and granules in neurons, which were shown by electron dispersive x-ray spectrophotometry to contain tellurium. Tellurium was found within lipofuscin granules, and these became more numerous with longer periods of dosing. Yuen, Agnew and Carregal (1975) found preferential uptake of tellurium into the choroid plexus of rats and rabbits. Increased numbers of lysosomes were found in choroidal epithelial cells, many containing needle-like crystals. Although tellurium persists in the brain parenchyma for many months after cessation of intake, it is cleared quite rapidly from choroid plexus cells, possibly by exocytosis of tellurium-laden lysosomes.

Industrial and environmental chemicals

Acrylamide

Exposure The main industrial use of acrylamide is as a grouting agent in tunnel construction and mining operations. Acrylamide monomer is poured into the soil and, with a catalyst, polymerizes making the soil stable. It is also used for separating solids from solution. Its use as a paper strengthener brings a possible hazard in the food industry because there is a theoretical danger from using paper so treated for packaging food. Acrylamide monomer is neurotoxic, but once polymerized it is no longer toxic. The greatest industrial exposure occurs with those involved in the polymerization process on a large scale and in workers handling large amounts of the monomer in the construction industry.

Neurological symptoms were recognized as a possible complication of acrylamide exposure when the substance was first manufactured commercially in the early 1960s (Fullerton and Barnes, 1966). A few workers developed paraesthesiae which disappeared when they were removed from contact with acrylamide. At the same time animal tests revealed its neurotoxic effects. Since then there have been several reports of groups of workers who have developed neurological disorders following occupational exposure (Garland and Patterson, 1967; Kesson, Baird and Lawson, 1977).

Clinical features The exact nature of the disease depends on the severity of exposure. Intoxication after prolonged low level exposure causes peripheral neuropathy with sensory involvement occurring first, followed by weakness. Mild or moderate neuropathy will disappear when exposure ceases. After heavier exposure ataxia is prominent in addition to sensorimotor peripheral neuropathy. Encephalopathy with psychotic manifestations and coma has been described in some individuals with heavy exposure (Igisu et al., 1975). These subjects developed peripheral neuropathy some days after the onset of encephalopathy.

Additional clinical manifestations are skin changes causing redness of the hands and marked sweating of the extremities. Weight loss, drowsiness and sphincter disturbances are other notable features.

Human pathology In view of the nature of the condition little information is available. Sural nerves obtained by biopsy from two patients during recovery showed that large diameter fibres had been predominantly affected (Fullerton, 1969). Many regenerating fibres were recognized but no further details of the pathological process were revealed.

Experimental studies Fullerton and Barnes (1966) studied peripheral neuropathy in rats after chronic administration of acrylamide. The neuropathy was recognized to be due to a dying-back type of axonal degeneration affecting particularly the large diameter fibres, and thus associated with a slight reduction of maximal nerve conduction velocity. By ultrastructural examination, Prineas (1969b) demonstrated that neurofilaments accumulate in the axons before they degenerate (Fig. 14.9), such changes being initially most marked distally. When degeneration starts, neurofilaments accumulate at nodes and in the paranodal regions more proximally.

Schaumburg, Wiśniewski and Spencer (1974) found the earliest morphological change to be loss of filopod processes in nerve terminals of pacinian corpuscles in toe pads. Primary and then secondary annulospiral endings of muscle spindles were affected before motor nerve terminals. These morphological changes correlate well with physiological studies by Sumner and Asbury (1975), showing failure of response of muscle stretch receptors at an early stage of intoxication.

Tsujihata, Engel and Lambert (1974) have described sequential ultrastructural changes at neuromuscular junctions in more detail. The nerve terminal becomes distended with neurofilaments and some terminals disappear. Mitochondria and synaptic vesicles are decreased. Although degeneration occurs in the longest motor nerve fibres before shorter ones, Jennekens et al. (1979) reported that enlarged terminal swellings occurred equally in fibres of the same diameter regardless of whether axons were short or long, these changes thus being independent of total axonal volume.

Souryi, Chretien and Droz (1981) studied axonal transport following acrylamide administration to chickens and found an increased ac-

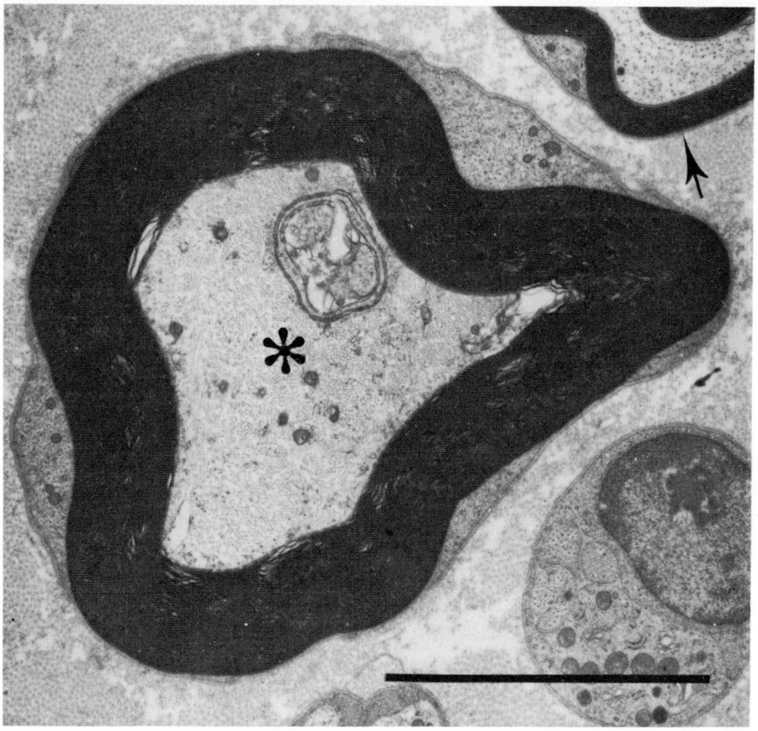

Fig. 14.9 Electron micrograph from the sciatic nerve of a rat dosed with acrylamide (20 mg/kg) for 27 weeks. The axon of a myelinated fibre contains an increased number of filaments (*); compare the filament density with that of an unaffected axon (arrow). Bar = 5 μm.

cumulation of fast transported protein preterminally with depletion at the nerve endings, suggesting a multifocal retention in the distal part of the axon. In a further electron microscopic radio-autographic study, Chretien et al. (1981) found intense labelling by fast axonally transported protein of tubulovesicular profiles of smooth endoplasmic reticulum, dense-cored vesicles and mitochondria preterminally. They suggested that the local disorganization of smooth endoplasmic reticulum which they observed distally could cause focal stasis of fast transported protein. However, these authors and Cavanagh and Gysbers (1981) have pointed out that similar changes in smooth endoplasmic reticulum have been seen in other conditions and the exact relevance of the observation to axonal degeneration in acrylamide neuropathy is uncertain.

Unmyelinated fibres are also involved when intoxication is severe (Post and McLeod, 1977). As in myelinated fibres, the largest and longest fibres degenerate first and neurofilaments accumulate before fibres degenerate completely.

Distal ends of central nerve fibres are involved to a lesser extent, with similar accumulation of neurofilaments (Prineas, 1969b; Spencer and Schaumburg, 1977). The latter authors also demonstrated involvement of mossy endings in the rostral cerebellar vermis.

Cavanagh (1982) studied sequential changes in rats in many regions of the nervous system, demonstrating widespread swelling and neurofilamentous accumulation in nerve terminals, only some of which eventually degenerate, and stressing the unique nature of this particular toxic lesion. In addition, there was acute degeneration of some Purkinje cells. A chromatolytic response was seen in some spinal ganglion cells before the onset of axonal degeneration, a finding confirmed by Sterman (1982a).

When exposure to acrylamide ceases there is functional, electrophysiological and histological evidence of regeneration. Fullerton and Barnes (1966) found regenerating nerves amongst degenerating fibres during continuous administration of low doses of acrylamide. Morgan-Hughes, Sinclair and Durston (1974), however, found that the capacity for regeneration following nerve crush was impaired during acrylamide administration. They demonstrated extensive degenerative changes proximal to the site of crush. Cavanagh and Gysbers (1980) also studied this phenomenon and found that the extent and degree of degeneration above the site of total degeneration produced by a tight ligature was dose-dependent and that it also occurred if acrylamide was given 1 week after nerve ligation. Changes could be found as high as 5 cm above the ligature. Ultrastructural examination (Cavanagh and Gysbers, 1981) revealed accumulation of smooth endoplasmic reticulum and vesicles, particularly proximal to nodes of Ranvier and in internodal regions, but without accumulation of neurofilaments, before degeneration occurred, in the segments above the ligature. The changes were similar to those described preterminally following acrylamide administration by Chretien et al. (1981) and to those seen above a ligature although over a shorter distance in normal nerves.

Carbon disulphide

Exposure The viscose rayon and viscose film industries are now the only known source of occupational exposure to carbon disulphide (CS_2); vapour of CS_2 is given off during the synthesis process. But the association between CS_2 and human neurological disease goes back to the 1950s when CS_2 was extensively used in the 'cold' vulcanization of rubber.

Carbon disulphide is toxic to many tissues, but its most important effects are on the cardiovascular and nervous systems. A comprehensive account of the neurotoxicity of CS_2 is given by Seppäläinen and Haltia (1980).

Clinical features Exposure to the high levels of CS_2 produced in the vulcanization process commonly caused acute psychotic symptoms of a maniacal or depressive type. This kind of exposure is now of historical interest only. As a result of chronic CS_2 exposure caused by poor working conditions in the viscose industry during World War II, symptoms of polyneuropathy were common, as were psychological disturbances with depression and an increased rate of suicide.

Clinical evidence of polyneuropathy may develop within 4–6 months of moderately heavy exposure (> 170 p.p.m.) or after several years of exposure to 65–100 p.p.m. As many as 80 per cent of exposed workers may show symptoms and signs of neuropathy; at lower levels, neuropathy may develop after many years of exposure. Paraesthesiae, sensory loss, and muscle pain and weakness occur distally in the limbs, particularly in the legs. In severe cases there may be difficulty in walking and absence of tendon reflexes at the ankle and/or knee. Corneal and pupillary reflexes are often lost and the cranial nerves, including the optic nerve, are frequently affected. Symptoms and signs of encephalopathy are non-specific and include general fatigue, headache, sleep disturbances and decreased libido; at moderately high exposure levels there may be signs of extrapyramidal involvement and a few cases show typical parkinsonism (Vigliani, 1954). Symptoms of both the neuropathy and the encephalopathy may worsen for 1–2 years following removal from exposure to CS_2; final recovery may be very slow but, in some cases, almost complete.

Human pathology Few detailed reports of post-mortem findings are available; several describe small, scattered foci of necrosis in the brain, possibly secondary to vascular change (Quensel, 1904; Bashore et al., 1938; Vigliani, 1954). Axonal degeneration and myelin loss of unspecified distribution were described by Gordy and Trumper (1940); 'peripheral neuritis' was noted by Bashore et al. (1938), and Lukas (1969) found evidence of segmental demyelination.

Experimental studies Rabbits and dogs are more susceptible to CS_2 than are rats (Seppäläinen and Linnoila, 1976). Daily exposure of dogs to CS_2 vapour caused loss of power in the hindlimbs; the forelimbs were affected later. Paralysis, which was sometimes flaccid, progressed to spasticity; behavioural changes were also observed. Rabbits developed loss of control of hindlimbs after several weeks' exposure; rats displayed weakness and ataxia but never paralysis.

Pathological changes were observed in the brains of various species after long-term exposure to CS_2; diffuse, non-specific nerve cell changes were described in the cerebral and cerebellar cortex and basal ganglia (Wiley, Hueper and von Oettingen, 1936; Baumann, 1939). Focal and symmetrical lesions were found in the globus pallidus in cats (Ferraro, Jervis and Flicker, 1941) and monkeys (Richter, 1945). More recent studies using rats (Szendzikowski et al., 1973) and rabbits (Linnoila et al., 1975) have failed to show degenerative changes in neurons.

Early descriptions of peripheral nerve changes are inconsistent but the studies of Szendzikowski et al. (1974) and Linnoila et al. (1975) have shown axonal changes characterized by large fusiform swellings containing accumulations of 10 nm filaments in axons of peripheral nerves and in the long tracts of the spinal cord. Juntunen, Linnoila and Haltia (1977) have shown that these axonal swellings developed first in the sciatic and tibial nerves with only occasional changes in the roots. Gottfried et al. (1984) report that the axonal swellings occur just proximal to the nodes of Ranvier. Some axons degenerate distal to the swellings. Clusters of regenerating axons were found after cessation of exposure to CS_2 but axonal regeneration was also a conspicuous feature in animals still being exposed.

A distal pattern of fibre degeneration was also seen in the spinal cord, affecting the lumbar and thoracic levels of the pyramidal tracts, and the cervical levels of the posterior columns and spinocerebellar tracts.

The focal nature of the axonal lesions, the normal morphology of associated perikarya and the capacity of axons to regenerate whilst still being intoxicated are features which suggest a local effect of CS_2 upon axons, resulting in a central-peripheral distal axonopathy which closely resembles the hexacarbon neuropathies. The mechanism of action of CS_2 is not known but it has been suggested that binding to free thiol groups of neurofilament protein may affect axonal transport (Makinen et al., 1977).

Fetal alcohol syndrome

Exposure Heavy alcohol consumption during pregnancy can cause abnormalities of fetal development. Although this association has long been known it is only fairly recently that a set of characteristic changes has been recognized and described (Jones and Smith, 1973). Features of the fetal alcohol syndrome include:

1. Persisting growth deficiency of length, body weight and brain weight, of prenatal origin.
2. Facial abnormalities, including short palpebral fissures, epicanthal folds, thin upper lip and growth retardation of jaw.
3. Cardiac defects, mostly septal.
4. Minor joint and limb abnormalities.
5. Delayed development and mental deficiency varying from borderline to severe, probably due in part to a lack of neuron numbers.

The full syndrome is likely to be the extreme end of a spectrum of prenatal damage. Its incidence is reported as 1 in 600 births in France and Sweden (see Pratt, 1982). The mechanism of action of alcohol is not known, but acetaldehyde, which is the first metabolite of ethanol, is toxic to embryonic cells and to dividing cells in culture, and can cause some of the features of fetal alcohol syndrome, including abnormalities of neuronal migration, in experimental animals (O'Shea and Kaufman, 1979).

A similar syndrome is seen in the children of phenylketonuric mothers and of epileptic mothers treated with hydantoins during pregnancy (see Pratt, 1982).

In adults, chronic alcoholism is associated with nutritional deficiencies (see Chapter 13). In the fetus, however, there seems to be clear evidence of a direct toxic effect of alcohol, although other factors such as malnutrition and exposure to other drugs may also be implicated.

Human pathology Examination of brains from fetuses and children of alcoholic mothers shows a wide spectrum of morphological changes. Four cases described by Clarren et al. (1978) had a fairly uniform type of abnormality caused by failure or interruption of neuronal and glial migration. Consistent abnormalities were cerebellar dysplasias and heterotopic cell clusters, found particularly in the meninges; microcephaly was an important feature. Brain stem malformations caused hydrocephalus in two cases. The first published case of the syndrome also showed agenesis of the corpus callosum (Jones and Smith, 1973). Peiffer et al. (1979) examined brains of three fetuses and three children of alcoholic mothers. Four of them showed microdysplasias and some spongiform change in the hypothalamic and thalamic regions. Partial fusion of the walls of the third ventricle and absence of convolutions in the dentate nucleus and inferior olives were both indications of a retardation or local disorder of brain development. In the most severe cases there was arhinencephaly with agenesis of the corpus callosum, porencephaly, incomplete cerebellocystomeningocele and syringomyelia. Nothing is known of the neuropathological changes in survivors of the fetal alcohol syndrome, in whom mental deficiency is the most debilitating handicap; neither is it clear how much alcohol must be consumed to produce changes in brain development. There is evidence that relatively small amounts of alcohol during pregnancy can cause growth retardation (Little, 1977), but this important aspect of the effects of alcohol upon the fetus is beyond the scope of this chapter.

Experimental studies A number of animal studies have shown that administration of alcohol during pregnancy can cause severe fetal malformations. Chernoff (1977) found malformations in fetal mice similar to those found in human cases.

There are also many reports of quantitative changes in the developing brains of animals born to mothers fed with alcohol during pregnancy. The findings are often difficult to interpret because of complicating factors such as malnutrition and reduced thyroxine levels (e.g. Kornguth et al., 1979). In studies using nutritionally controlled diets, where there was no reduction in the body weight of the young animals, there is nevertheless evidence that alcohol can affect brain growth.

Barnes and Walker (1981) found a 20 per cent reduction in numbers of CA1 pyramidal cells in the hippocampus of 60-day-old rats of alcohol-fed mothers. Neurogenesis of hippocampal pyramidal cells is complete before birth, when they are probably most susceptible to the toxic effects of alcohol.

Exposure of weanling rats to ethanol vapour caused a significant reduction of brain weight which persisted into adulthood; the cerebellum was particularly affected (Bauer-Moffatt and Altman, 1977). The Purkinje cell population in each vermis lobule was decreased after 5 days' treatment; no further decrement occurred and by 90 days the packing density was similar to that of controls, probably due to redistribution and the smaller size of the cerebellum. Loss of Purkinje cells was generally greater in the anterior lobe than in the posterior lobe, and may be related to the chronology of development of different lobes. Although granule cell production and migration was similar to that in the controls, the ethanol-treated rats consistently had fewer cells, with an ultimate and irreversible loss of 25 per cent of granule cells. Borges and Lewis (1982) showed a significant reduction in cerebellar weight and mid-sagittal cross-sectional area in the young of mothers given alcohol in their drinking water. An increase in the thickness of the external granular layer suggested retardation of maturation. Hammer and Scheibel (1981) also used rats to make a quantitative analysis of deep cortical pyramidal cell dendrites; they found less extensive arborizations of dendrites, and somata which were smaller and rounder than those of pair fed controls.

Hexacarbon solvents

Exposure Hexacarbon solvents have widespread industrial applications, one of the chief being as a solvent for adhesives and cement. Occupational exposure occurs in manufacturing processes where glueing is important, but it is dangerous only when hygienic conditions are poor.

n-Hexane neuropathy was recognized in Japan in the late 1960s (Yamamura, 1969), and there was one report of three affected workers in the USA in 1971 (Herskowitz, Ishii and Schaumburg, 1971). However, the condition received little attention until an outbreak of polyneuropathy due to another hexacarbon, methyl *n*-butyl ketone (MBK), occurred in a coated fabrics plant in Columbus, Ohio, in 1973: 86 employees were affected (Billmaier et al., 1974; Allen et al., 1975).

Following this, the cause of another hitherto obscure occupational neuropathy became clear: that occurring in shoemakers in Italy. Some workers were exposed to very high concentrations of *n*-hexane when they worked in hot unventilated rooms with solvents in wide open-mouthed containers (Abbritti et al., 1976). Further pathological and experimental studies established that *n*-hexane was responsible.

At about the same time glue-sniffing was becoming an addictive habit in the young, some of whom developed peripheral neuropathy (Korobkin et al., 1975). The solvent *n*-hexane was responsible. An epidemic of glue-sniffing neuropathy occurred in Berlin when the solvent for one of the common glues was changed to a particularly neurotoxic combination (Altenkirch et al., 1977). The reason for this epidemic revealed that some non-neurotoxic hexacarbons can potentiate the neurotoxicity of others.

The only commonly used hexacarbons which produce peripheral neuropathy are *n*-hexane and MBK.

Clinical features Although paraesthesiae in the extremities may be the first manifestation of neuropathy, sensory loss is not severe. Weakness develops distally and may become marked. Proximal muscles become involved only in severely affected sniffers. Ankle jerks are lost but other reflexes are usually preserved.

An unusual and characteristic feature of hexacarbon neuropathy, which initially led to diagnostic difficulties, is that the clinical condition frequently continues to deteriorate for some months after exposure ceases. In severely affected subjects some degree of spasticity may develop when the peripheral neuropathy has largely recovered (Korobkin et al, 1975).

Human pathology Nerve biopsies have been studied in a number of patients with neuropathies following a history of glue-sniffing or industrial exposure to hexacarbon solvents (see Spencer, Couri and Schaumburg, 1980). In mild cases the nerves may show no abnormalities; in more severe neuropathy a number of nerve fibres may appear swollen due to accumulations of 10-nm neurofilaments within the axons. Teased fibre preparations show that the swellings are focal, often forming in paranodal regions; there is associated thinning of myelin and in paranodal regions the myelin sheath may retract completely from the node (Korobkin et al., 1975). These myelin sheath changes are secondary to the axonal abnormalities and are the cause of marked slowing of conduction velocity found in many cases. Axonal loss in nerve biopsies is variable, the myelinated fibre density often remaining within normal limits or being only moderately reduced. Selective loss of large diameter fibres has been found in some cases. The degree of axonal loss is probably related to the duration and severity of exposure to the hexacarbon.

Similar giant axonal swellings are found in the genetically determined giant axonal neuropathy described by Asbury et al. (1972). Neurofilamentous accumulations within axons are also a marked feature of acrylamide and CS_2 neuropathy. No details are available of central nervous system pathology in human hexacarbon neurotoxicity.

Experimental studies The neurotoxicity of hexacarbon compounds was examined experimentally following the large outbreak of human peripheral neuropathy in Ohio in 1973, caused by industrial exposure to MBK. Neuropathy was produced by various hexacarbon compounds in a number of different species (see Spencer, Couri and Schaumburg, 1980), but rats have been the most widely used in these studies.

After exposure by inhalation to either *n*-hexane or MBK, the animals develop hindlimb weakness with foot drop and, later, forelimb weakness. The neuropathy is characterized by the appearance in peripheral nerves of giant axonal swellings (Spencer and Schaumburg, 1975); these closely resemble the swellings found in nerve biopsies from cases of human neuropathy. They appear to develop from a gradual increase in numbers of neurofilaments. As a secondary response to the axonal changes there is thinning of the myelin sheath, probably caused by slippage of the myelin lamellae (Saida, Mendell and Weiss, 1976). Spencer and Schaumburg (1976a) found axonal swellings to occur distally, but multifocally, first appearing in large fibres which supply the calf muscles and later involving the longer plantar nerves. The filament-containing swellings tend to develop in paranodal regions on the proximal side of nodes of Ranvier (Figs. 14.10 and 14.11); there is associated thinning or retraction of myelin from the nodes. Axonal degeneration may be seen, distal to the axonal swellings, and some regeneration may take place. Paranodal demyelination and remyelination perhaps indicate reversibility of the swellings, but are also possibly associated with atrophy of the axons distal to the swellings. With time, changes in the nerve extend to involve more proximal parts, sometimes spreading into the lumbar ventral roots. Sensory and motor neurons appear to be unaffected, although Sterman (1982b) described chromatolysis-like changes in dorsal root ganglion cells of rats exposed to 2,5-hexanedione.

Similar patterns of distal, focal axonal swellings are also found in the long ascending and descending tracts of the spinal cord. Gracile and, to a lesser extent, cuneate tracts are affected at cervical levels and spinocerebellar tracts as far as mid-thoracic regions. Descending pathways including the lateral columns containing corticospinal and rubrospinal fibres are more affected in caudal regions. In general, long tracts are affected first, with later involvement of shorter pathways (Spencer and Schaumburg, 1977). Giant axonal swellings (Fig. 14.11) were also seen in preterminal and terminal axons in spinal cord grey matter, particularly in Rexed's laminae V to VII and in relation to anterior horn cells.

Cats dosed with neurotoxic hexacarbons

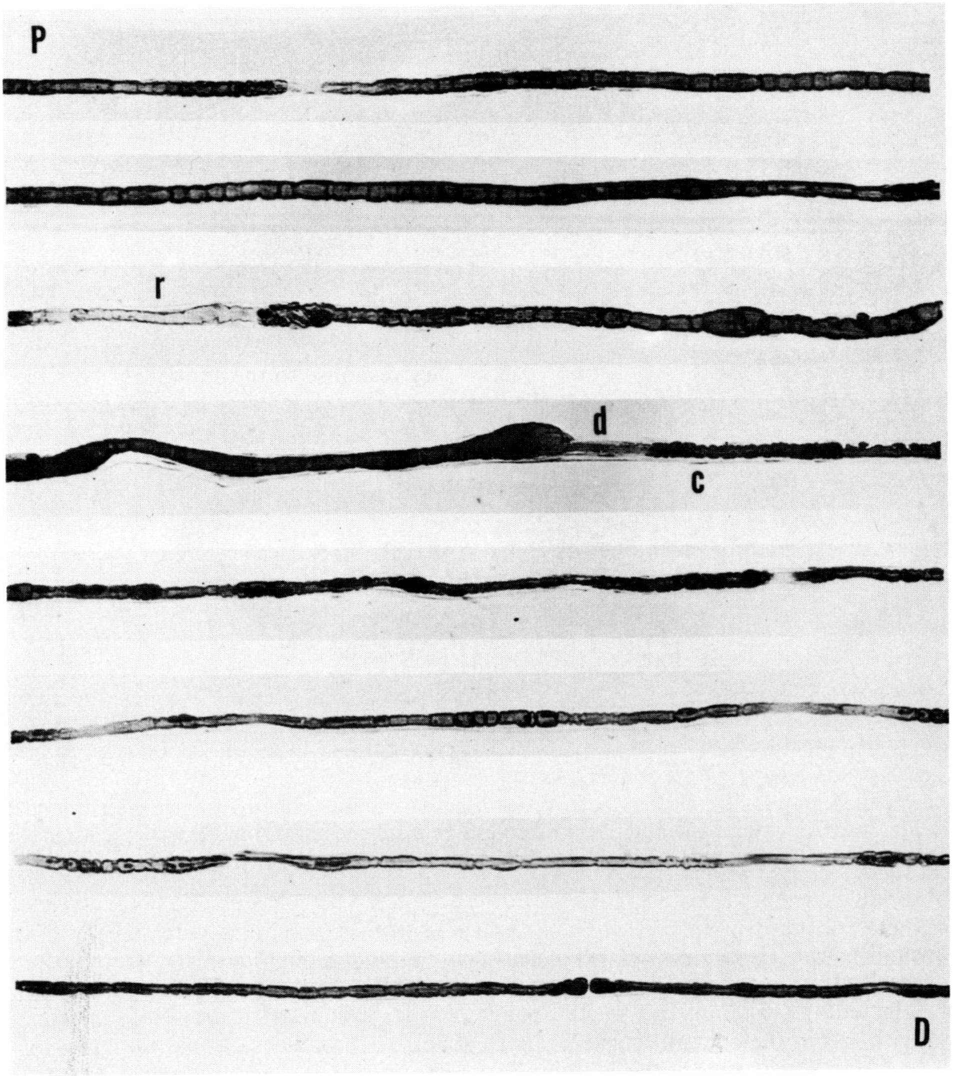

Fig. 14.10 Consecutive lengths of a teased single nerve fibre from a rat with 2,5-hexanedione neuropathy. Multifocal changes are present in the more proximal (P) parts of the fibre compared with distal (D). These include paranodal axonal swellings (third and fourth rows), segmental demyelination (r), paranodal demyelination (d) and irregularities of the myelin sheath (c). × 150. (Reproduced from Spencer and Schaumburg, 1977, by permission of the Editor of the *Journal of Neuropathology and Experimental Neurology*.)

showed changes similar to those found in rats (Spencer and Schaumburg, 1976b). In addition, axon swellings associated with widespread degeneration were found in the CNS in the mamillary body, lateral geniculate nucleus and superior colliculus; proximal parts of the optic nerve were spared (Schaumburg and Spencer, 1978). These lesions can be regarded as further examples of distal axonopathy; their late appearance relative to those in the spinal cord tracts may be a function of the short length of the pathways involved. Degenerative changes in the CNS were not accompanied by necrosis, macrophage accumulation or haemorrhage.

Cavanagh and Bennetts (1981) used conventional light microscopy to study the topography of lesions produced in rats by 2,5-hexanedione given in drinking water. Axon swellings and fibre degeneration were found in peripheral nerves as previously described by Spencer and his col-

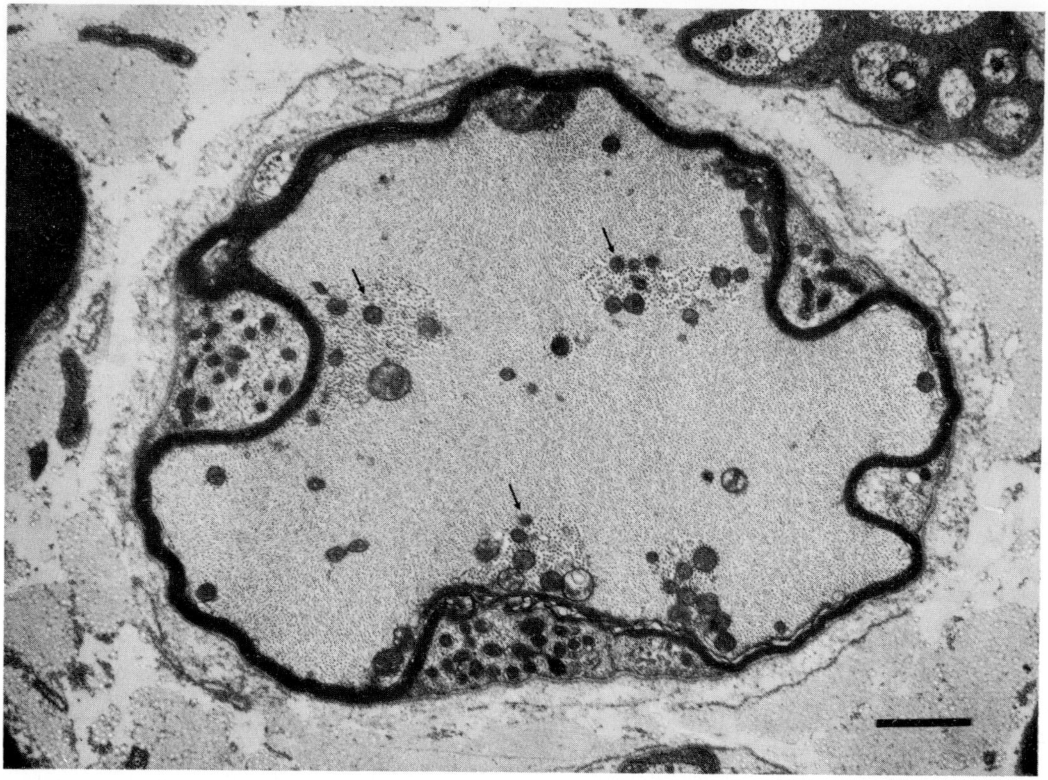

Fig. 14.11 Electron micrograph of sciatic nerve of a rat with hexacarbon neuropathy, showing a paranodal giant axonal swelling containing excessive numbers of 10-nm neurofilaments. Arrows point to clusters of neurotubules associated with mitochondria. Bar = 1 μm. (Reproduced, with permission, from Spencer, Couri and Schaumburg, 1980.)

leagues. However, swollen axons without evidence of fibre degeneration were found in many parts of the CNS, including most long fibre tracts in the cord, radial fibres in the cerebral cortex, the corpus callosum, in white matter of the cerebellar vermis, Purkinje cell axons and cerebellar roof nuclei; parts of the optic pathways were also affected. Although there was often a distal pattern to the localization of axon swellings, a number of exceptions were noted—e.g. pyramidal tract fibres were affected throughout their length.

Schwann cell changes have been described by Powell et al. (1978a) in rats exposed to 2,5-hexanedione. The cells were often hypertrophied, forming either focal expansions or a general increase in volume of cytoplasm. They contained accumulations of 10-nm cytoplasmic filaments (without the 'side-arms' seen in neurofilaments) and endoplasmic reticulum.

Hexacarbon and acrylamide both appear to produce a 'dying-back' type of neuropathy. Experimental studies show that degeneration does not begin at the nerve terminals as had been suggested in original theories of neuronal 'dying-back' (see later section, 'Organophosphorus compounds). Axonal neurofilamentous swellings, which may lead to degeneration, occur focally and distally but not terminally in motor fibres, and in both centrally and peripherally directed sensory fibres. Large but not necessarily the longest fibres are involved. Spencer and Schaumburg (1976a) have introduced the term 'central–peripheral distal axonopathy' to describe these particular types of neuropathy.

Biochemistry Studies on the principal metabolites of *n*-hexane and MBK indicate that 2,5-hexanedione is probably the active neurotoxic compound (DiVincenzo et al., 1980). The toxicity of a wider range of hexacarbons was studied by O'Donoghue and Krasavage (1979), who found that molecules with a γ-diketone configuration were neurotoxic, whereas those with a different diketone arrangement were not neurotoxic.

Sabri, Moore and Spencer (1979) have found that neurotoxic hexacarbons inhibit the glycolytic enzyme glyceraldehyde-3-phosphate dehydrogenase. Fast axonal transport, which is an energy-dependent process, decreases as clinical and histological signs of neuropathy develop (Mendell et al., 1977).

Graham (1980) has suggested that hexacarbons are toxic through an irreversible reaction with amino groups forming conjugated imines, which are orange in colour. Progressive covalent bridging of neurofilaments might result in aggregations too large to pass through nodes of Ranvier. Hair of chronically dosed albino rats becomes orange.

Methyl alcohol

Exposure The use, by alcoholics, of methanol-containing liquids as cheap intoxicants is probably the main source of poisoning. Methanol is present in a wide variety of products, including solvents and toiletries; its use in antifreeze and synthetic fuels is now being discontinued in some countries. Trace quantities of methanol are present in known brands of bourbon and vodka. Inhalation of methanol fumes can be fatal or lead to blindness.

Schneck (1979) has reviewed numerous outbreaks of methyl alcohol intoxication in the USA; these occurred particularly during periods of prohibition.

Although methyl alcohol was recognized as a poison in 1855, little heed was taken of this fact until a report by Wood and Buller (1904) of 275 cases of blindness and death related to methyl alcohol consumption. In 1953, Benton and Calhoun described 320 cases of methanol poisoning in Atlanta following drinking of bootleg whisky.

Clinical features Acute toxicity is associated with headache, extreme dilatation of the pupils, circulatory collapse; respiratory failure and blindness; death may occur very rapidly.

Chronic toxicity causes loss of visual acuity, oedema of the optic disc and surrounding retina and along the course of major retinal blood vessels (Hayreh et al., 1977). Other symptoms affecting the CNS, gastrointestinal and respiratory tracts are described by Schneck (1979).

Because of the wide range of tolerance to methanol, there is no correlation between severity of symptoms and quantities of methanol consumed.

Biochemistry Methanol is oxidized to formaldehyde by an alcohol dehydrogenase in the liver and kidney, with the final breakdown to formic acid often resulting in severe acidosis. The relative importance of acidosis and formate concentration in both ocular and systemic toxicity has recently been reviewed (*Lancet*, 1983).

Human pathology In most fatal cases congestion, oedema and petechial haemorrhages are found in many organs including the brain. Meningeal and subarachnoid petechiae may be prominent; petechiae have been particularly noted in the region of the third ventricle, the aqueduct of Sylvius and beneath the floor of the fourth ventricle. All three layers of the cerebellar cortex show ischaemic necrosis. Bilateral necrosis of the putamen, with cyst formation, appears to be a selective toxic effect of methanol (Orthner, 1953; Potts et al., 1955). Erlanson et al. (1965) described slit-like cysts in the putamen in a patient dying 1 year after intoxication. Evidence of a lesion in the putamen was seen on a CT scan of a survivor of methanol poisoning (Aquilonius et al., 1978) and in two surviving patients described by McLean, Jacobs and Mielke (1980). Cystic resorbed infarction of the putamen was confirmed *post mortem* in one of these cases (McLean, Jacobs and Mielke, 1980). Orthner (1950) suggested that putaminal necrosis might be due to decreased venous flow through the veins of Rosenthal. McLean, Jacobs and Mielke (1980) also found cystic areas of necrosis throughout subcortical white matter, especially in the frontal lobes. Microscopically there was scattered neuronal swelling and pyknosis in the third and deeper layers of the cortex and the medial nucleus of the thalamus. Swelling and chromatolysis were seen in the lateral geniculate bodies, scattered in many areas of central grey matter and in anterior horns and Clarke's column at all levels of the spinal cord. Marked loss of numbers of retinal ganglion cells was found, accompanied by gliosis, and there was almost complete absence of axons in the optic nerve, with intense astrocytic hyperplasia.

McGregor (1943) found no significant retinal changes in acute deaths due to methanol poisoning. Generally, however, degeneration of retinal ganglion cells is a common finding; the cells may also show chromatolytic change.

Experimental studies Potts et al. (1955) studied the ocular toxicity of methanol in monkeys. They found patchy demyelination in one animal out of eight given methanol. A further study showed 'cystoid' changes in the external nuclear layer, which were possibly artefactual; no significant alterations were seen in the retinal ganglion cells although the animals showed severe retinal oedema and apparent blindness.

In another study of methanol ocular toxicity in primates (Martin-Amat et al., 1977) tissues were fixed by *in vivo* glutaraldehyde perfusion to prevent fixation artefact (Baumbach et al., 1977). No changes were seen in the ganglion cells or in any other retinal tissue. Ophthalmoscopic examination showed oedema of the optic disc in these animals (Hayreh et al., 1977). Electron microscopy showed swelling of axons and accumulations of mitochondria in the optic nerve head, most marked in the lamina cribrosa (Baumbach et al., 1977). Hayreh et al. (1977) have suggested that these changes may be caused by stasis of axoplasmic flow, perhaps related to the diffusion of formic acid into the optic nerve head from the adjacent choroid which has fenestrated capillaries and a very large blood flow. Hayreh et al. (1977) are of the opinion that visual loss in human methanol toxicity is due to optic nerve lesions rather than retinal damage. This may be the explanation for the presence of chromatolytic cells in many cases. Other aspects of methanol toxicity to the central nervous system appear not to have been studied.

Organophosphorus compounds

Exposure Most organophosphates are used as insecticides. Exposure occurs in those manufacturing and formulating the compounds and those involved in large-scale spraying operations. Significant exposure does not follow domestic use of weak solutions. However, accidental or deliberate ingestion of concentrated solutions is not uncommon and is an important cause of toxicity.

Triorthocresyl phosphate is used as a plasticizer and lubricant. Human exposure is always accidental.

Organophosphates have also been developed as nerve gases, thus creating a potential source of exposure to these particular compounds.

Practically all organophosphates inhibit acetylcholinesterase. Symptoms due to anti-acetylcholinesterase effects from insecticide exposure have occurred commonly. For example, between 1953 and 1969 in Japan 19 436 cases of poisoning were recognized, approximately half occurring accidentally and half from attempted suicide or homicide. There were 9460 deaths (Namba et al., 1971).

Some organophosphates cause delayed neuropathy—i.e. symptoms of peripheral neuropathy developing from 1 to 3 weeks after a single dose. Triorthocresyl phosphate (TOCP) has been most commonly responsible for this syndrome. One of the best known epidemics resulted in 'ginger jake paralysis', which followed consumption of alcoholic extracts of ginger contaminated with TOCP during prohibition in the USA. About 20 000 people were affected in 1930 (J.G. Kidd and Langworthy, 1933). Other episodes have followed accidental contamination of cooking oil. About 10 000 people were affected in Morocco in 1959 when cooking oil was adulterated with aircraft lubricating oil (H.V. Smith and Spalding, 1959).

Although the organophosporus insecticides in current use are usually considered to be non-neuropathic, there have been several reports of peripheral neuropathy occurring after suicide attempts with massive doses of trichlorfon (Dipterex) (Hierons and Johnson, 1978; Shiraishi et al., 1983). These occur only if the patients are kept alive by energetic treatment of anticholinesterase effects.

Clinical features Acute anticholinesterase effects consist of headache, abdominal pain, vomiting, sweating, miosis and muscular twitching. These can be controlled with atropine or cholinesterase reactivators such as pralidoxime. There are no long-term effects.

Following ingestion of neurotoxic organophosphates, gastrointestinal symptoms are initially marked. There is then a latent interval of 1–3 weeks before neuropathy develops. Although there may be some sensory symptoms at the onset, the neuropathy is predominantly or entirely motor. Distal muscles are affected most, with flaccidity, wasting and loss of reflexes. There is often evidence of pyramidal tract involvement, with spasticity and increased reflexes at a later stage after regeneration of peripheral nerves. There is no specific treatment for delayed peripheral neuropathy.

Human pathology Post-mortem reports of cases from the 1930 'ginger jake' epidemic described degeneration of peripheral nerves, which was more extensive in leg nerves than in those from the arms (Goodale and Humphreys, 1931); no CNS changes were noted. Thirty-six patients who had survived this epidemic with residual paralysis for 10 years were examined *post mortem* by Aring (1942). Spinal meninges were thickened and there was nerve fibre degeneration at distal (cervical) levels of the long ascending gracile tracts whilst the shorter cuneate tracts were not affected. The lateral pyramidal tracts invariably showed distal degeneration of fibres, seen only in lower segments of the cord. Anterior horn cells were reduced in number and all the nerves and spinal roots examined showed fibre degeneration.

Experimental studies Following the identification of cresyl phosphate as the cause of the 'ginger jake' epidemic, experimental studies showed that several species were vulnerable although there was considerable variation in their susceptibility. These early studies were reviewed by Cavanagh (1964a). Chickens developed a reproducible paralysis following a single oral dose, and cats show much the same sensitivity as chickens. A comprehensive table of species sensitivity to various organophosphorus compounds has been assembled by C.S. Davis and Richardson (1980).

Essentially similar neurotoxic effects are produced in chickens by aryl- and alkyl-organophosphates (Cavanagh, 1954, Fenton, 1955). As in man, there is invariably a latent period of 8–12 days before the onset of functional disturbances. Cavanagh (1954) described the changes in hens which develop flaccid paralysis, death usually occurring by the 16th to 20th day. No histological changes are visible until the onset of paralysis, when axonal degeneration is seen in peripheral nerves, especially in their distal parts, and predominantly affecting large-diameter fibres. The spinal roots, dorsal root ganglion cells and anterior horn cells are unaffected. Degeneration of fibres in the long ascending spinal (spinocerebellar and gracile) tracts and in long descending (pyramidal) tracts occurs, always most marked at their distal ends. In a further study, in cats, Cavanagh (1964b) confirmed and extended his findings in chickens. Quantitative studies showed loss of large-diameter fibres with concomitant abnormalities in muscle spindle innervation, and Golgi tendon organs to a lesser degree. There was a pattern of spinal tract degeneration similar to that in chickens, with distal degeneration of longest, and also largest, fibres (Cavanagh and Patangia, 1965). At later stages, degeneration progressed towards the parent cell bodies but at no time was there involvement of entire fibres.

Baboons given TOCP showed little clinical evidence of neurological damage once they had recovered from the cholinergic effects (Hern, 1967, 1971). Although histological examination showed distal degeneration of peripheral nerve fibres there was no selective loss of large-diameter fibres. Few changes were found in baboon spinal cord but in squirrel monkeys given TOCP there was degeneration in the spinal cord, particularly affecting the ventrolateral columns.

Electron microscopy of peripheral nerves from TOCP-poisoned hens (Le Vay, Meier and Glees, 1971) and cats (Prineas, 1969a) showed collections of vesicles and tubules in distal parts of peripheral nerve axons. Similar vesicular and tubular profiles were seen in axons at distal ends of long fibre tracts in the spinal cord. Many presynaptic terminals were distended with small vesicles, and 10–20 per cent of axosomatic endings showed swelling and degenerative changes in synaptic vesicles (Bischoff, 1970). Prineas (1969a) found some alterations in anterior horn cells, probably of a chromatolytic type and which might be expected because of the peripheral nerve degeneration.

Of two studies on axoplasmic transport in TOCP intoxication, one showed no changes from normal (Pleasure, Mischler and Engel, 1969) whilst the other reported a reduced rate of slow axoplasmic transport (Bradley and Williams, 1973).

Awareness of the idea of distal degeneration of nerve fibres goes back to Gowers (1886); there was also recognition at that time that terminal parts of nerve fibres are farthest removed from the nerve cells 'on which their health depends' (Sharkey, 1896). Neuronal disease could become manifest by changes in the terminal regions of the fibres. In some diseases there may be a spread of degeneration beginning distally, then affecting nerve trunks and finally, perhaps, the nerve cells. Greenfield (1954) described this as 'dying-back' of the neuron.

Cavanagh considered that the pathology of TOCP poisoning supported the theory that dying-back was due to some impairment of perikaryal metabolism—extremities of axons being affected first, in particular those which are the longest and largest and which impose the greatest burden on the parent nerve cell body.

Whilst this explanation may hold true for some human conditions, there is now considerable evidence from experimental work that axons do not 'die back' from their ends, but develop local and often multifocal damage, tending to occur at their distal ends (Spencer and Schaumburg, 1976a).

Studies by Bouldin and Cavanagh (1979a, b) on cats given the alkyl organophosphate, di-isopropylfluorophosphonate (DFP) have indeed shown that there are focal and non-terminal abnormalities in the form of varicosities along fibres of the left recurrent laryngeal nerve whose axons do not branch. Ultrastructurally, the varicosities are seen to be associated with intra-axonal and/or intramyelin vacuoles and sometimes with accumulations of smooth endoplasmic reticulum. Varicosity formation appears to lead to axon degeneration. These studies refute the original proposition that organophosphates produce dying-back degeneration which spreads from the nerve terminals.

Biochemistry Considerable progress has been made in identifying some of the molecular events that occur after administration of neurotoxic organophosphorus compounds. Johnson (1975) has characterized a 'neurotoxic esterase' (NTE) whose inhibition is related to the development of neuropathy. A review of the present state of knowledge is given by Cremer (1981) and Johnson (1982). A number of compounds bind to NTE and inhibit its activity. Compounds which produce delayed neuropathy undergo a process of 'ageing' which is essential for the development of neuropathy. The degree of inhibition of NTE can be studied *in vitro* and this provides a valuable method of predicting the neurotoxicity of any particular compound.

Drugs

Clioquinol

Exposure Clioquinol (5-chloro-7-iodo-8-hydroxyquinoline) was originally marketed as an oral intestinal amoebicide, but has since been used in a wide range of intestinal disorders including non-specific and 'traveller's' diarrhoea. Its widespread consumption, mostly during the 1960s, was associated in Japan with the appearance of a new disease, subacute myelo-optic neuropathy (SMON), which reached epidemic proportions by the end of 1970. Although the causative agent of the disease has been in doubt, the rapid decrease in numbers of cases following a ban by the Japanese government on the sale of clioquinol in 1970 provides circumstantial evidence that it was an aetiological factor.

Clinical features The first neurological symptoms in almost all cases were of sensory disturbances in the legs; many patients also developed leg muscle weakness or paralysis. In his survey of clinical aspects of SMON, Sobue (1979) has described abnormalities of autonomic function and sphincter disturbances. Decreased visual acuity was found in more than 25 per cent of a series of 752 cases. Greenish discoloration of the tongue, faeces and urine is a characteristic sign of SMON, although not seen in all cases. It is caused by an iron chelate of clioquinol and provides strong evidence that the drug is aetiologically important in the disease.

Why SMON should have been so common in Japan and so rare in other countries in which clioquinol was used is a strange and unexplained feature of the disease. Baumgartner et al. (1979) have reviewed non-Japanese patients probably suffering from clioquinol neurotoxicity. Two neurological syndromes were described which were dose-related after high or prolonged treatment: an acute encephalopathy with features of transient global amnesia; and optic atrophy in children.

Human pathology The pathology of SMON has been reviewed by Shiraki (1979b); changes are generally restricted to the nervous system. Only minimal lesions are found rostral to the spinal cord; these include acute oedematous change in the cortex, and astrocytosis in the white matter of the cerebellum and the occipital pole, and in the substantia nigra and globus pallidus. In one patient with a clinical history of persistent amnesia, there was severe bilateral damage to Sommer's sector of Ammon's horn.

Symmetrical fibre loss was found in the posterior columns, the cervical (i.e. more distal) levels of the long gracile tracts being particularly involved. Spinocerebellar tracts were less severely affected. Descending tracts also showed distal degeneration with pronounced damage of anterior and/or lateral corticospinal tracts in the lumbar region. Spinal cord grey matter showed minimal changes of astrocytosis and gliosis; vacuolar changes in anterior horn cells at lumbosacral levels have also been described. Spheroids were noted in this region and elsewhere (e.g. lateral geniculate body). Loss of neurons and gliosis was found in the olivary nucleus in chronic cases.

Degeneration of ganglion cells with satellitosis was seen in dorsal root ganglia, particularly at lumbosacral levels, and in autonomic ganglia. Axonal degeneration was found in posterior roots at lumbosacral levels and in the cauda equina; anterior root changes were less obvious.

Biopsies and autopsy samples of sural and femoral nerves showed some evidence of axonal degeneration, and proliferation of Schwann cell nuclei; segmental demyelination has also been described. Baumgartner et al. (1979) have questioned the evidence of peripheral neuropathy in the Japanese cases, and P.K. Thomas (1982) decided that clinical signs and symptoms could all be due to CNS involvement; some peripheral nerve loss could be expected, however, due to loss of lumbosacral dorsal root ganglion and autonomic ganglion cells.

In the optic pathways there was often a distal pattern of degeneration with more severe damage in the optic tract near to the lateral geniculate bodies. Less frequently, focal lesions were found in the optic nerves and tracts. Cells of the inner ganglion cell layer were selectively damaged.

Experimental studies Shiraki (1979b) quotes a number of Japanese studies of clioquinol neurotoxicity in many species. Dogs and cats were the most sensitive: after oral administration of the drug they developed an ataxic gait, muscular weakness of the hindlimbs and impaired vision. Distal degeneration in the cord was found and optic tracts were often severely affected. Lumbosacral dorsal root ganglia and peripheral nerves were only mildly affected. Krinke et al. (1979) found similar changes in dogs given clioquinol; no peripheral nerve changes were observed. Schaumburg and Spencer (1980) have drawn attention to this unique pattern of distal axonal degeneration, affecting as it does the centrally directed fibres of sensory ganglion cells but apparently sparing the peripheral fibres; it is described as 'central distal axonopathy'.

Shiraki (1977) studied the distribution of isotopically labelled clioquinol using whole body autoradiography. There was not always a clear association between drug accumulation and neuronal damage.

Hexachlorophane*

Exposure Hexachlorophane was developed as an antiseptic in the 1940s and since then has been widely used for sterilizing the skin preoperatively and occasionally for treatment of burns and in vaginal douches. It is also a constituent of many cosmetic preparations.

Early reports of toxic effects in man have been reviewed by Lockhart (1972). During the 1960s toxicity developed in a few subjects following accidental ingestion or mistaken therapeutic oral use.

The dangers of the use of solutions containing hexachlorophane in the treatment of burns were then recognized because the substance is more easily absorbed through broken skin. Toxicity following absorption through the vaginal mucosa was also reported when impregnated packs were left in place for some days.

The greatest danger of toxicity has been in the use of powders and solutions containing hexachlorophane on the skin of premature infants. The drug is able to penetrate their skin more easily than that of full-term infants. Powell et al. (1973) found status spongiosus in the brain stem of seven out of 69 infants who had died in the neonatal period. These seven infants were all premature and had received multiple washings with a solution containing 3% hexachlorophane.

* Also known as *hexachlorophene*.

The greatest disaster attributable to hexachlorophane occurred in France in 1972, but was only recently reported in detail on account of legal complications (Martin-Bouyer et al., 1982): 204 children were affected, of whom 36 died as a result of treatment with a baby powder which accidentally contained 6.3% hexachlorophane.

Clinical features The clinical syndrome produced by hexachlorophane absorption consists of irritability, drowsiness and generalized convulsions. Confusion and coma follow. Papilloedema has been described. In those who have survived the acute episode, recovery has been complete.

Human pathology The lesions described in human brains are similar to those in the experimental studies discussed below. Intramyelinic oedema, most marked in the brain stem, was found in the seven premature infants who had been repeatedly washed in a solution containing 3% hexachlorophane (Powell et al., 1973). Similar white matter oedema was found in the infants affected in the outbreak in France (Martin-Bouyer et al., 1982).

Experimental studies Kimbrough and Gaines (1971) found that rats developed progressive paralysis of their hindlimbs when fed 25 mg/kg per day. Histological study revealed status spongiosus of the white matter of the brain and spinal cord. On stopping administration there was clinical and pathological recovery.

Lampert, O'Brien and Garrett (1973) demonstrated that the oedema was due to intramyelinic accumulation of fluid without damage to the blood–brain barrier, since there was no discoloration of the brain following intraperitoneal injection of trypan blue. Nor did intracerebrally injected Thorotrast (a proprietary preparation of thorium dioxide) penetrate into the oedematous vacuoles (Powell and Lampert, 1975). The lesion is similar to that produced by triethyl tin, but, in contrast to the triethyl tin lesion, peripheral nerve myelin is also affected (Towfighi, Gonatas and McCree, 1973). Maxwell and Le Quesne (1979) studied single peripheral nerve fibres of rats and noted that oedema first appeared in the middle of the internode, the nodes of Ranvier remaining normal. Several contiguous vacuoles were often present along the middle of a single internode (Fig. 14.12). Tabira et al. (1978) de-

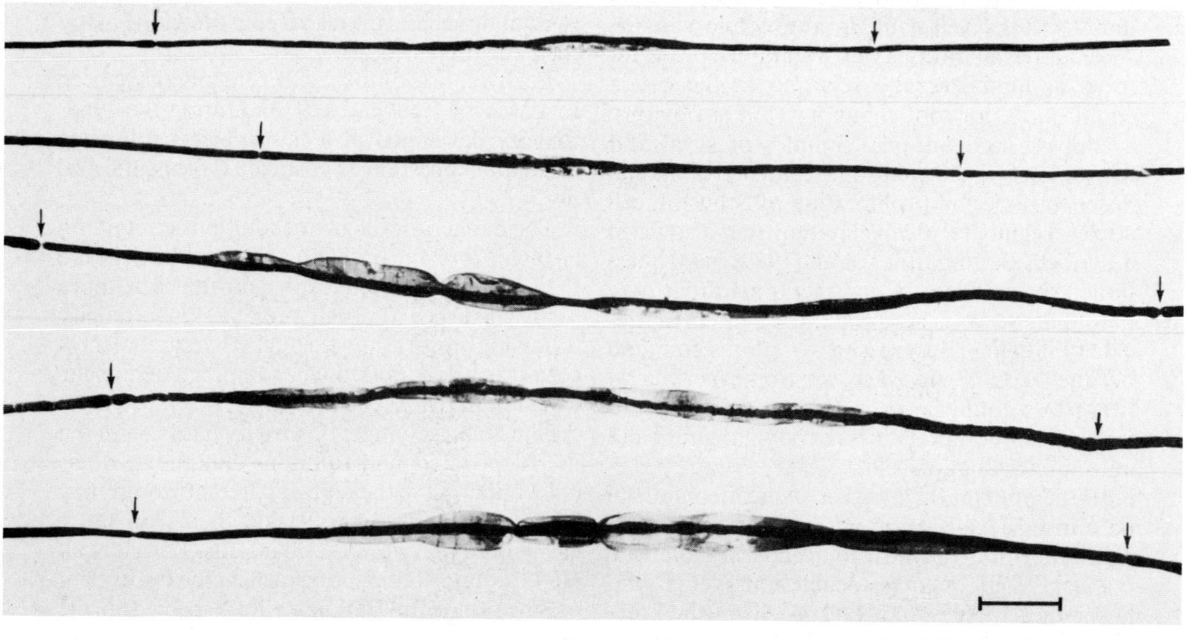

Fig. 14.12 Five single teased fibres from peripheral nerves of rats with hexachlorophane neuropathy, showing different degrees of internodal intramyelinic vacuolation. Arrows mark nodes of Ranvier. Bar = 100 μm. (Reproduced from Maxwell and LeQuesne, 1979, by permission of the Editor of the *Journal of the Neurological Sciences*.)

monstrated that the vacuole compartments were limited by intramyelinic tight junctions in tadpole optic nerves. In chronically poisoned animals which had received hexachlorophane for more than 3 months, Maxwell and Le Quesne (1979) found segmental demyelination and remyelination. In nerves from these animals much myelin irregularity was also present, even in the absence of oedema, suggesting that vacuoles in previously affected fibres had collapsed. A few fibres undergoing axonal degeneration have been described in all the morphological studies.

In animals poisoned for several months Maxwell and Le Quesne (1979) found interstitial oedema, particularly beneath the perineurium with an electron microscopic appearance suggesting that the fluid contained protein. Powell et al. (1978b) also described interstitial oedema during recovery from hexachlorophane neuropathy but not during the acute stage. It seems likely that this oedema is a non-specific late secondary effect unrelated to the essential intramyelin lesion.

Isoniazid

Exposure Isoniazid (isonicotinylhydrazide, INH) is used in the treatment of tuberculosis. Soon after its introduction in 1951, several papers appeared reporting peripheral neuropathy in patients taking the drug (see Cavanagh, 1973).

Clinical features Isoniazid therapy may produce many side-effects but toxic reactions affecting the liver and the nervous system are the most important. A total daily dose of 3–5 mg is usually given but higher doses are recommended in certain circumstances. Peripheral neuropathy may develop in up to 19 per cent of patients given 3–5 mg per day. Doses of 20 mg can produce neuropathy in more than 40 per cent of those treated (see Aita and Calame, 1972). The nutritional state of the patient, and genetic factors (see below), will influence the incidence of peripheral neuropathy. High doses may also produce a variety of CNS symptoms, including convulsions, stupor, ataxia, memory impairment and psychosis (Weinstein, 1975).

The first symptoms of neuropathy are paraesthesiae and numbness of the fingers and toes. Withdrawal of the drug at this stage is followed by rapid recovery within a few days to weeks (Biehl and Nimitz, 1954). With continuing dosing sensory symptoms extend to the knees and over the hands, and painful burning sensations may develop. There is superficial sensory loss, and vibration sensation in the limbs is reduced or lost (Le Quesne, 1975); deep sensation is less affected. Ochoa (1970) found hyperalgesia in the hands and feet in five out of nine cases of INH neuropathy. Symptoms of motor involvement such as distal muscle weakness, wasting and cramps often appear later than the sensory symptoms. Recovery may take many months if INH administration is continued for a few weeks beyond the first symptoms of neuropathy.

Acute and severe toxicity follows a single dose of 6–10 g INH, and 15 g is usually fatal (Sievers and Herrier, 1975).

Biochemistry INH is rapidly absorbed after oral or parenteral dosing. The first step in its metabolism is acetylation in the liver. In 1954 Hughes et al. noticed that one group of patients excreted 75% INH in the acetylated form, whilst another group excreted a higher proportion of free INH. High levels of free INH in blood and urine were associated with slow acetylation of the drug, and liver acetyltransferase was low. Slow acetylators tended to develop neuropathy and other signs of INH toxicity more frequently than did rapid acetylators.

The incidence of the two types of acetylators was found to vary in different racial groups (Harris, Knight and Selin, 1958), which suggested that rates of acetylation might be genetically determined. Slow acetylation is now known to be inherited as an autosomal recessive trait (Evans, Manley and McKusick, 1960).

The neurotoxic effects of INH originate from its disturbance of vitamin B_6 metabolism. Pyridoxine, pyridoxal and pyridoxamine, which comprise the vitamin B_6 group, must be phosphorylated in order to form the active coenzymes involved in many enzymatic reactions, including decarboxylations and transaminations. INH interferes with this essential phosphorylation by inhibiting pyridoxal phosphate kinase; INH also chelates with pyridoxal phosphate, forming an even more potent inhibitor of pyridoxal phosphate than INH alone.

The tryptophan load test (used in the detection of vitamin B_6 deficiencies) shows increased excretion of xanthurenic and kynurenic acids after dosing with INH, indicating pyridoxine deficiency (Biehl and Vilter, 1954a). Pyridoxal-phosphate is important as a cofactor in glutamate decarboxylase activity and the synthesis of gamma-aminobutyric acid (GABA). The convulsions which can occur in INH toxicity may result from reduced brain levels of GABA, an inhibitory transmitter.

The effectiveness of pyridoxine supplementation in reducing the incidence of INH was studied by Biehl and Vilter (1954b); no neuropathy occurred in patients given pyridoxine, whilst 40 per cent of those not receiving pyridoxine developed a neuropathy. Beneficial effects of pyridoxine were found by Ross (1958) and Ochoa (1970). The efficiency of INH as an antituberculosis drug is not affected by the administration of pyridoxine.

Human pathology Axonal degeneration in peripheral nerves, with associated atrophy of muscles, has been described in a number of *post mortem* studies of INH neuropathy (Klinghardt, 1954; Axt, Bunger and Lass, 1956; Ott, Rabinowicz and Morand, 1959). Changes in motor end-plates, axonal degeneration of intramuscular nerve fibres and collateral sprouting were found in the absence of clinical signs of motor involvement and without volumetric muscle changes of neurogenic origin. Presumably, as in the studies in the rat by Hildebrand, Joffroy and Coërs (1968), there was successful reinnervation of muscle by collateral sprouting. Axonal degeneration has also been described in the dorsal columns of the spinal cord.

Ochoa (1970) made an extensive study of nine patients with INH neuropathy; sural nerve biopsies showed loss of myelinated and unmyelinated fibres, with evidence of regeneration of both types of fibre in all nine cases. After careful correction for the presence of immature regenerating fibres, Ochoa found some correlation between the clinical and pathological findings.

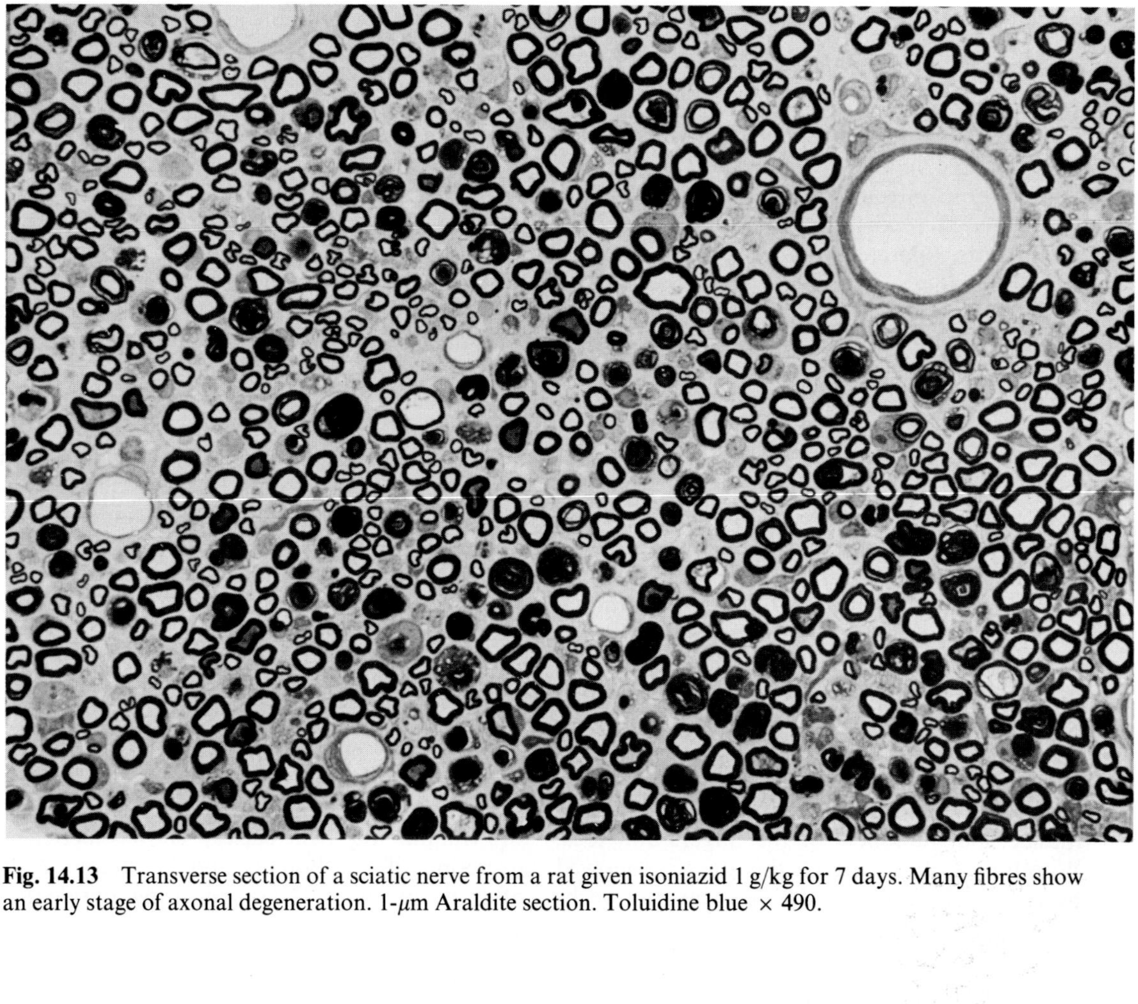

Fig. 14.13 Transverse section of a sciatic nerve from a rat given isoniazid 1 g/kg for 7 days. Many fibres show an early stage of axonal degeneration. 1-μm Araldite section. Toluidine blue × 490.

Experimental studies Chicks, ducklings and dogs, which are far more sensitive to INH than the rat as judged by the LD_{50}, develop lesions in the CNS with apparent sparing of peripheral nerves (Blakemore, 1980).

Peripheral neuropathy Rats fed daily on a diet containing INH 250 mg/kg develop axonal degeneration after 2 weeks, although functional disturbances may not become apparent for many weeks (Klinghardt, 1954; Zbinden and Studer, 1955; Cavanagh, 1967).

The pattern of nerve fibre degeneration was studied by Cavanagh (1967) who found that motor nerves were more severely affected than were sensory fibres; in addition, motor fibres degenerated along a major part of their length whilst sensory fibres tended only to be affected distally. Jacobs, Miller and Cavanagh (1979) confirmed these findings quantitatively; furthermore, they showed that, apart from some chromatolysis of ventral horn neurons, there was no ultrastructural evidence of primary damage to these cells, and the proximal parts of their axons were invariably spared although there might be extensive degeneration from the level of the spinal roots (Fig. 14.13). In severely affected animals there was distal degeneration of both central and peripheral fibres of sensory neurons. A striking feature of this neuropathy was the remarkable regenerative capacity of the damaged fibres despite continuing dosing with INH (Fig. 14.14).

These observations support the view that INH acts directly upon the axons, probably by causing local depletion of pyridoxal phosphate. Pyridoxal phosphate is most probably synthesized in the perikaryon; its transport into the axon would protect proximal parts of the fibres from the effects of enzyme depletion but leave the more distal parts deprived of the enzyme. The brisk regenerative response in the face of continuing dosing with INH is convincing evidence that the drug does not compromise perikaryal function.

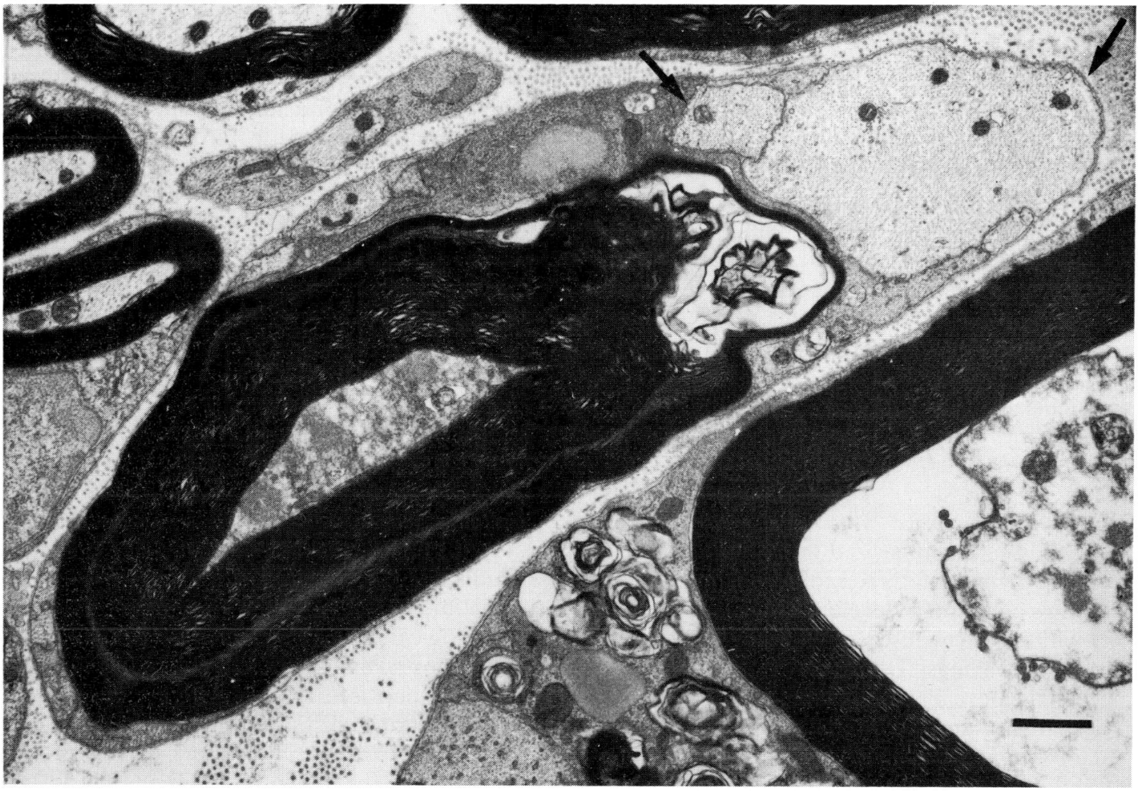

Fig. 14.14 Electron micrograph of the ventral root of a rat dosed with isoniazid 100 mg/kg for 7 days. Myelinated fibres show early axonal degeneration but already there are two regenerated axons (arrows) within the basal lamina of one fibre. Bar = 1 μm.

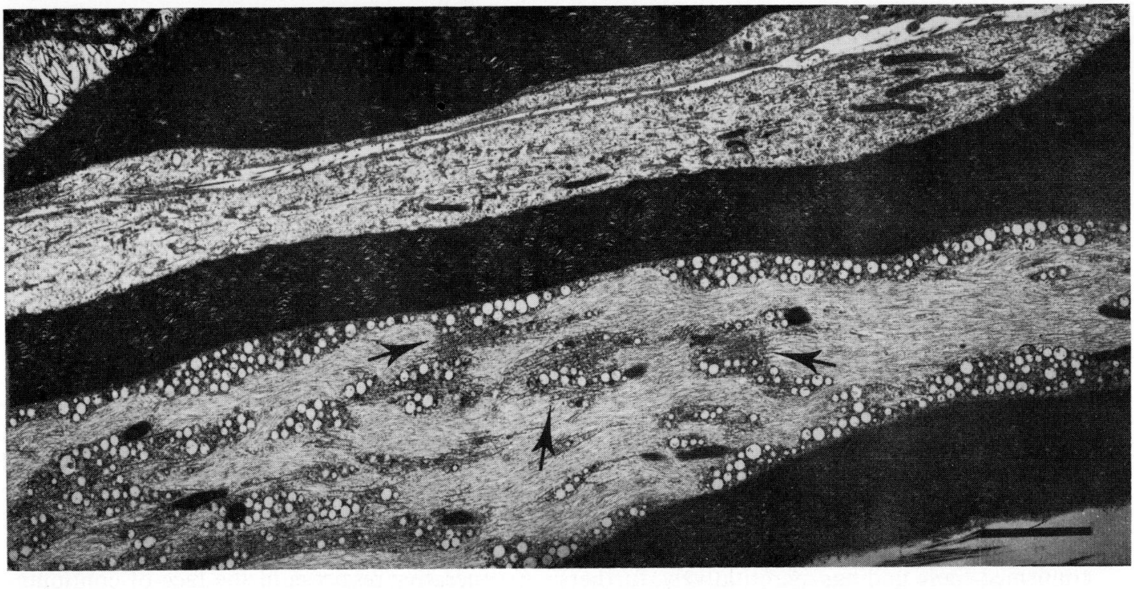

Fig. 14.15 Electron micrograph of the ventral root of a rat 2 days after dosing with isoniazid 1 g/kg. The longitudinal section of a myelinated fibre shows an accumulation of vesicles in the axon probably derived from smooth endoplasmic reticulum and associated with bundles of microtubules (arrows). Bar = 1 μm.

Several ultrastructural studies have demonstrated axonal degeneration in INH neuropathy (Schlaepfer and Hager, 1964; Schröder, 1975). Jacobs et al. (1979) studied acutely intoxicated rats for the earliest ultrastructural changes in the nerve fibres. Focal periaxonal swellings and accumulations of smooth endoplasmic reticulum were consistent findings which appeared to precede axonal degeneration (Fig. 14.15). Although there were some abnormalities in Schwann cells, these did not appear to be related to the axonal changes. It is not known how a deficiency of pyridoxal-phosphate-dependent enzymes is related to these ultrastructural changes.

Central nervous system lesions Blakemore (1980) has summarized the findings in the CNS in experimental INH intoxication. Chicks, ducklings and dogs develop vacuolated lesions in white matter caused, in most cases, by intramyelinic swellings. Ultrastructural studies in dogs (Blakemore, Palmer and Noel, 1972) have shown that the vacuoles generally arise at separations of the intraperiod line of the myelin sheath. In addition there may be distension of the periaxonal space, swelling of the inner tongue of oligodendroglial cytoplasm and focal swellings of axons. In dogs given high doses there were oligodendroglial changes such as nuclear pyknosis, loss of ribosomes and cytoplasmic swelling. Astrocytic swelling of a non-specific type was the predominating change in birds and dogs given large doses.

Methotrexate

Exposure Methotrexate is a folic acid antagonist used as a chemotherapeutic agent, particularly in the treatment of leukaemia. It is also used for some advanced solid tumours (e.g. of breast, and head and neck).

Since the treatment of acute leukaemia is now often successful, prophylaxis against CNS recurrence has become an important part of management. Intrathecal or intravenous methotrexate combined with cranial or craniospinal irradiation is often given. This combination has sometimes been responsible for producing neurological damage. Price and Jamieson (1975) have reported that cranial irradiation of 2000 rads or more increased the toxicity of methotrexate given intrathecally or intravenously. The syndrome can occasionally occur without cranial irradiation if the dose of intravenous methotrexate is sufficiently high. The syndrome may occur during treatment of recurrence with methotrexate alone following previous combined methotrexate and irradiation which appeared to have caused no neurological damage.

Neurological complications have also been described following intraventricular administration (Shapiro, Chernik and Posner, 1973).

Clinical features Symptoms of meningeal irritation may follow intrathecal methotrexate administration, but are thought to be due either to impurities in the methotrexate or to the vehicle in which it is dissolved.

The characteristic syndrome attributed to methotrexate is of subacute onset with drowsiness, irritability, ataxia and confusion. Fits may occur and spasticity may develop. The patient may recover if no further cytotoxic drugs are given, or the condition may progress to coma and death.

Human pathology Following intraventricular methotrexate, leucoencephalopathy affecting particularly the periventricular region with coagulative necrosis in this region has been described (Shapiro, Chernik and Posner, 1973).

Following irradiation and systemic or intrathecal methotrexate more widespread demyelination occurs. Rubinstein et al. (1975) described five cases with disseminated necrotizing lesions and extensive demyelination, particularly in the centrum ovale. Inflammatory cells were absent and there was a paucity of macrophage reaction in the demyelinated region, which was surrounded by status spongiosus with an astrocytic response. Axonal damage was marked and axonal swellings filled with mitochondria were prominent. Vascular fibrinoid necrosis was an inconstant feature. Price and Jamieson (1975) described similar pathological findings in 13 patients, stressing the multifocal nature of the lesions which then become confluent to produce extensive demyelination. Again, necrotizing or sclerotic microangiopathy was inconstantly present.

Similar multifocal lesions were found in the pons in four cases by Breuer, Blank and Schoene (1978). All had received cranial irradiation, three to the posterior fossa; three had received methotrexate and the fourth only methyl-CCNU. Thus the syndrome may not be uniquely caused by methotrexate, although this substance seems to have been the most important factor in practically all cases.

The mechanism of methotrexate toxicity is not known. It has been suggested on several occasions that irradiation may damage the blood–brain barrier so that larger amounts of methotrexate reach the white matter. The pathological changes do not suggest that the lesions have a primary vascular pathologenesis.

Nitroimidazoles

Misonidazole

Exposure Misonidazole, a 2-nitroimidazole (Ro-07-0582; 1-methoxy-3-(2-nitroimidazol-1-yl)-3-methoxypropan-2-ol) is a potent electron-affinic agent which sensitizes hypoxic cells to the lethal effects of ionizing radiation. Experimental studies have shown it to be highly effective in the control of animal tumours containing a significant proportion of hypoxic cells (Fowler, 1980).

Treatment of patients was begun using doses well below those found to produce neurotoxicity in dogs (Scharer, 1972) and primates (Parkes, personal communication to Dische et al., 1977). In clinical trials, however, peripheral neuropathy proved to be a limiting side effect, and convulsions sometimes occurred after treatment with high doses (Dische et al., 1977). Mamoli et al. (1979) refer to reports of polyneuropathy associated with misonidazole treatment. In their electrophysiological study they found neurological abnormalities to be dose-dependent; clinical and electrophysiological evidence of distal sensory disturbances was seen in six out of 13 patients; motor nerves were less affected.

Human pathology Urtasun et al. (1978) examined the sural nerve from a patient with symptoms of a peripheral sensory neuropathy after treatment with misonidazole. They found axonal degeneration with some segmental demyelination; electron microscopy showed axonal swelling and increased neurofilaments.

Experimental studies Mice given intraperitoneal misonidazole became alternately hyperactive and listless, and rotarod performances declined after 3–4 weeks of dosing; increased hindfoot splay and walking on tip toes appeared later. No significant electrophysiological or morphological changes were found in peripheral nerves and no gross changes were seen in the brain (Conroy et al., 1979).

Griffin et al. (1980) gave similar doses of misonidazole to rats. After 2–3 weeks, righting reflexes were reduced and the forelimbs became very weak. Some rats had a persistent tilt of the head, others repeatedly fell over to one side; there was no clinical evidence of peripheral neuropathy. Histological examination of the CNS showed sharply localized and symmetrical lesions in the vestibular nuclei and the superior olives; the coclear nuclei and cerebellar roof nuclei were sometimes involved. In severely affected rats there was necrosis of these nuclei, with haemorrhages and infiltration by phagocytic cells; in milder cases, extracellular oedema and swelling of astrocytic processes produced a spongiform change. The topography and pathological changes closely resembled those found in thiamine-deficient rats. However, administration of thiamine did not prevent the development of lesions. In peripheral nerves, distal axonal changes were seen with some loss of motor nerve terminals in hindfoot muscles but more severe loss of sensory endings in intrafusal fibres.

Metronidazole

Exposure Metronidazole, like misonidazole, is a nitroimidazole compound. Although well established as a protozoacide and bactericidal drug for the treatment of anaerobic infections, it has also been used as a potentiating agent in radiotherapy. Bradley, Karlsson and Rassol (1977) list various other conditions in which metronidazole has been used. Metronidazole is known to cross the blood–brain barrier.

Clinical features Neurological side effects associated with metronidazole therapy include convulsions (Frytak et al., 1978) and sensory polyneuropathy (Coxon and Pallis, 1976; Schipper et al., 1976; Bradley, Karlsson and Rassol, 1977). Kusumi et al. (1980) have reported encephalopathy, cerebellar dysfunction with ataxia and distal sensory neuropathy after treatment with high doses. The encephalopathy and cerebellar ataxia disappeared within 6 days following withdrawal of the drug; paraesthesiae persisted for several months but had gone within 7 months of cessation of treatment.

Human pathology Bradley, Karlsson and Rassol (1977) reported a case of peripheral neuropathy in detail. Electrophysiological investigations showed reduced amplitude of sensory nerve action potentials. In the sural nerve there was a marked loss of myelinated fibres of all sizes, with evidence of regeneration; unmyelinated fibres were less affected. All symptoms and signs of peripheral neuropathy had disappeared 7 months after withdrawal of metronidazole. Said, Goasguen and Laverdant (1978) found severe loss of myelinated fibres in a sural nerve biopsy; there was some evidence of demyelination secondary to axonal degeneration.

Experimental studies Rogulja, Kovac and Schmid (1973) dosed rats with metronidazole and noted behavioural and balance disturbances within 3 days. In the CNS, sharply defined, symmetrical, spongiform lesions were found in the vestibular and cochlear nuclei, the cerebellar roof nuclei, paramedially in the anterior colliculus and in the superior olive. The lesions resembled those seen in rats dosed with misonidazole in both their distribution and histological characteristics (Griffin et al. 1980). The metronidazole lesions have also been compared with B_1 avitaminosis in rats, and human Wernicke's encephalopathy.

Bradley, Karlsson and Rassol (1977) did not find neurotoxic changes in either the central or the peripheral nervous system of rats given daily doses of metronidazole approximating to those used in man for 16 weeks.

Perhexiline and other drugs causing lipidosis

A number of drugs are known to cause generalized lipidosis. A common structural feature of these drugs is the presence of a hydrophobic moiety in close association with a hydrophilic moiety which is positively charged; such drugs are described as amphiphilic. Apart from their amphiphilia these drugs have very varying chemical features and belong to different chemical classes. It is thought that these compounds interfere with lysosomal degradation, resulting in the accumulation of drug–lipid complexes within the lysosomes. In affected cells the enlarged lysosomes appear as inclusions with a lamellated or crystalline-like structure.

Experimental studies on drug-induced lipidosis in the nervous system have been reviewed by Drenckhahn and Lüllmann-Rauch (1979). Only those drugs known to cause neurotoxicity in man will be discussed further (see Table 14.1).

Table 14.1 Amphiphilic drugs known to induce lipidosis in the nervous system

Inducers of lipidosis in humans and animals	
Perhexiline maleate	Antianginal
Amiodarone	Antiarrhythmic
Chloroquine	Antimalarial
Inducers of lipidosis in animals	
Imipramine	Antidepressant
Clomipramine	Antidepressant
Iprindole	Antidepressant
Chlorphentermine	Anorectic
Chlorcyclizine	Antihistamine

Perhexiline maleate

Perhexiline maleate (dicyclohexyl-2,2′-ethyl-2-piperidine, Pexid) is used for the relief of angina pectoris and as an antiarrhythmic agent. In 1973, Abaza et al. described a case of peripheral neuropathy in a patient treated with perhexiline maleate; Laplane reviewed 35 cases in 1976 (Bousser et al., 1977), and numerous case reports have appeared since them.

Clinical features Peripheral neuropathy may develop from 3 weeks to 3 years after treatment has begun, usually at a dose of 200–300 mg daily. At first there is pain or numbness in the lower limbs, which is readily reversible if therapy is discontinued. The neuropathy is usually symmetrical and progresses to distal sensory loss in the extremities, and weakness affecting proximal and distal muscles. In severe cases dysaesthesias may occur in the perioral region and on the trunk. The presence of raised CSF protein and electrophysiological evidence of severe slowing of conduction velocities in many cases suggest a polyradiculoneuropathy (Bousser et al., 1977; Said, 1978; Wijesekera et al., 1980). Recovery takes place within weeks to months following withdrawal of the drug.

The rate of oxidation of several drugs is genetically controlled and can be assessed by measurement of oxidation of debrisoquine. In a study of 34 patients treated with perhexiline, Shah et al. (1982) found that drug oxidation was impaired in most patients who developed neuropathy but not in those without neuropathy, suggesting that the liability to perhexiline neuropathy is genetically determined.

Human pathology Sural nerve biopsies have been examined in a number of cases (Lhermitte et al., 1976; Mussini, Hauw and Escourolle, 1977; Said, 1978; Fardeau, Tomé and Simon, 1979). The neuropathy is of a demyelinating type. In a quantitative study of five patients, Said found segmental demyelination in 16–90 per cent of teased fibres; no onion bulbs were seen in these nerves although Mussini, Hauw and Escourolle (1977) found some small onion bulb formations. The extent of axonal loss varies considerably; in some cases myelinated fibre density remained within normal limits whilst in others it was severely reduced. Histograms of myelinated fibre diameter showed a shift to the left which might indicate a selective loss of large fibres but could also be due to reduced fibre size as a result of incomplete remyelination following demyelination. Numbers of unmyelinated fibres were decreased in some cases (Said, 1978; Fardeau, Tomé and Simon, 1979).

A striking ultrastructural feature in all the nerves was the presence of osmiophilic, membrane-bound inclusions, probably of lysosomal origin, having a paracrystalline or concentrically lamellated structure. These inclusions were abundant in Schwann cells and endothelial cells but were also seen in perineurial cells, pericytes, fibroblasts and phagocytes. The inclusions are 0.25–1.3 μm in diameter (Fardeau, Tomé and Simon, 1979), so some are visible by light microscopy as small dark granules in 1-μm plastic sections.

Experimental studies In a study on the effects of amphiphilic drugs on the CNS, Frisch and Lüllmann-Rauch (1980) showed that perhexiline produced conspicuous perikaryal lipidosis in the area postrema, a region of the lower brain stem lying outside the blood–brain barrier; axonal swellings containing large accumulations of polymorphic, osmiophilic materials, lamellated structures and autophagic vacuoles were also found in this area (Frisch and Lüllmann-Rauch, 1981). These may be caused by local action of perhexiline, or may result from lysosomal overloading of the perikarya. Inclusions accumulate in sensory and autonomic ganglion cells which also lie outside the blood–brain barrier.

When perhexiline was fed to suckling rats, osmiophilic inclusions were found in all types of cells in the CNS, although pyramidal neurons of the entorhinal cortex, cerebellar Purkinje cells and anterior horn cells were particularly affected. The inclusions were identical to those seen in biopsied nerve, skin and muscle from patients with perhexiline neuropathy (Jung and Suzuki, 1978). Presumably an incompletely formed blood–brain barrier facilitates passage of the drug into the immature rat brain.

Fardeau, Tomé and Simon (1979) found some inclusions in Schwann cells and perineurial cells in the nerves of adult mice dosed with perhexiline, but no other changes in nerve fibres were seen.

Amiodarone

Amiodarone is a di-iodinated benzofuran derivative used in the control of cardiac arrhythmias; it appears to act by prolonging the duration of the action potential in myocardial cells.

Clinical features Peripheral neuropathy associated with amiodarone treatment has been the subject of a number of papers (e.g. Kaeser, 1974; Lustman and Monseu, 1974; Kaeser, Ulrich and Wüthrich, 1976). The neuropathy is symmetrical and distal, often causing severe sensory and

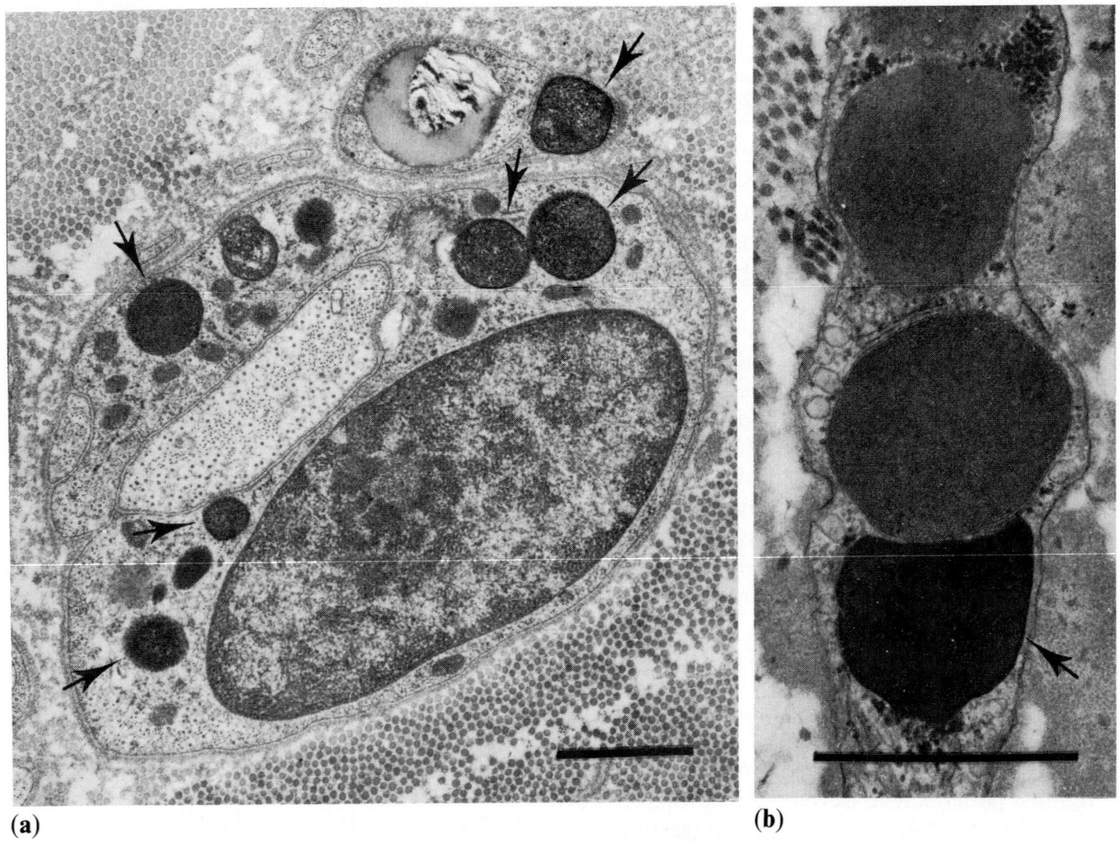

Fig. 14.16 (**a**) Electron micrograph of a sural nerve of a patient with amiodarone neuropathy. Numerous electron-dense inclusions (arrows) are seen in the cytoplasm of the Schwann cell enclosing an unmyelinated fibre. Bar = 1 μm. (**b**) Electron micrograph at a higher magnification showing inclusions in a fibroblast from a sural nerve of another case of amiodarone neuropathy. Two inclusions have a crystalline structure and one (arrow) has a finely lamellated form. Bar = 1 μm.

motor impairment, with muscle atrophy. Raised CSF protein levels have been found in many cases.

Human pathology Sural nerve biopsies examined by Meier et al. (1979) and Dudognon et al. (1979) showed severe loss of myelinated fibres. Three cases of amiodarone neuropathy studied by Kaeser, Ulrich and Wüthrich (1976) showed almost pure demyelination. Jacobs (unpublished observations, 1983) found a marked reduction of myelinated fibres in one patient but very mild loss in a second. Teased fibres from several cases showed axonal degeneration and demyelination and remyelination (Dudognon et al., 1979; Jacobs unpublished observations, 1983). Although unmyelinated fibre density was within normal limits in the case of Dudognon et al. (1979), many of the fibres were very small and probably represented regenerated fibres. Meier et al. and Jacobs noted loss of unmyelinated axons.

A common feature of amiodarone neuropathy was the presence of lipid-laden lysosomes in Schwann cells (particularly in unmyelinated fibres), endothelial cells, perineurial cells and fibroblasts (Fig. 14.16). Electron microscopy showed these dense bodies to have a paracrystalline or concentrically lamellated structure closely resembling the perhexiline-induced inclusions. Degenerative changes in Schwann cell cytoplasm were noted by Jacobs; in some cells no recognizable organelles were seen and only finely granular material remained, whilst the myelin sheath was intact or showed early evidence of disorganization (Fig. 14.17). Degenerative changes were also seen in endothelial cells and perineurial cells.

Although axonal loss may be severe in this neuropathy, it is apparent that amiodarone is toxic to Schwann cells; demyelination is therefore a primary event.

Chemical analysis of the nerve and muscle

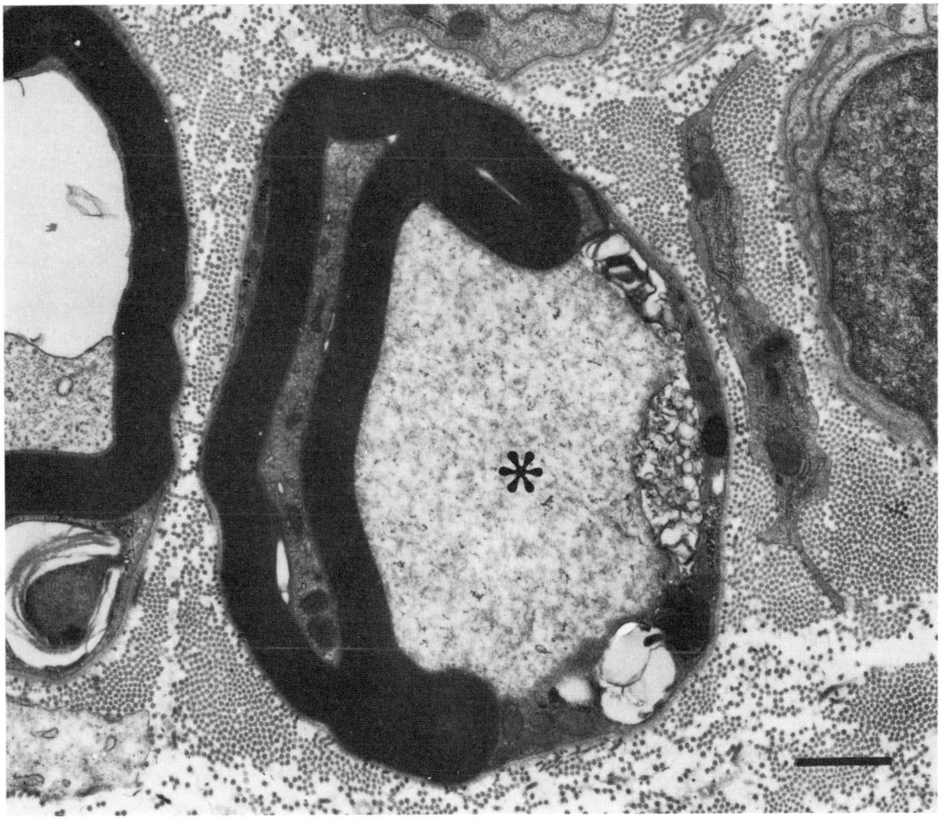

Fig. 14.17 Electron micrograph of the sural nerve of a patient with amiodarone neuropathy. The Schwann cell cytoplasm (*) consists of granular material. It has formed a 'vacuole' within the outermost lamellae of the myelin sheath. The axon is compressed. Bar = 1 μm.

biopsies from the case of Meier et al. (1979) showed levels of iodine 40 times that of normal.

Experimental studies There are no published studies of the neurotoxicity of amiodarone although it is known to produce a generalized lipidosis in rats (Bockhardt, Drenckhahn and Lüllmann-Rauch, 1978). Unpublished studies of neurotoxicity in the mouse and rat by Costa-Jussa and Jacobs have shown lipidosis in regions lying outside the blood barriers, including area postrema and sympathetic and dorsal root ganglia. Degeneration was seen in neurons of coeliac and superior cervical ganglia which accumulate particularly large numbers of inclusions.

Chloroquine

Chloroquine is used in the treatment of malaria and extraintestinal amoebiasis, and in chronic diseases such as rheumatoid arthritis and systemic lupus erythematosus.

Clinical features Vacuolar myopathy is a recognized side effect of chloroquine therapy, but electrophysiological examinations have shown a neuropathic component to the muscle weakness in some cases (Whisnant et al., 1963; Begg and Simpson, 1964; Gerard et al., 1973). Bischoff (1980) has described a patient with peripheral neuropathy who had sensory loss in the lower limbs in addition to muscle weakness, which was reversible after withdrawal of chloroquine treatment. Psychoses, epileptic seizures and acute extrapyramidal movements have also been reported as side effects of chloroquine therapy.

Human pathology A sural nerve from Bischoff's patient showed axonal degeneration and abundant inclusions of lysosomal origin within Schwann cells (see also chapter 21).

Experimental studies Chronic chloroquine intoxication in swine (Gleiser et al., 1968) and in rats and rabbits (Klinghardt, 1974) caused accumulations of concentrically lamellated inclusions in dorsal root ganglion cells. Klinghardt (1978) refers to other chloroquine studies in which inclusions have been found in terminal and preterminal axons and in a number of different neuronal types.

Vincristine

Exposure Vincristine was introduced in 1961 as a chemotherapeutic agent, being mainly used in the treatment of leukaemia, Hodgkin's disease and lymphomas.

Neurological complications were common initially when vincristine was used as the sole therapeutic agent. Because of its toxicity it is now usually used at a lower dose as one agent in a multiple chemotherapeutic regimen, often with intermittent administration. Neurological symptoms are now less common.

Clinical features Peripheral neuropathy occurs with initial paraesthesiae and sensory loss. All tendon reflexes are lost early. Weakness develops later and then often progresses rapidly to severe incapacity if administration continues, particularly in older people (Casey et al., 1973). Forearm extensor muscles may be particularly severely affected. Autonomic neuropathy may develop, with paralytic ileus and postural hypotension.

Human pathology Early studies of muscle biopsies in four patients by Hildebrand and Coërs (1965) demonstrated neurogenic atrophy with no evidence of collateral axonal sprouting of intramuscular nerves. McLeod and Penny (1969) found predominant axonal degeneration with only a few demyelinated fibres in sural nerves obtained at biopsy from patients treated with vincristine. Many regenerating fibres were present in a nerve examined several months after the drug was stopped. In a further study of muscle biopsies Bradley et al. (1970) found a few fibres showing spheromembranous changes similar to those seen in animal studies. They also found denervation atrophy in muscles and axonal degeneration in one sural nerve which was examined.

Neuronal changes in anterior horn cells of the spinal cord following intrathecal vincristine were described by Schochet, Lampert and Earle (1968), similar to those following intracisternal vincristine administration to rabbits. Following high doses of intravenous vincristine, Shelanski and Wiśniewski (1969) reported similar neuronal neurofilamentous proliferation in spinal ganglia, spinal cord, Purkinje cells, medulla and pons.

Experimental studies Slotwiner, Song and Anderson (1966) observed paralysis in rats given high doses of vincristine. Although the clinical syndrome in humans is characteristic of peripheral neuropathy, no abnormality was demonstrated in the rats' peripheral nerves, but spheromembranous degeneration of muscle fibres occurred. The spheromembranous bodies contained mitochondrial remnants, smooth-profiled vesicles and irregular dense bodies apparently arising from sarcoplasmic reticulum and transverse tubules (Anderson, Song and Slotwiner, 1967). Bradley (1970) produced similar muscle changes in guinea-pigs following a single large dose. When repeated smaller doses were given, some peripheral nerve fibres degenerated but the degree of nerve degeneration was never severe. No abnormality was seen in neuronal cell bodies.

Neuronal changes were described in the medulla and pons following a single intracisternal injection of vincristine to rabbits (Schochet, Lampert and Earle, 1968). These changes consisted of accumulations of neurofilaments in the cell body extending into the axons with an increase in free ribosomes and short fragments of granular endoplasmic reticulum. Crystalline osmiophilic masses were also present in neurons.

Schlaepfer (1971b) found loss of neurotubules and formation of microtubular crystals within axons following intraneural injection of vincristine. Neurofilaments and other axoplasmic organelles accumulated proximal to the site of injection and some were in continuity with the crystalline lattice. Axonal degeneration occurred distally. Intravenous injection of vincristine to cats produces massive swellings due to accumulation of neurofibrillary material in the proximal parts of axons, with secondary paranodal demyelination (Cho, Lowndes and Goldstein, 1980). Thus, accumulation of neurofilaments, with loss of neurotubules and formation of crystalline masses, is the characteristic pathological change produced by vincristine. However, the sites at which these changes occur depend on the dose and route of injection and the species of animal studied.

In vitro experiments have suggested that the neuronal crystalline masses are due to interaction of the Vinca alkaloid with microtubule protein (tubulin) (Bensch et al., 1969). Further *in vitro* work on the effect of Vinca alkaloids on tubulin from various sources has shown that polymerization of microtubules is inhibited but preformed microtubules are unaffected (Wilson, Creswell and Chin, 1975; Himes et al., 1976). Embryonic chick brain tubulin has two high-affinity binding sites per molecule. The antimitotic action of the drug is due to blocking of mitosis at metaphase.

In view of the effect of Vinca alkaloids on neurotubules it might be predicted that axonal transport would be disturbed. Indeed, Greet et al. (1977) studied the effect of vincristine on vagus nerves of the cat *in vitro* and found a dose-related partial block of fast transport with concurrent disappearance of microtubules and appearance of crystalline structures.

Other drugs

Disulfiram

Exposure Tetraethylthiuram disulphide (disulfiram) was introduced for the treatment of alcoholism in 1947 and has been widely used since then.

Clinical features Peripheral neuropathy is a rare complication of treatment. In 1978 Moddel et al. reviewed 26 reported cases, and a few further cases have since been described. Neuropathy occurs following high doses (500 mg or more daily) or prolonged treatment for several months. Sensory symptoms predominate. Optic neuritis is an occasional complication, but does not always occur in the same patients as those who develop neuropathy (Gardner-Thorpe and Benjamin, 1971).

Human pathology A few reports of sural nerve biopsies from affected subjects are available. Nukada and Pollock (1981) have described one patient in whom the diagnosis seemed certain with predominant segmental demyelination in the sural nerve. However, axonal degeneration has been the usual finding (Moddel et al., 1978). Bouldin, Hall and Krigman (1980) have described predominant involvement of large-diameter fibres; but both large and small fibres were degenerating in a nerve from one patient studied by Mokri, Ohnishi and Dyck (1981) at the height of the illness. There was no evidence of regenerating fibres in the nerve from the patient described by Bouldin, Hall and Krigman (1980) although she had stopped the drug some months before the biopsy and had improved clinically.

There had, however, been an increase in number of small fibres in one of the patients of Mokri, Ohnishi and Dyck (1981) nearly 2 years after stopping the drug, suggesting that regenerating fibres were present. These differences may reflect differing severity of disease.

Granular degeneration of axoplasmic organelles has been described, with no increase in neurofilaments. This observation is of some importance when considering the pathogenetic mechanism of the neuropathy. It has been argued that the primary toxic agent is carbon disulphide, which is produced during the metabolism of disulfiram (Casier and Merlevede, 1962). However, experimental studies have shown an increase in neurofilaments in carbon disulphide neuropathy, thus suggesting that this substance is not responsible for producing disulfiram neuropathy.

Experimental studies Anzil and Dozic (1978) found axonal degeneration in peripheral nerves of rats given disulfiram but there was no detailed study of the distribution of the lesion. Adachi and Solitaire (1979) have described primary mitochondrial changes in CNS and muscle in intoxicated rats. Following increased density of the matrix, mitochondria were lost and organelles degenerated.

Doxorubicin

Exposure Doxorubicin (Adriamycin) is a chemotherapeutic agent often used in multiple chemotherapy regimens for treating a wide variety of neoplastic conditions.

Clinical features The limiting factor in treatment is the danger of cardiomyopathy (Lefrak et al., 1973). No neurological abnormalities have been reported in humans, perhaps because of this limitation.

Human pathology Pathological changes in cardiac muscle have been described in patients dying of congestive cardiac failure (Lefrak et al., 1973). Many muscle cells had degenerated completely. Those that survived showed loss of contractile substance, mitochondrial swelling and intramitochondrial dense inclusion bodies.

Pathological studies have been reported on seven patients who died of acute leukaemia and who had been treated with rubidomycin, which is a hydroxylated derivative of doxorubicin (B. Smith, 1969). Degeneration of intracardiac neurons was seen, as were pathological changes in neurons in dorsal root ganglia.

Experimental studies A single intravenous dose of 10 mg/kg body weight to rats causes progressive ataxia after 11–12 days (Cho et al., 1980). Focal nuclear clearings due to loss of chromatin material have been described in dorsal root ganglion neurons as early as 3 hours after injection. By 9 days many of these nuclei were pyknotic and karyolytic. Cytoplasmic alterations consisted of perinuclear dense bodies, and neurofilaments separated by dense aggregations of cytoplasmic organelles; later many neurons and the associated nerve fibres in dorsal roots, dorsal columns of the spinal cord and sciatic nerve degenerated. Cho et al. (1980) have postulated that the effects were due to permanent disruption of nucleic acid metabolism in neurons resulting from the known action of doxorubicin on nucleic acids.

The site of action of doxorubicin on dorsal root ganglia may be related to the selective permeability of blood vessels in peripheral ganglia. Sahenk and Mendell (1979a) found fluorescent staining of nuclei of dorsal root ganglia and surrounding satellite cells 1 minute after intravenous injection of doxorubicin but no staining of dorsal or ventral roots. Bigotte, Arvidson and Olsson (1982) found that, following the injection in mice, drug fluorescence was localized to those parts of the nervous system which are outside the blood–brain barrier, including the circumventricular organs and cells of the choroid plexus and lamina cribrosa of the optic nerve.

In a study of axonal transport 48 hours after intravenous administration of doxorubicin to rats and before neuronal degeneration had started, Sahenk and Mendell (1979a) found normal rates of fast axonal flow but reduced neuronal processing of injected amino acid. This supports the idea that the primary defect is in the cell body and that axon functions remains normal until degeneration occurs.

Thalidomide

Exposure Thalidomide was a widely used sedative in UK and some European countries during the early 1960s. It was withdrawn from general use following the discovery of its teratogenic activity. However, it still has limited use in the prevention of erythema nodosum during the treatment of lepromatous leprosy.

Peripheral neuropathy due to thalidomide became a common condition at the time the drug was widely used (Fullerton and Kremer, 1961).

Clinical features Sensory symptoms and signs occur first, with prominent painful paraesthesiae. As the condition progresses, weakness develops often affecting proximal more than distal muscles. There may be signs of pyramidal tract involvement with brisk reflexes and extensor plantar responses. Recovery was poor after stopping the drug in many patients, residual paraesthesiae being a common complaint (Fullerton and O'Sullivan, 1968).

Human pathology Axonal degeneration in peripheral nerves and dorsal columns of the spinal cord of two patients with thalidomide neuropathy was described by Klinghardt (1965).

Fullerton and O'Sullivan (1968) and Krücke et al. (1971) examined sural nerve biopsies from a number of patients several years after they had stopped taking the drug. In both studies loss of large-diameter fibres was found. Evidence of regeneration was also found in both studies. Fullerton and O'Sullivan (1968) found an increase in numbers of small-diameter fibres and Krücke et al. (1971) found regenerating clusters on electron microscopic examination.

Experimental studies Diezel (1963) demonstrated pathological changes in posterior roots, spinal ganglion cells and posterior columns of the spinal cord in dogs given thalidomide for a year, but detailed studies of the nature of the changes were not undertaken.

Biological intoxication

Buckthorn toxin

Exposure Buckthorn poisoning is caused by ingestion of the fruit of *Karwinskia humboldtiana*, a shrub of the buckthorn family which grows in central and northern Mexico and the south western parts of the USA. Commonly known as the tullidora or coyotillo plant, this desert species flowers and produces a sweet-tasting, brownish-black fruit at any time of the year depending on the weather.

The oily seeds have been used as an anticonvulsant in epilepsy and tetanus, and an infusion of leaves was given for fever and toothache.

The toxic effects of eating buckthorn fruit were recorded as early as 1789 by Clavijeri (see Weller, Mitchell and Daves, 1980). One Indian tribe found that the fruit was safe to eat provided that the stones and seeds were removed. (Recent studies have shown that the stones and seeds contain most of the toxic components.) Buckthorn toxicity has recently been reviewed by Weller, Mitchell and Daves (1980).

In 1918, 106 soldiers were poisoned; 10 per cent of the cases died and many were still disabled after many months. Most cases of poisoning now occur in children, with more than a dozen fatal cases in Mexico each year.

Clinical features The clinical course in children suffering from buckthorn poisoning was described by Padron-Puyou and Velazquez in 1956 (see Weller, Mitchell and Daves, 1980). A delay of 5–20 days follows the ingestion of fruit, before the slow onset of flaccid quadriparesis and paralysis of bulbar and respiratory muscles which may lead to death. There is little evidence of loss of sensory modalities and this appears to be a predominantly motor neuropathy. Mental faculties are not affected. Some recovery may begin within a month (Calderon-Gonzales and Rizzi-Hernandez, 1967) although complete or near recovery may take many months to a year. The symptoms may resemble those of the Guillain–Barré syndrome but a distinguishing feature is the normal composition of the CSF.

Administration of thiamine hydrochloride was thought to cause some improvement in the condition of affected children; in rats, larger doses of buckthorn toxin were needed to produce effects when thiamine was given.

Ingestion of *K. humboldtiana* by livestock is an economic problem. Goats, cattle, pigs and sheep may die following consumption of the fruit; in less severe cases the animals develop progressive weakness of the legs with inco-ordination and ataxia, a condition called 'limberleg'. Death may then follow from starvation if the animals are unable to stand.

The active neurotoxic component of the coyotillo fruit is found mainly in the endocarp or stone. Four major toxins have been identified from the neurotoxic extract of the dried fruit (Dreyer et al., 1975); two of these are also present in root extracts.

Human pathology Reports on human pathology are scanty. Calderon-Gonzales and Rizzi-Hernandez (1967) described changes in a sural nerve biopsy from a child with severe polyneuropathy following ingestion of the fruit, including the stones. They reported segmental demyelination and axonal swelling. The relatively rapid onset of recovery in this patient and reports of eventual complete recovery in other cases support the view that buckthorn fruit causes a demyelinating neuropathy which predominantly affects motor nerves.

Experimental studies *K. humboldtiana* produces neurotoxic effects in a wide range of species, although their susceptibility varies considerably (see Weller, Mitchell and Daves, 1980).

Charlton, Claborn and Pierce (1971) studied goats fed with ground fruit; the goats developed hypersensitivity, cerebellar tremor and ataxia with increasing weakness, making them unable to stand. Conduction velocities in sciatic nerves were reduced, and histological examination showed swelling of Schwann cells, intramyelin vacuoles and segmental demyelination. Distal parts of long motor fibre tracts showed axonal degeneration thought to be associated with extensive demyelination. In the CNS the predominant change was chromatolysis, more marked in anterior horn cells than in dorsal root ganglion cells, and presumably secondary to the peripheral nerve changes. Axonal swelling and degeneration in the long tracts of the spinal cord were found in goats and also in monkeys which were accidentally poisoned by buckthorn fruit (Joiner et al., 1975). Goats with cerebellar symptoms were found to have swollen axons in cerebellar white matter.

Cats and rats were given a single dose of ground fruit by mouth; after a delay period of about a week a flaccid paresis of the hindlimbs developed, later affecting the forelimbs (Izquierdo and Nieto, 1965). Peripheral nerves showed demyelination, axon swelling and degeneration; chromatolysis was more obvious in anterior horn cells than in sensory ganglion cells.

In more recent studies in cats (Munoz-Martinez and Chavez, 1979), segmental demyelination was more marked in motor than in sensory nerves, whilst ventral root fibres were virtually unaffected. Axons showed accumulations of neurofilaments. Electrophysiological studies suggested a conduction block in the peripheral nerves with denervation-like changes in associated muscles.

Two neurotoxic compounds (T496 and T544) isolated from buckthorn fruit were dissolved in sesame seed oil and injected intraneurally into rat sciatic nerves (Mitchell et al., 1978). After a latent period of several days a flaccid paralysis developed in the limbs and extensive segmental demyelination was found; fibres showed increased nodal gap widening, indicating loss of paranodal regions of myelin as well as whole internodal breakdown. Buckthorn neuropathy has a number of features in common with diphtheritic neuropathy; both have a latent period before the onset of symptoms, and the pattern of clinical signs and segmental demyelination is similar.

Lathyrism

Exposure Neurolathyrism is caused by eating the chick pea, *Lathyrus sativus* or occasionally other related species, *L. clymenum* or *L. cicera.* The exact nature of the toxic agent is still not certain.

Osteolathyrism is an entirely different disease which results from feeding the sweet pea (*Lathyrus odoratus*) to animals. This was originally done during attempts to reproduce neurolathyrism experimentally, and has led to some confusion. Selye (1957) clearly differentiated the two conditions. Both types of lathyrism have been well reviewed by Barrow, Simpson and Miller (1974) and osteolathyrism will not be considered further.

The disease occurs when large quantities of plants containing the toxic substance are eaten, usually in times of famine when these hardy plants are the only ones to survive drought or flood. The occurrence of the disease and its cause have been recognized since the first century BC. An excellent history of the disease and accounts of various epidemics are to be found in Spencer et al. (1984).

Lathyrism occurs in countries liable to famines—e.g. India and parts of North Africa, particularly Ethiopia. There are histories of outbreaks in the Middle East, parts of Europe and Russia. Spencer et al. (1984) describe a well documented and followed up epidemic amongst Roumanian Jews in a labour camp in World War II.

Clinical features The characteristic feature of the disease is spastic paraplegia. Symptoms may be of acute or more gradual onset. Sphincter involvement is common, but significant abnormalities of the arms or the sensory system are rare. The condition does not progress after consumption of the toxic compound ceases, but there may be considerable residual disability.

Human pathology There have been few descriptions of the pathology of the condition. The scattered reports have been summarized by Spencer et al. (1984). Symmetrical degeneration of corticospinal tracts is characteristic. Patients examined many years after acquiring the disease have shown some degeneration of Betz cells and anterior horn cells. Spencer et al. (1983) consider the disease to be a central distal axonopathy.

Hirano et al. (1976) have described changes in anterior horn cells in the spinal cord of a man who had developed spastic paraplegia due to lathyrism 30 years before his death. On electron microscopic examination two types of inclusion were seen; one was composed of aggregates of filaments in small bundles and the other was composed of crystalloid structures of elements which were about 800 Å wide and hexagonal in cross-section. There was also loss of myelinated fibres in the posterior columns and pyramidal tracts.

Experimental studies The occurrence of lathyrism in domestic animals and attempts to establish an experimental model have been discussed in detail by Spencer et al. (1984). So far experimental studies have not been satisfactory.

There have been a number of attempts to isolate the toxic substance from species of *Lathyrus*. The substance at present considered most likely to be responsible is β-*N*-oxalylamino-L-alanine (BOAA) (Barrow, Simpson and Miller, 1974). This compound occurs only in those species of *Lathyrus* which produce lathyrism. It is acutely neurotoxic to certain species of young animals, producing convulsions. Intrathecal administration has produced flaccid or spastic paralysis in monkeys (Rao et al., 1967). Chronic feeding, however, has not yet produced a neurological syndrome like the human disease. The possibility of selective distribution due to the influence of the blood-brain barrier has been discussed. This topic is currently being actively investigated.

Other neurotoxic substances

Several substances produce neurotoxic effects which have been studied experimentally but are not known to have caused disease in humans. Some of those which produce distinctive neuropathological changes will be described briefly, because they widen the known range of structural changes that may occur in nervous tissue.

Acetyl ethyl tetramethyl tetralin (AETT)

This substance has been used in the cosmetic industry for its musk-like fragrance, particularly in soaps, aftershave lotions, perfumes and detergents. Since its neurotoxic properties were recognized it has been little used.

Application of AETT to rats, either dermally or parenterally, causes blue discoloration of tissues, including nervous tissue, thought to be due to the formation of a keto-AETT metabolite (Spencer et al., 1980). Blue discoloration does not occur in rabbits or monkeys.

Mild intoxication in rats results in hyperexcitability, and higher doses produce an abnormal gait with limb weakness. Spencer et al. (1979) have described both neuronal and myelin changes in the central and the peripheral nervous system. Ceroid-like pigment granules develop in cell bodies, particularly in pyramidal neurons, cells of the hypoglossal nuclei, anterior horn cells and dorsal root ganglion neurons. Their histochemical, autofluorescence and ultrastructural features are very like those seen in hereditary ceroid-lipofuscinoses in man. A second type of large inclusion, seen in severely affected regions, is similar to the Lafora bodies of the protein type. Schwann cells and oligodendrocytes also accumulate abnormal cytosomes.

Myelin changes begin with splitting of the sheaths at the intraperiod line and the formation of oedematous bubbles. Large-diameter fibres in both central and peripheral nerves are affected first. The changes occur along the length of the internode, in contrast to the myelin oedema produced by hexachlorophane which starts in the middle of the internodes (Maxwell and Le Quesne, 1979). Remyelination follows complete or partial demyelination.

6-Aminonicotinamide (6AN)

During studies on the inhibition of sulphonamide acetylation, 6-aminonicotinamide was noted to be extremely toxic to rabbits. After a delay period it caused loss of control of the hindlimbs (Johnson and McColl, 1955). Further studies showed it to be a potent antimetabolite of nicotinamide. A single intraperitoneal dose of 10 mg/kg produced consistent lesions in the CNS of rats, rabbits, dogs and cats. Light microscopy showed well defined and generally symmetrical spongy lesions in the anterior horn of the spinal cord (particularly affecting laminae VI and VII), the vestibular and cochlear nuclei, nuclei of cranial nerves V and VII, the medial reticular formation and the roof nuclei of the cerebellum (Wolf, Cowen and Geller, 1962; Schneider and Cervos-Navarro, 1974). The lesions showed cytoplasmic swelling of neuroglial cells, ballooned structures in the neuropil and some nerve cells shrunken and misshapen by vacuoles.

Schneider and Cervos-Navarro (1974) gave lower doses (5 mg/kg) to rats and found selective damage to neuroglial cells in affected areas; oligodendrocytes and astrocytes showed vacuolation and eventual necrosis 36 hours after giving 6AN. Involvement of neurons appeared to be a secondary event and was minimal in the lower-dosed animals but a significant feature after larger doses. They also developed cytoplasmic vacuolation leading to necrosis; in addition, dendritic and axonal swellings contributed to the spongy appearance of the lesions. Lipid phagocytes appeared within 24 hours. Blood vessels often collapsed due to surrounding oedema; others appeared to be obstructed by aggregations of red cells and thrombocytes. Twelve months after 6AN there was almost complete loss of neuropil in the cord lesions, with the formation of astrocytic scars.

Meyer-König (1973) described changes in the rat optic nerve and tract after injection of 6AN. In the orbital part of the nerve, progressive astrocytic swelling led to scar formation by fibrous astrocytes. In the optic tract and cerebral part of the nerve there was vacuolation of the myelin sheaths, usually due to splitting at the first and innermost intraperiod line.

When given to newborn rats, 6AN caused the formation of vacuoles between the axon and the inner lamella of myelin in peripheral nerves. This was due generally to swelling of the inner tongue of Schwann cell cytoplasm (Brzoska and Adhami, 1975); myelin formation was not affected.

Blakemore (1975) injected 6AN into the spinal cord of rats and observed a demyelinating lesion in which astrocytes as well as oligodendrocytes were damaged; the subsequent remyelination was largely of Schwann cell origin.

The CNS lesions following i.p. injection bear a close resemblance to those found in thiamine deficiency (Robertson, Wasan and Skinner, 1968), and in neurointoxications caused by 1-amino-3-chloro-2-propanol (Heywood, Sortwell and Prentice, 1978), 6-chloro-6-deoxyglucose (Jacobs and Ford, 1981), metronidazole (Rogulja, Kovac and Schmid, 1973) and misonidazole (Griffin et al., 1980). The regions affected all have a high rate of glucose utilization as shown by the uptake of ^{14}C-2-deoxyglucose from the blood (Schwartz and Sharp, 1978). There is evidence that 6AN inhibits phosphogluconate dehydrogenase, causing increased glucose utilization via pyruvate formation (Lange et al., 1970). In this case the morphological changes show some correlation with the biochemical abnormality.

Cuprizone

bis-Cyclohexanone oxalyldihydrazone (cuprizone) is a chelator used as a reagent for the detection of copper. No neurotoxic effects have been reported in man, but in some experimental animals it produces encephalopathy. Carlton (1966, 1969) observed that cuprizone produced a widespread status spongiosus which was particularly extensive in the cerebellar white matter and brain stem. Suzuki and Kikkawa (1969) showed that this status spongiosus was mainly due to vacuoles which formed within the myelin sheath by splitting at the intraperiod line. Similar vacuoles are found in triethyl tin intoxication (see the earlier section 'Tin'). Degenerate oligodendrocytes were identified in cuprizone-treated mice at all stages of intoxication (Blakemore, 1972); the subsequent appearance of large numbers of demyelinated axons suggested a direct action of cuprizone upon the myelin-forming cells in the brain. Astrocytic hypertrophy was one of the earliest changes to occur, particularly in regions of demyelination but also in parts not so affected.

A sequential study of the process of demyelination in the superior cerebellar peduncle of young mice was made by Blakemore (1973a). Almost all of the fibres were demyelinated after dosing for 5 weeks. Some remyelination was seen in these animals, but in mice taken off the cuprizone there was almost complete remyelination of the cerebellar peduncle within 6–7 weeks, although the myelin sheaths were thinner than normal (Blakemore, 1973b). The origin of the remyelinating oligodendroglia is not certain; the immaturity of the animals used may be an important factor since oligodendroglia of young animals are capable of dividing; moreover, the subependymal plate is active in young rodents.

Excitatory amino acid neurotoxins

During investigations into the effects of naturally occurring brain constituents on the electrical activity of the CNS, Curtis and Watkins (1963) discovered L-glutamate (Glu) and L-aspartate (Asp) to be neuronal excitants, acting by depolarizing the neuronal membrane. It has been suggested that Glu and Asp may be transmitters released at the majority of excitatory synapses in the CNS: probably more than one type of receptor is involved. Glu and Asp are normally found in high concentrations in the CNS, where they are known to have a role in intermediary metabolism in the brain, unrelated to transmission. When present in increased concentration, these amino acids have the potential to cause neuronal death, apparently by excessive stimulation of excitatory receptors on dendrosomal surfaces.

Neuronal degeneration was first described in the retina of mice after the subcutaneous administration of Glu; other toxic effects following systemic administration of Glu include convulsions in rats, cats and monkeys; vomiting in dogs, monkeys and man; and the Chinese restaurant syndrome in adult humans (Schaumburg et al., 1969). Reviews of excitatory amino acid neurotoxins are to be found by Olney (1978, 1980, 1981) and in the Neurosciences Research Program Bulletin (1981).

The blood–brain barrier largely prevents systemically administered acidic amino acids from entering the brain; they can, however, reach regions without a blood–brain barrier such as the area postrema, the arcuate nucleus of the hypothalamus and circumventricular organs (Perez and Olney, 1972). There they produce a distinctive type of neuronal damage; rapid swelling of neuronal perikarya and dendrites is followed by acute degenerative changes in intracellular organelles and clumping of nuclear chromatin; phagocytosis of necrotic neurons may occur within 3 hours of systemic administration of Glu. Axons within the affected area show no degenerative changes in the acute period of severe toxic reaction. Damage to the endocrine hypothalamus causes multiple endocrine disturbances in Glu-treated animals. Experimental studies show that infant animals are more susceptible than adults to Glu-induced changes in the circumventricular organs.

The potential risks of excitatory amino acid drugs and of additives, particularly monosodium glutamate, have been pointed out by Olney (1980) who has also suggested a possible role in certain human neurological conditions such as the aminoacidopathies, and basal ganglia disorders (e.g. Huntington's disease, drug-induced parkinsonism and tardive dyskinesias).

Many analogues of Glu have been tested for neuroexcitatory and neurotoxic activity; these two properties are found to be closely related. The most potent of the Glu analogues is kainic acid, which is more than 500 times as toxic as Glu.

Kainic acid is obtained from a seaweed, *Digenea simplex*; it was formerly used in the treatment of ascariasis. No CNS side effects have been reported in man although it has a strong emetic action in dogs. Systemically injected kainic acid causes convulsions and leads to destruction of neurons in the hippocampus, the olfactory cortex and certain amygdaloid, thalamic and septal regions; circumventricular organs are relatively spared.

When injected locally into the diencephalon, many excitotoxins, including kainic acid, cause neuronal and dendritic degeneration with sparing of axons and terminals of extrinsic origin. Coyle and Schwarcz (1976) and McGeer and McGeer (1976) both reported that microinjection of kainic acid into adult rat striatum produced morphological and biochemical changes resembling those of Huntington's chorea. Nadler, Perry and Cotman (1978) injected kainic acid intraventricularly and found selective destruction of cells in the hippocampus; CA3 and CA4 pyramidal cells were the most sensitive whilst dentate granule cells were very resistant. Injection of kainic acid into the cerebellum caused degeneration of Purkinje, Golgi II, basket and stellate cells, whilst granule cells (other than those in the vicinity of the injection) were spared (Herndon and Coyle, 1978). Granule cells are excitatory and probably use Glu as their transmitter; this result is therefore consistent with the view that kainic acid exerts its toxic action through Glu excitatory receptors. However, other experimental evidence suggests that this is not the only explanation of the action of kainic acid, although it is likely that receptors are implicated, as well as synaptic input. Because excitotoxins can produce degeneration of neurons and their dendrites whilst sparing axons, they are potentially useful tools for studying anatomical pathways in the CNS.

β,β'-iminodipropionitrile (IDPN)

The syndrome of 'waltzing' and head-rolling in rats produced by IDPN was recognized in 1952 (Delay et al., 1952). Hartmann, Lalich and Akert (1958) described large spherical structures in the anterior horns of the spinal cord and in the brain stem in a similar syndrome produced by the related compound, *bis-β*-cyanethylamine. Ule (1962) found the same structures following IDPN intoxication. Initially these structures were thought to be disintegrating nerve cells, but Chou and Hartmann (1964, 1965) recognized that the swellings were due to accumulation of neurofilaments in proximal axonal segments. The involvement of reticular and VIIIth nerve neurons is responsible for the disequilibrium producing the clinical signs.

Symptoms following intermittent administration of IDPN for 4 weeks are permanent and a progressive pathological lesion develops. Axonal swellings gradually spread distally, affecting the distal parts of the roots after about a year. Shimono, Izumi and Kuroiwa (1978) and Griffin and Price (1981a) have studied the myelin changes associated with the swellings. Demyelination occurs over the ballooned segments with eventual onion bulb formation. Griffin and Price (1981b) have described frequent Schwann cell and oligodendrocyte ingrowths into the giant swellings arising from Schmidt–Lanterman clefts in the internodes.

When low doses of IDPN are administered chronically (e.g. 0.5% in the drinking water) similar proximal axonal swellings develop, but after 6 months distal axons shrink (Clark, Griffin and Price, 1980). An associated reduction in nerve conduction velocity of up to 22 per cent was found by Höfinger, Le Quesne and Gajree (1982) after 13 months' chronic administration.

A defect in slow axoplasmic transport has been found in animals intoxicated with IDPN (Griffin et al., 1978) and this is thought to be the fundamental defect responsible for the subsequent pathological changes.

Lysophosphatidyl choline (LPC)

Lysophosphatidyl choline has been used to produce demyelination which is virtually free from axonal degeneration for electrophysiological and histological study. Any associated axonal degeneration has usually been thought to be due to trauma associated with local injection. Hall and Gregson (1971) injected LPC intraneurally into the sciatic nerve of mice. Rapid demyelination within 30 minutes was followed by remyelination within 14 days. Only whole internodes demyelinated and were replaced by two internodes, on average, during remyelination. Cellular proliferation, predominantly of Schwann cells, reached a maximum at 2–3 weeks (Gregson and Hall, 1973).

Injection into CNS white matter produces similar demyelination in the spinal cord of mice (Hall, 1972), rats (Blakemore, 1976), cats (Blakemore et al., 1977) and rabbits (Blakemore, 1978) and rabbit corpus callosum (Waxman, Kocsis and Nitta, 1979). Remyelination in all these species was by oligodendrocytes or Schwann cells depending on the site of the lesion. The degree of astrocytic response varies in different species, being intense in the cat and poor in the rabbit. In the rabbit spinal cord remyelination was incomplete even after 6 months and there was less Schwann cell invasion of the cord than in the other species (Blakemore, 1978). Internodal length of remyelinated segments was more variable in cat spinal cord than in peripheral nerve fibres, varying from short segments of 100 μm to segments whose length was appropriate for the fibre diameter (Blakemore and Murray, 1981).

Mitchell and Caren (1982) looked particularly for the effect on unmyelinated fibres of LPC injection into rat sciatic nerves. These fibres and their Schwann cells were lost at the site of injection. The authors suggest that the axons of myelinated fibres, which remained normal, are protected from LPC by their myelin sheaths but that for fibres without myelin sheaths LPC has a direct effect on the axon after lysis of Schwann cells.

Electrophysiological study of conduction during demyelination and remyelination in cat spinal cord has shown initial conduction block, then recovery of conduction at about the time of onset of remyelination, but with detectable electrophysiological change (delayed refractory period of transmission) for about 2 months (K.J. Smith, Blakemore and McDonald, 1981).

In mouse peripheral nerve, after initial conduction block, slow conduction was restored in some fibres when axons were associated with debris-free Schwann cells, but before remyelination had commenced (Smith and Hall, 1980). In a more recent study of rat ventral roots, Smith, Bostock and Hall (1982) demonstrated that blocked fibres began to conduct in a saltatory fashion as early as 4 days after LPC injection and 3 days before the onset of remyelination. These authors suggest that the electrophysiological findings may be due to aggregates of sodium channels appearing along the demyelinated axon before remyelination commences.

Zinc pyridinethione (ZPT)

This antibacterial and antifungal agent is widely used as an antiseborrhoeic in hair shampoos. There appears to be no danger to humans at the concentrations used and no human disease has been reported (Sahenk and Mendell, 1980a).

Chronic administration to rats and rabbits produces progressive hindlimb weakness due to central–peripheral distal axonopathy (Sahenk and Mendell, 1979b). Initial changes at motor nerve terminals consist of accumulation of branched interconnecting membrane arrays of tubulovesicular profiles 25–40 nm in diameter, probably originating from smooth endoplasmic reticulum, and irregular loosely packed membranous lamellae. Synaptic vesicles are reduced in number. Nerve terminal swelling and degeneration follow. Large-diameter fibres are earliest and most affected. These changes gradually spread proximally. Similar changes occur slightly later in the lateral funiculus of lumbar and sacral segments of the spinal cord and cerebellar vermis. Sensory nerves are much less affected.

Sahenk and Mendell (1980b) found no defect in anterograde transport in ZPT-intoxicated animals nor in the rate of retrograde transport, but they did find a delay in distal turn-around of rapidly transported membrane-associated proteins, which could account for the accumulation of tubulovesicular profiles. The exact relation of these data to the onset of degeneration is not clear.

References

Abaza, A., Cattan, D., Aziza, C. and Pappo, E. (1973) Effets secondaires mais réversibles à la prise perhexiline. *Nouvelle Presse Médicale* **2,** 2820.

Abbritti, G., Siracusa, A., Cianchetti, C., Coli, C.A., Curradi, F., Perticone, G.F. and De Rosa, F. (1976) Shoe-makers' polyneuropathy in Italy: the aetiological problem. *British Journal of Industrial Medicine* **33,** 92–9.

Adachi, M. and Solitaire, G.B. (1979) Histologic and ultrastructural studies of long term effects of disulfiram on the CNS and skeletal muscles of rats. *Journal of Neuropathology and Experimental Neurology* **38,** 301.

Agnew, W.F., Fauvre, F.M. and Pudenz, P.H. (1968) Tellurium hydrocephalus: distribution of tellurium-127m between maternal, fetal and neonatal tissues of the rat. *Experimental Neurology* **21,** 120–32.

Aita, J.F. and Calame, T.R. (1972) Peripheral neuropathy secondary to isoniazid-induced pyridoxine deficiency. *Maryland State Medical Journal* **21,** 68–70.

Akelaitis, A.J. (1941) Lead encephalopathy in children and adults: a clinicopathological study. *Journal of Nervous and Mental Diseases* **93,** 313–32.

Alajouanine, Th., Derobert, L. and Thieffry, S. (1958) Etude clinique d'ensemble de 210 cas d'intoxication par les sels organiques d'étain. *Revue Neurologique* **98,** 85–96.

Aleu, F.P., Katzman, R. and Terry, R.D. (1963) Fine structure and electrolyte analysis of cerebral edema induced by alkyl tin intoxication. *Journal of Neuropathology and Experimental Neurology* **22,** 403–13.

Alfrey, A.C., LeGendre, G.R. and Kaehny, W.D. (1976) The dialysis encephalopathy syndrome. Possible aluminium intoxication. *New England Journal of Medicine* **294,** 184–8.

Allen, N., Mendell, J.R., Billmaier, J., Fontaine, R.E. and O'Neill, J. (1975) Toxic polyneuropathy due to methyl *n*-butyl ketone. *Archives of Neurology* **32,** 209–18.

Altenkirch, H., Mager, J., Stoltenburg, G. and Helmbrecht, J. (1977) Toxic polyneuropathies after sniffing a glue thinner. *Journal of Neurology* **214,** 137–52.

Amore, F. (1974) Determination of cadmium, lead, thallium and nickel in blood by atomic absorption spectrometry. *Analytical Chemistry* **46,** 1597–9.

Anderson, F.H., Richardson, E.P., Okazaki, H. and Brody, J.A. (1979) Neurofibrillary degeneration on Guam. Frequency in Chamorros and non-Chamorros with no known neurological disease. *Brain* **102,** 65–77.

Anderson, P.J., Song, S.K. and Slotwiner, P. (1967) The fine structure of spheromembranous degeneration of skeletal muscle induced by vincristine. *Journal of Neuropathology and Experimental Neurology* **26,** 15–24.

Anzil, A.P. and Dozic, S. (1978) Disulfiram neuropathy: an experimental study in the rat. *Journal of Neuropathology and Experimental Neurology* **37,** 585.

Aquilonius, S.M., Askmark, H., Enoksson, P., Lundberg, P.O. and Mostrom, U. (1978) Computerised tomography in severe methanol intoxication. *British Medical Journal* **2,** 929–30.

Arena, J.M., Watson, G.A. and Sakhadeo, S.S. (1965) Fatal thallium poisoning: a plea for a safer pesticide. *Clinical Pediatrics* **4,** 267–70.

Aring, C.D. (1942) The systemic nervous affinity of triorthocresyl phosphate (Jamaica ginger palsy). *Brain* **65,** 34–47.

Arvidson, B. (1980) Regional differences in severity of cadmium-induced lesions in the peripheral nervous system in mice. *Acta Neuropathologica* **49,** 213–24.

Asbury, A.K., Gale, M.K., Cox, S.C., Baringer, J.R. and Berg, B.O. (1972) Giant axonal neuropathy: a unique case with segmental neurofilamentous masses. *Acta Neuropathologica* **20,** 237–47.

Axt, F., Bunger, P. and Lass, A. (1956) Vitamin-B-stoffwechsel und Polyneuritis bei Isoniazidbehandlung. *Fortschritte der Neurologie, Psychiatrie und ihrer Grenzgebiete* **24,** 369–91.

Bakir, F., Damluji, S., Amin-Zaki, L., Murtadha, M., Khalidi, A., Al-Rawi, N.Y. et al. (1973) Methylmercury poisoning in Iraq. *Science* **181,** 230–41.

Bank, W.J., Pleasure, D.E., Suzuki, K., Nigro, D.O. and Katz, R. (1972) Thallium poisoning. *Archives of Neurology* **26,** 456–64.

Barbeau, A., Inoue, N. and Cloutier, T. (1976) Role of manganese in dystonia. In *Advances in Neurology*, vol 14. (Eds. Eldridge, R. and Fahn, S.), pp. 339–52. Raven Press, New York.

Barnes, D.E. and Walker, D.W. (1981) Prenatal ethanol exposure permanently reduces the number of pyramidal neurons in the rat hippocampus. *Developmental Brain Research* **1,** 333–40.

Barrow, M.V., Simpson, C.F. and Miller, E.J. (1974) Lathyrism: a review. *Quarterly Review of Biology* **49,** 101–28.

Bashore, R.M., Hamilton, A., Lewy, F.H., Braceland, F.J., McDonald, R., Batson, O.V. et al. (1938) *Survey of Carbon Disulphide and Hydrogen Sulphide Hazards in the Viscose Rayon Industry*. Bulletin 46. Department of Labor and Industry, Pennsylvania, Harrisburg, Pa.

Bauer-Moffat, C. and Altman, J. (1977) The effect of ethanol chronically administered to preweanling rats on cerebellar development: a morphological study. *Brain Research* **119,** 249–68.

Baumann, C. (1939) Die Schwefelkohlenstoffvergiftungen des Nervensystems. *Zeitschrift fur die Gesamte Neurologie und Psychiatrie* **166,** 568–80.

Baumbach, G.L., Cancilla, P.A., Martin-Amat, G., Tephly, T.R., McMartin, K.E., Makar, A.B. et al. (1977) Methyl alcohol poisoning. IV. Alterations of the morphological findings of the retina and optic nerve. *Archives of Ophthalmology* **95,** 1859–65.

Baumgartner, G., Gawel, M.J., Kaeser, H.E., Pallis, C.A., Clifford Rose, F., Schaumburg, H.H. et al. (1979) Neurotoxicity of halogenated hydroxyquinolines: clinical analysis of cases reported outside Japan. *Journal of Neurology, Neurosurgery and Psychiatry* **42,** 1073–83.

Begg, T.B. and Simpson, J.A. (1964) Chloroquine neuromyopathy. *British Medical Journal* **1,** 770.

Bensch, K.G., Marantz, R., Wiśniewski, H. and Shelanski, M. (1969) Induction *in vitro* of microtubular crystals by vinca alkaloids. *Science* **165,** 495–6.

Benton, C.D. Jr and Calhoun, F.P. Jr (1953) The ocular effects of methyl alcohol poisoning. Report of a catastrophe involving 320 persons. *American Journal of Ophthalmology* **36,** 1677–85.

Biehl, J.P. and Nimitz, H.J. (1954) Studies on the use of a high dose of isoniazid: toxicity studies. *American Review of Tuberculosis and Pulmonary Diseases* **70,** 430–41.

Biehl, J.P. and Vilter, R.W. (1954a) Effects of isoniazid on pyridoxine metabolism. *Journal of the American Medical Association* **156,** 1549–52.

Biehl, J.P. and Vilter, R.W. (1954b) Effect of isoniazid on vitamin B_6 metabolism: its possible significance in producing isoniazid neuritis. *Proceedings of the Society for Experimental Biology and Medicine* **85,** 389–92.

Bigotte, L., Arvidson, B. and Olsson, Y. (1982) Cytofluorescence localization of adriamycin in the nervous system. I. Distribution of the drug in the central nervous system of normal adult mice after intravenous injection. *Acta Neuropathologica* **57,** 121–9.

Billmaier, D., Yee, H.T., Allen, N., Craft, B., Williams, N., Epstein, S. and Fontaine, R. (1974) Peripheral neuropathy in coated fabrics plant. *Journal of Occupational Medicine* **16,** 665–71.

Bischoff, A. (1970) Ultrastructure of tri-cresyl phosphate poisoning in the chicken. II. Studies on spinal cord alterations. *Acta Neuropathologica* **15,** 142–155.

Bischoff, A. (1980) Clinical and experimental work in neurotoxicity. In *Mechanisms of Toxicity and Hazard Evaluation* (Eds. Holmstedt, B., Lauwerys, R., Mercier, M. and Roberfroid, M.), pp. 39–51. Elsevier/North-Holland, Amsterdam.

Blackman, S. S. Jr (1937) The lesions of lead encephalitis in children. *Bulletin of the Johns Hopkins Hospital* **58,** 1–43.

Blakemore, W.F. (1972) Observations on oligodendrocyte degeneration, the resolution of status spongiosus and remyelination in cuprizone intoxication in mice. *Journal of Neurocytology* **1,** 413–26.

Blakemore, W.F. (1973a) Demyelination of the superior cerebellar peduncle in the mouse induced by cuprizone. *Journal of the Neurological Sciences* **20,** 63–72.

Blakemore, W.F. (1973b) Remyelination of the superior cerebellar peduncle in the mouse following demyelination induced by feeding cuprizone. *Journal of the Neurological Sciences* **20,** 73–83.

Blakemore, W.F. (1975) Remyelination by Schwann cells of axons demyelinated by intraspinal injection of 6-aminonicotinamide in the rat. *Journal of Neurocytology* **4,** 745–57.

Blakemore, W.F. (1976) Invasion of Schwann cells into the spinal cord of the rat following local injections of lysolecithin. *Neuropathology and Applied Neurobiology* **2,** 21–39.

Blakemore, W.F. (1978) Observations on remyelination in the rabbit spinal cord following demyelination induced by lysolecithin. *Neuropathology and Applied Neurobiology* **4,** 47–59.

Blakemore, W.F. (1980) Isoniazid. In *Experimental and Clinical Neurotoxicology* (Eds. Spencer, P.S. and Schaumburg, H.H.), pp. 476–89. Williams and Wilkins, Baltimore, Md.

Blakemore, W.F. and Murray, J.A. (1981) Quantitative examination of internodal length of remyelinated nerve fibres in the central nervous system. *Journal of the Neurological Sciences* **49,** 273–84.

Blakemore, W.F., Palmer, A.C. and Noel, P.R.B. (1972) Ultrastructural changes in isoniazid-induced brain oedema in the dog. *Journal of Neurocytology* **1,** 263–78.

Blakemore, W.F., Eames, R.A., Smith, K.J. and McDonald, W.I. (1977) Remyelination in the spinal cord of the cat following intraspinal injections of lysolecithin. *Journal of the Neurological Sciences* **33,** 31–43.

Bockhardt, H., Drenckhahn, D. and Lüllman-Rauch, R. (1978) Amiodarone-induced lipidosis-like alterations in ocular tissues of rats. *Graefes Archiv für klinische und experimentelle Ophthalmologie* **207,** 91–6.

Bonilla, E. and Diez-Ewald, M. (1974) Effect of *l*-DOPA on brain concentration of dopamine and homovanillic acid in rats after chronic manganese chloride administration. *Journal of Neurochemistry* **22,** 297–9.

Borges, S. and Lewis, P.D. (1982) A study of alcohol effects on the brain during gestation and lactation. *Teratology* **25,** 283–9.

Bouldin, T.W. and Cavanagh, J.B. (1979a) Organophosphorus neuropathy. I.A teased-fibre study of the spatiotemporal spread of axonal degeneration. *American Journal of Pathology* **94,** 241–52.

Bouldin, T.W. and Cavanagh, J.B. (1979b) Organophosphorus neuropathy. II. A fine-structure study of the early stages of axonal degeneration. *American Journal of Pathology* **94,** 253–70.

Bouldin, T.W., Hall, C.D. and Krigman, M.R. (1980) Pathology of disulfiram neuropathy. *Journal of Neuropathology and Experimental Neurology* **6,** 155–60.

Bouldin, T.W. and Krigman, M.R. (1975) Acute lead encephalopathy in the guinea pig. *Acta Neuropathologica* **33,** 185–90.

Bouldin, T.W., Goines, N.D., Bagnell, C.R. and Krigman, M.R. (1981) Pathogenesis of trimethyltin neuronal toxicity. *American Journal of Pathology* **104,** 237–49.

Bousser, M.-G., Bouche, P., Hauw, J.-J., Singlas, E., Touboul, P.-J. and Laplane, D. (1977) Neuropa-

thies périphériques au maléate de perhexiline. *Annales de Cardiologie et d'Angeiologie* **26,** 493–9.
Bradley, W.G. (1970) The neuromyopathy of vincristine in the guinea pig. An electrophysiological and pathological study. *Journal of the Neurological Sciences* **10,** 133–62.
Bradley, W.G., Karlsson, I.J. and Rassol, C.G. (1977) Metronidazole neuropathy. *British Medical Journal* **2,** 610–11.
Bradley, W.G. and Williams, M.H. (1973) Axoplasmic flow in axonal neuropathies. I. Axoplasmic flow in cats with toxic neuropathies. *Brain,* **96,** 235–46.
Bradley, W.G., Lassman, L.P., Pearce, G.W. and Walton, J.N. (1970) The neuromyopathy of vincristine in man. Clinical, electrophysiological and pathological studies. *Journal of the Neurological Sciences* **10,** 107–31.
Breuer, A.C., Blank, N.K. and Schoene, W.C. (1978) Multifocal pontine lesions in cancer patients treated with chemotherapy and CNS radiotherapy. *Cancer* **41,** 2112–20.
Brown, A.W., Aldridge, W.N., Street, B.W. and Verschoyle, R.D. (1979) The behavioral and neuropathologic sequelae of intoxication by trimethyl tin compounds in the rat. *American Journal of Pathology* **97,** 59–76.
Brzoska, H.R. and Adhami, H. (1975) Electron microscopic study of the effect of 6-AN on the sciatic nerve in newborn rats. *Acta Neuropathologica* **33,** 59–66.
Buchanan, W.D. (1962) *Toxicity of Arsenic Compounds.* Elsevier, Amsterdam.
Buchthal, F. and Behse, F. (1979) Electrophysiology and nerve biopsy in men exposed to lead. *British Journal of Industrial Medicine* **36,** 135–47.
Burks, J.S., Alfrey, A.C., Huddlestone, J., Norenberg, M.D. and Lewin, E. (1976) A fatal encephalopathy in chronic haemodialysis patients. *Lancet* **1,** 764–8.
Burns, R., Thomas, D.W. and Barron, V.J. (1974) Reversible encephalopathy possibly associated with bismuth subgallate ingestion. *British Medical Journal* **1,** 220–3.
Calderon-Gonzales, R. and Rizzi-Hernandez, H. (1967) Buckthorn polyneuropathy. *New England Journal of Medicine* **277,** 69–71.
Carbonneau, S.N., Munro, I.C., Nera, E.A., Willes, R.F., Kupier-Goodman, T., Iverson, F. et al. (1974) Subacute toxicity of methylmercury in the adult cat. *Toxicology and Applied Pharmacology* **27,** 569–81.
Carlton, W.W. (1966) Response of mice to the chelating agents sodium diethyldithiocarbamate, α-benzoinoxime and bicyclohexanone oxaldihydrazone. *Toxicology and Applied Pharmacology* **8,** 512–21.
Carlton, W.W. (1969) Spongiform encephalopathy induced in rats and guinea pigs by cuprizone. *Experimental and Molecular Pathology* **10,** 274–87.
Carmichael, N. and Cavanagh, J.B. (1976) Autoradiographic localisation of $_3$H-uridine in spinal ganglion neurons of the rat and the effects of methyl mercury poisoning. *Acta Neuropathologica* **34,** 137–48.
Carmichael, N., Cavanagh, J.B. and Rodda, R.A. (1975) Some effects of methyl mercury salts on the rabbit nervous system. *Acta Neuropathologica* **32,** 115–125.
Casey, E.B., Jelliffe, A.M., Le Quesne, P.M. and Millett, Y.L. (1973) Vincristine neuropathy—clinical and electrophysiological observations. *Brain* **96,** 69–86.
Casier, H. and Merlevede, E. (1962) On the mechanism of the disulfiram-ethanol intoxication symptoms. *Archives Internationales de Pharmacodynamie et de Thérapie* **139,** 165–76.
Cassells, D.A.K. and Dodds, E.C. (1946) Tetra-ethyl lead poisoning. *British Medical Journal* **2,** 681–5.
Cavanagh, J.B. (1954) The toxic effects of tri-ortho-cresyl phosphate poisoning in the cat. *Journal of Neurology, Neurosurgery and Psychiatry* **17,** 163–72.
Cavanagh, J.B. (1964a) The significance of the 'dying back' process in experimental and human neurological disease. *International Review of Experimental Pathology* **3,** 219–67.
Cavanagh, J.B. (1964b) Peripheral nerve changes in ortho-cresyl phosphate poisoning in the cat. *Journal of Pathology and Bacteriology* **87,** 365–83.
Cavanagh, J.B. (1967) On the pattern of changes in peripheral nerves produced by isoniazid intoxication in rats. *Journal of Neurology, Neurosurgery and Psychiatry* **30,** 26–33.
Cavanagh, J.B. (1973) Peripheral neuropathy caused by chemical agents. *CRC Critical Reviews in Toxicology* **2,** 365–417.
Cavanagh, J.B. (1979) The 'dying back' process. A common denominator in many naturally occurring and toxic neuropathies. *Archives of Pathology and Laboratory Medicine* **103,** 659–64.
Cavanagh, J.B. (1982) The pathokinetics of acrylamide intoxication: a reassessment of the problem. *Neuropathology and Applied Neurobiology* **8,** 315–36.
Cavanagh, J.B. and Bennetts, R.J. (1981) On the pattern of changes in the rat nervous system produced by 2,5-hexanediol. *Brain* **104,** 297–318.
Cavanagh, J.B. and Chen, F. C.-K. (1971) Amino acid incorporation in protein during the 'silent phase' before organo-mercury and β-bromophenylacetylurea neuropathy in the rat. *Acta Neuropathologica* **19,** 216–24.
Cavanagh, J.B. and Gregson, M. (1978) Some effects of a thallium salt on the proliferation of hair

follicle cells. *Journal of Pathology* **125,** 179–91.

Cavanagh, J.B. and Gysbers, M.F. (1980) 'Dying back' above a nerve ligature produced by acrylamide. *Acta Neuropathologica* **51,** 169–77.

Cavanagh, J.B. and Gysbers, M.F. (1981) Ultrastructural changes in axons caused by acrylamide above a nerve ligature. *Neuropathology and Applied Neurobiology* **7,** 315–26.

Cavanagh, J.B. and Patangia, G.N. (1965) Changes in the central nervous system in the cat as the result of tri-*o*-cresyl phosphate poisoning. *Brain* **88,** 165–80.

Cavanagh, J.B., Fuller, N.H., Johnson, H.R.M. and Rudge, P. (1974) The effects of thallium salts, with particular reference to the nervous system changes. *Quarterly Journal of Medicine* **43,** 293–319.

Chang, L.W. and Hartmann, H.A. (1972) Ultrastructural studies of the nervous system after mercury intoxication. II. Pathological changes in nerve fibres. *Acta Neuropathologica* **20,** 316–34.

Charlton, K.M. (1974) Experimental alkylmercurial poisoning in swine. Lesions in the peripheral and central nervous system. *Canadian Journal of Comparative Medicine* **38,** 75–81.

Charlton, K.M., Claborn, L.D. and Pierce, K.R. (1971) A neuropathy in goats caused by experimental coyatillo (*Karwinskia humboldtiana*) poisoning: clinical and neurophysiological studies. *American Journal of Veterinary Research* **32,** 1381–9.

Chernoff, G.F. (1977) The fetal alcohol syndrome in mice: an animal model. *Teratology* **15,** 223–9.

Chhuttani, P.N. and Chopra, J.S. (1979) Arsenic poisoning. In *Handbook of Clinical Neurology*, vol. 36 (Eds. Vinken, P.J. and Bruyn, G.W.), pp. 199–216. North-Holland, Amsterdam.

Cho, E.-S., Lowndes, H.E. and Goldstein, B.D. (1980) Vincristine induces proximal giant axonal neuropathy in cats. *Journal of Neuropathology and Experimental Neurology* **39,** 345.

Cho, E.S., Spencer, P.S., Jortner, B.S. and Schaumburg, H.H. (1980) A single intravenous infection of doxorubicin (adriamycin) induces sensory neuronopathy in rats. *Neurotoxicology* **1,** 583–91.

Chou, S.M. and Hartmann, H.A. (1964) Axonal lesions and waltzing syndrome after IDPN administration in rats. *Acta Neuropathologica* **3,** 428–50.

Chou, S.M. and Hartmann, H.A. (1965) Electron microscopy of focal neuroaxonal lesions produced by β,β'-iminodipropionitrile (IDPN) in rats. *Acta Neuropathologica* **4,** 590–603.

Chretien, M., Patey, G., Souyri, F. and Droz, B. (1981) 'Acrylamide-induced' neuropathy and impairment of axonal transport of proteins. II. Abnormal accumulations of smooth endoplasmic reticulum as sites of focal retention of fast transported proteins. Electron microscope radio-autographic study. *Brain Research* **205,** 15–28.

Christian, R.G. and Tryphonas, L. (1971) Lead poisoning in cattle: brain lesions and hematological changes. *American Journal of Veterinary Research* **32,** 203–16.

Clark, A.W., Griffin, J.W. and Price, D.L. (1980) The axonal pathology in chronic IDPN intoxication. *Journal of Neuropathology and Experimental Neurology* **39,** 42–55.

Clark, A.W., Parhad, I.M., Griffin, J.W. and Price, D.L. (1980) Neurotoxicity of *cis*-platinum: pathology of the central and peripheral nervous systems. *Neurology (New York)* **30,** 429.

Clarren, S.K., Alvord, E.C. Jr, Sumi, S.M., Streissguth, A.P. and Smith, D.W. (1978) Brain malformations related to prenatal exposure to ethanol. *Journal of Pediatrics* **92,** 64–7.

Clasen, R.A., Hartmann, J.F., Starr, A.J., Coogan, P.S., Pandolfi, S., Laing, I. et al. (1974) Electron microscopic and chemical studies of the vascular changes and oedema of lead encephalopathy. *American Journal of Pathology* **74,** 215–40.

Conroy, P.J., von Burg, R., Passalacqua, W., Penney, D.P. and Sutherland, R.M. (1979) Misonidazole neurotoxicity in the mouse: evaluation of functional, pharmacokinetic, electrophysiological and morphological parameters. *International Journal of Radiation Oncology, Biology, Physics* **5,** 983–91.

Cossa, P., Duplay, J., Fischgold, Arfel-Capdeville, Lafon, Passouant et al. (1958) Encéphalopathies toxiques au Stalinon. Aspects anatomocliniques et electroencephalographiques. *Revue Neurologique* **98,** 97–108.

Couper, J. (1837) On the effects of black oxide of manganese when inhaled into the lungs. *British Annals of Medical Pharmacology* **1,** 41–5.

Coxon, A. and Pallis, C.A. (1976) Metronidazole neuropathy. *Journal of Neurology, Neurosurgery and Psychiatry* **39,** 403–5.

Coyle, J.T. and Schwarcz, R. (1976) Lesion of striatal neurones with kainic acid provides a model for Huntington's chorea. *Nature (London)* **263,** 244–6.

Crapper McLachlan, D.R. and De Boni, U. (1980) Aluminum in human brain disease—an overview. *Neurotoxicology* **1,** 3–16.

Crapper McLachlan, D.R., Krishnan, S.S., Quittkat, S. and De Boni, U. (1980) Brain aluminum in Alzheimer's disease: influence of sample size and case selection. *Neurotoxicology* **1,** 25–32.

Cremer, J.E. (1981) The neurotoxic effects of environmental chemicals. In *The Molecular Basis of Neuropathology* (Eds. Davidson, A.N. and Thompson, R.H.S.), pp. 234–64. Edward Arnold, London.

Curtis, D.R. and Watkins, J.C. (1963) Acidic amino acids with strong excitatory actions on mammalian neurons. *Journal of Physiology* **166,** 1-14.

Davis, C.S. and Richardson, R.J. (1980) Organophosphorus compounds. In *Experimental and Clinical Neurotoxicology.* (Eds. Spencer, P.S. and Schaumburg, H.H.), pp. 527-44. Williams and Wilkins, Baltimore, Md.

Davis, L.E., Wands, J.R., Weiss, S.A., Price, D.L. and Girling, E.F. (1974) Central nervous system intoxication from mercurous chloride laxatives. *Archives of Neurology* **30,** 428-31.

Davies, LE., Standefer, J.C., Kornfeld, M., Abercrombie, D.M. and Butler, C. (1980) Acute thallium poisoning: toxicological and morphological studies of the nervous system. *Annals of Neurology* **10,** 38-44.

Davis, R.K., Horton, A.W., Larson, E.E. and Stemmer, K.L. (1963) Inhalation of tetramethyllead and tetraethyllead. *Archives of Environmental Health* **6,** 473-9.

Davison, A.M., Walker, G.S., Oli, H. and Lewins, A.M. (1982) Water supply aluminium concentration, dialysis dementia, and effect of reverse-osmosis water treatment. *Lancet* **2,** 285-7.

De Meio, R.H. and Henriques, F.C. (1947) Tellurium. IV. Excretion and distribution in tissues studied with a radioactive isotope. *Journal of Biological Chemistry* **169,** 609-23.

Delay, J., Pichot, P., Thuillier, J. and Marquiset, J.P. (1952) Action de l'aminodipropionitrile sur le comportement moteur de la souris blanche. *Comptes Rendus de la Société de Biologie* **146,** 533.

Diezel, P.B. (1963) Morphologische Veränderungen bei experimenteller Thalidomid-neuropathie und Thalidomid-bedingten Extremitätenmissbildungen. *Münchener medizinische Wochenschrift* **105,** 2265.

Dische, S., Saunders, M.I., Lee, M.E., Adams, G.E. and Flockhart, I.R. (1977) Clinical testing of the radiosensitizer Ro-07-0582: experience with multiple doses. *British Journal of Cancer* **35,** 567-79.

DiVicenzo, G.D., Hamilton, M.L., Kaplan, C.J. and Dedinas, J. (1980) Characterization of the metabolites of methyl *n*-butyl ketone. In *Experimental and Clinical Neurotoxicology* (Eds. Spencer, P.S. and Schaumburg, H.H.), pp. 846-55. Williams and Wilkins, Baltimore, Md.

Drenckhahn, D. and Lüllmann-Rauch, R. (1979) Drug-induced experimental lipidosis in the nervous system. *Neuroscience* **4,** 697-712.

Dreyer, D.L., Arai, I., Bachman, C.D., Anderson, W.R. Jr, Smith, R.G. and Daves, G.D. Jr (1975) Toxins causing non-inflammatory paralytic neuropathy. Isolation and structure elucidation. *Journal of the American Chemical Society* **97,** 4985-90.

Duckett, S. (1971) The morphology of tellurium-induced hydrocephalus. *Experimental Neurology* **31,** 1-16.

Duckett, S., Sandler, A. and Scott, T. (1971) The target period during fetal life for the production of tellurium hydrocephalus. *Experientia* **27,** 1064-5.

Duckett, S. and White, R. (1974) Cerebral lipofuscinosis induced with tellurium: electron dispersive x-ray spectrophotometry analysis. *Brain Research* **73,** 205-14.

Duckett, S., Said, G., Strelitz, L.G., White, R.G. and Galle, P. (1979) Tellurium-induced neuropathy: correlative physiological, morphological and electron microprobe studies. *Neuropathology and Applied Neurobiology* **5,** 265-78.

Dudognon, P., Hauw, J.-J., de Baecque, C., Derrida, J. P., Escourolle, R. and Nick, J. (1979) Neuropathie au chlorohydrate d'amiodarone. *Revue Neurologique* **135,** 527-40.

Dyck, P.J., O'Brien, P.C. and Ohnishi, A. (1977) Lead neuropathy. 2. Random distribution of segmental demyelination among 'old internodes' of myelinated fibres. *Journal of Neuropathology and Experimental Neurology* **36,** 570-5.

Dyck, P.J., Windebank, A.J., Low, P.A. and Baumann, W.T. (1980) Blood nerve barrier in rat and cellular mechanisms of lead-induced segmental demyelination. *Journal of Neuropathology and Experimental Neurology* **39,** 700-9.

Elliott, H.L., Dryburgh, F., Fell, G.S., Sabet, S. and MacDougall, A.I. (1978) Aluminium toxicity during regular haemodialysis. *British Medical Journal* **1,** 1101-3.

Endtz, L.J. (1958) Complications nerveuses du traitement aurique. Aperçu des symptomes neurologiques et psychiatriques; résultats du traitement par le B.A.L. *Revue Neurologique* **99,** 395-410.

Erlanson, P., Fritz, H., Hagstam, K.E., Liljenberg, B., Tryding, N. and Voigt, G. (1965) Severe methanol intoxication. *Acta Medica Scandinavica* **177,** 393-408.

Escourolle, R., Bourdon, R., Galli, A., Galle, P., Jaudon, M.C., Hauw, J.J. and Gray, F. (1977) Étude neuropathologique et toxicologique de douze cas d'éncephalopathie bismuthique. *Revue Neurologique* **133,** 153-63.

Evans, D.A.P., Manley, K.A. and McKusick, V.A. (1960) Genetic control of isoniazid metabolism in man. *British Medical Journal* **2,** 485-91.

Fardeau, M., Tomé, F.M.S. and Simon, P. (1979) Muscle and nerve changes induced by perhexiline maleate in man and mice. *Muscle and Nerve* **2,** 24-36.

Fenton, J.C.B. (1955) The nature of the paralysis in chickens following organophosphorus poisoning. *Journal of Pathology and Bacteriology* **69,** 181-9.

Ferraro, A. and Hernandez, R. (1932) Lead poisoning. A histopathological study of the nervous system of cats and monkeys in the acute and subacute stages. *Psychiatric Quarterly* **6,** 121–46.

Ferraro, A., Jervis, G.A. and Flicker, D.J. (1941) Neuropathologic changes in experimental carbon disulfide poisoning in cats. *Archives of Pathology* **32,** 723–38.

Foncin, J.F. and Gruner, J.E. (1979) Tin neurotoxicity. In *Handbook of Clinical Neurology*, vol. 36 (Eds. Vinken, P.J. and Bruyn, G.W.), pp. 279–90. North-Holland, Amsterdam.

Fortemps, E., Amand, G., Bomboir, A., Lauwerys, R. and Laterre, E.C. (1978) Trimethyltin poisoning. Report of two cases. *International Archives of Occupational and Environmental Health* **41,** 1–6.

Fowler, J.F. (1980) Animal experimental results with radiosensitizers of hypoxic cells. In *Progress in Radio-Oncology* (Eds. Karcher, K.-H., Kogelnik, H.D. and Meyer, H.-J.), pp. 95–108. Thieme, Stuttgart.

Friberg, L., Piscator, M., Nordberg, G. and Kjellstrom, T. (1974) *Cadmium in the Environment*, 2nd edn., pp. 137–95. CRC Press, Cleveland, Ohio.

Frisch, W. and Lüllmann-Rauch, R. (1980) Effects of several lipidosis-inducing drugs upon the area postrema and adjacent medullary nuclei of adult rats. I. Alterations in perikarya and dendrite. *Acta Neuropathologica* **52,** 179–87.

Frisch, W. and Lüllmann-Rauch, R. (1981) Effects of several lipidosis-inducing drugs upon the area postrema and adjacent medullary nuclei of adult rats. II. Axonal alterations. *Acta Neuropathologica* **53,** 41–50.

Frytak, S., Moertel, C.G., Childs, D.S. and Alpers, J.W. (1978) Neurologic toxicity associated with high-dose metronidazole therapy. *Annals of Internal Medicine* **88,** 361–2.

Fullerton, P.M. (1966) Chronic peripheral neuropathy produced by lead poisoning in guinea pigs. *Journal of Neuropathology and Experimental Neurology* **25,** 214–36.

Fullerton, P.M. (1969) Electrophysiological and histological observations on peripheral nerves in acrylamide poisoning in man. *Journal of Neurology, Neurosurgery and Psychiatry* **32,** 186–92.

Fullerton, P.M. and Barnes, J.M. (1966) Peripheral neuropathy in rats produced by acrylamide. *British Journal of Industrial Medicine* **23,** 210–21.

Fullerton, P.M. and Kremer, M. (1961) Neuropathy after intake of thalidomide (Distaval). *British Medical Journal* **2,** 855–8.

Fullerton, P.M. and O'Sullivan, D.J. (1968) Thalidomide neuropathy: a clinical, electrophysiological, and histological follow-up study. *Journal of Neurology, Neurosurgery and Psychiatry* **31,** 543–51.

Gabbiani, G., Baic, D. and Deziel, C. (1967) Toxicity of cadmium for the central nervous system. *Experimental Neurology* **18,** 154–60.

Gabbiani, G., Gregory, A. and Baic, D. (1967) Cadmium-induced selective lesions of sensory ganglia. *Journal of Neuropathology and Experimental Neurology* **26,** 498–506.

Gabbiani, G., Badonnel, M.C., Mathewson, S.M. and Graeme, B.R. (1974) Acute cadmium intoxication. Early selective lesions of endothelial clefts. *Laboratory Investigation* **30,** 686–95.

Gardner-Thorpe, C. and Benjamin, S. (1971) Peripheral neuropathy after disulfiram administration. *Journal of Neurology, Neurosurgery and Psychiatry* **34,** 253–9.

Garland, T.O. and Patterson, M.W.H. (1967) Six cases of acrylamide poisoning. *British Medical Journal* **4,** 134–8.

Garman, R.H., Weiss, B. and Evans, H.L. (1975) Alkylmercurial encephalopathy in the monkey (*Saimiri sciureus* and *Macaca arctoides*). *Acta Neuropathologica* **32,** 61–74.

Garro, F. and Pentschew, A. (1964) Neonatal hydrocephalus in the offspring of rats fed during pregnancy nontoxic amounts of tellurium. *Archiv für Psychiatrie und Nervenkrankheiten* **206,** 272–80.

Gerard, J.M., Stoupel, N., Collier, A. and Flament-Durand, J. (1973) Morphological study of a neuromyopathy caused by prolonged chloroquine treatment. *European Neurology* **9,** 363–79.

Gettler, A.O. and Weiss, L. (1943) Thallium poisoning. III. Clinical toxicology of thallium. *American Journal of Clinical Pathology* **13,** 422–9.

Gleiser, C.A., Bay, W.W., Dukes, T.W., Brown, R.S., Read, W.K. and Pierce, K.R. (1968) Study on chloroquine toxicity and a drug-induced cerebrospinal lipodystrophy in swine. *American Journal of Pathology* **53,** 27–45.

Globus, J.H. and Ginsburg, S.W. (1933) Pericapillary encephalorrhagia due to arsphenamine. *Archives of Neurology* **30,** 1226–47.

Goldstein, G.W., Asbury, A.K. and Diamond, I. (1974) Pathogenesis of lead encephalopathy. Uptake of lead and reaction of brain capillaries. *Archives of Neurology* **31,** 382–9.

Goldstein, N.P., McCall, J.T. and Dyck, P.J. (1975) Metal neuropathy. In *Peripheral Neuropathy* (Eds. Dyck, P.J., Thomas, P.K. and Lambert, E.H.), pp. 1227–62. W.B. Saunders, Philadelphia, Pa.

Gombault, M.* (1873) Contribution à l'histoire anatomique de l'atrophie musculaire saturnine. *Archives de Physiologie Normale et Pathologique* **5,** 592–7.

* A note on Gombault's initials.

In early French journals, authors were often referred to as Monsieur – hence M. Gombault (see ref. of 1873). Although the initial A. appears in a number of references (e.g. 1880) – his initials were A.F.

Gombault, A. (1880) Contribution a l'étude anatomique de la névrite parenchymateuse subaiguë et chronique-névrite segmentaire périaxile. *Archives de Neurologie* **1,** 11–38.

Goodale, R.H. and Humphreys, M.B. (1931) Jamaica ginger paralysis: autopsy observations. *Journal of the American Medical Association* **96,** 14–16.

Gordy, S.T. and Trumper, M. (1940) Carbon disulphide poisoning. Report of 21 cases. *Industrial Medicine* **9,** 231–4.

Gottfried, M.R., Graham, D.G., Morgan, J.M., Casey, H.W. and Bus, J.S. (1984) Morphological features of carbon disulfide intoxication. *Neurotoxicology* (in press).

Gowers, W.R. (1886). *A Manual of Diseases of the Nervous System*, vol 1, p. 329. Churchill, London.

Graham, D.G. (1980) Hexane neuropathy: a proposal for pathogenesis of a hazard of occupational exposure and inhalant abuse. *Chemicobiological Interactions* **32,** 339–45.

Graham, D.I. and Gonatas, N.K. (1973) Triethyltin sulphate induced splitting of peripheral myelin in rats. *Laboratory Investigation* **29,** 628–32.

Green, L.S., Donoso, J.A., Heller-Bettinger, I.E. and Samson, F.E. (1977) Axonal transport disturbances in vincristine-induced peripheral neuropathy. *Annals of Neurology* **1,** 255–62.

Greenfield, J.G. (1954) *The Spino-cerebellar Degenerations*, pp. 14–15. Blackwell, Oxford.

Gregson, N.A. and Hall, S.M. (1973) A quantitative analysis of the effects of the intraneural injection of lysophosphatidyl choline. *Journal of Cell Science* **13,** 257–77.

Griffin, J.W. and Price, D.L. (1981a) Segmental demyelination in experimental IDPN and hexacarbon neuropathies: evidence for an axonal influence. *Laboratory Investigation* **45,** 130–41.

Griffin, J.W. and Price, D.L. (1981b) Schwann cell and glial responses in β,β'-iminodipropionitrile intoxication. *Journal of Neurocytology* **10,** 995–1007.

Griffin, J.W., Hoffman, P.N., Clark, A.W., Carroll, P.T. and Price, D.L. (1978) Slow axonal transport of neurofilament proteins—impairment by β,β'-iminodipropionitrile administration. *Science* **202,** 633–5.

Griffin, J.W., Price, D.L., Kuethe, D.O. and Goldberg, A.M. (1980) Neurotoxicity of misonidazole in rats. 1. Neuropathology. *Neurotoxicology* **1,** 653–66.

Gruner, J.E. (1958) Lésions du névraxe secondaires à l'ingestion d'éthyl-étain (Stalinon). *Revue Neurologique* **98,** 109–16.

Grzycki, J. and Kobusowna, B. (1951) Histophysiological effects of arsenic and its derivatives on the central nervous system, and particularly on the third element of the central nervous system. *Journal of Neuropathology and Experimental Neurology* **10,** 325–37.

Hall, S.M. (1972) The effect of injections of lysophosphatidyl choline into white matter of the adult mouse spinal cord. *Journal of Cell Science* **10,** 535–46.

Hall, S.M. and Gregson, N.A. (1971) The *in vivo* and ultrastructural effects of injection of lysolecithin into myelinated peripheral nerve fibres of the adult mouse. *Journal of Cell Science* **9,** 769–89.

Hamada, T., Iwamasa, T., Tsuru, T., Sato, K. and Takeuchi, T. (1981) Mechanism of glycogenosome formation in axons of cadmium-induced neuropathy. Ultrastructural and biochemical studies. *Neurotoxicology* **2,** 33–41.

Hammer, R.P. and Scheibel, A.B. (1981) Morphological evidence for a delay of neuronal maturation in fetal alcohol exposure. *Experimental Neurology* **74,** 587–96.

Harris, H.W., Knight, R.A. and Selin, M.J. (1958) Comparison of isoniazid concentrations in the blood of people of Japanese and European descent. *American Review of Tuberculosis and Pulmonary Diseases* **78,** 944–8.

Hartfall, S.J., Garland, H.G. and Goldie, W. (1937) Gold treatment of arthritis. A review of 900 cases. *Lancet* **2,** 838–42.

Hartmann, H.A., Lalich, J.J. and Akert, K. (1958) Lesions in the anterior horn cells of rats after administration of *bis*-b-cyanoethylene. *Journal of Neuropathology and Experimental Neurology* **17,** 298–304.

Hayreh, M.S., Hayreh, S.S., Baumbach, G.L., Cancilla, P., Martin-Amat, G., Tephly, T.R. et al. (1977) Methyl alcohol poisoning. III. Ocular toxicity. *Archives of Ophthalmology* **95,** 1851–8.

Hemphill, M., Pestronk, A., Walsh, T., Parhad, I., Clark, A. and Rosenshein, N. (1980) Sensory neuropathy in *cis*-platinum chemotherapy. *Neurology (New York)* **30,** 429.

Harman, M.M. and Bensch, K.G. (1967) Light and electron microscopic studies of acute and chronic thallium intoxication in rats. *Toxicology and Applied Pharmacology* **10,** 199–222.

Herman, S.P., Klein, R., Talley, F.A. and Krigman, M.R. (1973) An ultrastructural study of methylmercury-induced sensory neuropathy in the rat. *Laboratory Investigation* **28,** 104–18.

Hern, J.E.C. (1967) Inhibition of true cholinesterase in TOCP poisoning with potentiation by 'Tween 80'. *Nature (London)* **215,** 963.

Hern, J.E.C. (1971) *Some effects of experimental organophosphorus intoxication in primates.* DMed thesis, University of Oxford.

Herndon, R.M. and Coyle, J.R. (1978) Glutamergic innervation, kainic acid, and selective vulnerability in the cerebellum. In *Kainic Acid as a Tool in Neurobiology* (Eds. McGeer, E.G., Olney, J.W.

and McGeer, P.L.), pp. 189–200. Raven Press, New York.

Herskowitz, A., Ishii, N. and Schaumburg, H.H. (1971) *n*-Hexane neuropathy. A syndrome occurring as a result of industrial exposure. *New England Journal of Medicine* **285,** 82–5.

Hertz, M.M., Bolwig, T.G., Grandjean, P. and Westergaard, E. (1981) Lead poisoning and the blood–brain barrier. *Acta Neurologica Scandinavica* **63,** 286–96.

Heyman, A., Pfeiffer, J.B., Willett, R.W. and Taylor, H.M. (1956) Peripheral neuropathy caused by arsenical intoxication. *New England Journal of Medicine* **254,** 401–9.

Heywood, R., Sortwell, R.J. and Prentice, D.E. (1978) The toxicity of 1-amino-3-chloro-2-propanol hydrochloride (CL 88,236) in the rhesus monkey. *Toxicology* **9,** 219–25.

Hierons, R. and Johnson, M.K. (1978) Clinical and toxicological investigations of a case of delayed neuropathy in man after acute poisoning by an organophosphorus pesticide. *Archives of Toxicology* **40,** 279–84.

Hildebrand, J. and Coërs, C. (1965) Etude clinique, histologique et électrophysiologique des neuropathies associées au traitement par la vincristine. *European Journal of Cancer* **1,** 51–8.

Hildebrand, J., Joffroy, A. and Coërs, C. (1968) Myoneural changes in experimental isoniazid neuropathy. Electrophysiological and histological study. *Archives of Neurology* **19,** 60–70.

Hillemand, P., Pallière, M., Laquais, B. and Bouvet, P. (1977) Traitement bismuthique et bismuthémie. *Semaine des Hôpitaux de Paris* **53,** 1663–9.

Himes, R.H., Kersey, R.N., Heller-Bettinger, I. and Samson, F.E. (1976) Action of the Vinca alkaloids vincristine, vinblastine and desacetyl vinblastine amide on microtubules *in vitro*. *Cancer Research* **36,** 3798–802.

Hirano, A. and Kochen, J.A. (1976) Experimental lead encephalopathy. In *Progress in Neuropathology*, vol. 3 (Ed. Zimmerman, H.M.), pp. 319–42 Grune and Stratton, New York.

Hirano, A., Llena, J.F., Streifler, M. and Cohn, D.F. (1976) Anterior horn cell changes in a case of neurolathyrism. *Acta Neuropathologica* **35,** 277–83.

Höfinger, E., Le Quesne, P.M. and Gajree, T. (1982) Conduction velocity in nerve fibres with axonal atrophy due to chronic β,β'-iminodipropionitrile (IDPN). *Journal of the Neurological Sciences* **53,** 159–67.

Hughes, H.B., Biehl, J.P., Jones, A.P. and Schmidt, L.H. (1954) Metabolism of isoniazid in man as related to the occurrence of peripheral neuritis. *American Review of Tuberculosis and Pulmonary Diseases* **70,** 266–73.

Hunter, D., Bomford, R.R. and Russell, D.S. (1940) Poisoning by methylmercury compounds. *Quarterly Journal of Medicine* **9,** 193–241.

Hunter, D. and Russell, D.S. (1954) Focal cerebral and cerebellar atrophy in a human subject due to organic mercury compounds. *Journal of Neurology, Neurosurgery and Psychiatry* **17,** 235–41.

Hurst, E.W. (1959) The lesions produced in the central nervous system by certain organic arsenical compounds. *Journal of Pathology and Bacteriology* **77,** 523–34.

Igisu, H., Goto, I., Kawamura, Y., Kato, M., Izumi, K. and Kuroiwa, Y. (1975) Acrylamide encephaloneuropathy due to well water pollution. *Journal of Neurology, Neurosurgery and Psychiatry* **38,** 581–4.

Izquierdo, A.E. and Nieto, D. (1965) Aspectos neuropatologicos de la intoxicacion con *Karwinskia humboldtiana*. Estudio experimental. *Gaceta Médica de México* **95,** 163–77.

Jacobs, J.M. (1980) Vascular permeability and neural injury. In *Experimental and Clinical Neurotoxicology* (Eds. Spencer, P.S. and Schaumburg, H.H.), pp. 102–17. Williams and Wilkins, Baltimore.

Jacobs, J.M., Carmichael, N. and Cavanagh, J.B. (1975) Ultrastructural changes in the dorsal root and trigeminal ganglia of rats poisoned with methyl mercury. *Neuropathology and Applied Neurobiology* **1,** 1–19.

Jacobs, J.M., Carmichael, N. and Cavanagh, J.B. (1977) Ultrastructural changes in the nervous system of rabbits poisoned with methyl mercury. *Toxicology and Applied Neurobiology* **39,** 249–61.

Jacobs, J.M., Cavanagh, J.B. and Carmichael, N. (1975) The effect of chronic dosing with mercuric chloride on dorsal root and trigeminal ganglia of rats. *Neuropathology and Applied Neurobiology* **3,** 321–37.

Jacobs, J.M., Cremer, J.E. and Cavanagh, J.B. (1977) Acute effects of triethyltin on the rat myelin sheath. *Neuropathology and Applied Neurobiology* **3,** 169–81.

Jacobs, J.M. and Ford, W.C.L. (1981) The neurotoxicity and antifertility properties of 6-chloro-6-deoxyglucose in the mouse. *Neurotoxicology* **2,** 405–17.

Jacobs, J.M., Miller, R.H. and Cavanagh, J.B. (1979) The distribution of degenerative changes in INH neuropathy: further evidence for focal axonal lesions. *Acta Neuropathologica* **48,** 1–9.

Jacobs, J.M., Miller, R.H., Whittle, A. and Cavanagh, J.B. (1979) Studies on the early changes in acute isoniazid neuropathy in the rat. *Acta Neuropathologica* **47,** 85–92.

Jennekens, F.G.I., Veldman, H., Schotman, P. and Gispen, W.H. (1979) Sequence of motor nerve terminal involvement in acrylamide neuropathy. *Acta Neuropathologica* **46,** 57–63.

Johnson, M.K. (1975) Organophosphorus esters causing delayed neurotoxic effects. Mechanism of action and structure/activity studies. *Archives of Toxicology* **34,** 259–88.

Johnson, M.K. (1982) Initiation of organophosphate-induced neuropathy. *Neurobehavioral Toxicology and Teratology* **4,** 759–65.

Johnson, W.J. and McColl, J.D. (1955) 6-Aminonicotinamide—a potent nicotinamide antagonist. *Science* **122,** 834.

Joiner, G.G., Russell, L.M., Bush, D.E., Gleiser, C.A., Johnston, T.D. and Fedigan, L. (1975) A spontaneous neuropathy of free-ranging Japanese macaques. *Laboratory Animal Science* **25,** 232–7.

Jones, K.L. and Smith, D.W. (1973) Recognition of the fetal alcohol syndrome in early infancy. *Lancet* **2,** 999–1001.

Jung, H.J. and Suzuki, K. (1978) Morphological changes in CNS of rats treated with perhexiline maleate (Pexid). *Acta Neuropathologica* **42,** 159–64.

Juntunen, J., Linnoila, I. and Haltia, M. (1977) Histochemical and electron microscopic observations on the myoneural junctions of rats with carbon disulfide polyneuropathy. *Scandinavian Journal of Work Environment and Health* **3,** 36–42.

Kaeser, H.E. (1962) Funktionsprufüngen peripherer Nerven bei experimentellen Polyneuritiden und bei der Wallerschen Degeneration. *Deutsche Zeitschrift für Nervenheilkunde* **183,** 268–304.

Kaeser, H.E. (1974) Amiodarone neuropathy. *Schweizerische medizinische Wochenschrift* **109,** 606–8.

Kaeser, H.E., Ulrich, J. and Wuthrich, R. (1976) Amiodarone neuropathy. *Praxis* **65,** 1121–2.

Kamerbeck, H.H., Rauws, A.G., ten Ham, M. and van Heijst, A.N.P. (1971) Prussian blue in therapy of thallotoxicosis. An experimental and clinical investigation. *Acta Medica Scandinavica* **189,** 321–4.

Katrak, S.M., Pollock, M., O'Brien, C.P., Nukada, H., Allpress, S., Calder, C. et al. (1980) Clinical and morphological features of gold neuropathy. *Brain* **103,** 671–93.

Kennedy, P. and Cavanagh, J.B. (1976) Spinal changes in the neuropathy of thallium poisoning. *Journal of the Neurological Sciences* **29,** 295–301.

Kennedy, P. and Cavanagh, J.B. (1977) Sensory neuropathy produced in the cat with thallous acetate. *Acta Neuropathologica* **39,** 81–8.

Kesson, C.M., Baird, A.W. and Lawson, D.H. (1977) Acrylamide poisoning. *Postgraduate Medical Journal* **53,** 16–17.

Kidd, J.G. and Langworthy, O.R. (1933) Paralysis following the ingestion of Jamaica ginger extract adulterated with tri-ortho-cresyl phosphate. *Johns Hopkins Medical Journal* **52,** 39–60.

Kidd, M. (1964) Alzheimer's disease—an electron microscopical study. *Brain* **87,** 307–19.

Kimbrough, R.D. and Gaines, T.B. (1971) Hexachlorophene effects on the rat brain: study of high doses by light and electron microscopy. *Archives of Environmental Health* **23,** 114–18.

Kirschner, D.A. and Sapirstein, V.S. (1982) Triethyl tin induced myelin oedema: an intermediate swelling state detected by x-ray diffraction. *Journal of Neurocytology* **11,** 559–69.

Klatzo, I., Wisniewski, H.M. and Streicher, E. (1965) Experimental production of neurofibrillary degeneration. I. Light microscopic observations. *Journal of Neuropathology and Experimental Neurology* **24,** 187–99.

Klinghardt, G.W. (1954) Experimentelle Nervenfaserschädigungen durch Isonicotinsäurehydrazid und ihre Bedeutung für die Klinik. *Verhandlungen der deutschen Gesellschaft für innere Medizin* **60,** 764–8.

Klinghardt, G.W. (1965) Ein Beitrag der experimentellen Neuropathologie zur Toxizitätsprüfung neurer Chemotherapeutica. *Mitteilungen aus der Max-Planck-Gesellschaft* **3,** 142–55.

Klinghardt, G.W. (1974) Experimentelle Schädigungen von Nervensystem und Musculatur durch Chlorochin: Modelle verschiedenartiger Speicherdystrophien. *Acta Neuropathologica* **28,** 117–41.

Klinghardt, G.W. (1978) Experimental neuropathology and clinical neurology of chloroquine side effects. *International Journal of Neurology* **11,** 331–41.

Kornguth, S.E., Rutledge, J.J., Sunderland, E., Siegel, F., Carlson, I., Smollens, J. et al. (1979) Impeded cerebellar development and reduced serum thyroxine levels associated with fetal alcohol intoxication. *Brain Research* **177,** 347–60.

Korobkin, R., Asbury, A.K., Sumner, A.J. and Nielsen, S.L. (1975) Glue-sniffing neuropathy. *Archives of Neurology* **32,** 158–62.

Krigman, M.R. and Hogan, E.L. (1974) Effect of lead intoxication on the postnatal growth of the rat nervous system. *Environmental Health Perspectives* **7,** 187–99.

Krigman, M.R., Druce, M.J., Traylor, T.D., Wilson, M.H., Newell, L.R. and Hogan, E.L. (1974) Lead encephalopathy in the developing rat: effect upon myelination. *Journal of Neuropathology and Experimental Neurology* **33,** 58–73.

Krinke, G., Schaumburg, H.H., Spencer, P.S., Thomann, P. and Hess, R. (1979) Clioquinol and 2,5-hexanedione induce different types of distal axonopathy in the dog. *Acta Neuropathologica* **47,** 213–21.

Krücke, W., von Hartrott, H.H., Schröder, J.M.,

Thomas, E., Gibbels, E. and Scheid, W. (1971) Licht- und elektronenmikroskopische Untersuchungen zum Spatstadium der Thalidomid-Pölyneuropathie. *Fortschritte der Neurologie, und ihner Grenzgebiete Psychiatrie* **39,** 15–50.

Kurland, L.T., Faro, S.N. and Siedler, H. (1960) Minamata disease. *World Neurology* **1,** 370–95.

Kusumi, R.K., Plouffe, J.F., Wyatt, R.H. and Fass, R.J. (1980) Central nervous system toxicity associated with metronidazole therapy. *Annals of Internal Medicine* **93,** 59–60.

Lampert, P.W. and Garrett, R.S. (1971) Mechanism of demyelination in tellurium neuropathy. *Laboratory Investigation* **25,** 380–8.

Lampert, P., Garro, F. and Pentschew, A. (1970) Tellurium neuropathy. *Acta Neuropathologica* **15,** 308–17.

Lampert, P., O'Brien, J. and Garrett, R. (1973) Hexachlorophene encephalopathy. *Acta Neuropathologica* **23,** 326–33.

Lampert, P.W. and Schochet, S.S. Jr (1968) Demyelination and remyelination in lead neuropathy. Electron microscopic studies. *Journal of Neuropathology and Experimental Neurology* **27,** 527–44.

Lancet (1900) Arsenical poisoning from beer drinking. **1,** 1600.

Lancet (1983) Methanol poisoning. **1,** 910–12.

Lange, K., Kolbe, H., Keller, K. and Henker, H. (1970) Der Kohlemhydratstoffwechsel des Gehirns nach Blockade des Pentose-phosphat-Weges durch 6-Aminonicotinsäureamid. *Hoppe Seylers Zeitschrift für physiologische Chemie* **351,** 1241–52.

Le Quesne, P.M. (1975) Neuropathy due to drugs. In *Peripheral Neuropathy* (Eds. Dyck, P.J., Thomas, P.K. and Lambert, E.H.), pp. 1263–80 Saunders, Philadelphia, Pa.

Le Quesne, P.M. (1981) Commentary on contemporary neurotoxicity. Toxic substances and the nervous system: the role of clinical observation. *Journal of Neurology, Neurosurgery and Psychiatry* **44,** 1–8.

Le Quesne, P.M., Damluji, S.F. and Rustam, H. (1974) Electrophysiological studies of peripheral nerves in patients with organic mercury poisoning. *Journal of Neurology, Neurosurgery and Psychiatry* **3,** 333–9.

Le Quesne, P.M. and McLeod, J.G. (1977) Peripheral neuropathy following a single exposure to arsenic. Clinical course in four patients with electrophysiological and histological studies. *Journal of the Neurological Sciences* **32,** 437–51.

Le Vay, S., Meier, C. and Glees, P. (1971) Effects of tri-ortho-cresyl phosphate on spinal ganglia and peripheral nerves of chicken. *Acta Neuropathologica* **17,** 103–13.

Lefrak, E.A., Pitha, J., Rosenheim, S. and Gottlieb, J.A. (1973) A clinicopathologic analysis of adriamycin cardiotoxicity. *Cancer* **32,** 302.

Lescher, C. (1936) Nervous complications following treatment by gold salts. *British Medical Journal* **2,** 1303–5.

Lhermitte, F., Fardeau, M., Chedru, F. and Mallecourt, J. (1976) Polyneuropathy after perhexiline maleate therapy. *British Medical Journal* **1,** 1256.

Liessens, J.L., Monstrey, J., Vanden Eeckhout, E., Djudzman, R. and Martin, J.J. (1978) Bismuth encephalopathy. A clinical and anatomo-pathological report of one case. *Acta Neurologica Belgica* **78,** 301–9.

Linnoila, I., Haltia, M., Seppäläinen, A.-M. and Palo, J. (1975) Experimental carbon disulphide poisoning: morphological and neurophysiological studies. In *Proceedings of the VIIth International Congress of Neuropathology, Budapest.* (Eds. Kornyey, St., Tariska, St. and Gosztonyi, G.), pp. 383–6. Excerpta Medica, Amsterdam.

Little, R.E. (1977) Moderate alcohol use during pregnancy and decreased infant birth weight. *American Journal of Public Health* **67,** 1154–6.

Lock, E.A. and Aldridge, W.N. (1975) The binding of triethyltin to rat brain myelin. *Journal of Neurochemistry* **25,** 871–6.

Lockhart, J.D. (1972) How toxic is hexachlorophene? *Pediatrics* **50,** 229–35.

Lukas, E. (1969) Leitgeschwindigkeit peripheren Nerven bei Schwefelkohlenstoff ausgesetzten Personen. *International Journal of Clinical Pharmacology and Biopharmacy* **2,** 354–8.

Lund, A. (1956) Distribution of thallium in the organism and its elimination. *Acta Pharmacologica et Toxicologica* **12,** 251–9.

Lustman, F. and Monseu, G. (1974) Amiodarone and neurological side effects. *Lancet* **1,** 568.

Lutier, F. (1963) Manganese poisoning in the electric battery industry. *Presse Médicale* **71,** 661–4.

McAlpine, D. and Araki, S. (1959) Minamata disease. Late effects of an unusual neurological disorder caused by contaminated fish. *Archives of Neurology* **1,** 522–30.

McCauley, P.T., Bull, R.J. and Lutkenhoff, S.D. (1979) Association of alterations in energy metabolism with lead-induced delays in rat cerebral cortical development. *Neuropharmacology* **18,** 93–101.

McDermott, J.R., Smith, A.I., Ward, M.K., Parkinson, I.S. and Kerr, D.N.S. (1978) Brain-aluminium concentration in dialysis encephalopathy. *Lancet* **1,** 901–3.

McGeer, P.L. and McGeer, E.G. (1976) Duplication of biochemical changes of Huntington's chorea by intrastriatal injections of glutamic and kainic acids. *Nature (London)* **263,** 517–19.

McGregor, I.S. (1943) A study of the histopathological changes in the retina and later changes in the visual field in acute methyl alcohol poisoning. *British Journal of Ophthalmology* **27,** 523-43.

McLaughlin, A.I.G., Kazantzis, G., King, E., Teare, D., Porter, R.J. and Owen, R. (1962) Pulmonary fibrosis and encephalopathy associated with the inhalation of aluminium dust. *British Journal of Industrial Medicine* **19,** 253-63.

McLean, D.R., Jacobs, H. and Mielke, B.W. (1980) Methanol poisoning: a clinical and pathological study. *Annals of Neurology* **8,** 161-7.

McLeod, J.G. and Penny, R. (1969) Vincristine neuropathy: an electrophysiological and histological study. *Journal of Neurology, Neurosurgery and Psychiatry* **32,** 297-304.

Magee, P.N., Stoner, H.B. and Barnes, J.M. (1957) The experimental production of oedema in the central nervous system of the rat by triethyl tin compounds. *Journal of Pathology and Bacteriology* **73,** 107-24.

Magos, L. (1975) Mercury and mercurials. *British Medical Bulletin* **31,** 241-5.

Makinen, A., Savolainen, H., Lehtonen, E. and Vaino, H. (1977) Reduced sulfhydryl groups of rat neurons, glial cells and neurofilaments. *Research Communications in Chemical Pathology and Pharmacology* **16,** 577-80.

Mamoli, B., Wessely, P., Kogelnik, H.D., Muller, M. and Rathkolb, O. (1979) Electroneurographic investigations of misonidazole polyneuropathy. *European Neurology* **18,** 405-14.

Marsh, D.O., Myers, G.J., Clarkson, T.W., Amin-Zaki, L., Tikriti, S. and Majeed, M.A. (1980) Fetal methylmercury poisoning: clinical and toxicological data on 29 cases. *Annals of Neurology* **7,** 348-53.

Martin-Amat, G., Tephly, T.R., McMartin, K.E., Makar, A.B., Hayreh, M.S., Hayreh, S.S. et al. (1977) Methyl alcohol poisoning. II. Development of a model for ocular toxicity in methyl alcohol poisoning using the rhesus monkey. *Archives of Ophthalmology* **95,** 1847-50.

Martin-Bouyer, G. (1978) Intoxication par les sels de bismuth administres par voie orale. *Gastroenterologie Clinique et Biologique* **2,** 349-56.

Martin-Bouyer, G., Lebreton, R., Toga, M., Stolley, P.D. and Lockhart, J. (1982) Outbreak of accidental hexachlorophane poisoning in France. *Lancet* **1,** 91-5.

Maxwell, I.C. and Le Quesne, P.M. (1979) Conduction velocity in hexachlorophane neuropathy. Correlation between electrophysiological and histological findings. *Journal of the Neurological Sciences* **43,** 95-110.

Meier, C., Kauer, B., Müller, U. and Ludin, H.P. (1979) Neuromyopathy during chronic amiodarone treatment. *Journal of Neurology* **220,** 231-9.

Mena, I. (1979) Manganese poisoning. In *Handbook of Clinical Neurology*, vol. 36 (Eds. Vinken, P.J. and Bruyn, G.W.), pp. 217-37. North-Holland, Amsterdam.

Mena, I., Court, J., Fuenzalida, S., Papavasiliou, P.S. and Cotzias, G.C. (1970) Modification of chronic manganese poisoning. Treatment with *l*-DOPA or 5-OH tryptophane. *New England Journal of Medicine* **282,** 5-10.

Mendell, J.R., Sahenk, Z., Saida, K., Weiss, H.S., Savage, R. and Couri, D. (1977) Alteration of fast axoplasmic transport in experimental methyl-*n*-butyl ketone neuropathy. *Brain Research* **133,** 107-18.

Meyer-König, E. (1973) Ultrastruktur der Glia und Axonschädigung durch 6-Aminonicotinamide (6-AN) am Sehnerv der Ratte. *Acta Neuropathologica* **26,** 115-26.

Michaelson, I.A. and Sauerhoff, M.W. (1974) Animal models of human disease. Severe and mild lead encephalopathy in the neonatal rat. *Environmental Health Perspectives* **7,** 201-25.

Mitchell, J. and Caren, C.A. (1982) Degeneration of non-myelinated axons in the rat sciatic nerve following lysolecithin injection. *Acta Neuropathologica* **56,** 187-93.

Mitchell, J., Weller, R.O., Evans, H., Arai, I. and Daves, G.D. Jr (1978) Buckthorn neuropathy: effects of intraneural injection of *Karwinskia humboldtiana* toxins. *Neuropathology and Applied Neurobiology* **4,** 85-97.

Moddel, G., Bilbao, J.M., Payne, D. and Ashby, P. (1978) Disulfiram neuropathy. *Archives of Neurology* **35,** 658-60.

Moeschlin, S. (1980) Thallium poisoning. *Clinical Toxicology* **17,** 133-46.

Mokri, B., Ohnishi, A. and Dyck, P.J. (1981) Disulfiram neuropathy. *Neurology* **31,** 730-5.

Morgan-Hughes, J.A., Sinclair, S. and Durston, J.H.J. (1974) The pattern of peripheral nerve regeneration induced by crush in rats with severe acrylamide neuropathy. *Brain* **97,** 235-59.

Munch, J.C. (1934) Human thallotoxicosis. *Journal of the American Medical Association* **102,** 1929-34.

Munch, J.C., Ginsburg, H.M. and Nixon, C.E. (1933) The 1932 thallotoxicosis outbreak in California. *Journal of the American Medical Association* **100,** 1315-19.

Munoz-Martinez, E.J. and Chavez, B. (1979) Conduction block and functional denervation caused by tullidora (*Karwinskia humboldtiana*). *Experimental Neurology* **65,** 255-70.

Murai, Y., Shiraishi, S., Yamashita, Y., Ohnishi, A. and Arimura, K. (1982) Neurophysiological effects of methyl mercury on the nervous system. *Electroencephalography and Clinical Neurophys-*

iology **36,** suppl. *Kyoto Symposium* (Eds. Buser, P.A., Cobb, W.A. and Okuma, T.), pp. 682–7. Elsevier Biomedical Press, Amsterdam.

Mussini, J.M., Hauw, J.-J. and Escourolle, R. (1977) Étude en microscopie électronique des lésions nerveuses, musculaires et cutanées déterminées par le maléate de perhexiline. *Acta Neuropathologica* **38,** 53–9.

Nadler, J.V., Perry, B.W. and Cotman, C.W. (1978) Preferential vulnerability of hippocampus to intraventricular kainic acid. In *Kainic Acid as a Tool in Neurobiology* (Eds. McGeer, E.G., Olney, J.W. and McGeer, P.L.), pp. 219–38. Raven Press, New York.

Namba, T., Nolte, C.T., Jackrel, J. and Grob, D. (1971) Poisoning due to organophosphate insecticides. *American Journal of Medicine* **50,** 475–92.

Neurosciences Research Program Bulletin (1981) Excitatory amino acid neurotoxins: selectivity, specificity and mechanisms of action. **19,** 335–427.

Noetzel, H. (1955) Schädigung und Verkalkung der Körnerschicht des Kleinhirns bei chronischer experimenteller Sublimatvergiftung. *Beiträge zur pathologischen Anatomie und zur allgemeinen Pathologie* **115,** 226–36.

Nukada, H. and Pollock, M. (1981) Disulfiram neuropathy—a morphometric study of sural nerve. *Journal of the Neurological Sciences* **51,** 51–67.

Ochoa, J. (1970) Isoniazid neuropathy in man: quantitative electron microscopic study. *Brain* **93,** 831–50.

O'Donoghue, J.L. and Krasavage, W.J. (1979) Hexacarbon neuropathy: a γ-diketone neuropathy? *Journal of Neuropathology and Experimental Neurology* **38,** 333.

Ohnishi, A., Schilling, W.S., Brimijoin, W.S., Lambert, E.H., Fairbanks, V.F. and Dyck, P.J. (1977) Lead neuropathy. I. Morphometry, nerve conduction and choline acetyltransferase transport: new finding of endoneurial oedema associated with segmental demyelination. *Journal of Neuropathology and Experimental Neurology* **36,** 499–518.

Okazaki, H., Aronson, S.M., DiMeio, D.J. and Olvera, J.E. (1963) Acute lead encephalopathy of childhood. *Transactions of the American Neurological Association* **88,** 248–50.

Olney, J.W. (1978) Neurotoxicity of excitatory amino acids. In *Kainic Acid as a Tool in Neurobiology* (Eds. McGeer, E.G., Olney, J.W. and McGeer, P.L.), pp. 95–122. Raven Press, New York.

Olney, J.W. (1980) Excitotoxic mechanisms of neurotoxicity. In *Experimental and Clinical Neurotoxicology* (Eds. Spencer, P.S. and Schaumburg, H.H.), pp. 272–94. Williams and Wilkins, Baltimore, Md.

Olney, J.W. (1981) Excitatory amino acid neurotoxins: selectivity, specificity and mechanisms of action. II. Historical perspective. *Neurosciences Research Program Bulletin* **19,** 337–46.

Orthner, H. (1950) *Die Methylalkoholvergiftung.* Springer, Berlin.

Orthner, H. (1953) Methylalkoholvergiftung mit besonders schweren Hirnveränderungen. *Virchows Archiv für pathologische Anatomie* **323,** 442–64.

Osetowska, E. (1971) Metals. In *Pathology of the Nervous System*, vol. 2 (Ed. Minckler, J.), pp. 1644–51. McGraw-Hill, New York.

O'Shea, K.S. and Kaufman, M.H. (1979) The teratogenic effect of acetaldehyde: implications for the study of the fetal alcohol syndrome. *Journal of Anatomy* **128,** 65–76.

Ota, M. (1970) Ultrastructure of sural nerve in a case of arsenic neuropathy. *Acta Neuropathologica* **16,** 233–42.

Ott, T., Rabinowicz, T. and Morand, B. (1959) Etude clinique et histopathologique d'un cas de polynevrite survenue au cours du traitement par l'isoniazide. *Revue Neurologique* **100,** 103–17.

Parkinson, I.S., Ward, M.K., Feest, T.G., Fawcett, R.W.P. and Kerr, D.N.S. (1979) Fracturing dialysis osteodystrophy and dialysis encephalopathy. An epidemiological survey. *Lancet* **1,** 406–9.

Peiffer, J., Majewski, F., Fischbach, H., Bierich, J.R. and Volk, B. (1979) Alcohol embryo- and fetopathy. *Journal of the Neurological Sciences* **41,** 125–37.

Pentschew, A. (1965) Morphology and morphogenesis of lead encephalopathy. *Acta Neuropathologica* **5,** 133–60.

Pentschew, A. and Garro, F. (1966) Lead encephalomyelopathy of the suckling rat and its implications on the porphyrinopathic nervous diseases. *Acta Neuropathologica* **6,** 266–78.

Pentschew, A., Ebner, F.F. and Kovatch, R.M. (1963) Experimental manganese encephalopathy in monkeys: a preliminary report. *Journal of Neuropathology and Experimental Neurology* **22,** 488–99.

Perez, V.J. and Olney, J.W. (1972) Accumulation of glutamic acid in the arcuate nucleus of the hypothalamus of the infant mouse following subcutaneous administration of monosodium glutamate. *Journal of Neurochemistry* **19,** 1777–82.

Perl, D.P. and Brody, A.R. (1980) Alzheimer's disease: x-ray spectrometric evidence of aluminum accumulation in neurofibrillary tangle-bearing neurons. *Science* **208,** 297–9.

Perl, D.P., Gajdusek, D.C., Yanagihara, R.T. and Gibbs, C.J. (1982) Intraneural aluminum accumulation in amyotrophic lateral sclerosis and Parkinsonism-dementia of Guam. *Science* **217,** 1053–5.

Peters, R.A., Bennett, J., King, A.J., Carlton, A.B.,

Dixon, M., Cameron, J.R. et al. (1947) British anti-lewisite. A report on its use and therapeutic value in arsenical intoxications, from the BAL conference, Medical Research Council. *British Medical Journal* **2,** 520–1.

Peterson, E.R. and Murray, M.R. (1965) Patterns of peripheral demyelination in vitro. *Annals of the New York Academy of Sciences* **122,** 39–50.

Pierce, P.E., Thompson, J.F., Likosky, W.H., Nickey, L.N., Barthel, W.F. and Hinman, A.R. (1972) Alkyl mercury poisoning in humans. Report of an outbreak. *Journal of the American Medical Association* **220,** 1439–42.

Pleasure, D.E., Mischler, K.C. and Engel, W.K. (1969) Axonal transport of proteins in experimental neuropathies. *Science* **166,** 524–5.

Post, E.J. and McLeod, J.G. (1977) Acrylamide autonomic neuropathy in the cat. 1. Neurophysiological and histological studies. *Journal of the Neurological Sciences* **33,** 353–74.

Potts, A.M., Praglin, J., Farkas, J., Orbison, L. and Chickering, D. (1955) Studies on the visual toxicity of methanol. VIII. Additional observations on methanol poisoning in the primate test object. *American Journal of Ophthalmology* **40,** 76–83.

Powell, H.C. and Lampert, P.W. (1975) Effects of hexachlorophene on the central and peripheral nervous systems. In *Proceedings of the VIIth International Congress of Neuropathology, Budapest* (Eds. Kornyey, St., Tariska, St. and Gosztonyi, G.), pp. 377–82. Excerpta Medica, Amsterdam.

Powell, H.C., Swarner, O., Gluck, L. and Lampert, P. (1973) Hexachlorophene myelinopathy in premature infants. *Journal of Pediatrics* **82,** 976–81.

Powell, H.C., Koch, T., Garrett, R. and Lampert, P. (1978a) Schwann cell abnormalities in 2,5-hexanedione neuropathy. *Journal of Neurocytology* **7,** 517–28.

Powell, H.C., Myers, R.R., Zweifach, B.W. and Lampert, P.W. (1978b) Endoneurial pressure in hexachlorophene neuropathy. *Acta Neuropathologica* **41,** 139–44.

Pratt, O.E. (1982) Alcohol and the developing fetus. *British Medical Journal* **38,** 48–52.

Press, M.F. (1977a) Lead encephalopathy in neonatal rats: morphological studies. *Journal of Neuropathology and Experimental Neurology* **36,** 169–93.

Press, M.F. (1977b) Neuronal development in the cerebellum of lead poisoned neonatal rats. *Acta Neuropathologica* **40,** 259–68.

Price, R.A. and Jamieson, P.A. (1975) The central nervous system in childhood leukemia. II. Subacute leukoencephalopathy. *Cancer* **35,** 306–18.

Prick, J.J.G. (1979) Thallium poisoning. In *Handbook of Clinical Neurology*, vol. 36 (Eds. Vinken, P.J. and Bruyn, G.W.), pp. 239–78. North-Holland, Amsterdam.

Prineas, J. (1969a) The pathogenesis of dying-back polyneuropathies. I. An ultrastructural study of experimental tri-ortho-cresyl phosphate intoxication in the cat. *Journal of Pathology and Experimental Neurology* **28,** 571–97.

Prineas, J. (1969b) The pathogenesis of dying-back polyneuropathies. II. An ultrastructural study of experimental acrylamide intoxication in the cat. *Journal of Neuropathology and Experimental Neurology* **28,** 598–621.

Quensel, F. (1904) Neue Erfahrungen über Geistesstörungen nach Schwefelkohlenstoffvergiftung. *Monatsschrift für Psychiatrie und Neurologie* **16,** 246–68.

Rao, S.L.N., Sarma, P.S., Mari, K.S., Raghunatha Rao, T.R. and Shiramachari, S. (1967) Experimental neurolathyrism in monkeys. *Nature (London)* **214,** 610–11.

Reuhl, K.R. and Chang, L.W. (1979) Effects of methylmercury on the development of the nervous system: a review. *Neurotoxicology* **1,** 21–55.

Richter, R. (1945) Degeneration of the basal ganglia in monkeys from chronic sulfide poisoning. *Journal of Neuropathology and Experimental Neurology* **4,** 324–53.

Robertson, D.M., Wasan, S.M. and Skinner, D.B. (1968) Ultrastructural features of early brain stem lesions of thiamine deficient rats. *American Journal of Pathology* **52,** 1081–8.

Rodier, J. (1955) Manganese poisoning in Moroccan miners. *British Journal of Industrial Medicine* **12,** 21–35.

Rogulja, P.R., Kovac, W. and Schmid, H. (1973) Metronidazol-encephalopathie der Ratte. *Acta Neuropathologica* **25,** 36–45.

Rosenblum, W.I. and Johnson, M. (1968) Neuropathological changes produced in suckling mice by adding lead to the maternal diet. *Archives of Pathology* **85,** 640–8.

Ross, R.R. (1958) Use of pyridoxine hydrochloride to prevent isoniazid toxicity. *Journal of the American Medical Association* **168,** 273–5.

Rothstein, A. (1973) Mercaptans, the biological targets for mercurials. In *Mercury, Mercurials and Mercaptans* (Eds. Miller, M.W. and Clarkson, T.W.), pp. 68–92. Thomas, Springfield, Ill.

Rubinstein, L.J., Herman, M.M., Long, T.F. and Wilbur, J.R. (1975) Disseminated necrotizing leukoencephalopathy: a complication of treated central nervous system leukemia and lymphoma. *Cancer* **35,** 291–305.

Sabri, M.I., Moore, C.L. and Spencer, P.S. (1979) Studies on the biochemical basis of distal axonopathies. I. Inhibition of glycolysis by neurotoxic hexacarbon compounds. *Journal of Neurochemistry* **32,** 683–9.

Sahenk, Z. and Mendell, J.R. (1979a) Analysis of fast

axoplasmic transport in nerve ligation and adriamycin-induced neuronal perikaryon lesions. *Brain Research* **171,** 414–53.

Sahenk, Z. and Mendell, J.R. (1979b) Ultrastructural study of zinc pyridinethione-induced peripheral neuropathy. *Journal of Neuropathology and Experimental Neurology* **38,** 532–50.

Sahenk, Z. and Mendell, J.R. (1980a) Zinc pyridinethione. In *Clinical and Experimental Neurotoxicology* (Eds. Spencer, P.S. and Schaumburg, H.H.), pp. 578–92. Williams and Wilkins, Baltimore, Md.

Sahenk, Z. and Mendell, J.R. (1980b) Axoplasmic transport in zinc pyridinethione neuropathy: evidence for an abnormality in distal turn-around. *Brain Research* **31,** 343–53.

Said, G. (1978) Perhexiline neuropathy: a clinicopathological study. *Annals of Neurology* **3,** 259–66.

Said, G. and Duckett, S. (1981) Tellurium-induced myelinopathy in adult rats. *Muscle and Nerve* **4,** 319–25.

Said, G., Goasguen, J., and Laverdant, Ch. (1978) Neuropathy in long term treatment with metronidazole. *Revue Neurologique* **134,** 515–21.

Saida, K., Mendell, J.R. and Weiss, H.S. (1976) Peripheral nerve changes induced by methyl *n*-butyl ketone and potentiation by methyl ethyl ketone. *Journal of Neuropathology and Experimental Neurology* **35,** 207–25.

Sato, K., Iwamasa, T., Tsura, T. and Takeuchi, T. (1978) An ultrastructural study of chronic cadmium chloride-induced neuropathy. *Acta Neuropathologica* **41,** 185–90.

Sauer, R., Zook, B.C. and Garner, F.M. (1970) Demyelinating encephalomyelopathy associated with lead poisoning in nonhuman primates. *Science* **169,** 1091–3.

Scharer, K. (1972) Selective alteration of Purkinje cells in the dog after oral administration of high doses of nitroimidazole derivatives. *Verhandlungen der deutscher Gesellschaft für Pathologie* **56,** 407–10.

Schaumburg, H.H. and Spencer, P.S. (1978) Experimental hydrocarbons produce degeneration in cat hypothalamus and optic tract. *Science* **199,** 199–200.

Schaumburg, H.H. and Spencer, P.S. (1980) Clioquinol. In *Experimental and Clinical Pathology* (Eds. Spencer, P.S. and Schaumburg, H.H.), pp. 395–406. Williams and Wilkins, Baltimore, Md.

Schaumburg, H.H., Wiśniewski, H.M. and Spencer, P.S. (1974) Ultrastructural studies of the dying-back process. I. Peripheral nerve terminal and axon degeneration in systemic acrylamide intoxication. *Journal of Neuropathology and Experimental Neurology* **33,** 260–84.

Schaumburg, H.H., Byck, R., Gerstl, R. and Mashman, J.H. (1969) Monosodium L-glutamate: its pharmacology and role in the Chinese restaurant syndrome. *Science* **163,** 826–9.

Schepers, G.W.H. (1964) Tetraethyllead and tetramethyllead. *Archives of Environmental Health* **8,** 277–95.

Schipper, H., Beale, F.A., Bush, R.S. and Fryer, C. (1976) Metronidazole as a radiosensitizer. *New England Journal of Medicine* **295,** 901.

Schlaepfer, W.W. (1969) Experimental lead neuropathy: a disease of the supporting cells in the peripheral nervous system. *Journal of Neuropathology and Experimental Neurology* **28,** 410–18.

Schlaepfer, W.W. (1971a) Sequential study of endothelial changes in acute cadmium intoxication. *Laboratory Investigation* **25,** 556–64.

Schlaepfer, W.W. (1971b) Vincristine-induced axonal alterations in rat peripheral nerve. *Journal of Neuropathology and Experimental Neurology* **30,** 488–505.

Schlaepfer, W.W. and Hager, H. (1964) Ultrastructural changes of INH-induced neuropathy in rats. 1. Early axonal changes. *American Journal of Pathology* **45,** 209–19.

Schneck, S.S. (1979) Methyl alcohol. In *Handbook of Clinical Neurology* vol. 37 (Eds. Vinken, P.J. and Bruyn, G.W.), pp. 351–60. North-Holland, Amsterdam.

Schneider, H. and Cervos-Navarro, J. (1974) Acute gliopathy in spinal cord and brain stem induced by 6-aminonicotinamide. *Acta Neuropathologica* **27,** 11–23.

Schochet, S.S., Lampert, P.W. and Earle, K.M. (1968) Neuronal changes induced by intrathecal vincristine sulfate. *Journal of Neuropathy and Experimental Neurology* **27,** 645–57.

Schröder, J.M. (1975) Zur Pathogenese der Izoniazid-Neuropathie. 1. Eine feinstrukturelle Differenzierung gegenüber der Wallerschen Degeneration. *Acta Neuropathologica* **16,** 301–23.

Schroeder, H.A. and Vinton, W.H. (1969) Hypertension induced in rats by small doses of cadmium. *American Journal of Physiology* **202,** 515–19.

Schwartz, W.J. and Sharp, F.R. (1978) Autoradiographic maps of regional brain glucose consumption in resting, awake rats using C14-2-deoxyglucose. *Journal of Comparative Neurology* **177,** 325–60.

Seawright, A.A., Brown, A.W., Aldridge, W.N., Verschoyle, R.D. and Street, B.W. (1980) Neuropathological changes caused by trialkyl lead compounds in the rat. In *Mechanisms of Toxicity and Hazard Evaluation* (Eds. Holmsted, B., Lauwerys, R., Mercier, M. and Roberfroid, M.), pp. 71–4. Elsevier/North Holland Biomedical Press, Amsterdam.

Selye, H. (1957) Lathyrism. *Revue Canadienne de Biologie* **16,** 1–82.

Seppäläinen, A.M. and Haltia, M. (1980) Carbon disulfide. In *Experimental and Clinical Neurotoxicology* (Eds. Spencer, P.S. and Schaumburg, H.H.), pp. 356–73. Williams and Wilkins, Baltimore, Md.

Seppäläinen, A.M. and Linnoila, I. (1976) Electrophysiological findings in rats with experimental carbon disulphide neuropathy. *Neuropathology and Applied Neurobiology* **2,** 209–16.

Shah, R.R., Oates, N.S., Idle, J.R., Smith, R.L. and Lockhart, J.D. (1982) Impaired oxidation of debrisoquine in patients with perhexiline neuropathy. *British Medical Journal* **1,** 295–9.

Shapiro, W.R., Chernik, N.L. and Posner, J.B. (1973) Necrotizing encephalopathy following intraventricular instillation of methotrexate. *Archives of Neurology* **28,** 96–102.

Sharkey, S.J. (1896) Peripheral neuritis. *British Medical Journal* **1,** 457–8.

Shelanski, M. and Wiśniewski, H. (1969) Neurofibrillary degeneration induced by vincristine therapy. *Archives of Neurology* **20,** 199–206.

Shimono, M., Izumi, K. and Kuroiwa, Y. (1978) 3,3-Iminodipropionitrile induced centrifugal segmental demyelination and onion bulb formation. *Journal of Neuropathology and Experimental Neurology* **37,** 375–86.

Shiraishi, S., Inoue, N., Murai, Y., Ohnishi, A. and Noda, S. (1983) Dipterex (trichlorfon) poisoning—clinical and pathological studies in humans and monkeys. *Journal UOEH (Japan)* **5,** 125–32.

Shiraki, H. (1977) The neuropathology of subacute myelo-opticoneuropathy, SMON, in humans with special reference to the experimental whole body ARG studies using labelled quinaform compounds. In *Neurotoxicology* (Eds. Roizin, L., Shiraki, H. and Grcevic, N.), pp. 327–44. Raven Press, New York.

Shiraki, H. (1979a) Neuropathological aspects off organic mercury intoxication, including Minamata disease. In *Handbook of Clinical Neurology*, vol. 36 (Eds. Vinken, P.J. and Bruyn, G.W.), pp. 83–145. North-Holland, Amsterdam.

Shiraki, H. (1979b) Neuropathological aspects of the etiopathogenesis of subacute myelo-optico-neuropathy (SMON). In *Handbook of Clinical Neurology*, vol. 37 (Eds. Vinken, P.J. and Bruyn, G.W.), pp. 141–98. North-Holland, Amsterdam.

Shiraki, H. and Nagashima, K. (1977) Essential neuropathology of alkylmercury intoxications in humans from the acute to the chronic stage with special reference to whole body autoradiographic study using labelled mercury compounds. In *Neurotoxicology* (Eds. Roizin, L., Shiraki, H. and Grcevic, N.), pp. 247–60. Raven Press, New York.

Sievers, M.L. and Herrier, R.N. (1975) Treatment of acute isoniazid toxicity. *American Journal of Hospital Pharmacy* **32,** 202–6.

Slotwiner, P., Song, S.K. and Anderson, P.J. (1966) Spheromembranous degeneration of muscle induced by vincristine. *Archives of Neurology* **15,** 172–6.

Smith, B. (1969) Damage to the intrinsic cardiac neurones by rubidomycin (daunorubicin). *British Heart Journal* **31,** 607–9.

Smith, H.V. and Spalding, J.M.K. (1959) Outbreak of paralysis in Morocco due to ortho-cresyl phosphate poisoning. *Lancet* **2,** 1019–21.

Smith, J.F., McLaurin, R.L., Nichols, J.B. and Asbury, A. (1960) Studies in cerebral oedema and cerebral swelling. 1. The changes in lead encephalopathy in children compared with those in alkyl tin poisoning in animals. *Brain* **83,** 411–24.

Smith, K.J., Blakemore, W.F. and McDonald, W.I. (1981) The restoration of conduction by central remyelination. *Brain* **104,** 383–404.

Smith, K.J., Bostock, H. and Hall, S.M. (1982) Saltatory conduction precedes remyelination in axons demyelinated with lysophosphatidyl choline. *Journal of the Neurological Sciences* **54,** 13–31.

Smith, K.J. and Hall, S.M. (1980) Nerve conduction during peripheral demyelination and remyelination. *Journal of the Neurological Sciences* **48,** 201–19.

Sobue, I. (1979) Clinical aspects of subacute myelo-optico-neuropathy (SMON). In *Handbook of Clinical Neurology*, vol. 37 (Eds. Vinken, P.J. and Bruyn, G.W.), pp. 115–39. North-Holland, Amsterdam.

Souryi, F., Chretien, M. and Droz, B. (1981) 'Acrylamide-induced' neuropathy and impairment of axonal transport of proteins. I. Multifocal retention of fast transported proteins at the periphery of axons as revealed by light microscope radioautography. *Brain Research* **205,** 1–13.

Specht, W. and Rohner, D. (1960) Determination of thallium traces in human hair by means of neutron activation analysis. *Archives of Toxicology* **18,** 359–67.

Spencer, P.S., Couri, D. and Schaumburg, H.H. (1980) *n*-Hexane and methyl *n*-butyl ketone. In *Experimental and Clinical Neurotoxicology* (Eds. Spencer, P.S. and Schaumburg, H.H.), Williams and Wilkins, Baltimore, Md.

Spencer, P.S. and Schaumburg, H.H. (1975) Experimental neuropathy produced by 2,5-hexanedione—a major metabolite of the neurotoxic industrial solvent methyl *n*-butyl ketone. *Journal of Neurology, Neurosurgery and Psychiatry* **38,** 771–5.

Spencer, P.S. and Schaumburg, H.H. (1976a) Central-peripheral distal axonopathy. The pathology of dying-back polyneuropathies. In *Progress in Neuropathology*, vol. 3 (Ed. Zimmerman, H.), pp. 253-95. Grune and Stratton, New York.

Spencer, P.S. and Schaumburg, H.H. (1976b) Feline nervous system response to chronic intoxication with commercial grades of methyl *n*-butyl ketone, methyl isobutyl ketone and methyl ethyl ketone. *Toxicology and Applied Pharmacology* **37**, 301-11.

Spencer, P.S. and Schaumburg, H.H. (1977) Ultrastructural studies of the dying-back process. IV. Differential vulnerability of PNS and CNS fibers in experimental central-peripheral distal axonopathies. *Journal of Neuropathology and Experimental Neurology* **36**, 300-20.

Spencer, P.S., Peterson, E.R., Madrid, R.A. and Raine, C.S. (1973) Effects of thallium salts on neuronal mitochondria in organotypic cord-ganglia- muscle combination cultures. *Journal of Cell Biology* **58**, 79-95.

Spencer, P.S., Sterman, A.B., Horoupian, D. and Bischoff, M. (1979) Neurotoxic changes in rats exposed to the fragrance compound acetyl ethyl tetramethyl tetralin. *Neurotoxicology* **1**, 221-37.

Spencer, P.S., Foster, G.V., Sterman, A.B. and Horoupian, D. (1980) Acetyl ethyl tetramethyl tetralin. In *Experimental and Clinical Neurotoxicology* (Eds. Spencer, P.S. and Schaumburg, H.H.), pp. 296-308. Williams and Wilkins, Baltimore, Md.

Spencer, P.S., Schaumburg, H.H., Cohn, D.F. and Seth, P.K. (1984) Lathyrism: a useful model of primary lateral sclerosis. In *Research Progress in Motor Neurone Disease* (Ed. Rose, F.C.), pp. 312-27. Pitman, London.

Sterman, A.B. (1982a) Acrylamide induces early morphologic reorganization of the neuronal cell body. *Neurology (New York)* **32**, 1023-6.

Sterman, A.B. (1982b) Cell body remodelling during dying back axonopathy: DRG changes during advanced disease. *Journal of Neuropathology and Experimental Neurology* **41**, 400-11.

Stumpf, W.E., Sar, M. and Grant, L.D. (1980) Autoradiographic localization of ^{210}Pb and its decay products in rat forebrain. *Neurotoxicology* **1**, 593-606.

Sumner, A.J. and Asbury, A.K. (1975) Physiological studies of the dying-back phenomenon. Muscle stretch afferents in acrylamide neuropathy. *Brain* **98**, 91-100.

Suzuki, K. (1971) Some new observations in triethyltin intoxication of rats. *Experimental Neurology* **31**, 207-13.

Suzuki, K. and Kikkawa, Y. (1969) Status spongiosus of CNS and hepatic changes induced by cuprizone (*bis*-cyclo-hexanone oxalydihydrazone). *American Journal of Pathology* **54**, 307-25.

Szendzikowski, S., Stetkiewicz, J., Wronska-Nofer, T. and Zdrajkowska, I. (1973) Structural aspects of experimental carbon disulfide neuropathy. I. Development of neurohistological changes in chronically intoxicated rats. *Internationales Archiv für Arbeits und Umweltmedizin* **31**, 135-49.

Szendzikowski, S., Stetkiewicz, J., Wronska-Nofer, T. and Karasak, M. (1974) Pathomorphology of the experimental lesion of the peripheral nervous system in white rats chronically exposed to carbon disulphide. In *Structure and Function of Normal and Diseased Muscle and Peripheral Nerve* (Eds. Hausmanowa-Petrusewicz, I. and Jedrzejowska, H.), pp. 319-26. Polish Medical Publishers, Warsaw.

Tabira, T., Cullen, M.J., Reier, P.J. and Webster, H. deF. (1978) An experimental analysis of interlamellar tight junctions in amphibian and mammalian CNS myelin. *Journal of Neurocytology* **7**, 489-503.

Takeuchi, T. (1977) Neuropathology of Minamata disease in Kumamoto: especially at the chronic stage. In *Neurotoxicology* (Eds. Roizin, L., Shiraki, H. and Grcevic, N.), pp. 235-46. Raven Press, New York.

Takeuchi, T., Eto, N. and Eto, K. (1979) Neuropathology of childhood cases of methylmercury poisoning (Minamata disease) with prolonged symptoms, with particular reference to the decortication syndrome. *Neurotoxicology* **1**, 1-20.

Tellenbach, H. (1949) Zur Pathogenese und Klinik der 'Salvarsankrankeit', insonderheit der Salvarsan-polyneuritis. *Deutsche Zeitschrift für Nervenheilkunde* **163**, 40-71.

Thomas, J.A., Dallenbach, F.D. and Thomas, I.M. (1971) Considerations on the development of experimental lead encephalopathy. *Virchow's Archiv für pathologische Anatomie und Physiologie* **352**, 61-74.

Thomas, P.K. (1982) Selective vulnerability of the centrifugal and centripetal axons of primary sensory neurons. *Muscle and Nerve* **5**, S117-21.

Toews, A.D., Kolber, A., Hayward, J., Krigman, M.R. and Morell, P. (1978) Experimental lead encephalopathy in the suckling rat: concentration of lead in cellular fractions enriched with brain capillaries. *Brain Research* **147**, 131-8.

Torack, R.M., Gordon, J. and Prokop, J. (1970) Pathobiology of acute triethyltin intoxication. In *International Review of Neurobiology*, vol. 12 (Eds. Pfeiffer, C. and Smythes, J.R.), pp. 45-86. Academic Press, New York.

Towfighi, J., Gonatas, N.K. and McCree, L. (1973) Hexachlorophene neuropathy in rats. *Laboratory Investigation* **29**, 428-36.

Tsujihata, M., Engel, A.G. and Lambert, E.H. (1974) Motor end-plate fine structure in acrylamide dying-back neuropathy: a sequential morphometric study. *Neurology* **24**, 849-56.

Ule, G. (1962) Zur Ultrastruktur der ghost-cells beim experimentellen Neurolathyrismus der Ratte. *Zeitschrift für Zellforschung und mikroskopische Anatomie* **56,** 130–42.

Urtasun, R.C., Chapman, J.D., Feldstein, M.L., Band, P.R., Rabin, H.R., Wilson, A.F. et al. (1978) Peripheral neuropathy related to misonidazole: incidence and pathology. *British Journal of Cancer* **37,** suppl. III, 271–5.

Valpey, R., Sumi, M., Copass, M.K. and Goble, G.J. (1978) Acute and chronic progressive encephalopathy due to gasoline sniffing. *Neurology (New York)* **28,** 507–10.

Vigliani, E.C. (1954) Carbon disulphide poisoning in viscose rayon factories. *British Journal of Industrial Medicine* **11,** 235–44.

Walsh, J.C. (1970) Gold neuropathy. *Neurology* **20,** 455–8.

Watanabe, I. (1977) Effect of triethyltin on the developing brain of the mouse. In *Neurotoxicology* (Eds. Roizin, L., Shiraki, H. and Grcevic, N.) pp. 317–26. Raven Press, New York.

Watanabe, I. (1980) Organotins (triethyltin). In *Experimental and Clinical Neurotoxicology* (Eds. Spencer, P.S. and Schaumburg, H.H.), pp. 545–57. Williams and Wilkins, Baltimore, Md.

Waxman, S.G., Kocsis, J.D. and Nitta, K.C. (1979) Lysophosphatidyl choline-induced focal demyelination in the rabbit corpus callosum. *Journal of the Neurological Sciences* **44,** 45–53.

Webb, M. (1975) Cadmium. *British Medical Bulletin* **31,** 246–50.

Webster, W.S. and Valois, A.A. (1981) The toxic effects of cadmium on the neonatal mouse CNS. *Journal of Neuropathology and Experimental Neurology* **40,** 247–57.

Weinstein, L. (1975) Drugs used in the chemotherapy of tuberculosis and leprosy. In *The Pharmacological Basis of Therapeutics* (Eds. Goodman, L.S. and Gilman, A.) pp. 1204–7. Macmillan, New York.

Weller, R.O., Mitchell, J. and Daves, J.D. Jr (1980) Buckthorn (*Karwinskia humboldtiana*) toxins. In *Experimental and Clinical Neurotoxicology* (Eds. Spencer, P.S. and Schaumburg, H.H.), pp. 336–47. Williams and Wilkins, Baltimore, Md.

Whisnant, J.P., Espinosa, R.E., Kierland, R.R. and Lambert, E.H. (1963) Chloroquine neuromyopathy. *Proceedings of the Mayo Clinic* **38,** 501–13.

Widy, W. (1959) Die Pigmentansammlungen in den Haarwurzeln bei Thalliumvergiftungen. *Hautarzt* **10,** 216–18.

Wijesekera, J.C., Critchley, E.M.R., Fahim, Y., Lynch, P.G. and Wright, J.S. (1980) Peripheral neuropathy due to perhexiline maleate. *Journal of the Neurological Sciences* **46,** 303–9.

Wiley, F.H., Hueper, W.C. and von Oettingen, W.F. (1936) On toxic effects of low concentrations of carbon disulfide. *Journal of Industrial Hygiene and Toxicology* **18,** 733–40.

Wilson, L., Creswell, K.M. and Chin, D. (1975) The mechanism of action of vinblastine. Binding of (acetyl-3H) vinblastine to embryonic chick brain tubulin and tubulin from sea urchin sperm tail outer doublet microtubules. *Biochemistry* **14,** 5586–92.

Windebank, A.J., McCall, J.T., Hunder, H.G. and Dyck, P.J. (1980) The endoneurial content of lead related to the onset and severity of segmental demyelination. *Journal of Neuropathology and Experimental Neurology* **39,** 692–9.

Winder, C., Garten, L.L. and Lewis, P.D. (1983) The morphological effects of lead on the developing central nervous system. *Neuropathology and Applied Neurobiology* **9,** 87–108.

Wiśniewski, H., Terry, R.D. and Hirano, A. (1970) Neurofibrillary pathology. *Journal of Neuropathology and Experimental Neurology* **29,** 163–76.

Wolf, A., Cowen, D. and Geller, L.M. (1962) Structural and functional effects of 6-aminonicotinamide and other antimetabolites on the central nervous system. In *IVth International Congress of Neuropathology*, vol. III (Ed. Jacobs, H.), pp. 447–53. Thieme, Stuttgart.

Wood, C.A. and Buller, F. (1904) Poisoning by wood alcohol. Cases of death and blindness from Columbian spirits and other methylated preparations. *Journal of the American Medical Association* **43,** 1289–96.

Yamamura, Y. (1969) *n*-Hexane polyneuropathy. *Folia Psychiatrica et Neurologica Japonica* **23,** 45–57.

Yuen, T.G.H., Agnew, W.F. and Carregal, E.J.A. (1975) Lysosomal handling of tellurium by the choroid plexus following chronic administration: an ultrastructural study. *Experimental Neurology* **47,** 213–28.

Zbinden, G. and Studer, A. (1955) Experimenteller Beitrag zur Frage der Izoniazid-Neuritis und ihre Beeinflussung durch Pyridoxin. *Zeitschrift für Tuberkulose und Heilstättenwesen* **107,** 97–107.

Zunker, E. (1880) Zur Pathologie der Bleilähmung. *Zeitschrift für klinische Medizin* **1,** 496–505.

15

Diseases of the basal ganglia, cerebellum and motor neurons

D. R. Oppenheimer

Most of the conditions discussed in this chapter are classified as *primary neuronal degenerations*; that is, diseases in which, for unknown reasons, nerve cells of a particular type or in a particular region successively shrivel and die. Excluded by this definition are diseases due to infections or poisons, or to the 'pathoclitic' effects of hypoxia or epilepsy, or to metabolic deficiencies or avitaminoses; also conditions ascribed to the remote effects of malignant disease elsewhere in the body.

The common characters of the degenerative diseases are: (1) they are selective, affecting one or more 'systems' of neurons in a more or less symmetrical pattern; (2) they are steadily progressive, though not necessarily fatal; and (3) they are variable in their clinical and pathological features and often appear to overlap with one another, making accurate classification difficult if not impossible. Some have a clear genetic basis, others not; in certain diseases with dominant inheritance—for instance, in Huntington's chorea—the disease tends to run a similar course in all the affected members of a family, whereas in other families, such as the one described by Schut and Haymaker (1951), it seems that a single dominant gene may produce a bewildering variety of lesions and syndromes in different individuals. Where a large number of nervous structures is at risk, as in multiple system atrophy of the pontocerebellar type, different combinations of lesions can give rise to a wide variety of clinical pictures, whereas a disease normally affecting very few systems, such as Werdnig–Hoffmann disease, has a fairly uniform clinical manifestation. Table 15.1 shows the structures at risk in a few of the commoner degenerative diseases.

For the most part, the histology of the lesions reveals no more than focal or systematic loss of neurons, with reactive gliosis. In many instances there is evidence of a 'dying-back' process, in which neuronal atrophy begins at the distal end of the axis cylinder, and proceeds centripetally towards the cell body (Spatz, 1938; Greenfield, 1954; Cavanagh, 1979). This is seen most convincingly in the pyramidal tracts in motor neuron disease, and in the middle cerebellar peduncles in pontocerebellar atrophy. In other cases one may find that the distal parts of long tracts have degenerated, without evidence of progressive degeneration of the proximal parts—for instance, in the long tracts of the spinal cord in Strümpell's familial spastic paraplegia, or the pyramidal tracts in Friedreich's ataxia. Here the impression is that the parent cell body does not die, but is incapable of maintaining the vitality of a long axon.

In many degenerative conditions there is an appearance of 'linked' or 'chain' (i.e. transneuronal) degeneration. Examples are the 'linked' degeneration of the pallidum and subthalamic nucleus in progressive supranuclear palsy; of striatum and substantia nigra, and of pontine nuclei and Purkinje cells, in multiple system atrophy; and of motor neurons and pyramidal tracts in motor neuron disease. Almost nothing is known of the mechanisms involved in such transneuronal degenerations—not even whether it occurs in anterograde or retrograde direction, or both. In any case, 'linked' degeneration does not account for all the combinations of lesions which are found in practice. For instance, in Friedreich's ataxia there is degeneration of the spinocerebellar tracts and of the dentate nuclei, but not of the Purkinje cells which presumably constitute the 'link' between these two.

A few degenerative diseases have peculiar histological features, other than simple neuronal

Table 15.1 Sites of neuronal degeneration in various diseases

	MND	PA	PSP	FA	MSA	DPLA
Cerebral cortex	(+)	(+)	–	–	(+)	–
Caudate nuclei	–	–	–	–	(+)	(+)
Putamen	–	–	–	–	++	(+)
Pallidum	–	–	++	+	(+)	++
Thalamus	–	–	+	–	–	–
Subthalamic nuclei (Luys)	–	–	++	+	(+)	+
Red nuclei	–	–	+	(+)	(+)	+
Substantia nigra	–	++	++	–	+	(+)
Locus ceruleus	–	++	+	–	+	–
Pontine nuclei	–	–	(+)	–	+	–
Inferior olives	–	–	(+)	–	+	(+)
Purkinje cells	–	–	(+)	–	+	(+)
Dentate nuclei	–	–	+	++	(+)	++
Dorsal vagal nuclei	–	+	–	–	+	–
Thoracic (Clarke's) nuclei	(+)	–	–	++	(+)	(+)
Intermediolateral columns	–	(+)	–	–	+	–
Onuf's nuclei	–	(+)	–	–	+	–
Motor nuclei	++	–	+	–	(+)	(+)
Sensory ganglia	(+)	–	–	++	(+)	(+)
Sympathetic ganglia	–	+	–	–	(+)	–
Vestibular nuclei	–	–	+	+	+	+
Optic nerves	–	–	–	+	(+)	–
Pyramidal tracts	+	–	–	++	+	(+)

MND, motor neuron disease (amyotrophic lateral sclerosis); PA, paralysis agitans (Parkinson's disease); PSP, progressive supranuclear palsy; FA, Friedreich's ataxia; MSA, multiple system atrophy (pontocerebellar or striatonigral); DPLA dentatopallidoluysian atrophy.
++, always or nearly always affected; +, commonly affected; (+), occasionally affected; –, not known to be affected.

loss and gliosis. Examples are the cytoplasmic inclusion bodies described by Lewy (1913) in Parkinson's disease, and the neurofibrillary tangles found in Alzheimer's disease, in progressive supranuclear palsy and in the Parkinson–dementia complex of Guam. Whether these special features indicate a different type of pathological process from that in the 'simple' neuronal degenerations is still not known. On the other hand there are diseases, of which Jakob–Creutzfeldt disease is an instance, having the histological features of a simple neuronal degeneration, in which it has been discovered that material from the diseased brain can be used to transmit a similar, progressive disorder to experimental animals (Beck et al., 1969). With the knowledge that these conditions are transmissible, it is now usual to remove them from the category of primary degenerations into that of 'slow virus diseases'. These are discussed in Chapters 7 and 20. It may well happen that other diseases, at present regarded as primary degenerations, may be found to belong to this group.

There is a much debated question, of medicolegal importance, whether a progressive neuronal degeneration can be caused, or its onset precipitated, by bodily or mental trauma. Evidence on this is mainly of an anecdotal kind, and generally unconvincing, except perhaps in the case of post-traumatic parkinsonian syndromes, which are discussed below.

In practice, it is often difficult to determine the extent of a neuronal degeneration affecting more than one group of cells. Undoubtedly, lesions are often missed through incomplete examination of the brain and spinal cord; on the other hand, the literature is cluttered with reports of 'slight cell loss' in this nucleus or that, where the reader is left uncertain whether this represents a genuine atrophy, or an ageing change, or a subjective impression on the part of the author. The examination of Nissl-stained sections is often insufficient, unless it is combined with laborious and carefully controlled cell counts. Where a nucleus has a well-defined efferent tract—for instance, the dentate nucleus—myelin-stained sections of this tract may be more informative than the Nissl preparation of the nucleus itself. In the striatum, where the nerve cells are frequently shrivelled and distorted by agonal ischaemic changes, the appearance of the myelinated bundles and of the myelin within the globus pallidus is often more revealing than that of the cell bodies. Positive evidence of disease, in the form of reactive gliosis or of fatty degeneration products, may be necessary as confirmation of the negative features of neuronal loss seen in Nissl and myelin preparations.

No attempt will be made here to classify the primary neuronal degenerations. They will be discussed, in this and other chapters, according to the topography of the principal lesions. Alzheimer's and Pick's diseases, in which the main lesions are in the cerebral cortex, are dealt with in Chapter 20; also Huntington's chorea, in which striatal and cortical lesions are combined. For a fuller discussion, see Seitelberger (1975).

Diseases of basal ganglia and brain stem

There is no agreed definition of the term 'basal ganglia'. For present purposes the term is used to cover the *striatum* (i.e. caudate nucleus and putamen), *pallidum* (globus pallidus), *claustrum*, *amygdala*, *substantia innominata*, *subthalamic nucleus* (corpus Luysii), *red nucleus* and *substantia nigra* (functionally closely related to the preceding structures, but usually classified as a midbrain nucleus). The *thalamus*, though not usually included among the basal ganglia, is included in this section for convenience.

Although much is already known about the anatomical connections of the basal ganglia (Mettler, 1968; Kemp and Powell, 1971; Carpenter, 1981), their functions are still poorly understood. Attempts to reproduce familiar clinical syndromes by means of stimulation or ablation in experimental animals have seldom been successful; and although it has been known for many years that various disturbances of movement and posture are associated with lesions in one or other of the basal ganglia, it is still not possible to account for individual symptoms, such as tremor, rigidity or athetosis, in terms of normal or abnormal functioning of a particular nucleus. In other words, one cannot speak confidently of striatal or pallidal or nigral syndromes. One reason for this may be that there are lesions of a biochemical kind, which are not shown by routine neurohistological methods. In Parkinson's disease, for example, routine methods show cell loss in the substantia nigra but not in the striatum. In experimental animals, destruction of the substantia nigra on one side gives rise, after a delay, to depletion of dopamine in the striatum of the same side, without apparent loss of striatal nerve cells. The dramatic effects of L-dopa in alleviating the parkinsonian disorder are probably exerted through the striatum and other structures, rather than through the remaining cells of the substantia nigra. In general, it is no longer justifiable to explain disorders of function in simple terms of neuronal circuits with excitatory and inhibitory synapses, and loss of component neurons. If the substantia nigra is regarded merely as part of a neuronal circuit, it is hard to explain why an attack of encephalitis lethargica, with destruction of the substantia nigra, commonly gave rise to a delayed, ingravescent parkinsonian syndrome rather than to an immediate full-blown parkinsonism.

Accounts of the clinical features of diseases of the basal ganglia include those of Denny-Brown (1962, 1968) and J.P. Martin (1967). Jellinger (1968a) has reviewed the pathology of a wide variety of degenerative, toxic, metabolic and vascular diseases affecting the striatum and pallidum. These include Wilson's disease and Hallervorden-Spatz disease, which are discussed in Chapter 13 of this book.

Parkinson's disease (paralysis agitans)

In his *Essay on the Shaking Palsy* Parkinson (1817) defined the disease which bears his name in these words: 'Involuntary tremulous motion, with lessened muscular power, in parts not in action and even when supported; with a propensity to bend the trunk forwards, and to pass from a walking to a running pace: the senses and intellects being uninjured'. Subsequent clinical descriptions have amplified this picture and emphasized the muscular stiffness, the immobile face and the mumbling speech of the sufferer.

The disease affects both sexes, and is slowly progressive, with onset most commonly in later middle age. No causative agent is known, and although some families show an undue incidence of the disease, there is no evidence of simple genetic transmission.

Pathology Trétiakoff (1919), writing a century after Parkinson, appears to have been the first to observe the characteristic lesions of the substantia nigra (Figs. 15.1 and 15.2). Earlier pathologists had described various changes in the basal ganglia, which have since frequently been found in the brains of old people not suffering from parkinsonism, but had failed to observe lesions in the brain stem. Among these was Lewy (1913), who first described the concentric hyaline cytoplasmic inclusions which bear his name (Fig. 15.3). These bodies, which can be seen in melanin-containing cells of the brain stem in almost every case of Parkinson's disease, were observed by Lewy in the nucleus of the substantia innominata. Following Trétiakoff, Foix (1921) studied seven cases of Parkinson's disease and one of the newly observed postencephalitic parkinsonism. In the latter, he found gross destructive lesions of the substantia nigra, with residual inflammatory changes. In the other seven, he found loss of pigmented cells from the substantia nigra in all cases; lesions of the striatum, pallidum and hypothalamus were present in some, absent in others.

Hassler (1938) in a study of nine cases of Parkinson's disease found lesions of the substantia nigra and locus ceruleus in every case. The most severe lesions were in the central part of the zona compacta, where some groups of pigmented cells had almost disappeared. The medial and lateral cell groups were less affected. Cell loss was also seen in the substantia innominata. Lesions of the striatum and pallidum were present in some cases, not in others. Klaue (1940) in a study of 32 cases of Parkinson's disease, with 22 controls from non-parkinsonian patients aged over 50, confirmed Hassler's findings. All 32 cases had nigral lesions, which were not present in the controls, the lesions consisting of cell loss, degenerative cell changes, inclusion bodies of Lewy type, and gliosis. Various lesions of the striatum and pallidum were present in the subjects and in the controls.

Subsequent studies have largely confirmed these findings. In Greenfield and Bosanquet's (1953) study, nigral cell loss and Lewy bodies were constant findings in Parkinson's disease, whereas striatal and pallidal lesions corresponded with those found in brains from non-parkinsonian elderly subjects. Greenfield and Bosanquet listed a number of staining reactions, which differentiated the Lewy bodies from other types of cell change and of cytoplasmic inclusions. This work was followed up by Bethlem and Jager (1960), who concluded that the central core of the bodies was composed of proteins containing aromatic alpha-amino acids, but did not contain any lipids, mucopolysaccharides or nucleic acids.

In a later report, based on histochemical studies, Jager (1969) claimed to have shown the presence of sphingomyelin in Lewy bodies; and in the following year (1970) the same author described inclusions in cells of the adrenal medulla of two patients with Parkinson's disease, not present in 10 controls. These are said to contain sphingomyelin, free fatty acids and polysaccharides. Whether this finding is peculiar to the disease remains to be established. Electron microscopy (Duffy and Tennyson, 1965; Roy and Wolman, 1969) has shown the bodies to consist of filaments, loosely packed in the outer zone, densely packed and mixed with granular material in the central core.

It is generally agreed that Lewy bodies are to be found in all, or nearly all, cases of Parkinson's disease, to the extent that it would be difficult to make this histological diagnosis without finding them; on the other hand, they have also been seen in a few cases of well-documented postencephalitic parkinsonism, and occasionally in 'control' material. Lipkin (1959) observed them in 5 per cent of 206 'control' brains, and Forno (1966) in 4 per cent of 400 controls. Whether such brains should be regarded as showing preclinical or subclinical Parkinson's disease is a matter of opinion. Regarding their distribution, they are not confined to the pigmented cells of the substantia nigra, locus ceruleus and dorsal vagal nucleus. Apart from the substantia innominata, which is not pigmented, Jager and Bethlem

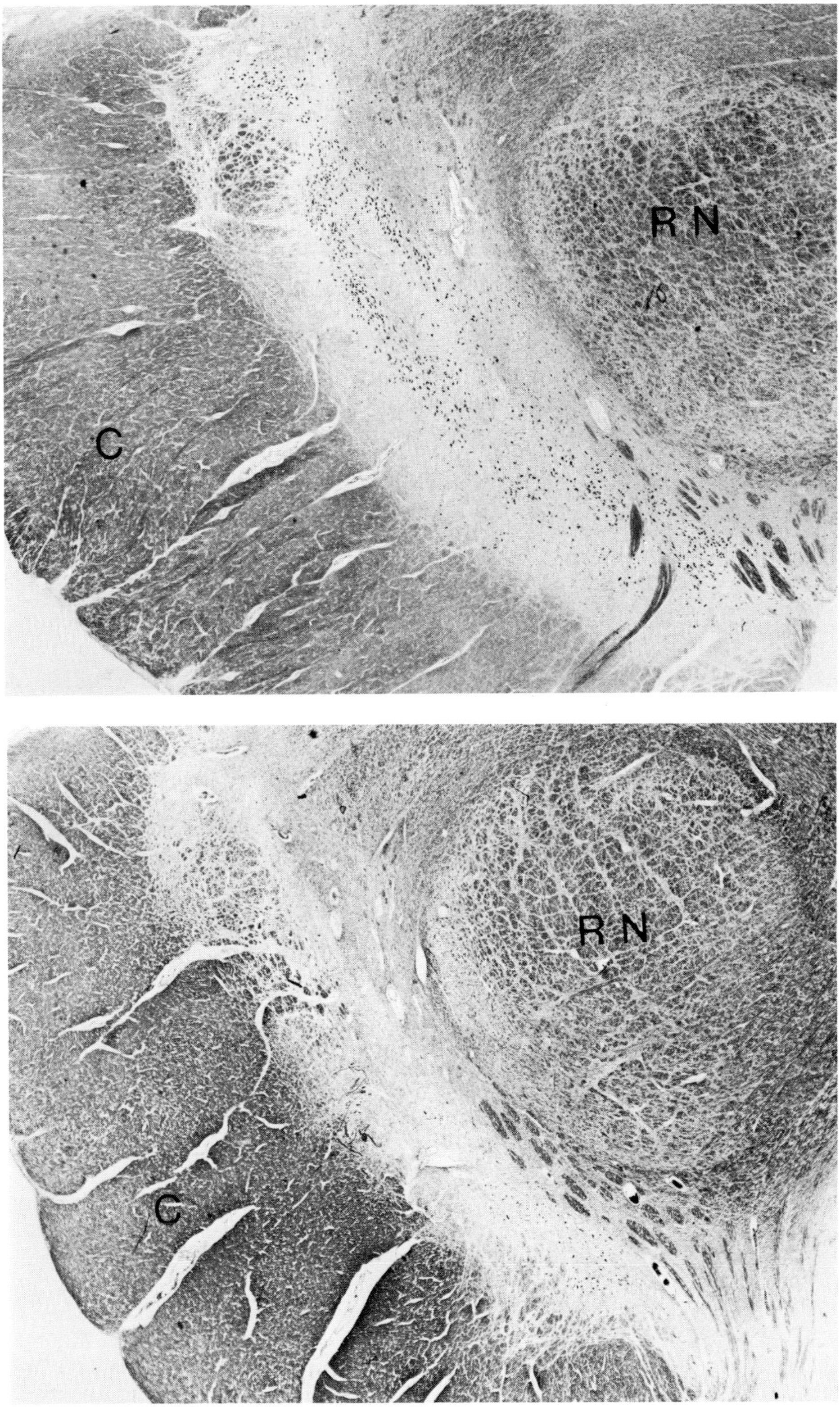

(a)

(b)

Fig. 15.1 Parkinson's disease. (**a**) A normal population of pigmented cells in the substantia nigra, in a 68-year-old man. (**b**) Depletion of these cells in a 69-year-old woman with Parkinson's disease. RN, red nucleus. C, crus cerebri. Klüver–Barrera stain, 20μm sections. ×10.

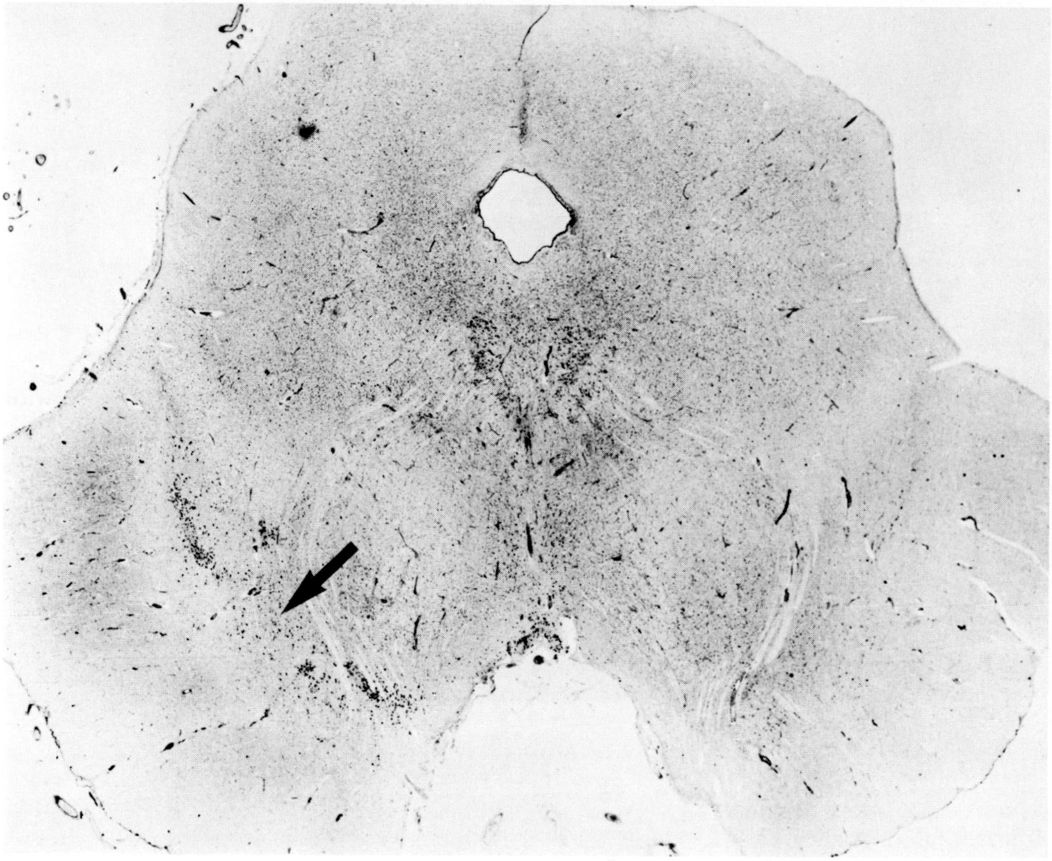

Fig. 15.2 Case of 'hemi-parkinsonism'. Male, aged 74. On the left of the picture there is a mild loss of pigmented cells in the middle zone of the substantia nigra (arrow), on the right, the loss is almost complete. Other basal ganglia appeared normal, and symmetrical. Nissl, 20μm section. ×7.5.

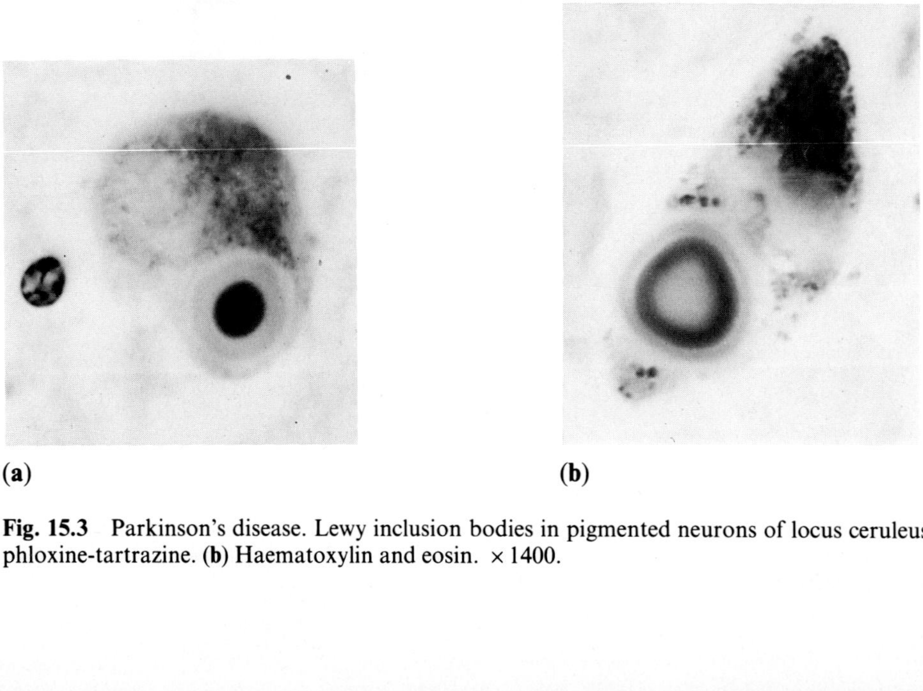

(a) **(b)**

Fig. 15.3 Parkinson's disease. Lewy inclusion bodies in pigmented neurons of locus ceruleus. (**a**) Lendrum's phloxine-tartrazine. (**b**) Haematoxylin and eosin. ×1400.

(1960) found them in numerous brain stem nuclei and in the lateral grey horns of the thoracic cord segments. They also observed bodies, having the same staining reactions but somewhat different shapes, in the cytoplasm and dendrites of nerve cells in sympathetic ganglia. These were not present in control material, and were not found in sensory ganglia. The only other histological report of lesions in the peripheral nervous system appears to be that of Byrnes (1926), who described degenerative changes in muscle spindles in 13 cases of Parkinson's disease, which were not present in controls nor in a case of postencephalitic Parkinsonism. This observation seems to have been neither confirmed nor refuted by subsequent work.

Although Parkinson's disease and Alzheimer's disease are generally regarded as quite separate conditions, a number of recent workers have observed a striking degree of overlap between the two. Hakim and Mathieson (1979), in a retrospective study of 34 cases of Parkinson's disease, of which over half were thought to have suffered some degree of dementia, observed neurofibrillary tangles and granulovacuolar degeneration in the hippocampus in nearly 90 per cent of cases, as against 21 per cent of age-matched controls. Only one case of Parkinson's disease was entirely free from lesions of Alzheimer type. In a similar study by Boller et al. (1980) on 36 cases of Parkinson's disease, of which 9 were severely demented, senile plaques and neurofibrillary tangles were present in 15 cases, including all those with severe dementia. These authors considered that lesions of Alzheimer type were six times as common in patients with Parkinson's disease as in age-matched controls. (See also Chap. 20.)

This is not the place to discuss the much-studied biochemical features of Parkinson's disease. Recent reviews of the histological and chemical pathology of the disease are those of Pearce (1979), Marsden (1981), Sourkes (1981) and Hornykiewicz (1982).

The association of Parkinson's disease with autonomic failure is discussed later in this chapter.

Postencephalitic parkinsonism

The pathology of the acute phase of *encephalitis lethargica* has been described in Chapter 7. Selective damage to the substantia nigra had been observed by various authors before Hallervorden (1933, 1935), in a study of 35 cases of postencephalitic parkinsonism, drew attention to the presence of neurofibrillary changes in nerve cells (Fig. 15.4), not only in the pigmented nuclei but also scattered through the cortex, basal ganglia, thalamus, hypothalamus, tegmentum and dentate nuclei. These changes were present in all

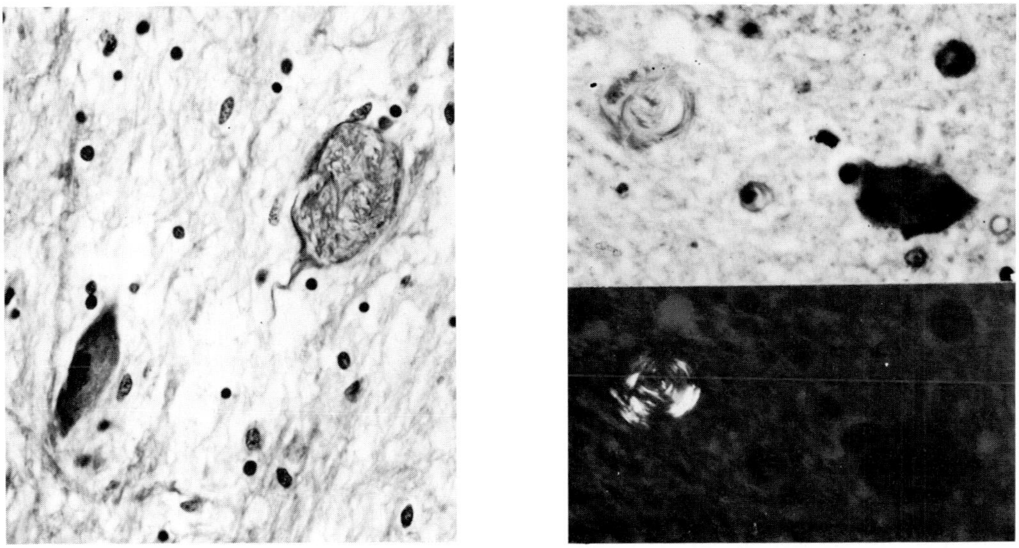

(a) **(b)**

Fig. 15.4 Postencephalitic parkinsonism. Neurofibrillary changes in midbrain. (**a**) Haematoxylin and van Gieson. (**b**) Congo red (the lower half is the same field viewed through crossed Nicol prisms).

cases. Subsequent studies (Klaue, 1940; Beheim-Schwarzbach, 1952; Greenfield and Bosanquet, 1953; Hirano and Zimmerman, 1962; Forno, 1966; Torvik and Meen, 1966; Earle 1968) comparing the findings in this condition with those in Parkinson's disease have confirmed that there is at least a statistical difference between the two; that is, Lewy bodies are always or nearly always present in Parkinson's disease, and are rare in controls and in postencephalitic cases, whereas neurofibrillary tangles are nearly always found in postencephalitic cases and are rare in controls and in Parkinson's disease. In a few cases, both changes have been observed; in a few others, neither. Other points of difference are that in postencephalitic cases the destruction in the substantia nigra tends to be more severe and uniformly distributed, and there may be widespread small glial scars, presumably dating from the acute stage of the disease. At present, most neuropathologists regard these two conditions as separate entities, with a small area of unexplained overlap, and would be prepared to make a diagnosis of 'idiopathic' or of postencephalitic parkinsonism on the basis of the histological findings. When the lesions are those of the postencephalitic disease, in the absence of a history of epidemic encephalitis, the question arises whether other neurotropic viruses may occasionally attack the substantia nigra. The development of immunofluorescent techniques may help to resolve this problem. Gamboa and colleagues (1974) announced the finding of influenza A antigen in the brains of six well-documented cases of postencephalitic parkinsonism. The antigen was not found in five patients with the 'idiopathic' disease, or in two controls. This work has not so far been confirmed.

Striatonigral degeneration

In 1961 and 1964 Adams, van Bogaert and Vander Eecken drew attention to a group of cases in which the clinical picture was indistinguishable from that of Parkinson's disease. They described four cases, in which the most striking pathological features were shrinkage, with discolouration, cell loss and gliosis, of the putamen (Fig. 15.5) and loss of pigmented cells from the substantia nigra. Lewy bodies were seen in only one case. Lesser degrees of cell loss were observed in many other structures including the caudate nucleus, globus pallidus, subthalamic and red nuclei; and

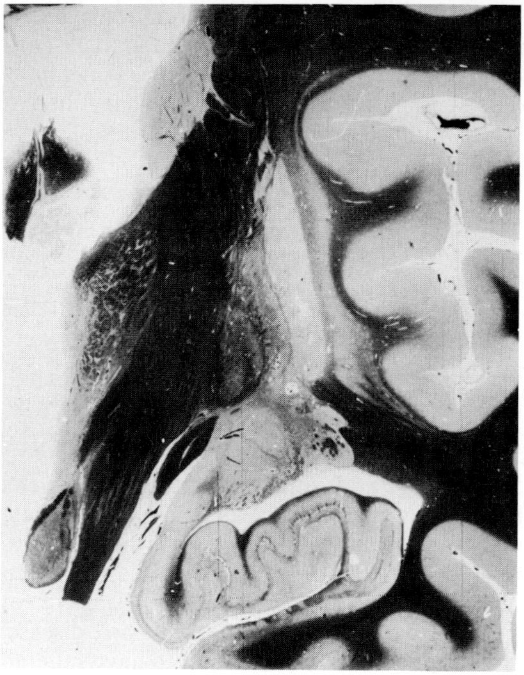

Fig. 15.5 Striatonigral degeneration (Case 1 of Bannister and Oppenheimer, 1972). Shrinkage and myelin loss in putamen. The pigmented nuclei and intermediolateral cell columns were also degenerate. Myelin stain. (Reproduced by courtesy of the Editor, *Brain*).

in one case there were also lesions typical of pontocerebellar atrophy. The authors discussed the nosological placing of the condition at great length, leaving open the question whether it was a new disease or an unfamiliar form of a familiar condition. There have been further case reports, and review articles by Jellinger and Danielczyk (1968) and by Takei and Mirra (1973). The latter authors indicate their view of the nosology in their title: 'Striatonigral degeneration: a form of multiple system atrophy with clinical parkinsonism'. They emphasize the frequent association, previously noted by Scherer (1933), Welte (1939) and Rosenhagen (1943), of lesions of the putamen and substantia nigra with those of pontocerebellar atrophy. More recently, a further association has been established, in the finding that the great majority of cases of progressive autonomic failure show the lesions of striatonigral degeneration, often combined with those of pontocerebellar atrophy (Oppenheimer, 1983); and the term *multiple system atrophy* is now commonly used to cover the whole of this group.

Patients with multiple system atrophy presenting clinically with parkinsonism rather than with ataxia or with autonomic failure are nearly always first diagnosed as having Parkinson's disease. The diagnosis of striatonigral degeneration may be suspected when the symptoms fail to respond to L-dopa, and when other neurological disturbances arise. Neurochemical differences between striatonigral degeneration and Parkinson's disease were reported by Sharpe et al. in 1973, and chemical studies have been made on four cases with autonomic failure by Spokes, Bannister and Oppenheimer (1979). Borit, Rubinstein and Urich (1975) have made observations on the various pigments which are found in the shrivelled, discoloured putamina in such cases. The pathology of autonomic failure is discussed later in this chapter.

Parkinsonism-dementia complex of Guam

Hirano, Kurland, Krooth and Lessell (1961) described the clinical features of an endemic disease confined to the Chamorro population of Guam, one of the Mariana Islands. It appeared to have a genetic basis, and in many families was associated with the locally prevalent amyotrophic lateral sclerosis described by Kurland and Mulder (1954). In some patients the two conditions are combined, and they are reasonably regarded as variants of a single disease. The onset is insidious, usually in the fifth and sixth decades, and progresses to death in about 4 years. About three males are affected to one female. The main clinical features are progressive dementia and parkinsonism, often with signs of upper motor neuron involvement. The pathological findings in 17 cases were described by Hirano, Malamud and Kurland (1961). To the naked eye there was cortical atrophy, particularly of the frontal and temporal lobes, and loss of pigment from the substantia nigra and locus ceruleus. The microscopic changes consisted in widespread loss of neurons and gliosis, especially in the hippocampus, cerebral cortex, amygdala, hypothalamus, globus pallidus, thalamus, substantia nigra and tegmentum; in the same areas there were numerous intraneuronal neurofibrillary tangles, resembling those seen in Alzheimer's disease, but not associated with 'senile' plaques.

Comparing this with other known diseases, the closest clinical resemblance is with some forms of Jakob-Creutzfeldt disease; these, however, usually run a much more rapid course. The histology of the condition is closer to that of progressive supranuclear palsy (see below).

Other causes of parkinsonism

Drugs, especially the phenothiazines, are today common causes of non-idiopathic parkinsonism. Schwab and England (1968) discuss these and other toxic causes such as manganese and carbon monoxide poisoning. Parkinsonism has also been induced by inadvertent use by drug addicts of 1-methyl-4-phenyl-1, 2, 3, 6-tetrahydropyridine and by its experimental administration to monkeys (Langston and Ballard, 1984; Burns et al, 1984).

Stress is often laid on arteriosclerosis as a cause of parkinsonism and the clinical diagnosis of 'arteriosclerotic parkinsonism' commonly made. While the scattered softenings and rarefactions, so frequently seen in the basal ganglia and thalamus of elderly partients may be causually related to bradykinesia, tremor and rigidity (Hassler, 1939) there is a dearth of neuropathological evidence that full-blown parkinsonism can be caused by such lesions. Schwab and England (1968) concluded that 'arteriosclerosis is not a cause of the disease but exists with it, and greatly adds to the burdens of the patient'.

The same authors discussed at great length the question whether trauma or other forms of stress can cause or precipitate a progressive parkinsonian disorder, and referred to a previous review of the subject by Grimberg (1934). Apart from the very rare instances in which parkinsonism was attributable to midbrain trauma, the published evidence is hard to interpret. The authors argue that since various kinds of stress may temporarily exacerbate the symptoms of parkinsonism, it is reasonable to suppose that stress may unmask symptoms in a case of incipient, subclinical disease. As an argument against trauma actually causing the disease, they note that trauma is not known to precipitate parkinsonism in young people. Counter to this, the writer once examined the brain of a previously healthy man who had fallen into a dry dock at the age of 21, suffering concussion and minor injuries. During his slow recovery in hospital he developed generalized muscular rigidity, weakness, and later a marked parkinsonian tremor, mask-like facies and mumbling dysarthria. All these slowly progressed; the patient became chairfast, and died at the age of 38. The findings were of severe striatonigral degeneration. There were no Lewy bodies or neurofibrillary tangles, and no traces of brain trauma. Since the usual age of onset in striatonigral degeneration is in the fifth to seventh decades (Adams, 1968), it is difficult not to conclude that in this instance the disease had been caused, or its onset prematurely 'triggered', by trauma.

Pallidoluysian degenerations

Ramsay Hunt (1917) described four patients in whom progressive symptoms typical of Parkinson's disease developed before the age of 30. In one case, with onset at age 15 and death at 40, he found a severe loss of large nerve cells from the caudate nucleus, putamen, globus pallidus and substantia innominata (nucleus basalis). No other lesions were observed. No mention was made of the substantia nigra. In 1930 van Bogaert described a similar case, with onset at age 7 and death at 30. There was degeneration and loss of large cells from the striatum and pallidum, with minor changes in the subthalamic nucleus (corpus Luysii) and substantia nigra.

Van Bogaert later (1946) described a series of cases of progressive pallidal and pallidoluysian degeneration, some of which were familial, and which differed clinically from the cases of juvenile parkinsonism described by Hunt in 1917. Since then, there have been several reports (Titica and van Bogaert, 1946; André-van Leeuwen and van Bogaert, 1949; Smith, Gonda and Malamud, 1958; Neumann, 1959; Iizuka, Hirayama and Maehara, 1980) of patients with various disorders of posture and movement, in whom pallidoluysian degeneration has been combined with atrophy of the dentate nuclei, superior cerebellar peduncles, red nuclei and various brain stem structures. Although there is a little overlap with the lesions of multiple system atrophy of the striatonigral and pontocerebellar types, these cases appear to belong to a different kind of multisystem degeneration (see Table 15.1). They are discussed by Jellinger (1968a, b), and by Smith (1975) under the forbidding label of *dentatorubropallidoluysian atrophy*. Naito and Oyanagi (1982) have described five kinships showing this combination of lesions, associated with myoclonus epilepsy and choreo-athetosis, with autosomal dominant inheritance. The relationship of this condition with others, such as Friedreich's ataxia and progressive supranuclear palsy, in which there is selective degeneration of the pallidum and subthalamic nucleus, remains obscure.

For the pathology of the other syndrome described by Ramsay Hunt—so-called *dyssynergia cerebellaris myoclonica*—see p. 723.

Progressive supranuclear palsy

In 1964 Steele, Richardson and Olszewski gave an account of nine patients (all male) with a syndrome of progressive paralysis of vertical eye movements, dysarthria, and muscular rigidity, most marked in the muscles of the neck. The disease started in the fifth to seventh decades, and usually led to death in 5–7 years. In four of these cases, detailed examination showed widespread symmetrical neuronal loss with gliosis, affecting most conspicuously the globus pallidus, subthalamic nucleus, red nucleus, substantia nigra, tectum and periaqueductal grey matter, and dentate nucleus (Fig. 15.6). In the same structures, and in many parts of the brain stem where cell loss was not appreciable, many of the nerve cells showed Alzheimer's neurofibrillary change. The cerebral cortex appeared unaffected, and the 'senile plaques' characteristic of Alzheimer's disease were not present.

Subsequent clinical reports on over 40 cases have shown that the disease is rather uniform in its manifestations. Males are affected more than twice as often as females. No familial cases are recorded. Pathological examinations (David, Mackey and Smith, 1968; Behrman et al., 1969; Steele, 1975 and others); have conformed very closely with the findings of Steele et al. (1964). Nothing is yet known of the aetiology. Electron microscopic studies (Tellez-Nagel and Wiśniewski, 1973; Powell, London and Lampert, 1974; Roy et al., 1974) have shown a consistent difference in the ultrastructure of the neurofibrillary tangles found in this disease and that of the tangles occurring in Alzheimer's disease, Down's syndrome, the parkinsonism–dementia of Guam, and postencephalitic parkinsonism, which resemble each other very closely.

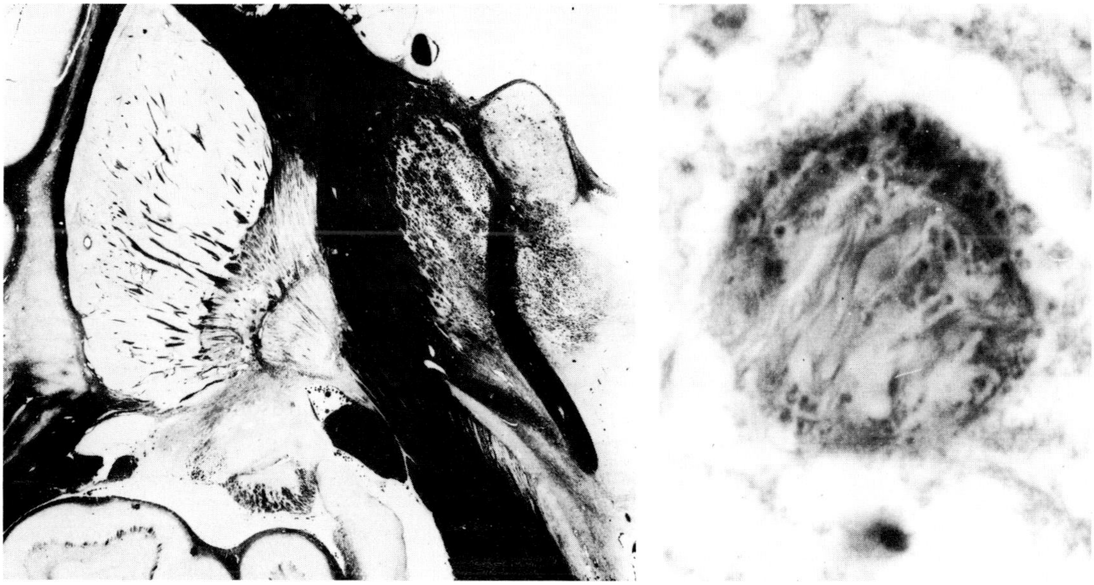

(a) **(b)**

Fig. 15.6 Progressive supranuclear palsy. Woman, dying at age 71 after 3 years' illness. (**a**) Myelin stain, showing atrophy and loss of myelin in globus pallidus and subthalamic nucleus. × 3. (**b**) Neurofibrillary tangle in globus pallidus. Hortega double impregnation. × 1700.

Calcification of the basal ganglia

A mild degree of calcification in and around blood vessels in the lentiform nucleus (less frequently in the hippocampus, dentate nucleus and striate cortex) is a common incidental finding, without associated symptoms, in elderly brains. A somewhat more severe degree of calcification in the basal ganglia, visible on computed tomography, again without associated symptoms, was an incidental finding in 42 out of 7000 tomograms reported by Harrington and colleagues in 1981. These authors list 24 different conditions which have at various times been associated with this finding. Calcification of far greater intensity and wider distribution, visible in plain x-rays of the skull, is an uncommon but very striking post-mortem finding (Figs. 15.7,8). The condition has been recognized since the middle of the nineteenth century (for references, see Löwenthal and Bruyn (1968). Over half of the patients with this condition suffer from a deficiency of parathyroid hormone, either 'idiopathic' or in consequence of radical thyroid surgery. Of the remainder, some have one or other form of Albright's hereditary osteodystrophy; others, including a number of familial cases, have no demonstrable endocrine or metabolic disorder. Clinical disturbances attributed to the lesions in the brain include epilepsy, dementia, abnormal movements, parkinsonism and ataxia. These symptoms are variable, may be slight or severe, and progress very slowly.

Whatever the underlying disease may be, the distribution of the lesions is rather stereotyped. The heaviest calcifications are found in the globus pallidus, putamen, caudate nucleus, internal capsule, the lateral parts of the thalamus and the dentate nuclei of the cerebellum (Figs. 15.7 to 15.10). Smaller concretions, which may however be visible in x-ray pictures, are present at the junction of cortex and white matter at the bases of cerebral sulci, and in parts of the cerebellar cortex. On slicing the brain, the smaller lesions are felt as a gritty resistance to the knife, whereas the larger concretions ('brain stones') are dislodged, and appear as solid lumps with an irregular rough surface. Microscopically, the lesions are more widespread than appears on gross inspection, and may be found in other basal and brain stem nuclei. Calcification occurs in two forms (Fig. 15.11). The first is seen as rows of tiny calcospherites lying along capillary vessels; in the second, calcium salts form tubular deposits

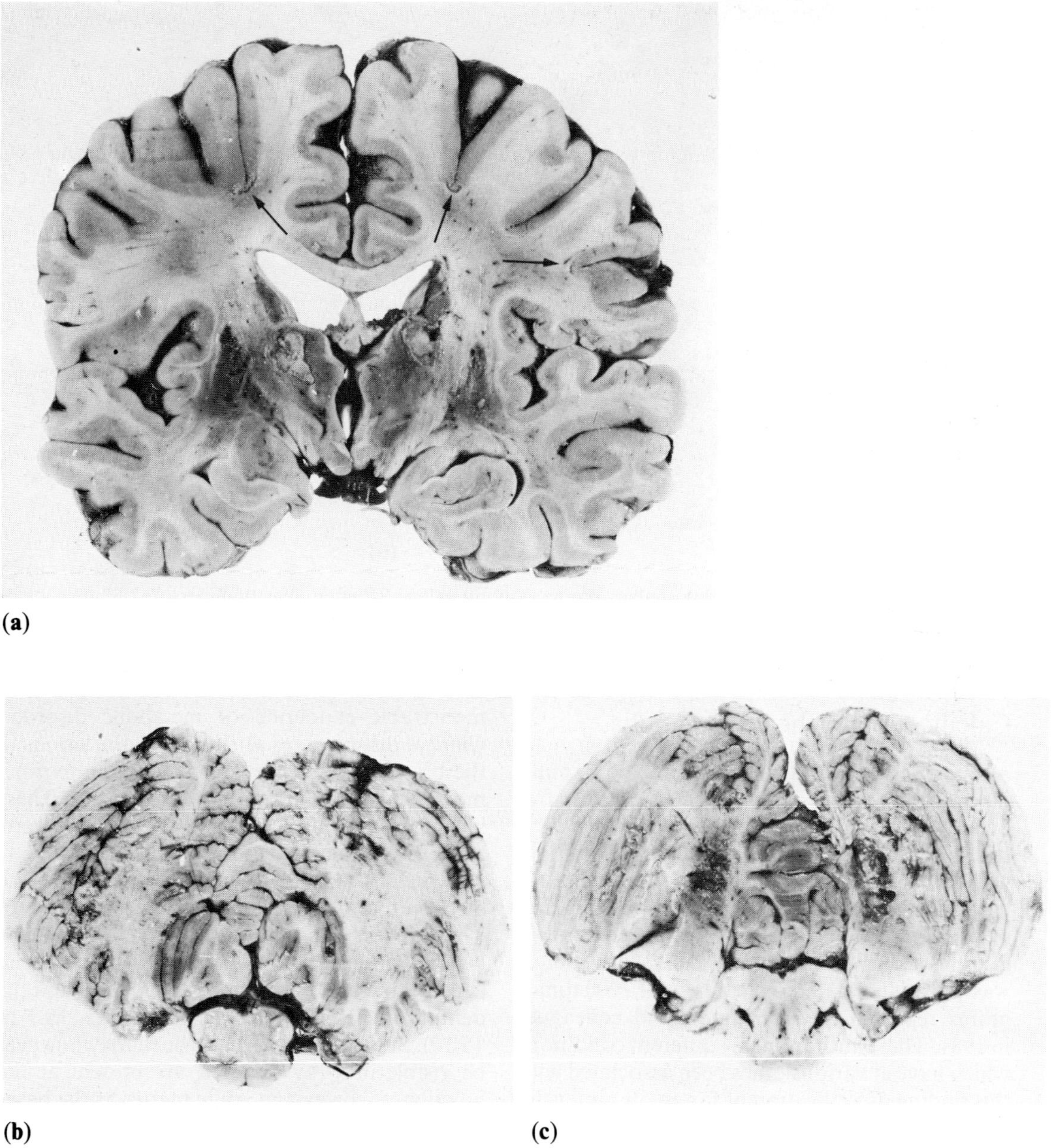

Fig. 15.7 Cerebral calcification in a case of hypoparathyroidism. Three slices showing 'brain stones' in thalamus and dentate nuclei, with more diffuse calcification in the lentiform nuclei, cerebellar cortex and white matter, and at the bases of cerebral sulci (arrows).

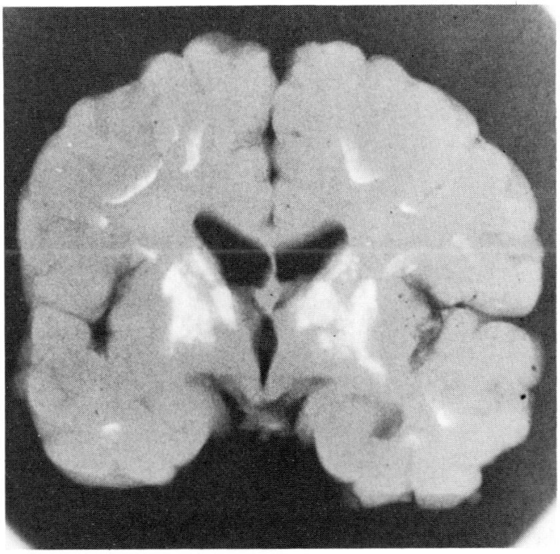

(a)

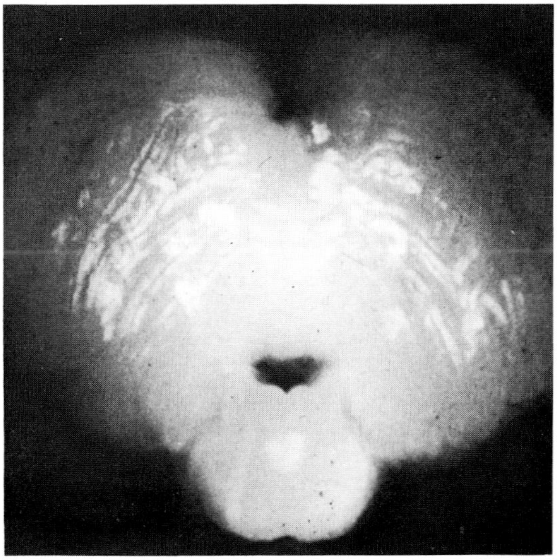

(b)

Fig. 15.8 Cerebral calcification. Case as in Fig. 15.7. (**a**) X-ray of a slice at the level of the mamillary bodies. (**b**) X-ray of pons and superior part of cerebellum. Note the small crescentic shadows cast by cortical calcifications.

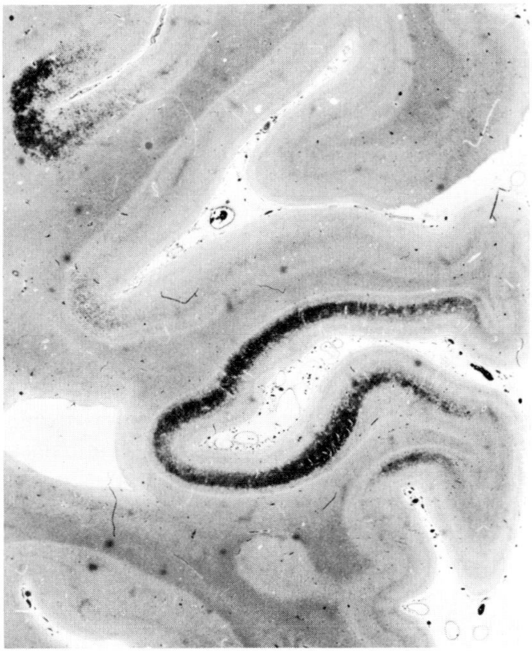

Fig. 15.9 Cerebral calcification. Case as in Fig. 15.7. Calcification of cortex in striate area. Haematoxylin and eosin $\times 3$.

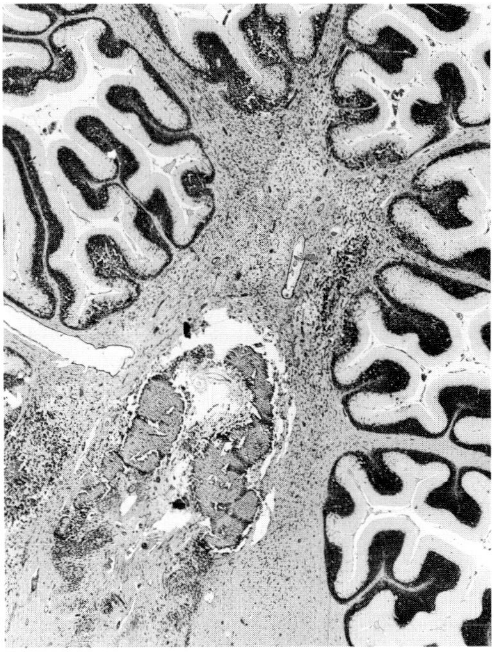

Fig. 15.10 Cerebral calcification. There is a 'brain stone' in the dentate nucleus, with more diffuse calcification in the cerebellar white matter and cortex. Haematoxylin and eosin $\times 5.6$.

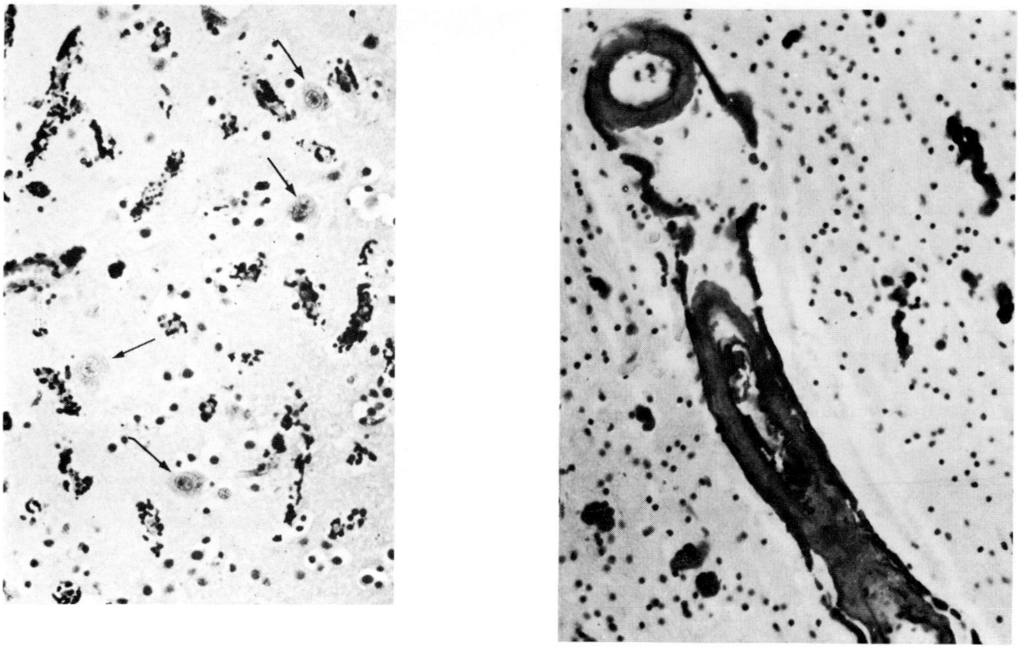

(a) **(b)**

Fig. 15.11 Cerebral calcification. (**a**) Layer 5 of cerebral cortex, showing pericapillary calcospherites. Note good preservation of nerve cells (arrows). PAS ×230. (**b**) Vessel in cerebellar white matter, showing medial calcification. Haematoxylin and eosin ×230.

in the medial walls of small or medium-sized arteries and veins. Lesions of the first type are seen mainly in grey matter, including the cerebral and cerebellar cortex. The larger concretions, or brain stones, appear to develop by coalescence of these pericapillary deposits. Calcification of the media of larger vessels is seen mainly in the cerebral and cerebellar white matter. As the lesions enlarge, nervous tissue is destroyed, but healthy-looking nerve cells are seen immediately alongside the deposits, and there is no inflammatory, and very little glial, reaction. Involvement of the internal capsules may lead to Wallerian degeneration of the pyramidal tracts. No abnormal calcification is seen in the meninges or choroid plexus.

Chemical analysis of brain stones has shown variable amounts of proteins, polysaccharides and metallic ions—in particular calcium, iron, magnesium and aluminium (Löwenthal and Bruyn 1968). The nature of the biochemical disturbances responsible for calcification is not known. Cerebral calcification associated with micrencephaly and other congenital diseases is discussed in Chapter 10.

Effects of focal thalamic and subthalamic lesions

Associations of well-defined clinical disturbances with focal lesions in one or other of the basal ganglia are uncommon. Exceptions are the association of *hemiballism* with lesions of the contralateral subthalamic nucleus, and the *thalamic syndrome* described by Dejerine and Roussy in 1906. In both cases the association is strong, but not absolute. Most cases of hemiballism show the expected lesion in the opposite subthalamic nucleus, but some do not; some have solitary lesions in other nuclei, including thalamus, pallidum and striatum (Schwarz and Barrows, 1960; Smith, 1971), and destructive lesions of a subthalamic nucleus have been found in patients who did not suffer from hemiballism during life. Reviews, with discussion of pathophysiology, include those of Whittier (1947) and Meyers (1968).

The main feature of the thalamic syndrome is a sensory disturbance affecting one side of the body, in which sensory thresholds are raised, but stimulation of the affected side evokes a delayed 'hyperpathic' response, referred to a large area of the body, and subsiding slowly. The lesion responsible for this is commonly an infarct or haemorrhage involving the posterior ventral nucleus of the opposite thalamus. In the original case descriptions, hemiplegia formed part of the 'syndrome'; but subsequent reports on cases with small lesions and no hemiplegia make it probable that hemiplegia occurs only when the lesions spread into the relevant part of the internal capsule. In a case examined by the writer, a lesion a few millimetres in diameter, involving only the medial part of the posterior ventral nucleus, was associated with hyperpathia affecting only the face on the opposite side. As with hemiballism, lesions in other sites, including the brain stem and parietal cortex and white matter, have been described as responsible for a sensory disorder indistinguishable from that of the thalamic syndrome (see Cassinari and Pagni, 1969), and lesions of the posterior ventral nucleus may be associated with sensory loss without hyperpathia. Small vascular lesions in other parts of the thalamus are a common finding in the brains of elderly subjects, and are generally not associated with a recognized clinical disturbance. It is also common to find cell loss and gliosis in the principal thalamic nuclei, associated with destructive lesions of areas of cerebral cortex to which they project. The participation of individual thalamic nuclei in a wide range of degenerative and other diseases has been reviewed in great detail by Martin (1969, 1970, 1975).

Neuropathology of various disturbances of muscular tone and movement

Although there is a rough correspondence between disorders of movement and demonstrable lesions in the basal ganglia, and although the clinically described disturbances—chorea, athetosis, myoclonus and so forth—are generally characteristic of particular diseases, there is a very poor correlation between the various types of dyskinesia and the various anatomical sites of lesions. The striatum, for instance, is severely affected in Huntington's disease, in Wilson's disease and in many cases of Jakob-Creutzfeldt disease; but the disorders of movement in these three are different. Chorea occurs in Huntington's disease and in rheumatic fever, but the lesions are different. The same applies to disorders of muscular tone. Zeman and Whitlock (1968) have reviewed a number of diseases of widely differing pathology giving rise to 'symptomatic' dystonia. These include various forms of perinatal brain damage, Wilson's and Huntington's diseases, Hallervorden-Spatz disease and other conditions in which lesions of the basal ganglia are consistently present. On the other hand, in *dystonia musculorum deformans*, which appears to be a specific disorder with autosomal dominant inheritance, Zeman and Dyken (1968) have maintained that no characteristic lesions have hitherto been demonstrated—reports to the contrary being attributed to overenthusiasm leading to self-deception on the part of the investigator, or to the fact that the subjects investigated were suffering from some other disease. Clinical, genetic and pathological aspects of dystonia musculorum were reviewed by Eldridge and Fahn (1976). Clinical manifestations of dystonia may complicate homocystinuria without apparent histological changes in the basal ganglia (Gale and Brenton, personal communication). Problems of this kind serve to emphasize the difficulties of central neurophysiology and the inadequacies of conventional neuropathological techniques.

Diseases of the cerebellum and its connections

Attempts to classify the cerebellar system degenerations have been unsatisfactory, for several reasons. Clinical classifications are of little use, as indistinguishable states of 'cerebellar ataxia' may result from a variety of different lesions. Even when the disease has a genetic basis, as in the family described by Schut and Haymaker (1951), there may be extreme variation in the clinical and in the pathological expression of the offending gene. The problems of classification and nomenclature have been discussed, with refreshing cynicism, by Netsky (1968). General reviews of the subject are those of Greenfield (1954) and Ule (1957). The genetic aspects have been discussed by Pratt (1967), and there is a detailed account by Bell and Carmichael (1939) of 242 families, with over 400 cases of hereditary ataxia.

In what follows, three well-known types of cerebellar system degeneration are described: first, cerebellar cortical atrophy, which is almost confined to the Purkinje cells and the inferior olives; second, pontocerebellar atrophy, a multisystem degeneration affecting a selection of cerebellar and other structures; and third, Friedreich's ataxia, in which many structures, including the heart and peripheral nerves, are involved. Brief reference will be made to cases which appear to fall somewhere between these three. Other conditions in which the cerebellum or its afferents degenerate, but in which the aetiology appears to be different, are dealt with in other chapters of this book. These include carcinomatous cerebellar degeneration (Chapter 13), toxic disorders, affecting mainly the Purkinje cells (Chapter 14), and forms of Jakob–Creutzfeldt disease in which the cerebellar cortex or dentate nuclei are particularly involved (Chapter 20). Atrophy of the granular layer of the cerebellum is described, with other congenital diseases, in Chapter 10.

Cerebellar cortical degeneration (cerebello-olivary degeneration)

Gordon Holmes (1907) reported a family in which three brothers and one sister became ataxic between the ages of 35 and 40. Four siblings remained well. Gait was first affected, then the finer hand movements. Dysarthria and tremor of the head and limbs appeared later. There was little alteration of deep or superficial reflexes. A post-mortem examination on one patient who reached the age of 70 showed considerable atrophy of the cerebellum, greatest in the superior parts of the vermis and hemispheres (Fig. 15.12). Histologically there was almost complete disappearance of Purkinje cells from the most affected areas, with proliferation of Bergmann nuclei and fibrous gliosis of the molecular layer. The granule cells were less damaged. There was some loss of myelinated fibres from the folia, proportionate to the loss of Purkinje cells, but no degeneration of the pontine or dentate nuclei or of the superior or middle cerebellar peduncles. The inferior and accessory olives had also undergone atrophy, associated with loss of olivocerebellar fibres. This spared to some extent the medial half of the ventral layer and the caudal end of the medial accessory olive. The latter parts of the olivary nucleus were found

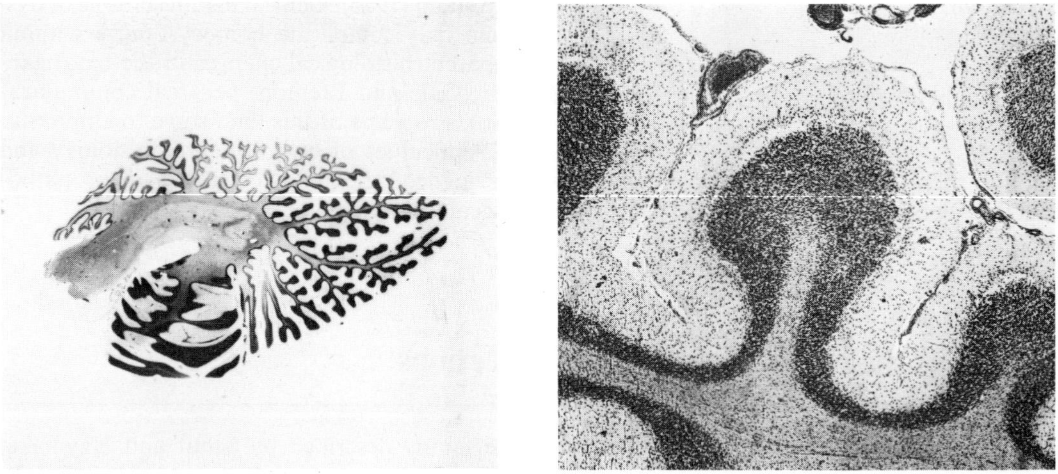

(a) (b)

Fig. 15.12 Familial cerebellar cortical degeneration (case of Weber and Greenfield, 1942). (**a**) Parasagittal section of cerebellum showing atrophy greatest in the superior folia. (**b**) Higher power view of less atrophied folia, showing disappearance of Purkinje cells. Haematoxylin and van Gieson.

(Stewart and Holmes, 1908) to project to the less affected parts of the cerebellum, whereas the dorsal folia projected to the superior surface. Holmes therefore considered that the olivary degeneration was secondary to atrophy of the cerebellar cortex.

A number of similar, isolated cases were collected by Marie, Foix and Alajouanine (1922) under the name *late cortical cerebellar atrophy*. In these the onset of the disease was usually later, with an average age of 57 years. In some the cerebellar atrophy was less widespread than in Holmes' case. When the distribution of atrophy in the inferior olives was reported it usually corresponded to that found in Holmes' case in being greater in the dorsal laminae.

Writing in 1942, Weber and Greenfield noted that among the 20 or so reported cases of this type about half were familial. Hall, Noad and Latham (1941, 1945) reported on a large family in which nine members in two generations were known to have been affected. Post-mortem examinations in two members of the older generation, who died aged 80 and 82, showed the atrophy to be limited to the cerebellar cortex and inferior olives. The condition does not generally or appreciably shorten life, but in a family recorded by Akelaitis (1938) the course of the disease was rapid and accompanied by mental confusion, and led to death in less than 2 years.

Victor (1980) has drawn attention to the close similarities, both clinical and pathological, between the Holmes type of cerebellar cortical degeneration and the cerebellar degeneration observed in chronic alcoholics by Victor, Adams and Mancall (1959).

Pontocerebellar atrophy (olivopontocerebellar atrophy)

Menzel (1891) described a form of generalized ataxia affecting three generations of a family. In one patient in the second generation, with three affected siblings, the disease began at the age of 28 and death occurred at 46. Post-mortem examination showed degeneration of the pyramidal and posterior spinocerebellar tracts, thoracic nuclei (Clarke's columns), and the posterior columns of the cord. In the brain stem, there was loss of nerve cells from the gracile, cuneate, hypoglossal, facial and trigeminal nuclei. There was also atrophy of the inferior olives, pontine nuclei and cerebellar cortex, with rarefaction of granule cells and great loss of Purkinje cells, and poverty of myelin in the white matter.

The name *olivopontocerebellar atrophy* was given to a similar, isolated, case by Dejerine and Thomas (1900). This name has persisted; but since the inferior olives normally react to lesions of the cerebellar cortex with retrograde cell loss, it is reasonable to abbreviate the name to *pontocerebellar atrophy*. Since 1900 many cases, both isolated and familial, have been described; and the subject has been reviewed at length by Scherer (1933), Welte (1939), Rosenhagen (1943) and Jellinger and Tarnowska-Dziduszko (1971).

In a typical case, the most striking naked-eye feature is a gross shrinkage of the ventral part of the pons, which on section may appear wedge-shaped, and of the middle cerebellar peduncles (Fig. 15.13). The cerebellar cortex and the inferior olives may also appear shrunken. In sections stained for myelin, the tegmentum of the pons appears normal or almost so, but there is pallor, which may amount to complete loss of staining, of the transverse fibres in the ventral half, among

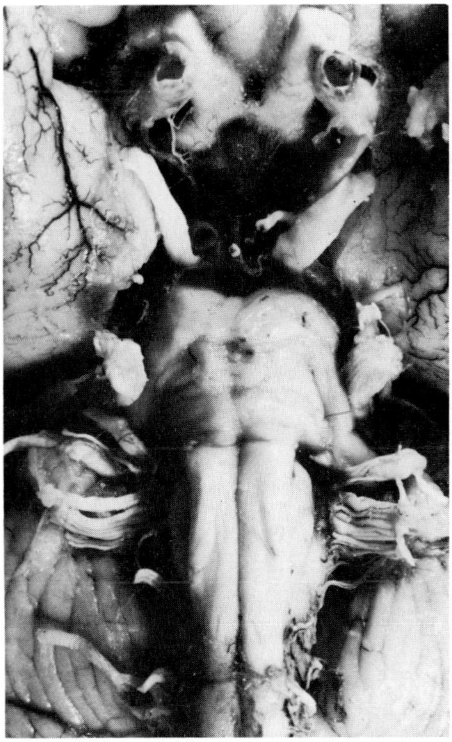

Fig. 15.13 Pontocerebellar atrophy. Sporadic case. Woman, dying at age 76. View of base, showing gross atrophy of pons.

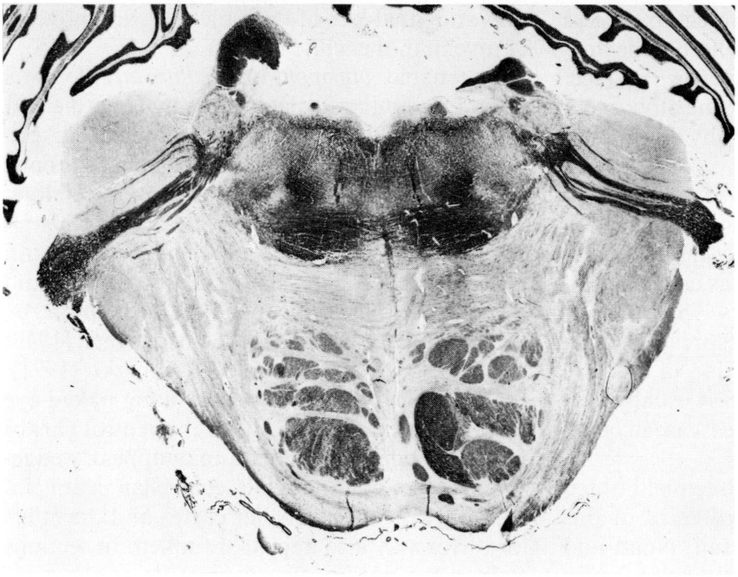

Fig. 15.14 Pontocerebellar atrophy. (Case 4 of Bannister and Oppenheimer, 1972). Section of pons, stained for myelin, showing degeneration of transverse fibres and middle cerebellar peduncles, with preservation of tegmentum, trigeminal fibres and pyramidal tracts.

which the pyramidal tract fibres stand out by their normal staining (Figs. 15.14 and 15.15). In the medulla, there is shrinkage and loss of neurons in the inferior olives, with loss of olivocerebellar fibres (Fig. 15.15). The cerebellar cortex shows a variable—rarely complete—loss of Purkinje cells, the gaps being marked, in silver impregnations, by empty basket formations. The vermis and flocculus tend to be spared, in contrast with the distribution of cell loss in cerebellar cortical atrophy. Granule cells are less affected. The dentate nuclei are gliotic, owing to loss of incoming Purkinje axons, but their cells, and the superior cerebellar peduncles, are well preserved. The cerebellar white matter is grossly deficient in myelinated fibres. It has been observed by several authors that the loss of fibres from the middle peduncles appears disproportionately great in relation to the loss of cells in the pontine nuclei, indicating a 'dying-back' process.

The lesions are not confined to the cerebellar system. There is commonly some degeneration, though not of the severity seen in Friedreich's ataxia, in the long tracts of the spinal cord, and sometimes a loss of motor cells from the anterior horns. In the brain, the commonest associated lesions are loss of cells, with fibrous gliosis, from the striatum (especially the putamen) and the substantia nigra. These features may make it possible to distinguish clinically between pontocerebellar atrophy and other degenerations of the cerebellar system. In cerebellar cortical degeneration, for instance, pyramidal signs and parkinsonian disturbances do not occur, whereas they are sometimes prominent in pontocerebellar atrophy.

The distribution and relative severity of the lesions in this condition vary considerably, even within a single family, such as the one described by Schut and Haymaker in 1951; for instance, there may be only minor changes in the pons, with severe cell loss from the putamen and substantia nigra. Rather than labelling such cases 'striatonigral degeneration', it is reasonable to include them, along with 'classic' cases of pontocerebellar atrophy, under the general heading of *multiple system atrophy* (p. 706).

Biochemical abnormalities in two cases of pontocerebellar atrophy with dominant inheritance have been reported by Perry et al. (1977).

A brave attempt has been made by Konigsmark and Weiner (1970) to classify the varieties of pontocerebellar atrophy, on the basis of reported autopsy-proven cases. They propose a sixfold division:

1. *Menzel type*, with dominant inheritance; sensory and upper motor neuron signs present.

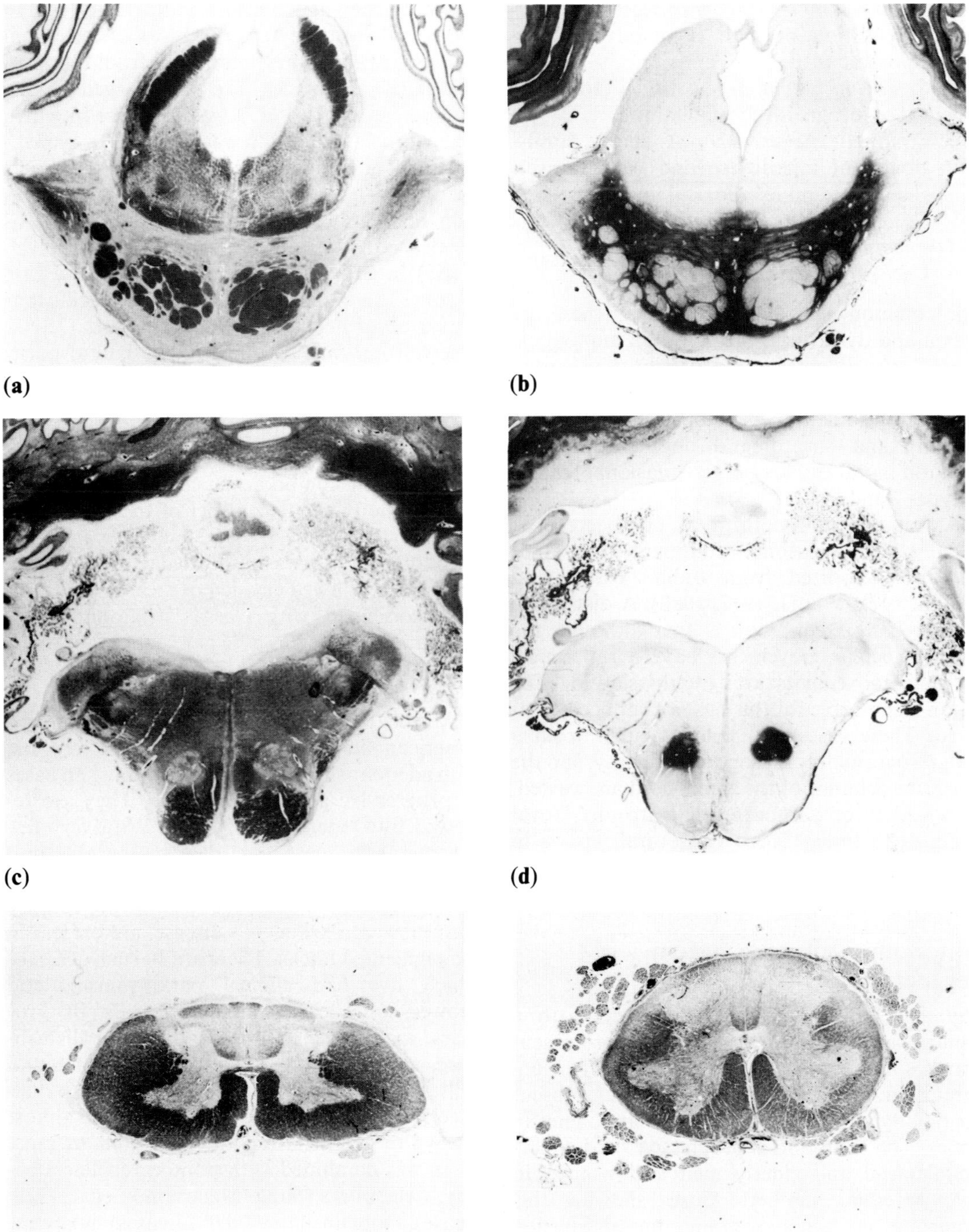

(a) (b) (c) (d) (e) (f)

Fig. 15.15 Pontocerebellar atrophy. (Case 10 of Oppenheimer, 1980). Man, aged 61. Familial case, with sensory neuropathy and slow eye movements. Sections of pons, medulla and cervical and lumbar cord. (**a**), (**c**), (**e**) and (**f**) stained for myelin; (**b**) and (**d**) Holzer stain for glia. There is gross atrophy, with gliosis and myelin loss, of the pontine nuclei and transverse fibres, middle cerebellar peduncles, inferior olives, olivocerebellar fibres and posterior columns. Pyramidal tract degeneration is apparent at the lumbar level. Tegmentum, dentate nuclei and superior cerebellar peduncles are well preserved.

2. *Fickler–Winkler type*, with recessive inheritance; sensation normal. (Probably includes many sporadic cases.)
3. *Cases with retinal degeneration*. Dominant inheritance, progressive visual failure.
4. *Schut–Haymaker type*. A single family, with dominant inheritance and very variable clinical pictures and histological findings.
5. *Cases with parkinsonism, ophthalmoplegia and dementia*. Dominant inheritance.
6. *Unclassified cases*.

The common clinical features in all these are ataxia and dysarthria; the common anatomical lesions are cell losses in the inferior olives, pontine nuclei and Purkinje cells. The authors do not discuss the relation between pontocerebellar atrophy and striatonigral degeneration, but mention nigral cell loss as an occasional feature in types 2 and 5.

A not uncommon form of pontocerebellar atrophy with autosomal dominant inheritance has been reported from India (Wadia and Swami, 1971; Wadia, 1977, 1983). A distinctive feature of this condition is that although the external ocular movements have a full range, saccadic movements are greatly slowed. The lesion responsible for this has not yet been identified. These cases also tend to suffer from a progressive, mainly sensory, neuropathy, and the posterior columns of the spinal cord are wasted. This variety of pontocerebellar atrophy is not confined to India. There are several reports in the European literature (see Wadia, 1983), and Fig. 15.15 is from a case of this type.

Autonomic failure in system degenerations

Shy and Drager (1960) drew attention to a clinical syndrome in which the prominent features are postural (orthostatic) hypotension, urinary incontinence, inability to sweat, muscular rigidity and tremor, and sexual impotence in males. The condition is progressive, and affects middle-aged and elderly men and women in roughly equal numbers. Cases showing this syndrome are usually sporadic, but an affected family has been described by Lewis (1964). Shy and Drager carried out the first neuropathological examination on a case of this type, and found widespread symmetrical neuronal degeneration affecting in particular the caudate nucleus, substantia nigra, locus ceruleus pontis, inferior olives, dorsal vagal nuclei, and Purkinje cells. In the spinal cord they observed loss of cells from the ventral and lateral horns and from the thoracic (Clarke's) nuclei. The second such report, by Fichefet et al. (1965), was of a case in which orthostatic hypotension was followed by parkinsonism. The findings were typical of Parkinson's disease, with loss of cells and Lewy-type inclusion bodies in the substantia nigra and locus ceruleus. In the following year Johnson et al. (1966) described two cases. The first was a case of 'pure' autonomic failure, without parkinsonian or other neurological disturbances. Detectable cell loss was confined to the lateral horns (intermediolateral cell columns) of the thoracic cord. Cell counts showed a loss of nearly 90 per cent of the preganglionic sympathetic neurons in this position. The only other positive finding was of Lewy inclusion bodies, unassociated with cell loss, in the pigmented nuclei of the brain stem and a few other sites. The second case, in which autonomic failure was associated with dyskinesia and ataxia, showed classic pontocerebellar atrophy, combined with classic striatonigral degeneration, as well as a 75 per cent loss of intermediolateral neurons. Inclusion bodes were not found.

At the time of writing, the European and American literature contains some 51 reports, with adequate histological descriptions, on cases of progressive autonomic failure. They are reviewed by Oppenheimer (1983). With very few exceptions the cases are clearly separable into two groups. In the first group are those in which Lewy inclusion bodies, identical in appearance with those of Parkinson's disease, are present in the pigmented nuclei. There are 10 such cases, of which five had clinical parkinsonism, and showed some loss of pigmented cells. In three cases, autonomic failure was the only disturbance, and there was no obvious loss of nigral cells. The second group comprises those with evidence of multiple system atrophy. This was almost always of the striatonigral type, and in most cases was combined with pontocerebellar atrophy. Cell counts (Sung, Mastri and Segal, 1979: 4 cases; Oppenheimer, 1980: 21 cases) have consistently shown loss of 50 per cent or more of the cells in the lateral horns. Other common sites of cell loss are the medial vestibular and dorsal vagal nuclei. Sung, Mastri and Segal (1979) have also reported loss of cells (presumably parasympathetic preganglionic cells) from the intermediolateral column and from Onuf's nucleus in the sacral cord in four cases of multiple system atrophy with autonomic failure. Sung (1979) gives evidence for the view that the cells of Onuf's nucleus (described by Onufrowicz in 1900), although morphologically similar to somatic motor neurons, form part of the parasympathetic system.

The lesions causing progressive autonomic failure, both in cases with Lewy bodies and in those with multiple system atrophy, are found in the central nervous system. Significant lesions in sympathetic ganglia have often been sought but very rarely found, and there are no reports of lesions in the peripheral parts of the autonomic system. This is clearly a major difference from autonomic disorders due to peripheral causes such as diabetic neuropathy. The extent to which the upper levels of the autonomic system are involved is not at present known. Neurochemical studies were carried out on the brains of four cases of multiple system atrophy, of striatonigral type, with autonomic failure, by Spokes, Bannister and Oppenheimer (1979). The main finding was of profound depletion of dopamine and noradrenaline in regions which are normally rich in these catecholamines. The neurochemistry of autonomic failure is reviewed by Spokes (1983).

A not infrequent component of the Shy–Drager syndrome, which has only recently attracted notice, is laryngeal stridor, caused by paralysis of the posterior cricoarytenoid muscles. Three cases of this type were examined by Bannister et al. (1981). The findings in all three were of multiple system atrophy, with intermediolateral cell loss, and gross selective atrophy of the posterior cricoarytenoid muscles. The microscopic changes in the latter were of myopathic type, with evidence of denervation in two cases. Cell counts in the nucleus ambiguus were inconclusive.

It has been the custom in some quarters to speak of the 'Shy–Drager syndrome' or of 'idiopathic orthostatic hypotension' as if these were alternative names for a distinct entity. Pathological studies do not support this usage. It seems, rather, that progressive autonomic failure results from degeneration of central autonomic structures which are at risk in two well-recognized conditions: (1) Lewy body disease, which includes classic Parkinson's disease, and (2) multiple system atrophy, particularly of the striatonigral variety.

Friedreich's ataxia

Friedreich, of Heidelberg, in 1863 and 1876 described a familial form of ataxia with onset under the age of 20. For many years there was reluctance to distinguish between this condition and tabes dorsalis, but the disease is now recognized as one of the commoner hereditary diseases of the nervous system. The proportion of familial cases to 'sporadic' ones is such as would be expected from an autosomal recessive heredity.

The usual presenting symptom is ataxia of gait. This progresses at a variable rate, but towards the end of their lives most patients are unable to walk, even with help. Sensory disturbances, when sought, are nearly always found, at least in the lower part of the body (Saunders, 1913–14). In particular there is loss of joint position sense, vibration sense and two-point discrimination. Other neurological disturbances, in descending order of frequency, include dysarthria, visual deterioration leading to blindness and usually associated with optic atrophy, deafness, dementia or other mental disorders, and epilepsy.

Skeletal deformities, in particular pes cavus and kyphoscoliosis, develop at an early stage of the disease. In over half of the cases the heart is clinically abnormal, and the commonest single cause of death is heart failure, often complicated by diabetes mellitus, of which the incidence is high in Friedreich's ataxia (Hewer, 1968).

The peak age of onset is about 10 years, with roughly equal numbers during the first and second decades. The duration of the disease ranges from under 5 to over 50 years; death occurs most commonly in the third and fourth decades. For more details, see Tyrer (1975) and Geoffroy et al. (1976).

The characteristic *pathological changes* are in the peripheral and central nervous system and in the heart.

Peripheral nervous system

The somatic motor fibres and their cells of origin are usually intact, but degeneration of sensory fibres, posterior roots and ganglion cells in the lower segments of the cord is a constant finding (Fig. 15.16). In a series of 18 necropsied and four biopsied cases, Hughes, Brownell and Hewer (1968) found severe loss (estimated at about 95 per cent) of thick myelinated fibres, with preservation of large numbers of fine unmyelinated

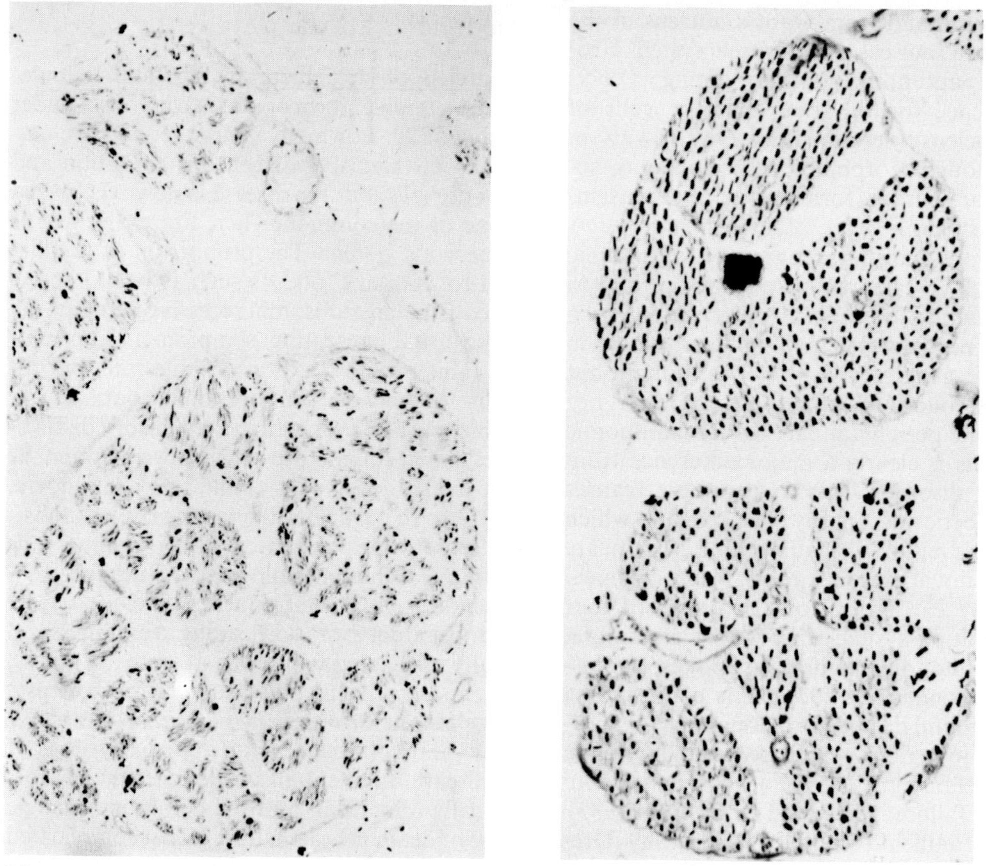

(a) **(b)**

Fig. 15.16 Friedreich's ataxia. Onset age 6, death age 10. Lumbar roots: (**a**) posterior; (**b**) anterior. There is gross loss, especially of thick fibres, in the posterior roots. Holmes silver stain × 120.

axons, and increase in interstitial fibrous tissue. In the ganglia there was widespread loss of ganglion cells, with proliferation of capsule cells (*Residualknötchen*), and abnormalities of intraganglionic nerve fibres. Loss of myelinated fibres from the posterior spinal roots corresponded with that in the peripheral nerves. Comparable data on the state of the trigeminal ganglia and nerves are not at present available.

Central nervous system

The most conspicuous lesions are in the spinal cord (Figs 15.17 to 15.19). The posterior columns are shrunken and degenerate, as is to be expected from the loss of incoming sensory fibres. Fibre loss from the gracile fasciculi is often almost complete, the cuneate fasciculi being affected later and less intensely. Whether there is a 'dying-back' of posterior column fibres towards their cells of origin in sensory ganglia is not known; but 'dying-back' is apparent in the pyramidal tracts, which are often relatively or completely intact at the level of the brain stem, and show progressive loss as they descend through the cord. Degeneration of the thoracic nuclei (Clarke's columns) and the posterior spinocerebellar tracts is constant, and sometimes almost complete. Anterior spinocerebellar tract degeneration is usual, but less marked. The degenerate tracts are shrunken and gliotic, and overall shrinkage of the cord in cross-section is easily seen by naked eye. In severe cases, there is also visible atrophy of the brain stem.

Lesions in the brain are more variable, and less well documented. Some idea of the relative frequency of such lesions came from a personal examination (Oppenheimer, 1979) of 15 brains

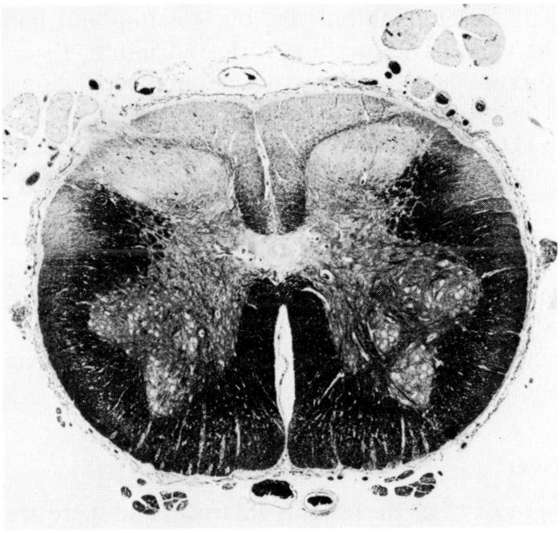

Fig. 15.17 Friedreich's ataxia. Death age 32. Sacral cord. Myelin stain, showing loss of myelin in posterior roots, posterior columns and pyramidal tracts.

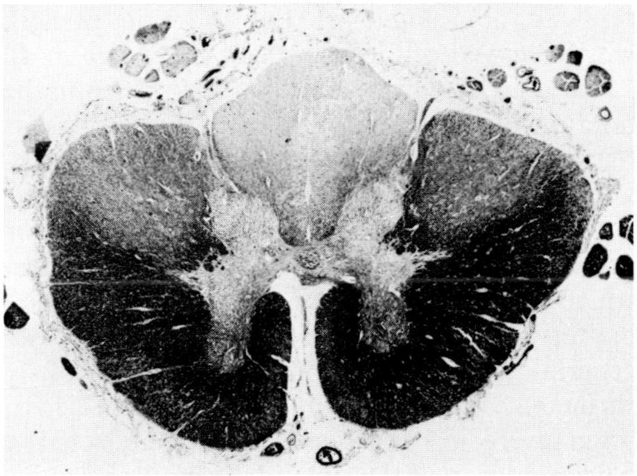

Fig. 15.18 Friedreich's ataxia. Death age 23. Thoracic cord. Myelin stain, showing pallor and shrinkage of posterior columns, and pallor of pyramidal and spinocerebellar tracts.

from cases of 'classic' Friedreich's ataxia. As some of the specimens were incomplete, the findings are given as fractions, in which the denominator denotes the number of specimens examined. In the *sensory system*, myelin pallor of the entering roots of the trigeminal nerves was seen in 8/9, and pallor of the descending trigeminal tracts in 11/15. Pallor of the glossopharyngeal and/or vagus nerves was seen in 7/13, and pallor of the solitary tracts in 7/15. There was heavy gliosis (attributable to degeneration of the posterior columns) in the gracile and cuneate nuclei in 13/13, the gracile nucleus being the most affected. Loss of secondary sensory neurons (apparent 'chain' degeneration) was detectable in the gracile nucleus in 9/13, and there was wasting and myelin pallor in the ventral (gracile) portion of the medial lemniscus in 12/15. In the *motor system*, there was some degree of myelin pallor in the medullary pyramids in 13/15, but in no case was there detectable pallor of the cerebral peduncles. Loss and/or shrinkage of giant pyramidal cells in the motor cortex was observed in 11/11. No changes were seen in cranial motor nuclei.

Of the cerebellar afferents, the most constantly affected were the accessory cuneate nuclei (the

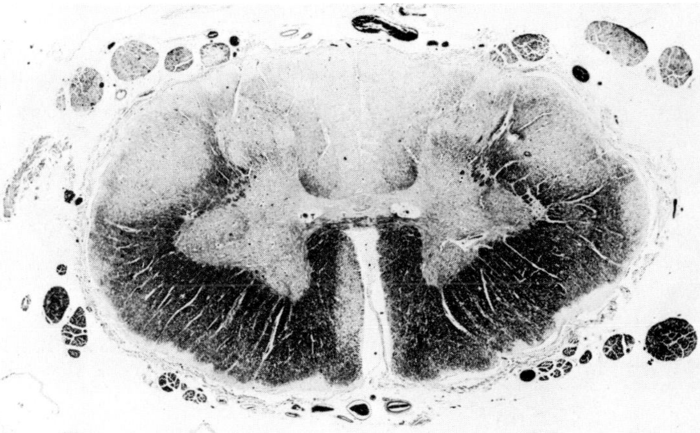

Fig. 15.19 Friedreich's ataxia. Death age 31. Cervical cord, showing pallor of posterior roots, posterior columns (gracile more than cuneate), crossed and uncrossed pyramidal tracts and anterior and posterior spinocerebellar tracts.

cephalic homologue of the thoracic nuclei), which showed cell loss and cell shrinkage in all 15 cases. Only five showed cell loss from the inferior olives, and in these cases there was reason to attribute the loss to circulatory disturbances. The pontine nuclei and middle cerebellar peduncles were never affected. The cerebellar cortex was normal apart from vascular lesions, which were not uncommon. The cerebellar white matter was always gliotic (presumably from degeneration of afferent fibres) but not obviously shrunken. The dentate nuclei showed cell loss, often severe, in 13/15 cases. This was reflected in a degeneration of the superior cerebellar peduncles, usually more marked in their ventral parts (Fig. 15.20). Cell loss and gliosis were also seen in the vestibular system (especially the medial vestibular nuclei) and in the auditory system (cochlear nuclei and superior olive) in over half the cases. The medial longitudinal bundles were not affected.

Loss of nerve fibres from the optic tracts was seen in about half the cases, and when severe was accompanied by cell loss from the lateral geniculate bodies (regarding the retinal changes occurring in Friedreich's ataxia, and their clinical manifestations, see André-van Leeuwen and van Bogaert, 1949). In the basal nuclei, there was cell loss in the external segment of the globus pallidus and subthalamic nucleus in about half the cases. The cerebral cortex, striatum, thalamus and substantia nigra were unaffected, apart from vascular lesions.

It is clear from this account that several lesions contribute to the dominant clinical feature of the disease—ataxia. They include lesions of sensory nerves, of various cerebellar afferents, and of the cerebellar outflow from the dentate nuclei. The most disabling of these is probably the first, which gives rise to the clinical resemblance, already mentioned, between Friedreich's ataxia and tabes dorsalis.

Heart

In most cases the heart is enlarged, and there are some pericardial adhesions. Microscopical examinations by a number of observers from Friedreich to Russell (1946) and Hewer (1969) have shown interstitial myocarditis, with necrosis or granular degeneration of some fibres and hypertrophy of others. This may be associated with diffuse or focal cellular infiltrations. Valvular lesions of congenital or acquired type are much less common. Intracardial thrombosis has repeatedly been observed at necropsy. Cerebral complications of the heart disease are not uncommon, and take the form either of diffuse

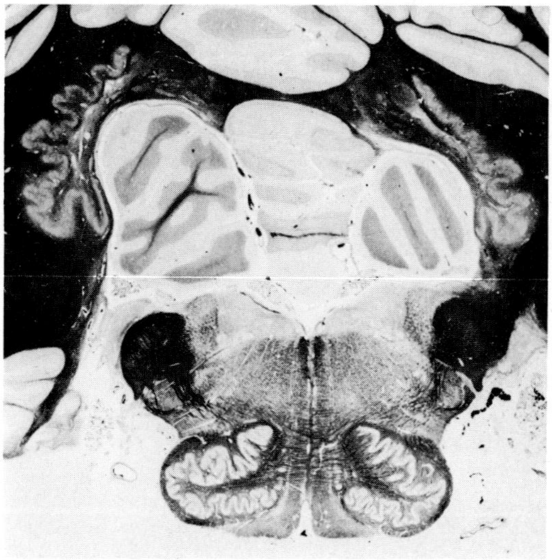

(a)

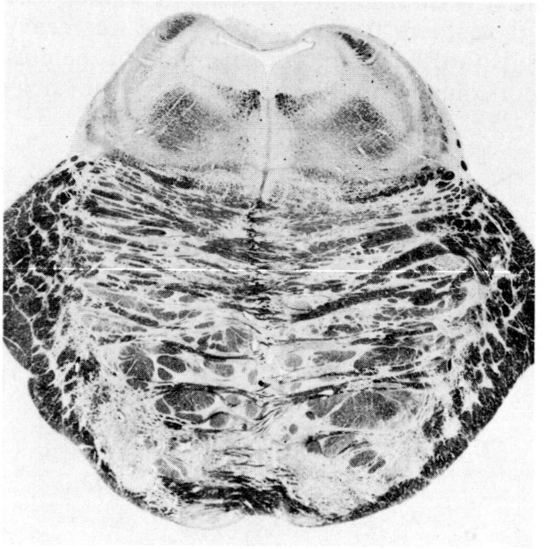

(b)

Fig. 15.20 Friedreich's ataxia. (**a**) Myelin stain, showing pallor of pyramids, solitary tracts, and hila of dentate nuclei. There is shrinkage of the pyramids and medial lemnisci. (**b**) Myelin stain, showing degeneration of the superior cerebellar peduncles in the upper pons.

hypoxic damage or of focal infarcts, presumably due to emboli from mural thrombi within the heart.

In recent years there has been an intensive study of Friedreich's ataxia in the Quebec province of Canada. Biochemical studies have been in the forefront. For details of these, see Barbeau (1982a, b).

A condition resembling Friedreich's ataxia in showing severe degeneration of the dentate nuclei was described by Hunt (1921) under the title of *dyssynergia cerebellaris myoclonica*, and is more euphoniously referred to as the Ramsay Hunt syndrome. This condition, and its claim to be considered as a separate disease, is discussed by Gilbert (1975). At the present time, it seems unwise to relate any particular disorder of posture or of movement to a lesion in any single structure such as the dentate nucleus. Degeneration of this nucleus usually occurs as part of a multisystem atrophy such as Friedreich's ataxia, pallidoluysian degeneration or progressive supranuclear palsy. Isolated dentate atrophy, if it occurs at all, is very rare.

Other forms of progressive ataxia

There have been numerous accounts of cases, both sporadic and familial, of progressive ataxia in which the most conspicuous lesions are in the long tracts of the spinal cord. Many of these give the impression of being incomplete manifestations of Friedreich's ataxia (Fig. 15.21). In these the disease tends to be milder, and the onset is at a later age than in Friedreich's ataxia, especially in cases with dominant inheritance (Bell and Carmichael, 1939). In several families (Biemond, 1928; Spillane, 1940), some siblings show the signs of Friedreich's ataxia and others those of peroneal atrophy. In other families, pes cavus, ataxia of gait and absence of knee and ankle jerks are combined in some members with atrophy of muscles below the knee and in the hands and forearms. This syndrome was described by Roussy and Lévy in 1926. A long list of similar 'unclassified' diseases could be compiled from published case reports. In the present state of knowledge it would be idle to invent a new name for each of these. Schut (1950) and others have pointed out the great variability, both clinical and anatomical, of these conditions within a single family, where presumably a single aberrant gene is responsible. Clinical and pathological accounts of a number of variations on the pontocerebellar and spinocerebellar themes are given by Eadie (1975a, b). Involvement of the optic, cochlear and vestibular pathways in various types of hereditary ataxia is discussed by van Bogaert and Martin (1974).

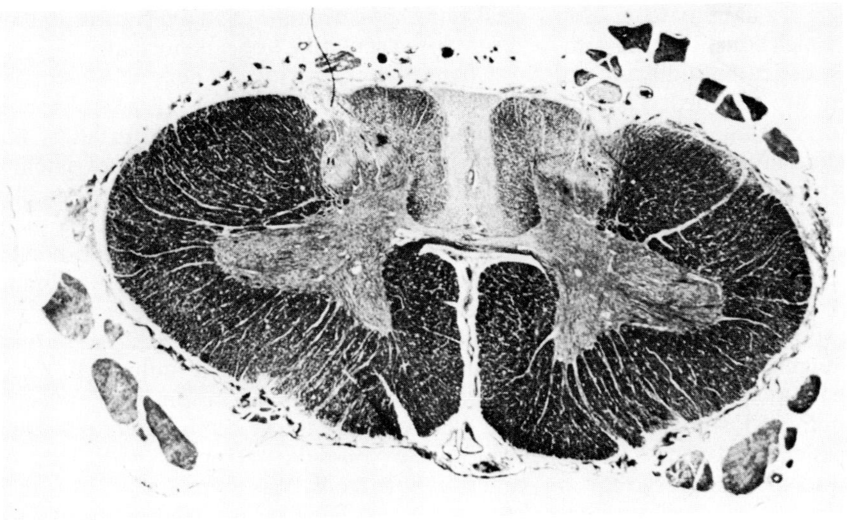

Fig. 15.21 Cervical cord from a sporadic case of progressive ataxia, with onset at age 14, death at age 40. Wassermann negative. Severe degeneration of posterior roots and posterior columns. Cerebellum, and its connections, unaffected. Myelin stain.

Ataxia-telangiectasia (Louis-Bar syndrome)

This familial disease of children, characterized by a progressive cerebellar ataxia, with symmetrical telangiectases of skin and conjunctiva, was described by Syllaba and Henner in 1926 and by Louis-Bar in 1941. Boder and Sedgwick (1958) described eight cases, one with necropsy, and named the condition *ataxia-telangiectasia*. Since that time many cases have been recorded, and much has been discovered about the clinical pathology of the condition. Sedgwick and Boder (1972) list 445 case reports up to that date, including 40 with necropsy. The condition is sometimes classified, along with von Recklinghausen's disease, Bournville's disease and the von Hippel-Lindau syndrome, as a *phacomatosis*.

Clinical features The incidence of the condition is suggestive of autosomal recessive inheritance (Sedgwick and Boder, 1972; Koch, 1972). In a typical case, the child appears normal at birth. The first signs of ataxia appear in infancy and progress steadily; the child learns to walk and talk, but by the second decade of life is chairfast and grossly dysarthric. Ataxia is often combined with involuntary movements of choreic or athetotic type. Most cases also show progressive abnormalities of eye movements. The appearance of telangiectases, in the conjunctivae and elsewhere, follows the onset of ataxia by a few years. From the beginning there is a liability to develop respiratory infections, which constitute the commonest immediate cause of death. Bodily growth and sexual development are retarded. The skin and hair show premature ageing. Mental deterioration sometimes occurs in the later stages of the disease. There is a strong tendency to develop malignant disease—most frequently a malignant lymphoma—this being the second commonest cause of death. Few patients survive into the third decade.

Laboratory investigations reveal abnormalities which serve to distinguish this disease from other causes of progressive ataxia, such as Friedreich's ataxia. Immunological studies, originally prompted by the patients' proneness to respiratory infections, led to the discovery that in ataxia-telangiectasia there is a consistent deficiency of IgA in serum and other body fluids, a defect of delayed hypersensitivity responses, aplasia or hypoplasia of the thymus and decreased blast cell transformation of lymphocytes cultured *in vitro* with phytohaemagglutinin (Peterson, Kelly and Good, 1964; Leikin, Bazelon and Park, 1966).

Pathological changes The *thymus* is absent, or rudimentary, without Hassall's corpuscles. *Lymphoid tissue* is reduced, with loss of lymphoid follicles, in tonsils, adenoids, lymph nodes and spleen; along with this, there is an apparent hyperplasia of reticulum cells. *Gonads* (particularly the ovaries) are hypoplastic. Other viscera are not abnormal, apart from the presence of scattered large cells with bizarre nuclei. Such cells have repeatedly been observed in the anterior lobe of the *pituitary*. The cutaneous and conjunctival *telangiectases* take the form of dilated, tortuous venules. The *lungs* show the expected changes due to chronic and recurrent infections.

In the *central nervous system*, the constant feature is atrophy of the cerebellar cortex, with extensive loss of Purkinje and granule cells (Fig. 15.22). Remaining Purkinje cells may show irregular dendritic expansions, and eosinophilic cytoplasmic inclusion bodies have been observed (Strich, 1966). In many cases (especially those of longer duration) there is degeneration in the posterior columns of the spinal cord, affecting the gracile more than the cuneate fasciculi. Apart from these features, there are no striking changes in the brain or cord. Abnormally dilated meningeal veins have been noted in a few cases, but as a rule the vasculature appears normal.

Changes in the peripheral nervous system are less well documented. Strich (1966) observed changes in posterior root ganglia in all of her three cases. These showed a paucity of satellite cells, and the ganglion cells appeared smaller than normal. Among the interstitial cells there were abnormal large cells with bizarre nuclei. Similar changes are reported by Amromin, Boder and Teplitz (1979) in a case with an unusually long survival, dying at age 32. Additional findings in this case included multiple tiny angiomatous vessels, with occlusion, haemorrhages and glial scarring, in the cerebral white matter. Neurogenic muscular atrophy, with loss of anterior horn cells, was observed, as in other reported cases. The liver was cirrhotic, and contained multiple telangiectases.

The condition has been exhaustively reviewed by Sedgwick and Boder (1972). These authors

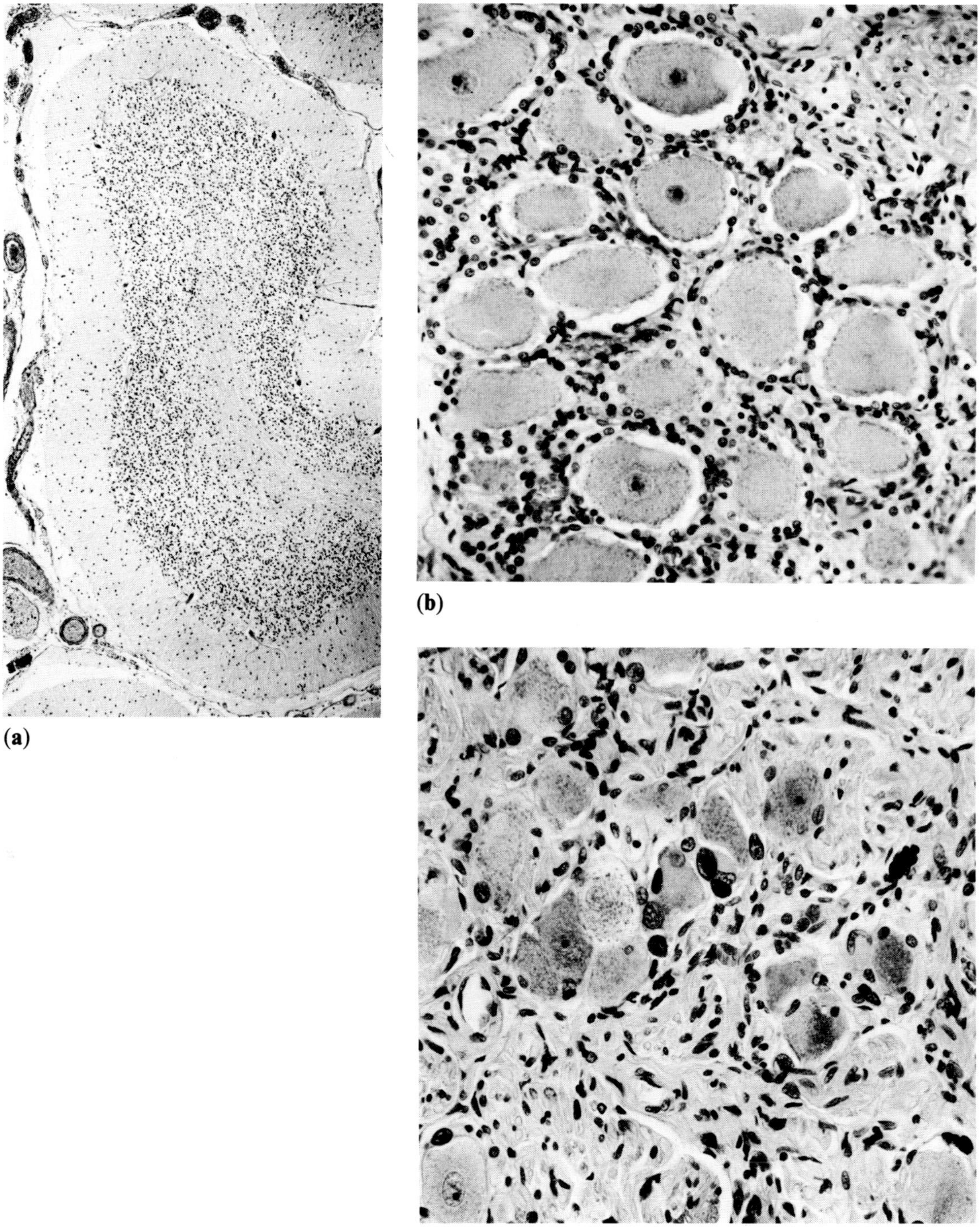

(a)

(b)

(c)

Fig. 15.22 Ataxia-telangiectasia. (**a**) Cerebellar cortex, showing severe loss of both Purkinje and granule cells. H & E ×42. (Case 1 of Strich, 1966). (**b**) Normal posterior root ganglion with satellite cells. Haematoxylin and eosin ×200. (**c**) Posterior root ganglion from case 1 of Strich (1966), showing reduction of satellite cells and abnormal nuclei. Haematoxylin and eosin ×200. (Reproduced by courtesy of the Editor, *Journal of Neurology, Neurosurgery and Psychiatry*.)

consider that the disease is underdiagnosed and is probably commoner than Friedreich's ataxia. Its prevalence has probably been much increased by the use of antibiotics in controlling the recurrent respiratory infections. For more recent research, see Bridges and Harnden (1982).

Diseases of motor neurons and pyramidal tracts

Selective destruction of lower motor neurons occurs in a variety of inflammatory and degenerative conditions. The best known of these are *acute anterior poliomyelitis*, which is described in Chapter 7, the various forms of *motor neuron disease*, and *Werdnig–Hoffmann disease*. Motor cells may also be lost in a number of multisystem degenerations, such as *pontocerebellar atrophy*; in *peroneal muscular atrophy* (see Chapter 18), which is generally regarded as a primary neuropathy, with 'dying-back' of motor root fibres; and in chronic (especially syphilitic) radiculopathies, which are discussed in Chapter 6.

It is doubtful whether a pure degeneration of the pyramidal tracts (the 'primary lateral sclerosis' of some authors) ever occurs. Severe pyramidal tract degeneration, without motor cell loss, is characteristic of *Friedreich's ataxia*. Concomitant pyramidal and motor cell lesions are typical of *motor neuron disease*, and of the amyotrophic form of *Jakob–Creutzfeldt disease*, in which the histology of the spinal cord may be indistinguishable from that of classic motor neuron disease. The simultaneous involvement of upper and lower motor neurons in these conditions strongly suggests a 'linked' degeneration; but the process can hardly be one of simple trans-synaptic degeneration, either anterograde or retrograde. Motor cells are not known to disappear in cases of long-standing cord transection, hemiplegia or Friedreich's ataxia; nor do the pyramidal tracts atrophy following an attack of poliomyelitis.

This section is concerned only with changes observed in the central nervous system. The changes in muscle resulting from denervation are described in Chapter 21.

Motor neuron disease (Progressive muscular atrophy; progressive bulbar palsy; amyotrophic lateral sclerosis)

The term *progressive muscular atrophy* was introduced by Aran (1850) and his teacher Duchenne (1853), who described a series of cases of progressive muscular weakness and wasting in middle-aged patients. They did not suspect damage to the nervous system. In 1860 Duchenne also described the syndrome which later became known as *progressive bulbar palsy*. In his paper of 1853 Duchenne mentioned the observation, made by Cruveilhier on one of his patients, of relative atrophy of the anterior spinal roots, but the involvement of the central nervous sytem in progressive muscular atrophy was first demonstrated in 1869 by Charcot and Joffroy, and in progressive bulbar palsy by Charcot (1870). The discovery of pyramidal tract lesions in cases of progressive muscular atrophy led Charcot (1874) to introduce the term *amyotrophic lateral sclerosis*.

During the next 30 years there were numerous neuropathological studies on such cases. Kojewnikow (1885) was able to trace pyramidal tract degeneration upwards through the brain stem and internal capsules to the cerebral cortex, and Probst (1898, 1903), using the Marchi technique, demonstrated a widespread but systematic fibre degeneration in the cerebral hemispheres, including parts of the corpus callosum. Dejerine (1883) put forward the view—hotly debated for many years but now generally accepted by both clinicians and pathologists—that progressive muscular atrophy, progressive bulbar palsy and amyotrophic lateral sclerosis are one and the same condition, with variations in the local distribution and relative severity of the lesions in grey matter and white. Since there is still no precise diagnostic marker for the condition, it is impossible to be sure whether these are in fact variants of a single disease. An idea of the range of variation can be gained from a number of recent accounts of series of cases with histological examination of the central nervous system by Lawyer and Netsky (1953; 53 cases), Brownell, Oppenheimer and Hughes (1970: 45 cases) and Castaigne et al. (1972: 61 cases). On the whole, the findings are similar from series to series; however, there appear to be regional differences—for instance in the sex incidence, which is said to be approximately equal in the British and French series, while in American series two or even three males are affected for every one female. Other variables—possibly due to selection errors—are the mean age of onset and the frequency of involvement of the pyramidal tracts. The clinical and pathological aspects of the condition have been reviewed by Colmant (1958a, c; 1975) and by Bonduelle (1975). As to nomenclature, the condition is generally called *motor neuron disease* in Britain, and *amyotrophic lateral sclerosis* in other countries.

Clinical features The disease occurs in all parts of the world. In general, it is not familial. In most series males are affected about 1.7 times as often as females. It is a disease of middle-aged and elderly people, rare before the age of 35, with a rapidly rising incidence rate in the fifth and later decades. The presenting symptom is weakness, often accompanied by pain, in one or two limbs, or in the bulbar musculature. The weakness progresses, involving more and more of the body, and though in the early stages it may be one-sided, it tends to become symmetrical. The external ocular muscles are not affected. Sensation is intact, and there is no sign of involvement of the cerebellar system. Physical signs include muscular wasting and fasciculation, with a very variable admixture of upper motor neuron signs. The cerebrospinal fluid is usually normal. The average duration from the first symptom till death is 2 or 3 years, but cases with a duration of 5 or more years are not uncommon and a benign, very chronic form was described by Pearce and Harriman (1966). The cause of death in most cases is respiratory failure, often with a terminal aspiration pneumonia.

Pathological changes To the naked eye, the most striking changes are in the affected muscles, which are pale and shrunken, and in the anterior spinal nerve roots (Fig. 15.23). In some cases there is selective atrophy of the precentral gyri

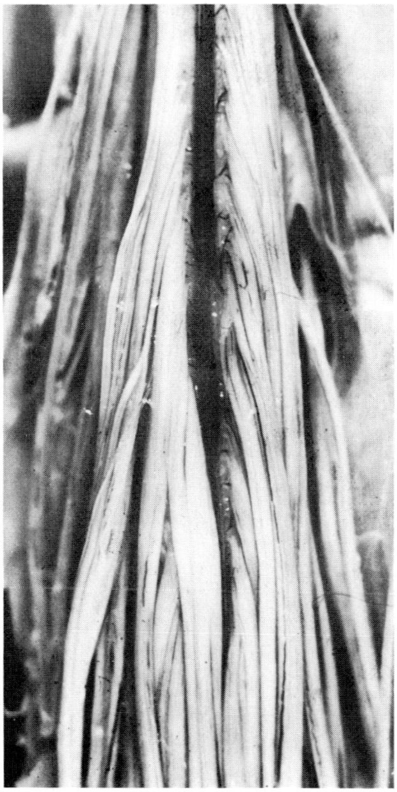

(a)

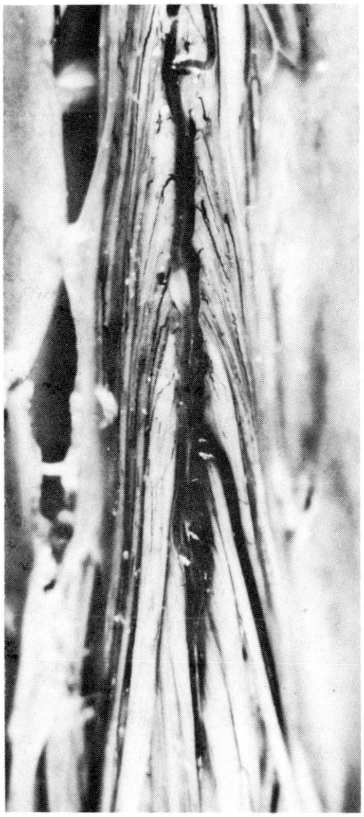

(b)

Fig. 15.23 Motor neuron disease. (**a**) Normal subject. (**b**) Atrophy of anterior roots in lumbosacral region.

(see Colmant 1958c), which becomes more apparent after stripping off the leptomeninges.

The essential histological change is a loss of large motor cells, with resulting gliosis (Figs. 15.24 and 15.25). This is most easily observed in the anterior horns of the lumbar and cervical enlargements and in the hypoglossal nuclei. Remaining motor neurons are commonly shrunken and pyknotic; but this change may be hard to distinguish from *post mortem* shrinkage. Large,

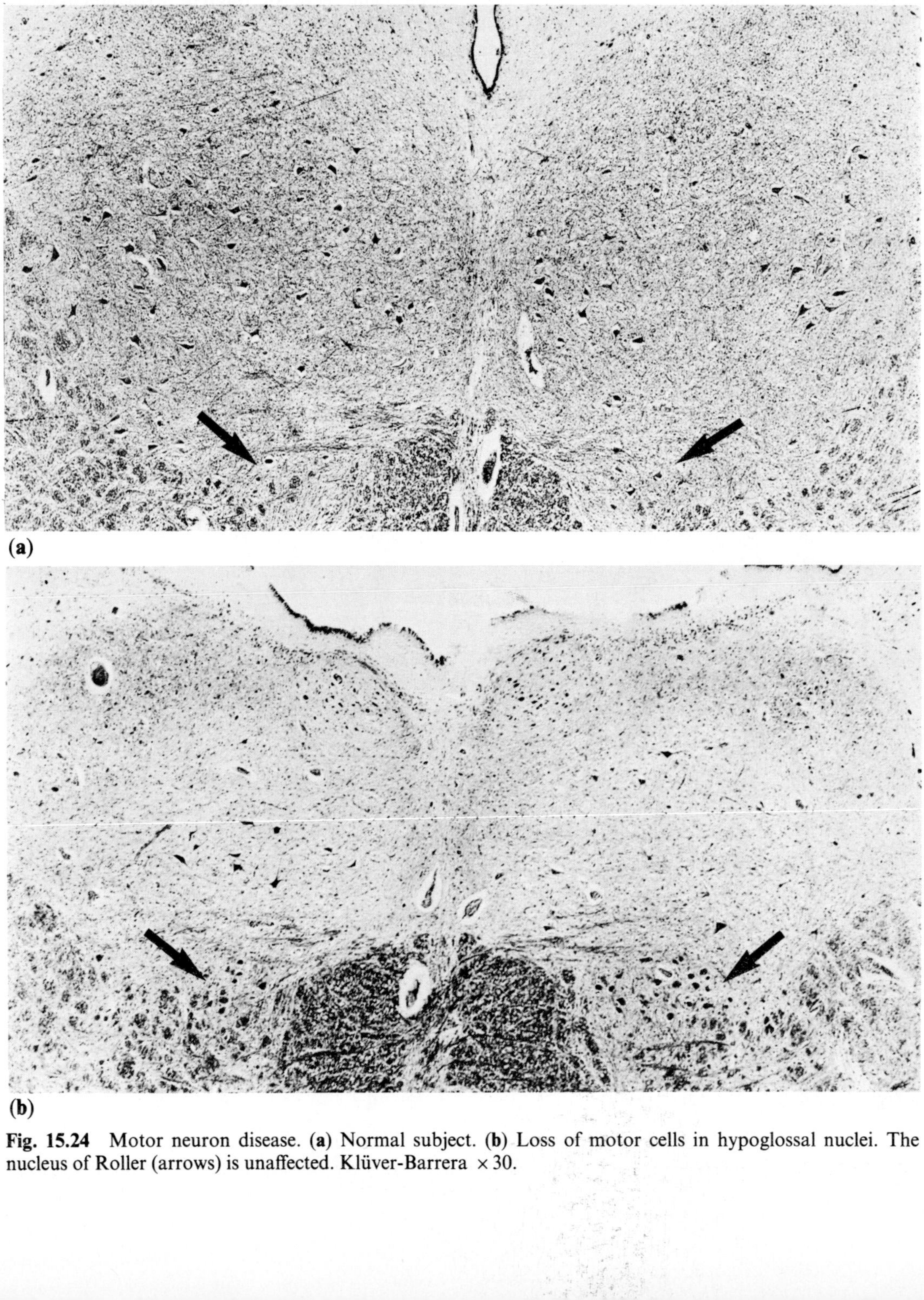

(a)

(b)

Fig. 15.24 Motor neuron disease. (**a**) Normal subject. (**b**) Loss of motor cells in hypoglossal nuclei. The nucleus of Roller (arrows) is unaffected. Klüver-Barrera ×30.

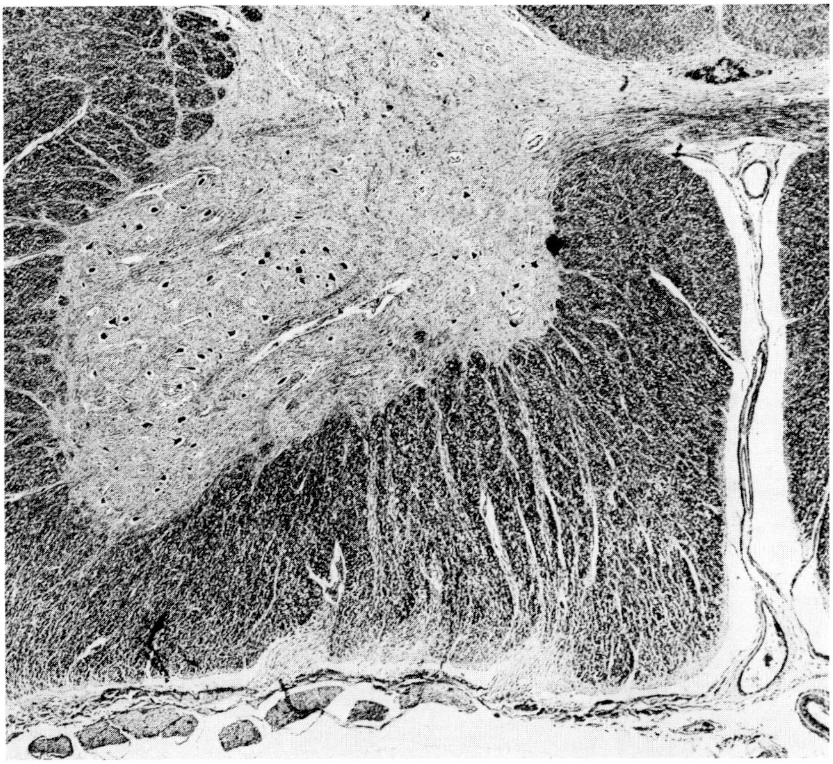

(a)

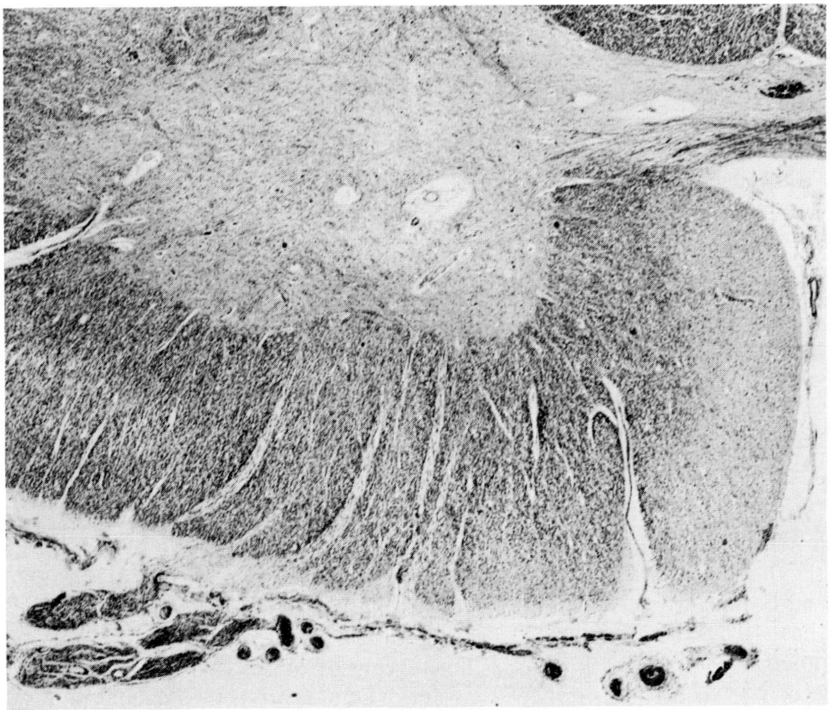

(b)

Fig. 15.25 Motor neuron disease. (**a**) Normal subject. (**b**) Loss of motor cells in anterior horn of sixth cervical segment. Klüver-Barrera ×25. In (**b**), the direct corticospinal tract shows loss of myelin.

pale 'ghost' cells may be present, but typical central chromatolysis is rarely seen. Figures of neuronophagia are often present, especially in cases running a rapid course (Fig. 15.26). In the motor nuclei of the facial and trigeminal nerves, and in the nuclei ambigui, it is often easier to find such changes than to demonstrate an actual loss of cells. The nuclei of the oculomotor, trochlear and abducent nerves are rarely if ever affected.

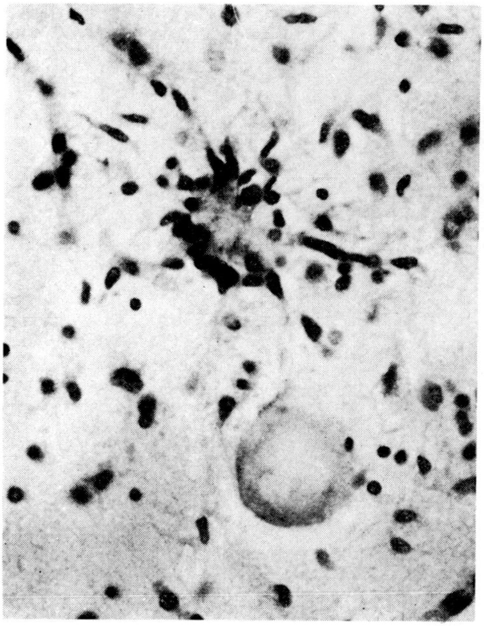

Fig. 15.26 Motor neuron disease. Neuronophagia and 'ghost' cell in anterior horn. Nissl ×345. (Case 2 of Brownell, Oppenheimer and Hughes, 1970). (Reproduced by courtesy of the Editor, *Journal of Neurology Neurosurgery and Psychiatry*).

Changes in the white matter of the spinal cord are variable. The commonest is a degeneration (sometimes asymmetrical) of the pyramidal tracts. When this is severe it can be traced upwards into the white matter of the cerebral hemispheres (Fig. 15.27). In other cases it may be undetectable above the medulla, or even the cervical cord (Davison, 1941). In a series of 45 necropsied cases Brownell *et al.* (1970) found degeneration extending into the hemispheres in under half: and in 10 cases they were unable to observe pyramidal degeneration at any level (it is worth remarking that these 10 cases, clinically and pathologically diagnosed as suffering from motor neuron disease, would be excluded by definition from the diagnosis of amyotrophic lateral sclerosis).

At higher levels, the degenerate tracts occupy the middle thirds of the crura of the cerebral peduncles. Above that, they form discrete bundles in the posterior part of the posterior limbs of the internal capsules (Bertrand and van Bogaert, 1925; Smith, 1960; Brownell *et al.*, 1970)—i.e. well behind the position usually assigned to the pyramidal tracts in textbooks of anatomy. Above this they fan out widely towards their origins in the precentral and postcentral gyri and beyond. There is also a discrete bundle of degenerate fibres running across the middle of the corpus callosum (Fig. 15.28). Loss of pyramidal cells from the pre- and postcentral gyri may be severe enough to be obvious without formal cell counts. Loss of the giant pyramidal cells of Betz from the precentral gyrus is often apparent, but may be due to shrinkage, rather than to disappearance, of these cells. Cell loss and astrocytic gliosis have been reported in other parts of the brain, in particular the basal ganglia and thalamus; as with Parkinson's disease, however, the significance of these changes in the brains of elderly subjects is doubtful.

In the spinal white matter, in addition to degeneration of the crossed and uncrossed pyramidal tracts, there is often a diffuse loss of stainable myelin in the anterior and lateral columns, with intact posterior columns (Fig. 15.29). Whether this is due to demyelination or to degeneration of axons is not known. In Marchi preparations, where the pyramidal tracts are clearly marked by degeneration products, these are rarely seen in the remainder of the anterior and lateral columns, and loss of axons is not detectable in silver impregnations. Degeneration of the dorsal spinocerebellar tracts, with loss of cells from the thoracic nuclei, has been described, but appears to be rare (Brownell *et al.* 1970). Loss of myelin in a narrow subpial zone is a common finding in elderly subjects, and may on occasion have been mistaken for specific tract degeneration. On the other hand, an average of 36 per cent cell loss in Clarke's (thoracic) nucleus has been reported in 12 cases of motor neuron disease by Averback and Crocker (1982).

The absence of sensory changes is a cardinal point in the clinical diagnosis of motor neuron disease, and routine histological examination does not reveal obvious changes in sensory ganglia, posterior spinal roots or posterior columns. Recently, however, systematic counting has shown some loss of both motor and sensory cells

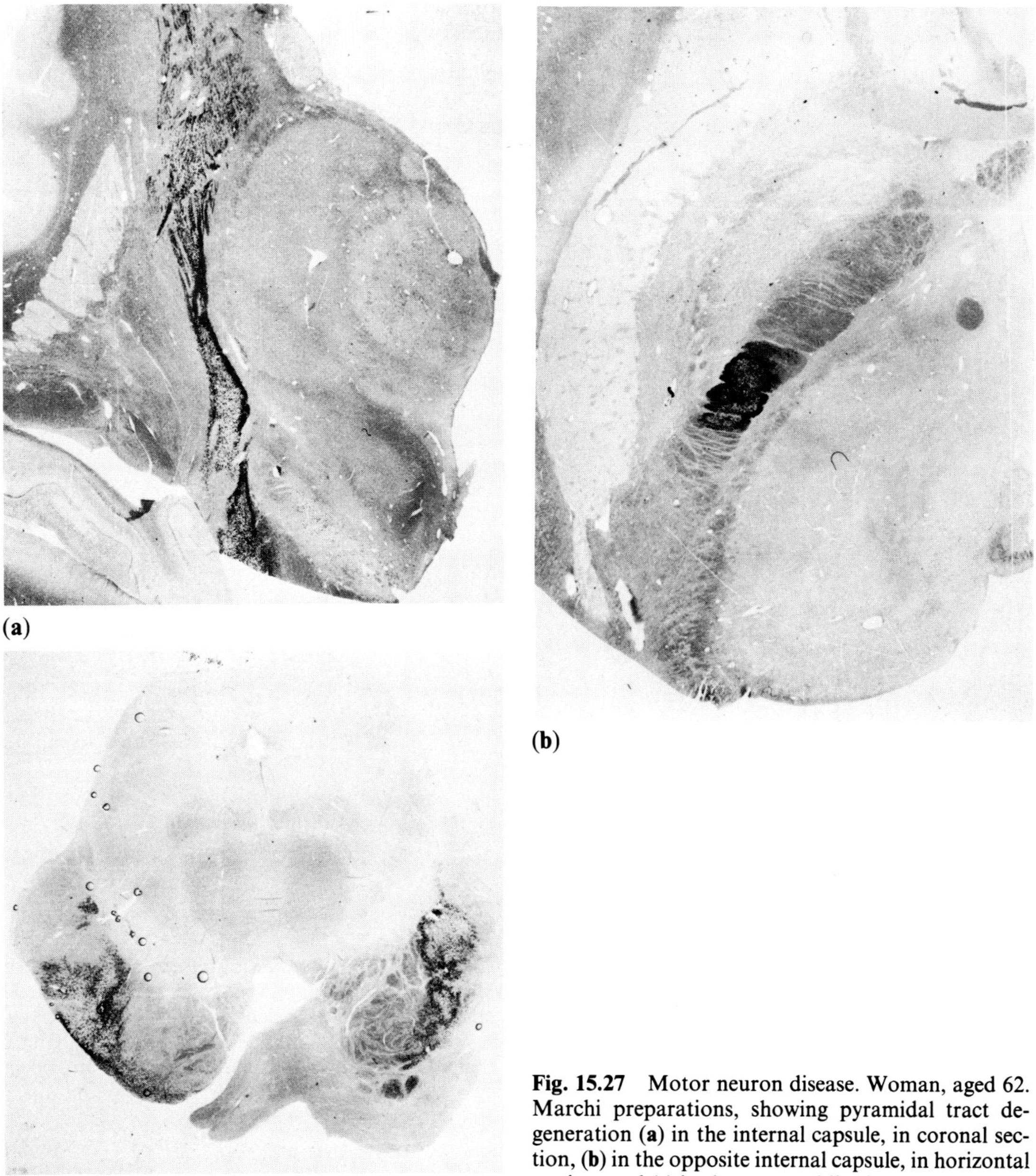

(a)

(b)

(c)

Fig. 15.27 Motor neuron disease. Woman, aged 62. Marchi preparations, showing pyramidal tract degeneration (**a**) in the internal capsule, in coronal section, (**b**) in the opposite internal capsule, in horizontal section, and (**c**) in the upper midbrain.

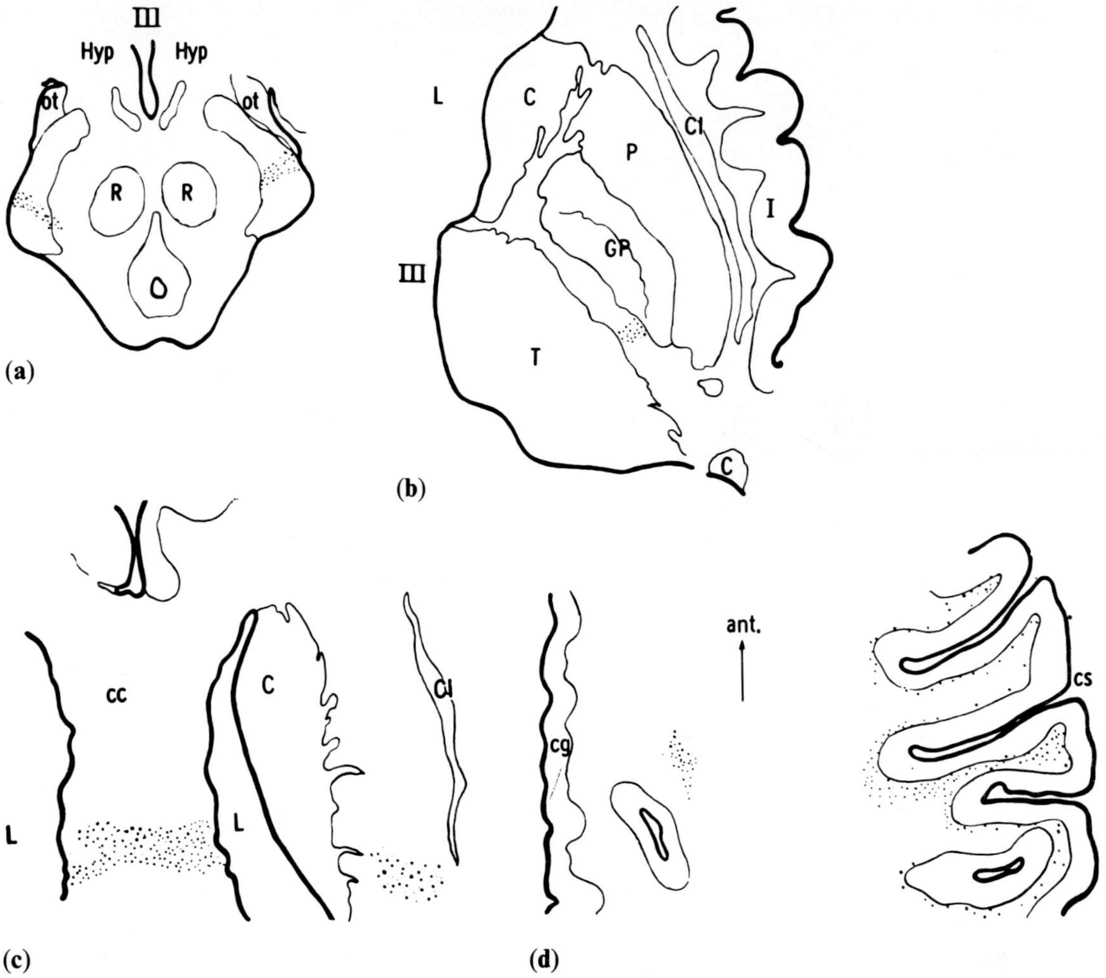

Fig. 15.28 Motor neuron disease. Camera lucida tracings from Marchi preparations of horizontal sections of (**a**) upper midbrain, (**b**) basal nuclei, (**c**) centrum ovale and corpus callosum, and (**d**) superior frontoparietal region. The stippled areas indicate positive Marchi degeneration. C, caudate nucleus; cc, corpus callosum; cg, cingulate gyrus; Cl, claustrum; cs, central sulcus, GP, globus pallidus; Hyp, hypothalamus; I, insula; L, lateral ventricle; ot, optic tract; P, putamen; R, red nucleus; T, thalamus; III, third ventricle. (Case 18 of Brownell, Oppenheimer and Hughes, 1970.) (Reproduced by courtesy of the Editor, *Journal of Neurology, Neurosurgery and Psychiatry*.)

and axons in cases of 'classic' motor neuron disease (Kawamura et al., 1981).

Problems of classification The search for genetic, metabolic and environmental causes for motor neuron disease has so far yielded nothing substantial. Cases in which some degree of dementia is present, or in which status spongiosus is observed in parts of the cerebral cortex, have suggested a relationship with Jakob–Creutzfeldt disease (Meyer, 1929; Brownell *et al.*, 1970); but repeated attempts to transmit the disease to experimental animals have been unsuccessful. Instances in which there is reason to suspect that a progressive atrophy of motor cells is caused by a virus, 'slow', latent or otherwise, are discussed below. The epidemiology of the disease is discussed by Kurtzke (1969) and Kurland (1977).

Motor neuron disease, if it is a single entity, is a very variable one. In the series of Brownell *et*

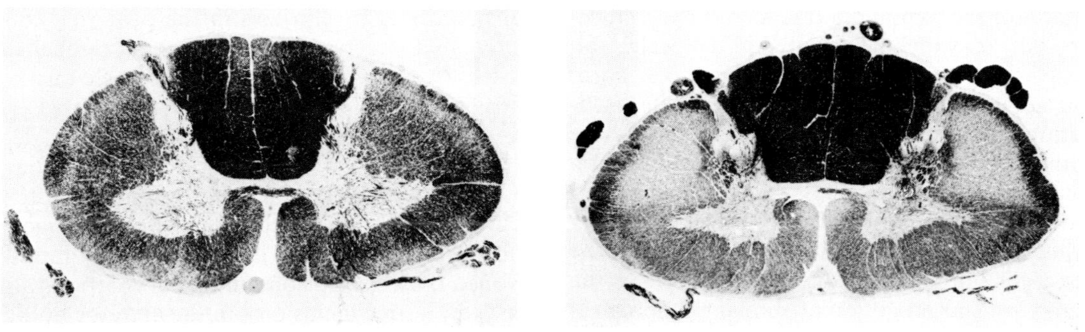

(a) (b)

Fig. 15.29 Motor neuron disease. Sections from the cervical enlargement. (**a**) Myelin stain from a case with 9 months' history of bulbar palsy. No abnormal physical signs in the arms or legs. (**b**) Myelin stain from a typical case with wasting of the small hand muscles and spastic paraplegia.

al. there were two cases in which muscular wasting progressed over 10 years. Post-mortem examination showed an almost total loss of motor cells from the anterior horns and hypoglossal nuclei; the pyramidal tracts were intact, and there were no other lesions in the central nervous system. In contrast, there were three cases of progressive spastic paraparesis, with death after 16, 22 and 30 months of illness. In these, motor cell loss was slight, but there was very heavy pyramidal tract degeneration, and intense gliosis in thalamus and basal ganglia. In the present state of knowledge it is impossible to decide whether these represent the extreme ends of a spectrum or two different diseases.

In addition to the acute destruction of motor cells in poliomyelitis, it has often been suspected that these cells may be progressively attacked by a 'slow' or latent infection. Zilkha (1962) presented figures showing a very high incidence of a past history of acute poliomyelitis in patients with motor neuron disease. Greenfield and Matthews (1954) and others have described cases of postencephalitic parkinsonism, later developing a progressive amyotrophy, with loss of motor cells. A number of authors (Brain, Croft and Wilkinson, 1965; Norris and Engel, 1965; Norris, McMenemey and Barnard, 1969) have maintained that there is an association, beyond what would be expected by chance, between a form of motor neuron disease and malignant disease. Here, too, the suggestion has been made of an 'opportunistic' virus infection. The evidence for the association of malignancy and motor cell disease in humans is hard to assess. An experimental approach to the subject was made by Klüver and Weil (1948), who, having observed loss and vacuolation of motor cells in a monkey with a carcinoma of the tongue, implanted carcinoma cells into the tongue of another monkey; the tumour grew apace, and the recipient subsequently showed a disease of the motor cells similar to that of the donor.

A possible association between motor neuron disease and pancreatic malfunction has been discussed by Quick (1969). Various toxic and metabolic conditions affecting motor cells and long tracts are dealt with in Chapter 14. Spontaneous diseases of motor neurons in other mammals have been reviewed by Andrews and Maxwell (1969).

Motor neuron disease in Guam

Following earlier reports of a high incidence of motor neuron disease in the island of Guam, Kurland and Mulder (1954) made a detailed epidemiological survey, which showed that among the Chamorro population (but not among other inhabitants of the island) the disease was at least 50 times commoner than in most parts of the world, and accounted for 8–10 per cent of adult deaths. Males were affected nearly twice as often as females. Dominant inheritance was suspected, but it is still uncertain whether genetic or environmental and cultural factors are the main cause. The pathology in 22 of these cases was described by Malamud, Hirano and Kurland in 1961. The consistent findings were loss of motor cells from the cervical and lumbar enlargements and hypoglossal nuclei, degeneration (usually severe) of the pyramidal tracts, and neurofibrillary tangles, widely distributed in the brain, and occasionally in motor cells of the spinal cord. The appearance of these tangles and their distribution corresponded closely with the same authors' findings in the parkinsonism–dementia complex of Guam (p. 707); and they concluded that the two conditions were different expressions of the same disease. An indication that the disease is not confined to the Chamorros is the report by Shiraki (1969) of similar pathological findings in patients from the Kii peninsula, in Japan, where the incidence of motor neuron disease is abnormally high. The subject is reviewed by Kurland and Brody (1975).

Other conditions affecting motor neurons

The separation of a degenerative motor neuropathy, with 'dying-back' of axons, from a primary degeneration of motor cells is somewhat artificial. In the case of *peroneal muscular atrophy* (Charcot–Marie–Tooth disease: see Chapter 18) the pathological changes in the motor cells of the spinal cord are indistinguishable from those in various conditions described above (Hughes and Brownell, 1972), and the concomitant degeneration of sensory ganglion cells and their processes resembles that found in Friedreich's ataxia (Hughes, Brownell and Hewer, 1968). The distinction appears even more unreal in view of reports of families in which some members show the clinical features of Friedreich's ataxia and others those of peroneal atrophy (p. 723).

Familial forms of motor neuron disease

There have been numerous reports (see Colmant 1958c; Bonduelle, 1975) of motor neuron disease occurring in several members of a family, with an apparently autosomal dominant inheritance. According to Kurland and Mulder (1954) such cases probably account for 5–10 per cent of all cases dying of motor neuron disease in the USA. Clinically, and in most instances pathologically, these cases are indistinguishable from the more usual sporadic cases. In 1959, however, Engel, Kurland and Klatzo described two families in which clinically typical motor neuron disease occurred as an autosomal dominant; in three cases with necropsy they found, in addition to motor cell loss and pyramidal degeneration, symmetrical patches of myelin loss in the posterior columns, and degeneration in the spinocerebellar tracts, with loss of cells from the thoracic nuclei. In 1967, Hirano, Kurland and Sayre reported on five familial cases (three from the families described by Engel, Kurland and Klatzo). In four of these they observed similar lesions of motor neurons, pyramidal tracts, spinocerebellar tracts and posterior columns; in addition, they found swollen motor cells, containing concentric hyaline cytoplasmic inclusions, in the anterior horns and hypoglossal nuclei. Whether this constitutes a distinct disease, and whether it occurs sporadically, is at present uncertain.

External ophthalmoplegia

In the degenerative conditions hitherto mentioned, other than progressive supranuclear palsy, there is a striking, and unexplained, tendency for the external ocular muscles to be spared. An exception to this rule is a family described by Woods and Schaumburg (1975), in which there is a clinical picture of ataxia, dysarthria, gaze palsy, rigidity and weakness, with dominant inheritance. Two necropsies have been performed. These showed widespread neurogenic muscle atrophy, with loss of spinal, bulbar and oculomotor neurons, combined with degeneration of the thoracic nuclei, spinocerebellar tracts, vestibular and pontine nuclei, substantia nigra and dentate nuclei. Cerebral hemispheres and pyramidal tracts were unaffected. Apart from such rare instances of involvement of oculomotor nuclei in multisystem degenerations, there are scattered reports of cases of *progressive external ophthalmoplegia* occurring sometimes in apparent isolation, sometimes associated with a generalized myopathy, and sometimes with evidence of disease of the peripheral or central nervous system. Muscle biopsies have been suggestive of myopathy in some cases, of denervation in others. Few such cases have had full neuropathological studies, and in these the interpretation of the findings has been difficult. The subject has been reviewed by Colmant (1958b), Drachman (1975) and Rowland (1975).

Infantile spinal muscular atrophy of Werdnig and Hoffmann

Various conditions, some of which are still poorly understood, may give rise to congenital amyotonia (the 'floppy baby' syndrome). Of these the best known, the most rapidly lethal and probably the commonest is the disease described by Werdnig (1891, 1894) and Hoffmann (1893, 1900). Clinically, a progressive muscular weakness, sparing only the diaphragm and the muscles supplied by the upper brain stem, usually leads to death in a matter of months from respiratory failure, often hastened by aspiration pneumonia. The floppiness is often detectable at birth, and the mother may have noticed feebleness of fetal movements. In general, the earlier the onset, the more rapid the course. The disease is transmitted by simple autosomal recessive inheritance. For a detailed discussion, see the monograph by Brandt (1950) and the review by Dubowitz (1975).

Pathological changes The changes in skeletal muscle are those of progressive denervation, as described in Chapter 21. They are widespread and severe, but there is marked sparing of the diaphragm, the 'strap' muscles of the neck, the external ocular and masticator muscles. Those supplied by the lower cranial nerves are not spared (Byers and Banker, 1961).

On naked-eye examination there is atrophy of the anterior spinal roots. Microscopically, there is loss of motor cells from most levels of the spinal cord (Fig. 15.30), from the nuclei ambigui and from the hypoglossal and facial nuclei. Among the remaining motor cells there are frequent figures of neuronophagia and pale, swollen cells, resembling the 'ghost' cells seen in motor neuron disease. These are commonly described as showing central chromatolysis, but it may be doubted whether the change is a true axonal reaction. A further point of resemblance with adult motor neuron disease is that the cells of the so-called Onuf's nucleus in the sacral cord, as well as the autonomic efferents of the thoracolumbar and sacral outflows, are spared (Mannen et al., 1977; Iwata and Hirano, 1978; Sung and Mastri, 1980). Long tracts in the brain stem and spinal cord appear intact. Gruner and Bargeton (1952) reported, as a constant finding in nine otherwise typical cases, a symmetrical loss of nerve cells, with 'ghost' cells and neuronophagia, from the posteroventral nucleus of the thalamus—a finding confirmed in other reported cases in which the thalamus has been carefully examined (Fig. 15.31). Lesions elsewhere in the brain tend to be of a non-specific kind, attributable to cerebral hypoxia.

There appears to be no distinct upper age limit for this disease. Late infantile, juvenile and adolescent forms of spinal amyotrophy, with autosomal recessive inheritance, have been described by Wohlfart, Fex and Eliasson (1955), Kugelberg and Welander (1956), Gardner-Medwin, Hudgson and Walton (1967) and others. In general, the later the onset the slower the progression and the more favourable the prognosis. In the juvenile and adolescent forms the proximal limb muscles are often affected, bulbar muscles are spared, and the disease may be mistaken for a muscular dystrophy. The diagnosis of neurogenic atrophy depends on electromyography and muscle biopsy. Because of the benign course of the disease, there is a dearth of anatomical reports on the central nervous system in these cases. The same is true of the neurogenic muscular atrophies with dominant inheritance (discussed by Gardner-Medwin, Hudgson and Walton, 1967, and by Fenichel 1969), in which the clinical course is even slower.

The condition of *arthrogryposis multiplex congenita* (deformed and rigid joints, associated with muscular wasting) results, according to Drachman (1969) from paralysis of, or interference with, muscular activity in the fetus. The causes of this are various, and include primary muscle disorders (Banker, Victor and Adams, 1957); most commonly, there is a primary disease of the central nervous system, which may be a gross malformation (such as meningomyelocele), or merely a deficit of anterior horn cells. Drachman (1969) has listed 21 necropsy reports, in 14 of which loss of motor cells was observed. In all but three of these, which showed some pyramidal tract degeneration, this was the only lesion in the central nervous system. On this basis, it is thought that Werdnig–Hoffmann disease, with early onset, constitutes a major cause of congenital arthrogryposis.

A number of cases, clinically diagnosed as Werdnig–Hoffmann disease, have been reported as showing lesions far more widespread than those described above. For the most part, these have been regarded as 'atypical' cases of the disease. Steiman, Rorke and Brown (1980) have reviewed 14 such cases. All showed the clinical picture of Werdnig–Hoffmann disease, but were found to have, in addition to the expected loss of motor neurons, lesions of the thoracic (Clarke's

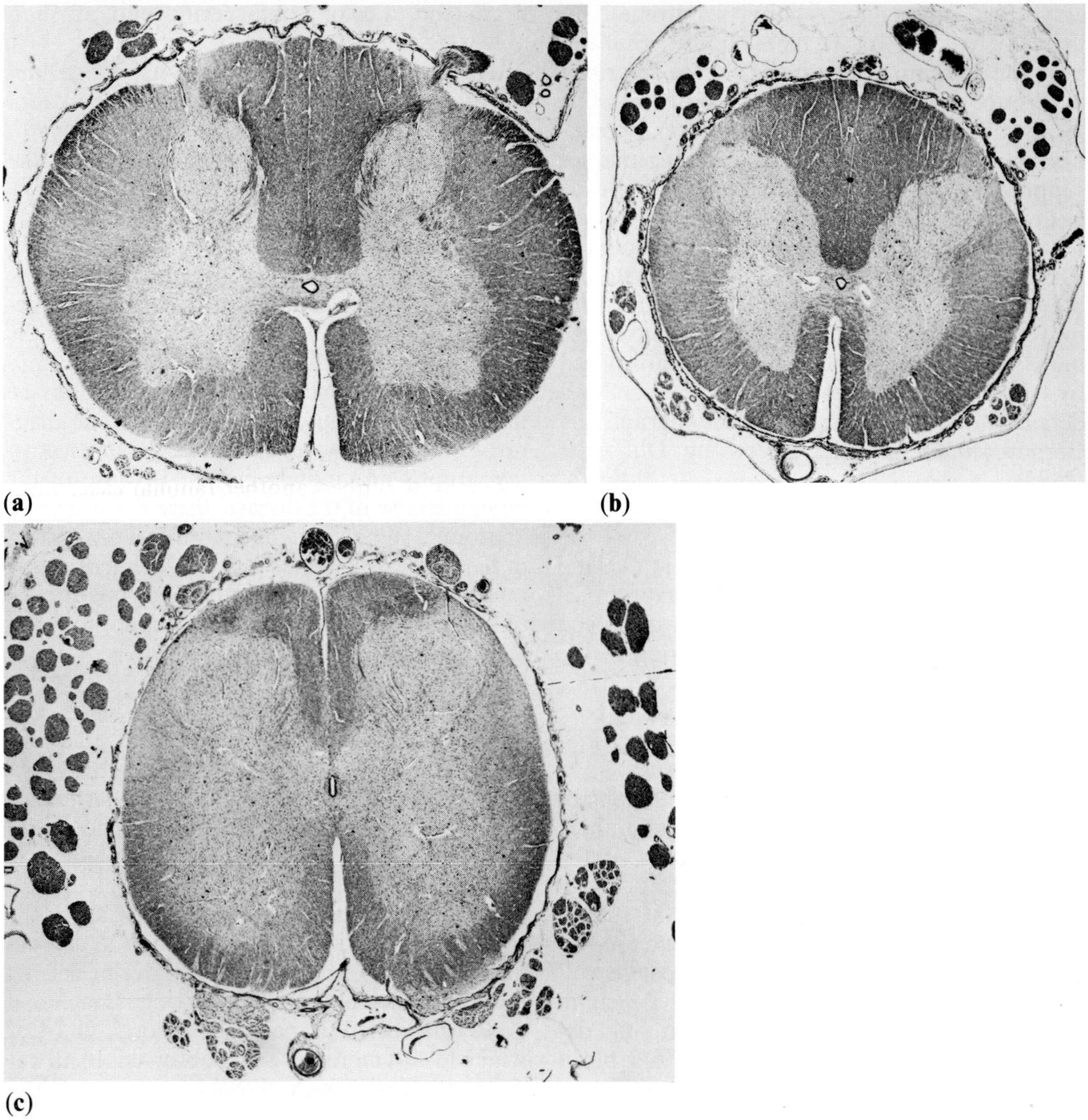

Fig. 15.30 Werdnig–Hoffmann disease. Three-month-old infant. Spinal cord: (**a**) cervical, (**b**) thoracic (note well-preserved cells in thoracic nuclei) and (**c**) sacral (note relative atrophy of anterior roots). There is a severe loss of motor cells at all levels. Klüver–Barrera. × 18.

column) nuclei, spinocerebellar and pyramidal tracts, posterior and lateral white columns, brain stem motor nuclei, olives, pontine nuclei, Purkinje cells, dentate nuclei, thalamus, basal ganglia, optic nerves and peripheral nerves, or a selection of these. Steiman, Rorke and Brown argue for the recognition of a disease, separate from Werdnig–Hoffmann disease, to which they give the title *infantile neuronal degeneration*.

There are at least two recognized diseases in which loss of motor cells affects principally the nuclei of the lower cranial nerves. Both are rare. In *Fazio–Londe disease* the onset of cranial nerve palsies is generally in early life; the clinical course is irregularly progressive, leading to death after intervals which have ranged from 9 months to over 8 years. Some cases are sporadic, others familial. In two cases with autopsy, loss of motor cells has been observed in the motor nuclei of cranial nerves III, IV, V, VI, VII, X, and XII (see Gomez, 1975; Alexander, Emery and Koerner, 1976). In the *Brown–Vialetto–van Laere syn-*

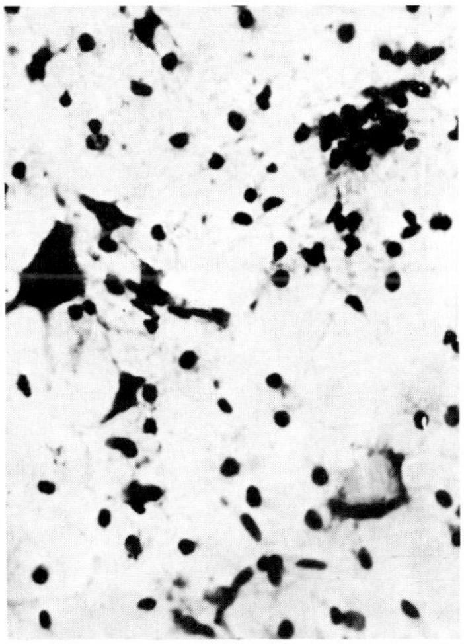

Fig. 15.31 Werdnig-Hoffmann disease. Thalamus, showing a degenerate nerve cell and a figure of neuronophagia. Carbol azure.

drome (pontobulbar palsy with deafness), the normal presenting symptom is a profound deafness, of abrupt onset, accompanied or followed by various cranial nerve palsies. The condition is often familial, with a pattern suggesting an autosomal recessive trait; but there is an unexplained 2:1 preponderance of females over males. The age of onset is most commonly in the second decade of life, but has varied between infancy and 31 years. Eighteen cases have been reported, with necropsy reports on four. The histological findings have been of cell loss in cranial nerve motor nuclei VII to XI, more rarely in the masticator and oculomotor nuclei and in the anterior horn cells; and of devastating fibre loss in the cochlear nerves, with heavy gliosis in the ventral cochlear nuclei. Affected muscles show the usual changes of denervation.

A peculiar feature of this condition is that the clinical course is often very irregular, with sudden dramatic episodes, and long periods in which progression appears to be arrested, though no true recovery occurs. This is in contrast with the relentless progression, whether rapid or slow, characteristic of motor neuron disease, Werdnig-Hoffmann disease and most of the other primary neuronal degenerations. In some cases there is a strong suspicion that episodes are provoked by intercurrent happenings, such as infectious fevers and pregnancies. For recent accounts, with reviews of the literature, see Gallai et al. (1981) and Brucher et al. (1981).

Familial spastic paraplegia

Strümpell (1880) described two brothers in whom spastic paraplegia, with very little involvement of the arms or face, developed in middle life. On post-mortem examination of the younger patient (1886) he found degeneration of the pyramidal tracts, beginning below their decussation and most definite in the lower thoracic and lumbar segments. Degeneration of the posterior columns was slight at the lumbar level but became more evident in the upper thoracic and cervical segments, in which the fasciculus gracilis was extensively, and the fasciculus cuneatus slightly, involved. Degeneration of the spinocerebellar tracts was also evident at these levels. In 1904 Strümpell described another familial case, with onset at 35, slow progression, and death at 69. The lesions in the cord were almost identical with those in the first case.

Since that time there have been many clinical, and a few pathological, reports on families affected with spastic weakness of the lower limbs. As in the case of familial ataxias, these families show a great variety of clinical syndromes, with various combinations of degenerative lesions; it is at present unprofitable to attempt to classify and name separate conditions. Within single families, there are wide variations in age of onset, severity of symptoms and associated disabilities. In some cases, spasticity and weakness are followed by loss of motor neurons and amyotrophy. In others (Bickerstaff 1950; van Bogaert 1952a) there is optic neuropathy, leading to blindness; and in a number of cases lesions of long motor tracts are combined with degeneration of parts of the cerebellar system. The subject has been reviewed by Schwarz (1952) and Schwarz and Liu (1956), and the genetic aspects discussed by van Bogaert (1952b). According to Schwarz (1952) the published reports constituted 'a hodgepodge of varied disorders of the nervous system, with paraparesis or paraplegia simply one of the occurrences in the illness, not the main or only factor'. Cases closely resembling those of Strümpell, with late onset, slow progression and degeneration practically confined to the long cord tracts, include the case of Schwarz and Liu (1956) and two cases reported by Behan and Maia (1974) (Figs. 15.32 and 15.33). Figure 15.32 is from an unpublished case of this type. Harding (1981) gives a clinical and genetic analysis of 22 families with 'pure' hereditary spastic paraple-

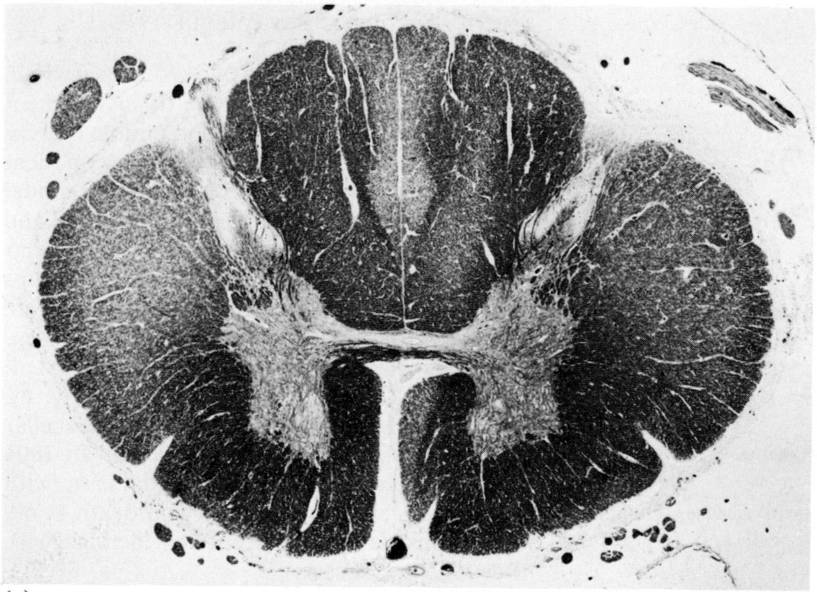

(a)

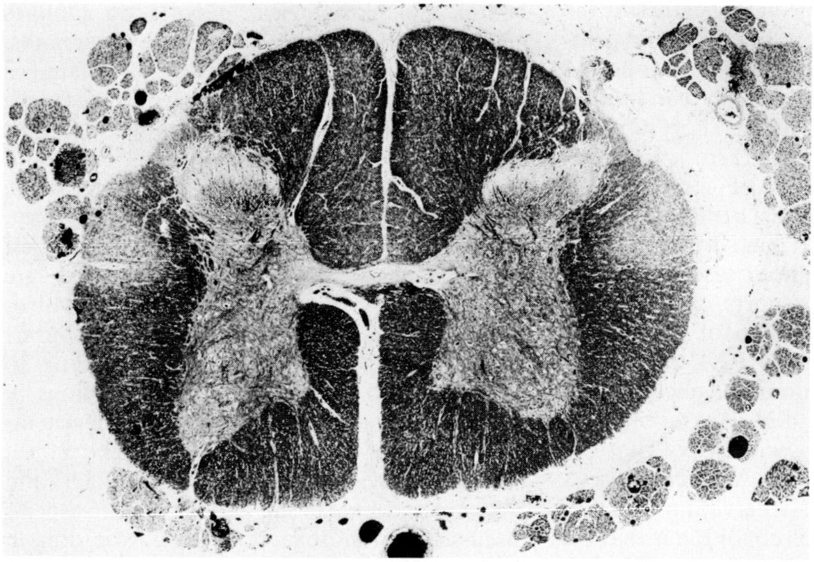

(b)

Fig. 15.32 Familial spastic paraplegia. Dominant inheritance. Early onset, death age 74. (**a**) Fourth cervical level. (**b**) Lower lumbar level. The posterior columns are more affected at the higher level, and the pyramidal tracts at the lower one. Myelin stain.

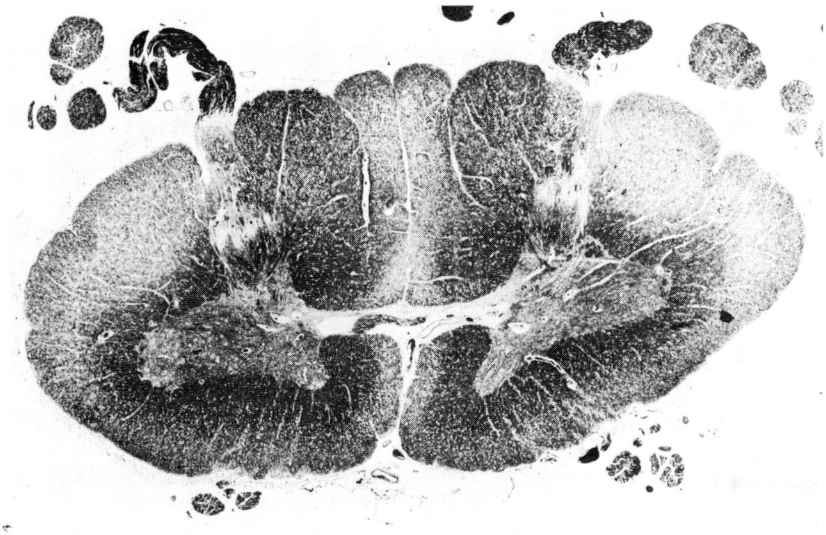

(a)

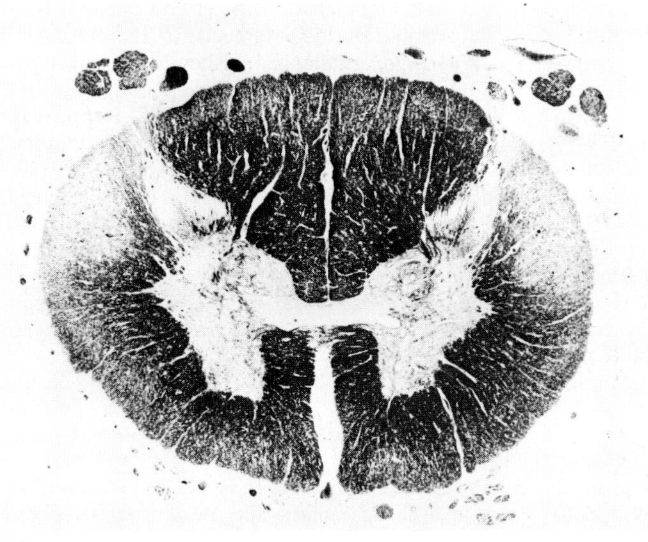

(b)

Fig. 15.33 Familial spastic paraplegia. (Case 2 of Behan and Maia, 1974). Dominant inheritance. Onset age 55, death age 66. (**a**) Cervical level. (**b**) Upper lumbar level. Tract degeneration as in Fig. 15.32 but more severe. Myelin stain. (Reproduced by courtesy of the Editor, *Journal of Neurology, Neurosurgery and Psychiatry*.)

gia. In 19 of these, inheritance was of autosomal dominant type; in three it appeared to be autosomal recessive.

Degeneration of the distal portions of long axons, without appreciable loss of parent cell bodies, is characteristic of these cases. It is uncertain whether or not this represents a retarded 'dying-back' process, of the kind seen in other degenerative conditions, where the parent cell body eventually disappears. An alternative explanation would be in terms of a generalized failure of nerve cells to maintain the vitality of the distal parts of long axons. It is also uncertain to what extent the spasticity and weakness in this condition are due to involvement of motor pathways other than the pyramidal tracts. It is noteworthy that, although posterior columns are involved, sensory loss is never severe and is often undetected.

References

Adams, R.D. (1968) The striatonigral degenerations. In *Handbook of Clinical Neurology* (Eds. Vinken, P.J. and Bruyn, G.W.), vol. 6, chapter 26, pp. 694–702. North-Holland, Amsterdam.

Adams, R.D., van Bogaert, L. and Vander Eecken, H. (1961) Dégénérescences nigro-striées et cérébello-nigro-striées. *Psychiatria et Neurologia* **142,** 219.

Adams, R.D., van Bogaert, L. and Vander Eecken, H. (1964) Striato-nigral degeneration. *Journal of Neuropathology and Experimental Neurology* **23,** 584–608.

Akelaitis, A.J. (1938) Hereditary form of primary parenchymatous atrophy of the cerebellar cortex associated with mental deterioration. *American Journal of Psychiatry* **94,** 1115–40.

Alexander, M.P., Emery, E.S. and Koerner, F.C. (1976) Progressive bulbar paresis in childhood. *Archives of Neurology* **33,** 66–8.

Amromin, G.D., Boder, E. and Teplitz, R. (1979) Ataxia-telangiectasia with a 32-year survival. A clinico-pathological report. *Journal of Neuropathology and Experimental Neurology* **38,** 621–43.

André-van Leeuwen, M. and van Bogaert, L. (1949) Hereditary ataxia with optic atrophy of the retrobulbar neuritis type, and latent pallido-luysian degeneration. *Brain* **72,** 340–63.

Andrews, J.M. and Maxwell, D.S. (1969) Motor neuron diseases in animals in *Motor Neuron Diseases* (Eds. Norris, F.H. and Kurland, L.T.), chapter 35. Grune and Stratton, New York.

Aran, F.A. (1850) Recherches sur une maladie non encore décrite du système musculaire (atrophie musculaire progressive). *Archives Générales de Médecine* **24,** 5–35, 172–214.

Averback, P. and Crocker, P. (1982) Regular involvement of Clarke's nucleus in sporadic amyotrophic lateral sclerosis. *Archives of Neurology* **39,** 155–6.

Banker, B.Q., Victor, M. and Adams, R.D. (1957) Arthrogryposis multiplex due to congenital muscular dystrophy. *Brain* **80,** 319–34.

Bannister, R. and Oppenheimer, D.R. (1972) Degenerative diseases of the nervous system associated with autonomic failure. *Brain* **95,** 457–74.

Bannister, R., Gibson, W., Michaels, L. and Oppenheimer, D.R. (1981) Laryngeal abductor paralysis in multiple system atrophy. A report on three necropsied cases, with observations on the laryngeal muscles and the nuclei ambigui. *Brain* **104,** 351–86.

Barbeau, A. (1982a) Friedreich's disease 1982: etiologic hypotheses. A personal analysis. *Canadian Journal of Neurological Sciences* **9,** 243–63.

Barbeau, A. (1982b) Pathophysiology of Friedreich's ataxia. In *Recent Advances in Clinical Neurology* (Eds. Matthews, W.B. and Glaser, G.H.), vol. 3, pp. 125–45. Churchill Livingstone, Edinburgh.

Beck, E., Daniel, P.M., Matthews, W.B., Stevens, D.L., Alpers, M.P., Asher, D.M., et al. (1969) Creutzfeldt-Jakob disease: the neuropathology of a transmission experiment. *Brain* **92,** 699–716.

Behan, W.M.H. and Maia, M. (1974) Strümpell's familial spastic paraplegia: genetics and neuropathology. *Journal of Neurology, Neurosurgery and Psychiatry* **37,** 8–20.

Beheim-Schwarzbach, D. (1952) Über Zelleibveränderungen im Nucleus coeruleus bei Parkinsonsymptomen. *Journal of Nervous and Mental Disease* **116,** 619–32.

Behrman, S., Carroll, J.D., Janota, I. and Matthews, W.B. (1969) Progressive supranuclear palsy: clinico-pathological study of four cases. *Brain* **92,** 663–77.

Bell, J. and Carmichael, E.A. (1939) On hereditary ataxia and spastic paraplegia. In *The Treasury of Human Inheritance* (Ed. Fisher, R.A.), vol. 4, part 3, Cambridge University Press, London.

Bertrand, I. and van Bogaert, L. (1925) Rapport sur la sclérose latérale amyotrophique (anatomie pathologique). *Revue Neurologique* **1,** 779–806.

Bethlem, J. and Jager, W.A. den H. (1960) The incidence and characteristics of Lewy bodies in idiopathic paralysis agitans. *Journal of Neurology, Neurosurgery and Pyschiatry* **23,** 74–80.

Bickerstaff, E.R. (1950) Hereditary spastic paraplegia. *Journal of Neurology, Neurosurgery and Psychiatry* **13,** 134–45.

Biemond, A. (1928) Neurotische Muskelatrophie und Friedreichsche Tabes in derselben Familie. *Deutsche Zeitschrift für Nervenheilkunde* **104,** 113–45.

Boder, E. and Sedgwick, R.P. (1958) Ataxia-telangiectasia: a familial syndrome of progressive cerebellar ataxia, oculocutaneous telangiectasia and frequent pulmonary infection. *Pediatrics* **21,** 526–54.

van Bogaert, L. (1930) Contribution clinique et anatomique à l'étude de la paralysie agitante juvénile primitive. *Revue Neurologique* **37,** 315–26.

van Bogaert, L. (1946) Aspects cliniques et pathologiques des atrophies pallidales et pallido-luysiennes progressives. *Journal of Neurology, Neurosurgery and Psychiatry* **9,** 125–57.

van Bogaert, L. (1952a) Etudes sur la paraplégie spasmodique familiale. V: Forme classique pure avec atrophie optique massive. *Acta Neurologica et Psychiatrica Belgica* **52,** 795–807.

van Bogaert, L. (1952b) Etude génétique sur les paraplégies spasmodiques familiales. *Journal de Génétique Humaine* **1,** 6–23.

van Bogaert, L. and Martin, L. (1974) Optic and cochleovestibular degenerations in the hereditary ataxias. *Brain* **97,** 15–40.

Boller, F., Mizutani, T., Roessmann, U. and Gambetti, P. (1980) Parkinson disease, dementia and Alzheimer disease: clinicopathological correlations. *Annals of Neurology* **7,** 329–35.

Bonduelle, M. (1975) Amyotrophic lateral sclerosis. In *Handbook of Clinical Neurology* (Eds. Vinken, P.J. and Bruyn, G.W.), vol. 22, pp. 281–338. North-Holland, Amsterdam.

Borit, A., Rubinstein, L.J. and Urich, H. (1975) The striatonigral degenerations: putaminal pigments and nosology. *Brain* **98,** 101–12.

Brain, Lord, Croft, P.B. & Wilkinson, M. (1965) Motor neurone disease as a manifestation of neoplasm. *Brain* **88,** 479–500.

Brandt, S. (1950) *Werdnig–Hoffmann's Infantile Progressive Muscular Atrophy*. Munksgaard, Copenhagen.

Bridges, B.A. and Harnden, D.G. (Eds.) (1982) *Ataxia–Telangiectasia. A cellular and molecular link between cancer, neuropathology and immune deficiency*. John Wiley, Chichester.

Brownell, B., Oppenheimer, D.R. & Hughes, J.T. (1970) The central nervous system in motor neurone disease. *Journal of Neurology, Neurosurgery and Psychiatry* **33,** 338–57.

Brucher, J.M., Dom, R., Lombaert, A. and Carton, H. (1981) Progressive pontobulbar palsy with deafness: clinical and pathological study of two cases. *Archives of Neurology* **38,** 186–90.

Burns, R.S., Markey, S.P., Phillips, J.M. and Chiueh, C.C. (1984). The neurotoxicity of 1-methyl-4-phenyl-1, 2, 3, 6-tetrahydropyridine in the monkey and man. *Canadian Journal of Neurological Sciences* **11,** 166–168.

Byers, R.K. and Banker, B.Q. (1961) Infantile muscular atrophy. *Archives of Neurology* **5,** 140–64.

Byrnes, C.M. (1926) A contribution to the pathology of paralysis agitans. *Archives of Neurology and Psychiatry* **15,** 407–43.

Carpenter, M.B. (1981) Anatomy of the corpus striatum and brain stem integrating systems. In *Handbook of Physiology: The Nervous System* (Eds. Brookhart, J.M., Mountcastle, V.B. and Brooks, V.B.), pp. 947–95. American Physiological Society, Bethesda.

Cassinari, V. and Pagni, C.A. (1969) *Central Pain: a Neurosurgical Survey*, Harvard University Press, Cambridge, Mass.

Castaigne, P., Lhermitte, F., Cambier, J., Escourolle, R. and Le Bigot, P. (1972) Etude neuropathologique de 61 observations de sclérose latérale amyotrophique: discussion nosologique. *Revue Neurologique* **127,** 401–14.

Cavanagh, J.B. (1979) The 'dying-back' process: a common denominator in many naturally occurring and toxic neuropathies. *Archives of Pathology and Laboratory Medicine* **103,** 659–64.

Charcot, J.-M. (1870) Note sur un cas de paralysie glosso-laryngée suivi d'autopsie. *Archives de Physiologie* **3,** 247–60.

Charcot, J.-M. (1874) De la sclérose latérale amyotrophique. *Progrès Médical* **2,** 325–27, 341–2, 453–5.

Charcot, J.-M. and Joffroy, A. (1869) Deux cas d'atrophie musculaire progressive avec lésions de la substance grise et des faisceaux antérolatéraux de la moelle épinière. *Archives de Physiologie (Paris)* **2,** 354–67, 629–49, 744–60.

Colmant, H.-J. (1958a) Die chronisch-progressive Bulbärparalyse. In *Handbuch der speziellen pathologischen Anatomie und Histologie* (Eds. Lubarsch, O., Henke, F. and Rössle, R.), vol. 13/2B, pp. 2571–84, Springer: Berlin.

Colmant, H.-J. (1958b) Die chronisch-progressive exteriore Ophthalmoplegie. In *Handbuch der speziellen pathologischen Anatomie und Histologie* (Eds. Lubarsch, O., Henke, F. and Rössle, R.), vol. 13/2B, pp. 2585–623. Springer, Berlin.

Colmant, H.-J. (1958c) Die myatrophische Lateralsklerose. In *Handbuch der speziellen pathologischen Anatomie und Histologie* (Eds. Lubarsch, O., Henke, F. and Rössle, R.), vol. 13/2B, pp. 2624–92. Springer, Berlin.

Colmant, H.J. (1975) Progressive bulbar palsy in adults. In *Handbook of Clinical Neurology* (Eds. Vinken, P.J. and Bruyn, G.W.), vol. 22, pp. 111–56. North-Holland, Amsterdam.

David, N.J., Mackey, E.A. and Smith, J.L. (1968) Further observations in progressive supranuclear palsy *Neurology* **18,** 349–356.

Davison, C. (1941) Amyotrophic lateral sclerosis. Origin and extent of the upper motor neuron lesion. *Archives of Neurology and Psychiatry* **46,** 1039–56.

Dejerine, J. (1883) Etude anatomique et clinique sur la paralysie labio-glosso-laryngée. *Archives de Physiologie Normale et Pathologique* Série 3, **2,** 180–227.

Dejerine, J. and Roussy, G. (1906) Le syndrome thalamique. *Revue Neurologique* **12,** 521–32.

Dejerine, J. and Thomas, A. (1900) L'atrophie olivo-ponto-cérébelleuse. *Nouvelle Iconographie de la Salpêtrière* **13,** 330–70.

Denny-Brown, D. (1962) *The Basal Ganglia and their Relation to Disorders of Movement*. Oxford Neurological Monographs. Oxford University Press, London.

Denny-Brown, D. (1968) Clinical symptomatology of diseases of the basal ganglia. In *Handbook of Clinical Neurology* (Eds. Vinken, P.J. and Bruyn, G.W.), vol. 6, chapter 5, pp. 133–72, North-Holland, Amsterdam.

Drachman, D.A. (1975) Ophthalmoplegia plus; a classification of the disorders associated with progressive external ophthalmoplegia. In *Handbook of Clinical Neurology* (Eds. Vinken, P.J. and Bruyn, G.W.), vol. 22, pp. 203–16. North-Holland, Amsterdam.

Drachman, D.B. (1969) Congenital deformities produced by neuromuscular disorders of the developing embryo. In *Motor Neuron Diseases* (Eds. Norris, F.H. and Kurland, L.T.), chapter 10, Grune and Stratton, New York.

Dubowitz, V. (1975) Infantile spinal muscular atrophy. In *Handbook of Clinical Neurology* (Eds. Vinken, P.J. and Bruyn, G.W.), vol. 22, pp. 81–101. North-Holland, Amsterdam.

Duchenne, G.B.A. (1853) Etude comparée des lésions anatomiques dans l'atrophie musculaire progressive et dans la paralysie générale. *Union Médicale* **7,** 246–7.

Duchenne, G.B.A. (1860) Paralysie musculaire progressive de la langue, du voile du palais et des lèvres. *Archives Générales de Médecine* **16,** 283–96, 431–45.

Duffy, P.E. and Tennyson, V.M. (1965) Phase and electron microscopic observations of Lewy bodies and melanin granules in the substantia nigra and locus ceruleus in Parkinson's disease. *Journal of Neuropathology and Experimental Neurology* **24,** 398–414.

Eadie, M.J. (1975a) Hereditary spastic ataxia. In *Handbook of Clinical Neurology* (Eds. Vinken, P.J. and Bruyn, G.W.), vol. 21, pp. 365–75. North-Holland, Amsterdam.

Eadie, M.J. (1975b) Olivopontocerebellar atrophy. In *Handbook of Clinical Neurology* (Eds. Vinken, P.J. and Bruyn, G.W.), vol. 21, Chapters 19, 20, 21, 22 and 23. North-Holland, Amsterdam.

Earle, K.M. (1968) Studies on Parkinson's disease, including X-ray fluorescent spectroscopy of formalin-fixed brain tissue. *Journal of Neuropathology and Experimental Neurology* **27,** 1–14.

Eldridge, R. and Fahn, S. (Eds.) (1976) Dystonia. In *Advances in Neurology*, vol. 14. Raven Press, New York.

Engel, W.K., Kurland, L.T. and Klatzo, I. (1959) An inherited disease similar to amyotrophic lateral sclerosis with a pattern of posterior column involvement. *Brain* **82,** 203–20.

Fenichel, G.M. (1969) The spinal muscular atrophies. In *Motor Neuron Diseases* (Eds. Norris, F.H. and Kurland, L.T.), chapter 11. Grune and Stratton, New York.

Fichefet, J.P., Sternon, J.E., Franken, L., Demanet, J.C. and Vanderhaeghen, J.J. (1965) Etude anatomoclinique d'un cas d'hypotension orthostatique 'idiopathique'. *Acta Cardiologica* **20,** 332–48.

Foix, M.C. (1921) Les lésions anatomiques de la maladie de Parkinson. *Revue Neurologique* **28,** 593–600.

Forno, L.S. (1966) Pathology of Parkinsonism: a preliminary report of 24 cases. *Journal of Neurosurgery* **24,** 266–71.

Friedreich, N. (1863) Ueber degenerative Atrophie der spinalen Hinterstränge. *Virchows Archiv für pathologische Anatomie* **26,** 391–419, 433–59; **27,** 1–26.

Friedreich, N. (1876) Ueber Ataxie mit besonderer Berücksichtigung der hereditären Formen. *Virchows Archiv für pathologische Anatomie* **68,** 145–245.

Gallai, V., Hockaday, J.M., Hughes, J.T., Lane, D.J., Oppenheimer, D.R. and Rushworth, G. (1981) Ponto-bulbar palsy with deafness (Brown–Vialetto–van Laere syndrome)—a report on three cases. *Journal of the Neurological Sciences* **50,** 259–75.

Gamboa, E.T., Wolf, A., Yahr, M.D., Harter, D.H., Duffy, P.E., Barden, H. and Hsu, K.C. (1974) Influenza virus antigen in postencephalitic Parkinsonism brain. *Archives of Neurology* **31,** 228–32.

Gardner-Medwin, D., Hudgson, P. and Walton, J.N. (1967) Benign spinal muscular atrophy arising in childhood and adolescence. *Journal of the Neurological Sciences* **5,** 121–58.

Geoffroy, G., Barbeau, A., Breton, G. Lemieux, B., Aube, M., Léger, C. and Bouchard, J.P. (1976) Clinical description and roentgenologic evaluation of patients with Friedreich's ataxia. *Canadian Journal of Neurological Sciences* **3,** 279–86.

Gilbert, G.J. (1975) Dyssynergia cerebellaris myoclonica. In *Handbook of Clinical Neurology* (Eds. Vinken, Vinken, P.J. and Bruyn, G.W.), vol. 21, pp. 509–18. North-Holland, Amsterdam.

Gomez, M.R. (1975) Progressive bulbar paralysis of childhood (Fazio–Londe disease). In *Handbook of Clinical Neurology* (Eds. Vinken, P.J. and Bruyn, G.W.), vol. 22, pp. 103–9. North-Holland, Amsterdam.

Greenfield, J.G. (1954) *The Spino-cerebellar Degenerations.* Blackwell, Oxford.

Greenfield, J.G. and Bosanquet, F.D. (1953) The brain-stem lesions in Parkinsonism. *Journal of Neurology, Neurosurgery and Psychiatry* **16,** 213–26.

Greenfield, J.G. and Matthews, W.B. (1954) Post-encephalitic parkinsonism with amyotrophy. *Journal of Neurology, Neurosurgery and Psychiatry* **17,** 50–6.

Grimberg, L. (1934) Paralysis agitans and trauma. *Journal of Nervous and Mental Diseases* **79,** 14–42.

Gruner, J.-E. and Bargeton, E. (1952) Lésions thalamiques dans la myatonie du nourrisson. *Revue Neurologique* **86,** 236–42.

Hakim, A. and Mathieson, G. (1979) Dementia in

Parkinson disease: a neuropathologic study. *Neurology* **29,** 1209–14.

Hall, B., Noad, K. B. and Latham, O. (1941) Familial cortical cerebellar atrophy. *Brain* **64,** 178–94.

Hall, B., Noad, K. B. and Latham, O. (1945) Familial cortical cerebellar atrophy: a contribution to the study of heredo-familial cerebellar disease in Australia. *Medical Journal of Australia* **1,** 101–8.

Hallervorden, J. (1933) Zur Pathogenese des postencephalitischen Parkinsonismus. *Klinische Wochenschrift* **12,** 692–4.

Hallervorden, J. (1935) Anatomische Untersuchungen zur Pathogenese des postencephalitischen Parkinsonismus. *Deutsche Zeitschrift für Nervenheilkunde* **136,** 68–77.

Harding, A. E. (1981) Hereditary 'pure' spastic paraplegia: a clinical and genetic study of 22 families. *Journal of Neurology, Neurosurgery and Psychiatry* **44,** 871–83.

Harrington, M. G., Macpherson, P., McIntosh, W. B., Allam, B. F. and Bone, I. (1981) The significance of the incidental finding of basal ganglia calcification on computed tomography. *Journal of Neurology, Neurosurgery and Psychiatry* **44,** 1168–70.

Hassler, R. (1938) Zur Pathologie der Paralysis agitans und des postenzephalitischen Parkinsonismus. *Journal für Psychologie und Neurologie* **48,** 387.

Hassler, R. (1939) Zur pathologischen Anatomie des senilen und des parkinsonistischen Tremor. *Journal für Psychologie und Neurologie* **49,** 193–230.

Hewer, R. L. (1968) Study of fatal cases of Friedreich's ataxia. *British Medical Journal* **3,** 649–52.

Hewer, R. L. (1969) The heart in Friedreich's ataxia. *British Heart Journal* **31,** 5–14.

Hirano, A., Kurland, L. T., Krooth, R. S. and Lessell, S. (1961) Parkinsonism-dementia complex, an endemic disease on the island of Guam. I. Clinical features. *Brain* **84,** 642–61.

Hirano, A., Kurland, L. T. and Sayre, G. P. (1967) Familial amyotrophic lateral sclerosis. *Archives of Neurology* **16,** 232–43.

Hirano, A., Malamud, N. and Kurland, L. T. (1961) Parkinsonism-dementia complex, an endemic disease on the island of Guam. II. Pathological features. *Brain* **84,** 662–79.

Hirano, A., and Zimmerman, H. M. (1962) Alzheimer's neurofibrillary change: a topographic study. *Archives of Neurology* **7,** 227–42.

Hoffmann, J. (1893) Ueber chronische spinale Muskelatrophie im Kindesalter auf familiäre Basis. *Deutsche Zeitschrift für Nervenheilkunde* **3,** 427–70.

Hoffman, J. (1900) Ueber die hereditäre progressive spinale Muskelatrophie im Kindesalter. *Münchener medizinische Wochenschrift* **47,** 1649–51.

Holmes, G. (1907) A form of familial degeneration of the cerebellum. *Brain* **30,** 466–89.

Hornykiewicz, O. (1982) Brain neurotransmitter changes in Parkinson's disease. In *Movement Disorders* (Eds. Marsden, C. D. and Fahn, S.), Butterworths International Medical Reviews, Neurology 2, pp. 41–58. Butterworth, London.

Hughes, J. T. and Brownell, B. (1972) Pathology of peroneal muscular atrophy. *Journal of Neurology, Neurosurgery and Psychiatry* **35,** 648–57.

Hughes, J. T., Brownell, B. and Hewer, R. L. (1968) The peripheral sensory pathway in Friedreich's ataxia. *Brain* **91,** 803–18.

Hunt, J. R. (1917) Progressive atrophy of the globus pallidus. *Brain* **40,** 58–148.

Hunt, J. Ramsay (1921) Dyssynergia cerebellaris myoclonica—primary atrophy of the dentate system. *Brain* **44,** 490–538.

Iizuka, R., Hirayama, K. and Maehara, K. (1980) A neuropathological observation of extrapyramidal components in spinocerebellar degeneration—a comparison of so-called dentato-rubro-pallido-luysian atrophy with OPCA. In *Spinocerebellar Degenerations* (Ed. Japan Medical Research Foundation), pp. 171–83. University of Tokyo Press, Tokyo.

Iwata, M. and Hirano, A. (1978) Sparing of the Onufrowicz nucleus in sacral anterior horn lesions. *Annals of Neurology* **4,** 245–9.

Jager, W. A. den H. (1969) Sphingomyelin in Lewy inclusion bodies in Parkinson's disease. *Archives of Neurology* **21,** 615–19.

Jager, W. A. den H. (1970) Histochemistry of adrenal bodies in Parkinson's disease. *Archives of Neurology* **23,** 528–33.

Jager, W. A. den H. and Bethlem, J. (1960) The distribution of Lewy bodies in the central and autonomic nervous systems in idiopathic paralysis agitans. *Journal of Neurology, Neurosurgery and Psychiatry* **23,** 283–90.

Jellinger, K. (1968a) Degenerations and exogenous lesions of the pallidum and striatum. In *Handbook of Clinical Neurology* (Eds. Vinken, P. J. and Bruyn, G. W.), vol. 6, chapter 25, pp. 632–93. North-Holland, Amsterdam.

Jellinger, K. (1968b) Progressive Pallidum-atrophie. *Journal of the Neurological Sciences* **6,** 19–44.

Jellinger, K. and Danielczyk, W. (1968) Striato-nigrale Degeneration. *Acta Neuropathologica* **10,** 242–57.

Jellinger, K. and Tarnowska-Dziduszko, E. (1971) Die ZNS-Veränderungen bei den olivo-ponto-cerebellaren Atrophien. *Zeitschrift für Neurologie* **199,** 192–214.

Johnson, R. H., Lee, G. de J., Oppenheimer, D. R. and Spalding, J. M. K. (1966) Autonomic failure with orthostatic hypotension due to intermediolateral column degeneration. *Quarterly Journal of Medicine* **35,** 276–92.

Kawamura, Y., Dyck, P. J., Shimono, M., Okazaki,

H., Tateishi, J. and Doi, H. (1981) Morphometric comparison of the vulnerability of peripheral motor and sensory neurons in amyotrophic lateral sclerosis. *Journal of Neuropathology and Experimental Neurology* **40,** 667–75.

Kemp, J.M. and Powell, T.P.S. (1971) The connections of the striatum and globus pallidus; synthesis and speculation. *Philosophical Transactions of the Royal Society, London* Series B, **262,** 441–57.

Klaue, R. (1940) Parkinsonsche Krankheit (Paralysis agitans) und postencephalitischer Parkinsonismus. *Archiv für Psychiatrie und Nervenkrankheiten* **111,** 251–321.

Klüver, H. and Weil, A. (1948) Carcinomas of the tongue in monkeys and pathologic changes in the central nervous system. *Journal of Neuropathology and Experimental Neurology* **7,** 144–53.

Koch, G. (1972) Genetic aspects of the phakomatoses. In *Handbook of Clinical Neurology* (Eds. Vinken, P.J. and Bruyn, G.W.), vol. 14, chapter 20, pp. 515–17. North-Holland, Amsterdam.

Kojewnikow, A. (1885) Ein Fall von lateraler amyotrophischer Sclerose. *Zentralblatt für Nervenheilkunde* **8,** 409–14.

Konigsmark, B.W. and Weiner, L.P. (1970) The olivopontocerebellar atrophies: a review. *Medicine* **49,** 227–41.

Kugelberg, E. and Welander, L. (1956) Heredofamilial juvenile muscular atrophy simulating muscular dystrophy. *Archives of Neurology and Psychiatry* **75,** 500–9.

Kurland, L.T. (1977) Epidemiology of amyotrophic lateral sclerosis, with emphasis on antecedent events, from case-control comparisons. In *Motor Neurone Disease* (Ed. Rose, F.C.), pp. 14–29. Pitman Medical, London.

Kurland, L.T. and Brody, J.A. (1975) Amyotrophic lateral sclerosis—Guam type. In *Handbook of Clinical Neurology* (Eds. Vinken, P.J. and Bruyn, G.W.), vol. 22, pp. 339–47. North-Holland, Amsterdam.

Kurland, L.T. and Mulder, D.W. (1954) Epidemiologic investigations of amyotrophic lateral sclerosis. I. *Neurology* **4,** 355–78, 438–48.

Kurtzke, J.F. (1969) Comments on the epidemiology of amyotrophic lateral sclerosis. In *Motor Neuron Diseases* (Eds. Norris, F.H. and Kurland, L.T.), chapter 8. Grune and Stratton, New York.

Langston, J.W. and Ballard, P. (1984) Parkinsonism induced by 1-methyl-4-phenyl-1, 2, 3, 6-tetrahydropyridine (MPTP): Implications for treatment and the pathogenesis of Parkinson's disease. *Canadian Journal of Neurological Sciences,* **11,** 160–165.

Lawyer, T. and Netsky, M. (1953) Amyotrophic lateral sclerosis: a clinico-anatomic study of 53 cases. *Archives of Neurology and Psychiatry* **69,** 171–92.

Leikin, S.L., Bazelon, M. and Park, K.H. (1966) In vitro lymphocyte transformation in ataxia-telangiectasia. *Journal of Pediatrics* **68,** 477–9.

Lewis, P. (1964) Familial orthostatic hypotension. *Brain* **87,** 719–28.

Lewy, F.H. (1913) Zur pathologischen Anatomie der Paralysis agitans. *Deutsche Zeitschrift für Nervenheilkunde* **50,** 50–5.

Lipkin, L.E. (1959) Cytoplasmic inclusions in ganglion cells associated with Parkinsonian states. *American Journal of Pathology* **35,** 1117–33.

Louis-Bar, D. (1941) Sur un syndrome progressif comprenant des télangiectasies capillaires cutanées et conjonctivales symétriques, à disposition naevoïde, et des troubles cérébelleux. *Confinia Neurologica* **4,** 32–42.

Löwenthal, A. and Bruyn, G.W. (1968) Calcification of the striopallidodentate system. In *Handbook of Clinical Neurology* (Eds. Vinken, P.J. and Bruyn, G.W.), vol. 6, chapter 27, pp. 703–25. North-Holland, Amsterdam.

Malamud, N., Hirano, A. and Kurland, L.T. (1961) Pathoanatomic changes in amyotrophic lateral sclerosis on Guam. *Archives of Neurology* **5,** 401–15.

Mannen, T., Iwata, M., Toyokura, Y. and Nagashima, K. (1977) Preservation of a certain motoneurone group of the sacral cord in amyotrophic lateral sclerosis: its clinical significance. *Journal of Neurology, Neurosurgery and Psychiatry* **40,** 464–9.

Marie, P., Foix, C. and Alajouanine, T. (1922) De l'atrophie cérébelleuse tardive à prédominance corticale. *Revue Neurologique* **29,** 849–85, 1082–11.

Marsden, C.D. (1981) Extrapyramidal diseases. In *The Molecular Basis of Neuropathology* (Eds. Davison, A.N. and Thompson, R.H.S.), pp. 345–83. Edward Arnold, London.

Martin, J.J. (1969) Thalamic syndromes. In *Handbook of Clinical Neurology* (Eds. Vinken, P.J. and Bruyn, G.W.), vol. 2, chapter 17, pp. 469–96, North-Holland, Amsterdam.

Martin, J.J. (1970) Contribution à l'étude de l'anatomie du thalamus et de sa pathologie au cours des maladies dégénératives dites abiotrophiques. *Acta neurologica Belgica* **70,** 5–212.

Martin, J.J. (1975) Thalamic degenerations. In *Handbook of Clinical Neurology* (Eds. Vinken, P.J. and Bruyn, G.W.), vol. 21, pp. 587–604. North Holland, Amsterdam.

Martin, J.P. (1967) *The Basal Ganglia and Posture.* Pitman Medical, London.

Menzel, P. (1891) Beitrag zur Kenntnis der hereditären Ataxie und Kleinhirnatrophie. *Archiv für Psychiatrie* **22,** 160–90.

Mettler, F.A. (1968) Anatomy of the basal ganglia. In *Handbook of Clinical Neurology* (Eds. Vinken,

P.J. and Bruyn, G.W.), vol. 6, chapter 1, pp. 1-55. North-Holland, Amsterdam.

Meyer, A. (1929) Ueber eine der amyotrophischen Lateralsklerose nahestehende Erkrankung mit psychischen Störungen. *Zeitschrift für die gesamte Neurologie und Psychiatrie* **121,** 107-38.

Meyers, R. (1968) Ballismus. In *Handbook of Clinical Neurology* (Eds. Vinken, P.J. and Bruyn, G.W.), vol. 6, chapter 19, pp. 476-90. North-Holland, Amsterdam.

Naito, H. and Oyanagi, S. (1982) Familial myoclonus epilepsy and choreoathetosis: hereditary dentatorubral-pallidoluysian atrophy. *Neurology* **32,** 798-807.

Netsky, M.G. (1968) Degenerations of the cerebellum and its pathways. In *Pathology of the Nervous System* (Ed. Minckler, J.), vol. I, chapter 87. McGraw-Hill, New York.

Neumann, M.A. (1959) Combined degeneration of globus pallidus and dentate nucleus and their projections. *Neurology* **9,** 430-8.

Norris, F.H. and Engel, W.K. (1965) Carcinomatous amyotrophic lateral sclerosis. In *The Remote Effects of Cancer on the Nervous System* (Eds. Brain, Lord and Norris, F.H.), chapter 4. Grune and Stratton, New York.

Norris, F.H., McMenemey, W.H. and Barnard, R.O. (1969) Anterior horn pathology in carcinomatous neuromyopathy compared with other forms of motor neuron disease. In *Motor Neuron Diseases* (Eds. Norris, F.H. and Kurland, L.T.), chapter 9. Grune and Stratton, New York.

Onufrowicz, B. (1900) On the arrangement and function of the cell groups of the sacral region of the spinal cord in man. *Archives of Neurology and Psychopathology* **3,** 387-412.

Oppenheimer, D.R. (1979) Brain lesions in Friedreich's ataxia. *Canadian Journal of Neurological Sciences* **6,** 173-6.

Oppenheimer, D.R. (1980) Lateral horn cells in progressive autonomic failure. *Journal of the Neurological Sciences* **46,** 393-404.

Oppenheimer, D.R. (1983) Neuropathology of progressive autonomic failure. In *Autonomic Failure* (Ed. Bannister, R.), pp. 267-83. Oxford University Press, Oxford.

Parkinson, J. (1817) *An Essay on the Shaking Palsy.* London. Reproduced in *James Parkinson* (Ed. Critchley, M.) (1955). Macmillan, London.

Pearce, G.W. (1979) The neuropathology of parkinsonism. In *Recent Advances in Neuropathology* (Eds. Smith, W.T. and Cavanagh, J.B.), pp. 299-320. Churchill Livingstone, Edinburgh.

Pearce, J. and Harriman, D.G.F. (1966) Chronic spinal muscular atrophy. *Journal of Neurology, Neurosurgery and Psychiatry* **29,** 509-20.

Perry, T.L., Currier, R.D., Hansen, S. and MacLean, J. (1977) Aspartate-taurine imbalance in dominantly inherited olivopontocerebellar atrophy. *Neurology* **27,** 257-61.

Peterson, R.D.A., Kelly, W.D. and Good, R.A. (1964) Ataxia-telangiectasia: its association with a defective thymus, immunological deficiency disease and malignancy. *Lancet* **1,** 1189-93.

Powell, H.C., London, G.W. and Lampert, P.W. (1974) Neurofibrillary tangles in progressive supranuclear palsy: electron microscopic observations. *Journal of Neuropathology and Experimental Neurology* **33,** 98-106.

Pratt, R.T.C. (1967) *The Genetics of Neurological Disorders.* Oxford University Press, London.

Probst, M. (1898) Zu der fortschreitenden Erkrankungen der motorischen Leitungsbahnen. *Archiv für Psychiatrie und Nervenkrankheiten* **30,** 766-844.

Probst, M. (1903) Zur Kenntnis der amyotrophischen Lateralsklerose. *Sitzungsberichte der Akademie der Wissenschaften in Wien* **112,** *Abt. 3,* 683-824.

Quick, D.T. (1969) Pancreatic dysfunction in amyotrophic lateral sclerosis. In *Motor Neuron Diseases* (Eds. Norris, F.H. and Kurland, L.T.), chapter 20. Grune and Stratton, New York.

Rosenhagen, H. (1943) Die primäre Atrophie des Brückenfusses und der unteren Oliven. *Archiv für Psychiatrie* **116,** 163-228.

Roussy, G. and Lévy, G. (1926) Sept cas d'une maladie familiale particulière. *Revue Neurologique* **33,** 427-50.

Rowland, L.P. (1975) Progressive external ophthalmoplegia. In *Handbook of Clinical Neurology* (Eds. Vinken, P.J. and Bruyn, G.W.), vol. 22, pp. 177-202. North-Holland, Amsterdam.

Roy, S. and Wolman, L. (1969) Ultrastructural observations in Parkinsonism. *Journal of Pathology* **99,** 39-44.

Roy, S., Datta, C.K., Hirano, A., Ghatak, N.R. and Zimmerman, H.M. (1974) Electron microscopic study of neurofibrillary tangles in Steele-Richardson-Olszewski syndrome. *Acta Neuropathologica* **29,** 175-9.

Russell, D.S. (1946) Myocarditis in Friedreich's ataxia. *Journal of Pathology and Bacteriology* **58,** 739-48.

Saunders, P.W. (1913-14) Sensory changes in Friedreich's ataxia. *Brain* **36,** 166-92.

Scherer, H.-J. (1933) Extrapyramidale Störungen bei der olivopontocerebellaren Atrophie. *Zeitschrift für die gesamte Neurologie und Psychiatrie* **145,** 406-19.

Schut, J.W. (1950) Hereditary ataxia: clinical study through six generations. *Archives of Neurology and Psychiatry* **63,** 535-68.

Schut, J.W. and Haymaker, W. (1951) Hereditary ataxia: a pathologic study of five cases of common ancestry. *Journal of Neuropathology and Clinical Neurology* **1,** 183-213.

Schwab, R.S. and England, A.C. (1968) Parkinson syndromes due to various specific causes. In *Handbook of Clinical Neurology* (Eds. Vinken, P.J. and Bruyn, G.W.), vol. 6, chapter 9, pp. 227–47. North-Holland, Amsterdam.

Schwarz, G.A. (1952) Hereditary (familial) spastic paraplegia. *Archives of Neurology and Psychiatry* **68,** 655–82.

Schwarz, G.A. and Barrows, L.J. (1960) Hemiballism without involvement of Luys' body. *Archives of Neurology* **2,** 420–34.

Schwarz, G.A. and Liu, C.-N. (1956) Hereditary (familial) spastic paraplegia. *Archives of Neurology and Psychiatry* **75,** 144–62.

Sedgwick, R.P. and Boder, E. (1972) Ataxia-telangiectasia. In *Handbook of Clinical Neurology* (Eds. Vinken, P.J. and Bruyn, G.W.), vol. 14, chapter 10, pp. 267–339. North-Holland, Amsterdam.

Seitelberger, F. (1975) General neuropathology of the degenerative diseases of the central nervous system. In *Handbook of Clinical Neurology* (Eds. Vinken, P.J. and Bruyn, G.W.), vol. 21, pp. 43–71. North-Holland, Amsterdam.

Sharpe, J.A., Rewcastle, N.B., Lloyd, K.G., Hornykiewicz, O., Hill, M. and Tasker, R.R. (1973) Striatonigral degeneration: response to levodopa therapy, with pathological and neurochemical correlation. *Journal of the Neurological Sciences,* **19,** 275–86.

Shiraki, H. (1969) The neuropathology of amyotrophic lateral sclerosis in the Kii peninsula and other areas of Japan. In *Motor Neuron Diseases* (Eds. Norris, F.H. and Kurland, L.T.), chapter 7. Grune and Stratton, New York.

Shy, G.M. and Drager, G.A. (1960) A neurological syndrome associated with orthostatic hypotension. *Archives of Neurology* **2,** 511–27.

Smith, J.K. (1975) Dentato-rubro-pallido-luysian atrophy. In *Handbook of Clinical Neurology* (Eds. Vinken, P.W. and Bruyn, G.W.), vol. 21, pp. 519–34. North-Holland, Amsterdam.

Smith, J.K., Gonda, V.E. and Malamud, N. (1958) Unusual form of cerebellar ataxia—combined dentato-rubral and pallido-luysian degeneration. *Neurology* **8,** 205–9.

Smith, M.C. (1960) Nerve fibre degeneration in the brain in amyotrophic lateral sclerosis. *Journal of Neurology, Neurosurgery and Psychiatry* **23,** 269–82.

Smith, M.C. (1971) Pathology of unilateral Parkinsonism and of hemiballismus. In *Symposium Bel-Air IV (Geneva)* (Ed. de Ajuriaguerra, J.), pp. 263–67. Georg, Geneva.

Sourkes, T.L. (1981) Parkinson's disease and other disorders of the basal ganglia. In *Basic Neurochemistry* (Eds. Siegel, G.J., Albers, R.W., Agranoff, B.W. and Katzman, R.), 2nd edn., pp. 719–33. Little, Brown, Boston.

Spatz, H. (1938) Die 'systemischen Atrophien'. *Archiv für Psychiatrie* **108,** 1–18.

Spillane, J.D. (1940) Familial pes cavus and absent tendon jerks; its relationship with Friedreich's disease and peroneal muscular atrophy. *Brain* **63,** 275–90.

Spokes, E.G.S. (1983) Neurochemistry of autonomic failure. In *Autonomic Failure* (Ed. Bannister, R.), pp. 284–309. Oxford University Press, Oxford.

Spokes, E.G.S., Bannister, R. and Oppenheimer, D.R. (1979) Multiple system atrophy with autonomic failure—clinical, histological and neurochemical observations on four cases. *Journal of the Neurological Sciences* **43,** 59–82.

Steele, J.C. (1975) Progressive supranuclear palsy. In *Handbook of Clinical Neurology* (Eds. Vinken, P.W. and Bruyn, G.W.), vol. 22, pp. 217–29. North-Holland, Amsterdam.

Steele, J.C., Richardson, J.C. and Olszewski, J. (1964) Progressive supranuclear palsy. *Archives of Neurology* **10,** 333–59.

Steiman, G.S., Rorke, L.B. and Brown, M.J. (1980) Infantile neuronal degeneration masquerading as Werdnig–Hoffmann disease. *Annals of Neurology* **8,** 317–24.

Stewart, T.G. and Holmes, G. (1908) On the connection of the inferior olives with the cerebellum in man. *Brain* **31.** 125–37.

Strich, S.J. (1966) Pathological findings in three cases of ataxia-telangiectasia. *Journal of Neurology, Neurosurgery and Psychiatry* **29,** 489–99.

Strümpell, A. (1880) Beiträge zur Pathologie des Rückenmarks. *Archiv für Psychiatrie* **10,** 676–717.

Strümpell, A. (1886) Ueber eine bestimmte Form der primären combinierten Systemerkrankung des Rückenmarks. *Archiv für Psychiatrie* **17,** 217–38.

Strümpell, A. (1904) Die primäre Seitenstrangsklerose (spastische Spinalparalyse). *Deutsche Zeitschrift für Nervenheilkunde* **27,** 291–339.

Sung, J.H. (1979) Autonomic neurons affected by lipid storage in Fabry's disease: distribution of autonomic neurons in the sacral cord. *Journal of Neuropathology and Experimental Neurology* **38,** 87–98.

Sung, J.H. and Mastri, A.R. (1980) Spinal autonomic neurons in Werdnig–Hoffmann disease, mannosidosis and Hurler's syndrome: distribution of autonomic neurons in the spinal cord. *Journal of Neuropathology and Experimental Neurology* **39,** 441–51.

Sung, J.H., Mastri, A.R. and Segal, E. (1979) Pathology of Shy–Drager syndrome. *Journal of Neuropathology and Experimental Neurology* **38,** 353–68.

Syllaba, L. and Henner, K. (1926) Contribution à l'indépendance de l'athétose double idiopathique et congénitale. Atteinte familiale, syndrome dystrophique, signe du réseau vasculaire conjonctival, intégrité psychique. *Revue Neurologique* **1,** 541–62.

Takei, Y. and Mirra, S.S. (1973) Striatonigral degeneration: a form of multiple system atrophy with clinical parkinsonism. *Progress in Neuropathology* **2,** 217–51.

Tellez-Nagel, I. and Wiśniewski, H.M. (1973) Ultrastructure of neurofibrillary tangles in Steele–Richardson–Olszewski syndrome. *Archives of Neurology* **29,** 324–7.

Titica, J. and van Bogaert, L. (1946) Heredo-degenerative hemiballismus: a contribution to the question of primary atrophy of corpus Luysii. *Brain* **69,** 251–63.

Torvik, A. and Meen, D. (1966) Distribution of the brainstem lesions in postencephalitic parkinsonism. *Acta Neurologica Scandinavica* **42,** 415–25.

Trétiakoff, C. (1919) Contribution à l'étude de l'anatomie pathologique du locus niger. Thesis, University of Paris.

Tyrer, J.H. (1975) Friedreich's ataxia. In *Handbook of Clinical Neurology* (Eds. Vinken, P.J. and Bruyn, G.W.), vol. 21, pp 319–64. North-Holland, Amsterdam.

Ule, G. (1957) Die systematischen Atrophien des Kleinhirns. In *Handbuch der speziellen pathologischen Anatomie und Histologie* (Eds. Lubarsch, O., Henke, F. and Rössle, R.), vol. XIII/1A, pp. 934–88. Springer, Berlin.

Victor, M. (1980) The spino-cerebellar degenerations; cerebellar and brain stem forms. In *Spino cerebellar Degenerations* (Ed. Japan Medical Research Foundation), pp. 53–66. University of Tokyo Press, Tokyo.

Victor, M., Adams, R.D. and Mancall, E.L. (1959) A restricted form of cerebellar cortical degeneration occurring in alcoholic patients. *Archives of Neurology* **1,** 579–688.

Wadia, N.H. (1977) Heredo-familial spinocerebellar degeneration with slow eye movements: another variety of olivopontocerebellar degeneration. *Neurology (India)* **25,** 147–60.

Wadia, N.H. (1983) A variety of olivopontocerebellar degeneration distinguished by slow eye movements and peripheral neuropathy. In *The Olivopontocerebellar Atrophies* (Eds. Duvoisin, R.C. and Plaitakis, A.), Raven Press, New York.

Wadia, N.H. and Swami, R.K. (1971) A new form of heredofamilial spinocerebellar degeneration with slow eye movements. *Brain* **94,** 359–74.

Weber, F.P. and Greenfield, J.G. (1942) Cerebello-olivary degeneration: an example of heredo-familial incidence. *Brain* **65,** 220–31.

Welte, E. (1939) Die Atrophie des Systems des Brückenfusses und der unteren Oliven. *Archiv für Psychiatrie* **109,** 649–98.

Werdnig, G. (1891) Zwei frühinfantile hereditäre Fälle von progressiver Muskelatrophie. *Archiv für Psychiatrie* **22,** 437–80.

Werdnig, G. (1894) Die frühinfantile progressive spinale Amyotrophie. *Archiv für Psychiatrie* **26,** 706–44.

Whittier, J.R. (1947) Ballism and the subthalamic nucleus. *Archives of Neurology and Psychiatry* **58,** 672–92.

Wohlfart, G., Fex, J. and Eliasson, S. (1955) Hereditary spinal muscular atrophy. *Acta Psychiatrica et Neurologica Scandinavica* **30,** 395–406.

Woods, B.T. and Schaumburg, H.H. (1975) Nigro-spinodentatal degeneration with nuclear ophthalmoplegia. In *Handbook of Clinical Neurology* (Eds. Vinken, P.V. and Bruyn, G.W.), vol. 22, pp. 157–76. North-Holland, Amsterdam.

Zeman, W. and Dyken, P. (1968) Dystonia musculorum deformans. In *Handbook of Clinical Neurology* (Eds. Vinken, P.J. and Bruyn, G.W.), vol. 6, chapter 21, pp. 517–43. North-Holland, Amsterdam.

Zeman, W. and Whitlock, C.C. (1968) Symptomatic dystonias. In *Handbook of Clinical Neurology* (Eds. Vinken, P.J. and Bruyn, G.W.), vol. 6, chapter 22, pp. 544–66. North-Holland, Amsterdam.

Zilkha, K.J. (1962) Discussion on motor neurone disease. *Proceedings of the Royal Society of Medicine* **55,** 1028–9.

16

The hypothalamus and pituitary gland

C.S. Treip

The pathology of the hypothalamus and pituitary gland are described in a single chapter because the two regions are anatomically in continuity and are physiologically interdependent; they are often spoken of as the *hypothalamic-pituitary axis*. Some acquaintance with the anatomy (Clark, 1938; Daniel, 1966a; Daniel and Prichard, 1975) and physiology (Harris, 1960; Greep and Astwood, 1974; Guyton, 1981) of the axis is necessary for the study of pathological processes in this region; the chapter has accordingly been prefaced by brief outlines of these topics. From a practical point of view, it is pertinent to note that the hypothalamus is easily damaged during removal of the brain at necropsy; care must therefore be taken in carrying out this procedure. In particular, traction on the optic nerves and pituitary stalk should be avoided by cutting through both as soon as the brain is lifted from the base of the skull. Similarly, the neurohypophysis can easily be damaged or destroyed during removal of the pituitary; this can be avoided by dissecting out the gland complete within its dural capsule and taking the dorsum sellae with the gland.

The most comprehensive review of the earlier literature on the pathology of the hypothalamus is by Orthner (1955). Other reviews have been published by Bauer (1954), Herzog (1955), Orthner (1961), Sheehan (1968) and, more recently, by Daniel and Treip (1977) and Plum and van Uitert (1978).

Hypothalamus

Anatomy of the hypothalamus

The hypothalamus is one of the more primitve parts of the central nervous system, with complex and extensive connections which are not yet fully understood (Clark, 1938; Rioch, Wislocki and O'Leary, 1940; Nauta and Haymaker, 1969; Raisman, 1970). Its extent is poorly defined, but may be said roughly to comprise the lateral walls and base of the third ventricle below the level of the hypothalamic sulcus. The *rostral* boundary in man is a coronal plane passing anteriorly to the anterior commissure and the optic chiasma, whilst the *caudal* boundary is a coronal plane passing posteriorly to the mamillary bodies (Fig. 16.1). The *lateral* boundary is variable; at different coronal planes the following structures are found: the inferior border of the thalamus, the internal capsule, the globus pallidus, the ansa lenticularis and the optic tract. *Inferiorly*, the lower walls and the floor of the third ventricle form, in man, a funnel-like structure, the *infundibulum* or *tuber cinereum*, which is visible as a protuberance (the median eminence) on the base of the brain and is continuous with the *stalk* and *neural* (*posterior*) *lobe* of the pituitary gland. The infundibulum, pituitary stalk and neural lobe together make up the *neurohypophysis* (see Fig. 16.19). Hypophyseal terminology remains a subject for discussion (Everett, 1978).

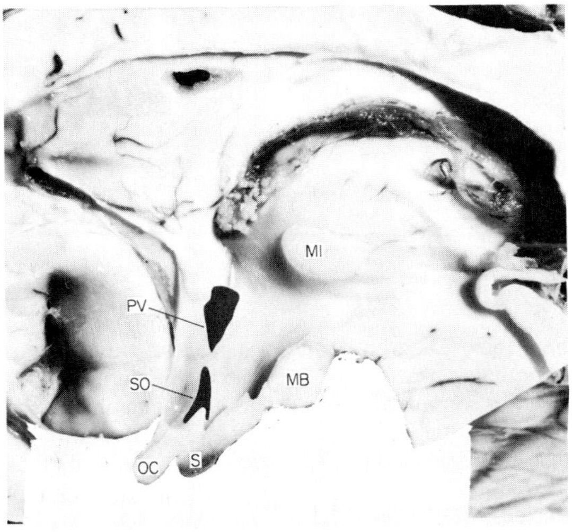

Fig. 16.1 View of the wall of the third ventricle, showing sites of supraoptic (SO) and paraventricular (PV) nuclei. MB, mamillary body; MI, massa intermedia; OC, optic chiasma; S, pituitary stalk.

Principal nuclei of the hypothalamus (Figs 16.2, 16.3)

The *supraoptic nucleus* is well defined and overlies the rostral extremity of the optic tract caudal to the optic chiasma; it tapers caudally for a considerable distance. The supraoptic neurons are large, with prominent eccentric nuclei which often have infoldings of the nuclear membrane and conspicuous nucleoli (Fig. 16.4). The Nissl substance is largely peripheral, the neurons having a clear central zone which resembles superficially central chromatolysis. The human supraoptic nucleus contains between 50 000 and 76 000 large cells (Rasmussen 1938; Maccubbin and van Buren, 1963; Morton, 1970).

The *paraventricular nucleus* lies adjacent to the ependymal lining of the third ventricle, parallel to the lateral wall and dorsal and caudal to the supraoptic nucleus; like the supraoptic nucleus it has a considerable anteroposterior extent. The large neurons, similar to those in the supraoptic nucleus, number from 30 000 to 54 000 (Maccubbin and van Buren, 1963) and are intermingled with many small neurons. The supraoptic and paraventricular nuclei are known as the *magnocellular neurosecretory nuclei* of the hypothalamus (see 'Hypothalamic neurosecretion', below).

Other hypothalamic nuclei are less clearly demarcated in the adult brain, but may be more prominent in the fetal brain. The *ventromedial and dorsomedial nuclei* are found between the tuber cinereum and the paraventricular nucleus, and are composed of small cells with poorly

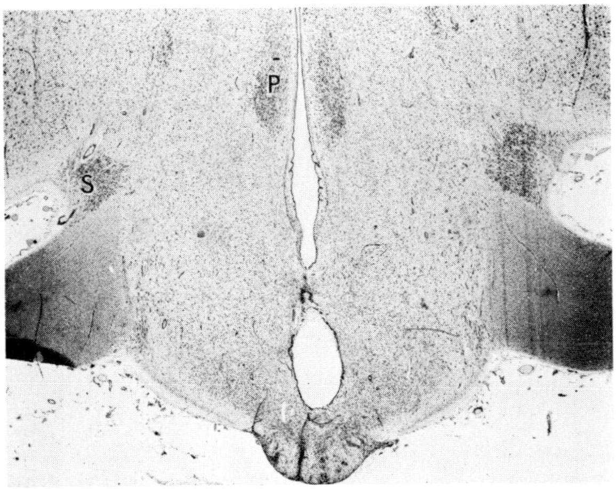

(a)

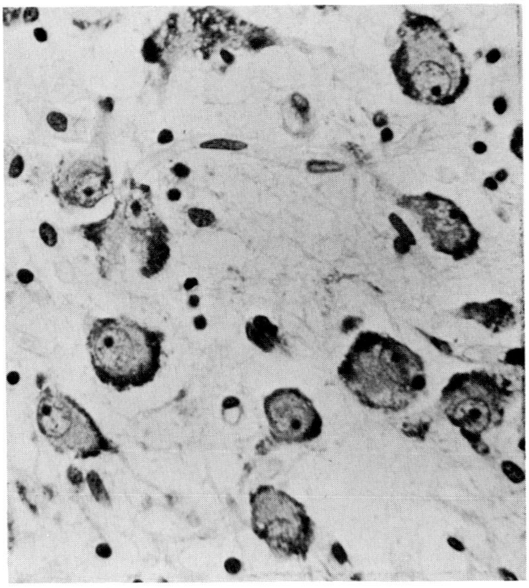

(b)

Fig. 16.2 (**a**) Coronal section through the hypothalamus, showing supraoptic (S) and paraventricular (P) nuclei. Luxol fast blue–cresyl violet × 6. (**b**) Cells of supraoptic nucleus, with eccentric nuclei and peripheral Nissl substance. Cresyl violet × 400.

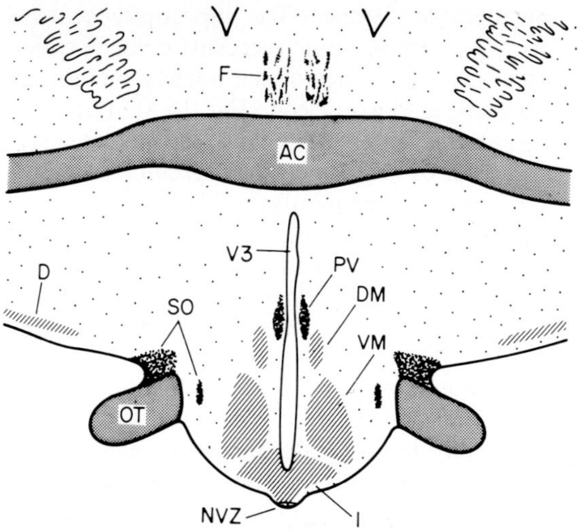

Fig. 16.3 Diagram of coronal section through the hypothalamus, to show the principal structures. AC, anterior commissure; D, nucleus of the diagonal band; DM, dorsomedial nucleus; F, fornix; I, infundibular (arcuate) nucleus; NVZ, neurovascular zone of the-median eminence; OT, optic tract; PV, paraventricular nucleus; SO, supraoptic nucleus; VM, ventromedial nucleus; V3, third ventricle.

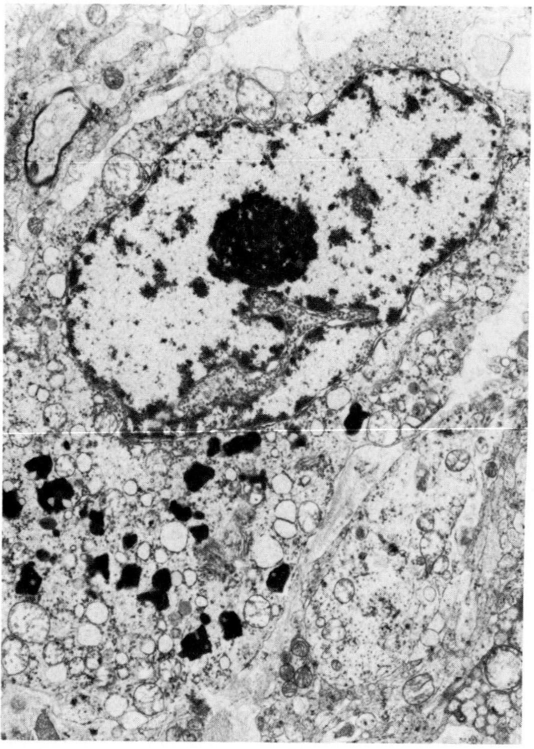

Fig. 16.4 Magnocellular neuron of the supraoptic nucleus. The nucleus is indented and the nucleolus is large. Little secretion is present in the cell. ×4590.

staining cytoplasm. The *arcuate* (*infundibular*) *nucleus* lies between the ventromedial nucleus and the base of the third ventricle. Neurons of the arcuate nucleus and the periventricular grey matter are called *parvicellular neurosecretory* cells, and the area in which they are found the *hypophysiotrophic area* (see 'Hypothalamic neurosecretion', below).

The poorly defined *posterior hypothalamic nucleus* lies above the *mamillary nuclei*, prominent nuclear masses surrounded by a capsule of myelinated nerve fibres. The mamillary nuclei are divided into a large medial and a small lateral portion, with a lateral and inferior *nucleus intercalatus* composed of larger, darker, angulated cells. In the lateral part of the hypothalamus are the poorly demarcated *lateral hypothalamic nucleus* (lateral to the fornix) and the inferiorly situated *tuberal nuclei*, present only in man. The *suprachiasmatic nuclei* are prominent in rodents.

Hypothalamic neurosecretion

There are two types of secretory neurons (transducer neurons) in the hypothalamus: large (magnocellular) in the supraoptic and paraventricular nuclei (Defendini and Zimmerman, 1978); and small (parvicellular), which have an uncertain distribution in the arcuate nucleus, tubero-infundibular area (hypophysiotrophic area) and preoptic area. Whereas the secretion of the magnocellular neurons can be identified by conventional histological staining, using Gömöri's chrome alum haematoxylin or aldehyde fuchsin, the parvicellular neurons can be identified as secretory only by electron microscopy or by specific immunological reactions, using immunofluorescence, or by immunohistochemical staining using horseradish peroxidase or similar techniques (Hökfelt et al., 1978). The secretions from the two types of cell, to which antibodies can be raised, differ in their function, although their structure is closely similar.

Magnocellular neurons synthesize the hormones *vasopressin* (*antidiuretic hormone*) and *oxytocin*; both are cyclic octapeptides and the cells are therefore called *peptidergic neurons*. It is probable that each nucleus produces both hormones, though the supraoptic nucleus produces more vasopressin and the paraventricular nucleus more oxytocin respectively. A single cell, however, can produce only one hormone. The cells also synthesize a carrier protein, *neurophysin*, which is bound to the peptide, and the secretion is transported in the form of membrane-bound granules by axoplasmic flow—seen by light microscopy as bead-like swellings (Fig. 16.5)—to the neural lobe where it is stored in the Hering bodies (accumulations of granules) and later released into the circulation.

Parvicellular neurons secrete substances which stimulate the trophic cells of the anterior lobe of the pituitary (pars distalis) to secrete and release their endocrine products—growth hormone (GH), thyrotrophic hormone (TSH), adrenocorticotrophic hormone (ACTH), luteinizing hormone (LH) and gonadotrophic hormone (GnH). Mammotrophic hormone or prolactin (PRL) differs in its control in that hypothalamic secretion *inhibits* rather than stimulates its production. The hypothalamic secretions that produce these effects are known as *releasing* (*or inhibiting*) *hormones* if their structure is known, or *releasing* (*or inhibiting*) *factors* if the structure is as yet unknown (McCann and Porter, 1969; Porter et al., 1973). So far, thyrotrophin-releasing hormone (TRH), luteinizing-hormone-releasing hormone (LHRH) and gonadotrophic-hormone-releasing hormone (GnHRH) and somatostatin (somatotrophin release-inhibiting factor, SRIF) have been isolated; all have a peptide structure of varying size. More recently, corticotrophin-releasing factor (CRF) has been synthesized (Sueiraz Diaz et al.; cited by Grossman et al., 1982) as a peptide with 41 amino acid residues. The secretions of parvicellular neurons are visible under the electron microscope as membrane-bound granules which travel down the axons of the cells to the median eminence, where they pass by exocytosis into the portal capillaries of the neurohaemal zone of the median eminence and are thereby conveyed to the adenohypophysis (see 'Blood supply of the hypothalamus and pituitary', below). The inhibition

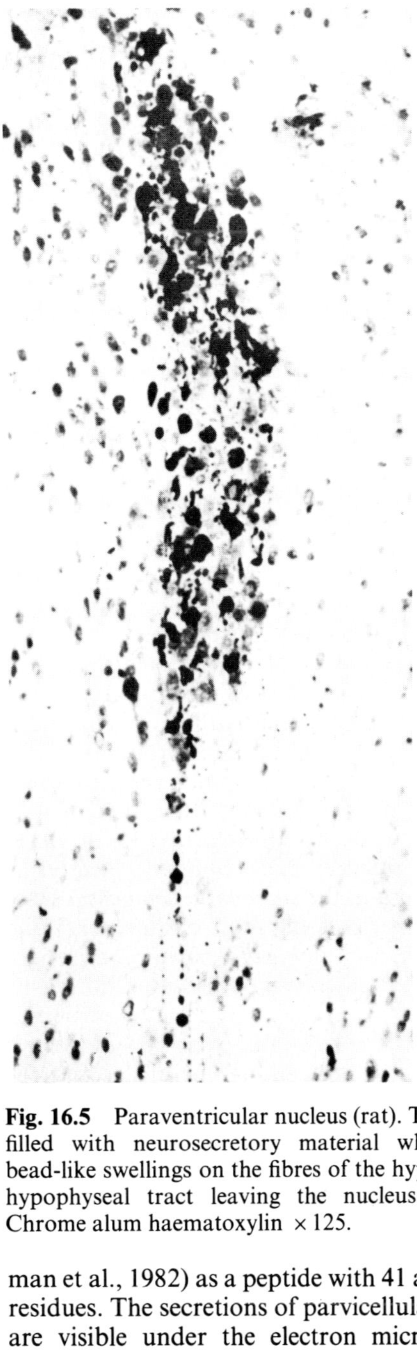

Fig. 16.5 Paraventricular nucleus (rat). The cells are filled with neurosecretory material which forms bead-like swellings on the fibres of the hypothalamo-hypophyseal tract leaving the nucleus inferiorly. Chrome alum haematoxylin ×125.

of prolactin by the hypothalamus seems to be effected by the arcuate nucleus, in which the neurons secrete dopamine (DA)—these neurons are therefore *aminergic* and not peptidergic. Control of the hypothalamic secretory neurons seems to be partly autonomous, partly by inputs from extrahypothalamic areas such as the limbic system, thalamus and midbrain, and partly by endocrine feedback (Hutchinson, 1978). Many neurotransmitters, such as adrenaline, noradrenaline, 5-hydroxytryptamine and dopamine, as well as acetylcholine and gamma-aminobutyric acid, appear to be involved in the transfer of stimuli to peptidergic neurons (Langevin and Iversen, 1980; Peters et al., 1982).

Principal connections of the hypothalamus

Hypothalamic neural pathways fall into two groups—myelinated and non-myelinated; some of the latter pathways are neurosecretory (Raisman, 1966). The most conspicuous myelinated tracts are the *fornix*, the *mamillothalamic tract* and the *anterior commissure* (see Fig. 16.3). The fornix is an afferent limbic pathway ending in the mamillary body which then projects to the anterior nucleus of the thalamus via the mamillothalamic tract and thence to the cingulate gyrus (Meyer, Beck and McLardy, 1947). Other myelinated tracts are the *mamillotegmental tract* to the midbrain, the *supraoptic commissures* (of which Meynert's is the most conspicuous) and the *medial forebrain bundle*, an important fibre system in the lateral hypothalamus not easily identified in man. The medial forebrain bundle receives fibres from the olfactory nuclei, the precommissural fornix, the septal nuclei and the midbrain reticular system; efferent fibres pass as short transverse fibres to many parts of the medial hypothalamus. The optic chiasma sends a *retinohypothalamic* projection to the suprachiasmatic nucleus.

Many fibres within the hypothalamus are *unmyelinated*, such as the subependymal *periventricular fibres*, which connect with the thalamus, and may interconnect the ventromedial and dorsomedial hypothalamic nuclei with other hypothalamic nuclei. The efferent fibres of the magnocellular neurosecretory nuclei are unmyelinated and form a combined tract passing down through the anterior part of the infundibulum into the pituitary stalk and thence to the neural lobe—the *tractus hypophyseus or hypothalamohypophyseal tract*. The tract is demonstrable by Gomori's method (see Fig 16.5). Its significance as a *peptidergic pathway* has been mentioned and is discussed further in this chapter in the section on diabetes insipidus.

The peptidergic and aminergic fibres of the parvicellular neurosecretory nuclei pass through the median eminence to release their secretions into the portal hypophyseal vessels. These diffusely scattered myelinated fibres are derived mainly from the periventricular fibres and arcuate nucleus (Szentágothai et al., 1968) and are known collectively as the *tuberoinfundibular tract*. The ependymal cells of the median eminence, known as tanycytes ('stretched' cells; Horstmann, 1954) may be considered as part of the connecting system of the hypothalamus in view of the theory (Knigge and Scott, 1970; Knigge et al., 1976) that hypothalamic hormones are secreted into the third ventricle, are absorbed at the ependymal surface of the tanycytes and pass through them to the portal capillaries of the neurohaemal zone by their long basal processes, which extend through the thickness of the median eminence (Millhouse, 1971).

Blood supply of the hypothalamus

The vascular supply of the hypothalamus derives from small arterial branches of the circle of Willis (Dawson, 1958; Daniel, 1966b). The finer vascular pattern resembles that seen elsewhere in the grey and white matter of the brain except in the magnocellular nuclei, which have a richer capillary supply than the other nuclei (Finley, 1940). The magnocellular neurons are closely apposed to the capillaries, which occasionally give the appearance of passing through the cell. The median eminence contains well-developed capillary loops, part of the neurohaemal contact system which is an extension of the hypophyseal portal system (Duvernoy, 1972).

Functions of the hypothalamus

Much of what is known about hypothalamic function has been gained from animal experiments, but an increasing amount is being derived from the study of normal physiology and pathological conditions in man (Besser, 1974). The hypothalamus is placed at the centre of the *limbic system* with which it has connections through the mamillary bodies and preoptic area, and of which it is a major efferent path (Guyton, 1981). The functions of the hypothalamus may therefore be divided roughly into *endocrine*, through the neurosecretory pathway, and *vegetative*, through the limbic pathways.

Control of endocrine activity

Neurohypophysis The neurohypophyseal hormones *vasopressin* and *oxytoxin* are formed in the magnocellular secretory nuclei and pass down the hypothalamohypophyseal tract to be stored in the neurohypophysis. Vasopressin (antidiuretic hormone) controls water balance by inducing reabsorption of water by the renal tubules. The neurosecretory cells are stimulated by a rising concentration of body fluid electrolytes, mainly sodium. The sensitive neurons are therefore acting as *osmosodium receptors* (Jewell and Verney, 1957). Oxytocin produces uterine contraction and also milk ejection, the latter being induced by sensory stimuli (suckling) from the nipple.

Adenohypophysis (pars distalis) The production of the adenohypophyseal hormones referred to above is triggered by the arrival in the adenohypophysis, via the portal hypophyseal system, of the various hypothalamic releasing factors or hormones which stimulate (or inhibit) the appropriate trophic cells (McCann and Porter, 1969). Some of these hypophysiotrophic peptides have been isolated from the hypothalamus and synthesized, and their presence in hypophyseal portal blood has been demonstrated. The earlier evidence for hypothalamic neurohumoral control of adenohypophyseal function is summarized by Harris (1955), a pioneer in the field; more recent reviews of the subject are those by Blackwell and Guillemin (1973), Porter et al. (1973), and Jeffcoate and Hutchinson (1978). The hypothalamic areas which control specific adenohypophyseal secretion are poorly delineated but may be described approximately as follows: anterior hypothalamus—thyrotrophic hormone and luteinizing hormone; median eminence—adrenocorticotrophic hormone, follicle-stimulating hormone (FSH); arcuate nucleus—prolactin inhibition by dopamine; posterior hypothalamus—adrenocorticotrophic hormone; ventromedial nucleus and medial basal hypothalamus—growth hormone.

Control of vegetative functions

Feeding Stimulation of the lateral hypothalamic area causes hyperphagia and obesity, as does destruction of the ventromedial nucleus (Kennedy, 1966). Conversely, stimulation of the ventromedial nucleus (the satiety centre) causes abolition of appetite, as does destruction of the lateral hypothalamic area. Obesity in patients with tumours or other lesions of the hypothalamus is well known, although precise location of such lesions is rarely possible by the time the patient comes to necropsy. In the case of hyperphagia described by Reeves and Plum (1969), however, there was localized destruction of the ventromedial hypothalamus by a hamartoma.

The *diencephalic syndrome* of infancy, in which the ventromedial hypothalamus is destroyed by a neoplasm (Fig. 16.6), paradoxically produces wasting despite the child's having a good appe-

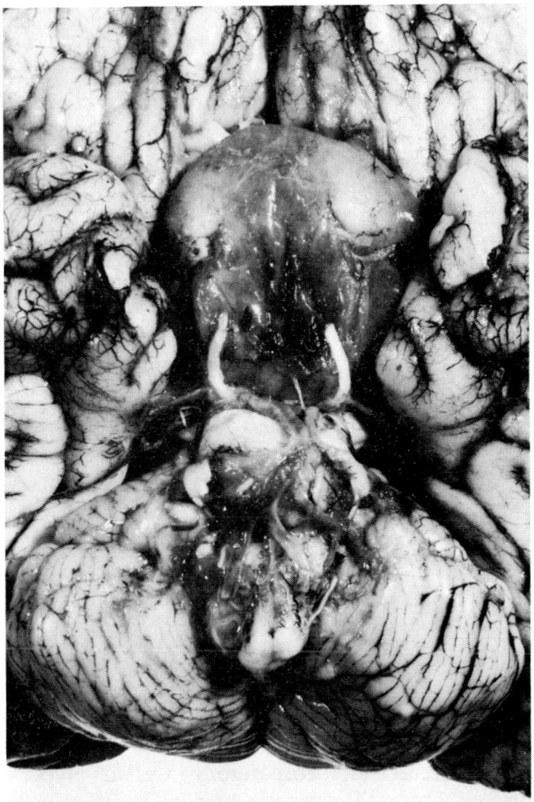

Fig. 16.6 The hypothalamus of a young child, replaced by a large pilocytic astrocytoma. This resulted in the diencephalic syndrome.

tite (Russell, 1951; Braun and Forney, 1959). Plum and van Uitert (1978) have suggested that the mechanisms of metabolic control in the immature hypothalamus differ from those in the adult brain. Kamalian, Keesey and ZuRhein (1975), commenting on a case of cachexia associated with demyelination of the lateral hypothalamus by multiple sclerosis, have suggested that widespread hypothalamic disease has to be present for aphagia to occur.

Drinking Apart from the magnocellular nuclei, which control the absorption and excretion of water, a thirst centre with osmosodium receptors exists in the lateral hypothalamus, as adipsia occurs after lesions of this area. Fitzsimons (1966, 1972) proposed that the limbic system as well as the hypothalamus is involved in the control of drinking. Most human cases of abnormal thirst of central nervous origin are associated with abnormalities of the magnocellular secretory system and pathway (see 'Diabetes insipidus', later in this chapter).

Control of body temperature There are thermosensitive neurons in the anterior (preoptic) hypothalamus which increase their rate of firing in response to a rise in local blood temperature (Hardy, Hellon and Sutherland, 1964). Thermoregulatory disturbances in man may occur with lesions within and around the third ventricle.

Cardiovascular regulation In experimental animals vasodilatation can be produced in skeletal muscle by stimulation of the hypothalamus (Abrahams, Hilton and Zbrozyna, 1964), but other cardiovascular responses—such as an increase of 25–100 per cent in cerebral blood flow—can be elicited by hypothalamic stimulation (Hilton, 1966). The efferent path is through the reticular substance of the medulla and pons.

Behaviour and affect Complex behavioural and emotional patterns may result from experimental stimulation or lesions of certain hypothalamic areas. Bilateral ventromedial lesions may produce hyperactivity and rage as well as hyperphagia. Lateral lesions produce passivity as well as aphagia. Stimulation of the medial forebrain bundle, and of the lateral and ventromedial nuclei produces feelings of 'reward'. When the periventricular grey matter is stimulated, feelings of 'punishment' are elicited; when the stimulus is strong, a rage pattern is produced. Neurohypophyseal hormones seem to be involved in cognition, and patients with cranial diabetes insipidus may have deficits in attention, concentration and memory (de Wied, 1980).

Diseases of the hypothalamus

Congenital malformations

Hamartoma Hamartomas are not uncommon in the hypothalamus, and usually take the form of nodules either attached by a pedicle to the tuber cinereum or the mamillary bodies or merging with these structures (Fig. 16.7). They rarely

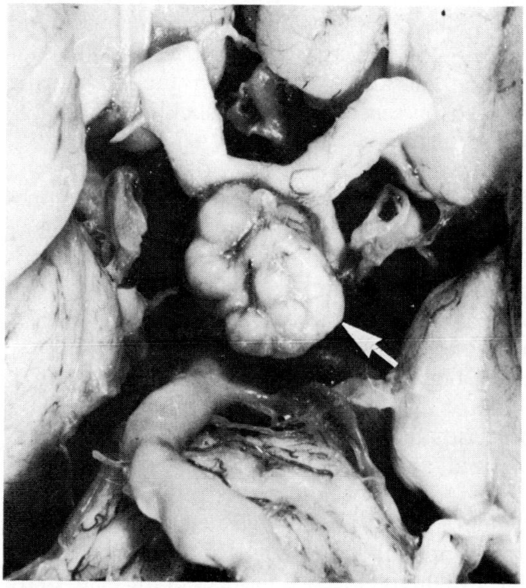

Fig. 16.7 Hamartoma (arrow) involving the tuber cinereum and hypothalamus.

reach a diameter of more than 1 cm but they may be much larger (Lange-Cosack, 1951, 1952). The pituitary gland is usually, but not invariably, normal (Asa et al., 1980). Other malformations (such as polydactyly) may be present, as in the Pallister–Hall syndrome (Haas et al., 1980; Huff and Fernandes, 1982). The histological pattern is one of groups of small cells (Schmidt, Hallervorden and Spatz, 1958) scattered in a haphazard fashion through glial tissue in which there may be myelinated nerve fibres (Fig. 16.8). Ependymal rests may be present. Other varieties of

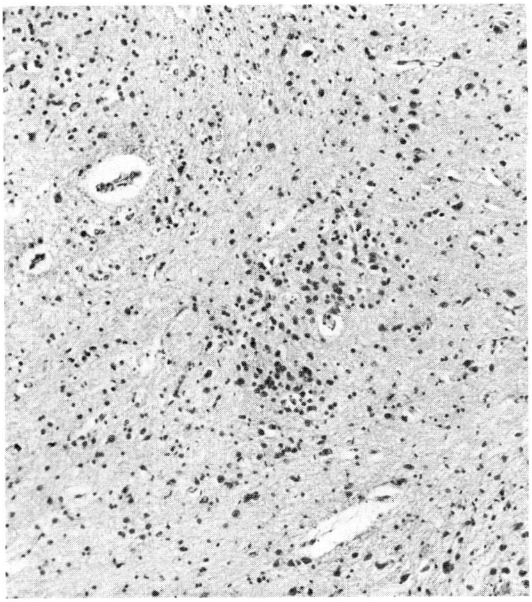

Fig. 16.8 Groups of small, uniform cells in a hypothalamic hamartoma. Haematoxylin and eosin ×80.

hamartoma may be lipomatous (Orthner, 1961, case 13), osteolipomatous (Friede, 1977) or of the type associated with tuberous sclerosis (Krabbe, 1922).

Clinical interest in these lesions, which may be found incidentally at necropsy, arises when they are associated with endocrine dysfunction, most commonly *precocious puberty* (le Marquand and Russell, 1934–35; Weinberger and Grant, 1941; Lange-Cosack, 1951, 1952; Northfield and Russell, 1967). Gonadotrophic secretion is normally subject to hypothalamic inhibition before puberty (Donovan and van der Werff ten Bosch, 1965; Critchlow and Bar-Sela, 1967). Experimental damage to the rostral hypothalamus can advance puberty by reduction of inhibition; in the same way the presence of a hamartoma, though at a different site, may have the same effect.

Inflammatory conditions involving the hypothalamus

Acute infections Hypothalamic hypopituitarism may follow acute viral meningoencephalitis (Glanzmann and Wegelin, 1942; Levy and Notkins, 1971; Kupari, Pelkonen and Valtonen, 1980; Lichtenstein, Tilley and Sandler, 1982), but few reports have been published of the structural changes in the hypothalamus in such patients. Baker, Cornwell and Brown (1952) described inflammation of the supraoptic and other hypothalamic nuclei in poliomyelitis. Lipsett, Dreifuss and Thomas (1962) found lymphocytic infiltration of the supraoptic nuclei and tuber cinereum in a patient with hypothalamic obesity and hypothyroidism following varicella. As a time lapse is necessary for the development of endocrine symptoms (other than diabetes insipidus), the state of the hypothalamus at the onset of the disease in such cases cannot be ascertained.

Chronic inflammatory disease of the hypothalamus There are many causes of such disease (Orthner, 1961): giant cell granuloma (Rickards and Harvey, 1954), sarcoidosis (Kraemer and Paarmann, 1956; Scadding, 1967), syphilis, tuberculosis (Smith and Daniel, 1947), cryptococcal infection, non-lipid reticuloendotheliosis (Hewer and Heller, 1949), Hand–Schüller–Christian disease, and the granuloma localized to the neurohypophysis and floor of the third ventricle (Gagel, 1941) which has been identified with histiocytosis X (Kepes and Kepes, 1969; Schneider and Güthert, 1975). The lesions may be localized or spread throughout the hypothalamohypo-

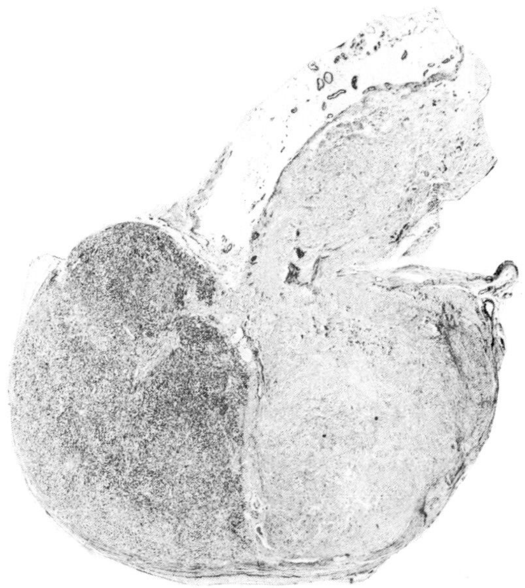

Fig. 16.9 Gagel type of granuloma. Sagittal section of the pituitary showing enlargement of the stalk and posterior lobe (right of picture) by granulomatous infiltration. Haematoxylin and eosin ×5.5.

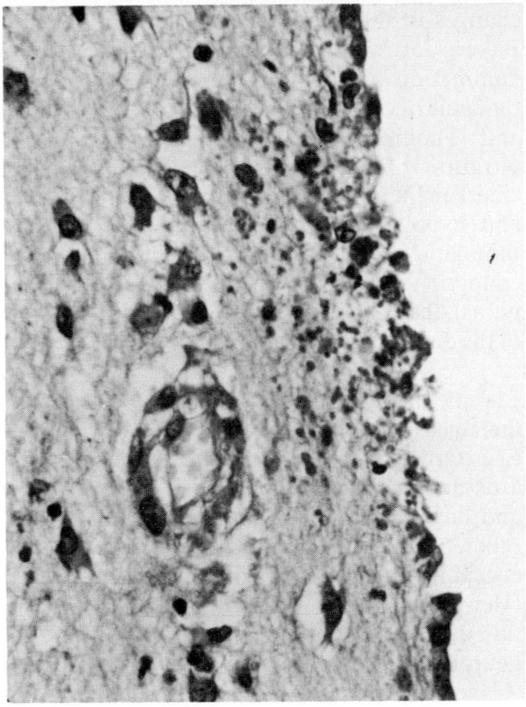

Fig. 16.10 Toxoplasmosis involving the ependyma of the third ventricle, adjacent to the paraventricular nucleus. Haematoxylin and eosin ×480.

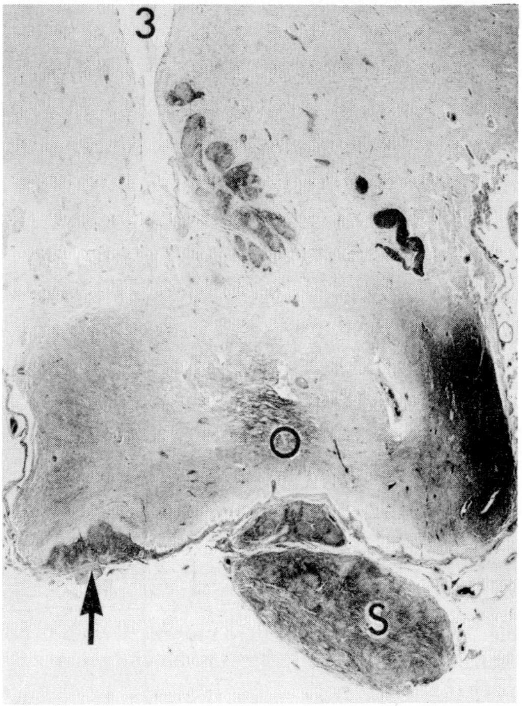

Fig. 16.11 Coronal section of the hypothalamus in a case of sarcoidosis. The pituitary stalk (S) is replaced and expanded by granuloma. A small granulomatous plaque (arrow) is present on the inferior surface of the optic chiasma (O) and other foci are present to the right of the lower part of the third ventricle (3). Luxol fast blue–cresyl violet ×6.5.

physeal system (including the pars distalis). Spread may occur through the portal vessels or via the systemic circulation (Wilke, 1956). Rarely, suppuration may spread directly to the pituitary and hypothalamus from the accessory sinuses (Mohr, 1975). The aetiology of granulomatous lesions may be obscure and not traceable to a micro-organism. The hypothalamus may be less involved than the neurohypophysis and pituitary stalk in the Gagel type of granuloma (Fig. 16.9). In this condition lymphocytes and plasma cells, but not giant cells, are found. Permanent diabetes insipidus may result from involvement of the magnocellular nuclei. The possibility of an autoimmune pathogenesis should be considered (see 'Lymphocytic and autoimmune hypophysitis' later in this chapter). Specific chronic infections of the central nervous system may involve the hypothalamus; for example, *toxoplasmosis* in the immunologically compromised patient may produce ependymal lesions in the ventricles (Fig. 16.10), infiltrate the hypothalamus and spread to the anterior lobe of the pituitary. *Sarcoidosis* usually has a leptomeningeal predilection, but may spread into the adjacent brain, tracking along blood vessels (Wilke, 1956); diabetes insipidus is the commonest symptom (Rickards and Harvey, 1954). A personally observed case, a man aged 33 years, suffered from both diabetes insipidus and panhypopituitarism for 3.5 years. Sarcoid granulomas were present in the major hypothalamic nuclei, the pituitary stalk and both lobes of the pituitary gland (Fig. 16.11). Vascular involvement was a striking feature of this case (Fig. 16.12).

Vascular lesions of the hypothalamus

Vascular lesions in the hypothalamus usually occur only in association with more generalized cerebrovascular disease or a stroke, such as intracerebral or, more commonly, subarachnoid haemorrhage. Crompton (1963) described hypothalamic lesions associated with the rupture of intracranial aneurysms. He found lesions in the hypothalamus in about 60 per cent of

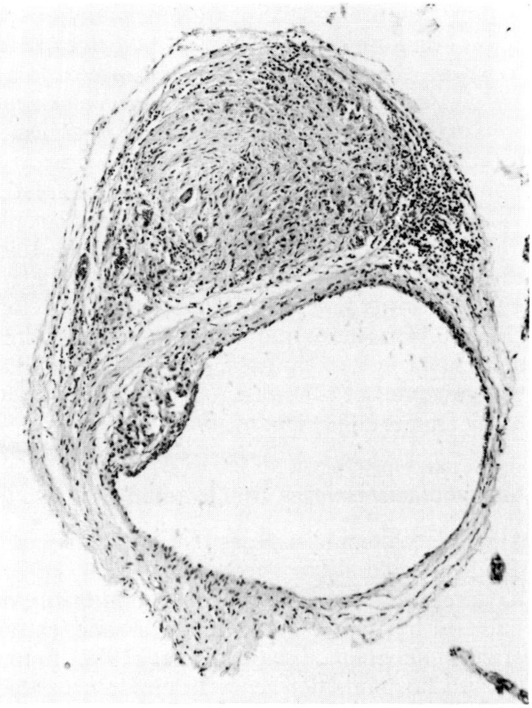

Fig. 16.12 Sarcoidosis involving a meningeal vessel. There is granulomatous infiltration of the medial and intimal coats of a small artery in the hypothalamic area. Haematoxylin and eosin ×75.

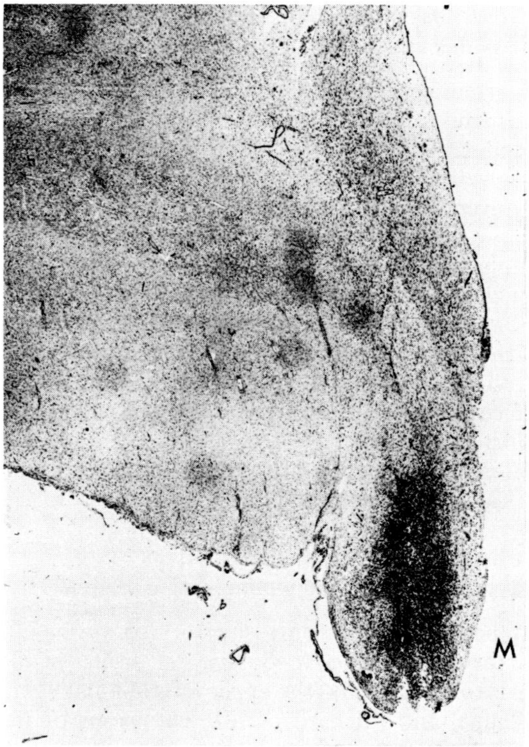

Fig. 16.13 Wernicke's encephalopathy. There are haemorrhages in the mamillary body (M). Haematoxylin and eosin ×5.

patients, most often in those with aneurysms of the anterior and posterior communicating arteries. Areas of ischaemic necrosis (up to 5 mm across) were the commonest finding and were accompanied by infarcts elsewhere in the brain. Small haemorrhages were also seen, often in the paraventricular and supraoptic nuclei; occasionally the haemorrhages became confluent and destroyed the nuclei, but such large destructive haemorrhages were not common. Crompton considered that the haemorrhages had been caused by venous back-pressure produced by bleeding into the chiasmatic cistern. Similar infarcts and haemorrhages may occur in head injury (Fig. 16.30b).

Petechial haemorrhages of the 'ring' and 'ball' types are typically seen in Wernicke's encephalopathy, most commonly in the mamillary bodies (Fig. 16.13) but also throughout the hypothalamic periventricular grey matter. The pathogenesis of these haemorrhages is obscure.

Septic emboli may occasionally involve the hypothalamus and cause infarction (Fig. 16.14). Fat emboli may be found in cases of fracture of long bones (Sevitt, 1971, personal communication). Traumatic lesions of the hypothalamus are mainly of a vascular nature and will be considered together with traumatic lesions of the pituitary (see p. 767).

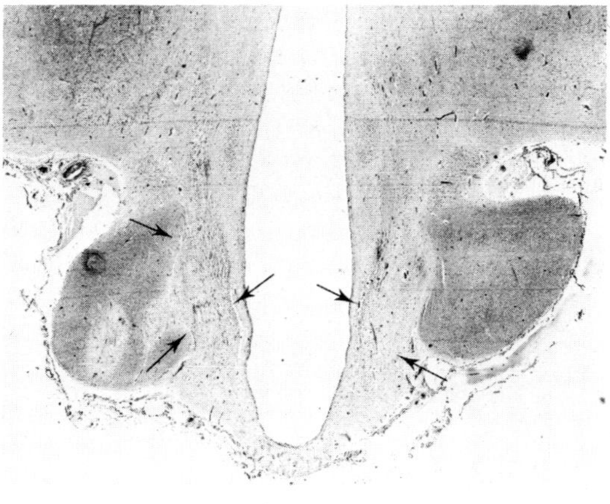

Fig. 16.14 Widespread infarction of the inferior hypothalamus (arrows) and optic tract, caused by septic emboli. Haematoxylin and eosin ×6.

Miscellaneous conditions affecting the hypothalamus

Certain generalized diseases of the nervous system may involve the hypothalamus and produce endocrine or hypothalamic symptoms; such involvement is analogous to hypothalamic involvement by inflammatory disease. Scrapie, a slow virus infection of sheep, occasionally involves the supraoptic and paraventricular nuclei, which results in clinical diabetes insipidus (Beck, Daniel and Parry, 1964). Demyelination of the lateral hypothalamus in multiple sclerosis has resulted in aphagia and cachexia (Kamalian, Keesey and ZuRhein, 1975), and Lewy neuronal inclusion bodies have been found in the hypothalamic nuclei of patients with parkinsonism (Langston and Forno, 1978).

Changes in the hypothalamus after hypophysectomy and pituitary stalk section

When hypophysectomy is performed, or the pituitary stalk cut, a venous infarct occurs in the proximal cut stalk (the upper infundibular stem; Daniel and Prichard, 1972). The axons of the supraopticohypophyseal tract are severed and, within 2 months of the operation, many of the cells of the supraoptic nucleus, which give rise to most of the severed axons, disappear (Fig. 16.15). A smaller number of magnocellular neurons in the paraventricular nucleus are lost (Daniel and Prichard, 1975). Neurosecretory material is increased in the surviving neurons and greatly increased in the tuber cinereum and in the stalk above the level of transection, suggesting that there is a damming back of secretion (Muller, 1955). Fibrous gliosis of the nucleus may develop (Fig. 16.16). The supraopticohypophyseal fibres show some evidence of regeneration in man, but to a much lesser extent than in animals (Sloper, 1966; Daniel and Prichard, 1975).

Hypothalamic changes after irradiation

The hypothalamus is sensitive to therapeutic doses of irradiation. Perry-Keene et al. (1976) have reported hypothalamic hypopituitarism in patients irradiated for both intra- and extracranial malignant disease. Shalet (1982) found growth hormone deficiency in children treated by therapeutic irradiation for brain tumours and by prophylactic irradiation of the neuraxis for

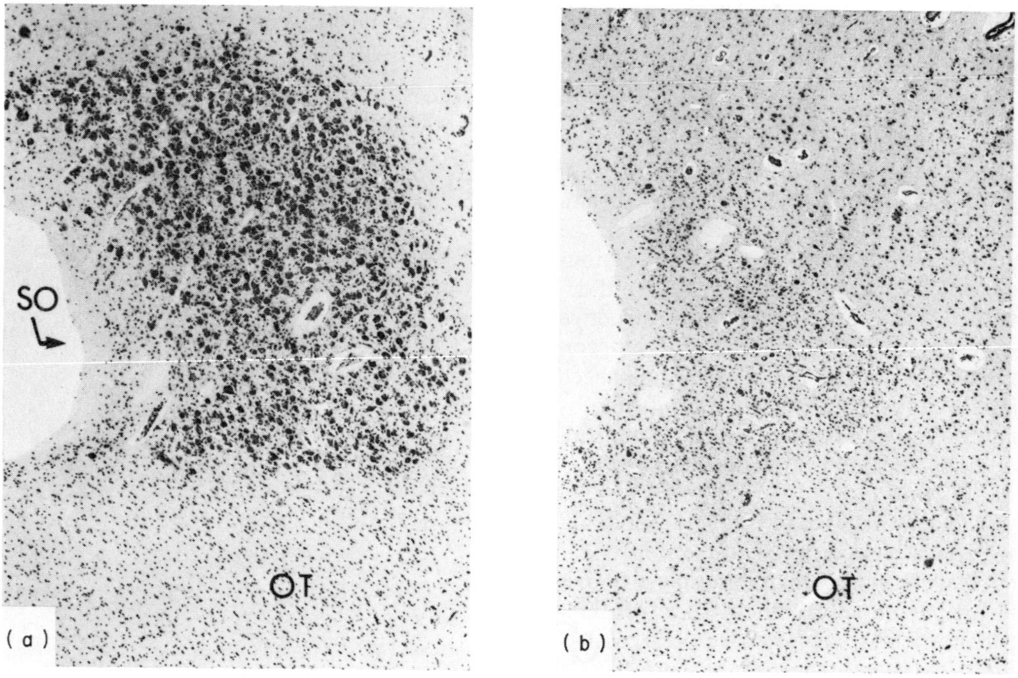

Fig. 16.15 (**a**) Coronal section of the normal supraoptic nucleus (SO). OT, optic tract. (**b**) Supraoptic nucleus 4 months after hypophysectomy, showing almost total loss of neurons and shrinkage of the nucleus. Cresyl violet ×40.

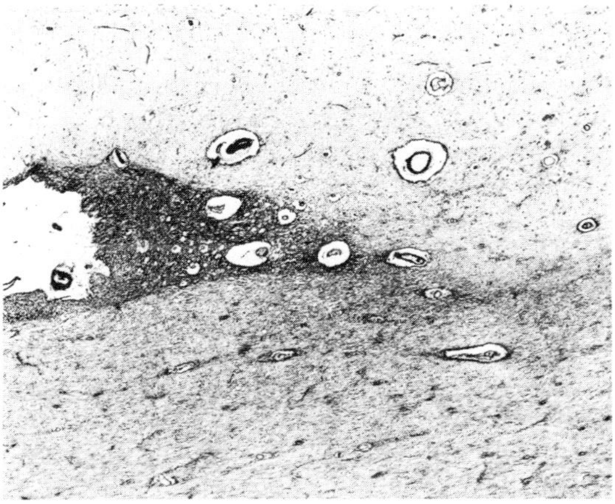

Fig. 16.16 Supraoptic nucleus 10 months after hypophysectomy. The entire nucleus is gliotic. The neurons have disappeared. The optic tract lies inferiorly. Holzer ×30.

acute lymphoblastic leukaemia, and considered the hypothalamus to be the major site of damage. Hypothalamic damage may occur when ablation of the pituitary by implantation of yttrium-90 is attempted. Accidental damage may result from displacement of radioactive implants into the third ventricle (Fig. 16.17). The lesions in the hypothalamus range from some loss of neurons (including those of the supraoptic nucleus), occasional glial stars and cuffing of vessels with round cells, to necrosis of considerable areas. Crompton and Layton (1961) found astrocytic reaction in the surviving tissue around the necrotic areas.

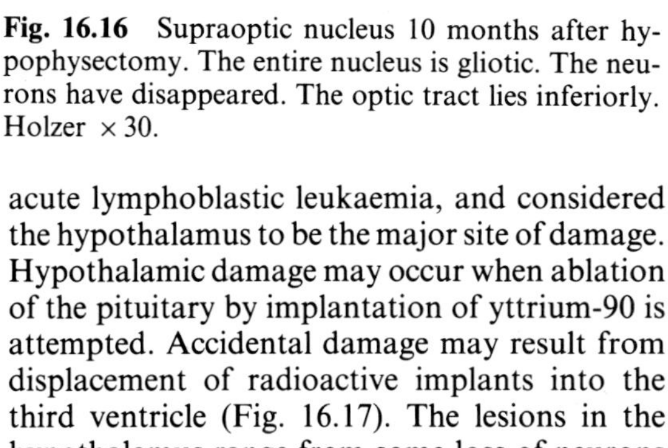

Fig. 16.17 Necrosis and gliosis of the walls of the third ventricle caused by the accidental displacement of a needle of yttrium-90 into the ventricular cavity. Haematoxylin and eosin ×4.

Diabetes insipidus

Diabetes insipidus may be defined as polydipsia and polyuria occurring as the result either of failure of production by the magnocellular secretory nuclei of the antidiuretic hormone arginine vasopressin—cranial diabetes insipidus—or of failure of the normal renal tubular absorptive response to vasopressin—nephrogenic diabetes insipidus. Antibodies to vasopressin in human patients treated with vasopressin are of low titre and affinity (Edwards, 1975). More recently autoantibodies to hypothalamic vasopressin-producing cells have been found in patients with idiopathic diabetes insipidus (Scherbaum and Bottazzo, 1983). Only the cranial form of diabetes insipidus is considered in this chapter.

Pathogenesis of cranial diabetes insipidus Three principal mechanisms may operate to produce cranial diabetes insipidus:

1. *Primary failure of production of vasopressin.* Such failure may occur as the result either of defective function of the magnocellular secretory neurons or of primary absence or atrophy of these cells. Both mechanisms appear to operate, but in different mammalian species. Rats with familial hypothalamic diabetes insipidus (the Brattleboro' strain of Long-Evans hooded rats), first described by Valtin and Schroeder (1964), have a normal complement of magnocellular neurons but they cannot, however, synthesize vasopressin (Valtin, 1967). The trait is autosomal recessive and could be the product of an enzyme deficit. A study of vasopressin function in human familial cranial diabetes insipidus by Baylis and Robertson (1981) showed that small increases of vasopressin could be produced by osmotic or non-osmotic stimuli, suggesting that vasopressin-synthesizing neurons were present but were few or degenerate.

2. *Failure of the osmoreceptor response in the thirst centre of the preoptic hypothalamus.* Spontaneous isolated lesions causing such failure have not, as far as the author is aware, been demonstrated in man.

3. *Destruction of the magnocellular neurosecretory nuclei or axons, or interruption of the neurosecretory pathway to the neurohypophysis.* Fisher, Ingram and Ransom (1938) were able to produce permanent diabetes insipidus in dogs by stereotaxic destruction of both supraoptic nuclei, thus demonstrating that the supraoptic nucleus

is the principal source of vasopressin. Such isolated bilateral destructive lesions are found only rarely in man; diffuse lesions are more likely to occur. Interruption of the neurosecretory pathway is a common cause of diabetes insipidus in man; the lesion may be found at several levels—in the infundibulum, the pituitary stalk, or the neurohypophysis—at which the final common path of neurosecretion is blocked, and release of vasopressin into the circulation is prevented (Fig. 16.18). If the neurosecretory axons are severed at a point at which retrograde atrophy and disappearance of the neurosecretory perikarya occurs, diabetes insipidus will be permanent (see Fig. 16.15). More frequently, it is temporary, either because damage to the neurosecretory neurons or path is transient or because axons of surviving neurosecretory neurons are able to regenerate to some extent and transmit their secretion to the circulation even if the neurohypophysis is absent (Daniel and Prichard, 1975). This form of cranial diabetes insipidus is known as the secondary form.

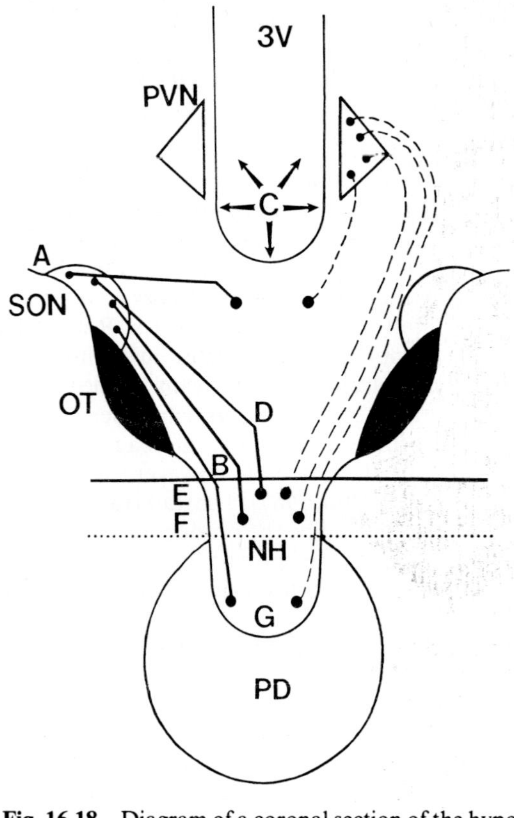

Fig. 16.18 Diagram of a coronal section of the hypothalamus to illustrate the pathogenesis of diabetes insipidus. The positions of various lesions which could interrupt magnocellular neurosecretion are shown (A–G). A, supraoptic nucleus; B, hypothalamohypophyseal tract; C, third ventricle; D, median eminence; E, high pituitary stalk section (solid line); F, low pituitary stalk section (dotted line); G, lower infundibular stem (posterior lobe); NH, posterior lobe; OT, optic tract; PD, pars distalis (anterior lobe); PVN, paraventricular nucleus; SON, supraoptic nucleus; 3V, third ventricle.

Pathology of cranial diabetes insipidus *Familial* This is very rare (Forssman, 1945); according to Baylis and Robertson (1981) only 1 per cent of all cases are familial. The condition may be isolated (DI), or may occur in association with other disabilities such as diabetes mellitus (DM), optic atrophy (OA), deafness (D)—Wolfram's syndrome or the DIDMOAD syndrome (Page, Asmal and Edwards, 1976; Cremers, Wijdeveld and Pinckers, 1977)—and with Friedreich's ataxia. Isolated diabetes insipidus is inherited as an autosomal dominant, whereas inheritance of the DIDMOAD syndrome is autosomal recessive. Few autopsy reports have been recorded of isolated familial cranial diabetes insipidus (Gaupp, 1941; Braverman, Mancini and McGoldrick, 1965; Green et al., 1967). All reports agree that there is a reduction in the number of magnocellular neurons, with an accompanying gliosis, affecting the supraoptic nucleus more severely than the paraventricular. The neurohypophysis may be small. In the necropsy reported on one case of DIDMOAD syndrome (Cremers, Wijdeveld and Pinckers, 1977) the pituitary and hypothalamus were said to be normal, but a precise description of the state of the supraoptic nucleus was not given.

Idiopathic cranial diabetes insipidus Edwards (1975) gives an incidence of 12.2 per cent (5 out of 41 cases). The pathological changes are similar to those found in the isolated familial type of the disease.

Secondary cranial diabetes insipidus Edwards (1975) gives the incidence as 72 per cent of all his cases. Many different causes of secondary cranial diabetes insipidus have been recorded. The incidence of the various causes may have changed during the past 50 years, if the series of Fink (1928) and of Edwards (1975) are compared (Table 16.1).

Table 16.1 Causes of secondary cranial diabetes insipidus

Aetiology	1928 (Fink) (%)	1975 (Edwards) (%)
Head injury	10	5
Neurosurgery		29
Tumours (total)	64	26
Primary		19
Secondary		7
Histiocytosis X		10
Tuberculosis	5	2
Syphilis	13	
Other inflammations	8	

Edwards' series is small (41 patients) in comparison with Fink's (107 cases collected from the literature) but certain trends may nevertheless be seen; for example, the increase of postsurgical cranial diabetes insipidus and the decline of syphilis as a cause. Histiocytosis X, a relatively modern concept, may account for some of the 'other inflammations' in Fink's series. Sarcoidosis is a well-known cause of cranial diabetes insipidus, as is metastatic tumour in the neurohypophysis. The mode of action of the lesions varies; there may be diffuse inflammatory or neoplastic infiltration involving the whole infundibulum, including the magnocellular nuclei, but without neurohypophyseal involvement (a rare event); similar lesions may involve the hypothalamus and neurohypophysis together (as in the case of sarcoidosis reported on p. 756); or there may be a traumatic rupture of the pituitary stalk or a metastatic tumour within the stalk, interrupting the neurosecretory path and causing retrograde atrophy of the supraoptic nuclei—only if such atrophy takes place will permanent diabetes insipidus ensue (see Fig. 16.15). Dense gliosis of the supraoptic nucleus may occur in such cases (see Fig 16.16).

Lesions of parvicellular neurons

There is as yet little morphological evidence of primary disorders of hypothalamic neurons producing endocrine effects. Hirabayashi et al. (1979) have described hypertrophy of neurons of the arcuate nucleus in patients in which the pituitary gland was destroyed by tumour, but this was presumably a secondary effect. Cerebral gigantism with mental retardation (Sotos' syndrome) has a familial background and is probably a genetic disorder; in a case which came to necropsy (Sugarman, Heuser and Reed, 1977) no abnormality was found in the hypothalamus.

The pituitary gland

Anatomy

The pituitary gland lies within the sella turcica (pituitary fossa) which is lined by dura; because the human sella has a dural roof (diaphragma sellae), the gland is completely enclosed. Considerable variation in the morphology of the sella is, however, possible (Busch, 1951). The pituitary stalk passes through the diaphragma sellae, which tethers the gland in the sella and may thus render the stalk more vulnerable to traction, either traumatic or surgical. The adult human gland is about 15 mm in transverse diameter and weighs from 0.5 to 0.9 g (Doniach, 1977). The gland is heavier in females and increases in weight during pregnancy. The sphenoid sinus lies below and anterior to the sella, the anterior clinoid processes lie above and anteriorly, and the posterior clinoid processes lie posteriorly. The lateral walls of the sella are formed by the cavernous sinuses and the structures passing through them. The pituitary stalk is continuous with the tuber cinereum and is surrounded by the basal cisterns of the subarachnoid space.

The nomenclature of Rioch, Wislocki and O'Leary (1940) is used to describe the constituent parts of the pituitary gland (Fig. 16.19). In the fetus a neural downgrowth from the brain forms the median eminence, the upper and lower infundibular stem (pituitary stalk) and the infundibular process (posterior lobe); the pituitary stalk and posterior lobe together form the *neurohypophysis.* An epithelial upgrowth from the pharynx gives rise, from its rostral wall, to the *pars distalis* (anterior lobe) or *adenohypophysis.* A caudal pharyngeal outgrowth gives rise to the *pars in-*

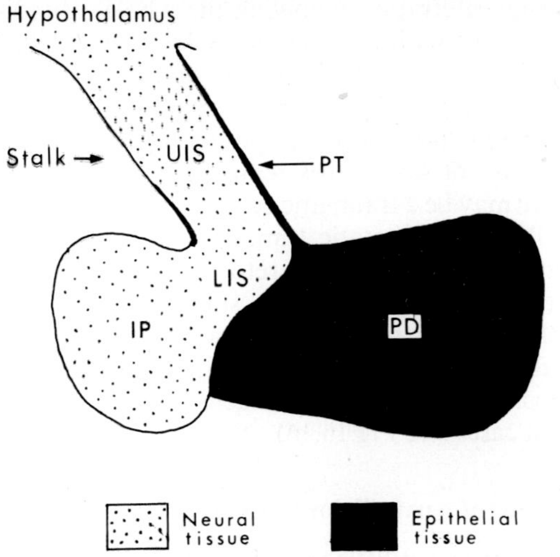

Fig. 16.19 Diagram of the anatomical subdivisions of the pituitary gland. Black: adenohypophysis. Stippled: neurohypophysis. IP, infundibular process (posterior lobe); LIS, lower infundibular stem; PD, pars distalis (anterior lobe); PT, pars tuberalis; UIS, upper infundibular stem.

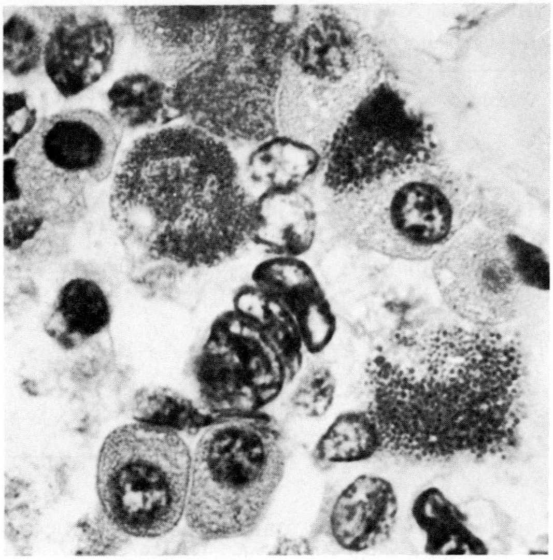

Fig. 16.20 Normal adenohypophysis. Four basophil cells (dark) containing granules of different sizes. The lightly staining granulated cells are acidophils. Thin section (resin-embedded; 1 μm). Haematoxylin and eosin × 700.

termedia, which is not readily identifiable in man. A thin layer of cells of the pars distalis projects upwards around the stalk as far as the inferior surface of the median eminence to form the *pars tuberalis*.

Adenohypophysis (pars distalis)

The pars distalis is composed of epithelial glandular cells, sometimes arranged in an acinar manner, supported by a framework of reticulin and permeated by vascular sinusoids. Colloid material may be seen in the acinar lumina. In the simplest histological terms, three principal cell types are found with haematoxylin and eosin staining: acidophil, basophil and chromophobe (Romeis, 1940). Acidophil cells are more numerous in the posterolateral part of the lobe; they are typically large cells with abundant cytoplasm containing a variable number of coarse acidophil granules. Basophil cells are more numerous in the anteromedial part of the lobe (though both cell types are found scattered throughout the adenohypophysis). The cytoplasm of basophils contains haematoxophil granules which vary considerably in size as well as in number. The variation in size can be seen in resin-embedded sections 1–2 μm thick examined with an oil-immersion lens (Fig. 16.20). The cytoplasm of chromophobe cells, which make up at least half of the adenohypophyseal population, has no special tinctorial affinity; under the light microscope their cytoplasm appears to contain few or no granules.

Functional differentiation of adenohypophyseal cells The knowledge that the three cell types of the adenohypophysis secrete at least six hormones (growth hormone, prolactin, adrenocorticotrophic hormone, follicle-stimulating hormone, luteinizing hormone and thyrotrophic hormone) has made the functional differentiation of these cells a major problem for histologists for many years (Purves, 1966). Various classifications have been proposed, representing different attempts, using histological or histochemical methods to correlate cell type with secretion (Romeis, 1940; Ezrin and Murray, 1963; Conklin, 1968). For accurate histochemical identification it is necessary to obtain tissue within 3 hours of death; this requirement can rarely be fulfilled with human material. The principal techniques available for the differentiation of cell types are:

1. *Histological staining*—haematoxylin and eosin; Mallory's trichrome (Mallory, 1900).
2. *Histochemical staining*—periodic acid

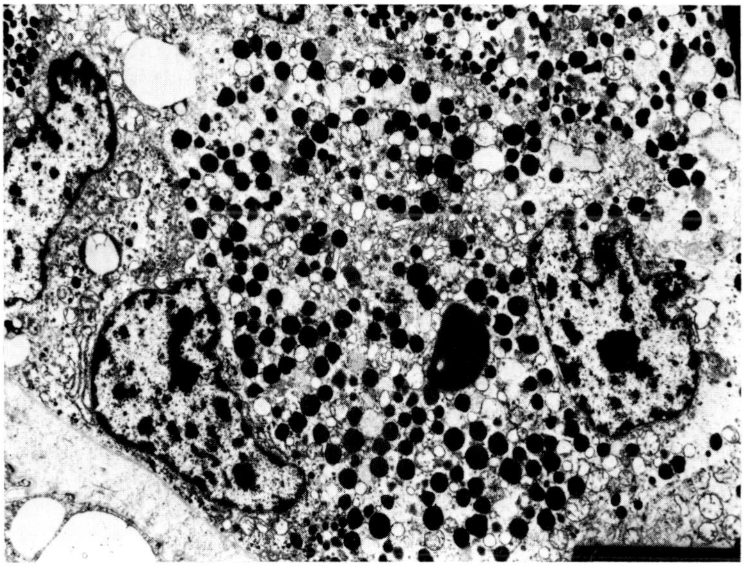

Fig. 16.21 Normal adenohypophysis. Differing granule sizes of pituitary basophils. The largest granules are growth hormone or prolactin, the smallest thyrotrophin (below left) and the intermediate (upper right) adrenocorticotrophin or gonadotrophin. ×4600.

Schiff/orange G (PAS/OG) (Pearse, 1952); erythrosin/orange G (Herlant, 1960); performic acid/alcian blue/PAS/OG (PFAB/PAS/OG) (Adams and Swettenham, 1958).

3. *Electron microscopy* to measure granule size (Bergland and Torack, 1969; Gray, 1977).

4. *Immunocytochemistry* (using perodixase staining or immunofluorescence) for the identification of hormones as specific antigens, which also demonstrate the size and shape of the cells and their distribution within the gland.

Immunocytochemistry is the only specific method of identification, given the purity of the antigens and antibodies used; with other methods cell function can only be inferred. Electron microscopy shows variation of granule size within single cells which are presumed to secrete a single hormone (Fig. 16.21); there is therefore an overlap of size between granules of different hormones (Bergland and Torack 1969; Doniach, 1977; Gray, 1977). The results of these methods are summarized in Table 16.2. The number of true chromophobe (agranular) cells in the human adenohypophysis is low (McCormick and Halmi, 1971); electron microscopy shows that most of the cells, including the chromophobes, contain secretory granules (Doniach, 1982).

Table 16.2 Cytological identification of adenohypophyseal hormones

Hormone	Trichrome (Mallory, 1900)	PAS/OG (Pearse, 1952)	Erythrosin/OG (Herlant, 1960)	PFAB/PAS/OG (Adams and Swettenham, 1958)	EM-granule diameter (nm) (Gray, 1977)
'Acidophil' cells					
Growth hormone	Red	Yellow	Orange	Yellow	452 ±23.8
Prolactin	Red	Yellow	Red	Yellow	559 ±38.0
'Basophil' cells					
Thyrotrophic hormone	Blue	Magenta	—	Blue	135.5±13.6
Luteinizing hormone	Blue	Magenta	—	Blue	181.6± 9.3
Follicle-stimulating hormone	Blue	Magenta	—	Blue	226.0±19.4
Adrenocorticotrophic hormone	Blue	Magenta	—	Magenta	356.8±30.5

OG, orange G; PFAB, performic acid/alcian blue; PAS, periodic acid Schiff.

Neurohypophysis (pars nervosa)

The human neurohypophysis is composed of the nerve fibres (axons) and terminals of the hypothalamohypophyseal tract, pituicytes and blood vessels, together with some collagenous connective tissue (Christ, 1966). The axons have bead-like swellings which contain variable amounts of neurosecretory material stainable by Gomori's chromalum haematoxylin, and probably represent vasopressin and oxytocin bound to neurophysin (see Fig. 16.5). Herring bodies are larger aggregates of Gomori-positive material. Under the electron microscope (Lederis, 1965) both axons and Herring bodies are seen to contain membrane-bound secretory granules (90–200 nm in diameter). Some small vesicles and multilamellar bodies are also present (Fig. 16.22). The *pituicytes* are modified glial cells,

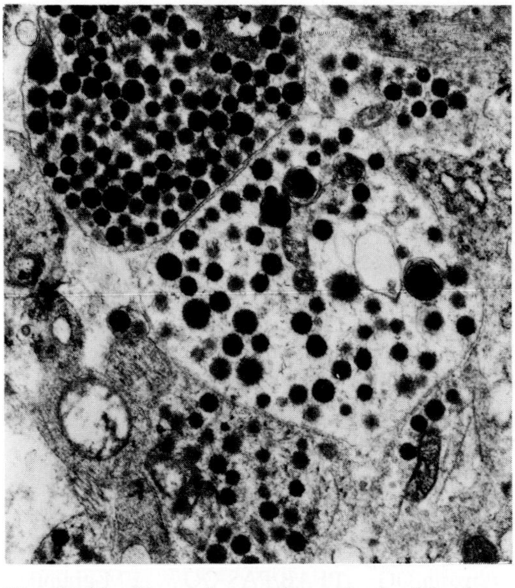

Fig. 16.22 Normal neurohypophysis. Membrane-bound neurosecretory granules within axons of the pituitary stalk. The pale axon contains vacuoles and lamellar bodies. ×7700.

containing glycogen, with processes ending near or within the perivascular space. The pars nervosa is often infiltrated by basophil cells with advancing age (Doniach, 1982).

Blood supply of the pituitary gland

The pars distalis (adenohypophysis), as in most vertebrates, is supplied solely by portal blood (Xuereb, Prichard and Daniel, 1954a, b; Daniel and Prichard, 1975) apart from the trabecular artery supplying connective tissue. The blood is carried mainly by the long portal vessels, originating in the coiled capillaries (gomitoli) of the tuber cinereum and ending distally in the sinusoids of the pars distalis (Fig. 16.23). The pars

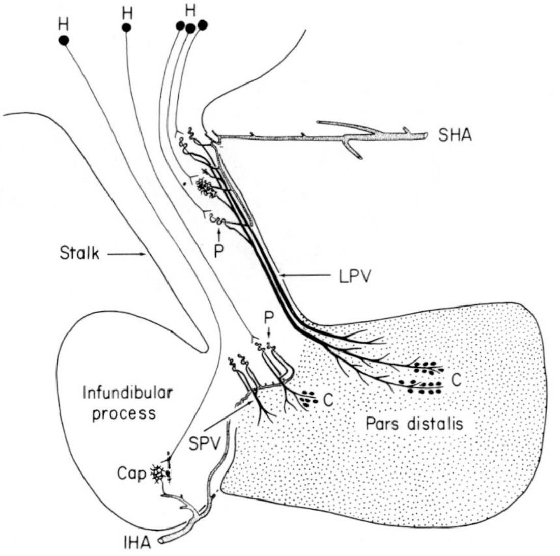

Fig. 16.23 Diagram of the blood supply of the pituitary gland. C, adenohypophyseal cells of the pars distalis; H, hypothalamic neurosecretory cells; IHA, inferior hypophyseal artery; LPV, long portal vessels; P, primary capillary bed; SHA, superior hypophyseal artery; SPV, short portal vessels.

distalis adjacent to the lower infundibular stem (lower part of the pituitary stalk) is supplied by short portal vessels originating from the primary capillary bed of simple coiled vessels in the lower infundibular stem (Fig. 16.24). The portal blood transports the hypothalamic releasing or inhibiting factors (entering the blood from neurosecretory fibres) to the appropriate adenohypophyseal trophic cells.

The posterior lobe has a separate and direct arterial supply from the inferior hypophyseal artery, a fact which is of great importance in the pathogenesis of pituitary infarction (see 'Ischaemic necrosis of the pituitary gland', later in this chapter). The capillaries of the neurohypophysis, where the blood–brain barrier is absent, are fenestrated (Peters, Palay and Webster, 1976).

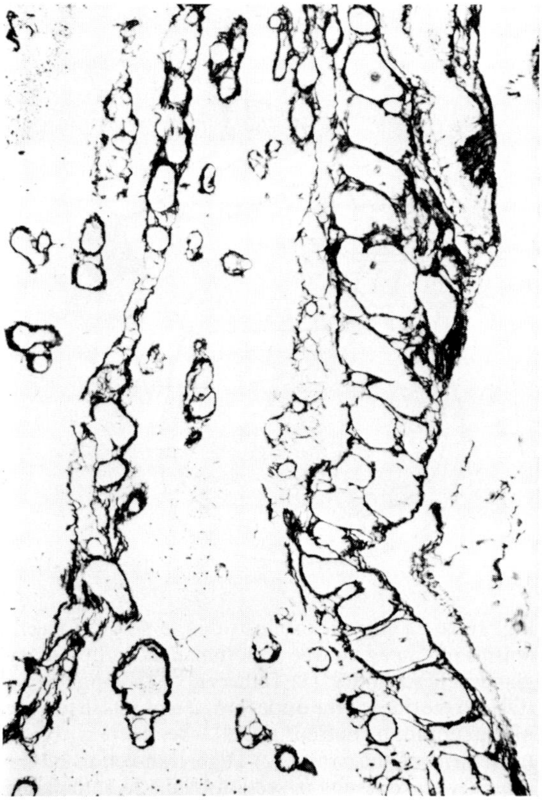

Fig. 16.24 Normal pituitary stalk. The helical nature of the primary capillaries produces a septate appearance on section. Reticulin × 120.

Diseases of the pituitary gland

Agenesis and hypoplasia

Complete absence of the pituitary gland is very rare and is usually incompatible with life; in the case of Sadeghi-Nejad and Senior (1974), in which the patient survived on hormone replacement, absence of the gland must have been putative. Agenesis of the gland is usually associated with severe cranial and neural developmental abnormalities such as cyclopia and holoprosencephaly (Brewer, 1957; Johnson et al., 1973) but cases with normal cranial and cerebral development have been recorded (Moncrieff et al., 1972; Johnson et al., 1973). The association between anencephaly and pituitary hypoplasia is well known; both pars distalis and pars nervosa are usually present, but in reduced amount (Salazar et al., 1969). Identifiable trophic cells were present in their two cases; as the hypothalamus was absent they suggested that differentiation of trophic cells is independent of hypothalamic neurosecretion. Atrophy of the suprarenal and thyroid glands is almost always present in anencephalic fetuses (Potter, 1961) and in other cases of pituitary dysgenesis. The pharyngeal pituitary was not identified in any of the cases recorded above.

Specific inflammatory diseases of the pituitary gland

A metastatic *abscess* of the pars distalis may be seen, though it is rare (Mohr, 1975) and must be distinguished from the collections of pus commonly seen on the diaphragma and around the stalk in cases of acute bacterial meningitis. *Tuberculous infiltration* is likewise uncommon although the author has seen an example. The pituitary may be involved in *toxoplasmosis* spreading from the brain.

Non-specific inflammatory disease

Sarcoidosis may spread to the pituitary from the meninges and usually involves the neurohypophysis, causing diabetes insipidus (already discussed in this chapter); the adenohypophysis may also be involved, with the production of hypopituitarism.

Giant cell granuloma usually involves the adenohypophysis (Doniach and Wright, 1951) and is composed of epithelioid cells, giant cells, lymphocytes and other chronic inflammatory cells (Fig. 16.25). Similar granulomas may be found in other endocrine organs, notably the adrenal gland (Rickards and Harvey, 1954). The cause is unknown, but it may be an autoimmune lesion (Doniach, 1977).

Lymphocytic and autoimmune hypophysitis

Lymphocytic hypophysitis was described by Goudie and Pinkerton (1962), who were the first to suggest that it might represent an autoimmune reaction to pituitary antigens released (in the case they reported) during puerperal involution of the hypophysis. There was extensive lymphocytic infiltration of the adenohypophysis in this and in the few other cases described subsequently (Lack, 1975). There seems to be an association with organ-specific autoimmunity to other en-

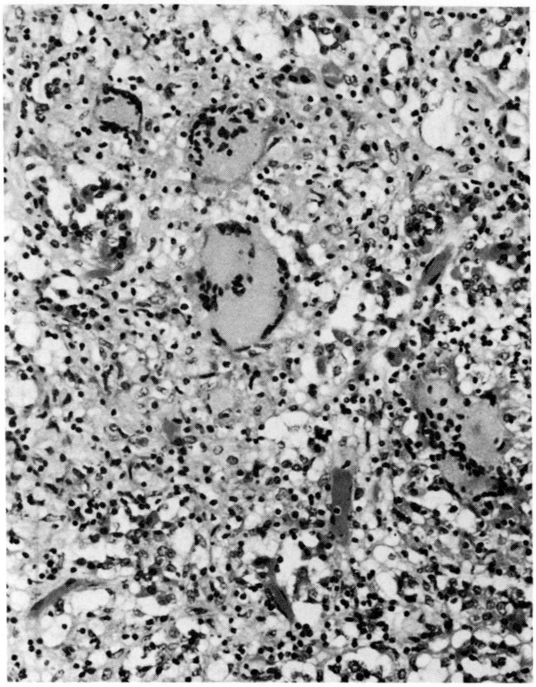

Fig. 16.25 Giant cell granuloma of the pituitary. Much of the glandular tissue has been replaced by chronic inflammatory cells. Four giant cells are present. Haematoxylin and eosin × 150.

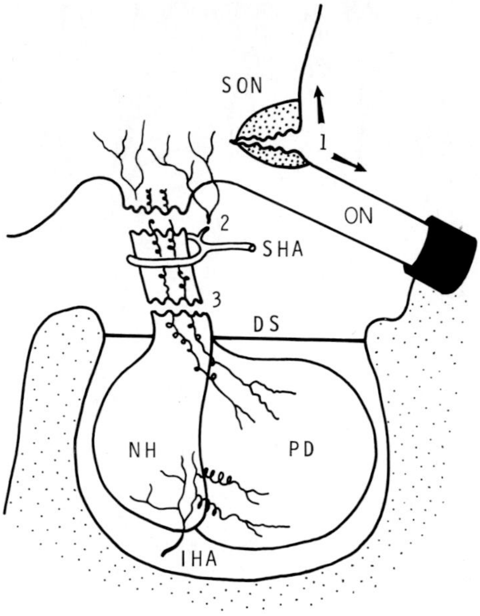

Fig. 16.26 Diagram to illustrate the possible mechanisms of damage to the hypothalamus and pituitary gland in head injury. (1) Tethering of the optic nerve (ON) to the dura at the optic foramen results in tearing of the supraoptic nucleus (SON) when there is abrupt movement of the brain. (2) High transection of the pituitary stalk results in section of the hypothalamic branches of the arterial ring, but leaves the pituitary branches intact. (3) Low transection of the stalk sections the long pituitary portal vessels, but leaves the hypothalamic branches intact. DS, diaphragma sellae; IHA, inferior hypophyseal artery; NH, neurohypophysis; PD, pars distalis; SHA, superior hypophyseal artery.

docrine organs and to gastric mucosa (Davis and Hipkin, 1977). The finding of antiprolactin antibodies in patients with polyendocrinopathy (Bottazzo et al., 1975) and of pituitary antibodies in patients with diabetes mellitus (Mirakian et al., 1982) suggests that pituitary autoimmunity may occur either in isolation or as part of a spectrum of endocrine autoimmunity.

Ischaemic necrosis of the pituitary gland

Understanding of the effects of ischaemia on the human pituitary gland has come about partly from anatomical studies of the pituitary blood supply (Xuereb, Prichard and Daniel, 1954a, b), partly from experimental work (Daniel and Prichard, 1975) and partly from the study of therapeutic pituitary stalk section in man carried out in patients with metastatic carcinoma (Adams, Daniel and Prichard, 1966). In such cases necrosis involving up to 90 per cent of the anterior lobe (pars distalis) was found. The reason for this large infarct is that most of the blood supply of the anterior lobe is carried by the long portal vessels in the stalk, which are severed at operation. The surviving portion of the lobe receives blood from the short portal vessels originating below the transection (Figs. 16.26 and 16.29). A thin rim of tissue, possibly nourished by diffusion of oxygen from blood surrounding the gland, also commonly survives.

Postpartum pituitary necrosis

Simmonds (1914) described the finding of a shrunken fibrotic pituitary in a woman suffering from hypopituitarism many years after a complicated labour. Such a pituitary gland is shown in Fig. 16.27. Sheehan (1937), Sheehan and Summers (1949) and Sheehan and Davis (1968) reported that in many fatal cases of postpartum

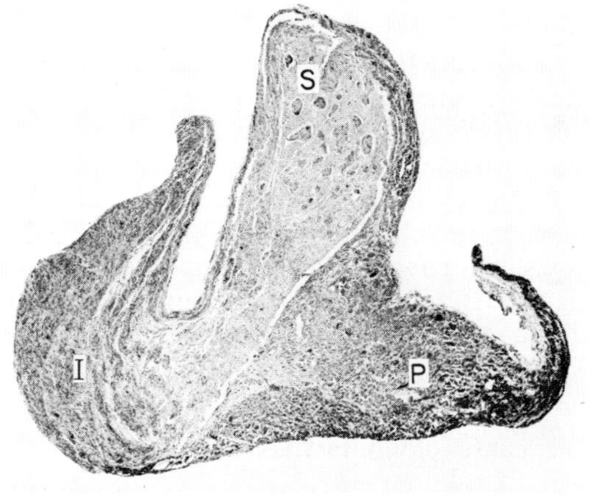

Fig. 16.27 Severely shrunken pituitary gland from a case of Sheehan's syndrome (Simmonds' disease). Both pars distalis (P) and the infundibular process (I) are atrophic. S, pituitary stalk. Haematoxylin and eosin × 12.

haemorrhage and shock there was a large infarct in the pars distalis, which clearly could have led to subsequent hypopituitarism in surviving patients (Sheehan's syndrome). The cause of the pituitary infarct in these cases must have been something other than transection of the portal vessels—slowing or cessation of flow due to hypotensive shock are possible explanations. Thrombi are not usually found in the pituitary vessels (Sheehan and Davis, 1968). Scarring of the posterior lobe may also be present in these cases (Sheehan and Whitehead, 1963); concomitant diabetes insipidus occurs occasionally (Aguiló et al., 1969).

Traumatic infarction and haemorrhage in the pituitary and hypothalamus

Damage to the pituitary gland may occur in head injury when, for example, a fracture passes through the floor of the sella. More commonly, there is shearing or avulsion of the pituitary stalk, with consequent interruption of the blood supply (Ceballos, 1966; Daniel and Treip, 1966a; Orthner and Meyer, 1967). Haemorrhage into the neural lobe often occurs, but may not be extensive (Fig. 16.28). Diabetes insipidus after head injury is often transient; if long-lasting or permanent it is probably related to hypothalamic damage involving the infundibulum or neurosecretory nuclei rather than to neurohypophyseal

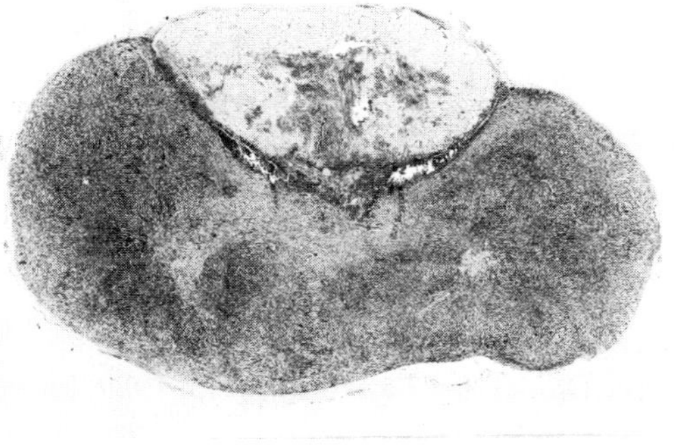

Fig. 16.28 Haemorrhages into the posterior (neural) lobe of the pituitary in a case of head injury. Haematoxylin and eosin × 6.

damage (see p. 760). Infarction of the posterior lobe is rare, occurring in cases of severe hypoxia (see p. 769). Traumatic section of the pituitary stalk may be followed by a large infarct (Daniel, Prichard and Treip, 1959; Daniel and Treip, 1966a), but not all large infarcts are associated with transection (Fig. 16.29); mechanisms such as vascular spasm following stretching or shearing of the stalk vessels due to tethering of the pituitary in the sella (Kornblum and Fisher, 1969), or hypotensive shock analogous to that occurring in postpartum haemorrhage (Orthner and Meyer, 1967) have been proposed. Few patients survive injuries of this severity for long,

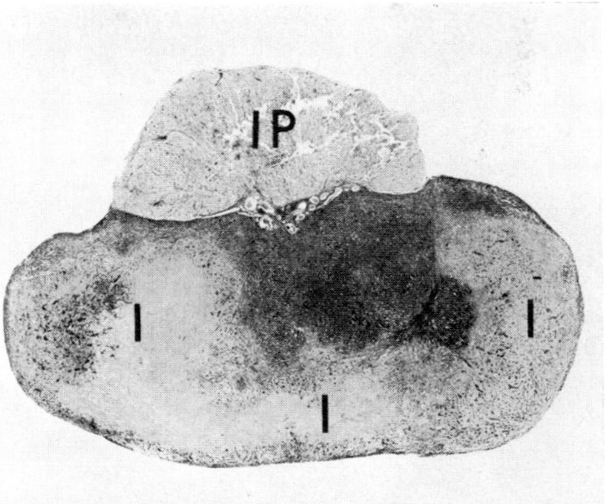

Fig. 16.29 Infarction of the anterior lobe (adenohypophysis) caused by traumatic rupture of the pituitary stalk (15 days' survival). A considerable proportion of the adenohypophyseal cells has survived (central dark area) as the cells in this area are supplied by the short portal vessels derived from the inferior hypophyseal artery (see Fig. 16.23). I, infarct; IP, infundibular process (posterior lobe). × 6.

but a few cases of post-traumatic hypopituitarism, with varying degrees of pituitary atrophy, have been recorded (Marañon, 1926; Lerman and Means, 1945; Henzi, 1952; Goldman and Jacobs, 1960; Cabellos, 1966; Orthner and Meyer, 1967). The various hypotheses for the mechanisms of infarction have been discussed by Kovacs (1969), Daniel, Spicer and Treip (1973) and Davis and Hipkin (1977). Occasional cases occur in which the stalk is transected but no pituitary infarct is found (Daniel, Prichard and Treip, 1959, case 6; Orthner and Meyer, 1967, case 3). This may be the result of high transection of the stalk above the hypophyseal arterial ring, sparing the long portal vessels, but involving the infundibular branches, so that a hypothalamic infarct occurs (see Figs. 16.26 and 16.31).

Hypothalamic damage occurs with some regularity in severe head injury, but few reports are available (Vonderahe, 1940; Henzi, 1952; Goldman and Jacobs, 1960; Orthner and Meyer, 1967; Treip, 1970). The supraoptic nucleus is the most vulnerable part and damage to it may be associated with macroscopic tearing of the optic tract (Fig. 16.30a), with haemorrhage into and disruption of the nucleus (Fig. 16.30b). This vulnerability may be explained by the tethering of the optic nerves to the optic foramen and the consequent shearing strain imposed by sudden cerebral deceleration on the angle in which the supraoptic nucleus lies (see Fig. 16.26). There are often petechial haemorrhages and oedema in the paraventricular nuclei. Infundibular infarction, the mechanism of which may be high stalk transection or stretching or spasm of the infundibular vessels, is not uncommon and may be widespread (Fig. 16.31). Fibrosis may be the long-term result of such infarction (Goldman and Jacobs, 1960).

Other causes of pituitary necrosis

Therapeutic pituitary stalk section has been used as a method of inhibiting pituitary trophic stimulation in cases of hormone-dependent carcinoma, usually mammary, but is seldom undertaken now. Up to 90 per cent of the pars distalis may be destroyed by the procedure; the infarct shrinks rapidly and is ultimately represented by a small scar (Adams, Daniel and Prichard, 1966). The surviving cells are mainly prolactin-secreting (Turkington, Underwood and Judson, 1971). No regeneration of pars distalis occurs in man. The posterior lobe also shrinks and be-

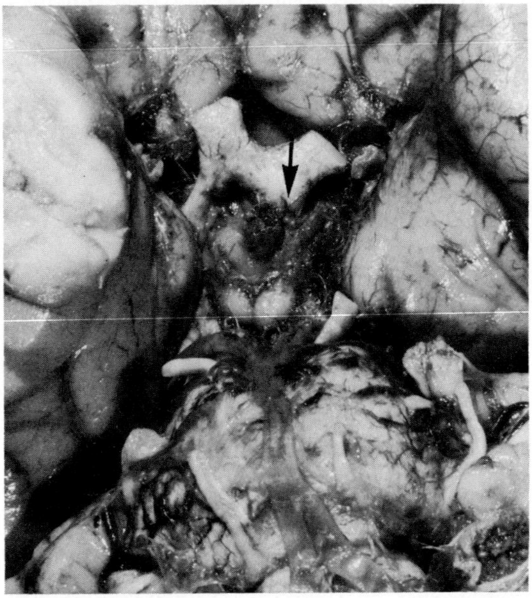

(a)

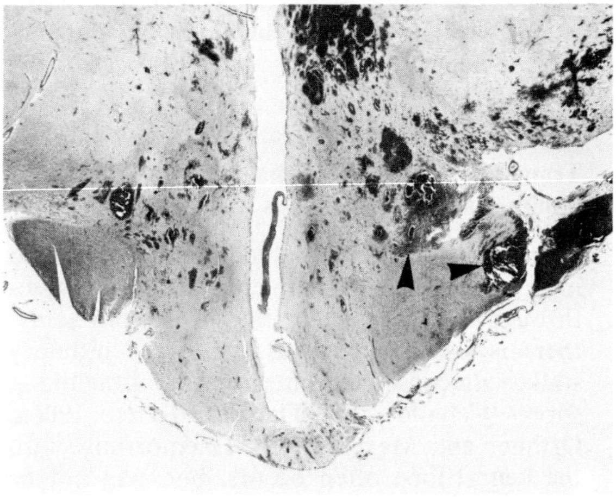

(b)

Fig. 16.30 (**a**) Tearing of the left optic tract (arrow) in a case of head injury. The transected pituitary stalk is immediately below and to the left. (**b**) Coronal section through the hypothalamus (same case), showing recent haemorrhages in the left optic tract and both supraoptic nuclei (arrowheads), as well as in the periventricular region. Luxol fast blue–cresyl violet ×4.

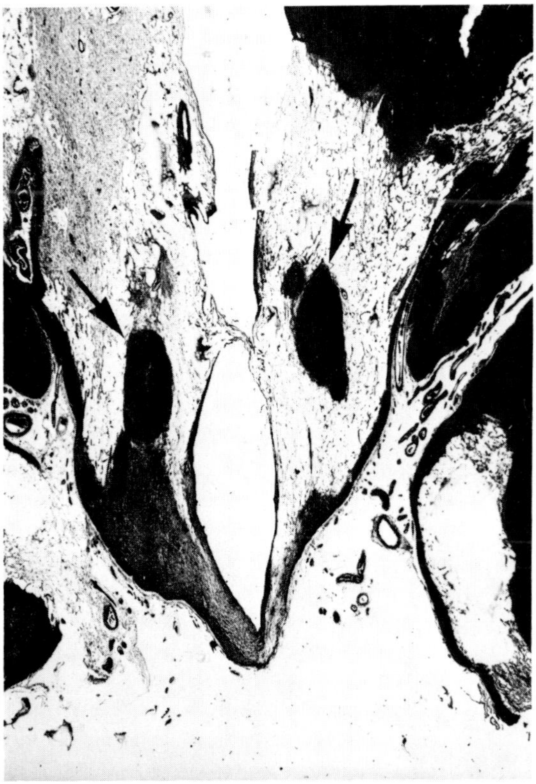

Fig. 16.31 Traumatic infarction of the infundibulum. Extensive old (pale) infarcts are present, involving the wall of the third ventricle but sparing the fornices (arrows). Survival of 110 days; persistent hypothermia. Loyez ×5.5.

comes more densely cellular (Daniel and Treip, 1966b).

Extensive necrosis of the pars distalis may occur in patients who have been kept on mechanical respirators for more than a few days (Daniel, Spicer and Treip, 1973). It is not uncommon in cases of subarachnoid haemorrhage; the cause of ischaemia in such patients may be spasm of the superior hypophyseal arteries, related to raised intracranial pressure. Infarction of the pars nervosa is also sometimes seen in these cases.

Infarcts of the anterior pituitary, sometimes large, may develop in patients with diabetes mellitus (Brennan, Malone and Weaver, 1956); the mechanism is obscure. Haemorrhagic necrosis may occur in some types of virus infection such as Korean fever (Hullinghorst and Steer, 1953). Small infarcts are not infrequently seen in patients with raised intracranial pressure (Wolman, 1956). Spontaneous anterior lobe infarction or pituitary apoplexy (Brougham, Heussner and Adams, 1950) almost always occurs within a pituitary adenoma; it may cause the sudden onset of hypopituitarism and even sudden death (Sachdev et al., 1981). Therapeutic irradiation of the pituitary, by implantation of yttrium-90, is sometimes carried out for metastatic carcinoma, pituitary adenoma, diabetes mellitus and, occasionally, for exophthalmic ophthalmoplegia. The glandular tissue undergoes necrosis, is replaced by scar tissue, and the pituitary gland shrinks (Fig. 16.32). Viable glandular cells

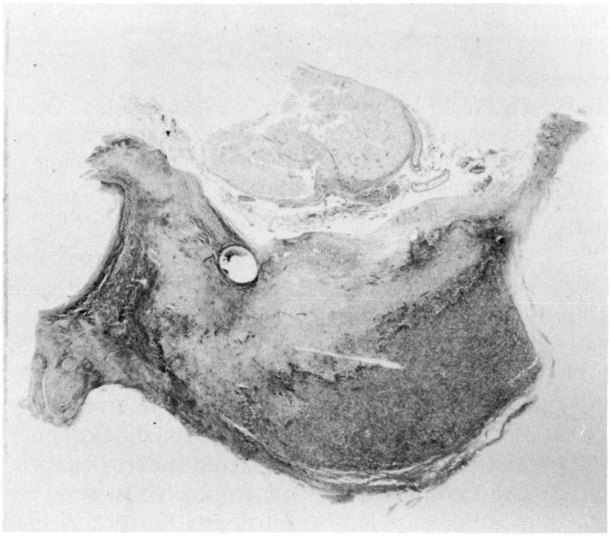

Fig. 16.32 Radiation necrosis. Horizontal section of pituitary gland in which an yttrium-90 seed had been implanted for the treatment of an acidophil adenoma. The ovoid clear space is the site of the implant. About half of the pars distalis has survived (dark area to right and below). Haematoxylin and van Gieson ×6.

usually remain in the periphery of the gland (Oppenheimer, 1959).

The empty sella syndrome

Busch (1951), in a study of the sella turcica in 788 necropsies, noted that considerable defects of the diaphragma sellae were present in 20 per cent of his cases. In 5 per cent of cases the sella appeared at first sight to be empty, but on closer examination was found to contain thinned out anterior pituitary tissue. Busch described several such cases of 'empty sella' in which the finding was incidental at necropsy, with no history of hypopituitarism during life; as the adenohypophysis has a functional reserve of 90 per cent there is no pathophysiological anomaly requiring explanation in such cases.

More recent interest has arisen from the radiological finding of an 'empty' (air-filled) sella in patients with hypopituitarism. The patients are usually female and middle-aged, but young, and male, patients have been reported (Farber, Turksoy and Rogers, 1977; Boyden and Hanson, 1981). The pathogenesis of the condition has been the subject of considerable discussion (Busch, 1951; Sachdev et al., 1976; Farber, Turksoy and Rogers, 1977). If the diameter of the sellar opening is more than 5 mm, or if the diaphragma sellae is incomplete, intracranial pressure, whether normal or abnormal, may cause herniation of arachnoid into the sella and consequent pressure atrophy of the anterior pituitary. Such cases may be considered as empty sellae arising as a result of congenital defect. In other patients the condition may be the result of necrosis, with consequent scarring and shrinkage, of the adenohypophysis (the neurohypophysis is often spared). Necrosis of this type may occur postpartum, after irradiation (see Fig. 16.32), or in an adenoma (pituitary apoplexy, which rarely may be a clinically silent event). A further example of collapse and shrinkage may be the result of rupture of an intrasellar cyst, perhaps of Rathke pouch origin (Raiti et al., 1976). Some pituitary tissue is usually present in the sella (though few necropsy reports are available); in patients with hypopituitarism either the functioning tissue is presumably less than the necessary minimum 10 per cent or the hypothalamic and vascular connections have been lost.

Abnormal depositions in the pituitary gland

The pituitary may be involved in a number of conditions in which there is widespread deposition of abnormal substances. Deposits of amyloid may be found in capsular vessels and in the trabecular connective tissue. In Hurler's syndrome (gargoylism) the pars distalis may contain enlarged, faintly PAS-positive cells and interstitial amorphous material (Fig. 16.33). In a study by Bergeron and Kovacs (1978), patients suffering from diseases of iron overloading, such as haemochromatosis and haemosiderosis, showed abnormal amounts of haemosiderin in the pituitary. All the trophic cell types of the adenohypophysis contained pigment, irregularly distributed. Electron microscopy showed both ferritin aggregates and haeomosiderin clumps. The finding that gonadotrophic cells were the most affected led Bergeron and Kovacs to spe-

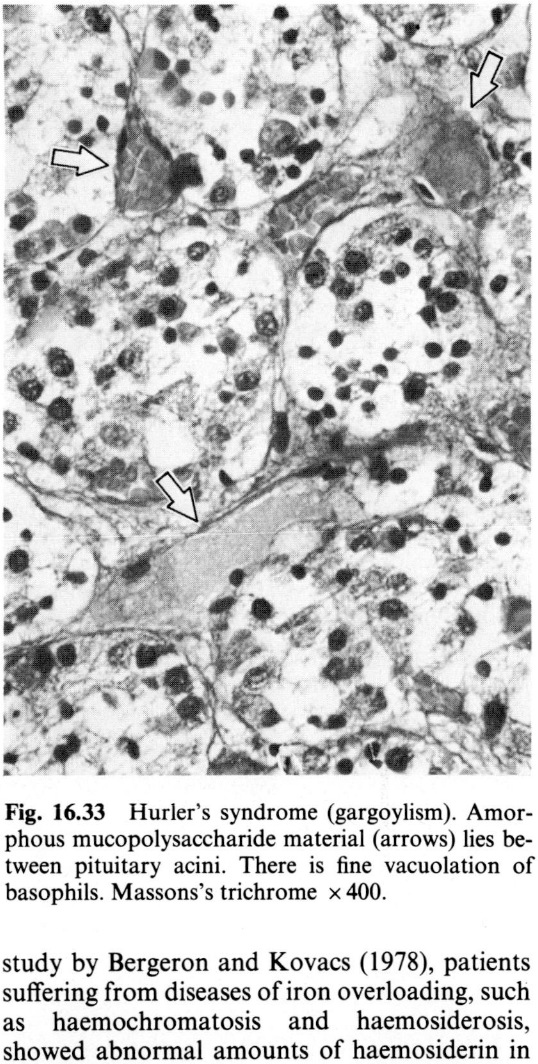

Fig. 16.33 Hurler's syndrome (gargoylism). Amorphous mucopolysaccharide material (arrows) lies between pituitary acini. There is fine vacuolation of basophils. Massons's trichrome ×400.

culate whether the gynaecomastia and testicular atrophy found in male patients with haemochromatosis might be attributable to functional failure caused by the iron deposition; it might equally be argued that failure of hepatic inactivation of oestrogens in cirrhosis could play a part by stimulating prolactin production.

Pituitary changes in endocrine disease

The changes seen in the adenohypophysis in physiological and pathological states are the morphological expression of changes in the balance between the hypothalamus, the pituitary gland and the target endocrine glands. The servo mechanisms involved have been discussed by Hutchinson (1978). Physiological changes are seen most commonly during pregnancy and the menopause. In *pregnancy* the pituitary gland enlarges, as a result of the proliferation of prolactin-secreting cells (Doniach, 1977). The stimulus is probably oestrogenic, either directly on pituitary cell receptors or possibly via the hypothalamus (which also contains oestrogen receptors), by an inhibitory effect on the dopaminergic cells of the arcuate nucleus, although the latter mechanism is open to question (Treip, 1983). The fall in ovarian oestrogens in the *menopause* is associated, perhaps by negative feedback, with increased gonadotrophin production, but without apparent morphological change in the pituitary gland.

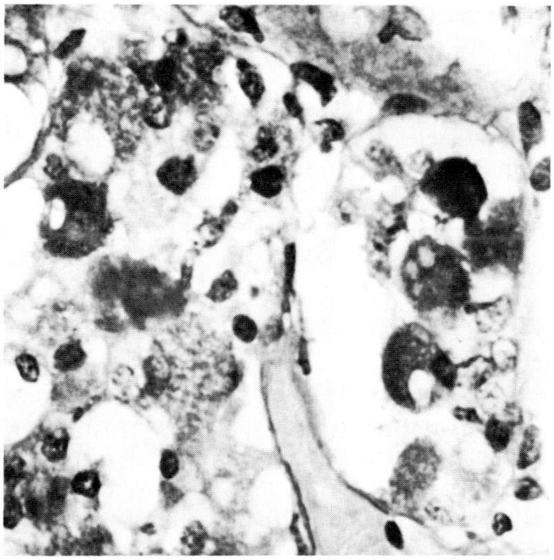

Fig. 16.34 Myxoedema. Four vaculoted basophils (thyrotrophs) are present in a section of pars distalis. Masson's trichrome ×600.

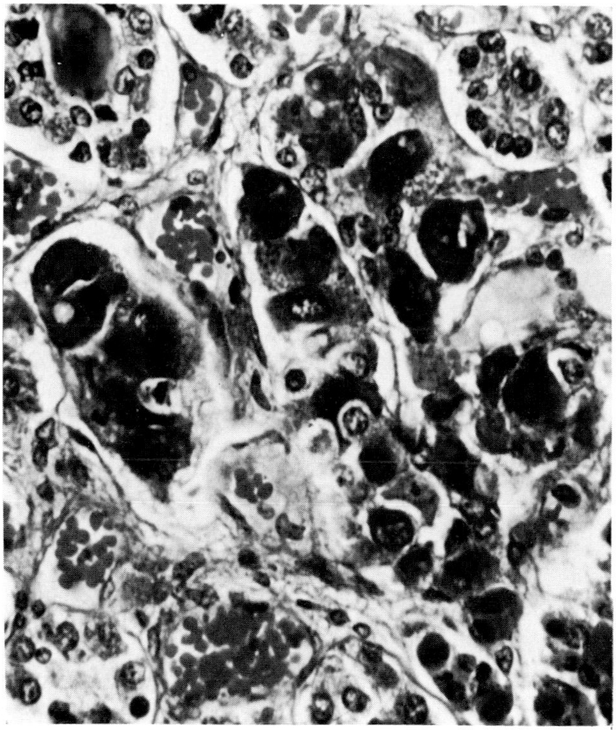

Fig. 16.35 Crooke's hyaline change. Enlarged adrenocorticotrophs which have lost their cytoplasmic granules. From a patient who had been treated with large doses of glucocorticoids. Masson's trichrome ×650.

Changes in the adenohypophysis may be seen in *thyroid disease*. In myxoedema the pituitary enlarges owing to an increase in thyrotrophic cells (Fig. 16.34), which have lipoprotein-containing vesicles (Thornton, 1959); there is an associated degranulation and loss of acidophils. This would seem to be, by analogy with pituitary TSH-secreting tumours in thyroidectomized rats (Furth and Clifton, 1966), a product of negative feedback. In hyperthyroidism there is a converse loss of thyrotrophs (Murray and Ezrin, 1966).

Changes in the pituitary gland occur in disease of the *suprarenals* (Ezrin and Murray, 1963). Cushing's syndrome is associated with Crooke's hyaline change (Crooke, 1935) in adrenotrophic cells—the cytoplasm of these cells is agranular with vacuolation. This change is also seen in patients who have received large doses of glucocorticoids (Fig. 16.35) and is thought to indicate loss of function, possibly by a negative feedback caused by a high level of circulating glucocorticoids. Partial degranulation of adrenotrophs can occur in Addison's disease (Crooke and Russell, 1935).

A well-known example of hypothalamic feedback occurs in *Nelson's syndrome* in which an ACTH-secreting pituitary tumour, with skin pigmentation, develops after bilateral adrenalectomy for Cushing's disease (Nelson, Meakin and Thorn, 1960). Despite maintenance doses of corticosteroids the plasma level of cortisol remains low enough to stimulate secretion of hypothalamic corticotrophin-releasing factor and induce pituitary tumour formation. Pigmentation results from the stimulation of melanocyte-stimulating-hormone activity by ACTH (Davis and Hipkin, 1977).

References

Abrahams, V.C., Hilton, S.M. and Zbrozyna, A.W. (1964) The role of active muscle vasodilatation in the alerting stage of the defence reaction. *Journal of Physiology* **171,** 189-202.

Adams, C.W. and Swettenham, K.V. (1958) The histochemical identification of two types of basophil cell in the normal human adenohypophysis. *Journal of Pathology and Bacteriology* **75,** 95-103.

Adams, J.H., Daniel, P.M. and Prichard, M.M.L. (1966) Transection of the pituitary stalk in man; anatomical changes in the pituitary glands of 21 patients. *Journal of Neurology, Neurosurgery and Psychiatry* **29,** 545-55.

Aguiló, F., Vega, L.A., Haddock, L. and Rodriguez, O. (1969) Diabetes insipidus syndrome in hypopituitarism of pregnancy. *Acta Endocrinologica* **60,** suppl. 137, 1-32.

Asa, S.L., Bilbao, J.M., Kovacs, K. and Linfoot, J.A. (1980) Hypothalamic neuronal hamartoma associated with pituitary growth hormone cell adenoma and acromegaly. *Acta Neuropathologica* **52,** 231-4.

Baker, A.B., Cornwell, S. and Brown, I.A. (1952) Poliomyelitis. VI. The hypothalamus. *Archives of Neurology and Psychiatry* **68,** 16-36.

Bauer, H.G. (1954) Endocrine and other manifestations of hypothalamic disease. *Journal of Clinical Endocrinology* **14,** 13-31.

Baylis, P.H. and Robertson, G.L. (1981) Vasopressin function in cranial diabetes insipidus. *Postgraduate Medical Journal* **57,** 36-40.

Beck, E., Daniel, P.M. and Parry, H.B. (1964) Degeneration of the cerebellar and hypothalamo-neurohypophysial systems in sheep with scrapie and its relationship to human system degenerations. *Brain* **87,** 153-76.

Bergeron, C. and Kovacs, K. (1978) Pituitary siderosis. *American Journal of Pathology* **93,** 295-310.

Bergland, R.M. and Torack, R.M. (1969) An ultrastructural study of follicular cells in the human anterior pituitary. *American Journal of Pathology* **57,** 273-97.

Besser, G.M. (1974) Hypothalamus as an endocrine organ. *British Medical Journal* **2,** 560-4; 613-15.

Blackwell, R.E. and Guillemin, R. (1973) Hypothalamic control of adenohypophysial secretions. In *Annual Review of Physiology*, vol. 35 (Eds. Comroe, J.H., Edelman, I.S. and Sonnenschein, R.R.), pp. 357-90. Annual Reviews, Palo Alto, Cal.

Bottazzo, G.F., Pouplard, A., Florin-Christensen, A. and Doniach, D. (1975) Autoantibodies to prolactin-secreting cells of human pituitary. *Lancet* **2,** 97-101.

Boyden, T.W. and Hanson, F. (1981) Hypopituitarism, delayed growth and an empty sella turcica. *American Journal of the Medical Sciences* **282,** 75-9.

Braun, F.C. and Forney, W.R. (1959) Diencephalic syndrome of early infancy associated with brain tumor. *Pediatrics* **24,** 609-15.

Braverman, L.E., Mancini, J.P. and McGoldrick, D.M. (1965) Hereditary idiopathic diabetes insipidus. A case report with autopsy findings. *Annals of Internal Medicine* **63,** 503–8.

Brennan, C.F., Malone, R.G.S. and Weaver, J.A. (1956) Pituitary necrosis in diabetes mellitus. *Lancet* **2,** 12–16.

Brewer, D.B. (1957) Congenital absence of the pituitary gland and its consequences. *Journal of Pathology and Bacteriology* **73,** 59–67.

Brougham, M., Heussner, A.P. and Adams, R.D. (1950) Acute degenerative changes in adenomas of the pituitary body—with special reference to pituitary apoplexy. *Journal of Neurosurgery* **7,** 421–39.

Busch, W. (1951) Die Morphologie der Sella Turcica und ihre Beziehungen zur Hypophyse. *Virchows Archiv für pathologische Anatomie und Physiologie* **320,** 437–58.

Ceballos, R. (1966) Pituitary changes in head trauma (analysis of 102 consecutive cases of head injury). *Alabama Journal of Medical Sciences* **3,** 185–98.

Christ, J.F. (1966) Nerve supply, blood supply and cytology of the neurohypophysis in *The Pituitary Gland,* vol. 3 (Eds. Harris, G.W. and Donovan, B.T.), Butterworths, London. pp. 62–130.

Clark, W.E. Le Gros (1938) Morphological aspects of the hypothalamus. In *The Hypothalamus* (Eds. Clark, W.E. Le Gros, Beattie, J., Riddoch, G. and Dott, N.M.), pp. 1–68. Oliver and Boyd, Edinburgh.

Conklin, J.L. (1968) A histochemical study of mucoid cells in the pars distalis of the human hypophysis. *Anatomical Record* **160,** 59–78.

Cremers, C.W.R.J., Wijdeveld, P.G.A.B. and Pinckers, A.J.L.G. (1977) Juvenile diabetes mellitus, optic atrophy, hearing loss, diabetes insipidus, atonia of the urinary tract and bladder and other abnormalities (Wolfram syndrome). *Acta Paediatrica Scandinavica* suppl. **264,** 1–16.

Critchlow, V. and Bar-Sela, M.E. (1967) Control of the onset of puberty. In *Neuroendocrinology*, vol. 2 (Eds. Martini, L. and Ganong, W.F.), pp. 101–62. Academic Press, New York and London.

Crompton, M.R. (1963) Hypothalamic lesions following the rupture of cerebral berry aneurysms. *Brain* **86,** 301–14.

Crompton, M.R. and Layton, D.D. (1961) Delayed radionecrosis of the brain following therapeutic X-irradiation of the pituitary. *Brain* **84,** 85–101.

Crooke, A.C. (1935) A change in the basophil cells of the pituitary gland common to conditions which exhibit the syndrome attributed to basophil adenoma. *Journal of Pathology and Bacteriology* **41,** 339–49.

Crooke, A.C. and Russell, D.S. (1935) The pituitary gland in Addison's disease. *Journal of Pathology and Bacteriology* **40,** 255–83.

Daniel, P.M. (1966a) The anatomy of the hypothalamus and pituitary gland. In *Neuroendocrinology*, vol. 1 (Eds. Martini, L. and Ganong, W.F.), pp. 15–80. Academic Press, New York and London.

Daniel, P.M. (1966b) The blood supply of the hypothalamus and pituitary gland. *British Medical Bulletin* **22,** 202–8.

Daniel, P.M. and Prichard, M.M.L. (1972) The human hypothalamus and pituitary stalk after hypophysectomy or pituitary stalk section. *Brain* **95,** 813–24.

Daniel, P.M. and Prichard, M.M.L. (1975) Studies of the hypothalamus and the pituitary gland: with special reference to the effects of transection of the pituitary stalk. *Acta Endocrinologica* **80,** suppl. 201, 1–216.

Daniel, P.M., Prichard, M.M.L. and Treip, C.S. (1959) Traumatic infarction of the anterior lobe of the pituitary gland. *Lancet* **2,** 927–31.

Daniel, P.M., Spicer, E.J.F. and Treip, C.S. (1973) Pituitary necrosis in patients maintained on mechanical respirators. *Journal of Pathology* **111,** 135–8.

Daniel, P.M. and Treip, C.S. (1966a) Lesions of the pituitary gland associated with head injuries. In *The Pituitary Gland,* vol. 2 (Eds. Harris, G.W. and Donovan, B.T.), pp. 535–44. Butterworths, London.

Daniel, P.M. and Treip, C.S. (1966b) The regenerative capacity of pars distalis of the pituitary gland. In *The Pituitary Gland,* vol. 2 (Eds. Harris, G.W. and Donovan, B.T.), pp. 519–34. Butterworths, London.

Daniel, P.M. and Treip, C.S. (1977) The pathology of the hypothalamus. *Clinics in Endocrinology and Metabolism* **6,** 3–19.

Davis, J.C. and Hipkin, L.J. (1977) *Clinical Endocrine Pathology.* Blackwell Scientific, Oxford.

Dawson, B.H. (1958) The blood vessels of the human optic chiasma and their relation to those of the hypophysis and hypothalamus. *Brain* **81,** 207–17.

Defendini, R. and Zimmerman, E.A. (1978) the magnocellular neurosecretory system of the mammalian hypothalamus. *Research Publications of the Association for Research in Nervous Mental Disease* **56,** 137–52.

Doniach, I. (1977) Histopathology of the Anterior Pituitary. In *Clinics in Endocrinology and Metabolism* **6,** 21–52.

Doniach, I. (1982) The pathology of adenomas of the pituitary gland. In *Current Endocrine Concepts* (Ed. Besser, G.M.), pp. 205–31. Praeger, Eastbourne.

Doniach, I. and Wright, E.A. (1951) Two cases of giant-cell granuloma of the pituitary gland. *Journal of Pathology and Bacteriology* **63,** 67–9.

Donovan, B.T. and van der Werff ten Bosch, J.J. (1965) *Physiology of Puberty.* Edward Arnold, London.

Duvernoy, H. (1972) The vascular architecture of the median eminence. In *Brain-endocrine Interaction. Median Eminence: Structure and Function* (Eds. Knigge, K.M., Scott, D.E. and Weindl, A.), pp. 79–108. Karger, Basel.

Edwards, C.R.W. (1975) Diabetes insipidus. In *Advanced Medicine, Symposium 11* (Ed. Lant, A.F.), pp. 276–88. Pitman Medical, London.

Everett, J.W. (1978) The mammalian hypothalamus-hypophysial system. In *The Endocrine Hypothalamus* (Eds. Jeffcoate, S.L. and Hutchinson, J.S.M.), pp. 1–33. Academic Press, London.

Ezrin, C. and Murray, S. (1963) The cells of the human adenohypophysis in pregnancy, thyroid disease and adrenal cortical disorders. In *Cytologie de l'Adénohypophyse* (Eds. Benoit, J. and Da Lage, C.), pp. 183–99. Centre Nationale de la Recherche Scientifique, Paris.

Farber, M., Turksoy, R.N. and Rogers, J. (1977) The primary empty sella syndrome. *Obstetrics and Gynecology* **49,** 2s–5s.

Fink, E.B. (1928) Diabetes insipidus. *Archives of Pathology* **6,** 101–20.

Finley, K.H. (1940) Angio-architecture of the hypothalamus and its peculiarities. *Research Publications of the Association for Research in Nervous and Mental Disease* **20,** 286–309.

Fisher, C., Ingram, W.R. and Ransom, S.W. (1938) *Diabetes Insipidus and the Neuro-hormonal Control of Water Balance.* Edwards, Ann Arbor, Mich.

Fitzsimons, J.T. (1966) The hypothalamus and drinking. *British Medical Bulletin* **22,** 232–7.

Fitzsimons, J.T. (1972) Thirst. *Physiological Reviews* **52,** 468–561.

Forssman, H. (1945) Hereditary diabetes insipidus. *Acta Medica Scandinavica* suppl. **159,** 41–2.

Friede, R.L. (1977) Osteolipomas of the tuber cinereum. *Archives of Pathology and Laboratory Medicine* **101,** 369–72.

Furth, J. and Clifton, K.H. (1966) Experimental pituitary tumours. In *The Pituitary Gland,* vol. 2 (Eds. Harris, G.W. and Donovan, B.T.), pp. 460–497. Butterworths, London.

Gagel, O. (1941) Eine Granulationgeschwulst im Gebiete des Hypothalamus. *Zeitschrift für die gesamte Neurologie und Psychiatrie* **172,** 710–22.

Gaupp, R. (1941) Über den Diabetes Insipidus. *Zeitschrift für die gesamte Neurologie und Psychiatrie* **171,** 514–46.

Glanzmann, E. and Wegelin, C. (1942) Diabetes insipidus und Simmonds Syndrom nach Encephalitis. *Schweizerische medizinische Wochenschrift* **72,** 1401.

Goldman, K.P. and Jacobs, A. (1960) Anterior and posterior pituitary failure after head injury. *British Medical Journal* **2,** 1924–6.

Goudie, R.B. and Pinkerton, P.H. (1962) Anterior hypophysitis and Hashimoto's disease in a young woman. *Journal of Pathology and Bacteriology* **83,** 584–5.

Gray, A.B. (1977) Analysis of diameters of human pituitary hormone secretory granules. *Acta Endocrinologica* **85,** 249–55.

Green, J.R., Buchan, G.C., Alvord, E.C. and Swanson, A.G. (1967) Hereditary and idiopathic types of diabetes insipidus. *Brain* **90,** 707–14.

Greep, R.O. and Astwood, E.B. (1974) The pituitary gland and its neuroendocrine control. *Handbook of Physiology,* vol. 4, parts 1 and 2. American Physiological Society, Washington DC.

Grossman, A., Nieuwhuyzen-Kruseman, A.C., Perry, L., Tomkin, S., Schally, A.V., Coy, D.H., et al. (1982) New hypothalamic hormone, corticotropin-releasing factor, specifically stimulates the release of adrenocorticotropic hormone and cortisol in man. *Lancet* **1,** 921–2.

Guyton, A.C. (1981) *Textbook of Medical Physiology.* Saunders, London.

Haas, J.E., Clarren, S.K., Beckwith, J.B. and Hall, J.G. (1980) Hypothalamic hamartoblastoma, hypoendocrinism and hypomelia: a new syndrome? *Laboratory Investigation* **42,** 172.

Hardy, J.D., Hellon, R.F. and Sutherland, K. (1964) Temperature-sensitive neurones in the dog's hypothalamus. *Journal of Physiology* **175,** 242–53.

Harris, G.W. (1955) *Neural Control of the Pituitary Gland.* Edward Arnold, London.

Harris, G.W. (1960) Central control of pituitary secretion. *Handbook of Physiology,* section 1, Neurophysiology, vol. 2, pp. 1007–38. American Physiological Society, Washington DC.

Henzi, H. (1952) Zur pathologischen Anatomie des Diabetes insipidus. *Monatsschrift für Psychiatrie und Neurologie* **123,** 292–316.

Herlant, H. (1960) Étude critique de deux techniques nouvelles destinées à mettre en évidence les différentes catégories cellulaires présentes dans la glande pituitaire. *Bulletin de Microscopie Appliquée* **10,** 37–44.

Herzog, E. (1955) Histopathologie des vegetativen Nervensystems. In *Handbuch der speziellen pathologischen Anatomie und Histologie,* vol. 13, part 5 (Eds. Lubarsch, O., Henke, F. and Rössle, R.), pp. 361–75. Springer, Berlin.

Hewer, T.F. and Heller, H. (1949) Non-lipid reticulo-endotheliosis with diabetes insipidus: report of a case with estimation of posterior pituitary hormones. *Journal of Pathology and Bacteriology* **61,** 499–505.

Hilton, S.M. (1966) Hypothalamic regulation of the cardiovascular system. *British Medical Bulletin* **22,** 243–8.

Hirabayashi, K., Eins, S., Spaar, F.W. and Olthner, H. (1979) Über die neuronale Hypertrophie der

Pars Subventricularis nuclei infundibularis bei Hypophysentumoren. *Acta Neuropathologica* **47,** 223–30.

Hökfelt, T., Elde, R., Fuxe, K., Johansson, O., Ljungdahl, Å., Goldstein, M. et al. (1978) Aminergic and peptidergic pathways in the nervous system with special reference to the hypothalamus. *Research Publications of the Association for Research in Nervous and Mental Disease* **56,** 69–135.

Horstmann, E. (1954) Die Faserglia des Selachiergehirns. *Zeitschrift für Zellforschung und mikroskopische Anatomie* **39,** 588–617.

Huff, D.S. and Fernandes, M. (1982) Two cases of congenital hypothalamic hamartoblastoma, polydactyly and other congenital anomalies (Pallister–Hall syndrome). *New England Journal of Medicine* **306,** 430–1.

Hullinghorst, R.L. and Steer, A. (1953) Pathology of epidemic hemorrhagic fever. *Annals of Internal Medicine* **38,** 77–101.

Hutchinson, J.S.M. (1978) Control of the endocrine hypothalamus. In *The Endocrine Hypothalamus* (Eds. Jeffcoate, S.L. and Hutchinson, J.S.M.), pp. 75–106. Academic Press, London.

Jeffcoate, S.L. and Hutchinson, J.S.M. (1978) *The Endocrine Hypothalamus.* Academic Press, London.

Jewell, P.A. and Verney, E.B. (1957) An experimental attempt to determine the site of the neurohypophysial osmoreceptors in the dog. *Philosophical Transactions of the Royal Society, B* **240,** 197–324.

Johnson, J.D., Hansen, R.C., Albritton, W.L., Werthemann, U. and Christiansen, R.O. (1973) Hypoplasia of the anterior pituitary and neonatal hypoglycemia. *Journal of Pediatrics* **82,** 634–41.

Kamalian, N., Keesey, R.E. and ZuRhein, G.M. (1975) Lateral hypothalamic demyelination and cachexia in a case of 'malignant' multiple sclerosis. *Neurology* **25,** 25–30.

Kennedy, G.C. (1966) Food intake, energy balance and growth. *British Medical Bulletin* **22,** 216–20.

Kepes, J.J. and Kepes, M. (1969) Predominantly cerebral forms of histiocytosis-X. *Acta Neuropathologica* **14,** 77–98.

Knigge, K.M. and Scott, D.E. (1970) Structure and function of the median eminence. *American Journal of Anatomy* **129,** 223–44.

Knigge, K.M., Joseph, S.A., Sladek, J.R., Notter, M.F., Morris, M., Sundberg, D.K. et al. (1976) Uptake and transport activity of the median eminence of the hypothalamus. *International Review of Cytology* **45,** 383–408.

Kornblum, R.N. and Fisher, R.S. (1969) Pituitary lesions in craniocerebral injuries. *Archives of Pathology* **88,** 242–8.

Kovacs, K. (1969) Necrosis of anterior pituitary in humans. *Neuroendocrinology* **4,** 170–99; 201–41.

Krabbe, K.H. (1922) La sclérose tubéreuse du cerveau. *Encéphale* **17,** 281–9.

Kraemer, W. and Paarmann, H.F. (1956) Beitrag zur cerebralen Form der Besnier-Boeck-Schaumannschen Krankheit unter Berücksichtigung hypothalamischen Regulationsstörungen. *Nervenarzt* **27,** 160–165.

Kupari, M., Pelkonen, R. and Valtonen, V. (1980) Post-encephalitic hypothalamic-pituitary insufficiency. *Acta Endocrinologica* **94,** 433–8.

Lack, E. (1975) Lymphoid hypophysitis with end-organ insufficiency. *Archives of Pathology* **99,** 215–19.

Lange-Cosack, H. (1951) Verschiedene Gruppen der hypothalamischen Pubertas praecox (1). *Deutsche Zeitschrift für Nervenheilkunde* **166,** 499–545.

Lange-Cosack, H. (1952) Verschiedene Gruppen der hypothalamischen Pubertas praecox (2). *Deutsche Zeitschrift für Nervenheilkunde* **168,** 237–66.

Langevin, H. and Iversen, L.L. (1980) A new method for microdissection of the human hypothalamus, with mapping of cholinergic, GABA and catecholamine systems in twelve nuclei and areas. *Brain* **103,** 623–38.

Langston, J.W. and Forno, L.S. (1978) The hypothalamus in Parkinson disease. *Annals of Neurology* 3, 129–33.

Lederis, K. (1965) An electron microscopical study of the human neurohypophysis. *Zeitschrift für Zellforschung* **65,** 847–68.

Le Marquand, H.S. and Russell, D.S. (1934–35) A case of pubertas praecox (macrogenitosomia praecox) in a boy associated with a tumour in the floor of the third ventricle. *Royal Berkshire Hospital Reports* **3,** 31–61.

Lerman, J. and Means J.H. (1945) Hypopituitarism associated with epilepsy following head injury. *Journal of Clinical Endocrinology* **5,** 119–31.

Levy, N.L. and Notkins, A.L. (1971) Viral infections and diseases of the endocrine system. *Journal of Infectious Diseases* **124,** 94–103.

Lichtenstein, M.J., Tilley, W.S. and Sandler, M.P. (1982) The syndrome of hypothalamic hypopituitarism complicating viral meningoencephalitis. *Journal of Endocrinological Investigation* **5,** 111–15.

Lipsett, M.B., Dreifuss, F.E. and Thomas, L.B. (1962) Hypothalamic syndrome following varicella. *American Journal of Medicine* **32,** 471–5.

McCann, S.M. and Porter, J.C. (1969) Hypothalamic pituitary stimulating and inhibiting hormones. *Physiological Reviews* **49,** 240–84.

McCormick, W.F. and Halmi, N.S. (1971) Absence of chromophobe adenomas from a large series of pituitary tumours. *Archives of Pathology* **92,** 231–8.

Maccubbin, D.A. and van Buren, J.M. (1963) A quantitative evaluation of hypothalamic degeneration and its relation to diabetes insipidus following interruption of the human hypophysial stalk. *Brain* **86,** 443–64.

Mallory, F.B. (1900) A contribution to staining methods. *Journal of Experimental Medicine* **5,** 15–20.

Marañon, G. (1926) Über die hypophysäre Fettsucht. *Deutsches Archiv für klinische Medizin* **151,** 129–53.

Meyer, A., Beck, E. and McLardy, T. (1947) Prefrontal leucotomy: a neuroanatomical report. *Brain* **70,** 18–49.

Millhouse, O.E. (1971) A Golgi study of third ventricle tanycytes in the adult rodent brain. *Zeitschrift für Zellforschung* **121,** 1–13.

Mirakian, R., Cudworth, A.G., Bottazzo, G.F., Richardson, C.A. and Doniach, D. (1982) Autoimmunity to anterior pituitary cells and the pathogenesis of insulin-dependent diabetes mellitus. *Lancet* **1,** 755–9.

Mohr, P.D. (1975) Hypothalamic-pituitary abscess. *Postgraduate Medical Journal* **51,** 468–71.

Moncrieff, M.W., Hill, D.S., Archer, J. and Arthur, L.J.H. (1972) Congenital absence of pituitary gland and adrenal hypoplasia. *Archives of Disease in Childhood* **47,** 136–7.

Morton, A. (1970) The time course of retrograde neuron loss in the hypothalamic magnocellular nuclei of man. *Brain* **93,** 329–36.

Muller, A. (1955) Neurosekretstauung im Tractus supraopticophyophyseus des Menschen durch einen raumbeengenden Prozess. *Zeitschrift für Zellforschung* **42,** 439–42.

Murray, S. and Ezrin, C. (1966) Effect of Graves' disease on the 'thyrotroph' of the adenohypophysis. *Journal of Clinical Endrocrinology and Metabolism* **26,** 287–93.

Nauta, W.J.H. and Haymaker, W. (1969) Hypothalamic nuclei and fiber connections. In *The Hypothalamus* (Eds. Haymaker, W., Anderson, E. and Nauta, W.J.H.), pp. 136–209. Thomas, Springfield, Ill.

Nelson, D.H., Meakin, J.W. and Thorn, G.W. (1960) ACTH-producing pituitary tumours following adrenalectomy for Cushing's syndrome. *Annals of Internal Medicine* **52,** 560–9.

Northfield, D.W.C. and Russell, D.S. (1967) Pubertas praecox due to hypothalamic hamartoma: report of two cases surviving surgical removal of the tumour. *Journal of Neurology, Neurosurgery and Psychiatry* **30,** 166–73.

Oppenheimer, D.R. (1959) Some pathological findings in cases with radioactive pituitary implants. *Journal of Laryngology and Otology* **73,** 670–8.

Orthner, H. (1955) Pathologische Anatomie und Physiologie der hypophysär-hypothalamischen Krankheiten. In *Handbuch der speziellen pathologischen Anatomie und Histologie*, vol. 13 (Eds. Lubarsch, O., Henke, F. and Rössle, R.), part 5, pp. 543–939. Springer, Berlin.

Orthner, H. (1961) Tumoröse Veränderungen im Sellabereich. *Beiträge zur modernen Therapie* **3,** 313–72.

Orthner, H. and Meyer, E. (1967) Der posttraumatische Diabetes insipidus. *Acta Neurovegetativa* **30,** 216–50.

Page, M.McB., Asmal, A.C. and Edwards, C.R.W. (1976) Recessive inheritance of diabetes: the syndrome of diabetes insipidus, diabetes mellitus, optic atrophy and deafness. *Quarterly Journal of Medicine* **45,** 505–20.

Pearse, A.G.E. (1952) Observations on the localisation, nature and chemical constitution of some components of the anterior hypophysis. *Journal of Pathology and Bacteriology* **64,** 791–826.

Perry-Keene, D.A., Connolly, J.F., Young, R.A., Wettenhall, H.N.B. and Martin, F.I.R. (1976) Hypothalamic hypopituitarism following external radiotherapy for tumours distant from the adenohypophysis. *Clinical Endocrinology* **5,** 373–80.

Peters, A., Palay, S.L. and Webster, H. de F. (1976) *The Fine Structure of the Nervous System*. Saunders, Philadelphia.

Peters, J.R., Rodriguez-Arnao, M.D. Foord, S.M. and Scanlon, M.F. (1982) Aminergic control of hypothalamic-pituitary function. In *Current Endocrine Concepts* (Ed. Williams, E.D.), pp. 173–93. Praeger, Eastbourne.

Plum, F. and van Uitert, R. (1978) The non-endocrine diseases and disorders of the hypothalamus. *Research Publications of the Association for Research in Nervous and Mental Disease* **56,** 415–73.

Porter, J.C., Mical, R.S., Ben-Jonathan, N. and Ondo, J.G. (1973) Neurovascular regulation of the anterior hypophysis. In *Recent Progress in Hormone Research*, vol. 29 (Ed. Greep, R.O.), pp. 161–98. Academic Press, New York and London.

Potter, E.L. (1961) *Pathology of the Fetus and the Newborn*, 2nd edn. Yearbook, Chicago.

Purves, H.D. (1966) Cytology of the adenohypophysis. In *The Pituitary Gland*, vol. 1 (Eds. Harris, G.W. and Donovan, B.T.), pp. 147–232. Butterworths, London.

Raisman, G. (1966) Neural connexions of the hypothalamus. *British Medical Bulletin* **22,** 197–201.

Raisman, G. (1970) Some aspects of the neural connections of the hypothalamus. In *The Hypothalamus* (Eds. Martini, L., Motta, M. and Fraschini, F.), pp. 1–15. Academic Press, New York and London.

Raiti, S., Albrink, M.J., Maclaren, M.K., Chadduck, W.M., Gabriele, O.F. and Chou, S.M. (1976)

Empty sella syndrome secondary to intrasellar cyst in adolescence. *American Journal of Diseases of Children* **130,** 1009–12.

Rasmussen, A.T. (1938) Innervation of the hypophysis. *Endocrinology* **23,** 263–78.

Reeves, A.G. and Plum, F. (1969) Hyperphagia, rage and dementia accompanying a ventromedial hypothalamic neoplasm. *Archives of Neurology* **20,** 616–24.

Rickards, A.G. and Harvey, P.W. (1954) 'Giant-cell granuloma' and the other pituitary granulomata. *Quarterly Journal of Medicine* **23,** 425–39.

Rioch, D.McK., Wislocki, G.B. and O'Leary, J.L. (1940) A précis of preoptic, hypothalamic and hypophysial terminology with atlas. *Research Publications of the Association for Research in Nervous and Mental Diseases* **20,** 3–30.

Romeis, B. (1940) Hypophyse. In *Handbuch der mikroskopischen Anatomie des Menschen* vol. 6 (Ed. von Möllendorff, W.), part 3, pp. 1–625. Springer, Berlin.

Russell, A. (1951) A diencephalic syndrome of emaciation in infancy and childhood. *Archives of Disease in Childhood* **26,** 274.

Sachdev, Y., Evered, D.C., Appleby, A. and Hall, R. (1976) The empty sella syndrome. *Postgraduate Medical Journal* **52,** 703–5.

Sachdev, Y., Gopal, K., Garg, V. and Mongia, S.S. (1981) Pituitary apoplexy (spontaneous pituitary necrosis). *Postgraduate Medical Journal* **57,** 289–93.

Sadeghi-Nejad, A. and Senior, B. (1974) A familial syndrome of isolated 'aplasia' of the anterior pituitary. *Journal of Pediatrics* **84,** 79–84.

Salazar, H., MacAulay, M.A., Charles, D. and Pardo, M. (1969) The human hypophysis in anencephaly. *Archives of Pathology* **87,** 201–11.

Scadding, J.G. (1967) *Sarcoidosis.* Eyre and Spottiswoode, London.

Scherbaum, W.A. and Bottazzo, G.F. (1983) Autoantibodies to vasopressin cells in idiopathic diabetes insipidus. *Lancet* **1,** 897–901.

Schmidt, E., Hallervorden, J. and Spatz, H. (1958) Die Entstehung der Hamartom am Hypothalamus mit und ohne Pubertas praecox. *Deutsche Zeitschrift für Nervenheilkunde* **177,** 235–62.

Schneider, J. and Güthert, H. (1975). Histiozytosis X des Hypothalamus. *Zentralblatt für allgemeine Pathologie* **119,** 49–55.

Shalet, S.M. (1982) Iatrogenic hypothalamic-pituitary disease. In *Clinical Endocrinology*, vol. 1 (Eds. Beardwell, C. and Robertson, G.L.), pp. 175–210. Butterworths, London.

Sheehan, H.L. (1937) Post-partum necrosis of the anterior pituitary. *Journal of Pathology and Bacteriology* **45,** 189–214.

Sheehan, H.L. (1968) Neurohypophysis and hypothalamus. In *Endocrine Pathology* (Ed. Bloodworth, J.M.B. Jr), pp. 12–74. Williams and Wilkins, Baltimore, Md.

Sheehan, H.L. and Davis, J.C. (1968) Pituitary necrosis. *British Medical Bulletin* **24,** 59–70.

Sheehan, H.L. and Summers, V.K. (1949) The syndrome of hypopituitarism. *Quarterly Journal of Medicine* **18,** 319–78.

Sheehan, H.L. and Whitehead, R. (1963) The neurohypophysis in post-partum hyopituitarism. *Journal of Pathology and Bacteriology* **85,** 145–69.

Simmonds, M. (1914) Ueber Hypophysisschwund mit tödlichem Ausgang. *Deutsche medizinische Wochenschrift* **40,** 322–3.

Sloper, J.C. (1966) Hypothalamic neurosecretion. *British Medical Bulletin* **22,** 209–15.

Smith, H.V. and Daniel, P.M. (1947) Some clinical and pathological aspects of tuberculosis of the central nervous system. *Tubercle* **28,** 64–80.

Sugarman, G.I., Heuser, E.T. and Reed, W.B. (1977) A case of cerebral gigantism and hepatocarcinoma. *American Journal of Diseases of Children* **131,** 631–3.

Szentágothai, J., Flerkó, B., Mess, B. and Halász, B. (1968) *Hypothalamic Control of the Anterior Pituitary.* Akadémiai Kiado, Budapest.

Thornton, K.R. (1959) The cytology of the pituitary gland in myxoedema. *Journal of Pathology and Bacteriology* **77,** 249–55.

Treip, C.S. (1970) Hypothalamic and pituitary injury. In *The Pathology of Trauma. Journal of Clinical Pathology* **23,** Suppl. (Royal College of Pathologists) **4,** 178–86.

Treip, C.S. (1983) The regression of oestradiol-induced pituitary tumours in the rat. *Journal of Pathology* **141,** 29–40.

Turkington, R.W., Underwood, L. E. and Judson, J. van Wyk (1971) Elevated serum prolactin levels after pituitary stalk section in man. *New England Journal of Medicine* **285,** 707–10.

Valtin, H. (1967) Hereditary hypothalamic diabetes insipidus in rats (Brattleboro strain). A useful experimental model. *American Journal of Medicine* **42,** 814–27.

Valtin, H. and Schroeder, H.A. (1964) Familial hypothalamic diabetes insipidus in rats (Brattleboro strain). *American Journal of Physiology* **206,** 425–30.

Vonderahe, A.R. (1940) Changes in the hypothalamus in organic disease. *Research Publications of the Association for Research in Nervous and Mental Disease* **20,** 689–712.

Weinberger, L.M. and Grant, F.C. (1941) Precocious puberty and tumors of the hypothalamus. *Archives of Internal Medicine* **67,** 762–92.

de Wied, D. (1980) Behavioural actions of neurohypophysial peptides. *Proceedings of the Royal Society of London, B* **210,** 183–95.

Wilke, G. (1956) Die granulomatöse Encephalitis mit

Bezug auf bekannte oder unbekannte Ätiologie. *Nervenarzt* **27,** 244–51.
Wolman, L. (1956) Pituitary necrosis in raised intracranial pressure. *Journal of Pathology and Bacteriology* **72,** 575–86.
Xuereb, G.P., Prichard, M.M.L. and Daniel, P.M. (1954a) The arterial supply and venous drainage of the human hypophysis cerebri. *Quarterly Journal of Experimental Physiology* **39,** 199–217.
Xuereb, G.P., Prichard, M.M.L. and Daniel, P. M. (1954b) The hypophysial portal system of vessels in man. *Quarterly Journal of Experimental Physiology* **39,** 219–30.

17

Disorders of the spine and spinal cord

J. Trevor Hughes

The conditions described in this chapter are divided into: (1) traumatic lesions of the spine and spinal cord; (2) diseases of the spine affecting the spinal cord; and (3) vascular disorders of the spinal cord.

Traumatic lesions of the spinal cord

The spinal cord is protected from injury by the complex bony structure forming the spinal canal and, except in the cervical region, a considerable degree of force is needed to damage this to such an extent as to injure the spinal cord. Fracture-dislocation of the lower thoracic or lumbar spine is, nevertheless, a well-recognized lesion in mining accidents due to roof falls, and may be caused in many other ways. The cervical spine is much more vulnerable and a fracture or fracture-dislocation at this level is a common cause of death or quadriparesis. Direct injuries to the spinal cord by stab wounds, bullets or fragments of shell or bomb casing are common both at the thoracic and at the cervical level. Wounds of the spine and spinal cord by high-velocity bullets have special pathological features due to the severity of the jarring injury to the spinal column.

Traumatic lesions of the spinal cord may be classified as: (1) direct, from injury to the cord by stab wounds or penetrating missiles; (2) indirect, due to fractures or fracture-dislocations, or subluxations of the spine; or (3) a combination of direct and indirect violence as in wounds with high-velocity missiles, or in cases of fracture dislocation where the cord is lacerated or pierced by a piece of bone.

Direct injuries to the spinal cord

The spinal cord may be directly injured without obvious or serious injury to the spine by discrete stab wounds or by tiny fragments of high-velocity missiles which pass between the vertebral laminae. Stab wounds are of special interest to clinicians owing to the close correlation which may be traced between the lesions and the symptoms they cause. Three of the cases showing his syndrome, in the series which Brown-Sequard published in 1868, were of this kind. Their chief interest to the neuropathologist is the opportunity they may give for the study of the course and termination of the long spinal tracts and the phenomena of Wallerian degeneration.

As the imbrication of the spines of the thoracic vertebrae protects the spinal canal on its posterior surface, stab wounds enter it lateral to the midline. The severance of nerve tracts in the spinal cord is therefore greater on one side than the other and the posterior columns are usually more severely damaged than the anterolateral. Often, however, the damage to the spinal cord is greater and the cord may be more or less completely severed. In most cases there is little bleeding except from the epidural veins and there is comparatively slight bruising of the tissues of the cord. The spinal cord lesion is therefore circumscribed and, unless complicated by sepsis or an injury to the anterior spinal artery, is limited to the level of the wound and a few millimetres on either side of this where the nervous tissue is contused and damaged.

Indirect injuries of the spinal cord

These involve subluxations and fracture dislocations of the spine. In civil life these are the most common form of traumatic lesions of the spinal cord and may be caused by road or industrial accidents, frequently from diving into shallow water, and also by a variety of falls and accidents in other sports and games. In some cases head injuries are complicated by an associated fracture or subluxation of the cervical spine. Indeed, when the slenderness of the cervical spine is considered in relation to the weight of the head and the stresses to which it is commonly subjected, it is surprising that it is not more often the site of fracture-dislocation or subluxation. Sudden hyperflexion of the cervical spine in a forward direction may tear the interspinous and posterior common ligaments of the vertebrae as well as the annulus fibrosus of one or more intervertebral discs without causing any fracture of bone. Lateral and backward hyperflexion is more likely to be associated with bony fracture but this may be limited to a pedicle or lamina or to the avulsion of an articular process. After these slighter degrees of injury, the spine returns to its normal alignment, and the fracture may not be easily visible in radiographs. Whether or not there is fracture-dislocation, the injury to the spinal cord is caused chiefly at the time of the accident by the sudden mechanical stresses to which the neural tissue is subjected. But when there is dislocation with pressure on the cord, or continuous stretching of the cord over a bony or cartilaginous protrusion, the ischaemia caused in this way produces additional lesions. In some cases herniation and protrusion of the nucleus pulposus, causing serious compression of the spinal cord, results immediately from an injury to the spine (Schneider, 1951). There are important differences, depending on the level of spinal injury.

Fracture-dislocations of the cervical spine These are most common at the level of the C5–6 vertebrae. In these injuries the cord is moved over a bony or cartilaginous prominence and the effects of pressure and ischaemia are added to the immediate mechanical trauma. Occasionally the cord may be pierced by spicules of bone, but in most cases it is protected from penetrating injury by the dura. One or more nerve roots are also commonly compressed by the dislocation, and this may contribute to the amyotrophy caused by the destruction of motor nerve cells in the cord.

Fracture-dislocations of the thoracic and lumbar spine These are most common at the lower thoracic level (Fig. 17.1). They are more often caused by crushing, as by an excessive weight on the shoulders in roof falls in mines, or by extreme forward or backward flexion of the spine in falls or road accidents. The damage to the spinal cord is less sudden than in fracture-dislocations of the neck, and the effects on the cord are due more to compression and less to the sudden jar of the accident. The degree of damage to the spinal cord varies greatly. As the space between it and the bony canal is greater at the thoracic than at the cervical level, the cord is less constantly damaged, and its injury is often incomplete and compatible with some recovery of function. In severe cases, however, there may be complete of almost complete destruction of neural tissue at the level of the lesion. Lesions of the lumbar spine may damage the conus, with permanent effects, or may compress the less vulnerable roots of the cauda equina. In the latter case, considerable recovery of function is possible if the compression is relieved without delay.

Direct and indirect spinal injuries from high-velocity missiles

High-velocity bullets or portions of shell or bomb casing which pass at speed through the vertebral bodies or spinous lamina cause severe jars to the spinal column. Even when they do not touch either the dura mater or the spinal cord they may cause extensive damage at the level of impact and minor lesions for a distance of several spinal cord segments above and below this.

Pathological findings following spinal cord trauma

The extent of the damage seen at necropsy depends on the degree and type of injury, but the histological appearances vary strikingly depending on the period of survival. The pathological

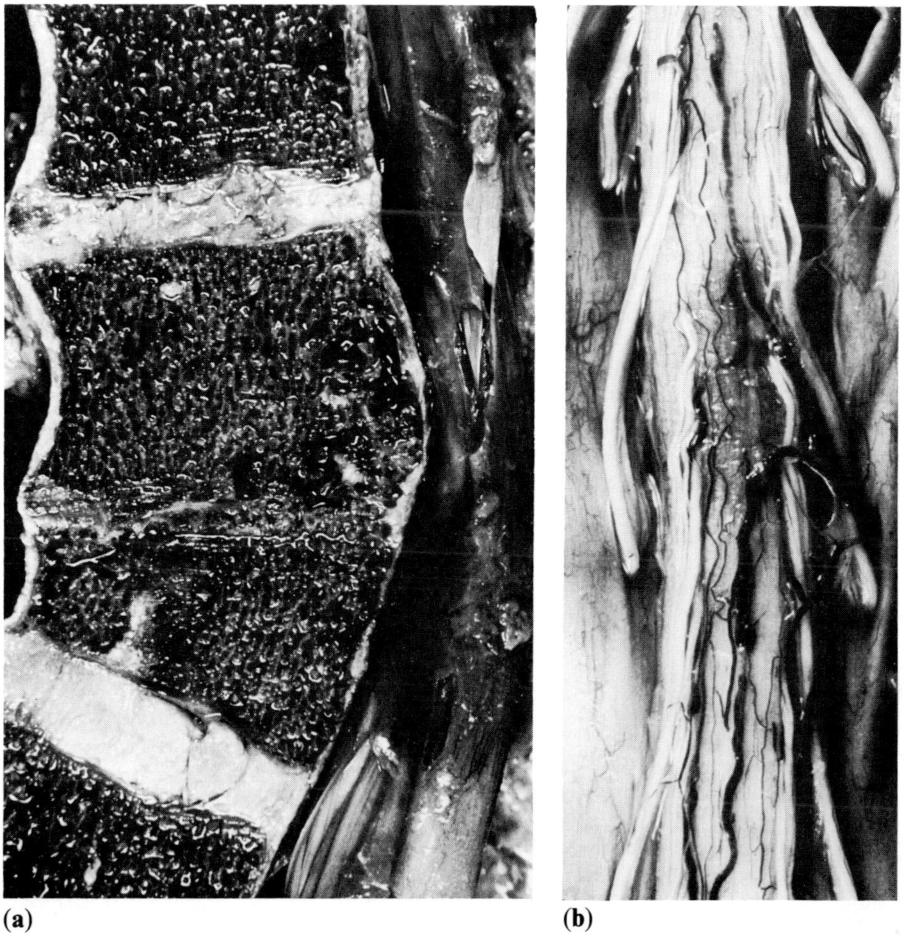

Fig. 17.1 Traumatic paraplegia. Findings several years after trauma. (**a**) Sagittally sawn spine showing T11, T12, L1 and L2 vertebral bodies. There is traumatic angulation at T12 with impaction of L1. The intervertebral disc between T12 and L1 has prolapsed backwards and the disc space is largely obliterated by fibrosis and bony overgrowth. (**b**) The posterior aspect of the spinal cord is shown with the dura reflected. Note the discoloration and atrophy level with the kyphos in (**a**). The posterior spinal veins and a major radicular vein are distended.

changes are therefore considered under the headings early, intermediate and late changes. Some terms currently used require definition. *Concussion*, used in the sense of a reversible physiological disturbance of spinal cord function caused by sudden jarring of the spine, is a valuable term for a phenomenon analogous to cerebral concussion. By definition, concussion is benign and, for obvious reasons, the histopathology of the human condition has not been investigated. In experimental studies it is clear that minor reversible changes of blood supply occur. *Contusion* means a crushing injury to the spinal cord, and may range in severity from a trivial lesion to one in which the cord is pulped. Contusion is more common than a complete tear through the spinal cord. *Haematorrhachis* means haemorrhage into the spinal canal; the blood may be in the extradural, subdural or subarachnoid spaces. *Haematomyelia* means a definite collection of blood in the spinal cord and should not be confused with the more common haemorrhagic pulping seen in severe contusion.

Early pathological changes

The immediate consequences of a spinal cord contusion or laceration are damaged or severed nerve fibres, effects on neuronal cell bodies, and exudative phenomena. The macroscopic appearance of the acutely damaged cord is shown in Fig. 17.2.

Both the axon and its myelin sheath become swollen and disintegrate. The axons when mildly damaged show beading; a more severe state is a line of droplets of axonal material in the former position of the axon, whilst in grossly contused specimens appropriate methods demonstrate only a silver-impregnated dust of scattered displaced axonal fragments. The point where an axon is completely torn may develop a terminal swelling (end-bulb). The myelin sheaths show corresponding changes ranging from a bubbly appearance in the myelin, detected only under high magnification, to complete fragmentation of the myelin giving abundant fatty droplets scattered amid the axonal material. The cell bodies of the neurons are either disrupted or show the axonal reaction (central chromatolysis).

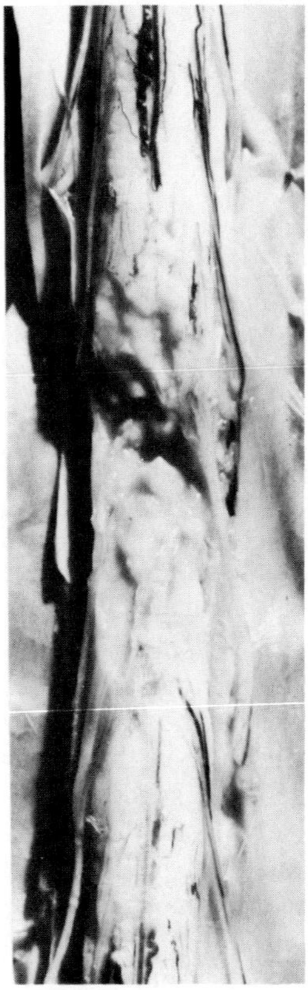

Fig. 17.2 Spinal cord 10 days after injury. Anterior aspect of the spinal cord, with the dura opened and reflected. Note the softened state of the destroyed part of the cord. (Reproduced, with permission, from J. Trevor Hughes, 1978, *Pathology of the Spinal Cord*, 2nd edn, Lloyd-Luke (Medical Books), London.)

The early exudative changes are oedema, red cell diapedesis, and an inflammatory cellular reaction of polymorphs and lymphocytes. These changes are best sought a little distance from the main site of injury at which they are obscured by the haemorrhage and haemorrhagic necrosis caused directly. Oedema, when slight, may be perivascular but often affects the whole cross-sectional area of the cord. As in the cerebrum, it is seen microscopically as rounded perivascular spaces in the white matter and perineuronal spaces in the grey matter. All these changes cause swelling of the spinal cord which becomes rounded and tense within the leptomeninges and dura, the subarachnoid and subdural spaces being obliterated. In addition to the swelling there is purple discoloration arising from the initial haemorrhage and later from venous stasis. This oedematous swollen state of the acutely damaged cord has provoked much speculation. Examination of the spinal arteries in human cases of spinal trauma (Hughes, 1981) has shown proliferative intimal lesions suggestive of former spasm in the arteries. Whatever its cause, the cord swelling enlarges the region of traumatic damage and the final form is usually in the shape of a spindle. This comprises a fusiform region of softening which affects one or more segments and tapers to end above and below as a small round area of necrosis usually situated in the posterior columns. This round area is considered to be a core of damaged tissue forced up or down by pressure and may be exaggerated by post-mortem handling which also may push softened material into the dural root sleeves. Measures in the immediate post-traumatic period to combat this cord swelling have frequently been advocated, but the majority opinion favours conservative measures. Decompression by laminectomy and opening the dura is hazardous, and violent extrusion of a considerable amount of softened cord may result.

Apart from the oedema, the exudative phenomena include the diapedesis of red cells and the appearance of leucocytes. Red cell extravasation, when marked, forms petechial haemorrhages; this feature, together with hyperaemia due to vascular dilatation, is attributable to venous stasis, an accompaniment of the swollen state of the cord. The cellular reaction is at first of polymorphonuclear leucocytes but later lymphocytes predominate.

For an account of the appearances in experimental trauma to the spinal cord the reader is referred to Wagner, Dohrmann and Bucy (1971), and the ultrastructural changes are described by Dohrmann, Wagner and Bucy (1971).

Intermediate pathological changes

The acute changes described above subside and are gradually replaced after 2–3 weeks by a reparative phase which may continue for up to 2 or more years. The pathological changes in this phase are very different from those in the early and late stages.

The oedema has now largely subsided and the smaller haemorrhages have been absorbed. The larger haemorrhages lead to the formation of cysts and these, if of considerable longitudinal extent, have the form of a syrinx. The polymorphs of the acute reaction are replaced by lymphocytes and large macrophages. The most striking cell everywhere is the lipid phagocyte. These phagocytes are present wherever necrosis has destroyed neurons, nerve fibres and other elements with the liberation of breakdown products. The phagocytes are frequently clustered around small vessels, forming rosette-like aggregates. In grossly damaged areas, there are countless closely apposed lipid phagocytes; where the damage was slight, as in the margins of the injury, fewer scattered phagocytes are found. The presence of a reactive astrocytic gliosis in any particular part of the lesion depends on the degree of damage, and occurs when this is slight. In the severely damaged areas the glia will have been destroyed along with the parenchyma, and here organization is by young fibroblasts. Changes in remaining neurons consist of central chromatolysis. These neurons, with their swollen cytoplasm and eccentric nuclei, may persist for up to 3 years.

Late pathological changes

Gradually the pathological picture changes, and when the survival period is 5–10 years or more a different histological state is found at necropsy (Fig. 17.3). There is now a traumatic scar with acellular collagenous connective tissue uniting meninges to the spinal canal and to the spinal cord and, in this fibrous scar, anatomical planes are often indistinct (Fig. 17.4).

The histological features are well seen with the van Gieson stain. The grossly damaged regions of the cord are replaced by connective tissue occupying the position of the former blood clot and the severe parenchymal necrosis. The less damaged regions of the cord and always a zone above and below the main damage show an intense astrocytic fibrous gliosis. A glial network with occasional astrocyte cell bodies replaces the damaged nerve fibres and the destroyed cell bodies. An interesting regenerative phenomenon is frequently seen in these traumatic scars. The cell bodies of the posterior root ganglia regenerate their central processes into the region of the connective tissue scar. These fibres, which are myelinated by Schwann cells, ramify in the connective tissue in the manner of an amputation neuroma of peripheral nerve. They do not enter the glial scar nor penetrate intact nervous tissue.

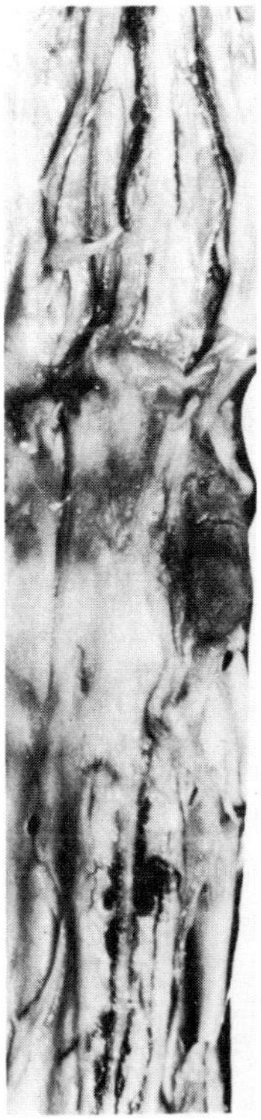

Fig. 17.3 Spinal cord 12 years after injury. Anterior aspect of spinal cord, with the dura opened and reflected. Above and below, the spinal cord can be made out but in the region of the injury a connective tissue scar replaces the damaged spinal cord and blends with the thickened dura mater. (Reproduced, with permission, from J. Trevor Hughes, 1978, *Pathology of the Spinal Cord*, 2nd edn, Lloyd-Luke (Medical Books), London.)

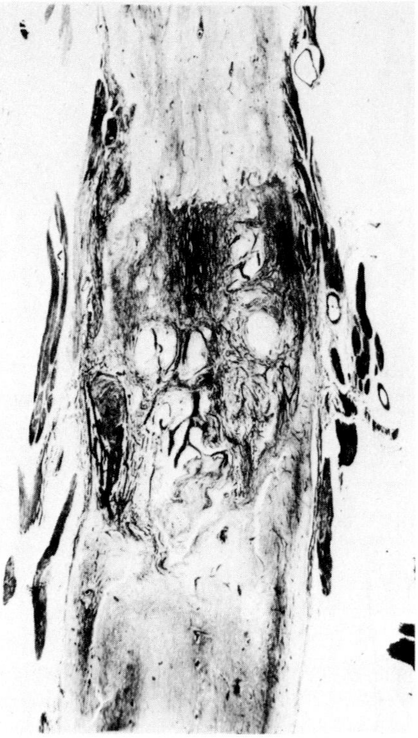

Fig. 17.4 Spinal cord 16 years after injury. Longitudinal histological section through the traumatic scar of a case with long survival after a spinal cord injury. The injured spinal cord segments are telescoped and three occupy the space of one. The centre of the scar is connective tissue which is invaded by regenerating fibres from the posterior roots. (Reproduced, with permission, from J. Trevor Hughes, 1978, *Pathology of the Spinal Cord*, 2nd edn, Lloyd-Luke (Medical Books), London.)

The significance of this phenomenon was reviewed in the report by Hughes and Brownell (1963) and by Hughes (1974).

Post-traumatic syringomyelia

It was mentioned earlier in this chapter that a longitudinal cavity in the form of a syrinx commonly forms in the intermediate stage of a severe injury to the spinal cord. This cavity replaces the zone of haemorrhagic necrosis seen in the acute stage of the injury, and later comes to have a glial and connective tissue lining which sometimes forms a thick wall. The interest in this common feature of spinal cord trauma is that occasionally a progressive post-traumatic syringomyelia develops.

Long after the initial injury and at a time when the neurological state has been stable for several months there are signs of an upward extension of the spinal cord lesion. This development can progress rapidly and may reach the level of the medulla. The central part of the spinal cord is the most affected, with neurological signs and myelographic appearances similar to those seen in idiopathic syringomyelia. Whilst in the majority of cases the syringomyelia is an upward cavitation from the original trauma, downward cavitation can also occur but is clinically silent because of the existing cord lesion above. A combination of upward and downward syringomyelia extending from the trauma may be found. The anatomical extent of these post-traumatic syringes can be demonstrated *post mortem* provided that many sections are examined. In some cases personally studied by the writer there appear to be a communication or communications between the syrinx and the subarachnoid space, usually laterally and near the posterior root entry zone. The clinical and pathological features of post-traumatic syringomyelia have been discussed by Barnett, Foster and Hudgson (1973).

Diseases of the spine affecting the spinal cord

The complicated bony, cartilaginous and fibrous components of the vertebral column normally protect the spinal cord but disease or malformation of the spine may cause local or widespread pressure either on the neural parenchyma or on the blood vessels which supply it. The effects of this type of pressure resemble those of slowly growing tumours. In some cases the pressure is widely spread, in others it is sharply localized, but in most cases the onset is insidious and progressive. In the early stage of cases with an acute onset the loss of function often seems greater than can easily be explained by the lesions found. The reverse is true in long-standing cases, in which the lower limbs retain useful function in spite of severe distortion of the cord. Mechanical pressure is more likely to compress blood vessels than solid tissue, and veins more than arteries. Many of the effects of pressure have been attributed to venous stasis in which oedema is an important component. There may be compression or spasm of small arteries. Myelin is more vulnerable to mechanical pressure and to hypoxia than are nerve cells or axons, and in the spinal cord the effects of pressure are seen particularly in the myelin. Movement of the cord over bony prominences on the posterior surface of the spinal canal seems to have a specially deleterious effect on neural tissue. This effect may be arterial and ischaemic, or venous and secondary to vascular stasis.

The differing types of pathology which are found in the spinal cord under conditions either of acute or of chronic compression are well established. The earliest lesion is usually a rounded or wedge-shaped area of spongy degeneration in the posterior part of the lateral columns. This may be unilateral or bilateral and consists of distended myelin sheaths many of which contain swollen axons. In more advanced cases these lesions become more extensive and similar areas often appear in the deeper parts of the posterior columns. The anterior third of the white matter usually remains intact. Areas of more frank necrosis in which the neuroglia also suffers may appear in the centre of the older areas and there may also be areas of necrosis in the grey matter, most often near the base of the anterior horns. Cavitation often appears in the deeper parts of the posterior columns or in the region of the grey commissure. In chronic cases the myelin is replaced by an overgrowth of neuroglial and connective tissue fibres, among which many axons still persist. Experimental studies have shown that some degree of remyelination can occur. There is usually shrinkage of the anterior horns associated with atrophy and loss of nerve cells, and hyaline thickening of the small intramedullary vessels.

Although this progressive type of degeneration is very common in cases of subacute or chronic compression of the cord, many cases of sudden paraplegia due to pressure are associated in their early stages with necrotic changes in the cord which may involve all or part of it in a transverse plane. In such cases a vascular cause is probable and it seems likely that there is compression of an important radicular vessel in or close to the intervertebral foramen. Examples of this are seen in extensive tumour infiltration in and around the spine.

Osteitis deformans (Paget's disease of bone)

The skull and vertebral column are common sites of osteitis deformans, and this may produce lesions in the brain, spinal cord or spinal nerve roots. The rarefaction of the bony trabeculae, which constitutes the early stage of the disease, makes the bone less able to resist the effects of gravity in spite of its increased thickness, so that, as it thickens, it becomes moulded into new shapes.

In osteitis deformans of the spine there is usually some degree of kyphosis, and in some cases this may be a sharp curvature. But the paraplegia, which sometimes results, is more often due to a general reduction in the size of the lumen of the canal or to local pressure by bony prominences which may form on the dorsal surfaces of the vertebral bodies. In two cases reported by Wyllie (1923) laminectomy showed a loss of the space which normally exists between the cord and the bone, and absence of pulsation in the cord.

Bony abnormalities in the region of the foramen magnum

Abnormalities in the floor of the posterior fossa, or in the articulation of the skull with the atlas or of the atlas with the axis, may be the cause of serious neurological symptoms. There are three common abnormalities: (1) occipitalization or assimilation of the atlas, in which there is partial or complete bony fusion of the atlas with the ring of the foramen magnum; (2) basilar invagination or impression; and (3) anomalies either of the odontoid process itself or in its relation to the atlas. In over 100 patients with bony abnormalities in the region of the foramen magnum, McRae (1953) found 28 instances of the first type, 21 of the second, and 17 of the third, and others with combinations of these. Because in most cases these are congenital abnormalities, symptoms often begin in childhood or early adult life. In some cases they follow an injury involving the head or neck.

Assimilation or fusion of the atlas with the margin of the foramen magnum does not cause compression or abnormal angulation of the medulla but it may be combined with other abnormalities such as an odontoid process which is abnormally long, angulated backwards, or placed unusually high. In these cases the size of the foramen magnum may be reduced. In McRae's (1953) series, neurological signs were always present if the anteroposterior diameter of the spinal canal behind the odontoid process was less than 20 mm. The lack of movement between the skull and atlas may also throw an abnormal strain on the atlantoaxial joint and produce excessive movement of the odontoid process in relation to the arch of the atlas or actual dislocation at this joint. This strain may be increased by fusion of the C2 and 3 vertebrae. Assimilation of the atlas may also be associated with platybasia or basilar invagination.

Basilar invagination or impression has been defined by means of lateral radiographs of the skull

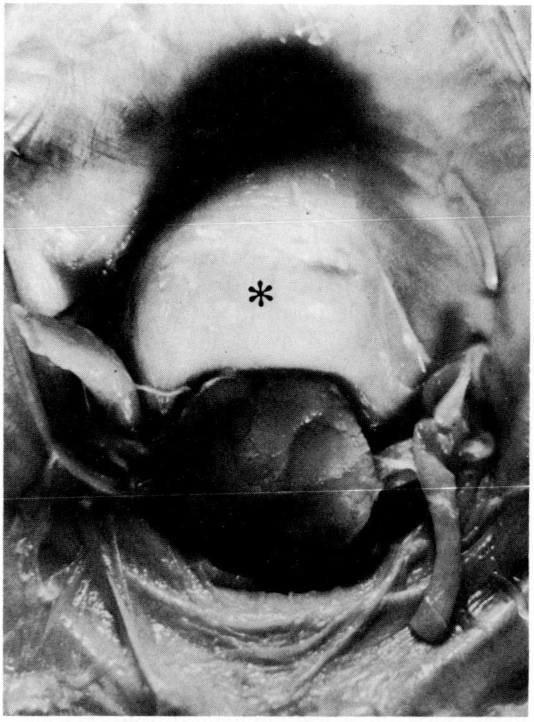

Fig. 17.5 Rheumatoid arthritis. Base of skull, showing foramen magnum from above. There is upward dislocation of the odontoid process of the axis which is seen as a bony protuberance (*) in the foramen magnum anteriorly and pushing the medulla and spinal cord backwards.

as an abnormal protrusion of the tip of the odontoid process above Chamberlain's line, which is a line drawn from the back of the hard palate to the posterior margin of the foramen magnum. The malformation is usually developmental but more rarely can result from softening of the base of the skull by osteitis deformans, rickets, osteomalacia or osteogenesis imperfecta. The severe destruction caused by rheumatoid arthritis may also cause upward movement of the odontoid process (Fig. 17.5). In most cases the atlas is tilted in relation to the skull, so its anterior arch, carrying the odontoid process with it, may lie at a higher level than the spinous process. Basilar invagination is not uncommonly accompanied by fusion of two or more cervical vertebrae. It may produce abnormal angulation of the lowest part of the medulla, or the first cervical segment over the prominence formed by the odontoid process and transverse ligament. This angulation and pressure vary with the position of the head, and some patients relate their symptoms to head movements. Thickening of the transverse ligament of the atlas and of the dural sheath is often present and increases the constriction of the cord and medulla. The effect of these structures is usually gradual but eventually there is degeneration of white matter and reduction in the size of the cord, especially in its anteroposterior diameter. In some cases the cord has been compressed to a fibrous ribbon.

Separation of the odontoid process from the axis may result either from a fracture across the base of the odontoid or from tearing of a persistent cartilaginous union at this level. Separations which result from slight strains or injuries may be explained most easily on the basis of a congenital abnormality. In these cases the inferior surface of the separated odontoid usually has a smooth horizontal line. Other congenital anomalies may be present. In two of McRae's cases, the tip of the odontoid was fused to the anterior lip of the foramen magnum. The separated odontoid process, which is often shorter and smaller than normal, retains its relation to the anterior arch of atlas, but the separation allows abnormal anteroposterior movement of the atlas on the axis and in many cases there is permanent forward dislocation of the head and atlas at this level. In some cases the appearance of neurological symptoms and signs may be delayed for weeks (Wallace and Bruce, 1910) or even years

(Bachs et al., 1955), and three of McRae's (1953) cases were asymptomatic. In most cases, however, there is a more rapid onset of signs of compression of the spinal cord.

In *atlantoaxial dislocation*, the atlas is displaced forward, in relation to the axis and lower cervical spine, and the odontoid process is separated from the anterior arch of the atlas. In cases of this type McRae found little or no glid ing of the atlas on the axis and little anteroposterior movement of the skull on the atlas; flexion and extension movements occurred chiefly at lower levels of the cervical spine. In his cases the odontoid lay from 5 to 17 mm behind the arch of the atlas and the anteroposterior diameter of the spinal canal at this level was correspondingly reduced. In spite of this, four of his six cases showed no signs of spinal compression.

Intervertebral disc protrusion

Protrusion of intervertebral discs appears to have been first recognized by Luschka (1858), who also described the small neurocentral joints of the cervical vertebrae which play an important part in the pathology of cervical discs. Cases of spinal compression due to this cause were described by Goldthwait (1911) and Middleton and Teacher (1911).

Anatomical considerations The anatomy of intervertebral discs was studied by Luschka (1858), Schmorl and Junghans (1959), Andrae (1929) and Beadle (1931). The central part of the disc consists of soft cellular fibrocartilage, with very fine collagenous fibres, forming the *nucleus pulposus*. This is surrounded by a ring of much firmer fibrocartilage, the *annulus fibrosus*, which is attached directly to the margin of the vertebral bodies. Between the nucleus pulposus and the spongiosa of the bone there is a thin layer of hyaline cartilage. These three forms of cartilage merge into one another without any abrupt transition. In the central part of the nucleus pulposus, in addition to numerous cartilage cells, there may be a few myxomatous or physaliphorous cells which are vestigial remains of the notochord. The ring of the annulus fibrosus is thicker anteriorly than posteriorly, so the nucleus pulposus lies eccentrically. This may explain why disc herniations only occasionally take place in a forward direction.

In the child, the nucleus pulposus constitutes by far the greater part of the disc, but as age advances it becomes gradually encroached on centripetally by the annulus fibrosus. After middle age it also becomes considerably dehydrated and shrinks in its vertical diameter. In children and young adults the disc is under considerable tension, so that on sawing through the vertebral bodies in a sagittal plane the nuclei bulge out from the surface. When bearing the weight of the body, this intradisc tension must be even greater. The normal disc has been compared to a fully inflated tyre; it allows rocking and, to a minor degree, torsion movements between the vertebral bodies, while at the same time it absorbs jars in the longitudinal direction. At the thoracic level the ribs and intercostal muscles limit the forward and backward flexion of the spine, and very little rotation is possible. The thoracic intervertebral discs are thus protected from many of the stresses and strains to which those at higher and lower levels are subject, and protrusions at this level are less common.

Pathology Intervertebral discs may be the subject of: (1) horizontal tearing; and (2) herniation of the nucleus pulposus.

1. *Disc tearing* may occur at the lower thoracic and lumbar levels in spinal trauma which is often the cause of dislocation. Spondylolisthesis at the lumbosacral or lower lumbar level is also associated with horizontal tearing of the disc and tearing or more gradual stretching of the anterior and posterior longitudinal ligaments. At the cervical level, tearing, usually of a single disc, is found in the sudden traumatic subluxations which will be described later. Such tears, without herniation of the nucleus, are most often seen in middle-aged or elderly subjects in whom the nucleus is less tense.

2. *Herniation of the nucleus pulposus* occurs almost always in a backward direction because the annulus fibrosus is thinner posteriorly. The nucleus may herniate through a weakened or torn part of the annulus, or between annulus and bone or, in rare cases, through the spongy bone to its posterior or posterolateral surface. The herniations through the hyaline cartilage into the spongy tissue of the vertebral body, which may be seen near the centre of the disc in about 38 per cent of normal subjects, are called Schmorl's nodes and are of themselves of little importance, but by reducing tension in the nucleus pulposus

they may lead to bulging of the annulus fibrosus and to osteophytosis. Their effects are therefore similar to those of degeneration of the nucleus pulposus. (The appearance of a Schmorl's node is seen incidentally in Fig. 17.8a.) This Schmorl's node has ruptured upwards into the T9 vertebral body from the T9/10 intervertebral disc. Herniation of the nucleus pulposus is most common in young adults in whom the nucleus is more tense, and the annulus is thinner than in older subjects. The herniation may be caused either by trauma or by a sudden severe muscular strain. Posterior or posterolateral herniations may burst through the annulus into the spinal canal either as a single mass or in several fragments, but more commonly they are checked by the outer fibres of the annulus and the posterior longitudinal ligament and so form a localized bulge into the spinal canal or intervertebral foramen. Owing to the firm central strands of the posterior longitudinal ligament in the lumbar region, herniations here are usually posterolateral rather than posteromedian. They may be unilateral or bilateral.

Spondylosis deformans

Degeneration of the intervertebral discs is very common after about the age of 50. The nucleus pulposus progressively loses water with increasing age and the proportion of water in its composition falls from 88 per cent at birth to 70 per cent at the age of 70. This loss of water of the nucleus is associated with shrinkage and an increase in its fibrous tissue so that the transition from nucleus to annulus fibrosus becomes more gradual. There is also loss of tension which allows of some bulging of the annulus fibrosus in all directions when any pressure is put on the disc. The condition then resembles that of a partially deflated tyre. This is commonly followed by bony outgrowths from the margins of the upper and lower surfaces of the vertebral bodies, forming the lipping which is very commonly seen after middle age especially on the ventral surface of the lower thoracic and lumbar vertebral bodies. Schmorl found this condition in 10 per cent of young adults in the third decade, in 35 per cent in the fourth decade, in 70 per cent in the fifth decade and in 90 per cent of men over 50 and women over 60 years of age (Collins, 1950). In most cases it remains slight at the cervical and upper thoracic levels where the pressure on the discs in the erect posture is less. But if for any reason (such as the occurrence of Schmorl's intraosseous herniations) there is considerable loss of nuclear substance in a disc, lipping tends to occur above and below it. At the cervical level, some loss of disc space associated with ventral lipping is recognized by radiologists as an early sign of degeneration of a disc. Schmorl recognized this process to be degenerative and distinguished it from rheumatic and inflammatory conditions by the term *spondylosis deformans*. Collins (1950) recommended the term *osteophytosis*, but it is probable that formation of osteophytes is secondary to the bulging of the annulus fibrosus which is itself secondary to loss of disc substance, and that bone formation follows the curve which the annulus assumes when pressure is applied to the disc. Anterior lipping causes no neurological symptoms and many cases with minor degrees of posterior lipping are also asymptomatic. In a minority of cases, however, bony transverse ridges on the dorsal surface of the cervical vertebrae (Fig. 17.6) associated with protrusions of disc substance are the cause of paraparesis or tetraparesis. Osteophytes in relation to the neurocentral joints of the lower cervical vertebrae also may cause signs of pressure on the roots of the brachial plexus. Degeneration of discs and osteophytosis are thus common causes of neurological symptoms at the cervical level whereas herniation of nuclear substance is the usual cause of symptoms at the lumbar level.

Because the causes and effects of protrusions of intervertebral discs differ in this and other ways according to the level at which they are situated, those at the cervical, thoracic and lumbar levels will be considered separately.

Cervical disc disease

Anatomical considerations The lower five cervical vertebrae differ from all the others in the shape of their bodies which are considerably wider in the transverse than in the anteroposterior direction and are saddle-shaped. When viewed from the front the lateral margins of the upper surface are seen to be curved sharply upwards, and the upper edges of these 'uncinate processes' come into contact through fibrocartilage with recesses on the outer margins of the inferior surface of the body of the upper vertebra, and thus form a joint in which there is usually a cavity (Bull, 1948; Frykholm, 1951).

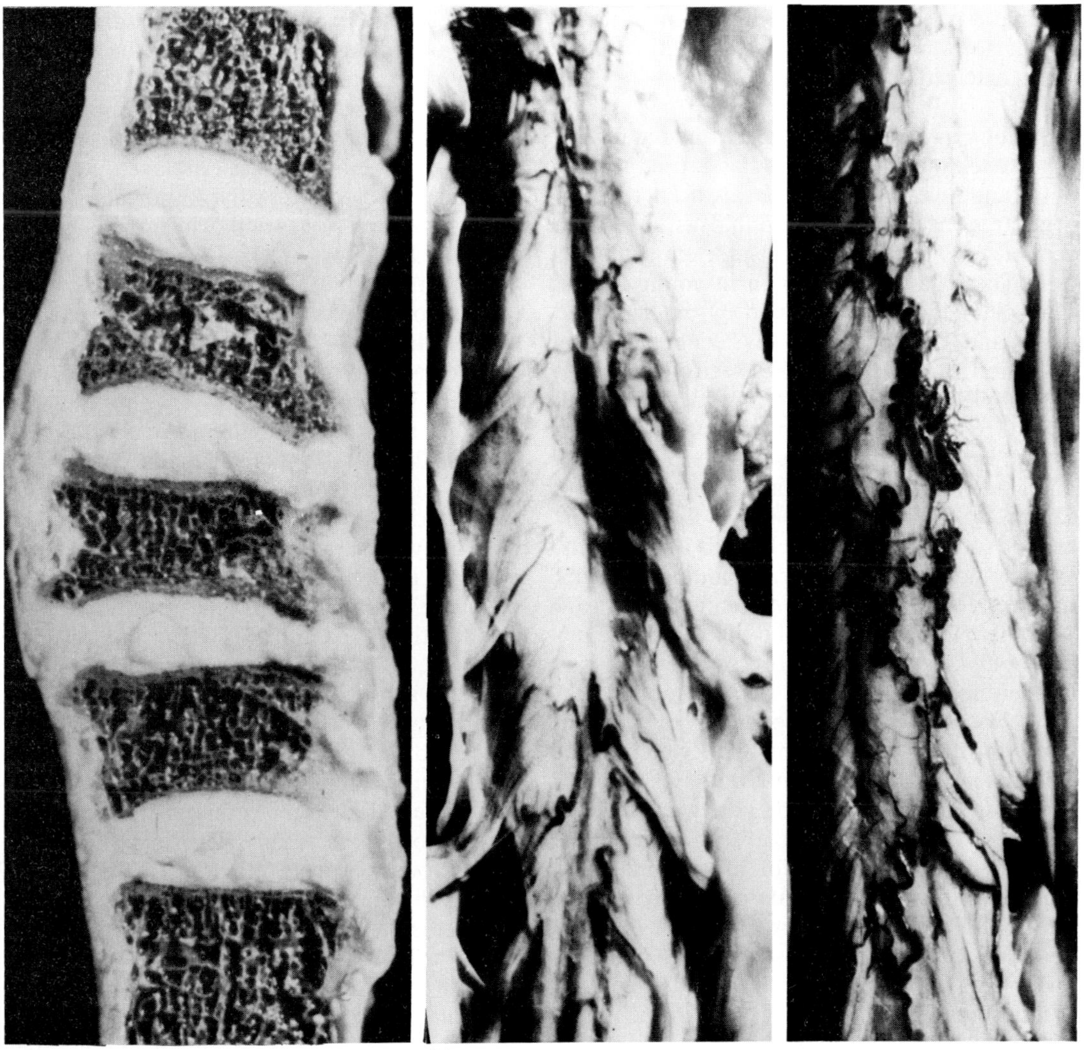

(a) (b) (c)

Fig. 17.6 Cervical spondylosis. (**a**) Right half of sagittally sawn specimen showing cervical spine from C4 to 8. Severe spondylosis affects C4/5, C5/6, C6/7 disc spaces. This results in a huge posterior protrusion from C5 to 7, seen directed to the left of the picture. (**b**) The spinal cord is viewed from the anterior aspect. Note the deep indentation of the cord at C6/7 corresponding to the cervical spondylosis seen in the spine in (**a**). (**c**) Posterior aspect of the cord in (**b**). Note the dilatation of the posterior spinal veins.

These neurocentral joints prevent lateral displacement of the vertebral bodies and also ensure that in flexion and extension movements of the neck the vertebral bodies rock on a pivot near their centre. The superior surfaces of the vertebral bodies are slightly convex in the anteroposterior direction, and the inferior surfaces correspondingly concave, with their anterior lips slightly overhanging the body of the subjacent bone. The shortness of the spinous processes at the cervical level allows more backward movement (extension) than at the thoracic level where the spines are imbricated. Forward flexion also is more free. Lateral flexion and rotation are limited by the neurocentral joints and articular processes, but the joint between the latter is rather lax and allows some movement. These movements are associated with moulding of the intervertebral discs. Owing to the position of the neurocentral joints there is little difference between the tensions produced within the discs by full flexion and those produced by full (backward) extension of the neck.

Pathology A few cases in which sudden flexion of the neck by external force has caused tearing of the annulus fibrosus and backward herniation of a large mass of nucleus pulposus have been verified by operation or post-mortem examination. These have usually been in young adults. The spinal cord is compressed by the herniated tissue, and when this tissue has been removed by operation there has sometimes been considerable or complete restoration of its function. Small central or posterolateral protrusions which encroach on the canal or the intervertebral foramina are more common. Many of these cases are caused by trauma such as blows by which the head is suddenly jerked backwards or forwards. When sudden pain in the arm, shoulder or trunk has been felt at the time of the injury it is probably that there has been a herniation of the nucleus pulposus through a torn or stretched part of the annulus. Operation or post-mortem examination shows a posteromedian or posterolateral protrusion of disc material which in the early stages may be fairly soft, but later becomes firmer and often fibrous or partly calcified or may be covered with a thin layer of bone. In the cervical region the posterior longitudinal ligament is rather weaker at its centre than more laterally, and therefore herniations are likely to be either median or in close relation to the intervertebral foramina (Brain, Northfield and Wilkinson, 1952). The age of onset in such cases is usually below 40.

In cases of disc degeneration, symptoms come on more gradually. There may be no history of injury, or trauma, often of minor degree, may have occurred several months or years previously. X-ray examination in these cases may show some loss of the disc space at one or more levels, often associated with anterior and posterior osteophytosis, and this osteophytosis may also be seen by oblique views in the intervertebral canals. In some cases paraplegia may develop suddenly after a minor degree of flexion or extension of the neck. Paraplegia has occurred after tooth extraction or tonsillectomy. In such cases there is often radiological evidence of previous degeneration of one or more discs. It is in fact doubtful whether paraplegia can follow such minor strains unless there is already degeneration of a disc. In patients over middle life, the backward protrusion of the annulus fibrosus, which is the chief cause of pressure on the cord, may be visualized by myelography, but may not be visible at operation with the head in the normal position and the muscles relaxed. Surgeons therefore tend to stress the importance of the transverse bony ridges with which the bulging is associated. On post-mortem examination no distinct protrusion may be visible, but a more diffuse narrowing of the spinal canal by several disc degenerations.

Whereas nuclear herniations at the cervical level are most often found between either the fifth and sixth or the sixth and seventh bodies, chronic degenerations are equally common in the two discs next above these (Brain, Northfield and Wilkinson, 1952). Their incidence at these levels may be partly explained by their tendency to occur immediately below congenitally fused vertebrae, usually the second and third or the second, third and fourth. The strong leverage which the fused segments exert on such a vulnerable disc is probably the cause of its premature degeneration. In cases of severe degeneration limited to one disc the vertebrae above it may tend to move forward out of line with those below it, especially on flexion or extension of the neck. In other cases bony ridges may be seen at several levels, or in myelograms the column of contrast medium is seen to be indented opposite several discs.

Protrusions of intervertebral discs, whether due to herniation or to degeneration, give rise to hyperplasia of the fibrous tissue in their neighbourhood. The dura mater becomes thickened and adherent to the posterior longitudinal ligament and there is also thickening and fibrosis of the pia-arachnoid, especially around the roots. Narrowing of one or more intervertebral foramina by cartilaginous protrusion and osteophytosis, along with the thickening of the fibrous tissue of the dural sleeve (Frykholm, 1951), may cause degeneration of the nerve roots that pass through them. This is most common between the fifth and sixth and the sixth and seventh vertebrae and is usually bilateral but may be greater on one side. Although in most cases both anterior and posterior components of the root are damaged, in some cases the position of the protrusion is such that it presses chiefly on the anterior root.

The effects of disc protrusion on the spinal

cord vary in different cases according to variations in the causative factors.

Lesions of roots in the intervertebral foramina show themselves by wedge-shaped areas of degeneration in the dorsal columns which pass medially and become narrower in successively higher segments. When a ventral root is severely damaged there is an outgrowth of fresh axons from proximal to the level of damage and these may form a stump neuroma at the entrance to the intervertebral foramen or, more commonly, leashes of fine myelinated fibres (clothed with Schwann cells) which run in the meninges or pass along the walls of blood vessels into the tissues of the cord. Such regenerative phenomena are common in chronic cases with lesions of cervical discs.

Posteromedial or posterolateral protrusions may press on the anterior surface of the cord, and encroach on the restricted space of the spinal canal. Normally the anteroposterior diameter of the spinal canal from C3 to C7, with the neck in the neutral position, as measured by radiographs, is 17 mm (Wolf, Khilnani and Malis, 1956) but in cases of cervical spondylosis with myelopathy this measurement averages 14 mm (Payne and Spillane, 1957). When the neck is extended, this distance, from the spur on the posteroinferior aspect of one vertebra to the base of the spinous process of the vertebra below, may be reduced by 2 mm, and if there is any posterior movement of one vertebra upon the other (Penning, 1962) the distance is even further reduced. Posteriorly, in hyperextension, the ligamentum flavum may be infolded and press upon the cord (Nugent, 1959). The effects of pressure by the firm boss of cartilage on the anterior spinal artery are probably even more important than pressure on the cord itself because at the cervical level this vessel supplies not only the anterolateral white columns and grey matter but also the anterior third or quarter of the posterior columns (Bolton, 1939). The tension of the ligamentum denticulatum adds to this pressure because by its attachment to the dura mater which is itself anchored by the root sleeves, it prevents the cord from moving backwards. Allen (1952) observed that flexion of the neck during operations might produce blanching of the cord at the level of a disc protrusion, and it is possible that the mechanical effects of compression are supplemented by spasm of the artery. To these effects may be added in some cases those of compression of the nutrient arterial branches in their course through the intervertebral foramina. These branches are very variable both in position and importance, but a common arrangement is for a fairly large branch, which may be unilateral or bilateral, to enter along with the root of C6 or C7. Blood flow in the anterior spinal artery is caudal and, as Bolton (1939) showed, a valvular arrangement at the junction of branches with the main vessel prevents them from supplying the cord above the level at which they join it. These factors explain the ischaemic changes in the anterior horns, which are frequently seen in one or two segments below the level of compression. For example, loss of nerve cells and ischaemic changes in those that remain may be found in the T1 segment when the cord has been compressed by protrusion of the disc between the C5 and 6 vertebrae (C7 segment) (Mair and Druckman, 1953).

The most severe changes seen in the spinal cord are at the level of compression (Höök, Lidvall and Åstrom, 1960; Wilkinson, 1960). Here the cord is flatter than normal because of compression in its anteroposterior diameter. Not infrequently there is some demyelination of the white matter at the point of attachment of the thickened ligamentum denticulatum in a line passing inwards from this towards the base of the ventral horns, suggesting the lines of tension to which the cord has been subjected. Ill-defined areas of demyelination are also commonly found in the ventral parts of the posterior columns, either in the midline or at one or both sides. These are not so easily explained. They have been ascribed to ischaemia in the terminal area of supply of the anterior spinal artery or to venous stasis.

In cases of severe disc lesions there is the further factor of abnormal mobility of the spine and consequent abnormal bending of the spinal cord and this is most likely to occur in cases with fusion of vertebrae. In all these cases hyaline changes are often found in the vessel walls within the spinal cord.

Thoracic discs

Protrusions of intervertebral discs at the thoracic level are, for the reasons stated above, comparatively rare. Some are due to trauma, but in a few cases the spinal injury has been masked by other severe injuries or, more rarely, the onset of paraplegia is delayed for some weeks or even months. The great majority of protrusions at this level begin as herniations of nuclear tissue which later becomes fibrous and may undergo calcification or ossification. The normal slight kyphosis at the thoracic level brings the spinal cord into constant contact with these hard projections, and upward and downward movements cause some frictional injury.

Logue (1952), from a review of the literature and his own experience, considered that protrusions at this level constituted only about 2–3 per cent of all disc protrusions. Most occurred in patients of middle or later age and only a few appeared to be related to trauma. Thoracic disc protrusions were found only in the lower nine discs and seldom above the level of T6. In his cases the damage to the cord appeared to be disproportionate to the degree of protrusion, suggesting that some factor such as ischaemia was more important than pressure.

Lumbar discs

Although the lumbar spine is robust and well supported by muscles it has to withstand very heavy compressive strains, especially in athletic young adults. This is probably the reason why lesions of lumbar discs are common in those under the age of 40. These may be caused by external violence, such as a fall on the sacrum, but in many cases they can be attributed to severe muscular strain, especially lifting heavy weights in a stooping position. Because the majority of protrusions at this level occur between the lower lumbar vertebrae or between the lowest of these and the sacrum, they do not damage the spinal cord and their effects are those of compression of the roots of the cauda equina. Almost all are due to herniation of the nucleus pulposus, but spondylolisthesis due to tearing of the disc may occur between the lowest lumbar vertebra and the sacrum or between the two lowest lumbar vertebrae. Herniations are usually posterolateral. When they project chiefly into the intervertebral foramen they compress only one root, the most common being L4 or L5. These disc protrusions are usually associated with thickening of the connective tissue around the articular joints and this may contribute to the narrowing of the intervertebral foramina. When the disc protrudes into the canal the roots which are descending to a lower level are affected. Usually only a few roots are involved, but in some cases there is severe damage to most of the lower roots of the cauda equina. In these exceptional cases, flaccid paralysis and anaesthesia of the ankles and feet, and loss of sphincter control, may come on suddenly or progressively over a few days. In 17 cases of this kind, Jennett (1956) found large herniations of the nucleus pulposus which almost filled the spinal canal. In a further eight cases the herniation was not so large but the nerve roots were bound together by thickened arachnoid.

Degeneration of lumbar discs with osteophytosis is also very common at the lumbar level, but prominent bony ridges on the posterior surface of the vertebral bodies are rarer than at the cervical level. In severe cases osteophytes may occlude the intervertebral foramen which contains the important *arteria radicis anterior magna* going to the lumbosacral cord. These vessels are unpaired and their occlusion may lead to partial or even complete necrosis of the spinal cord at this level. Suh and Alexander (1939) found that the arteria radicis anterior magna most often entered along with the L2 root, but in different subjects it has ranged from the T8 to the L4.

Spillane (1952) drew attention to the frequency of severe protrusions at the lumbar level in achondroplasia, and related it to the dorsolumbar kyphosis which is common in these dwarfs.

Lumbar puncture and radiography

In cases of cervical disc protrusion there is very seldom any increase in the cell count in the cerebrospinal fluid but some excess of protein is found in about one-third of the cases and partial or complete spinal block in a similar proportion. When no block can be demonstrated by the usual technique, 'postural manometry'—i.e. compressing the jugular veins with the neck fully flexed or fully extended—has been recommended (Clarke and Robinson, 1956). By using the latter position those authors demonstrated spinal block in ten cases in which none was found in the normal position.

When the site of the protruded disc is at the thoracic level, an increased protein and spinal block become more common. Protrusions in the lumbar region are most often below the usual level of puncture, through the third interspace, so no spinal block is found unless there are considerable arachnoidal adhesions. But there is often a considerable rise in protein in the cerebrospinal fluid. In severe lesions of the cauda equina Jennett (1956) constantly found a complete spinal block and considerable excess of protein when the puncture was made below the level of the protrusion; in two of his cases the fluid was yellow and clotted spontaneously.

The diagnosis of disc disease rests chiefly on radiography, both by direct views and by myelograms with opaque media. At the cervical level, anteroposterior views are of little value owing to the shape of the vertebral bodies but oblique views outlining the intervertebral foramina are useful especially in cases with root symptoms. As some degree of degeneration of cervical discs is very common in middle-aged patients, slight indentation of the contrast medium, usually at several levels, may be seen in many normal cervical spines, especially when the myelogram is taken with the neck fully extended. This appearance may usually be discounted. Deeper indentations, especially if associated with posterior lipping, are more important. Protrusions at a single level are less common and are more often the result of trauma. Some, especially those between C3 and 4, may be secondary to fusion of vertebrae.

Rheumatoid arthritis involving the spinal cord

Rheumatoid arthritis is an arthropathy in which there is destruction not only of the articular joint

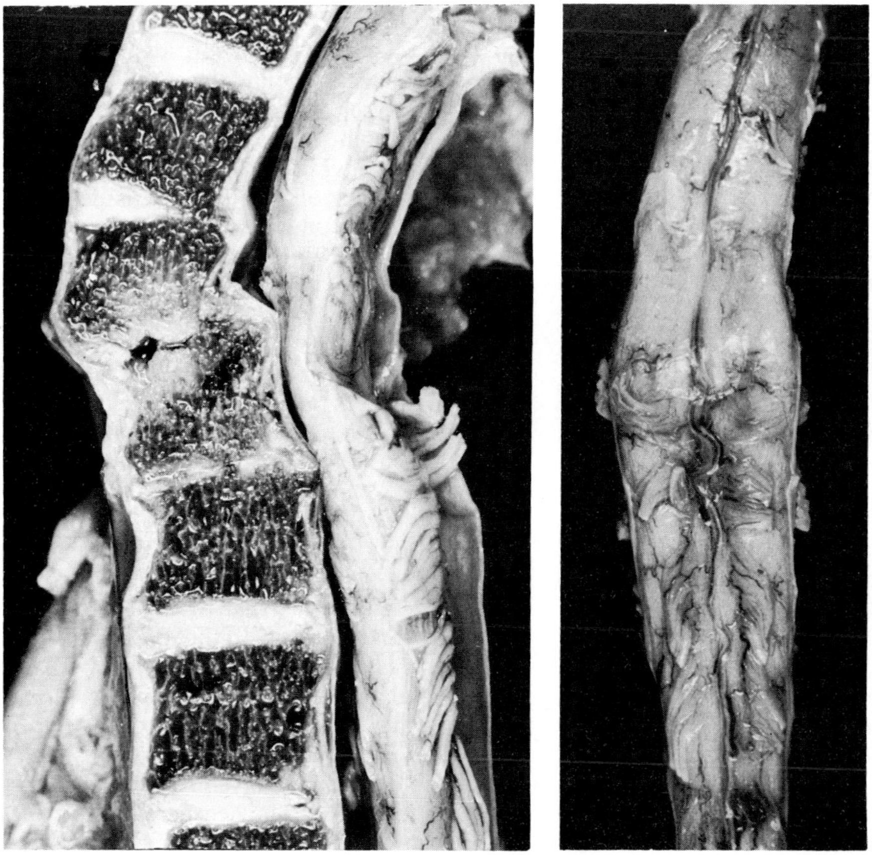

(a) **(b)**

Fig. 17.7 Rheumatoid arthritis with myelopathy. **(a)** Right half of a sagittally sawn spine at C3 to 7. There is subluxation forward of the spine down to C4 with respect to the part from C5 downwards. Note the deformity produced in the spinal cord. **(b)** Anterior aspect of spinal cord, showing compression at C4 spinal cord segment. (Reproduced, with permission, from J. Trevor Hughes, 1978, *Pathology of the Spinal Cord*, 2nd edn, Lloyd-Luke (Medical Books), London.)

surfaces and joint capsules but also of the ancillary ligaments which support the joints. It is characteristic of this disease that there is relatively little reactive bone formation and that, in the intervals when the disease is inactive, little bony repair takes place. When rheumatoid arthritis affects the spine, the arthritis does not itself create the osteophytes characteristic of spondylosis deformans, although this disorder may co-exist. Rheumatoid arthritis involving the spine produces a myelopathy by cervical dislocations which may occur between C1 and 2 (atlantoaxial) or below C2 (subaxial). Subaxial dislocations are less common, and in neither has the pathological abnormality of the spinal cord been studied in more than a few cases. Hughes (1977) described two cases with severe long-standing rheumatoid arthritis involving the cervical spine. A progressive spinal cord syndrome developed in which spastic paraparesis was combined with a lower motor neuron paresis affecting the upper limbs. In both cases necropsy showed the cause to be subluxation between the C4 and 5 vertebral bodies and backward encroachment into the spinal canal of the upper and posterior part of the C5 vertebral body (Fig. 17.7). A feature of the spinal cord abnormality was central infarction, apparently caused by an effect on a patent anterior spinal artery and manifested not only at the site of spinal cord compression but also for several spinal cord segments caudal to this level.

Pott's paraplegia (paraplegia associated with spinal caries)

The name Pott's disease should be reserved for the association of paraplegia with spinal curvature due to tuberculous caries, since Percival Pott in 1779 was the first to draw attention to this association in the English literature. But as the name is often used for the spinal disease alone (although this was described by Galen) the term Pott's paraplegia is here used to avoid ambiguity. A fuller account of the condition was published in France in the same year by David, and indeed Pott did not recognize the tuberculous nature of the spinal disease until 1782.

Pott's paraplegia occurs in from 5 to 20 per cent of all cases of spinal caries involving the cervical and thoracic vertebrae. As is well known, spinal caries is most common in the thoracic vertebrae and paraplegia is therefore most often due to lesions at this level, but caries of cervical vertebrae carries an equal risk of paraplegia (Butler, 1935). Paraplegia may precede obvious disease of the spine, especially in adults, but usually follows very soon after the appearance of spinal disease. In cases with angular kyphosis due to caries of one or more vertebral bodies three factors may combine to damage the spinal cord: (1) the presence of granulation tissue or a cold abscess in the epidural space; (2) pressure on the cord; and (3) compression or disease of its nutrient vessels. The first of these factors is probably the most important and has received most attention, but either or both of the latter may contribute to cause the more severe and permanent forms of paraplegia.

1. *Granulation tissue*. Whether the primary disease is in the vertebral bodies or, as rarely occurs, in the laminae, granulation tissue tends to reach the epidural space, where it spreads both up and down the canal and around the cord. It soon fills the space between the spinal theca and bone, and becomes adherent to the dura mater. The dura usually resists invasion and becomes thickened by the formation of new fibrous tissue on its outer surface. The tuberculous granulation tissue compresses the cord and produces oedema by impeding venuous drainage. This compression of the cord is the probable cause of the minor degrees of paraplegia which improve after treatment. In some such cases improvement coincides with, and appears to be due to, the tracking of a cold abscess into the soft paravertebral tissues.

The most usual lesion in early cases is a vacuolar type of myelin degeneration in the lateral or anterolateral columns. This is often more diffuse than that seen in ischaemic lesions and may be secondary to venous obstruction. It can sometimes be demonstrated that the myelin is more damaged than the axons. In three cases of Pott's paraplegia, associated with sharp kyphosis and epidural granulation tissue, Holmes (1906) could find no evidence of Wallerian degeneration of long tracts above or below the lesion in spite of considerable damage to myelin at this level. In a few cases there are severe degenerative and necrotic lesions in the white and grey matter with long tract degeneration.

2. *Angulation pressure*. Prolonged angulation of the cord over a sharp kyphosis usually results in thinning of the cord at that level, especially in its anteroposterior diameter (Fig. 17.8). This may not be associated with much damage to the

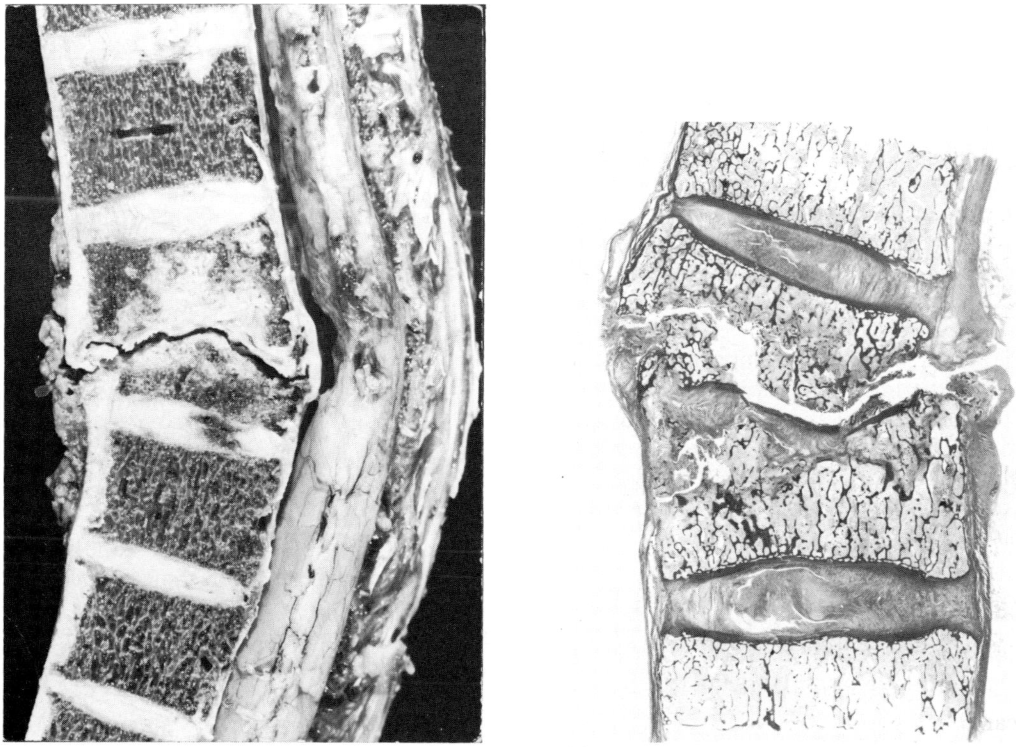

(a) **(b)**

Fig. 17.8 Pott's paraplegia. (**a**) Right half of the sagittally sawn specimen of thoracic cord. There is collapse of T7 and 8 vertebral bodies due to a tuberculous osteitis which has spread into the T7/8 intervertebral disc. The anterior aspect of the spinal cord is compressed by the kyphosis. (There is, incidentally, a Schmorl's node in the lower part of T9 body.) (**b**) Section of decalcified spine seen in (**a**); the histological appearances are a mirror image. Haematoxylin and van Gieson stain for connective tissue. (Reproduced, with permission, from J. Trevor Hughes, 1978, *Pathology of the Spinal Cord*, 2nd edn, Lloyd-Luke (Medical Books), London.)

white columns of the cord, but there is evident loss of tissue and, in many cases, definite demyelination at this level. Acute and severe lesions of the cord may be produced in cases of rapid collapse of a vertebral body, when the cord is bent over a relatively intact intervertebral disc between two diseased vertebrae, or when a sequestrum is pushed backwards into the spinal canal by the angulation (Seddon, 1935). Dislocation of the spine is also liable to produce sudden severe damage to the cord.

3. *Vascular effect*. In all these cases an important radicular artery may be compressed in the intervertebral foramen or may be the seat of tuberculous arteritis before it enters the dural sheath. This may account for some cases of paraplegia of rapid onset in cases in which the vertebral and epidural disease is not usually severe.

Compression of the spinal cord in other inflammatory diseases of the spine

A number of other micro-organisms may cause osteomyelitis of the vertebral bodies or laminae with spread of inflammatory granulation tissue into the epidural space. Of these the most common is *Staphylococcus pyogenes*, which may produce an epidural abscess which tracks down the spinal canal, or a more localized mass of granulomatous tissue which compresses the cord. Subacute cases of this kind may occur after one or more attacks of staphylococcal infection in other parts of the body.

Vascular disorders of the spinal cord

Anatomy

Thomas Willis in 1664, in his book *Cerebri Anatome*, made the first important anatomical description of the vessels of the human spinal cord (Hughes, 1982). Many subsequent writers copied Willis' drawings, which were not bettered until those of Albrecht von Haller (1708–1777). The modern literature begins with the publications of Adamkiewicz (1881, 1882), then professor at the Institute of Experimental Pathology at Krakow, and his pupil Kadyi (1889), who together laid the foundations of our modern understanding of the blood supply of the human spinal cord.To this has been added the findings of injection studies (Bolton, 1939; Herren and Alexander, 1939; Suh and Alexander, 1939) and of experimental work on the spinal cord of the monkey (Sahs, 1942; Yoss, 1950). The vasculature of the human spinal cord has been described in detail by Corbin (1961), Jellinger (1966) and Hughes (1967).

Embryology

In the embryo, the arterial supply of the spinal cord accurately follows the segmental arrangement of vertebrate development. The aorta, which first appears as a capillary ventral to the neural tube, gives off branches to each spinal cord segment and these arteries are among the first in the body to develop and for a time are the largest and the most important vessels. At this stage, each spinal cord segment is supplied by a pair of anterior and a pair of posterior radicular arteries. Each radicular artery gives off an ascending and a descending branch which anastomose with the corresponding branches belonging to adjacent segments. With the passage of time many of these radicular arteries become rudimentary or disappear, but the anastomotic channels increase in calibre and importance, resulting in one large anterior anastomotic channel, or anterior spinal artery, and two smaller posterior anastomotic channels, or posterior spinal arteries. The adult arterial vasculature is based on these three vessels of which the first described is by far the most important.

Arteries

The anterior spinal artery arises by the union of the anterior spinal branches of each vertebral artery, which usually takes place at the level of the foramen magnum. In about 10 per cent of cases this union is delayed as far down as the lower cervical region. Very rarely, the anterior spinal artery is duplicated throughout most of its length but small parts of the artery are commonly double. The anterior spinal artery lies in approximate relation to the anterior median sulcus but pursues a slightly zigzag course determined by the entry of the radicular tributaries. The calibre of the artery is widest in the lumbosacral region and narrowest in the thoracic region but also varies at various segments, being wider just caudal to the entry of a large tributary artery. From this observation, from the results of injection experiments, from some radiological evidence, and from certain case reports, it is thought that during life the blood flow in the human anterior spinal artery is in the caudal direction. The artery throughout the length of the spinal cord is maintained by successive contributions of the various radicular arteries which enter the anterior spinal artery in a caudal direction and supply the spinal cord below the point of their entry.

The two posterior spinal arteries arise from the vertebral arteries or, more rarely, from the posterior inferior cerebellar arteries. The continuity of the channel of a posterior spinal artery is much less distinct than that of the anterior spinal artery and each posterior spinal artery may appear as more than a single vessel. When, as is usual, the artery can be recognized as a single structure it is tortuous and often moves medially or laterally away from its usual position at the region of entry of the posterior nerve roots. Frequently the arteries are discontinuous and sometimes one artery moves across to supply the other side. It is rare for the posterior radicular tributaries to be seen easily, as they frequently end in a plexus of small arteries. The blood flow of the posterior spinal arteries is probably caudal in the cervical and thoracic regions and in an upward direction in the lumbosacral region. There is a good anastomosis around the cauda equina between the anterior spinal artery and the posterior spinal arteries.

Of the radicular tributary arteries, those accompanying the anterior spinal nerve roots (the anterior radicular arteries) are of considerable importance. Anterior radicular tributaries accompany nearly every anterior spinal nerve root but some of these provide a blood supply only for the root itself. A small and variable number are large and supply the anterior spinal artery. The larger tributaries usually number from three to nine. The largest anterior tributary is usually a substantial vessel and has been called the artery of Adamkiewicz. In 12 out of 40 human cords (Hughes, 1967) this artery accompanied the left T10 anterior nerve root. In most of the remainder of the cases this major artery accompanied one of the anterior roots from T9 to L1. These radicular tributaries may be subdivided into two groups, the first being those derived from the subclavian artery and the second directly from the aorta. It follows that somewhere in the region of the second thoracic spinal cord segment there is a change of arterial supply from a subclavian supply to a direct aortic supply, and this anatomical feature is sometimes of clinical importance.

The sulcal arteries arise from the anterior spinal artery and pass backwards in the anterior median sulcus. They enter the grey commissure and, by turning either left or right, supply the grey matter and central white matter of one side. These vessels and their branches form what is termed the centrifugal arterial system. The centripetal arterial system, of lesser importance, is formed by radial arteries proceeding inwardly as branches from the coronal arterial plexus surrounding the spinal cord.

It is remarkable that certain vascular diseases affect the vessels of the spinal cord much less than those of the brain. Atherosclerosis is very rare, and hypertensive arterial and arteriolar changes are much less severe in the spinal cord than in the brain of the same patient. The blood pressure in the spinal arteries is probably lower than elsewhere in the vascular system.

Veins

The spinal venous system is prominent on the posterior aspect of the spinal cord, particularly in the lumbosacral region. The venous network is irregular and there is considerable anastomosis between the large venous trunks. There is, however, with regularity a single large median posterior vein, applied to the posterior aspect of the spinal cord in the region of the posterior median septum, and this vessel appears to have no arterial counterpart. The posterior spinal vein receives draining veins from the posterior columns and parts of the posterior horns. The anterior spinal vein accompanies the anterior spinal artery and receives small veins corresponding to the sulcal arteries arising from the anterior spinal artery. Both the anterior spinal veins and the median posterior vein are themselves drained by radicular veins, which accompany the anterior or posterior spinal nerve roots. These radicular veins are commoner than the corresponding radicular arteries, and, like them, some are especially large. These large veins can be termed major radicular veins but often are independent of the major arterial tributaries. The radicular veins drain into the paravertebral and intervertebral plexus, which caudally communicate with the pelvic venous plexuses.

Pathological changes

Occlusion of the anterior spinal artery

The upper part of the anterior spinal artery supplies the anterior and median portion of the lower medulla, in which the following structures are present: the pyramids and pyramidal decussations; the medial lemnisci; the medial longitudinal fasciculi; the caudal portions of the hypoglossal and posterior vagal nuclei; the nucleus and tractus solitarius on each side (at the level of the decussation); the lateral spinothalamic and ventral spinocerebellar tracts (Gower's tracts); the olivocerebellar fibres as they cross the midline; part of the inferior olivary nuclei; and the internal and ventral external arcuate fibres and nuclei. In the spinal cord this artery supplies about two-thirds of the cross-sectional area of the cord, excluding the posterior parts of the posterior white columns and the posterior grey columns.

Obstruction of the upper part of the anterior spinal artery to involve the medulla is uncommon. The occlusion of the spinal part of the anterior spinal artery, commonly by thrombosis, causes a well-recognized clinical syndrome. In obstruction of the upper spinal part the onset is sudden with pain in the back and in the neck and with paraesthesiae experienced in the upper limbs. In a few hours the condition progresses to a flaccid paralysis of both arms with loss of pain and temperature sensation below a sensory level.

Touch, joint and position sense are preserved. The lower limbs may develop a spastic paraplegia, and paralysis of the bowel and/or bladder is common. The prognosis is reasonably good, with considerable improvement in the neurological deficit except for the lower motor neuron paralysis in the arms which is usually permanent.

Published accounts of this syndrome with confirmation of the pathology by necropsy are surprisingly few. The account of Margulis (1930) referred to three cases (cases 1, 2 and 7) in which syphilitic arteritis caused anterior spinal artery thrombosis, and these cases were similar to several described earlier in this century. Syphilis is no longer the common predisposing cause of the condition. In the case of Schott (1915) the thrombosis was attributed to minor trauma, and this was also the cause in the report of Grinker and Guy (1927). In their case, a 15-year-old boy developed thrombosis of the upper part of the anterior spinal artery, apparently caused by subluxation of the cervical spine. Similar minor trauma was postulated in the case of Hughes and Brownell (1964) in which cervical spondylosis was present. That part of the anterior spinal artery affected by thrombosis was adjacent to a large spondylotic protrusion. This case, in which cervical spondylosis was complicated by anterior spinal artery thrombosis, is relevant to the problem of chronic myelopathy due to spondylosis. In these cases, Mair and Druckman (1953) considered that the changes which occur in the spinal cord, in association with protrusion of cervical intervertebral discs, are secondary to compression of the anterior spinal artery and its branches.

Proven cases of occlusion of the caudal portion of the anterior spinal artery are also few and were reviewed by Zeitlin and Lichtenstein (1936). All were due to syphilis. Their own case was unusual in that the extent of the lesion was in the middle segment of the cord from C5 to T10, being maximal at T7. This case was also exceptional in that the thrombosis occurred in an anterior spinal artery which was affected by atheroma. Atheroma has very rarely been reported in the anterior spinal artery, and most authors comment on its rarity.

Occlusion of the posterior spinal artery

The syndrome of anterior spinal artery occlusion is well known, but that of obstruction of the posterior spinal arteries is scarcely recognized. Hughes (1970), in describing a case with necropsy confirmation of the diagnosis, could find only seven previous case reports. Clinically, the onset begins with pain or dysaesthesia but paresis or paralysis of the lower limbs and trunk rapidly supervenes. The bladder and bowel are also paralysed. This description refers to the period immediately following the onset of the neurological syndrome when, because of swelling and oedema, there is a temporary disability of the spinal cord amounting to a cord transection. If the patient survives this acute phase, considerable neurological improvement may occur, and recovery may be almost complete. The lower limb and trunk paresis may disappear, and normal control of bladder and bowel can be regained. Only a moderate sensory deficit may persist, demonstrable on careful neurological examination and causing no symptons. This would be the expected loss of function from destruction of the spinal cord in the territories of the posterior spinal arteries. The predisposing cause of the occlusion of the posterior spinal artery is usually apparent in the case history, and in the case of Hughes (1970) the thrombosis was caused by an intrathecal phenol injection. Thrombosis is generally present, and in the earlier reports this occurred in the setting of syphilitic arteritis. In the case of Stone and Roback (1937), the onset of the neurological syndrome followed minor indirect trauma. Two cases were described by Perier et al. (1960), and the second of these was exceptional in that the posterior spinal arteries were obstructed by embolic atheromatous material.

Neurological complications of the adult type of coarctation of the aorta

Coarctation of the aorta, first described by Morgagni in 1761, is a congenital stenosis of the isthmus of the aorta, which is that part of the aorta between the origin of the left subclavian artery and the ductus arteriosus. It has been customary to divide cases into two types: 'infantile' with extensive obliteration of the aortic isthmus; and 'adult' type in which there is a small segment of narrowing which may be before, at or (the usual situation) beyond the origin of the left subclavian artery. In the adult type the ductus arteriosus closes and there is an extensive anastomotic circulation between the arteries supplying the upper trunk and limbs and those arising beyond the aortic constrictions which supply the lower trunk and lower limbs. These 'adult' type cases alone concern us in a consideration of neurological complications. An important factor is the arterial hypertension in the upper parts of the body, which contrasts with the hypotension in the lower parts of the body.

In the combined figures of Abbott (1928) and Reifenstein, Levine and Gross (1947), which covered 304 cases of the adult type of coarctation, death was considered on clinical grounds to be due to an intracranial haemorrhage in 36 cases and this diagnosis was confirmed *post mortem* in 29 of them. In 10 cases a ruptured saccular aneurysm of the circle of Willis was found and this mechanism is probably a common cause of intracranial haemorrhage complicating coarctation of the aorta.

Complications affecting the spinal cord are fewer and are of two types:

1. *Those due to a reduced blood supply to the more caudal part of the spinal cord.* These complications formed the majority of the case reports recorded by Tyler and Clark (1958). The symptoms and signs of paresis and sensory and sphincteric disturbance were attributed by these authors to ischaemia and hypotension of that part of the spinal cord supplied by arteries derived from the aorta distal to the constriction.
2. *Complications due to the hypertension present in the body in arteries arising proximal to the aortic constriction.* The anastomotic circulation mentioned above includes the anterior spinal artery. The blood passes from the heart to the subclavian arteries, then via the vertebral arteries into the upper part of the anterior spinal artery, and via the ascending cervical branches of the thyrocervical trunks into the upper radicular tributaries of the anterior spinal artery. The blood bypasses the aortic obstruction by flowing down the anterior spinal artery to reach the spinal branches of the aortic intercostals below the obstruction. In such cases the anterior spinal artery becomes enlarged and tortuous and may compress the spinal cord.

Neurological complications of dissecting aneurysm of the aorta

In dissecting aneurysms of the aorta there is an extensive haemorrhage into the tunica media of the aorta, and within this plane the aortic wall is forced apart into two layers. The dissection by this haemorrhage may extend along the tunica media to involve the innominate, carotid or femoral arteries, narrowing the lumen and impairing the blood flow. It may surround, stretch or even tear the intercostal and lumbar arteries and obliterate their lumen. Thrombosis may occur in these narrowed arteries. Accounts of the pathology of the condition were listed by Braunstein (1963). In its commonest form the condition is associated with arteriosclerosis in which systemic hypertension and aortic dilatation probably predispose to the dissection. The commonest finding at necropsy is severe atherosclerosis and a tear through the intima of the aorta often sited on an atheromatous plaque. More rarely, dissecting aneurysm of the aorta is seen in Marfan's syndrome and there is also an uncommon association with pregnancy, aortic stenosis and myxoedema. Syphilitic aortitis does not seem to be linked to dissection of the aorta.

Neurological complications are common in dissecting aneurysm of the aorta. Shennan (1934) found them in 45 out of 317 cases, and Lindsay and Hurst (1967) in 26 out of 62. Weismann and Adams (1944) divided the neurological complications into three groups:

1. *Ischaemic necrosis of peripheral nerves.* This is the commonest neurological complication and is usually associated with extension of the haemorrhage into the subclavian or iliac arteries, thus causing impairment of blood supply to the nerves of the limbs.
2. *Ischaemic necrosis of the brain.* This is the least common complication. It is usually associated with extension of the dissection into the innominate or carotid arteries. The effects are similar to occlusion of the carotid artery, which has already been considered.
3. *Ischaemic necrosis of the spinal cord.* The involvement of the spinal cord in cases of dissecting aneurysm of the aorta requires more detailed comment. Reviewing the literature of this association and considering only the accounts with necropsy, about 11 case reports are readily accessible. It is evident from these reports that the dissection of the aorta causes more extensive spinal damage in some cases than in others. In some case reports, as in the case of Kalischer (1914) and the first case of Lange-Cosack and Köhn (1962), it is probable that death supervened before the changes in the spinal cord became evident. This explanation will not suffice for all

these instances and, for example, in the case of Moersch and Sayre (1950), despite a sufficient interval to death, no changes were found. Several cases have had complete necrosis of the whole cross-sectional area of the spinal cord affecting several consecutive spinal cord segments. To this group belong the cases of Schwartz, Shorey and Anderson (1950), Ballentine (1952), and Hills and Vasquez (1962).

The striking differences in the extent of spinal cord involvement can be explained by the pattern of blood supply to the spinal cord. The obstructive effect of the dissecting aneurysm, which may involve a variable extent of the aortic media, may occlude one or several of the intercostal and lumbar arteries. The degree of interference with the blood flow in these spinal branches accounts for the variations in the extent of the spinal cord infarction. The other complicating factor is the importance to the spinal cord of these spinal branches and, in particular, whether a large tributary or small insignificant tributaries are affected.

In general, the portion of the spinal cord which is severely damaged is the mid- and lower thoracic region, and this is the region supplied by the intercostal arteries. The upper part of the cord, which derives its blood supply from branches of the vertebral arteries, is seldom involved. The lumbosacral cord, which is supplied by the lumbar, iliolumbar and lateral sacral arteries, is sometimes damaged when the aneurysmal dissection has been extensive. The ischaemic necrosis always involves the grey matter and the adjacent white matter. The white matter at the periphery of the cord is sometimes spared but, in severe cases, the whole cross-section of the cord may be necrotic at certain levels.

Arteriovenous malformation of the spinal cord

In 1926 Foix and Alajouanine described two cases under the title 'La myélite nécrotique subaigue'. These male patients, aged 19 and 27, had developed a progressive ascending paralysis and anaesthesia. The paralysis was initially of the upper motor neuron type but later became flaccid, and the anaesthesia, initially dissociated in character, later became complete. The spinal fluid was remarkable in that a massive protein increase was accompanied by only a slight lymphocytosis. In both cases the progressive course of the illness led to a fatal issue, in 2 years 9 months in the first case and in 11 months in the second case. The necropsy findings in both cases were distinctive. The lower thoracic, lumbar and sacral parts of the spinal cord were affected by large areas of necrosis. The grey matter was completely destroyed but the white matter damage, although extensive, was incomplete. The histological picture in the severely affected spinal cord segments was remarkable not only for the necrosis and numerous lipid phagocytes but also because of the striking vascular changes. In both cases the authors observed enlargement and thickening of the extramedullary and of the intramedullary vessels of the spinal cord, the veins being chiefly affected. These vascular changes were termed 'endomesovascularitis' and were attributed to some toxic or infective agent which had also caused the parenchymal destruction in the spinal cord.

This paper, containing the two case reports described above, directed attention to a condition which is sometimes called Foix–Alajouanine disease and was renamed *angiodysgenetische nekrotisierende Myelopathie* by Scholtz and Manuelidis (1951). The underlying pathology in many of these cases is now considered (Antoni, 1962) to be a spinal arteriovenous malformation (aneurysm) or fistula. The numerous case reports of the condition have been reviewed by Wyburn-Mason (1943), Corbin (1961), Jellinger (1966), Neumayer (1967).

Spinal cord angiography The great advance in our understanding of these cases has come from the development of angiographic procedures directed at the spinal cord. Formerly, angiomatous malformations were recognized by myelography but this technique added little to our knowledge of the type of malformation present. In 1962 Djindjian and his co-workers (Djindjian, 1970) reported their first angiographic investigation of an intraspinal arteriovenous aneurysm, and in 1966 this group (Djindjian, Faure and Hurth, 1966) reported 12 cases of intraspinal arteriovenous aneurysms examined by this technique. An important part of the technique depends on removing the opacity of overlying bone structure by cancelling the image components common to the preliminary and subsequent (contrast-filled) radiographs. These radiographic studies, now widely employed (Di Chiro and Wener, 1973), have shown that the commonest type of spinal angioma is an arteriovenous communication in which one or more of the spinal arteries forms a cluster of vessels which allow blood flow through into one or more of the draining veins without the blood passing in the normal way through the capillary bed of the spinal cord. The feeding artery (or arteries) to one of these angiomatous malformations has a normal origin and direction but is enormously enlarged. If this arterial pedicle can be identified and ligated the progressive enlargement of the malformation can be arrested. These angiographic observations, which have so elegantly demonstrated the haemodynamics of these spinal angiomas, now direct attention to the pathological findings which are consistent with the presence of abnormal arteriovenous communication in the spinal vessels.

Morbid anatomy The macroscopic appearances at necropsy (Fig. 17.9) are remarkably

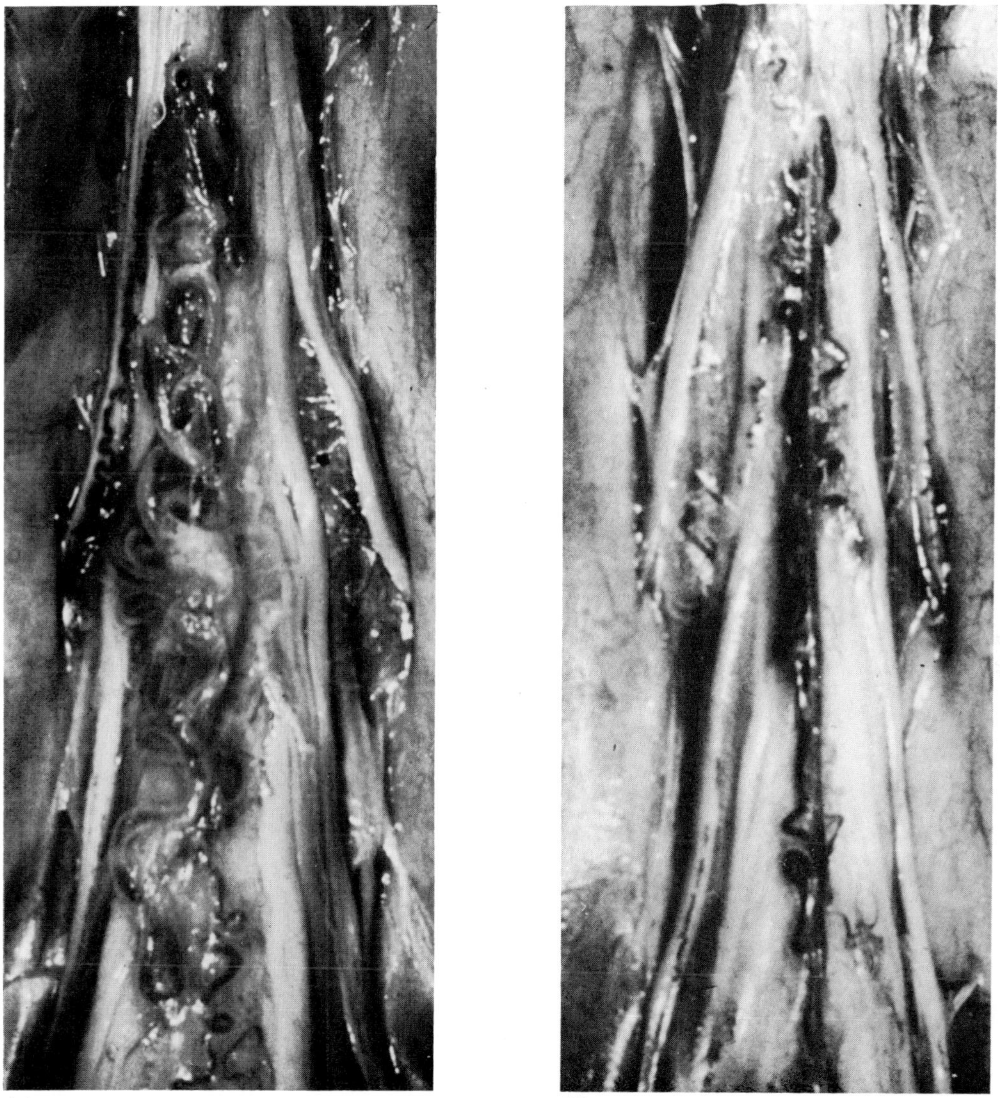

(a) **(b)**

Fig. 17.9 Arteriovenous angiomatous malformation. (**a**) Posterior aspect of lower thoracic and lumbar regions of the spinal cord. There is a large tortuous vessel additional to the normal venous system. (**b**) Anterior aspect of the lower thoracic and lumbar regions of the spinal cord of case seen in (**a**). The anterior spinal artery is normal but the anterior spinal vein is enlarged and tortuous.

uniform in these cases. However, the complexity of the various components of the spinal cord vasculature makes a complete assessment difficult even for the expert and very confusing to the inexperienced pathologist.

The anterior spinal artery is normal or slightly enlarged. The posterior spinal arteries are normal. The spinal venous system is normal in its fundamental anatomy but abnormal in the hypertrophy and distension of most of the spinal veins. The anterior spinal vein, for example, is always normally situated. A constant finding is a very abnormal large thick-walled tortuous vessel pursuing an irregular course longitudinally on the posterior surface of the spinal cord. At necropsy (and by some surgeons during life) this tortuous convoluted vessel can be dissected away from the spinal cord as a single continuous vascular channel greatly exceeding in length that of the whole spinal cord. This abnormal vessel is now known from angiographic studies during life to be part of an abnormal vascular communication between the arterial and venous systems of the spinal cord. It is difficult at necropsy, but easy during life with the angiographic techniques mentioned, to determine the artery or arteries feeding into this large complex vessel and the veins which drain it.

Histological findings The microscopical findings (Fig. 17.10) are so unusual that, in many of the published reports, attention has been directed away from the more informative macroscopic appearances. Furthermore, the anatomy of the malformation described above becomes difficult to eludicate after the spinal cord is cut transversely and tissue blocks are taken. The histological changes are more advanced in the caudal part of the spinal cord, being very evident in the lumbosacral enlargement. There are many capillaries and other small thick-walled channels, the size and position of which suggest that they are altered capillaries and veins. These vessels have thick hyaline walls which are sometimes calcified. Recent thrombosis may be seen within these intramedullary vessels and others show changes indicative of the organization of earlier thrombus. Thrombosis may also be seen in the large extramedullary vessels. The examination by elastin stains of the tunica media of the large abnormal vessels shows them to have the structure of arterialized veins.

The substance of the spinal cord is affected by an unusual form of incomplete necrosis (Fig. 17.10) which involves grey and white matter but particularly the central parts of the cord. The majority of the neuronal cell bodies are lost but

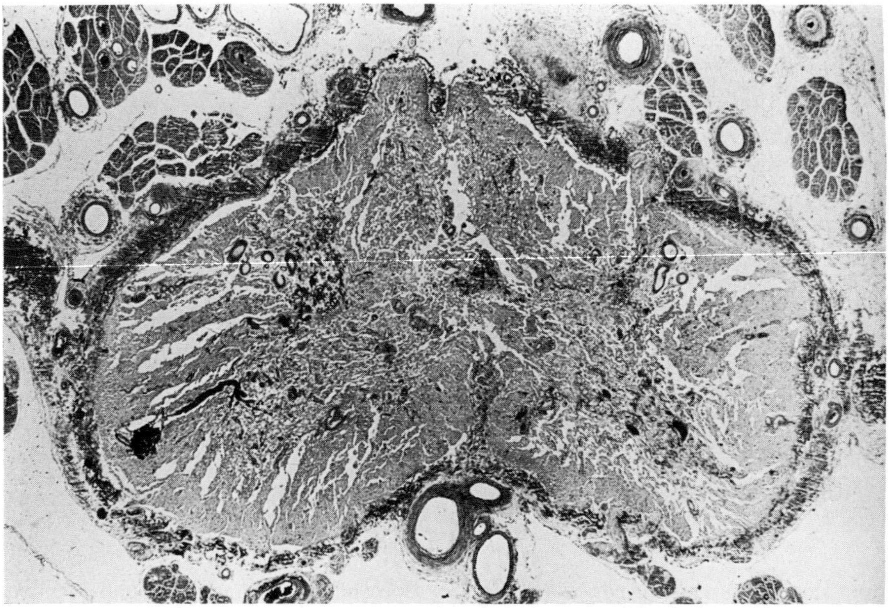

Fig. 17.10 Transverse section (at S1) of the cord in Fig. 17.9, showing the enlarged vessels and partial necrosis of the parenchyma of the cord.

some, although apparently dead, are encrusted with material that stains for iron and calcium. Lipid phagocytes are common but acute inflammatory cells are usually absent. The upper parts of the spinal cord show Wallerian degeneration of the upward-directed long tracts.

Spinal thrombophlebitis Proven cases of a syndrome caused by spinal thrombophlebitis are extremely rare. In the reported cases, the occlusion of the spinal veins has led to an acute haemorrhagic venous infarction of the spinal cord which has caused the rapid development of an acute syndrome of the spinal cord destruction. The name 'spinal thrombophlebitis' has also been applied to cases which now would be recognized as an angiomatous malformation of the spinal cord with thrombosis in some of the abnormal vessels. This condition has been described above. Only acute thrombophlebitis is considered here.

One of the earliest cases of this type of venous infarction of the spinal cord was that reported by Wyss (1898) under the name 'acute haemorrhagic myelitis'. In this report extensive haemorrhagic infarction of the spinal cord was associated with thrombosis of the veins of the spinal cord and those of the spinal meninges. The cause of the venous thrombosis was a tumour of the spinal cord which was said to be a gliosarcoma. In the same year, Petren (1898) described spinal cord infarction due to venous thrombosis associated with extensive generalized septicaemia. There are now at least seven case reports (Hughes, 1971) in which necropsy has shown venous infarction of the spinal cord caused by acute thrombophlebitis. In these case reports the clinical features and the pathological findings are remarkably constant.

Clinical features The onset of the condition is rapid and invariably associated with pain which is felt in the back, the legs or the abdomen. After 1 or 2 days, weakness and loss of sensation in the legs and trunk develop, and these symptoms are usually combined with paralysis of the bladder and bowel. The spinal fluid shows an elevation of cells and of protein but these changes may be slight or absent. If myelography is performed it gives findings indicative of moderate swellings of the spinal cord with a partial hold-up of the column of contrast medium rather than a complete obstruction. In all cases the illness has been rapidly progressive and the outcome has been death in the first or second week of the neurological illness. In these reviewed cases the poor prognosis has been due to the gravity of the associated illness which causes the venous infaction of the spinal cord. The actual prognosis of the condition may be less grave because only cases verified by necropsy have been diagnosed. It is possible that a milder form of the condition exists but is not recognized clinically.

Pathological findings In nearly all the cases there is an obvious causative disease to explain this extensive venous thrombosis. The commonest causative condition has been generalized sepsis but other causes have been a spinal cord tumour and a generalized thrombotic syndrome.

The spinal veins are always greatly distended and are usually extensively thrombosed. The venous obstruction may, however, be sited in the plexus of veins in the spinal canal or in the veins in the pelvis and abdomen. The spinal cord itself is disrupted by severe haemorrhagic necrosis in which small haematomas are conspicuous. The worst-affected parts of the spinal cord are the central areas, and the infarction is much more haemorrhagic than after arterial occlusion. The extent of the infarct both longitudinally and in its cross-sectional area is greater even than that caused by an extensive thrombosis of the anterior spinal artery.

Subacute and chronic spinal thrombophlebitis. The above description refers to acute infarction caused by an acute thrombophlebitis. Cases do occur of a subacute or chronic spinal cord syndrome produced by either a more gradual venous thrombotic occlusion or a recurrence of episodes of spinal cord deficit due to recurrent thrombosis. These cases require careful separation from case of spinal vascular malformations. The finding of thrombosed veins either around the spinal cord or in the abdomen and pelvis is not conclusive. These obscure myelopathies invariably suffer from a paraplegic syndrome in which pressure sores and urinary tract infection in a recumbent patient commonly lead to venous thrombosis. In many of these cases the venous thrombosis demonstrated at necropsy is likely to have been caused by the paraplegia rather than to be itself the primary condition.

References

Abbott, M.E. (1928) Coarctation of aorta of adult type; statistical study and historical retrospect of 200 recorded cases with autopsy, of stenosis or obliteration of descending arch in subjects above age of 2 years. *American Heart Journal* **3,** 574-618.

Adamkiewicz, A. (1881) Die Blutgefässe des menschlichen Rückenmarkes. 1. Die Gefässe der Rückenmarkssubstanz. *Sitzungsberichte der Akademie der Wissenschaften in Wien. Mathematisch-naturwissenschaftliche Klasse* **84,** 469-502.

Adamkiewicz, A. (1882) Die Blutgefässe des menschlichen Rückenmarkes. 2. Die Gefässe der Rückenmarksoberfläche. *Sitzungsberichte der Akademie der Wissenschaften in Wien. Mathematisch-naturwissenschaftliche Klasse* **85,** 101-30.

Allen, K.L. (1952) Neuropathies caused by bony spurs in the cervical spine with special reference to surgical treatment. *Journal of Neurology, Neurosurgery and Psychiatry* **15,** 20-36.

Andrae, R. (1929) Ueber Knorpelknötchen am hinteren Ende der Wirbelbandscheiben im Bereich des Spinal-kanals. *Beiträge zur pathologischen Anatomie und zur allgemeinen Pathologie* **82,** 464-74.

Antoni, N. (1962) Spinal vascular malformation (angiomas) and myelomalacia. *Neurology* **12,** 795-804.

Bachs, A., Barraquer-Bordas, L., Barraquer-Ferre, L., Canadell, J.M. and Modolell, A. (1955) Delayed myelopathy following atlanto-axial dislocation by separated odontoid process. *Brain* **78,** 537-53.

Ballentine, H.T. (1952) Case records of the Massachusetts General Hospital. *New England Journal of Medicine* **247,** 326-9.

Barnett, H.J.M., Foster, J.B. and Hudgson, P. (1973) *Syringomyelia.* Saunders, London.

Beadle, O.C. (1931) *Special Report Series of the Medical Research Council, London* **161.**

Bolton, B. (1939) Blood supply of the human spinal cord. *Journal of Neurology and Psychiatry* **2,** 137-48.

Brain, W.R., Northfield, D. and Wilkinson, M. (1952) The neurological manifestations of cervical spondylosis. *Brain* **75,** 187-225.

Braunstein, H. (1963) Pathogenesis of dissecting aneurysm. *Circulation* **28,** 1071-80.

Bull, J.W.D. (1948) Discussion on rupture of the intervertebral disc in the cervical region. *Proceedings of the Royal Society of Medicine* **41,** 513-16.

Butler, R.W. (1935) Paraplegia in Pott's disease with special reference to pathology and aetiology. *British Journal of Surgery* **22,** 738-68.

Clarke, E. and Robinson, P.K. (1956) Cervical myelopathy: a complication of cervical spondylosis. *Brain* **79,** 483-510.

Collins, D.H. (1950) *The Pathology of Articular* and *Spinal Diseases.* Edward Arnold, London.

Corbin, J.L. (1961) *Anatomie et Pathologie Artérielles de la Moelle.* Masson, Paris.

Di Chiro, G. and Wener, L. (1973) Angiography of the spinal cord. *Journal of Neurosurgery* **39,** 1-29.

Djindjian, R. (1970) *Angiography of the Spinal Cord.* University Park Press, Baltimore.

Djindjian, R., Faure, C. and Hurth, M. (1966) Explorations artériographiques des anéurismes artério-veineux de la moelle épinière. *Annales de Radiologie*, Monograph No. 1.

Dohrmann, G.T., Wagner, F.C. Jr and Bucy, P.C. (1971) The microvasculature in transitory traumatic paraplegia. An electron microscopic study in the monkey. *Journal of Neurosurgery* **35,** 263-71.

Foix, C. and Alajouanine, T. (1926) La myélite nécrotique subaiguë. *Revue Neurologique* **2,** 1-42.

Frykholm, R. (1951) Lower cervical vertebrae and intervertebral discs. Surgical anatomy and pathology. *Acta Chirurgica Scandinavica* **101,** 345-59.

Goldthwait, J.E. (1911) The lumbo-sacral articulation; an explanation of many cases of 'lumbago', sciatica and paraplegia. *Boston Medical and Surgical Journal* **164,** 365-72.

Grinker, R. and Guy, C. (1927) Sprain of cervical spine causing thrombosis of the anterior spinal artery. *Journal of the American Medical Association* **88,** 1140-2.

Herren, R.Y. and Alexander, I. (1939) Sulcal and intrinsic blood vessels of human spinal cord. *Archives of Neurology and Psychiatry* **41,** 678-87.

Hills, S. and Vasquez, J.M. (1962) Massive infarction of spinal cord and vertebral bodies as a complication of dissecting aneurysm of the aorta. *Circulation* **25,** 997-1000.

Holmes, G. (1906) On the relation between loss of function and structural change in focal lesions of the central nervous system, with special reference to secondary degeneration. *Brain* **29,** 514-23.

Höök, O., Lidvall, H. and Åstrom, K.E. (1960) Cervical disk protrusions with compression of the spinal cord. *Neurology* **10,** 834-41.

Hughes, J.T. (1967) The Blood Supply and Vascular Disorders of the Human Spinal Cord. DPhil thesis, University of Oxford.

Hughes, J.T. (1970) Thrombosis of the posterior spinal arteries. A complication of an intrathecal injection of phenol. *Neurology* **20,** 659-64.

Hughes, J.T. (1971) Venous infarction of the spinal cord. *Neurology* **21,** 794-800.

Hughes, J.T. (1974) Pathology of spinal cord damage

in spinal injuries. In *Brock's Injuries of the Brain and Spinal Cord*, 5th edn (Ed. Feiring, E.H.), pp. 668–87. Springer, New York.

Hughes, J.T. (1977) Spinal cord involvement by C4–C5 vertebral subluxation in rheumatoid arthritis. A description of 2 cases examined at necropsy. *Annals of Neurology* **1,** 575–82.

Hughes, J.T. (1981) Cerebral arterial changes following acute head/spinal trauma. In *Cerebral Microcirculation and Metabolism* (Eds. Cervós-Navarro, J. and Fritschka, E.), pp. 359–60. Raven Press, New York.

Hughes, J.T. (1982) Spinal cord arteries described by Willis. In *Historical Aspects of the Neurosciences* (Eds. Rose, F.C. and Bynum W.F.), pp. 195–203. Raven Press, New York.

Hughes, J.T. and Brownell, B. (1963) Aberrant nerve fibres within the spinal cord. *Journal of Neurology, Neurosurgery and Psychiatry* **26,** 528–34.

Hughes, J.T. and Brownell, B. (1964) Cervical spondylosis complicated by anterior spinal artery thrombosis. *Neurology* **14,** 1073–7.

Jellinger, K. (1966) *Zur Orthologie und Pathologie der Rückenmarksdurchblutung*. Springer, Berlin.

Jennett, W.B. (1956) A study of 25 cases of compression of the cauda equina by prolapsed intervertebral discs. *Journal of Neurology, Neurosurgery and Psychiatry* **19,** 109–16.

Kadyi, H. (1889) *Ueber die Blutgefässe des nenschlichen Rückenmarkes*. Gubrynowicz and Schmidt, Lemberg.

Kalischer, O. (1914) Demonstration eines Präparates (Aneurysma dissecans der Aorta mit Paraplegie). *Berliner klinische Wochenschrift* **51,** 1286–8.

Lange-Cosack, H. and Köhn, K. (1962) Ischämische Rückenmark-schädigung bei Aneurysm dissecans der Aorta. *Münchener medizinische Wochenschrift* **104,** 410–13.

Lindsay, J. and Hurst, J.W. (1967) Clinical features and prognosis in dissecting aneurysm of the aorta. *Circulation* **35,** 880–8.

Logue, V. (1952) Thoracic intervertebral disc prolapse with spinal cord compression. *Journal of Neurology, Neurosurgery and Psychiatry* **15,** 227–41.

von Luschka, H. (1858) *Die Halbgelenke des Menschlichen Körpers*. Reiner, Berlin.

McRae, D.L. (1953) Bony abnormalities in region of foramen magnum: correlation of anatomic and neurologic findings. *Acta Radiologica* **40,** 335–55.

Mair, W.G.P. and Druckmann, R. (1953) The pathology of spinal cord lesions and their relation to clinical features in protrusions of cervical intervertebral discs. *Brain* **76,** 70–91.

Margulis, M.W. (1930) Pathologische Anatomie und Klinik der akuten thrombotischen Erweichungen bei spinaler Lues. *Deutsche Zeitschrift für Nervenheilkunde* **113,** 113–45.

Middleton, G.S. and Teacher, J.H. (1911) Injury of the spinal cord due to rupture of an intervertebral disc during muscular effort. *Glasgow Medical Journal* **76,** 1–6.

Moersch, F.P. and Sayre, G. (1950) Neurologic manifestations associated with dissecting aneurysm of the aorta. *Journal of the American Medical Association* **144,** 1141–8.

Neumayer, E. (1967) *Die vasculäre Myelopathie*. Springer, Berlin.

Nugent, G.R. (1959) Clinicopathologic correlations in cervical spondylosis. *Neurology* **9,** 273–81.

Payne, E.E. and Spillane, J.D. (1957) The cervical spine. An anatomico-pathological study of 70 specimens (using a special technique) with particular reference to the problem of cervical spondylosis. *Brain* **80,** 571–96.

Penning, L. (1962) Some aspects of plain radiography of the cervical spine in chronic myelopathy. *Neurology* **12,** 513–19.

Perier, O., Demanet, J.C., Henneaux, J. and Nunès-Vincénte, A. (1960) Existe-t-il un syndrome des artères spinales posterieures? *Revue Neurologique* **113,** 396–409.

Petren, K. (1898) Ein Fall von akuter Infektionskrankheit mit Thrombosen in den pialen Gefässen des Rückenmarks. *Nordiskt Medicinskt Arkiv* **7,** 1–48.

Reifenstein, G.H., Levine, S.A. and Gross, R.E. (1947) Coarctation of aorta: review of 104 autopsied cases of 'adult type', 2 years of age or older. *American Heart Journal* **33,** 146–68.

Sahs, A.L. (1942) The vascular supply of the spinal cord in monkeys. *Journal of Comparative Neurology* **76,** 403–15.

Schmorl, G. and Junghans, H. (1959) *The Human Spine in Health and Disease*, 1st American edn. (Trans. and Ed. Wilk, S.P.). Grune and Stratton, New York.

Schneider, R.C. (1951) Syndrome in acute cervical spine injuries for which early operation is indicated. *Journal of Neurosurgery* **8,** 360–7.

Scholtz, W. and Manuelidis, E.F. (1951) Angiodysgenetische nekrotisierende Myelopathie. *Deutsche Zeitschrift für Nervenheilkunde* **165,** 56–71.

Schott, E. (1915) Schwere Rückenmarksläsion nach leichtem Trauma. *Medizinische Klinik* **9,** 43–5.

Schwartz, G.A., Shorey, W.K. and Anderson, N.S. (1950) Myelomalacia secondary to dissecting aneurysm of the aorta. *Archives of Neurology and Psychiatry* **64,** 401–16.

Seddon, H.J. (1935) Pott's paraplegia, prognosis and treatment. *British Journal of Surgery* **22,** 769–99.

Shennan, T. (1934) *Special Report Series of the Medical Research Council, London* **193.**

Spillane, J.D. (1952) Three cases of achondroplasia with neurological complications. *Journal of Neurology, Neurosurgery and Psychiatry* **15,** 246–52.

Stone, L. and Roback, H.N. (1937). Myelomalacia

without thrombosis following indirect trauma (strain). *Journal of the American Medical Association* **108,** 1698–701.

Suh, T.H. and Alexander, L. (1939) Vascular system of the human spinal cord. *Archives of Neurology and Psychiatry* **41,** 659–77.

Tyler, H.R. and Clark, O.B. (1958) Neurological complications in patients with coarction of aorta. *Neurology* **8,** 712–18.

Wagner, F.C. Jr, Dohrmann, G.J. and Bucy, P.C. (1971) Histopathology of transitory traumatic paraplegia in the monkey. *Journal of Neurosurgery* **35,** 272–6.

Wallace, D. and Bruce, A. (1910) Case of dislocation between the atlas and the axis vertebrae, with probable fracture of the odontoid process, reduction, recovery. *Review of Neurology and Psychiatry* **8,** 1–7.

Weismann, A.D. and Adams, R.A. (1944) The neurological complications of dissecting aortic aneurysm. *Brain* **67,** 69–92.

Wilkinson, M. (1960) The morbid anatomy of cervical spondylosis and myelopathy. *Brain* **83,** 589–617.

Wolf, B.S., Khilnani, M. and Malis, L.I. (1956) Sagittal diameter of bony cervical canal and its significance in cervical spondylosis. *Journal of Mount Sinai Hospital* **23,** 283–92.

Wyburn-Mason, R. (1943) *The Vascular Abnormalities and Tumours of the Spinal Cord and its Membranes*. Kimpton, London.

Wyllie, W.G. (1923) The occurrence in osteitis deformans of lesions of the central nervous system with a report of four cases. *Brain* **46,** 336–51.

Wyss, O. (1898) Über acute hämorrhagische Myelitis. *Deutsche medizinische Wochenschrift* **24,** 81V.

Yoss, R.E. (1950) Vascular supply of the spinal cord: the production of vascular syndromes. *University of Michigan Medical Bulletin* **16,** 333–45.

Zeitlin, H. and Lichtenstein, B.W. (1936) Occlusion of the anterior spinal artery. *Archives of Neurology and Psychiatry* **36,** 96–111.

18

Diseases of the peripheral nerves

P.K. Thomas, D.N. Landon and R.H.M. King

Normal structure of peripheral nerve

Introduction

The peripheral nerves of vertebrates are composite structures containing nerve fibres, blood vessels and collagenous connective tissue, all enclosed within continuous cellular and connective tissue sheaths. The nerve fibres are themselves composite, each consisting of an axon or axons, greatly elongated processes of a neuron and a longitudinal chain of satellite cells which closely envelop the greater part of the external surfaces of the axons. The axons of peripheral nerves arise from neuron somata lying within the grey matter of the ventral lamina of the brain stem and the ventral horns of the spinal cord, and from others situated more peripherally within the sensory ganglia of the cranial and spinal nerves, and the ganglia of the autonomic nervous system. They end either in synaptic contact with other neurons in the dorsal horns of the spinal cord or autonomic ganglia or with secretory or muscular effector cells; or in the case of sensory axons, as free terminal arborizations, or specialized terminals within a variety of encapsulated sense organs. Neither the cells of origin of peripheral axons nor the details of their terminations will be described in this chapter, which will be concerned solely with the structure, function and pathology of the cellular elements which constitute the peripheral nerve fibres and their immediate integuments. More detailed treatments of all of these topics will be found in a number of recent texts (e.g. Landon, 1976; Peters, Palay and Webster, 1976; Dyck et al., 1984).

The general arrangement of the constituent components of a peripheral nerve trunk is illustrated in Fig. 18.1. The nerve fibres are readily

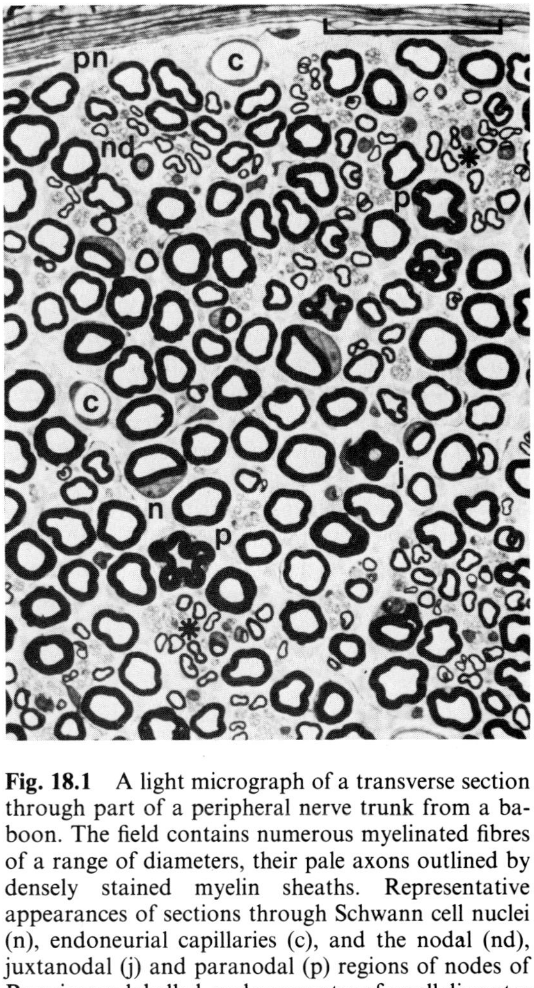

Fig. 18.1 A light micrograph of a transverse section through part of a peripheral nerve trunk from a baboon. The field contains numerous myelinated fibres of a range of diameters, their pale axons outlined by densely stained myelin sheaths. Representative appearances of sections through Schwann cell nuclei (n), endoneurial capillaries (c), and the nodal (nd), juxtanodal (j) and paranodal (p) regions of nodes of Ranvier are labelled, and aggregates of small diameter myelinated fibres and unmyelinated fibres are marked with *. Above, the nerve fascicle is bounded by the multilayered perineurial sheath (pn). Bar = 50 μm.

distinguishable into two classes, myelinated and unmyelinated, according to the presence or absence of a densely staining sheath of myelin around the axon; this is a proteophospholipid material, a product of the satellite or Schwann cells, and is produced only by those chains of satellite cells which enclose a single axon. Myelinated fibres are further distinguished by their generally much larger calibre, having diameters ranging from 1 to 20 μm in human peripheral nerves. Unmyelinated fibres are always of small diameter, and pass through the nerve trunk in groups of 8–15 within a common chain of satellite cells.

All axonal satellite cells are generally included under the term 'Schwann cells', but some writers distinguish those which surround unmyelinated fibres as Remak cells. The spaces between individual nerve fibres are packed with longitudinally orientated collagen fibrils and an amorphous extracellular matrix material, and together these constitute the endoneurium. This compartment also contains capillaries and a sparse population of other cell types. The latter include the fibroblasts responsible for producing the endoneurial connective tissues, mast cells and occasional macrophages of haematogenous origin. The whole assemblage of nerve fibres and connective tissue is enclosed and isolated from surrounding tissue elements by a multilayered sheath which consists of alternating layers of flattened cells and fine collagen fibrils, the perineurium. Large nerve trunks consist of a number of funiculi, each enclosed within an individual perineurial sheath, and these are frequently subdivided into two or more fascicles by extensions of the inner aspect of their perineurial sheath.

Classification

Nerve fibres have been categorized according to their calibre into three groups—A, B and C. Group A includes the largest fibres with the fastest conduction velocities (i.e. the myelinated somatic afferent and efferent fibres); group B includes myelinated preganglionic fibres of the autonomic nervous system; and group C is composed of the smallest diameter slowly conducting fibres, the unmyelinated visceral and somatic afferent fibres, and the postganglionic autonomic efferent fibres. Group A fibres can be subdivided according to their calibre and function into the afferent groups I, II and III, and efferent groups α, β and γ. The values obtained for conduction velocity and fibre diameter vary with species, but Boyd and Davey (1968) showed that in the adult cat group I fibres (10–20 μm, 50–100 metres per second) include the primary sensory fibres from muscle spindles and tendon organs; that group II (5–15 μm, 20–70 metres per second) contains fibres from the secondary sensory endings on the intrafusal muscle fibres within muscle spindles, and cutaneous afferent receptors; and that group III (1–7 μm, 5–30 metres per second) includes the fibres responsible for nociceptive activity and some aspects of cutaneous sensibility. The efferent α-fibres (9–20 μm, 50–100 metres per second) are exclusively skeletomotor; the β-fibres (9–15 μm, 50–85 metres per second) are both skeletomotor and fusimotor; and the γ-fibres (4.5–8.5 μm, 20–40 metres per second) are exclusively fusimotor. Unmyelinated axons have diameters ranging from 0.2–3.0 μm, and in normal human nerves show a unimodal distribution with a peak at around 1.5 μm (Ochoa, 1976).

The axon

The **axon** of a peripheral nerve is a more or less cylindrical extension of the nerve cell body bounded externally by a prolongation of its cell membrane, the **axolemma**. Due to its great length (which may exceed 1 metre in nerves to the human lower limb), when compared to the dimensions of the cell soma, the axonal cytoplasm will in most instances contribute by far the largest component to the total mass of the neuron. Furthermore, this cytoplasm, the **axoplasm**, lacks any of the cellular structures usually associated with protein synthetic activity or assembly (i.e. ribosomes, rough endoplasmic reticulum and Golgi membranes) and this feature, in conjunction with the length of peripheral nerve axons, has important consequences for their growth, long-term maintenance and the mechanisms of intracellular communication. In myelinated fibres the first part of the axon is a short, relatively narrow, unmyelinated initial segment, but acquisition of a myelin sheath distal to this region is accompanied by an abrupt increase in axon diameter to that which characterizes the greater part of the subsequent peripheral course of the fibre. The myelin sheath is segmented, the junctions between adjacent segments corresponding to the edges of adjacent Schwann cell territories, and these interruptions to the myelin are known as the *nodes of Ranvier*. Passage of the axon through these regions is accompanied by systematic changes in calibre and external contour, which will be described in greater detail below. Most of the branching of peripheral myelinated axons occurs within a few millimetres of their termination by way of a series of di- or trichotomous subdivisions at nodes of Ranvier, but a small amount of branching may also occur along the course of their passage through the nerve trunks. Such divisions are accompanied by some reduction in the calibre of the individual daughter branches relative to that of the parent axon, but a substantial increase in total cross-sectional area (Zenker and Hohberg, 1973a).

Axoplasm

The axoplasm of a peripheral nerve has a somewhat simple structure and internal organization when compared with the cytoplasm of its parent neuron. The predominant component of the axoplasm is an electron-lucent amorphous matrix within which is suspended a characteristic population of filamentous and membranous organelles (see Figs. 18.4 and 18.7a). The smallest of the axoplasmic constituents which can be distinguished morphologically are 5–7 nm diameter **microfilaments**, each of which is thought to be composed of paired helical chains of actin. They appear to be homologous with the thin filaments of muscle cells and contribute approximately 10 per cent to the total complement of axonal protein. They are most conspicuous in the growth cones of actively elongating neurites, but are less evident in unmyelinated axons and in the internodal portions of myelinated axons, where they appear to be confined to the cortical zone of axoplasm immediately subjacent to the axolemma. Their numbers are probably underestimated in conventional electron microscopical preparations, due to the destructive effect of both glutaraldehyde and osmium tetroxide on the stability of filamentous actin. The observed association of microfilaments with the plasma membrane, and less frequently with other formed elements of the axoplasm, has led to suggestions that they may have contractile function and play a part in the mechanisms responsible for intra-axonal transport (Schwartz, 1979), a process discussed in greater detail below.

A far more obvious and ubiquitous component of axoplasm are the **neurofilaments**. These are longitudinally orientated filaments of 8–11 nm diameter and indefinite length, linked by ill-defined lateral interconnections of a less dense axoplasmic component into an irregular polygonal lattice. In normal nerves this lattice fills the axoplasm not occupied by other organelles, and has a packing density of the order of 100–300 filaments/μm^2 of axon cross-sectional area (i.e. a minimum average interfilament spacing of 30–40 nm). The filament density remains constant along the length of individual axons and is not affected by changes in axon diameter. Biochemical studies indicate that neurofilaments are composed of four or five chains of globular protein subunits, and are akin to, but not identical with, the 10 nm 'intermediate filaments' of other cell types. The three principal constituent proteins have been identified, and have molecular weights of 68 000, 150 000 and 200 000, the latter two being considerably larger than the proteins 'skeletin' or 'desmin' and 'vimentin' which are believed to constitute the 'intermediate filaments' of other cells. Neurofilaments are generally well preserved by aldehyde fixatives in conventional fine structural preparations, but they have been shown to be susceptible to digestion by an intrinsic axonal calcium-activated protease (Schlaepfer and Hasler, 1979), and this finding may account for the rapid disappearance of neurofilaments from damaged axons (Schlaepfer, 1983). Clusters of neurofilaments provide the anatomical basis for the neurofibrillae visible in axons and neurons in silver-stained light microscopical preparations.

Axoplasm also contains an additional class of larger diameter filamentous structures usually referred to by the specific term **neurotubules**, although they do not seem to differ in any important respect from the **microtubules** of other cells. They are longitudinally orientated and occur singly, or in parallel arrays, and, in nerves prepared for electron microscopy by conventional techniques, appear to be unbranched 23–25 nm 'hollow' cylinders of indefinite length. In cross-section the microtubular walls can be seen to be composed of 13 globular 4-nm subunits of the protein *tubulin*, arranged in a simple 4 × 5 nm lattice. This material has been shown to exist in two distinct monomeric forms, alpha and beta, having molecular weights of 57 000 and 54 000 respectively, and each microtubule is composed of helically arranged chains of alternating alpha and beta monomers. Microtubules are labile structures and will tend to disaggregate into their monomeric components if subjected to low temperature, increased hydrostatic pressure or treatment with the drug colchicine or its analogues. It was originally inferred from the absence of branching that a finite population of microtubules extended along the length of the axon without interruption, from the neuron soma to its peripheral terminations (Weiss and Mayr, 1971). It has since been shown that the sum of the numbers of tubules in the terminal branches of some large mammalian axons can be at least ten times the number found more centrally in the parent axon (Zenker and Hohberg, 1973b); the increase may represent branching of individual microtubules, but as this phenomenon has never been observed it appears more likely that additional axonal microtubules are assembled locally from centrally synthesized molecules of tubulin monomer, in numbers necessary to match the increased total axoplasmic mass of the distal axon branches (Zenker and Hohberg, 1973a). More marked fluctuations in the numbers of microtubules along the length of individual axons have been described in invertebrate species, in which individual microtubules may be no more than 10–20 μm in length, and in the axons of cultured rat sensory neurons in which microtubules appear to be only 100 μm long (Bray and Bunge, 1981).

The frequency of occurrence of microtubules differs among different classes of nerve fibres (Friede and Samorajski, 1970), with proportionately larger numbers being found in unmyelinated nerve fibres, in which there are between 50 and 100/μm^2 of axonal cross-sectional area, in contrast with a more sparse distribution in large myelinated fibres where there may be only 10–20/μm^2. Differences have also been described in the concentrations of microtubules in different classes of myelinated fibre, small motor axons containing the most microtubules and large sensory axons the least (Zenker, Mayr and Gruber, 1974). Microtubules appear to be scattered at random throughout the axoplasm of unmyelinated, and the internodal regions of smaller myelinated, fibres, but in large myelinated fibres there is a tendency for the majority to be arranged around the periphery of the axon, and at some sites these are consistently grouped into parallel arrays, or small fascicles, having a minimum lateral spacing of around 25 nm. The most common sites of occurrence of such microtubule groups are the initial segments of the ventral horn motor neurons (Palay et al., 1968), and the dorsal root ganglion cells (Lieberman, 1976), in which they are commonly cross-linked by short electron-dense projections; at the nodes of Ranvier where they frequently form extensive palisades around the larger intra-axonal organelles and beneath the axolemma (Landon and Hall, 1976); and in the internodal regions of large myelinated fibres of the dorsal and ventral roots, in which small groups of microtubules are distributed in a semiregular fashion throughout the axonal cross-section. Groups of microtubules are always separated from their surrounding neurofilament-rich matrix by an electron-lucent interval; this may well represent an artefact of preparation, but it could, alternatively, signify some special organization of the axoplasmic matrix adjacent to the microtubule groups, perhaps associated with the presence of the large molecular weight microtubule-associated proteins (MAPs) which are known to be capable of influencing the assembly of microtubules *in vitro*. Circumferential bundles of marginal microtubules arranged at right angles to the long axis of the nerve fibre have been observed around the periphery of the swollen nodal axon of nerve fibres from several sites (Gray and Westrum, 1979; Mohammed, 1983), and it has been suggested that these may have a function in maintaining the shape of the nodal axon, a role similar to that ascribed to the circumferential microtubules of the blood platelets.

The axoplasm also contains a variety of types of membranous organelle, including mitochondria, smooth endoplasmic reticulum, lysosomes, and empty and dense-cored vesicles of a range of sizes. **Axonal mitochondria** are characteristically long and thread-like, 0.1–0.3 μm in diameter and up to 10 μm or more in length, and are constructed of concentric funnel-shaped cristae surrounded by the usual double external envelope. The number of mitochondria present is inversely related to the diameter of the axon, being 2–5/μm^2 of cross-sectional area in the smallest fibres, and 0.1/μm^2 in the internodal regions of large fibres (Berthold, 1968; Zenker, Mayr and Gruber, 1974). In normal mammalian axons, mitochondria usually appear to be randomly scattered throughout the axoplasmic matrix and they commonly have a close association with one or more microtubules. Observations using dark-field time-lapse cinematography have demonstrated that, in both amphibian (Cooper and Smith, 1974) and mammalian (Forman, Padjen and Siggins, 1977) axons, rod-like bodies of mitochondrial dimensions travel along the axon by saltatory motion in both proximal and distal directions and in approximately equal numbers (Zelena, 1968). The inference that these objects are indeed mitochondria is supported by experimental evidence of rapid distal transport of mitochondrial protein along peripheral axons (Droz, Rambourg and Koenig, 1975), and the observation that mitochondria tend to accumulate on either side of a crush lesion (Smith, 1980). In large myelinated fibres increased numbers of mitochondria are often found in the narrowed nodal and juxtanodal regions of the axon (Landon and Hall, 1976; Berthold, 1978), points at which the presumed mitochondria often seem to be arrested in time-lapse films. The nose-to-tail arrangement of mitochondria and other membranous structures in these regions, and the tendency for mitochondria to occur in chains in damaged axons (Martinez and Friede, 1970; Smith, 1980) have led to suggestions that such organelles follow definite pathways or 'streets' within the axon, and it is possible that such pathways may be defined by the clusters of microtubules with which they often appear to be associated (see below).

The **smooth endoplasmic reticulum** is a far less conspicuous component of normal axons when examined by standard methods of transmission electron microscopy, being represented in sections by short discontinuous segments of narrow angular spaces surrounded by a trilaminar membrane, and occupying less than 2.5 per cent of the cross-sectional area of the axon (Zenker, Mayr and Gruber, 1974). However, Droz, Rambourg and Koenig (1975), who have used metal impregnation techniques combined with high voltage electron microscopy to demonstrate the three-dimensional arrangement of the smooth endoplasmic reticulum, have shown it to consist of a continuous network of tubules extending from the neuron soma to its distal terminations, with regional specializations in the form of locally flattened expansions, subaxolemmal sacs or plates, and elaborate primary and secondary preterminal networks. They have suggested that the last may give rise to secretory vesicles, including the synaptic vesicles at nerve terminals, and that the membrane system as a whole may play an important role in the transport of materials along the axon, but it appears that the reticulum is not itself transported rapidly (Ellisman and Lindsey, 1983).

Vesicles with diameters varying from 40 to 100 nm may be found at any point along the length of peripheral axons (Berthold, 1978), occurring either singly or as short chains, but they are most common at the nodes of Ranvier (Landon and Hall, 1976) and at nerve terminals. Secondary **lysosomes** containing dense laminated material are also found within peripheral axons, and are seen most commonly on the distal side of the nodes of Ranvier of myelinated fibres (Smith, 1980). Large and small **dense-cored vesicles** can be found occasionally in most peripheral axons and appear to have no preferred locations, but the small variety with diameters of 50–70 nm are more common in postganglionic unmyelinated autonomic fibres, where they appear to be involved in the transport of catecholamines. Lastly, endocytotic **'coated' vesicles** have been observed at the axolemma of both myelinated and unmyelinated fibres (Ochoa, 1976). They are common at the neuromuscular junction, where they appear to play a part in the recycling of synaptic vesicle membrane from the axon plasmalemma to the smooth endoplasmic reticulum (Heuser and Reese, 1973; Holtzman, 1977), and they also occur at nodes of Ranvier where they may function to transport extracellular material from the axon surface to local regions of the smooth endoplasmic reticulum (Singer, Krishnan and Fyfe, 1972).

Axoplasmic flow and intra-axonal transport

The problems of maintenance and communication presented to a cell such as the neuron, in which the large majority of its cytoplasm is at a considerable distance from the cell soma and its nuclear-controlled metabolic systems, have been alluded to above, and have attracted considerable attention in recent years. The movement of material along axons was first demonstrated by Weiss and Hiscoe (1948), and the phenomenon has since been extensively explored, predominantly by techniques involving radioisotopic tracers pioneered by Droz and LeBlond (1963). As a result of this work it is now firmly established that there are well-organized transport mechanisms within axons capable of moving material both towards and away from the cell body

(Zelena, 1968; Lubińska and Niemierko, 1971), concurrently and at a variety of rates (Lasek, 1982). The somatofugal or anterograde transport mechanisms have been the most extensively studied (Schwartz, 1979; Wilson and Stone, 1979; Grafstein and Forman, 1980; Ochs, 1982), and have been found to operate at a minimum of two, and probably in excess of five different rates, which for the purposes of description are usually divided into a slow transport component moving at 0.25–4 mm per day, and a fast transport component which may reach speeds in excess of 400 mm per day. Transport at an intermediate velocity of approaching 100 mm per day has also been described but its characteristics, and the materials transported, are as yet ill-defined.

Anterograde transport

Slow transport The slow anterograde transport system appears to be a mass movement of axoplasm in a distal direction, with a rate equivalent to that of regrowing severed axons (Wilson and Stone, 1979). In mammalian peripheral motor axons 75 per cent of the dry weight of the material transported, slow component 'a', appears to consist of tubulin and neurofilament proteins which travel as a coherent neurotubule–neurofilament network at a rate of 0.25–1 mm per day (Tytell et al., 1981). The remainder of the slow component, slow component 'b', is composed of actin microfilaments, proteins complexed to these, and soluble enzymes, which collectively move at the somewhat higher rate of 2–4 mm per day. The ease with which neurofilaments can be isolated from mammalian axons (Schlaepfer and Freeman, 1978) and the reported finding that 98 per cent of the neurofilament protein in squid axons is in a stable polymeric form (Morris and Lasek, 1982) support the suggestion that the neurofilament protein of slow component 'a' travels in the form of polymerized filaments (Lasek, 1982). Isotope labelling experiments (Black and Lasek, 1980) have demonstrated that the neurofilament and microtubule proteins remain closely associated during their passage along the axon for periods of at least several months. The slow 'a' component of the axoplasm thus represents a linear record of the protein synthetic activity of the parent neuron, and material entering the most distal terminals of human peripheral nerves may have commenced its journey as much as three years previously. From a microscopical standpoint, however, the movement of axoplasm is surprisingly rapid, the content of each 1–2 mm internodal segment being replaced once per day in axons in the intermediate to upper range of myelinated fibre diameters. Furthermore, the packing density of neurofilaments is unaltered along the course of any individual axon, despite the major changes in axon calibre which occur at the nodes of Ranvier of larger fibres (see below), suggesting that transit of the column of axoplasm through the node involves disaggregation of the neurotubule–neurofilament network, with depolymerization of the neurofilaments proximal, and repolymerization distal, to each node. The microtubules appear not to be involved in this process and pass through the nodes in unaltered numbers. The mechanism responsible for neurofilament disaggregation at the nodes is not at present obvious, but may involve local concentrations of calcium-activated proteases similar to those postulated to be responsible for the degradation of the cytoskeletal network at nerve terminals (Lasek and Black, 1977; Schlaepfer, 1983).

Fast transport Fast anterograde axonal transport is an energy-utilizing, ATP-dependent and temperature-sensitive process (Grafstein and Forman, 1980). It does not appear to require that the axon be in continuity with the neuron soma, and will continue unimpaired in extruded squid axoplasm. Furthermore, transport will persist in this preparation after the axoplasm has been stirred with a needle, but with changed orientation, indicating its dependence upon intrinsic pathways defined by the axonal cytoskeleton (Lasek, 1982). It is concerned with the transport of particulate constituents of the axoplasm, including the mitochondria and transmitter storage vesicles, and materials such as some transmitter-synthesizing enzymes and glycoproteins, as well as membrane components (Droz et al., 1979; Griffin et al., 1981) for supply to both the nerve terminals and to the intra-axonal membrane systems. No differences have been detected between the materials carried, and rates of transport, in sensory and motor axons (Barker, Neale and Gainer, 1976). The speeds of transport quoted above are average values, but the movement of large particles such as mitochondria, and other membrane-bound structures which can be visualized *in vivo* by dark-field illumination and time-lapse cinematography, have been shown to be saltatory (Forman, Padjen and Siggins, 1977); it is at present not known whether the other, smaller, elements carried by the fast anterograde transport system behave in a similar manner.

Retrograde transport

Retrograde or somatopetal axonal transport consists primarily of the fast transport of membrane-bound structures towards the cell body, at a speed of around 200 mm per day—i.e. at approximately half the rate of the fast component of orthograde transport. The structures carried include secondary lysosomes, multivesicular bodies and a heterogeneous collection of smaller vesicles; these represent a mixture of superfluous or degraded axonal constituents originally transported to the distal terminals by fast orthograde transport, and now returned to the soma for recycling or destruction, together with exogenous materials absorbed at the nerve terminal (Holtzman, 1971; Bunt and Hasche, 1978), in many instances (e.g. nerve growth factor) by active receptor-mediated absorptive pinocytosis (Dumas, Schwab and Thoenen, 1979). A slow component of retrograde transport has also been described recently in mammalian peripheral nerve fibres (Gainer and Fink, 1982). This material has a molecular weight of 68 000 and moves at some 3–6 mm per day; it has been tentatively identified as serum albumin. Heavy metal ions may also be transported retrogradely to the cell soma, in the case of lead at a rate of some 10 mm per day (Baruah et al., 1981).

Retrograde transport mechanisms, although they have as yet been less thoroughly investigated than those of anterograde transport, are clearly quite as important to the cell as the latter, in that they appear to provide the means by which unutilized or degraded materials synthesized in the cell are 'turned around' and made available to the cell soma for recycling or disposal. Their return to the cell body also probably provides a part of the necessary 'feedback signal' which will enable the cell to modulate the balance of its anabolic and catabolic activities in response to the needs of its far distant axon terminals. Retrograde transport is thus of considerable interest in studies of nerve regeneration following injury (Forman, 1983), and defective turnaround of materials at nerve terminals and reduction in the rate of retrograde transport have recently been suggested as primary defects in some experimental neuropathies, such as those caused by 2,5-hexanedione and acrylamide (Sahenk and Mendell, 1981), and in the peripheral neuropathy of diabetes (Brimijoin, 1982a; Jakobsen, Brimijoin and Sidenius, 1983).

Possible mechanisms of fast transport

A number of explanations have been proposed for the mechanisms which may be responsible for fast axonal transport (Schwartz, 1979; Grafstein and Forman, 1980; Bray and Gilbert, 1981). One suggestion is that movement is generated by interactions between actin and myosin, both of which are known to be present within neurons (Trifaro, 1978), and that this may result in the establishment of cytoplasmic streaming capable of transporting particulate components (Isenberg, Schubert and Kreutzberg, 1980). Some support for this proposal is provided by the requirement of the transport mechanism for calcium ions (Ochs, 1983), and by the observations that the substance cytochalasin B, well known for its ability to inhibit cell movements, including that of neurite growth cones, also inhibits axonal fast transport systems (Fernandez and Samson, 1974), and that a synthetic derivative, dihydrochalasin B, binds to actin and inhibits its polymerization (Brown and Spudich, 1979). An alternative explanation for fast transport which has received much attention in recent years is that axonal and dendritic microtubules are capable of generating movement of adjacent structures, either by interacting with them directly (Schmitt and Samson, 1968) or via an intermediate carrier mechanism (Smith, 1970; Ochs, 1971, 1982; Smith, Jarlfors and Cameron, 1975). Evidence supporting this proposal has included numerous observations of dense cross-links between organelles such as mitochondria or synaptic vesicles and the microtubules within fixed and sectioned axons and at synaptic boutons, and the sensitivity of the fast component of protein transport to mitotic inhibitors such as colchicine (Hanson and Edström, 1978) and cold (Tsukita and Ishikawa, 1980), both of which are known to disaggregate microtubules *in vivo*. Interaction between adjacent microtubules which results in movement is a well-established phenomenon in motile structures such as the flagella of invertebrates, where it is mediated by the high molecular weight protein dynein. It is therefore of interest that preparations of brain microtubules have recently been shown to contain an ATPase having a molecular size, affinity for microtubules and requirements for enzyme activation which resemble those of axonene dynein. Such circumstantial evidence must be evaluated in the context of other experimental observations that fast transport can be dissociated from the presence of microtubules (Fernandez, Burton and Samson, 1971; Byers, 1974) and that, where such transport persists after dissolution of the tubules by treatment with high concentrations of calcium ions, it is itself sensitive to colchicine (Brady et al., 1980); but the validity of these findings has been disputed by others (Brimijoin, 1982b). Other mechanisms proposed include: the 'microstream concept' of Gross (1975) in which organelles are postulated to be carried on annular streams of axoplasm surrounding the microtubules, which would generate a vectorial shear force powered by the hydrolysis of ATP; and the suggestion that the continuous membrane-bound spaces of the smooth endoplasmic reticulum may provide a potential channel for the fast intra-axonal movement of some materials (Droz et al., 1979; Brady et al., 1980), but the speed of movement within these channels and whether the system can sustain simultaneous bidirectional transport have yet to be determined. For recent reviews of the structure and function of the neuronal cytoskeleton, see Schwartz (1979), Wilson and Stone (1979), Grafstein and Forman (1980), Bray and Gilbert (1981), Ochs (1982) and Schlaepfer (1983); and Anderton (1982) for its involvement in peripheral nerve pathology.

Transmission of the nerve impulse

The aspect of axonal function of greatest general interest is its capacity to transmit signals over considerable distances in the form of propagated action potentials. The basis of this property lies in the polarization of the axolemma, the internal surface of which is maintained at a negative potential of around −70 mV by energy-dependent, ATP-utilizing, ionic-pumping mechanisms which are integral components of the membrane. The principal partitioned ion is sodium, and this is pumped outwards into the extracellular space. Electrical or mechanical disturbance of the axolemma at any point along its course will result in a transient increase in permeability to sodium ion, which then flows into the cell down its concentration and voltage gradients. The advance of current through the axoplasm causes depolarization of adjacent segments of the axoplasm, resulting in a continuously propagated wave of depolarization which spreads along the axon. In unmyelinated fibres the large capacitance of the axon membrane attenuates forward axial flow of current within the axoplasm, and limits conduction to a speed of around 1 metre per second. In myelinated fibres, on the other hand, electrical activity is restricted to the narrow spaces between the myelin segments, the nodes of Ranvier, the myelin insulating the much more extensive intervening portions of the axon membrane from depolarization, with the effect that ionic activity leaps from one node to the next in series. The principal functional implication of this saltatory activity is a considerable enhancement of conduction velocity over that achieved by non-myelinated fibres—i.e. to between 20 and 70 metres per second, depending upon fibre diameter and myelin sheath thickness. Loss of one or more myelin segments from a myelinated axon, as a consequence of either naturally occurring pathology or localized experimental injury, will result acutely in conduction block, but the axon subsequently develops the capacity to sustain continuous conduction, in a manner comparable to that seen in normal unmyelinated fibres (Bostock and Sears, 1978; Sears and Bostock, 1981).

Satellite cells of peripheral axons

All axons of the peripheral nervous system are ensheathed by cords of satellite or *Schwann cells* along the greater part of their length; the term *Remak cell* is occasionally used to distinguish those which surround unmyelinated fibres (Ochoa, 1976). Specialized forms of satellite cells are found at several locations within the peripheral nervous system. Examples are the satellite cells of peripheral nerve ganglia, in which they provide multilayered capsules around individual neuron somata and the initial segments of their axons (Lieberman, 1976); at the neuromuscular junctions of striated muscle, where their flattened processes provide a superficial covering for the unmyelinated terminal arborizations of the axon as it lies within the primary postsynaptic cleft of the motor end-plate; and within encapsulated sensory receptors—e.g. the inner-core cells of Pacinian corpuscles in which they provide a series of overlapping lamellae immediately surrounding the terminal region of the axon (Spencer and Schaumburg, 1973).

Development

Schwann cells are believed to be derived during development from the neural crest and to a lesser extent from the neural tube, and they accompany, or possibly precede (Gamble, 1976), the outgrowing neurites of the primitive peripheral nerves arising from the primordial dorsal root ganglia and ventral horn neurons. At the earliest identifiable stages in the formation of peripheral nerves—i.e. between 10 and 15 weeks of gestation in man (Cravioto, 1965; Gamble, 1966; J.S. Dunn, 1970)—each Schwann cell possesses several flattened processes which enwrap large clusters of fine axons (Fig. 18.2). Further development is accompanied by continuing Schwann cell proliferation and the progressive division of the large communally enclosed bundles of axons into smaller groups by the invasion of new processes from the increasing Schwann cell population (Friede and Samorajski, 1968; Webster, 1971; Webster, Martin and O'Connell, 1973). Beyond 14–15 weeks of gestation in man, increasing numbers of the largest diameter (1–2 μm) axons become enwrapped individually within the processes of a single column of Schwann cells and are distinguishable as promyelin fibres (Friede

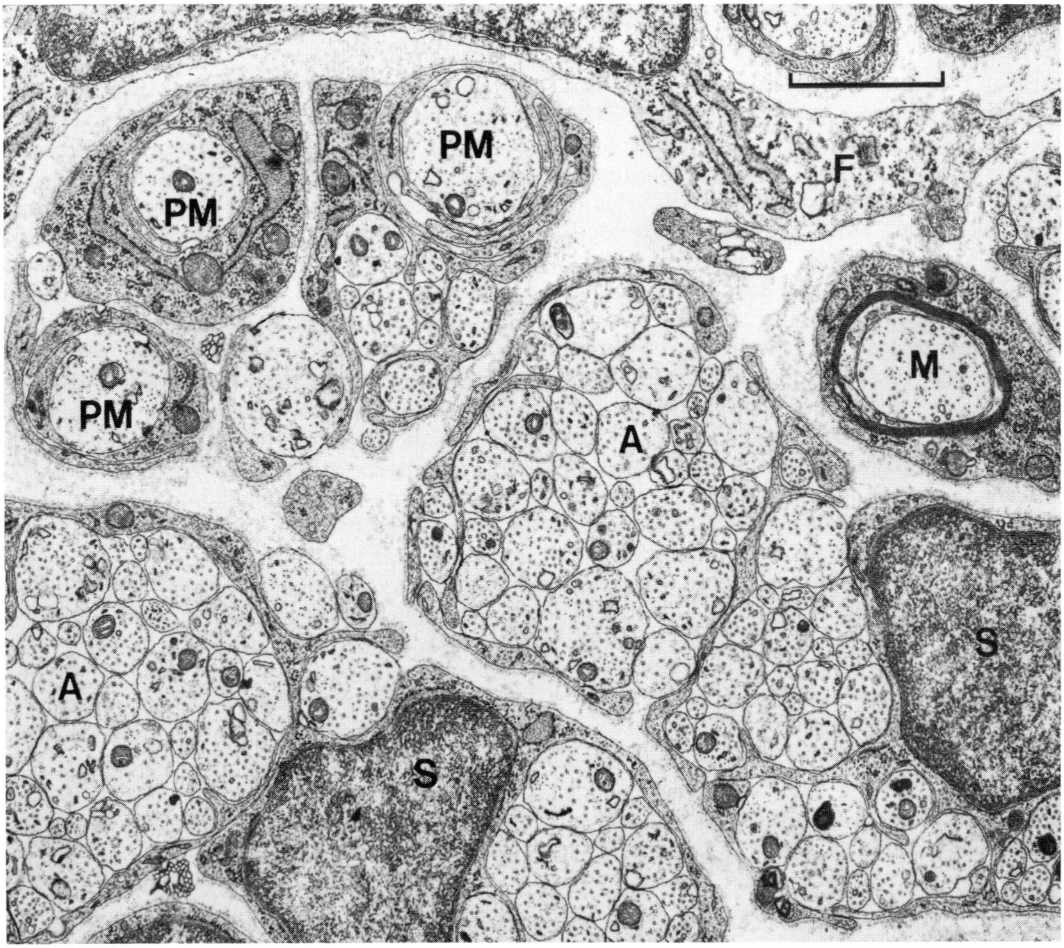

Fig. 18.2 An electron micrograph of a transverse section through a muscle nerve from a newborn rat. Bundles of primitive unmyelinated axons (A) are enwrapped by the processes of adjacent Schwann cells (S). A few larger diameter 'promyelin' fibres (PM) are enclosed within individual Schwann cell sheaths, and myelination has commenced around another fibre (M). An endoneurial fibroblast is also visible (F). Bar = 1 μm.

and Samorajski, 1968) (Fig. 18.2). Later circumferential extension of the overlapping Schwann cell processes and their compaction give rise to the first few lamellae of the future myelin sheath (Webster, 1971; Martin and Webster, 1973). The persisting groups of smaller diameter axons, amounting to between 50 and 80 per cent of the total within the nerve (Ochoa, 1976), also become segregated into smaller groups of between 8 and 15, and these in turn come to lie within individual longitudinal pockets in the surface of chains of Schwann (or Remak) cells, each of such assemblies of several unmyelinated axons with a column of satellite cells constituting one unmyelinated fibre. The factors which lead to the selection of some axons for myelination and not others are still largely unknown, but experimental studies have shown that all Schwann cells, including those of normally wholly unmyelinated autonomic nerve trunks, are competent to produce myelin (Simpson and Young, 1945; Weinberg and Spencer, 1975, 1976; Aguayo et al., 1976b), and that the necessary stimulus is provided by the axon (Aguayo et al., 1978a), and is to some extent, but not entirely, related to axon calibre (Fraher, 1972). The processes which lead to the final mature pattern of axon calibre and ensheathment by satellite cells also involve the spontaneous loss of some axons (Aguayo, Terry and Bray, 1973) and Schwann cells (Berthold, 1973), but the bases of such selection remain a matter for speculation. Schwann cells respond acutely to loss of their contained axon by proliferation within the pre-existing basal lamina tube, to form the *bands of Büngner* characteristic of wallerian degeneration (see below), but in chronically demyelinated nerve trunks the Schwann cells dwindle in number and are replaced by connective tissue, indicating their trophic dependence on innervation in the longer term (Weinberg and Spencer, 1978).

Unmyelinated nerve fibres

The principal structural features of a typical unmyelinated nerve fibre are illustrated in Fig. 18.3. Each small diameter axon lies recessed within a separate cleft in the surface of the Schwann cell, itself one of a chain of similar cells arranged end to end. Measurements of internuclear distance along unmyelinated fibres have indicated that individual cells in the chain are between 100 μm (Peyronnard, Aguayo and Bray, 1973) and 200–500 μm (Carlsen, Knappeis and Behse, 1974; Carlsen and Behse, 1980) in length. The apposed cell membranes which form the wall of the cleft containing the axon and connect it to the surface of the Schwann cell are known as the *mesaxon*, by analogy with the arrangement of the peritoneal membrane of the intestinal mesentery. A single basal lamina surrounds the entire fibre. The Schwann cells of unmyelinated fibres form branching and anastomosing cords of cells (Gasser, 1955; Aguayo et al., 1976a; Carlsen and Behse, 1980), with some overlap and interdigitation of the terminal processes at their points of junction (Carlsen, Knappeis and Behse, 1974), points at which their complement of axons is passed on to the next member of the chain. Increased electron density of the cytoplasm of one or other of the cells at such a point of contact has been reported by Eames and Gamble (1970), but the increase in staining may extend to the whole cell (Morris, Hudson and Weddell, 1972; Carlsen and Behse, 1980) and cannot be taken to indicate the presence of specialized regions of intercellular contact (Ochoa, 1976); small puncta adhaerentia are, however, not uncommon at points of contact between overlapping processes of the same Schwann cell in human, and other primate, unmyelinated fibres (Fig. 18.3). In some species, including man, each individual Schwann cell may split into a number of smaller cords in their abnuclear regions (Fig. 18.3), each of which provides ensheathment for only one or two members of the total axonal complement of the cell (Gamble and Eames, 1964). Such arrangements permit the transfer of individual axons between the different Schwann cell cords and ensure that few unmyelinated axons maintain a consistent relationship with their neighbours for any significant distance.

Fig. 18.3 A transverse section of a human sural nerve biopsy showing a group of unmyelinated axons lying within the endoneurial collagen matrix (C). Some axons (A) lie within pockets in the surface of the nuclear region of their ensheathing Schwann cell (S), while others (A′) are enclosed singly or as small groups within slender cytoplasmic cords derived from the same or neighbouring Schwann cells. A collagen pocket (P) is also visible within one of these cords, and arrowheads mark the sites of maculae adhaerentes between contiguous Schwann cell processes. Bar = 2 μm.

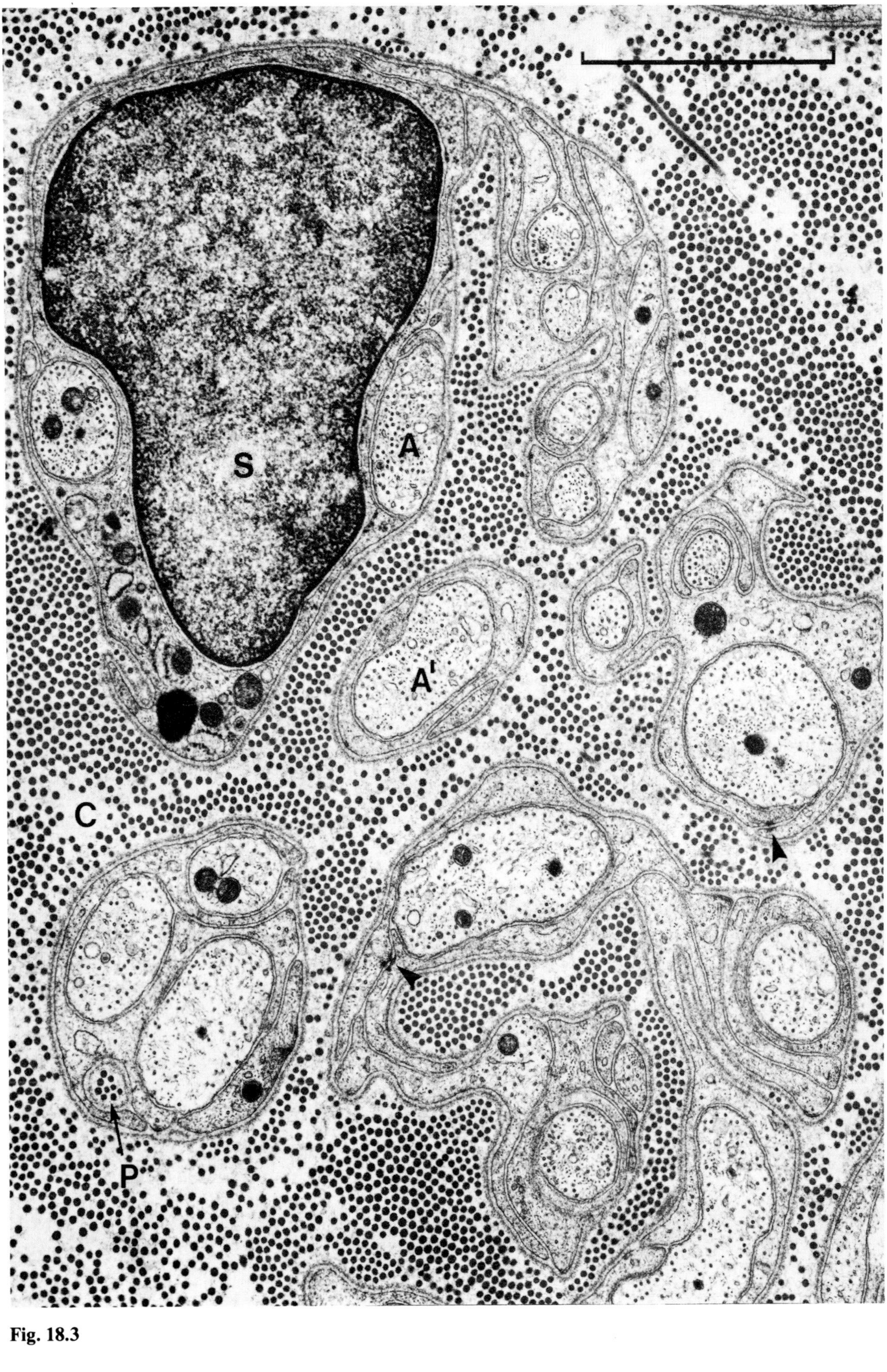

Fig. 18.3

A not uncommon feature of unmyelinated fibres in many mammalian species, and in human subjects of all ages, is the enclosure of bundles of endoneurial collagen fibrils within a longitudinal furrow in the surface of the Schwann cell, as if the fibrils collectively constituted an additional axon, but with the difference that the furrow is usually lined by an extension of the Schwann cell basal lamina (Fig. 18.3). Such **collagen pockets** (Gamble, 1964; Gamble and Eames, 1964) appear to be formed only by the Schwann cells of unmyelinated fibres, and their apparent increase following loss of non-myelinated axons in some neuropathies has led to the proposal that newly formed collagen may fill clefts formerly occupied by axons which have degenerated (Thomas, 1973). However, reconstructions from serial sections of human cutaneous nerve have shown that such pockets are seldom longer than 6 μm, recurring at intervals of about 20 μm, and it has been suggested that they may serve to anchor the unmyelinated fibre to the adjacent endoneurial connective tissue (Carlsen and Behse, 1980).

The axons of unmyelinated nerve fibres are small, ranging in diameter from 0.2 to 3.0 μm in man, with a unimodal size distribution having its peak at around 1.5 μm (Gasser, 1955; Ochoa, 1976). Even smaller diameter axons (i.e. <0.1 μm) may be seen in pathological material, and such small profiles are usually considered to represent regrowing axonal sprouts. The axoplasm of unmyelinated fibres shows no evidence of regional specialization and contains representatives of all of the subcellular components listed in the general description of axoplasm given above. The only general features which distinguishes them from the axons of myelinated fibres are the much higher proportion of axonal microtubules compared with neurofilaments (Friede and Samorajski, 1970) and the frequent presence of dense-cored vesicles in autonomic efferent fibres. Similarly, neither transmission nor freeze-fracture studies have shown any evidence of local specializations of the axolemma of unmyelinated fibre axons, dispersed E- and P-face particles being present at concentrations equivalent to those found over the major part of the internodal regions of myelinated axons (Black, Foster and Waxman, 1981). ^{3}H-saxitoxin binding studies have shown that the axolemma of unmyelinated fibres possesses sodium channels at a density of around 110/μm^2 (Ritchie, Rogart and Strichartz, 1976), compared with the rather lower value of 25/μm^2 found in the internodal axolemma of myelinated fibres (Ritchie and Rogart, 1977; Ritchie, 1979).

No structural differences have been reported between the unmyelinated fibres of sensory and of motor nerves, but the numbers present do differ considerably, myelinated and unmyelinated axons being found in the ratio of around 1:1 in muscle nerves, and 1:4 in cutaneous nerves (Ranson et al., 1935; Ochoa, 1976). In both classes of nerve the distribution of unmyelinated fibres is markedly non-uniform, with small groups of non-myelinated fibres occurring close together, usually in association with a number of small diameter myelinated fibres, these groups appearing in cross-section as scattered islands between the larger myelinated fibres.

Myelinated fibres

Myelin and its formation The characteristic features of myelinated axons which distinguish them from their unmyelinated neighbours are their larger diameter (which may occasionally exceed 20 μm), the enclosure of each within its own individual chain of Schwann cells, and the presence of a myelin sheath, a proteophospholipid multilayered spiral derived from the apposed and compacted membranes of a greatly elaborated Schwann cell mesaxon (Geren, 1954). During development the process of myelination is initiated by increase in the length of the mesaxon connecting the periaxonal space to the surface of its chain of Schwann cells. At first this may take the form of a few incomplete and irregular folds (see Fig. 18.2), but thereafter the elongated mesaxon becomes rearranged into a regular spiral around the axon perimeter. The thin layer of cytoplasm between the pairs of membranes is extruded, and the membranes themselves then compact, to give rise to the radially repeating structure of alternate dense and less dense lines characteristic of compact myelin in electron micrographs. The dense lines are derived from the cytoplasmic aspect of each pair of membranes, and the less dense lines (which often appear double in micrographs of aldehyde-fixed myelin) from the apposed outer surfaces of each pair of membranes. The spacing between each dense line of the myelin seen in electron micrographs, the myelin period, varies with the methods used to prepare the tissue, but in aldehyde-fixed, ethanol-dehydrated nerves embedded in epon or araldite epoxy resins, the observed periodicity is usually within the range of 14.0–15.0 nm. This compares with the values of 17.0–18.4 nm obtained by x-ray diffraction from fresh wet myelin by Schmitt, Bear and Palmer (1941), implying a maximum shrinkage of around 20 per cent relative to the fresh state. Myelin is thus an integral part of the Schwann cell, a sequestered elaboration of its surface plasma membrane and, as will be seen, its persistence is dependent upon the viability of both the axon and the Schwann cell.

Internodal length

The origin of myelin within a chain of separate cells results in its segmentation along the length of any individual axon, with interruptions at the points of junction of adjacent Schwann cell territories—the nodes of Ranvier. In mammalian fibres the internodal segments range in size from 200–250 μm to up to 1500 μm (Williams and Wendell-Smith, 1971), and a fairly close and direct relationship exists between axon diameter and internodal length, small fibres having short internodes and large fibres longer ones. The precise values for this relationship vary between species, however, and also between fibres from different nerves within the same species (Williams and Wendell-Smith, 1971; Friede, Meier and Diem, 1981), but in mammals internodal lengths are remarkably consistent when measured along the length of any one axon. Where short ('intercalated') myelin segments occur they represent a manifestation of previous Schwann cell damage with subsequent regeneration (see below). The origin of the relationship between internodal length and axon diameter has been attributed to the earlier onset of myelination in fibres destined to have the largest final diameter. This event is considered to fix the total number of Schwann cells along the length of the axon by inhibiting further cell division, subsequent growth in length of the fibre necessitated by continued growth of the surrounding tissues being accommodated by elongation of this finite population of Schwann cells and their contained myelin segments (Boycott, 1904; Vizoso and Young, 1948; Vizoso, 1950; Schlaepfer and Myers, 1973).

Myelin sheath thickness

The thickness of the myelin sheath also varies in fibres of differing axonal diameter, large fibres having thicker sheaths than smaller diameter fibres. The relationship between axon diameter, d, and fibre diameter, D (i.e. d plus twice the myelin sheath thickness), is usually expressed as the ratio d/D, or g (Schmitt and Bear, 1937). Values for g obtained from light microscope observations of osmium-stained or fresh-frozen nerves indicated that g was lowest for small diameter fibres, which thus appeared to have relatively thick myelin sheaths, and increased to around 0.6 in the middle range of diameters in both sensory and motor fibres. This value was predicted by Rushton (1951) and Hodgkin (1971) on biophysical grounds, and later by Smith and Koles (1970) using computer simulation techniques, to be the energetically most efficient for saltatory conduction; thereafter it remained more or less constant regardless of further increase in axon diameter (Schmitt and Bear, 1937; Sanders, 1948; Evans and Vizoso, 1951; Williams and Wendell-Smith, 1971). Dorsal and ventral spinal nerve roots showed a similar tendency for the smaller diameter fibres to have thicker myelin sheaths, but the larger fibres were found to have proportionally somewhat thinner sheaths, in which the *g ratio* exceeded 0.7 (Williams and Wendell-Smith, 1971). Rather different results were reported by Sunderland and Roche (1958) who found that the *g ratio* increased continuously with increase in fibre diameter throughout the observed range of fibre sizes, and by Buchthal and Rosenfalck (1966) who found, on the contrary, that the value for g fell in the largest fibres. Despite majority agreement that there is a general trend for g values to increase with fibre size, Williams and Wendell-Smith (1971) found consistent differences between sensory and motor nerves. Whilst the rate of increase of sheath thickness with increasing axon diameter was similar in skin and muscle nerves, the myelin sheath was always thicker in a muscle nerve for any given axon diameter. The dorsal and ventral spinal nerve roots, which have a much greater range of axon diameters, showed a much slower increase in sheath thickness with increase in axon calibre.

Such light microscopical observations are subject to a number of sources of error, of which two in particular—the lens effect of the refractile myelin on the apparent diameter of its enclosed axon in teased preparations, and the difficulty of determining the true internal diameter of a narrow tube of myelin when viewed end-on in osmicated transverse sections several micrometres in thickness—tended to lead to overestimates of the thickness of the myelin sheath, particularly that around the smaller myelinated fibres. The availability of electron microscopy during the last 30 years has led to further studies of the parametric relationships between axon and myelin sheath, in which accurate measurements of axon perimeter and counts of numbers of lamellae have taken the place of optical measurements of mean axon and fibre diameters (Friede and Samorajski, 1967, 1968; Friede, 1972). These and many later studies have shown that axon circumference is linearly related to myelin sheath thickness, or cross-sectional area in normal fibres (Yates, Bouchard and Wherrett, 1976), and that the value for the ratio *g* remains constant at around 0.7 throughout the entire fibre diameter range. These relationships do not hold, however, where the internodal length is substantially below the normal range for a particular axon diameter, as may occur naturally at the initial segments of dorsal root ganglion neurons (Lieberman, 1976) or as a consequence of remyelination following the loss of one or more myelin segments. In such situations the myelin sheath is thinner than would be expected from the diameter of the contained axon, and it has therefore been proposed recently that the relationship with the most general application is likely to be that between the area of axolemma exposed to each Schwann cell and myelin thickness or volume (Landon and Hall, 1976; Friede and Bischhausen, 1980; Smith et al., 1982), but how these are related in a causal sense has yet to be determined. Explanations range from proposals that there is a direct intercellular signal to which the Schwann cell responds by producing myelin, a signal originating from specific surface macromolecules in the axolemma (Spencer and Weinberg, 1978), to quasimechanical models in which distension and elongation of the myelin sheath by the growing axon provide the necessary stimulus for growth in sheath thickness and length respectively (Friede, 1972). None of these hypotheses offers any explanation for the observed discontinuity in the scaling factor relating conduction velocity to axon diameter for myelinated afferent fibres, which Boyd and Kalu (1979) and Arbuthnott, Boyd and Kalu (1980) have shown to be 5.6–5.7 for the larger (group I) fibres, and 4.6 for the remainder (groups II and III). It appears probable, therefore, that this functional difference between large and small diameter myelinated fibres cannot be referred to the passive properties of myelin as an electrical insulator, but resides in some other aspect of their structure, and may possibly be related to differences in conductance at the nodes of Ranvier (Jack, 1976).

The structure and chemical composition of myelin This has received intensive study during the past 30 years, both for its inherent neurobiological interest and as a model of the structure of biological membranes in general, and such work has been frequently and extensively reviewed (e.g. Gregson, 1976; Morell, 1977; Davison and Dobbing, 1978; Norton, 1981). The majority of the original observations concerning the composition of myelin were performed on material obtained from the white matter of the central nervous system, due to the greater ease with which it could be extracted uncontaminated by other tissue components. Such mammalian CNS myelin was shown to possess a number of features which differentiated it from other cellular membranes, the most notable of which were its much higher ratio of lipid to protein, its possession of a large proportion of cholesterol and galactosphingolipid, the predominance of relatively saturated long chain fatty acids and a simple protein composition in which two or three major proteins contributed over 80 per cent of the total. Later studies have shown that whereas both central and peripheral nervous system myelins are individually broadly similar in their constitution across a range of animal species and phyla, consistent differences can be found between central and peripheral myelin obtained from any one animal and that these are of a surprisingly fundamental kind in the context of their apparently very similar structure and function. Examples are the finding that peripheral and central myelin have only one protein in common, and that their lipid compositions differ, PNS myelin containing a much larger proportion of sphingomyelin. PNS myelin is also much richer in glycoprotein.

The metabolism of myelin has also been much studied in recent years (Davison and Dobbing, 1978; Norton, 1981). Both the synthesis and the assembly of myelin appear to be performed wholly within the sheath cells, but there is evidence (Rawlins, 1973; Droz et al., 1978; Haley and Ledeen, 1979) that some low molecular weight lipid constituents may be obtained from the axon. Whilst it is clear that the synthesis and assembly of myelin are subject to a general overall level of metabolic control, synthesis of its individual components can be dissociated, inhibition of protein synthesis with puromycin, for example, having no effect upon the rate of synthesis or incorporation of lipids (Benjamins et al., 1971). There is also evidence that individual protein components of myelin are under separate synthetic control at different loci within the satellite cell, and that they may reach the myelin via different intracellular transport routes.

Once myelin has been laid down around an axon it shows remarkable metabolic stability when its rate of turnover is compared with those of other constituents of neural tissue (Davison and Dobbing, 1978); as this property appeared to be shared by all of its components, it was initially assumed that myelin was metabolized as a unit. Later experimental results have indicated that there is considerable variation in the metabolic turnover rates of each of the individual myelin components, both lipid and protein, and that these range from a few weeks to several months (Smith, 1967), suggesting that in catabolism, as in synthesis, the individual chemical subunits of myelin are handled separately. The slow rate of turnover as a whole may be attributed in part to metabolic inaccessibility of the deeper turns of the myelin spiral, as there is evidence that during myelination the new myelin constituents are added to the outer aspect of the sheath and then become buried beneath later-formed turns of the membrane spiral (Gould, 1977).

The Schwann cell

Myelinated fibres are commonly portrayed as if they were cylinders, but in reality very few are truly cylindrical at any point along their internodal regions and all depart from circularity in cross-section at the level of the Schwann cell nucleus (Fig. 18.4) and in the regions abutting upon the nodes of Ranvier. For many years much of this variation in cross-sectional profile was attributed to artefacts of preparation, but fine structural observations have now made it clear that the views of Ranvier (1878) and other early histologists, that there are systematic changes in the shape and dimensions of the myelin sheath along each internode, were fully justified. It can also be demonstrated that there are differences in shape between large and small diameter myelinated fibres, the latter (with thinner sheaths) having consistently more irregular contours in cross-section (Arbuthnott et al., 1980). In all myelinated fibres the Schwann cell is effectively divided into two portions by the presence of the myelin spiral within its cytoplasm. At the inner, adaxonal, end of the spiral the apposed membranes 'decompact' to enclose a slender band of cytoplasm which represents the tip of the original spiral process from which the myelin was derived (Fig. 18.4). In large diameter fibres of larger mammals the inner pair of membranes may also split at one or two other points around the axon perimeter to give additional adaxonal Schwann cell bands. These may indent the axon surface and occasionally contain small mitochondria and lysosomes. The gap between the innermost Schwann cell membrane and the axolemma is known as the periaxonal space. Over the greater part of the internode it is represented by a uniform interval of 20–25 nm between the two membranes; this gap is obliterated at either end of the myelin segment by close attachment of the proximal and distal margins of the myelin spiral to the axolemma immediately adjacent to each node; the structural details of this region will be described below. Apart from this specialized myelin attachment zone, no specific contacts have been described between the axolemma and the adaxonal Schwann plasma membrane, but the regularity of the 'gap' between the two indicates that there is, under normal circumstances, a negligible extracellular space, and that the two membranes are effectively in contact via cell-surface components unstained by conventional electron microscopical techniques.

The external compartment of the Schwann cell is more substantial and more complex in its arrangement. Major accumulations of material occur adjacent to both poles of the longitudinally orientated ellipsoidal nucleus, which generally lies slightly distal to the mid-point of the internodal segment. This perinuclear cytoplasm contains conspicuous accumulations of rough endoplasmic reticulum, Golgi membrane systems

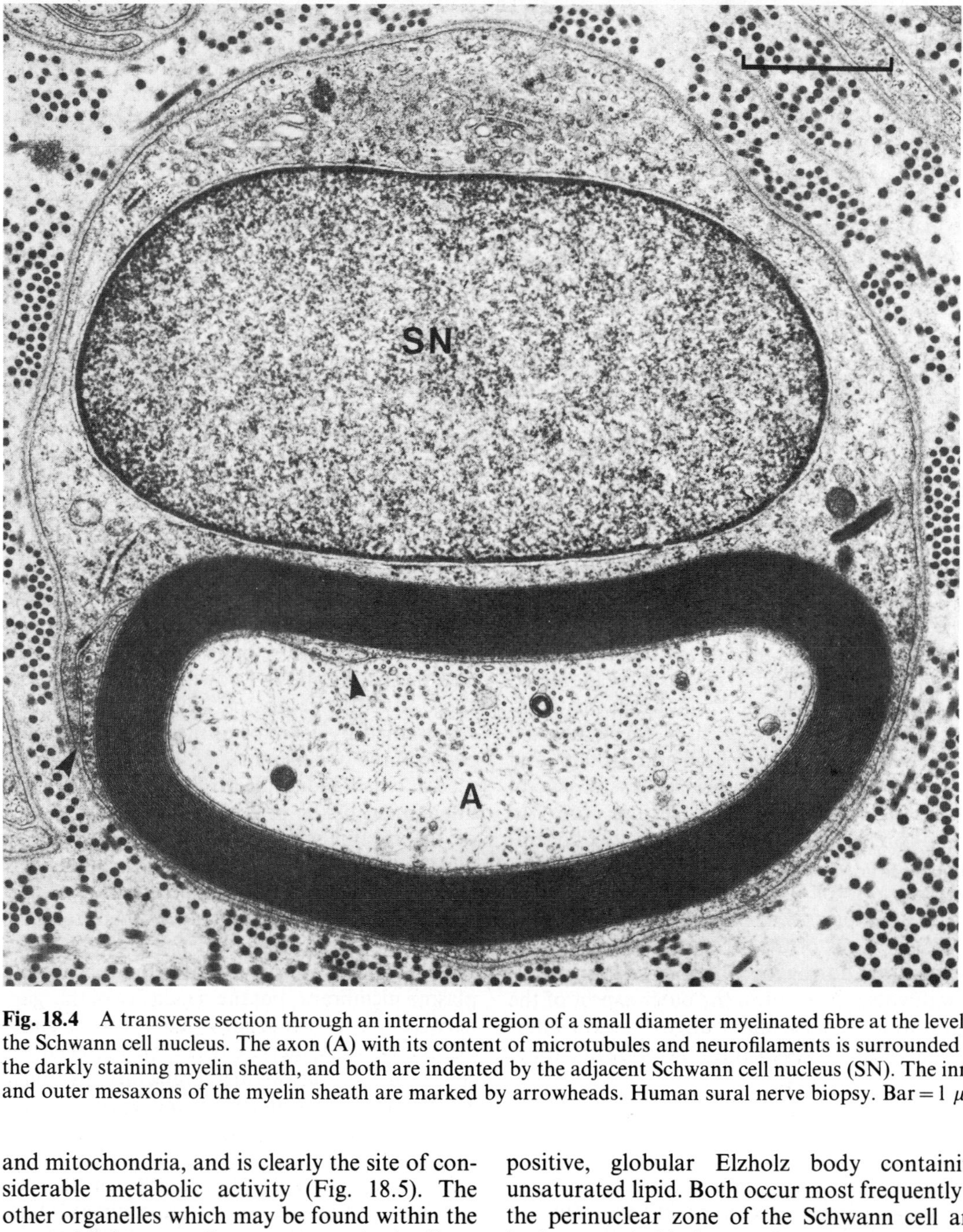

Fig. 18.4 A transverse section through an internodal region of a small diameter myelinated fibre at the level of the Schwann cell nucleus. The axon (A) with its content of microtubules and neurofilaments is surrounded by the darkly staining myelin sheath, and both are indented by the adjacent Schwann cell nucleus (SN). The inner and outer mesaxons of the myelin sheath are marked by arrowheads. Human sural nerve biopsy. Bar = 1 μm.

and mitochondria, and is clearly the site of considerable metabolic activity (Fig. 18.5). The other organelles which may be found within the external Schwann cell compartment in the fibres of larger mammals and man are, the Reich or pi granule, a metachromatic rod-shaped body about 1 μm long containing fine granular material stacked in regular lamellae with a spacing of 5-6 nm (Thomas and Slatford, 1964; Tomonaga and Sluga, 1970), and the Marchi-positive, globular Elzholz body containing unsaturated lipid. Both occur most frequently in the perinuclear zone of the Schwann cell and both are probably forms of secondary lysosome. Additional collections of mitochondria-rich Schwann cytoplasm occur in the paranodal regions at either end of the Schwann cell, where they lie within grooves on the external surface of the myelin sheath. They will be discussed in greater detail below in the context of the node

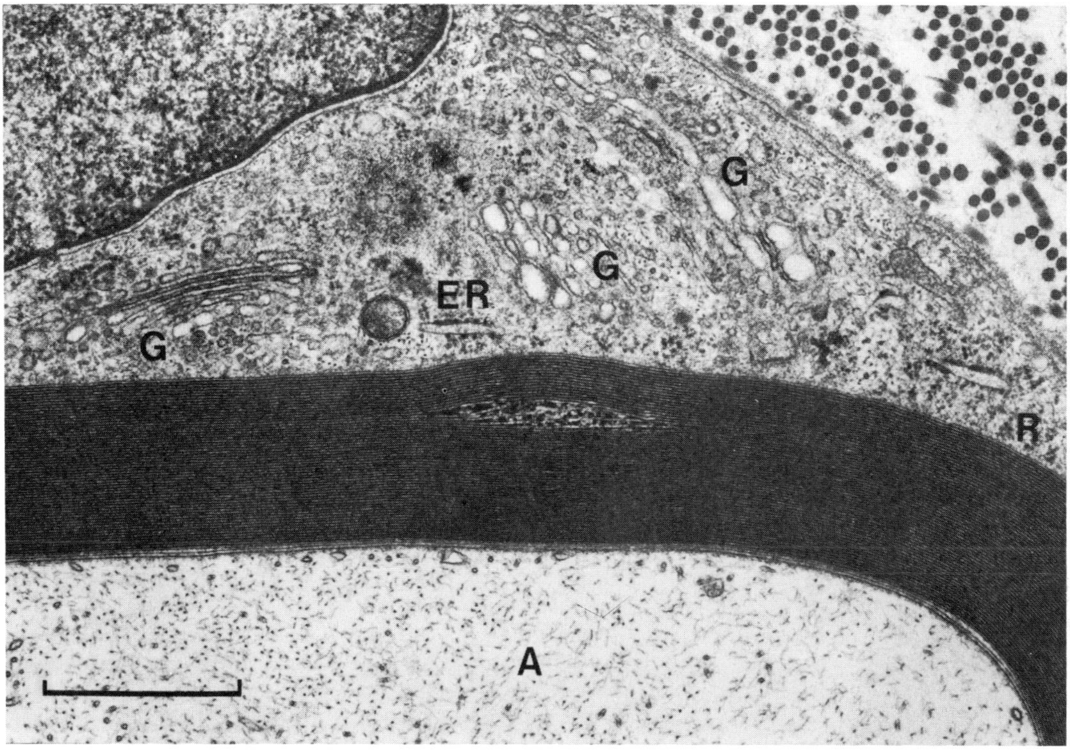

Fig. 18.5 A transverse section through part of the perinuclear cytoplasm of a Schwann cell on a large diameter myelinated axon (A), to illustrate the content of organelles: rough endoplasmic reticulum (ER), Golgi membranes (G) and free ribosomes (R). Human sural nerve biopsy. Bar = 1 μm.

and its adjacent structures. These perinuclear and paranodal components of the external Schwann cell compartment are connected along the length of the remaining, and major, part of the internodal myelin segment by slender spiral or reticular bands of cytoplasm (Fig. 18.6), some of which lie within shallow indentations in the external surface of the myelin. Their presence leads to minor irregularities in the contour of many transversely sectioned myelin sheaths (see Fig. 18.1), causing a cogwheel appearance (Berthold, 1968), but their arrangement is best illustrated by histochemical techniques which display their content of mitochondria (Berthold and Skoglund, 1967), by autoradiography following the uptake of labelled metabolites (Gould and Sinatra, 1981), or in freeze-fracture preparations (Mugnaini et al., 1977; Abrahams, Day and Allt, 1980).

Schmidt–Lanterman incisures

In small diameter fibres the only connection between the inner and outer Schwann cell compartment is via the continuous spiral of Schwann cytoplasm within the expanded end of each layer of the myelin sheath where these make contact with the axolemma at the margins of the nodes of Ranvier. In larger diameter fibres the compact myelin is interrupted at intervals by the presence of oblique clefts at an angle of about 9 degrees to the long axis of the sheath (Friede and Samorajski, 1969), the incisures of Schmidt–Lanterman, with the result that the sheath is divided into a series of interlocking cylindricoconical segments. Electron microscopy (Fig. 18.7) shows the incisures to be narrow oblique zones at which the myelin lamellae are less tightly compacted than elsewhere along the sheath. Lamellar continuity is maintained, but the major dense line, the fused cytoplasmic surfaces of the paired membranes which constitute each lamella, is replaced by a continuous spiral of Schwann cytoplasm which thus connects the outer, nuclear, and inner, adaxonal, Schwann cell compartments (Hall and Williams, 1970); the spiral of

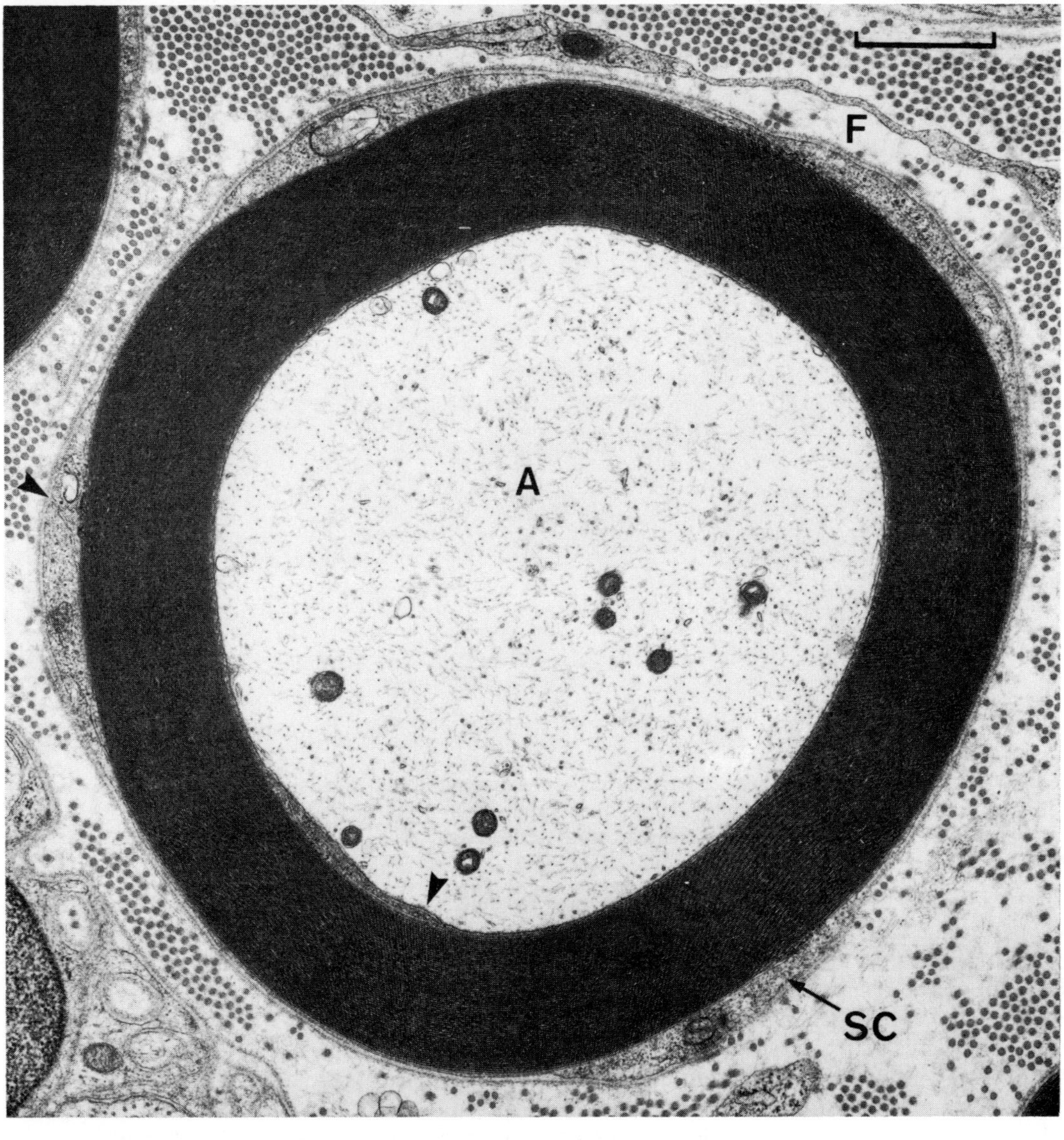

Fig. 18.6 A transverse section through an internodal region of a 7 μm diameter myelinated fibre. The axon (A) and surrounding myelin sheath are cylindrical, and the external compartment of the Schwann cell (SC) is reduced to four shallow bands external to the sheath. The internal and external mesaxons are marked with arrowheads, and the process of an endoneurial fibroblast is also visible (F). Human sural nerve biopsy. Bar = 1 μm.

Golgi–Rezzonico of light microscopy. The intraperiod line of the myelin to either side of the cytoplasmic spiral also separates at the incisure, creating potential paired spiral extracellular connections between the endoneurium and the periaxonal space beneath the myelin sheath. The longitudinal extent of myelin decompaction usually increases towards the external end of the incisure, and the outermost sets of membranes are often linked by a radial series of puncta adhaerentia (Hall and Williams, 1970). Incisures are labile structures, readily responding by swelling to trauma or a reduction in the tonicity of their immediate environment (Hall and Williams, 1970; Landon and Hall, 1976), a property which has in the past led to some dispute

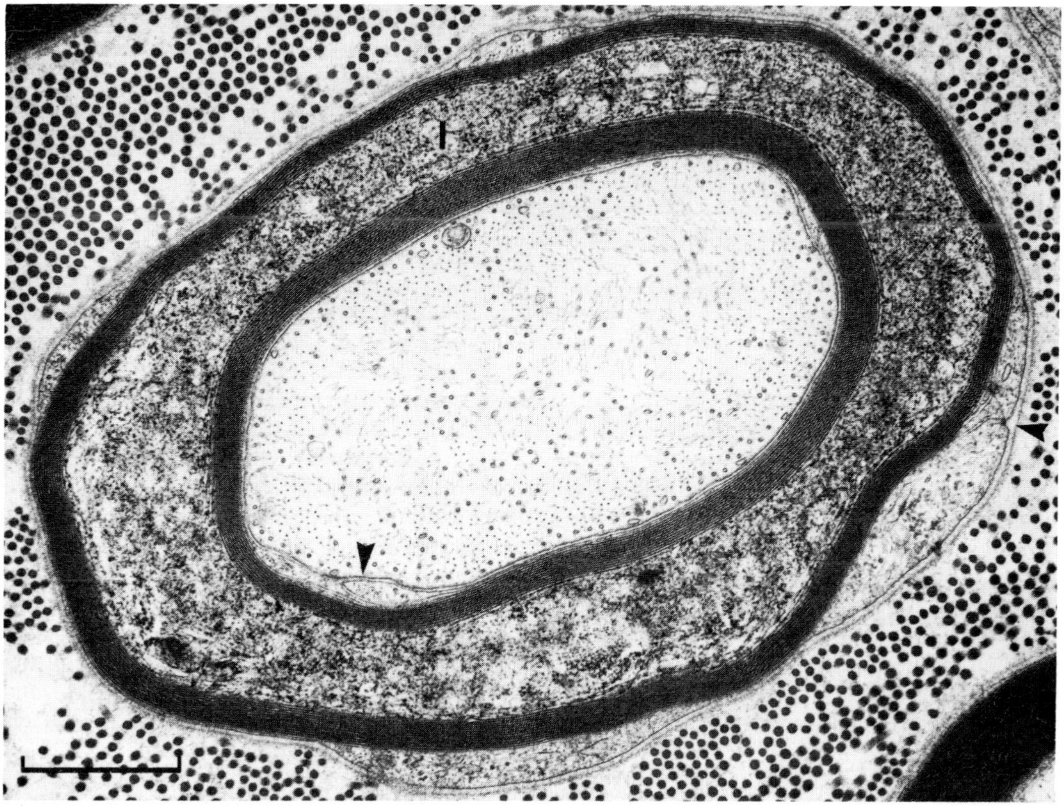

(a)

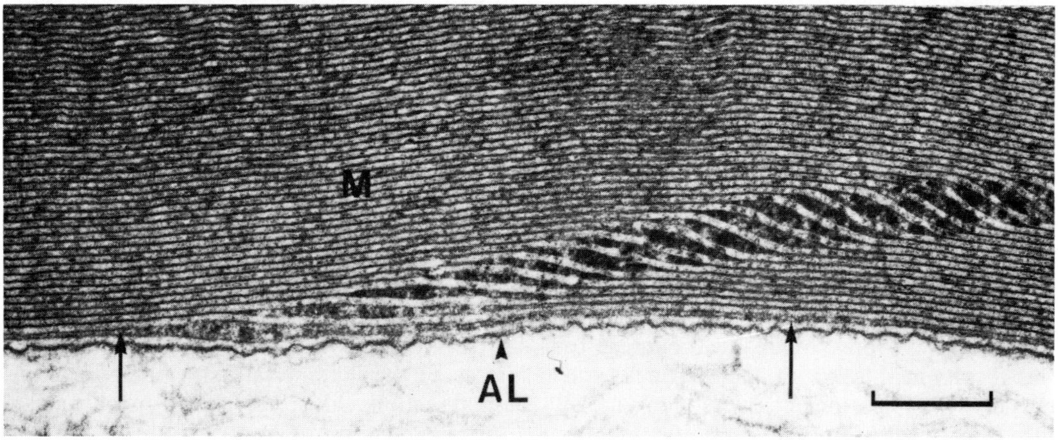

(b)

Fig. 18.7 (**a**) A transverse section through a myelinated axon at the site of an incisure of Schmidt–Lanterman. The compact myelin is separated into inner and outer components by the granular cytoplasm of the incisure (I). Arrowheads mark the inner and outer mesaxons. Human sural nerve biopsy. Bar = 1 μm. (**b**) A longitudinal section passing through the inner, axonal, end of an incisure of Schmidt–Lanterman. Each major dense line of the compact myelin (M) divides at the incisure to include a short segment of dense granular cytoplasm; these represent successive sections through a continuous cytoplasmic spiral linking the internal and external Schwann cell compartments. The former is visible as a thin layer lining the inner aspect of the myelin sheath (arrows), and is separated from the axolemma (AL) by a narrow periaxonal space. Human sural nerve biopsy. Bar = 0.25 μm.

concerning their reality as permanent components of the myelin sheath, and their incidence in large and small diameter fibres. It is now well established that the incisures are fixed components of the myelin sheath and not artefacts of preparation, and that their numbers correlate positively with fibre diameter and sheath thickness, larger diameter fibres having more, and more closely spaced, incisures in their myelin sheaths, both in the normal state and also in the shortened internodes which follow nerve regeneration (Hiscoe, 1947; Hall and Williams, 1970; Ghabriel and Allt, 1979a, b).

The functional significance of the Schmidt–Lanterman incisures is still an open question. It is clear that they provide a pathway for protoplasmic connections between the inner and outer compartments of the Schwann cell, and it has been suggested that this may be the route by which metabolic materials may pass between these two parts of the cell (Rawlins, 1973), and possibly onwards to the axon—a transport function which is supported by the near universal presence of one or more microtubules within the cytoplasmic spiral of the incisures. The adjacent extracellular spirals at the intraperiod line to either side of the cytoplasmic component may also permit interchange of ions between the periaxonal space and the exterior of the fibre (Hall and Williams, 1971; Krishnan and Singer, 1973; Landon and Hall, 1976; Mugnaini et al., 1977; Ghabriel and Allt, 1981), although it is claimed that both the outer and the inner ends of this cleft are sealed by tight junctions (Schnapp and Mugnaini, 1975). Equally little is known for certain of the role of the incisures in the normal metabolism of myelin sheaths or in their growth in length or thickness during development, or to what extent the presence or absence of incisures may influence the electrical properties of myelinated nerve fibres. Mechanical damage to nerves results in dilation of the incisures, and where nerve degeneration occurs distal to a nerve section (i.e. in wallerian degeneration) the fragmentation of the myelin sheath into primary ovoids appears to be initiated at the sites of the swollen incisures (Williams and Hall, 1971) which have been shown to be rich in acid phosphatase and esterases (Gould and Holt, 1961).

The node of Ranvier

At the ends of each internodal segment the myelin sheath increases in diameter, a swelling which is asymmetric in larger fibres, the bulb on the proximal side of each node of Ranvier being consistently the larger in most peripheral nerves (Lubińska, 1954; Williams and Landon, 1963), but the direction of asymmetry has been reported to reverse in the ascending limb of the recurrent laryngeal nerve in mammals (Williams and Kashef, 1968). The sheath as a whole also develops a series of longitudinal grooves and ridges, which often adopt a spiral configuration (Hess and Young, 1952), and extend back some 20–40 μm from the nodal margin, to give the paranodal bulb a crenated appearance in transverse section (Ranvier, 1878; Williams and Landon, 1963; Berthold, 1968). The external contour of the contained axon conforms to that of the inner aspect of the myelin sheath, and is thus reciprocally ridged and grooved, whereas the outer surface of the paranodal bulb is returned to a more or less cylindrical profilc by the presence of columns of Schwann cell cytoplasm within the grooves on the external surface of the myelin (Fig. 18.8), the marginal protoplasmic network (Nageotte, 1922). These paranodal accumulations of Schwann cell cytoplasm contain large aggregations of small rod-shaped mitochondria (Hess and Lansing, 1953; Williams and Landon, 1963; Berthold and Skoglund, 1967) in concentrations at least ten- to twentyfold larger than that found elsewhere along the internode, with up to 100 or more being visible within a single cross-section through a large diameter paranodal bulb (Williams and Landon, 1963). In the immediate vicinity of the node the ridges and grooves of the myelin sheath become shallower and eventually disappear, and the myelin lamellae turn inwards to run more or less radially towards the underlying axolemma. The lamellae of the myelin sheath end as a continuous spiral of Schwann cell cytoplasm closely applied to the surface of the juxtanodal axolemma. In longitudinal sections this spiral has the appearance of a series of loops or pockets, each of which is formed by an expansion of the end of a major dense line of the myelin, in a manner analogous to that described above for the Schmidt–Lanterman incisures. As at the incisure, the continuous cytoplasmic spiral which fills the terminal pockets of the sheath serves to link the external and internal compartment of the Schwann cell at its proximal and distal margins, and can generally be seen to contain one or more microtubules.

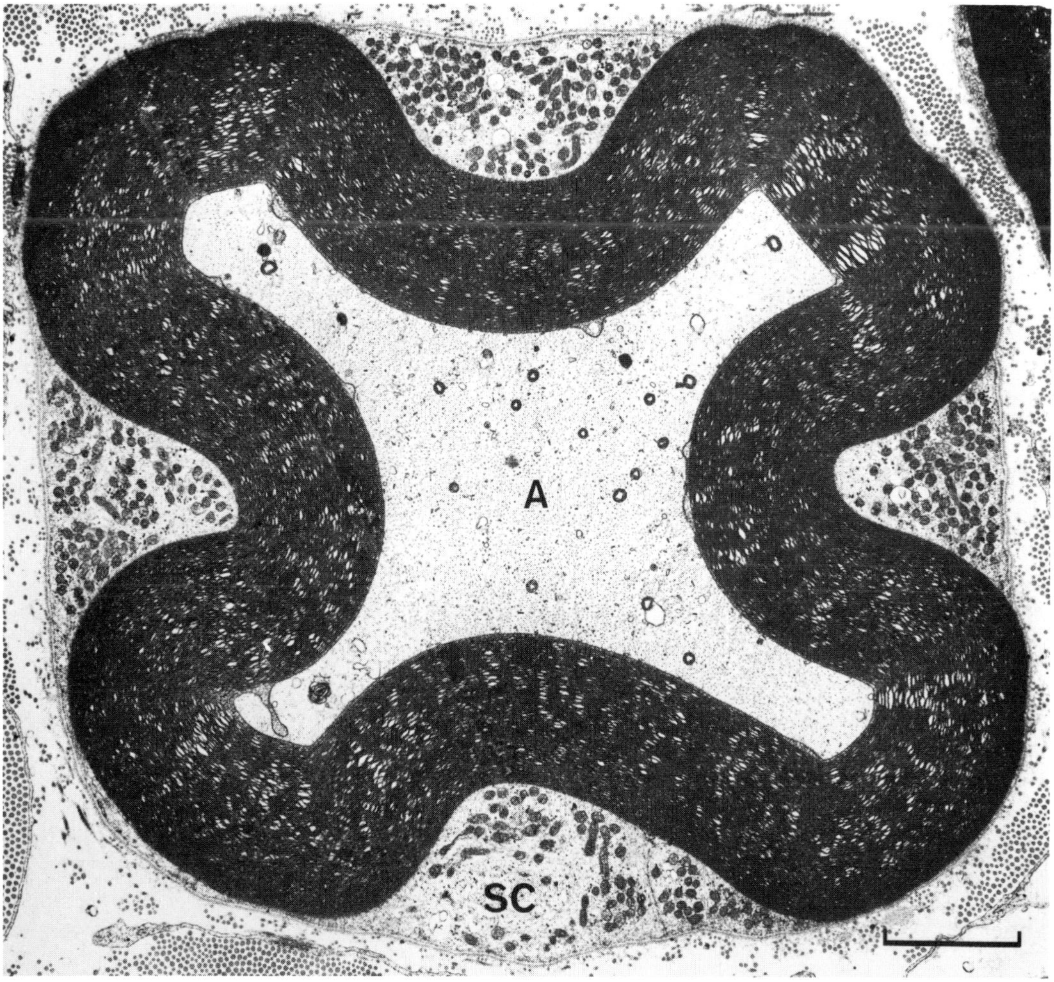

Fig. 18.8 A transverse section through the paranodal region of a large myelinated fibre from a cutaneous nerve of a baboon. The fluted axon (A) is surrounded by a thick crenated myelin sheath, the grooves in the external surface of which are filled by columns of Schwann cell cytoplasm (SC) containing large numbers of mitochondria. Bar = 2 μm.

The apposed membranes on the external aspect of the outermost terminal pockets are frequently linked by a series of puncta adhaerentia (Harkin, 1964), and at their inner ends adjacent to the axolemma they are united by a continuous tight junction (Schnapp and Mugnaini, 1975). In small diameter myelinated fibres every turn of the spiral, and thus every pocket, is in close apposition to the axolemma; in larger fibres, however, only some of the loops may make contact with the axon, the remainder being stacked in sets, resembling ears of barley in longitudinal sections, which project back into the compact myelin of the end of the sheath (Berthold, 1968; Landon and Hall, 1976). These sets of unattached myelin loops are probably responsible for the light microscopical appearance at the nodal end of the myelin sheath known as the *spiny bracelet of Nageotte* (Nageotte, 1922).

The juxtanodal flattening of the pleats in the myelin sheath is accompanied by confluence of the columns of Schwann cell cytoplasm into a complete circumferential collar immediately adjacent to the node. It contains a few mitochondria, and in larger fibres small dense membrane-bound bodies, the latter of which may be lysosomal or represent precursors of the gap substance (Berthold, 1968), and gives rise to

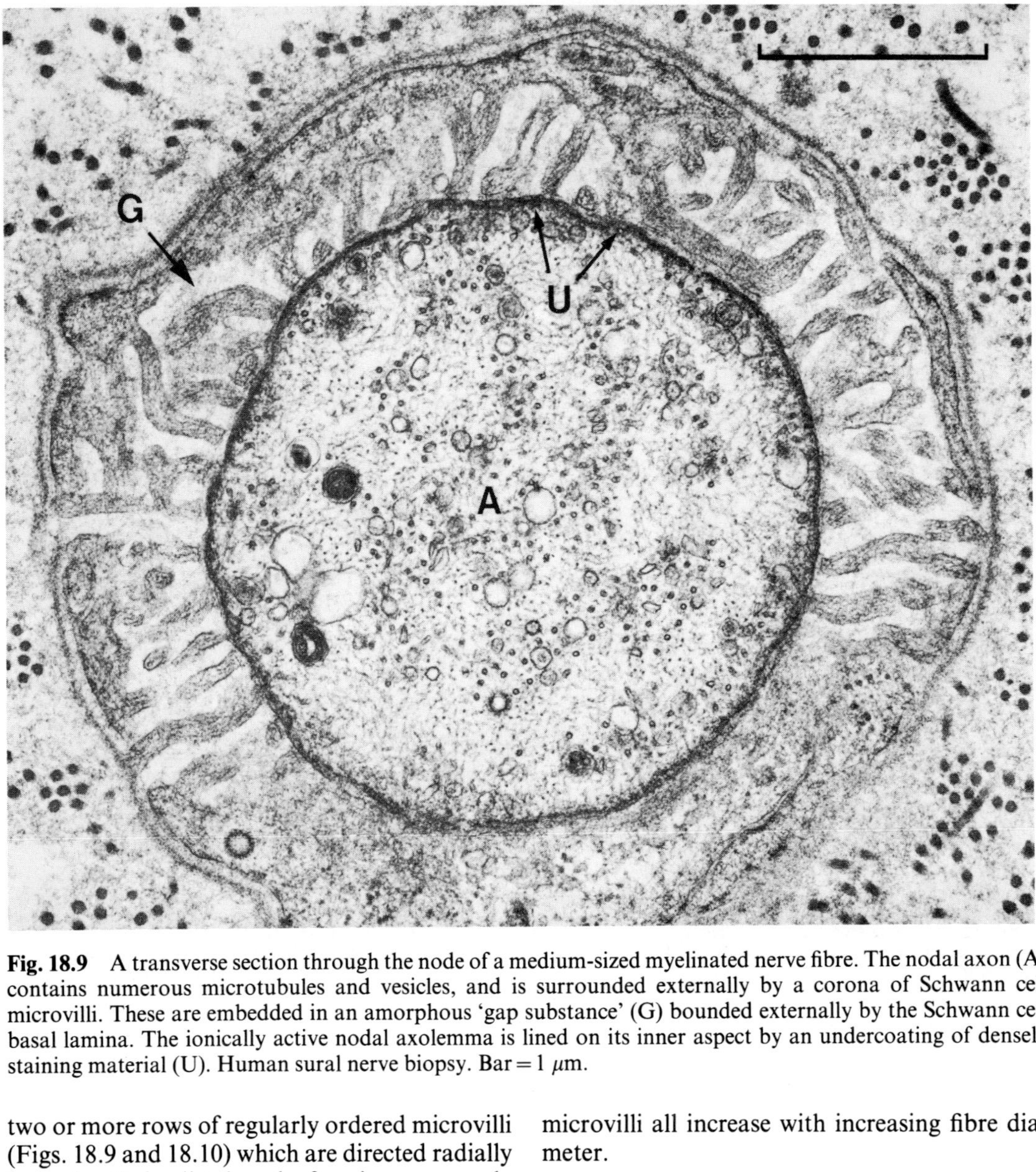

Fig. 18.9 A transverse section through the node of a medium-sized myelinated nerve fibre. The nodal axon (A) contains numerous microtubules and vesicles, and is surrounded externally by a corona of Schwann cell microvilli. These are embedded in an amorphous 'gap substance' (G) bounded externally by the Schwann cell basal lamina. The ionically active nodal axolemma is lined on its inner aspect by an undercoating of densely staining material (U). Human sural nerve biopsy. Bar = 1 μm.

two or more rows of regularly ordered microvilli (Figs. 18.9 and 18.10) which are directed radially inwards, their distal ends forming an evenly spaced hexagonal array in contact with the external surface of the nodal axolemma. These microvilli each contain six to eight parallel longitudinal microfilaments, and are embedded in an amorphous or finely flocculent, moderately electron-dense gap substance (Fig. 18.9). This material is distinguishable structurally from the overlying Schwann cell basal lamina, which is continuous from one Schwann cell to the next, and thus bridges the nodal gap. The number, length and regularity of the arrangement of the microvilli all increase with increasing fibre diameter.

The nodal axon and axolemma

The axon also varies in its form and calibre as it passes through the nodal and paranodal regions, changes which reflect, and may well be determined by, the morphology and organization of their ensheathing Schwann cells. The variation in axon calibre is slight in small diameter fibres (below 4 μm) in which there are no paranodal bulbs, with the axon being very slightly constricted as it passes under the myelin attachment zone, and returning to a cylinder of approximately the same diameter as that of the internodal axon at the node itself. In fibres of greater internodal diameter having paranodal bulbs, the axon first adopts the wider fluted form described above as it passes through the paranodal region, and then shrinks to one-third to one-fifth of its internodal calibre and resumes a cylindrical shape as it passes through the constricted myelin attachment zone. At the outer limit of the zone of myelin attachment axon diameter again increases to give the nodal axon a barrel-like shape with a biconical profile, and a mid-nodal diameter of between one-half and one-quarter that of its internodal value, the precise dimensions being related to fibre size. The true longitudinal extent of axon exposed at the node proved difficult to assess by light microscopy (Hess and Young, 1952), due to the refractility of the outward-bulging ends of the paranodal myelin, but recent electron microscopy studies have demonstrated that it varies little with fibre calibre, and ranges between 1 and 1.25 μm in the peripheral nerves of both cats (Rydmark and Berthold, 1983) and frogs (Mohammed, Landon and Love, 1983). The importance of the role of the node in the biophysical events responsible for the propagation of the axon potential in saltatory conduction has prompted a number of attempts to assess the area of axolemma exposed to the external medium, or rather to the annulus of microvilli and gap substance which intervene between the axolemma and the endoneurial tissue space. Electron microscopy has yielded little reliable information on this point until recently, due to the labour and difficulties involved in reconstructing sufficiently large numbers of nodes from serial ultrathin sections, but it is now clear that in both cats (Rydmark and Berthold, 1983) and frogs (Mohammed, Landon and Love, 1983) the nodal axolemmal area increases linearly with internodal fibre calibre, from 4–5 μm^2 in small to 25–30 μm^2 in large diameter fibres. A somewhat higher figure (30–60 μm^2) has been obtained from individually teased, large diameter frog fibres (Uhrik and Stämpfli, 1981). Cat and frog peripheral nerve nodes have been found to differ, however, in that mid-nodal axon diameter appears to correlate positively with internodal axon diameter throughout the range of fibre diameters in the cat (Rydmark, 1981), permitting nodal area and diameter values to be estimated from internodal diameter measurements, whereas in the frog *Rana temporaria* such a correlation is restricted to fibres of below 6 μm internodal diameter, there being little increase in mid-nodal diameter with further increase in fibre size. Nodal axolemmal area therefore increases steadily with increasing fibre diameter in the cat, but in the frog it appears to reach a maximum value in the middle range of fibre diameters and thereafter remains relatively constant regardless of further increase in fibre calibre (Mohammed, Landon and Love, 1983). The values quoted above have been obtained from fixed and plastic-embedded tissues subject to an unknown degree of shrinkage during their preparation. However, even if the shrinkage overall equals that of the myelin sheath, which shows a 20 per cent reduction in periodicity relative to fresh myelin, the values given above are considerably less than the minimum predicted from previous physiological studies (Chiu and Ritchie, 1981; Ritchie and Chiu, 1981; Stämpfli, 1981; Uhrik and Stämpfli, 1981).

The nodal axolemma

The axolemma of the nodal and juxtanodal regions possesses structural features which distinguish it from the internodal axolemma elsewhere along the course of the nerve fibre. At the node the inner surface of the axolemma is lined with a patchy electron-dense 'undercoating' of amorphous osmiophilic material some 20–30 nm thick (Peters, 1966), an arrangement which is also characteristic of both the spike-generating regions of the initial axon segment and the axolemma of some sensory receptor terminals. This cytoplasmic density (see Fig. 18.9) beneath the axon membrane is strictly confined to the nodal region, and ceases abruptly at the point of attachment of the outermost turn of the Schwann cell spiral to the axolemma at the region of myelin termination. On its deep surface the undercoating merges with a more diffuse increase in the density of the nodal and juxtanodal axoplasmic matrix. It has been demonstrated that under certain staining conditions (Quick and Waxman, 1977a) the nodal axoplasm, and particularly the subaxolemmal osmiophilic layer, has a high affinity for both ferric iron and ferrocyanide ions, a property also shared by the initial axon segment of the ventral horn motor neurons (Waxman and Quick, 1978). It has been proposed that the increased staining and ion-binding properties of these regions reflect functional specializations of the adjacent axolemma associated with its role as a site of high ionic current density during impulse initiation or transmission. Circumstantial support for this suggestion is provided by the finding that only the excitable nodes of *Sternarchus albifrons* electrocyte fibres both possess a dense undercoating material beneath the axolemma and are stained with ferric ion ferrocyanide (Waxman, Pappas and Bennett, 1972; Quick and Waxman 1977b).

Studies of nodes in both the peripheral and the central nervous system by the freeze-fracture technique (Rosenbluth, 1976, 1981; Sandri, Van Buren and Akert, 1977) have shown that the nodal axolemma is characterized by the possession of greatly increased numbers of large intramembranous E-face particles at around 1200/μm^2, when compared with either the internodal or the juxtanodal membranes in which E-face particle density averages approximately 100 μm^2 (Kristol, Sandri and Akert, 1978). It has been proposed that such particles represent the voltage-sensitive ionic channels of the nodal axolemma, a suggestion supported by the finding that only the excitable nodes of *Sternarchus* electrolyte fibres possess large concentrations of E-face particles (Kristol et al., 1977). The numbers of particles observed also match the predicted density of sodium ion channels based upon current fluctuation analysis (Conti et al., 1976; Sigworth, 1980) and gating current studies (Chiu, 1980), although saxitoxin-binding studies have yielded values an order of magnitude higher (Ritchie and Rogart, 1977). The nodes of all mammalian myelinated fibres (Kocsis and Waxman, 1980; Sherratt, Bostock and Sears, 1980; Chiu and Ritchie, 1982), and small diameter myelinated frog fibres (Smith and Schauf, 1981) have been shown to lack physiologically detectable potassium ion channels under normal circumstances, although potassium conductance can be detected in such fibres following damage to the paranodal regions (Chiu and Ritchie, 1982). These findings suggest that if potassium channels are visible in membrane fracture faces they must be sought among the P-face particles, which have as yet been studied much less intensively (Rosenbluth, 1983).

The myelin attachment zone

The juxtanodal axolemma corresponding to the zone of myelin termination also shows specific regional specialization in both sectioned and freeze-fracture replicated preparations. In the former the external leaflet of the axolemma beneath the terminal pockets of the myelin lamellae frequently shows a regular sequence of alternating dense and pale regions, which in favourable tangential views can be seen to form a continuous shallow helix of increased electron density within the outer leaflet of the juxtanodal axolemma (Bargmann and Linder, 1964; Andres, 1965; Peters, 1966; Hirano and Dembitzer, 1969). Freeze-fracture images of this region show a helical pattern of comparable dimensions and pitch (Livingston et al., 1973; Rosenbluth, 1976; Schnapp and Mugnaini, 1978) in which lines of fine particles alternate with narrow particle-free zones. This arrangement appears to represent an unique form of intercellular attachment, not corresponding to any type of gap or close junction described between other classes of cells. It has been suggested that the junction may have functions that go beyond mere physical attachment of the myelin to the axolemma, and that it may be concerned with interchange of ions and/or metabolites, or the transfer of the information needed to initiate and maintain the co-operative interaction of axon and Schwann cell which results in the complex morphology of the mature node of Ranvier. A similar role in metabolic communication has been ascribed to some recently reported associations of particle aggregates in the juxtaparanodal axon and apposed adaxonal Schwann cell membrane in rat peripheral nerve fibres (Stolinski et al., 1981). The juxtanodal axolemma is largely free of large E-face particles but small aggregates can occur at locations which appear to coincide with areas lacking attachment to myelin terminal pockets (Rosenbluth, 1981).

Experimental evidence that ions such as lanthanum can penetrate between the terminal pockets of the myelin and the juxtanodal axolemma at the myelin attachment zone (Hirano and Dembitzer, 1969; Revel and Hamilton, 1969) have led to suggestions that extracellular ions and small macromolecules (Hall and Williams, 1971) may under normal circumstances be able to obtain access to the periaxonal space via a helical low-resistance pathway defined by the particle-free zones of membrane attachment. However, it is probable that, within the context of the time-course of ionic movements involved in impulse transmission, the nature of the attachment of the myelin loops to the axon is such that the internodal axolemma is effectively isolated from ionic events at the node (Rosenbluth, 1983).

The nodal axon

Both the arrangement and content of organelles within the nodal and juxtanodal axon show consistent differences from those seen elsewhere along the internode. Mitochondria are approximately five times more numerous (Berthold, 1978), from one to five being visible in a mid-nodal transverse section, depending upon the size of fibre, and these are often situated close to the nodal axolemma. The vesicle content of the nodal axoplasm is also increased, and may take the form of longitudinally aligned strings of round or ovoid vesicles having diameters in the range of 50–200 nm. Elements of the axonal smooth endoplasmic reticulum, lamellated autophagic vesicles, dense lysosome-like granules of varying size and glycogen granules are also found in greater numbers in the nodal axon (see Fig. 18.9). Microtubules are present in much higher density than in the internodal axoplasm, as a consequence of their compression into a much smaller volume as they pass through the narrow nodal and juxtanodal regions, and they tend to be arranged in a series of small bundles associated with membranous organelles or as a peripheral palisade (Landon and Hall, 1976). Circumferential microtubules running at right angles to the long axis of the fibre have been described within the axoplasm underlying the maximum outward convexity of the nodal axon in both rat (Gray and Westrum, 1979) and frog (Mohammed, 1983) nodes.

Relatively few neurofilaments are evident in transverse sections of the nodal axon, and these retain the same packing density as in the internodal regions; the implications of this finding for the mechanisms responsible for the transport of the slow component of axoplasm have been discussed above. A number of metabolic poisons, such as *n*-hexane and its analogues, and carbon disulphide and acrylamide, induce axonal swellings in peripheral nerves in which large masses of axoplasm containing whorls of neurofilaments appear proximal to some nodes of Ranvier. These appearances have been interpreted to indicate that the agents act directly upon the neurofilaments to induce their aggregation, and that the resultant 'filamentous masses' obstruct the normal flow of axoplasm along the fibre (Cavanagh, 1982). There is, however, no evidence that the filaments within the 'masses' are either morphologically abnormal or more tightly packed than in normal axoplasm, and it is possible that the accumulation of axoplasm seen in these forms of intoxication is a consequence of impaired transnodal axoplasmic transport rather than its cause, being brought about by failure of the system normally responsible for solubilizing the neurofilaments proximal to each node.

The consistent and characteristic difference in organelle content and staining characteristics between the nodal and paranodal axon on the one hand and the internodal axon on the other imply that the nodal axon is not merely a narrowed portion of an otherwise homogeneous cylinder, and that it has specific cytological properties which depend for their expression on a co-operative interaction between axon and Schwann cell.

The perinodal space

The perinodal space, or nodal periaxonal space, is an annular interval around the axon, defined longitudinally by the abutting ends of the adjacent Schwann cells, and internally and externally by the nodal axolemma and the Schwann cell basal lamina respectively. The material within this space has been shown to have a high affinity for metal ions, a fact recognized by Ranvier (1878), who reported the appearance of a black cross at the nodes of frog nerve fibres which had been soaked in diluted silver nitrate and exposed to light. This cross of Ranvier consists of two components: the first a longitudinal bar corresponding to the nodal and juxtanodal axon, and the second a transverse component, the cementing disc. Light microscopic observations of the latter showed it to be a moderately refractile annulus surrounding the nodal axon and stainable with methylene blue (the Nemiloff ring). Adhesive properties were ascribed to it as it was considered to be responsible for holding the ends of the adjacent myelin segments together to strengthen the narrowest, and ostensibly weakest, portions of the nerve fibre from the effects of longitudinal tension. It was subsequently recognized that the disc could also constitute a barrier to the free diffusion of ions between the endoneurial tissue space and the nodal axolemma, as a consequence of its location and its capacity to bind metal ions (Hess and Young, 1952). Electron microscopy has shown that the ultrastructural counterpart of the cementing disc is the complex of Schwann cell microvilli and the extracellular gap substance which immediately surround the nodal axolemma. Histochemical studies at a fine structural level (Landon and Langley, 1971; Langley, 1971; Landon and Hall, 1976) have demonstrated that the gap substance contains glycosaminoglycans having cation binding and exchange properties analogous to those of an ion exchange resin.

Functional implications of nodal structure

The form and arrangement of the various cellular elements which constitute the node of Ranvier of a large myelinated nerve fibre are shown diagrammatically in Fig. 18.10. It is evident that the region possesses a far more complex structure than is apparent by light microscopy or is required by most contemporary theories of saltatory conduction. A short length of axon is indeed exposed free of myelin ensheathment at the node, but it is related externally to a complex arrangement of Schwann cell microvilli embedded in a matrix of material rich in fixed anionic charges and not to tissue fluid in the sense in which the term is usually applied. This arrangement must be expected to influence the concentrations and kinetics of ions in the vicinity of the nodal axolemma, and it has been suggested that the gap substance may act as an ion exchange buffer with a capacity to concentrate and maintain a high, but osmotically inactive, concentration of sodium ions immediately adjacent to the axolemma (Landon and Langley, 1971; Landon and Hall, 1976), and to limit diffusion away from the axolemma of the potassium ions which have passed outwards through the membrane during the passage of an action potential. A similar function to the latter has been proposed for the glycocalyx of muscle fibres (Bennett, 1963), and potassium ion accumulation in the nodal gap has been reported to occur in voltage-clamped frog myelinated fibres (Moran et al., 1980).

The conspicuous aggregations of mitochondria present within the paranodal Schwann cell cytoplasm (see Fig. 18.8) have also invited

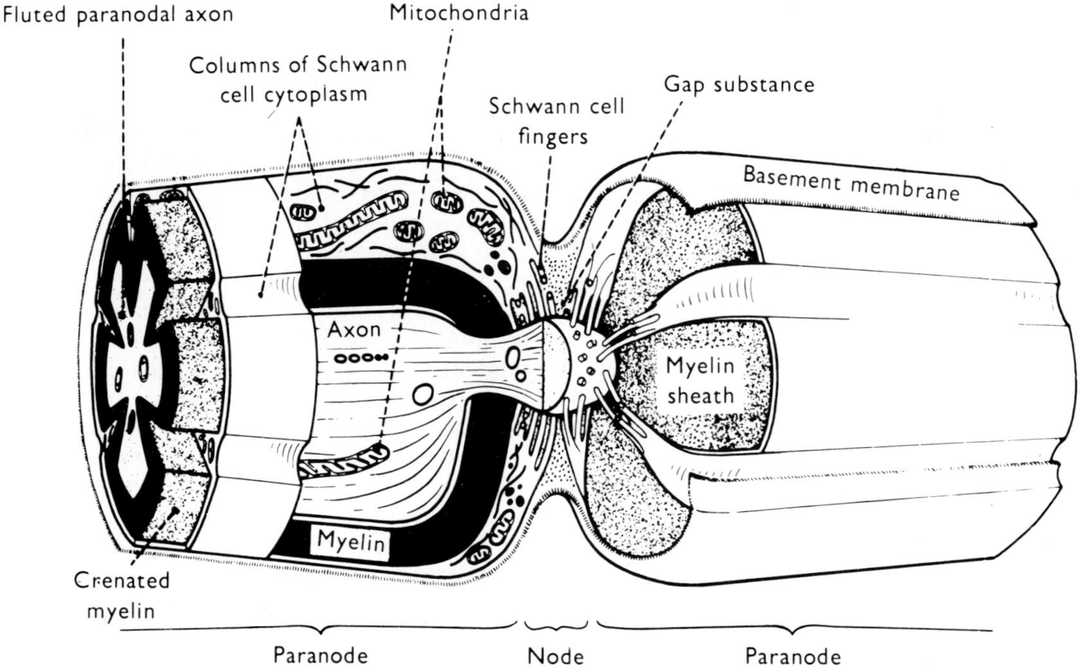

Fig. 18.10 A diagrammatic representation of the principal features of the fine structure of a node of Ranvier on a large mammalian myelinated fibre. (Reproduced, with permission, from R. Warwick and P.L. Williams (eds), 1973, *Gray's Anatomy*, 35th edn, Churchill Livingstone, Edinburgh.)

speculation concerning their function, as mitochondrial numbers and mass are in general closely geared to the energy requirements of a cell. In large diameter mammalian fibres their numbers may exceed those of the mitochondria visible within the corresponding section of the underlying axon by at least 100-fold, and there can be little doubt that such a concentration must reflect the existence of continuing energy-consuming activity in this region of the Schwann cell. As a consequence it has been suggested that the paranodal portion of adjacent Schwann cells at each node, including their nodal microvilli and gap substance, should be regarded as a functional unit—the paranodal apparatus (Landon and Williams, 1963; Williams and Landon, 1963)—which could function to provide a source of energy-rich compounds to fuel the ion translocation mechanisms necessary to maintain the polarization of the nodal axolemma, either directly or by controlling the ionic milieu within the nodal gap (Landon and Langley, 1971; Landon and Hall, 1976; Landon, 1981).

The connective tissues and sheaths of peripheral nerves

The endoneurium

As noted previously, the interstices between the fibres of peripheral nerves are packed with collagen fibrils in a mucopolysaccharide ground substance, and this interfibre matrix constitutes the endoneurium. The great majority of the collagen fibrils run longitudinally in parallel with the nerve fibres (see Fig. 18.3), and have relatively uniform diameters in the range of 30–65 nm (Thomas 1963; Gamble and Eames, 1964). In addition, each nerve fibre is surrounded immediately outside the Schwann cell basal lamina by a thin sleeve of much finer and more irregularly disposed reticulin fibres (Thomas, 1963). When a nerve funiculus is teased apart for microscopic examination, each fibre carries with it its own reticulin sheath together with a variable portion of the immediately adjacent, larger diameter, interstitial collagen fibrils, and these two components were formerly distinguished histologically as the sheaths of Plenk and Laidlaw, and of Key and Retzius, respectively. These terms are, however, of little significance or utility in describing the arrangements of the connective tissue in an intact nerve, and are now seldom used in the context of descriptions of fine structure. The principal cellular constituents of the endoneurium are fibroblasts (Fig. 18.11). In section these are angular cells lacking a basal lamina which lie free between the endoneurial collagen fibrils. They possess pale angular nuclei, often with a prominent nucleolus, and their cytoplasm contains conspicuous stacks of Golgi membranes and cisterns of rough endoplasmic reticulum, the latter having a moderately electron-dense, finely granular content. The endoplasmic reticulum extends out into the extensive flattened processes which radiate from the cell body between the adjacent bundles of endoneurial collagen fibrils. The endoneurial fibro-

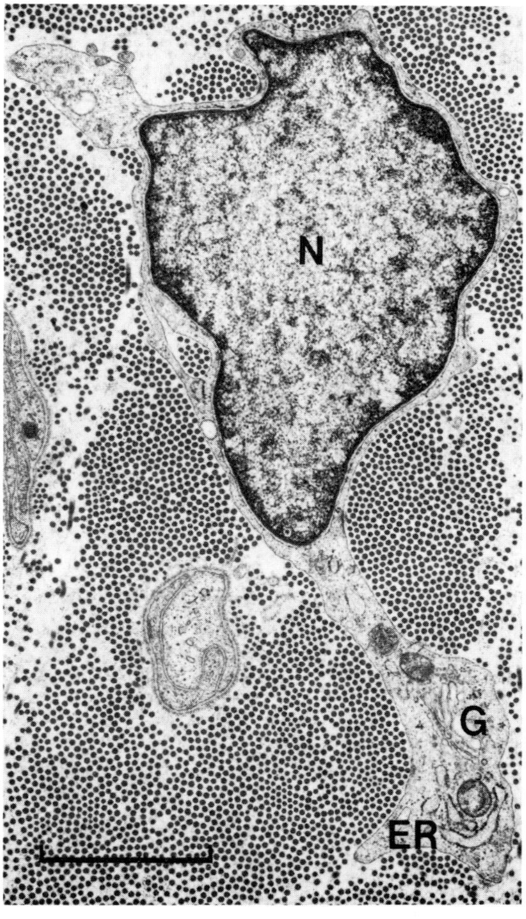

Fig. 18.11 An example of an endoneurial fibroblast from a human sural nerve biopsy. A thin shell of cytoplasm surrounds the angular nucleus (N), and from this arise flattened processes containing Golgi membranes (G) and rough endoplasmic reticular cisterns (ER). Bar = 2 μm.

blast population has been reported to range from 5 to 25 per cent of the nuclear profiles visible in transversely sectioned peripheral nerves (Causey and Barton, 1959; Thomas, 1963), and they are believed to be responsible for the production of the major part of the extracellular endoneurial connective tissue.

Other cells which may be found within the endoneurium are mast cells and macrophages. The former are the more common and are encountered quite frequently in the limb nerves of amphibia, and of small mammals such as rats and mice (Gamble, 1964; Olsson, 1968), but are rarely seen in human nerves; they have been reported to be absent from spinal nerve dorsal roots (Gamble, 1964). In appearance they are characterized by dense nuclei with clumped chromatin; dense cytoplasm packed with numerous large vesicles having a dense, finely granular or irregularly lamellated content, the latter being more common in human mast cells; and a conspicuously folded cell surface. Macrophages are very seldom seen in normal peripheral nerves, but when present may be of haematogenous origin; they have cytological features resembling those of mononuclear leucocytes.

The perineurium

The endoneurium and its contained nerve fibres are enclosed within a tubular cellular and connective tissue sheath, the perineurium or sheath of Henle. This structure consists of layers of sheets of extremely flattened, squame-like cells, interleaved by thin layers of fine collagen fibrils aligned parallel to the axis of the nerve. The number of layers is highest proximally, and may amount to 12 or more in large funiculi, progressively diminishing to a single layer at the finest distal cutaneous and intramuscular nerve branches. In larger nerves septa composed of two or three layers of perineurial cells arising from the inner aspect of the sheath may serve to subdivide individual funiculi into two or more subsidiary fascicles. Blood vessels penetrating the perineurium to supply the endoneurial capillary plexus also carry sleeves of perineurial cells with them into the endoneurium for short distances (Burkel, 1967; Lieberman, 1968).

In sections the individual perineurial cells appear as extremely thin sheets of cytoplasm, often no more than 0.1 μm thick, which contain occasional small cisterns of endoplasmic reticulum, and numerous pinocytotic vesicles which open on to both the external and internal surfaces of the cell (Fig. 18.12). The cells are somewhat thicker in their central zones (1.0–1.5 μm) where two equally thin layers of cytoplasm enclose a thin discoid nucleus. Both faces of the perineurial cells are covered by basal lamina, which in man may become much thickened when compared to the basal laminae of other cells, even in quite young subjects, and to which the cell membrane may be anchored by scattered hemidesmosomes (Thomas and Jones, 1967; Lieberman, 1968). The connective tissue between these layers of cells consists of collagen fibrils of comparable dimensions to those of the endoneurium (40–80 nm; Gamble and Eames, 1964) and occasional elastic fibrils (Thomas 1963; Thomas and Jones, 1967). The outer layers may also contain occasional fibroblasts and mast cells. At their margins the individual perineurial cells overlap and interdigitate and are linked by tight junctions between their apposed membranes. Peripherally the ends of the perineurial tubes merge with the outer capsular layers of encapsulated sensory terminals (Shantha and Bourne, 1968; Schoultz and Swett, 1972; Spencer and Schaumburg, 1973; Low, 1976) but at the neuromuscular junction they terminate as an open-ended sleeve (Burkel, 1967), providing a potential connection between the endoneurial compartment and the general connective tissue space between the muscle fibres. The same arrangement may pertain at the ends of the perineurial sheaths of unencapsulated sensory nerve branches but their detailed anatomy has yet to be defined.

Fig. 18.12 A transverse section through the perineurial sheath of a human peripheral nerve. It consists of seven layers of flattened cells having flattened discoid nuclei (N), interleaved by layers of slender collagen (C), and more substantial elastin (E), fibrils. The individual perineurial cells are linked by complex interdigitating junctions (J) at their contiguous margins: they contain numerous small pinocytotic vesicles (V) and are attached to the thickened basal laminae on their two surfaces by scattered hemidesmosomes (arrowheads). The endoneurial space (EN) contains fibroblast processes (F), elastin and fine longitudinal collagen fibrils; the last contrast with the thicker and more irregularly disposed fibrils of the epineurial collagen (EP) on the external aspect of the sheath. Bar = 2 μm.

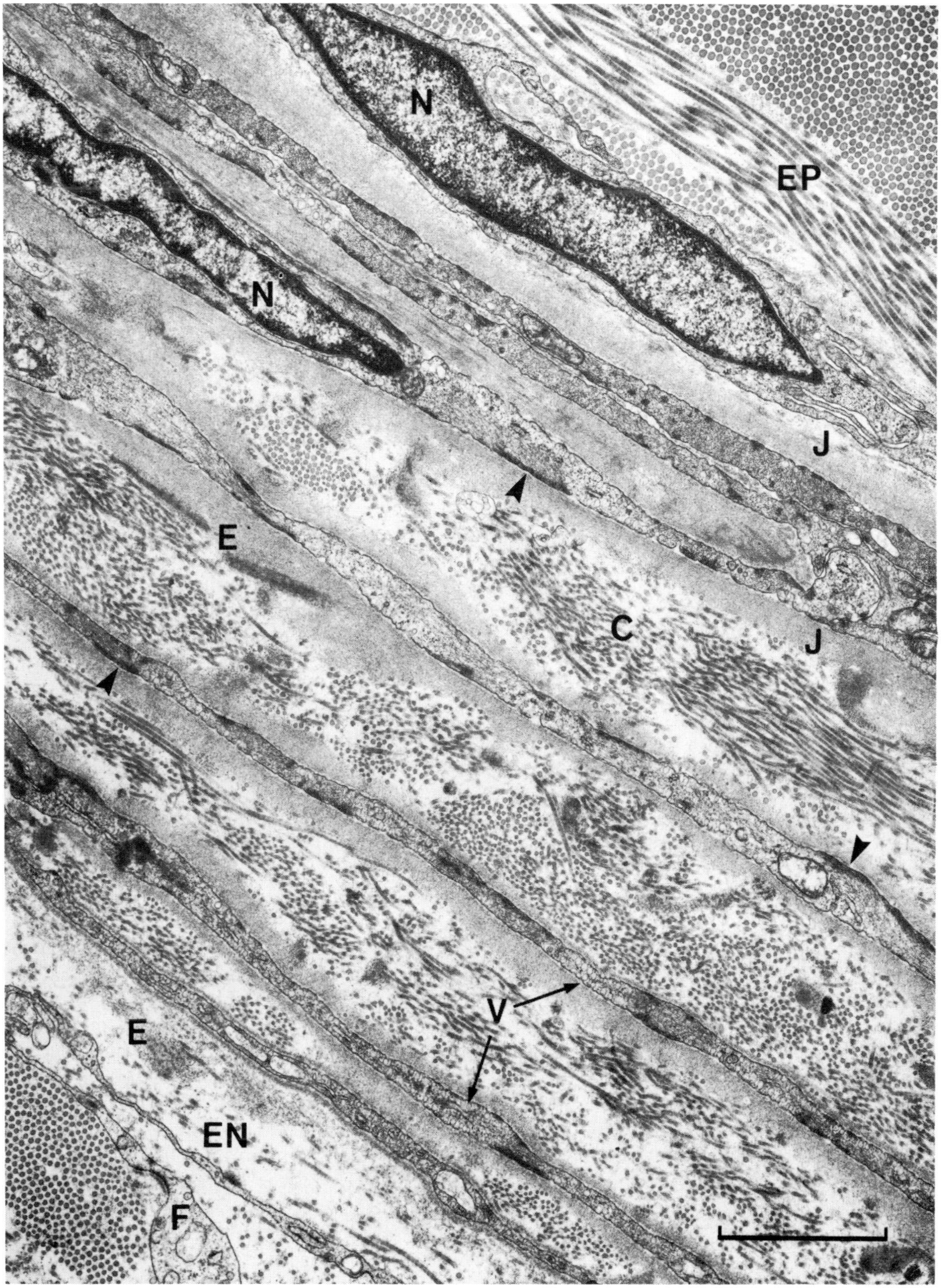

Fig. 18.12

The epineurium

The outermost of the peripheral nerve sheaths is the epineurium. It consists of massed collagen fibrils with a longitudinal or shallow spiral orientation, interspersed with occasional elastin fibres, fibroblasts, mast cells, and the small arterial and venous vessels which supply the capillary plexus of the underlying nerve. The individual collagen fibrils are both larger and more variable in size than those of the inner two layers of the nerve sheath (see Fig. 18.12), and range from 60 to 100 nm in human sural nerve (Gamble and Eames, 1964). Superficially the epineurium merges with the surrounding areolar connective tissue of the deep fascia, and on its deep surface with the outermost layer of the perineurium. It is distinguishable as a separate sheath only in the largest nerves and nerve trunks; its thickness diminishes as the nerves pass distally, and a distinct epineurial layer cannot usually be identified around the smaller peripheral branches in most species.

Function of peripheral nerve sheaths

A primary and obvious function of the connective tissues which contribute to the structure of the peripheral nerve sheaths is a mechanical one, the massed array of collagen in parallel with the nerve fibres having considerable mechanical strength and resilience which may serve to protect the nerve fibres from the stresses imposed by movement of the bodily parts through which they run. The sheaths of peripheral nerves have also long been known to be extremely resistant to penetration by foreign materials and infective agents. A considerable body of experimental work has demonstrated conclusively that the principal barrier to the entry of materials into the peripheral nerve is the perineurial sheath, and particularly its innermost layers in which (as has been noted above) the constituent cells are linked by a continuous series of tight junctional complexes (Burkel, 1967). Tracer materials such as lanthanum salts, ferritin, horseradish peroxidase and other exogenous proteins readily penetrate the epineurium and outer layers of the perineurium, but are thereafter excluded from the endoneurial compartment for many hours by the innermost layers of cells. Such material as does enter the endoneurium appears to be transported actively across the perineurial cells via the pinocytotic vesicles (Waggener, Bunn and Beggs, 1965; Olsson and Reese, 1969; Klemm, 1970). The perineurial barrier may be disrupted by mechanical trauma or osmotic shock (Olsson and Kristensson, 1972; Kristensson and Olsson, 1976), and may be circumvented at the sites of penetration of the perineurium by blood vessels, and at the peripheral open ends of the perineurial tubes, particularly at the neuromuscular junction (Burkel, 1967; Zacks and Saito, 1969); the last has been suggested to be an important portal of entry for viruses and toxins into the peripheral nervous system. The perineurial permeability barrier has also been found to be incomplete in newborn rats and mice, and does not appear to become fully effective until the end of the third postnatal week (Kristensson and Olsson, 1971).

Vasculature of peripheral nerves

Peripheral nerves are supplied by branches from their local regional vessels which ramify and branch within the epineurium. Precapillary vessels penetrate the perineurium at an oblique angle and are ensheathed for a short distance within the endoneurial compartment by internal prolongations of the innermost layers of the perineurial sheath. They then divide to supply the endoneurial plexus which appears to consist exclusively of capillaries. The plexus has a predominantly longitudinal orientation, and is said to drain directly to collecting vessels situated outside the perineurium, few if any venules being found within the endoneurium.

The contacts between the edges of adjacent capillary endothelial cells of the endoneurial circulation have been shown to be completely sealed by tight junctions, and in most species this arrangement provides a second and effective barrier to the penetration of higher molecular weight materials into the endoneurial compartment (Waksman, 1961; Olsson, 1971; Olsson and Reese, 1971; Kristensson and Olsson, 1973). This blood–nerve barrier is, however, much less effective in the spinal nerve roots, and in the dorsal root and autonomic ganglia, to which plasma proteins and exogenous tracer molecules such as horseradish peroxidase appear to have relatively unimpeded access (Olsson, 1971; Arvidsson, Kristensson and Olsson, 1973; Lieberman, 1976). The anatomical basis for this difference has been attributed to a lack of tight junctions between the capillary endothelial cells of the endoneurial compartment at these sites and the presence of 'fenestrated' capillaries within the dorsal root ganglia of some species (Olsson, 1971).

Pathological classification of peripheral neuropathies

Disorders of the peripheral nerves can be classified in terms of the component of the peripheral nervous system that is primarily affected. Classifications are necessarily approximations but can be useful in emphasizing general principles. *Neuronopathies* consist of conditions in which there is loss of neurons that contribute axons to the peripheral nerves: the cranial and spinal lower motor neurons, the preganglionic autonomic neurons and the sensory and autonomic ganglion cells. In *axonopathies*, axonal degeneration occurs but the neuronal cell bodies survive. In generalized axonopathies there is usually a distal axonal degeneration which advances proximally towards the cell body in a 'dying-back' manner. Occasionally the degenerative process may begin proximally in the axons. Axonopathies may also be focal, related to localized neural damage. Other conditions primarily affect the Schwann cells or myelin, leading to a *demyelinating neuropathy*. Demyelination may also be a consequence of axonal disease (secondary demyelination). These processes are considered in greater detail in the succeeding sections. Finally, disorders that primarily affect the supporting tissues and blood vessels may have secondary effects on the nerve fibres.

General pathology of peripheral nerve disorders

Neuronal degeneration

The pathology of anterior horn cells and preganglionic sympathetic neurons is considered in Chapter 15. In sensory neuronopathies (ganglioneuropathies), loss of dorsal root ganglion cells occurs. This may be preceded by cytoplasmic vacuolation, followed by cell necrosis and neuronophagia. An accompanying proliferation of satellite cells takes place. This is an early event, and is often discernible before disappearance of the ganglion cells. After loss of the ganglion cells, compact groups of satellite cells remain—the residual nodules of Nageotte (Fig. 18.13). In chronic disorders they probably gradually disappear. The loss of dorsal root ganglion cells may be selective. Thus in Friedreich's ataxia (Chapter 15) there is a predominant loss of the larger cells, whereas in Fabry's disease it is the smaller cells which degenerate (Ohnishi and Dyck, 1974). Specific intracellular inclusions are observable in some conditions, including Fabry's disease (Ohnishi and Dyck, 1974). Inflammatory infiltrates accompany some ganglion cell degenerations, such as carcinomatous sensory neuropathy (Horwich et al., 1977).

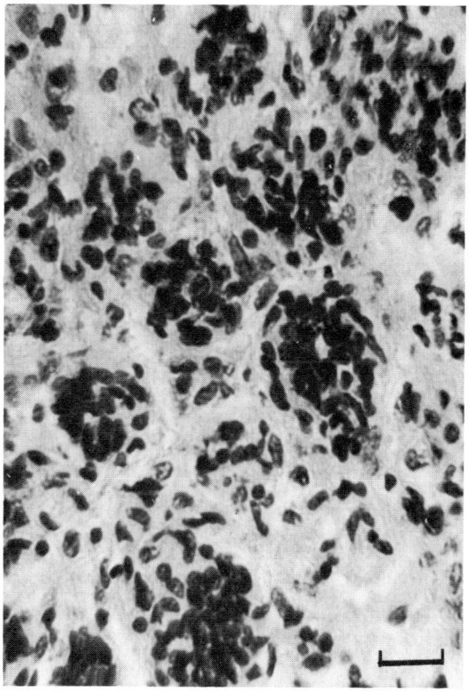

Fig. 18.13 Group of residual nodules of Nageotte. Haematoxylin and eosin. Bar = 20 μm.

Loss of autonomic ganglion cells in neuropathies produces changes similar to those which occur in the dorsal root ganglia. Proliferation of satellite cells again leads to the formation of residual nodules. Fibrosis and skeins of fine regenerating axons derived from the surviving cells may be observed. In diabetic and alcoholic neuropathies, enlargement of cells (which show PAS-positive inclusions and displaced nuclei) has been described (Appenzeller and Richardson, 1966).

Axonal degeneration and regeneration

Wallerian degeneration

The consequences of nerve section were first adequately studied by Waller in 1850, although there had been less-complete earlier descriptions. Despite the fact that the observations were made on fresh unfixed material, Waller was able to recognize the initial 'coagulation' of fibres distal to the site of interruption, followed by their segmentation into linear rows of granules. Definitive studies by light microscopy were undertaken by Cajal (1928), Nageotte (1932) and Holmes and Young (1942), who demonstrated the breakdown and interruption of the axons and the segmentation of the myelin into ellipsoids ('digestive chambers') which contain axonal debris (Fig. 18.14A,B). This occurs within the endoneurial connective tissue sheaths. The axonal and myelin debris was considered to be removed by macrophages. Schwann cell proliferation was observed to occur within the persisting endoneurial sheaths, resulting in longitudinally continuous cell columns, the bands of Büngner.

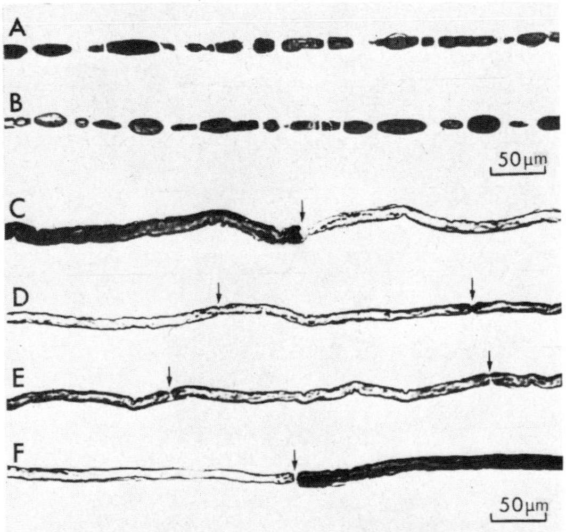

Fig. 18.14 Teased single fibres. A and B show wallerian degeneration with linear rows of osmiophilic droplets. C–F show remyelination after segmental demyelination; five short internodes with thin myelin are interposed between internodes with normal myelin. The position of the nodes of Ranvier is indicated by the arrows.

The details of the changes were illuminated by subsequent ultrastructural studies. The earliest axoplasmic changes are the accumulation of mitochondria, multivesicular bodies and lamellar osmiophilic bodies at nodes of Ranvier, especially on the distal side. This occurs after 12 hours in the region of the nerve 2–4 cm from the site of axonal interruption (Webster, 1962; Ballin and Thomas, 1969). By 24 hours, the axoplasmic reticulum breaks up into rows of vesicles. This is followed by the disappearance of the microtubules, fragmentation of the neurofilaments (Fig. 18.15) and swelling of the mitochondria (Schlaepfer and Micko, 1978), changes which become advanced by 48 hours (Vial, 1958; Honjin, Nakamura and Imura, 1959). Accumulations

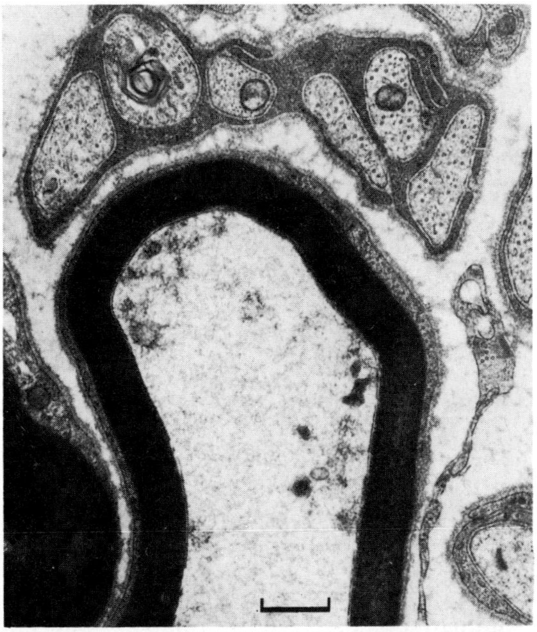

Fig. 18.15 Wallerian degeneration, 24 hours after nerve section. The myelinated fibre shows granular disintegration of the microtubules and neurofilaments which are still present in some of the unmyelinated axons. Bar = 1 μm.

of glycogen particles may occur. The axons become filled with clumps of granular debris.

The chemical changes which take place during wallerian degeneration have been reviewed by Gerstl and Eng (1981). The loss of proteins is correlated with increased neutral and acid proteinase activity (Hallpike, Adams and Bayliss, 1970) which may be related to calcium influx into the axons (Schlaepfer and Hasler, 1979).

By light microscopy, an early change seen in the myelin sheath is the development of an unduloid outline and a retraction from the nodes of Ranvier prior to its segmentation into ellipsoids. Webster (1965) showed that the incisures of Schmidt–Lanterman become more obvious because of an increase in the amount of Schwann cell cytoplasm which they contain. It was believed that their number increases, but this is simply because they enlarge and become more readily visible (Ghabriel and Allt, 1979a). Interruption of the myelin occurs immediately adjacent to the incisures (Ghabriel and Allt, 1979b), and the interrupted regions seal off at either end to form the ellipsoids. These contain axonal debris. This process takes place within the Schwann cell basal laminal tubes, proceeds more rapidly in the fibres of smaller diameter, and has occurred in all fibres within 3–4 days. Segmentation into increasingly shorter ellipsoids and finally spherical droplets follows, this again occurring at the Schmidt–Lanterman incisures. Some of these ellipsoids are situated within Schwann cell cytoplasm; others lie within the basal laminal tubes. At the nodes of Ranvier, the

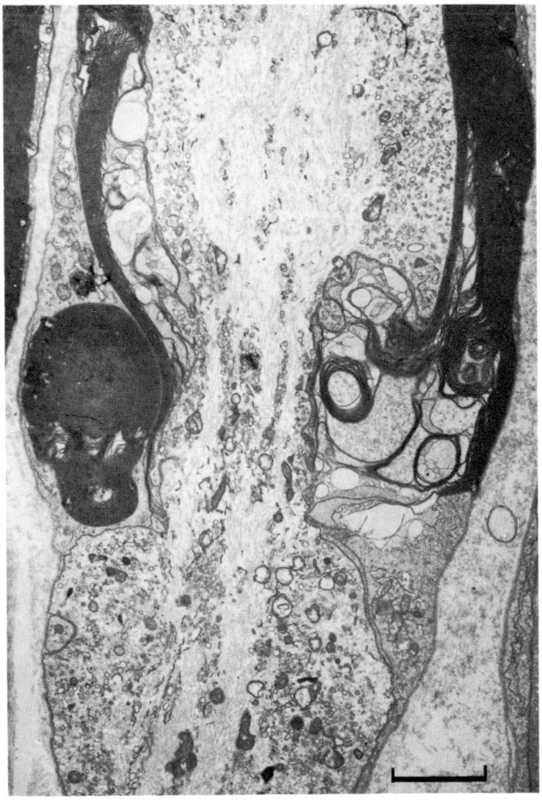

Fig. 18.16 Wallerian degeneration, 24 hours after nerve section. This longitudinal section shows myelin retraction from the node of Ranvier. The axon contains numerous peripherally situated vesicular structures, together with dense lamellar bodies and degenerating mitochondria. Bar = 2 μm.

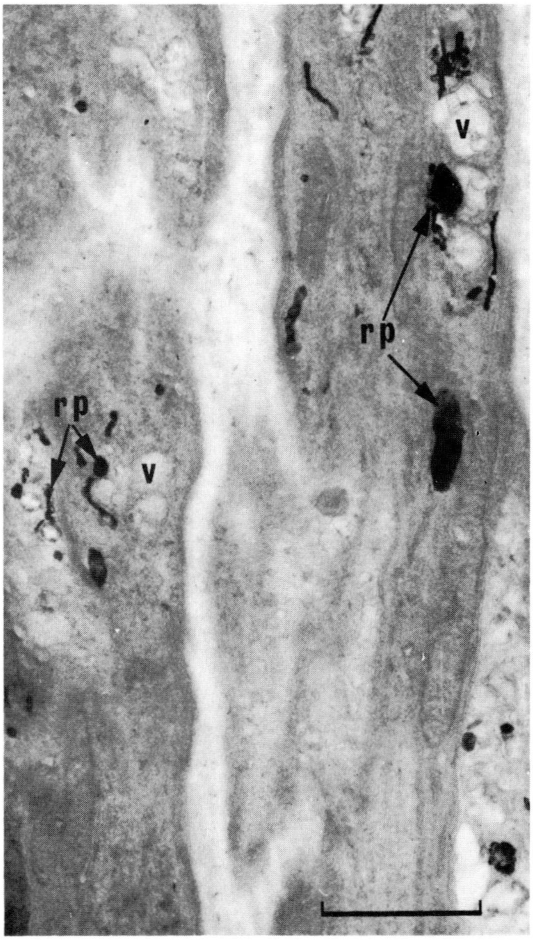

Fig. 18.17 Wallerian degeneration, 7 days after nerve section. Following Gomori incubation, reaction product (rp) for acid phosphatase is present in relation to vacuoles (v) derived from degenerating myelin within Schwann cell cytoplasm. Bar = 1 μm.

collar of Schwann cell cytoplasm sends out processes which separate from the axolemma the nodal processes and the terminal helical attachment of the myelin in the paranodal region (Ballin and Thomas, 1969). This leads to the retraction of the myelin from the node (Fig. 18.16). When interruption of the nodal axon occurs, the myelin seals itself off to form the ends of adjacent ellipsoids. Myelin breakdown occurs within Schwann cells by lysosomal activity (Fig. 18.17) (Holtzman and Novikoff, 1965), so these cells come to contain multiple vacuoles.

There has been little unanimity in the literature as to the longitudinal distribution of the changes during wallerian degeneration. Cajal (1928) considered that axonal breakdown occurs simultaneously throughout the length of the degenerating nerve, whereas Causey and Palmer (1953) and Lubińska (1982) reported a proximodistal gradient of change. Possibly the divergences of opinion are related to the criteria employed. Those who have used axonal changes as criteria—such as Cajal (1928), Donat and Wiśniewski (1973) and Malbouisson, Ghabriel and Allt (1984)—have found a simultaneous onset and evolution proximally and distally; those who have examined myelin and Schwann cell changes (Causey and Palmer, 1953; Lubińska, 1982) have found a proximodistal gradient. While myelin breakdown is taking place the Schwann cells proliferate within the basal laminal tubes, the extent of the proliferation being greater for nerves with a higher proportion of large myelinated fibres than in those with predominantly small fibres (Thomas, 1948). Myelin breakdown occurs within Schwann cells but the debris is transferred to vacuolated macrophages which appear within the endoneurium. They accumulate subperineurially and around small blood vessels and then disappear. Their origin is disputed. Possible sources are blood-borne monocytes, local tissue histiocytes

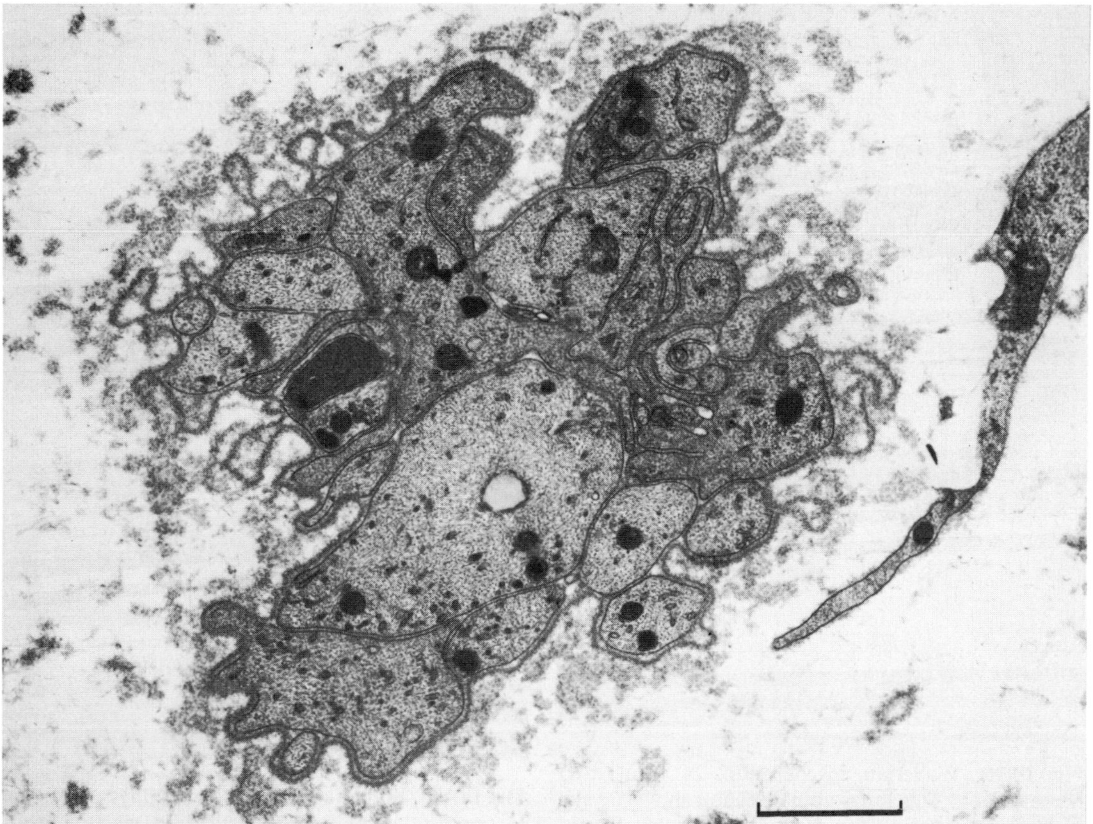

Fig.18.18 Late wallerian degeneration. Büngner band composed of multiple Schwann cell processes surrounded by a corrugated basal lamina. Bar = 1 μm.

or 'transformed' Schwann cells. The latter origin is unlikely (Gibson, 1979). After disappearance of the myelin debris, the Schwann cell basal laminal tubes persist and are filled with longitudinally continuous columns of tightly packed Schwann cells and their processes, constituting the bands of Büngner (Fig. 18.18). Collagen fibrils are deposited external to the persisting basal laminal tubes, at least in the region near the site of axonal interruption or nerve section (Thomas, 1964).

Degeneration of unmyelinated axons

Following nerve section, degeneration of unmyelinated axons proceeds rapidly. Within 24 hours, loss of microtubules and break-up of the endoplasmic reticulum occurs, followed by gradual disintegration of the neurofilaments (Fig. 18.19) and swelling of the mitochondria. The axons on both sides of the interruption react to transection by producing large club-shaped swellings filled with mitochondria, dense lamellar bodies and other organelles (Fig. 18.20). Most of the axons disappear within 2–3 days. The debris is removed

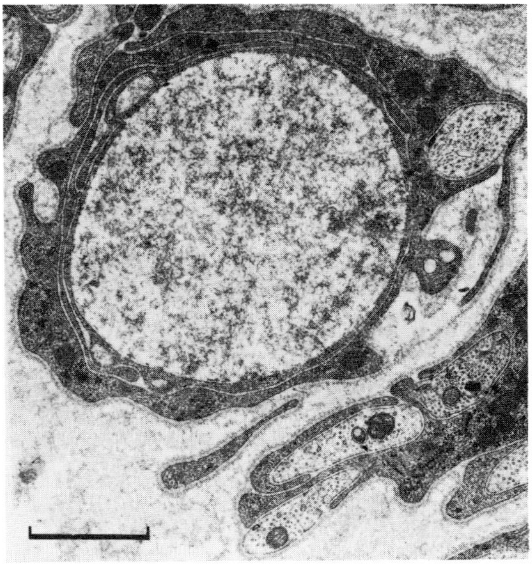

Fig. 18.19 Wallerian degeneration. Electron micrograph showing a degenerating unmyelinated axon 7 days after nerve section. The axon is filled with fine fibrillar material. Bar = 1 μm.

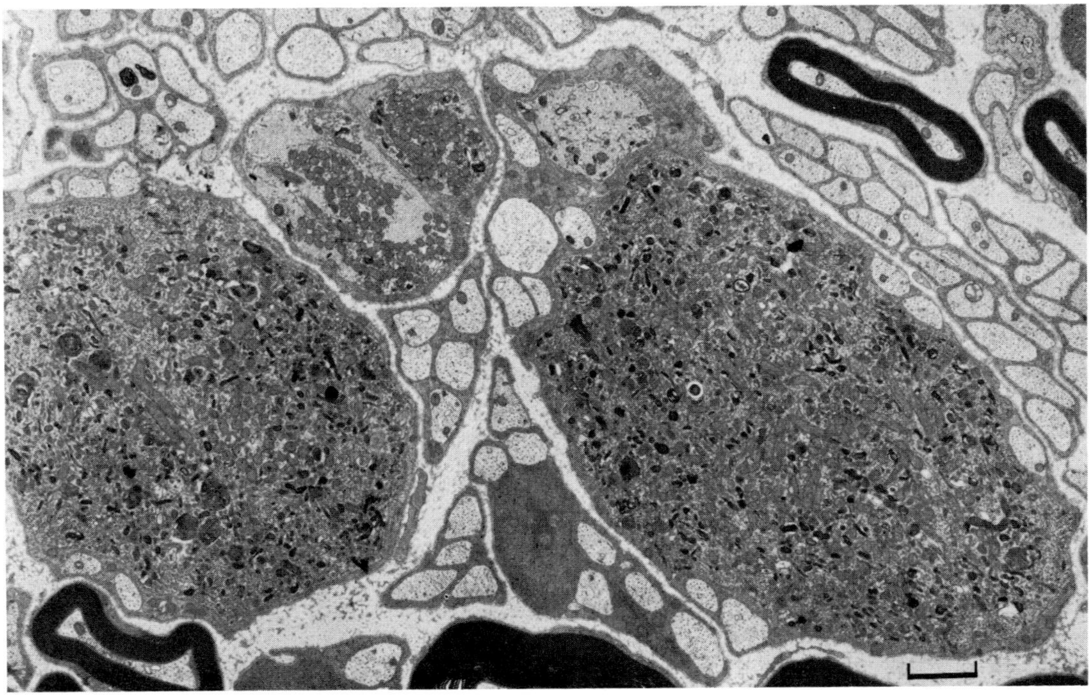

Fig. 18.20 Wallerian degeneration, 48 hours after nerve section. Club-like expansions of unmyelinated axons close to the site of transection are filled with numerous mitochondria, dense lamellar bodies and other organelles. Bar = 1 μm.

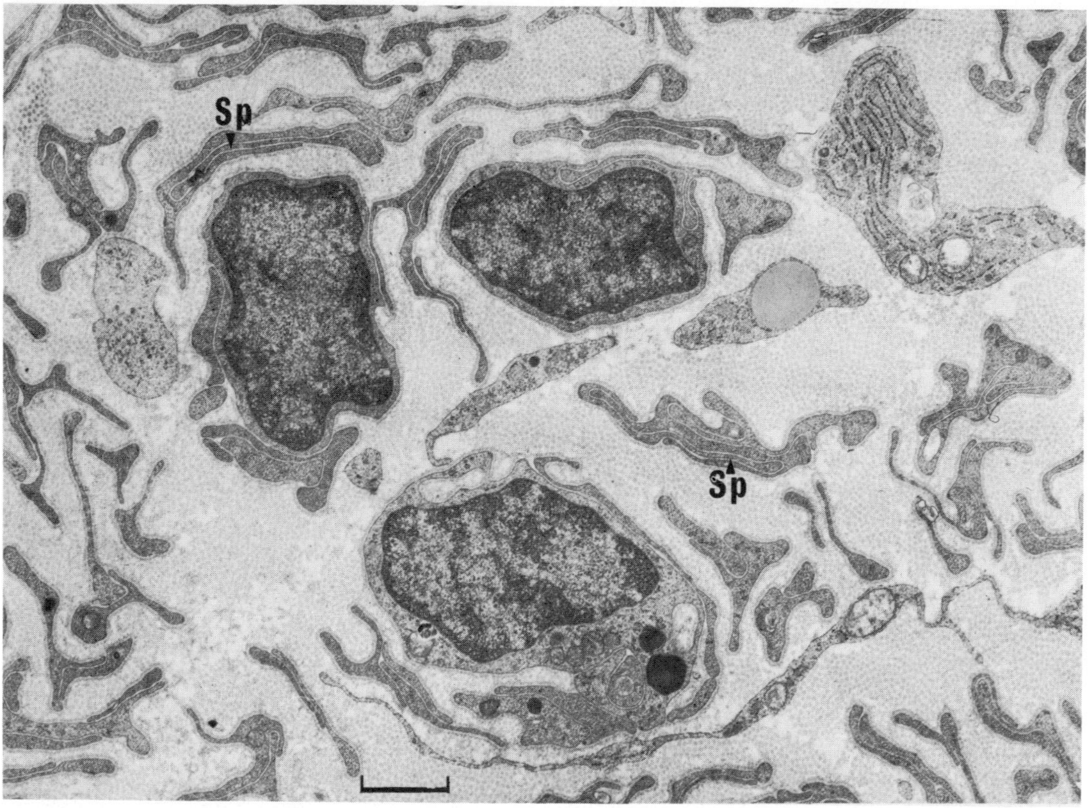

Fig. 18.21 Late wallerian degeneration showing groups of flattened cell processes (Sp) derived from Schwann cells previously associated with unmyelinated axons. Bar = 1 μm.

by Schwann cells and macrophages. Schwann cell proliferation occurs, but is less extensive than for myelinated fibres. The degenerating axons become encircled by overlapping Schwann cell processes. When the axons disappear, the Schwann cell processes come together to produce flattened stacks surrounded by a basal laminal ensheathment (Fig. 18.21). It is probable that longitudinally continuous columns, comparable to the bands of Büngner, do not develop.

Retrograde effects of axon section

Immediately following interruption, the axon retracts for a short distance to adopt a spiral configuration. The myelin sheath of the terminal internode breaks down either completely or in its distal part, depending upon the level of the injury in relation to the Schwann cell nucleus (Lubińska, 1961). Over the course of the ensuing 3 months, axon diameter decreases, this being associated with a relative increase in myelin thickness. If satisfactory regeneration takes place, axonal diameter recovers; should regeneration not occur, axonal atrophy progresses (Cragg and Thomas, 1961; Aitken and Thomas, 1962). Demyelination associated with such axonal atrophy is considered later.

Transection of proximal axons leads to chromatolysis ('axon reaction') in the neuronal perikaryon (see Chapter 1). Depending upon the type of lesion and the proximity to the cell body, neuronal death may ensue. This is more likely to happen the nearer the site of the axon transection is to the perikaryon.

Axonal regeneration

After axonal interruption, abortive sprouting occurs from the region of the cut end as early as 7 hours after injury (Duce and Keen, 1976), but definitive sprouts do not appear until 4 days after nerve transection (Duce and Keen, 1976) although they develop earlier after a nerve crush

(Haftek and Thomas, 1968). They are always accompanied by Schwann cells and arise either from the terminal axons or by collateral sprouting from nodes of Ranvier immediately proximal to the site of injury. The growth cones possess multiple finger-like processes ('microspikes') (O'Daly and Imaeda, 1967). After nerve transection, as many as 25 sprouts may arise from a single axon.

When a nerve is transected and only a short gap exists between the two cut ends, groups of regenerating axons and their associated Schwann cells cross the gap and become surrounded by cells with the morphological appearance of fibroblasts which assume the features of perineurial cells. A multicompartmental arrangement ensues. In the distal stump the axon sprouts enter the Büngner bands and are thence guided to the periphery. After nerve transection and suture, in chronic neuropathies with continuing axonal degeneration and regeneration and following repeated experimental crush injuries, each Büngner band comes to contain large numbers of myelinated and unmyelinated regenerating axons ('clusters') (Thomas, 1968). Satisfactory maturation of the regenerating fibres depends upon the establishment of appropriate connections (Aitken, Sharman and Young, 1947), although even if this is achieved fibre diameter is not fully restored. Axon sprouts which do not attain an appropriate peripheral connection probably ultimately disappear. Internodal length in regenerated unmyelinated fibres (in the adult) is uniformly short on fibres of all sizes, instead of displaying the normal positive correlation with fibre size (Vizoso and Young, 1948).

In the regeneration of unmyelinated nerves, large groups of regenerating axonal sprouts are observed within a basal laminal envelope, together with Schwann cell processes. With time, they become directly associated with the processes but, in experimental studies (Dyck and Hopkins, 1972), may remain in groups unassociated with Schwann cell processes, even as late as 3 months after nerve injury. In nerves with a mixed population of myelinated and unmyelinated axons, there is evidence that the regenerating unmyelinated axons preferentially become diverted so that they accompany regenerating myelinated axons (King and Thomas, 1971).

Other types of axonal degeneration

Distal axonopathy Many neuropathies related to toxic or metabolic causes are characterized by a distal axonal degeneration that, with advance of the disease process, spreads in a progressive manner towards the cell body. Such neuropathies have been characterized by Cavanagh (1964, 1979) as of 'dying-back' type. The phenomenon has been studied in greater detail by Spencer and Schaumburg (1976, 1977) in hexacarbon-induced neuropathy. This gives rise to multifocal preterminal intra-axonal neurofilamentous accumulations, initially observed on the proximal sides of nodes of Ranvier, distal to which axonal degeneration occurs. The process then spreads sequentially to more and more proximal nodes. For the primary sensory neurons, it was observed that degeneration also occurs in the centrally directed axons in the spinal cord. Thus in the dorsal columns, degeneration begins in the rostral portions of the gracile fasciculi and then advances caudally. The combined involvement of axons in the peripheral and central nervous systems was encapsulated in the term *central-peripheral distal axonopathy*. Neuropathies other than those which give rise to focal neurofilamentous accumulations, such as those related to triorthocresyl phosphate and isoniazid intoxication, also give rise to this pattern of degeneration.

Proximal axonopathy Other neuropathies in which focal neurofilamentous accumulations are a feature may initially exhibit these in proximal axons, below which axonal atrophy or degeneration may occur. Such proximal axonopathies have been most closely studied in the experimental model produced by intoxication with β,β'-iminodipriopionitrile (IDPN) (Clark, Griffin and Price, 1980).

Axonal sequestration In neuropathies in which there is a slowly evolving axonal degeneration, such as the distal and proximal axonopathies just described, prominent axon–Schwann cell networks develop, particularly in the paranodal regions (Fig. 18.22). These are related to the ingrowth of processes from the adaxonal Schwann cell which branch and enclose multiple small compartments of the axon (Fig. 18.23). Spencer and Thomas (1974) have suggested that this constitutes a mechanism for the sequestration and

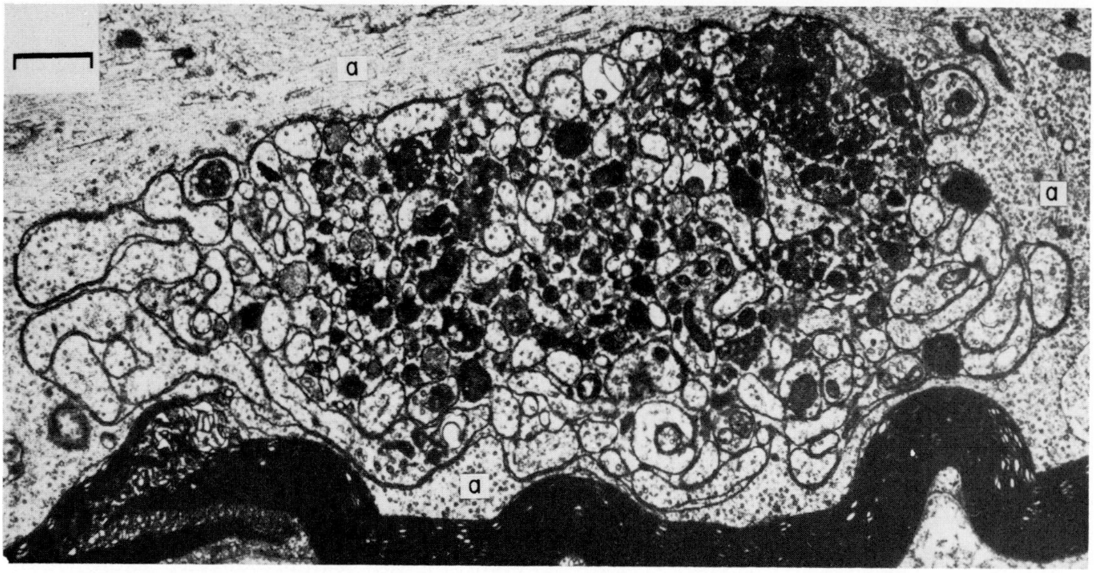

Fig. 18.22 Experimental methyl isobutyl ketone intoxication. Complex axon–Schwann cell network. Sequestered areas of axon (a) contain pleomorphic debris. (Reproduced, with permission, from Spencer and Thomas, 1974.) Bar = 1 μm.

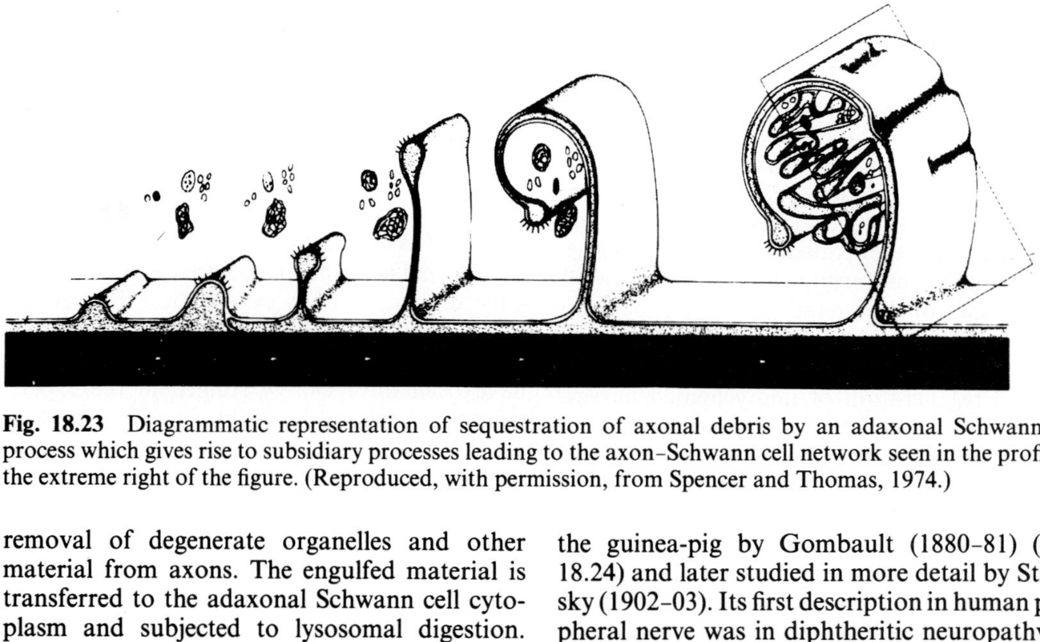

Fig. 18.23 Diagrammatic representation of sequestration of axonal debris by an adaxonal Schwann cell process which gives rise to subsidiary processes leading to the axon–Schwann cell network seen in the profile at the extreme right of the figure. (Reproduced, with permission, from Spencer and Thomas, 1974.)

removal of degenerate organelles and other material from axons. The engulfed material is transferred to the adaxonal Schwann cell cytoplasm and subjected to lysosomal digestion. Such appearances are seen in normal nerve but become much more evident in neuropathies.

Segmental demyelination

The process of segmental demyelination was first recognized in experimental lead neuropathy in the guinea-pig by Gombault (1880–81) (Fig. 18.24) and later studied in more detail by Stransky (1902–03). Its first description in human peripheral nerve was in diphtheritic neuropathy by Meyer (1881). Surprisingly it then received little attention from neuropathologists until about 25 years ago when the use of teased fibre studies to examine nerve was revived. Since then the process has been studied in detail, particularly in experimental diphtheritic neuropathy which produces a relatively pure demyelinating pathology

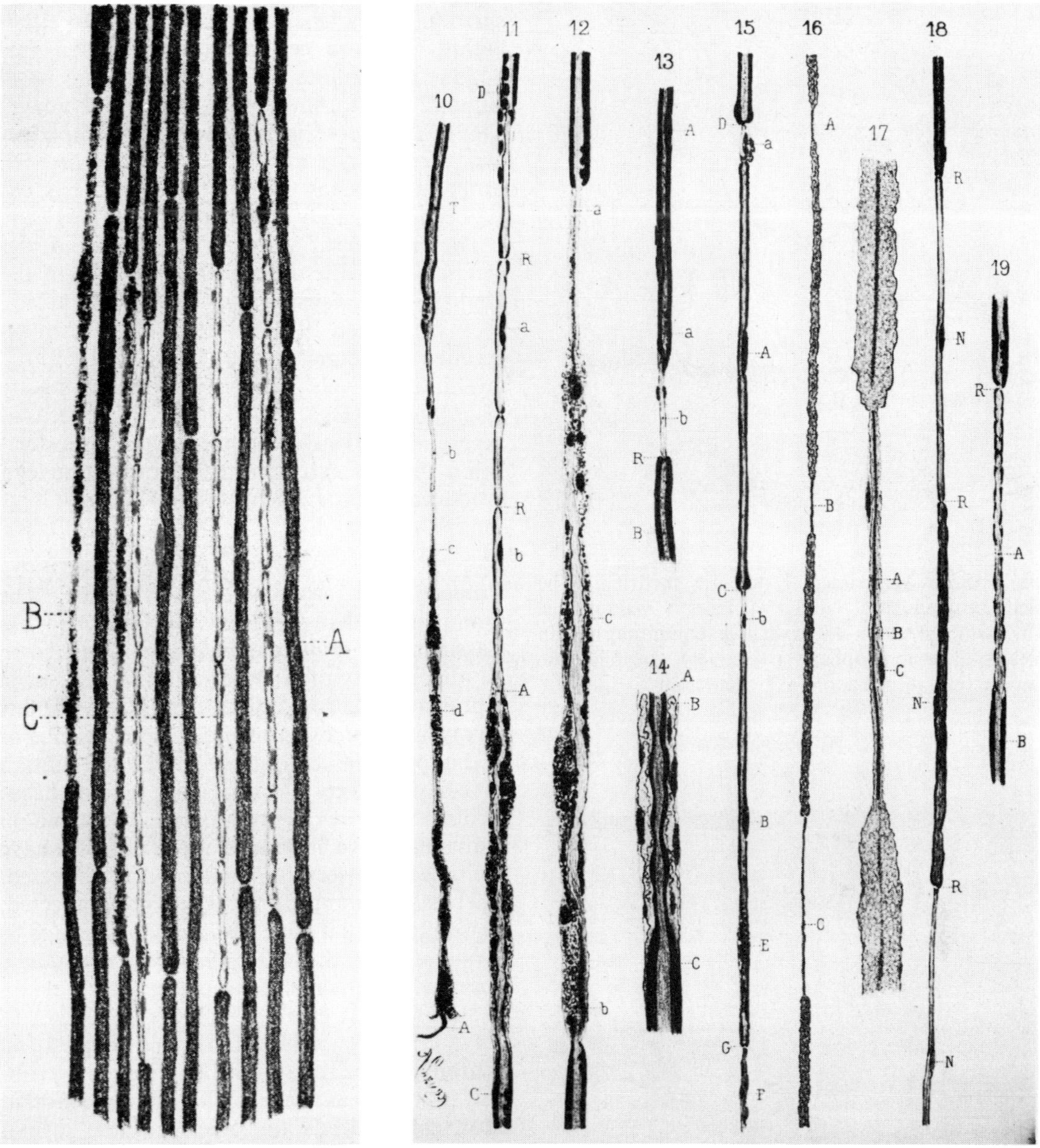

Fig. 18.24 Experimental lead neuropathy. Teased fibre preparations showing segmental demyelination and remyelination. Osmium tetroxide and picrocarmine. (From Gombault, 1880–81.)

with little axonal degeneration, in various other experimental neuropathies including experimental allergic neuritis and the intraneural injection of lysophosphatidyl choline (lysolecithin), and in numerous human disorders.

Primary segmental demyelination is a disturbance of Schwann cell function or of myelin itself. The appearances in experimental diphtheritic neuropathy (Webster et al., 1961; Cavanagh and Jacobs, 1964; Weller, 1965) can be taken as a model. The initial changes are observed at the nodes of Ranvier. The terminal helical cytoplasmic rim of the myelin separates from the axolemma and leads to myelin retraction and a widening of the nodal gap. The myelin then breaks down in the region of the node (paranodal demyelination) or the process extends to the whole of the internode, leaving a denuded axon

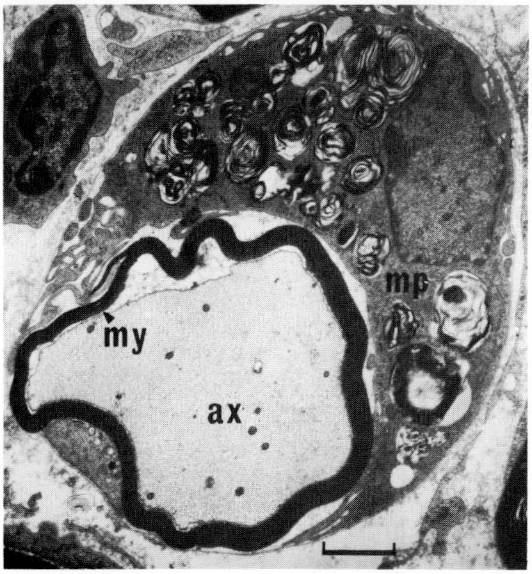

Fig. 18.25 Experimental allergic neuritis. The Schwann cell basal lamina encloses a macrophage (mp) which shows multiple vacuoles containing myelin debris. The macrophage is actively stripping the myelin (my) off the axon (ax). Bar = 2 μm.

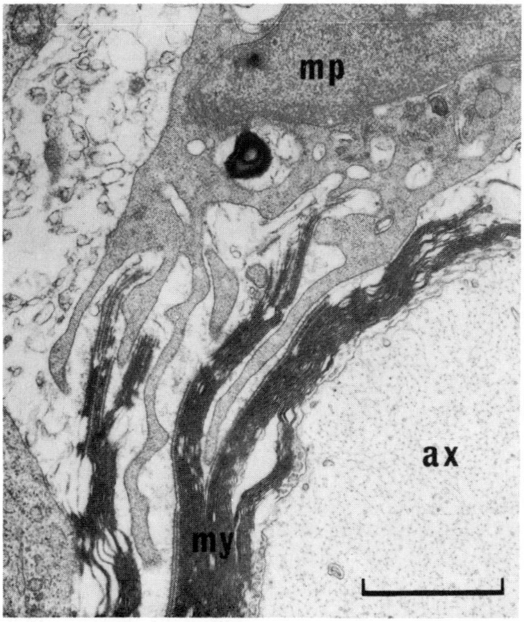

Fig. 18.26 Experimental allergic neuritis. Myelin (my) is being stripped off the axon (ax) by a macrophage (mp). Bar = 1 μm.

surrounded by small globules of myelin either within Schwann cell processes or lying free within the confines of the Schwann cell basal laminal ensheathment (Allt and Cavanagh, 1969). The nerve is invaded by macrophages which engulf the myelin debris. Schwann cell proliferation takes place, although this has not yet been adequately quantified.

The mechanism of demyelination varies, depending upon the disease process. Thus in the Guillain-Barré syndrome (Wiśniewski et al., 1969; Carpenter, 1972; Prineas, 1972) and in experimental allergic neuritis (Lampert, 1969) the myelin is actively stripped off the axons by macrophages (Figs. 18.25 and 18.26), whereas in experimental demyelination induced by lysolecithin there is extensive dissolution of myelin produced by its detergent action (Hall and Gregson, 1971).

Primary and secondary demyelination The examples of demyelination just described are classifiable as *primary demyelination*, related to an abnormality of Schwann cell function, as in diphtheritic neuropathy, or from a direct effect on myelin, as in experimental allergic neuritis or in that produced by lysolecithin. Demyelination of this type affects internodes on a random basis. In other instances, demyelination is clustered on individual nerve fibres so that one fibre will have multiple consecutive internodes affected, whereas neighbouring fibres remain unaffected. This suggests that the demyelination is related to axonal disease. Such *secondary demyelination* is observed in uraemic neuropathy (Dyck et al., 1971a; Thomas et al., 1971), and proximal to nerve crush (Lubińska, 1961) and amputation neuromas (Dyck et al., 1981a), where it is probably caused by axonal atrophy. The reduction in axon calibre leads to collapse of the myelin sheath, which becomes wrinkled and corrugated and then undergoes demyelination, initially paranodally and then of whole internodes (Fig. 18.27). Secondary demyelination is also observed in relation to the paranodal axonal swellings in giant axonal neuropathy (Spencer and Schaumburg, 1977), where the myelin becomes attenuated around the swellings.

Remyelination Remyelination after restricted paranodal demyelination may occur by extension of myelin from the neighbouring intact in-

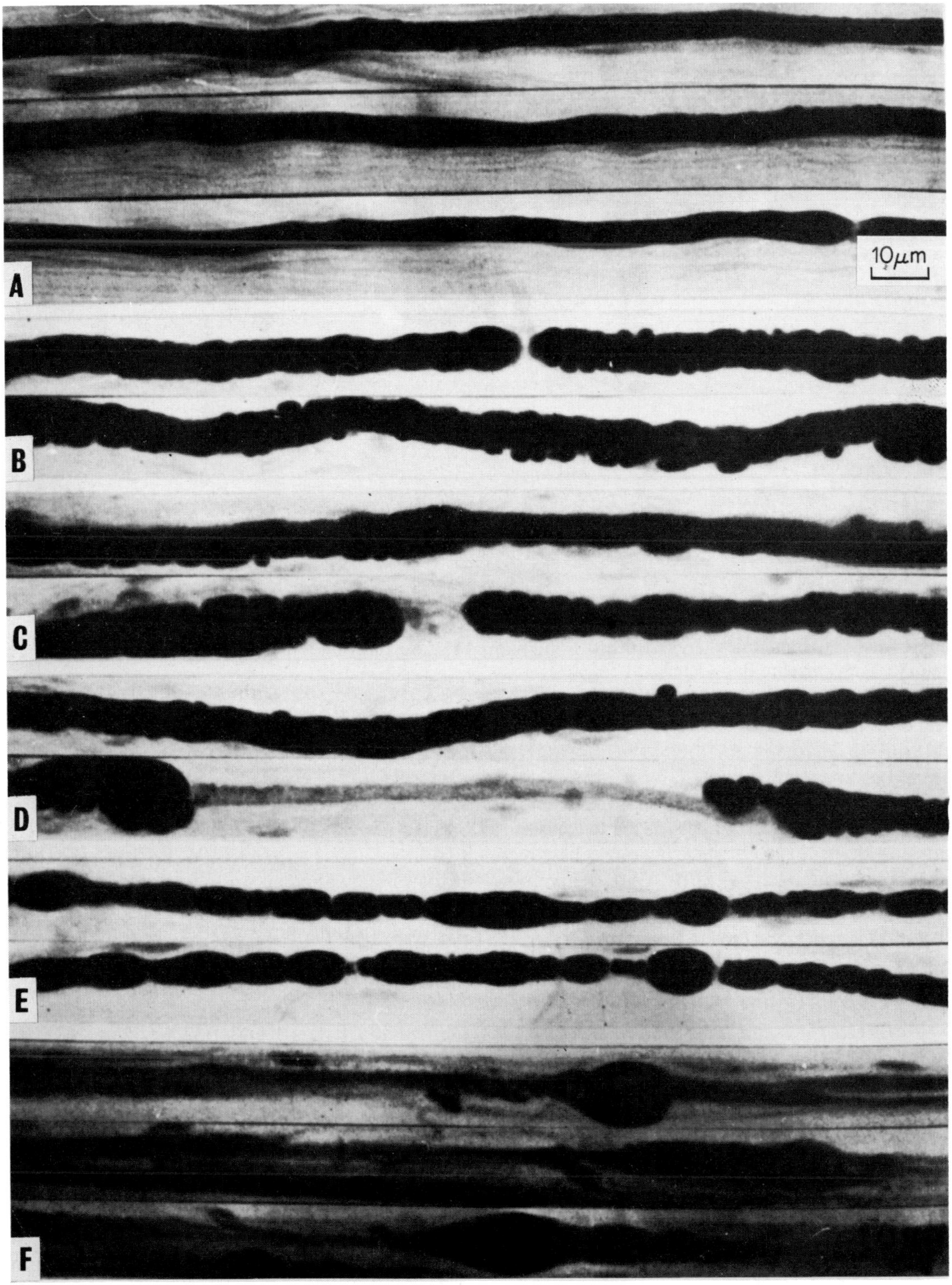

Fig. 18.27 Graded pathological abnormalities in teased fibres encountered in uraemic neuropathy ranging from normal appearances in A, through myelin corrugation in B, nodal widening and paranodal demyelination in C and D, to axonal degeneration and myelin breakdown in E and F. (Reproduced, with permission, from Dyck et al., 1981a.)

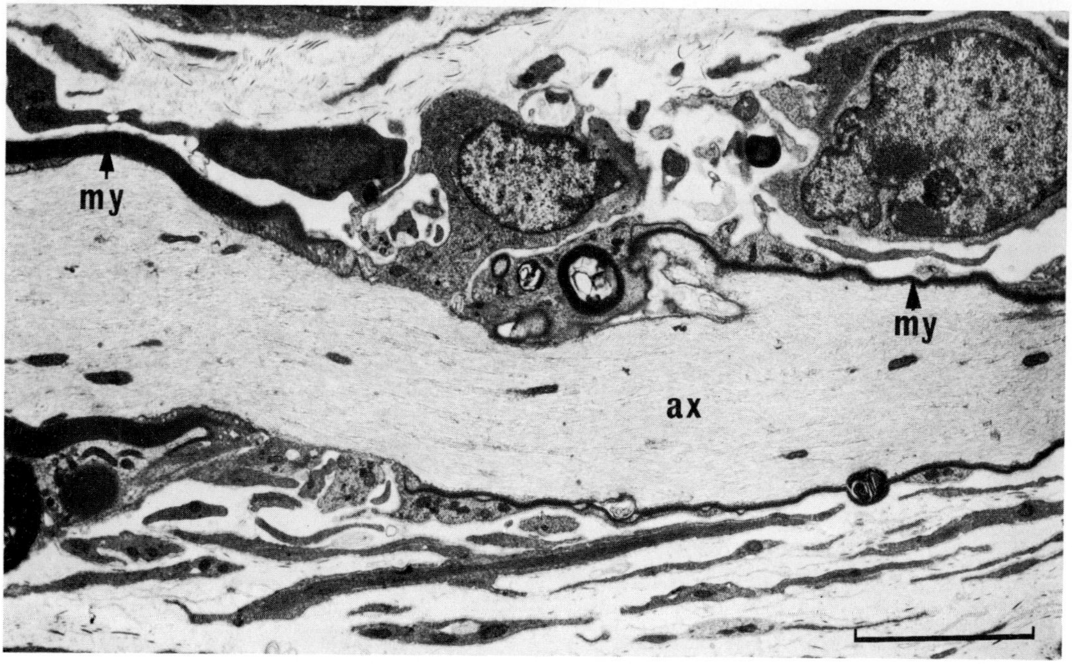

Fig. 18.28 Experimental allergic neuritis. Longitudinal section showing a thinly remyelinated portion of an axon (ax). my, myelin. Bar = 5 μm.

ternodes. Alternatively, Schwann cells may migrate into the denuded portion of the fibre and the axon becomes remyelinated by a single short 'intercalated segment'. The source of the Schwann cells is uncertain, as the evidence is that division does not occur in Schwann cells which are supporting myelin sheaths. With demyelination of whole internodal segments Schwann cell proliferation takes place and a number of Schwann cells migrate into demyelinated regions and give rise to several short internodal segments (Fig. 18.28 and see Fig. 18.14C–F).

Hypertrophic neuropathy

Concentric proliferation of Schwann cells around axons produces appearances that are perhaps the most striking amongst the repertoire of reactions encountered in peripheral nerve pathology. They have been likened to cross-sections through onions. Such 'onion bulb' formations (Fig. 18.29), originally recognized by Gombault and Mallet (1889), were considered to be a specific type of pathological reaction and became associated with the names of Dejerine and Sottas (1893) who described these appearances in a pair of siblings with an inherited peripheral neuropathy (see p. 879). It is now realized that hypertrophic neuropathy is the non-specific consequence of repeated demyelination and remyelination and that it is encountered in a wide range of inherited and acquired disorders (Thomas and Lascelles, 1967). Demyelination leads to Schwann cell proliferation; an excess of Schwann cells results and those which are not involved in remyelinating the axon accumulate around the fibre. Hypertrophic changes are usually observed in ongoing demyelinating neuropathies such as hereditary motor and sensory neuropathy (types I and III), Refsum's disease and chronic idiopathic inflammatory neuropathy. Hypertrophic changes have been produced in a variety of experimental demyelinating neuropathies, including lead neuropathy (Lampert and Schochet, 1968), recurrent compression (Dyck, 1969) and experimental allergic neuritis (Pollard, King and Thomas, 1975). Whether such changes are permanent once they have arisen is not established, and studies on Schwann cell kinetics in experimental neuropathies in which this type of change occurs would be of interest. After demyelination produced by the repeated inoculation of lysophosphatidyl choline, the supernumerary Schwann cells persisted

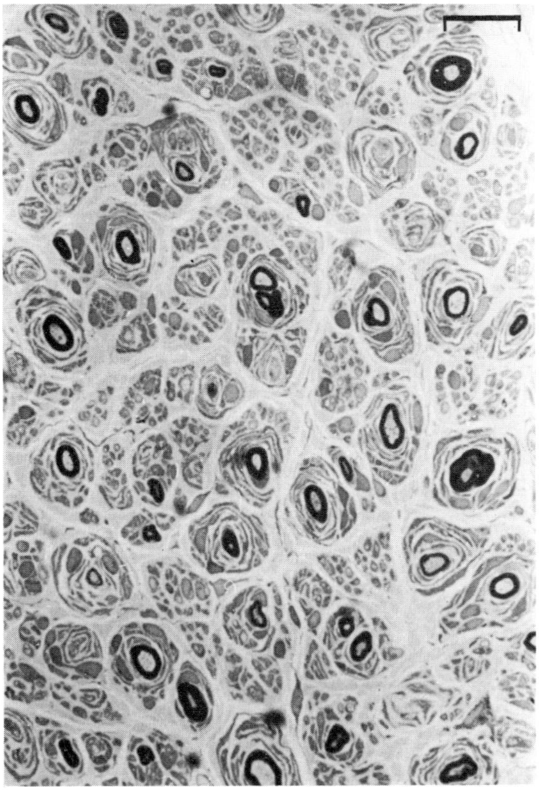

Fig. 18.29 Hypertrophic neuropathy. Transverse section through sural nerve from a case of type I hereditary motor and sensory neuropathy showing myelinated axons surrounded by concentrically proliferated Schwann cells. Semithin section; thionin and acridine orange. Bar = 20 μm.

only temporarily and hypertrophic changes did not develop (Hall, 1983).

Hypomyelination and hypermyelination

Under normal circumstances, myelin thickness is correlated with axon diameter (see p. 820). In certain neuropathies, myelin sheaths of appropriate thickness do not develop, the sheaths being thin on fibres of all diameters (Fig. 18.30). Such hypomyelination is a feature of hereditary motor and sensory neuropathy type III (Dyck et al., 1971b), congenital hypomyelination neuropathy (Guzzetta, Ferrière and Lyon 1982) and in the *Trembler* mouse mutant (Low, 1976a, b).

Other neuropathies are characterized by focal areas of hypermyelination, observed as sausage-shaped expansions of the myelin sheath (tomaculi) in teased fibre preparations. Electron

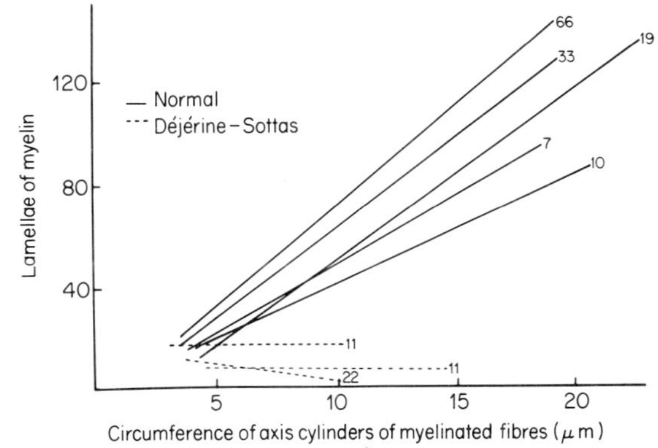

Fig. 18.30 Regression lines showing the relationship between the number of myelin lamellae and axon circumference for sural nerve of healthy subjects and Dejerine–Sottas disease. (Reproduced, with permission, from Dyck et al., 1971b.)

scopy demonstrates that these are due to abnormal numbers of myelin lamellae often related to folding and reversals in the direction of the myelin spiral (Fig. 18.31). Such appearances are non-specific but they are most characteristic of hereditary pressure-sensitive neuropathy (Behse et al., 1972; Madrid and Bradley, 1975; Meier and Moll, 1982); they are considered in greater detail on p. 883.

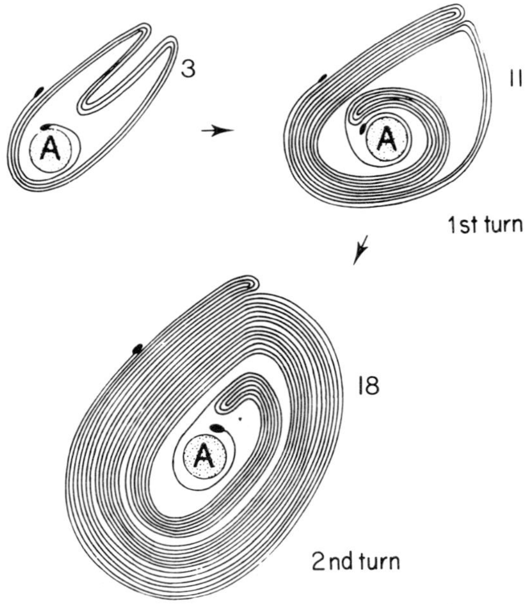

Fig. 18.31 Diagrammatic representation of mode of formation of redundant folds of myelin in tomaculous neuropathy. (Reproduced, with permission, from Madrid and Bradley, 1975.)

Pathological changes in specific neuropathies

Neuropathies due to nerve injury

Classifications of nerve injury

It has been recognized for more than a century (Mitchell, 1872; Erb, 1876) that localized mechanical injury to peripheral nerve can give rise to either temporary or persisting paralysis. It was also realized that the degree of damage at the site of injury has a profound influence on the quality of recovery. The two classifications that have mainly been advocated for the types of localized nerve injury that may be encountered are those of Seddon (1943) and Sunderland (1951). The term *neurapraxia* was introduced by Seddon to describe a localized conduction block with preservation of conduction distal to the lesion. Signs of denervation do not develop and full recovery takes place within 6–8 weeks, occurring more or less simultaneously throughout the whole territory of the nerve. *Axonotmesis* denotes the type of injury which causes axonal interruption but with preservation of the connective tissue framework of the nerve. Wallerian degeneration takes place distal to the lesion and signs of denervation develop. Recovery occurs by axonal regeneration, and as the endoneurial connective tissue framework is preserved the axons regain their former connection at the periphery. Recovery is therefore satisfactory, so long as regeneration distance is not too great. Evidence of reinnervation is initially detectable in the territory of the nerve closest to the site of injury. Finally, *neurotmesis* describes injuries in which the axons are interrupted but, in addition, the nerve is partially or completely transected. Recovery also has to take place by axonal regeneration but is never fully satisfactory because of misrouting of fibres at the site of injury.

Sunderland (1951) devised a more elaborate classification with subdivision into five degrees, the first two of which corresponded to neurapraxia and axonotmesis in Seddon's classification. The third to fifth degrees represented subdivisions of neurotmesis. Third degree injuries consist of rupture of endoneurial sheaths and intrafascicular haemorrhage, but with preservation of the fascicular architecture of the nerve. In fourth degree injuries perineurial rupture also occurs, but the epineurium remains intact. In fifth degree injuries, the epineurium is ruptured with loss of nerve continuity. The merit of this more elaborate subdivision is debatable. It is clear that crush injury and nerve injury related to penetrating wounds will not follow this pattern, and Haftek (1970) failed to confirm this temporal sequence in experimental stretch injury.

A classification which corresponds to currently available information is given in Table 18.1. The first category comprises lesions which do not give rise to severance of axons and which are due to a local conduction block. They are subdivisible into those which are purely transient and related to temporary ischaemia, and those which persist for days or weeks. The second category comprises lesions which interrupt axonal continuity, either with preservation of the Schwann cell basal laminal sheaths (axonotmesis) or with partial or complete severance of the neural connective tissues (neurotmesis). The underlying pathological changes are considered in more detail in the following section.

Table 18.1 Classification of focal mechanical nerve injury

Focal conduction block
Transient:
Ischaemic
Other
More persistent:
Demyelinating
Axonal constriction (?)
Axonal degeneration
With preservation of nerve fibre basal laminal sheaths
With partial nerve section
With complete nerve transection

Mechanical injury

Acute demyelinating conduction block Familiar examples of this type of lesion are 'Saturday-night paralysis' of the radial nerve and tourniquet paralysis, in which a focal conduction block related to an acute compression injury persists for several weeks. Direct confirmation of the pathological changes in man is not available but can be inferred from the results of animal ex-

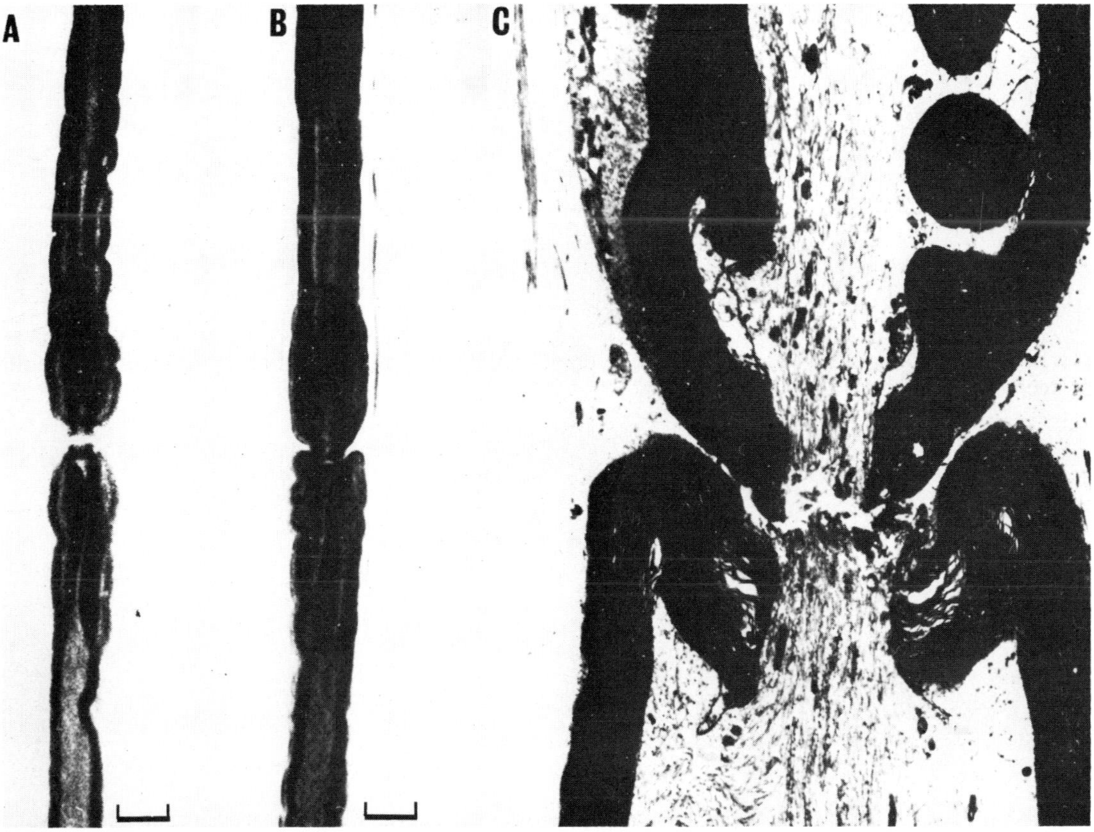

Fig. 18.32 Experimental tourniquet paralysis. In (A) is shown a normal node of Ranvier. Bar = 10 μm. In (B) there is a mild degree of invagination of the upper paranode into the lower, with obliteration of the nodal gap. Bar = 10 μm. (C) is an electron micrograph of the node illustrated in (B). (Reproduced, with permission, from Ochoa, Fowler and Gilliatt, 1972.)

periments. Studies in cats with pressure cuffs showed that conduction block is related to focal demyelination and that recovery is associated with remyelination (Denny-Brown and Brenner, 1944a). It was originally assumed that the demyelination is due to ischaemia, but subsequent studies in baboons (Ochoa, Fowler and Gilliatt, 1972) demonstrated that it is mechanical in origin and related to displacement of axoplasm to either side from under the compressed region. This is accompanied by outward dislocation of myelin internodes with invagination of their outer ends into the adjacent internodes (Figs. 18.32 and 18.33). This involves obliteration of the nodal gaps, the original position of the nodes of Ranvier being indicated by the persisting collars of Schwann cell nodal processes. Larger diameter fibres are preferentially affected. Presumably this is the result of the physical resistance

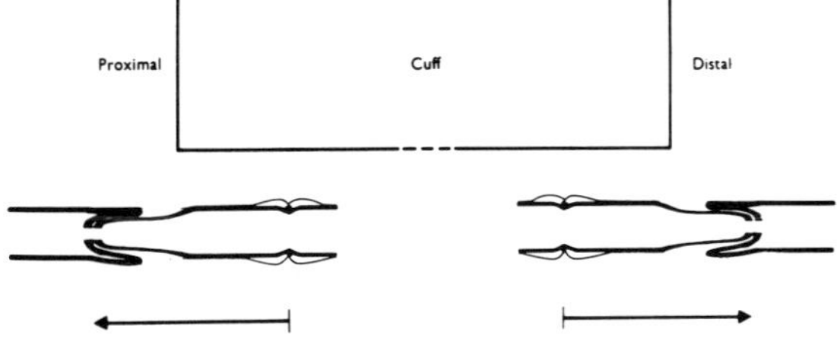

Fig. 18.33 Experimental tourniquet paralysis. Diagram showing direction of displacement of the nodes of Ranvier in relation to the compression cuff. There is an outward invagination at the nodes in both directions. (Reproduced, with permission, from Ochoa, Fowler and Gilliatt, 1972.)

offered by the axonal constriction at the nodes of larger fibres, although the narrower calibre of the axons of small fibres also might impede axoplasmic displacement. Demyelination occurs at

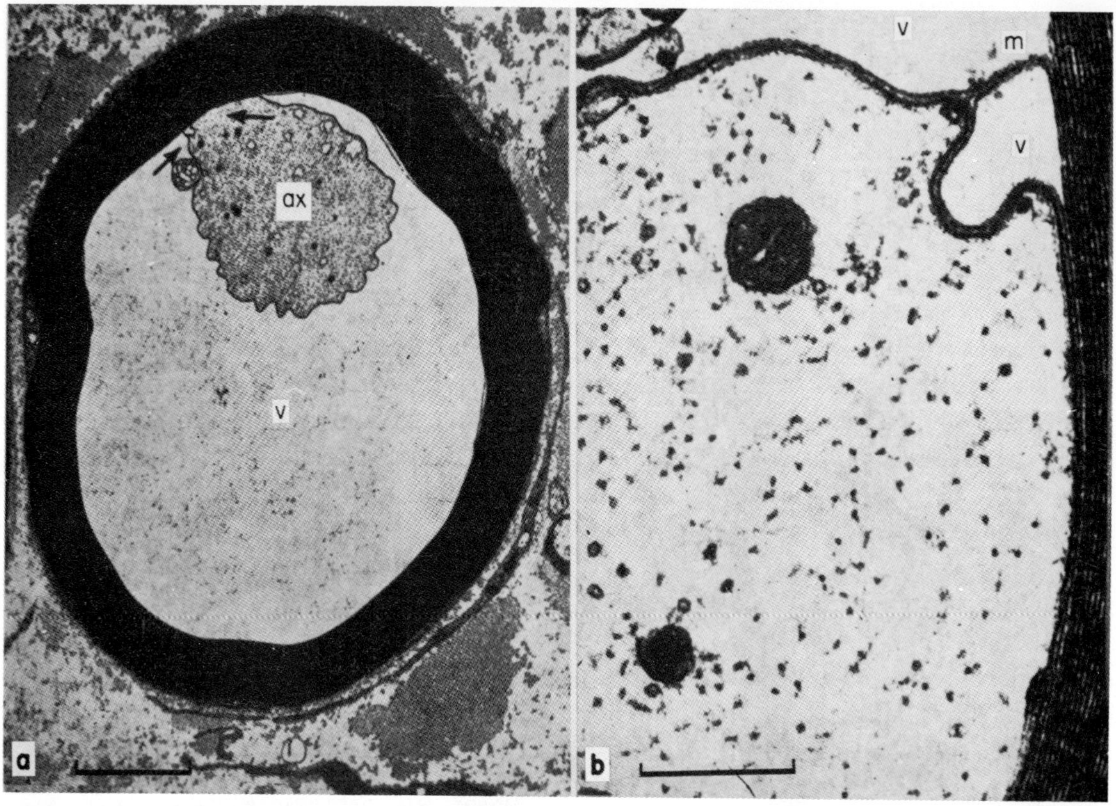

Fig. 18.34 Experimental tourniquet paralysis, 6 weeks after compression. (**a**) The swollen adaxonal Schwann cell process (v) separates most of the surface of the axon (ax) from the myelin sheath. Attached sector arrowed. Bar = 5 μm. (**b**) The mesaxon (m) is seen with swollen Schwann cell cytoplasm (v) to either side of it. Bar = 0.5 μm. (Reproduced, with permission, from Ochoa, Fowler and Gilliatt, 1972.)

the displaced nodes and recovery takes place by remyelination.

In occasional instances of conduction block in 'Saturday-night' radial nerve palsy, recovery is protracted, failing to begin before 7 weeks or to reach any substantial degree until 15–17 weeks after injury. The explanation is uncertain, as the experimental studies of Ochoa and colleagues did not suggest that demyelination is ever a persistent phenomenon. Possibly axonal constriction related to oedema of the adaxonal Schwann cell process could be the explanation. This may persist for long periods (Fig. 18.34).

Crush and percussion injury Again, direct information for man is not available. The usual animal model for focal compression injury has been squeezing the nerve with smooth-tipped forceps. Haftek and Thomas (1968) showed that the axons are interrupted within the Schwann cell basal laminal tubes which remain intact (Fig. 18.35). Axonal and myelin debris is displaced to either side but flows back into the region which was compressed. This region is quickly invaded by Schwann cells and crossed by regenerating axons within a few days. They are therefore guided back to their former peripheral connections by the surviving basal laminal tubes. Recovery is thus satisfactory, provided the regenerating distance is not too great.

No information is available for man as to the consequences of percussion injury to nerve sustained, for example, by a blow from a blunt object, compressing the nerve against underlying bony structures. Experimental studies have indicated a combination of segmental demyelination, periaxonal and intramyelinic oedema, and axonal interruption (Denny-Brown and Brenner, 1944b; Richardson and Thomas, 1979).

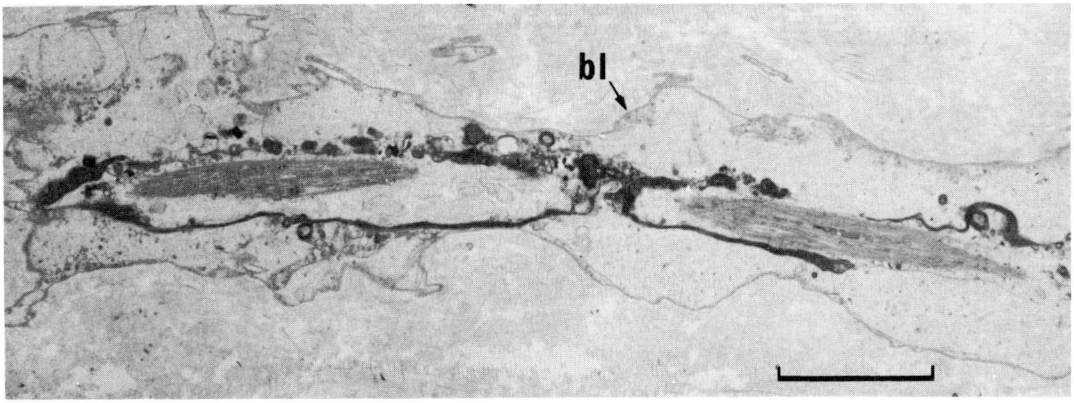

Fig. 18.35 Experimental crush injury. Longitudinal section through region of crush 1 hour after injury. The persisting basal lamina (bl) of a compressed fibre contains axonal and myelin debris. Bar = 5 μm.

Chronic nerve compression and entrapment In human entrapment neuropathies, the compressed region is narrowed and the nerve is expanded on the proximal side and, to a lesser extent, on the distal side of the constricted segment. The swelling is mainly the consequence of expansion of the intrafascicular area with only slight perineurial thickening (Neary and Eames, 1975). Numbers of Renaut bodies are often seen. Myelinated fibre size is diminished in the compressed region (Thomas and Fullerton, 1963) and evidence of axonal degeneration and regeneration may be present. Teased fibre studies have shown segmental demyelination and remyelination, together with paranodal bulbous swellings (Neary and Eames, 1975). The nature of this appearance was elucidated from observations on the naturally occurring compression of the median nerve in the carpal tunnel. Ochoa and Marotte (1973) found that the myelin segments were distorted, being tapered away from the compressed region and heaped up at the bulbous paranodal swellings at the further ends of the internodes, which assumed a tadpole-like configuration. More advanced distortion led to demyelination and axonal degeneration (Fig. 18.36). These changes have been confirmed in cases of subclinical entrapment of the median nerve at the wrist, the ulnar nerve at the elbow and the lateral cutaneous nerve of the thigh (Neary, Ochoa and Gilliatt, 1975; Jefferson and Eames, 1979).

Observations on the pathological effects of chronic or recurrent external pressure on nerves have not been made in man. Morton's neuroma is likely to be related to repeated compression injury, although the precise mechanisms involved are uncertain. A fusiform swelling develops at the region of bifurcation of a plantar interdigital nerve. Histologically there is epineurial, perineurial and endoneurial fibrosis with nerve fibre loss and proliferation of Schwann cells and fibroblasts. Deposits of mucopolysaccharide may be present and the accompanying plantar digital artery may be fibrosed or occluded (Lassmann, Lassmann and Stockinger, 1976; Asbury and Johnson, 1978).

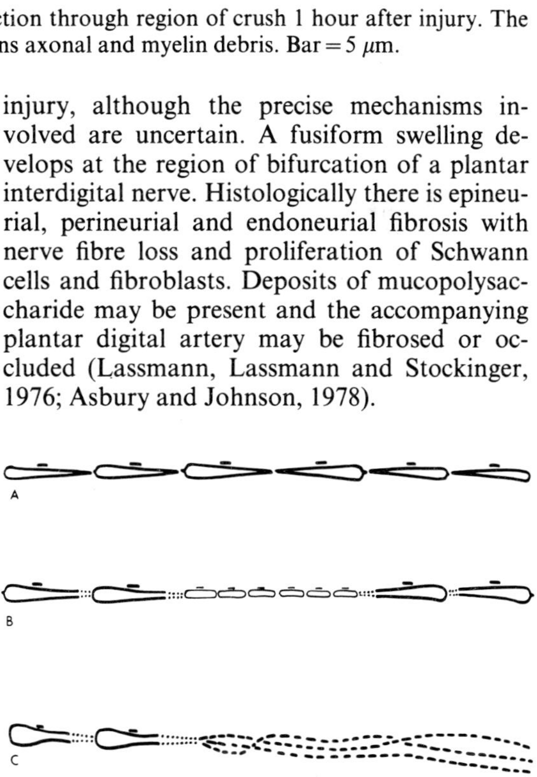

Fig. 18.36 Diagrammatic representation of entrapment neuropathy (median nerve of guinea-pig). (A) shows distorted myelin segments which reverse in direction on either side of the compressed region. In (B) demyelination and remyelination has taken place in the compressed region, together with paranodal demyelination in the distorted segments to either side. In (C) is shown an advanced stage in which axonal degeneration and regeneration have taken place. The surviving internodes proximal to the site of compression show massive bulbous expansions proximally and paranodal demyelination distally. (Reproduced, with permission, from Ochoa, 1980.)

Examples of focal 'hypertrophic neuropathy' have been documented affecting the posterior interosseous nerve of the forearm (Lallemand and Weller, 1973; Hawkes et al., 1974) and other nerves. These may be of traumatic origin (Ochoa and Neary, 1975).

Penetrating wounds Peripheral nerves may be partially or completely severed by incised wounds or lacerations. If the nerve is completely divided the cut ends draw apart. Outgrowths develop on both cut ends. That on the proximal stump, often referred to as a neuroma (Fig. 18.37), consists of groups of intertwined regenerating axon sprouts and associated Schwann cells, each surrounded by a perineurial ensheathment resulting in a multicompartmented arrangement. The outgrowth from the distal stump is composed of interlacing columns of Schwann cells, continuous with the Büngner bands in the distal stump, and associated connective tissue of endoneurial type (Thomas, 1966).

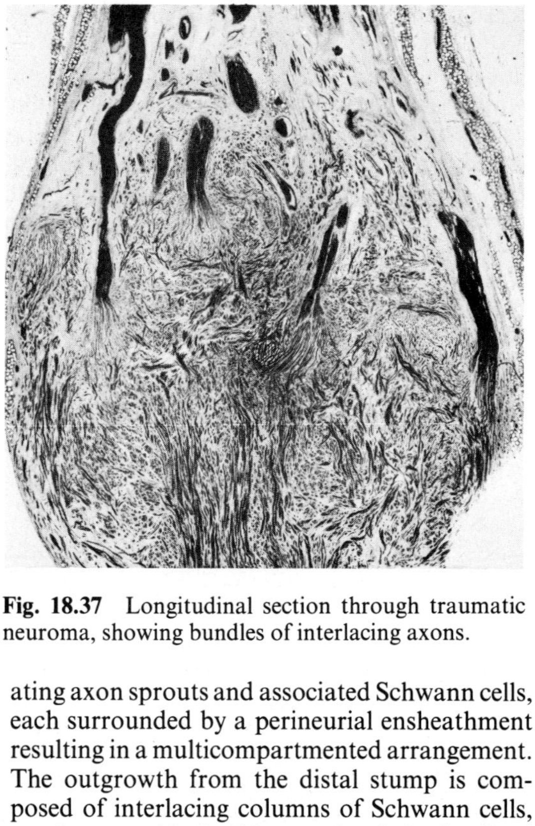

Fig. 18.37 Longitudinal section through traumatic neuroma, showing bundles of interlacing axons.

With partial severance, or following nerve suture, regenerating axons from the proximal stump are able to regain the peripheral stump and to invade the Schwann cell Büngner bands. Recovery is always unsatisfactory to a greater or lesser extent because of misrouting of fibres, leading to failure of reinnervation or aberrant reinnervation, although the extensive sprouting from the axons in the proximal stump will increase the chances of appropriate reconnection to peripheral sites. The various factors involved in the failure to achieve full recovery have been considered in detail by Sunderland (1978).

Stretch injury Traction injuries of the peripheral nerve trunks, limb girdle plexuses and spinal nerve roots occur in a variety of ways. The brachial plexus may be injured by forcible depression of the shoulder or traction on the arm. This can also result in avulsion of nerve roots from the spinal cord. In that eventuality, the motor axons in the peripheral nerves degenerate while the sensory axons remain because the lesion is central to the posterior root ganglia. Injuries to the lumbosacral plexus and lumbosacral roots are commonly associated with fractures of the pelvis. Avulsion of roots from the spinal cord does not occur. Stretch injury of peripheral nerves usually results from displacement secondary to fractures and joint dislocations, but may occur during operative or other surgical procedures. Except when nerves are directly involved, nerve injury from missile wounds results from displacement caused by rapid tissue expansion in the track of the missile.

Minor traction injury may simply produce a reversible conduction block (Seddon, 1975). The explanation of paralysis which recovers within a matter of hours is uncertain, as the time lapse is too short for demyelination and remyelination. More severe degrees of stretch injury tend to give rise to damage over considerable lengths of the nerve, with interruption of axons, disruption of the neural connective tissues and intraneural haemorrhage (Highet and Holmes, 1943). Extensive intraneural fibrosis may impede regeneration.

Cold injury

Freezing injury (frostbite) leads to necrosis of all tissues involved, including peripheral nerve. Non-freezing cold injury ('trench foot', 'immersion foot') occurs as the result of exposure to ambient temperature above $-2.5°C$ and usually below $10°C$ for several hours. The peripheral nerves are more vulnerable than other tissues (Blackwood, 1944). Sural nerve biopsy from a more recently studied case (Peyronnard, Pedneault and Aguayo, 1978) demonstrated myelinated fibre damage.

Experimental studies in animals on localized non-freezing cold injury have demonstrated focal conduction block and cessation of axonal transport in the acute stage with early recovery of function but followed by axonal degeneration, particularly of large myelinated fibres, after a few days (Basbaum, 1973; Nukada, Pollock and Allpress, 1981). The mechanism is uncertain. The blood–nerve barrier has been shown to become defective and extensive endoneurial oedema occurs. This is progressive, probably related to the absence of endoneurial lymphatics. If raised intraneural pressure secondary to the oedema is the mechanism of the fibre degeneration, this could explain the greater vulnerability of peripheral nerve.

Radiation neuropathy

Radiation neuropathy is uncommon but is most often observed in the brachial plexus following irradiation for the treatment of carcinoma of the breast. The lumbosacral plexus may also be affected. It tends to develop with a peak latency of 3–4 years after irradiation and never earlier than 6 months. The mechanism is unclear. Pathologically, fibre loss is demonstrable, in association with extensive fibrosis (see Thomas and Holdorff, 1984).

Experimental studies in animals were undertaken by Cavanagh (1968a, b). It is important that peripheral nerves are a non-mitotic tissue. After early development, Schwann cells do not multiply unless they are injured. Cell division is impaired by prior irradiation. This is a persisting defect which will lead to greater vulnerability of nerves to subsequent injury. Myelination is retarded (Love, 1983).

Neuropathies due to nutritional deficiency

Neuropathic beriberi

The common aetiology of the 'dry' and 'wet' forms of beriberi, originally considered to be separate conditions, was recognized about 150 years ago, and was established during the first decade of the present century as being the result of nutritional deficiency. The historical aspects of these developments have been comprehensively reviewed by Victor (1984). Peripheral nerve involvement consists of a distal symmetrical sensorimotor neuropathy, sometimes accompanied by pain, dysaesthesiae and cutaneous hyperaesthesia. The onset is insidious. Cranial nerve manifestations are rare, except for dysphonia from involvement of the vagus nerve.

As emphasized by Victor (1984), the classic account of the pathology in peripheral nerve made by Pekelharing and Winkler (1887) clearly demonstrated the salient neuropathological features. More recent contributions are those of Vedder (1938) and Takahashi and Nakamura (1976). The most constant changes were demonstrated in distal limb nerves and the vagus and phrenic nerves. Axonal degeneration and loss predominated distally. Segmental demyelination was observed more proximally and is therefore likely to be of the secondary variety. Chromatolysis in dorsal root ganglion and anterior horn cells was observed. Degeneration also occurs in the gracile columns in the spinal cord. The process is thus a central–peripheral distal axonopathy. A relative preservation of small myelinated and unmyelinated axons was observed in a nerve biopsy study by Ohnishi et al. (1980), who pointed out the occurrence of intraneural oedema.

It is likely that thiamine deficiency is implicated in the causation of neuropathic beriberi but it is uncertain whether this is the complete explanation. Coexistent additional vitamin deficiencies may contribute. Thiamine, as thiamine pyrophosphate (TPP), acts as a cofactor in the decarboxylation of α-ketoacids and the formation and degradation of α-ketols. TPP is involved in the former reaction of pyruvate to acetyl-CoA; this is catalysed by the pyruvate dehydrogenase complex. Its precise role in the metabolism of peripheral nerve is not clear. It has been difficult to produce neuropathy by experimental thiamine deficiency, but this was demonstrated by Swank (1940) and North and Sinclair (1956). In an ultrastructural study in the rat, Prineas (1970) reported the accumulation of flattened membrane-bound sacs and a depletion of neurofilaments and microtubules in the distal branches of peripheral axons and in the centrally directed axons of the primary sensory neurons.

Neuropathy related to pyridoxine deficiency is discussed later (p. 859). A deficiency of pantothenic acid, a constituent of coenzyme A, has also been implicated as a cause of neuropathy but requires confirmation. Bean, Hodges and Daum (1955) reported that a sensory neuropathy developed in human volunteers on a diet deficient in pantothenic acid and peripheral nerve degeneration was found by Follis and Wintrobe (1945) in pantothenic acid-deficient pigs.

Pellagra

Pellagra comprises a combination of cutaneous lesions, gastrointestinal disturbances and manifestations affecting the nervous system. The last comprise behavioural changes and dementia, spinal cord involvement and variable peripheral neuropathy. Some authors have maintained that peripheral nerve involvement, although mild, is relatively frequent (Lewy, Spies and Aring, 1940); others have found it to be rare (Spillane, 1947). The clinical features resemble those of beriberi (Aring et al., 1941). Pathological studies on peripheral nerve are sparse, but fibre degeneration and loss have been documented (Wilson, 1913–14; Aring et al., 1941). Pellagra is considered to be due to a deficiency of nicotinic acid (niacin) and its precursor, tryptophan, but it is not established that nicotinic acid deficiency results in neuropathy.

Victor (1984) has argued that a syndrome of amblyopia, orogenital dermatitis and painful neuropathy is distinct from pellagra (Strachan's syndrome). Fisher (1955) studied the neuropathological changes and concluded that degeneration in the rostral portion of the gracile fasciculi predominated over changes in peripheral nerve, but extensive studies of this syndrome have not been undertaken.

Alcoholic neuropathy

The recognition and early descriptions of alcoholic neuropathy have been reviewed by Victor (1984). It occurs in a context of chronic and usually severe alcohol abuse, develops insidiously, and consists of a distal symmetrical sensorimotor neuropathy which may be painful. Bilateral footdrop and later weakness of the small hand muscles and finger extensors ensue. Weakness of the anterior thigh muscles may be prominent. Dysphonia from vagal involvement sometimes occurs, as do autonomic symptoms, although the latter are uncommon apart from distal anhidrosis in the legs. The sensory loss affects all modalities and may be associated with prominent hyperaesthesia of the soles of the feet and tenderness of the calf muscles.

Denny-Brown (1958) believed segmental demyelination to be the primary lesion in the peripheral nerves and it was found with some frequency by Bischoff (1971), together with axonal degeneration. Subsequent studies have made it clear that the major effect is a distal axonal degeneration (Walsh and McLeod, 1970; Behse and Buchthal, 1977; Said and Landrieu, 1978).

The close clinical and pathological similarities of alcoholic neuropathy to beriberi and the constant association with a defective nutritional status (Victor, 1984) have led to the view that alcoholic neuropathy is the result of B vitamin deficiency and not to a direct toxic effect of alcohol. A contribution from the latter is nevertheless not excluded (Behse and Buchthal, 1977), but a clear demonstration of this has not been made, nor is a satisfactory animal model of alcoholic neuropathy currently available.

Vitamin B_{12} deficiency

A symmetrical sensory polyneuropathy may result from a deficiency of vitamin B_{12}, from whatever cause, which may or may not be associated with a myelopathy ('subacute combined degeneration of the cord'). Although the neuropathology of the myelopathy has been examined in some detail (Chapter 13), this is not true of the neuropathy. Few studies by contemporary techniques have been published. No autopsy report is available in which the peripheral nervous system has been examined in its full extent. In a biopsy study from the anterior tibial nerve, Carmichael and Greenfield (1935) recorded loss of myelin sheaths but no loss of axons. Coërs and Woolf (1959) described changes in the terminal innervation of muscle. There are earlier autopsy descriptions of degenerative changes in a variety of nerves; others have failed to find changes, despite the presence of neurological symptoms (see Victor, 1984). Electrophysiological studies indicate that the central processes of the primary sensory neurons are more vulnerable than peripheral sensory axons (Fine and Hallett, 1980).

Recent experimental studies (Scott et al., 1981) suggest that the neurological deficit resulting from vitamin B_{12} deficiency is due to a deficiency of methyl groups related to inadequate methionine and S-adenosyl methionine synthesis. Prolonged exposure of monkeys to nitrous oxide inactivates methylcobalamin and leads to the development of subacute combined degeneration of the cord. This can be prevented by oral methionine supplements.

Vitamin E deficiency

A spinocerebellar degeneration and a sensory neuropathy may develop in relation to chronic intestinal fat absorption. This has been described for children with congenital biliary atresia and fibrocystic disease (Rosenblum et al., 1981) and in adults with chronic malabsorption (Harding et al., 1982). There is now good evidence that it is related to vitamin E deficiency (Muller, Lloyd and Wolff, 1983). The neurological syndrome associated with abetalipoproteinaemia is likely to have the same basis and can be improved or prevented by vitamin E supplementation. No studies on the peripheral nerves in man are yet available. Observations in monkeys (Nelson et al., 1981) and rats (Towfighi, 1981) indicate that this is a central–peripheral distal axonopathy.

Toxic neuropathies

Neuropathies due to environmental agents

Acrylamide This compound is important as a flocculator and grouting agent, employing catalytic polymerization of the monomer, which is neurotoxic. The polymer is non-toxic. Most examples of neuropathy have been related to industrial exposure by skin contact. It is characterized by distal sensorimotor changes with accompanying limb ataxia. Sural nerve biopsy during the recovery stage has shown loss of myelinated nerve fibres of large diameter (Fullerton, 1969). Extensive experimental studies have been undertaken in animals (Fullerton and Barnes, 1966; Spencer and Schaumburg, 1974), which have established that acrylamide gives rise to a central–peripheral distal axonopathy. This preferentially affects both the longer and the larger myelinated fibres in the peripheral nerves and in central long tracts. With more advanced disease, progressively shorter and thinner myelinated fibres are affected. Unmyelinated fibres are involved only with severe intoxication. The earliest detectable change is the multifocal occurrence of paranodal neurofilamentous accumulations, distal to which axonal degeneration takes place. As with other distal axonopathies of this pattern, the process spreads to progressively more proximal internodes. Regeneration may occur despite continued administration of acrylamide. The mechanism of nerve damage is not understood, but it is discussed below in relation to hexacarbon neurotoxicity.

Carbon disulphide This agent is used in the manufacture of viscose rayon fibres and cellophane films. Prolonged low-level atmospheric exposure gives rise to a peripheral neuropathy. Satisfactory observations on the pathological changes in man are not available. Experimental studies in animals have demonstrated the occurrence of a central–peripheral distal axonopathy with focal neurofilamentous accumulations of the type described for acrylamide intoxication (Seppäläinen and Haltia, 1980).

Carbon monoxide Focal peripheral lesions following coma related to carbon monoxide intoxication are probably due to compression, possibly complicated by hypoxia. Symmetrical neuropathies have been described, the explanation for which is uncertain. An experimental study has shown axonal and paranodal myelin changes (Grunnet and Petajan, 1976).

Dimethylaminopropionitrile (DMAPN) Workers exposed to this substance, which is used as a catalyst in the manufacture of polyurethane foam, have developed a distinctive distal sensory neuropathy in the legs with, additionally, sensory symptoms in the lower sacral dermatomes, bladder dysfunction and impotence. Sural nerve biopsy has shown loss of both myelinated and unmyelinated fibres with nonspecific axonal changes (Pestronk, Keogh and Griffin, 1979).

Hexacarbons *n*-Hexane has been widely used as a solvent in glues and methyl *n*-butyl ketone (M*n*BK) in the manufacture of PVC. Both are metabolized to 2,5-hexanedione (2,5-HD), which is their major neurotoxic product. *n*-Hexane neurotoxicity has been encountered in the shoe manufacturing industry and as the result of solvent abuse (glue-sniffing) and M*n*BK neurotoxicity in factory workers engaged in the manufacture of PVC. In affected individuals, a slowly progressive distal sensorimotor neuropathy has developed. An interesting clinical feature is the phenomenon of 'coasting', that is, the continued progression of the neuropathy for up to 4 months after withdrawal from exposure.

Nerve biopsies from patients have shown loss of larger myelinated fibres. Surviving fibres have displayed 'giant axonal' changes, with focal en-

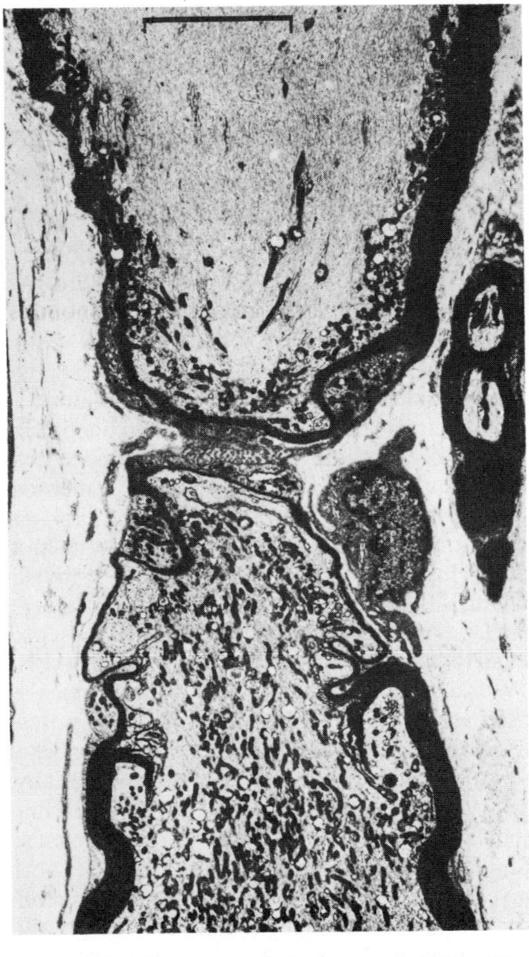

Fig. 18.38 Hexacarbon-induced neuropathy. The proximal paranode (upper) is enlarged and contains an accumulation of neurofilaments. The distal paranode (lower) contains multiple mitochondria. (Reproduced, with permission, from Spencer and Schaumburg, 1978.) Bar = 5 μm.

largements containing 10 nm neurofilaments associated with localized thinning of the myelin sheath (Korobkin et al., 1975; Altenkirch et al., 1977; Rizzuto, Terzian and Galiazzo-Rizzuto, 1977). Giant axonal changes have also been noted in the fasciculus gracilis at post-mortem in a fatal case (Schaumburg and Spencer, 1984). The appearances duplicate those which have been found experimentally (Fig. 18.38) where, as for acrylamide and carbon disulphide, a distal multifocal giant axonal neuropathy is produced which initially affects the preterminal portions of the larger and longer myelinated fibres (Schaumburg and Spencer, 1984).

The mechanism by which *n*-hexane and M*n*BK and their metabolite 2,5-HD produce their effect is not understood. It has been suggested that this could be through interference with glycolysis by inhibition of the enzyme glyceraldehyde-3-phosphate dehydrogenase, as it is also inhibited by acrylamide and carbon disulphide (Spencer et al., 1979). An alternative suggestion has been abnormal cross-linking between axonal neurofilaments (Graham et al., 1982).

Metals Peripheral neuropathy is the main neurological fcaturc of intoxication with inorganic *arsenic*, currently most often encountered as a consequence of attempted suicide or homicide. Arsenic is present in indigenous medicines in some parts of the world, and exposure from the accidental contamination of beverages has led to outbreaks. Neuropathy may develop acutely after a massive intake or gradually after chronic low dose or repeated exposure. Gastrointestinal disturbances develop after acute intake. An additional effect of chronic administration is cutaneous pigmentation and hyperkeratosis. In both, a distal, predominantly sensory, neuropathy develops, sometimes accompanied by severe painful dysaesthesiae. The pathological changes are not well characterized. Axonal degeneration has been demonstrated in biopsies from cases with acute exposure and from chronic cases (Dyck et al., 1968; Ohta, 1970). Le Quesne and McLeod (1977) have shown loss of myelinated fibres of all sizes with sparing of unmyelinated axons and little segmental demyelination. An autopsy study revealed loss of anterior horn cells (Erlicki and Rybalkin, 1892). A major histochemical effect of arsenic is to bind with sulphydryl groups. This may lead to interference with pyruvate dehydrogenase activity through conversion of the cofactor lipoic acid, which contains a dithiol group, to lipoate arsenate. The conversion of pyruvate to acetyl-CoA is thus inhibited (Schoental and Cavanagh, 1977; Politis, Schaumburg and Spencer, 1980). The effect of arsenic may thus be similar to that of thiamine, as thiamine pyrophosphate is also a cofactor for pyruvate dehydrogenase.

Lead neuropathy is now rare and usually occurs in adults rather than children, in whom lead intoxication is more likely to lead to encephalopathy. The typical clinical picture is of a predominantly motor neuropathy which affects the upper limbs to a greater extent than the lower, resulting in weakness and atrophy of the wrist and finger extensor muscles, and to footdrop. Sources of intoxication include industrial exposure, lead drinking-water pipes and lead-containing paints. Although the original demonstration of experimental segmental demyelination by Gombault (1880–81) was in lead-intoxicated guinea-pigs, the observations that have been performed on lead neuropathy in man (reviewed by Windebank, McCall and Dyck, 1984) have shown mainly axonal degeneration. A study on industrial workers subjected to chronic low-level exposure, however, revealed predominantly paranodal demyelination and internodal remyelination (Buchthal and Behse, 1979). Experimental studies in recent years have shown species differences in the proportion of demyelination and axonal degeneration which occurs, and have demonstrated that endoneurial oedema may be a prominent finding (Fullerton, 1966; Ohnishi et al., 1977; Myers et al., 1980). The precise cellular effects of lead are not understood, but an interference with mitochondrial function has been proposed (Walton and Buckley, 1977).

The major neurotoxic effects both of organic *mercury* (usually methyl mercury) and inorganic mercury salts are on the central nervous system (see Chapter 14), but a sensory neuropathy may occur. In cases of methyl mercury intoxication, loss of axons in peripheral nerves has been demonstrated (Takeuchi and Eto, 1977) and, from animal experiments, the primary site of the lesion appears to be the dorsal root ganglia (Jacobs, Carmichael and Cavanagh, 1975). Mercury may interfere with cellular function by binding with sulphydryl groups (Windebank, McCall and Dyck, 1984).

Thallium intoxication is currently most often encountered following administration with homicidal intent. A predominantly sensory and often painful distal polyneuropathy occurs, later followed by distal motor involvement. Gastro-intestinal disturbances are produced after acute ingestion, and if large amounts are given, mental confusion, coma and seizures occur. Alopecia is a characteristic feature, but it does not develop until 2–4 weeks after intake.

Studies on autopsied cases have shown distal axonal degeneration in the peripheral nerves with chromatolytic changes in anterior horn cells (Cavanagh et al., 1974). From observations on animals, the earliest change is the occurrence of large intra-axonal vacuoles, first seen in the region of the nodes of Ranvier. These may represent ballooned mitochondria. This may occur because of the binding of thallium with mitochondrial thiol groups (Goldstein, McCall and Dyck, 1975).

Neuropathy related to *gold* is considered below.

Organophosphorus esters Most examples of peripheral neuropathy caused by organophosphates have been attributable to contamination of food or beverages by triorthocresyl phosphate (TOCP) which is used both as a high temperature lubricant and as a softener in the manufacture of plastics. Absorption through the skin may also be responsible. After a latent interval of 1–3 weeks following exposure, a subacutely evolving distal neuropathy appears, which is predominantly motor. After recovery from the neuropathy, lower limb spasticity may become evident. Autopsy studies at the time of 'ginger jake' paralysis in the USA documented axonal degeneration in the peripheral nerves, in the cervical regions of the gracile fasciculi and in the corticospinal tracts of the lumbar spinal cord (Aring, 1942). This pattern is thus consistent with a central–peripheral distal axonopathy. This was also observed in animal studies (Cavanagh, 1954) which, as for the neuropathies with focal neurofilamentous accumulations, displays a multifocal preterminal distribution (Bouldin and Cavanagh 1979a, b). Larger and longer fibres are preferentially affected.

Toxic oil syndrome An outbreak of a toxic syndrome related to denatured rapeseed oil occurred in Spain in 1981. The toxic agent has not been identified. The disease was ushered in with fever, constitutional symptoms, skin rashes and respiratory embarrassment. This was followed by neuromuscular features, consisting of patchy muscle weakness and wasting, and by sensory loss. Peripheral nerve involvement was the most severe pathological change. An inflammatory perineuritis and, later, perineurial fibrosis were conspicuous changes with accompanying degeneration of myelinated axons (Ricoy et al., 1983). There was denervation atrophy of muscle, together with some inflammatory changes.

Trichlorethylene This solvent and anaesthetic agent (or an impurity) may give rise to a cranial neuropathy, predominantly affecting the fifth and seventh cranial nerves. An autopsied case showed axonal degeneration in the trigeminal nerve and root (Buxton and Hayward, 1967).

Iatrogenic neuropathies

Amiodarone The antiarrhythmic drug amiodarone, a diiodinated benzofuran derivative, occasionally gives rise to a sensorimotor neuropathy after prolonged administration. Nerve biopsy has shown loss of myelinated fibres of all sizes and probably of unmyelinated axons. Lysosomal bodies containing lamellar material were present in Schwann cells, fibroblasts and perineurial cells. They were also present in muscle fibres (Meier et al., 1979). The iodine content of the tissues was greatly increased and it was suggested that the lipid storage in nerve and muscle was secondary to the accumulation of the drug or its metabolites.

Disulfiram (tetraethylthiuram disulphide) A distal sensorimotor neuropathy may be produced by this drug, used in the treatment of alcoholism. Nerve biopsies have shown axonal degeneration (Bradley and Hewer, 1966) as have animal studies (Zuccarello and Anzil, 1979). As disulfiram is metabolized to carbon disulphide in the body, it has been suggested that this may explain the neuropathy. This is unlikely, as the giant axonal swellings that are a feature of carbon disulphide neuropathy are not seen in that due to disulfiram.

Gold It is now accepted that gold salts, used in the treatment of rheumatoid arthritis, may cause peripheral neuropathy. A complicating factor is that neuropathy may also occur as a manifestation of rheumatoid disease. An acute distal polyneuropathy, sometimes with prominent myokymia, characterizes that due to chrysotherapy. Nerve biopsy studies from human cases, and in an animal study, have shown a combination of segmental demyelination and axonal degeneration (Katrack et al., 1980). It is not certain whether this is the direct result of toxicity or whether gold salts induce a hypersensitivity reaction.

Isoniazid (isonicotinic acid hydrazide) A distal symmetrical and predominantly sensory neuropathy may be produced by this antituberculous agent, particularly in slow acetylators in whom blood levels of the drug are abnormally high (Evans, Manley and McKusick, 1960). Nerve biopsy studies have shown degeneration of both myelinated and unmyelinated axons (Ochoa, 1970). Experimental observations in the rat established that isoniazid produces a distal multifocal neuropathy which is characterized by periaxonal vacuolation and the occurrence of proliferated intra-axonal agranular reticulum and vacuoles which progress to axonal degeneration (Jacobs, Miller and Cavanagh, 1979; Jacobs et al., 1979).

The drug causes neuropathy mainly or entirely by interference with pyridoxine metabolism. Isoniazid combines with the cofactor pyridoxal phosphate, producing an inactive compound. The precise role which pyridoxal plays in axons is uncertain. Peripheral neuropathy has been produced in pigs (Wintrobe et al., 1943; Swank and Adams, 1948) by a pyridoxine-deficient diet, and in monkeys (Victor and Adams, 1956) and human volunteers (Vilter et al., 1953) by the administration of the antagonist desoxypyridoxine.

Metronidazole Neuropathy is a rare complication of treatment with this chemotherapeutic preparation, and in the treatment of protozoal and Gram-negative infections. Nerve biopsy has shown axonal loss (Bradley, Karlsson and Rasso, 1977). The chemically related radiation sensitizer *misonidazole* frequently produces a peripheral neuropathy. A combination of axonal degeneration and demyelination has been described on nerve biopsy (Urtasun et al., 1978).

Nitrofurantoin This preparation is used in the treatment of urinary infections. Neuropathy usually occurs only if renal failure is present, leading to excessively high blood levels of the drug (Collings, 1960). Widespread axonal degeneration in the peripheral nerves has been documented in an autopsied case (Lhermitte et al., 1963).

Perhexilene A mixed sensorimotor neuropathy, sometimes with autonomic features, and bulbar involvement, develops in occasional individuals receiving perhexilene maleate, a preparation which has been employed in the treatment of angina pectoris. Neuropathy is probably more likely to occur in individuals who are at risk because of a genetically determined defect in the metabolism of perhexilene (by hydroxylation), this leading to excessive blood levels of the drug (Cooper, Evans and Whibley, 1984). As well as axonal degeneration there is extensive segmental demyelination, an unusual feature for a toxic neuropathy (Lhermitte et al., 1976; Said, 1978). The Schwann cells contain lamellar and crystalloid inclusions, which are also present in skeletal and smooth muscle cells and fibroblasts. There is an accumulation of gangliosides in nerve. Administration of perhexilene to rats gives rise to a generalized lipidosis with membrane-bound lamellar and crystalloid inclusions in several organs (Lüllmann and Lüllmann-Rauch, 1978). Perhexilene is a cationic amphiphilic substance and it may form complexes with polar lipids. This possibly interferes with their degradation.

Sodium cyanate This substance has been used in the treatment of sickle cell anaemia. It binds to the terminal NH_2 groups of haemoglobin. Prolonged administration has been found to cause neuropathy with axonal degeneration and segmental demyelination, assumed to be of the secondary type, in nerve biopsies (Ohnishi, Petersen and Dyck, 1975). In rats, this substance has produced giant intramyelinic vacuolation and demyelination in spinal roots (Tellez-Nagel et al., 1977).

Thalidomide (γ-phthalimidoglutarimide) Cases of a distal predominantly sensory polyneuropathy occurred in patients given this drug as a hypnotic. Clinical signs of corticospinal tract damage were sometimes also present. This drug is still used in the treatment of erythema nodosum leprosum. Nerve biopsies taken in the recovery phase have shown loss of large myelinated axons and increased numbers of small fibres which were probably regenerating axons (Fullerton and O'Sullivan, 1968).

Vincristine The *Vinca* alkaloid vincristine is widely used as an antimitotic agent. A distal sensory polyneuropathy may develop in patients receiving therapeutic doses. This may be followed by distal weakness if administration is continued. Nerve biopsy and autopsy studies have demonstrated distal axonal degeneration in the peripheral nerves (Bradley et al., 1970). Vincristine binds to tubulin, its antimitotic effect being dependent on interference with the mitotic spindle. Animal studies have demonstrated the accumulation of neurofilaments and paracrystalline material in neuronal cell bodies and axons (Shelanski and Wiśniewski, 1969), and it has been proposed that the neuropathy results from an interference with axonal transport.

Diphtheritic neuropathy

A generalized or a focal neuropathy may be related to infection with *Corynebacterium diphtheriae*. It is now rare in Western countries. With faucial diphtheria, palatal paralysis develops between the fifth and the twelfth days of the disease and, when diphtheria was prevalent, occurred in about 20 per cent of cases (Rolleston, 1904). Shortly after this, other cranial nerve palsies appear, in particular paralysis of the ciliary muscle, leading to blurred vision with defective accommodation. Recovery occurs after about 3 weeks. In a minority of cases a generalized polyneuropathy, predominantly motor in pattern, develops at between 5 and 8 weeks after the acute illness. If death does not supervene from respiratory failure or myocardial involvement, full recovery occurs within weeks or months.

In patients with cutaneous diphtheria, it has been stated that local paralysis may occur, related to the site of the infection (Walshe, 1918–19). This view is likely to be correct, despite the failure of Gaskill and Korb (1946) to confirm such a relationship. Weakness of the ciliary muscles may develop, as may generalized polyneuropathy identical to that occurring after faucial infection (Walshe, 1918–19).

In a very early teased fibre study, Meyer (1881) demonstrated segmental demyelination with sparing of axons, and the finding was substantiated by observations in more recent years (Veith, 1949; Scheid and Peters, 1952; Fisher and Adams, 1956). It was emphasized by Fisher and Adams that the demyelination tended to be concentrated in the spinal roots and dorsal root ganglia and that it was not associated with infiltration by inflammatory cells, as had been claimed by some of the early observers.

Diphtheritic neuropathy has been studied experimentally by the inoculation of diphtheria toxin into animals (Waksman, Adams and Mansmann, 1957; Webster et al., 1961; McDonald, 1963; Weller, 1965) and by intraneural injection (Cavanagh and Jacobs, 1964). These observations confirmed selective paranodal and segmental demyelination with preservation of axonal continuity.

Diphtheritic neuropathy in man is due solely to diphtheria toxin, as was inadvertently demonstrated following the accidental injection of toxin into 14 children, four of whom developed neuropathy within a month (Jakovleva, 1927). Experimental studies have demonstrated that the toxin becomes fixed to Schwann cells within 1 hour, and that the latency of development of neuropathy varies with the dose and species. The toxin inhibits Schwann cell protein synthesis, including myelin basic protein and proteolipid (Pleasure, Feldmann and Prockop, 1973). It has been suggested that the demyelination is the result of failure of replacement of proteins lost during the normal metabolic turnover of myelin.

Neuropathies related to systemic metabolic disorders

Diabetes mellitus

The peripheral nerve disorders related to diabetes mellitus are complex. The most satisfactory subdivision is into symmetrical polyneuropathies, predominantly sensory and autonomic, on the one hand, and focal and multifocal neuropathies on the other. The latter comprise cranial nerve lesions, particularly of the third and seventh, thoracoabdominal neuropathy, focal lesions of limb nerves and the syndrome of proximal motor neuropathy (diabetic amyotrophy) (see Thomas and Eliasson, 1984).

Symmetrical polyneuropathy Loss of axons has been clearly established (Greenbaum et al., 1964; Thomas and Lascelles, 1966), affecting both myelinated and unmyelinated (Behse, Buchthal and Carlsen, 1977) axons. It is most prominent distally but may also affect the spinal roots, particularly the dorsal roots. Loss of dorsal root ganglion cells and anterior horn cells may occur (Bosanquet and Henson, 1957; Greenbaum et al., 1964). In cases of acute painful neuropathy, active fibre breakdown is demonstrable in teased fibre preparations (Archer et al., 1983), and in chronic cases regenerative activity is prominent. Fibre degeneration also occurs in the posterior columns, possibly secondary to loss of dorsal root ganglion cells (Olsson et al., 1968) or, conceivably, reflecting a central-peripheral distal axonopathy.

Selective loss of small myelinated axons and degeneration of unmyelinated axons has been shown in cases of painful diabetic neuropathy (Brown, Martin and Asbury, 1976). In more severe cases of diabetic pseudosyringomyelic neuropathy, Said, Slama and Selva (1983) have found a predominant loss of small myelinated and unmyelinated axons. It has been proposed (Brown, Martin and Asbury, 1976) that there is a spectrum ranging between selective small fibre neuropathies of this type to others with selective large fibre loss, although the latter has not yet been documented by morphometric studies. In cases of acute painful diabetic neuropathy, Archer et al. (1983) have found loss of myelinated fibres of all diameters, as did Behse, Buchthal and Carlsen (1977) in more chronic cases.

The nature of the axonal pathology is not fully established. Loss of dorsal root ganglion cells and anterior horn cells is not an important cause. A distal axonal degeneration has been demonstrated in teased fibre studies (Said, Slama and Selva, 1983), indicating that distal axonopathy of 'dying-back' type may occur in some instances. A symmetrical neuropathy may also be related to multifocal proximal lesions (Sugimura and Dyck, 1982). The occurrence of axonal atrophy has not been detected (Sugimura and Dyck, 1981).

Segmental demyelination may be a feature in diabetic neuropathy (Thomas and Lascelles, 1965; Behse, Buchthal and Carlsen, 1977). Said, Slama and Selva (1983) have reported demyelination of secondary type proximal to distal degeneration, together with more widespread primary demyelination. Small 'onion bulbs' are occasionally seen (Ballin and Thomas, 1968), indicating recurrent demyelination and remyelination. The correlation between the severity of axonal loss and demyelination is not strong (Behse, Buchthal and Carlsen, 1977), suggesting independent effects of the diabetic state on axonal and Schwann cell function. Dyck et al.

(1980) correlated the type and extent of teased fibre abnormalities with the duration of diabetes and the severity of neuropathy. In untreated diabetics without symptoms of neuropathy, segmental demyelination and remyelination were the salient abnormality.

Excessive numbers of Schwann cell pi granules have been described (Bischoff, 1968), but this has not been assessed quantitatively. Thickening of the Schwann cell basal lamina is sometimes observable (Bischoff, 1968; Asbury and Johnson, 1978; Guy et al., 1984).

Autonomic system The autonomic nervous system has not so far been studied extensively in cases of diabetic autonomic neuropathy. Degenerative changes have been described in autonomic ganglia (Olsson and Sourander, 1968) and enlargement of sympathetic ganglion cells that contained PAS-positive material was noted by Appenzeller and Richardson (1966). Duchen et al. (1980) have noted the occurrence of inflammatory changes in autonomic ganglia and around small nerve bundles in the walls of viscera. Axonal loss and segmental demyelination have been observed in the white communicating rami and the greater splanchnic nerve (Low et al., 1975), and loss of axons in the vagus (Kristensson et al., 1971). Guy et al. (1984) have reported severe loss of axons in the abdominal vagus in a case of diabetic gastroparesis. Grover-Johnson et al. (1981) have documented reduced innervation of lower limb arterioles, and abnormalities in the innervation of the bladder wall and corpora cavernosa were recorded by Faerman et al. (1971) and Faerman et al. (1974).

Focal and multifocal nerve lesions Variable fibre loss in component fascicles may be evident in patients with multifocal neuropathy (Thomas and Lascelles, 1966). Focal lesions, probably of a demyelinating nature, have been demonstrated in cases with isolated third cranial nerve lesions (Dreyfus, Hakim and Adams, 1957; Asbury et al., 1970). In a patient with lower limb multiple mononeuropathy, Raff, Sangalang and Asbury (1968) described ischaemic changes. The interpretation of these is difficult. One change was the presence of areas of 'pallor', mainly involving bridging fascicles. Appearances described as infarcts were subsequently realized to be Renaut bodies.

Connective tissue changes Endoneurial area is often increased (Behse, Buchthal and Carlsen, 1977) and endoneurial collagen deposition may be extensive (Thomas and Eliasson, 1984). The perineurial basal laminae may be thickened (Asbury and Johnson, 1978) and perineurial calcification has been described (Paetau and Haltia, 1976).

Vascular changes Thickening and hyalinization of the walls of small neural blood vessels was originally noted by Fagerberg (1959) and shown to be due to reduplication of the basal

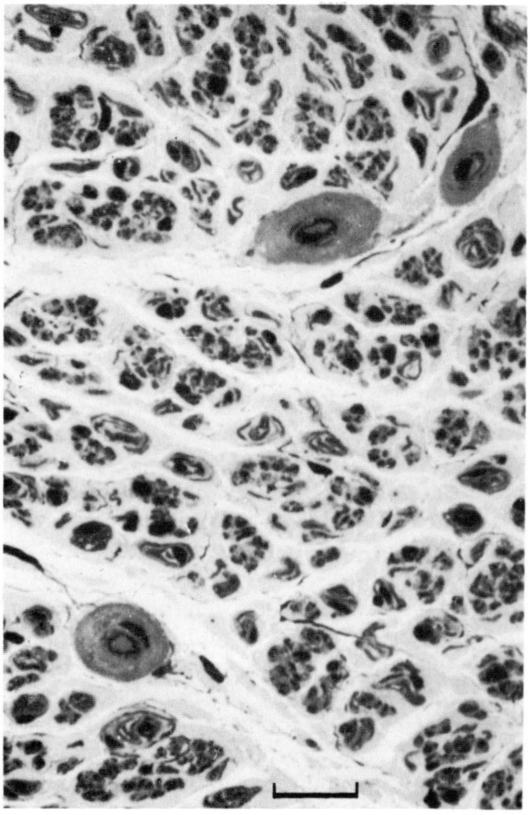

Fig. 18.39 Diabetic neuropathy. Nerve biopsy showing gross loss of myelinated nerve fibres and thickening of the walls of endoneurial capillaries. Semithin sections; thionin and acridine orange. Bar = 20 μm.

lamina (Bischoff, 1967) (Figs. 18.39 and 18.40). Hyperplasia of the basal lamina of endoneurial vessels is common in chronic neuropathies but is statistically more frequent in diabetics (Vital et al., 1974).

Intraluminal vascular changes have received

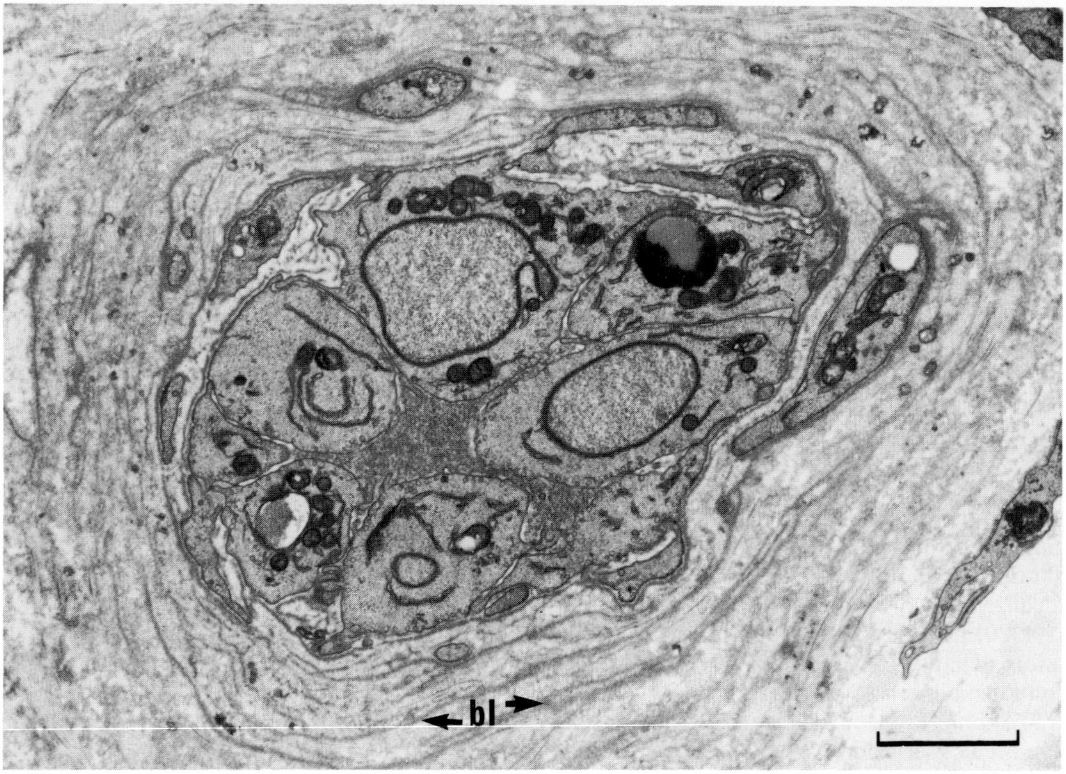

Fig. 18.40 Diabetic neuropathy. Electron micrograph of endoneurial capillary showing reduplicated basal lamina (bl). Bar = 2 μm.

comment from Timperley et al. (1976) and Williams et al. (1980). Occlusion of intraneural vessels by deposits of fibrin was noted.

Pathogenesis The clinical heterogeneity of diabetic neuropathy suggests multifactorial causation. Some focal lesions, such as those of the third cranial nerve, may be ischaemic in origin. An ischaemic basis for the totality of diabetic neuropathy is now generally considered to be unlikely, although this possibility has been raised in the recent experimental studies of Tuck, Schmelzer and Low (1984). Abnormal susceptibility to external pressure may explain some focal lesions.

The symmetrical polyneuropathies are likely to have a metabolic basis. A depression of Na^+,K^+-ATPase activity secondary to a reduced concentration of *myo*-inositol, and to which elevated neural sorbitol levels may contribute (Finegold et al., 1983), is currently being considered. This might lead to neuropathy by interfering with axonal transport. This topic has been reviewed by Brown and Greene (1984) and by Thomas and Eliasson (1984).

Hypoglycaemia

Loss of anterior horn cells may occur as a consequence of hypoglycaemia. This is considered in Chapter 4.

Uraemic neuropathy

A symmetrical distal sensorimotor polyneuropathy may develop as a consequence of severe chronic renal failure (Asbury, Victor and Adams, 1963; Thomas et al., 1971). It is considered that it is likely to be due to a retained metabolite but this has not been identified.

An autopsy study (Asbury, Victor and Adams, 1963) demonstrated a distally accentuated axonal degeneration in the peripheral nerves with chromatolytic changes in anterior horn cells. In addition to axonal loss, nerve biopsies have demonstrated demyelination which is of the secondary type (Dyck et al., 1971a; Thomas et al., 1971). In milder cases the axonal loss predominantly affects myelinated fibres of larger diameter, with relative sparing of small myelinated and unmyelinated axons.

Neuropathy related to liver disease

Peripheral neuropathy does not constitute a clinical problem in patients with either acute or chronic liver disease, except in conditions such as alcoholism which also cause neuropathy or when the Guillain–Barré syndrome follows acute viral hepatitis, and sometimes in primary biliary cirrhosis. In nerve biopsies from an unselected series of cases with chronic liver disease, Knill-Jones et al. (1972) found evidence of segmental demyelination and remyelination, and the suggestion was made that a demyelinating neuropathy may be a consequence of chronic liver disease. Interpretation of these results is difficult because a high proportion of the cases were alcoholic or had impaired glucose tolerance.

Occasional patients with primary biliary cirrhosis develop a sensory neuropathy in which nerve biopsies show xanthomatous deposits mainly situated in the perineurium (Thomas and Walker, 1965). In a recent autopsied case of drug-induced hepatic disease, such deposits were confined to nerves in the hilum of the liver (Ludwig, Dyck and LaRusso, 1982). Some patients with primary biliary cirrhosis and neuropathy do not demonstrate xanthomatous infiltration, and the neuropathy may have an immunological basis (Charron, Peyronnard and Marchard, 1980).

Neuropathy in hypothyroidism

The commonest type of peripheral nerve involvement is a focal compression neuropathy, usually the carpal tunnel syndrome. Rarely, a distal symmetrical sensorimotor polyneuropathy develops which recovers with treatment of the hypothyroidism. Nerve biopsies were studied by Dyck and Lambert (1970) who concluded that segmental demyelination was the predominant abnormality. Excessive amounts of glycogen were present, both within Schwann cell cytoplasm and in axons, and were also observed within Schwann cells by Pollard et al. (1982). These authors and Meier and Bischoff (1977) concluded that axonal degeneration rather than demyelination is the main lesion. Deposition of 'mucoid' material, emphasized in some earlier reports (e.g. Nickel et al., 1961), is not a feature.

Neuropathy in acromegaly

The carpal tunnel syndrome is the commonest form of peripheral nerve involvement in acromegaly. A generalized neuropathy independent of the presence of diabetes is also relatively frequent (Low et al., 1974). The peripheral nerves show an expanded fascicular area with an increase in subperineural and endoneurial connective tissue and a reduction in the density of myelinated and unmyelinated axons. This is probably related both to fibre loss and to expanded endoneurial area. Teased fibre preparations demonstrate a combination of axonal degeneration and segmental demyelination.

Amyloid neuropathy

Peripheral nerve involvement may be encountered in primary amyloidosis, in amyloidosis related to myeloma and Waldenström's macroglobulinaemia, and in a number of hereditary amyloid syndromes in which neuropathy is the salient feature. In the first three conditions, immunoamyloid (AL), derived from immunoglobulin light chains, is deposited. In the Swedish and Japanese forms of hereditary amyloid neuropathy the amyloid is closely similar to prealbumin. The precursor substances undergo a physicochemical alteration, within or induced by macrophages or cells of the reticuloendothelial system, to yield a beta-pleated sheet configuration. It is the beta-pleated molecular structure that confers the characteristic staining properties of amyloid, the most important of which is lime-green fluorescence when viewed in polarized light after staining with Congo red. Neuropathy does not occur in secondary amyloidosis where there is deposition of AA amyloid. In all types of amyloidosis the deposits, at the ultrastructural level, consist of 10 nm unbranched 'rigid' fibrils, either in an irregular array or organized into parallel or fan-shaped bundles (Figs. 18.41 and 18.42) or sometimes radiating stellate clusters.

The deposits regularly contain small quantities of a second component, P component or AP. Ultrastructurally, this consists of thick 9 nm pentagonal discs when examined in extracts from

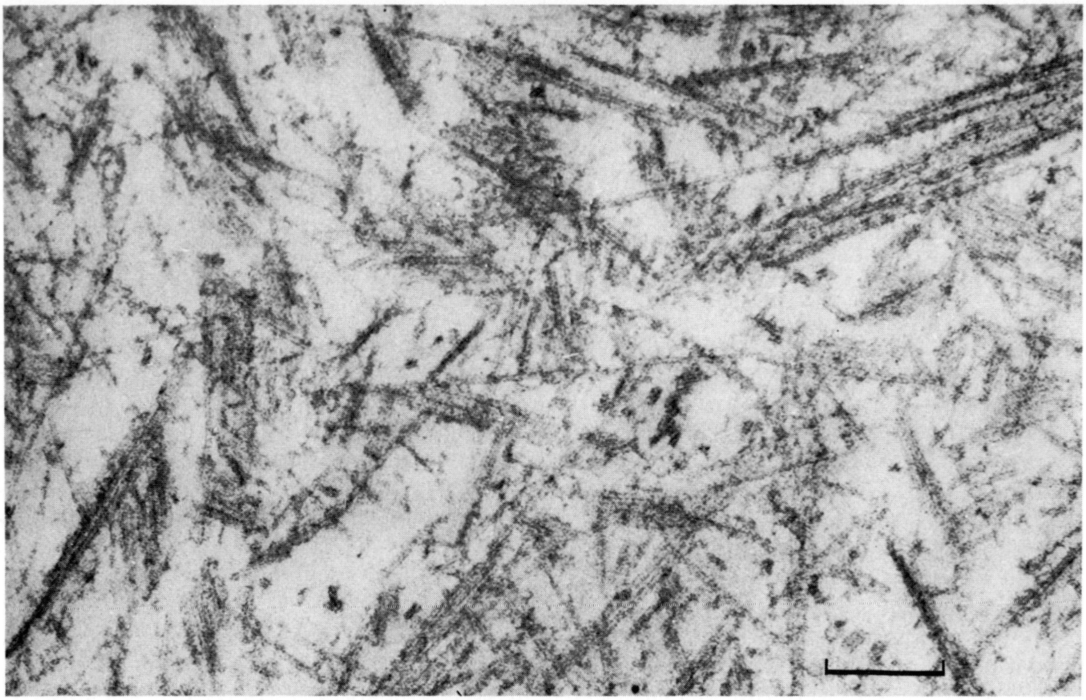

Fig. 18.41 Amyloid neuropathy. Electron micrograph of amyloid fibrils in endoneurium. Bar = 0.1 μm.

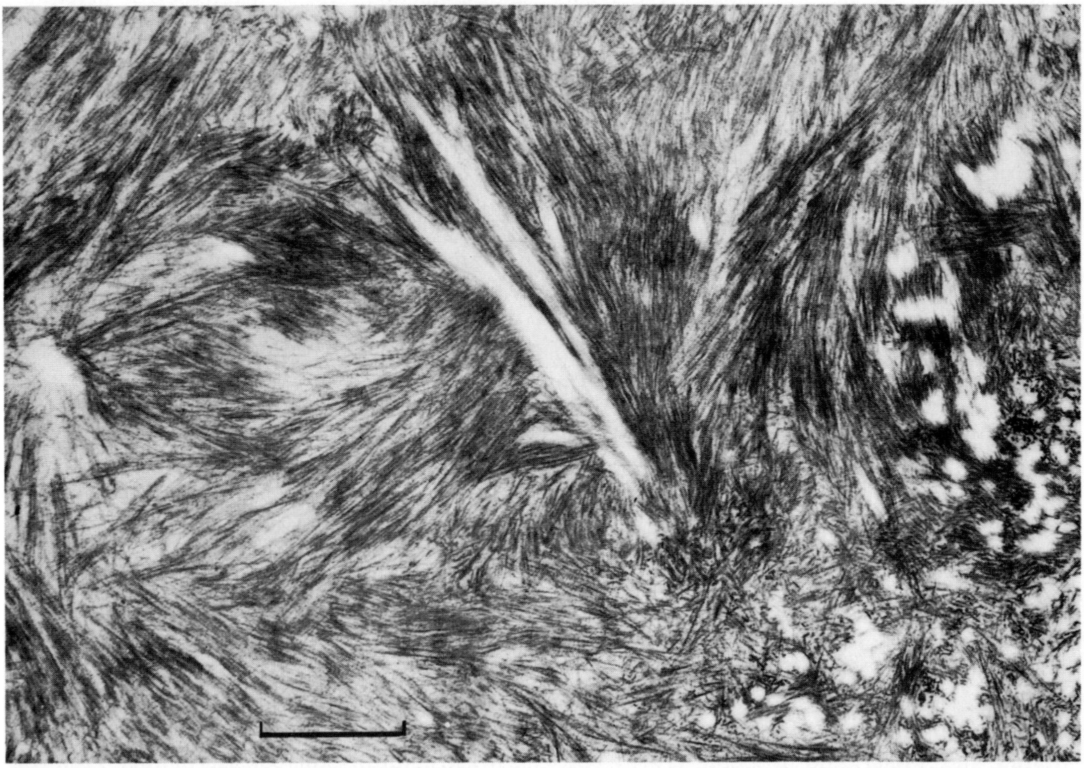

Fig. 18.42 Amyloid neuropathy. Electron micrograph of amyloid fibrils in endoneurium. Bar = 0.5 μm.

amyloid deposits. It has been shown to be identical to a circulating α-glycoprotein (serum amyloid protein, SAP) which becomes non-specifically adsorbed to the amyloid deposits, together with other substances such as polysaccharide, complement components, lipoprotein and fibrinogen. The nature of amyloid has been reviewed by Glenner, Ignaczak and Page (1978).

The neuropathy which may be associated with primary amyloidosis usually consists of a slowly progressive distal symmetrical sensorimotor polyneuropathy with an onset in the lower limbs. Spontaneous pain is often a feature. Sensory loss occurs before motor features appear, and commonly affects pain and temperature sensibility to a greater extent than large fibre modalities. There is often an accompanying autonomic neuropathy. Distal motor involvement ensues later. The peripheral nerves may be thickened. Cases associated with myeloma may begin with the carpal tunnel syndrome.

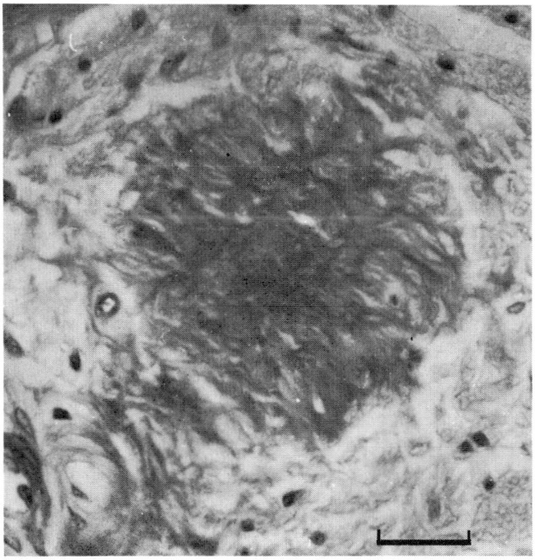

Fig. 18.43 Amyloid neuropathy. Endoneurial amyloid deposit. Congo red. Bar = 20 μm.

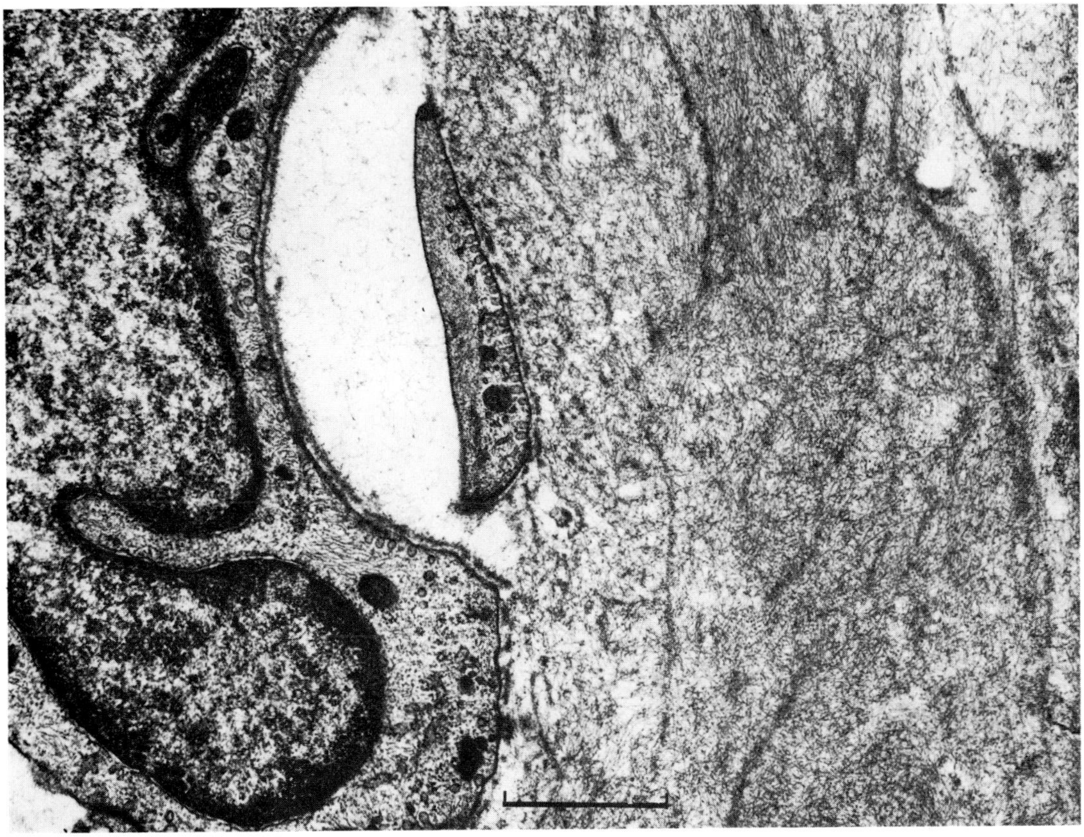

Fig. 18.44 Amyloid neuropathy. Electron micrograph showing amyloid fibrils surrounding an endoneurial capillary. Bar = 1 μm.

Four main types of hereditary amyloid neuropathy are recognized (Thomas, 1975). All are inherited as autosomal dominant traits. Type I (Portuguese) was originally recognized by Andrade (1952) and is common in northern Portugal. Its clinical features resemble those of neuropathy associated with sporadic primary amyloidosis just described. Similar cases occur in Japan. The Swedish and British cases are comparable but display minor differences. Type II (Rukavina or Indiana form) is characterized by presentation with the carpal tunnel syndrome. The type III (Van Allen or Iowa form) consists of a symmetrical polyneuropathy which is frequently accompanied by renal involvement and duodenal ulceration. The distinguishing features of type IV (Meretoja or Finnish form) are cranial neuropathy, lattice corneal dystrophy and only minor limb involvement.

Amyloid deposits are present in the peripheral nerves in all these disorders. In type II hereditary amyloid neuropathy and in some cases with myeloma, presentation with the carpal tunnel syndrome is related to deposits in the flexor retinaculum. The pathological changes in peripheral nerve have been most extensively studied in neuropathy related to primary amyloidosis and in the type I hereditary form (Thomas and King, 1974). Widespread deposits are found in the peripheral nerves, limb girdle plexuses and in the sensory and autonomic ganglia. Diffuse infiltration of the peripheral nerves is known to be present in some patients with myeloma or Waldenström's macroglobulinaemia (Bigner, Olson and McFarlin, 1971; Davies-Jones and Esiri, 1971), although most cases of neuropathy associated with these disorders are not related to amyloidosis.

In peripheral nerve, the amyloid deposits are present in the epineurium and endoneurium and in relation to blood vessels (Figs. 18.43 and 18.44). On electron microscopy, the amyloid fibrils in the endoneurium are often observed to be closely associated with the basal lamina of

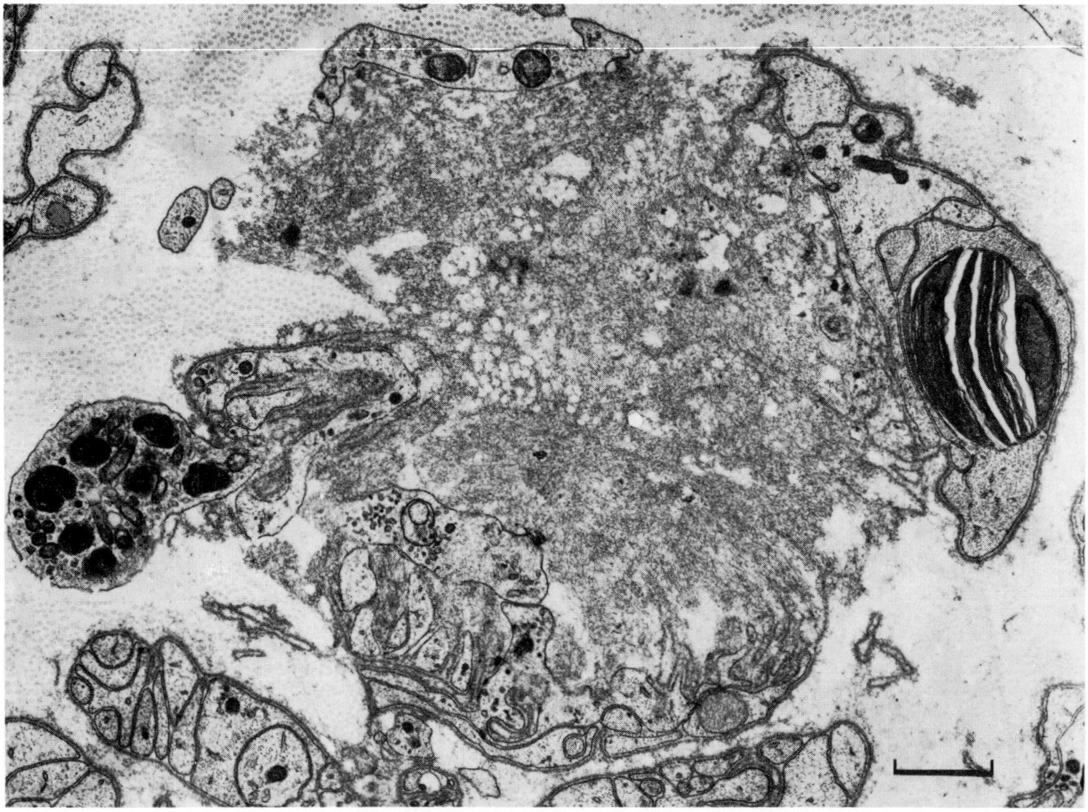

Fig. 18.45 Amyloid neuropathy. Endoneurial amyloid deposit in relation to Schwann cells associated with unmyelinated axons. Bar = 1 μm.

Schwann cells (Fig. 18.45). Morphometric studies show that in the early stages there is a preferential loss of small myelinated and unmyelinated axons (Dyck and Lambert, 1969; Thomas and King, 1974). Later a diffuse loss occurs. Teased fibre studies demonstrate predominant axonal degeneration with some segmental demyelination and remyelination. In sensory and autonomic ganglia, the deposits again may occur in the connective tissues or in relation to blood vessels. In the sensory ganglia, they may surround the capsule cells, particularly those of smaller size.

The mechanism of the neuropathy is uncertain. Ischaemia related to the perivascular deposits has been proposed as an explanation but is considered to be unlikely. Mechanical distortion may play some part (Dyck and Lambert, 1969). The close apposition of the amyloid fibrils in relation to Schwann cell basal laminae raises the possibility that they may have a deleterious effect on the activity of these cells. Coimbra and Andrade (1971) believed that nerve fibre degeneration antedated amyloid deposition, but their observations were made on nerve biopsies which did not preclude earlier amyloid deposition in the more proximal nerve trunks or in the sensory and autonomic ganglia.

Hereditary neuropathies

Neuropathy may occur as the salient manifestation of a variety of inherited disorders, in association with involvement of the central nervous system, or as part of a multisystem disorder. It is convenient to separate those conditions with and without a specific metabolic basis. A classification of these terms is given in Table 18.2.

Table 18.2 Classification of hereditary neuropathies

Neuropathies associated with specific metabolic defects

- Disturbance of lipid metabolism
  - Leucodystrophies:
    - metachromatic
    - globoid cell (Krabbe's disease)
    - adrenomyeloneuropathy
  - Refsum's disease
  - Fabry's disease
  - Lipoprotein deficiencies:
    - Tangier disease
    - abetalipoproteinaemia
  - Other disorders:
    - cholestanolosis, Farber disease, gangliosidosis, Gaucher's disease, multisystem degeneration with reduced tissue arachidonic acid, Niemann–Pick disease, Wolman's disease
- Porphyrias
  - Hepatic porphyria
  - Variegate porphyria
  - Hereditary coproporphyria
- Disorders with defective DNA repair
  - Xeroderma pigmentosum
  - Ataxia telangiectasia
  - Cockayne syndrome
- Mucopolysaccharidoses
- Primary hyperoxaluria
- Hereditary amyloidoses
  - Type I (Andrade)
  - Type II (Rukavina)
  - Type III (Van Allen)
  - Type IV (Meretoja)

Neuropathies of unknown causation

- Hereditary motor neuronopathies (spinal muscular atrophies)
- Hereditary motor and sensory neuropathies
  - Type I (hypertrophic)
  - Type II (neuronal)
  - Type III (Dejerine–Sottas disease, congenital hypomyelination neuropathy)
  - Complex forms
- Hereditary sensory and autonomic neuropathies
  - Type I (dominant)
  - Type II (recessive)
  - Type III (familial dysautonomia, Riley–Day syndrome)
  - Type IV (congenital sensory neuropathy with anhidrosis)
  - Hereditary sensory neuropathy with spastic paraplegia
- Hereditary pressure-sensitive neuropathy
- Giant axonal neuropathy
- Chorea–acanthocytosis syndrome
- Chediak–Higashi disease
- Neuropathy in hereditary ataxias and spastic paraplegias
- Other conditions:
  - ceroid lipofuscinosis, Leigh's disease, mitochondrial myopathy

Metachromatic leucodystrophy (MLD, sulphatide lipidosis)

MLD consists of a group of recessively inherited disorders characterized by the occurrence of demyelination in both the central and the peripheral nervous systems, associated with the storage of sulphatides. Late-infantile, juvenile and adult onset forms are recognized, all related to a deficiency of aryl sulphatase A. A rare form, the MLD variant, is associated with multiple sulphatase deficiencies; in a further variety, the AB variant, aryl sulphatase activity is normal, the disorder probably being due to a deficiency of activator protein. In all forms of MLD, central nervous system involvement usually predominates (see Chapter 12), but most cases show clinical or electrophysiological evidence of peripheral nerve involvement, and occasional cases present with neuropathy. The pathological changes in peripheral nerve are similar in all forms of MLD but minor variations, some probably related to the degree of chronicity of the disorder, are apparent (Thomas et al., 1977; J.-J. Martin et al., 1982). This is also true of multiple sulphatase deficiency (Bischoff and Ulrich, 1967) and the AB variant (Hahn et al., 1981).

The peripheral nerves in the commonest form, the late-infantile variety, show a reduction in myelinated fibre numbers and evidence of segmental demyelination and remyelination (Dayan, 1967). Fibre loss is usually less obvious in the juvenile and adult onset cases, but in these evidence of demyelination and remyelination ultimately becomes greater and hypertrophic neuropathy may be more obtrusive (Percy, Kaback and Herndon, 1977). The characteristic feature is the accumulation of granules of 0.5–1 μm diameter in the perinuclear region of the Schwann cell cytoplasm which stain metachromatically with cresyl violet or toluidine blue (Fig. 18.46). Such granules are present within Schwann cells associated with myelinated and unmyelinated axons and in macrophages. By electron microscopy they can be equated with membrane-bounded lamellated inclusions with a periodicity of 5.6–5.8 nm (Figs. 18.47 and 18.48b). They are associated with acid phosphatase activity and are therefore classifiable as lysosomes. Such material is present in prismatic stacks, in 'tuffstone bodies' (Fig. 18.48a) so termed because of their resemblance to volcanic limestone and in striated 'zebra bodies' (Bischoff, 1975) (Fig. 18.49). Myelin figures composed of concentric lamellar material with a major periodicity of 8 nm are also present in Schwann cells associated with myelinated axons (Webster, 1962; Thomas et al., 1977) and are possibly derived from myelin breakdown.

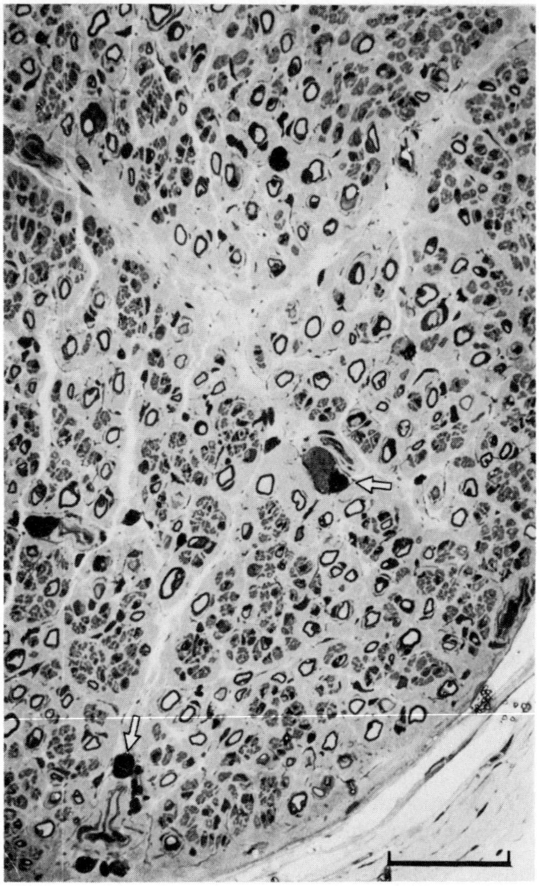

Fig. 18.46 Late-infantile metachromatic leucodystrophy. Transverse section through sural nerve showing deposits of metachromatic material (arrowed). Semithin section; thionin and acridine orange. Bar = 50 μm.

The explanation of the demyelination is uncertain. It is not clearly correlated with the presence of metachromatic inclusions in Schwann cells (Dayan, 1967). These inclusions are not derived from myelin breakdown as they are present in Schwann cells associated with unmyelinated axons and in fetal nerves before demyelination is evident. A possible cause of the demyelination is the existence of abnormalities in the lipid composition of myelin (O'Brien and Sampson, 1965)

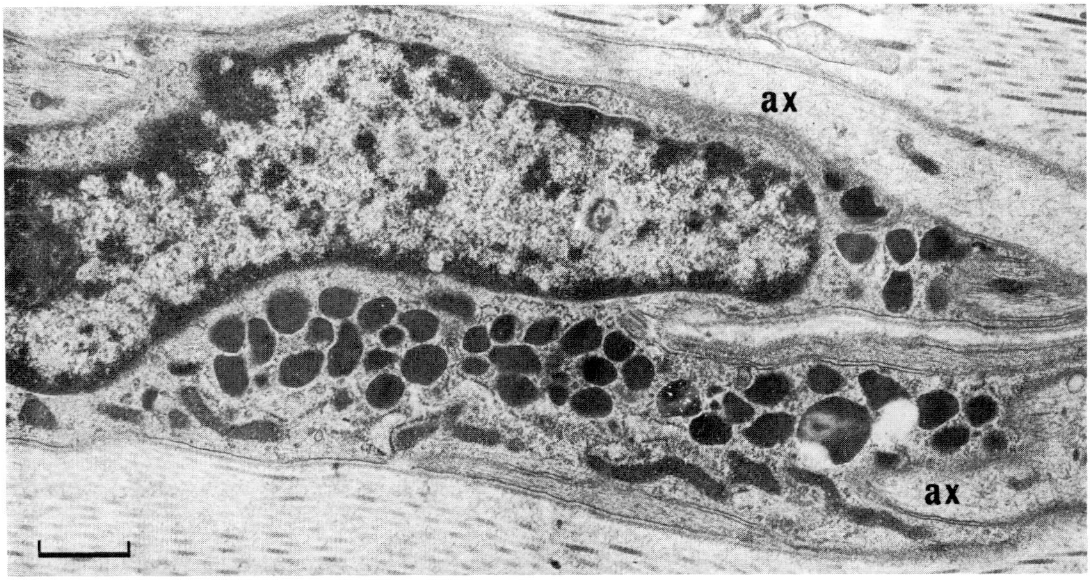

Fig. 18.47 Late-infantile metachromatic leucodystrophy. Schwann cells associated with unmyelinated axons (ax) containing multiple electron-dense inclusions. Bar = 1 μm.

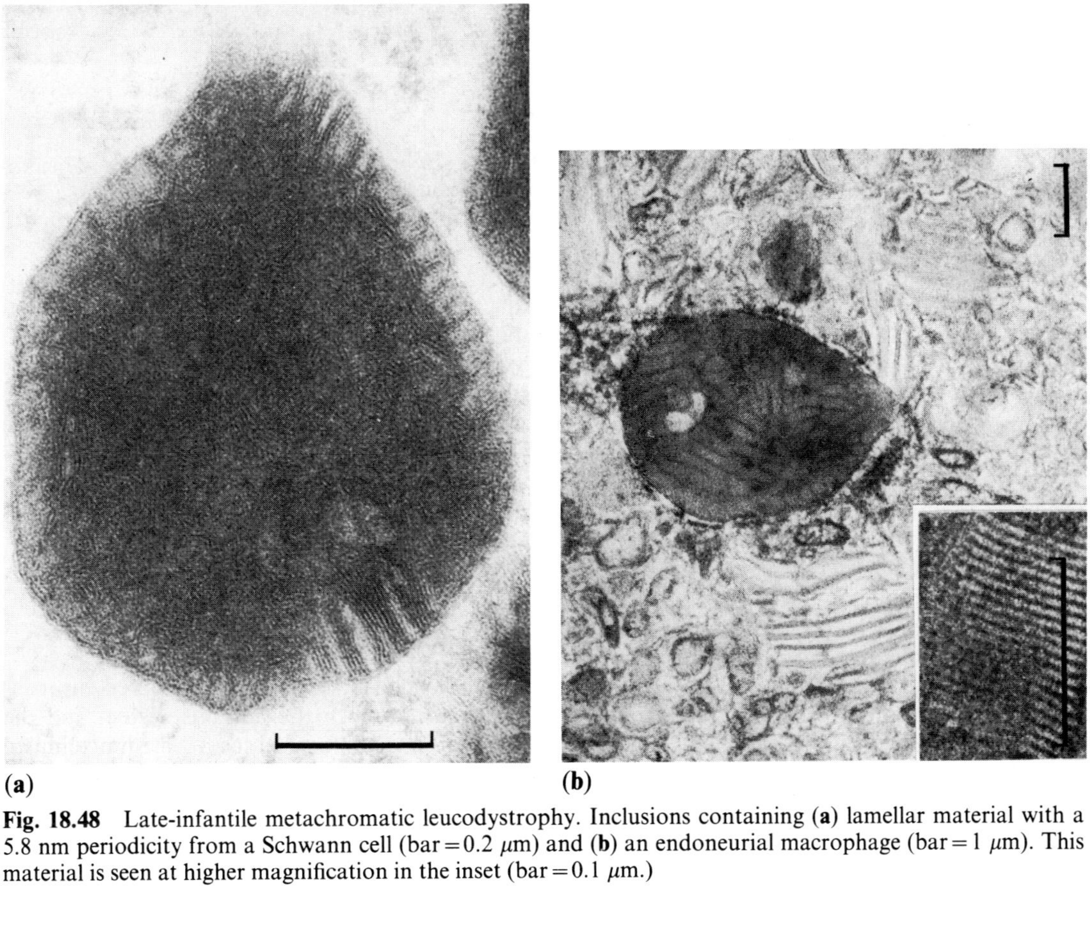

(a) **(b)**

Fig. 18.48 Late-infantile metachromatic leucodystrophy. Inclusions containing (**a**) lamellar material with a 5.8 nm periodicity from a Schwann cell (bar = 0.2 μm) and (**b**) an endoneurial macrophage (bar = 1 μm). This material is seen at higher magnification in the inset (bar = 0.1 μm.)

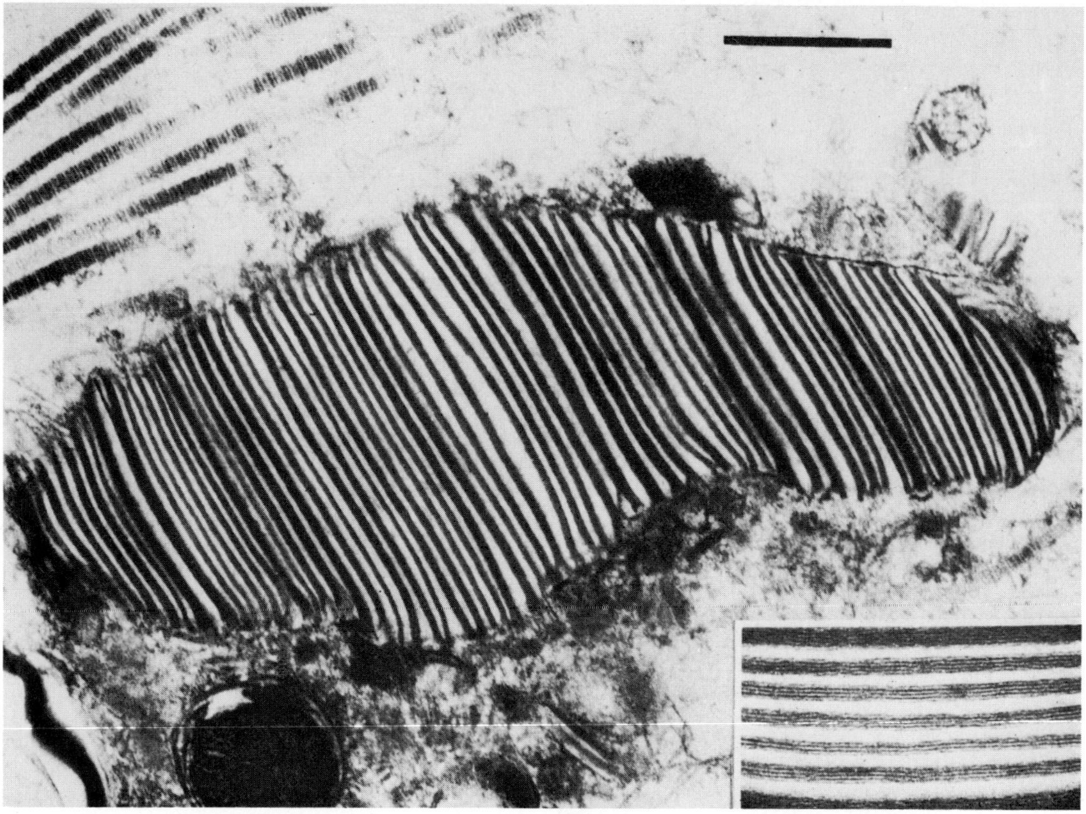

Fig. 18.49 Late-infantile metachromatic leucodystrophy. A zebra body is visible in a disintegrating macrophage. The inclusion material is shown at higher magnification in the inset. The groups of lamellae have a periodicity of 5.8 nm. Bar = 0.5 μm. (Reproduced, with permission, from Thomas et al., 1977.)

or the presence of cytotoxic substances such as sulphogalactosylsphingosine (Dulaney and Moser, 1978).

Globoid cell leucodystrophy (galactosylceramide lipidosis, Krabbe's disease)

This autosomal recessive disorder also generally produces predominant central nervous system manifestations (see Chapter 12), but accompanying peripheral nerve involvement is usual. Most cases have an onset in infancy, but late-infantile, juvenile and even adult onset cases are occasionally encountered.

The peripheral nerves show a moderate reduction in the myelinated fibre population, together with segmental demyelination and remyelination. The Schwann cells of both myelinated and unmyelinated fibres contain non-orientated straight or curved prismatic or tubular inclusions in a clear matrix (Figs. 18.50 and 18.51) (Bischoff and Ulrich, 1969), which are also present in macrophages. They are similar to those observed in the globoid cells in the brain.

The disorder is due to a deficient activity of the enzyme galactocerebroside-β-galactosidase, which converts galatocerebroside to ceramide and galactose. The damage to oligodendrocytes and Schwann cells may be directly related to the accumulation of galactocerebroside or its precursor, psychosin.

Adrenoleucodystrophy and adrenomyeloneuropathy

Adrenoleucodystrophy is an X-linked disorder which affects both the nervous system and the adrenal cortex. In typical cases there is no clinical involvement of the peripheral nerves but inclusions are demonstrable in Schwann cells. Other cases, with predominant spinal cord and peripheral nerve rather than cerebral involvement,

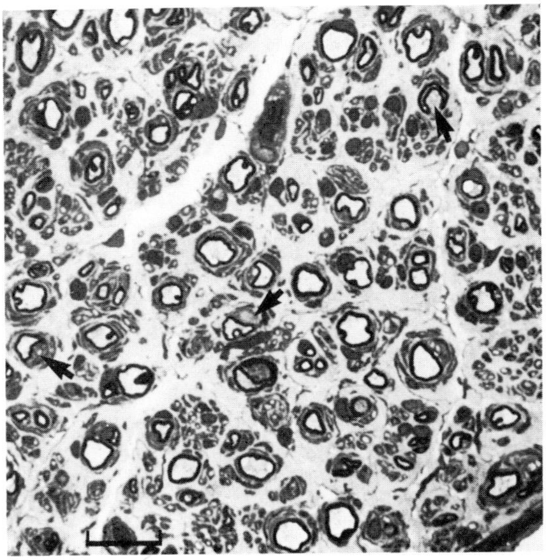

Fig. 18.50 Krabbe's disease. Transverse section through sural nerve. The axons all possess inappropriately thin myelin sheaths, indicating remyelination. Some of the Schwann cells contain inclusion material (arrowed). Semithin section; thionin and acridine orange. Bar = 20 μm.

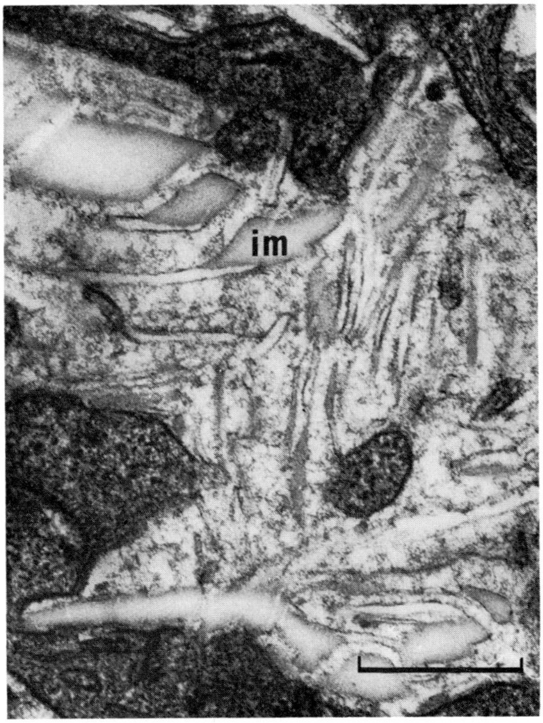

Fig. 18.51 Krabbe's disease. Electron micrograph showing inclusion material (im) in Schwann cell cytoplasm. Bar = 0.5 μm.

termed adrenomyeloneuropathy, are probably phenotypic variants related to the same abnormal gene. The peripheral nerves in such cases show loss of both myelinated and unmyelinated axons, evidence of demyelination and remyelination and minor hypertrophic changes. On electron microscopy, Schwann cells may contain lamellar inclusions, each lamella consisting of two parallel electron-dense 2- to 5-nm leaflets separated by a clear space varying from 2 to 7 nm in width (Griffin et al., 1977).

The salient biochemical change in adrenoleucodystrophy is the accumulation of very long chain fatty acids, especially hexacosanate, a 26-carbon unbranched fatty acid. This is demonstrable in brain and adrenal cortex, and in cultured skin fibroblasts. The metabolic abnormality may involve the beta-oxidation of these very long chain fatty acids (Moser et al., 1980).

Refsum's disease (phytanic acid storage disease, heredopathia atactica polyneuritiformis)

A chronic distal symmetrical sensorimotor neuropathy associated with ataxia and pigmentary retinal degeneration are the salient neurological features in this autosomal recessive disorder which usually develops in the second or third decades. The peripheral nerves may be enlarged. Sensorineural deafness is sometimes an additional feature, as are ichthyosis and cardiomyopathy. The course can be steadily progressive or relapsing and remitting. The long chain fatty acid 3,7,11,15-tetramethylhexadecanoic acid (phytanic acid) accumulates in the serum and a variety of tissues. It is derived from dietary phytol and accumulates because of a block in its alpha-oxidation to α-hydroxyphytanic acid. The clinical, biochemical and neuropathological features have recently been reviewed by Refsum et al. (1984).

Autopsy studies have demonstrated that the nerve hypertrophy is maximal proximally and most evident in the limb girdle plexuses. The enlargement may be diffuse or nodular and may also affect the spinal nerve roots and sensory ganglia. The endoneurial spaces are increased and contain material of 'mucoid' appearance. The number of myelinated nerve fibres is reduced and hypertrophic changes, sometimes with extremely large 'onion bulb' formations, may be present (Cammermeyer, 1956). Such hypertrophic changes may be seen in nerve biopsies

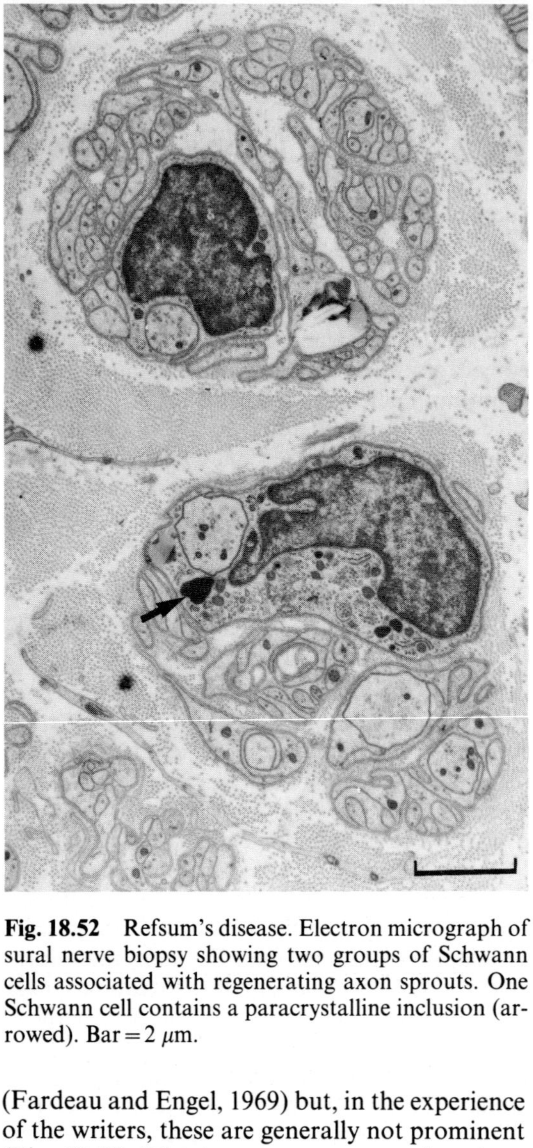

Fig. 18.52 Refsum's disease. Electron micrograph of sural nerve biopsy showing two groups of Schwann cells associated with regenerating axon sprouts. One Schwann cell contains a paracrystalline inclusion (arrowed). Bar = 2 μm.

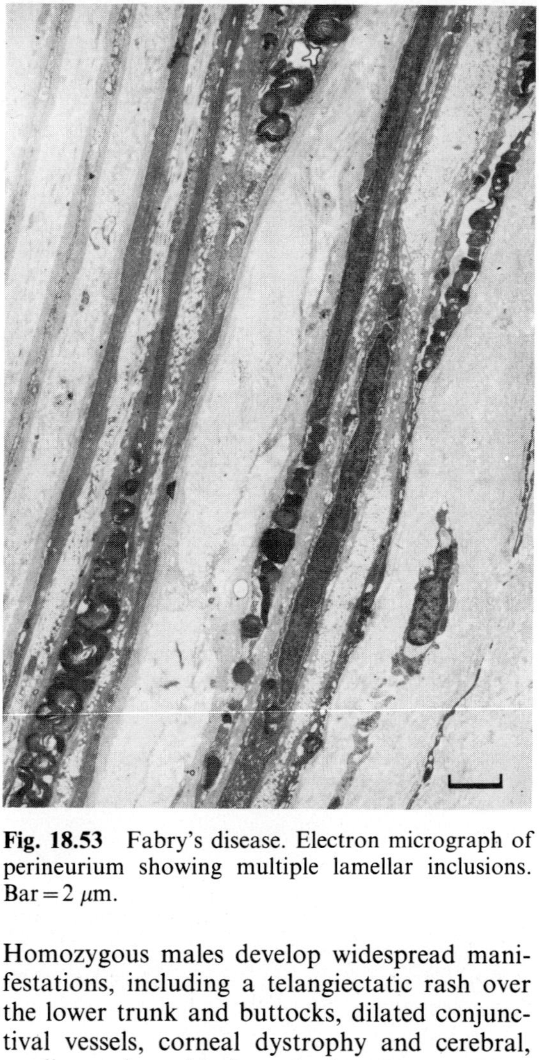

Fig. 18.53 Fabry's disease. Electron micrograph of perineurium showing multiple lamellar inclusions. Bar = 2 μm.

(Fardeau and Engel, 1969) but, in the experience of the writers, these are generally not prominent (Fig. 18.52). Distal sensory nerves tend to show loss of myelinated fibres, together with cluster formation, indicating regenerative activity. Fardeau and Engel (1969) commented upon the presence of rounded paracrystalline inclusions in Schwann cells. These are a non-specific feature but they were particularly numerous in the cases examined by Fardeau and Engel.

Fabry's disease (angiokeratoma corporis diffusum)

This condition is of X-linked recessive inheritance related to a deficiency of α-galactosidase A. Homozygous males develop widespread manifestations, including a telangiectatic rash over the lower trunk and buttocks, dilated conjunctival vessels, corneal dystrophy and cerebral, cardiac and renal lesions. An important component of the disease is a mild sensory and autonomic neuropathy, but this is accompanied by severe paroxysmal pain in the extremities (Fabry crises). These begin in childhood or adolescence. Heterozygous females may display minor manifestations but do not develop neuropathic symptoms.

Nerve biopsies have demonstrated a loss of small myelinated and unmyelinated axons and the presence of lamellated inclusions in perineurial and vascular endothelial cells (Bischoff et al., 1968; Kocen and Thomas, 1970) (Fig. 18.53). This material consists of glycosphingolipid, and ultrastructurally displays alternate light and dark lines with a periodicity of approximately 5 nm (Fig. 18.54). The inclusions are either in the

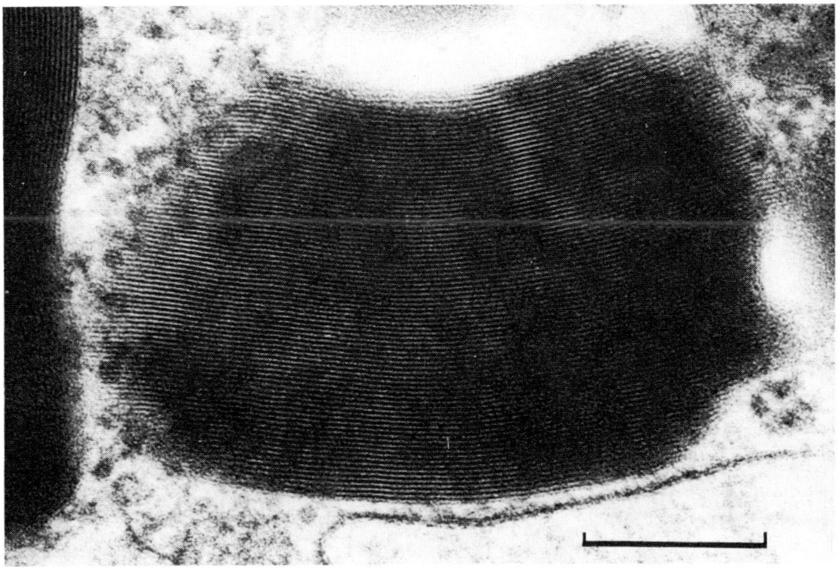

Fig. 18.54 Fabry's disease. Electron micrograph showing lamellar inclusion in a perineurial cell. The periodicity is approximately 5 nm. Bar = 0.2 μm.

form of flattened stacks or concentric lamellar bodies.

Autopsy studies have shown that the storage material is present in dorsal root ganglion cells. The numbers of these are reduced, particularly those of small size (Ohnishi and Dyck, 1974).

Hereditary high density lipoprotein deficiency (Tangier disease)

Tangier disease is named after an island in the Chesapeake Bay. The salient clinical manifestation, apart from peripheral nerve involvement, is the deposition of cholesteryl esters in various tissues, particularly in the tonsils (which become enlarged and yellowish in colour), in the spleen, bone marrow, lymph glands, intestinal submucosa and skin. Approximately half of the reported cases have developed a neuropathy, which may be of two differing patterns. The first is a pseudosyringomyelic syndrome with an adult onset. Affected individuals develop weakness of the facial and small hand muscles, generalized tendon areflexia and sensory loss which involves the trunk and proximal parts of the limbs, initially predominantly affecting pain and temperature sensibility (Kocen et al., 1967). The second consists of a relapsing multifocal neuropathy (Pollock et al., 1983).

The serum concentrations of high density lipoprotein are severely reduced, and the small quantities which are present are abnormal. Plasma cholesterol levels are usually reduced, triglyceride levels being normal or increased (Yao et al., 1978). The disorder is of autosomal recessive inheritance. It is as yet uncertain whether the two clinical forms are genetically distinct, although this appears likely.

Nerve biopsies from pseudosyringomyelic cases (Kocen et al., 1973; Dyck et al., 1978a) show a severe depletion of unmyelinated axons, and also of myelinated fibres, particularly those of smaller size. Teased fibre studies reveal no significant demyelination. The most striking abnormality is the presence of numerous lipid droplets and pleomorphic inclusions in the cytoplasm of Schwann cells (Fig. 18.55). These consist of neutral lipid and cholesteryl esters. The reason for the lipid accumulation in Schwann cells is uncertain. Possibly it is the result of nerve fibre degeneration and an inability of these cells to eliminate the products of axonal and myelin breakdown. Nerve biopsies from cases with multifocal neuropathy show prominent demyelination and remyelination and a restriction of the lipid droplets to Schwann cells associated with unmyelinated axons (Pollock et al., 1983).

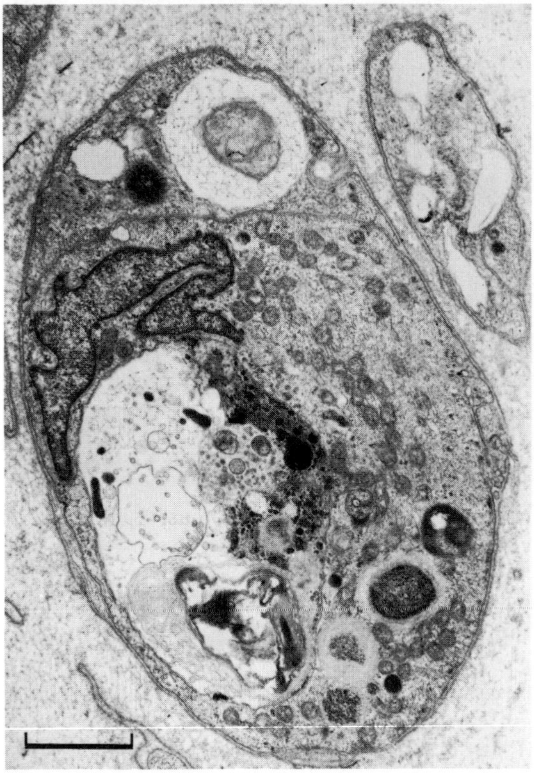

Fig. 18.55 Tangier disease. Schwann cell showing pleomorphic inclusion material. Bar = 1 μm.

Abetalipoproteinaemia (Bassen–Kornzweig disease)

The neurological manifestations of this autosomal recessive disorder are those of a spinocerebellar degeneration accompanied by symmetrical distal peripheral neuropathy and pigmentary retinal degeneration. Symptoms develop within the first two decades and are associated with intestinal malabsorption and abnormal erythrocytes (acanthocytes).

Detailed studies on the peripheral nervous system have not yet been reported. Demyelination and loss of axons in the peripheral nerves have been described, as has inconstant loss of anterior horn cells (Schwartz et al., 1963; Sobrevilla, Goodman and Kane, 1964; Dische and Porro, 1970). There is now good evidence that the neurological changes are secondary to severe vitamin E deficiency consequent upon the intestinal malabsorption (Muller, Lloyd and Wolff, 1983).

Other disorders of lipid metabolism

Peripheral neuropathy has been documented in a number of rare conditions, including cerebrotendinous xanthomatosis (cholestanolosis) (Ohnishi et al., 1979), Farber disease (Moser, 1983) and a multisystem degeneration associated with reduced tissue arachidonic acid (Dyck et al., 1981b). Histological or ultrastructural abnormalities are also evident in a variety of other disorders, usually without clinically evident peripheral neuropathy. These have been reviewed by Thomas (1984) and include G_{M1} and G_{M2} gangliosidosis, and Gaucher's, Niemann–Pick and Wolman's diseases.

Porphyria

Peripheral nerve involvement may occur in the hepatic porphyrias, either in the acute intermittent or variegate forms or in the much rarer hereditary coproporphyria. The features of the neuropathy are similar in all three disorders. Attacks with predominantly motor involvement occur which may be proximal, distal or generalized in distribution and which sometimes begin in the upper limbs or may be focal or asymmetrical. Sensory impairment may affect the trunk rather than the limbs and there can be associated autonomic involvement with abdominal pain, vomiting, tachycardia and hypertension. Accompanying behavioural changes are common. The attacks are frequently precipitated by drug ingestion, particularly barbiturates. Recovery is slow and often incomplete.

Although there were early suggestions that demyelination is an important aspect of the peripheral nerve pathology (Denny-Brown and Sciarra, 1945; Gibson and Goldberg, 1956), it is now generally agreed that the changes are predominantly those of a distal axonopathy of dying-back type (Cavanagh and Mellick, 1965; Sweeney, Pathak and Asbury, 1970). Some loss of anterior horn cells may occur, and chromatolysis may be observed in the cells of the coeliac ganglion (Hierons, 1957).

The hepatic porphyrias, which are all of autosomal dominant inheritance, are disorders of haem synthesis. In acute intermittent porphyria there is a deficiency of uroporphyrin I synthetase and of coproporphyrinogen oxidase in hereditary coproporphyria. The defect in variegate porphyria has not yet been established with certainty. The mechanism by which the accumulation of haem precursors or other secondary consequences of the metabolic change leads to neuronal dysfunction is not known.

Disorders with defective DNA repair

The pathology of *ataxia telangiectasia* is considered in Chapter 15. The manifestations predominantly involve the central nervous system but in this and in *xeroderma pigmentosum* there is a loss of larger sensory fibres in the peripheral nerves and a depletion of the larger dorsal root ganglion cells (Goodman et al., 1969; Thrush et al., 1974). Lewis (1977) has speculated on a possible relationship between the defective DNA repair known to exist in these disorders and the development of the neurological deficits.

Cockayne syndrome

This disorder comprises growth retardation, progeria, cutaneous photosensitivity, microcephaly, mental retardation, pigmentary retinopathy, deafness and ataxia. The cerebral changes are those of a leukodystrophy. Nerve biopsies have demonstrated that demyelination is a frequent finding (Moosa and Dubowitz, 1970; Vos et al., 1983). Granular lysosomal inclusions are present in Schwann cells (Grunnet, Zimmerman and Lewis, 1983).

Mucopolysaccharidoses

The mucopolysaccharidoses (see Chapter 12) are a group of inherited disorders in which glycosaminoglycans (mucopolysaccharides) are stored within lysosomes in various tissues. Entrapment neuropathies may be encountered in Hurler's and Scheie's syndromes, and Schwann cell inclusions, in the absence of clinically evident neuropathy, may be found in the Hurler, Hunter and Sanfilippo syndromes, and also in I-cell disease (see Thomas, 1984).

Primary hyperoxaluria

This encompasses two disorders of glyoxalate metabolism, the commoner of which is glycolic aciduria. Massive tissue deposition of oxalate occurs, including involvement of the peripheral nerves. The resulting neuropathy may be predominantly motor or mainly sensory. A combination of segmental demyelination and axonal loss has been described. Oxalate crystals are present in the walls of epineurial arterioles, in sensory and sympathetic ganglia and in peripheral nerve trunks. Crystals are also encountered within axons (Moorhead, Cooper and Timperley, 1975; Hall et al., 1976).

Hereditary motor and sensory neuropathy

The use of nerve conduction studies and nerve biopsy in conjunction with genetic analysis has, in recent years, brought a semblance of order to a confused group of conditions which included peroneal muscular atrophy (Charcot–Marie–Tooth disease), Dejerine–Sottas disease, the Roussy–Lévy syndrome, and a number of other eponymous conditions (Dyck and Lambert, 1968a, b; Harding and Thomas, 1980a). The term 'hereditary motor and sensory neuropathy' (HMSN) was introduced to cover this group of conditions (Thomas, Calne and Stewart, 1974; Dyck, 1975). Disorders with a clinical diagnosis of peroneal muscular atrophy are broadly divisible into cases of distal spinal muscular atrophy (Harding and Thomas, 1980b) and HMSN types I and II. Further categories include cases of congenital or childhood onset hypomyelinating neuropathy (HMSN III) and more complex forms.

Hereditary motor and sensory neuropathy type I (hypertrophic form of Charcot–Marie–Tooth disease) This is the commonest variant of Charcot–Marie–Tooth disease. The onset is commonly during the first or second decades with foot deformity or difficulty in walking. Examination reveals distal weakness and wasting in the lower limbs, tendon areflexia, minor distal sensory impairment and foot deformity, usually pes cavus. Slow advance takes place with later distal weakness, wasting and sensory impairment in the upper limbs. Some cases exhibit ataxia and upper limb postural tremor. They have been designated the Roussy–Lévy syndrome but are not genetically distinct. Scoliosis may be present. Nerve conduction velocity is usually markedly reduced.

Nerve biopsies demonstrate reduced numbers of myelinated nerve fibres and extensive segmental demyelination and remyelination. Intrafascicular area is increased. Hypertrophic changes with concentric Schwann cell proliferation are frequently encountered (Fig. 18.56 and see Fig. 18.29) these having led to the use of the term

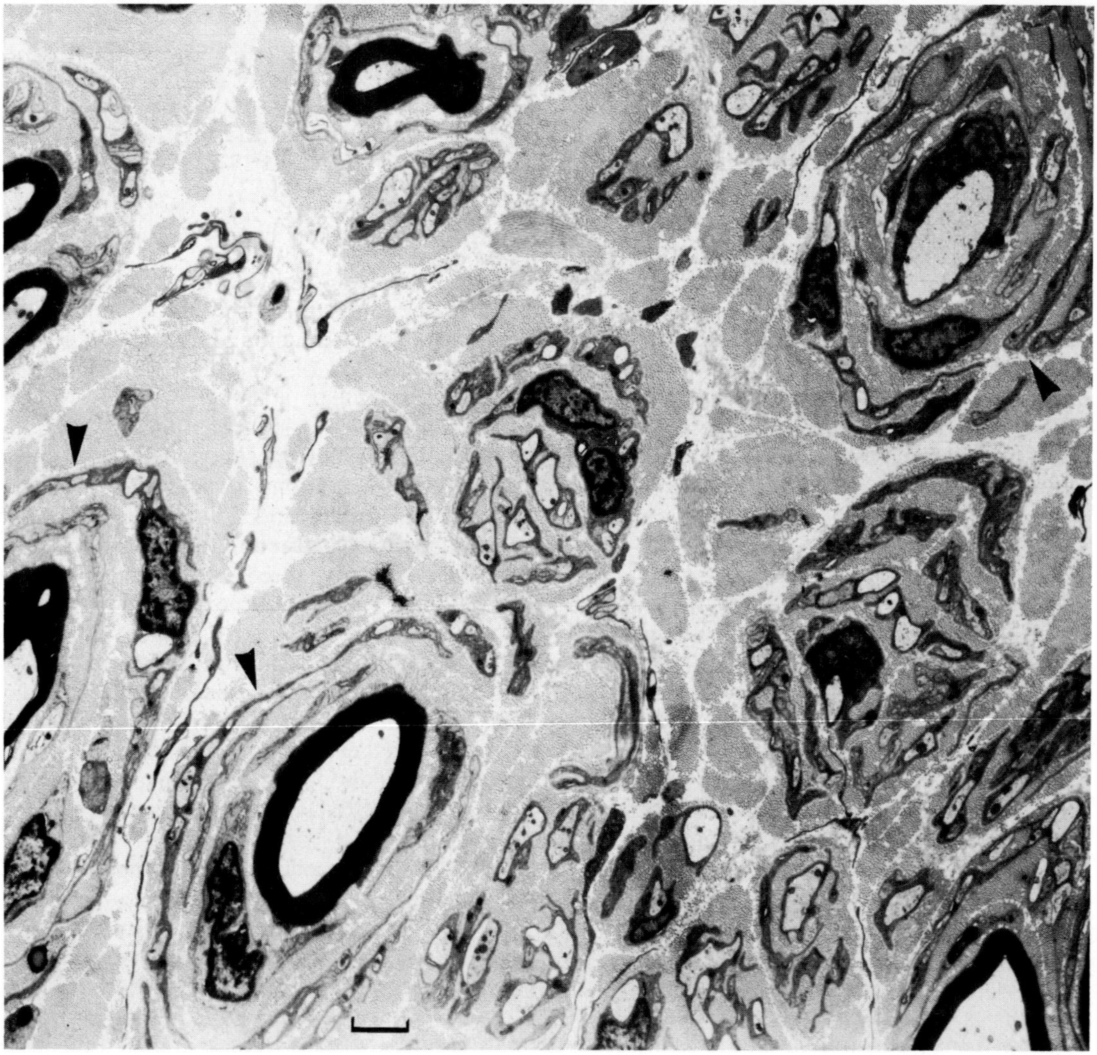

Fig. 18.56 Hereditary motor and sensory neuropathy, type 1. Electron micrograph showing myelinated axons surrounded by concentrically arranged proliferated Schwann cells (arrowed). A totally demyelinated axon is visible in the top right of the figure. Bar = 2 μm.

'hypertrophic form of Charcot–Marie–Tooth disease' (Dyck and Lambert, 1968a; Buchthal and Behse, 1977b; Low, McLeod and Prineas, 1978). These cases are probably equivalent to Hoffmann's syndrome in the older literature. Morphometric studies on sural nerve biopsies by Nukada, Dyck and Karnes (1983) have indicated that in HMSN I, transverse axonal area is reduced in relation to the length of the myelin spiral, suggesting a primary axonal defect, axonal atrophy leading to secondary segmental demyelination and remyelination and to the development of hypertrophic changes. The fact that the pathological changes are more marked peripherally supports this interpretation (Smith, 1980). Nerve grafting studies have yielded conflicting results. Aguayo et al. (1978b) found that Schwann cells in xenografts from patients with HMSN transplanted into immunosuppressed mice failed to myelinate axons as effectively as controls. Dyck, Lais and Low (1978), on the other hand, found no difference between grafts from such patients and controls.

Reports of complete post-mortem studies have been infrequent in recent years. Those recorded in the past are difficult to interpret in view of the fact that investigative techniques did not permit distinction between HMSN I and II or between the various types of chronic demyelinating neuropathy which give rise to hypertrophic changes. They have been collected by Thomas, Lascelles and Stewart (1975). The two autopsied cases reported by T.W. Smith et al. (1980) are acceptable as HMSN I. Both show loss of myelinated nerve fibres, prominent hypertrophic changes and endoneurial fibrosis maximal distally and greater in the lower limbs. Bundles of fibrillary astrocytes in the proximal portions of the spinal roots were an interesting finding. There was some loss of anterior horn and dorsal root ganglion cells without chromatolysis in surviving cells, together with degeneration in the posterior columns, particularly the gracile fasciculi.

The inheritance is usually autosomal dominant. Linkage with Duffy blood group has been established in some but not all families (Bird, Ott and Giblett, 1982; Guiloff et al., 1982), indicating that the responsible gene for such cases is on chromosome I near the centromere. Families exhibiting linkage to Duffy have been designated HMSN Ib. Those without linkage, HMSN Ia, tend to have slightly less severely reduced nerve conduction velocity (Bird et al., 1983). They may be equivalent to the intermediate form described by Davis, Bradley and Madrid (1978) in which the severity of the demyelination and the extent of the hypertrophic changes are less. Harding and Thomas (1980a) also have provided evidence of genetic heterogeneity from intrafamilial correlation of motor nerve conduction velocity within HMSN I. Cases of autosomal recessive inheritance have been described (Harding and Thomas, 1980c) in whom the condition tends to be more severe and nerve conduction velocity more markedly reduced. The appearances on nerve biopsy are similar to those of dominantly inherited cases.

Hereditary motor and sensory neuropathy type II (neuronal form of Charcot–Marie–Tooth disease) The genetic distinction of this form of peroneal muscular atrophy from HMSN I has been established by intrafamiliar correlation studies of nerve conduction velocity (Dyck and Lambert, 1968b; Buchthal and Behse, 1977a; Harding and Thomas, 1980a) and (from HMSN Ib) by the absence of linkage with Duffy blood group (Guiloff et al., 1982). Both autosomal dominant and autosomal recessive families have been described. The clinical features of the dominant cases resemble those of HMSN I but in general have a later onset, and less prominent upper limb involvement, ataxia, tendon areflexia and sensory loss. Associated skeletal deformity is also less evident, this presumably being related to the later age of onset. Autosomal recessive cases tend to be more severely affected, particularly a variety described by Ouvrier et al. (1981) which is possibly genetically distinct.

Dyck and Lambert (1968b) noted that in HMSN II, nerve conduction was either within normal limits or only modestly reduced. Nerve biopsies showed axonal loss with little demyelination. The variant was therefore termed the 'neuronal' form of Charcot–Marie–Tooth disease. Quantitative studies on sural nerve biopsies by Buchthal and Behse (1977b) showed fibre loss and regenerative clusters. Demyelination and hypertrophic changes were rare or absent. The number of unmyelinated axons was reduced in occasional nerves. The endoneurial space was normal or slightly increased.

Since hypertrophic changes were not described it is likely that the autopsied cases of peroneal muscular atrophy reported by Hughes and Brownell (1972) represented HMSN II. Chromatolysis and loss of anterior horn cells with numerous corpora amylacea in the anterior horns, loss of dorsal root ganglion cells and distally accentuated axonal loss in the spinal roots and peripheral nerves were described. The central nervous system was intact except for axonal loss in the dorsal columns considered to be secondary to loss of dorsal root ganglion cells. An autopsy study of a definite case of autosomal dominant HMSN II was reported by Dupuis, Brucher and Gonsette (1983). This showed some loss of anterior horn cells and relative preservation of the posterior columns and anterior and posterior spinal roots. Unfortunately, the peripheral nerves were not examined, but a sural nerve biopsy had shown a loss of myelinated fibres without hypertrophic changes.

Hereditary motor and sensory neuropathy, type III Cases of autosomal recessive hypertrophic neuropathy with onset in childhood and characterized by hypomyelination have been designated HMSN III (Dyck, 1975). It has been suggested that the term Dejerine–Sottas disease should be restricted to this form. The clinical features are of a sensorimotor neuropathy, often with associated ataxia and skeletal deformity and with markedly enlarged peripheral nerves, which has a more aggressive course than in HMSN I. Nerve conduction velocity is very severely reduced. Nerve biopsies show that myelin sheaths are abnormally thin on fibres of all diameters (Figs. 18.57 and 18.58) and that many fibres with an axon diameter in the normal myelinated range are amyelinate. Hypertrophic changes are prominent.

Some cases of hypomyelination neuropathy are congenital. Guzzetta, Ferrière and Lyon (1982) have demonstrated that these show a higher frequency of axons totally devoid of myelin sheaths than cases with onset later in childhood. They also show a higher frequency of 'onion bulbs' composed of double layers of basal lamina from which the Schwann cell processes have presumably disappeared (Fig. 18.59). It is

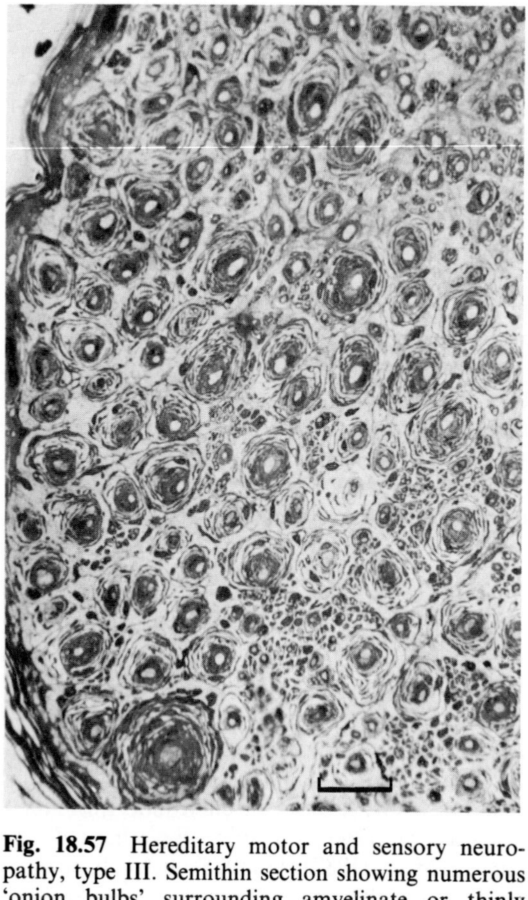

Fig. 18.57 Hereditary motor and sensory neuropathy, type III. Semithin section showing numerous 'onion bulbs' surrounding amyelinate or thinly myelinated fibres. Thionin and acridine orange. Bar = 20 μm.

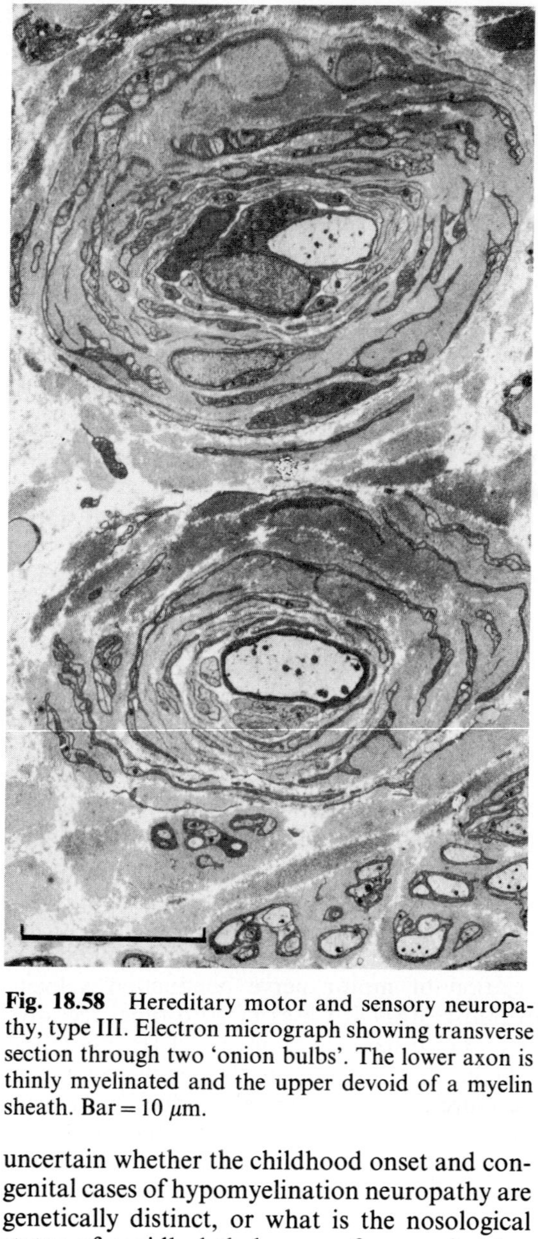

Fig. 18.58 Hereditary motor and sensory neuropathy, type III. Electron micrograph showing transverse section through two 'onion bulbs'. The lower axon is thinly myelinated and the upper devoid of a myelin sheath. Bar = 10 μm.

uncertain whether the childhood onset and congenital cases of hypomyelination neuropathy are genetically distinct, or what is the nosological status of rapidly lethal cases of congenital hypomyelination neuropathy in which 'onion bulbs' have not been present (Karch and Urich, 1975; Palix and Coignet, 1978).

Complex forms of HMSN Disorders with the clinical features of peroneal muscular atrophy combined with pyramidal signs or with optic atrophy, optic atrophy and deafness, or pigmentary retinal degeneration, have been described. The pathological changes in the peripheral

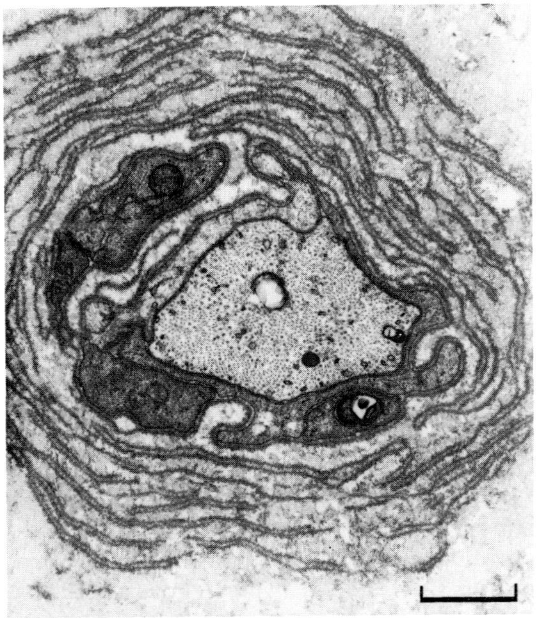

Fig. 18.59 Hereditary motor and sensory neuropathy, type III. Electron micrograph showing transverse section through an 'onion bulb' largely composed of concentrically arranged paired basal laminae unassociated with Schwann cell processes. Bar = 1 μm.

nervous system are so far poorly characterized, but have been reviewed by Dyck (1984).

Hereditary sensory and autonomic neuropathies

As for hereditary motor and sensory neuropathy, inherited neuropathies of unknown causation in which the major manifestations are related to sensory loss are also genetically heterogeneous. Autonomic involvement may be associated and it has therefore been proposed that this group of conditions should be categorized as hereditary sensory and autonomic neuropathy (HSAN) (Dyck et al., 1983).

Hereditary sensory and autonomic neuropathy, type I (dominantly inherited sensory neuropathy) This disorder was first adequately described by Denny-Brown (1951) under the title hereditary sensory radicular neuropathy. Symptoms begin in the second, third or fourth decades with sensory loss, particularly for pain and temperature sensibility, with initial involvement distally in the lower limbs and later in the upper limbs. Spontaneous pain may be a troublesome feature, and neuropathic ulceration and atrophy may develop. Slight distal muscle weakness and wasting are often evident. There is distal anhidrosis in the limbs but autonomic function is otherwise preserved. Inheritance is by an autosomal dominant gene.

Peripheral nerve biopsies have shown axonal loss without significant demyelination. This affects unmyelinated and small myelinated fibres to a greater extent than large fibres and is accentuated distally in the limbs (Dyck and Ohta, 1975). Dorsal root ganglion cells are lost (Denny-Brown, 1951), with a depletion in the number of fibres entering the spinal cord, particularly in Lissauer's tract (Fig. 18.60).

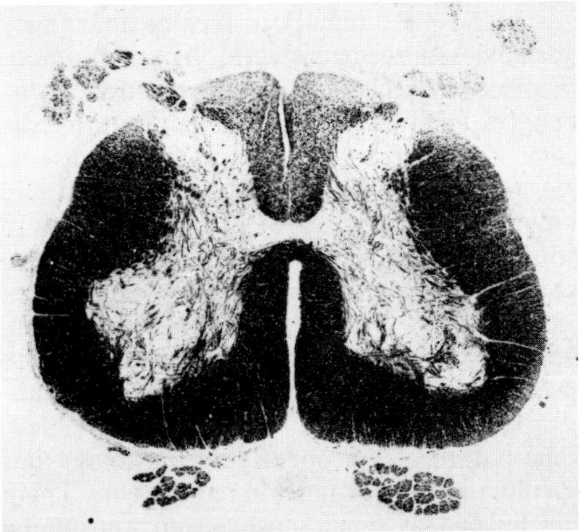

Fig. 18.60 Hereditary sensory and autonomic neuropathy, type I: lumbar cord. The degeneration is greatest in Lissauer's tract and slightly less in the posterior root zone. The middle root zone is relatively intact.

Hereditary sensory and autonomic neuropathy, type II In this variety, the neuropathy is congenital and is of autosomal recessive inheritance. There is distal sensory loss for all modalities. The disorder is slowly progressive and distal mutilating changes are frequent. Demonstrable autonomic involvement is restricted to anhidrosis and to the occurrence of gustatory facial sweating. Sural nerve biopsy has shown profound fascicular atrophy and severe loss of myelinated fibres of all sizes with a relative preservation of unmyelinated axons (Ohta et al., 1973; Nukada, Pollock and Haas, 1982). Giant vacuolated fibroblasts may be prominent in the endoneurium (Asbury, Cox and Baringer, 1971), although they are not confined to this condition.

Sural nerve fascicles from patients with HSN II grafted into the sciatic nerve of mice showed normal myelination of regenerating axons by the donor Schwann cells (Dyck et al., 1979). This indicates that the absence of myelinated axons in patients with this disorder is likely to be related to a failure of axonal development or axonal degeneration *in utero* rather than the operation of any Schwann cell abnormality.

Hereditary sensory and autonomic neuropathy, type III (Riley–Day syndrome, familial dysautonomia) This disorder is also recessively inherited and congenital, and occurs most often on an Ashkenazi Jewish background. The clinical features include difficulty in feeding in infancy associated with recurrent vomiting and pulmonary infections and a variety of autonomic disturbances such as diminished lacrimation, defective temperature regulation, episodic hypertension and postural hypotension, skin blotching and excessive sweating in response to emotional stimuli. There is tendon areflexia and loss of pain sensibility present from birth. Fungiform papillae on the tongue fail to develop. Kyphoscoliosis may be present and large fibre sensory modalities become affected in older subjects.

The nature of the underlying pathology has been illuminated by studies in recent years. There is an aplasia of small sensory and autonomic neurons affecting the sympathetic system to a greater extent than the parasympathetic, but with a slow continued postnatal neuronal degeneration. Sensory nerve biopsies have shown a loss of small myelinated axons (Aguayo, Nair and Bray, 1971) with a lesser depletion of larger myelinated axons. The number of neurons is reduced in sensory ganglia and Lissauer's tract is hypoplastic (Pearson et al., 1978). Sympathetic ganglia have a markedly reduced population of neurons and there is a less severe reduction of preganglionic neurons in the spinal cord (Pearson and Pytel, 1978a). Parasympathetic ganglia are variably affected (Pearson and Pytel, 1978b). Smaller anterior horn cells may also be depleted (Dyck et al., 1978b).

Hereditary sensory and autonomic neuropathy, type IV (congenital sensory neuropathy with anhidrosis) Of autosomal recessive inheritance, this rare disorder is first recognized within a few months of birth by failure to thrive, retarded motor development and unexplained pyrexia. Affected children fail to respond normally to painful stimuli. Cutaneous ulceration, bone fractures and sometimes self-mutilation may occur. Depressed tendon reflexes and a widespread loss of pain, temperature and, to a lesser extent, tactile sensation, are demonstrable. Sweating is absent or considerably reduced. Swanson, Buchan and Alvord (1965) reported an absence of small dorsal root ganglion cells and of small fibres in the dorsal roots, and also of Lissauer's tract. The spinal tract of the fifth cranial nerve was small. The virtual absence of unmyelinated axons in peripheral sensory nerves was confirmed by Goebel, Veit and Dyck (1980).

Congenital indifference to pain Cases with a universal or widespread lack of response to noxious stimuli who fail to show clinical evidence of neuropathy and in whom non-quantitative studies on the peripheral nervous system or examination of the central nervous system have failed to reveal abnormalities have been categorized under titles such as congenital indifference to pain or asymbolia for pain. The use of quantitative morphometric studies has now demonstrated that at least some of these cases are examples of sensory neuropathy. In one case studied by Dyck et al. (1983), there was a severe decrease in the number of sural nerve A delta-fibres and a small reduction in C-fibres. Abnormalities of sudomotor function were demonstrable. A similar case was reported by Low, Burke and McLeod (1978). The preservation of large calibre sensory fibres means that sensory nerve action potentials recorded by standard techniques are normal.

Hereditary sensory neuropathy with spastic paraplegia A severe sensory neuropathy of probable autosomal recessive inheritance has been described by Cavanagh et al. (1979). Onset was in childhood and the disorder gave rise to a severe mutilating acropathy. Autopsy in one case showed a severe loss of dorsal root ganglion cells, and loss of myelinated fibres in the peripheral nerves and dorsal columns. A sural nerve biopsy in another case demonstrated a profound loss of unmyelinated axons and of myelinated axons of all diameters.

Hereditary pressure-sensitive neuropathy

The occurrence of recurrent peripheral nerve palsies often related to mechanical compression but frequently with minimal trauma characterizes this dominantly inherited disorder. Nerve conduction studies show evidence of an underlying generalized neuropathy. The condition has been reviewed by Meier and Moll (1982).

Behse et al. (1972) first demonstrated the presence of focal regions of hypermyelination, which were termed tomaculi by Madrid and Bradley (1975) from their resemblance to sausages in teased fibre preparations. Ultrastructural studies indicate that in the swellings there are excessive numbers of myelin lamellae for axonal diameter. The most important mechanism for this is the formation of redundant folds and loops of myelin (Figs. 18.61 and 18.62, and see Fig. 18.31) often resulting in an asymmetric expansion of the sheath. Branching of lamellae has also been described (Madrid and Bradley, 1975), as have other types of abnormality, including transnodal myelination. Redundant myelin loop formation may occur during normal development with subsequent elimination by remodelling. Possibly this fails to occur in this condition (Meier and Moll, 1982). Nerve biopsies also show evidence of paranodal and segmental demyelination and remyelination, and axonal loss.

Familial recurrent brachial plexus neuropathy (Jacob, Andermann and Robb, 1961) may be a separate entity, although tomaculi are also found in the peripheral nerves in such patients (Bradley et al., 1975).

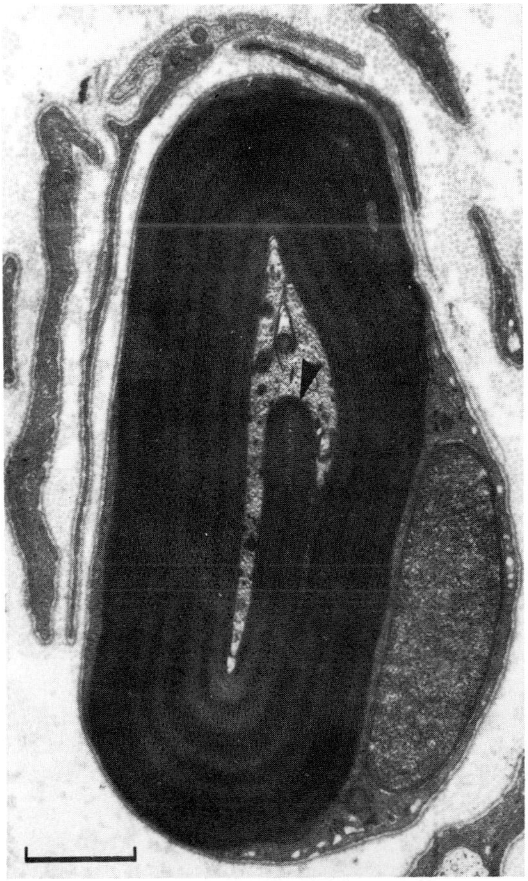

Fig. 18.61 Tomaculous neuropathy. Electron micrograph of transverse section through a myelin swelling showing folding of myelin lamellae (arrowed). Bar = 1 μm.

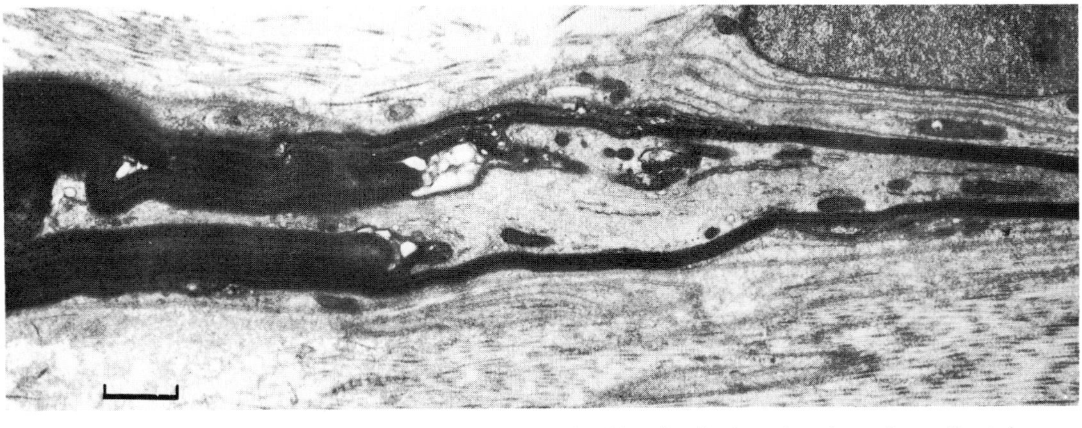

Fig. 18.62 Tomaculous neuropathy. Electron micrograph of longitudinal section through myelinated nerve fibre showing folding and overlapping of redundant myelin lamellae in region of thickened myelin. Bar = 1 μm.

Giant axonal neuropathy

Berg, Rosenberg and Asbury (1972) originally recognized an unusual distal sensorimotor neuropathy which develops in childhood, characterized by the presence of segmental swellings on axons. The condition is probably of autosomal recessive inheritance. Affected children may also show signs of central nervous system involvement, including optic atrophy, abnormal eye movements, nystagmus and pyramidal signs in the limbs, and most have abnormally kinky hair. Asbury et al. (1972b) and later writers have shown that the swellings contain increased numbers of neurofilaments (Fig. 18.63). Focal demyelination occurs in relation to the swellings and minor hypertrophic changes may be observable. A concomitant proliferation of filaments within Schwann cells, endothelial cells, perineurial cells and endoneurial and endomysial fibroblasts (Prineas et al., 1976; Koch et al., 1977) suggests a generalized disorder of cytoplasmic intermediate filaments. The giant axonal swellings resemble those which occur in a number of toxic neuropathies, such as those produced by hexacarbons and acrylamide.

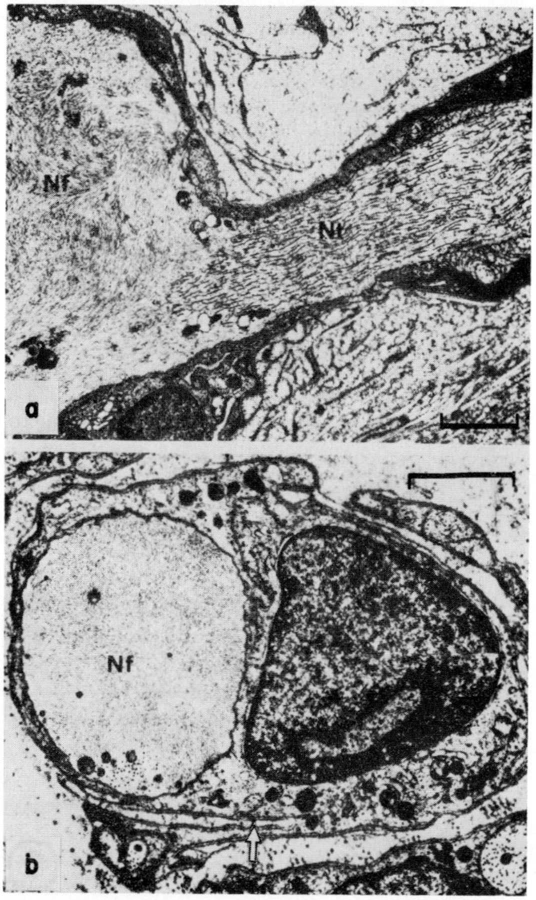

Fig. 18.63 Giant axonal neuropathy. Electron micrographs showing (**a**) longitudinal and (**b**) transverse sections through axonal neurofilamentous swellings. Nf, neurofilaments; Nt, neurotubules. Bar = 2 μm. (Reproduced, with permission, from Asbury et al., 1972.)

Chorea-acanthocytosis syndrome

Adult onset chorea without significant dementia is the salient feature of this disorder, but affected individuals may also show depressed tendon reflexes, and variable neurogenic muscle atrophy and sensory loss in the legs. There is loss of larger myelinated fibres in sensory nerves (Ohnishi et al., 1981).

Chediak-Higashi disease

This autosomal recessive childhood disorder causes defective hair pigmentation, pancytopenia and mental retardation, together with an increased incidence of infection and lymphoreticular malignancy (Blume and Wolff, 1972). It may be accompanied by neuropathy, the distinguishing feature of which is the presence of giant lysosomes in Schwann cells (Lockman, Kennedy and White, 1967).

Neuropathy in hereditary ataxia

The hereditary ataxias are considered in Chapter 15. Loss of larger dorsal root ganglion cells with consequent depletion of larger myelinated fibres in the peripheral nerves occurs in Friedreich's ataxia (McLeod, 1971). There is some segmental demyelination, considered by Dyck and Lais (1973) to be secondary to axonal atrophy. There is also slight loss of anterior horn cells.

Depletion of larger sensory fibres in the peripheral nerves also occurs in other hereditary ataxias, including Behr's syndrome (Thomas, Workman and Thage, 1984), olivopontocerebellar atrophy (McLeod and Evans, 1981), and a dominantly inherited syndrome with parkinsonism and ataxia (Byrne, Thomas and Zilkha, 1982).

Other conditions

Chronic progressive external ophthalmoplegia consists of a heterogeneous group of conditions that includes oculopharyngeal myopathy, the Kearns–Sayre syndrome and mitochondrial myopathy. Demyelinating neuropathy has been recorded in the Kearns–Sayre syndrome (Groothuis et al., 1980), and a neuropathy characterized by axonal degeneration in association with mitochondrial myopathy (Peyronnard et al., 1980). Peripheral nerve involvement may also occur in Leigh's disease (see Chapter 13); demyelination and axonal loss have been described (Dunn and Dolman, 1969). Inclusions are demonstrable in Schwann cells, histiocytes and endothelial cells in peripheral nerve in ceroid lipofuscinosis (see Chapter 12), both in the childhood variants (Batten's disease) and the later onset cases (Kufs' disease). They have the same appearance as the intraneural inclusions (see Thomas, 1984).

Inflammatory neuropathies

Acute idiopathic inflammatory polyneuropathy (Guillain–Barré syndrome)

The precise limits of acute inflammatory polyneuropathy (AIP) are unsettled, but it is generally accepted (Asbury, 1981) that it is an acute or subacute monophasic illness which gives rise to predominant motor involvement. The distribution of the weakness may be proximal, distal or generalized. Assisted ventilation may be necessary. Facial weakness is frequent and bulbar involvement may occur. Papilloedema is observed in a small proportion of cases. Distal sensory symptoms with tingling paraesthesiae and sensory loss are less obtrusive than muscle weakness. The tendon reflexes are depressed or lost. Autonomic abnormalities may develop, including atonic weakness of the bladder, cardiac dysrhythmias, hypertension or postural hypotension, and also distal anhidrosis. The cerebrospinal fluid protein content is characteristically elevated, although not always in the early stages. Nerve conduction velocity is reduced, but this may only be detectable proximally, from F wave latencies, in the early stages of the disease. Conduction block is demonstrable, as are signs of denervation. Evolution to maximal severity may occur rapidly within days, or more gradually over 2–4 weeks.

The earlier study of Haymaker and Kernohan (1949) emphasized oedema of the spinal roots as a prominent early finding, and they considered that invasion by inflammatory cells and Schwann cell proliferation were secondary to myelin breakdown. Other writers have not been impressed by inflammatory changes (Scheinker, 1947). The extensive autopsy study performed by Asbury, Arnason and Adams (1969) concluded that inflammatory infiltration, not only in the spinal roots but throughout the peripheral nervous system, was a regular initial event and that widespread demyelination with variable associated axonal degeneration was a consistent subsequent feature. Ultrastructural studies (Wiśniewski et al., 1969; Carpenter, 1972; Prineas, 1972) have confirmed invasion of the peripheral nerves by mononuclear cells and have demonstrated stripping of myelin off the axons by macrophages. Focal lysis of myelin has also been observed. Schwann cell proliferation ensues as a prelude to remyelination. Changes in the central nervous system are restricted to chromatolysis of anterior horn cells and fibre degeneration in the posterior columns in some cases, considered to be secondary to axonal destruction in the dorsal roots and spinal ganglia.

The causation of AIP is still not established, but current views have been discussed by Leibowitz and Hughes (1983). Approximately two-thirds of patients have a history of an antecedent infection within the preceding 2–3 weeks. The range of organisms implicated is wide, including cytomegalovirus, Epstein–Barr virus and mycoplasma, but most commonly the disorder follows relatively trivial upper respiratory or gastrointestinal infections. It may also follow immunizing procedures, such as occurred in relation to the influenza A/New Jersey vaccination programme in the USA in 1976 (Schonberger et al., 1981). It may follow surgical operations (Arnason and Asbury, 1968) or treatment with hyperthermia. There is also a probable association with Hodgkin's disease. No association with particular HLA antigens has been established.

Studies of cell-mediated immunity show that circulating lymphocytes are sensitized to peripheral nerve antigens, but the precise antigen has not been identified. The histological appearances suggest a cell-mediated process. Nevertheless there are also indications that humoral factors may be implicated. Circulating antibodies to nervous tissues are demonstrable, but again the nature of the responsible antigens is uncertain. Serum from patients with AIP, if added to myelinated tissue cultures or if injected intraneurally, will produce demyelination. It is not known, however, whether such effects are implicated in the production of the demyelinating lesions in the human disease.

Parallels have been drawn with the animal disease, experimental allergic neuritis (EAN). Inoculation of animals with homologous or heterologous peripheral nerve together with Freund's adjuvant gives rise to an acute demyelinating neuropathy after 2–3 weeks (Waksman and Adams, 1955), with histological features similar to those of AIP. The nerves are invaded by mononuclear cells and myelin is stripped off the axons by macrophages (Lampert, 1969) (see Figs. 18.25 and 18.26). EAN can be induced by purified myelin P_2 protein, and is associated with the development of both cell-mediated hypersensitivity and antibodies to P_2 (Hughes et al., 1981). A further animal model has been produced in rabbits by repeated inoculation with galactocerebroside (Saida et al., 1981). Serum containing antigalactocerebroside antibodies from such animals will produce demyelination if injected intraneurally into other animals.

Chronic relapsing and chronic progressive inflammatory polyneuropathy

Cases exist with features similar to those of acute inflammatory polyneuropathy except that they pursue a chronic relapsing (Thomas et al., 1969) or chronic progressive (Dyck et al., 1975) course. The chronic relapsing cases have an association with the HLA-A1-B8,-DRw3 haplotype (Adams et al., 1979).

As for AIP, focal inflammatory infiltrates are demonstrable, particularly in the chronic progressive cases, together with widespread segmental demyelination. Prominent hypertrophic changes may be present, the hallmark of a chronic demyelinating neuropathy.

Leprous neuropathy

Infection with *Mycobacterium leprae* produces manifestations predominantly in the skin, mucous membranes and peripheral nerves. The early stages of the infective process are uncertain but prolonged exposure is usually necessary. After a lengthy incubation period, the initial manifestations are generally cutaneous lesions or, less commonly, peripheral neuropathy. Classification of leprosy depends on differences in the host–parasite relationships, which cover a spectrum from individuals with little cellular immunity (lepromatous leprosy) in whom the organisms proliferate in the infected cells with a scanty inflammatory reaction to individuals with high cellular immunity (tuberculoid leprosy) who display a vigorous inflammatory response and in whom few organisms are demonstrable. Between these two polar forms are borderline or dimorphous cases which have been subdivided into borderline leptomatous, borderline intermediate and borderline tuberculoid (Ridley and Jopling, 1966). There is also an indeterminate group comprised of early cases which do not show the characteristic features of the polar types. They may evolve towards either. The borderline cases tend to be unstable and to progress towards one or other of the polar types. The immunological aspects of these various forms of leprosy were examined by Turk and Waters (1971). Typically, the lepromin skin test is positive in tuberculoid leprosy and negative in the lepromatous form.

Lepromatous leprosy Clinical involvement occurs late in the evolution of lepromatous leprosy. Entry is probably through the skin, and spread of the bacilli throughout the body is now considered to be haematogenous. A symmetrical polyneuropathy develops. The distribution is initially distal in the limbs but also affects other sites such as the ears, nose, supraorbital regions and the skin over the zygomatic arches. This pattern depends upon temperature gradients, as leprosy bacilli proliferate more readily at lower temperatures (Sabin and Ebner, 1969). Sensory loss initially affects temperature and pain sensation and is accompanied by anhidrosis. The loss of pain sensibility frequently leads to mutilating lesions because of tissue destruction from unheeded injury. The peripheral nerves are thickened and this may lead to the occurrence of superimposed entrapment neuropathies.

The histological changes have been examined by Job and Desikan (1968), Job (1970), Pedley et al. (1980) and others, and have been reviewed by Weddell and Pearson (1975), including the ultrastructural appearances. It is clear that the Schwann cells become colonized by the bacilli at an early stage, particularly those associated with unmyelinated axons (Fig. 18.64), where they are

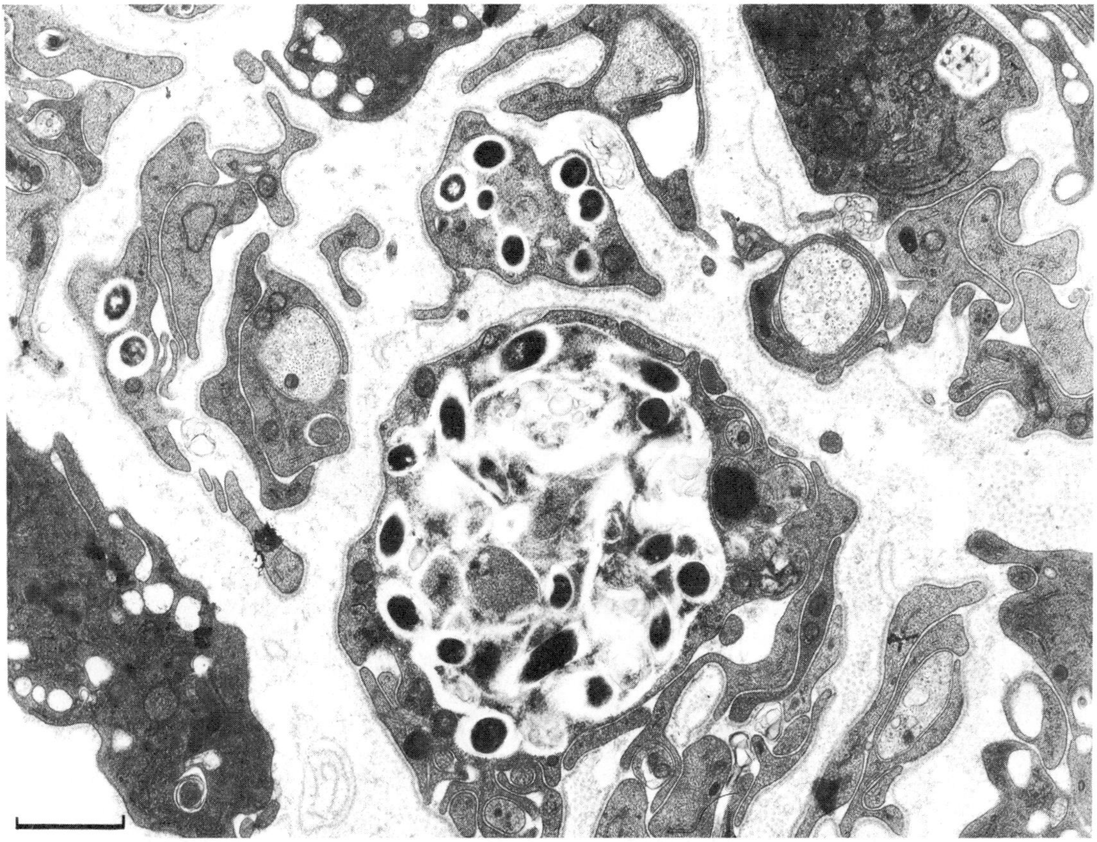

Fig. 18.64 Borderline lepromatous leprosy. Electron micrograph of Schwann cells, associated with unmyelinated axons, containing multiple leprosy bacilli. Bar = 1 μm.

present in large numbers, as they are in macrophages. Bacilli are also seen in fibroblasts, capillary endothelial cells and perineurial cells, and rarely in axons (Yoshizumi and Asbury, 1974). When detected in axons they are usually surrounded by double membranes, suggesting their invagination by a tongue of adaxonal Schwann cell cytoplasm. In macrophages, degenerating bacteria are surrounded by a clear space (Fig. 18.65), which may enlarge to form large vesicles, the vacuolated 'lepra cells' seen by light microscopy. Both demyelination and axon loss occur, the latter initially predominantly involving unmyelinated and small myelinated fibres. The precise mechanism of the axonal damage is not clear. The endoneurium is oedematous in the early stages, this being followed by dense fibrosis. The perineurium is also involved, and is invaded by foamy macrophages. Destruction of perineurial cells occurs, abolishing the normal perifascicular barrier (Fig. 18.66).

Tuberculoid leprosy In contrast to the lepromatous form, this tends to pursue a more benign and less progressive course. Localized anaesthetic skin lesions occur, the margins of the sensory loss being sharply defined and coinciding with the cutaneous changes. Such lesions are also anhidrotic. Local cutaneous nerves are often irregularly thickened and focal intraneural 'cold abscesses' may develop. The pattern of involvement in tuberculoid leprosy may depend upon the bacilli being restricted to the region of their portal of entry.

The basic pathological lesion in tuberculoid leprosy is an inflammatory granuloma (Fig. 18.67a), composed of epithelioid cells (macrophages), multinucleate giant cells and lymphocytes, the latter usually being situated at the periphery. Bacilli are very rarely discernible. Such granulomas are found mainly in cutaneous and subcutaneous nerves in proximity to the skin lesion and are associated with severe disorgani-

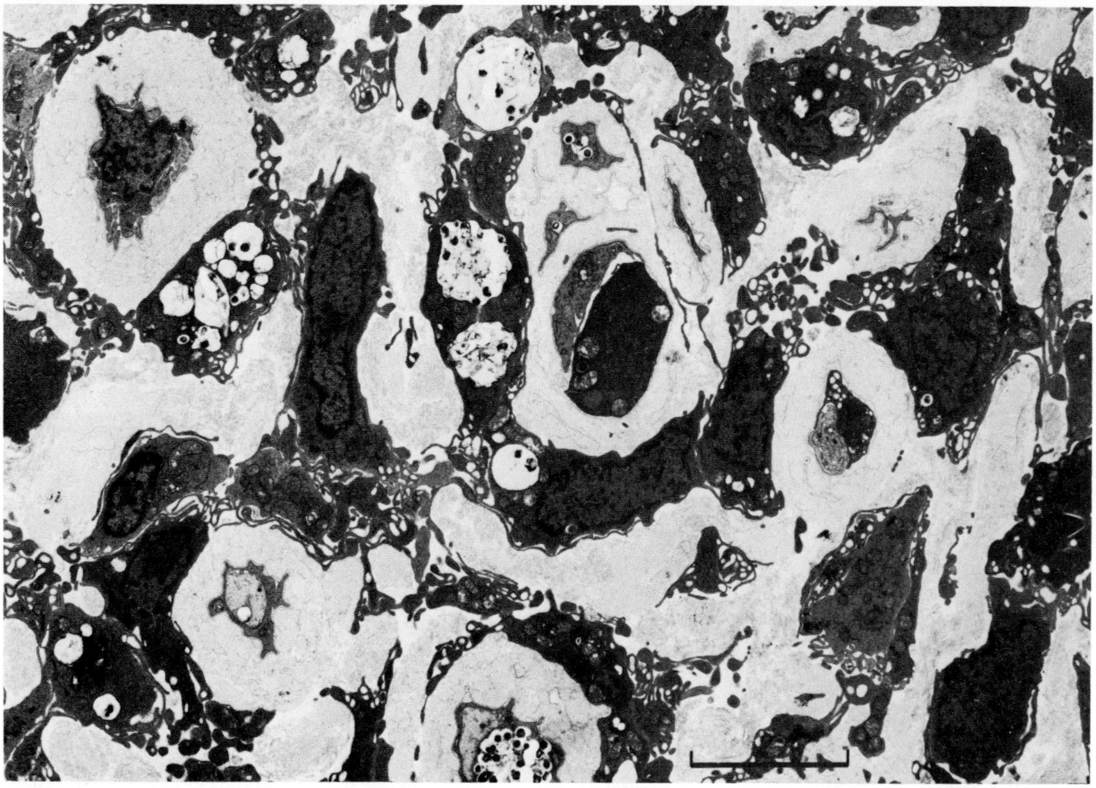

Fig. 18.65 Borderline lepromatous leprosy. Electron micrograph showing network of vacuolated endoneurial macrophages containing leprosy bacilli. Bar = 5 μm.

zation of the neural architecture. Some fascicles become totally destroyed with few surviving nerve fibres; other neighbouring fascicles may be relatively normal. Central necrosis may occur in the granulomas (Fig. 18.67b), leading to the formation of caseous abscesses. In the late stages of the disease there is extensive endoneurial fibrosis with few recognizable normal neural components. During the process, the perineurium becomes thickened and the perineurial cells are frequently destroyed. The fibrotic reaction often involves the epineurial and surrounding connective tissues.

Borderline (dimorphous leprosy) Here the histological features are variable, and both lepromatous and tuberculoid features are present, sometimes within different regions of the same nerve. The precise features define whether the cases are classifiable as intermediate, borderline lepromatous or borderline tuberculoid. Cases of so-called pure neural leprosy are usually of the borderline category on histological criteria. For cases of indeterminate leprosy, there are minimal inflammatory infiltrates in cutaneous nerves; small numbers of bacteria are detectable.

'Reversal reactions' are important in the production of neural damage. These are seen in borderline and tuberculoid leprosy. There is a sudden appearance of large numbers of bacilli and the occurrence of new lesions. Existing lesions become acutely inflamed. The process, which may be precipitated by treatment, subsides, but leaves epithelioid granulomas and endoneurial scarring in its wake. In erythema nodosum leprosum, arteritic lesions from involvement of the vasa nervorum may lead to neural damage (Karat et al., 1969).

Transfer of human leprosy to immunosuppressed mice has confirmed that Schwann cell colonization is an early event in peripheral nerve involvement (Rees et al., 1967). Histological changes mimicking human leprous neuropathy have not been reproduced. This has been

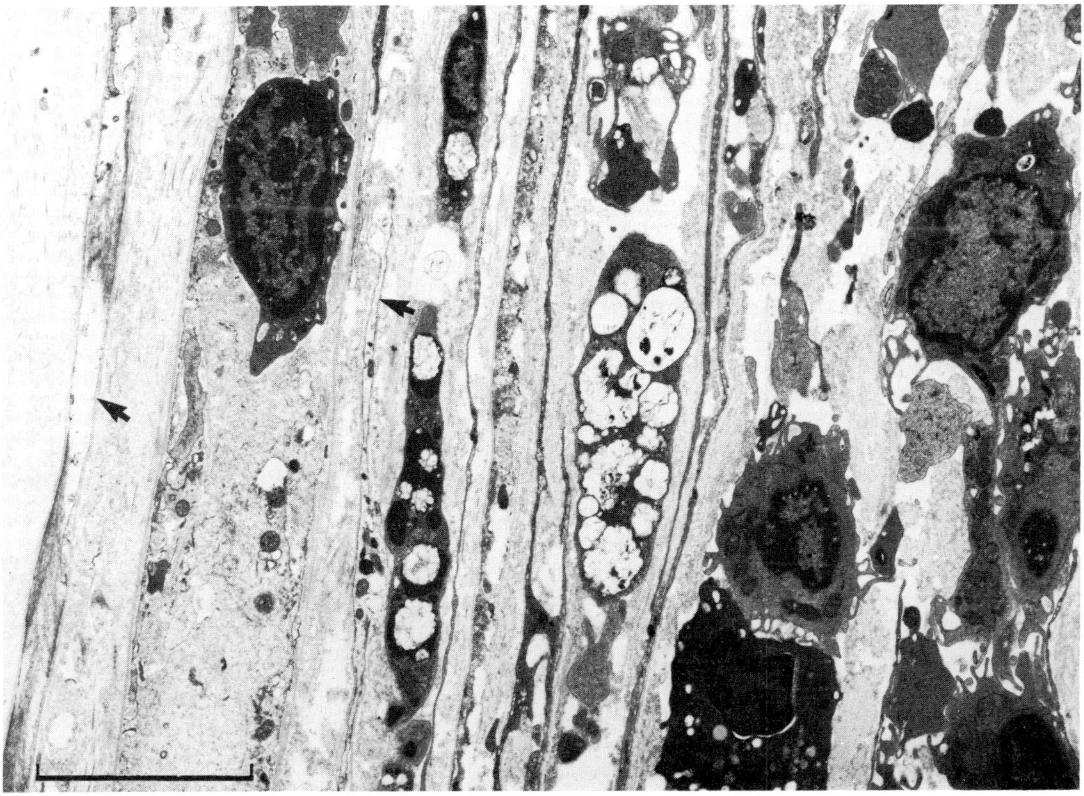

Fig. 18.66 Borderline lepromatous leprosy. Electron micrograph through perineurium which is infiltrated with vacuolated macrophages containing leprosy bacilli. Some of the perineurial cells are necrotic; others have disappeared, leaving paired basal laminae (arrowed). Bar = 5 μm.

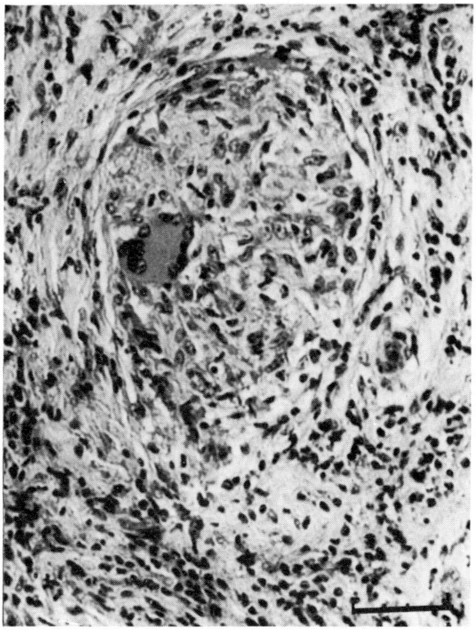

(a)

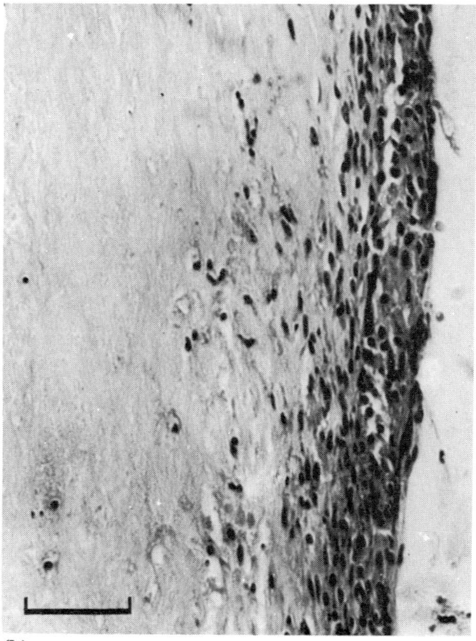

(b)

Fig. 18.67 Tuberculoid leprosy. (**a**) Epithelioid and giant cell granuloma. (**b**) Necrotic fascicle with rim of granulation tissue. Haematoxylin and eosin. Bars = 50 μm.

achieved by injection of the armadillo with human *M. leprae*, the features of which closely resemble lepromatous leprosy in man (Yoshizumi, Kirchheimer and Asbury, 1974).

Neuropathy in sarcoidosis

Peripheral nerve involvement in sarcoidosis may occur on a background of more widespread multisystem involvement or pathology may be substantially confined to the peripheral nerves. The most characteristic pattern of involvement is a fluctuating 'polyneuritis cranialis' with the seventh nerve being most often affected. Either in association with cranial nerve lesions or independently, a multifocal neuropathy affecting the limbs and trunk or, less commonly, a generalized distal symmetrical polyneuropathy may be encountered. The latter may sometimes be of relatively acute onset, resembling the Guillain–Barré syndrome.

The mechanisms involved in the production of peripheral nerve damage are poorly understood. Nerve biopsies in most instances have failed to reveal specific changes (see Matthews, 1984). Sometimes multiple endoneurial granulomas have been detected (Nemni et al., 1981) or a granulomatous periangiitis affecting endoneurial arterioles (Vital et al., 1982). A combination of demyelination and axonal loss has been observed.

Sensory perineuritis

A single report (Asbury, Picard and Baringer, 1972a) described two cases of a patchy lower limb sensory neuropathy with pain as a prominent symptom. Tinel's sign was produced by tapping affected nerves. The pathological changes were those of a chronic inflammatory cellular reaction and fibrosis largely restricted to the perineurium with variable fibre loss in the component fascicles of the nerve. Some giant cells were present. It was not considered to represent tuberculoid leprosy or sarcoidosis and no vasculitic lesions were detected. The appearances are similar to those which were observed in the nerves from cases of the toxic neuromuscular syndrome related to adulterated rapeseed oil reported from Spain (Ricoy et al., 1983).

Chagas disease

This disorder is the result of infection with *Trypanosoma cruzi* and is endemic in Brazil. An acute septicaemic stage usually occurs in childhood. The chronic state is the result of the destruction of ganglion cells in the peripheral autonomic system which has occurred in the acute stage. This may be the consequence of the liberation of a neurotoxin from the parasites. The main effects are on the parasympathetic innervation of the heart, gut and, sometimes, the genitourinary tract. The common gut lesions are megaoesophagus and megacolon, less commonly of other parts of the alimentary tract. The nature of the lesions of the myenteric plexus has been described by Smith (1967).

Herpes zoster ganglionitis

This is considered in Chapter 7.

Paraneoplastic neuropathy

Carcinomatous neuropathy

The occurrence of peripheral neuropathy not related to direct invasion by malignant cells was first clearly recognized by Denny-Brown (1948). The clinical features of non-metastatic carcinomatous neuropathy have recently been reviewed by Henson and Urich (1982) and McLeod (1984). It is most often encountered in relation to bronchial carcinoma, and can be subdivided into a subacute sensory form and examples of sensorimotor neuropathy. The latter are further subdivisible into acute and subacute or chronic forms; relapsing cases also occur (McLeod, 1984). These are all symmetrical polyneuropathies and are usually distal in distribution. Direct invasion of spinal roots, the limb girdle plexuses or isolated peripheral nerves by carcinoma may occur. The malignant cells penetrate the perineurium and tend to accumulate in a subperineurial position or as sheets in the endoneurial septa.

In cases of non-metastatic subacute sensory neuropathy (Croft et al., 1965; Horwich et al., 1977) there is a loss of fibres in sensory roots and peripheral nerves. This may be virtually total in sensory nerves, and partial in mixed nerves related to the presence of preserved motor fibres. Changes in anterior horn cells and anterior roots are only mild. In the dorsal root ganglia there is extensive depletion of ganglion cells and a proliferation of capsule cells with the formation of residual nodules of Nageotte (Fig. 18.68a). Peri-

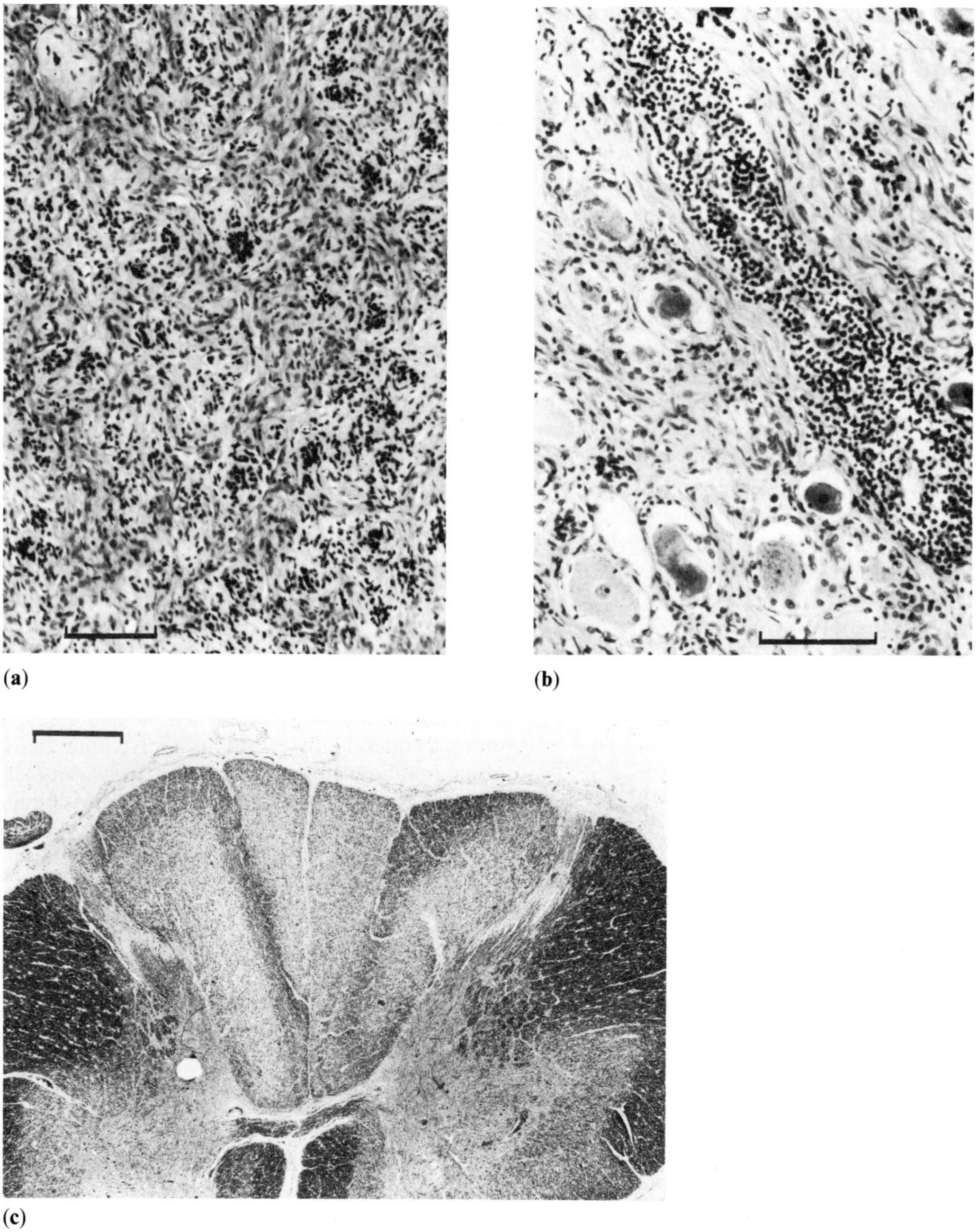

Fig. 18.68 Carcinomatous sensory neuropathy. (**a**) Almost total loss of neurons in a posterior root ganglion and replacement by nodules of Nageotte. Haematoxylin and eosin. Bar = 100 μm. (**b**) Perivascular lymphocytic infiltration in posterior root ganglion. Haematoxylin and eosin. Bar = 100 μm. (**c**) Degeneration of posterior columns. Klüver–Barrera. Bar = 1 mm.

vascular lymphocytic infiltrates are found in most affected ganglia (Fig. 18.68b). These usually do not extend into the roots. The cervical and lumbar sensory ganglia are more severely affected than are those in the thoracic region, and a somewhat random involvement of the ganglia is not uncommon. Single ganglia sometimes escape from an otherwise diffuse destruction. The posterior columns show secondary axon degeneration (Fig. 18.68c). Concomitant inflammatory lesions elsewhere in the nervous system may be associated with carcinomatous ganglioradiculitis including limbic encephalitis, a diffuse encephalomyelitis or a restricted myelitis (see Chapter 13). The responsible tumour is usually oat cell bronchial carcinoma.

In patients with carcinomatous sensorimotor neuropathy, the predominant change in the peripheral nerves is axonal loss although there may be some associated segmental demyelination (Croft, Urich and Wilkinson, 1967). There are sometimes sparse inflammatory infiltrates. Loss of dorsal root ganglion cells occurs, but not to the extent seen in carcinomatous sensory ganglioradiculitis, together with degeneration in the posterior columns. There is some degeneration of anterior horn cells.

The mechanism of non-metastatic carcinomatous neuropathy is not understood. Possibilities have been discussed by Henson and Urich (1982) and McLeod (1984). The pathological changes which occur in the dorsal root ganglia in cases of sensory neuropathy (see below) suggest that the mechanism in such cases may differ from that (or those) operating in cases of sensorimotor neuropathy.

Neuropathies related to lymphoreticular proliferative disorders

Lymphoma The cranial nerves and spinal nerve roots may be directly invaded in cases where there is involvement of the leptomeninges, as may occur in the limb girdle plexuses or individual peripheral nerve trunks (Jellinger and Radiaszkiewicz, 1976). Spinal roots may be damaged by compression from meningeal deposits or vertebral collapse. In addition, as for carcinoma, a number of types of non-metastatic neuropathy have been recognized. These are subdivisible into subacute sensory neuropathy, acute or chronic relapsing demyelinating neuropathy and subacute motor neuropathy.

Subacute sensory neuropathy is a rare association of lymphoma, but its clinical and pathological features resemble those of carcinomatous sensory neuropathy (Horwich et al., 1977). Either an acute demyelinating neuropathy with clinical and pathological features identical to those of the Guillain-Barré syndrome (Cameron, Howell and Hutchinson, 1958) or a chronic relapsing demyelinating neuropathy may occur in patients with Hodgkin's disease with sufficient frequency to indicate that this is not a spurious association (Lisak et al., 1977). Subacute motor neuropathy constitutes a rare but distinct syndrome. At autopsy, neuronal degeneration restricted to anterior horn cells, together with mild posterior column demyelination, has been described (Schold et al., 1979).

Leukaemia The usual explanation for peripheral nerve involvement in both acute and chronic leukaemia is direct invasion of spinal roots or peripheral nerve trunks. Occasional cases without such an explanation are encountered, sometimes with features resembling the Guillain-Barré syndrome (Vital et al., 1975).

Myeloma Peripheral nerve involvement occurs more frequently in relation to myeloma than other malignancies and may take a variety of forms. Compression of cranial nerves and spinal roots by plasmacytomas or secondary to vertebral collapse may occur, and sparse endoneurial infiltration with plasma cells has been described. Amyloidosis related to myeloma may lead to a generalized neuropathy or to compression of the median nerve in the carpal tunnel. A sensorimotor neuropathy with predominant axonal degeneration may be encountered with features resembling the sensorimotor neuropathy that is seen as a non-metastatic complication of carnoma. The changes are more pronounced in distal nerves and this therefore is probably a distal axonopathy of dying-back type (Victor, Banker and Adams, 1958). A chronic demyelinating neuropathy, predominantly motor, is usually related to osteosclerotic myeloma (Kelly et al., 1981). This may be accompanied by additional features which include papilloedema, widespread oedema, cutaneous changes and endocrine dysfunction. Most such cases have been reported from Japan (Iwashita et al., 1977).

Polycythaemia vera A generalized sensorimotor neuropathy is a rare accompaniment of polycythaemia vera (Yiannikas, McLeod and Walsh, 1983). In a personally observed case, sural nerve biopsy showed a severe loss of myelinated fibres of all diameters.

Dysproteinaemic neuropathy

Benign paraproteinaemias A chronic sensorimotor neuropathy is encountered in relation to a variety of benign gammopathies. Nerve biopsies usually demonstrate a predominantly axonal degeneration with some demyelination unaccompanied by inflammatory cellular infiltrates. A distinctive demyelinating distal sensorimotor neuropathy has recently been defined in relation to *benign IgM paraproteinaemia*, usually with a kappa light chain. Most cases are male and in the older age groups. Ataxia and tremor are often prominent associated features. Nerve conduction velocity is severely reduced (Smith et al., 1983). Nerve biopsies show loss of myelinated fibres and evidence of chronic demyelination and remyelination with hypertrophic changes. An interesting feature is the occurrence of abnormally widely spaced myelin with approximately twice the normal periodicity (King and Thomas, 1984). The widening is related to separation at the intraperiod line. The density of unmyelinated axons in biopsy specimens is normal. The serum contains monoclonal IgM antibodies which react with peripheral nerve myelin and monoclonal IgM is demonstrable on surviving myelin sheaths by immunofluorescence (Fig. 18.69) (Latov et al., 1980; Smith et al., 1983). The antigen has been shown to be myelin-associated glycoprotein (Braun, Frail and Latov, 1981) but whether the deposition of antibody on myelin is directly responsible for the demyelination has not been established. It is also deposited on the perineurium.

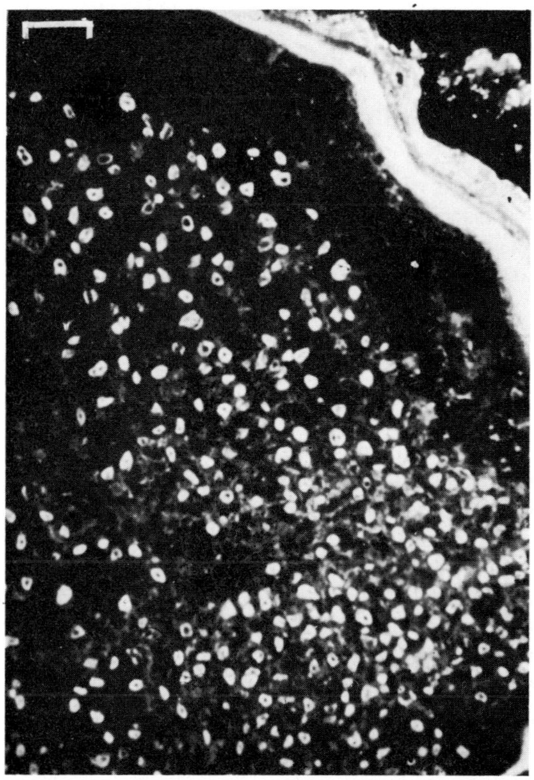

Fig. 18.69 IgM paraproteinaemic neuropathy. Photomicrograph with dark ground illumination showing attachment of fluorescein-conjugated anti-human IgM antibody to surviving myelin sheaths and perineurium. Bar = 50 μm. (Reproduced, with permission, from I.S. Smith et al., 1983.)

Waldenström's macroglobulinaemia This is a chronic lymphoreticular proliferative disorder which is associated with a circulating monoclonal IgM paraprotein. An underlying lymphoma is usually present. A chronic distal sensorimotor neuropathy may occur (Iwashita et al., 1974), in which there is either predominantly axonal degeneration or segmental demyelination. Foci of lymphocytes may be present in the endoneurial spaces, and deposits of IgM may be demonstrable in the endoneurium and on myelin (Propp et al., 1975). Abnormal widely spaced myelin may also be a feature (King and Thomas, 1984) (Fig. 18.70).

Cryoglobulinaemia Lower limb neuropathy may develop in both essential and secondary cryoglobulinaemia. A vasculitis affecting the vasa nervorum, possibly related to cryoglobulin deposition and activation of the complement system, has been demonstrated (Cream et al., 1974). Otherwise, ischaemia of the nerves caused by intravascular cryoglobulin deposition has been postulated. Vallat et al. (1980) have shown, in a case related to myeloma, the presence of masses of closely packed tubular structures in the endoneurium, in the walls of vasa nervorum and within the lumen of some vessels. The appearances of this material were identical to cryoprecipitates extracted from the serum.

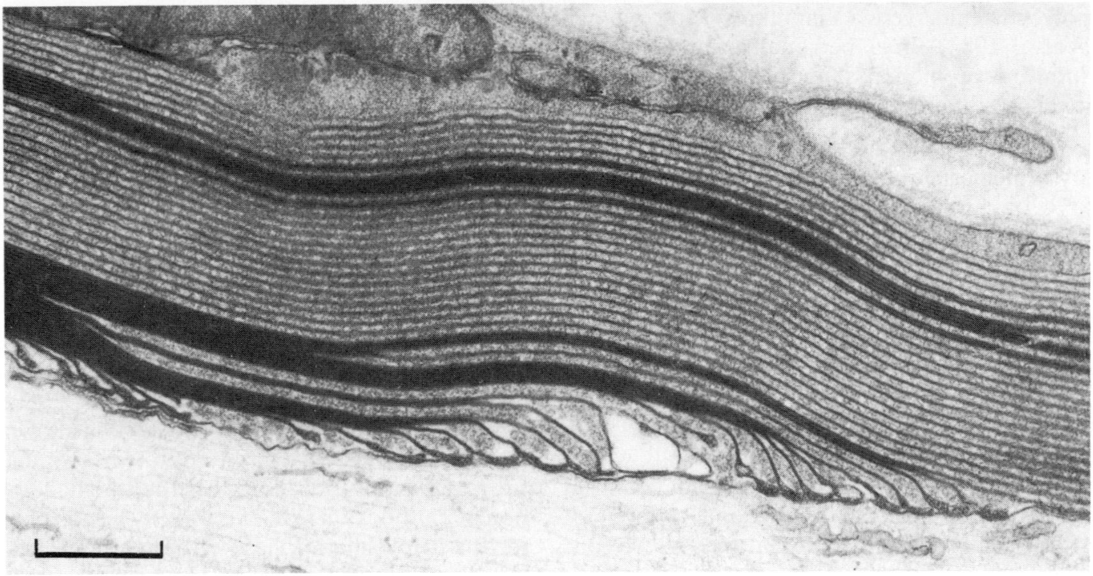

Fig. 18.70 Waldenström's macroglobulinaemia. Electron micrograph of longitudinal section through a myelin sheath displaying abnormally wide periodicity. Bar = 0.5 μm.

Neuropathy related to peripheral vascular disease

Occlusion of large vessels

Ischaemia related to occlusion of large arteries is encountered as a result of atherosclerosis, embolism, thromboangiitis obliterans (Buerger's disease), compression (trauma, masses, tourniquets) and compartment syndromes (such as the anterior tibial syndrome). The consequences have been most closely studied in relation to lower limb atherosclerotic disease but so far even these have not been extensively examined using contemporary techniques. Hutchinson and Liversedge (1956) found neurological abnormalities in nearly 60 per cent of their series of cases. Garven, Gairns and Smith (1962) documented myelinated fibre loss, particularly for those of larger diameter. Eames and Lange (1967) and Chopra and Hurwitz (1967) reported widespread segmental demyelination and remyelination, and the latter authors considered that this was the initial pathological response to ischaemia. Recent experimental studies employing embolization with arachidonic acid, on the other hand, have suggested that the predominant change is axonal degeneration and that the small myelinated and unmyelinated axons are more vulnerable (Parry and Brown, 1982).

Vasculitic neuropathy

Asbury and Johnson (1978) defined 11 forms of vasculitis with which peripheral neuropathy may be associated: (1) polyarteritis nodosa; (2) allergic granulomatosis (Churg–Strauss syndrome); (3) hypersensitivity angiitis; (4) rheumatoid arthritis; (5) vasculitis with systemic lupus erythematosus; (6) vasculitis with progressive systemic sclerosis; (7) vasculitis in Sjögren's syndrome; (8) vasculitis in Wegener's granulomatosis; (9) cranial (giant cell) arteritis; (10) Köhlmeier–Degos arteritis (malignant atrophic papulosis); (11) microvasculitis of nerve with ganglionitis as a remote effect of carcinoma (Johnson et al., 1979). To this list must now be added the vasculitic lesions which were observed in peripheral nerve in the neuromuscular syndrome related to the ingestion of adulterated rapeseed oil in Spain (Ricoy et al., 1983). Reference has also already been made to neural vasculitic lesions in mixed cryoglobulinaemia (Cream et al., 1971).

Polyarteritis nodosa This condition is commonly accompanied by peripheral nerve involvement. It was found in half of Lovshin and Kernohan's (1948) series of 25 patients. The occurrence of progressive multifocal peripheral nerve lesions ('mononeuritis multiplex'), affect-

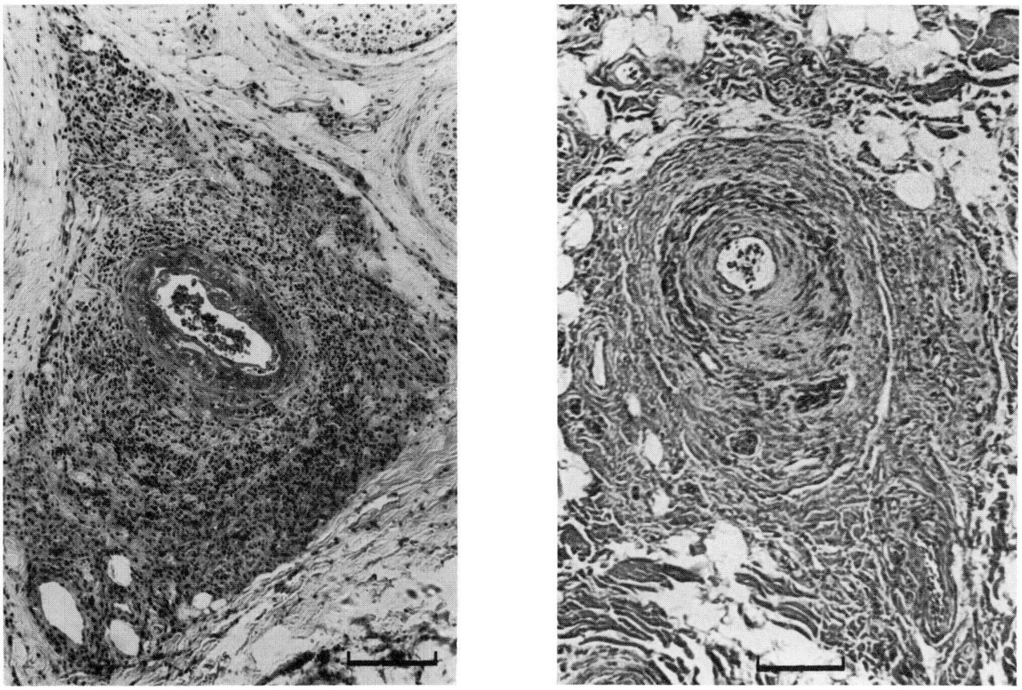

(a) (b)

Fig. 18.71 Polyarteritis nodosa. (**a**) Acute lesion with fibrinoid necrosis of an epineurial arteriole and inflammatory infiltration of the adventitia. Haematoxylin and eosin. (**b**) Healed lesion with fibrosis of all coats of an epineurial arteriole and total loss of internal elastic lamina. Elastic van Gieson. Bars = 100 μm.

ing both motor and sensory function and often accompanied by pain, was established as the characteristic clinical picture by Kernohan and Woltman (1938). The onset of individual lesions can be abrupt or gradual. They tend to summate to produce a symmetrical disturbance. The lesions are those of a necrotizing arteritis of the vasa nervorum (Fig. 18.71). They resemble those which occur in other parts of the body. The predominant lesion is axonal degeneration, although foci of demyelination without axonal loss have been observed (Bignami, 1961). Clear descriptions of nerve infarction are not available.

Allergic granulomatosis (Churg-Strauss syndrome) This is a variant of polyarteritis nodosa. The salient clinical features are a marked eosinophilic leucocytosis, pulmonary involvement with asthma and extravascular granulomas. Of the 13 cases originally reported by Churg and Strauss (1951), nine had neuropathy. Vasculitis affecting vasa nervorum was documented. A further variant of polyarteritis nodosa is lymphomatoid granulomatosis (Liebow, Carrington and Friedman, 1972) in which the vascular path-

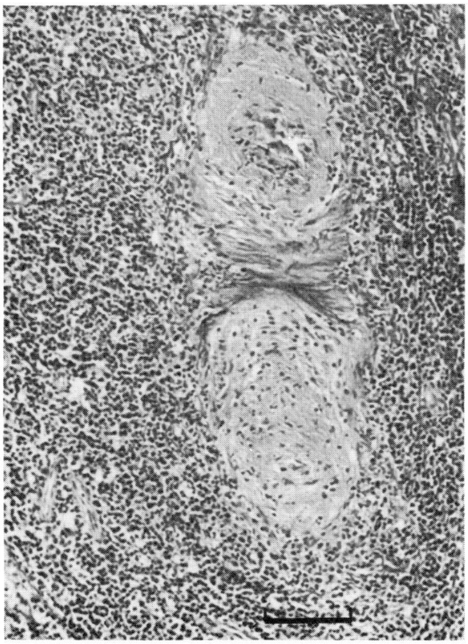

Fig. 18.72 Lymphomatoid granulomatosis. Necrotizing arterial lesion surrounded by massive lymphocytic infiltrate. Elastic van Gieson. Bar = 100 μm.

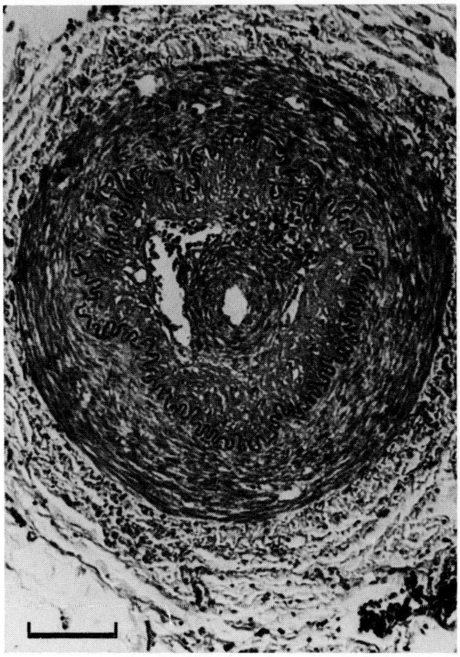

(a)

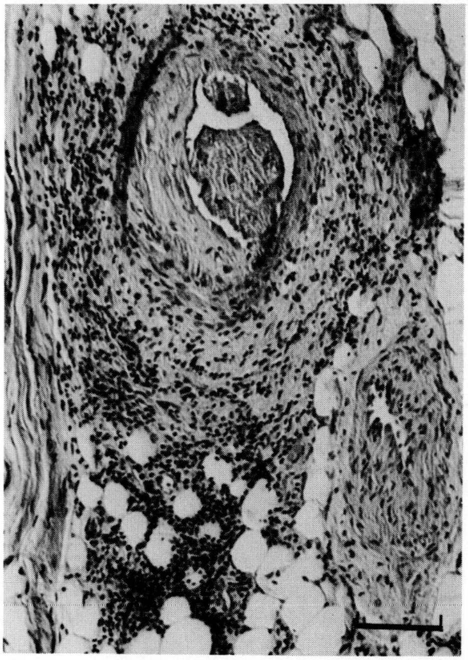

(b)

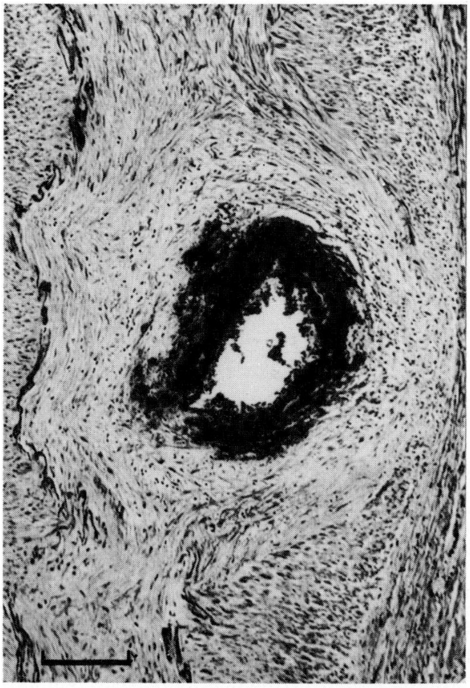

(c)

Fig. 18.73 Rheumatoid neuropathy. (**a**) Intimal fibrosis with otherwise intact vessel wall. Haematoxylin and eosin. (**b**) Arteritis with lymphocytic infiltration. Haematoxylin and eosin. (**c**) Arteritis with deposition of fibrinoid. Mallory's PTAH. Bars = 100 μm.

ology is characterized by a necrotizing arteritis with an infiltration predominantly with lymphocytes and plasmacytoid cells (Fig. 18.72).

Rheumatoid arthritis A variety of different peripheral nerve abnormalities are encountered in this disorder. Median nerve compression in the carpal tunnel, secondary to tenosynovitis and arthritis of the carpal bones, is common, and other nerve entrapments related to joint involvement may be observed. Digital mononeuropathies are also well recognized, as is a relatively benign distal sensory neuropathy predominantly affecting the lower limbs (Pallis and Scott, 1965). The digital mononeuropathies may have a vasculitic basis; the explanation of the symmetrical sensory neuropathy is unclear but it is probably also related to vasculitis. The most devastating type of neuropathy is a progressive multifocal neuropathy with features similar to those of polyarteritis nodosa. It is not necessarily associated with severe or active joint disease. Pathological studies have largely been confined to the severe cases. A spectrum of vascular lesions can be defined (Fig. 18.73), ranging from acute necrotizing lesions indistinguishable from those of polyarteritis nodosa to a bland intimal proliferation with preservation of the internal elastic lamina leading to partial or total occlusion of the vascular lumen (Bywaters, 1957). Other vessels show mild inflammatory infiltration with some deposition of fibrinoid material. Dyck, Conn and Okazaki (1972) undertook an extensive study with serial sections on a young adult with severe vasculitic multifocal neuropathy. Localized areas of damage were defined which were mainly sited in the centre of fascicles, beginning in major nerves at mid-femoral and mid-humeral level and spreading to more diffuse axonal degeneration at more distal sites. An ischaemic basis, possibly at watershed areas, was considered the probable explanation. Frank infarction was not observed.

Systemic lupus erythematosus (SLE) This disorder may again be associated with several different types of peripheral neuropathy, although the peripheral nervous system is less commonly affected than in rheumatoid disease. The most frequent manifestation is a progressive multifocal neuropathy related to vasculitis (Hughes, Cameron and Hall, 1982). A symmetrical distal sensorimotor neuropathy and an acute predominantly motor neuropathy with features resembling the Guillain–Barré syndrome (R.T. Johnson and Richardson, 1968) have also been described for which the pathological basis is less clear.

Progressive systemic sclerosis Scleroderma rarely causes neuropathy, but focal and multifocal lesions may develop (Kibler and Rose, 1960). Arteritis is demonstrable on nerve biopsy (Asbury and Johnson, 1978).

Sjögren's syndrome This syndrome comprises the combination of keratoconjunctivitis sicca and/or xerostomia with rheumatoid arthritis, SLE or other connective tissue disorder. A trigeminal sensory neuropathy and a mild distal sensory neuropathy in the limbs have been found to be related to arteritis (Kaltreider and Talal, 1969).

Wegener's granulomatosis A combination of granulomas in the respiratory tract, arteritis and nephropathy characterize this disorder. The peripheral nerves may be directly involved by granulomas (Drachman, 1963) or a diffuse multifocal neuropathy similar to that seen in polyarteritis nodosa may develop (Stern, Hoffbrand and Urich, 1965) (Fig. 18.74).

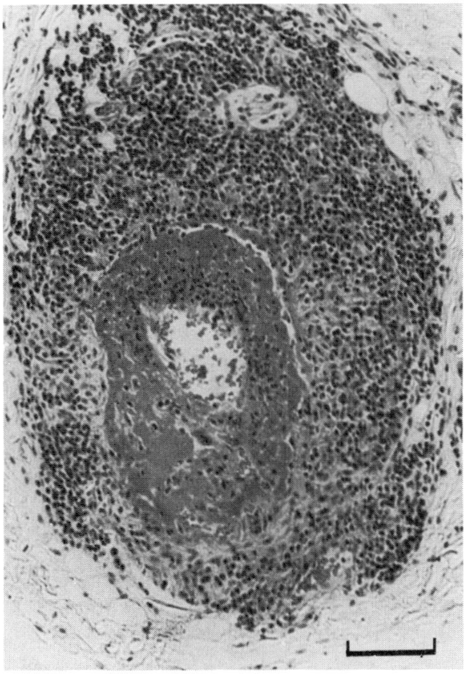

Fig. 18.74 Wegener's granulomatosis. Acute necrotizing arteritis. Haematoxylin and eosin. Bar = 100 μm.

References

Abrahams, P.H., Day, A. and Allt, G. (1980) Schwann cell plasma membrane changes induced by nerve crush. *Acta Neuropathologica* **50,** 85–90.

Adams, D., Festenstein, H., Gibson, J.D., Hughes, R.A.C., Jaraquemada, J., Papasteriadis, C. et al. (1979) HLA antigens in chronic relapsing idiopathic inflammatory polyneuropathy. *Journal of Neurology, Neurosurgery and Psychiatry* **42,** 184–6.

Aguayo, A.J., Bray, G.M., Terry, L.C. and Sweezey, E. (1976a) Three-dimensional analysis of unmyelinated fibres in normal and pathologic autonomic nerves. *Journal of Neuropathology and Experimental Neurology* **35,** 136–51.

Aguayo, A.J., Dickson, R., Trecarten, J., Attiwell, M., Bray, G.M. and Richardson, P.R. (1978a) Ensheathment and myelination of regenerating PNS fibres by transplanted nerve glia. *Neuroscience Letters* **9,** 97–104.

Aguayo, A.J., Epps, J., Charron, L. and Bray, G.M. (1976b) Multipotentiality of Schwann cells in cross-anastomosed and grafted myelinated and unmyelinated nerves: quantitative microscopy and autoradiography. *Brain Research* **104,** 1–20.

Aguayo, A.J., Nair, C.P.V. and Bray, G.M. (1971) Peripheral nerve abnormalities in the Riley–Day syndrome; findings in a sural nerve biopsy. *Archives of Neurology* **24,** 106–16.

Aguayo, A.J., Perkins, S., Bray, G.M. and Duncan, I. (1978b) Transplantation of nerves from patients with Charcot-Marie-Tooth (CMT) disease into immune-suppressed mice. *Journal of Neuropathology and Experimental Neurology* **37,** 582.

Aguayo, A.J., Terry, L.C. and Bray, G.M. (1973) Spontaneous loss of axons in sympathetic unmyelinated nerve fibres of the rat during development. *Brain Research* **54,** 360–4.

Aitken, J.T., Sharman, M. and Young, J.Z. (1947) Maturation of regenerating fibres with various peripheral connexions. *Journal of Anatomy* **81,** 1–22.

Aitken, J.T. and Thomas, P.K. (1962) Retrograde changes in fibre size following nerve section. *Journal of Anatomy* **96,** 121–9.

Allt, G. and Cavanagh, J.B. (1969) Ultrastructural changes in the region of the node of Ranvier in the rat caused by diphtheria toxin. *Brain* **92,** 459–68.

Altenkirch, H., Mager, J., Stoltenburg, G. and Helmbrecht, J. (1977) Toxic polyneuropathies after sniffing a glue thinner. *Journal of Neurology* **214,** 137–52.

Anderton, B.H. (1982) The neuronal cytoskeleton: proteins and pathology. In *Recent Advances in Neuropathology*, vol. 2 (Eds. Thomas-Smith, W. and Cavanagh, J.B.), pp. 29–51. Churchill Livingstone, Edinburgh.

Andrade, C. (1952) A peculiar form of peripheral neuropathy: familial atypical generalised amyloidosis with special involvement of the peripheral nerves. *Brain* **75,** 408–27.

Andres, K.H. (1965) Uber die Feinstruktur besonderer Einrichtungen in Markhaltigen Nervenfasern des Kleinhirns der Ratte. *Zeitschrift für Zellforschung und mikroskopische Anatomie* **65,** 701–12.

Appenzeller, O. and Richardson, E.P. Jr (1966) The sympathetic chain in patients with diabetic and alcoholic polyneuropathy. *Neurology* **16,** 1205–9.

Arbuthnott, E.R., Ballard, K.J., Boyd, I.A. and Kalu, K.U. (1980) Quantitative study of the non-circularity of myelinated peripheral nerve fibres in the cat. *Journal of Physiology* **308,** 99–123.

Arbuthnott, E.R., Boyd, I.A. and Kalu, K.U. (1980) Ultrastructural dimensions of myelinated peripheral nerve fibres in the cat and their relation to conduction velocity. *Journal of Physiology* **308,** 125–57.

Archer, A.G., Watkins, P.J., Thomas, P.K., Sharma, A.K. and Payan, J. (1983) The natural history of acute painful neuropathy in diabetes mellitus. *Journal of Neurology, Neurosurgery and Psychiatry* **46,** 491–9.

Aring, C.D. (1942) The systemic nervous affinity of triorthocresyl phosphate (Jamaica ginger palsy). *Brain* **65,** 34–47.

Aring, C.D., Bean, W.B., Roseman, E., Rosenbaum, M. and Spies, T.D. (1941) The peripheral nerves in cases of nutritional deficiency. *Archives of Neurology and Psychiatry* **45,** 772–87.

Arnason, B.G. and Asbury, A.K. (1968) Idiopathic polyneuritis after surgery. *Archives of Neurology* **18,** 500–7.

Arvidsson, B., Kristensson, K. and Olsson, Y. (1973) Vascular permeability to fluorescent protein tracer in trigeminal nerve and gasserian ganglion. *Acta Neuropathologica* **26,** 199–205.

Asbury, A.K. (1981) Diagnostic considerations in Guillain–Barré syndrome. *Annals of Neurology* **9,** suppl., 1–5.

Asbury, A.K., Aldridge, H., Hershberg, R., Fisher, C.M. (1970) Oculomotor palsy in diabetes mellitus: a clinico-pathological study. *Brain* **93,** 555–66.

Asbury, A.K., Arnason, B.G. and Adams, R.D. (1969) The inflammatory lesion in idiopathic polyneuritis: its role in pathogenesis. *Medicine* **48,** 173–215.

Asbury, A.K., Cox, S.C. and Baringer, J.R. (1971) The significance of giant vacuolation of endoneurial fibroblasts. *Acta Neuropathologica* **18,** 123–31.

Asbury, A.K., Gale, M.K., Cox, S.C., Baringer, J.R. and Berg, B.O. (1972b) Giant axonal neuropathy: a unique case with segmental neurofilamentous masses. *Acta Neuropathologica* **20,** 237–47.

Asbury, A.K. and Johnson, P.C. (1978) *Pathology of Peripheral Nerve.* W.B. Saunders, Philadelphia.

Asbury, A.K., Picard, E.H. and Baringer, J.R. (1972a) Sensory perineuritis. *Archives of Neurology* **26,** 302–12.

Asbury, A.K., Victor, M. and Adams, R.D. (1963) Uremic polyneuropathy. *Archives of Neurology* **8,** 413–28.

Ballin, R.H.M. and Thomas, P.K. (1968) Hypertrophic changes in diabetic neuropathy. *Acta Neuropathologica* **11,** 93–102.

Ballin, R.H.M. and Thomas, P.K. (1969) Changes at the nodes of Ranvier during Wallerian degeneration: an electron microscope study. *Acta Neuropathologica* **14,** 237–49.

Bargmann, W. and Linder, E. (1964) Uber den Feinbau des Nebennierenmarkes des Igels (*Erinaceus europaeus* L.). *Zeitschrift für Zellforschung und mikroskopische Anatomie* **64,** 868–912.

Barker, J.L., Neale, J.H. and Gainer, H. (1976) Rapidly transported proteins in sensory, motor and sympathetic nerves of the isolated frog nervous system. *Brain Research* **105,** 497–515.

Baruah, J.K., Rasool, C.G., Bradley, W.G. and Munsat, T.L. (1981) Retrograde axonal transport of lead in rat sciatic nerve. *Neurology* **31,** 612–16.

Basbaum, C.B. (1973) Induced hypothermia in peripheral nerve: electron microscopic and electrophysiological observations. *Journal of Neurocytology* **2,** 171–87.

Bean, W.B., Hodges, R.E. and Daum, K.E. (1955) Pantothenic acid deficiency induced in human subjects. *Journal of Clinical Investigation* **34,** 1073–84.

Behse, F. and Buchthal, F. (1977) Alcoholic neuropathy: clinical, electrophysiological, and biopsy findings. *Annals of Neurology* **2,** 95–110.

Behse, F., Buchthal, F. and Carlsen, F. (1977) Nerve biopsy and conduction studies in diabetic neuropathy. *Journal of Neurology, Neurosurgery and Psychiatry* **40,** 1072–82.

Behse, F., Buchthal, F., Carlsen, F. and Knappeis, G.G. (1972) Hereditary neuropathy with liability to pressure palsies. Electrophysiological and histopathological aspects. *Brain* **95,** 777–94.

Benjamins, J.A., Herschkowitz, N., Robinson, J. and McKhann, G.M. (1971) The effect of inhibitors of protein synthesis on incorporation of lipids into myelin. *Journal of Neurochemistry* **18.** 729–38.

Bennett, H.S. (1963) Morphological aspects of extracellular polysaccharides. *Journal of Histochemistry and Cytochemistry* **11,** 14–23.

Berg, B.O., Rosenberg, S.H. and Asbury, A.K. (1972) Giant axonal neuropathy. *Pediatrics* **49,** 894–9.

Berthold, C.-H. (1968) Ultrastructure of the node-paranode region of mature feline ventral lumbar spinal-root fibres. *Acta Societatis Medicorum Upsaliensis* **73,** suppl. 9, 37–78.

Berthold, C.-H. (1973) Local demyelination of developing feline nerve fibres. *Neurobiology* **3,** 339–52.

Berthold, C.-H. (1978) Morphology of normal peripheral axons. In *Physiology and Pathobiology of Axons* (Ed. Waxman, S.G.) pp. 3–63. Raven Press, New York.

Berthold, C.-H. and Skoglund, S. (1967) Histochemical and ultrastructural demonstration of mitochondria in the paranodal region of developing feline spinal roots and nerves. *Acta Societatis Medicorum Upsaliensis* **72,** 37–70.

Bignami, A. (1961) Le neuriti nella periarterite nodosa. *Il Policlinico* **68,** 577–95.

Bigner, D.D., Olson, W.H. and McFarlin, D.E. (1971) Peripheral polyneuropathy, high and low molecular weight IgM and amyloidosis. *Archives of Neurology* **24,** 365–73.

Bird, T.D., Ott, J. and Giblett, E.R. (1982) Evidence for linkage of Charcot–Marie–Tooth neuropathy to the Duffy locus on chromosome 1. *American Journal of Human Genetics* **34,** 388–94.

Bird, T.D., Ott, J., Giblett, E.R., Chance, P.F., Sumi, S.M. and Kraft, G.H. (1983) Genetic linkage evidence for heterogeneity in Charcot–Marie–Tooth neuropathy (HMSN type I). *Annals of Neurology* **14,** 679–84.

Bischoff, A. (1967) Die Ultrastruktur peripherer Nerven bei der diabetischen Neuropathie. *Verhandlungen der deutschen Gesellschaft für Innere Medizin* **72,** 1138–41.

Bischoff, A. (1968) Diabetische Neuropathie: pathologische Anatomie, Pathophysiologie und Pathogenese auf Grund elekronenmikroskopische Untersuchungen. *Deutsche Medizinische Wochenschrift* **93,** 237–41.

Bischoff, A. (1971) Die alkoholische Polyneuropathie: klinische, ultrastrukturelle und pathogenetische Aspekte. *Deutsche Medizinische Wochenschrift* **96,** 317–22.

Bischoff, A. (1975) Neuropathy in leukodystrophies. In *Peripheral Neuropathy* (Eds. Dyck, P.J., Thomas, P.K. and Lambert, E.H.), pp. 891–913. W.B. Saunders, Philadelphia.

Bischoff, A., Fierz, U., Regli, F. and Ulrich, J. (1968) Peripherneurologische Störungen bei der Fabryschen Krankheit (Angiokeratoma corporis diffusum universale). Klinische-elektronenmikroskopische Befunde bei einem Fall. *Klinische Wochenschrift* **46,** 666–71.

Bischoff, A. and Ulrich, J. (1967) Amaurotische Idiotie in Verbindung mit metachromatischer Leukodystrophie. Uebergangsform oder Kombination? *Acta Neuropathologica* **8,** 292–308.

Bischoff, A. and Ulrich, J. (1969) Peripheral neuropathy in globoid cell leucodystrophy (Krabbe's disease). Ultrastructural and histochemical findings. *Brain* **92,** 861–70.

Black, J.A., Foster, R.E. and Waxman, S.G. (1981) Freeze-fracture ultrastructure of rat CNS and PNS nonmyelinated axolemma. *Journal of Neurocytology* **10,** 981–93.

Black, M.M. and Lasek, R.J. (1980) Slow components of axonal transport: two cytoskeletal networks. *Journal of Cell Biology* **86,** 616–23.

Blackwood, W. (1944) Studies in the pathology of human 'immersion foot'. *British Journal of Surgery* **31,** 329–50.

Blume, R.-S. and Wolff, S.M. (1972) The Chediak-Higashi syndrome: studies in four patients and a review of the literature. *Medicine* **51,** 247–80.

Bosanquet, F.D. and Henson, R.A. (1957) Sensory neuropathy in diabetes mellitus. *Folia Psychiatrica, Neurologica et Neurochirurgica Neerlandica* **60,** 107–17.

Bostock, H. and Sears, T.A. (1978) The internodal axon membrane: electrical excitability and continuous conduction in segmental demyelination. *Journal of Physiology* **280,** 273–301.

Bouldin, T.W. and Cavanagh, J.B. (1979a) Organophosphorous neuropathy. I. Teased-fibre study of the spatio-temporal spread of axonal degeneration. *Journal of Pathology* **94,** 241–52.

Bouldin, T.W. and Cavanagh, J.B. (1979b) Organophosphorous neuropathy. II. A fine structural study of the early stages of axonal degeneration. *Journal of Pathology* **94,** 253–70.

Boycott, A.E. (1904) On the number of nodes of Ranvier in different stages of the growth of nerve fibres in the frog. *Journal of Physiology* **30,** 370–80.

Boyd, I.A. and Davey, M.R. (1968) *Composition of Peripheral Nerves.* Livingstone, Edinburgh.

Boyd, I.A. and Kalu, K.U. (1979) Scaling factor relating conduction velocity and diameter for myelinated afferent nerve fibres in the cat hind limb. *Journal of Physiology* **289,** 277–97.

Bradley, W.G. and Hewer, R.L. (1966) Peripheral neuropathy due to disulphiram. *British Medical Journal* **2,** 449–50.

Bradley, W.G., Karlsson, I.J. and Rasso, I.C.G. (1977) Metronidazole neuropathy. *British Medical Journal* **2,** 610–11.

Bradley, W.G., Lassman, L.P., Pearce, G.W. and Walton, J.N. (1970) The neuromyopathy of vincristine in man. Clinical, electrophysiological and pathological studies. *Journal of the Neurological Sciences* **10,** 107–31.

Bradley, W.G., Madrid, R., Thrush, D.C. and Campbell, D.J. (1975) Recurrent brachial plexus neuropathy. *Brain* **98,** 381–98.

Brady, S.T., Crothers, S.D., Nosal, C. and McClure, W.O. (1980) Fast axoplasmic transport in the presence of high Ca^{2+}: evidence that microtubules are not required. *Proceedings of the National Academy of Sciences of the USA* **77,** 5909–13.

Braun, P.E., Frail, D.E. and Latov, N. (1981) Myelin-associated glycoprotein is the antigen for a monoclonal IgM in polyneuropathy. *Journal of Neurochemistry* **39,** 1261–5.

Bray, D. and Bunge, M.B. (1981) Serial analysis of microtubules in cultured rat sensory axons. *Journal of Neurocytology* **10,** 589–605.

Bray, D. and Gilbert, D. (1981) Cytoskeletal elements in neurons. *Annual Review of Neuroscience* **4,** 505–23.

Brimijoin, W.S. (1982a) Mictotubules and the capacity of the system for rapid axonal transport. *Federation Proceedings* **41,** 2312–16.

Brimijoin, W.S. (1982b) Abnormalities of axonal transport. Are they a cause of peripheral nerve disease? *Mayo Clinic Proceedings* **57,** 707–14.

Brown, M.J. and Greene, D.A. (1984) Diabetic neuropathy: pathophysiology and management. In *Peripheral Nerve Disorders. A Practical Approach* (Eds. Asbury, A.K. and Gilliatt, R.W.), pp. 126–53. Butterworths, London.

Brown, M.J., Martin, J.R. and Asbury, A.K. (1976) Painful diabetic neuropathy: a morphometric study. *Archives of Neurology* **33,** 164–71.

Brown, S.S. and Spudich, J.A. (1979) Cytochalasin inhibits the rate of elongation of actin filament fragments. *Journal of Cell Biology* **83,** 657–62.

Buchthal, F. and Behse, F. (1977a) Peroneal muscular atrophy (PMA) and related disorders. I. Clinical manifestations as related to biopsy findings, nerve conduction and electromyography. *Brain* **100,** 41–66.

Buchthal, F. and Behse, F. (1977b) Peroneal muscular atrophy (PMA) and related disorders. II. Histological findings in sural nerves. *Brain* **100,** 67–85.

Buchthal, F. and Behse, F. (1979) Electrophysiology and nerve biopsy in men exposed to lead. *British Journal of Industrial Medicine* **36,** 135–47.

Buchthal, F. and Rosenfalck, A. (1966) Evoked action potentials and conduction velocity in human sensory nerves. *Brain Research* **3,** 1–119.

Bunt, A.H. and Hasche, R.H. (1978) Features of foreign proteins affecting their retrograde transport in axons of the visual system. *Journal of Neurocytology* **7,** 665–78.

Burkel, W.E. (1967) The histological fine structure of the perineurium. *Anatomical Record* **158,** 177–90.

Buxton, P.H. and Hayward, M. (1967) Polyneuritis cranialis associated with industrial trichlorethylene poisoning. *Journal of Neurology, Neurosurgery and Psychiatry* **30,** 511–18.

Byers, M.A. (1974) Structural correlates of rapid axonal transport: evidence that microtubules may not be directly involved. *Brain Research* **75,** 97–113.

Byrne, E., Thomas, P.K. and Zilkha, K.J. (1982) Familial extrapyramidal disease with peripheral neuropathy. *Journal of Neurology, Neurosurgery and Psychiatry* **45,** 372–4.

Bywaters, E.G.L. (1957) Peripheral vascular obstruction in rheumatoid arthritis and its relationship to other vascular lesions. *Annals of the Rheumatic Diseases* **16,** 84–103.

Cajal, S., Ramón y (1928) *Degeneration and Regeneration in the Nervous System*, vol. 1. Oxford University Press, London.

Cameron, D.G., Howell, D.A. and Hutchinson, J.L. (1958) Acute peripheral neuropathy in Hodgkin's disease. Report of a fatal case with histologic features of allergic neuritis. *Neurology* **8,** 575–7.

Cammermeyer, J (1956) Neuropathological changes in hereditary neuropathies: manifestation of the syndrome heredopathia atactica polyneuritiformis in the presence of interstitial hypertrophic neuropathy. *Journal of Neuropathology and Experimental Neurology* **15,** 340–61.

Carlsen, F. and Behse, F. (1980) Three dimensional analysis of Schwann cells associated with unmyelinated nerve fibres in human sural nerve. *Journal of Anatomy* **130,** 545–57.

Carlsen, F., Knappeis, G.G. and Behse, F. (1974) Schwann cell length in unmyelinated fibres of human sural nerve. *Journal of Anatomy* **117,** 463–7.

Carmichael, E.A. and Greenfield, J.G. (1935) Peripheral nerves in combined degeneration of the cord. *Brain* **58,** 483–91.

Carpenter, S. (1972) An ultrastructural study of an acute fatal case of the Guillain–Barré syndrome. *Journal of the Neurological Sciences* **15,** 125–40.

Causey, G. and Barton, A.A. (1959) The cellular content of the endoneurium of peripheral nerve. *Brain* **82,** 594–8.

Causey, G. and Palmer, E. (1953) The centrifugal spread of structural changes at the nodes in degenerating mammalian nerves. *Journal of Anatomy* **87,** 185–91.

Cavanagh, J.B. (1954) The toxic effect of tri-ortho-cresyl phosphate on the nervous system. *Journal of Neurology, Neurosurgery and Psychiatry* **17,** 163–72.

Cavanagh, J.B. (1964) The significance of the 'dying-back' process in experimental and human neurological disease. *International Review of Experimental Pathology* **7,** 219–67.

Cavanagh, J.B. (1968a) Effects of x-irradiation on the proliferation of cells in peripheral nerve during Wallerian degeneration in the rat. *British Journal of Radiology* **41,** 275–81.

Cavanagh, J.B. (1968b) Prior x-irradiation and the cellular response to nerve crush: duration of effect. *Experimental Neurology* **22,** 253–8.

Cavanagh, J.B. (1979) The 'dying-back' process. A common denominator in many naturally occurring and toxic neuropathies. *Archives of Pathology and Laboratory Medicine* **103,** 659–64.

Cavanagh, J.B. (1982) Mechanisms of axon degeneration in three toxic 'neuropathies' organophosphorus, acrylamide and hexacarbon compared. *Advances in Neuropathology* **2,** 213–42.

Cavanagh, J.B., Fuller, N.H., Johnson, H.R.M. and Rudge, P. (1974) The effects of thallium salts, with particular reference to the nervous system changes. *Quarterly Journal of Medicine* **43,** 293–320.

Cavanagh, J.B. and Jacobs, J.M. (1964) Some quantitative aspects of diphtheritic neuropathy. *British Journal of Experimental Pathology* **45,** 309–22.

Cavanagh, J.B. and Mellick, R.S. (1965) On the nature of the peripheral nerve lesions with acute intermittent porphyria. *Journal of Neurology, Neurosurgery and Psychiatry* **28,** 320–72.

Cavanagh, N.P.C., Eames, R.A., Galvin, R.J., Brett, E.M. and Kelly, R.E. (1979) Hereditary sensory neuropathy with spastic paraplegia. *Brain* **102,** 79–94.

Charron, L., Peyronnard, J.-M. and Marchard, L. (1980) Sensory neuropathy associated with primary biliary cirrhosis. Histologic and morphometric studies. *Archives of Neurology* **37,** 84–7.

Chiu, S.Y. (1980) Asymmetry currents in the mammalian myelinated nerve. *Journal of Physiology* **309,** 499–519.

Chiu, S.Y. and Ritchie, J.M. (1981) Ionic and gating currents in mammalian myelinated nerve. In *Demyelinating Disease: Basic and Clinical Electrophysiology* (Eds. Waxman, S.G. and Ritchie, J.M.), pp. 313–28. Raven Press, New York.

Chiu, S.Y. and Ritchie, J.M. (1982) Evidence for the presence of potassium channels in the internode of frog myelinated fibres. *Journal of Physiology* **322,** 485–500.

Chopra, J.S. and Hurwitz, L.J. (1967) Internodal length of sural nerve fibres in chronic occlusive vascular disease. *Journal of Neurology, Neurosurgery and Psychiatry* **30,** 207–14.

Churg, J. and Strauss, L. (1951) Allergic granulomatosis, allergic angiitis, and periarteritis nodosa. *American Journal of Pathology* **27,** 277–301.

Clark, A.W., Griffin, J.W. and Price, D.L. (1980) The axonal pathology in chronic IDPN intoxication. *Journal of Neuropathology and Experimental Neurology* **39,** 42–55.

Coërs, C. and Woolf, A.L. (1959) *The Innervation of Muscle*, pp. 87–90. Blackwell Scientific, Oxford.

Coimbra, A. and Andrade, C. (1971) Familial amyloid polyneuropathy: an electron microscope study of the peripheral nerve in five cases. II. Nerve fibre changes. *Brain* **94,** 207–12.

Collings, H. (1960) Polyneuropathy associated with

nitrofuran therapy. *Archives of Neurology* **3,** 656–60.

Conti, F., Hille, B., Neumcke, B., Nonner, W. and Stämpfli, R. (1976) Conductance of the sodium channels in myelinated nerve fibres with modified sodium inactivation. *Journal of Physiology* **262,** 729–42.

Cooper, P.D. and Smith, R.S. (1974) The movement of optically detectable organelles in myelinated axons of *Xenopus laevis*. *Journal of Physiology* **242,** 77–97.

Cooper, R.G., Evans, D.A.P. and Whibley, E.J. (1984) Polymorphic hydroxylation of perhexilene maleate in man. *Journal of Medical Genetics* **21,** 27–33.

Cragg, B.G. and Thomas, P.K. (1961) Changes in conduction velocity and fibre size proximal to peripheral nerve lesions. *Journal of Physiology* **157,** 315–27.

Cravioto, H. (1965) The role of Schwann cells in the development of human peripheral nerves. An electron microscope study. *Journal of Ultrastructure Research* **12,** 634–51.

Cream, J.J., Hern, J.E.C., Hughes, R.A.C. and Mackenzie, I.C.K. (1974) Mixed or immune complex cryoglobulinaemia and neuropathy. *Journal of Neurology, Neurosurgery and Psychiatry* **37,** 82–7.

Croft, P.B., Henson, R.A., Urich, H. and Wilkinson, P.C. (1965) Sensory neuropathy with bronchial carcinoma; a study of four cases showing serological abnormalities. *Brain* **88,** 501–14.

Croft, P.B., Urich, H. and Wilkinson, M. (1967) Peripheral neuropathy of sensorimotor type associated with malignant disease. *Brain* **90,** 31–66.

Davies-Jones, G.A.B. and Esiri, M.M. (1971) Neuropathy due to amyloid in myelomatosis. *British Medical Journal* **2,** 444.

Davis, C.J.F., Bradley, W.G. and Madrid, R. (1978) The peroneal muscular atrophy syndrome (clinical, genetic, electrophysiologic and nerve biopsy studies). *Journal de Génétique Humaine* **26,** 311–49.

Davison, A.N. and Dobbing, J. (1978) *Applied Neurochemistry*. Davis, Philadelphia.

Dayan, A.D. (1967) Peripheral neuropathy of metachromatic leucodystrophy: observations on segmental demyelination and remyelination and the intracellular distribution of sulphatide. *Journal of Neurology, Neurosurgery and Psychiatry* **30,** 311–18.

Dejerine, J. and Sottas, J. (1893) Sur la névrite interstitielle hypertrophique et progressive de l'enfance. *Comptes Rendus des Séances de la Société de Biologie et de ses Filiales* **45,** 63–96.

Denny-Brown, D. (1948) Primary sensory neuropathy with muscular changes associated with carcinoma. *Journal of Neurology, Neurosurgery and Psychiatry* **11,** 73–87.

Denny-Brown, D. (1951) Hereditary sensory radicular neuropathy. *Journal of Neurology, Neurosurgery and Psychiatry* **14,** 237–52.

Denny-Brown, D. (1958) The neurological aspects of thiamine deficiency. *Federation Proceedings* **17,** suppl. 2, 35–9.

Denny-Brown, D. and Brenner, C. (1944a) Paralysis of nerve induced by direct pressure and by tourniquet. *Archives of Neurology and Psychiatry* **51,** 1–26.

Denny-Brown, D. and Brenner, C. (1944b) The effect of percussion on nerve. *Journal of Neurology, Neurosurgery and Psychiatry* **7,** 76–95.

Denny-Brown, D. and Sciarra, D. (1945) Changes in the nervous system in acute porphyria. *Brain* **68,** 1–16.

Dische, M.R. and Porro, R.S. (1970) The cardiac lesions in Bassen–Kornzweig disease. *American Journal of Medicine* **49,** 568–71.

Donat, J.R. and Wiśniewski, H. (1973) The spatio-temporal pattern of Wallerian degeneration in mammalian peripheral nerves. *Brain Research* **53,** 41–53.

Drachman, D.A. (1963) Neurological complications of Wegener's granulomatosis. *Archives of Neurology* **8,** 145–55.

Dreyfus, P.M., Hakim, S. and Adams, R.D. (1957) Diabetic ophthalmoplegia. *Archives of Neurology and Psychiatry* **77,** 337–49.

Droz, B., Di Giamberardino, L., Koenig, H.L., Boyenval, J. and Hassig, R. (1978) Axon-myelin transfer of phospholipid components in the course of their axonal transport as visualized by radioautography. *Brain Research* **155,** 347–53.

Droz, B., Koenig, H.L., Di Giamberardino, L., Couraud, J.Y. and Souyri, F. (1979) The importance of axonal transport and endoplasmic reticulum in the function of the cholinergic synapse in normal and pathological conditions. In *The Cholinergic Synapse* (Ed. Tucek, S.), *Progress in Brain Research*, vol. 49, pp. 23–44. Elsevier, Amsterdam.

Droz, B. and LeBlond, C.P. (1963) Axonal migration of proteins in the central nervous system and peripheral nerves as shown by radioautography. *Journal of Comparative Neurology* **121,** 325–37.

Droz, B., Rambourg, A. and Koenig, H.L. (1975) The smooth endoplasmic reticulum: structure and role in the renewal of axon membrane and synaptic vesicles by fast axonal transport. *Brain Research* **93,** 1–13.

Duce, I.R. and Keen, P. (1976) A light and electron microscope study of changes occurring at the cut ends following section of the dorsal roots of rat spinal nerves. *Cell and Tissue Research* **170,** 491–505.

Duchen, L.W., Anjorin, A., Watkins, P.J. and Mackay, J.D. (1980) Pathology of autonomic neuropathy in diabetes. *Annals of Internal Medicine* **92,** 301–3.

Dulaney, J.T. and Moser, H.W. (1978) Sulfatide lipidosis: metachromatic leukodystrophy. In *The Metabolic Basis of Inherited Disease*, 4th edn (Eds. Stanbury, J.B., Wyngaarden, J.B. and Fredrickson, D.S.), pp. 770–809. McGraw-Hill, New York.

Dumas, M., Schwab, M.E. and Thoenen, H. (1979) Retrograde axonal transport of specific macromolecules as a tool for characterizing nerve terminal membranes. *Journal of Neurobiology* **10,** 179–97.

Dunn, H.G. and Dolman, C.L. (1969) Necrotizing encephalomyelopathy. Report of a case with relapsing polyneuropathy and hyperalaninemia and with manifestations resembling Friedreich's ataxia. *Neurology* **19,** 536–50.

Dunn, J.S. (1970) Developing myelin in human peripheral nerves. *Scottish Medical Journal* **15,** 108–17.

Dupuis, M., Brucher, J M. and Gonsette, R. (1983) Etude anatomoclinique d'une forme neuronale de la maladie de Charcot–Marie–Tooth. *Revue Neurologique* **139,** 643–9.

Dyck, P.J. (1969) Experimental hypertrophic neuropathy. Pathogenesis of onion-bulb formations produced by repeated tourniquet applications. *Archives of Neurology* **21,** 73–95.

Dyck, P.J. (1975) Inherited neuronal degeneration and atrophy affecting peripheral motor, sensory, and autonomic neurons. In *Peripheral Neuropathy* (Eds. Dyck, P.J., Thomas, P.K. and Lambert, E.H.), pp. 825–67. W.B. Saunders, Philadelphia.

Dyck, P.J. (1984) Inherited neuronal degeneration and atrophy, affecting peripheral motor, sensory, and autonomic neurons. In *Peripheral Neuropathy*, 2nd edn (Eds. Dyck, P.J., Thomas, P.K., Lambert, E.H. and Bunge, R.), pp. 1600–55. W.B. Saunders, Philadelphia.

Dyck, P.J., Conn, D.L. and Okazaki, H. (1972) Necrotizing angiopathic neuropathy: three-dimensional morphology of fiber degeneration related to sites of occluded vessels. *Mayo Clinic Proceedings* **47,** 461–75.

Dyck, P.J., Ellefson, R.D., Yao, J.K. and Herbert, P.N. (1978a) Adult-onset of Tangier disease. I. Morphometric and pathological studies suggesting delayed degradation of neutral lipids after fiber degeneration. *Journal of Neuropathology and Experimental Neurology* **37,** 119–37.

Dyck, P.J., Gutrecht, J.A., Bastron, J.A., Karnes, W.E. and Dale, A.J. (1968) Histologic and teased fiber measurements of sural nerve in disorders of lower motor and primary sensory neurons. *Mayo Clinic Proceedings* **43,** 81–123.

Dyck, P.J. and Hopkins, A.P. (1972) Electron microscopic observations on degeneration and regeneration of unmyelinated fibres. *Brain* **95,** 223–34.

Dyck, P.J., Johnson, W.J., Lambert, E.H. and O'Brien, P.C. (1971a) Segmental demyelination secondary to axonal degeneration in uremic neuropathy. *Mayo Clinic Proceedings* **46,** 400–31.

Dyck, P.J., Kawamura, Y., Low, P.A. and Shimono, M. (1978b) The numbers and sizes of reconstructed peripheral autonomic neurons in a case of dysautonomia. *Journal of Neuropathology and Experimental Neurology* **37,** 741–55.

Dyck, P.J. and Lais, A.C. (1973) Evidence for segmental demyelination secondary to axonal degeneration in Friedreich's ataxia. In *Clinical Studies in Myology* (Ed. Kakulas, B.A.), pp. 253–63. Excerpta Medica, Amsterdam.

Dyck, P.J., Lais, A.C., Karnes, J.L., Sparks, M., Hunder, H., Low, P.A. and Windebank, A.J. (1981a) Permanent axotomy, a model of axonal atrophy and secondary segmental demyelination and remyelination. *Annals of Neurology* **9,** 575–83.

Dyck, P.J., Lais, A.C. and Low, P.A. (1978) Nerve xenografts to assess cellular expression of the abnormality of myelination in inherited neuropathy and Friedreich ataxia. *Neurology* **28,** 261–5.

Dyck, P.J., Lais, A.C., Ohta, M., Bastron, J.A., Okazaki, H. and Groover, R.V. (1975) Chronic inflammatory polyradiculoneuropathy. *Mayo Clinic Proceedings* **50,** 621–37.

Dyck, P.J., Lais, A.C., Sparks, M.F., Oviatt, K.F., Hexum, L.A. and Steinmuller, D. (1979) Nerve xenografts to apportion the role of axon and Schwann cell in myelinated fiber absence in hereditary sensory neuropathy, type II. *Neurology* **29,** 1215–21.

Dyck, P.J. and Lambert, E.H. (1968a) Lower motor and primary sensory neuron diseases with peroneal muscular atrophy. I. Neurologic, genetic and electrophysiologic findings in hereditary polyneuropathies. *Archives of Neurology* **18,** 603–18.

Dyck, P.J. and Lambert, E.H. (1968b) Lower motor and primary sensory neuron diseases with peroneal muscular atrophy. II. Neurologic, genetic and electrophysiologic findings in various neuronal degenerations. *Archives of Neurology* **18,** 619–25.

Dyck, P.J. and Lambert, E.H. (1969) Dissociated sensation in amyloidosis. *Archives of Neurology* **20,** 490–507.

Dyck, P.J. and Lambert, E.H. (1970) Polyneuropathy associated with hypothyroidism. *Journal of Neuropathology and Experimental Neurology* **29,** 631–58.

Dyck, P.J., Lambert, E.H., Sanders, K. and O'Brien, P.C. (1971b) Severe hypomyelination and marked abnormality of conduction in Dejerine–Sottas hypertrophic neuropathy: myelin thickness and compound action potential of sural nerve in vitro. *Mayo Clinic Proceedings* **46,** 432–6.

Dyck, P.J., Mellinger, J.F., Reagan, T.J., Horowitz, S.J., McDonald, J.W., Litchy, W.J. et al. (1983) Not 'indifference to pain' but varieties of hereditary sensory and autonomic neuropathy. *Brain* **106,** 373–90.

Dyck, P.J. and Ohta, M. (1975) Neuronal atrophy and degeneration predominantly affecting peripheral sensory neurons. In *Peripheral Neuropathy* (Eds. Dyck, P.J., Thomas, P.K. and Lambert, E.H.), pp. 791–824. W.B. Saunders, Philadelphia.

Dyck, P.J., Sherman, W.R., Hallcher, L.M., Service, F.J., O'Brien, P.C., Grina, L.A. et al. (1980) Human diabetic endoneurial sorbitol, fructose and myo-inositol related to sural nerve morphometry. *Annals of Neurology* **8,** 590–6.

Dyck, P.J., Thomas, P.K., Lambert, E.H. and Bunge, R. (1984) *Peripheral Neuropathy*, 2nd edn. W.B. Saunders, Philadelphia.

Dyck, P.J., Yao, J.K., Knickerbocker, D.E., Holman, R.T., Gomez, M.R., Hayles, A.B. and Lambert, E.H. (1981b) Multisystem neuronal degeneration, hepatosplenomegaly, and adrenocortical deficiency associated with reduced tissue arachidonic acid. *Neurology* **31,** 925–34.

Eames, R.A. and Gamble, H.J. (1970) Schwann cell relationships in normal human cutaneous nerves. *Journal of Anatomy* **106,** 417–35.

Eames, R.A. and Lange, L.S. (1967) Clinical and pathological study of ischaemic neuropathy. *Journal of Neurology, Neurosurgery and Psychiatry* **30,** 215–26.

Ellisman, M.H. and Lindsey, J.D. (1983) The axoplasmic reticulum within myelinated axons is not transported rapidly. *Journal of Neurocytology* **12,** 393–411.

Erb, W.H. (1876) Diseases of the peripheral cerebrospinal nerves. In *Cyclopaedia of the Practice of Medicine*, vol. XI (Ed. Van Ziemssen, H.) William Wood, New York.

Erlicki, A. and Rybalkin, J. (1892) Ueber Arseniklähmung. *Archiv für Psychiatrie und Nervenkrankheiten* **23,** 861–95.

Evans, D.A.P., Manley, K.A. and McKusick, V.A. (1960) Genetic control of isoniazid metabolism in man. *British Medical Journal* **2,** 485–91.

Evans, D.H.L. and Vizoso, A.D. (1951) Observations on the mode of growth of motor nerve fibers in rabbits during postnatal development. *Journal of Comparative Neurology* **95,** 429–61.

Faerman, I., Glocer, L., Fox, D., Jadzinsky, M. and Rapaport, M. (1974) Impotence and diabetes: histological studies of the autonomic nervous fibers on the corpora cavernosa in impotent diabetic males. *Diabetes* **23,** 971–6.

Faerman, I., Maler, M., Jadzinsky, M., Alvarez, E., Fox, D., Zilbervarg, J. et al. (1971) Asymptomatic neurogenic bladder in juvenile diabetes. *Diabetologia* **7,** 168–72.

Fagerberg, S.E. (1959) Diabetic neuropathy: a clinical and histological study on the significance of vascular affections. *Acta Medica Scandinavica* suppl. 345.

Fardeau, M. and Engel, W.K. (1969) Ultrastructural study of peripheral nerve biopsy in Refsum's disease. *Journal of Neuropathology and Experimental Neurology* **28,** 278–94.

Fernandez, H.L., Burton, P.R. and Samson, F.E. (1971) Axoplasmic transport in the crayfish nerve cord. The role of fibrillar constituents of neurons. *Journal of Cell Biology* **51,** 176–92.

Fernandez, H.L. and Samson, F.E. (1974) Axoplasmic transport: differential inhibition by cytochalasin. *Journal of Neurobiology* **4,** 201–6.

Fine, E.J. and Hallett, M. (1980) Neurophysiological study of subacute combined degeneration. *Journal of the Neurological Sciences* **45,** 331–6.

Finegold, D., Lattimer, S.A., Nolle, S., Bernstein, M. and Greene, D.A. (1983) Polyol pathway activity and myo-inositol metabolism. A suggested relationship in the pathogenesis of diabetic neuropathy. *Diabetes* **32,** 988–92.

Fisher, C.M. (1955) Residual neuropathological changes in Canadians held prisoners of war by the Japanese. *Canadian Services Medical Journal* **11,** 157–99.

Fisher, C.M. and Adams, R.D. (1956) Diphtheritic polyneuritis—a pathological study. *Journal of Neuropathology and Experimental Neurology* **15,** 243–68.

Follis, R.H. and Wintrobe, M.M. (1945) A comparison of the effects of pyridoxine and pantothenic acid deficiency in swine. *Journal of Experimental Medicine* **81,** 539–52.

Forman, D.S. (1983) Axonal transport and nerve regeneration: a review. In *Spinal Cord Reconstruction* (Eds. Kao, C.C., Bunge, R.P. and Reier, P.J.), pp. 75–86. Raven Press, New York.

Forman, D.S., Padjen, A.L. and Siggins, G.R. (1977) Axonal transport of organelles visualized by light microscopy: cinematographic and computer analysis. *Brain Research* **136,** 197–213.

Fraher, J.P. (1972) A quantitative study of anterior root fibres during early myelination. *Journal of Anatomy* **112,** 99–124.

Friede, R.L. (1972) Control of myelin formation by axon calibre (with a model of the control mechanism). *Journal of Comparative Neurology* **144,** 233–52.

Friede, R.L. and Bischhausen, R. (1980) The precise geometry of large internodes. *Journal of the Neurological Sciences* **48,** 367–81.

Friede, R.L., Meier, T. and Diem, M. (1981) How is

the exact length of an internode determined? *Journal of the Neurological Sciences* **50,** 217–28.

Friede, R.L. and Samorajski, T. (1967) Relation between the number of myelin lamellae and axon circumference in fibers of vagus and sciatic nerves of mice. *Journal of Comparative Biology* **130,** 223–32.

Friede, R.L. and Samorajski, T. (1968) Myelin formation in the sciatic nerve of the rat—a quantitative electron microscopic, histochemical and radioautographic study. *Journal of Neuropathology and Experimental Neurology* **27,** 546–70.

Friede, R.L. and Samorajski, T. (1969) The clefts of Schmidt-Lanterman: a quantitative electron microscopic study of their structure in developing and adult sciatic nerves of the rat. *Anatomical Record* **165,** 379–88.

Friede, R.L. and Samorajski, T. (1970) Axon caliber related to neurofilaments and microtubules in sciatic nerve fibers of rats and mice. *Anatomical Record* **167,** 379–87.

Fullerton, P.M. (1966) Chronic peripheral neuropathy produced by lead poisoning in guinea-pigs. *Journal of Neuropathology and Experimental Neurology* **25,** 214–36.

Fullerton, P.M. (1969) Electrophysiological and histological observations on peripheral nerves in acrylamide poisoning in man. *Journal of Neurology, Neurosurgery and Psychiatry* **32,** 186–92.

Fullerton, P.M. and Barnes, J.M. (1966) Peripheral neuropathy in rats produced by acrylamide. *British Journal of Industrial Medicine* **25,** 210–21.

Fullerton, P.M. and O'Sullivan, D.J. (1968) Thalidomide neuropathy: a clinical, electrophysiological, and histological follow-up study. *Journal of Neurology, Neurosurgery and Psychiatry* **31,** 543–51.

Gainer, H. and Fink, D.J. (1982) Evidence for slow retrograde transport of serum albumin in rat sciatic nerve. *Brain Research* **233,** 404–8.

Gamble, H.J. (1964) Comparative electron-microscopic observations on the connective tissues of a peripheral nerve and a spinal nerve root in a rat. *Journal of Anatomy* **98,** 17–25.

Gamble, H.J. (1966) Further electron microscope studies of human foetal peripheral nerves. *Journal of Anatomy* **100,** 487–502.

Gamble, H.J. (1976) Spinal and cranial nerve roots. In *The Peripheral Nerve* (Ed. Landon, D.N.), pp. 330–54. Chapman and Hall, London.

Gamble, H.J. and Eames, R.A. (1964) An electron microscope study of the connective tissues of human peripheral nerve. *Journal of Anatomy* **98,** 655–63.

Garven, H.S.D., Gairns, F.W. and Smith, G. (1962) The nerve fibre populations of the nerves of the leg in chronic occlusive arterial disease in man. *Scottish Medical Journal* **7,** 250–65.

Gaskill, H.S. and Korb, M. (1946) Occurrence of multiple neuritis in cases of cutaneous diphtheria. *Archives of Neurology and Psychiatry* **55,** 559–72.

Gasser, H.S. (1955) Properties of dorsal root unmedullated fibers on the two sides of the ganglion. *Journal of General Physiology* **38,** 709–28.

Geren, B.B. (1954) The formation from the Schwann cell surface of myelin. *Experimental Cell Research* **7,** 558–62.

Gerstl, B. and Eng, L.F. (1981) Wallerian degeneration and molecular aspects of experimental allergic encephalomyelitis and peripheral neuritis. In *The Molecular Basis of Neuropathology* (Eds. Davison, A.N. and Thompson, R.H.S.), pp. 44–80. Edward Arnold, London.

Ghabriel, M.N. and Allt, G. (1979a) The role of Schmidt-Lanterman incisures in Wallerian degeneration. I. A quantitative teased fibre study. *Acta Neuropathologica* **48,** 83–93.

Ghabriel, M.N. and Allt, G. (1979b) The role of Schmidt-Lanterman incisures in Wallerian degeneration. II. An electron microscope study. *Acta Neuropathologica* **48,** 95–103.

Ghabriel, M.N. and Allt, G. (1981) Incisures of Schmidt-Lanterman. *Progress in Neurobiology* **17,** 25–58.

Gibson, J.B. and Goldberg, A. (1956) The neuropathy of acute porphyria. *Journal of Pathology and Bacteriology* **71,** 495–510.

Gibson, J.D. (1979) The origin of the neural macrophage: a quantitative ultrastructural study of cell population changes during Wallerian degeneration. *Journal of Anatomy* **129,** 1–19.

Glenner, G.C., Ignaczak, T.F. and Page, D.L. (1978) The inherited systemic amyloidoses and localized amyloid deposits. In *The Metabolic Basis of Inherited Disease* (Eds. Stanbury, J.B., Wyngaarden, J.B. and Fredrickson, D.S.), pp. 1308–39. McGraw-Hill, New York.

Goebel, H.H., Veit, S. and Dyck, P.J. (1980) Confirmation of virtual unmyelinated fiber absence in hereditary sensory neuropathy type IV. *Journal of Neuropathology and Experimental Neurology* **39,** 670–5.

Goldstein, N.P., McCall, J.T. and Dyck, P.J. (1975) Metal neuropathy. In *Peripheral Neuropathy* (Eds. Dyck, P.J., Thomas, P.K. and Lambert, E.H.), pp. 1227–62. W.B. Saunders, Philadelphia.

Gombault, A. (1880–81) Contribution à l'étude anatomique de la névrite parenchymateuse subaiguë et chronique: névritre segmentaire périaxile. *Archives de Neurologie (Paris)* **1,** 11–38, 177–190.

Gombault, A. and Mallet (1889) Un cas de tabès ayant débuté dans l'enfance. *Archives de Médecine Expérimentale* **1,** 385–415.

Goodman, W.N., Cooper, W.C., Kessler, G.B.,

Fischer, M.S. and Gardner, M.B. (1969) Ataxia telangiectasia, a report of two cases in siblings presenting a picture of progressive muscular atrophy. *Bulletin of the Los Angeles Neurological Society* **34,** 1-22.

Gould, R.M. (1977) Incorporation of glycoprotein into peripheral nerve myelin. *Journal of Cell Biology* **75,** 326-38.

Gould, R.M. and Holt, S.J. (1961) Observations on acid phosphatase and esterases in the rat sciatic nerve undergoing Wallerian degeneration. *Journal of Anatomy* **95,** 45-8.

Gould, R.M. and Sinatra, R.S. (1981) Internodal distribution of phosphatidylcholine biosynthetic activity in teased peripheral nerve fibres: an autoradiographic study. *Journal of Neurocytology* **10,** 161-7.

Grafstein, B. and Forman, D.S. (1980) Intracellular transport in neurons. *Physiological Reviews* **60,** 1167-283.

Graham, D.G., Anthony, D.C., Boekelheide, K., Maschmann, N.A., Richards, R.G., Wolfram, J.W. and Shaw, B.R. (1982) Studies of the molecular pathogenesis of hexane neuropathy. II. Evidence that pyrrole derivatization of lysyl residues leads to protein cross linking. *Toxicology and Applied Pharmacology* **64,** 415-22.

Gray, E.G. and Westrum, L.E. (1979) Marginal bundles of axoplasmic microtubules at nodes of Ranvier within muscle. *Cell and Tissue Research* **199,** 281-8.

Greenbaum, D., Richardson, P.C., Salmon, M.V. and Urich, H. (1964) Pathological observations on six cases of diabetic neuropathy. *Brain* **87,** 201-14.

Gregson, N.A. (1976) The chemistry and structure of myelin. In *The Peripheral Nerve* (Ed. Landon, D.N.), pp. 512-604. Chapman and Hall, London.

Griffin, J.W., Goren, E., Schaumburg, H., Engel, W.K. and Loriaux, L. (1977) Adrenomyeloneuropathy: a probable variant of adrenoleukodystrophy. I. Clinical and endocrinologic aspects. *Neurology* **27,** 1107-13.

Griffin, J.W., Price, D.L., Drachman, D.B. and Morris, J. (1981) Incorporation of axonally transported glycoproteins into axolemma during nerve regeneration. *Journal of Cell Biology* **88,** 205-14.

Groothuis, D.R., Schulman, S., Wollman, R., Frey, J. and Vick, N.A. (1980) Demyelinating radiculopathy in the Kearns-Sayre syndrome: a clinicopathological study. *Annals of Neurology* **8,** 373-80.

Gross, G.G. (1975) The microstream concept of axoplasmic and dendritic transport. In *Advances in Neurology* (Ed. Kreutzberg, G.W.), pp. 283-96. Raven Press, New York.

Grover-Johnson, N.M., Baumann, F.G., Imparato, A.M., Kim, G.E. and Thomas, P.K. (1981) Abnormal innervation of lower limb epineurial arterioles in human diabetes. *Diabetologia* **20,** 31-8.

Grunnet, M.L. and Petajan, J.H. (1976) Carbon monoxide induced neuropathy in the rat. Ultrastructural changes. *Archives of Neurology* **33,** 158-63.

Grunnet, M.L., Zimmerman, A.W. and Lewis, R.A. (1983) Ultrastructure and electrodiagnosis of peripheral neuropathy in Cockayne's syndrome. *Neurology* **33,** 1606-12.

Guiloff, R.J., Thomas, P.K., Contreras, M., Armitage, S., Schwarz, G. and Sedgwick, E.M. (1982) Evidence for linkage of type I hereditary motor and sensory neuropathy with the Duffy locus on chromosome 1. *Annals of Human Genetics* **46,** 25-9.

Guy, R., Watkins, P.J., Sharma, A.K., Thomas, P.K. and Dawson, J.L. (1984) Symptomatic gastroparesis diabeticorum: the role of surgery. *Journal of Neurology, Neurosurgery and Psychiatry* **47,** 686-91.

Guzzetta, F., Ferrière, G. and Lyon, G. (1982) Congenital hypomyelination polyneuropathy: pathological findings compared with polyneuropathies starting in later life. *Brain* **105,** 395-416.

Haftek, J. (1970) Stretch injury of peripheral nerve. Acute effects of stretching on rabbit nerve. *Journal of Bone and Joint Surgery* **52B,** 354-65.

Haftek, J. and Thomas, P.K. (1968) Electron-microscope observations on the effects of localized crush injuries on the connective tissues of peripheral nerve. *Journal of Anatomy* **103,** 233-43.

Hahn, A.F., Gordon, B.A., Gilbert, J.J. and Hinton, G.G. (1981) The AB variant of metachromatic leukodystrophy (postulated activator protein deficiency). Light and electron microscope findings in a sural nerve biopsy. *Acta Neuropathologica* **55,** 218-27.

Haley, J.E. and Ledeen, R.W. (1979) Incorporation of axonally transported substances in myelin lipids. *Journal of Neurochemistry* **32,** 735-42.

Hall, B.M., Walsh, J.C., Horvath, J.S. and Lytton, D.G. (1976) Peripheral neuropathy complicating primary hyperoxaluria. *Journal of the Neurological Sciences* **29,** 343-9.

Hall, S.M. (1983) The response of the (myelinating) Schwann cell population to multiple episodes of demyelination. *Journal of Neurocytology* **12,** 1-12.

Hall, S.M. and Gregson, N.A. (1971) The *in vivo* and ultrastructural effects of injection of lysophosphatidyl choline into myelinated peripheral nerve fibres of the adult mouse. *Journal of Cell Science* **9,** 769-89.

Hall, S.M. and Williams, P.L. (1970) Studies on the incisures of Schmidt and Lanterman. *Journal of Cell Science* **6,** 767-92.

Hall, S.M. and Williams, P.L. (1971) The distribution

of electron-dense tracers in peripheral nerve fibres. *Journal of Cell Science* **8,** 541–55.

Hallpike, J.F., Adams, C.W.M. and Bayliss, O.B. (1970) Histochemistry of myelin. IX. Neutral and acid proteinases in early Wallerian degeneration. *Histochemical Journal* **2,** 209–18.

Hanson, M. and Edström, A. (1978) Mitosis inhibitors and axonal transport. *International Review of Cytology* suppl. 7, 373–402.

Harding, A.E., Muller, D.P.R., Thomas, P.K. and Willison, H.J. (1982) Spinocerebellar degeneration secondary to chronic intestinal malabsorption: a vitamin E deficiency syndrome. *Annals of Neurology* **12,** 419–24.

Harding, A.E. and Thomas, P.K. (1980a) The clinical features of hereditary motor and sensory neuropathy types I and II. *Brain* **103,** 259–80.

Harding, A.E. and Thomas, P.K. (1980b) Hereditary distal spinal muscular atrophy. A report on 34 cases and a review of the literature. *Journal of the Neurological Sciences* **45,** 337–48.

Harding, A.E. and Thomas, P.K. (1980c) Autosomal recessive forms of hereditary motor and sensory neuropathy types I and II. *Journal of Neurology, Neurosurgery and Psychiatry* **43,** 669–78.

Harkin, J.C. (1964) A series of desmosomal attachments in the Schwann cell sheath of myelinated mammalian nerves. *Zeitschrift für Zellforschung und mikroskopische Anatomie* **64,** 189–95.

Hawkes, C.H., Jefferson, J.M., Jones, E.L. and Smith, W.T. (1974) Hypertrophic mononeuropathy. *Journal of Neurology, Neurosurgery and Psychiatry* **37,** 76–81.

Haymaker, W. and Kernohan, J.W. (1949) Landry-Guillain-Barré syndrome: 50 fatal cases and a critique of the literature. *Medicine* **28,** 59–141.

Henson, R.A. and Urich, H. (1982) *Cancer and the Nervous System.* Blackwell Scientific, Oxford.

Hess, A. and Lansing, A.J. (1953) The fine structure of peripheral nerve fibers. *Anatomical Record* **117,** 175–200.

Hess, A. and Young, J.Z. (1952) The nodes of Ranvier. *Proceedings of the Royal Society of London B* **140,** 301–20.

Heuser, J.E. and Reese, T.S. (1973) Evidence for recycling of synaptic vesicle membrane during transmitter release at the frog muscular junction. *Journal of Cell Biology* **57,** 315–44.

Hierons, R. (1957) Changes in the nervous system in acute porphyria. *Brain* **80,** 176–92.

Highet, W.B. and Holmes, W. (1943) Traction injuries to the lateral popliteal nerve and traction injuries to peripheral nerves after suture. *British Journal of Surgery* **30,** 212–33.

Hirano, A. and Dembitzer, H.M. (1969) The transverse bands as a means of access to the periaxonal space of the central myelinated nerve fibers. *Journal of Ultrastructure Research* **28,** 141–9.

Hiscoe, H.B. (1947) Distribution of nodes and incisures in normal and regenerated nerve fibers. *Anatomical Record* **99,** 447–76.

Hodgkin, A.L. (1971) *The Conduction of the Nervous Impulse.* University Press, Liverpool.

Holmes, W. and Young, J.Z. (1942) Nerve regeneration after immediate and delayed suture. *Journal of Anatomy* **77,** 63–96.

Holtzman, E. (1971) Cytochemical studies of protein transport in the nervous system. *Philosophical Transactions of the Royal Society of London, B* **261,** 407–21.

Holtzman, E. (1977) The origin and fate of secretory packages, especially synaptic vesicles. *Neuroscience* **2,** 327–55.

Holtzman, E. and Novikoff, A.B. (1965) Lysosomes in the rat sciatic nerve following crush. *Journal of Cell Biology* **27,** 651–69.

Honjin, R., Nakamura, T. and Imura, M. (1959) Electron microscopy of peripheral nerve fibres. III. On the axoplasmic changes during Wallerian degeneration. *Okajimas Folia Anatomica Japonica (Tokyo)* **33,** 131–56.

Horwich, M.S., Cho, L., Porro, R.S. and Posner, J.B. (1977) Subacute sensory neuropathy: a remote effect of carcinoma. *Annals of Neurology* **2,** 7–19.

Hughes, J.T. and Brownell, B. (1972) Pathology of peroneal muscular atrophy (Charcot-Marie-Tooth disease). *Journal of Neurology, Neurosurgery and Psychiatry* **35,** 648–57.

Hughes, R.A.C., Cameron, J.S. and Hall, S.M. (1982) Multiple mononeuropathy as the initial presentation of SLE. *Journal of Neurology* **228,** 239–47.

Hughes, R.A.C., Kadlubowski, M., Gray, I.A. and Leibowitz, S. (1981) Immune responses in experimental allergic neuritis. *Journal of Neurology, Neurosurgery and Psychiatry* **44,** 565–9.

Hutchinson, E.C. and Liversedge, L.A. (1956) Neuropathy in peripheral vascular disease. *Quarterly Journal of Medicine* **25** (NS), 267–74.

Isenberg, G., Schubert, P. and Kreutzberg, G.W. (1980) Experimental approach to test the role of actin in axonal transport. *Brain Research* **194,** 588–93.

Iwashita, H., Argyrakis, A., Lowitzsch, K. and Spaar, F.W. (1974) Polyneuropathy in Waldenström's macroglobulinaemia. *Journal of the Neurological Sciences* **21,** 341–54.

Iwashita, H., Ohnishi, A., Asada, Y., Kanazawa, Y. and Kuroiwa, Y. (1977) Polyneuropathy, skin hyperpigmentation, edema and hypertrichosis in localized osteosclerotic myeloma. *Neurology* **7,** 675–81.

Jacob, J.C., Andermann, F. and Robb, J.P. (1961) Heredofamilial mononeuritis multiplex with brachial predeliction. *Brain* **83,** 113–37.

Jacobs, J.M., Carmichael, N. and Cavanagh, J.B. (1975) Ultrastructural changes in the dorsal root and trigeminal ganglia of rats poisoned with methylmercury. *Neuropathology and Applied Neurobiology* **1,** 1–19.

Jacobs, J.M., Miller, R.H. and Cavanagh, J.B. (1979) The distribution of degenerative changes in INH neuropathy. Further evidence for focal axonal lesions. *Acta Neuropathologica* **48,** 1–9.

Jacobs, J.M., Miller, R.H., Whittle, A. and Cavanagh, J.B. (1979) Studies on the early changes in acute isoniazid neuropathy in the rat. *Acta Neuropathologica* **47,** 85–92.

Jack, J.J.B. (1976) Electrophysiological properties of peripheral nerve. In *The Peripheral Nerve* (Ed. Landon, D.N.), pp. 740–818. Chapman and Hall, London.

Jakobsen, J., Brimijoin, W.S. and Sidenius, P. (1983) Axonal transport in neuropathy. *Muscle and Nerve* **6,** 164–6.

Jakovleva, J. (1927) Diphtheriepolyneuritis nach (versehentlicher) Einspritzung von Diphtherietoxin (Abstr.). *Zentralblatt für die gesamte Neurologie und Psychiatrie* **47,** 203.

Jefferson, D. and Eames, R.A. (1979) Subclinical entrapment of the lateral femoral cutaneous nerve: an autopsy study. *Muscle and Nerve* **2,** 145–54.

Jellinger, K. and Radiaszkiewicz, T. (1976) Involvement of the central nervous system in malignant lymphomas. *Virchows Archiv Abteilung A. Pathologische Anatomie* **370,** 345–62.

Job, C.K. (1970) *Mycobacterium leprae* in nerve lesions in lepromatous leprosy: an electron-microscopic study. *Archives of Pathology* **89,** 195–207.

Job, C.K. and Desikan, K.V. (1968) Pathologic changes and their distribution in peripheral nerves in lepromatous leprosy. *International Journal of Leprosy* **36,** 257–70.

Johnson, P.C., Rolak, L.A., Hamilton, R.H. and Laguna, J.F. (1979) Paraneoplastic vasculitis of nerve: a remote effect of cancer. *Annals of Neurology* **5,** 437–44.

Johnson, R.T. and Richardson, E.P. (1968) The neurological manifestations of systemic lupus erythematosus: a clinicopathological study of 24 cases and a review of the literature. *Medicine* **47,** 337–69.

Kaltreider, H.B. and Talal, N. (1969) The neuropathy of Sjögren's syndrome: trigeminal nerve involvement. *Annals of Internal Medicine* **70,** 751–62.

Karat, A.B.A., Furness, M.A., Karat, S. and Rao, P.S.S. (1969) Patterns of neurological involvement in relation to chronic and/or recurrent erythema nodosum leprosum. *Leprosy Review* **40,** 49–53.

Karch, S.B. and Urich, H. (1975) Infantile polyneuropathy with defective myelination: an autopsy study. *Developmental Medicine and Child Neurology* **17,** 504–11.

Katrak, S.M., Pollock, M., O'Brien, C.P., Nukada, H., Allpress, S., Calder, C. et al. (1980) Clinical and morphological features of gold neuropathy. *Brain* **103,** 671–93.

Kelly, J.J., Kyle, R.A., Miles, J.M., O'Brien, P.C. and Dyck, P.J. (1981) The spectrum of peripheral neuropathy in myeloma. *Neurology* **31,** 24–31.

Kernohan, J.W. and Woltman, H.W. (1938) Periarteritis nodosa: a clinicopathologic study with special reference to the nervous system. *Archives of Neurology and Psychiatry* **39,** 655–86.

Kibler, R.F. and Rose, F.C. (1960) Peripheral neuropathy in the 'collagen diseases'. A case of scleroderma neuropathy. *British Medical Journal* **1,** 1781–4.

King, R.H.M. and Thomas, P.K. (1971) Electron microscope observations on aberrant regeneration of unmyelinated axons in the vagus nerve of the rabbit. *Acta Neuropathologica* **18,** 150–9.

King, R.H.M. and Thomas, P.K. (1984) The occurrence and significance of myelin with unusually large periodicity. *Acta Neuropathologica* **63,** 319–29.

Klemm, H. (1970) Das Perineurium als Diffusionsbarriere gegenüber Peroxydase bei epi- und endoneuraler Applikation. *Zeitschrift für Zellforschung und mikroskopische Anatomie* **108,** 431–5.

Knill-Jones, R.P., Goodwill, C.J., Dayan, A.D. and Williams, R. (1972) Peripheral neuropathy in chronic liver disease; clinical, electrodiagnostic and nerve biopsy findings. *Journal of Neurology, Neurosurgery and Psychiatry* **35,** 22–30.

Kocen, R.S., King, R.H.M., Thomas, P.K. and Haas, L.F. (1973) Nerve biopy findings in two cases of Tangier disease. *Acta Neuropathologica* **26,** 317–27.

Kocen, R.S., Lloyd, J.K., Lascelles, P.T., Fosbrooke, A.S. and Williams, D. (1967) Familial α-lipoprotein deficiency (Tangier disease) with neurological abnormalities. *Lancet* **1,** 1341–5.

Kocen, R.S. and Thomas, P.K. (1970) Peripheral nerve involvement in Fabry's disease. *Archives of Neurology* **22,** 81–8.

Koch, T., Schultz, P., Williams, R. and Lampert, P. (1977) Giant axonal neuropathy: a childhood disorder of microfilaments. *Annals of Neurology* **1,** 138–51.

Kocsis, J.D. and Waxman, S.G. (1980) Absence of potassium conductance in central myelinated axons. *Nature* (*London*) **287,** 348–9.

Korobkin, R., Asbury, A.K., Sumner, A.J. and Nielsen, S.L. (1975) Glue-sniffing neuropathy. *Archives of Neurology* **32,** 158–62.

Krishnan, N. and Singer, M. (1973) Penetration of peroxidase into peripheral nerve fibers. *American Journal of Anatomy* **136,** 1–14.

Kristensson, K., Nordborg, C. Olsson, Y. and Sourander, P. (1971) Changes in the vagus nerve in diabetes mellitus. *Acta Pathologica et Microbiologica Scandinavica (A)* **79,** 684–5.

Kristensson, K. and Olsson, Y. (1971) The perineurium as a diffusion barrier to protein tracers. Differences between mature and immature animals. *Acta Neuropathologica* **17,** 127–38.

Kristensson, K. and Olsson, Y. (1973) Diffusion pathways and retrograde axonal transport of protein tracers in peripheral nerves. In *Progress in Neurobiology*, vol. 1 (Eds. Kerkut, G.A. and Phillis, J.W.), pp. 85–109. Pergamon Press, Oxford.

Kristensson, K. and Olsson, Y. (1976) Osmotic opening of perineurial diffusion barrier in peripheral nerve. *Neuropathology and Applied Neurobiology* **2,** 479–88.

Kristol, C., Akert, K., Sandri, C., Wyss, U.R., Bennett, M.V.L. and Moor, H. (1977) The Ranvier nodes in the neurogenic electric organ of the knife fish *Sternarchus*: a freeze-etching study on the distribution of membrane associated particles. *Brain Research* **125,** 197–212.

Kristol, C., Sandri, C. and Akert, K. (1978) Intramembranous particles at the nodes of Ranvier of the cat spinal cord: a morphometric study. *Brain Research* **142,** 391–400.

Lallemand, R.C. and Weller, R.O. (1973) Intraneural neurofibromas involving the posterior interosseous nerve. *Journal of Neurology, Neurosurgery and Psychiatry* **36,** 991–6.

Lampert, P. (1969) Mechanism of demyelination in experimental allergic neuritis. *Laboratory Investigation* **20,** 127–38.

Lampert, P.W. and Schochet, S.S.Jr (1968) Demyelination and remyelination in lead neuropathy—electron microscopic studies. *Journal of Neuropathology and Experimental Neurology* **27,** 527–45.

Landon, D.N. (Ed.) (1976) *The Peripheral Nerve*. Chapman and Hall, London.

Landon, D.N. (1981) Structure of normal peripheral myelinated nerve fibres. In *Demyelinating Disease: Basic and Clinical Electrophysiology* (Eds. Waxman, S.G. and Ritchie, J.M.), pp. 25–49. Raven Press, New York.

Landon, D.N. and Hall, S. (1976) The myelinated nerve fibre. In *The Peripheral Nerve* (Ed. Landon, D.N.), pp. 1–105. Chapman and Hall, London.

Landon, D.N. and Langley, O.K. (1971) The local chemical environment of nodes of Ranvier. A study of cation binding. *Journal of Anatomy* **108,** 419–32.

Landon, D.N. and Williams, P.L. (1963) Ultrastructure of the node of Ranvier. *Nature (London)* **199,** 575–7.

Langley, O.K. (1971) A comparison of the binding of Alcian blue and inorganic cations to polyanions in peripheral nerve. *Histochemical Journal* **3,** 251–60.

Lasek, R.J. (1982) Translation of the neuronal cytoskeleton and axonal locomotion. *Philosophical Transactions of the Royal Society of London, B* **229,** 313–27.

Lasek, R.J. and Black, M.M. (1977) How do axons stop growing? Some clues from the metabolism of the proteins in the slow component of axonal transport. In *Mechanisms, Regulation and Special Function of Protein Synthesis in the Brain* (Eds. Roberts, S., Lajtha, A. and Gispen, W.H.), pp. 161–70, Elsevier, Amsterdam.

Lassmann, G., Lassmann, H. and Stockinger, L. (1976) Morton's metatarsalgia. Light and electron microscope observations and their relation to entrapment neuropathies. *Virchows Archiv Abteilung A. Pathologische Anatomie* **370,** 307–21.

Latov, N., Sherman, W.H., Nemni, R., Galassi, G., Shyong, J.S., Penn, A.S. et al. (1980) Plasma cell dyscrasia and peripheral neuropathy with a monoclonal antibody to peripheral nerve myelin. *New England Journal of Medicine* **303,** 618–21.

Leibowitz, S. and Hughes, R.A.C. (1983) *Immunology of the Nervous System*, pp. 101–30. Edward Arnold, London.

Le Quesne, P.M. and McLeod, J.G. (1977) Peripheral neuropathy following a single exposure to arsenic. Clinical course in four patients with electrophysiological and histological studies. *Journal of the Neurological Sciences* **32,** 437–51.

Lewis, P.D. (1977) Abiotrophy revisited. In *Motor Neurone Disease* (Ed. Clifford Rose, F.), pp. 30–5. Pitman Medical, London.

Lewy, F.H., Spies, T.D. and Aring, C.D. (1940) Incidence of neuropathy in pellagra: effect of cocarboxylase upon its neurologic signs. *American Journal of the Medical Sciences* **199,** 840–9.

Lhermitte, F., Fardeau, M., Chedru, F. and Mallecourt, J. (1976) Polyneuropathy after perhexilene maleate therapy. *British Medical Journal* **1,** 1256.

Lhermitte, F., Fritel, D., Cambier, J., Marteau, R., Gautier, J.C. and Nocton, F. (1963) Polynévrites au cours des traitements par la nitrofurantoine. *Presse Médicale* **71,** 767–70.

Lieberman, A.R. (1968) The connective tissue elements of the mammalian nodose ganglion. *Zeitschrift für Zellforschung und mikroskopische Anatomie* **89,** 95–111.

Lieberman, A.R. (1976) Sensory ganglia. In *The Peripheral Nerve* (Ed. Landon, D.N.), pp. 188–278. Chapman and Hall, London.

Liebow, A.A., Carrington, C.R.B. and Friedman, P.J. (1972) Lymphomatoid granulomatosis. *Human Pathology* **3,** 457–558.

Lisak, R.P., Mitchell, M., Zweiman, B., Orrechio, E. and Asbury, A.K. (1977) Guillain-Barré syndrome and Hodgkin's disease: three cases with immunological studies. *Annals of Neurology* **1,** 72–8.

Livingston, R.B., Pfenniger, K., Moor, H. and Akert, K. (1973) Specialized paranodal and interparanodal glial-axonal junctions in the peripheral and central nervous system: a freeze-etching study. *Brain Research* **58,** 1-24.

Lockman, L.A., Kennedy, W.R. and White, J.G. (1967) The Chediak-Higashi syndrome. *Journal of Pediatrics* **79,** 942-51.

Love, S. (1983) An experimental study of peripheral nerve regeneration after x-irradiation. *Brain* **106,** 39-54.

Lovshin, L.L. and Kernohan, J.W. (1948) Peripheral neuritis in periarteritis nodosa: a clinicopathologic study. *Archives of Internal Medicine* **82,** 321-38.

Low, F.N. (1976) The perineurium and connective tissue of peripheral nerve. In *The Peripheral Nerve* (Ed. Landon, D.N.), pp. 159-87. Chapman and Hall, London.

Low, P.A. (1976a) Hereditary hypertrophic neuropathy in the trembler mouse. 1. Histopathological studies: light microscopy. *Journal of the Neurological Sciences* **30,** 327-41.

Low, P.A. (1976b) Hereditary hypertrophic neuropathy in the trembler mouse. 2. Histopathological studies: electron microscopy. *Journal of the Neurological Sciences* **30,** 343-68.

Low, P.A., Burke, W.J. and McLeod, J.G. (1978) Congenital sensory neuropathy with selective loss of small myelinated fibers. *Annals of Neurology* **3,** 179-82.

Low, P.A., McLeod, J.G. and Prineas, J.W. (1978) Hypertrophic Charcot-Marie-Tooth disease: light and electron microscope studies of the sural nerve. *Journal of the Neurological Sciences* **35,** 93-115.

Low, P.A., McLeod, J.G., Turtle, J.R., Donnelly, P. and Wright, R.E. (1974) Peripheral neuropathy in acromegaly. *Brain* **97,** 139-52.

Low, P., Walsh, J.C., Huang, C.Y. and McLeod, J.G. (1975) The sympathetic nervous system in diabetic neuropathy—a clinical and pathological study. *Brain* **98,** 357-64.

Lubińska, L. (1954) Form of myelinated nerve fibres. *Nature (London)* **173,** 867-9.

Lubińska, L. (1961) Demyelination and remyelination in the proximal parts of regenerating nerve fibres. *Journal of Comparative Neurology* **117,** 275-89.

Lubińska, L. (1982) Patterns of Wallerian degeneration of myelinated fibres in short and long peripheral stumps and in isolated segments of rat phrenic nerve. Interpretation of the role of axoplasmic flow of the trophic factor. *Brain Research* **233,** 227-40.

Lubińska, L. and Niemierko, S. (1971) Velocity and intensity of bidirectional migration of acetylcholinesterase in transected nerves. *Brain Research* **27,** 329-42.

Ludwig, J., Dyck, P.J. and LaRusso, N.F. (1982) Xanthomatous neuropathy of the liver. *Human Pathology* **13,** 1049-51.

Lüllmann, H. and Lüllmann-Rauch, R. (1978) Perhexilene induces generalized lipidosis in rats. *Klinische Wochenschrift* **56,** 309-10.

McDonald, W.I. (1963) The effects of experimental demyelination on conduction in peripheral nerve: a histological and electrophysiological study. I. Clinical and histological observations. *Brain* **86,** 481-524.

McLeod, J.G. (1971) An electrophysiological and pathological study of peripheral nerves in Friedreich's ataxia. *Journal of the Neurological Sciences* **12,** 333-49.

McLeod, J.G. (1984) Carcinomatous neuropathy. In *Peripheral Neuropathy*, 2nd edn (Eds. Dyck, P.J., Thomas, P.K., Lambert, E.H. and Bunge, R.), pp. 2180-91. W.B. Saunders, Philadelphia.

McLeod, J.G. and Evans, W.A. (1981) Peripheral neuropathy in spinocerebellar degenerations. *Muscle and Nerve* **4,** 51-61.

Madrid, R. and Bradley, W.G. (1975) The pathology of neuropathies with focal thickening of the myelin sheath (tomaculous neuropathy): studies on the formation of the abnormal myelin sheath. *Journal of the Neurological Sciences* **25,** 415-48.

Malbouisson, A.M.B., Ghabriel, M.N. and Allt, G. (1984) The non-directional pattern of axonal changes in Wallerian degeneration: a computer-aided morphometric analysis. *Journal of Anatomy* **139,** 159-74.

Martin, J.-J., Ceuterick, C., Mercelis, R. and Joris, C. (1982) Pathology of peripheral nerves in metachromatic leucodystrophy: a comparative study of ten cases. *Journal of the Neurological Sciences* **53,** 95-112.

Martin, J.R. and Webster, H. de F. (1973) Mitotic Schwann cells in developing nerve: their changes in shape, fine structure and axon relationships. *Developmental Biology* **32,** 417-31.

Martinez, A.J. and Friede, R.L. (1970) Accumulation of axoplasmic organelles in swollen nerve fibres. *Brain Research* **19,** 183-98.

Matthews, W.B. (1984) Sarcoid neuropathy. In *Peripheral Neuropathy*, 2nd edn (Eds. Dyck, P.J., Thomas, P.K., Lambert, E.H. and Bunge, R.), pp. 2018-26. W.B. Saunders, Philadelphia.

Meier, C. and Bischoff, A. (1977) Polyneuropathy in hypothyroidism—clinical and nerve biopsy study of 4 cases. *Journal of Neurology* **213,** 103-14.

Meier, C., Kauer, B., Müller, U. and Ludin, H.P. (1979) Neuromyopathy during chronic amiodarone treatment. A case report. *Journal of Neurology* **220,** 231-9.

Meier, C. and Moll, C. (1982) Hereditary neuropathy with liability to pressure palsies. Report of two families and review of the literature. *Journal of Neurology* **228,** 73–95.

Meyer, P. (1881) Anatomische Untersuchungen über diphtheritische Lähmung. *Virchows Archiv für pathologische Anatomie* **85,** 181–226.

Mitchell, S. Weir (1872) *Injuries of Nerves and their Consequences*, p. 92. J.B. Lippincott, Philadelphia.

Mohammed, U.H.M. (1983) Quantitative Light and Electron Microscopic Studies of Peripheral Nerve Fibres in the Frog *Rana temporaria:* with particular reference to the nodes of Ranvier. PhD Thesis, University of London.

Mohammed, U.H.M., Landon, D.N. and Love, S. (1983) Ultrastructural morphometry of frog nodes of Ranvier. *Journal of Anatomy* **137,** 822–3.

Moorhead, P.J., Cooper, D.J. and Timperley, W.R. (1975) Progressive peripheral neuropathy in a patient with primary hyperoxaluria. *British Medical Journal* **2,** 312–13.

Moosa, A. and Dubowitz, V. (1970) Peripheral neuropathy in Cockayne's syndrome. *Archives of Disease in Childhood* **45,** 674–7.

Moran, N., Palti, Y., Levitan, E. and Stämpfli, R. (1980) Potassium ion accumulation at the external surface of the nodal membrane in frog myelinated fibres. *Biophysical Journal* **32,** 939–54.

Morell, P. (1977) *Myelin.* Plenum Press, New York.

Morris, J.H., Hudson, A.R. and Weddell, G. (1972) A study of degeneration and regeneration in the divided rat sciatic nerve based on electron microscopy. I. The traumatic degeneration of myelin in the proximal stump of the divided nerve. *Zeitschrift für Zellforschung und mikroskopische Anatomie* **124,** 86–102.

Morris, J.R. and Lasek, R.J. (1982) Stable polymers of the cytoskeleton: the axoplasmic ghost. *Journal of Cell Biology* **92,** 192–8.

Moser, H.W. (1983) Ceramidase deficiency: Farber's lipogranulomatosis. In *The Metabolic Basis of Inherited Diseases*, 5th edn (Eds. Stanbury, J.B., Wyngaarden, J.B., Fredrickson, D.S., Goldstein, J.L. and Brown, M.S.), pp. 820–30. McGraw-Hill, New York.

Moser, H.W., Moser, A.B., Kawamura, M., Migeon, B., O'Neill, B., Fenselau, B. and Kishimoto, Y. (1980) Adrenoleukodystrophy: studies in the phenotype, genetics and biochemistry. *Johns Hopkins Medical Journal* **147,** 217–24.

Mugnaini, E., Osen, K.K., Schnapp, B. and Friedrich, V.L. (1977) Distribution of Schwann cell cytoplasm and plasmalemmal vesicles (caveolae) in peripheral myelin sheaths. An electron microscopic study with thin sections and freeze-fracturing. *Journal of Neurocytology* **6,** 647–68.

Muller, D.P.R., Lloyd, J.K. and Wolff, O.H. (1983) Vitamin E and neurological function. *Lancet* **1,** 225–8.

Myers, R.R., Powell, H.C., Shapiro, H.M., Costello, M.L. and Lampert, P.W. (1980) Changes in endoneurial fluid pressure, permeability, and peripheral nerve ultrastructure in experimental lead neuropathy. *Annals of Neurology* **8,** 392–401.

Nageotte, J. (1922) *L'Organisation de la Matière.* Felix Alcan, Paris.

Nageotte, J. (1932) Sheaths of the peripheral nerves, nerve degeneration and regeneration. In *Cytology and Cellular Pathology of the Nervous System* vol. 1 (Ed. Penfield, W.), pp. 189–239. Hoeber, New York.

Neary, D. and Eames, R.A. (1975) The pathology of ulnar compression in man. *Neuropathology and Applied Neurobiology* **1,** 69–88.

Neary, D., Ochoa, J. and Gilliatt, R.W. (1975) Subclinical entrapment neuropathy in man. *Journal of the Neurological Sciences* **24,** 283–98.

Nelson, J.S., Fitch, C.D., Fischer, V.W., Broun, G.O. and Chou, A.C. (1981) Progressive neuropathologic lesions in a vitamin E-deficient rhesus monkeys. *Journal of Neuropathology and Experimental Neurology* **40,** 166–86.

Nemni, R., Galassi, G., Cohen, M., Hays, A.P., Gould, R., Singh, N. et al. (1981) Symmetric sarcoid polyneuropathy: analysis of a sural nerve biopsy. *Neurology* **31,** 1217–23.

Nickel, S.N., Frame, B., Bebin, J., Tourtellotte, W.W., Parker, J.A. and Hughes, B.R. (1961) Myxedema neuropathy and myopathy—A clinical and pathological study. *Neurology* **11,** 125–37.

North, J.D.K. and Sinclair, H.M. (1956) Nutritional neuropathy: chronic thiamine deficiency in the rat. *AMA Archives of Pathology* **62,** 341–53.

Norton, W.T. (1981) Biochemistry of myelin. In *Demyelinating Disease: Basic and Clinical Electrophysiology* (Eds. Waxman, S.G. and Ritchie, J.M.), *Advances in Neurology* **31,** 93–121.

Nukada, H., Dyck, P.J. and Karnes, J.L. (1983) Thin axons relative to myelin spiral length in hereditary motor and sensory neuropathy, type I. *Annals of Neurology* **4,** 648–55.

Nukada, H., Pollock, M. and Allpress, S. (1981) Experimental cold injury to peripheral nerve. *Brain* **104,** 779–811.

Nukada, H., Pollock, M. and Haas, L.F. (1982) The clinical spectrum and morphology of type II hereditary sensory neuropathy. *Brain* **105,** 647–66.

O'Brien, J.S. and Sampson, E.L. (1965) Metachromatic leucodystrophy: myelin analysis. *Science* **150,** 1613–14.

Ochoa, J. (1970) Isoniazid neuropathy in man: quantitative electron microscope study. *Brain* **93,** 831–50.

Ochoa, J. (1976) The unmyelinated nerve fibre. In *The*

Peripheral Nerve (Ed. Landon, D.N.), pp. 106–58. Chapman and Hall, London.

Ochoa, J. (1980) Nerve fiber pathology in acute and chronic compression. In *Management of Peripheral Nerve Problems* (Eds. Omer, G.E. and Spinner, M.), pp. 487–501. W.B. Saunders, Philadelphia.

Ochoa, J., Fowler, T.J. and Gilliatt, R.W. (1972) Anatomical changes in peripheral nerves compressed by a pneumatic tourniquet. *Journal of Anatomy* **113,** 433–55.

Ochoa, J. and Marotte, L. (1973) The nature of the nerve lesion caused by chronic entrapment in the guinea pig. *Journal of the Neurological Sciences* **19,** 491–5.

Ochoa, J. and Neary, D. (1975) Localized hypertrophic neuropathy, intraneural tumour or chronic nerve entrapment. *Lancet* **1,** 632–3.

Ochs, S. (1971) Characteristics and a model for fast axoplasmic transport in nerve. *Journal of Neurobiology* **2,** 331–45.

Ochs, S. (1982) *Axoplasmic Transport and its Relation to Nerve Function.* John Wiley, New York.

Ochs, S. (1983) Calcium and the mechanism of axoplasmic transport in nerve fibers. In *Spinal Cord Reconstruction* (Eds. Kao, C.C., Bunge, R.P. and Reier, P.J.), pp. 87–98. Raven Press, New York.

O'Daly, J.A. and Imaeda, T. (1967) Electron microscopic study of Wallerian degeneration in cutaneous nerves caused by mechanical injury. *Laboratory Investigation* **17,** 744–66.

Ohnishi, A. and Dyck, P.J. (1974) Loss of small peripheral sensory neurons in Fabry's disease. *Archives of Neurology* **31,** 120–7.

Ohnishi, A., Petersen, C.M. and Dyck, P.J. (1975) Axonal degeneration in sodium cyanate-induced neuropathy. *Archives of Neurology* **32,** 530–4.

Ohnishi, A., Sato, Y., Nagara, H., Sakai, T., Iwashita, H., Kuroiwa, Y. et al. (1981) Neurogenic muscular atrophy and low density of large myelinated fibres of sural nerve in chorea-acanthocytosis. *Journal of Neurology, Neurosurgery and Psychiatry* **44,** 645–8.

Ohnishi, A., Schilling, K., Brimijoin, W.S., Lambert, E.H., Fairbanks, V.F. and Dyck, P.J. (1977) Lead neuropathy. I. Morphometry, nerve conduction, and choline acetyltransferase transport: new finding of endoneurial edema associated with segmental demyelination. *Journal of Neuropathology and Experimental Neurology* **36,** 499–518.

Ohnishi, A., Tsuji, S., Igisu, H., Murai, Y., Goto, I., Kuroiwa, Y. et al. (1980) Beriberi neuropathy. Morphometric study of sural nerve. *Journal of the Neurological Sciences* **45,** 177–90.

Ohnishi, A., Yamashita, Y., Goto, I., Kuroiwa, Y., Murakami, S. and Ikeda, M. (1979) De- and remyelination and onion bulb in cerebrotendinous xanthomatosis. *Acta Neuropathologica* **45,** 43–5.

Ohta, M. (1970) Ultrastructure of sural nerve in a case of arsenical neuropathy. *Acta Neuropathologica* **16,** 233–42.

Ohta, M., Ellefson, R.D., Lambert, E.H. and Dyck, P.J. (1973) Hereditary sensory neuropathy type II. Clinical, electrophysiologic, histologic and biochemical studies of a Quebec kinship. *Archives of Neurology* **29,** 23–37.

Olsson, Y. (1968) Mast cells in the nervous system. *International Review of Cytology* **24,** 27–79.

Olsson, Y. (1971) Studies on vascular permeability in peripheral nerves. 4. Distribution of intravenously injected protein tracers in the peripheral nervous system of various species. *Acta Neuropathologica* **17,** 114–26.

Olsson, Y. and Kristensson, K. (1972) The perineurium as a diffusion barrier to protein tracers following trauma to nerves. *Acta Neuropathologica* **23,** 105–11.

Olsson, Y. and Reese, T.S. (1969) Inaccessibility of the endoneurium of mouse sciatic nerve to exogenous proteins. *Anatomical Record* **163,** 318–19.

Olsson, Y. and Reese, T.S. (1971) Permeability of vasa nervorum and perineurium in mouse sciatic nerve studied by fluorescence and electron microscopy. *Journal of Neuropathology and Experimental Neurology* **30,** 105–17.

Olsson, Y., Säve-Söderbergh, K., Sourander, P. and Angervall, L. (1968) A pathoanatomical study of the central and peripheral nervous system in diabetes of early onset and long duration. *Pathologia Europaea* **3,** 62–79.

Olsson, Y. and Sourander, P. (1968) Changes in the sympathetic nervous system in diabetes mellitus. A preliminary report. *Journal of Neuro-Visceral Relations* **31,** 86–95.

Ouvrier, R.A., McLeod, J.G., Morgan, G.J., Wise, G.A. and Conchin, T.E. (1981) Hereditary motor and sensory neuropathy of neuronal type with onset in early childhood. *Journal of the Neurological Sciences* **51,** 181–97.

Paetau, A. and Haltia, M. (1976) Calcification of the perineurium. *Acta Neuropathologica* **36,** 185–91.

Palay, S.L., Sotelo, C., Peters, A. and Orkand, P.M. (1968) The axon hillock and initial segment. *Journal of Cell Biology* **38,** 193–201.

Palix, C. and Coignet, J. (1978) Un cas de polyneuropathie périphérique neonatale par amyelinisation. *Pédiatrie* **33,** 201–7.

Pallis, C.A. and Scott, J.T. (1965) Peripheral neuropathy in rheumatoid arthritis. *British Medical Journal* **1,** 1141–7.

Parry, G.J. and Brown, M.J. (1982) Selective fiber vulnerability in acute ischemic neuropathy. *Annals of Neurology* **11,** 147–54.

Pearson, J. and Pytel, B. (1978a) Quantitative studies of sympathetic ganglia and spinal cord intermedio-lateral grey columns in familial dysautonomia. *Journal of the Neurological Sciences* **39,** 47–59.

Pearson, J. and Pytel, B. (1978b) Quantitative studies of ciliary and sphenopalatine ganglia in familial dysautonomia. *Journal of the Neurological Sciences* **39,** 123–30.

Pearson, J., Pytel, B., Grover-Johnson, N., Axelrod, F. and Dancis, J. (1978) Quantitative studies of dorsal root ganglia and neuropathologic observations on spinal cords in familial dysautonomia. *Journal of the Neurological Sciences* **35,** 77–92.

Pedley, J.C., Harman, D.J., Waudby, H. and McDougall, A.C. (1980) Leprosy in peripheral nerves: histopathological findings in 119 untreated patients in Nepal. *Journal of Neurology, Neurosurgery and Psychiatry* **43,** 198–204.

Pekelharing, C.A. and Winkler, C. (1887) Mittheilung über die Beriberi. *Deutsche medizinische Wochenschrift* **13,** 845–8. [Beriberi: researches concerning its nature and cause, and the means of its arrest. Translated by J. Canthe. John Bale Sons and Danielson, London. 1893.]

Percy, A.K., Kaback, M.M. and Herndon, R.M. (1977) Metachromatic leukodystrophy: comparison of early and late-onset forms. *Neurology* **27,** 933–41.

Pestronk, A., Keogh, J.P. and Griffin, J.W. (1979) Dimethylaminopropionitrile (DMAPN) intoxication: a new industrial neuropathy. *Neurology* **29,** 540.

Peters, A. (1966) The node of Ranvier in the central nervous system. *Quarterly Journal of Experimental Physiology* **51,** 229–36.

Peters, A., Palay, S.L. and Webster, H. de F. (1976) *The Fine Structure of the Nervous System: the Neurons and Supporting Cells*. W.B. Saunders, London.

Peyronnard, J.-M., Aguayo, A.J. and Bray, G.M. (1973) Schwann cell internuclear distances in normal and regenerating unmyelinated nerve fibers. *Archives of Neurology* **24,** 56–9.

Peyronnard, J.-M., Charron, L., Bellavance, A. and Marchand, L. (1980) Neuropathy and mitochondrial myopathy. *Annals of Neurology* **7,** 262–8.

Peyronnard, J.-M., Pedneault, M. and Aguayo, A.J. (1978) Neuropathies due to cold: quantitative studies of structural changes in human and animal nerves. In *Neurology* (Eds. Hartog Jager, W.A. den, Bruyn, G.W. and Heijstee, A.P.J.), International Congress Series 434, 308–29. Excerpta Medica, Amsterdam.

Pleasure, D.E., Feldmann, B. and Prockop, D.J. (1973) Diphtheria toxin inhibits the synthesis of myelin proteolipid and basic proteins by peripheral nerve *in vitro*. *Journal of Neurochemistry* **20,** 81–90.

Politis, M.J., Schaumburg, H.H. and Spencer, P.S. (1980) Neurotoxicity of selected chemicals. In *Experimental and Clinical Neurotoxicology* (Eds. Spencer, P.S. and Schaumburg, H.H.), pp. 613–30. Williams & Wilkins, Baltimore.

Pollard, J., King, R.H.M. and Thomas, P.K. (1975) Recurrent experimental allergic neuritis: an electron microscope study. *Journal of the Neurological Sciences* **24,** 365–83.

Pollard, J.D., McLeod, J.G., Honnibal, T.G.A. and Verheijden, M.A. (1982) Hypothyroid polyneuropathy. Clinical, electrophysiological and nerve biopsy findings in two cases. *Journal of the Neurological Sciences* **53,** 461–71.

Pollock, M., Nukada, H., Frith, R.W., Simcock, J.P. and Allpress, S. (1983) Peripheral neuropathy in Tangier disease. *Brain* **106,** 911–28.

Prineas, J. (1970) Peripheral nerve changes in thiamine-deficient rats. *Archives of Neurology* **23,** 541–8.

Prineas, J.W. (1972) Acute idiopathic polyneuritis. An electron microscope study. *Laboratory Investigation* **26,** 133–47.

Prineas, J.W., Ouvrier, R.A., Wright, R.G., Walsh, J.C. and McLeod, J.G. (1976) Giant axonal neuropathy—a generalized disorder of cytoplasmic microfilament formation. *Journal of Neuropathology and Experimental Neurology* **9,** 458–70.

Propp, R.P., Means, E., Diebel, R., Sherer, G. and Barron, K. (1975) Waldenström's macroglobulinaemia and neuropathy. Deposition of M-component on myelin sheaths. *Neurology* **25,** 980–8.

Quick, D.C. and Waxman, S.G. (1977a) Ferric ion, ferrocyanide and inorganic phosphate as cytochemical reactants at peripheral nodes of Ranvier. *Journal of Neurocytology* **6,** 555–70.

Quick, D.C. and Waxman, S.G. (1977b) Specific staining of the axon membranes at nodes of Ranvier with ferric ion and ferrocyanide. *Journal of the Neurological Sciences* **31,** 1–11.

Raff, M.C., Sangalang, V. and Asbury, A.K. (1968) Ischemic mononeuropathy multiplex associated with diabetes mellitus. *Archives of Neurology* **18,** 487–99.

Ranson, S.W., Droegemuller, W.H., Davenport, H.K. and Fisher, C. (1935) Number, size and myelination of sensory fibers in the cerebrospinal nerves. *Research Publications of the Association for Research in Nervous and Mental Diseases* **15,** 3–34.

Ranvier, L.A. (1878) *Leçons sur l'Histologie du Système Nerveux*. Savy, Paris.

Rawlins, F.A. (1973) A time-sequence autoradiographic study of the *in vivo* incorporation of [1,2-^{3}H] cholesterol into peripheral nerve myelin. *Journal of Cell Biology* **58,** 42–53.

Rees, R.J.W., Waters, M.F.R., Weddell, A.G.M. and Palmer, E. (1967) Experimental lepromatous leprosy. *Nature* (*London*) **215,** 599–602.

Refsum, S., Stokke, O., Eldjarn, L. and Fardeau, M. (1984) Heredopathia atactica polyneuritiformis (Refsum's disease). In *Peripheral Neuropathy*, vol. II (Eds. Dyck, P.J., Thomas, P.K., Lambert,

E.H. and Bunge, R.), pp. 1680–1703. W.B. Saunders, Philadelphia.

Revel, J.P. and Hamilton, D.W. (1969) The double nature of the intermediate dense line in peripheral nerve myelin. *Anatomical Record* **163,** 7–16.

Richardson, P.M. and Thomas, P.K. (1979) Percussive injury to peripheral nerve in rat. *Journal of Neurosurgery* **51,** 178–87.

Ricoy, J.R., Cabello, A., Rodriguez, J. and Téllez, I. (1983) Neuropathological studies on the toxic syndrome related to adulterated rapeseed oil in Spain. *Brain* **106,** 817–35.

Ridley, D.S. and Jopling, W.H. (1966) Classification of leprosy according to immunity. *International Journal of Leprosy* **34,** 255–73.

Ritchie, J.M. (1979) Sodium channels in muscle and nerve. In *Current Topics in Nerve and Muscle Research* (Eds. Aguayo, A.J. and Karpati, G.), pp. 210–19. Excerpta Medica, Amsterdam.

Ritchie, J.M. and Chiu, S.Y. (1981) Distribution of sodium and potassium channels in mammalian myelinated nerve. In *Demyelinating Disease: Basic and Clinical Electrophysiology* (Eds. Waxman, S.G. and Ritchie, J.M.), pp. 329–42. Raven Press, New York.

Ritchie, J.M. and Rogart, R.B. (1977) Density of sodium channels in mammalian myelinated nerve fibers and nature of the axonal membrane under the myelin sheath. *Proceedings of the National Academy of Sciences of the USA* **74,** 211–15.

Ritchie, J.M., Rogart, R.B. and Strichartz, G. (1976) A new method for labelling saxitoxin and its binding to nonmyelinated fibers in the rabbit vagus, lobster walking leg and garfish olfactory nerves. *Journal of Physiology* **261,** 477–94.

Rizzuto, W., Terzian, H. and Galiazzo-Rizzuto, S. (1977) Toxic polyneuropathies in Italy due to leather cement poisoning in shoe industries. A light and electron-microscopic study. *Journal of the Neurological Sciences* **31,** 343–54.

Rolleston, J.D. (1904) Clinical observations on diphtheritic paralysis. *Practitioner* **73,** 597–623.

Rosenblum, J.L., Keating, J.P., Prensky, A.L. and Nelson, J.S. (1981) A progressive neurologic syndrome in children with chronic liver disease. *New England Journal of Medicine* **304,** 503–8.

Rosenbluth, J. (1976) Intramembranous particle distribution at the node of Ranvier and adjacent axolemma in myelinated axons of the frog brain. *Journal of Neurocytology* **5,** 731–45.

Rosenbluth, J. (1981) Freeze-fracture approaches to ionophore localization in normal and myelin-deficient nerves. In *Demyelinating Disease: Basic and Clinical Electrophysiology* (Eds. Waxman, S.G. and Ritchie, J.M.), pp. 391–418. Raven Press, New York.

Rosenbluth, J. (1983) Structural studies of the node of Ranvier. In *Structure and Function in Excitable Cells* (Eds. Chang, D.C., Tasaki, I., Adelman, W.J. and Leuchtag, H.R.). Plenum Press, New York.

Rushton, W.A.H. (1951) A theory of the effects of fibre size in medullated nerve. *Journal of Physiology* **115,** 101–22.

Rydmark, M. (1981) Nodal axon diameter correlates linearly with internodal axon diameter in spinal roots of the cat. *Neuroscience Letters* **24,** 247–50.

Rydmark, M. and Berthold, C.-H. (1983) Electron microscopic serial sections analysis of nodes of Ranvier in lumbar spinal roots of the cat. A morphometric study of nodal compartments in fibres of different sizes. *Journal of Neurocytology* **12,** 537–65.

Sabin, T.D. and Ebner, J.D. (1969) Patterns of sensory loss in lepromatous leprosy. *International Journal of Leprosy* **37,** 239–48.

Sahenk, Z. and Mendell, J.R. (1981) Acrylamide and 2,5-hexanedione neuropathies: abnormal bidirectional transport rate in distal axons. *Brain Research* **219,** 397–405.

Said, G. (1978) Perhexilene neuropathy: a clinicopathological study. *Annals of Neurology* **3,** 259–66.

Said, G. and Landrieu, P. (1978) Etude quantitative des fibres nerveuses isolées dans les polynévrites alcooliques. *Journal of the Neurological Sciences* **35,** 317–30.

Said, G., Slama, G. and Selva, J. (1983) Progressive centripetal degeneration of axons in small fibre type diabetic polyneuropathy. A clinical and pathological study. *Brain* **106,** 791–807.

Saida, T., Saida, K., Silberberg, D.H. and Brown, M.J. (1981) Experimental allergic neuritis induced by galactocerebroside. *Annals of Neurology* **9,** suppl., 87–101.

Sanders, F.K. (1948) The thickness of the myelin sheath of normal and regenerating peripheral nerve fibres. *Proceedings of the Royal Society of London, B* **135,** 323–57.

Sandri, C., Van Buren, J.M. and Akert, K. (1977) Membrane morphology of the vertebrate nervous system: a study with freeze-etch technique. *Progress in Brain Research* **46,** 1–384.

Schaumburg, H.H. and Spencer, P.S. (1984) Human toxic neuropathy due to industrial agents. In *Peripheral Neuropathy*, 2nd edn (Eds. Dyck, P.J., Thomas, P.K., Lambert, E.H. and Bunge, R.) p. 2124. W.B. Saunders, Philadelphia.

Scheid, W. and Peters, G. (1952) Über die tödlich verlaufenden Diphtherielähmungen unter besonderen Berücksichtigung der anatomische Befunde. *Deutsche Zeitschrift für Nervenheilkunde* **167,** 355–90.

Scheinker, M. (1947) Pathology and pathogenesis of infectious polyneuritis. *Transactions of the American Neurological Association* **72,** 141–3.

Schlaepfer, W.W. (1983) Neurofilaments and the

axonal cytoskeleton as determinants of stability and growth in regenerating axons. In *Spinal Cord Reconstruction* (Eds. Kao, C.C., Bunge, R.P. and Reier, P.J.), pp. 59–73. Raven Press, New York.

Schlaepfer, W.W. and Freeman, L.A. (1978) Neurofilament proteins of rat peripheral nerve and spinal cord. *Journal of Cell Biology* **78**, 653–62.

Schlaepfer, W.W. and Hasler, M.B. (1979) Characterization of the calcium-induced disruption of neurofilaments in rat peripheral nerve. *Brain Research* **168**, 299–309.

Schlaepfer, W.W. and Micko, S. (1978) Chemical and structural changes in neurofilaments in transected rat sciatic nerve. *Journal of Cell Biology* **78**, 269–78.

Schlaepfer, W.W. and Myers, F.K. (1973) Relationship of myelin internode elongation and growth in the rat sural nerve. *Journal of Comparative Neurology* **147**, 255–66.

Schmitt, F.O. and Bear, R.S. (1937) The optical properties of vertebrate nerve axons as related to fiber size. *Journal of Cellular and Comparative Physiology* **9**, 261–73.

Schmitt, F.O., Bear, R.S. and Palmer, K.J. (1941) X-ray diffraction studies on the structure of the nerve myelin sheath. *Journal of Cellular and Comparative Physiology* **18**, 31–41.

Schmitt, F.O. and Samson, F.E. (1968) Neuronal fibrous proteins. *Neurosciences Research Program Bulletin* **6**, 113–219.

Schnapp, B. and Mugnaini, E. (1975) The myelin sheath: electron microscopic studies with thin sections and freeze-fracture. In *Golgi Centennial Symposium Proceedings* (Ed. Santini, M.), pp. 209–33. Raven Press, New York.

Schnapp, B. and Mugnaini, E. (1978) Membrane architecture of myelinated fibers as seen by freeze-fracture. In *Physiology and Pathobiology of Axons* (Ed. Waxman, S.G.), pp.83–122. Raven Press, New York.

Schoental, R. and Cavanagh, J.B. (1977) Mechanisms involved in dying-back process—hypothesis implicating coenzymes. *Neuropathology and Applied Neurobiology* **3**, 145–60.

Schold, S.C., Cho, E.-K., Somasundaram, M. and Posner, J.B. (1979) Subacute motor neuropathy: a remote effect of lymphoma. *Annals of Neurology* **5**, 271–87.

Schonberger, L.B., Hurwitz, E.S., Katona, P., Holman, R.C. and Bregman, D.J. (1981) Guillain-Barré syndrome: its epidemiology and associations with influenza vaccination. *Annals of Neurology* **9**, suppl., 31–8.

Schoultz, T.W. and Swett, J.E. (1972) The fine structure of the Golgi tendon organ. *Journal of Neurocytology* **1**, 1–26.

Schwartz, J.A. (1979) Axonal transport: components, mechanisms, and specificity. *Annual Review of Neurosciences* **2**, 467–504.

Schwartz, J.F., Rowland, L.P., Eder, H., Marks, P.A., Osserman, E.F., Hirschberg, E. and Anderson, H. (1963) Bassen-Kornzweig syndrome. *Archives of Neurology* **8**, 438–54.

Scott, J.M., Dinn, J.J., Wilson, P. and Weir, D.G. (1981) Pathogenesis of subacute combined degeneration: a result of methyl group deficiency. *Lancet* **2**, 334–7.

Sears, T.A. and Bostock, H. (1981) Conduction failure in demyelination: is it inevitable? In *Demyelinating Disease: Basic and Clinical Electrophysiology* (Eds. Waxman, S.G. and Ritchie, J.M.), pp. 357–75. Raven Press, New York.

Seddon, H.J. (1943) Three types of nerve injury. *Brain* **66**, 237–88.

Seddon, H.J. (1975) *Surgical Disorders of the Peripheral Nerves*, 2nd edn. Churchill Livingstone, Edinburgh.

Seppäläinen, A.M. and Haltia, M. (1980) Carbon disulfide. In *Experimental and Clinical Neurotoxicology* (Eds. Spencer, P.S. and Schaumburg, H.H.), pp. 356–73. Williams and Wilkins, Baltimore.

Shantha, T.R. and Bourne, G.H. (1968) The peripheral epithelium—a new concept. In *The Structure and Function of Nervous Tissue* (Ed. Bourne, G.H.), pp. 379–459. Academic Press, New York.

Shelanski, M.L. and Wiśniewski, H. (1969) Neurofibrillary degeneration induced by vincristine therapy. *Archives of Neurology* **20**, 199–206.

Sherratt, R.M., Bostock, H. and Sears, T.A. (1980) Effects of 4-aminopyridine on normal and demyelinated mammalian nerve fibres. *Nature (London)* **283**, 570–2.

Sigworth, F.J. (1980) The variance of sodium current fluctuations at the node of Ranvier. *Journal of Physiology* **307**, 97–129.

Simpson, S.A. and Young, J.Z. (1945) Regeneration of fibre diameter after cross-unions of visceral and somatic nerves. *Journal of Anatomy* **79**, 48–65.

Singer, M., Krishnan, N. and Fyfe, D.A. (1972) Penetration of ruthenium red into peripheral nerve fibers. *Anatomical Record* **173**, 375–90.

Smith, B. (1967) The myenteric plexus in Chagas' disease. *Journal of Pathology and Bacteriology* **94**, 462–3.

Smith, D.S. (1970) Bridges between vesicles and axoplasmic microtubules. *Journal of Cell Biology* **47**, 195–6A.

Smith, D.S., Järlfors, U. and Cameron, B.F. (1975) Morphological evidence for the participation of microtubules in axonal transport. *Annals of the New York Academy of Sciences* **253**, 472–506.

Smith, I.S., Kahn, S.N., Lacey, B.W., King, R.H.M., Eames, R.A., Whybrew, D.J. and Thomas, P.K. (1983) Chronic demyelinating neuropathy associated with IgM paraproteinaemia. *Brain* **106,** 169–95.

Smith, K.J., Blakemore, W.F., Murray, J.A. and Patterson, R.C. (1982) Internodal myelin volume and axon surface area. A relationship determining myelin thickness? *Journal of the Neurological Sciences* **55,** 231–46.

Smith, K.J. and Schauf, C.L. (1981) Size-dependent variation of nodal properties in myelinated nerve. *Nature (London)* **293,** 297–9.

Smith, M.E. (1967) The metabolism of myelin lipids. *Advances in Lipid Research* **5,** 241–78.

Smith, R.S. (1980) The short term accumulation of axonally transported organelles in the region of localized lesions of single myelinated axons. *Journal of Neurocytology* **9,** 39–65.

Smith, R.S. and Koles, Z.J. (1970) Myelinated nerve fibers: computed effect of myelin thickness on conduction velocity. *American Journal of Physiology* **219,** 1256–8.

Smith, T.W., Bhawan, J., Keller, R.B. and De Girolami, U. (1980) Charcot–Marie–Tooth disease associated with hypertrophic neuropathy. A neuropathologic study of two cases. *Journal of Neuropathology and Experimental Neurology* **39,** 420–40.

Sobrevilla, L.A., Goodman, M.L. and Kane, C.A. (1964) Demyelinating central nervous disease, macular atrophy and acanthocytosis (Bassen–Kornzweig syndrome). *American Journal of Medicine* **37,** 821–32.

Spencer, P.S., Sabri, M., Schaumburg, H.H. and Moore, C.L. (1979) Hypothesis: does a defect of energy metabolism in the nerve fiber underlie axonal degeneration in polyneuropathies. *Annals of Neurology* **5,** 501–7.

Spencer, P.S. and Schaumburg, H.H. (1973) An ultrastructural study of the inner core of the Pacinian corpuscle. *Journal of Neurocytology* **2,** 217–35.

Spencer, P.S. and Schaumburg, H.H. (1974) A review of acrylamide neurotoxicity. II. Experimental animal neurotoxicity and pathologic mechanisms. *Canadian Journal of Neurological Science* **1,** 152–69.

Spencer, P.S. and Schaumburg, H.H. (1976) Central–peripheral distal axonopathy—the pathology of dying-back polyneuropathies. *Progress in Neuropathology* **3,** 253–95.

Spencer, P.S. and Schaumburg, H.H. (1977) Ultrastructural studies of the dying-back process. III. The evolution of experimental peripheral giant axonal degeneration. *Journal of Neuropathology and Experimental Neurology* **36,** 276–99.

Spencer, P.S. and Schaumburg, H.H. (1978) Pathobiology of neurotoxic axonal degeneration. In *Physiology and Pathobiology of Axons* (Ed. Waxman, S.), pp. 265–82. Raven Press, New York.

Spencer, P.S. and Thomas, P.K. (1974) Ultrastructural studies of the dying-back process. II. The sequestation and removal by Schwann cells and oligodendrocytes of organelles from normal and diseased axons. *Journal of Neurocytology* **3,** 763–83.

Spencer, P.S. and Weinberg, H.J. (1978) Axonal specification of Schwann cell expression and myelination. In *Physiology and Pathobiology of Axons* (Ed. Waxman, S.G.), pp. 385–405. Raven Press, New York.

Spillane, J.D. (1947) *Nutritional Disorders of the Nervous System.* Williams & Wilkins, Baltimore.

Stämpfli, R. (1981) Overview of studies on the physiology of conduction in myelinated nerve fibers. In *Demyelinating Disease: Basic and Clinical Electrophysiology* (Eds. Waxman, S.G. and Ritchie, J.M.), pp. 11–23. Raven Press, New York.

Stern, G.M., Hoffbrand, A.V. and Urich, H. (1965) The peripheral nerves and skeletal muscles in Wegener's granulomatosis: a clinico-pathological study of four cases. *Brain* **88,** 151–64.

Stolinski, C., Breathnach, A.S., Martin, B., Thomas, P.K., King, R.H.M. and Gabriel, G. (1981) Associated particle aggregates in juxtaparanodal axolemma and adaxonal Schwann cell membrane of rat peripheral nerve. *Journal of Neurocytology* **10,** 679–91.

Stransky, E. (1902–03) Über discontinuierliche Zerfallsprozesse an der peripheren Nervenfaser. *Journal für Psychologie und Neurologie* **1,** 169–99.

Sugimura, K. and Dyck, P.J. (1981) Sural nerve myelin thickness and axis cylinder caliber in human diabetes. *Neurology* **31,** 1087–91.

Sugimura, K. and Dyck, P.J. (1982) Multifocal fiber loss in proximal sciatic nerve in symmetric distal diabetic neuropathy. *Journal of the Neurological Sciences* **53,** 501–9.

Sunderland, S. (1951) A classification of peripheral nerve injuries producing loss of function. *Brain* **74,** 491–516.

Sunderland, S. (1978) *Nerves and Nerve Injuries.* Churchill Livingstone, Edinburgh.

Swank, R.L. (1940) Avian thiamine deficiency. *Journal of Experimental Medicine* **71,** 683–702.

Swank, R.L. and Adams, R.D. (1948) Pyridoxine and pantothenic acid deficiency in swine. *Journal of Neuropathology and Experimental Neurology* **7,** 274–86.

Swanson, A.G., Buchan, G.C. and Alvord, E.C. Jr (1965) Anatomic changes in congenital insensitivity to pain. Absence of small primary sensory neurons in ganglia, roots and Lissaeur's tract. *Archives of Neurology* **12,** 12–18.

Sweeney, V.P., Pathak, M.H. and Asbury, A.K. (1970) Acute intermittent porphyria. Increased

ALA-synthetase activity during an acute attack. *Brain* **93,** 369–80.

Takahashi, K. and Nakamura, H. (1976) Axonal degeneration in beriberi neuropathy. *Archives of Neurology* **33,** 836–41.

Takeuchi, T. and Eto, K. (1977) Pathology and pathogenesis of Minamata disease. In *Minamata Disease: Methylmercury Poisoning in Minamata and Nigata Japan* (Eds. Tsubaki, T. and Irukayama, K.), p. 103. Elsevier, Amsterdam.

Tellez-Nagel, I., Korthals, J.K., Vlassara, H.V. and Cerami, A. (1977) An ultrastructural study of chronic sodium cyanate-induced neuropathy. *Journal of Neuropathology and Experimental Neurology* **36,** 351–63.

Thomas, G.A. (1948) Quantitative histology of Wallerian degeneration. II. Nuclear population in two nerves of different fibre spectrum. *Journal of Anatomy* **82,** 135–45.

Thomas, P.K. (1963) The connective tissue of peripheral nerve: an electron microscopic study. *Journal of Anatomy* **97,** 35–44.

Thomas, P.K. (1964) Changes in the endoneurial sheaths of peripheral myelinated nerve fibres during Wallerian degeneration. *Journal of Anatomy* **98,** 175–82.

Thomas, P.K. (1966) The cellular response to nerve injury. I. The cellular outgrowth from the distal stump of transected nerve. *Journal of Anatomy* **100,** 287–303.

Thomas, P.K. (1968) The effect of repeated regenerative activity on the structure of peripheral nerve. In *Research in Muscular Dystrophy* (Eds. Research Committee of the Muscular Dystrophy Group), pp. 413–16. Pitman, London.

Thomas, P.K. (1973) The ultrastructural pathology of unmyelinated nerve fibres. In *New Developments in Electromyography and Clinical Neurophysiology*, vol. 2 (Ed. Desmedt, J.E.), pp. 227–39. Karger, Basel.

Thomas, P.K. (1975) Genetic factors in amyloidosis. *Journal of Medical Genetics* **12,** 317–26.

Thomas, P.K. (1984) Other inherited neuropathies. In *Peripheral Neuropathy* 2nd edn (Eds. Dyck, P.J., Thomas, P.K., Lambert, E.H. and Bunge, R.), pp. 1745–72. W.B. Saunders, Philadelphia.

Thomas, P.K., Calne, D.B. and Stewart, G. (1974) Hereditary motor and sensory polyneuropathy (peroneal muscular atrophy). *Annals of Human Genetics* **88,** 111–53.

Thomas, P.K. and Eliasson, S.G. (1984) Diabetic neuropathy. In *Peripheral Neuropathy*, 2nd edn (Eds. Dyck, P.J., Thomas, P.K., Lambert, E.H. and Bunge, R.), pp. 1773–1810. W.B. Saunders, Philadelphia.

Thomas, P.K. and Fullerton, P.M. (1963) Nerve fibre size in the carpal tunnel syndrome. *Journal of Neurology, Neurosurgery and Psychiatry* **26,** 520–7.

Thomas, P.K. and Holdorff, B. (1984) Neuropathy due to physical agents. In *Peripheral Neuropathy*, 2nd edn (Eds. Dyck, P.J., Thomas, P.K., Lambert, E.H. and Bunge, R.), pp. 1479–511. W.B. Saunders, Philadelphia.

Thomas, P.K., Hollinrake, K., Lascelles, R.G., O'Sullivan, D.J., Baillod, R.A., Moorhead, J.F. and Mackenzie, J.C. (1971) The polyneuropathy of chronic renal failure. *Brain* **94,** 761–80.

Thomas, P.K. and Jones, D.G. (1967) The cellular response to nerve injury. 2. Regeneration of the perineurium after nerve section. *Journal of Anatomy* **101,** 45–55.

Thomas, P.K. and King, R.H.M. (1974) Peripheral nerve changes in amyloid neuropathy. *Brain* **97,** 395–406.

Thomas, P.K., King, R.H.M., Kocen, R.S. and Brett, E.M. (1977) Comparative ultrastructural observations on peripheral nerve abnormalities in the late infantile, juvenile and late onset forms of metachromatic leukodystrophy. *Acta Neuropathologica* **39,** 237–45.

Thomas, P.K. and Lascelles, R.G. (1965) Schwann cell abnormalities in diabetic neuropathy. *Lancet* **1,** 1355–7.

Thomas, P.K. and Lascelles, R.G. (1966) Pathology of diabetic neuropathy. *Quarterly Journal of Medicine* **35** (NS), 489–509.

Thomas, P.K. and Lascelles, R.G. (1967) Hypertrophic neuropathy. *Quarterly Journal of Medicine* **36** (NS), 223–38.

Thomas, P.K., Lascelles, R.G., Hallpike, J.F. and Hewer, R.L. (1969) Recurrent and chronic relapsing Guillain–Barré polyneuritis. *Brain* **92,** 589–606.

Thomas, P.K., Lascelles, R.G. and Stewart, G. (1975) Hypertrophic neuropathy. In *Handbook of Clinical Neurology* (*System Disorders and Atrophies*, part 1), vol. 21 (Eds. Vinken, P.J. and Bruyn, G.W.), pp. 145–70. North-Holland, Amsterdam.

Thomas, P.K. and Slatford, J. (1964) Lamellar bodies in the cytoplasm of Schwann cells. *Journal of Anatomy* **98,** 691.

Thomas, P.K. and Walker, J.G. (1965) Xanthomatous neuropathy in primary biliary cirrhosis. *Brain* **88,** 1079–88.

Thomas, P.K., Workman, J.M. and Thage, O. (1984) Behr's syndrome: a family exhibiting pseudodominant inheritance. *Journal of the Neurological Sciences* **64,** 137–48.

Thrush, D.C., Holt, I.G., Bradley, W.G., Campbell, M.J. and Walton, J.N. (1974) Neurological manifestations of xeroderma pigmentosum in two siblings. *Journal of the Neurological Sciences* **22,** 91–104.

Timperley, W.R., Ward, J.D., Preston, F.G., Duckworth, T. and O'Malley, B.C. (1976) A reassessment of vascular factors in relation to intravascular coagulation. *Diabetologia* **12,** 237–43.

Tomonaga, M. and Sluga, E. (1970) Zur Ultrastruktur der π-Granula. *Acta Neuropathologica* **15,** 56–9.

Towfighi, J. (1981) Effects of chronic vitamin E deficiency on the nervous system of the rat. *Acta Neuropathologica* **54,** 261–8.

Trifaro, J.M. (1978) Contractile proteins in tissues originating in the neural crest. *Neuroscience* **3,** 1–24.

Tsukita, S. and Ishikawa, H. (1980) The movement of membranous organelles in axons. Electron microscopic identification of anterogradely and retrogradely transported organelles. *Journal of Cell Biology* **84,** 513–30.

Tuck, R.R., Schmelzer, J.D. and Low, P.A. (1984) Endoneurial blood flow and oxygen tension in the sciatic nerves of rats with experimental diabetic neuropathy. *Brain* in press.

Turk, J.L. and Waters, M.F.R. (1971) Immunological significance of changes in lymph nodes across the leprosy spectrum. *Clinical and Experimental Immunology* **8,** 363–76.

Tytell, M., Black, M.M., Garner, J. and Lasek, R.J. (1981) Axonal transport: each rate component reflects the movement of distinct macromolecular complexes. *Science* **214,** 179–81.

Uhrik, B. and Stämpfli, R. (1981) Ultrastructural observations on nodes of Ranvier from isolated single frog peripheral nerve fibres. *Brain Research* **215,** 93–102.

Urtasun, R.C., Chapman, J.D., Feldstein, M.L., Band, R.P., Rabin, H.R., Wilson, A.P. et al. (1978) Peripheral neuropathy related to misonidazole: incidence and pathology. *British Journal of Cancer* **37,** suppl. III, 271–5.

Vallat, J.M., Desproges-Gotteron, R., Leboutet, M.J., Loubet, A., Gualde, N. and Treves, R. (1980) Cryoglobulinemic neuropathy: a pathological study. *Annals of Neurology* **8,** 179–85.

Vedder, E.B. (1938) The pathology of beriberi. *Journal of the American Medical Association* **110,** 893–6.

Veith, G. (1949) Untersuchungen über die Histologie der Polyneuritis diphtheritica. *Beiträge zur pathologischen Anatomie* **110,** 567–606.

Vial, J.D. (1958) The early changes in the axoplasm during Wallerian degeneration. *Journal of Biophysical and Biochemical Cytology* **4,** 551–6.

Victor, M. (1984) Polyneuropathy due to nutritional deficiency and alcoholism. In *Peripheral Neuropathy*, 2nd edn (Eds. Dyck, P.J., Thomas, P.K., Lambert, E.H. and Bunge, R.), pp. 1899–940. W.B. Saunders, Philadelphia.

Victor, M. and Adams, R.D. (1956) Neuropathology of experimental vitamin B_6 deficiency in monkeys. *American Journal of Clinical Nutrition* **4,** 346–53.

Victor, M., Banker, B.Q. and Adams, R.D. (1958) The neuropathy of multiple myeloma. *Journal of Neurology, Neurosurgery and Psychiatry* **21,** 73–8.

Vilter, R.W., Mueller, J.F., Glazer, H.S., Jarrold, T., Abraham, J., Thompson, C. and Hawkins, V.R. (1953) The effect of vitamin B_6 deficiency induced by desoxypyridoxine in human beings. *Journal of Laboratory and Clinical Investigation* **42,** 335–57.

Vital, C., Aubertin, J., Ragnault, J.M., Amiques, H., Mouton, L. and Bellance, R. (1982) Sarcoidosis of peripheral nerve: a histological and ultrastructural study of two cases. *Acta Neuropathologica* **58,** 111–14.

Vital, C., Bonnaud, E., Arne, L., Barrat, M. and Le Blanc, M. (1975) Polyradiculonévrité au cours d'une leucémie lymphoide chronïque. Étude ultrastructurale d'une biopsie de nerf periphérique. *Acta Neuropathologica* **32,** 169–72.

Vital, C., LeBlanc, M., Vallat, J.M., Coquet, M., Vallat, M. and Roques, J.C. (1974) Études ultrastructurale du nerf périphérique chez 16 diabétiques sans neuropathie clinique. Comparison avec 16 neuropathies diabétiques et 16 neuropathies non diabétiques. *Acta Neuropathologica* **30,** 63–72.

Vizoso, A.D. (1950) The relationship between internodal length and growth in human nerves. *Journal of Anatomy* **84,** 342–53.

Vizoso, A.D. and Young, J.Z. (1948) Internode length and fibre diameter in developing and regenerating nerves. *Journal of Anatomy* **82,** 110–34.

Vos, A., Gabreëls-Festen, A., Joosten, E., Gabreëls, F., Renier, W. and Mullaart, R. (1983) The neuropathy of Cockayne syndrome. *Acta Neuropathologica* **61,** 153–6.

Waggener, J.D., Bunn, S.M. and Beggs, J. (1965) The diffusion of ferritin within the peripheral nerve sheath: an electron microscopy study. *Journal of Neuropathology and Experimental Neurology* **24,** 430–43.

Waksman, B.H. (1961) Experimental study of diphtheritic polyneuritis in the rabbit and guinea pig. *Journal of Neuropathology and Experimental Neurology* **21,** 35–77.

Waksman, B.H. and Adams, R.D. (1955) Allergic neuritis: an experimental disease of rabbits induced by the injection of peripheral nervous tissue and adjuvants. *Journal of Experimental Medicine* **102,** 213–35.

Waksman, B.H., Adams, R.D. and Mansmann, H.C. Jr (1957) Experimental study of diphtheritic polyneuritis in the rabbit and guinea pig. I. Immunologic and histopathologic observations. *Journal of Experimental Medicine* **105,** 591–614.

Waller, A. (1850) Experiments on the section of the glossopharyngeal and hypoglossal nerves of the frog, and observations on the alterations produced thereby in the structure of their primitive fibres. *Philosophical Transactions of the Royal Society of London, B* **140,** 423–9.

Walsh, J.C. and McLeod, J.G. (1970) Alcoholic neuropathy. An electrophysiological and histological study. *Journal of the Neurological Sciences* **10,** 459–69.

Walshe, F.M.R. (1918–19) On the pathogenesis of diphtheritic paralysis. II. Clinical observations on the paralysis of faucial and extrafaucial diphtheria with an analysis of 30 cases following skin and wound infections. *Quarterly Journal of Medicine* **13,** 14–37.

Walton, J. and Buckley, I.K. (1977) The lead-poisoned cell: a fine structural study using cultured kidney cells. *Experimental and Molecular Pathology* **27,** 167–82.

Waxman, S.G., Pappas, G.D. and Bennett, M.V.L. (1972) Morphological correlates of functional differentiation of nodes of Ranvier along single fibers in the neurogenic electric organ of the knife fish *Sternarchus*. *Journal of Cell Biology* **53,** 210–24.

Waxman, S.G. and Quick, D.C. (1978) Functional architecture of the initial segment. In *Physiology and Pathobiology of Axons* (Ed. Waxman, S.G.), pp. 125–130. Raven Press, New York.

Webster, H. de F. (1962) Schwann cell alterations in metachromatic leucodystrophy: preliminary phase and electron microscopic observations. *Journal of Neuropathology and Experimental Neurology* **21,** 534–41.

Webster, H. de F. (1965) The relationship between Schmidt–Lanterman incisures and myelin segmentation during Wallerian degeneration. *Annals of the New York Academy of Sciences* **122,** 29–38.

Webster, H. de F. (1971) The geometry of peripheral myelin sheaths during their formation and growth in rat sciatic nerves. *Journal of Cell Biology* **48,** 348–67.

Webster, H. de F., Martin, J.R. and O'Connell, M.F. (1973) The relationships between interphase Schwann cells and axons before myelination: a quantitative electron microscope study. *Developmental Biology* **32,** 401–16.

Webster, H. de F., Spiro, D., Waksman, B. and Adams, R.D. (1961) Phase and electron microscopic studies of experimental demyelination. 2. Schwann cell changes in guinea pig sciatic nerves during experimental diphtheritic neuritis. *Journal of Neuropathology and Experimental Neurology* **20,** 5–34.

Weddell, A.G.M. and Pearson, J.M.H. (1975) Leprosy—histological aspects of nerve involvement. In *Topics on Tropical Neurology* (Ed. Hornabrook, R.W.), pp. 17–19. F.A. Davis, Philadelphia.

Weinberg, H.J. and Spencer, P.S. (1975) Studies on the control of myelinogenesis. I. Myelination and regenerating axons after entry into a foreign unmyelinated nerve. *Journal of Neurocytology* **4,** 395–418.

Weinberg, H.J. and Spencer, P.S. (1976) Studies on the control of myelinogenesis. II. Evidence for neuronal regulation of myelin production. *Brain Research* **113,** 363–78.

Weinberg, H.J. and Spencer, P.S. (1978) The fate of Schwann cells isolated from axonal contact. *Journal of Neurocytology* **7,** 555–69.

Weiss, P.A. and Hiscoe, H.B. (1948) Experiments of the mechanism of nerve growth. *Journal of Experimental Zoology* **107,** 315–95.

Weiss, P.A. and Mayr, R. (1971) Neuronal organelles in neuroplasmic ('axonal') flow. II. Neurotubules. *Acta Neuropathologica* suppl. 5, 198–206.

Williams, E., Timperley, W.R., Ward, J.D. and Duckworth, T. (1980) Electron microscopical studies of vessels in diabetic peripheral neuropathy. *Journal of Clinical Pathology* **33,** 462–70.

Weller, R.O. (1965) Diphtheritic neuropathy in the chicken: an electron-microscope study. *Journal of Pathology and Bacteriology* **89,** 591–8.

Williams, P.L. and Hall, S.M. (1971) Chronic Wallerian degeneration—an *in vivo* and ultrastructural study. *Journal of Anatomy* **109,** 487–503.

Williams, P.L. and Kashef, R. (1968) Asymmetry of the node of Ranvier. *Journal of Cell Science* **3,** 341–56.

Williams, P.L. and Landon, D.N. (1963) Paranodal apparatus of peripheral nerve fibres of mammals. *Nature (London)* **198,** 670–3.

Williams, P.L. and Wendell-Smith, C.P. (1971) Some additional parametric variations between peripheral nerve fibre populations. *Journal of Anatomy* **109,** 505–26.

Wilson, D.L. and Stone, G.C. (1979) Axoplasmic transport of proteins. *Annual Review of Biophysics and Bioengineering* **8,** 27–45.

Wilson, S.A.K. (1913–14) The pathology of pellagra. *Proceedings of the Royal Society of Medicine* **7** (part 2), 31–41.

Windebank, A.J., McCall, J.T. and Dyck, P.J. (1984) Metal neuropathy. In *Peripheral Neuropathy*, 2nd edn (Eds. Dyck, P.J., Thomas, P.K., Lambert, E.H. and Bunge, R.), pp. 2133–61. W.B. Saunders, Philadelphia.

Wintrobe, M.M., Follis, R.H. Jr, Miller, M.H., Stein, H.J., Alcayaga, R., Humphreys, S. et al. (1943) Pyridoxine deficiency in swine with particular reference to anaemia, epileptiform convulsions and fatty liver. *Bulletin of the Johns Hopkins Hospital* **72,** 1–25.

Wiśniewski, H., Terry, R.D., Whitaker, J.N., Cook, S.D. and Dowling, P.C. (1969) Landry-Guillain-Barré syndrome: a primary demyelinating disease. *Archives of Neurology* **21,** 269–76.

Yao, J.K., Herbert, P.N., Fredrickson, D.S., Ellefson,

R.D., Heinen, R.J., Forte, T. and Dyck, P.J. (1978) Biochemical studies in a patient with a Tangier syndrome. *Journal of Neuropathology and Experimental Neurology* **37,** 138–54.

Yates, A.J., Bouchard, J.-P. and Wherrett, J.R. (1976) Relation of axon membrane in myelin membrane in sciatic nerve during development—comparison of morphological and chemical parameters. *Brain Research* **104,** 261–71.

Yiannikas, C., McLeod, J.G. and Walsh, J.C. (1983) Peripheral neuropathy associated with polycythaemia vera. *Neurology* **33,** 139–43.

Yoshizumi, M.O. and Asbury, A.K. (1974) Intra-axonal bacilli in lepromatous leprosy: a light and electron microscopic study. *Acta Neuropathologica* 27, 1–10.

Yoshizumi, M.O., Kirchheimer, W.F. and Asbury, A.K. (1974) A light and electron microscope study of peripheral nerves in an armadillo with disseminated leprosy. *International Journal of Leprosy* **42,** 251–9.

Zacks, S.I. and Saito, A. (1969) Uptake of exogenous horseradish peroxidase by coated vesicles in mouse neuromuscular junctions. *Journal of Histochemistry and Cytochemistry* **17,** 161–70.

Zelena, J. (1968) Bidirectional movements of mitochondria along axons of an isolated nerve segment. *Zeitschrift für Zellforschung und mikroskopische Anatomie* **92,** 186–96.

Zenker, W. and Hohberg, E. (1973a) A-α-Motorische Nervenfaser: Axonquerschnittsfläche von Stammfaser und Endästen. *Zeitschrift für Anatomie und Entwicklungsgeschichte* **139,** 163–72.

Zenker, W. and Hohberg, E. (1973b) A-α-nerve fibre: number of neurotubules in the stem fibre and in the terminal branches. *Journal of Neurocytology* **2,** 143–8.

Zenker, W., Mayr, R. and Gruber, H. (1974) Neurotubules: different densities in peripheral motor and sensory nerve fibres. *Experientia* **31,** 318–20.

Zuccarello, M. and Anzil, A.P. (1979) A localized model of experimental neuropathy by topical application of disulfiram. *Experimental Neurology* **64,** 699–703.

19

Epilepsy

B.S. Meldrum and J.A.N. Corsellis

Epilepsy is an episodic disorder of the nervous system, arising from the excessively synchronous and sustained discharge of a group of neurons. Seizures which arise only as the result of a generalized metabolic or toxic disorder, such as recurrent hypoglycaemia or a febrile illness, do not constitute epilepsy.

The clinical expression of an epileptic attack can range from a transient arrest of movement, an episode of disordered thought or an 'absence', to sustained, generalized, clonic or tonic movements. The aetiology of epilepsy is poorly understood and so the classifications currently in use (Commission on Classification and Terminology, 1981; Gastaut, 1983) are based on the clinical features, without reference to a pathological process. Nevertheless it is customary to think in terms of symptomatic or 'secondary' epilepsy and of primary or idiopathic epilepsy, this latter form also being known as cryptogenic epilepsy. In the former group a pathological condition such as a malformation, trauma, neoplasm, infection or a metabolic disorder is found in the brain; the epilepsy therefore is considered to be secondary. This relationship, however, is not always simple because similar lesions may be found in patients without epilepsy. In the idiopathic form there may be no gross or microscopic abnormalities. However, there is often some neuronal loss and gliosis to a degree which exceeds the normal range for the patient's age, and the question arises whether these changes are secondary to the epileptic attacks or are part of an antecedent process that has triggered the development of the attack. This problem is particularly troublesome in evaluating the significance of pathological findings in temporal lobe epilepsy.

The neuropathologist's contribution to the study of epilepsy concerns either the examination of fragments of neural tissue removed surgically during life or the post-mortem examination of the whole brain, both at gross and at microscopical levels, to identify lesions and evaluate their relationship to the epilepsy.

Incidence

Population studies in Europe and North America indicate a lifetime prevalence rate of epilepsy, defined as two or more recurrent afebrile convulsions of between 7 per 1000 (Hauser and Kurland, 1975) and 17 per 1000 (Goodridge and Shorvon, 1983). The rates are higher in South America and Africa (Chiofalo et al., 1979). The incidence is highest in the first decade of life and after the age of 60 years. Approximately 40 per cent of cases are of primary generalized seizures (absence, myoclonic or tonic–clonic) and 60 per cent are of partial seizures (simple or complex, with a presumed focal origin). In the population studied in Minnesota, 1935–67, a cause of the epilepsy was identified in only a quarter of the patients (Hauser and Kurland, 1975).

Genetic aspects

Reviews of the genetics of epilepsy have been provided by Metrakos and Metrakos (1974) and by Newmark and Penry (1979). Three aspects merit consideration.

First there are some 150 *genetic syndromes* in which myoclonus or epilepsy are either characteristically or commonly observed. These have been divided by McKusick (1983) into three groups. The first consists of 15 syndromes with an autosomal dominant inheritance. These include conditions such as familial cavernous angioma, acute intermittent porphyria, neurofibromatosis and tuberous sclerosis. The second, and largest, group consists of nearly 100 autosomal recessive phenotypes. They are for the most part rare, some to the point of obscurity, but they also include the various forms of Batten's disease, glycogen storage disease, Krabbe's disease and maple syrup urine disease. In the third, smallest, group the inheritance is X-linked. Although many of these syndromes are usually diagnosed on the basis of clinical and biochemical observations, others can be diagnosed definitively only on the basis of histological appearances. The confirmation of such a diagnosis, even when made after death, can be of great help both to the family and to their medical advisers. At the same time the characteristic histological appearances of a number of disorders have not yet been established although current developments in immunohistochemical techniques may well alter this in the future.

Second, several forms of *primary generalized epilepsy*, have a strong genetic element which may be carried on a single locus but is more probably polygenic. Thus generalized seizures of the absence type appear to be due to an autosomal dominant gene with variable penetrance. Although only 8 per cent of siblings of children with petit mal are clinically affected, nearly 50 per cent between the ages of 4 and 16 years show paraxysmal EEG abnormalities when tested with provocation techniques (Metrakos and Metrakos, 1966, 1974). Febrile convulsions have been found to occur in excess in the first degree relatives of infants with febrile convulsions. The expression of the gene or genes involved depends strongly on age, being greatest between 1.5 and 4.5 years of age. Photosensitive epilepsy has a strong genetic basis, the expression of which is age- and sex-dependent, and photoconvulsive responses can be elicited in up to 15 per cent of 15-year-old girls, as well as in up to 50 per cent of mothers of children with photosensitive epilepsy (Newmark and Penry, 1979).

Third, a genetic component has been found in partial or *focal epilepsy* which is secondary to a non-specific but primary abnormality such as a tumour or a traumatic lesion. For example, the incidence of epilepsy in the relatives of patients with cerebral tumours is higher for probands with epilepsy than for those who are epilepsy-free (Kirstein, 1942; Lund, 1952).

This generalized genetic susceptibility to epilepsy applies to those with febrile convulsions, primary generalized seizures and focal seizures secondary to a pathological process. Thus there is an increased proclivity for 3 Hz spike and wave activity to occur in the near relatives of patients with febrile or focal convulsions (Metrakos and Metrakos, 1974). In probands with idiopathic seizures the risk of epilepsy among their siblings or children is three times greater than in the general population (Annegers et al., 1982).

Neuroimaging in epilepsy

For many years established radiographic techniques, including the use of contrast media for ventriculography or angiography, have made possible the clinical identification of many causes of focal epilepsy, such as calcified tumours and vascular malformations. The introduction of computerized tomographic techniques has led to focal lesions being identified in a substantially greater number of patients with epilepsy—for example, the incidence of organic lesions in one large series went up from under a third to over a half (Gastaut and Gaustaut, 1976), although in other studies the increase has been less dramatic (MGahan, Dublin and Hill, 1979; Young, et al., 1982). Tumours have been detected at times in children and adults suffering from either focal or generalized seizures even though they had produced no clinical or electroencephalographic focal signs (Gastaut and Gastaut, 1976; Blume, Girvin and Kaufmann, 1982).

The improved anatomical resolution of the newer techniques has made possible the more accurate study of ventricular size and shape, although the underlying significance of variations is not clear. For example, on the one hand, a subgroup of patients with epilepsy has been identified in which the cerebral ventricles were abnormally small (Awa et al., 1979). In contrast, in a population of epileptic patients with high psychiatric morbidity, nearly half showed an abnormality of the ventricular system, which was commonly that of enlarged lateral ventricles, usually being asymmetrical (Fenwick, Master and Brown, 1981). CT scans, particularly with metrizamide enhancement, may be used to demonstrate both mesial temporal sclerosis and trans-tentorial herniation of mesial temporal structures (Bolender and Wyler, 1982). The introduction of nuclear magnetic resonance

(NMR) imaging is likely to widen the scope of studies of this kind.

Positron emission tomography, using an isotope with a very short half-life, has been used to study regional glucose or oxygen consumption. Interictal studies of this kind have revealed zones of reduced metabolism in the temporal lobe in patients with partial complex seizures. These zones are substantially more extensive than the gross pathology identified at subsequent anterior temporal lobectomy (Engel et al., 1982; Bernardi et al., 1983).

Symptomatic epilepsy

Systemic disorders which may precipitate convulsions are listed in standard textbooks of neurology (eg Walton, 1977). Metabolic, endocrine and toxic factors have been reviewed by Millichap (1974) and Meldrum (1982). They include derangements of body fluids and electrolytes, renal failure, hypoglycaemia, hypocalcaemia, various other endocrine and metabolic disturbances and poisonings, both medicinal (eg antidepressants and antibiotics) and industrial (eg organophosphorus insecticides). Febrile convulsions are a separate group, discussed in the next section.

Almost any pathological process involving the brain may be associated with epilepsy. The more common local causes of symptomatic epilepsy include congenital abnormalities (vascular malformations, hamartomas, etc.) primary and secondary tumours, encephalitis, meningitis, cerebral abscess, parasitic infections, trauma, vascular accidents and degenerative processes.

It is difficult to be precise about the incidence of the different types of abnormality because the figures vary not only according to the source but also according to the age range of the patients being studied. Bridge (1949) in his analysis of 742 children attending an epileptic clinic considered that birth and neonatal injuries were the commonest causes since they accounted for nearly 25 per cent of the cases. Vascular accidents and head injury after the neonatal period accounted for 12 per cent and 7 per cent respectively, whilst acute infection, malformation and cerebral tumour were all considerably lower. In 20 per cent of the cases cerebral injury of uncertain cause was suspected and in nearly one-third no evidence of brain disease was found.

A study (Rose and Lombroso, 1970) confined to seizures in the neonatal period (full-term infants, 0–21 days old) suggests that metabolic disorders (hypocalcaemia and hypoglycaemia) account for 25 per cent of seizures, and intracranial birth injury (especially subarachnoid haemorrhage) and CNS infection for another 25 per cent. Congenital malformations and perinatal anoxia each appeared to be responsible for less than 10 per cent of seizures.

When fits develop in the adult, tumour and trauma become the most important of the identifiable factors. Almost 50 per cent of patients with intracranial tumours suffer from epileptic attacks at some time during the illness (Ketz, 1974). In 60–80 per cent of tumour patients with fits the epileptic attacks are the presenting symptom. Tumours are more likely to give rise to an epileptic fit when they are situated in the cerebral hemispheres than when they lie below the tentorial opening. Within the hemispheres the position of the tumour and its nearness to the cortex are important. Lund (1952), for example, in his study of 'epilepsy with intracranial tumour' found that the most sensitive region was the frontal and parietal cortex around the central fissure, either generalized or focal attacks being recorded in 75 per cent of patients with a tumour in this area. The figure for the temporal lobes was 50 per cent and for other regions it was still lower. Patients with slowly growing tumours develop fits more often than those with rapidly invasive tumours. A survey by Ketz (1974) of the relationship between the occurrence of epilepsy and the type of tumour gave 71 per cent in cases of oligodendroglioma, 59 per cent in astrocytoma, 37 per cent in meningioma and 29 per cent in glioblastoma, the last-named being particularly associated with focal seizures. These figures are not a true indication of the difference in epileptogenicity of the type of tumour, but they do reflect the important role in epileptogenesis of elapsed time following the onset of any pathological change in the brain (Penfield, Erickson and Tarlov, 1940).

The reason why some patients with tumours have seizures and others do not is obscure. The patient's genetic predisposition to epilepsy can play a role but is probably critical in only a minority of cases. Kirstein (1942) found that 7 per cent of tumour patients with seizures had a relative with epilepsy, whilst among those without seizures only 2 per cent had such a relative. Lund (1952), on similar grounds, concluded that a hereditary tendency to epilepsy possibly contributed to the occurrence of seizures in 10 per cent of patients with tumours.

The immediate pathogenetic mechanism is often broadly described as 'hypoxia' or 'ischaemia' of the grey matter adjacent to the tumour but this should not be interpreted in any direct sense. Although generalized cerebral hypoxia may trigger off epileptic seizures, there is little reason to believe that a degree of focal cortical hypoxia, which is too slight to result in cellular damage, will have the same effect. It is well established that the occurrence of fits, symptomatic of tumours, is little related to the general physiological state of the patient (Janz, 1964) and this would suggest that they are unrelated to acute fluctuations in the oxygen tension around the tumour. The failure of fast-growing and invasive tumours to show any excess of seizures also argues against the acute effects of hypoxia. On the contrary, slowly developing neuronal and glial changes are more likely to be the important factors. Because cellular mechanisms of this kind are, however, common to many forms of epilepsy they are discussed later in a separate section.

Neurosurgical excision of the tumour abolished the seizures in about 50 per cent of cases, but according to Ketz (1974) about 10 per cent of patients who had no seizures before operation develop them subsequently.

Epilepsy following head injury is more likely to occur with open than with closed wounds. Russell and Whitty (1952) found that attacks had developed in 40 per cent of their patients during the 5-year period after a penetrating injury to the skull. As with tumours, the most sensitive region was the cerebral cortex adjacent to the central fissure. There seems to be no evident difference in the incidence of traumatic epilepsy in the two world wars, in spite of the improved methods of treatment and of combating infection. In closed head injuries the incidence is much lower. Jennett (Jennett and Lewin, 1960; Jennett, 1965) gave the overall figure as less than 10 per cent, but he emphasized that the risk varied greatly according to the severity of the injury and the nature of the complications. Thus prolonged post-traumatic amnesia when combined with a depressed skull fracture carried a higher risk than on its own. Jennett (1969) later emphasized that 'early fits', or those occurring during the first week after an injury, are commonly of the focal motor variety and it is only after this period that temporal lobe attacks are liable to develop.

The damage responsible for fits during the first few hours after cerebral trauma is likely to be a combination of shearing of nerve cell processes and of capillaries, cerebral oedema and other early consequences of focal ischaemia. The late seizures which may occur 10 or more years after the trauma are presumably due to cellular changes, similar to those occurring in relation to tumours and abscesses (see Chapter 6.)

Of 1000 patients with non-missile depressed skull fracture, 10 per cent developed early epilepsy (1–7 days) and 15 per cent developed late epilepsy (Jennett, Miller and Braakman, 1974). The risk of late epilepsy is increased if the dura is torn or if there are focal signs. Indeed in a recent study of 233 head trauma patients all ten who developed late post-traumatic epilepsy had evidence of focal damage on a CT scan performed within 48 hours of the trauma (D'Alessandro et al., 1982).

Acute infections, especially viral meningoencephalitides, are not infrequent causes of focal or generalized seizures. Protozoal infections such as toxoplasmosis or cerebral malaria (in tropical countries) are causes of seizures which may be diagnosed sometimes only after death. Among metazoan parasitic disorders, cysticercosis is the most important cause of epilepsy in Mexico (Escobedo, Garcia-Ramos and Sotelo, 1983). Intracranial infections are also liable to give rise to epileptic attacks after the acute episode. Legg, Gupta and Scott (1973) found that in 72 per cent of patients with a history of cerebral abscess, occasional fits occurred which commonly started during the first year although in many there was an interval of 3 or more years.

In later adult life and in old age, epilepsy may occur in association with various degenerative conditions of the brain (reviewed by Radermecker, 1974). Alzheimer's disease, Huntington's chorea and, occasionally, senile dementia are examples. Cerebrovascular disease is also an important cause of seizures in later life. Fits occur in 13 per cent of patients with cerebral haemorrhage or infarct (Richardson, Dodge and Victor, 1954). Venous thrombosis and subdural haematomas may cause seizures at any age but are commonest at the two extremes of life.

At all ages, however, there are some epileptic patients in whom no underlying disturbance is to be found either within the nervous system or outside it. The figures quoted earlier from Bridge (1949) strongly substantiate this, for aetiological factors could be identified in only about half the children. Similarly, in a clinical study of late onset epilepsy in adults, Serafetinides and Dominian (1963) found no cause for the fits in as many as three-quarters of the patients. The pathological findings in this cryptogenic group, however, are bound up with the type of brain damage which may occur in association with, or as a result of, convulsions particularly in early life and when status epilepticus develops. The main features of these conditions will therefore be described first.

Febrile convulsions and status epilepticus

The incidence of febrile convulsions is much higher than that of epilepsy.

In North America in 1960, 3.2 per cent of children less than 5 years of age experienced one or more febrile seizures (Hauser and Kurland, 1975), which is consistent with mean figures from six population studies in temperate climates, of 29 per 1000 (Lennox-Buchthal, 1973). The incidence is apparently higher in tropical countries (Lessell, Torres and Kurland, 1962; Hall, 1964; Edgell and Stanfield, 1972). About 10 per cent of patients showing febrile convulsions subsequently experience afebrile seizures (Juul-Jensen and Foldspang, 1983). Conversely, of patients with epilepsy, about 12 per cent have had febrile convulsions (Hauser and Kurland, 1975). Population studies have not shown any preferential relationship between febrile convulsions and complex partial (temporal lobe) seizures.

'Febrile convulsions', in which the primary infection does not involve the brain, are usually distinguished from seizures secondary to meningitis and encephalitis (Millichap, 1968; Lennox-Buchthal, 1973). In practice the distinction is not easily made, partly because the primary infection in many febrile illnesses is not identified (exanthem subitum is commonly not recognized); even when a viral agent is identified, the degree of direct cerebral involvement is hard to ascertain (Wallace and Zealley, 1970).

Febrile convulsions are important because of the risk of status epilepticus and of damage to the brain, particularly if the episode is prolonged. The cerebral consequences may be graded as:

1. Generalized damage, but involving principally those areas vulnerable to any form of cerebral hypoxia (neocortex, cerebellum, thalamus, hippocampus) (Zimmerman, 1938; Fowler, 1957).
2. Cerebral hemiatrophy, associated with hemiparesis and sometimes hemiconvulsions (Gastaut et al., 1960; Isler, 1969; Aicardi and Chevrie, 1970; Aicardi and Baraton, 1971).
3. Ammon's horn sclerosis or other 'ischaemic' pathology of the hippocampus and temporal lobe. This may be a more restricted form of (2). It is the lesion found in 50 per cent of anterior temporal specimens when the operation is performed for temporal lobe epilepsy (Falconer, 1974).

'Minimal changes'. Approximately one-third of children show EEG abnormalities 1 week or more after the convulsion, usually asymmetrical slowing in the occipital or temporal regions, which is sometimes replaced by a spike focus (Lennox-Buchthal, 1973).

One-third of 208 children followed up for up to 7 years after febrile convulsions showed behavioural disturbance or educational retardation (Frantzen, 1971). The nature of the brain damage underlying this has not been demonstrated, but a similar behavioural disorder was described pior to the onset of temporal lobe epilepsy (Aird, Venturini and Spielman, 1967) in which it was suggested that the abnormality is similar to, but milder than, that of sclerosis of the medial temporal areas.

Analysis of the neurological and pathological sequelae of febrile convulsions is complicated by two factors: (1) pre-existing brain damage (commonly arising from perinatal asphyxia or trauma) predisposes to febrile convulsions (Peterman, 1950, 1952; Millichap, 1968; Wallace, 1972; Lennox-Buchthal, 1973); and (2) viral infections (even when signs of encephalitis are not present) may give rise to neurological sequelae whether or not convulsions occur (Wallace and Zealley, 1970).

Although these two factors may introduce a variable bias into collected series, there is a good correlation between seizure duration and incidence and severity of sequelae both within and between reported series. Furthermore prompt medical care of febrile convulsions leads to fewer severe sequelae, including non-febrile convulsions, although it possibly has less effect on minor sequelae (Frantzen, 1971; Lennox-Buchthal, 1973).

Status epilepticus may be defined broadly as a convulsive episode lasting over an hour, without an intervening period of consciousness. It has long been recognized as a serious danger to life at any age (Hunter, 1959), but it offers a special threat in the early years. Aicardie and Chevrie (1970) found that, of a series of children under 15 years with an episode of status, about 40 per cent were young infants in whom mortality was high. In 85 per cent the status occurred before the age of 5 years. Three out of four affected children who survived for more than a year had further epileptic attacks. Aicardi and Chevrie considered that in 50 per cent of their patients the status was due to organic cerebral disease. In more than half of those in whom no cause could be identified the status had developed following a non-specific febrile episode.

Oxbury and Whitty (1971) made a comparable study of status epilepticus in adults and found it to have been symptomatic in 63 per cent of their series. Tumours, vascular disease, infections and trauma, all involving the brain, were the most common causes and, in so far as any localization was identified, the abnormalities tended to involve the frontal lobes. Whitty (1961) had earlier observed this association in relation to trauma whilst Janz (1964, 1983) has described status epilepticus as the particular presenting sign of a frontal tumour. Oxbury and Whitty emphasized that status may also affect patients with long-established cryptogenic epilepsy.

In such patients non-compliance with drug therapy is the commonest cause of status epilepticus (Aminoff and Simon, 1980). In patients without a history of epilepsy, cerebrovascular disease and drug overdose are the commonest causes, but tumour, cardiac arrest and alcohol are also significant factors (Aminoff and Simon, 1980). These authors emphasized that hyperpyrexia commonly occurred secondarily to the status and was associated with an unfavourable outcome.

The prognosis of symptomatic status depends more on the underlying disease than on damage resulting from the attack, status associated with cerebral trauma or with cardiac arrest having a particularly unfavourable outcome. However, Aminoff and Simon (1980) have estimated the morbidity associated with the status itself as 12.5 per cent, with a duration greater than 2 hours carrying a less favourable prognosis.

The prognosis in an attack of symptomatic status usually depends more on the underlying cerebral disease than on damage resulting from the attack itself. When, therefore, the status has no known cause the immediate outlook is better, but the risk of permanent brain damage or even death is always there.

Since, as already mentioned, the risk is much greater in the earlier years of life, it is not surprising that the neuropathological aspects have been studied most intensively in the brains of young children (Zimmerman, 1938; Meyer, Beck and Shepherd, 1955). Norman (1964) and Ounsted, Lindsay and Norman (1966), in a study of 11 cases, found that the brain is usually, but not always, slightly swollen; some congestion is common and occasional petechial haemorrhages may occur. There is often a striking difference between the relatively normal appearance of a fixed brain and the structural devastation seen under the microscope, or even that seen by the naked eye on the stained slide. In the latter, using a cell stain such as cresyl violet, wide expanses of the cortical ribbon stand out as abnormally pale (Fig. 19.1). Sometimes the outer, or less often the deeper, layers are affected. This is due to the extensive neuronal necrosis which tends to follow a pattern. Thus the calcarine cortex and the parahippocampal gyri are usually spared whereas the hippocampus (see Fig. 19.3b) and uncus appear blanched. The hippocampus in particular may have a swollen outline in the region of the Sommer sector and the dentate fascia. Other cortical regions are affected to a more variable degree. The deep grey matter, and particularly the thalamus, may be patchily necrotic. In the affected parts the neuronal changes are similar to those commonly seen in severe hypoxia or ischaemia (see Chapter 4). The 'ischaemic nerve cell change' of Spielmeyer is common. In this the cell body becomes scarcely visible with a Nissl stain, but is eosinophilic in haematoxylin and eosin preparations. At the same time both the cell outline and the cell nucleus take on a triangular shape while the nucleus becomes small and darkly stained so that the nucleolus can no longer be identified. Many other nerve cells disappear, only small tags of eosinophilic cytoplasm and distintegrating nuclei being visible. In the cerebellum the Purkinje cells are commonly affected in many folia or lobules. The cytoplasm

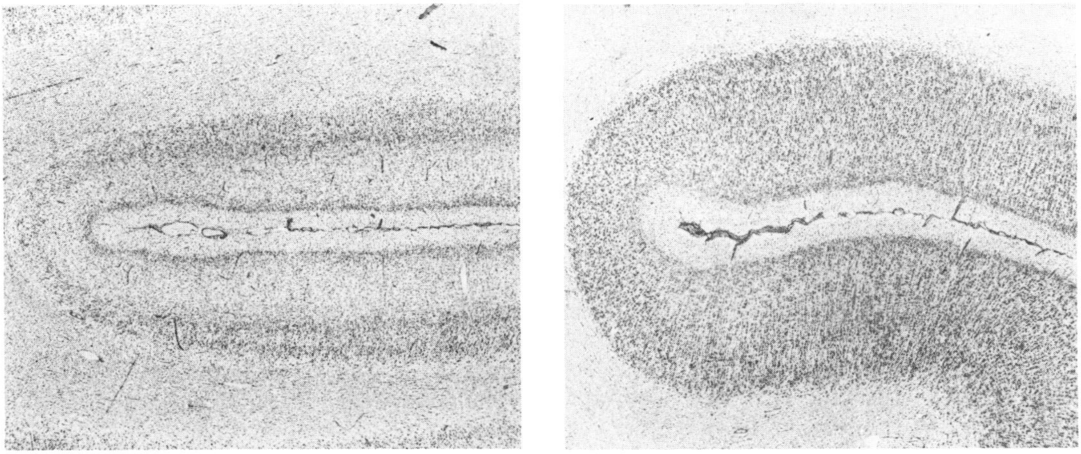

(a) (b)

Fig. 19.1 (**a**) Cerebral cortex of an infant dying shortly after an episode of status epilepticus. Extensive neuronal necrosis has destroyed the middle layers, and particularly the third. The resulting pallor is seen when compared with the normal cortex in (**b**). Cresyl violet × 12.

then loses its Nissl substance and becomes eosinophilic, while the nucleus may be dark and shrunken or at times it may stain faintly.

In any of the affected parts of the brain a microglial and astrocytic reaction occurs. The microglia are the more prominent in the early stages and neutral fat may be seen in their processes if survival has lasted for more than a few days. As the length of survival increases, the astrocytic reaction becomes more noticeable and eventually a dense fibrous gliosis may be laid down. The necrosis is rarely extensive enough to result in the breakdown of tissue or cyst formation. The white matter may show slight diffuse pallor in the more oedematous brains.

Although pathological changes similar to those found in children can occur in the brains of adults dying acutely after status epilepticus (Corsellis and Bruton, 1983) the incidence and severity of the lesion is less. Indeed, seven out of 12 adults showed no acute pathological changes. Status epilepticus lasting 6 days in a 52-year-old woman produced symmetrical haemorrhagic lesions in the hippocampus and amygdala (Noel et al., 1977)—lesions apparently similar to those originally reported by Pfleger (1880).

The neuronal necrosis and glial reaction following severe serial convulsions or an episode of status are acute and tend to be considerably more extensive than the chronic scarring found when an epileptic patient has died after many years of recurrent epileptic fits, that is to say in an adult patient with cryptogenic epilepsy.

Cryptogenic epilepsy

The absence of any clear-cut cause for the epilepsy in the cryptogenic group does not mean that all pathological change is absent. Three main types of pathology will be considered here: (1) minor dysgenetic lesions; (2) lesions secondary to trauma; and (3) diffuse neuronal loss and gliosis which may be secondary to epilepsy or may have an independent origin.

Minor dysgenetic lesions These have been an enduring focus of comment and speculation. They were remarked upon at the beginning of the century by Alzheimer (Alzheimer and Vogt, 1907).

The most recent report concerns eight patients whose epilepsy began with absence attacks in childhood evolving to awakening grand mal in adolescence (Meencke and Janz, 1984). The microdysgenesis was evident in cortex, hippocampus and cerebellum, with nerve cells lying in rows subpially and an increased density of nerve cells in the stratum moleculare in the neocortex, an increase in nerve cells in the stratum radiatum of the hippocampus and Purkinje cell dystopia in the cerebellum.

Such minor developmental abnormalities could reflect the genetic component of primary generalized epilepsy or could be a consequence of an exogenous pathological process affecting morphogenesis which is of aetiological significance for epilepsy.

Lesions secondary to trauma Stauder (1935) observed superficial erosion and scarring of the orbital, frontal and temporal cortex in 25 per cent of a series of chronic epileptic brains. He also pointed out that 16 of 77 contused brains investigated by Spatz had come from epileptic patients, and he suggested that such damage was considerably commoner in chronic epilepsy than was generally recognized. Sano and Malamud (1953) found the incidence as high as 36 per cent but the figure given by Margerison and Corsellis (1966) was lower (11 per cent). The impression of the present writers is that this damage has become less common in recent years. It is clearly of the contrecoup type and although it may occasionally be the result of a closed head injury preceding the onset of the epilepsy, it is much more commonly the result of a fall during a fit. This can at times be obvious when both old and recent damage is seen in the same brain (Fig. 19.2).

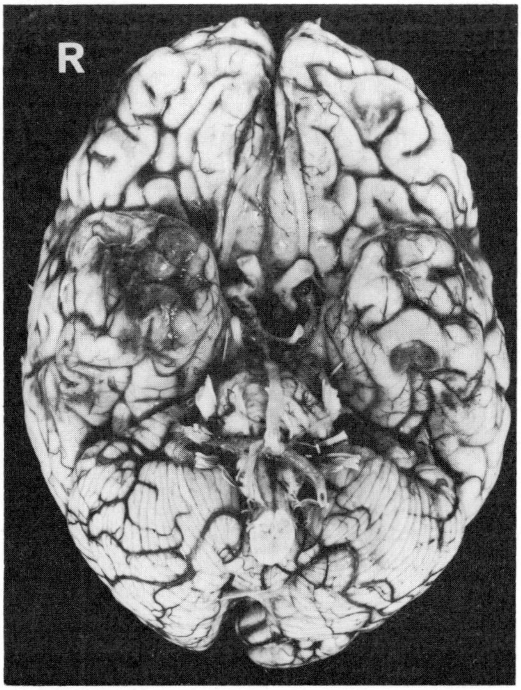

Fig. 19.2 The undersurface of the brain, showing contrecoup bruising and scarring in an adult patient with life-long epilepsy. The right temporal lobe has suffered in a recent fall whereas there is older cortical scarring at a more posterior level in both temporal lobes. The left orbital area also shows a shallow cortical 'ulcer' due to past trauma and scarring. × 0.5.

Neuronal loss and gliosis Reports of major series of patients with idiopathic or cryptogenic epilepsy have consistently described an appreciable degree of neuronal loss accompanied by a glial reaction in more than half of the patients. Not all parts of the brain are equally vulnerable. As first described by Bouchet and Cazauvieilh (1825), areas damaged most often are the Ammon's horn and the cerebellum. Spielmeyer (1927) observed that 80 per cent of the 125 epileptic brains he had examined were damaged in one or both of these regions. Later studies, and particularly those of Scholz (1951) and Pieffer (1963), extended the range of vulnerability to include the thalamus and the cerebral neocortex, whilst Meyer and Beck (1955) added the amygdaloid nucleus and the grey matter adjacent to it to the list. The striatum and pallidum seem rarely to be affected. In the brain stem the most vulnerable areas are the inferior olives.

The damage, wherever it occurs, looks much the same. The acute stages are found at their most severe in the brains of young children who have died during or shortly after a bout of status epilepticus, and have been described in the previous section. In the great majority of people with long-standing cryptogenic epilepsy, however, the histological abnormality, when present, is one of scarring and appears to be the result of one or more insults well in the past, for acute damage of this kind is rarely seen in such people even if they have died shortly after an attack.

The histological minutiae of the process may be particularly well studied in the hippocampus. The final stage of scarring in this region is the lesion known as Ammon's horn or hippocampal sclerosis. The normal structure is illustrated in Fig. 19.3a in which the ribbon of nerve cells has been divided into the simplified areas as proposed by Scholz (1951). The first part is the Sommer sector or the h1 field, and is the commonest site for severe neuronal loss and gliosis (Fig. 19.3c). The end-folium, or h3 field, is also highly vulnerable whilst a remarkably constant and inexplicable feature is the marked tendency for a short run of nerve cells lying between these two fields to be relatively spared—this is the resistant part or h2. The small, dark, densely packed neurons of the dentate fascia are also often more or less erased. In its chronic stage the atrophy is usually obvious to the naked eye (Fig. 19.4). It can, with some exceptions (Bodechtel, 1930), be seen running through the full length of the hip-

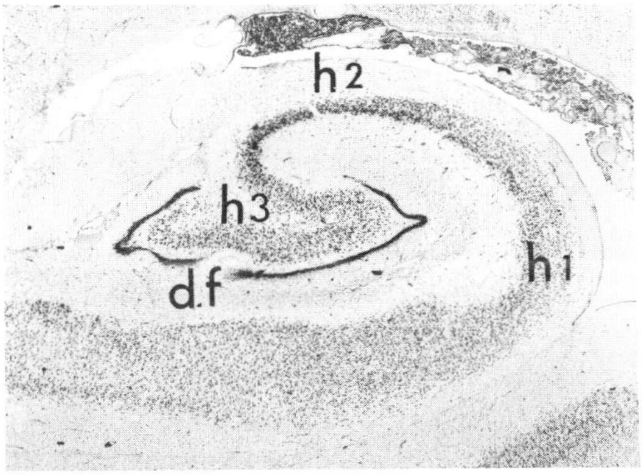

(a)

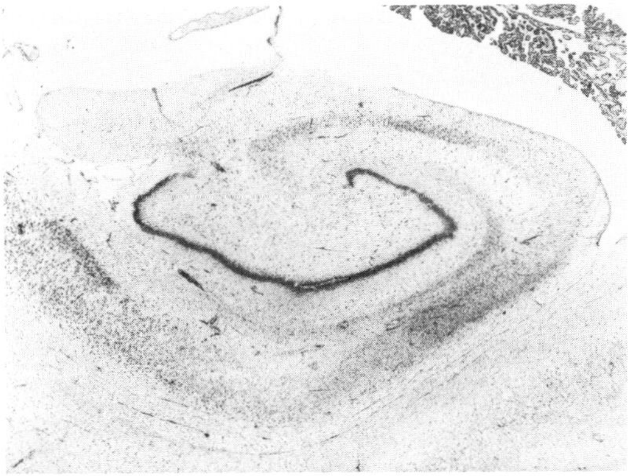

(b)

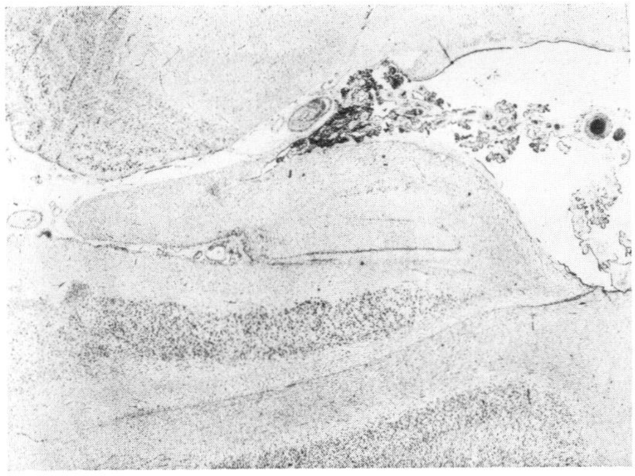

(c)

Fig. 19.3 (**a**) The normal hippocampus (see text); (**b**) acute selective necrosis of hippocampus following status epilepticus; (**c**) the classic Ammon's horn, or hippocampal sclerosis. Cresyl violet × 7.

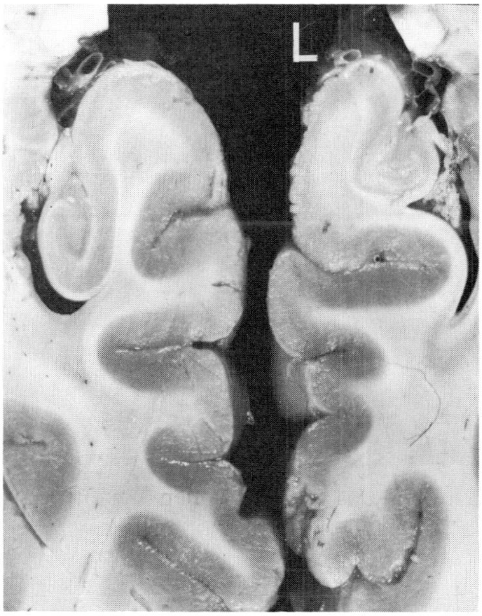

Fig. 19.4 Naked-eye coronal view of the two hippocampi from an epileptic brain with the adjacent gyri placed side by side. The right side is normal; on the left the hippocampus and the parahippocampal gyrus are greatly shrunken and sclerosed. × 1.4.

pocampal formation, although it becomes more patchy anteriorly in the pes and is then less easily identified.

In the cerebellum the Purkinje cells are the most vulnerable and their numbers may be greatly reduced over many folia. Along the line of the Purkinje cell loss, the astrocytes (or Bergmann glia) proliferate and spread out into the overlying molecular layer which can become heavily gliosed (Fig. 19.5). Considerable destruction of the granular layer sometimes occurs as well; and dense fibrous gliosis of the deep white matter spreads into the dentate nucleus which may also lose nerve cells. The severity of the cerebellar damage, therefore, ranges from the gross atrophy of many or most folia easily seen with the naked eye (Fig. 19.6) to the restricted loss of nerve cells in the occasional folium, often then around its base and detectable only with the microscope (Fig. 19.7).

The same process of selective neuronal necrosis and gliosis can affect one or both cerebral hemispheres more widely, and occasionally an entire hemisphere is smaller than the other leading to a clear-cut hemiatrophy (Fig. 19.8). More often the damage is less marked and is

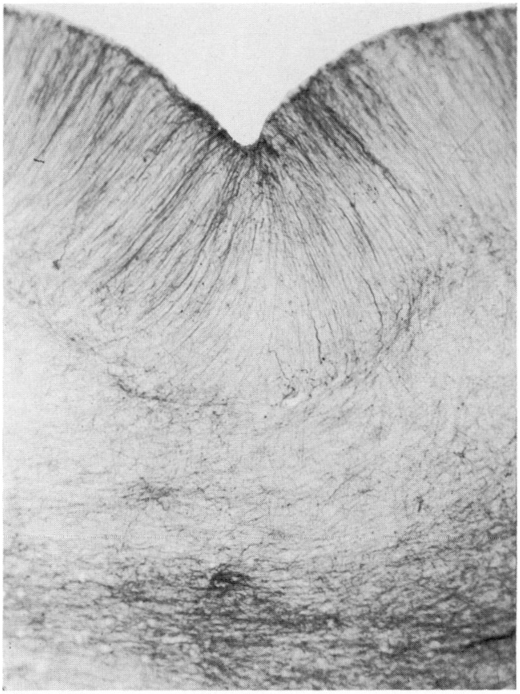

Fig. 19.5 Cerebellar cortex and subadjacent white matter showing an intense fibrous gliosis spreading through the molecular layer, less in the granular layer and more intense in the white matter. Holzer stain × 110.

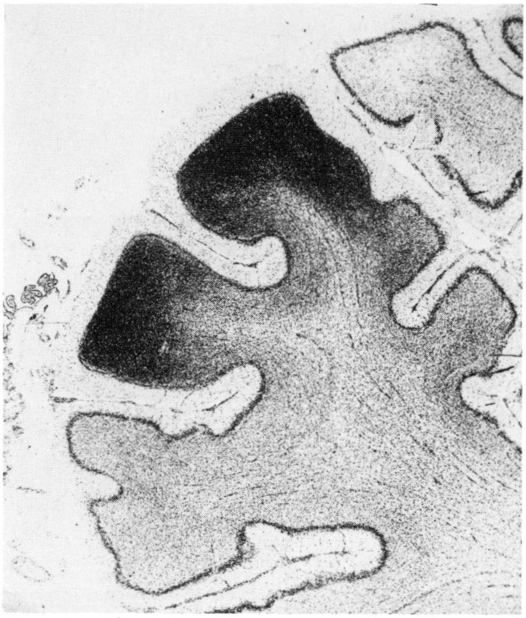

Fig. 19.7 Cerebellar folia with extensive loss of Purkinje cells and almost complete destruction of the granular layer. A few deeply stained patches of surviving granular cells are seen. Cresyl violet × 18.

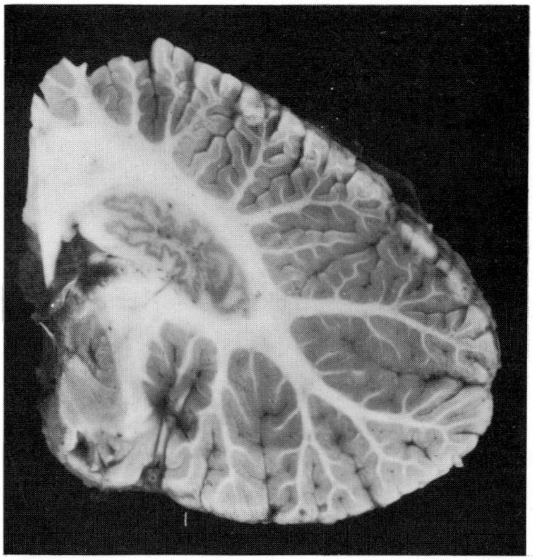

(a)

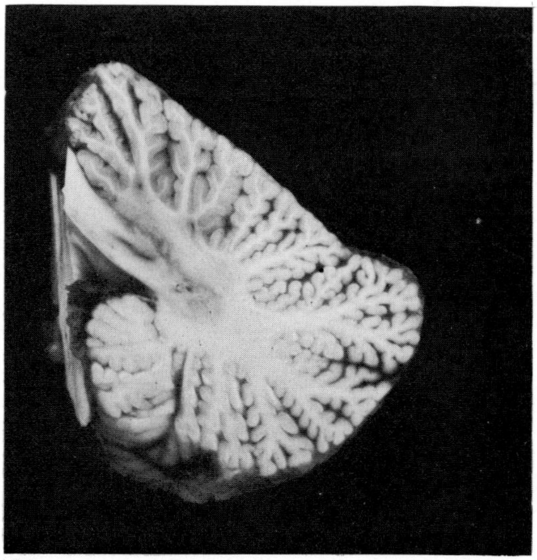

(b)

Fig. 19.6 (**a**) The normal cerebellum for comparison with (**b**), which shows the naked-eye appearance of atrophy which is not infrequently seen in chronic epileptic patients. In this case the folial atrophy is most marked in the posterior and inferior parts of the lateral lobe × 1.25.

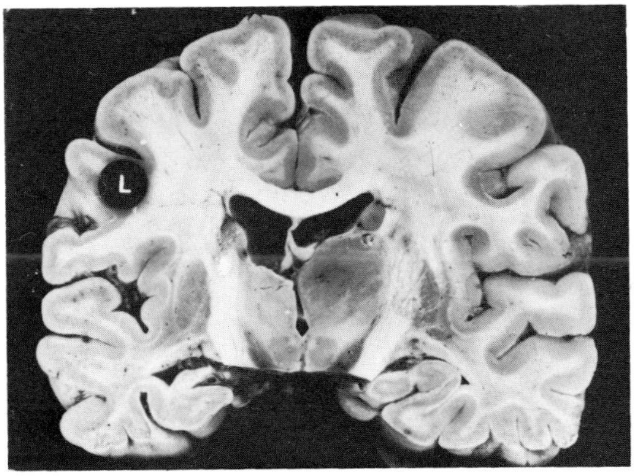

Fig. 19.8 Coronal view of the brain from a patient with long-standing epilepsy. The left hemisphere is smaller than the right, the hippocampus and the thalamus being particularly severely affected ×0.5.

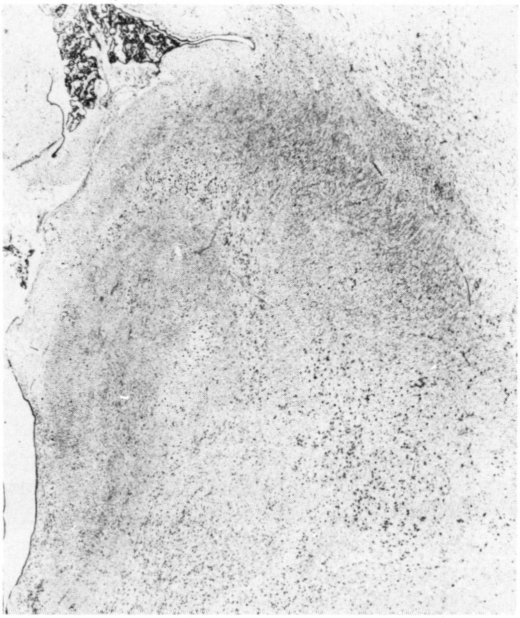

Fig. 19.10 Medial part of the thalamus, showing irregular areas of neuronal loss and dense glial proliferation, which has stained darkly. Cresyl violet × 15.

patchy, ranging from localized neuronal loss (Fig. 19.9) and gliosis scattered through the cerebral neocortex to more extensive damage which runs horizontally, in a laminar way, mainly through the intermediate layers of the cortex. In the deep grey matter of the hemisphere the area most frequently affected is the thalamus and, particularly in the presence of hemiatrophy, a gross inequality between the two thalami may be seen. The neuronal loss in the thalamus is distributed throughout the different nuclei and shows no systematic or anatomical preference (Fig. 19.10). The mamillary body may also be grossly shrunken (Fig. 19.11).

The incidence of damage in the vulnerable areas was studied by Peiffer (1963) and by Mar-

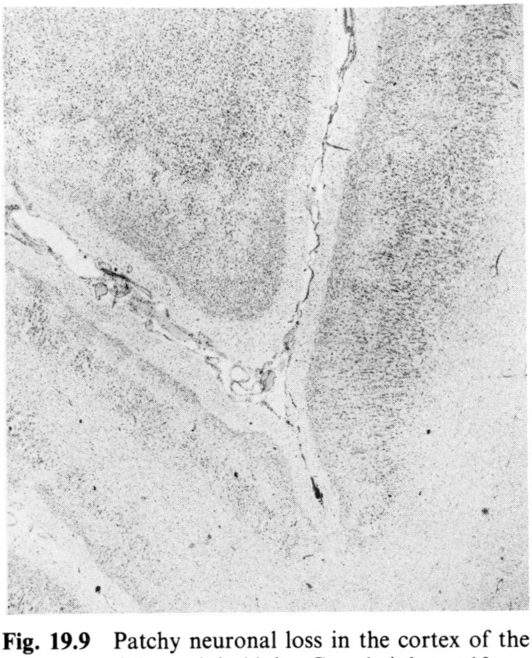

Fig. 19.9 Patchy neuronal loss in the cortex of the convexity of the occipital lobe. Cresyl violet × 10.

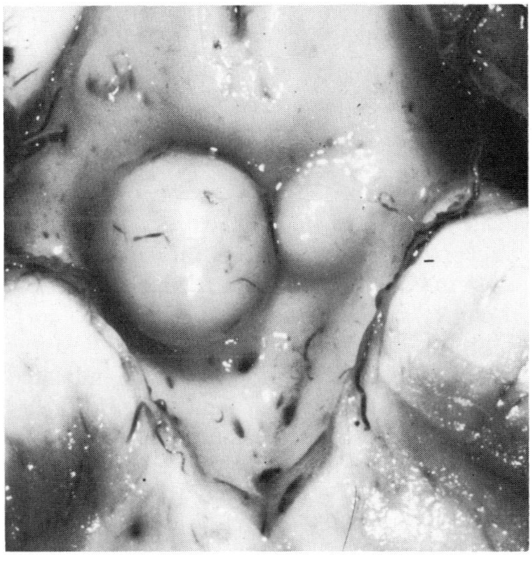

Fig. 19.11 Severe atrophy of the left mamillary body in the same specimen as shown in Fig. 19.8 × 5.

gerison and Corsellis (1966). The latter study found that one or both hippocampi were affected in 50–60 per cent of cases of chronic cryptogenic epilepsy, and that the unilateral damage was far the commoner, a classic Ammon's horn sclerosis being found bilaterally in only 3 per cent. The cerebellum was damaged in 45 per cent of the cases and the thalamus, the amygdaloid nucleus and the cerebral cortex each, not necessarily together, in about 25 per cent. Nearly all cases in which the hippocampus was affected showed some damage elsewhere in the brain. In several cases the cerebellum was affected although the hippocampi were not. It should be emphasized that most, if not all, studies in this field have been based on patients whose epileptic illness has been severe enough to bring them into the long-stay hospitals. Considerably less is therefore known about the incidence and extent of cerebral damage in those less seriously afflicted.

Pathogenesis of 'epileptic' brain damage

The origin of the kind of damage just described has long been discussed and there is still controversy over the extent to which it is the result of seizures and the extent to which it is the cause of seizures. Sommer, in 1880, unequivocally expressed the view that the sclerotic lesions in the hippocampus were the cause of epilepsy (with generalized seizures). In the same year, in the same journal, Pfleger, observing haemorrhagic lesions in the limbic system (apparently similar to those described by Noel et al. (1977) in patients dying shortly after status epilepticus), concluded that the neuronal necrosis arose from local circulatory or metabolic disturbances related to the seizures.

Chaslin described in 1889 the way in which the delicate network of fine glial fibres covering the surface of the normal cerebral cortex could thicken in epileptic brains to form a dense subpial 'carpet' spreading down into the deeper cortical layers. Chaslin saw this 'marginal gliosis' as a primary proliferation of fibres which indicated the presence of a pathological process underlying the epilepsy and could be compared to the formation of glial tumours. Alzheimer (1898), however, considered the gliosis to be a secondary reaction following the loss of nerve cells from the cortex. The controversy, like that about the hippocampus, continued for many years, and, as Scholz (1959) emphasized, the hypothesis of a progressive cerebral process as the cause of idiopathic epilepsy was widely accepted until the major contribution from Spielmeyer in 1927. He had analysed both the nature and the pathogenesis of the neuronal and of the glial abnormalities in many epileptic brains and came down firmly on the side of those who saw the changes as secondary to the fits or, more precisely in his view, to the vascular spasm believed to occur at the onset of an epileptic attack. Although the precise mechanism proposed by Spielmeyer proved unacceptable, the view that the scarring and atrophy were the consequence of interference with the blood and oxygen supply to certain parts of the brain persisted and was supported by Scholz (1951) and by Peiffer (1963). Because the damage was, therefore, described as a result of the fits there was no contradiction in the fact that although this change was present the epilepsy was classified as cryptogenic.

This view of the inertness of the cerebral scarring was accepted for some years and it only began to be questioned, particularly in so far as the hippocampus was concerned, after psychomotor attacks—and the electrical abnormalities associated with them—had been found to occur in many patients with atrophy of the medial temporal grey matter (which includes the parahippocampal gyrus, the hippocampus, the uncus and the amygdaloid nucleus).

It was then postulated by Earle, Baldwin and Penfield (1953) that the neuronal hypoxia leading to the sclerosis was not the consequence of fits but that the initial damage had occurred during the process of birth, by deformation of the skull and herniation of the medial temporal gyri through the incisura of the tent. According to this view, such distortion of the brain impedes the blood supply via the branches of the posterior cerebral artery to the grey matter in and around the hippocampus, and the resultant scar, or 'incisural sclerosis' as it was called, becomes liable to ripen after months or years into an epileptogenic focus. Penfield and his colleagues, however, did not regard birth as the only time during which this damage could occur, and Gastaut (1956) extended the concept to include other pathological events, such as head injury or cerebral infarction. According to this view, the common factor was the development of cerebral oedema which led to transtentorial herniation with compression of the anterior choroidal and posterior cerebral arteries. This hypothesis was given added weight by Lindenberg (1955), who concluded that 'a typical vascular sclerosis of the Ammon's horn generally signifies at least one phase of increased supratentorial pressure during the life of the individual'.

Although the hypotheses of Penfield and Gastaut were soon preferred by many to that of the German school there are cogent reasons why they should be questioned. First, Ounsted, Lindsay and Norman (1966) pointed out that the distribution of the damage, with the emphasis on the hippocampus and the almost invariable sparing of the calcarine cortex, is radically different from that which usually results from an obstruction of the posterior cerebral artery. Furthermore, the explanation also fails to take into account that damage of a similar nature is often encountered in other parts of the brain, well away from the tentorial opening and not lying in the territory of any vessel manifestly at risk in the same way as the posterior cerebral artery. Although the evidence quoted both for and against such hypotheses is too often drawn from studies of the mature rather than the developing brain, there is little doubt that the so-called hypoxic cerebral changes seen in epileptic children and in adults can develop in the absence of brain swelling; conversely, the changes which usually result from brain swelling are not merely those of hypoxia. Secondly, Veith (1970) found no evidence that herniation of the temporal lobes at birth could be held responsible for the neuronal changes he had occasionally encountered in a histological study of several hundred infant brains. The reasons just given not only make Penfield's theory of the origin of incisural sclerosis difficult to accept, at least as the common causal mechanism, but also militate against the unqualified acceptance of that proposed by Gastaut.

The important fact in both hypotheses is the emphasis that they lay on the occurrence of some initial catastrophe at birth or in the first few years of life. Insults such as a severe infection or a head injury may well be important factors in some cases, but the most sinister event commonly found to have occurred in epileptic patients with 'hypoxic' brain damage is the onset of fits in infancy or in childhood (Falconer, Serafetinides and Corsellis, 1964; Veith, 1970). If the fits are serial or if status supervenes the outlook is particularly ominous, for there is then a good chance that irretrievable destruction of nerve cells will result and in due course scar tissue will form. A widely held view, which is essentially that taught by Scholz and by Norman, attributes the selective damage in the brain to the hypoxia occurring during the course of these attacks. This remains compatible with the view that the scarring, however caused, is liable to perpetuate the attacks and, by its localization, to influence their clinical pattern (Margerison and Corsellis, 1966).

The need remains, however, to define more precisely the course of the physiological events by which the pathological changes are produced. As McMenemey (1940) put it in another context, the morbid anatomist has only the battlefield to work on after the battle has been lost.

Experimental studies have provided clear evidence that sustained seizures can produce the classic patterns of epileptic brain damage.

Experiments in primates (Meldrum and Brierley, 1973; Meldrum and Horton, 1973; Meldrum, Vigouroux and Brierley, 1973) have emphasized systemic changes which tend to impair cerebral energy metabolism.

Measurements of the physiological changes during drug-induced status epilepticus and the incidence and severity of ischaemic cell change in the perfusion-fixed brain a few hours after the episode of status, failed to show any correlation between the early transient systemic hypoxia and brain damage. On the other hand, physiological events occurring after 30 minutes of sustained seizure activity did show a relation to brain damage. Hyperpyrexia and arterial hypotension appeared to play a critical role in producing cerebellar damage (i.e. ischaemic cell change in Purkinje and basket cells, especially in the boundary zone between the arterial territories of the superior cerebellar artery and the posterior inferior cerebellar artery). The incidence of ischaemic cell change in the neocortex, hippocampus and thalamus was related to the total duration of seizure activity in the range 1.5–5 hours. An impaired neuronal energy metabolism results from the combination of excessive neuronal activity and the cumulative effects of secondary changes such as hypoxia, hypoglycaemia, arterial hypotension and hyperpyrexia. If the secondary changes are prevented or markedly diminished by peripheral muscular paralysis, neuronal changes still occur in the neocortex, thalamus and hippocampus but only after relatively more prolonged seizures (3–8 hours) (Meldrum, Vigouroux and Brierley, 1973). These experiments in subhuman primates have provided a good model in physiological and pathological terms for studying the lesions in man resulting from status epilepticus.

It is also possible experimentally to produce a pattern of damage which involves predominantly the hippocampus, and more closely resembles the lesions found in chronic epileptic patients and especially those with temporal lobe epilepsy (see below). In experimental primates this has been achieved by using allylglycine (an inhibitor of the cerebral enzyme glutamate decarboxylase (Horton and Meldrum, 1973)) to produce recurrent brief seizures (Meldrum and Brierley, 1972; Meldrum, Horton and Brierley, 1974). The generalized physiological changes associated with a sequence of 26–62 brief tonic-clonic seizures in 8–13 hours are relatively mild, and the baboons appear neurologically normal 1–2 days later. However, examination of the hippocampus after a 1- to 6-week survival period showed neuronal loss in the Sommer sector (CA_1) and the endfolium (CA_4), and an associated proliferation of fibrous astrocytes and microglia. As in temporal lobe epileptics, the CA_1 (h1) lesions tended to be unilateral whereas the CA_4 (h3-5) lesions were symmetrical. Systemic factors such as hypoxia and arterial hypotension appear to be less important than local factors secondary to the local epileptic activity.

The importance of the local seizure activity is supported by a wide range of recent studies on the pathological consequences of limbic seizures. Such seizures may be induced by systemic administration of kainic acid or pilocarpine or dipiperidinoethane (Ben-Ari et al., 1980; Olney et al., 1980; Turski et al., 1983) or by focal injection into the amygdala of various convulsants (kainic acid, picrotoxin, bicuculline, opiates or pilocarpine) (Menini et al., 1980; Turski et al., 1984). After local seizure activity has been strongly maintained for 2–5 hours, ischaemic cell change and subsequently neuronal loss and gliosis become demonstrable in the hilus, CA_3, CA_1 and, sometimes, the subiculum and entorhinal cortex. This hippocampal pathology appears to be primarily due to the local seizure activity. Systemic changes are commonly minimal. Somewhat similar early pathological changes involving the hilar (GABAergic) neurons and the CA_3 pyramidal neurons are seen after electrical stimulation of the perforant path (either continuous for 2 hours or intermittent for 24 hours) (Sloviter, 1983).

Ultrastructural studies of the early changes in vulnerable regions of the hippocampus provide important indications of the mechanisms involved (Olney, Fuller and de Gubareff, 1979; Evans, Griffiths and Meldrum, 1983, 1984; Griffiths, Evans and Meldrum, 1983, 1984). Swelling of perineuronal astrocytic processes occurs early in seizures throughout the pyramidal cell layer. Swollen mitochondria are seen in neuronal perikarya and in focal dendritic swellings, especially in the outer third of the basal dendrites in CA_3 and CA_1 (Evans, Griffiths and Meldrum, 1983; Griffiths, Evans and Meldrum, 1984). The oxalate pyroantimonate method shows these swollen mitochondria to be densely loaded with calcium (Griffiths, Evans and Meldrum, 1983). Although this calcium overload is acutely reversible (Griffiths, Evans and Meldrum, 1984), it is potentially a lethal lesion if energy metabolism becomes impaired and mitochondrial calcium sequestration is finally overwhelmed so that the cystosolic free calcium concentration rises to cytotoxic levels (Farber, 1981; Meldrum, 1983).

Epilepsy and the temporal lobes

During the initial period in which the interpretation of the various histological abnormalities in the brains of epileptic patients was the subject of controversy, Hughlings Jackson and his colleagues (Anderson, 1886; Jackson and Beevor, 1889) described a complex pattern of epileptic attacks in which auras of smell or taste occurred. Feelings of unreality or familiarity and dream-like illusory experiences were also common. Visual hallucinations could display an organized scenic character. In the brains of several people with such symptoms, focal abnormalities were found lying close to the hippocampus, but centred on the region of the uncus and the amygdaloid nucleus. Other workers confirmed these observations, and the existence of a focal form of symptomatic epilepsy became established which was linked to the temporosphenoidal regions, much as the motor attacks of jacksonian epilepsy had been associated with the frontal, and particularly with the precentral, cortex.

In 1935 Stauder claimed to have made a comparable correlation based on the hippocampus. He carefully analysed the nature of the attacks in 53 patients with long-standing epilepsy and found the Ammon's horn, or hippocampus, to be sclerotic in 36 of them. In all but three of these

36 the clinical picture had pointed to a lesion in the temporal lobes although in some brains there was also frontotemporal scarring of the contrecoup type. None of the 17 patients in whose brains the Ammon's horns were normal had shown signs of a temporal lobe disturbance.

Less attention was paid to Stauder's observations than to the more notable contribution by Hughlings Jackson, but both took on a new importance when the neurosurgical treatment of the focal epilepsies began to be combined with the use of the electroencephalogram. The introduction of this technique led to the identification of abnormal paroxysmal electric discharges in tracings obtained from epileptic patients and one particular type of these was claimed by Gibbs, Gibbs and Lennox in 1937 to be characteristic of what had, by them, come to be known as 'psychomotor epilepsy'. In 1951 Jasper, Pertuisset and Flanigin introduced the term 'temporal lobe seizures' to embrace the wide spectrum of complex attacks which could range from the dreamy states of Hughlings Jackson to the psychomotor epilepsies.

The common factor in the EEG records of patients suffering from temporal lobe seizures was the occurrence, during the interictal period, of spikes or sharp waves thought to originate in the affected temporal lobe (Jasper and Kershman, 1941). This was an observation of great practical as well as theoretical importance since about half the epileptic patients living in long-stay hospitals were found to fall into the category of temporal lobe epilepsy (Liddell, 1953; Gastaut, 1956), even if the precise incidence depends on the definition of its clinical and electrical criteria (Margerison and Liddell, 1961).

In recent years the use of stereotactically implanted recording electrodes has clarified the relationship between the focal onset and spread of seizure activity and the experiential phenomena and clinical signs of temporal lobe epilepsy (Gloor et al., 1982; Wieser, 1983; Bossi et al., 1984). Experiential phenomena, such as perceptual hallucinations or illusions of familiarity, occur only when the ictal discharge involves the limbic system. Impairment of consciousness may occur with bilateral temporal discharges. Somatomotor manifestations such as facial clonic jerks are associated with spread of ictal activity to the parietal cortex.

At the beginning of the 1950s reports appeared on the neurosurgical removal of anterior portions of the affected temporal lobe (Pensfield and Flanigin, 1950; Green, Duisberg and McGrath, 1951). According to what was already known from post-mortem studies it was reasonable to expect that the resected tissue might contain either the kind of focal abnormalities described by Hughlings Jackson or a sclerotic hippocampus. At first, however, there was little apparent incidence of any kind of lesion. In 1951 Bailey and Gibbs reported that they had failed to find anything abnormal in about half the 25 temporal lobes they had resected. The figure given by Morris (1956) was of the same order, whilst Haberland (1958) observed histopathological changes in only 19 out of 47 specimens; in 6 of the 19 the lesion was a typical Ammon's horn sclerosis. In 1953 Earle, Baldwin and Penfield claimed to have found macroscopical or histological abnormalities in all the temporal lobes removed from 157 epileptic patients. In 57 of these cases a postnatal abnormality was found which was usually tumorous in nature or had occurred as a sequele to trauma or infection. In the remaining 100 cases, however, a variable degree of atrophy was found which ranged from the shrinkage of a single convolution to that of the entire temporal lobe. The uncus, amygdaloid nucleus and the parahippocampal gyrus were the areas most often affected but the extent could not be precisely defined. This was partly because no systematic histological investigations had been undertaken and partly because the more medial grey matter, and particularly the hippocampus, was not included in the resected tissue. Nevertheless, the distribution and the nature of the atrophic changes seemed similar to those seen when an Ammon's horn sclerosis was present. Penfield and his colleagues, however, preferred to label the condition 'incisural sclerosis' since its origin, in their view, depended on the medial parts of the temporal lobes being displaced through the incisura during birth. Meyer, Falconer and Beck (1954) followed these positive observations with the statement that they, too, had found some kind of abnormality in all the 14 specimens they had examined. Crome (1955) was loath to accept that the degree of gliosis described in some of the cases was beyond the range of normal and further suggested that the epileptogenic significance of the sclerotic changes was doubtful. By 1958 Cavanagh, Falconer and Meyer had increased the number of cases to 50. They agreed that in about 30 per cent the glial reaction was relatively slight, and as Meyer commented in 1963 'it is certainly justifiable to doubt its value as a substrate of the psychomotor attacks and in not a few cases it was of doubtful pathological significance altogether'. Other studies reported since then (Falconer, Serafetinides and Corsellis, 1964; Green and Scheetz, 1964; Jann-Brown, 1973) report a clean-cut abnormality in about 75 per cent of the specimens examined.

Although there are exceptions, there is a marked tendency for the abnormalities, irrespective of their nature, to lie deep in the temporal lobe and less often towards the convexity. It is these deep limbic parts—which include the uncus, the amygdaloid nucleus and the hippocampus—that lie on the edge of most resections and are therefore liable to be sucked away or lost during the operation, or remain *in situ*. The tissue available for examination can therefore range from the full coronal extent of the temporal lobe with a major part of the amygdala and the hippocampus to no more than some part of the three temporal gyri. Abnormalities will therefore be found less often if only the latter, neocortical, areas are examined. This helps to explain the variable incidence of sclerosis which has been reported by different observers. It is also important to emphasize that not all lesions can be seen, or even suspected, with the naked eye. A few may therefore be overlooked if the tissue is not sampled histologically at several levels, or occasionally by an interrupted run of serial sections.

The abnormalities may be divided into those which tend to be focal and those which are more diffuse. In the former there is a small number with cortical scarring following trauma (Cavanagh, Falconer and Meyer, 1958; Corsellis, 1970), with a patch of old infarction or with evidence of past infection such as an abscess or, rarely, an encephalitis (Aguilar and Rasmussen, 1960). The main focal group comprises abnormalities which range from small discrete masses, obvious to the naked eye, to aggregations of bizarre neurons and glia identifiable only under the microscope. The label of tumour is often inappropriate in this connection, at least without qualification, because the lesions appear to replace rather than to expand and indeed in most series patients suffering primarily from a cerebral tumour have been deliberately excluded. The masses which are found, even in patients with an epileptic history lasting for many years, are small, measuring a few millimetres to about 2 cm across. They may not be identified at operation; very occasionally they are calcified. The lesions are usually single, but multiple islets of abnormal cells may be found. The histological picture varies greatly; the cellular population is usually mainly glial, appearing as an astrocytoma, an oligodendroglioma or as a mixed glial tumour (Cavanagh, 1958) (Fig. 19.12). Not infrequently,

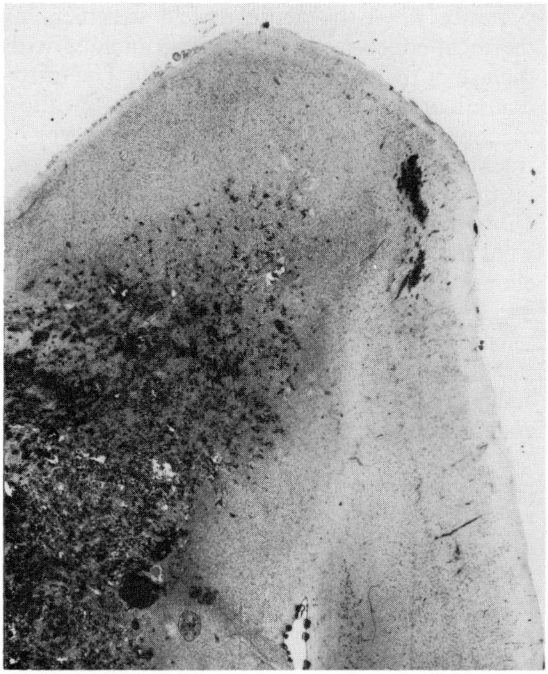

Fig. 19.12 Atypical glioma in the region of the uncus and amygdaloid complex. Haematoxylin and eosin × 8.

abnormal neurons are present and the overall picture resembles that of a ganglioglioma; less often the growth is predominantly vascular (Edgar and Baldwin, 1960). There is usually little or no evidence of recent growth or of infiltration. Many of the masses seem, therefore, to be more in the nature of malformation than of neoplasm. The term 'hamartoma' is applicable in many instances, although not invariably, since sometimes the mass appears frankly neoplastic while at others the lesion is clearly that of a malformation or 'hamartia'. Very occasionally, patches of typical heterotopic grey matter are seen deep in the white matter. Another, and more common, abnormality is a form of cortical dysplasia in which large, and even giant, malformed neurons are scattered through one or more short runs of

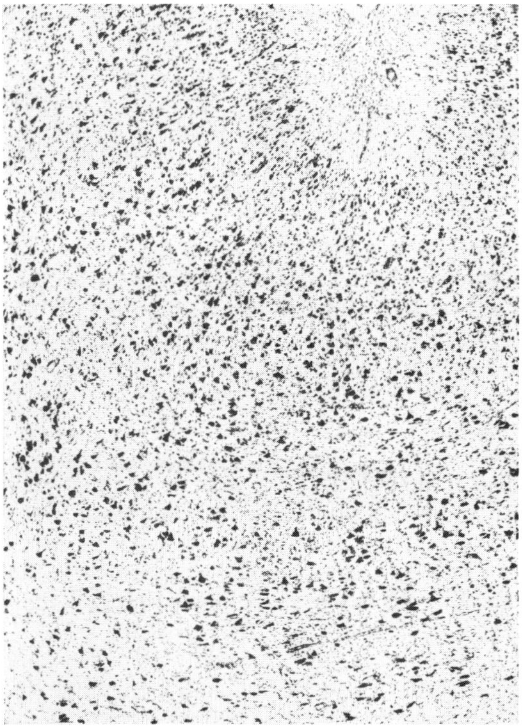

Fig. 19.13 Cortical dysplasia—a population of large anomalous neurons scattered through all but the first cortical layer. The cortical ribbon is widened and the lamination is lost. Cresyl violet × 30.

cortex and may be accompanied by bizarre glial cells spreading into the subjacent white matter (Fig. 19.13). These can at times be reminiscent histologically of the tuber in tuberous sclerosis, but there are usually many clinical and histological points of difference which make this diagnosis unacceptable (Taylor et al., 1971). Perot, Weir and Rasmussen (1966) and others have, however, described classic tuber formation in tissue resected from epileptic patients with tuberous sclerosis. Taylor (1975) has reported that the incidence of schizophrenia-like psychosis is significantly higher when 'alien' tissue (i.e. small tumours, hamartomas or focal dysplasia) is found in the resected lobe (23 per cent of 47 patients) than when mesial temporal sclerosis is present (5 per cent of 41 patients). Although alien tissue was more often found in the right hemisphere, it was most common in the left hemisphere in the psychotic patients in accordance with the known association between left-sided epileptogenesis and schizophreniform psychosis (Flor-Henry, 1969; Sherwin, 1981).

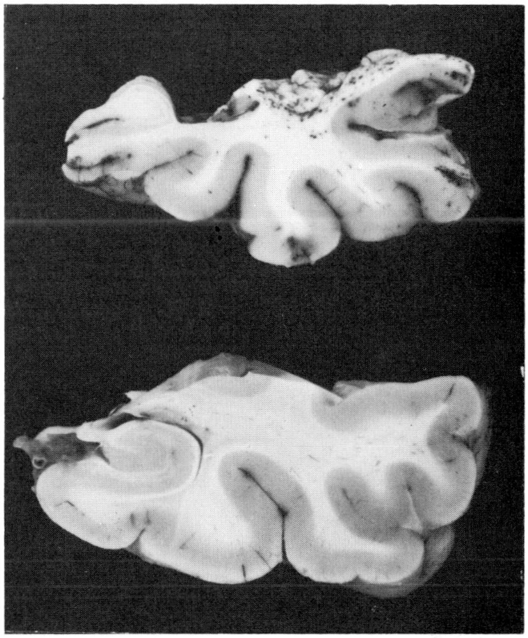

Fig. 19.14 The upper view is of a temporal lobectomy specimen which has been cut coronally. A typical hippocampal sclerosis can be seen when compared with the normal picture in the lower view.

Ammon's horn, or hippocampal sclerosis, is the diffuse type of abnormality (Fig. 19.14). This has been identified in 50–60 per cent of resected temporal lobes and it is therefore the commonest lesion found. Its pathological features and its pathogenesis have been discussed in the previous sections and they will be reconsidered here only in so far as they may throw light on the role in epilepsy of the sclerotic hippocampus, or more correctly sclerosis of the medial temporal areas, since the scarring tends to spread out anteriorly to the amygdaloid nucleus (Fig. 19.15). and uncus as well as laterally into the parahippocampal gyrus and beyond. It is important to emphasize that there are other ways in which the hippocampus may be damaged besides the classic Ammon's horn sclerosis. Thus the hippocampus may be largely destroyed by atheromatous occlusion of the posterior cerebral artery or less severely by microinfarcts due to the degeneration of its small vessels. It is also peculiarly liable to disintegrate with the almost total loss of the Sommer sector in senile dementia of the Alzheimer type (Morel and Wildi, 1956; Corsellis, 1957). Haymaker et al. (1958) found no history of epilepsy in 21 infants with kernicterus in all of

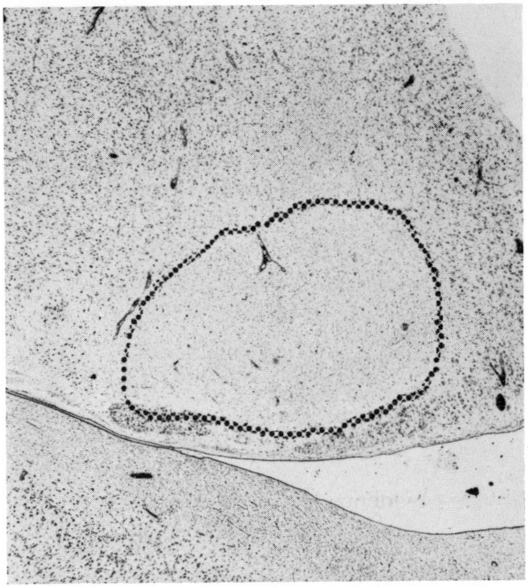

Fig. 19.15 Part of the amygdaloid nucleus in a lobectomy specimen. A sizeable patch of neuronal loss is outlined. The edge of the resection is seen at the top right hand corner. Cresyl violet ×20.

whose brains the large hippocampal neurons were destroyed. Similarly, they found that fits were a far from constant feature in a large series of infants with inclusion body encephalitis which had damaged the temporal lobes. In none of these conditions is the sporadic convulsion, let alone any form of long-standing epilepsy, particularly liable to appear. It is only when 'hypoxic' damage occurs, but does not kill during the acute stages, that the classic sclerosis will have time to develop and, as Penfield put it, ripen into a scar. It is in this situation, which is particularly prone to occur in the first few years of life, that the risk of an epilepsy becoming permanently established is greatest, whether or not fits or status epilepticus had occurred as a feature of the initial hypoxic episode. The hippocampal sclerosis may then be seen as part of a posthypoxic scarring process which preferentially, but not exclusively, affects the medial temporal grey matter and which, like scarring elsewhere in the brain, may sooner or later lead to epileptic attacks which tend to be of a particular kind or constellation because of the pattern of localization. This hypothesis does not require either that temporal lobe seizures should inevitably follow development of the scarring or that such damage should be the only determining factor. The genetic side is also important since a family history of epilepsy was found in nearly 40 per cent of a group of epileptic patients with sclerosis of the Ammon's horn (Margerison and Corsellis, 1966).

Recently, quantitative techniques for cell counting have been applied to the hippocampus, both *post mortem* in patients with epilepsy of various kinds (Dam, 1980, 1982) and in temporal lobectomy specimens from patients with complex partial seizures (Babb et al., 1984). Postmortem study shows a loss of hippocampal neurons which is correlated with the frequency of tonic–clonic seizures and the total duration of epilepsy. It is most marked in the end-folium, where the loss associated with normal ageing is greatly accentuated. The dentate granule cells also show significant loss. In Dam's study the type of epilepsy (i.e. primary generalized, or simple or complex partial epilepsy) appeared not to determine the extent of cell loss. Babb and colleagues made cell counts in the anterior and posterior regions of their lobectomy specimens and reported that a good postoperative outcome (relief from seizures) was associated with a predominantly anterior cell loss. This loss was significant in the dentate fascia and in pyramidal cells in regions CA_3 and CA_2 (but not in CA_4) and in the prosubiculum and subiculum, and the hippocampal gyrus. When cell loss predominated in the posterior portion of the resected tissue it involved all hippocampal zones (including dentate gyrus, CA_2 and CA_4), and was associated with an unsatisfactory postoperative outcome, indicating that significant epileptogenic tissue remained *in situ*.

The clinicopathological problem is further complicated by the fact that no clear-cut structural abnormality can be found in about every fifth temporal lobe that is fully resected, but there are other possibilities. Sometimes the specimen is incomplete; it is also conceivable that lateralization was wrong, whilst both Falconer, Driver and Serafetinides (1962) and Schneider, Crosby and Farhat (1965) reported instances of temporal lobe epilepsy due to distant extratemporal lesions.

The postoperative prognosis with regard to seizures is unfavourable when no pathology is found, whereas it is particularly good when mesial temporal sclerosis is identified (Falconer, Serafetinides and Corsellis, 1964; Green, 1967; Bengzon et al., 1970; Jann-Brown, 1973; Falconer, 1974; Turner and Wyler, 1981; Babb et al., 1984). This observation is sometimes presented as conclusive evidence that the hippocampal sclerosis is the focal cause of the seizure activity, whereas it remains possible that the sclerosis is secondary either to focal or to generalized seizure activity, and that the favourable outcome arises because of the removal of epileptogenic tissue in the anterior part of the temporal lobe.

A difficult histological problem is set by findings which lie in the borderlands between normal and abnormal. The commonest of these is an apparent astrocytic proliferation with some degree of fibrous gliosis similar to that described by Chaslin (1889). This is usually seen most clearly in the subpial surface of the cortex and spreading into the deeper cortical layers, but the white matter and the amygdaloid nucleus may also be affected. This kind of glial reaction is most often seen when a typically sclerosed hippocampus is present and there is then no special problem. The difficulty arises when no hippocampal tissue is present, or when this is normal, or at least no more gliotic than the rest of the lobe. Crome (1955) was particularly critical of attributing any special importance to such uncertain changes which can vary from person to person with age and are not specific either to the temporal lobes or to the epileptic brain. It seems wisest, therefore, to accept as abnormal only a gliosis which is both unquestionably severe and accompanied by neuronal loss. Unfortunately, this is also notoriously difficult to estimate both in the neocortex and in the complex architecture of the uncus and the amygdaloid nucleus. In other words, these changes lie along a continuum and the point at which they become abnormal is an arbitrary one.

Cytological changes and epileptogenesis

Cerebral grey matter, when it is the focus of origin of epileptic discharges, shows a variety of cytological changes irrespective of the primary cause of the lesion (e.g. underlying tumour, infection, trauma, febrile convulsion, local ischaemia). Similar cytological changes are found in damaged grey matter which is not the substrate of epileptic activity. Some of these changes may be involved in epileptogenesis but in no case is definite proof available.

It is natural to enquire if the reactive or fibrous astrocytes which are so abundant in these lesions could play a role in epileptogenesis. Normal astrocytes are believed to (1) transport glucose and various metabolic precursors from capillaries to neurons, (2) take up and metabolize various amino acid transmitters and (3) participate in the regulation of the ionic composition of the extracellular fluid. A failure in the latter function could be critical, as an increase in the extracellular fluid content of potassium can lead to local epileptiform discharges (Zuckermann and Glaser, 1970). However, the resting potential of reactive astrocytes (in a freezing lesion) is very high (Grossman and Rosman, 1971), indicating a high intracellular, and a low extracellular potassium concentration. Physiological studies of glial membrane properties in a focus have also provided evidence against the hypothesis of a disorder in potassium transport (Glötzner, 1973).

A loss of neurons is also characteristic of epileptogenic tissue. Although this is obviously non-selective in the centre of a traumatic lesion or abscess, in some situations there are elements of selectivity, especially when ischaemia is the intermediate agent. This creates the possibility of a partially selective destruction of inhibitory interneurons. There is evidence that the spasticity which follows a period of spinal cord ischaemia results from the preferential destruction of inhibitory interneurons containing glycine (Werman, Davidoff and Aprison, 1968). In the cerebellum the two types of cells (Purkinje and basket cells) which are selectively vulnerable to ischaemia (Brierley, Meldrum and Brown, 1973) are inhibitory (Curtis and Johnston, 1974).

Experimental evidence for a selective loss of inhibitory nerve terminals after hypoxia has been presented by Sloper, Johnson and Powell (1980). In the motor cortex of infant monkeys examined electron microscopically 7 days after a 30-minute episode of hypoxia, 85 per cent of degenerating terminals were of symmetrical type, indicating a highly selective vulnerability of inhibitory interneurons. Such a phenomenon could explain why fetal or neonatal hypoxia in man increases the incidence of epilepsy in childhood fivefold (Bergamasco et al., 1984).

As mentioned above, there is a preferential involvement of GABAergic interneurons in the hilus of the hippocampus in the acute neuronal pathological changes following status epilepticus induced by allylglycine or kainic acid in rats (Griffiths, Evans and Meldrum, 1983; Evans. Griffiths and Meldrum, 1984).

A selective loss of GABAergic nerve terminals has also been described in the epileptogenic focus induced in monkey neocortex by alumina cream (Ribak, Bradburne and Harris, 1982). Neurons around such a focus show a reduction in dendritic branching and a loss of dendritic spines (Westrum, White and Ward, 1965; Ward, 1969; Ribak, 1983).

A loss of dendritic spines identified in Golgi impregnations of cortical sections has been described in epilepsy and in various degenerative disorders (DeMoor, 1898). This may be an indication of deafferentation (Globus and Scheibel, 1966). Traumatic or space-occupying lesions can partially deafferent areas of cortex. Experimental undercutting of the cortex prolongs the after-discharge which can be induced by electrical stimulation (Halpern, 1972), suggesting that deafferentation could be a significant factor in the genesis of a cortical focus.

A similar shrinkage of the apical dendrite system with loss of dendritic spines and the appearance of terminal nodules has been described in hippocampal pyramidal neurons and dentate granular cells in temporal lobectomy specimens from patients with temporal lobe epilepsy (Scheibel and Scheibel, 1973; Scheibel, Crandall and Scheibel, 1974). The nodular dendritic swellings in an epileptogenic focus have been described as containing microtubules arranged in whirls (Vaquero et al., 1982).

Myoclonus epilepsy

Brief myoclonic contractions may affect a small group of muscle fibres, an individual muscle or many different muscles. The effect may therefore be too slight for a limb to move or it may throw a person to the ground.

Myoclonic contractions are common in epileptic patients; Muskens (1909) observed them in about two-thirds of all patients suffering from convulsions. Epilepsy and myoclonus, occurring together as a progressive familial illness, were first reported by Unverricht (1891) and Lundborg (1903). Similar cases were described by Lafora and Glück (1911), Westphal and Sioli (1921), Ostertag (1925), Hodskins and Yakovlev (1930) and van Bogaert (1949). More recent studies, including detailed chemical and electron microscopical analyses, have been made by Seitelberger et al. (1964), Seitelberger (1968), Kraus-Ruppert (1969) and Bergener and Gerhard (1970). There are at least two pathologically distinct, genetically determined, syndromes: myoclonus epilepsy of Lafora or 'Lafora body disease', and 'Baltic myoclonus' (Unverricht-Lundborg disease, progressive myoclonus epilepsy without Lafora bodies).

Lafora body disease is an inborn error of carbohydrate metabolism with autosomal recessive inheritance. Storage of a polyglucosan in brain and liver produces the characteristic histological feature, which permits diagnosis on the basis of a liver biopsy in the presymptomatic phase (Baumann, Kocoshis and Wilson, 1983). The clinical disorder usually begins between the ages of 10 and 16 years. The first sign is the onset of generalized and often nocturnal convulsions. Myoclonic jerks develop during the next few years and may gradually render the patient helpless. Dementia supervenes, usually within 2 years, always within 5 years. The patient wastes away, death usually occurring within 10 years of the onset. During the later stages the epilepsy may disappear while the myoclonus persists.

The brain appears only slightly atrophic and there is some diffuse neuronal loss with a mild fibrous gliosis. The salient feature is the presence of Lafora inclusion bodies. These appear as concentric rounded inclusions of varying size lying in the neuronal cytoplasm. Davison and Keschner (1940) described two types—homogeneous and concentric. The homogeneous bodies are separated from the other contents of the cell body by a narrow capsule of unstainable material; some have a central core of cruciform or stellate shape. The concentric bodies have a deeply stained core with paler rings around this or with dark radial striae in the pale outer zone. Their size ranges from about 1 to 30 μm in diameter; there may be several in a single cell. Lafora and Glück (1911) pictured a cell of the vagal nucleus with one large and seven small inclusions, but so many is exceptional. They may be found in dendrites, axons or apparently free in the tissue. This last may indicate the loss of the parent cell, although their presence does not necessarily lead to cell degeneration and death, as Nissl granules are often normally present in the surrounding cytoplasm. Harriman and Millar (1955), in a careful histochemical study of these bodies, first showed them to contain an acid mucopolysaccharide. They are readily distinguished from the Lewy inclusions of paralysis agitans in being basophilic with all stains, in giving gamma-metachromasia with methyl violet and toluidine blue, and in staining with the PAS method for one to two glycol groupings after extraction with solvents for lipid, hyaluronic acid and glycogen. Both the intraneuronal bodies and those found by Harriman and Millar in heart muscle and liver differ from amyloid, as commonly seen in tissue, in being basophilic and in failing to stain with Congo red or to be anisotropic after this stain.

The distribution of Lafora bodies in the brain varies considerably (Seitelberger, 1968). They occur throughout the cerebral cortex but are usually best seen in the central gyrus and the anterior frontal cortex. The thalamus, globus pallidus and both zones of the substantia nigra tend to be heavily involved. The number drops lower down the brain stem, only scattered bodies being seen in the superior and inferior olives. The cerebellar cortex contains many and there may also be a patchy loss of Purkinje cells and granule cells with some glial increase. The dentate nucleus is one of the most severely affected regions, because of both the number of large Lafora bodies and the neuronal loss. Few bodies are seen below the medulla.

'*Baltic myoclonus*', or progressive myoclonus epilepsy without Lafora bodies (Koskiniemi et al., 1974), has an earlier age of onset (mean 10 years) than Lafora body disease. It is an autosomal recessive disorder whose biochemical basis is uncertain. The only identified abnormality is an enhanced urinary excretion of indican, a metabolite of tryptophan (Koskiniemi, 1975). The presenting symptom is either myoclonus or generalized tonic–clonic seizures. Photic stimulation triggers the myoclonus and EEG spike and wave discharges. Baltic myoclonus differs from Lafora body disease in the slower clinical course and the intellectual preservation seen in some cases. Indeed it has been suggested that deterioration is accelerated by treatment with phenytoin (Eldridge et al., 1983). The myoclonus responds to valproate and to L-tryptophan. The cerebral pathology has been described by Haltia, Kristensson and Sourander (1969), Matthews, Howell and Stevens (1969), Koskiniemi et al. (1974) and Eldridge et al. (1983). The most consistent finding is a marked loss of Purkinje cells in the cerebellum, with proliferation of Bergmann glia. There may also be a loss of cells in the granular cell layer. Other nuclear groups are not obviously affected (although degeneration in the medial thalamic nuclei has been described).

A third group of cases consists of those in which the myoclonus is part of another cerebral disorder. It is, for example, common in subacute sclerosing panencephalitis and is seen in some cases of Creutzfeldt–Jakob disease. It is also encountered occasionally in the lipidoses, the leucodystrophies, in gliotic encephalopathy and in tuberous sclerosis (Crome and Stern, 1972).

Myoclonus epilepsy (familial or sporadic) has also been found together with spinocerebellar degeneration. Dentatorubral atrophy, which Greenfield (1954) named the Ramsay Hunt syndrome, is an important example. Hunt (1921) described two clinical syndromes. In one, myoclonic epilepsy appeared in adolescence and progressive cerebellar ataxia developed subsequently. In the other, represented by two twin brothers, a spinocerebellar disorder was present from childhood and myoclonus developed in adult life. At post-mortem in the latter case the cerebellar cortex was intact, the dentate nucleus was atrophic and the myelin was rarefied in the superior cerebellar peduncle. In a similar case of Louis-Bar and van Bogaert (1947) there was severe neuronal loss in the cerebellar nuclei with some loss of granule cells in the cortex. The superior olives, superior vestibular nuclei and the spinal root of the trigeminal nucleus were also atrophic; the superior cerebellar peduncle were palely stained. In an earlier case of Hänel and Bielschowsky, quoted by Greenfield, the cerebellar cortex and the medullary olives were affected more severely than either the dentate nucleus or the superior cerebellar peduncles.

An autosomal dominant disorder with deafness, ataxia and myoclonus has been described by May and White (1968) and by Baraitser et al. (1984). At post-mortem there is nerve cell loss in the dentate nucleus and cerebellar cortex and pallor of the gracile tracts in the spinal cord. Myoclonus and cerebellar ataxia may also occur in association with mitochondrial myopathy and lactacidaemia (Fitzsimons, Clifton-Bligh and Wolfenden, 1981).

Action or intention myoclonus is sometimes a prominent feature of the 'Ramsay Hunt syndrome'. It is also seen in patients with ischaemic brain damage following cardiac arrest, asphyxia or blunt head injury (Lance and Adams, 1963; Boudin et al., 1963). Correleative clinicopathological studies of myoclonus and hypoxic encephalopathy are lacking. Cerebellar damage is, of course, common after cerebral hypoxia, and it is found in other myoclonic syndromes. However, conventional neurological signs of cerebellar damage are often lacking. Clinical features such as chorea, athetosis and parkinsonism, which suggest basal ganglia disease, may be present. The syndrome sometimes responds dramatically to the oral or intravenous administration of 5-hydroxytryptophan, the immediate precursor of serotonin (Lhermitte, Marteau and Degos, 1972). This does not necessarily indicate, however, that the primary abnormality lies in the serotoninergic system. Neurons containing serotonin, the cell bodies of which lie in the nuclei of the median raphe, have terminals within the basal ganglia and their influence could be critically modified by pathological changes in either the cerebellum or the basal ganglia.

The pathological basis of myoclonus is thus both aetiologically diverse and anatomically varied. Electrophysiological studies in patients (and in animals treated with excitant drugs) have been reviewed by Halliday (1967). Myoclonic activity can be differentiated according to the level showing abnormal responsiveness. In some cases of familial myoclonic epilepsy there is an apparent excessive responsiveness of the cortex which yields exceptionally high voltage responses to peripheral nerve stimulation. Pyramidal tract activity determines the myoclonus. In other patients the abnormality is within the extrapyramidal system, or can be demonstrated at the segmental or spinal level.

Convulsive treatment

The wide employment of convulsive therapy in psychiatry calls for a description of its pathology. In recent years the provocation of convulsions by chemical substances such as pentetrazol and related drugs has been almost universally superseded by electroconvulsive treatment.

Fatalities from both chemical and electroconvulsive treatment have been in the main due to complications, particularly independent disease of the cardiovascular system. This emerges clearly in the review by Maclay (1953) and in the reports of Paarmann and Veltin (1955), Madow (1956), Gaitz, Pokorny and Mills (1956) and Stensrud (1958). A rare complication is fat embolism following bone fracture or mobilization of other fat depots (Meyer and Teare, 1945; Paarman and Veltin, 1955). In electrically induced convulsions death may be due to faulty placing of the electrodes, allowing the current to flow through the hindbrain (Alexander and Löwenbach, 1944). The prior injection of muscle relaxants may in certain circumstances act cumulatively with the anoxia resulting from the convulsions and thus prove dangerous or fatal (Maclay, 1953).

Much discussion and experimental work has been directed to the question whether uncomplicated convulsive therapy, particularly electroconvulsive therapy, causes brain damage. The problem has been reviewed by Alpers (1946), Will, Rehfeldt and Neumann (1948), Corsellis and Meyer (1954), Madow (1956) and most recently and comprehensively by Weiner (1984). These reviewers agree that irreversible damage in uncomplicated cases is improbable. Where experimental conditions approximated to 'therapeutic' dosage, histological findings in the brains of animals were negative. The problem was investigated and comprehensively discussed also by Hartelius (1952), who found significant changes in nerve cells, blood vessels and glia, although by far the greater proportion of these seemed to be reversible. This does not preclude the possibility that occasionally, particularly after a large number of convulsions or after intensive treatment, mild changes of the kind seen after spontaneous convulsions may occur both in human patients and in experimental animals (Ferraro and Roizin, 1949; Corsellis and Meyer, 1954). Such changes may take the form of a marginal gliosis and astrocytic proliferation within the white matter. In a large number of brains of patients who had previously undergone electric shock treatment and had died from intercurrent disease, Ammon's horn sclerosis and lobular sclerosis of the cerebellum were never seen by Meyer (1963). In the literature only one worker, Zeman (1950), observed necrosis in Ammon's horn and the cerebellum, but in the few cases he studied the effect of the convulsions was aggravated by serious complications (endocarditis and pneumonia). Corsellis and Meyer (1954) concluded that the absence of appreciable neuronal loss in Ammon's horn, cerebellum and cerebral cortex was a further indication of the mildness of the sequelae which, rarely, may follow electrically induced convulsions. Measurement of serum myelin basic protein immunoreactivity, which provides a sensitive indication of brain damage following trauma or stroke, shows no change acutely after ECT or during the prolonged course of treatment (Hoyle, Pratt and Thomas, 1984).

A recent computed tomographic study of elderly depressives showed a correlation between frontal lobe atrophy and exposure to ECT (Calloway et al., 1981). An earlier study employing air ventriculography found abnormally large ventricles in 3 out of 8 patients over 60 years of age with schizoaffective illness (Van Boxel et al., 1978). Ventricular enlargement did not correlate with past ECT exposure. Obviously in any given retrospective series a correlation between cortical atrophy and ECT exposure could arise through the use of ECT in the drug-resistant depressive disorders with an organic basis.

The suggestion that ECT can facilitate the onset of epilepsy has not been confirmed in a careful study of the incidence of epilepsy in 166 patients having received ECT (Blackwood et al., 1980).

References

Aguilar, M.J. and Rasmussen, T. (1960) Role of encephalitis in pathogenesis of epilepsy. *Archives of Neurology* **2,** 663–76.

Aicardi, J. and Baraton, J. (1971) A pneumonencephalographic demonstration of brain atrophy following status epilepticus. *Developmental Medicine and Child Neurology* **13,** 660–7.

Aicardi, J. and Chevrie, J.J. (1970) Convulsive status epilepticus in infants and children. A study of 239 cases. *Epilepsia* **11,** 187–97.

Aird, R.B., Venturini, A.M. and Spielman, P.M. (1967) Antecedents of temporal lobe epilepsy. *Archives of Neurology* **16,** 67–73.

Alexander, L.& Löwenbach, H. (1944) Experimental studies on electroshock treatment: the intracerebral vascular reaction as an indicator of the path of the current and the threshold of early changes within the brain tissue. *Journal of Neuropathology and Experimental Neurology* **3,** 139–71.

Alpers, B.J. (1946) The brain changes associated with electrical shock treatment: a critical review. *Digest of Neurology and Psychiatry* **14,** 136–7.

Alzheimer, A. and Vogt, H. (1907) Die Gruppierung der Epilepsie. *Allgemeine Zeitschrift für Psychiatrie* **64,** 418–48.

Alzheimer, A. and Vogt, H. (1907) Die Gruppierung der Epilepsie. *Allgemeine Zeistschrift für Psychiatrie* **64,** 418–48.

Aminoff, M.J. and Simon, R.O. (1980) Status epilepticus. Causes, clinical features and consequences in 98 patients. *American Journal of Medicine* **69,** 657–66.

Anderson, J. (1886) On sensory epilepsy. *Brain* **9,** 385–95.

Annegers, J.F., Hauser, W.A., Anderson, V.E. and Kurland, L.T. (1982). The risks of seizure disorders among relatives of patients with childhood onset epilepsy. *Neurology* **32,** 174–9.

Awa, H., Niiro, M., Gondo, M., Yamamoto, K., Kobayashi, E., Mihara, T. and Asakura, T. (1979) Small ventricles detected by CT-scanning in epileptic patients. *Folia Psychiatrica et Neurologica Japonica* **33,** 297–303.

Babb, T.L., Brown, W.J., Pretorius, J., Davenport, C., Lieb, J.P. and Crandall, P.H. (1984) Hippocampal cell densities in temporal lobe epilepsy. *Epilepsia* (In press).

Bailey, P. and Gibbs, F.A. (1951) Surgical treatment of psychomotor epilepsy. *Journal of the American Medical Association* **145,** 365–70.

Baraitser, M., Gooddy, W., Halliday, A.M., Harding, A.E., Rudge, P. and Scaravilli, F. (1984) Autosomal dominant late onset cerebellar ataxia with myoclonus, peripheral neuropathy and sensorineural deafness: a clinicopathological report. *Journal of Neurology, Neurosurgery and Psychiatry* **47,** 21–5.

Baumann, R.J., Kocoshis, S.A. and Wilson, D. (1983) Lafora disease: liver histopathology in presymptomatic children. *Annals of Neurology* **14,** 86–9.

Ben-Ari, Y., Tremblay, E., Ottersen, O.P. and Meldrum, B.S. (1980) The role of epileptic activity in hippocampal and 'remote' cerebral lesions induced by kainic acid. *Brain Research* **191,** 79–97.

Bengzon, A.R.A., Rasmussen, T., Gloor, R., Dusault, J. and Stephens, M. (1968) Prognostic factors in the surgical treatment of temporal lobe epileptics. Neurology **18,** 717–31.

Bergamasco, B., Benna, P., Ferrero, P. and Gavinelli, R. (1984) Neonatal hypoxia and epileptic risk: a clinical prospective study. *Epilepsia* **25,** 131–6.

Bergener, M. and Gerhard, L. (1970) Myoklonuskörperkrankheit und progressive Myoklonusepilepsie. *Nervenarzt* **41,** 166–73.

Bernardi, S., Trimble, M.R., Frackowiak, R.S.J., Wise, R.J.S. and Jones, T. (1983) An interictal study of partial epilepsy using positron emission tomography and the oxygen-15 inhalation technique. *Journal of Neurology, Neurosurgery and Psychiatry* **46,** 473–7.

Blackwood, D.R.R., Cull, R.E., Freeman, C.P., Evans, J.I. and Mawdsley, C. (1980) A study of the incidence of epilepsy following ECT. *Journal of Neurology, Neurosurgery and Psychiatry* **43,** 1098–102.

Blume, W.T., Girvin, J.P. and Kaufmann, J.C.E. (1982) Childhood brain tumors presenting as chronic uncontrolled focal seizure disorders. *Annals of Neurology* **12,** 538–41.

Bodechtel, G. (1930) Die Topik der Ammonshornschädigung. *Zeitschrift für die gesamte Neurologie und Psychiatrie* **123,** 485–535.

van Bogaert, L. (1949) Sur l'épilepsie myoclonie progressive d'Unverricht-Lundborg; étude d'un cas anatomique et de la semiologie du syndrome amyostatique terminal. *Monatsschrift für Psychiatrie und Neurologie* **118,** 170–91.

Bolender, N-F. and Wyler, A.R. (1982) CT measurements of mesial temporal lobe herniation in epileptics. *Epilepsia* **23,** 409–16.

Bossi, L., Munari, C., Stoffels, C., Bonis, A., Bacia, T., Talairach, J. and Bancaud, J. (1984) Somatomotor manifestations in temporal lobe seizures. *Epilepsia* **25,** 70–6.

Bouchet, C. and Cazauveilh (1825) De l'épilepsie considerée dans ses rapports avec l'aliénation mentale. *Archives Générales de Médecine* **9,** 510–42.

Boudin, G., Pepin, B., Lauras, A., Masson, S. and Barraine, R. (1963) Myoclonies intentionelles persistantes après réanimation cardiaque. *Revue Neurologique* **109,** 468–72.

Bridge, E.M. (1949) *Epilepsy and Convulsive Disorders in Childhood.* McGraw-Hill, New York.

Brierley, J.B., Meldrum, B.S. and Brown, A.W. (1973) The threshold and neuropathology of cerebral 'anoxic-ischaemic' cell change. *Archives of Neurology* **29,** 367–74.

Calloway, S.P., Dolan, R.J., Jacoby, R.J. and Levy, R. (1981) ECT and cerebral atrophy: a computed tomographic study. *Acta Psychiatrica Scandinavica* **64,** 442–5.

Cavanagh, J.B. (1958) On certain small tumours encountered in the temporal lobe. *Brain* **81,** 389–405.

Cavanagh, J.B., Falconer, M.A. and Meyer, A. (1958) Some pathogenic problems of temporal lobe epilepsy. In *Temporal Lobe Epilepsy* (Eds. Baldwin, M. and Bailey, P.), pp. 140–8. Thomas, Springfield.

Chaslin, P. (1889) Note sur l'anatomie pathologique de l'épilepsie dite essentielle—la sclérose nevroglique. *Comptes Rendus des Séances de la Société de Biologie* **1,** 169–71.

Chiofalo, N., Kirschbaum, A., Fuentes, A., Cordero, M.L. and Madsen, J. (1979) Prevalence of epilepsy in children of Melipilla, Chile. *Epilepsia* **20,** 261–6.

Commission on Classification and Terminology of the International League Against Epilepsy (1981) Proposal for revised clinical and electroencephalograh classification of epiletic seizures. *Epilepsia* **22,** 489–501.

Corsellis, J.A.N. (1957) The incidence of Ammon's horn sclerosis. *Brain* **80,** 193–208.

Corsellis, J.A.N. (1970) The neuropathology of temporal lobe epilepsy. In *Modern Trends in Neurology* (Ed. Williams, D.), pp. 254–70. Butterworths, London.

Corsellis, J.A.N. and Bruton, C.J. (1983) Neuropathology of status epilepticus in humans. In *Status Epilepticus: mechanisms of brain damage and treatment.* (Eds. A.V. Delgado-Escueta, A.V., Wasterlain, C.G., Treiman, D. and Porter, R.J.), pp. 129–39. Raven Press, New York.

Corsellis, J.A.N. and Meyer, A. (1954) Histological changes in the brain after uncomplicated ECT. *Journal of Mental Science* **100,** 375–83.

Crome, L. (1955) A morphological critique of temporal lobectomy. *Lancet* **1,** 882–4.

Crome, L. and Stern, J. (1972) *Pathology of Mental Retardation.* Churchill Livingstone, Edinburgh and London.

Curtis, D.R. and Johnston, G.A.R. (1974) Amino acid transmitters in the mammalian central nervous system. *Ergebnisse der Physiologie* **69,** 98–188.

D'Alessandro, R., Tinuper, P., Ferrara, R., Cortelli, P., Pazzaglia, P., Sabattini, L. et al. (1982) CT scan prediction of late post-traumatic epilepsy. *Journal of Neurology, Neurosurgery and Psychiatry* **45,** 1153–5.

Dam, A.M. (1980) Epilepsy and neuron loss in the hippocampus. *Epilepsia* **21,** 617–29.

Dam, A.M. (1982) Hippocampal neuron loss in epilepsy and after experimental seizures. *Acta Neurologica Scandinavica* **66,** 601–42.

Davison, C. and Keschner, M. (1940) Myoclonus epilepsy. *Archives of Neurology and Psychiatry* **43,** 524–46.

DeMoor, J. (1898) Le méchanisme et la signification de l'état moniliforme des neurones. *Annales de la Société Royale des Sciences Médicales et Naturelles de Bruxelles* **7,** 205–50.

Earle, K.M., Baldwin, M. and Penfield, W. (1953) Incisural sclerosis and temporal lobe seizures produced by hippocampal herniation at birth. *Archives of Neurology and Psychiatry* **69,** 27–42.

Edgar, R. and Baldwin, M. (1960) Vascular malformation associated with temporal lobe epilepsy. *Journal of Neurosurgery* **17,** 638–56.

Egdell, H.P. and Stanfield, J.P. (1972) Paediatric neurology in Africa: a Ugandan report. *British Medical Journal* **1,** 548–52.

Eldridge, R., Iivanainen, M., Stern, R., Koerber, T. and Wilder, B.J. (1983) 'Baltic' myoclonus epilepsy: hereditary disorder of childhood made worse by phenytoin. *Lancet* **2,** 838–42.

Engel, J., Brown, W.J., Kuhl, D.E., Phelps, M.E., Mazziotta, J.C. and Crandall, P.H. (1982) Pathological findings underlying focal temporal lobe hypometabolism in partial epilepsy. *Annals of Neurology* **12,** 518–28.

Escobedo, F., Garcia-Ramos, G. and Sotelo, J. (1983) Parasitic disorders and epilepsy. In *Epilepsy: an update on research and therapy* (Eds., Nistico, G., Di Perri, R. and Meinardi, H.), pp. 227–33. Alan R. Liss, New York.

Evans, M., Griffiths, T. and Meldrum, B.S. (1983) Early changes in the rat hippocampus following seizures induced by bicuculline or L-allylglycine: a light and electron microscope study. *Neuropathology and Applied Neurobiology* **9,** 39–52.

Evans, M.C., Griffiths, T. and Meldrum, B.S. (1984). Kainic acid seizures and the reversibility of calcium loading in vulnerable neurons in the hippocampus. *Neuropathology and Applied Neurobiology* **10,** 285–302.

Falconer, M.A. (1974) Mesial temporal (Ammon's horn) sclerosis as a common cause of epilepsy. Aetiology, treatment and prevention. *Lancet* **2,** 767–70.

Falconer, M.A., Driver, M.V. and Serafetinides, E.A. (1962) Temporal lobe epilepsy due to distant lesions: two cases relieved by operation. *Brain* **85,** 521–34.

Falconer, M.A., Serafetinides, E.A. and Corsellis, J.A.N. (1964) Etiology and pathogenesis of temporal lobe epilepsy. *Archives of Neurology* **10,** 233–48.

Farber, J.L. (1981) The role of calcium in cell death. *Life Sciences* **29,** 1289–95.

Fenwick, P.B.C., Master, D. and Brown, D. (1981) Relationship between ventricular volume, cortical atrophy, and epilepsy. In *Advances in Epileptoloty: XIIth Epilepsy International Symposium* (Eds., M. Dam, M., Gram, L. and Penry, J.K.), pp. 483–91. Raven Press, New York.

Ferraro, A. and Roizin, L. (1949) Cerebral morphologic changes in monkeys subjected to a large number of electrically induced convulsions (32–100). *American Journal of Psychiatry* **106,** 278–84.

Fitzsimons, R.B., Clifton-Bligh, P. and Wilfenden, W.H. (1981) Mitochondrial myopathy and lactic acidaemia with myoclonic epilepsy, ataxia and hypothalamic infertility: a variant of Ramsay-Hunt syndrome? *Journal of Neurology, Neurosurgery and Psychiatry* **44,** 79–82.

Flor-Henry, P. (1969) Schizophrenic-like reactions and affective psychoses associated with temporal lobe epilepsy: etiological factors. *American Journal of Psychiatry* **126,** 148–52.

Fowler, M. (1957) Brain damage after febrile convulsions. *Archives of Disease in Childhood* **32,** 67–76.

Frantzen, E. (1971) Round table discussion on febrile convulsions. *Epilepsia* **12,** 191–4.

Gaitz, C.M., Pokorny, A.D. and Mills, M. (1956) Death following electroconvulsive therapy. *Archives of Neurology and Psychiatry* **75,** 493–9.

Gastaut, H. (1956) In *Colloque sur les problèmes d'anatomie normale et pathologique posés par les décharges épileptiques*, pp. 5–20, Editions Acta Medica Belgica, Bruxelles.

Gastaut, H. (1983) A proposed completion of the current international classification of the epilepsies. In *Research Progress in Epilepsy* (Ed. Rose, F.C.), pp. 8–13. Pitman, London.

Gastaut, H. and Gastaut, J.L. (1976) Computerized transverse axial tomography in epilepsy. *Epilepsia* **17,** 325–36.

Gastaut, H., Poirier, H., Salamon, G., Toga, M. and Vigouroux, M. (1960) H.H.E. syndrome. Hemiconvulsions, hemiplegia, epilepsy. *Epilepsia* **1,** 418–47.

Gibbs, F.A., Gibbs, E.L. and Lennox, W.G. (1937) Epilepsy: a paroxysmal cerebral dysrhythmia. *Brain* **60,** 377–88.

Globus, A. and Scheibel, A.B. (1966) Loss of dendritic spines as an index of pre-synaptic terminal patterns. *Nature (London)* **212,** 463–5.

Gloor, P., Olivier, A., Quesney, L.F., Andermann, F. and Horowitz, S. (1982) The role of the limbic system in experiential phenomena of temporal lobe epilepsy. *Annals of Neurology* **12,** 129–44.

Glötzner, F.L. (1973) Membrane properties of neuroglia in epileptogenic gliosis. *Brain Research* **55,** 159–71.

Goodridge, D.M.G. and Shorvon, S.D. (1983) Epileptic seizures in a population of 6000. I. Demography, diagnosis and classification, and role of the hospital services. *British Medical Journal* **287,** 641–4.

Green, J.R. (1967) Temporal lobectomy with special reference to selection of epileptic patients. *Journal of Neurosurgery* **26,** 584–93.

Green, J.R., Duisberg, R.E.H. and McGrath, W.B. (1951) Focal epilepsy of psychomotor type. A preliminary report of observations on effects of surgical therapy. *Journal of Neurosurgery* **8,** 157–72.

Green, J.R. and Scheetz, D.G. (1964) Surgery of epileptogenic lesions of the temporal lobe. *Archives of Neurology* **10,** 135–48.

Greenfield, J.G. (1954) *The Spino-cerebellar Degenerations*. Blackwell Scientific, Oxford.

Griffiths, T., Evans, M.C. and Meldrum, B.S. (1983) Intracellular calcium accumulation in rat hippocampus during seizures induced by bicuculline or L-allylglycine. *Neuroscience* **10,** 385–95.

Griffiths, T., Evans, M.C. and Meldrum, B.S. (1984).

Status epilepticus. The reversibility of calcium loading and acute neuronal pathological changes in the rat hippocampus. *Neuroscience* **12,** 557–67.

Grossman, R.G. and Rosman, L.J. (1971) Intracellular potentials of inexcitable cells in epileptogenic cortex undergoing fibrillary gliosis after a local injury. *Brain Research* **28,** 181–201.

Haberland, C. (1958) Histological studies in temporal lobe epilepsy based on biopsy materials. *Pychiatria et Neurologia* **135,** 12–29.

Hall, J. (1964) A pattern of convulsions in childhood. *West Indian Medical Journal* **13,** 244–8.

Halliday, A.M. (1967) The electrophysiological study of myoclonus in man. *Brain* **90,** 241–84.

Halpern, L.M. (1972) *Experimental Models of Epilepsy. Chronic isolated aggregates of mammalian cerebral cortical neurons studied in situ.* Raven Press, New York.

Haltia, M., Kristensson, K. and Sourander, P. (1969) Neuropathological studies in three Scandinavian cases of progressive myoclonus epilepsy. *Acta Neurologica Scandinavica* **45,** 63–77.

Harriman, D.G.F. and Millar, J.H. (1955) Progressive familial myoclonic epilepsy in three families: its clinical features and pathological basis. *Brain* **78,** 325–49.

Hartelius, U. (1952) Cerebral changes following electrically induced convulsions. An experimental study on cats. *Acta Psychiatrica et Neurologica Scandinavica* suppl. 77, 3–128.

Hauser, W.A. and Kurland, L.T. (1975) The epidemiology of epilepsy in Rochester, Minnesota, 1935 through 1967. *Epilepsia* **16,** 1–66.

Haymaker, W., Pentschew, A., Margoles, C. and Bingham, W.G. (1958) Occurrence of lesions in the temporal lobe in the absence of convulsive seizures. In *Temporal Lobe Epilepsy* (Eds. Baldwin, M. and Bailey, P.), pp. 166–202. Thomas, Springfield.

Hodskins, M.B. and Yakovlev, P.I. (1930) Anatomico-clinical observations on myoclonus in epileptics and on related symptom complexes. *American Journal of Psychiatry* **9,** 827–48.

Horton, R.W. and Meldrum, B.S. (1973) Seizures induced by allylglycine, 3-mercaptopropionic acid and 4-deoxypyridoxine in mice and photosensitive baboons, and different modes of inhibition of cerebral glutamic acid decarboxylase. *British Journal of Pharmacology* **49,** 52–63.

Hoyle, N.R., Pratt, R.T.C. and Thomas, D.G.T. (1984) Effect of electroconvulsive therapy on serum myelin basis protein immunoreactivity. *British Medical Journal* **220,** 1110–11.

Hunt, J.R. (1921) Dyssynergia cerebellaris myoclonica—primary atrophy of the dentate system. *Brain* **44,** 490–538.

Hunter, R.A. (1959) Status epilepticus. History, incidence and problems. *Epilepsia* **1,** 162–88.

Isler, W. (1969) *Akute Hemiplegien und Hemisyndrome im Kindesalter*. Thieme, Stuttgart.

Jackson, H. and Beevor, C.E. (1889) Case of tumour of the right temporo-sphenoidal lobe bearing on the localization of the sense of smell and on the interpretation of a particular variety of epilepsy. *Brain* **12,** 346–57.

Jann-Brown, W. (1973) Structural substrates of seizure foci in the human temporal lobe. *UCLA Forum in Medical Sciences* **17,** 339–74.

Janz, D. (1964) Status epilepticus and frontal lobe lesions. *Journal of the Neurological Sciences* **1,** 446–57.

Janz, D. (1983) Etiology of convulsive status epilepticus. In *Status Epilepticus: mechanisms of brain damage and treatment* (Eds. Delgado-Escueta, A.V., Wasterlain, C.G., Treiman, D.M. and Porter, R.J.), pp. 47–54. Raven Press, New York.

Jasper, H. and Kershaman, J. (1941) Electroencephalographic classification of the epilepsies. *Archives of Neurology and Psychiatry* **45,** 903–43.

Jasper, H., Pertuisset, B. and Flanigin, H. (1951) EEC and cortical electrograms in patients with temporal lobe seizures. *Archives of Neurology and Psychiatry* **65,** 272–90.

Jennett, W.B. (1965) Predicting epilepsy after blunt head injury. *British Medical Journal* **1,** 1215–16.

Jennett, W.B. (1969) Early traumatic epilepsy. *Lancet* **1,** 1023–5.

Jennett, W.B. and Lewin, W. (1960) Traumatic epilepsy after closed head injury. *Journal of Neurology, Neurosurgery and Psychiatry* **23,** 295–301.

Jennett, B., Miller, J.D. and Braakman, R. (1974) Epilepsy after non-missile depressed skull fracture. *Journal of Neurosurgery* **41,** 108–216.

Juul-Jensen P. and Foldspang, A. (1983) Natural history of epileptic seizures. *Epilepsia* **24,** 297–312.

Ketz, E. (1974) Brain tumours and epilepsy. In *Handbook of Clinical Neurology*, vol. 16 (Eds. Vinken, P.J. and Bruyn, G.W.), pp. 254–69. North-Holland, Amsterdam.

Kirstein, L. (1942) Epilepsie bei intrakraniellen expansiven Processen. *Acta Medica Scandinavica* **110,** 56–68.

Koskiniemi, M. (1975) Findings in routine laboratory examination in progressive myoclonus epilepsy. *Acta Neurologica Scandinavica* **51,** 12–20.

Koskiniemi, M., Donner, M., Majuri, H., Haltia, M. and Norio, R. (1974) Progressive myoclonus epilepsy. A clinical and histopathological study. *Acta Neurologica Scandinavica* **50,** 307–32.

Kraus-Reppert, R. (1969) Zur Frage der idiopathischen Randzonensiderose (Rosenthal) im Tierversuch. *Zentralblatt fur die allgemeine Pathologie* **112,** 332–4.

Lafora, G.R. and Glück, B. (1911) Beitrag zur Kenntnis der Alzheimerschen Krankheit oder präsenilen

Demenz mit Herdsymptomen. *Zeitschrift für die gesamte Neurologie und Pyschiatrie* **6,** 120.

Lance, J.W. and Adams, R.D. (1963) The syndrome of intention or action myoclonus as a sequel to hypoxic encephalopathy. *Brain* **86,** 111-36.

Legg, N.J., Gupta, P.C. and Scott, D.F. (1973) Epilepsy following cerebral abscess—a clinical and EEG study of 70 patients. *Brain* **96,** 259-68.

Lennox-Buchthal, M.A. (1973) *Febrile Convulsions.* Elsevier, Amsterdam.

Lessell, S., Torres, J.M. and Kurland, L.T. (1962) Seizure disorders in a Guanamanian village. *Archives of Neurology* **7,** 37-44.

Lhermitte, F., Marteau, R. and Degos, C.F. (1972) Analyse pharmacologique d'un nouveau cas de myoclonies d'intention et d'action post-anoxiques. *Revue Neurologique* **126,** 107-14.

Liddell, D.W. (1953) Observations on epileptic automatism in a mental hospital population. *Journal of Mental Science* **99,** 732-48.

Lindenberg, R. (1955) Compression of brain arteries as pathogenetic factor for tissue necroses and their areas of predilection. *Journal of Neuropathology and Experimental Neurology* **14,** 223-43.

Louis-Bar, D. and van Bogaert, L. (1947) Sur la dyssynergie cérébelleuse myoclonique (Hunt). *Monatsschrift für Psychiatrie und Neurologie* **113,** 215-47.

Lund, M. (1952) Epilepsy in association with intracranial tumour. *Acta Psychiatrica et Neurologica Scandinavica* suppl. 81, 3-149.

Lundborg, H. (1903) *Die Progressive Myoklonus-Epilepsie* (*Unverricht's Myoklonie*). Almquist and Wiksell, Uppsala.

McGahan, J.P., Dulbin, A.B. and Hill, R.P. (1979) The evaluation of seizure disorders by computerized tomography. *Journal of Neurosurgery* **50,** 328-32.

Maclay, W.S. (1953) Death due to treatment. *Proceedings of the Royal Society of Medicine* **46,** 13-20.

McMenemey, W.H. (1940) Alzheimer's disease. *Journal of Neurology and Psychiatry* **3,** 211-40.

Madow, L. (1956) Brain changes in electro-shock therapy. *American Journal of Psychiatry* **113,** 337-47.

Margerison, J.H. and Corsellis, J.A.N. (1966) Epilepsy and the temporal lobes. A clinical, electroencephalographic and neuropathological study of the brain in epilepsy, with particular reference to the temporal lobes. *Brain* **89,** 499-530.

Margerison, J.H. and Liddell, D.W. (1961) The incidence of temporal lobe epilepsy among a hospital population of long-stay female epileptics. *Journal of Mental Science* **107,** 909-20.

Matthews, W.B., Howell, D.A. and Stevens, D.L. (1969) Progressive myoclonus epilepsy without Lafora bodies. *Journal of Neurology, Neurosurgery and Psychiatry* **32,** 116-22.

May, D.L. and White, H.H. (1968) Familial myoclonus, cerebellar ataxia and deafness. Specific genetically determined disease. *Archives of Neurology* **19,** 331-8.

McKusick, R. (1983) *Mendelian Inheritance in Man*, 6th edn. Heinemann Medical, London.

Meenke, H.J. and Janz. D. (1984) Neuropathological findings in primary generalized epilepsy: a study of eight cases. *Epilepsia* **25,** 8-21.

Meldrum, B.S. (1982) Pathophysiology. In *Textbook of Epilepsy*, 2nd edn (Eds. Laidlaw, J. and Richens, A.), pp. 456-87. Churchill Livingstone, Edinburgh.

Meldrum, B.S. (1983). Metabolic factors during prolonged seizures and their relation to nerve cell death. In *Advances in Neurology*, vol. 34, *Status Epilepticus: Mechanism of Brain and Treatment* (Eds. A.V. Delgado-Escueta, C.G., Wasterlain, D.M. Treiman and Porter, R.J.), pp. 261-75. Raven Press, New York.

Meldrum, B.S. and Brierley, J.B. (1972) Neuronal loss and gliosis in the hippocampus following repetitive epileptic seizures induced in adolescent baboons by allylglycine. *Brain Research* **48,** 361-5.

Meldrum, B.S. and Brierley, J.B. (1973) Prolonged epileptic seizures in primates: ischaemic cell change and its relation to ictal physiological events. *Archives of Neurology* **28,** 10-17.

Meldrum, B.S. and Horton, R.W. (1973) Physiology of status epilepticus in primates. *Archives of Neurology* **28,** 1-9.

Meldrum, B.S., Horton, R.W. and Brierley, J.B. (1974) Epileptic brain damage in adolescent baboons following seizures induced by allylglycine. *Brain* **97,** 407-18.

Meldrum, B.S., Vigouroux, R.A. and Brierley, J.B. (1973) Systemic factors and epileptic brain damage. *Archives of Neurology* **29,** 82-7.

Menini, C., Meldrum, B.S., Riche, D., Silva-Comte, C. and Stutzmann, J.M. (1980). Sustained limbic seizures induced by intraamygdaloid kainic acid in the baboon: symptomatology and neuropathological consequences. *Annals of Neurology* **8,** 501-9.

Metrakos, K. and Metrakos, J.D. (1974) Genetics of epilepsy. In *Handbook of Clinical Neurology*, vol. 15 (Eds. Vinken, P.J. and Bruyn, G.W.), pp. 429-39. North-Holland Amsterdam.

Meyer, A. (1963) Epilepsy. In *Greenfield's Neuropathology*, 2nd edn. Edward Arnold, London.

Meyer, A. and Beck, E. (1955) Hippocampal formation in temporal lobe epilepsy. *Proceedings of the Royal Society of Medicine* **48,** 457-62.

Meyer, A., Beck, E. and Shepherd, M. (1955) Unusually severe lesions in the brain following status epilepticus. *Journal of Neurology and Psychiatry* **18,** 24-33.

Meyer, A., Falconer, M.A. and Beck, E. (1954) Pathological findings in temporal lobe epilepsy. *Journal of Neurology and Psychiatry* **17,** 276–85.

Meyer, A. and Teare, D. (1945) Cerebral fat embolism after electric convulsion therapy. *British Medical Journal* **2,** 42–4.

Millichap, J.G. (1968) *Febrile Convulsions.* Macmillan, New York.

Millichap, J.G. (1974) Metabolic and endocrine factors. In *Handbook of Clinical Neurology*, vol. 15. (Eds. Vinken, P.J. and Bruyn, G.W.), pp. 311–24. North-Holland, Amsterdam.

Morel, F. and Wildi, E. (1956) Sclérose ammonienne et épilepsies (Étude anatomopathologique et statistique). *Acta Neurologica Belgica* **2,** 61–74.

Morris, A.A. (1956) Temporal lobectomy with removal of uncus, hippocampus and amygdala. *Archives of Neurology and Psychiatry* **76,** 479–96.

Muskens, L.J.J. (1909) Regional and myclonic convulsions. *Epilepsia* **1,** 161–78.

Newmark, M.E. and Penry, J.K. (1979) *Genetics of Epilepsy: a review*, pp. 1–130. Raven Press, New York.

Noel, P., Cornil, A., Chailly, P. and Flament-Durand, J. (1977) Mesial temporal haemorrhage; consequence of status epilepticus. *Journal of Neurology, Neurosurgery and Psychiatry* **40,** 932–5.

Norman, R.M. (1964) The neuropathology of status epilepticus. *Medicine, Science and the Law* **4,** 46–51.

Olney, J.W., Fuller T. and de Gubareff, T. (1979) Acute dendrotoxic changes in the hippocampus of kainate treated rats. *Brain Research* **176,** 91–100.

Olney, J.W., Fuller, T.A., Collins, R.C. and de Gubareff, T. (1980) Systemic dipiperidinoethane mimics the convulsant and neurotoxic actions of kainic acid. *Brain Research* **200,** 231–5.

Ostertag, B. (1925) Zur Histopathologie der Myoklonusepilepsie (Eine weitere Studie über die intragangliocellulären, corpusculären Einlagerungen). *Archiv für Psychiatrie und Nervenkrankheiten* **73,** 633–56.

Ounsted, C., Lindsay, J. and Norman, R. (1966) *Biological Factors in Temporal Lobe Epilepsy.* Clinics in Developmental Medicine, 22. Heinemann Medical, London.

Oxbury, J.M. and Whitty, C.W.M. (1971) Causes and consequences of status epilepticus in adults. A study of 86 cases. *Brain* **94,** 733–44.

Paarmann, H.F. and Veltin, A. (1955) Zur Frage tödlicher Komplikationen nach Elektroschock (Bericht über 3 Beobachtungen). *Nervenarzt* **26,** 106–11.

Peiffer, J. (1963) *Morphologische Aspekte der Epilepsien.* Springer, Berlin.

Penfield, W., Erickson, T.C. and Tarlov, J. (1940) Relation of intracranial tumors and symptomatic epilepsy. *Archives of Neurology and Psychiatry* **44,** 300–15.

Penfield, W. and Flanigin, H. (1950) Surgical therapy of temporal lobe seizures. *Archives of Neurology and Psychiatry* **64,** 491–500.

Perot, P., Weir, B. and Rasmussen, T. (1966) Tuberous sclerosis. *Archives of Neurology* **15,** 498–506.

Peterman, M.G. (1950) Febrile convulsions in children. *Journal of the American Medical Association* **143,** 728–30.

Peterman, M.G. (1952) Febrile convulsions. *Journal of Pediatrics* **41,** 536–40.

Pfleger, L. (1880) Beobachtungen über Schrumpfung und Sklerose des Ammonshorns bei Epilepsie. *Allgemeine Zeitschrift für Psychiatre* **36,** 359–65.

Radermecker, J. (1974) Epilepsy in the degenerative diseases. In *Handbook of Clinical Neurology*, vol. 15 (Eds. Vinken, P.J. and Bruyn, G.W.), pp. 325–72. North-Holland, Amsterdam.

Ribak, C.E. (1983) Morphological, biochemical and immunocytochemical changes of the cortical GABAergic system in epileptic foci. In *Epilepsy* (Eds. Ward, A.A., Penry, J.K. and Purpura, D.), pp. 109–30. Raven Press, New York.

Ribak, C.E., Bradburne, R.M. and Harris, A.G. (1982) A preferential loss of GABAergic inhibitory synapses in epileptic foci: a quantitative ultrastructural analysis of monkey neocortex. *Journal of Neuroscience* **2,** 1725–35.

Richardson, E.P., Dodge, P.R. and Victor, M. (1954) Recurrent convulsive seizures as a sequel to cerebral infarction: a clinical and pathological study. *Brain* **77,** 610–38.

Rose, A.L. and Lombroso, C.T. (1970) Neonatal seizure states. *Pediatrics* **45,** 404–25.

Russell, W.R. and Whitty, C.W.M. (1952) Studies in traumatic epilepsy. I. Factors influencing the incidence of epilepsy after brain wounds. *Journal of Neurology, Neurosurgery and Psychiatry* **15,** 93–8.

Sano, K. and Malamud, N. (1953) Clinical significance of sclerosis of the cornu ammonis. *Archives of Neurology and Psychiatry* **70,** 40–53.

Scheibel, M.E., Crandall, P.H. and Scheibel, A.B. (1974) The hippocampal-dentate complex in temporal lobe epilepsy. *Epilepsia* **15,** 55–80.

Scheibel, M.E. and Scheibel, A.B. (1973) Hippocampal pathology in temporal lobe epilepsy. A Golgi survey. *UCLA Forum in Medical Sciences* **17,** 311–37.

Schneider, R.C., Crosby, E.C. and Farhat, S.M. (1965) Extratemporal lesions triggering the temporal lobe syndrome. The role of association bundles. *Journal of Neurosurgery* **22,** 246–63.

Scholz, W. (1951) *Die Krampfschädigungen des Gehirns.* Springer, Berlin.

Scholz, W. (1959) The contribution of patho-anatomical research to the problem of epilepsy. *Epilepsia* **1,** 36–55.

Seitelberger, F. (1968) Myoclonus body disease. In *Pathology of the Nervous System*, vol. 1 (Ed. Minckler, J.), pp. 1121–34. McGraw-Hill, New York.

Seitelberger, F., Jacob, J., Peiffer, J.J. and Colmant, H.T. (1964) Die Myoklonuskörperkrankheit. Eine angeborene Störung des Kohlenhydratstoffwechsels. Klinisch-pathologische Studie an fünf Fällen. *Fortschritte der Neurologie und Psychiatrie* **32,** 305–45.

Serafetinides, E.A. and Dominian, J. (1963) A follow-up study of late-onset epilepsy. I. Neurological findings. *British Medical Journal* **1,** 428–31.

Sherwin, I. (1981) Psychosis associated with epilepsy: significance of the laterality of the epileptogenic lesion. *Journal of Neurology, Neurosurgery and Psychiatry* **44,** 83–5.

Sloper, J.J., Johnson, P. and Powell, T.P.S. (1980) Selective degeneration of interneurons in the motor cortex of infant monkeys following controlled hypoxia: a possible cause of epilepsy. *Brain Research* **198,** 204–9.

Sloviter, R.S. (1983) Epileptic brain damage in rats induced by electrical stimulation of the perforant path. 1. Acute electrophysiological and light microscopic studies. *Brain Research Bulletin* **10,** 675–97.

Sommer, W. (1880) Erkrankung des Ammonshornes als aetiologisches Moment der Epilepsie. *Archiv für Psychiatrie und Nervenkrankheiten* **10,** 631–75.

Spielmeyer, W. (1927) Die Pathogenese des epileptischen Krampfes. *Zeitschrift für die gesamte Neurologie und Psychiatrie* **109,** 501–20.

Stauder, K.H. (1935) Epilepsie und Schläfenlappen. *Archiv für Psychiatrie und Nervenkrankheiten* **104,** 181–211.

Stensrud, P.A. (1958) Cerebral complications following 24,562 convulsion treatments in 893 patients. *Acta Psychiatrica Scandinavica* **33,** 115–26.

Taylor, D.C. (1975) Factors influencing the occurrence of schizophrenia-like psychosis in patients with temporal lobe epilepsy. *Psychological Medicine* **5,** 249–54.

Taylor, D.C., Falconer, M.A. Bruton, C.J. and Corsellis, J.A.N. (1971) Focal dysplasia of the cerebral cortex in epilepsy. *Journal of Neurology, Neurosurgery and Psychiatry* **34,** 369–87.

Turner, D.A. and Wyler, A.R. (1981) Temporal lobectomy for epilepsy: mesial temporal herniation as an operative and prognostic finding. *Epilepsia* **22,** 623–9.

Turski, W.A., Cavalheiro, E.A., Schwarz, M., Czuczwar, S.J., Kleinrok, Z. and Turski, L. (1983) Limbic seizures produced by pilocarpine in rats. A behavioral, electroenecephalographic and neuropathological study. *Behavioral Brain Research* **9,** 315–35.

Turski, W.A., Cavalheiro, E.A., Calderazzo-Filho, L.S., Kleinroh Z., Czuczwar, S.J. and Turski, L. (1984) Injections of picrotoxin and bicuculline into the amygdaloid complex of the rat: an electroencephalographic, behavioural and morphological analysis. *Neuroscience* in press.

Unverricht, H. (1891) *Die Myoklonie.* Deuticke, Leipzig and Vienna.

Van Boxel, P., Bridges, P.K., Bartlett, J.R. and Trauer, T. (1978) Size of cerebral ventricles in 66 psychiatric patients. *British Journal of Psychiatry* **133,** 500–6.

Vaquero, J., Oya, S., Cabezudo, J.M. and Bravo, G. (1982) Morphological study of human epileptic dendrites. *Neurosurgery* **10,** 720–4.

Veith, G. (1970) Anatomische Studie über die Ammonshornsklerose im Epileptikergehirn. *Deutsche Zeitschrift für Nervenheilkunde* **197,** 293–314.

Wallace, S.J. (1972) Aetiological aspects of febrile convulsions. Pregnancy and perinatal factors. *Archives of Disease in Childhood* **47,** 171–8.

Wallace, S.J. and Zealley, H. (1970) Neurological, electroencephalographic and virological findings in febrile children. *Archives of Disease in Childhood* **45,** 611–23.

Walton, J.N. (1977) *Brain's Diseases of the Nervous System*, 8th edn, pp. 1095–6. Oxford University Press, Oxford.

Ward, A.A. (1969) The epileptic neuron: chronic foci in animals and man. In *Basic Mechanisms of the Epilepsies* (Eds. Jasper, H.H., Ward, A.A. and Pope, A.), pp. 263–88. Little, Brown, Boston.

Weiner, R.D. (1984) Does electroconvulsive therapy cause brain damage? *Behavioral and Brain Sciences* **7,** 1–54.

Werman, R., Davidoff, R.A. and Aprison, M.H. (1968) Inhibitory action of glycine on spinal neurons in the cat. *Journal of Neurophysiology* **31,** 81–95.

Westphal, A. and Sioli, F. (1921) Weitere Mitteilung über den durch eigenartige einschliessende Ganglienzellen (Corpora amylacea) ausgezeichneten Fall von Myoklonusepilepsie. *Archiv für Psychiatrie und Nervenkrankheiten* **63,** 1–36.

Westrum, L.E., White, L.E. and Ward, A.A. (1965) Morphology of the experimental epileptic focus. Journal of Neurosurgery **21,** 1033–46.

Whitty, C.W.M. (1961) Focal epilepsy and the study of cortical function. *Medical Journal of Australia* **1,** 1–8.

Wieser, H.G. (1983) Depth recorded limbic seizures and psychopathology. *Neuroscience and Biobehavioral Reviews* **7,** 427–40.

Will, O.A., Rehfeldt, F.C. and Neumann, M.A. (1948) A fatality in electroshock therapy. *Journal of Nervous and Mental Disease* **107,** 105–26.

Young, A.C., Costanzi, J.B., Mohr, P.D. and Forbes, W.StC. (1982) Is routine computerized axial tomography in epilepsy worth while? *Lancet* **2,** 1446–7.

Zeman, W. (1950) Zur Frage der Hirngewebeschädigung durch Heilkrampfbehandlung. *Archiv für Psychiatrie und Nervenkrankheiten* **184,** 440–57.

Zimmerman, H.M. (1938) Histopathology of convulsive disorders in children. *Journal of Pediatrics* **13,** 859–90.

Zuckermann, E.C. and Glaser, G.H. (1970) Slow potential shifts in dorsal hippocampus during 'epileptogenic' perfusion of the inferior horn with high-potassium CSF. *Electroencephalography and Clinical Neurophysiology* **18,** 236–46.

20

Ageing and the dementias

B.E. Tomlinson and J.A.N. Corsellis

Dementia

Dementia has been recognized for many years, but it has never been easy to define. Late in the seventeenth century the physician William Salmon wrote of 'defects of the imagination, reason and memory in a man superannuated' whom he aptly described as 'decayed in his intellectuals' (Hollander, 1974). Esquirol in 1838 saw the dement as 'a man deprived of possessions that he once enjoyed, he is a rich man becoming poor'. More recently, and with more precision, Lishman (1978) has epitomized the syndrome 'as an acquired global impairment of intellect, reason and personality but without impairment of consciousness'.

Already in the 1840s Webster had made careful observations on patients with this clinical pattern of deterioration, and the main features of 'general paralysis of the insane' began to be delineated at much the same time (Hare, 1959). Improvements in microscopy near the turn of the century led to more detailed analysis of the various neurohistological abnormalities which were being identified. Alzheimer in 1898 confirmed Virchow's insistence on the general importance of vascular degeneration by demonstrating its relevance to the brain in the insanities of the aged. Within the next few years the histological basis of Pick's lobar atrophy and Huntington's chorea, as well as cerebral arteriosclerosis and the senile form of cerebral degeneration, were established under Alzheimer's influence. All these conditions were associated with dementia and all tended to develop in middle or later life. General paralysis of the insane proved to be the result of an infection but the others came to be linked through age to the process of senile involution, an association which was strengthened by the demonstration of neurohistological stigmata, such as the senile plaque and the neurofibrillary tangle, both of which occurred to a degree in 'normal' ageing but became particularly prominent in certain diseases.

These observations fitted in with Gowers' (1902) hypothesis that in some people a premature degeneration, or ageing, of tissue took place which was particularly liable to affect the nervous system. This concept of heredodegenerative disease has proved immensely valuable in unravelling the various genetic and enzymic deviations which lie at the root of many disorders in the nervous system.

The pattern of the degenerative process, however, varies according to the condition. In some, such as the presenile or senile forms of Alzheimer's disease, it tends to be diffuse; in others, such as Huntington's chorea or Pick's disease, the brunt of the pathological process falls on defined areas and pathways. The reasons why certain components of nervous tissue are more vulnerable than others in one condition and not in another remain unknown; some, however, are beginning to be identified. Thus the pigmented cells in the substantia nigra degenerate in idopathic parkinsonism for no known reason and yet the same cells may also be vulnerable following a viral infection and even as a result of repeated cerebral trauma. Kuru, which on clinical and on histological grounds, could well be, and indeed at one time was, placed in the heredodegenerative category, is now established as a transmissible illness. The same is equally true of the Creutzfeldt–Jakob form of presenile or senile dementia which has now many times been passaged to animals.

This fundamental discovery that hitherto unrecognized kinds of transmissible agent could lead to a cerebral disorder such as Creutzfeldt–Jakob disease, in which there is no evidence of an inflammatory reaction, has inevitably led to the intensive investigation of many other chronic diseases of the nervous system in the, as yet unfulfilled, hope that other bizarre forms of virus or transmissible agent might be found to be responsible.

Again, increasing efforts are now going into the search for biochemical defects in a similarly wide range of illnesses—an activity which was stimulated initially by the discovery that the degeneration of dopaminergic neurons in the substantia nigra could lead to reduced levels of dopamine in the corpus striatum and, because of this, that patients with Parkinson's disease could respond dramatically to treatment with dopamine.

Knowledge, therefore, is now increasing so rapidly in virology and chemistry, particularly when combined with genetics, that the treatment and even the prevention of the commoner dementing disorders of adult life may eventually become possible. For example, defects in the cholinergic pathways in the Alzheimer type of dementia have been identified, even if attempts to replace the missing substance by giving large doses of acetylcholine have not emulated the success of the dopamine story.

The causes of dementia and their prevalence

Although there are exceptions, dementia is commonly held to be the result of a more or less extensive destruction or disorganization of the cerebral cortex and its connections by one or other pathological process. Both the concomitant neurological picture and the salient clinical features of the dementia may, however, be influenced by the nature of the process, by the speed with which it develops and the extent to which the tissue damage is localized.

The common conditions in which dementia is most liable to occur at the present time are the two degenerative processes which tend to affect the brain in later life. In the first, the cerebral tissue generally, but particularly the cerebral grey matter, is liable to disintegrate more or less diffusely; the various parenchymatous changes involved in it are usually considered together as the 'senile form of cerebral degeneration'. In the second, it is the blood vessels which degenerate and, as the brain loses its blood supply, softening and the destruction of tissue, particularly in the area supplied by the affected vessel, will follow.

The age at which both the senile and the vascular forms begin to appear varies considerably, and, as with other rarer conditions, both young and old may be affected. Nevertheless, as a general rule, the prevalence of both increases rapidly after the 60s have been reached and there seems little justification for imposing an arbitary age of 65 years in order to separate the presenile from the senile period of life, particularly when the pathological changes in the two periods remain essentially the same. This is specially relevant to the so-called 'senile' degenerative process, which, when presenting clinically in the pre-senile period, used to be known as 'Alzheimer's disease' but became transformed into 'senile dementia' if the onset was after the age of 65 years. For this reason, it is now usual to fuse the two into senile dementia of the Alzheimer type (SDAT) or even merely to refer to the whole gamut as Alzheimer's disease.

It is as well to emphasize that both the Alzheimer and the vascular forms of degeneration may be found in the same brain although one or other is usually dominant, the Alzheimer type often occurring in the presence of negligible vascular degeneration while the converse is also true at times, particularly in the less elderly in whom the emphasis may be entirely on the vascular side.

It is now generally recognized that the most important single neuropathological cause of dementia at any adult age is the Alzheimer type of degeneration. This is indicated in Table 20.1, which outlines the results of a study by Marsden and Harrison (1972) on 84 patients, all of whom had been established, on clinical grounds, as examples of presenile dementia. The largest group, 48 in number, were attributed to cerebral atrophy, the cause of which was unknown

Table 20.1 Causes of dementia in adults

Intracranial space-occupying mass	8
Arteriosclerotic dementia	8
Dementia in alcoholics	6
Possible normal pressure communicating hydrocephalus	5
Creutzfeldt–Jakob disease	3
Huntington's chorea	3
Post-traumatic cerebral atrophy	1
Postsubarachnoid haemorrhage	1
Limbic encephalitis	1
Cerebral atrophy of unknown cause	48

because no biopsies were taken. Nevertheless, as Marsden and Harrison suggested, the great majority were in all probability suffering from Alzheimer's disease, particularly as several earlier comparable studies, in which biopsies had been performed, found a high proportion of the cases to have been of the Alzheimer type (Sim, Turner and Smith, 1966; Coblenz et al., 1973).

Clinicopathological studies of older patients dementing during the senile period have shown the same trend for Alzheimer's disease to be the commonest pathological diagnosis, followed in second place by one or other variant of cerebrovascular change, now often combined under the title of arteriosclerotic or multi-infarct dementia. Autopsy studies by Tomlinson, Blessed and Roth (1970) on dementia in old age demonstrated that about 50 per cent of the cases showed the features of Alzheimer's disease in a pure form; in 15 per cent extensive evidence of cerebral softening was the only major pathological lesion to be found; and in about 10 per cent the two degenerative processes were combined. In a further 15 per cent the senile changes were present to an extent which fell short of that on which to base a firm diagnosis and yet, particularly when accompanied by cerebral softenings, they were the only lesions to which the dementia could reasonably have been attributed. In about 4 per cent specific abnormalities such as Pick's disease or a tumour were found whilst no adequate morphological basis for dementia was found in the remaining 6 per cent. Jellinger (1976a) reported on a larger group of patients which included those dying over the age of 55 years and therefore spread into both the presenile and senile periods. Nevertheless, dementia of the Alzheimer type accounted for just over half the cases, whilst nearly a quarter belonged to the vascular group; the two disorders were combined in 13 per cent. Cerebral tumours, Pick's disease and other rarer conditions accounted for the remaining 12 per cent. Even among the elderly, however, the incidence of the different conditions is bound to vary with the kind of clinic or hospital in which the investigations are carried out. For example, patients in a neurological unit who are suspected of dementia will tend inevitably to be suffering from a greater variety of conditions such as a tumour or hydrocephalus, or from an extreme rarity such as Creutzfeldt–Jakob disease, than will those in serial post-mortem studies carried out in a long-stay psychiatric or geriatric hospital. Nevertheless, as already noted, the conditions which commonly lead to dementia are the vascular and the senile degenerative processes. Neither poses great diagnostic difficulty when one is present in the absence of the other, but when both occur together the assessment may be more difficult. Corsellis (1962) and many others, including Tomlinson, Blessed and Roth (1970), have all found that in about 15 per cent of cases the combined lesions of Alzheimer's disease and cerebral infarction have occurred together to an extent which requires them to be seen as cases of dementia due to mixed senile and vascular changes. The relative weight to put on each category of change can be no more than speculative unless both are present to a roughly equal degree of severity. It should be remembered, moreover, that small infarcts, particularly within the basal ganglia, can be found in some 60 per cent of intellectually normal people (Tomlinson, Blessed and Roth, 1968) so that a few such softenings in the striatum or in the thalamus, in the presence of extensive evidence of Alzheimer's disease, does not justify invoking the vascular component. In retrospect, it may well be that laying too much emphasis on such vascular changes could account for the higher incidence of arteriosclerotic disease recorded in the earlier studies on dementia, such as those by Rothschild (1942). Taking both the senile and the vascular degeneration together these two conditions account for between 75 and 95 per cent of cases of dementia over the age of 65. Moreover, in elderly women senile dementia of the Alzheimer type predominates over the vascular form to the extent that it alone accounts for around 80 per cent. Indeed, Escourolle and Poirier (1973) regarded Alzheimer's disease as responsible for 80 per cent of all cases of dementia in old age, an observation which may well reflect the fact that far fewer demented men, who in any case seem more prone to vascular disease than demented women, survive into the 80s for most have died before the 90s are reached. The Alzheimer type of cerebral degeneration is therefore now generally accepted as the most important single cause of dementia in western Europe and beyond. Consequently, as more and more people survive into old, and very old, age the concomitant spread of this devastating condition lays an ever-increasing burden on hospital services and has aptly come to be called the 'silent epidemic'.

Diagnosis of dementia

Dementia may develop at any time during adult life, or even in childhood. Many disorders can lead to it; Slaby and Wyatt (1974) and Tomlinson (1980) have listed the most important, the latter author showing the distribution of the common conditions according to the emphasis of damage within the cerebral hemispheres.

Dementia, however, does not always imply structural changes in the brain. As a rare example, a person with myxoedema may gradually become demented, and may die if the illness is not treated and yet the structure of the brain may appear no different from that of others who have died with a sound mind at a similar age. The same problem, moreover, may arise whenever disease outside the nervous system so disturbs the normal activity of the brain that the patient appears, at least for a time, to be demented even though the cerebral structure has remained histologically intact. Thus a person dying after an acute, or even a more lasting, confusional state, may be found to have no destructive cerebral changes. The position is further complicated by the ever-present risk of a primarily psychological disorder imitating an organic one for it is only in the last few decades that a diagnosis of dementia has been effectively separated from other psychiatric disorders of the same period (Roth and Morrisey, 1952). Thus depressive and schizophrenic illnesses, although not uncommon throughout adult life, continue on as a major problem into old age. In particular, the profound depression of an elderly person may be impossible to distinguish from someone who is irretrievably demented as a consequence of cerebral degeneration (Post, 1965). Another complicating factor is the increasing likelihood, as age advances, of a degree of vascular or other degenerative change and it then becomes difficult even to hazard the extent to which the clinical picture is the result of organic rather than psychological factors. This can be an important distinction because the less severe the cerebral degeneration the longer is the patient likely to survive.

Finally, individuals faced with organic disease either of the body or of the brain vary greatly in their liability to develop clinical evidence of this, and the disorganization of cerebral tissue can seemingly be far advanced in some people before an effect on the intellect or on behaviour becomes apparent. The converse is also true at times and, although extreme discordance between clinical and pathological observations on the brain is exceptional, too precise a connection between the two is scarcely to be expected, at least until more subtle methods both of psychological and of pathological measurement are established.

The brain in ageing

Changes in brain size during adult life The weight and the volume of the brain usually reach their highest figures in the early teens and little of either is lost for the first five or six decades; some evidence exists that atrophy begins earlier in women than men (Hatazawa et al., 1982; Hubbard and Anderson, 1983). Davis and Wright (1977) have found that the ratio of skull to brain volume remains at about 93 per cent until middle age, and falls only slightly in the 60s. From then on, however, in intellectually normal people, although the variation is considerable, the ratio between the seventh and tenth decades may fall to around 80 per cent.

Davis and Wright (1977) took no account of changing ventricular volume but there is evidence that this increases slowly until the 60s and then more dramatically in many, although not all, subjects after the seventh decade (Barron, Jacobs and Kinkel, 1976; Hubbard and Anderson, 1981a). Morel and Wildi (1955) found that the ventricular system in men is slightly larger than in women, whilst it was shown many years ago that the left lateral ventricle in both sexes tends to be slightly larger than the right. Miller, Alston and Corsellis (1980), working on fixed brains and using an image analysing system, have found that although the cerebral hemispheres consisted of roughly equal amounts of grey and white matter any loss through adult life tended to be slightly greater in the latter. Hubbard and Anderson (1981b) have further defined the reduction in volume of cerebral grey and white matter in old age.

The reduction in the size of the brain fits well with the long-known fact that brain weight tends to start its decline in middle life or even earlier. It should be accepted, though, that the weighing is rarely accurate and, like volume, the figures should be looked on as no more than a useful pointer to abnormality unless the deviation is extreme. As Cobb (1965) put it, ‘only very small brains are inadequate and very large brains have no advantage over medium-sized ones’. Indeed,

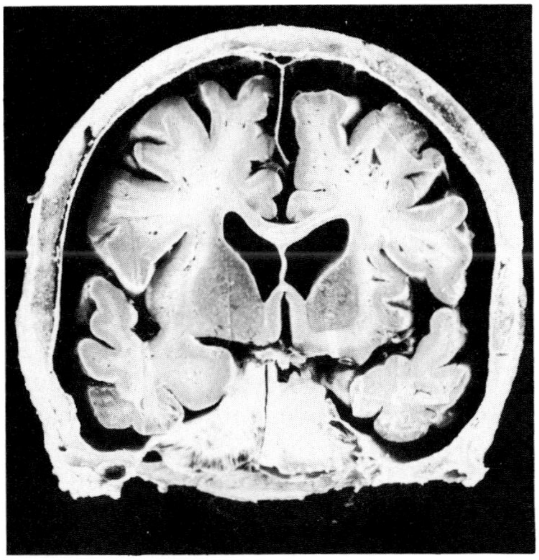

Fig. 20.1 A coronal cut through the skull and brain, showing the marked loss of cerebral tissue that occurs in the presence of atrophy.

too large or 'macrocephalic' a brain is often associated with mental retardation and epilepsy. Both weight and volume normally change noticeably during fixation in 10% formalin, an increase in weight and in volume of about 10 per cent being usual after a few weeks. In the present context the weight of the brain of a normal young adult male may be taken as 1400 g, and this may in later life drop to the 1200–1300 g level. The average female brain weight is roughly 100 g lower throughout adult life. Further details and references are included in Chapter 1.

In contrast, the brain often becomes considerably smaller in the dementias of old age. The hemispheres shrink away from the skull and the loss of tissue becomes obvious (Fig. 20.1). As a reflection of this loss, which affects both grey and white matter, the sulci (Fig. 20.2) and the ventricles (Fig. 20.3) tend to enlarge. As with all other changes linked to age, however, individual variations are considerable.

These gross alterations are reflected in the histological picture and they are most clearly seen in the severer degrees of cortical atrophy. In this

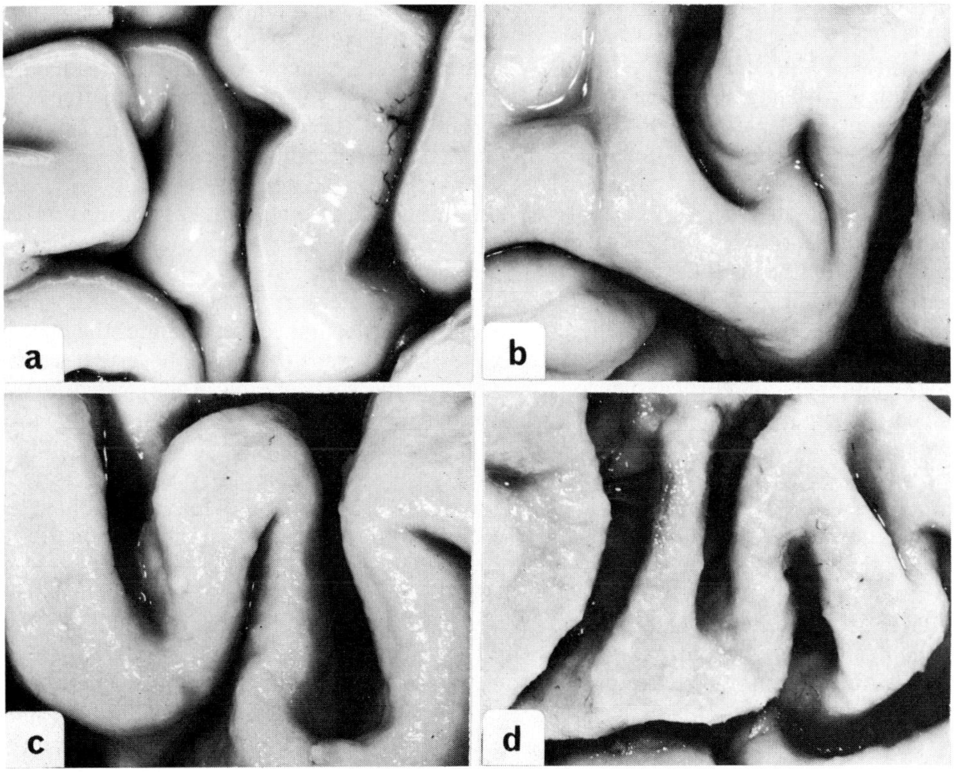

Fig. 20.2 The operculum of the frontal convexity enlarged ×3.25 (**a**) shows the normal appearance, with the degree of atrophy increasing through (**b**) and (**c**) to severe in (**d**).

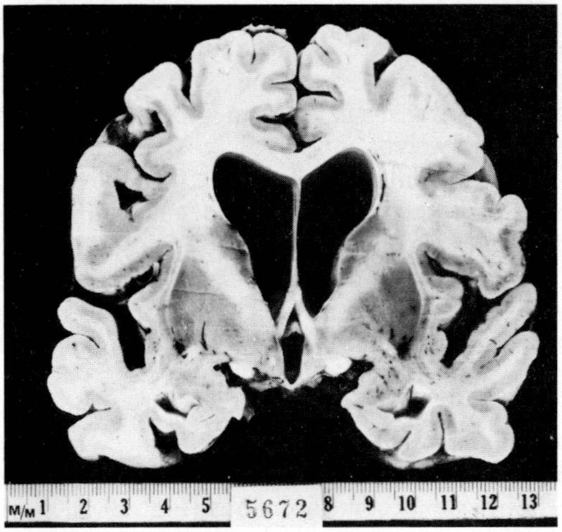

Fig. 20.3 Coronal view of the brain of a demented woman aged 78, showing considerable atrophy and enlargement of the anterior horns of the lateral ventricles.

the nerve cells get smaller, their cytoplasm contains less Nissl substance and it stains less intensely. Although traces of lipofuscin may be found in some neurons in the inferior olives of infants (Brody, 1960) and in the spinal cords of children (Humphrey, 1944), the typical pigment begins to accumulate with increasing age both in neurons and in many other cells in the body. Brizzee, Ordy and Kaack (1974) found in the macaque that the pigment first appeared regularly in the inferior olives and later in the motor and sensory nuclei of the brain stem. The amounts were greatest in the medulla and gradually decreased in a rank order of the hippocampus, midbrain, pons, neocortex and cerebellum. In man, Brody (1960) found a sharp increase with age in the numbers of cortical neurons which contained scattered pigment but in only a minority were large clumps formed. The highest percentage of heavily pigmented cells was found in the precentral gyrus, in which nerve cells tend to be large; the figure was lowest in the occipital cortex, in which there is a high proportion of small cells. The amount varied greatly elsewhere in the brain. The Purkinje cells, for example, and some of the small-celled groups in the brain stem showed little or none, and may be described as 'lipophobic'. In contrast, large amounts can be found in the cells of the cranial and spinal motor nuclei, in the red nucleus, in parts of the thalamus and in the globus pallidus; the inferior olives and the dentate nucleus of the cerebellum are exceptionally 'lipophilic'. Lipofuscin is an acid-fast lipid pigment containing protein. Its constitution has not so far been precisely defined and may vary within the same brain. Its chemical nature and its origin have been discussed by Horrocks, van Rollins and Yates (1981). The laying down of the pigment and the effect of its accumulation on cell metabolism are not clear although, as discussed later, Mann and Yates (1974) have produced evidence that it could lead to cell death. Against this, as a general statement, is the observation by Monagle and Brody (1974) who found no loss with age in the numbers of the heavily pigmented neurons in the inferior olives.

Neither the function nor the possible effect of lipofuscin accumulation is known, therefore, and it seems merely to be one of the inevitable consequences of ageing. The idea that it may occur in excess in dementia has been discounted by Mann and Sinclair (1978), whose controlled study showed no differences between the brains of their demented and non-demented groups. Zeman (1971) has described the condition of xeroid-lipofuscinosis in which excessive accumulation of lipofuscin and severe neuronal loss occur in the absence of the other common features of senescence. These include the argyrophilic (i.e. the senile or neuritic) plaque, the neurofibrillary tangles, granulovacuolar and other more recondite degenerative changes which are outlined later.

In addition to the neuronal alterations in the ageing and atrophic grey matter, a degree of neuronal loss is also likely. There is, however, no exact way of measuring the extent of cortical atrophy either by naked eye or under the microscope. The severer degrees are nevertheless obvious, for the cortical ribbon narrows and the histological picture is that of a considerable loss of nerve cells. Indeed, as already mentioned, it is this loss and the concomitant disorganization of interneuronal connections which probably lie at the root of the disintegration of the life and the mind of the dement.

For many years it was less certain whether there is a general trend for the neuronal population either in the cerebral cortex or elsewhere in the brain to diminish insidiously throughout life. The answer, however, has gradually, and not without controversy, become more clearly established during the last three decades, at least for certain parts of the brain. Brody (1955), in a pioneering study, found a loss of cortical neurons varying from 15 to 35 per cent between early and late adult life in counts carried out by eye on several carefully selected regions of the cerebral cortex, the most vulnerable area being the superior temporal gyrus. Burns (1958) concluded from studies such as these, and from the knowledge that the brain weight tends to drop with age, that 'every day of our adult life more than 100 000 neurons die'. This dubious calculation has not been accepted without question. Thus, Konigsmark and Murphy (1970) found no evidence of a drop with age in the neuronal numbers of the ventral cochlear nucleus and they emphasized that up to that time there was no conclusive evidence that the loss of brain weight, volume or function in the later decades of life was due to neuronal loss. Others also failed to identify a loss in some areas either in man or in animals and, in his review in 1974, Hanley concluded that the various 'negative results seem to dispose of neuronal fall-out with ageing as a *universal* effect, but leaves open the possibility that a particular animal species, or nervous tissue from particular regions of the brain, could be especially vulnerable'.

Subsequent studies have gone a long way to confirming this possibility. Hall, Miller and Corsellis (1975) have found that, although the number of Purkinje cells in a human cerebellum varied greatly at a given age from person to person, there was a reduction of about 2.5 per cent per decade with the greater loss occurring after the 60s had been reached. Tomlinson and Irving (1977) have established that about 20 per cent of the motor neurons in the lumbar and sacral levels of the spinal cord disappeared during later adult life, the figure often reaching 40 per cent by the tenth decade. Cell loss in the locus ceruleus as age advances has been shown by Brody (1976), and by Tomlinson, Irving and Blessed (1981). In contrast, other nuclear groups seem more resistant. Monagle and Brody (1974) found no evidence of neuronal loss in the inferior olive, whilst the abducent nucleus and nucleus of the trochlear nerve were found to remain intact by Vijayashankar and Brody (1971, 1973). It has been claimed, on the one hand, that the nerve cells in the human mamillary bodies become smaller in normal old age but retain their number (Wilkinson and Davis, 1978) whereas neuronal loss may occur in both the corpus striatum and the lentiform nucleus (Bugiani et al., 1978). All these observations, however, apart perhaps from that on the locus ceruleus, would seem to have little relevance to the unfolding of dementia in which the cerebral cortex is usually thought to play the dominant role. Here again, Hanley's (1974) conclusion about regional variation is pertinent, since as foreshadowed by Brody's work in 1955, increasing neuronal loss with age occurs normally in the superior temporal and frontal gyri but not in the occipital cortex. The possibility remains, therefore, that an increased loss of cortical (or other) neurons may be an important factor in the development of dementia. These problems are considered further in the section on Alzheimer's disease.

The mere loss of neurons, however, is not the only mechanism whereby cortical function can be impaired, for, even if the cell body survives, a diminution in the dendritic branching or a loss of synapses may interfere with proper cortical activity. There is now evidence that both these changes can occur in old age. Scheibel and his colleagues have described extensive qualitative changes in the dendritic trees of pyramidal cells in the temporal and the frontal cortex, including the ageing Betz cell (Scheibel, Tomiyasu and Scheibel, 1977), and in parts of the limbic areas (Scheibel, 1979b). These changes include the loss of dendritic spines, swellings, varicosities and distortions of the horizontal dendritic branches, followed by progressive swelling of the cell body and the loss of basilar dendrites and of branches of the apical shaft and the terminal arches. Finally the shaft is lost, the cell body disappears and gliosis follows. These changes have been based on the study of Golgi-impregnated sections and have not so far been quantified. It would be particularly interesting, therefore, to investigate systematically a series of intellectually normal, as well as impaired, individuals because severe dendritic changes have at times been found in the former (Scheibel, 1978, 1979a).

Moreover, difficulties in the preparation and in the interpretation of the Golgi picture, particularly on human tissue with its variable delays in fixation, are well known and Williams, Ferrante and Caviness (1978) have found neurons with similar appearances in young subjects. Nevertheless, Feldman and Down (1974), Feldman (1976) and Williams, Ferrante and Caviness (1978), working with rats, have demonstrated a progressive loss with age of dendritic spines in pyramidal neurons in the fifth layer of the visual cortex. In experimental animals, immediate fixation prevents artefact and many neurons remain normal without dendritic loss, although a quarter of the spines disappeared from the terminal tuft and nearly half from the oblique branching dendrites. The possibility has been raised that dendritic loss in man occurs in those cells with neurofibrillary degeneration. If dendritic loss should occur in normal old age, the latter possibility seems remote, since, as discussed later, neurofibrillary change in the neocortex is either absent or is present in very small numbers in intellectually normal old people (Tomlinson, Blessed and Roth, 1968; Tomlinson, 1972).

Further important histological features of the ageing brain include the formation of senile plaques and certain changes mainly affecting the nerve cells. The latter include Alzheimer's neurofibrillary degeneration, granulovacuolar degeneration and Hirano bodies. Each is discussed in the following sections.

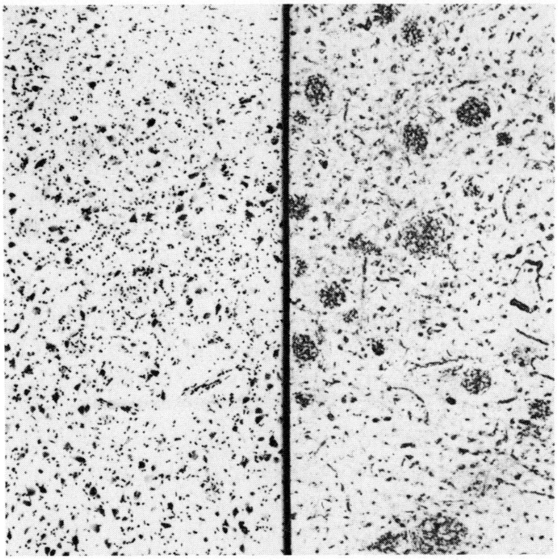

Fig. 20.4 The section of cerebral cortex on the left has been stained with cresyl violet. The view on the right is from the same brain but of an adjacent section which has been impregnated with silver. The plaque formation is shown clearly only by the latter method. Both views × 70.

Senile plaques

Senile, argyrophilic or, as they are now often called, neuritic plaques are the most striking, if inconsistent, feature of the ageing brain. They are difficult to see in sections stained with haematoxylin and eosin or with cresyl violet (Fig. 20.4), but are easily demonstrated in frozen sections of formalin-fixed tissue using the silver impregnation method described by von Braunmühl. Other effective techniques include a method for nitrocellulose sections described by Hirano and Zimmerman (1962a) and one by Cross (1982) for paraffin sections. The PAS reaction may be used. For comparative studies on the numbers of plaques, the present writers have found it advisable to rely on the use of a single method.

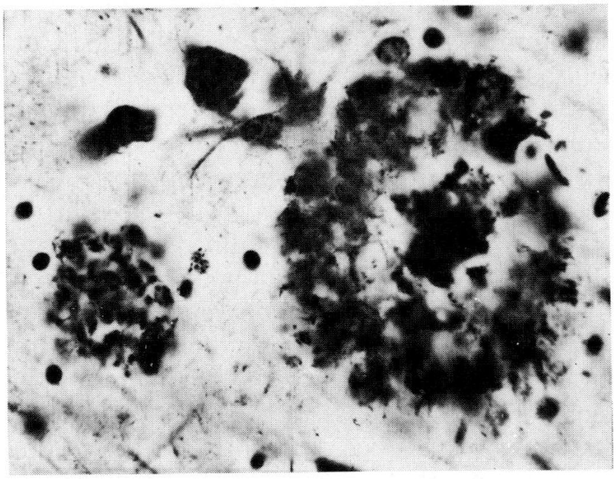

Fig. 20.5 Argyrophilic or 'senile' plaque formation in cortex. von Braunmühl silver impregnation.

Plaques are most often found in the cerebral cortex, but they also occur in the deeper grey matter, including the amygdaloid nucleus, the corpus striatum, the diencephalon generally and, to a lesser extent, along the brain stem. The cerebellum is rarely affected. They are not found in the depths of the white matter.

Many varieties of plaque have been described. The classic form consists of a dark central core surrounded by an irregular clear halo and beyond this, by a ring of granular, filamentous or rod-like material which, like the core, is argyrophilic (Fig. 20.5). Most plaques are roughly spherical and range from 5 to 200 μm across but their appearance and size can vary because, among other things, of the plane in which they have been cut. Some may therefore lack the central core or the clear halo, but consist merely of an irregular mass of fragmented tissue, while plagues adjacent to each other may coalesce into larger irregularly shaped patches; other single plaques appear as discrete homogeneous spheres which displace the nerve fibres to one side (Fig. 20.6). Plaques in the depths of the cortex tend to

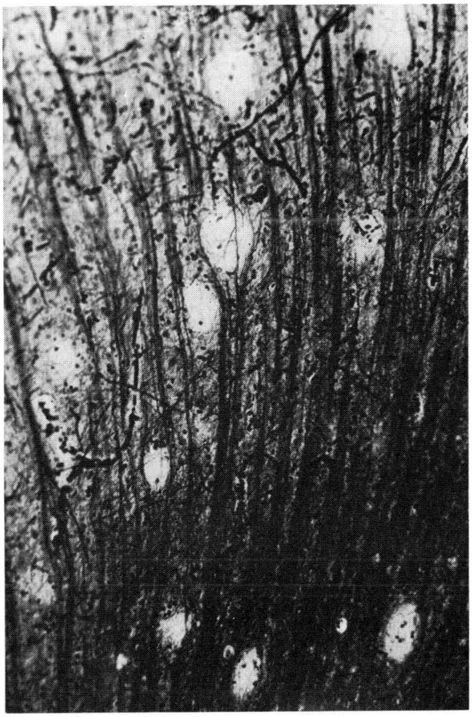

Fig. 20.6 Senile plaques in deeper layers of cortex, shown up by Heidenhain's stain for myelin.

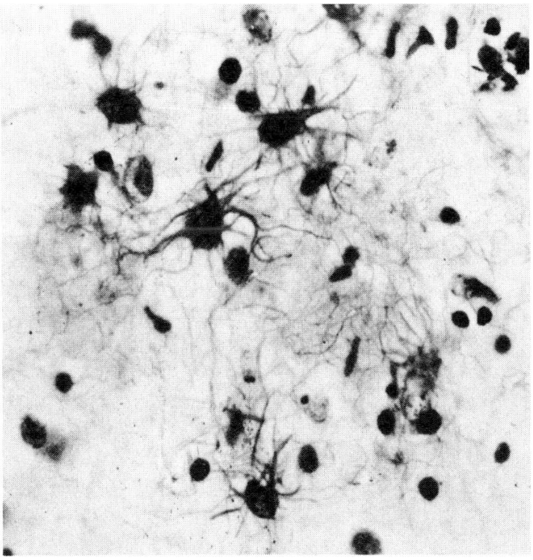

Fig. 20.7 Astrocytes encircling a plaque. Holzer stain ×225.

be larger, with the classic core and halo, than the more fragmented patches seen in the outer layers. Occasionally, discrete plaques are absent and ill-defined areas of faintly granular background are all that can be seen. Glial reaction in the vicinity of plaques varies. At times a few astrocytic nuclei may collect around the edge, the processes of the cell penetrating more deeply (Fig. 20.7); this can also be well shown in Cajal preparations or by the immunohistological demonstration of glial fibrillary acidic protein; the occasional rod-shaped microglial nucleus may lie within the plaque.

Pathogenesis Blocq and Marinesco first identified the senile plaque in 1892. Its origin, however, has remained in doubt, at least until the 1960s. Redlich (1898) thought that the plaques developed in a disintegrating glial reticulum. Bonfiglio (1908) claimed that they sprang from degenerating neurons, and since then nearly every component has been invoked as their source. Soniat (1941) and, later, Liss (1960) found them to develop in relation to degenerating neurofibrils. Neumann (1960) considered an axonal origin to be more likely. Ferraro (1931) suggested that oligodendroglial and microglial elements were responsible. But von Braunmühl (1931) had other ideas; he elaborated Marinesco's (1911) earlier contention that plaques derived from the condensation of a hypothetical intercellular ground substance. This hypothesis foreshadowed the work by Divry (1927), who showed that the centre of many plaques resembled amyloid in its histochemical reactions and in particular its congophilia, or affinity for the dye Congo red, the effect of which was to produce birefringence. Divry believed that the first trace of the 'primitive plaque' was the condensation of minute areas of ground substance into a 'substance trichosique' which acted as a foreign body attracting microglial cells containing amyloid, fat and perhaps a trace of iron. Astrocytes proliferated later around the periphery. Morel and Wildi (1952) demonstrated that enzyme activity increased in and around the plaque. Friede and Magee (1962) and Friede (1965) studied the increased concentration of oxidative and hydrolytic enzyme activity in relation to plaques whilst Johnson and Blum (1970) added that of nucleotide phosphatase and so destroyed the belief that a passive degenerative process was at work.

Light microscopy had gone so far but the more notable contributions were now coming from the use of the electron microscope. In 1964 both Kidd, and Terry, Gonatas and Weiss showed

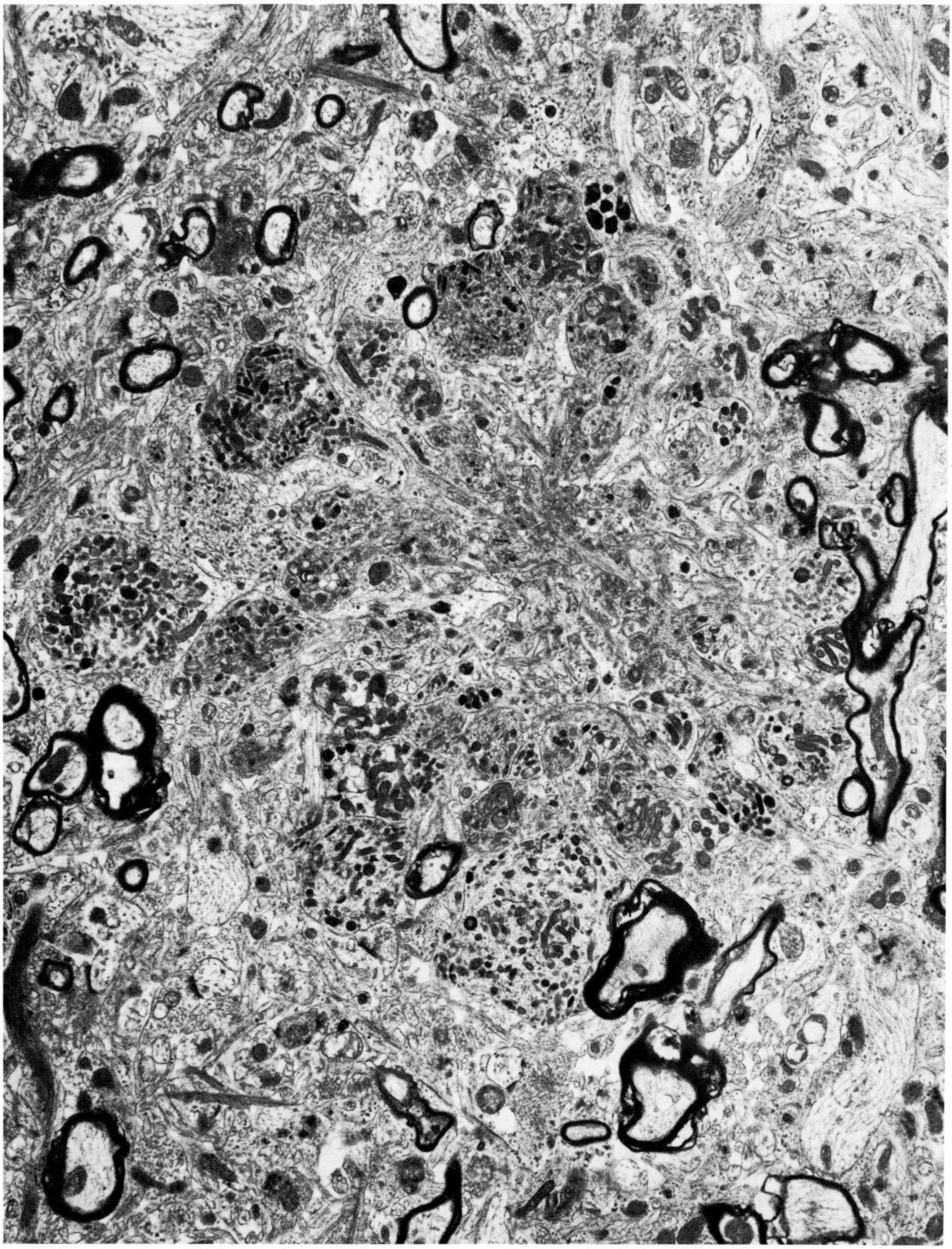

Fig. 20.8 Cerebral cortex in Alzheimer's disease. Neuritic plaque surrounded by neuropil. The distended cell processes (neurites) seen in the periphery of the plaque contain numerous mitochondria, dense bodies and membranous structures. $\times 7850$. (Courtesy of Dr Luis H. Carrasco.)

that, although variable, the ultrastructure of the typical senile plaque consists of large numbers of altered neuronal processes, designated as neurites, which are intermingled with glial processes, an occasional microglial cell and a central core of amyloid fibrils. Krigman, Feldman and Bensch (1965) and Gonatas, Anderson and Evangelista (1967) rapidly confirmed these observations. In 1972 Terry and Wisniewski brought together the results of their pioneering work by postulating that the earliest ultrastructural manifestations of the plaque is the enlarged abnormal neurite, many of which were shown to be related to presynaptic terminals. These become distended to five to ten times their normal diameter by large numbers of rounded dense bodies, many of which had probably originated from degenerating mitochondria (Fig. 20.8). Although these bodies make up the bulk of the distended terminal neurites, groups of helically wound fibrils may also be found which closely resemble those occurring in nerve cells affected by neurofibrillary degeneration.

This description greatly influenced ideas on the origin of senile plaques. Terry and Wisniewski (1972) saw the development of the plaque in three stages, their appearances at each stage being not unlike those of the main categories of plaque long recognized by light microscopists. The primitive plaque, which was seen as the earliest stage, consists of a small number of distended neurites, largely presynaptic or axonal in origin (Gonatas, Anderson and Evangelista, 1967; Gonatas and Gambetti, 1970), with either no or a few associated amyloid fibrils, demonstrable only by electron microscopy. A few astrocytic fibres or the odd microglial cell might also be present. The second stage (see Fig. 20.5) is that of the mature plaque with a dense amyloid core surrounded by many distended neurites, astrocytic processes and occasional microglial or astrocytic cell bodies. The last stage is the so-called burnt-out plaque consisting of little more than the core of amyloid. With the recognition of the neurite as a major component of the plaque, the term 'neuritic', instead of 'senile', came into use. A crucial part of Terry and Wisniewski's observations was the fact that the first wisps of amyloid appeared only after a cluster of four or five abnormal neurites had collected together, an observation which seemed to eliminate amyloid as the precursor of the abnormal neurites. The cause, therefore, both of neurite degeneration and of amyloid formation remains obscure.

Nothing is at present known about the particular neurons on whose processes the plaque begins to form nor is it known whether a single plaque, with its large number of abnormal neurites, arises from a single neuron or from several neurons. Indeed, the relation of neuronal loss to plaque, or to tangle, formation is equally obscure although the loss of nerve cells could scarcely be seen merely as the result of either plaque or tangle formation since neither occurs to more than a minor degree in early to late middle age—that is, at a time when progressive cortical neuronal loss is already being identified as a widespread phenomenon.

At this time of life, plaques may be present but in very small numbers in any part of the cortex. As sites of predilection, a few are usually to be found in the hippocampus, the parahippocampal gyrus and the amygdaloid nucleus, all being areas which tend to be most severely affected, both by plaques and by tangles, in the brain of the normal elderly person. In these old people, as in the young, plaques tend to cluster around the base of a sulcus; if, however, there are more than a handful, others are likely to be found spread widely, if sparsely, throughout the cortex. By the age of 70 years over half the population will show small, or even moderate, numbers in the cerebral cortex (Tomlinson, Blessed and Roth, 1968; Tomlinson, 1972) although not all individuals accumulate plaques even when extremely old (Dayan, 1970). Those brains with cortical plaques may well show them also scattered in the deep grey matter and particularly in the hypothalamus, including the mamillary bodies, the striatum and, at times, in the upper brain stem. Exceptionally, remarkably large numbers of plaques are evident throughout the neocortex and the hippocampus to a degree which is indistinguishable from that seen in demented patients (Tomlinson, 1980; D.M. Hollander and Corsellis, 1974, unpublished observations). In intellectually normal subjects, however, even when many plaques are seen, intracortical neurofibrillary tangles are either rare or absent.

Alzheimer's neurofibrillary degeneration

Alzheimer (1907a, b) described for the first time a change he had found in roughly every fourth nerve cell in the cerebral cortex of a 51-year-old

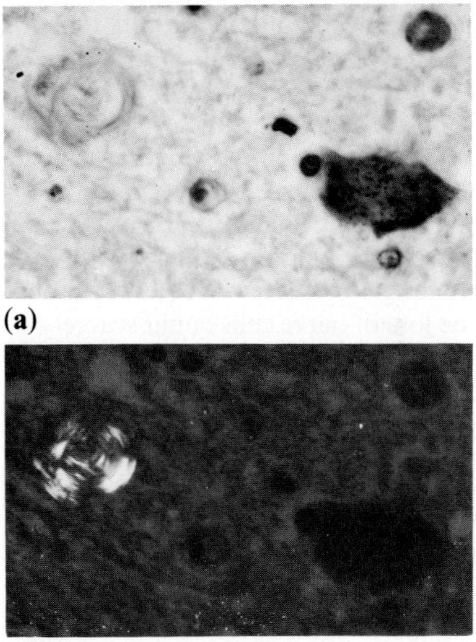

(a)

(b)

Fig. 20.9 Neurofibrillary changes in a pigmented cell of the substantia nigra: (**a**) stained with Congo red; (**b**) the same field under polarized light.

woman who had been suffering from the form of dementia named after him (and discussed at length in a later section). The alteration is not easy to see in preparations stained with haematoxylin and eosin or in Nissl, but it is clearly shown by the same methods as those described for plaques, one of the best being that developed by Cross (1982). Congo red provides a particularly valuable way to identify the change in any form of embedded or frozen tissue because not only do the altered fibrils take up the pink dye deeply but this also renders them intensely birefringent under polarized light (Fig. 20.9).

The essential change consists of the thickening and tortuosity of fibrils within the neuronal cytoplasm (Fig. 20.10). The configuration may vary according to the site and to the type of nerve cell affected, and probably according to the stage of its development. In the smaller pyramidal neurons of the cortex the change first appears as a single, sharply defined, dark band running or curving through the cytoplasm of the cell from the base towards the apical dendrite. In the larger, but not the largest, pyramidal cells the more mature thickened bands or loops (Fig. 20.11) come to resemble a skein of wool. Cortical neurons mostly show the simpler triangular or looped shapes while spool- or torch-like patterns are often seen in the hippocampus (Fig. 20.12). A globose form, with tightly wound thickened fibres, reminiscent of a ball of string, occurs in affected cells of the substantia nigra (see Fig. 20.9), the substantia innominata, the locus ceruleus and other neuronal groups in the lower brain stem (Ishii, 1965). In most cells with neurofibrillary change the nucleus can still be identified and, when appropriate to the cell, pigments such as melanin or lipofuscin may also be present. Sometimes, and presumably in the final stages, the nucleus and the cell outline disappear and only the contorted fibrils remain.

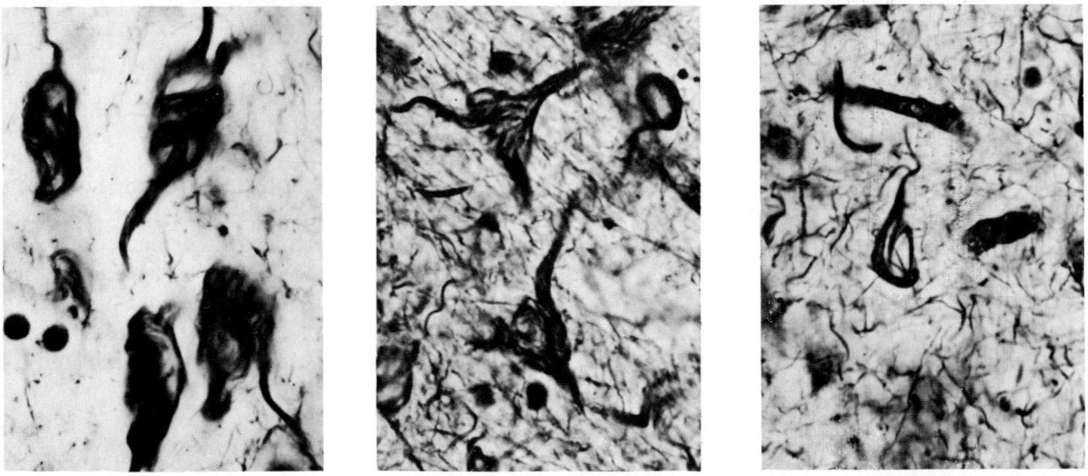

(a) **(b)** **(c)**

Fig. 20.10 Neurofibrillary change in presenile dementia (Alzheimer's disease): (**a**) from pyramidal layer of cornu Ammonis; (**b**) from parahippocampal gyrus; (**c**) from temporal cortex. All views Bielschowsky ×600.

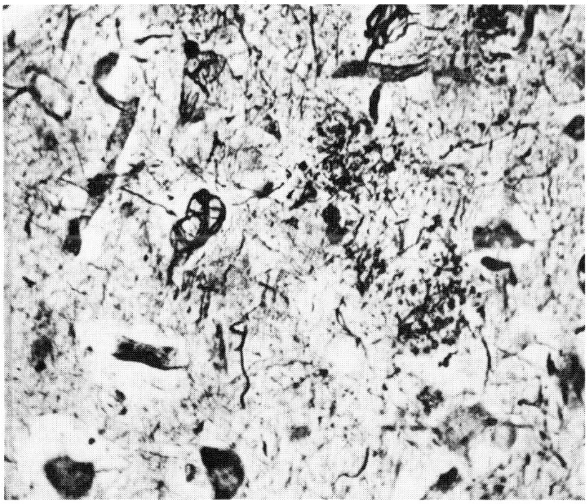

Fig. 20.11 Cortex showing Alzheimer tangles adjacent to an argyrophilic plaque. Bielschowsky silver impregnation.

Fig. 20.12 Neurofibrillary tangles in the cortex of the parahippocampal gyrus. von Braunmühl × 325.

Pathogenesis The nature and origin of the tangle have long been debated but the demonstration of their ultrastructure has helped to solve many, if not all, the problems. Alzheimer considered that the change developed in neurofibrils normally present in the nerve cell. Bielschowsky (1932) opposed this view because the altered and fragmented fibrils have little resemblance to the normal arrangement. Divry (1934), on the basis of the congophilic properties of tangles, considered that they were amyloid in nature

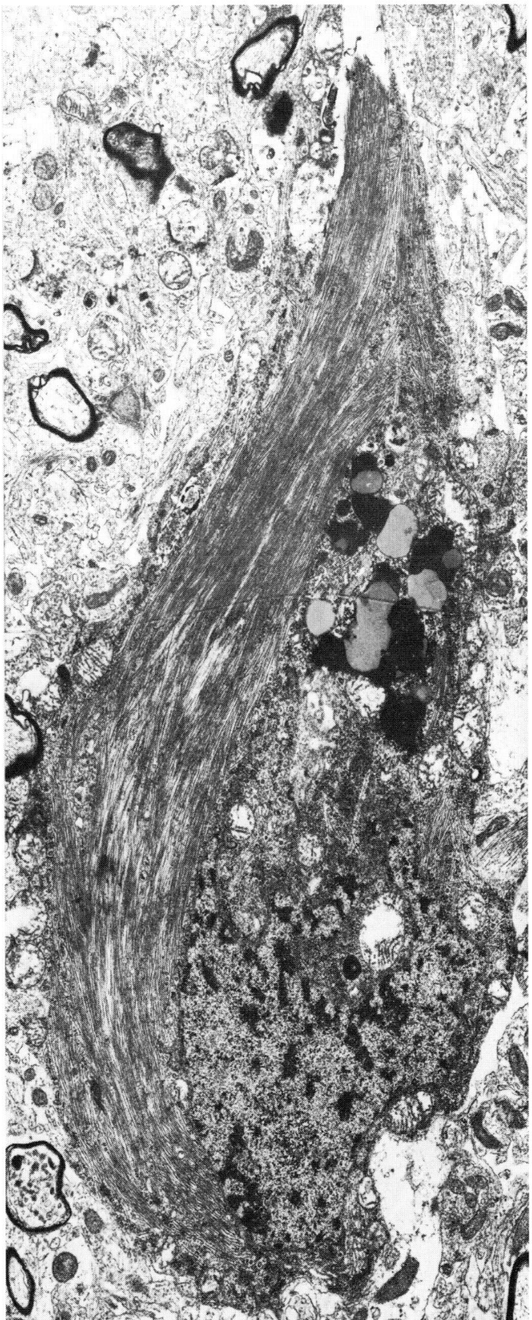

Fig. 20.13 Advanced neurofibrillary degeneration in a cortical neuron in Alzheimer's disease. Intracytoplasmic twisted filaments have displaced the cellular organelles and the atrophic mis-shapen nucleus × 7720. (Courtesy of Dr Luis H. Carrasco.)

and suggested a common origin with senile plaques since the core of these structures, which is also congophilic, appeared to consist of amyloid fibrils.

Electron microscopy (Fig. 20.13), however, although confirming that the fibrillary substance in the plaque core was a form of amyloid, indicated that the ultrastructure of the neurofibrillary tangle was not. Terry (1963) considered the tangle to consist almost exclusively of a mass of twisted tubules each measuring about 20 nm wide with periodic narrowing every 80 nm to about 10 nm (Fig. 20.14). Kidd (1964) suspected that this appearance was the product of paired filaments wound in a double helix which resulted in the intermittent narrowing. This was confirmed by Wisniewski, Narang and Terry (1976), who, using a tilting table, were able to analyse the curvilinear profile which results when such structures are cut transversely. The appearances were found to be identical with those produced by constrictions due to the spiral winding of fibres rather than to the narrowing of tubules. Since that time, descriptions of neurofibrillary tangles have been largely consistent although their interpretation as twisted tubules, as against helically wound fibrils, is disinterred from time to time. Gibson, Stones and Tomlinson (1976) illustrated abnormally large numbers of apparently straight tubules, as well as apparently twisted tubules, within a single neuron, whilst Shibayama and Kitoh (1978) saw both straight and paired helical filaments in a case of atypical senile dementia. Oyanagi (1979) observed 15-nm straight filaments in some dendrites, and Yagashita et al. (1981) found tangles which consisted of a mixture of straight and twisted filaments as well as some tangles of each variety. These variations, which must be borne in mind in the chemical and immunological study of tangles, are nevertheless infrequent. The great majority of tangles in the Alzheimer type of degeneration and in most, but not all, other human conditions in which they are prone to occur,

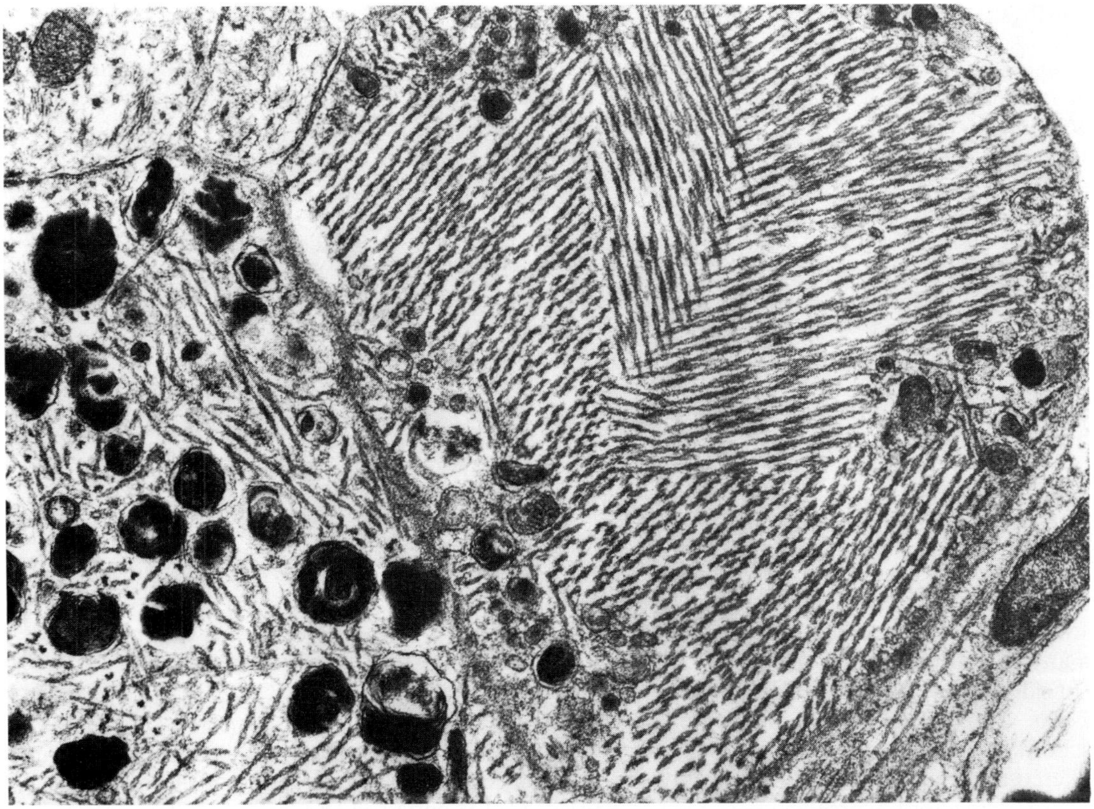

Fig. 20.14 Cerebral cortex in Alzheimer's disease. Bundles of paired filaments fill the dendritic processes and can also be seen on the left among electron-dense bodies. ×27 750. (Courtesy of Dr Luis H. Carrasco.)

consist predominantly of helically wound filaments.

Distribution Neurofibrillary tangles occur to a greater or lesser extent in ageing but also in various cerebral disorders. Some regions of the brain are more susceptible than others but although there are exceptions, such as in supranuclear palsy (discussed later), there is a tendency for the distribution to follow a common pattern (Simchowicz, 1911; Hirano and Zimmerman, 1962b).

The emphasis is usually more on the anterior frontal and the temporal cortex than on the posterior parts of the hemispheres; the pre- and postcentral gyri are usually less involved. Within the affected areas, cells in the outer and middle cortical layers are altered in greater numbers than those lying more deeply. The brunt of the process, however, tends to fall on the neurons in the anteromedial temporal grey matter, including the uncal cortex, the corticomedial part of the amygdaloid nucleus, the hippocampus and the adjacent parts of much of the parahippocampal gyrus (Morel and Wildi, 1952; Jamada and Mehraein, 1968). Neurons in the subcortical regions are less often affected, but the pigmented cells of the substantia nigra and of the locus ceruleus are also vulnerable. Ishii (1965) studied the distribution in the hypothalamus and brain stem and pointed out that the vulnerable nuclear groups showed certain metabolic features in common, including a high content of monamines and an early accumulation of lipofuscin. Some categories of cell are curiously resistant, and Purkinje cells, as well as the large motor neurons (including the Betz cells), all but escape this form of degeneration.

Prevalence A few tangles may be found in the brains of many intellectually normal people as they get older. Although later on they tend to be distributed in the areas just delineated, the change is usually confined initially to the hippocampal region, an area of the brain in which some altered cells are to be found in virtually all people over the age of 50 years (Ball, 1976). When more widespread, a few neurons scattered more generally through the cortex may be affected (Tomlinson, Blessed and Roth, 1968). Small numbers may also be found in non-demented people in the uncal area, the corticomedial part of the amygdaloid nucleus, the subiculum and a major part of the parahippocampal gyrus (Jamada and Mehraein, 1968). The number of affected cells in the hippocampus increases further with advancing age and sizeable clusters may be found at this time in intellectually normal old people. By systematic cell counting, Tomlinson and colleagues (Tomlinson, Blessed and Roth, 1968; Tomlinson and Kitchener, 1972) established that marked tangle formation was present in the anteromedial temporal grey matter in about 5 per cent of normal people dying as early as their 40s. By the seventh decade the proportion had risen to about 50 per cent and all the nonagenarians examined showed some affected neurons. Further studies by Morimatsu et al. (1975) and Ball (1976) confirmed the tendency in normal adults for the tangles to increase in number through middle or later life while remaining significantly fewer than those found in dementia of the Alzheimer type. In this pathological condition the neurons of the hippocampus, particularly in the posterior half of that structure, usually show the largest increase, while vast numbers of nerve cells throughout the rest of the neocortex may also be affected (see later).

Tangles and plaques, identical to those found in the ageing brain, are liable to occur prematurely in adults with Down's syndrome. Jervis identified this tendency in 1948, although Struwe had reported the presence of plaques alone as early as 1929. Several studies have confirmed that such patients dying in their 30s, and occasionally in their 20s or younger, may develop plaques although the tangles tend to appear later in adult life (Solitaire and Lamarche, 1966). Malamud (1972) found these changes in all 35 cases he had examined who died above the age of 40 years. One of Olson and Shaw's three patients (1969) who had all died in their 30s had developed the clincial picture of Alzheimer's disease but the other two had not, and it seems clear that there is no inevitable trend to mental deterioration, as distinct from defect, in such patients (Ropper and Williams, 1980). Thase et al. (1982) nevertheless found that neuropsychiatric status 'tended to worsen with advancing age and 45 per cent of patients with Down's syndrome were demented when over the age of 45'. This remains an interesting and unsolved clinicopathological problem.

In other disorders the ratio of plaques to tangles is reversed, the latter becoming dominant with the plaques scanty or absent. Thus classic tangles are found in vast numbers in the parkinsonism-dementia complex of Guam (Hirano, Malamud and Kurland, 1961) and in the amyotrophic lateral sclerosis of Guam (Malamud, Hirano and Kurland, 1961) as well as in other instances of motor neuron disease and its allied disorders (Hirano and Zimmerman, 1962b). Fényes (1932) and Hallervorden (1933) found neurofibrillary changes in neurons in the brain stem in patients with encephalitis lethargica in which, as in postencephalitic parkinsonism, the cells of the substantia nigra and locus ceruleus are particularly vulnerable as well as other cell groups in the reticular and midline regions (Greenfield and Bosanquet, 1953). Wisniewski, Terry and Hirano (1970) demonstrated that the ultrastructure of neurofibrillary changes seen in these conditions is identical to those found in the ageing brain. Malamud, Haymaker and Pinkerton (1950) and Corsellis (1951) made similar observations on the presence in the brain stem and cerebral cortex of tangles in subacute sclerosing panencephalitis. The classic ultrastructure of paired helical filaments in such altered neurons has been confirmed by Mandybur et al. (1977) and Paula-Barbosa et al. (1979).

Neurofibrillary tangles, again in large numbers, and usually, though not always, without plaque formation, have occurred as a late sequel to cerebral trauma. Possible examples are the rare cases of post-traumatic dementia following a single head injury, in which the histological features have proved to be those of Alzheimer's disease (Claude and Cuel, 1939; Corsellis and Brierley, 1959).

Repeated blows to the head as a possible triggering mechanism in the formation of plaques and tangles was considered by Brandenberg and Hallervorden (1954), who had found intense changes of both kinds in the brain of an amateur boxer who had died demented at the age of 51. In a second boxer Grahmann and Ule (1957) found only the neurofibrillary change, and in a third Constantinidis and Tissot (1967) emphasized strongly that tangles had occurred in the complete absence of senile plaques. Corsellis, Bruton and Freeman-Browne (1973), in a detailed account of 15 retired boxers, found that neurofibrillary changes, usually in the absence of plaques, were a major pathological feature of most brains. Tangle formation, the ultrastructure of which was later shown to be typical (Wisniewski et al., 1976), was particularly severe in the substantia nigra and locus ceruleus, but at its most intense in the vulnerable parts of the medial temporal grey matter. The frontal cortex was more affected than the parieto-occipital regions. The formation of tangles as a consequence of repeated blows to the head seems therefore undeniable even if the nature of the relationship remains obscure.

Neurofibrillary tangles have been reported as an occasional finding in many other conditions (see Hirano and Zimmerman, 1962b), but when they occur in small numbers only, particularly in the sites in which they are to be found in normal elderly people, it should be borne in mind that in any patient dying above the age of 60 years their appearance may be no more than the tangle formation of old age unrelated to the presence of some other specific disorder.

In summary, neurofibrillary tangles consisting of paired helical filaments have been found to develop to an intense degree in various cerebral disorders and to a slight extent merely as a factor in ageing. In only two human conditions have neurofibrillary changes been described in which the ultrastructural appearance has differed from those related to ageing and to dementia of the Alzheimer type. One is in some instances of sporadic motor neuron disease and the other is progressive supranuclear palsy in which the tangles consist predominantly of straight fibrils rather than paired helical filaments. These conditions are further considered in Chapter 15. It is curious that tangles consisting of paired helical filaments appear never, so far, to have been found either in old or in experimental animals.

Granulovacuolar degeneration

Whilst the neuritic plaque and the neurofibrillary tangle are the two major, and easily demonstrated, histological features of the ageing human brain, a third, which is less obvious, is 'granulovacuolar degeneration' (Fig. 20.15).

This neuronal change, which is largely confined to the cytoplasm of the pyramidal cells of the hippocampus, appears as one or more vacuoles, 3–5 μm in diameter. Each vacuole contains a central dot or granule; if there are several vacuoles the cell outline may bulge and become irregular with the nucleus becoming eccentric. The change is easily seen in haematoxylin and eosin and in many silver impregnations. Electron microscopy has added little to an understanding of the nature of the origin of the change, the

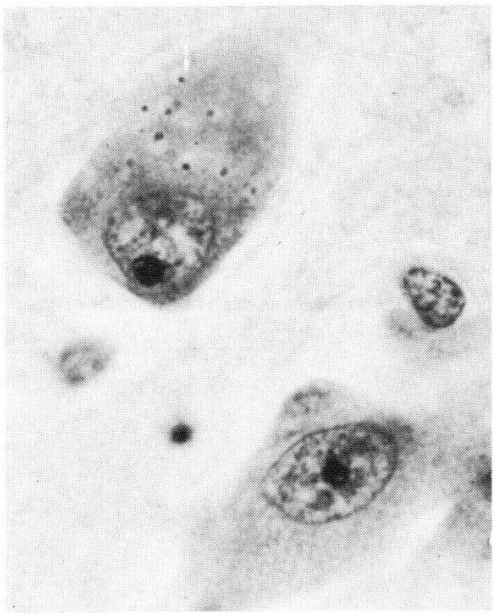

Fig. 20.15 Granulovacuolar degeneration in the pyramidal cells of the hippocampus. Lendrum's phloxine tartrazine stain.

appearances being described as cytoplasmic membrane-bound inclusions each with a translucent matrix containing an electron-dense granular core (Hirano, Malamud and Kurland, 1961).

The term was first applied by Simchowicz in 1911 to this kind of change which he had observed in cases of senile dementia. For many years its study was confined to this condition but Woodard (1962, 1966) broadened the scope. He examined the pyramidal cells in the ventrolateral quadrant of the hippocampus (roughly the Sommer sector or Rose's H-l field) in a series of patients from non-psychiatric hospitals or from county coroners, and found that, at the most, fewer than 7 per cent of the cells were affected. In contrast, more than 9 per cent were found diseased in cases of presenile or senile dementia of the Alzheimer type—a figure which was never reached in the non-dementia series. Tomlinson and Kitchener (1972) examined 30 non-demented and 50 demented elderly subjects, as well as 219 routinely autopsied patients from an acute general hospital, who had died between the ages of 20 and 95 years. The change was rarely found in those below the age of 65 but after that it occurred increasingly often in the non-demented until, by the ninth decade, it could be identified in three out of four cases. In the normal subjects the change was usually restricted to the run of hippocampal pyramidal cells in the area described above, but spreading at times into the adjacent subiculum. Only occasionally were more than a few vacuoles present in a single cell and only rarely were more than 9 per cent of cells in the Sommer sector affected. This contrasted markedly with the series of demented patients in which over 20 per cent of cells in the Sommer sector were commonly involved; sometimes the figure reached 50 per cent. Ball and Lo (1977) calculated, on serial sections, the number of cells affected and found that those with granulovacuolar degeneration were present in all patients dying over the age of 47 years. In other reports the findings were similar to those of Tomlinson and Kitchener, with the number of cells involved in the demented groups being on average many times greater than that of the age-related control. Its significance to hippocampal function is unknown and its rarity in cells outside this region may suggest that it has little or no part to play in the overall dementia of Alzheimer's disease, although it might conceivably be related to the memory disorder that is so common, possibly by interfering with nerve cells which lie along pathways linking the hippocampus to other parts of the brain. At present, perhaps, it is best looked on simply as a further marker of an ageing process, the intensity of which follows the usual trend to differ quantitatively rather than qualitatively from that found in the brains of intact, as compared with demented, old people.

Granulovacuolar degeneration has been reported in various disorders. In most it has affected the hippocampus and, as just described, may then be related more to age than to any specific disease. However, in progressive supranuclear palsy (Steele, Richardson and Olszewski, 1964) identical changes occur in neurons of the red nucleus and in other brain stem cell groups. This condition therefore constitutes a major exception to the rule that only cells within the hippocampal complex are vulnerable. The occurrence of affected hippocampal cells in youngish adults with Down's syndrome (Malamud, 1972) and in the amyotrophic lateral sclerosis and Parkinson-dementia of Guam may reflect a particular association with these disorders (Hirano, Malamud and Kurland, 1961; Hirano et al, 1968). Hirano, Tuazon and Zimmerman (1968) noted the change in the neurons of a parietally placed tuber in tuberous sclerosis.

Hirano bodies

These structures were first identified by Hirano et al. in 1966 in a study of the Parkinson-dementia syndrome of Guam. They are inconspicuous, and commonly either go unrecognized or are mistaken for single or short columns of red cells. They are shown up well by haematoxylin and eosin staining, when they tend to be brightly eosinophilic, ovoid in shape and 10–30 μm in length by 8 μm across. In rounded form they are usually hyaline in appearance, but when elongated, faint longitudinal striations are often visible. They are most often found among, and usually adjacent to, the hippocampal pyramidal cells; less frequently they are present in the *stratum lacunosum* in which there are no nerve cells. Gibson and Tomlinson (1977) have described their occurrence in intellectually normal old people, and in demented old people with the Alzheimer type of degeneration. They occur from youth into old age and become increasingly noticeable in the sixth and seventh decades of life. Up to middle age only the very occasional body is found in a single section, but in the elderly as many as 60 or 70 may be seen. Although there is a considerable overlap between the normal and the demented, the latter group are significantly more involved. Since their original description in 1966, Hirano et al. (1968), Schochet and McCormick (1972) and Tomonoga (1974) have observed them in many different disorders and it is now clear that they can be seen in almost every category of nerve cell or process within the central nervous system both in humans and in experimental animals (Gibson and Tomlinson, 1977), whether or not cerebral disease is present. Ogata, Budzilovich and Cravioto (1972) have made similar observations while confirming that they are particularly common in the elderly hippocampus.

Ultrastructurally they consist of parallel filaments 60–100 nm in length which alternate with longer sheet-like material (Hirano et al., 1968; Schochet and McCormick, 1972). The site at which they occur in relation to the neuron is debatable. In stained sections of the hippocampal Sommer sector they commonly seem to lie within the neuronal perikaryon, although this is clearly impossible in the neuron-free stratum lacunosum; here, however, they may still be included in neuronal processes. At electron microscope level they often seem to indent, rather than to occupy the perikaryon. In no condition have their pathogenesis or their significance been understood.

Congophilic angiopathy

As described in the section on senile plaques, Divry showed in 1927 that their core often consisted of an amyloid-like substance. In 1938 Scholz demonstrated that a similar material was laid down in the small cerebral vessels of about 10 per cent of people dying over the age of 70. In this change an affected arteriole appears at low power as a thickened homogeneous tube (Fig. 20.16a) which stains pink with eosin or cresyl violet and yellowish-brown with the van Gieson method. The alteration lies outside the elastic lamina, which is usually attenuated or split, and the muscle fibres of the middle coat have a blurred outline with nuclei which are indistinct or absent. Around this, in the advanced stages, an amorphous substance develops which under higher power has a reticulated or radial structure (Fig. 20.16b). With Congo red such a vessel stains pink and then becomes doubly refractile (Fig. 20.16c, d). Pantelakis (1954) called the change 'congophilic angiopathy'. Morel and Wildi (1955) and Surbeck (1961) went further in order to emphasize the importance of the way in which, in exceptional cases, small amyloid 'warts' would erupt on the edge of the degenerating vessels and fragments might then come to lie free in the tissue. It was this phenomenon which Scholz had interpreted as a possible origin of the senile plaque.

The change affects the small pial and intracortical arterioles, the leptomeningeal vessels and at times the intracortical capillaries. The parieto-occipital cortex is usually more affected than that in the frontal and temporal lobes and the change is often most easily identified in the striate cortex in the occipital lobe. The small vessels in the cerebellar cortex and in the deep grey matter of the cerebral hemispheres are affected occasionally; the brain stem seems always to be spared.

In contrast, the central nervous system rarely shows vascular changes of this kind in the primary, secondary or familial forms of secondary amyloidosis (Mandybur, 1975) whilst the presence of neuritic plaques in the brain in any of these conditions is also extremely rare (Krücke, 1950). On the other hand, Pantelakis (1954) and Schwartz et al. (1967) observed a mild degree of vascular amyloidosis in the internal organs, including the heart and pancreas, in some patients with cerebral congophilic angiopathy.

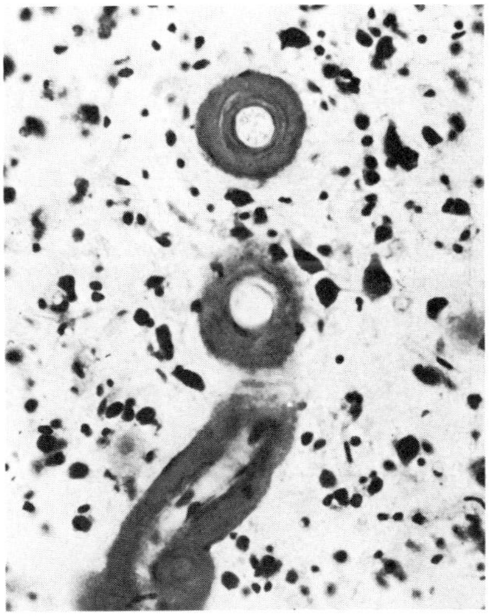

(a)

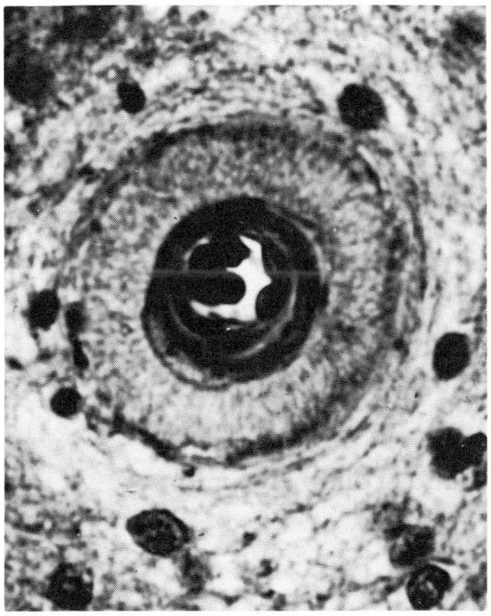

(b)

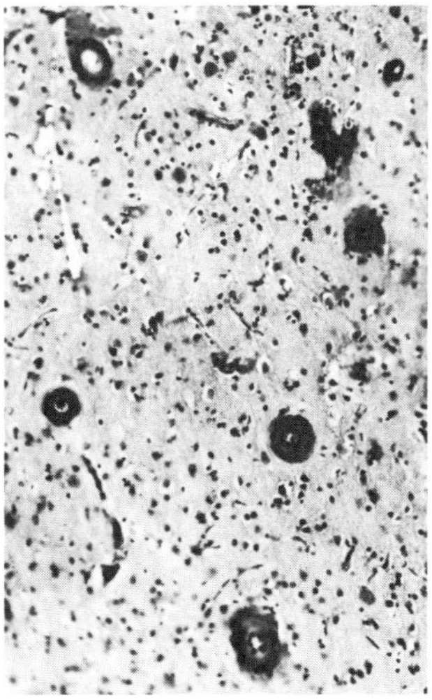

(c)

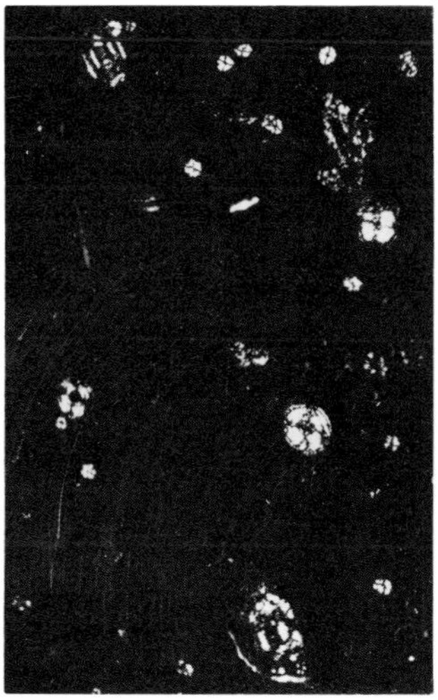

(d)

Fig. 20.16 (**c**) Cortical arteriole with the appearances of congophilic angiopathy. Cresyl violet ×240. (**b**) Higher power view of such an arteriole, showing gross thickening of the middle coat with a surrounding radial fibrillar structure. Iron haematoxylin and van Gieson ×550. (**c**) Small cortical vessels stained with Congo red. ×100. (**d**) The same as (**c**) but taken under polarized light. ×100.

As with the core of the senile plaque, the origin of the substance is still obscure. Schlote (1965) confirmed that its ultrastructure was similar to that of amyloid, and Terry and Wisniewski (1972) have described how congophilic angiopathy involves primarily the perithelial cells and the basement membrane, the latter being widened and replicated by the amyloid fibrils (Fig. 20.17). There is, however, some evidence that different mechanisms may be involved in the formation of amyloid within the plaque and within the vessel. Torack and Lynch (1981) have demonstrated immunoglobulins in the vascular form in three patients but consider that an endogenous substrate was more probable in the plaque.

Ishii and Haga (1976) have obtained positive reactions to immunoglobulin in amyloid fibrils in plaques but Powers and Spicer (1977) and Powers and Skeen (1980) have demonstrated similarities between plaques and APUD amyloid. Johnson et al. (1981) have produced evidence that plaque and vessel amyloid share a common antigen with neurofibrillary tangles.

It is not clear, however, at this time, that the amyloid found in the normal ageing brain, in blood vessels and in plaques in Alzheimer's disease is identical nor whether it is the product of

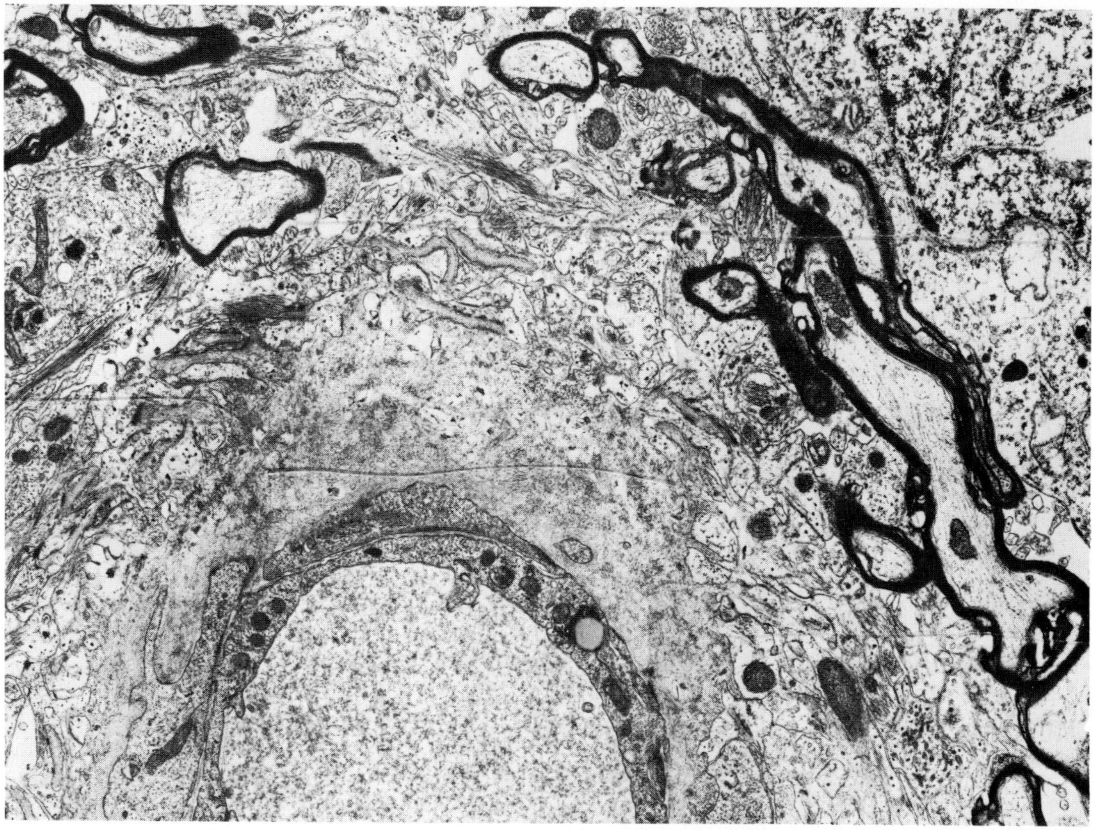

Fig. 20.17 Congophilic angiopathy in a terminal arteriole of the cerebral cortex in Alzheimer's disease. Note the great increase in thickness of the basal lamina in which amyloid has begun to develop. The material from which the basal lamina is made can be seen penetrating between the perivascular glial processes. ×10 000. (Courtesy of Dr Luis H. Carrasco.)

an immunological reaction or a secretion comparable to that which occurs in some endocrine tumours (Glenner, Terry and Isersky, 1973). In studying plaque amyloid, particularly after chemical extraction, it is essential to establish whether the resulting substances are not a combination of vascular and plaque amyloid since, as stated above, it is not certain that the two kinds have the same origin or chemical constitution. Although vascular amyloid is often present in Alzheimer's disease it may nevertheless be absent, even when there are many plaques (Mandybur, 1975; Mountjoy, Tomlinson and Gibson, 1982). There is therefore no constant relationship between the two. It is even possible that plaque amyloid is heterogeneous both in origin and in chemical constitution in a way similar to that which seems likely with the two types of amyloid already identified in the senile heart (Cornwell and Westermark, 1980). To establish whether this is so is fundamental because, whatever the connection between plaque amyloid and the surrounding neurites, the close association cannot be coincidental. As just mentioned, Glenner's statement (Glenner, Terry and Isersky, 1973) of amyloid being produced, and apparently secreted in certain endocrine tumours such as the medullary thyroid carcinoma, raises the possibility that plaque amyloid may result from neurosecretion, or even from a modification of one or more neuropeptides. These last have at this time no known morphological characteristics, but their ubiquitous presence within cerebral tissue means that they cannot be excluded as precursors of amyloid in the brain or even as constituents of neurofibrillary tangles. Recently Perry et al. (1981) have demonstrated that one neuropeptide, substance

P, can be induced to form polyuric fibrillary aggregates with ultrastructural dimensions similar to those reported for amyloid fibrils. There is a similar uncertainty about the origin of the paired helical filaments of the neurofibrillary tangle because there is evidence both of a possible derivation from human neurotubules (Iqbal et al., 1978; Schlaepfer, 1978; Grundke-Iqbal et al., 1979) and of a derivation from neurofilaments (Gambetti et al, 1980; Gambetti, Autilio-Gambetti and Shecket, 1981; Anderton et al., 1982). These diverse observations suggest that not all paired helical filaments are produced in the same way and that they may even derive from more than one component of the normal neuron.

Presenile and senile dementia of the Alzheimer type (Alzheimer's disease)

Alzheimer (1907a, b) reported the case of a 51-year-old woman whose memory began to deteriorate rapidly. She was excitable, she misnamed objects and was soon unable to manage at home. In hospital the patient was found to be disorientated, dysphasic and paranoid. She became mute and incontinent, and died, profoundly demented, 4 years later. The brain was generally atrophic but without focal emphasis. Using the Bielschowsky silver method, Alzheimer identified many argentophilic plaques in the cerebral cortex similar to those originally described in epilepsy by Blocq and Marinesco in 1892 and by Redlich in senile atrophy in 1898. A hitherto unrecorded form of widespread neuronal degeneration was also found which, as described in an earlier section, has come to be known as Alzheimer's neurofibrillary change or as neurofibrillary tangles.

The unusual severity of the degenerative process, as well as its early age of onset, impressed Alzheimer greatly; within a few years further examples had been reported by Bonfiglio (1908) and Perusini (1910). They believed that this disorder should be excluded from the category of senile dementia, and Kraepelin (1910), agreeing with this, called it Alzheimer's disease.

This separation, however, has never been fully accepted. Grünthal (1930b), who, like Mutrux (1958), favoured keeping the two conditions apart, stated that they were virtually the same clinically apart from the greater tendency in the presenile form for focal symptoms such as apraxia, aphasia and epileptic attacks to occur. Larsson, Sjögren and Jacobsen (1963) commented on, but did not define, clear-cut differences, at least in the advanced stages of the two disorders. Their genetic evidence, however, suggested that the senile form is connected neither with senility nor with the presenile dementia. On the pathological side Rothschild and Kasanin (1936) claimed that the pathological process tended to be more severe in Alzheimer's disease than in senile dementia, whilst many other subtle, and even trivial, differences in the local emphasis of the various histological changes were lucidly summarized by McMenemey (1963).

In summary, it seems at present to be generally agreed that the presenile form differs from the senile variety mainly in the greater likelihood of parietal lobe symptoms whilst the pathological changes vary only in the tendency for the brain in the younger form to be more consistently atrophied and for the plaque and tangle formation to be invariably widespread and severe. In extreme old age the pattern changes to the extent that the cerebral atrophy may be only slight and, while the formation of senile plaques remains intense, neurofibrillary tangles can be remarkably few in number and even, on occasions, absent. In other words, patients dying before their 80s resemble more closely the presenile group than do those which survive into their 90s. These differences are interesting and need to be studied further.

In the presenile group the illness usually appears between the ages of 50 and 60, although an occasional case in childhood has been identified (Løken and Cyvin, 1954). It is the commonest form of presenile dementia (McMenemey, 1940; Newton, 1948; Schenk, 1955; Smith, Turner and Sim, 1966; Marsden and Harrison, 1972); in later life when the incidence of dementia in the general population rises dramatically from about 5 per cent in the 60s to as high as 15 per cent in the 80s to 90s, the Alzheimer type of degeneration remains the commonest pathological process to be identified (Tomlinson, 1977). Inevitably the incidence based on studies of the general population will vary from those based on the admissions to a general or a psychiatric hospital. Nevertheless, it now seems clear that throughout Europe, the American continent and Japan this condition accounts for around 50 per cent of all demented people and contributes to another 25 per cent or so in which it is combined with the effects of cerebrovascular disease.

Women are affected more often than men, the proportion being about 2:1 until the late 70s are reached. After this the relative number of women affected becomes constantly higher. A family history of the illness is found in only a minority of patients. Pratt (1970) and Roth (1971) have both confirmed the view of Sjögren, Sjögren and Lindgren (1952) that multifactorial inheritance is probable. There is, however, a small group of cases in which the genetic factor is exceptionally strong. These are considered separately, particularly as the clinical and pathological findings tend to be atypical.

The illness lasts for an average of 5 years, but a course of only a few months (Abely, Guiraud and Dechosal, 1958) and one as long as 21 years (Newton, 1948) have been recorded.

Clinically, Alzheimer's disease shows a slowly progressive mental deterioration, almost invariably accompanied by an insidious failure of memory. Often those closest to the patient have noted this defect for even 1 or 2 years before the general deterioration has led them to seek clinical help. By the time such patients reach hospital they are commonly disorientated and confused and may be finding it increasingly difficult to look after themselves. In the earlier stages there may be periods of restlessness and excitement, sometimes with delusions and hallucinations, but apathy and inertia are the more common. A degree of agnosia or apraxia and even the occasional convulsion are not uncommon. At times there is evidence of involvement of the pyramidal or extrapyramidal pathways. Eventually past memories are all but lost, relatives and friends can no longer be recognized, and speech becomes largely incomprehensible; this extreme deterioration may be worsened by partial or complete incontinence. On the whole, the course is relentlessly downward and many, but not all, patients tend to waste away. A terminal bronchopneumonia is the commonest post-mortem finding to which death is immediately attributable. The total body weight may be as low as 30 kg in women and 35 kg in men. Inevitably all the viscera are then small, the heart weighing as little as 180 g, the liver 800 g and the kidneys each about 75 g. No constant abnormality has so far been found outside the central nervous system, although Averback (1983) has recently reported finding intracytoplasmic adrenal medullary inclusion bodies in six consecutive cases, these bodies being less frequent in normal, age-matched controls.

The brain is usually small, and particularly in the presenile period the weight may be less than 1000 g, having fallen from the expected level of 1200–1450 g. Atherosclerosis of the large cerebral vessels can be strikingly absent and is usually no more than mild. In about 20 per cent of cases, however, and especially in the elderly, a moderate degree of vascular disease develops and softenings sometimes occur. Those who adhere to the view that atherosclerosis is reversible attribute its remarkable absence in so many dements to the extreme wasting which is so often a late feature of the illness. The leptomeninges may be a little thickened and opaque; it has never been shown, however, that the thickening is greater than that in others of the same age. At autopsy the gyral atrophy is often obvious as soon as the cranial vault is removed, for the leptomeninges are seen to be lax, with pools of CSF separating them from the retracted cortex. In severe cases a gap of 1 cm or more may separate the brain from the inner table of the skull. In the brain the salient feature is the considerable, and usually symmetrical, atrophy which, although to some degree generalized, tends to affect most the frontal and temporal lobes (Fig. 20.18). Less often, according to Brun and Englund (1981), the parieto-occipital atrophy may be more marked. Although the undersurfaces of the hemispheres often appear to be relatively spared, in coronal section the widening of sulci as well as the enlarged horns of the lateral ventricles point to a more widespread atrophy. The degree of shrinkage, however, is far from constant for at one

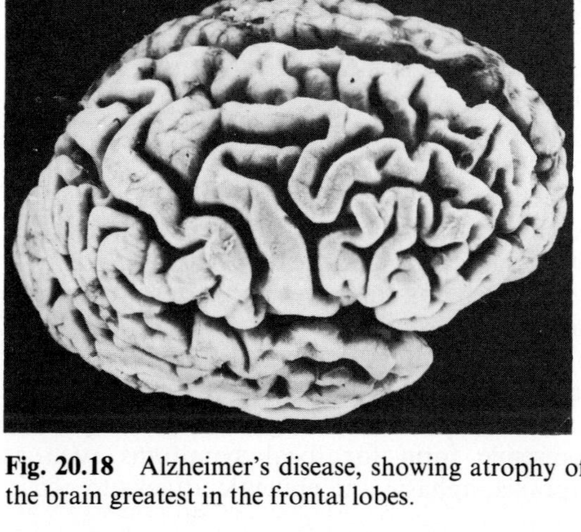

Fig. 20.18 Alzheimer's disease, showing atrophy of the brain greatest in the frontal lobes.

extreme it can be absent even though widespread histologically evident degeneration of the Alzheimer type is found. At the other extreme the macroscopic shrinkage can be so severe, and so localized, as to suggest Pick's disease although the striking 'knife-blade' atrophy of this latter condition is rarely seen.

Within these extremes an overall pattern can be recognized although there can be anomalies. Thus Corsellis (1976), using an image-analysing system, found that the average drop in volume in the cerebral hemispheres of elderly women with Alzheimer's disease was 18 per cent. Hubbard and Anderson (1981a), in a quantitative study, found that generalized cortical atrophy occurred in patients up to the age of 80 years but that the cerebral volume and degree of atrophy above that age were not uncommonly within normal limits. In other words, to generalize can be misleading. Such atrophy as was present in the older cases largely affected the temporal cortex, in comparison with the younger group in which the trend to a more diffuse gyral atrophy was significantly greater.

Ventricular size in the demented group also varies, and although at times it may be within normal limits, in the older dements particularly (Hubbard and Anderson, 1981b) a considerable degree of dilatation is usually found (Fig. 20.19). Tomlinson, Blessed and Roth (1970) estimated that the mean size of the ventricles in a series of patients with the Alzheimer type of degeneration was roughly twice that of intellectually well-preserved individuals of the same age. Exceptionally, however, the ventricular volume in the older demented group rose from the normal figure of 20–25 ml in middle age to as high as 120 ml even in normal old age, a figure of 30–50 ml being not uncommon in both the control and the demented groups. In short, the brains of most people with Alzheimer's disease, in either the presenile or the senile periods, have exceptionally large ventricles but occasionally they do not. Conversely, large ventricles are at times encountered in the intellectually intact person.

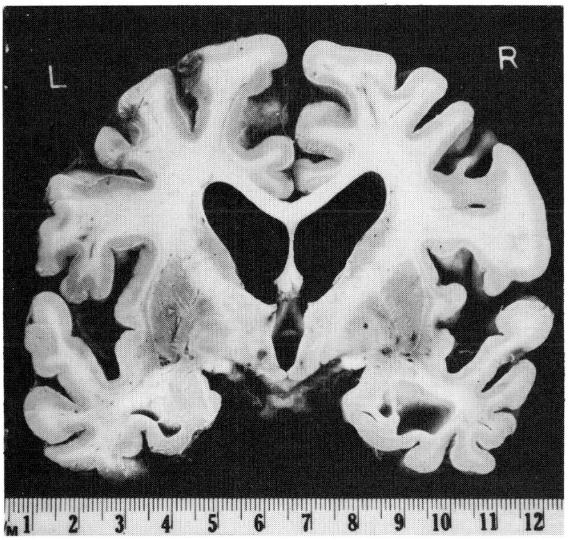

Fig. 20.19 Alzheimer's disease, showing general shrinkage of the brain in a coronal cut.

Although the great majority of cases therefore show considerable atrophy, its absence does not exclude the diagnosis because widespread microscopic change can occur without obvious shrinkage of the tissue.

Microscopically the striking feature of the cerebral cortex in Alzheimer's disease is the presence of neuritic plaques which may occur in such vast numbers as to occupy up to between one-third and one-half of the extent of the cortex in silver stained preparations (Fig. 20.20). In advanced cases no area of cerebral cortex is spared, although concentrations of plaques in the parahippocampal and temporal gyri often appear to be greater than elsewhere in the brain. Plaques occur in any or all layers of the cortex although commonly they are relatively few in the subpial, or first cortical, layer. They are often present in vast numbers in the cortex around the bottoms of sulci and may appear to spread into the subjacent parts of the white matter. They can be

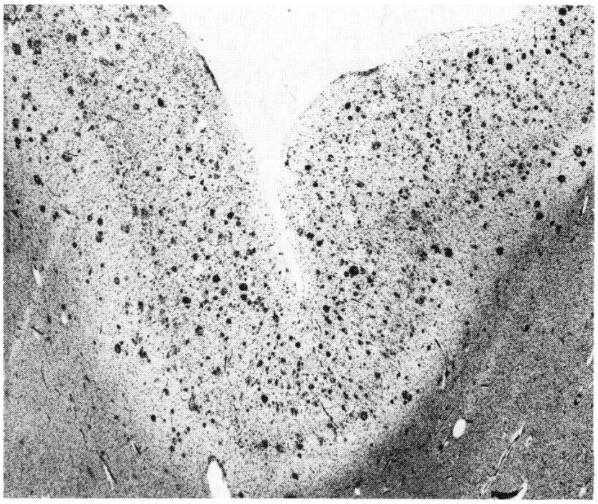

Fig. 20.20 Alzheimer's disease, showing many argyrophilic plaques in the cerebral cortex. King's silver method for amyloid.

found within all subcortical grey matter structures and may be very numerous throughout the hypothalamus, in the lateral walls of the third ventricle and mamillary bodies, and much less numerous but quite striking in the tegmentum of the midbrain and to a lesser extent the tegmentum of the pons; very occasionally they occur in the medulla and rarely in the cerebellar cortex. They vary in individual cases in size and in clarity of staining in silver, as compared with other preparations, and in the prominence of an amyloid core. In many instances in which silver impregnations have been used, individual plaques may coalesce to form irregular masses of abnormal fibrillary and granular material from 0.5 to 1 mm across. As already outlined, electron microscopy shows that the plaques consist of vast numbers of grossly enlarged neuritic processes mingled with astrocytes and microglia and with, in the majority, a demonstrable central deposit of amyloid. The recently developed immunoperoxidase technique for glial acidic protein clearly demonstrates the focal tangles of astrocytic fibres which are associated with a plaque both in this condition and at times in a normal old person.

Intermingled with the plaques is the second striking microscopic change found in this condition, for a variable number of nerve cells will show neurofibrillary degeneration. In most cases very large numbers of cortical neurons are affected by this change, and in well-stained preparations 'entangled' cells will usually be found in every field of the neocortex. It should be emphasized that different silver staining techniques show differing numbers of neurofibrillary tangles and that within any such technique, however standardized, the vagaries of the method occasionally result in difficulty in recognition of the tangles. In the present writers' experience von Braunmühl's method and King's procedure for amyloid demonstrate plaques and tangles uniformly well. Other methods, such as the Bielschowsky technique, and perhaps particularly the Glees–Marsland method, which is often used on paraffin sections, are unreliable in terms of showing total numbers of plaques and tangles even when these can be demonstrated by other techniques. The recently described variation of the Palmgren method using paraffin-embedded tissues (Cross, 1982) gives a particularly elegant picture of neurofibrillary tangles. Again, although tangles are commonly present in every section taken from the neocortex, the change is often most intense in the hippocampus (Fig.

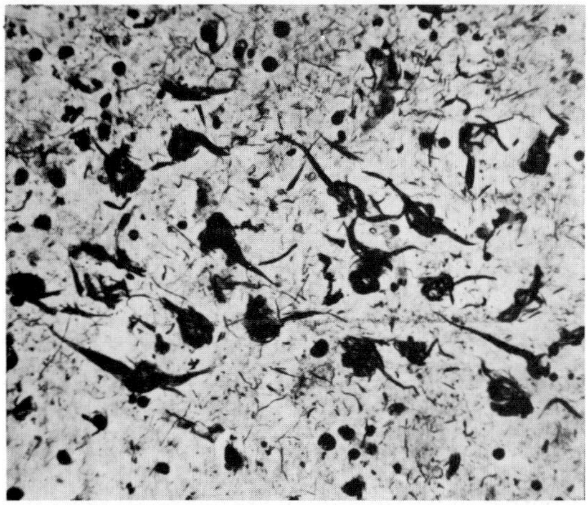

Fig. 20.21 Alzheimer's disease. Hippocampus showing neurofibrillary change in many neurons. von Braunmühl ×120.

20.21), the parahippocampal gyrus and the amygdaloid nucleus. In the last-named site they are often accompanied by particularly intense plaque formation. Despite large numbers of tangles shown up by special techniques, the neocortex in particular may look strikingly less abnormal when haematoxylin and eosin is used. Tangles are less readily visualized by this method or indeed by cresyl violet.

Neurofibrillary tangles can occur in the neurons of the deep grey matter but are relatively uncommon in the basal ganglia and thalamus. In contrast, they are often strikingly visible in the periventricular tissues along the wall of the third ventricle and in the brain stem. Here the midline septal nuclei and the neurons in the periaqueductal grey matter of the midbrain tegmentum may be heavily involved (see Fig. 20.22). This involvement of brain stem neurons by neurofibrillary tangle formation may be as striking a marker of Alzheimer's disease as is plaque and tangle formation in the neocortex. Tangles are also typically present in immense numbers in the Sommer sector of the hippocampus and throughout the medial nuclei of the amygdaloid complex and its overlying cortex. Indeed, as stated earlier, Ball (1976) has identified a significantly greater number of tangles in the diseased hippocampus than in that of the normal person of the same age.

As already noted, many experienced microscopists have long considered that, by using cells stains such as an aniline dye or haematoxylin and eosin, considerable reductions in the numbers of cortical nerve cells can be demonstrated in this condition—an observation, moreover, which is compatible with the manifest reduction in the amount of cortical tissue as shown by the gyral shrinkage. However, the position has become less clear following systematic neuronal counts being made on standard area or volumes of cortex taken from both demented and non-demented subjects. Tomlinson and Henderson (1976), for example, were unable to demonstrate any significant differences between age-matched controls and aged dements. Terry et al. (1977) at first seemed to agree with them. More recently, however, both Terry and his co-workers (1981) and Mountjoy et al. (1983) have used computerized image-analysing systems for cell counting and have demonstrated a significant loss of larger neurons in a given unit volume of tissue, particularly in the frontal and temporal cortices. Both of these groups of workers found that the loss, which is restricted to larger neurons in the deeper cortical layers, may reach 30–40 per cent but it was emphasized that such a reduction is not a constant feature in relation either to the different layers of the cerebral cortex or to different cortical areas.

Abnormalities in nerve processes Significant changes in nerve cell processes also are widespread in the neocortex in Alzheimer's disease though these changes are not readily appreciated without special techniques. Senile plaques largely consist of abnormal nerve endings, principally axonal; dendritic changes in old age have already been mentioned but evidence now exists through quantitative studies (Mehraein et al, 1975) that bouton and dendritic loss is greater in the cortical pyramidal cells in Alzheimer's disease than in age matched controls and that the loss is more severe in presenile cases. Buell and Coleman (1979) confirmed this loss of dendritic spines and branching and also demonstrated that plasticity of dendritic arborization persists in normal old age but is greatly diminished in senile dementia of Alzheimer type. Thus all aspects of the neuronal system are morphologically grossly disturbed in this disorder and since cell loss is not as extreme as was previously thought and the swollen axon terminals in senile plaques presumably increase cortical volume, the diminution of the latter in Alzheimer's disease may be very significantly contributed to by dendritic loss.

Reduction in nucleolar size and neuronal RNA Although knowledge of some neuronal populations in the normal and the ageing brain and in Alzheimer's disease has expanded greatly over the last two decades, other quantitative studies are still needed. On subjective examination many hypothalamic nuclei, neurons of the basal ganglia, thalamus and the majority of those in the midbrain and stem appear unaffected by the disorder. They certainly show no gross loss of cell numbers. Neurofibrillary degeneration is uncommon in the majority of such cell groups although occurring almost anywhere to a slight extent. In a series of investigations (Mann, Yates and Barton, 1977; Mann and Sinclair, 1978; Mann, Lincoln and Yates, 1981; Mann, 1982) evidence has been produced that neurons throughout the many parts of the brain thought to be subjectively normal show two important differences by comparison with age-matched controls: a nucleolus of reduced size and a reduction of cytoplasmic RNA. Pyramidal cells of the cortex and hippocampus are said to show both these features in Alzheimer's disease but, additionally, neurons sited in structures not thought to be affected by the pathological process of Alzheimer's disease, such as Purkinje cells of the cerebellum and the cells of the inferior olive, also have small nucleoli and an abnormally small quantity of cytoplasmic RNA. The authors have deduced from these findings two major and important conclusions: first, that in Alzheimer's disease the whole of the central nervous system is involved and, secondly, that the process involves neuronal protein metabolism. Evidence that neuronal protein metabolism is affected in the disorder is confirmed by the knowledge that neurofibrillary tangles are an abnormal form of fibrillary protein, but the possibility that protein metabolism is affected throughout the whole of the central nervous system is a revolutionary suggestion which requires confirmation or rebuttal. Little confirmation has been so far published of the findings of Mann and his colleagues on morphological grounds, and indeed Uemura and Hartmann (1978), using different techniques, failed to confirm loss of cytoplasmic RNA. Some chemical evidence for reduction of total protein in grey matter of brains in cases of Alzheimer's disease has existed for some time.

Suzuki, Katzman and Korey (1965) demonstrated decreased total protein in the cortex in Alzheimer's disease and a decline in protein lipid ratio. Bowen et al. (1977) have reported a reduction in the contents of temporal lobe RNA and a reduction in the ratio of RNA to DNA. Crapper, Quittkat and De Boni (1979) have reported a reduction in the transcriptionally active euchromatic fraction of neuronal chromatin in cases of Alzheimer's disease, suggesting a possible defect in the level of transcription. These studies, therefore, add to the indirect evidence that protein synthesis may be defective in this disorder. More recently, Sajdel-Sulkowska et al. (1983) have produced more direct evidence of defective protein production by the isolation and characterization of functionally active mRNA from post-mortem tissues, the yield of mRNA being significantly lower from cases of SDAT than from normal age-matched controls. Additionally, the translational activity of the mRNA as judged by *in vitro* reticulocyte protein synthesis was significantly less than that of controls, and Alzheimer's diseased brains synthesized lesser amounts of nearly all neuropeptides, including tubulin, by comparison with normal brains.

At this stage it needs to be pointed out that the latter impressive studies were done on samples of cerebral cortex which in Alzheimer's disease contain vast numbers of neurons with neurofibrillary tangle formation. It has been known for over 10 years (Dayan and Ball, 1973) and confirmed more recently by Uemura and Hartmann (1978) and Mann, Lincoln and Yates (1981) that tangle-bearing neurons have a very considerable reduction in nucleolar size and, it is said, in content of RNA than non-tangle bearing neurons, so the results reported by Sajdel-Sulkowska et al. (1983) could to some extent have been anticipated. What is now urgently required is a similar investigation of protein synthesis from neurons in sites such as the cerebellum, thalamus and nuclei of the stem where the characteristic changes, and particularly neurofibrillary degeneration, are not to be found.

In an occasional case the formation of plaques and of tangles appears to be part of a general disintegration of the neuronal population, particularly in the outer cortical layers, and this may lead to a degree of vacuolation. Brun and Englund (1981) have emphasized the severity of this change in the parietal lobe and posterior cingular gyrus. In the present writers' experience such alterations have been found to only a relatively minor degree, even when both the dementia and the cortical atrophy have been severe. Nevertheless, the findings, even if novel, emphasize that a great deal is still to be learned about the relationships, and the relative importance to intellectual deterioration, of neuronal change and loss, and the presence of tangles and plaques. Indeed, although these massive abnormalities of structure would be expected to interfere with neuronal activity and synaptic transmission, remarkably little is known about their precise role in Alzheimer's disease. In relation to plaques, even though the presynaptic terminals within them may be abnormal, the synapse itself may appear to retain its normal structure. It is therefore conceivable that if the formation of plaques were to be prevented or reversed by some pharmacological influence, and the amyloid were to be reabsorbed, a return to more normal activity might be achieved. Tangles, too, might be imagined to be reversible. However, until the millenium, the position remains that many studies, starting with that of Corsellis in 1962, have demonstrated the association of dementia with the presence of large numbers of neocortical plaques and tangles by comparison with non-demented subjects. As a consequence, the conclusion has been drawn (Roth, Tomlinson and Blessed, 1966; Blessed, Tomlinson and Roth, 1968; Tomlinson, Blessed and Roth, 1970; Constantinidis, 1978) that it is both the distribution and the quantity of these structures which distinguish Alzheimer's disease from non-demented subjects. Constantinides found that cases in which numerous neocortical tangles were present tended more often to have been aphasic, apraxic and agnosic, whereas this was not usually the case when only plaques were found. Such cases, in which neocortical plaques are present without tangles, form an interesting group but they have been generally considered to be restricted to only a small minority of elderly dements, although Terry et al. (1982) found the figure to be as high as 50 per cent.

Until the last few years, interest concentrated on the cerebral cortex to the neglect of other areas. Now, however, the importance of structural, and particularly neurochemical, changes in the deeper grey matter is becoming recognized. Thus there are several neurotransmitter substances which have so far been identified as having a role to play in the pathological process. These include the serotoninergic, noradrenergic and cholinergic groups. With regard to the first, the distribution of many neurofibrillary tangles in the brain stem, and particularly in the periventricular grey and midline raphe nuclei (Ishii, 1965), has raised the possibility of a specific involvement of serotoninergic neurons. Perhaps one of the most interesting areas is the locus ceruleus, which is considered to be the major source of noradrenergic fibres to the cerebral hemispheres. It has been known for some time that its neuronal population tends not only to drop with normal ageing (Vijayashankar and Brody, 1973) but also for the drop to be particularly severe in Alzheimer's disease (Forno, 1978; Mann et al., 1980). Tomlinson et al. (1980) have confirmed these observations but have gone on to produce quantitative evidence that the severity of the neuronal loss was associated with the degree of plaque formation in the brain. Bondareff, Mountjoy and Roth (1982) have been unable to confirm this but have found nevertheless evidence to suggest that the greater the cell loss the more profound was the dementia. No corresponding drop, however, in cortical noradrenaline levels has so far been demonstrated in the relevant cases because assays on post-mortem or on biopsy tissue have proved impracticable, the latter because of its rarity. Perry et al. (1981) have nevertheless been able to record a drop in the metabolites of noradrenaline within the cerebral hemispheres although this was not correlated with the loss of neurons from the locus ceruleus.

The most widely known of the neurochemical abnormalities in Alzheimer's disease are those which affect the cholinergic system and which are probably associated with a diminution in other neurotransmitter systems as well as in the levels of certain neuropeptides in various parts of the brain. The cholinergic deficits in the cerebral cortex were first demonstrated by three groups working in the UK (Bowen et al., 1976; Davies and Maloney, 1976; Perry et al., 1977). The origin of cholinergic fibres running to the cerebral cortex appears to be largely, if not solely, from the basal nucleus of Meynert. This is an anatomical area which has neuronal elements in relation to the substantia innominata, the anterior septal nuclei and the diagonal band of Broca. Many cells within this nuclear complex show neurofibrillary tangles in Alzheimer's disease, and Whitehouse et al. (1981) have reported massive neuronal loss, although Candy et al. (1983) have found in this condition that cell numbers overlapped to some extent with those found in normal old age.

Arendt et al. (1983) have reported, from an extensive study, that patients with Alzheimer's disease had a mean neuronal loss of 67 per cent compared with controls. This loss, however, was slightly less than that found in idiopathic Parkinsonism—a condition in which, if dementia occurs, it is of a milder degree than in Alzheimer's disease. The relation of the cholinergic deficit to the dementia in Alzheimer's disease seems, therefore, to be left in doubt. For a more comprehensive review of the neurochemical findings, the reader is referred to Bowen (1981) and Marchbanks (1982).

Familial cases A family history of the illness has been reported many times. Schottky (1932) described the disease in father and daughter with seven presumed cases in four generations. English (1942) reported it in four siblings and in the daughter of one of them. Wheelan (1959) recorded two proved and four presumed cases in a family of ten, including the mother. The parents of the juvenile case described by Løken and Cyvin (1954) were first cousins. Lowenberg and Waggoner (1934) described a man who was considered to have developed the illness at the age of 32, and four of whose five children developed the same clinical conditions at much the same age. One was proved histologically; the father's parents were first cousins.

A first-cousin marriage was also reported in a family studied by McMenemey et al. (1939). Only one necropsy was performed but the condition had affected clinically three out of four siblings and one child. Grünthal and Wenger (1939) described four clinical examples in two generations with pathological confirmation in a sister and brother, whilst Essen-Möller (1946) reported on a father, son and daughter with the disease. Marconi and Piazzesi (1965) reported on the genetic and cytogenetic aspects of an affected family. Davidson and Robertson (1955) encountered it in one of identical twins; this patient, whose symptoms began at the age of 50 and who died 19 years later, had spent her life in Edinburgh, while the sister, living mostly in Australia, was still healthy aged 73. Hunter, Dayan and Wilson (1972) reported the illness, lasting 15 years, in a woman of 64 whose monozygotic twin sister was clinically not affected and who died 2 years later of carcinoma. These authors pointed out that not a single pair of twins of whom both were affected has so far been reported and they, like Davidson and Robertson, suggested that the study of exogenous rather than inborn factors may prove more fruitful.

In the last few years, however, at least two pairs of identical twins have been reported. Sharman et al. (1979) described and illustrated two identical brothers who, when aged 38, developed a dementing illness within 3 months of each other. Genetic studies were not done but the authors quoted the statement by Shields (1962) that 'the fact that they were frequently mistaken for each other was the best single piece of evidence in favour of monozygosity'. The dementia ran a curiously similar course for nearly 4 years and they died within 3 months of each other. The histological findings in the atrophied brains confirmed the diagnosis of Alzheimer's disease. Their mother had died demented when aged 42; her brain had been considered atrophied but no microscopy was done. In 1983 Kilpatrick, Burns and Blumbergs described and illustrated an instance of genetically proven identical twin sisters who both began to dement when aged 50. Frontal biopsies, which showed the typical Alzheimer changes, including congophilic angiopathy, confirmed the diagnosis but, although deteriorating for 6 years, both were still alive in 1983. They also quoted Cook, Schneck and Clark's (1981) pair of identical twins in whom the onset of the disease was separated by 9 years. Kilpatrick Burns and Blumbergs considered that 'at least in cases of familial Alzheimer's disease, the disorder is inherited by a single mutant gene'.

It is noteworthy that Alzheimer's disease was found to be more common in Gothenburg than in Stockholm, whereas the prevalence was reversed in Pick's disease (Sjögren, Sjögren and Lindgren, 1952). The literature on the genetics of Alzheimer's disease was reviewed by Pratt (1970). Slater and Cowie (1971) concluded—mainly from the comprehensive studies by Sjögren and his colleagues, quoted above, and by Constantinidis, Garrone and de Ajuriaguerra (1962)—that the mode of inheritance is compatible with a polygenic basis but that in a few pedigrees a dominant inheritance has occurred. In the former there is evidence of female sex preponderance and in the latter of sex equality.

Apart from the familial instances of Alzheimer's disease, it is not unusual to encounter psychiatric illness in the families of affected patients. Schenk (1955), for example, found a history of dementia in the near relative in 10 out of 35 cases and of severe neurological disease in 15.

Atypical cases A small number have been recorded in which the clinical, and particularly the pathological, picture has been unusual. Sometimes it is the sporadic case which is affected; more often, and in a more striking way, there is a familial factor.

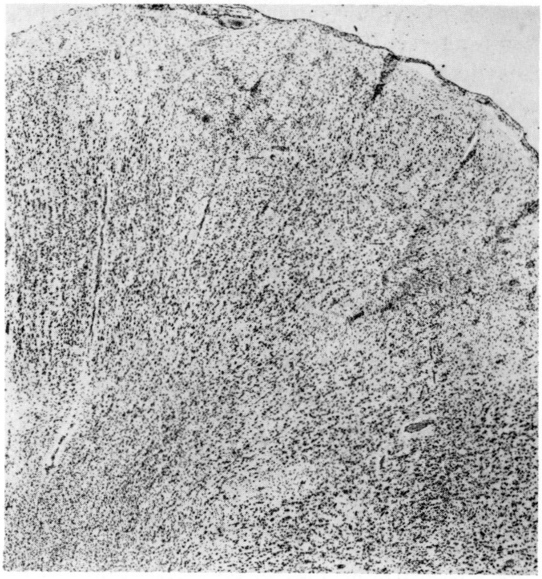

Fig. 20.22 Atypical Alzheimer's disease. Frontal cortex showing patchy neuronal necrosis and gliosis due to hyaline arteriolar degeneration and congophilic angiopathy. Nissl ×25.

Sporadic cases Schnitzler (1911) reported on a 37-year-old woman who died demented and in whom neurofibrillary tangles were plentiful but senile plaques were not seen. Weimann (1921), Goodman (1953) and Raskin and Ehrenberg (1956) reported similar instances. A second group of atypical cases are those in which the usual features of Alzheimer's disease are combined with those of Pick's disease. Liebers (1933, 1939) described two cases with severe Pick-like atrophy—one in which the parieto-occipital regions were involved whilst the other affected the frontal lobes. Other examples include those reported by Seitelberger and Jellinger (1958), Kreindler, Hornet and Appel (1959) and Smith and Lantos (1983) (see also Smith and Lantos (1983) for further references). Thirdly, a degree of congophilic, or amyloid, angiopathy (as described earlier in this chapter), and usually accompanied by atypical plaque formation (Fig. 20.22), has long been known to occur not only in the occasional case of typical Alzheimer's disease but also in the brains of some non-demented people (Neumann, 1960). At times, however, the amyloid vascular component is so obtrusive as to overshadow the other alzheimerian features; because the plaque formation which tends to occur with it can also be strikingly bizarre, an aberrant group of patients, usually with a family history, have come to be identified. The first two families reported were those of Worster-Drought, Greenfield and McMenemy (1940, 1944). Several others have followed and all have been reviewed by Griffiths et al. (1982). The usual clinical picture has been one of progressive dementia coupled with the onset of a spastic paralysis. At first the neuropathological picture, at least in some cases or to some authors, was reminiscent of Alzheimer's disease but its earlier attachment to this disorder is now considered untenable and its stands at present apart in a separate, if unnamed, category (Griffiths et al., 1982).

A further complicating factor, however, has now been added by the identification of vascular congophilia in other disorders. One is the occurrence of amyloid angiopathy in association with giant cell arteritis (Reid and Maloney, 1974). Another is the 'hereditary cerebral haemorrhage with amyloidosis' reported from Iceland by Gudmundsson et al. (1972), and there are several similar, but non-familial, examples reported from other countries in which congophilic angiopathy has led to intracranial bleeding (Jellinger, 1976b; Griffiths et al., 1982). Furthermore, amyloid vascular change with plaques was described in a 14-year-old demented boy by Shaw (1979) whilst the same phenomenon was recently identified in a form of familial cerebellar ataxia with dementia by Love and Duchen (1982). The last report, together with that of the family reported by Adam et al. (1982), brings to mind the complex Gerstmann–Sträussler syndrome of spinocerebellar ataxia with dementia for which Scheinker described the pathological basis (Gerstmann, Sträussler and Scheinker, 1936). This consisted, in effect, of intense amyloid plaque deposits, an amyloid-like vascular change and a vacuolar state in the cerebral grey matter. Other reports of this obscure condition have gradually accumulated and in 1981 Masters, Gajdusek and Gibbs were able to conclude, from their inoculation work, that 'at least some cases of the Gerstmann–Sträussler syndrome are variants of Creutzfeldt–Jakob disease'.

This short section therefore began by discussing 'atypical Alzheimer's disease' and has imperceptibly ended in the even more complex problem of the atypical forms of Creutzfeldt–Jakob disease.

Experimental production of tangles and plaques

Alzheimer's disease is not known to occur spontaneously in any animal species, and, so far, no experimental model has been developed in which the histological changes are reproduced. A small number of plaques may occur in ageing dogs (Wisniewski et al., 1970) and rhesus monkeys (Wisniewski, Ghetti and Terry, 1973); helical filaments were found in the distended neurites of the plaques in the monkeys but not the dogs, but in neither were neurons with tangles found.

Light-microscopic tangles consisting of straight but not helically twisted filaments have been produced in a range of experimental models by a variety of techniques, none of which seems likely to have direct relevance to Alzheimer's disease. Klatzo, Wisniewski and Streicher (1965) and Terry and Pena (1965) produced large numbers of intracerebral tangles by direct inoculation of aluminium phosphate. Intracerebral injection of colchicine (Wisniewski and Terry, 1967) and of mitotic spindle inhibitors (Schochet, Lampert and Earle, 1968) also produced large numbers of tangles. Mitotic spindle inhibitors and other substances capable of producing tangles experimentally are tubulin-binding agents (Ghetti, 1980). The possibility that aluminium is more directly related to Alzheimer's disease has been raised by the finding of Crapper, Krishnan and Quittkat (1976) of raised brain aluminium levels in patients with Alzheimer's disease; furthermore, De Boni et al, (1976), have successfully produced tangles by the use of systemic aluminium. However, a dispute has developed around the question of aluminium concentrations in the brain in Alzheimer disease, and McDermott et al. (1977) have failed to confirm the increased aluminium concentrations. Peri and Brody (1980) have demonstrated by the use of x-ray spectrometry that the nuclei of tangle-bearing neurons contained foci of aluminium; Duckett and Galle (1980), however, have found no evidence of any role for aluminium in the pathogenesis of tangles in electron microprobe studies. Furthermore, greatly increased brain concentrations of aluminium, which may occur in patients on haemodialysis, are not associated with either plaque or tangle formation (McDermott et al., 1978). Further study of this problem will continue, and includes the necessity to determine not only whether raised aluminium levels are consistent findings in Alzheimer's disease but also whether they are primary or secondary events.

Until 1975 plaques had not been demonstrated in any animal experimental model but Bruce and Fraser (1975) and Bruce, Dickinson and Fraser (1976) have demonstrated plaque formation in certain strains of mice infected with particular strains of scrapie agent. Many of these plaques consisted of massive deposits of amyloid but Wisniewski, Bruce and Fraser (1975) have shown that some were ultrastructurally similar to human plaques in that the amyloid was surrounded by swollen neurites of similar constitution to those found in the human plaque although not containing paired helical filaments. Dickinson, Meikel and Fraser (1968, 1969) demonstrated that the incubation period of scrapie was dependent on the genetic constitution of particular mice, and it seems possible that the particular features of scrapie agents which induce plaque formation in genetically susceptible mice may well be identified. These observations, however, along with the similarities which exist between scrapie and the disorders of kuru and Creutzfeldt-Jakob disease have raised speculation on the possibility that a transmissible agent may be responsible for Alzheimer's disease. Nevertheless, attempts to transmit Alzheimer's disease to experimental animals have been reported in only two cases of familial Alzheimer's disease (Gibbs, Gadjusek and Amyer, 1979) and have not been successful in any case of non-familial Alzheimer's disease nor so far have they been reported in any other instance of the familial variety. Paired helical filaments have, however, been produced in cultured fetal neurons treated with high dilutions of extract of cerebral cortex from cases of Alzheimer's disease (De Boni and Crapper, 1978; Crapper-McLachlan and De Boni, 1980). The latter authors also reported production of paired helical filaments in cultured human fetal neurons exposed to cerebrospinal fluid from cases of Alzheimer's disease. The same finding also occurred in one case exposed to normal cerebrospinal fluid. These findings clearly raise the possibility that some substance capable of stimulating the development of paired helical filaments may occur in the human brain and possibly in the normal human brain. It must, however, be stressed that, despite the intense interest and investigation into the possibility that Alzheimer's disease may be due to a transmissible agent of similar nature to that which produces Creutzfeldt-Jakob disease, kuru or scrapie, there is so far no direct evidence of this (as further discussed below).

Dementia in Parkinson's disease

Many patients with parkinsonism become depressed or demented (Mayeux, 1982). The former is the more frequent, and it is usually unrelated either to the severity of the parkinsonian features or to the age, sex or treatment (Horn, 1974; Robins, 1976; Mayeux et al., 1981). Studies of the prevalence of dementia in Parkinson's disease, although not numerous, have demonstrated some degree of mental deterioration in between 20 per cent (Pollack and Hornabrook, 1966) and 40 per cent (Celesia and Wanamaker, 1972). In a study of 520 patients, and with the criteria and methods for assessing dementia described, Liebermann et al. (1979) found 29 per cent to have been demented.

Descriptions of the features of the dementia in Parkinson's disease have frequently emphasized disturbances of visuospatial discrimination, with lesser evidence of memory or language disorder. Whether or not these unusual defects of perceptual-motor performance justify a diagnosis of dementia is discussed by Mayeux (1982). Nevertheless, evidence of intellectual deficits have usually been considered to have a close relationship with the severity of the physical disability of the patients (Celesia and Wanamaker, 1972; Liebermann et al., 1979; Mayeux et al., 1981), and in a number of studies, dementia has been particularly associated with increased age. Thus Liebermann et al. (1979) found demented parkinsonian patients to be, on average, 5 years older than non-demented patients, to have poorer response to levodopa and to have a shorter illness. Garron, Klawans and Narin (1972) observed a similar association between the later onset of parkinsonism and an increased tendency to intellectual deterioration. Sroka et al. (1981) have reported that two groups existed: 'typical' parkinsonism patients in whom impairment of cognition, reasoning and memory occurred in 15 per cent; and 'atypical' patients who, though of similar age, had an illness of shorter duration with a high incidence of dementia (68 per cent).

Developing from clinical studies of progressive supranuclear palsy and of parkinsonism has come the concept of a recognizable clinical syndrome which includes a milder degree of dementia than that which occurs in Alzheimer's disease and lacks the aphasic, apraxic and agnostic features common in that disorder. The term 'subcortical dementia' has been coined for this condition (Albert, Feldman and Willis, 1974; Albert, 1978; Mayeux et al., 1981). Mayeux et al. (1981) found a consistently less severe dementia in Parkinson's disease by comparison with cases diagnosed as Alzheimer's disease; indeed the dementia in the former was never as severe as the least demented of the Alzheimer group. Additionally, the language disorders, so common and severe in Alzheimer's disease, were absent in the parkinsonian patients.

These observations on the clinical features of the dementia of Parkinson's disease are of importance in relation to the pathological considerations because they have concentrated attention on the probability that disorders of the basal ganglia, or midbrain, without definable neuropathological changes in the cortex (though not necessarily without chemical changes) or white matter, may give rise to a recognizable dementia. This concept has been challenged in relation to Parkinson's disease by the assertion, in a retrospective study, that the dementia in that disorder was due to coexistent Alzheimer's disease (Hakim and Mathiewson, 1978). Boller et al. (1980) found neuropathological evidence of Alzheimer's disease in nine severely demented cases of Parkinson's disease, though a less certain relationship of such changes to the milder intellectual deterioration in seven other patients. These recent studies, both clinical and pathological, have therefore raised the controversial possibility of a close relationship between Parkinson's disease and Alzheimer's disease, although, so far, this relationship can only be regarded as unproven. Nevertheless, some neuropathological features of the two disorders are similar, and, in view of their neurochemical implications, need review now and much more detailed future study.

Idiopathic Parkinson's disease (see also Chapter 15), much the commonest type of parkinsonism, is overwhelmingly characterized by substantial nigral pigmented cell loss and gliosis, with Lewy body formation in some remaining nigral cells and elsewhere (Lipkin, 1959; Forno, 1982); cell loss is also heavy in the locus ceruleus and nucleus of Meynert. In a small minority of cases severe diffuse cell loss in the substantia nigra is accompanied by neurofibrillary degeneration, a finding typical of postencephalitic parkinsonism, although occasionally found in the absence of a history of encephalitis lethargica (Forno, 1982). These appearances contrast strongly with the findings in the substantia nigra in Alzheimer's disease at any age, for in that disorder there is usually no obvious loss of pigmented cells and neurofibrillary tangles are few in number. Moreover, the majority of tangled neurons in SDAT are clustered in a small group at the most medial extremity of the nucleus and not distributed throughout the pigmented cells (Tomlinson et al., 1984). The changes in the substantia nigra in the two disorders are therefore distinct. The possibility that Lewy bodies are present in greater numbers in the substantia nigra in Alzheimer's disease than in age-matched controls has been raised (Woodard, 1962), and in a recent examination (Tomlinson et al., 1984) of 81 cases of SDAT the incidence was found to be slightly higher than in control material; this interesting possibility needs further investigation.

The majority of reports on Parkinson's disease present no evidence of cortical changes suggestive of Alzheimer's disease. In a recent study (Tomlinson et al., 1984) of 36 cases of clinically typical parkinsonism with classic focal neuron loss, gliosis and Lewy body formation in the substantia nigra, 24 cases showed no suggestion of Alzheimer's disease neuropathologically, although in six (four commencing as Parkinson's disease and becoming severely demented) neuropathological changes of both disorders were present, a surprisingly large number if the association was coincidental. Six cases showed numerous cortical plaques although without tangle formation there or in other sites expected in Alzheimer's disease. These findings certainly deny any regular association between idiopathic Parkinson's disease and Alzheimer's disease, but suggest, as did the findings of Boller et al. (1980), that a severe dementia developing in Parkinson's disease is frequently due to Alzheimer's disease, and an association between the diseases, not explicable as coincidence, may exist.

Alzheimer's disease certainly does not account, however, for the frequency with which dementia, usually of a mild variety, is found in Parkinson's disease. Loss of cells from the locus ceruleus in both Parkinson's disease and Alzheimer's disease has been recorded for many years, and quantification in Alzheimer's disease (Tomlinson, Irving and Blessed, 1981; Bondareff,

Mountjoy and Roth, 1982) has established that this cell loss, at least in SDAT, is not always severe although may be as great as 90 per cent. This nucleus is considered to be the site of origin of cortical noradrenergic innervation, but no correlation between the degree of cell loss and cortical BDH (a principal metabolite of noradrenaline) has been found (Perry et al., 1981) Quantitative studies of the locus ceruleus neuron population in Parkinson's disease do not appear to be available, but subjectively the destruction of cells appears as great in many instances.

Recent studies have demonstrated that cell loss from the nucleus of Meynert, the nucleus of origin of cortical cholinergic fibres, is probably greater in Parkinson's disease than in SDAT (Arendt et al., 1983). Loss of cortical choline acetyltransferase (CAT) has been a consistent finding in Alzheimer's disease, and although originally recorded as normal in Parkinson's disease, recent studies have demonstrated a considerable diminution in cortical CAT in a small number of cases of demented Parkinson's disease. The possibility therefore exists that the shared common features of cell loss from the locus ceruleus and (particularly) the nucleus of Meynert, may contribute to the dementia to be found in Parkinson's disease and Alzheimer's disease. The difference in incidence, character and severity of the dementia in the two disorders clearly indicates that the changes in these nuclei do no more than contribute to the dementia; indeed, if cell loss in the two nuclei is found to be as severe in non-demented as in demented Parkinson's disease, changes in both nuclei can be eliminated as the primary source of the dementia in both disorders, as may the loss of cholinergic input to the cortex. This last would be an interesting addition to knowledge of the significance of cholinergic innervation and its relevance (or lack of it) to the dementia of Alzheimer's disease, since it has arisen from the study of Parkinson's disease. Finally, in Alzheimer's disease, involvement of raphe nuclei of the upper stem (probably serotoninergic neurons) and elsewhere by tangle formation is usually intense. A similar but less intense involvement by Lewy bodies occurs in Parkinson's disease. Whether or not the neurons in these cell groups are diminished in either disorder appears to be unknown but it is not obviously present to subjective assessment.

A summary of the present position of Parkinson's disease and the dementia which frequently develops and its relationship to the neuropathology of the disorder is as follows. The common mild dementia of Parkinson's disease is not explained by the presence of Alzheimer's disease or Alzheimer-type cortical changes because the cortex in Parkinson's disease is usually normal in appearance. Cell loss from the locus ceruleus and nucleus of Meynert, similar in quantity to that found in Alzheimer's disease, may contribute to the dementia, but the demonstration of severe cell loss from these nuclei in non-demented cases of Parkinson's disease would clearly throw doubt on even that possibility. Substantial nigral damage and the consequential striatal disturbances of function, possibly combined with the other nuclear damage in Parkinson's disease, may be the explanation of the so-called 'subcortical dementia'. Severe dementia, however, in most cases of Parkinson's disease is probably due to Alzheimer's disease, and the association of the two disorders may prove to be too frequent to be coincidental.

Arteriosclerotic or multi-infarct dementia

Cerebral softening is the second commonest cause of dementia in the elderly, accounting for 10–20 per cent of cases over the age of 65 years, and, combined with SDAT, contributing to a further 10 per cent (Tomlinson, Blessed and Roth, 1970; Jellinger, 1976a). In total, in 25–35 per cent of demented old subjects cerebral ischaemic lesions are a factor in the dementing process. Over the past 10 years the term multi-infarct dementia has become widely accepted as the most appropriate designation for that form of severe emotional, intellectual and memory disturbance which results from ischaemic damage to the brain. Not only do the subjects concerned frequently have historical evidence of one or more strokes, but also neurological evidence compatible with such occurrences is usually found and the presence of infarcts or focal enlarged sulci is demonstrated by CT scans (Radue et al., 1978); one or more softenings of variable size in the cerebral hemispheres is the characteristic finding in the brain at autopsy (Tomlinson, Blessed and Roth, 1970).

The diagnosis in life of multi-infarct, as opposed to a degenerative (Alzheimer type), dementia is made on the basis of the sudden onset of dementia, the occurrence of one or more strokes, a tendency for a fluctuating course with some day-to-day variation as well as some evidence of spontaneous improvement in the early part of the illness, a stepwise progression with sudden worsening of the mental state, hypertension, evidence of coronary or other major arterial disease, a labile emotional state and a tendency for a degree of insight to be retained for much longer than occurs in the degenerative group. The presence of these features is frequently used to construct an 'ischaemic' score as a diagnostic aid to the differentiation of the vascular dementias (Hachinski, Lassen and Marshall, 1974; Hachinski et al., 1975); such a procedure has been tested and generally validated by post-mortem studies (Rosen et al., 1980) although total accuracy in clinical diagnosis is not achieved, occasional cases of apparent multi-infarct dementia having Alzheimer's disease with one or more minor strokes, and occasional cases of multi-infarct dementia being free from the clinical evidence of stroke disease. The most frequent cause of diagnostic confusion is the presence of strokes in patients with Alzheimer's disease—a mixed dementia. Because of the severe vascular disease which frequently complicates diabetes and hypothyroidism, dementia in such subjects is frequently of this type.

Pathological changes Few descriptions of post-mortem findings in cases of proven arteriopathic dementia have appeared in recent years although evidence of the multiplicity of the infarcts in this disorder and their distribution as demonstrated by computerized radiography is growing rapidly (Frackowiak et al., 1981; Ladurner, Sager and Floch, 1982). Details of the areas of softening to be found in a demented and a non-demented group of old people were given by Tomlinson, Blessed and Roth (1968, 1970). Small softenings and some considerable infarcts were found in patients, who, though neurologically disabled, were intellectually well preserved. The patients were all in hospital and some were selected for study because of stroke disease, and it was not claimed that the findings in the 'control' group were representative of that which would be found in age-matched and non-demented people living in the community. Sixty per cent of the non-demented group showed some evidence of cerebral softening; in many this consisted of one or more very small lesions (often 5 μm or less across) in the white matter or basal ganglia, the total volume of destroyed cerebral tissue being less than 1 ml. A small number had scattered softenings amounting to less than 5 ml of destroyed brain, but three had lesions of considerable magnitude with destroyed brain twice around 50 ml and one about 90 ml. In the latter, the lesions represented areas of destruction up to $5 \times 4 \times 4$ cm at the cortical surface and several centimetres in depth to involve the white matter or basal ganglia. Basal ganglia were more frequently found to be affected by small, and sometimes numerous, softenings; the thalamus was less severely affected, but nevertheless showed small (1–10 mm foci) in around 20 per cent of cases. Middle and posterior cerebral artery territory (particularly the former) was most frequently involved, with anterior parts of the cerebral hemispheres least affected.

The differentiation of the appearances of the brain in the cases of multi-infarct dementia from those of the non-demented group lay largely in the more severe and widespread destruction of the cerebral hemispheres by softening; on these cases and others coming to autopsy since, the following description of the brain in multi-infarct dementia is based.

The brain may or may not be reduced in weight by comparison with age-matched controls. Frequently it is of normal size, shows no obvious generalized cortical atrophy and no abnormality of the meninges. The vessels of the circle of Willis show numerous patches of atheroma and not infrequently the basilar artery is tortuous and markedly atheromatous. Complete occlusion of a major intracranial artery is rare and only likely to be found if the patient has had a recent infarct. Furthermore, the brain shows some obvious evidence of softening with visible lesions affecting the cortex in the territory of the middle or the posterior cerebral artery. In the cortex these vary in size from many centimetres to a few millimetres across. Occasionally they may be massive, with destruction of much of one hemisphere. Considerable infarcts on the inferior temporo-occipital lobe may pass unnoticed at autopsy unless that area is deliberately examined. In half the cases multiple lesions are palpable or visible and usually both hemispheres are affected.

Multiple sections of the fixed brain often show enlarged ventricles; this may be unequal on the two sides or particularly involve one part (e.g. a posterior horn) more than elsewhere, thus reflecting the retraction of adjacent softened tissue. There is great variation in the amount and siting of the softenings, which are usually multiple and involve both hemispheres in over 90 per cent of cases; the exceptions have a single massive unilateral softening. In the commoner *multiple infarct* form, most cases have softenings which spread through the cerebral cortex, white matter and basal ganglia; in around 20 per cent the thalamus shows small softenings which are occasionally bilateral; in about the same number there are one or more softenings in the brain stem, most commonly in the pons. One or several softenings of considerable size may constitute the only lesion; more usually, large softenings are accompanied by several or many small ones in other parts of the hemispheres. Very large lesions involve middle cerebral artery territory or the temporo-occipital territory of the posterior cerebral artery, the damage here extending to much of the hippocampal gyrus and hippocampus. Bilateral occipitotemporal softenings may be the principal lesions found.

In approximately 40 per cent of cases, numerous softenings of 0.5–2 cm across involve cortex, white matter and basal ganglia predominantly, and in roughly half of these, scattered white matter softenings predominate with little involvement of other structures. Cortex or basal ganglia are, however, always involved to some extent. Subcortical arteriosclerotic encephalopathy (Binswanger's disease) involves particular hemisphere white matter and will be commented on later.

The individual softenings vary almost as much in appearance as they do in size, number and site. Many are areas of total destruction of grey and white matter. Some in the white matter and basal ganglia, and of considerable age, are sharply defined, clearly delineated and cystic, and filled with clear fluid; often, however, in many lesions the white and grey matter are only partly destroyed. In the white matter this may consist of loss of myelin with microcystic foci and some glial response; in the cortex, laminar necrosis or linear microscopic cortical scars running alongside penetrating cortical arteries at right angles to the pial surface are present. Microscopy invariably shows evidence of lesions outside the territory visibly damaged.

Small softenings may be found unilaterally in almost any cerebral structure in intellectually well-preserved elderly subjects, and no case of dementia has been seen in which only a single small ischaemic lesion was found. Bilateral ischaemic destruction of the dorsomedial thalamus has been recorded as producing a severe amnesic syndrome with symptoms of subcortical dementia, such as apathy, lack of spontaneity, diminished facial expression, slowness of thought and response but relatively preserved intellect on testing (Segara, von Stockert and Curtis, 1973). The diagnosis of this condition in life, of sudden onset and resulting from occlusion of a thalamosubthalamic perforating artery which supplies both thalami, has been reported by Guberman and Stuss (1983) using computerized tomography. The lesions usually centre on the dorsomedial nucleus, but also involve the ventral anterior and intralaminar nuclei and the mamillothalamic tracts (Castaigne et al., 1981).

Instances of bilateral thalamic degeneration of unknown aetiology producing dementia have also been recorded rarely (Stern, 1939; Schulman, 1956). In a comparison between the non-demented group with cerebral softenings and patients with multi-infarct dementia, the major differences in relation to the softenings were as follows.

The total volume of the softenings in the demented group greatly exceeded that in the non-demented group. All cases with softening estimated at more than 100 ml in volume were demented and only in two cases was destruction of tissue in excess of 50 ml not associated with dementia. Significant evidence also exists that the severity of the clinical features of the dementia increases with the volume of tissue destroyed (Blessed, Tomlinson and Roth, 1968). There are other differences of probable importance. Over 90 per cent of the demented group have bilateral hemisphere softenings, compared with the smaller softenings in the non-demented group which were unilateral in 60 per cent. Unilateral destruction of the hippocampus was found in only one of 28 non-demented cases with cerebral softening but was present in seven of 18 cases of multi-infarct or mixed multi-infarct SDAT; in two the damage was bilateral and severe. The corpus callosum was the site of a small softening in one of 28 non-demented patients, but in five of 18 dements. Basal ganglia softening was more frequent in the demented group, but common and frequently as severe in the non-demented subjects, strikingly the number with thalamic softening was almost identical in the two groups;

six of 28 non-demented patients showed thalamic softenings, in two cases bilateral and in one of these of considerable severity. In the dements, five of 18 showed thalamic softenings, bilateral in three cases and one involving all areas of thalamus with multiple softenings except the pulvinar. In both groups the lateral thalamus nuclei were usually affected with sparing of the dorsomedial thalamus.

In rare instances (probably less than 10 per cent), the ischaemic lesions involve wide areas of cerebral cortex, largely to the exclusion of other parts of the hemispheres. The cortex has a granular surface and is thinned. Microscopically, numerous cortical scars are mostly associated with small blood vessels, but patches of laminar scarring also occur whilst large stretches of affected cortex will be largely or totally replaced by proliferating glia and scattered lipid-filled macrophages with severe depletion of neurons.

Investigation of demented patients by computerized tomography is adding important information about the differences between non-demented and demented patients with stroke disease. Ladurner, Iliff and Lechner (1982) have found bilateral lesions, involvement of the dominant hemisphere, involvement of the thalamus and cerebral atrophy more common in a demented group than in non-demented patients with strokes; unfortunately, this type of investigation cannot take account of mixed cases of vascular and Alzheimer's disease, so some reservations must remain about conclusions drawn solely from such studies.

Subcortical arteriosclerotic encephalopathy was the name given by Olszewski (1962) to a condition in which multiple small total or partial softenings and extensive demyelination affect the cerebral hemisphere white matter, usually with sparing of the cortex although not infrequently with accompanying basal ganglia softening. The original description of eight cases of the disorder was given by Binswanger (1894), who attributed the white matter lesions to reduced blood supply but did not report on the histological lesions.

Patients with this form of cerebral ischaemic destruction may be hypertensive, and usually between 50 and 60 years of age, and undergo a slowly progressive dementia with some partial remissions; strokes, from which some recovery may occur, may be a feature and neurological deficits including pseudobulbar palsy and motor signs are frequent (Caplan and Schoene, 1978). Of particular importance when there is a clinical suspicion of the disorder is the presence of subacute neurological deficits in a slowly dementing patient (Loizou, Kendall and Marshall, 1981); some, however, present as multi-infarct dementia and others may be mistaken for Alzheimer's disease. Confirmation of the disorder as subacute arteriosclerotic encephalopathy in life is now possible by the demonstration in CT scans of low white matter attenuation in the cerebral hemispheres, often accompanied by some atrophy and ventricular dilatation and obvious infarcts (Rosenberg et al., 1979; Zeumer, Schonsky and Sturm, 1980).

How frequently dementia occurs which is due to ischaemic lesions limited largely to the white matter is not known. Previously regarded as uncommon, the identification of cases of this type by CT scan may well result in many more being identified. Almost certainly more will be identified in neurological clinics to which middle-aged, mildly and slowly dementing subjects with neurological signs are likely to be sent, rather than among the severely demented population of psychogeriatric wards. The numbers affected are also partly dependent on the attitude of clinicians and pathologists. The authors regard the disorder as a variant of multi-infarct dementia, which, on pathological and physiological grounds (Frackowiack et al., 1981), is distinguished from the more common cases only by the dominant lesions being in the white matter. In our experience, however, cases totally limited to white matter infarction are most unusual, the great majority being accompanied by some cortical or, more usually, obvious basal ganglia ischaemic foci.

The brain externally may be of normal appearance and weight, though in approximately half the cases some degree of atrophy is present, and occasionally a small cortical infarct is visible. The ventricles are, however, almost always considerably dilated. Coronal sections show numerous and sometimes confluent greyish foci of softening in the white matter of the frontal and parietal lobes, these areas being much more frequently involved than the temporal and occipital white matter. The involved white matter usually presents a mixture of total ischaemic lesions, with cyst formation, and partial ischaemic lesions represented by greyish gelatinous zones mingled or surrounded by cystic or honeycomb foci of more complete destruction.

Obvious small ischaemic foci are present in basal ganglia or brain stem, and in cortex in less than 50 per cent, although extensive histological examination will usually identify small ischaemic cortical foci. Confluent lesions of varying appearance, particularly in the frontal and parietal lobes, may extend from the ventricle wall or the lateral margins of the basal ganglia, to the subcortical arcuate fibres which are usually spared.

Histologically the lesions have the typical appearances of white matter infarcts of varying age and severity (De Reuck et al., 1980; Janota, 1981; see also Chapter 4).

The major blood vessels at the brain base are commonly atheromatous; intracranial arteries, particularly the perforating vessels of the white matter, show thickening of the wall from medial hypertrophy and lipohyalinosis, changes which are probably consequent on hypertension. These vessels in consequence show narrowing, or actual occlusion of the lumina, particularly at the origin of capillaries (Farnell and Globus, 1932; Davison, 1942; Iglesias-Rozas and Ebhardt, 1974). Blood flow studies and pathological studies show involvement of cortical arteries in the arteriosclerotic process, and Loizou, Kendall and Marshall (1981) have suggested that the lesions result from chronic ischaemia in the watershed territory between the long perforating arteries of the white matter and the cortical medullary arteries.

Changes in the blood vessels supplying the brain in dementia of vascular origin are obviously frequent. The most striking and common change demonstrable at autopsy is severe atheroma of the basal cerebral arteries, which may be accompanied by irregular dilatation and tortuosity, particularly of the basilar artery. Such an appearance cannot, however, be taken to indicate that dementia is of vascular origin since atheroma of the basal arteries is present to some degree, and may be severe in many intellectually normal old subjects, who may or may not have one or more cerebral softenings. A similar statement applies to the state of the extracranial cerebral arteries. Stenosis or even occlusion of the carotid and vertebral arteries in the neck is an important factor in stroke disease (Yates and Hutchinson, 1961), but examination of the entire vascular tree in patients with dementia of vascular origin and non-demented patients of a similar age range shows that stenosis of the arteries in the neck and within the skull is rarely found in the absence of comparable degeneration of the cerebral vessels (Corsellis and Evans, 1965; Worm-Petersen and Pakkenberg, 1968). Thus, in the majority of cases cortical and intracerebral arteries are affected, the former by atherosclerosis and the latter by fibrous and muscular thickening or hyalinization of the wall. The changes in the small vessels are similar to those which occur in other organs of the body in hypertension which is present to some degree in the majority of patients with stroke disease and multi-infarct dementia. The detailed pathology of the arteries in these conditions is described in Chapter 4.

Naturally, many patients with dementia of vascular origin have widespread vascular changes in other organs, particularly the heart and kidneys. Myocardial hypertrophy from hypertension is not uncommon, nor is infarction. In some cases, emboli from left ventricular or atrial thrombi are responsible for vascular dementia. A more favoured site for multiple cerebral emboli in stroke disease is thought by many clinicians to be thrombi superimposed on atheromatous plaques in the carotid arteries in the neck. In our experience, however, multi-infarct dementia is almost always associated with intracerebral arterial disease even when embolization is likely to have played a role. Very occasionally, bilateral embolic strokes, often involving the larger cerebral arteries and resulting from embolization associated with atrial fibrillation accompanying rheumatic heart disease, or of other origin, may cause dementia (Marsden, 1984).

On rare occasions, dementia may result from multiple infarcts associated with other causes of arterial occlusion or thrombosis, such as collagen vascular disease, or meningovascular syphilis. All severe meningeal infections tend to be associated with some degree of vasculitis or endarteritis obliterans which may lead to cerebral infarction, but the development of dementia following meningitis always raises the possibility of obstructive hydrocephalus from fibrosis of the basal meninges.

It should not be forgotten that cases of dementia following rupture of intracranial aneurysms, with or without operative interference, are likely to be due to cerebral infarction. The latter has been recognized for many years as a frequent complication of aneurysmal rupture (Robertson, 1949; Tomlinson, 1959; Birse and Tom, 1960; Crompton, 1964), and the serious sequelae in survivors (Logue et al., 1968) are largely of this origin. Detailed neuropathological examination of the brain in fatal cases undoubtedly reveals a greater incidence of infarction than does computerized tomography but the latter procedure revealed 19 per cent of cases with recent infarctions in a series of 59 patients investigated by Ladurner, Sager and Floch (1982). Significant cerebral infarction also occurs in many cases of closed head injury (see Chapter 3); its role in the severe intellectual and neurological disorders of the ever-growing number of permanently brain damaged subjects involved in road traffic accidents is difficult to assess because severe diffuse cerebral damage of other types also occurs in the majority of cases. Severe acute anoxia such as accompanies cardiac arrest or the lesions which follow severe hypotension (see Chapter 4) may also result in permanent intellectual and emotional damage from focal or more diffuse ischaemic lesions. No good evidence exists, however, for a dementing syndrome resulting from chronic global cerebral ischaemia, whether on clinical grounds (Hachinski, Lassen and Marshall 1974) or on neuropathological studies, or as a result of detailed studies of cerebral blood flow or cerebral oxygen utilization (Frackowiak et al., 1981). The latter article and that of Meyer and Shaw (1984) give up-to-date information on important neurophysiological studies which are complementary to the neuropathology of the dementia of Alzheimer or multi-infarct type.

Pick's disease

Some years before Alzheimer's studies on presenile dementia had been completed, Pick had been working on another dementing condition which he had found occasionally to affect older people but in which the neurological picture was more pronounced than that usually associated with the dementias of middle and later life. When Pick, together with the pathologist Chiari, examined the brains of his patients macroscopically they found within the usual setting of mild generalized atrophy a much more striking shrinkage of certain lobes and the condition became known as 'progressive circumscribed cerebral atrophy'.

As comprehensive reviews by Lüers and Spatz (1957), Delay and Brion (1962) and Jervis (1971a) have shown, the illness is rare and is encountered considerably less often than Alzheimer's disease. It occurs most often during later middle life, with a peak around 60. It has, however, been encountered well before this with an onset as early as the 30s and 40s, and even at 21. At the other extreme, several patients over the age of 80 or 90 have been recorded. The length of illness varies greatly but it is rarely less than 1 year and seldom runs to more than 10 years. There is some evidence that the duration tends to be shorter when the onset is early. Women seem to be affected a little more often than men. In the comprehensive survey by van Mansvelt (1954) the ratio was 5:4.

No major variations have been established in the geographic incidence of Pick's disease, although in Sweden Sjögren, Sjögren and Lindgren (1952) found that most proved examples of the illness came from Stockholm whilst those of Alzheimer's disease originated in Göteborg. Verhaart (1936) described the disease in Chinese and Malayans in Indonesia.

Grünthal (1930a) described the occurrence of Pick's disease in two brothers. This confirmed the observation by Reich (1927) and von Braunmühl (1928) that the condition could be familial. Since that time numerous other examples have been reported. Sjögren, Sjögren and Lindgren (1952) concluded from their genetic survey in Sweden that the condition is probably transmitted by a dominant major gene with polygenic modification. Schenk, in 1959, reported on a 20-year follow-up of a Swedish family in which 26 of the 51 endangered sibships were affected (Slater and Cowie, 1971).

The clinical story in most cases suggests the beginnings of frontal lobe damage. Insidious intellectual deterioration with difficulty in concentration occurs and perhaps some disturbance of memory (Lishman, 1978). The patient may become depressed, restless and apathetic. He loses insight, becomes untidy and may behave in a bizarre or socially disturbing way. As the intellect worsens, the patient becomes disorientated, and possibly dysphasic, dyslexic or dyspraxic. Repetitive utterances or actions are not uncommon. Occasionally a patient becomes mute at an early stage. Epileptic attacks are rare, at least in the early stages, and choreiform or athetotic movements are very unusual. Disturbances of gait are not uncommon towards the end of the illness. The disease progresses slowly but relentlessly into a stage of advanced dementia. Occasionally the symptoms are masked. Winkelman and Book's (1949) patient, for instance, who died aged 34, was thought to have been schizophrenic. Death is usually attributable to bronchopneumonia. There are no known abnormal *post mortem* findings in organs other than the brain.

Appearances of the brain The most striking feature in the typical case is the extreme shrinkage of relatively circumscribed parts of both cerebral hemispheres. The severity of the atrophy is best seen in the fixed brain after the leptomeninges, which are usually thickened but not adherent, have been stripped away and the underlying convolutions have been exposed (Fig. 20.23). These

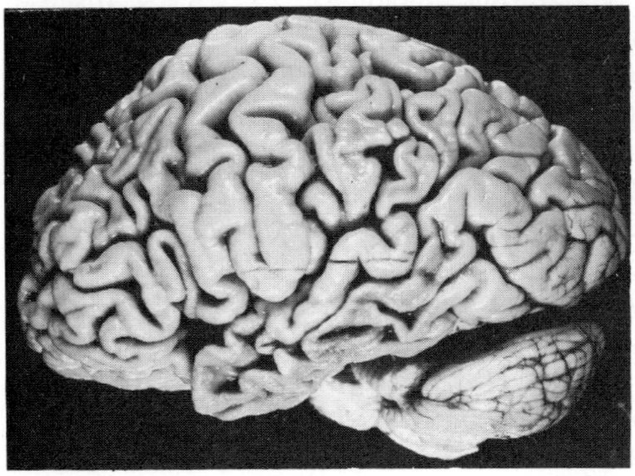

Fig. 20.23 Pick's disease. There is atrophy in the parietal as well as in the frontal and temporal lobes. The sparing of the posterior two-thirds of the superior temporal gyrus is noteworthy.

are then seen to be separated by widely gaping sulci; their roughened surface is yellow-brown with the crowns of the gyri often shrivelled up to the so-called 'walnut' or even 'knife-edge' appearance (Fig. 20.24). This marked loss of tissue is reflected in the brain weight which may fall to 1000 g or less in either sex. Lindgren (Sjögren, Sjögren and Lindgren, 1952) found the mean value for women to be 1005 g; for men it was 1075 g. van Mansvelt (1954) considered that the longer the illness, the greater the atrophy. In the typical case the diagnosis can be made with some certainty on the macroscopical appearances. The atrophy apparent to the naked eye can, however, be less obvious and may be overlooked, whilst it should not be forgotten that unusually severe degrees of atrophy may be found in dementia of the Alzheimer type.

The atrophy is usually frontotemporal in distribution, but at times the brunt of the process falls mainly on the frontal lobes and at others on

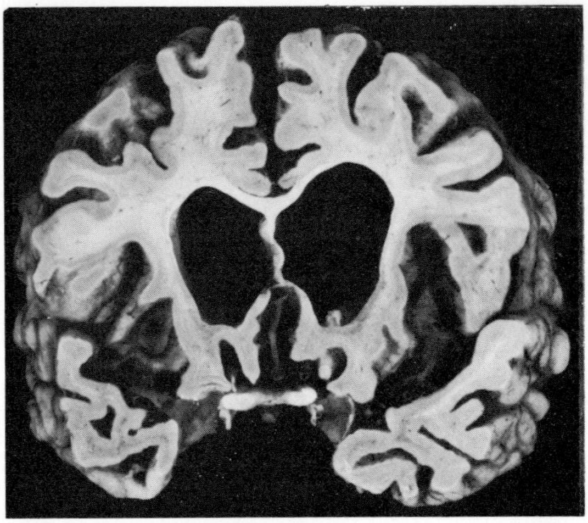

Fig. 20.24 Pick's disease. Coronal cut showing gross frontal and temporal atrophy with marked enlargement of lateral ventricles and atrophy of the caudate nuclei.

the temporal lobes. The figures given by van Mansvelt (1954) in his analysis of the degree of atrophy of the two hemispheres were that it was symmetrical in about a third, whilst in nearly a half of the cases the left hemisphere was the more affected and in only a fifth was the emphasis on the right side. In only one instance was the discrepancy very marked and in this case it is interesting that the illness had started after a head injury (Reich, 1927). The distribution of the lobar atrophy was frontal and temporal in 54 per cent, mainly frontal in 25 per cent, and mainly temporal in 17 per cent. Parietal and frontoparietal atrophy were rare. In one case the occipital lobe was heavily involved (Urechia, Dragomir and Elekes, 1935); slighter degrees of occipital atrophy have also occasionally been reported (Jakob, 1960).

The patterns of atrophy within the different lobes were analysed by Lüers and Spatz (1957). They described two main types of frontal involvement. In the commoner type the atrophy is focused on the medial orbital regions, including the gyrus rectus, spreading round on to the frontal pole with the marked atrophy extending along the inferior frontal gyrus towards the insula and into the pars opercularis but tending to spare the adjacent pars triangularis. In the less common type the emphasis is on the frontal convexity, in which the pole and the dorsal half of the frontal lobes are the more affected. At times the precentral gyrus is also involved, or indeed the whole convexity may be.

When the temporal lobe is affected the focus is always around the pole. The atrophy then spreads back to involve the whole of the middle and inferior temporal gyri, but a curiously characteristic feature of the disease is the way in which the anterior third of the superior temporal gyrus is more affected than the posterior part (see Figs. 20.23 and 20.24). Jakob (1969) reported two cases of pure temporal lobe involvement and analysed the clinicopathological implications in detail. Cummings and Duchen (1981) have examined an interesting series of five patients with severe anterior temporal atrophy which included the amygdaloid nuclei. Abnormal neurons and Pick bodies were abundant. Interestingly, in view of the anterior temporal localization, and as discussed previously by Pilleri (1966) and others, the oral and the affective components of the Klüver–Bucy syndrome were prominent features, as well as disorientation and aphasia, whilst memory disorder ended to show up later in the illness; hypersexuality was not a feature. The authors drew attention to this particular clinical presentation which could point early on to the diagnosis of this variant of Pick's disease.

On the rarer occasions in which the parietal lobe is affected the atrophy is usually in the region of the supramarginal and angular gyri. In contrast, other areas or gyri are relatively resistant. These include the occipital lobes, the posterior part of the paracentral lobule and the anterior transverse gyrus of Heschl.

Pick had already in 1906 noted that the atrophy tended to involve association areas, and Spatz (1952) and others emphasized that it is those parts of the hemispheres which develop late that tend to be picked out. A major exception to this, however, and one which conflicts with the above concept, is the fact that the hippocampus and the parahippocampal gyrus are at times considerably atrophied. Lüers and Spatz (1957) mentioned a small group in which the hippocampus has been severely, and even selectively, affected.

The atrophic process affects the white matter as well as the cortex. The junction between the two becomes blurred to the naked eye, the white matter turns greyish and the affected lobes feel like indiarubber, the condition at one time being known as 'lobar sclerosis'.

The deep grey matter may also be involved. Occasionally the atrophy of the caudate nucleus is severe and may resemble that seen in Huntington's chorea. Dewulf (1935) and Akclaitis (1944) reported cases in which the caudate nucleus had all but disappeared whilst the globus pallidus, but not the putamen, was also severely atrophied. van Mansvelt (1954) considered that some degree of caudate atrophy occurred in about two-thirds of cases, but others have estimated a lower figure (von Bagh, 1941). The brain stem, cerebellum and spinal cord usually appear normal to the naked eye.

Histology The first account was given by Alzheimer (1911). The findings consist essentially of an intense loss of nerve cells in the affected areas, accompanied by cortical and subcortical gliosis.

The neuronal loss is often greatest in the outer cortical layers but the pattern is variable and the full depth of the ribbon may be affected. Vogt (1928) and Schiffer (1955) contended that there is a sequence to the cell loss, layer 3 being the first to degenerate followed by layers 2 and 5. Schenk and van Mansvelt (1955), however, found many exceptions to this rule. Many of the surrounding nerve cells appear small and stain faintly. Pigment may accumulate in the cytoplasm, which contains a reduced amount of Nissl substance. These changes are not specific. There is, however, a more distinct type of degeneration which is found in many but not all cases. This consists of the swelling of the cell body which rounds up or becomes pear shaped. The Nissl substance disintegrates, the cytoplasm become homogeneous and weakly acidophilic whilst the nucleus is displaced towards the cell membrane (Fig. 20.25).

With Nissl's method the swollen area of the cell remains colourless or stains a pale matt blue whilst a few Nissl granules may still be seen adjacent to the nucleus or at the apex of the cell. With Mallory's phosphotungstic acid–haematoxylin the affected cells stand out as pale oval areas against the diffusely stained background. This appearance, combined as it often is with the fibrous gliosis of the cortex, is distinctive and may be of diagnostic value in cases in which the cortical and subcortical atrophy is less striking than that usually seen in Pick's disease.

Although a greater proportion of small than of large neurons in the cortex is generally affected

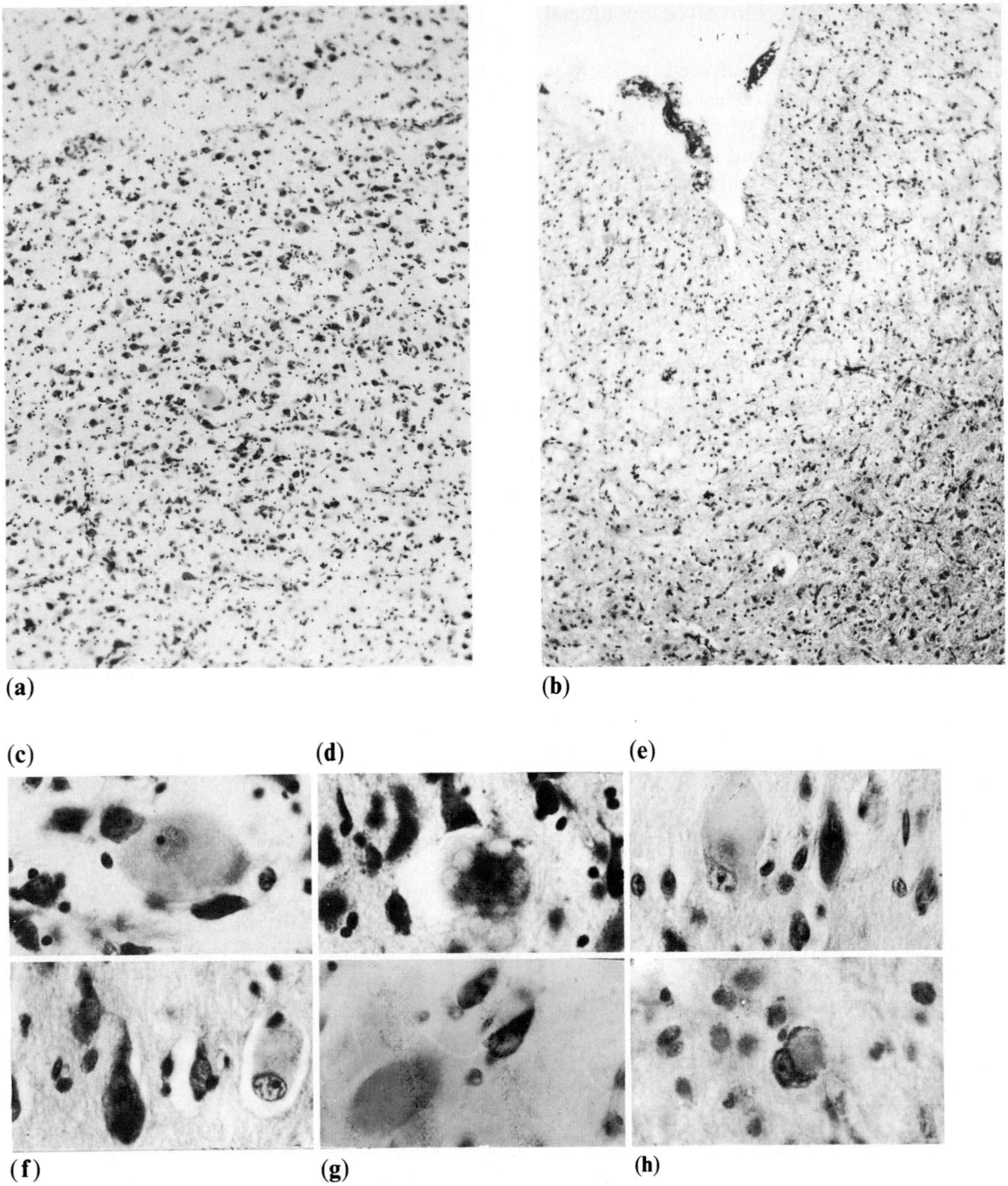

Fig. 20.25 Pick's disease. (**a**) Superior temporal gyrus. There is widespread neuronal degeneration with disalignment of neurons; note pale globose forms (Pick's cells). Near the foot is the line of a sulcus. Cresyl violet ×90. (**b**) Second temporal gyrus, showing widespread atrophy of the cortex with resulting status spongiosus. The section is taken in the depth of a sulcus. Celloidin. Haematoxylin and eosin ×90. (**c**) An enlargement of the cell seen in the centre of (**a**). (**d–h**) Nerve cells in various stages of degeneration. The nucleus is not visible in the large cell in (**g**). Cresyl violet ×400.

by this change, individual large pyramidal cells in the deeper layers may become severely distended. A similar change may be seen in some neurons of the basal ganglia and in the pigmented cells of the brain stem. In such cells the nucleus moves to one pole and often has an eccentric nucleolus which lies against the nuclear membrane. With Bielschowsky's silver impregnation the swollen part of the cytoplasm may contain a globular homogeneous well-defined mass which stains with varying intensity. In others the entire cytoplasm of the base of the cell may appear to consist of homogeneous argyrophilic material. In either case some intact neurofibrils may lie at the periphery of the cell.

Onari and Spatz (1926) recognized the resemblance of these Pick cells to those undergoing axonal degeneration, and Spatz (1952) reaffirmed his belief that the degenerative process in Pick's disease begins in the periphery of the neuron or in the white matter (Freeman, 1933). Jakob (1961), however, in a study of 12 cases opposed his view, holding that the neuronal changes start at the level of the cell body.

Electron microscopy of the ballooned cells (Schochet, Lampert and Earle, 1968; Wisniewski, Coblenz and Terry, 1972) has revealed no substantial qualitative difference between swollen cells with and without Pick bodies. In both, proliferating loss material of neurofilaments and some tubules were found, the endoplasmic reticulum tending to become vesiculated. Wisniewski et al. 1972 saw the Pick body as a cytoplasmic accumulation of filaments, tubules or twisted tubules which is possibly the secondary response of a neuron to damage to its processes or is the consequence of trans-synaptic degeneration.

The globular masses seen with the light microscope in this form of degeneration have sometimes been called inclusions, but they are less hyaline than those occurring in association with paralysis agitans and they do not have the concentric structure seen both in these and in Lafora inclusions.

Wechsler et al. (1982) have reported on the clinical and tomographic features of one case with bilateral, but especially left, frontotemporal atrophy. The histological features were typical for the condition but the use of Golgi impregnations demonstrated an almost complete absence of dendritic spines on pyramidal neurons, and although the apical dendrites appeared largely normal the basal ones had long thin primary and secondary dendrites with virtually no tertiary branching.

The astroglial proliferation is marked in the atrophic cortical and subcortical areas and the cortex may develop a spongy appearance (see Fig. 20.25b). Microglia and oligodendroglia play no special part, although fat phagocytes may at times be seen, particularly in the demyelinated and gliotic subcortical white matter. A lesser degree of neuronal loss and gliosis may be seen in cortical areas which are not grossly atrophic. The deep grey matter in the hemispheres may also be affected and, as already described at the macroscopic level, the caudate nucleus may be almost totally degenerate. Neuronal change and loss have also been reported in the putamen and pallidum, the thalamus and pons. Purkinje cell changes have been recorded at times but are usually absent or minor (Jervis, 1971b).

Senile plaques and neurofibrillary changes do not occur as a rule, even in elderly patients. They are, however, seen at times and have been reported by Liebers (1939), Smith, Turner and Sim (1966) and Terry and Wisniewski (1971). Moyano (1932) described five cases of Pick's disease in which the histological picture of Alzheimer's disease was also present in the atrophic areas. Berlin (1949) reported two cases with the typical features of both Pick's and Alzheimer's diseases and suggested that 'these may be conditions which are intermediate between the two'. Granulovacuolar degeneration, mainly in the pyramidal cells of the hippocampus, may also be seen in Pick's disease.

The cause of Pick's disease is unknown. van Mansvelt (1954) and others have emphasized the possible importance in some cases of exogenous factors, including trauma (Reich, 1907; Crezee, 1949). No vascular or other abnormality of aetiological significance has, however, so far been identified and the disease still remains best described, but not explained, as a heredodegenerative condition of middle and later life.

Bowen (1981) has touched on the limited information about the chemical aspects. He and his colleagues (White et al., 1977) have drawn attention to Ball's (1979) observation on the tendency for Pick bodies to occur in the hippocampus in a way similar to the pathological and chemical predilection of this area in ageing and in Alzheimer's disease. No transmitter studies appear so far to have been made in Pick's disease nor is there any evidence to support the possibility of a slow virus infection.

Progressive subcortical gliosis Neumann (1949) and Neumann and Cohn (1967) described several cases of insidious progressive dementia clinically resembling Alzheimer and Pick's diseases in which the most prominent histological feature was a pronounced subcortical gliosis without severe involvement of the cerebral cortex and with no significant myelin loss. Astrocytic and some microglial proliferation were also marked in the basal ganglia, thalamus, brain stem and ventral horns of the spinal cord. Neumann and Cohn referred to similar cases in the literature and considered that they should be taken together as forming Pick's disease type II or 'progressive subcortical gliosis'. The interest in this condition lies in the overwhelming subcortical proliferation of glia with a relatively intact neuronal population.

Huntington's chorea

In 1872, a year after George Huntington had qualified in medicine, he wrote about a hereditary chorea with mental deterioration which comes on in middle life and progresses remorselessly until 'the helpless sufferer is but a quivering wreck of his former self'. Lund (1860) and Lyon (1863) had already described a similar disease but it was Huntington's report, based on his father's and his own experiences in their family practice on Long Island, that gave the condition its solid foundation. Heathfield (1973) and Barbeau (1973) have reviewed the historical and other aspects of the disease at length. *Huntington's Disease*, edited by Chase, Wexler and Barbeau (1979), provides a comprehensive text.

The illness has occasionally been reported in children of 5 years or even younger; it has rarely appeared after the age of 75. The first manifestation is usually between 25 and 45 years. Bell (1934) found the average age of onset to be 35 but Wendt, Landzettel and Solth (1960) considered the mid-40s to be more accurate because, as argued by Slater and Cowie (1971), studies before the 1960s had tended to exclude cases with a late onset.

The disease lasts about 15 years on average, although survival as short as 5 and as long as 30 years has been recorded. Death usually occurs in the early 50s. It is a rare disorder but affects all races, the incidence in Europe, America and Australia being around 4–7 per 10 000 (Myrianthopoulos, 1966). In Japan the figure was found to be one-tenth of this (Kishimoto, Nakamura and Sotokawa, 1959). Local pockets of the disease may occur in which the figure is exceptionally high. These include the Moray Firth (Lyon, 1962), Tasmania (Brothers, 1949) and north Sweden (Sjögren, 1935).

The disease is linked to a single major gene, which manifests dominantly in the heterozygote with a penetrance negligibly less than 100 per cent. Half of any one generation may be expected to inherit the illness. Wendt, Landzettel and Unterreiner (1959), Bruyn (1967) and others have found that the father was the affected parent nearly four times as often as the mother when the illness began before the age of 21 years.

Bird, Caro and Pilling (1974) have shown that affected offspring of a male tend to die at an earlier age than the father, whereas the offspring of females with the disease die at an age not significantly different from that of their mother. No chromosome abnormalities have been found (Benirsche and Höfnagel, 1961). In spite of the major genetic factor, failure to obtain a family history of the illness is not uncommon.

In the typical form of Huntington's chorea an initial fidgetiness grows over several years into jerking and choreiform movements. At the same time, or even before this, the patient may become irritable, truculent and perhaps paranoid. Other patients are apathetic and slovenly. Depression is liable to be profound and suicide is a risk. Eventually lack of concentration, confusion and memory impairment merge into dementia. Instances have been recorded in families prone to chorea in which the dementia has progressed and the illness run its course without the development of choreiform movements (Curran, 1929; Worster-Drought and Allen, 1929; Bolt, 1970). It is because of the absence of chorea that the title of Huntington's disease is sometimes preferred (Whittier, 1963). Conversely, the chorea may progress with little or no evidence of mental disorder at any stage (Heathfield, 1967). Schizophrenia and depressive illness, psychopathic traits or mental subnormality may be found in affected patients and sometimes in other members of the family. Davenport (1915) maintained that the disease may follow a pattern within a family; Heathfield (1973) encountered one in which the father and one son both died with Huntington's chorea and schizophrenia, another son was merely schizophrenic whilst the third had only the chorea and was mentally normal. Pleydell (1954) found dyslalia was a premonitory sign in one of the families known to him.

A rare, though important, variant of Huntington's chorea is the juvenile form. This occurs with onset between 10 and 20 years in about 8 per cent of cases; it is much rarer in the first decade (Bruyn, 1967). The illness differs clinically from the adult form in that choreiform movements are rare whilst akinesia and extrapyramidal rigidity are usual (Campbell et al., 1961). The dementia becomes severe and epileptic attacks are common. Lindenberg (1960) reported on a man with typical Huntington's chorea, whose daughter died aged 29 with a diagnosis of 'juvenile parkinsonism'.

The disease progresses relentlessly, sometimes with intervals of little change, until death occurs, commonly from an intercurrent infection. The pathological changes in Huntington's chorea are generally considered to be restricted to the central nervous system.

Macroscopic appearances of brain There may be slight fibrous thickening of the leptomeninges and occasional mononuclear infiltrates. These changes, however, are seldom striking and are usually consistent with the age of the patient. The brain itself may look normal, but it is usually small and commonly weighs less than 1100 g; more rarely it falls below 1000 g. Cortical atrophy may appear uniform on the surface and is usually most easily discernible in the frontal and parietal lobes. It may be severe, but is usually only moderate. Changes in the basal vessels are usually compatible with the age of the patient. The cardinal feature (Fig. 20.26) in coronal sections of the fixed brain is the striking and usually severe atrophy of the corpus striatum to a degree rarely seen except in the very occasional case of Pick's disease. The head of the caudate nucleus, instead of bulging into the floor of the ventricle, shrinks to a narrow, and even concave, brownish ribbon with its volume dropping possibly to less than half the normal. This, and the affected putamen and pallidum, often turn deep blue in ferrocyanide solution. The anterior horn of the lateral ventricle is consequently much enlarged and widened with rounding and elongation of the dorsolateral angle due to the selective striatal atrophy. The putamen is commonly much reduced in size and a milder degree of atrophy of the globus pallidus may be visible. The internal capsule may appear unusually broad, but loss of white matter can also be considerable and is reflected by the thinning of the corpus callosum. The degree of gyral atrophy is variable, but many gyri look narrow and the sulci are widened; the thickness of the cortical ribbon may appear thinned and, according to Bruyn, Bots and Dom (1979), reduction in total cortical volume may be 20 per cent—a figure which would account for the greater part of the loss of brain weight. The brain stem, including the substantia nigra, usually appears normal but the midbrain, pons and medulla may be on the small side; the cerebellum usually appears normal. In summary, a diagnosis of Huntington's chorea can often be confidently asserted on the macroscopic appearance alone. Exceptions do occur, however, in which the striated atrophy is relatively slight even though severe degenerative changes are later seen under the microscope.

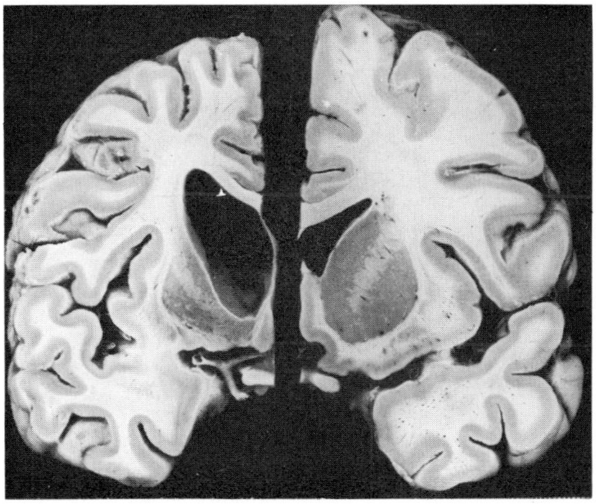

Fig. 20.26 Hungtington's chorea. The hemisphere on the left is from a case of this disease in a woman aged 49 (brain weight 1065 g). That on the right is from a normal woman aged 69 (brain weight 1415 g).

Histology The most easily recognized abnormalities are in the caudate nucleus and putamen (Fig. 20.27), in which there is extensive loss of small neurons with relative, though not total, preservation of large ones (Fig. 20.28). This is most easily seen in the striatum, in which severe shrinkage crowds the surviving neurons and glial cells together so that several large neurons may be present in a single field. Dom, Baro and Brucher (1973) and Lange et al. (1976), in morphometric studies, have shown that small to large neuron ratio is normally around 160:1 and this is reduced to 40:1 or less, the major loss being of the Golgi II neurons which may be depleted by 70–80 per cent. Dom, Baro and Brucher divided the population of small neurons into two groups of small and smaller neurons, and in the rigid Westphal variant of the disorder found that the smaller small cell population was almost elimi-

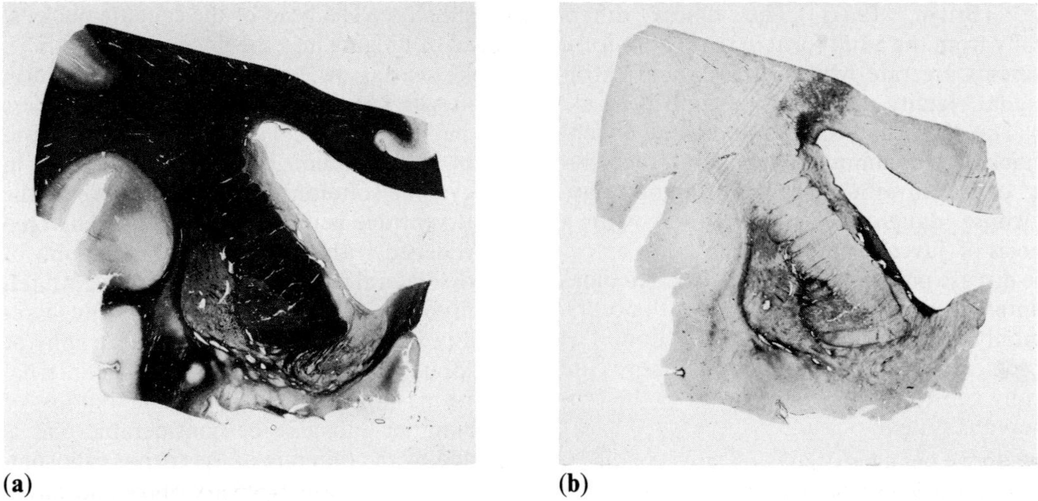

Fig. 20.27 Huntington's chorea. Coronal sections of the corpus striatum: (**a**) myelin stain; (**b**) Holzer's neuroglial fibre stain.

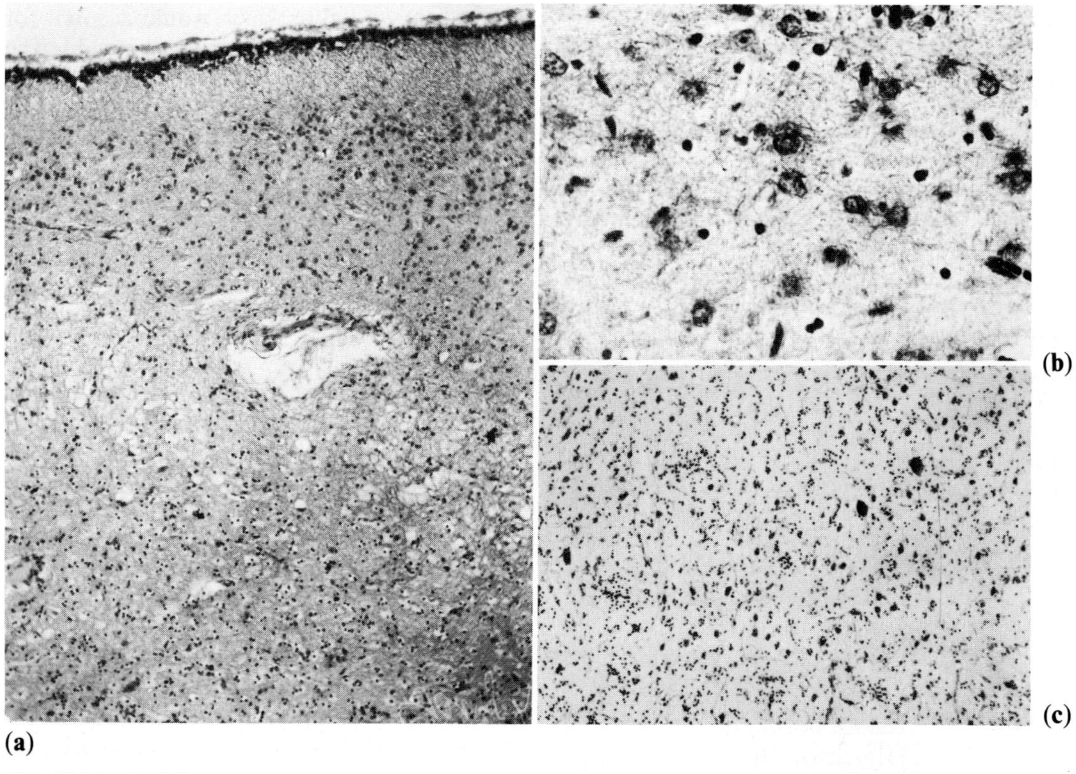

Fig. 20.28 Huntington's chorea. (**a**) Caudate nucleus showing a spongy state due to almost complete disappearance of neurons. Proliferation of astrocytes is most noticeable deep to the subependymal layer. Celloidin. Haematoxylin and eosin ×90. (**b**) Proliferating astrocytes near the ventricular surface of caudate nucleus showing only scanty fibre formation. Celloidin. Mallory's phosphotungstic acid–haematoxylin ×400. (**c**) Putamen. The small neurons have largely disappeared but occasional large ones are to be seen. Celloidin. Cresyl violet ×90.

nated. The appearances of the striatum suggest a considerable degree of astrocytic proliferation as well as fibrillary gliosis. The astrocytes may be clustered, and have large nuclei and abundant cytoplasm. Fibrillary gliosis undoubtedly occurs and is particularly intense in the subependymal tissues and around blood vessels, but quantitative studies have shown that glial loss also occurs from the striatum, being of the order of 25 per cent, the apparent increase of astrocytes being accounted for by this packing into a greatly reduced volume (Lange et al., 1976). The changes in neurons and glia result in an increase of the normal neuron to glial cell ratio of 1 : 3.5 to 1 : 10, this being produced by the severe loss of neurons.

The above changes occur in both the caudate head and the putamen. Usually the caudate is more severely involved, but occasionally the putamen suffers most. McCaughey (1961) found the rostral and inferior parts of the striatum to be less affected than the rest, and Dunlap (1927) considered the putamen to be most involved in its middle and posterior thirds. In the most extreme cases of striatal atrophy a spongy state results, an appearance reminiscent of Pick's disease.

The globus pallidus is less atrophied than the striatum. The external segment is most severely involved, with loss of large neurons; in some instances the internal segment is similarly affected. Demyelination may affect the border between the inner segment of the pallidum and adjacent internal capsule (Hallervorden, 1957), and the ansa and fasciculus lenticularis tend to be pale.

The thalamus shows a degree of neuronal loss (Forno and Jose, 1973), and Dom, Malfroid and Baro (1976) have calculated that the small internuncial neurons in ventrolateral basal thalamus are reduced to 50 per cent although the macroneuronal population is unaltered. Neuronal loss has also been reported in the lateral hypothalamic nuclei as well as neuronal hyperchromasia and cell loss in the supraoptic and hypothalamic nuclei (Bruyn, 1973). According to Lange et al. (1976), cell loss of up to 30 per cent of the Golgi II neurons occurs in the lateral and medial parts of the subthalamic nucleus, although only in rapidly progressive choreic cases; this nucleus is probably normal when the disease runs a chronic course.

In the brain stem only mild changes are usually found. The substantia nigra is usually darkly pigmented to the naked eye because the cell loss, which is present to some degree in many cases (Forno and Jose, 1973), is more severe in the zona reticularis than that of the compacta (Bird, 1978). Fibrillary gliosis is present particularly in the zona reticularis.

Other changes which are found at times consist of loss of Purkinje cells in the cerebellum, especially in juvenile cases in which almost total depletion may occur (Bittenbender and Quadfasel, 1962; Castaigne, Escourolle and Gray, 1976; Rodda, 1981). Cell loss in the dentate nucleus of the cerebellum may also occur, and superior olivary neuron loss is frequently severe (Weisschedel, 1938). According to Bruyn, Bots and Dom (1979), cell loss and fibrillary gliosis is the rule in the inferior olive and the central tegmental tracts, and the cerebro-olivary fibres and olivocerebellar fibres regularly show demyelination. Involvement of the lateral ventricular dorsal vagal and hypoglossal nuclei is common, as is subependymal gliosis in the brain stem. The spinal cord shows pallor of the lateral and anterior tracts; occasional cells in the ventral horn, Clarke's column and in the intermediolateral group of cells are vacuolated.

Cerebral cortical degeneration was reported by Alzheimer in 1911 and confirmed on many occasions since. Neuronal loss is then more prominent in the third cortical layer, but also involves the fourth and the fifth; it varies from slight to considerable and is accompanied by an apparent increase in astrocytes, although this may be the drawing together of the cells from atrophy as in the striatum. Neuronal loss may be focal or diffuse. The frontal lobes are usually most affected. Many remaining neurons are shrunken, some with bizarre shapes, ghost-like or misaligned in relation to the cortical surface. Many show marked accumulation of lipofuscin, as do glial cells, a feature confirmed by electron microscopy (Tellez-Nagel, Johnson and Terry, 1974; Roizin et al., 1976). Tellez-Nagel, Johnson and Terry (1974) have also demonstrated perinuclear increased astrocytic adenosinetryphosphatase. Other features noted by the above authors include increased smooth endoplasmic reticulum and vesicles in association with Golgi complexes, disruption of and diminished numbers of cristae in mitochondria, degeneration of presynaptic terminals with preservation of postsynaptic terminals and synaptic junctions, axon degeneration and some astrocytic proliferation. Various qualitative and quantitative alterations in the granular and fibrillary components of the nucleolus of the neurons have also been described by Roizin, Stellar and Liu (1979) as well as cytoplasmic changes similar to those described above. The significance of these ultrastructural changes, however, is not clear.

The very presence of such severe lesions in the basal ganglia and cerebellum would seem to be a guarantee of neurochemical abnormalities in the affected areas and their connecting pathways, but, although many abnormalities do indeed occur, it would be misleading to imply that they necessarily represent the basic defect of the disease. The most important neurochemical findings in the disease are summarized below; more detailed accounts have been given elsewhere (Chase, Wexler and Barbeau (1979).

The reduced levels which have been found in the substances mentioned below can be interpreted in two ways. Either they are an effect of selective neuronal degeneration and loss in the basal ganglia, or they reflect a functional, and presumably compensatory, change secondary to the losses in other systems. Neurochemical increases may also be due to such functional changes, but they may then represent merely a *relative* increase due to the degeneration and loss of tissue in other systems.

Gamma-aminobutyric acid (GABA), the first amino acid to be identified as a neurotransmitter, is markedly reduced in the substantia nigra and striatum in Huntington's chorea (Perry, Hansen and Kloster, 1973). The enzyme glutamic acid decarboxylase (GAD), which converts glutamic acid to GABA, is also reduced in these structures (Bird, MacKay and Rayner, 1973; Bird and Iversen, 1974). The activity, however, of this enzyme in post-mortem tissue is particularly sensitive to the agonal state prior to death (Spokes, 1979) and this may be responsible for conflicting data in respect of other brain regions. Bird (1976a) failed to find evidence for abnormal GAD function in non-neural tissue, indicating that a loss of enzyme was unlikely to be the primary specific defect in Huntington's chorea.

Measurement of dopamine concentrations in the brain has produced variable results and this transmitter appears to have no primary role in the disease. Bernheimer et al. (1973) and Bird and Iversen (1976) found slight reductions in the caudate nucleus and Mattson (1974) reported no change, whereas Spokes (1979) found an increase above control values within the striatum, the nucleus accumbens and in the pars compacta of the substantia nigra. Enzymes involved in the synthesis and degradation of dopamine have been reported to be normal (Bird and Iversen, 1974).

Choline acetyltransferase (CAT), the enzyme responsible for acetylcholine synthesis, is markedly reduced in the striatum (Bird and Iversen, 1974) and presumably represents a relative loss of cholinergic interneurons. Serotonin has been consistently reported as normal, but various changes among the more recently identified neuropeptide transmitters have been found. Kanazawa et al. (1977, 1979) have reported a decrease of substance P in the substantia nigra and globus pallidus. Angiotensin-converting enzyme, which is responsible for synthesis of the active form of angiotensin, has been shown to be 80–90 per cent reduced in the striatum globus pallidus and nucleus accumbens, and methionine-enkephalin concentrations are also reported decreased in the globus pallidus and substantia nigra (Arregui et al., 1979). Other neuropeptides—notably somatostatin and vasoactive intestinal polypeptide—are found to be normal (Arregui et al., 1979) although cholecystokinin is said to be reduced in the substantia nigra and globus pallidus (Emson et al., 1980).

Neurotransmitter receptor abnormalities have also been extensively investigated. Within the striatum, reductions in the binding capacity of receptors for muscarinic acetylcholine (Hiley and Bird, 1974), serotonin (Enna et al, 1976a, b), GABA (Lloyd, Dreksler and Bird, 1977; Olsen, Van Ness and Tourtellotte, 1979), dopamine (Reisine et al, 1978) and benzodiazepine (Reisine et al., 1979) have been reported, although Enna et al. (1976a, b) found GABA receptors to be normal. Beta-adrenergic receptors have been reported as normal by Enna et al. (1976a, b). Some of these findings do not distinguish between a reduction in receptor sites and decreased affinity for the binding agent. Subpopulations of striatal dopamine receptors are known to exist (Weiner et al., 1979) and the effects of drug therapy may vary in relation to these specific subpopulations. Findings such as the above, which may only be secondary to the basic defect of Huntington's chorea, may yet be important in relation to pharmacological responses in the disease and in the understanding of the complicated interactions of the neuropeptides and transmitters.

Creutzfeldt–Jakob disease (subacute spongiform encephalopathy)

'Creutzfeldt-Jakob disease' is now the most common name for a rare transmissible disorder of the central nervous system which presents, usually in the presenile period, as a progressive dementia and which runs a subacute or chronic course, ending in death in many cases within 3–12 months of the onset.

Creutzfeldt (1921) described the first, albeit atypical, case. The girl had two retarded sisters and her behaviour had been bizarre for many years. At 16 years she began to walk clumsily, but a few months before her death at 22 she ran an intermittent fever and developed a fluctuating psychotic disorder with jerky movements of hands and feet. She died demented with spastic limbs and in status epilepticus. She had a moderately atrophic brain in which there was no evidence of inflammation but patches of neuronal necrosis, gliosis and some capillary proliferation were present throughout the cortical ribbon particularly around the bases of the sulci and in the diencephalon, brain stem and spinal cord. A year later (1921) Alfons Jakob described three middle-aged patients who died a few months to 2 years after the onset with illnesses which he likened to that of Creutzfeldt's patient; he combined the four cases under the title of spastic pseudosclerosis because of a certain similarity with both Wilson's disease and amyotrophic–lateral sclerosis. The principal pathological findings in his cases were neuronal degeneration and loss, and astrocytic proliferation which was most marked in the frontal and temporal cortex, in the medial part of the thalamus and in the cerebellum, brain stem and spinal cord. By 1923 Jakob had described two more cases and others followed later from the same laboratory.

The term 'Creutzfeldt–Jakob disease', which is now often referred to as a subacute spongiform encephalopathy, was coined by Spielmeyer and has remained in common use, although the priority was reversed by Kirschbaum (1968) in recognition of the definitive contribution made by Jakob and because of the atypical nature of Creutzfeldt's case; indeed subsequent authors (Richardson, 1977; Masters and Gajdusek, 1982) have affirmed that Creutzfeldt's case cannot be placed within any of the presently accepted variants of the disease. Masters and Gajdusek (1982) were able to re-examine histological preparations from Jakob's first five cases. They concluded that the third and the fifth showed the features of a spongiform encephalopathy and probably represent the first acceptable examples of the condition. In contrast, two of the original cases no longer appeared to be classifiable as any variant of the disorder, although the first case, which combined dementia, motor neuron disease and extrapyramidal signs, would fit into the amyotrophic form of Creutzfeldt–Jakob disease (Meyer, 1929). In 1968, Kirschbaum summarized all the cases published up to that time and demonstrated both the widening range of the clinical and pathological features and the confusion which could result from introducing further names to cover each new variant.

In this way the concept of a complex of disorders grew up which, within the setting of dementia, could span the features of amyotrophic lateral sclerosis, cortical blindness, myoclonic epilepsy and bulbar myoclonus, as well as the predominant involvement of various combinations of the cerebral cortex, thalamus, striatum, cerebellum or spinal cord. The more precise morphological variants, with their many different names, have been summarized by Corsellis (1976) and some are considered briefly in the next section.

The demonstration by Gibbs et al. (1968) that Creutzfeldt–Jakob disease is a transmissible disorder with close similarities to scrapie in sheep, goats and mink, and to kuru in man, added a new dimension to the literature, and the inclusion, particularly of unusual cases, within the spectrum of the disorder since that time has usually depended on the demonstration of their transmissibility by the production of a spongiform encephalopathy in an inoculated animal. (See later and Chapter 7.)

Clinical features Creutzfeldt–Jakob disease has been recorded in most parts of the world. It leads to about one death a year for every 2–4 million of the population of the USA, and the figures seem not materially different in other countries (Masters et al., 1979). Curiously higher rates, however, have been reported among Libyan Jews by Kahana et al. (1974) and in their families by Neugut et al. (1979), and also in central Slovakia and neighbouring parts of Hungary by Mayer, Orolin and Mitrova (1977). Attempts by Matthews (1975) to trace every histologically diagnosed case over a number of years in the UK found the annual incidence to be around one case per 2 million of the population.

The disorder occurs mostly in middle life, affects both sexes equally and may be familial. It usually presents as a vague prodromal illness which may include confusion, inattention and forgetfulness, depression, periods of dizziness and fatigue or numbness or pain and weakness in the legs. The patient, however, is soon found to be dementing and the dementia itself, which may become profound within a few weeks to several months, is accompanied by the development of pyramidal, extrapyramidal and, often, cerebellar signs. Not infrequent, and particularly helpful in the diagnosis, is the onset of myoclonus, accompanied by an EEG showing periodic sharp-wave complexes (Traub, Gajdusek and Gibbs, 1977). As already mentioned, the emphasis on particular clinical features of marked severity in a given case has led to many subtypes being recognized. Two examples are an ataxic form with prominent cerebellar signs (Boudin, Pépin and Milhaud, 1965; Brownell and Oppenheimer, 1965) and a variety named after Heidenhain (1929) with severe occipital cortical involvement (Meyer, Leigh and Bagg, 1954). A review of these and other cases, however, convincingly demonstrates that these polyonymous variants lie within the broad spectrum of the disorder, so much overlapping of pathological and clinical features is evident from case to case and the continuation of subtypes in the clinical or pathological descriptions of the disorder would appear to be unjustified. Emphasis is laid by many investigators on the EEG and periodic sharp-wave complexes which are said to occur in around 70 per cent of cases (Traub, Gajdusek and Gibbs, 1977). Such changes might often be used as confirmatory findings in a suspected case but they are not diagnostic of the disorder. On clinical grounds, probably the most frequent confusion arises with cases of rapidly progressive Alzheimer's disease in which myoclonus may also occur. The final several days or weeks of the illness are usually dominated by deepening coma, often with rapidly developing cachexia.

Pathology No important pathological changes outside the nervous system have so far been reported. The neuropathological features vary considerably and may be influenced by the length of the illness. The mean period from the onset of symptoms to death is usually about 10 months but it may last only a few weeks or the patient may survive for a number of years. When death is rapid the fixed (or even the fresh) brain will show little or no macroscopic change and the weight will probably be normal. In patients surviving several years a moderate, or even considerable, degree of cerebral atrophy is more likely and the weight may fall to as low as 850 g. No gross evidence of inflammation is present and the vessels and meninges usually appear normal for the age. Those who have died rapidly tend to show fewer abnormalities although the ventricles may be slightly enlarged. In those who have died after months or years of the illness the brain is more likely to be more atrophic with visible shrinkage of the cortex and enlarged ventricles. At times the atrophy may affect the corpus striatum and thalamus; the brain stem itself may appear considerably diminished in size; as a rule the white matter shows no abnormality.

In most cases, histological examination will reveal evidence of a triad of changes which together make up the hallmark of the disorder and again are present to a degree which tends to reflect the length of the illness.

With regard to the *first* of the changes, a spongy appearance of the cerebral cortex and of the deeper subcortical grey matter is often the most obvious, and is certainly the most helpful, of the changes which help make up the histological diagnosis. The sponginess, which cannot be seen with the naked eye, comes in two forms which can usually be distinguished (Masters and Richardson, 1978). The first is now generally known as 'spongiform change' and is made up of many small, usually rounded or oval, vacuoles in the neuropil. Although they do not appear under the light microscope to be confined within a cell's limits, electron microscopy has shown that they lie in neuronal, or glial processes. The smallest vacuoles measure as little as 1–2 μm across but they may coalesce into confluent areas up to 50 μm or, rarely, more across. Electron microscopy of the vacuoles (Chou et al., 1980) has shown them to contain alterations in the membranes in which ulceration, focal thickening and splitting may occur. Small blisters containing minute particulates have also been described, but the possible relation of these structures to any transmitting agent was left, and remains, open. The vacuolation is seen in all layers of the cortex and may at times spread almost uniformly

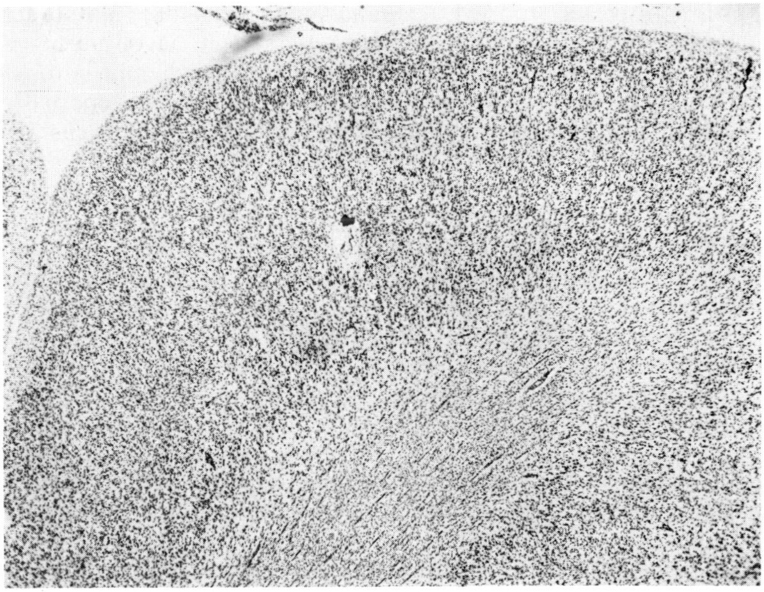

(**a**)

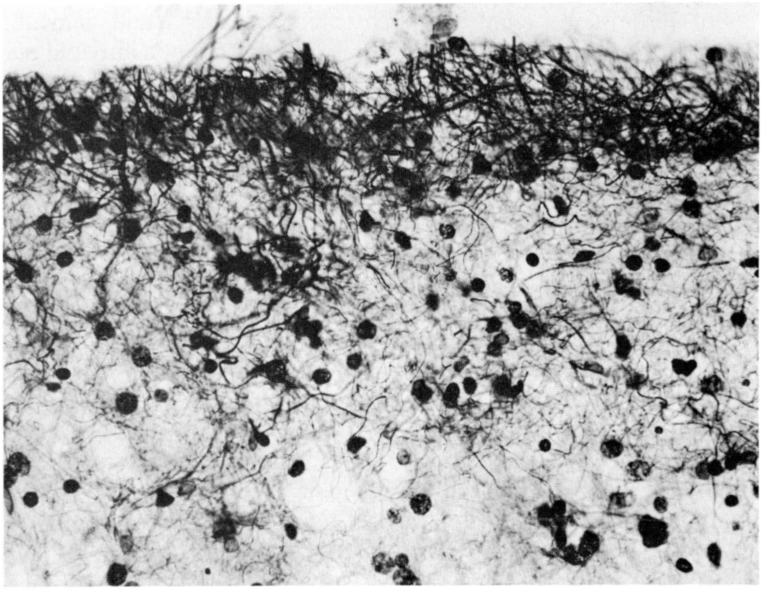

(**b**)

Fig. 20.29 Creutzfeldt–Jakob disease. (**a**) Frontal cortex showing almost complete disappearance of large pyramidal cells. Nissl ×20. (**b**) Subpial layer of frontal cortex. Holzer ×350.

through the thalamus, the striatum and the grey matter of the brain stem, as well as the molecular layer of the cerebellum. Most often it is patchy with stretches of apparently normal cortex or grey matter which alternate and intermingle with discrete patches of typical vacuolation. This change is usually readily identifiable (Fig. 20.29), but it is always advisable to keep in mind the possibility of processing artefact such as perineuronal vacuolation. Personal experience of a few cases, however, helps greatly in confident interpretation, although there always remains the need to distinguish as far as practicable this spongiform type of change from the looser and coarser 'microcystic' cavitation of cortex or other grey matter in which the tiny cysts or vacuoles are enmeshed in glial fibrils. This second form of sponginess is usually called 'status spongiosus' or 'spongy state'. This is a non-specific change and may for example, be found not uncommonly in the cerebral cortex and particularly in its outer layer in the brains of elderly people, in patients with Alzheimer's disease and in many other organic conditions, including those in which death has followed severe terminal anoxia.

The *second* change, that of neuronal loss, is also present in the great majority of cases. It may, however, be difficult to detect, particularly in those in whom the illness had been rapidly fatal or when a cortical biopsy has been taken early in the course of the illness. In either instance, areas of neuronal loss may be defined but they can at times be slight enough as to be unconvincing, and, particularly when spongiform change is not detectable, the diagnosis may become difficult. After death the degree of neuronal loss in the cortex, thalamus and striatum varies from severe and widespread, being most prominent in the third and deeper layer of the cortex, to irregular patchy loss of cells in the different layers; at times groups of abnormally shrunken, and often pale-staining, ghost-like remnants of cells may be seen to lie among other apparently normal neurons. This loss of nerve cells is accompanied by the third type of change: astrocytic proliferation. This may well be the dominant feature, particularly in long-standing cases. The affected areas are largely occupied by hypertrophied and often gemistocytic astrocytes among which vacuolation is commonly seen, interspersed with small numbers of surviving neurons, which may be shrunken or swollen and show cytoplasmic vacuoles. When the astrocytic proliferation is severe, it may spread over into areas of nerve cells which do not show obvious neuronal destruction or vacuolation; it may even reach into the adjacent parts of the white matter.

In spite of the transmissible nature of the disorder (which is discussed later, and also in Chapter 7) evidence of an inflammatory reaction is strikingly absent. The leptomeninges are normal and the very occasional cluster of perivascular lymphocytes in the occasional case is no more common than similar minor changes which occur in ageing generally. Even microglial proliferation is not prominent at any stage of the disease although an occasional microglial star or cluster can be found, particularly in the deeper layer of the cortex.

Cases which have presented unusual symptoms or pathological findings continue to be reported. Khurana and Garcia (1981) have found autonomic nervous system involvement in Creutzfeldt–Jakob disease, and optic atrophy with loss of retinal ganglion cells was reported in a single case by Lesser et al. (1979). Llena and Hirano (1979) have described a case of Creutzfeldt–Jakob disease with numerous eosinophilic rod-like bodies (Hirano bodies), a finding probably best interpreted as a secondary phenomenon. Occasional cases have presented and progressed with the clinical features of progressive supranuclear palsy (Russell, 1980); here spongiform change, neuronal loss and gliosis are concentrated in, or restricted to, the brain stem, the striatum and thalamus.

Some of the other occasional findings in Creutzfeldt–Jakob disease have produced evidence of pathological changes which may be looked on as notable variants. One example is the complex group of cases which closely resembles the Gerstmann–Sträussler syndrome (also mentioned on p. 979). This condition presents clinically with cerebellar ataxia and dementia whilst the brain is found to contain amyloid plaques accompanied at times by a spongiform change (Masters et al., 1981a). Masters and Gajdusek (1982) have reported on 17 examples, whilst others have been described by Boellaard and Schlote (1980) and by Schlote et al. (1980). The plaques which occur in this syndrome are said to have a structure intermediate between those seen in Alzheimer's disease and those in kuru. It may be relevant that Masters and Gajdusek (1982) consider that only those cases of the Gerstmann–Sträussler syndrome with spongiform change have proved to be transmissible. In general, typical neuritic (or senile) plaques have been found in small numbers in roughly 10 per cent of cases of Creutzfeldt–Jakob disease and may well be related more to ageing than to any direct link with the disease process itself.

Recently a material degree of myelin loss (Park, Kleinman and Richardson, 1980; Mizutani et al., 1981) has been recognized in some cases of Creutzfeldt–Jakob disease whilst infective agents have been isolated from white matter in experimentally infected rodents by Tateishi et al. (1979) and Sato, Ohta and Tateishi (1980). Extensive white matter degeneration has been reported involving the cerebellum, brain stem and spinal cord (Masters and Gajdusek, 1982).

The existence of an amyotrophic form of Creutzfeldt–Jakob disease is best regarded, at

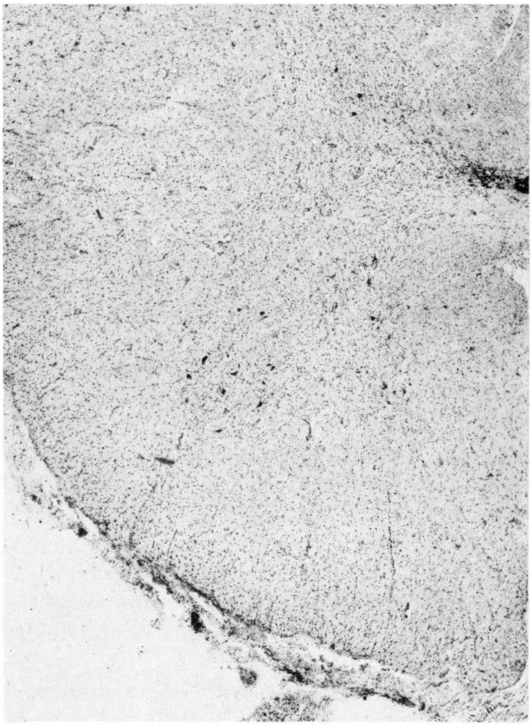

Fig. 20.30 Creutzfeldt-Jakob disease. Section of spinal cord at level L3 showing almost complete disappearance of motor nerve cells. Nissl ×25 reduced to 92%.

this stage, as unproven. Roughly 20 per cent of otherwise typical cases show muscle atrophy and fasciculation in the late stages of the illness but few, and possibly merely secondary, changes have been found in the spinal cord (Masters and Richardson, 1978). As first described by Jakob (1921) in his first case, those patients who present with motor neuron disease and dementia do not show the features of a spongiform disorder in the brain but the changes consist mainly of the loss of motor neurons in the cord (Fig. 20.30), brain stem and, commonly, in the substantia nigra, with some neuronal loss and gliosis in the cortex. This condition has not so far been transmitted to experimental animals (Salazar et al., 1983) and this fact, coupled with the atypical pathological picture, suggests that it should be provisonally looked on as a variant of motor neuron disease rather than as an unusual form of Creutzfeldt-Jakob disease.

Familial cases of Creutzfeldt-Jakob disease have been reported many times, and according to Masters et al. (1981b) there is a family history of the disease in about 15 per cent. The best known is the Backer family, first reported by Kirschbaum (1924) in which six histologically proven cases had occurred in three generations. Kirschbaum (1968) later traced the further ramifications of this remarkably family tree. Davison and Rabiner (1940) described the disease in two brothers and a sister. This family, however, has been considered by some as suffering from amyotrophic lateral sclerosis with a psychiatric illness resembling that reported by Meyer (1929). Friede and DeJong (1964) and May, Itabishi and DeJong (1968) have identified the illness in its typical form in three siblings and possibly in the father of the family. Masters et al. (1981b) have reviewed the familial occurrence of the disease, which occurs in affected families in a way consistent with autosomal dominance and transmission. The onset of symptoms is noticeably earlier than in sporadic cases whilst the incubation period was found to range from 1 to 40 years. The death of affected siblings, which tends to occur at the same age but not at the same time, suggests a form of vertical transmission which may be either pre- or postnatal, at least if a uniform incubation period is assumed. Within the affected families, however, the mechanism of spread has not been identified. The data from such families suggest that those acquiring the disease have a genetically determined susceptibility to the disorder which it probably acquired in early infancy or childhood. In affected families no evidence has been found of a maternal effect or a prenatal vertical transmission of the agent.

Transmissibility of Creutzfeldt–Jakob disease

This question is also considered in Chapter 7. Only three aspects most relevant to the problem of dementia are considered here.

Creutzfeldt-Jakob disease was looked on for many years as a rare, sometimes familial, form of dementia in adult life. Nothing in its clinical or neuropathological features suggested that it might be transmissible. The position changed, however, following the percipient observation by Hadlow in 1959 on the histological similarities between scrapie in sheep and the rare human disease of kuru. Although in both these conditions the changes appeared degenerative in nature, the former disease had already been recognized as transmissible and in due course kuru also proved to be (Gajdusek, Gibbs and Alpers,

1966). Meanwhile, Klatzo, Gajdusek and Zigas (1959) had compared kuru to Creutzfeldt–Jakob disease and the similarities were confirmed by Beck et al. in 1966. In the same year, cerebral biopsy taken from a proven case of Creutzfeldt–Jakob disease by Daniel, Beck & Matthews was injected into the brain of a chimpanzee, which 18 months later developed a similar illness (Gibbs et al., 1968; Beck et al., 1969). In due course the range of vulnerable animals has come to include New World and other monkeys, cats, rats, mice and guinea-pigs. The incubation period has been found to vary from months to years; other routes of transmission such as intravenous, intramuscular, subcutaneous and corneal have proved effective. The oral route has also been found to be effective for Creutzfeldt–Jakob disease, kuru and scrapie (Gibbs et al., 1980).

The agent has been isolated from human cases of Creutzfeldt–Jakob disease in lymph nodes, lungs, liver, kidney, CSF and possibly blood (Masters et al., 1979). The agent, moreover, may be detected in the various organs of an animal originally infected by intracerebral injection.

Creutzfeldt–Jakob disease, kuru and scrapie (with mink encephalopathy) have therefore been grouped together as the transmissible subacute spongiform encephalopathies. The nature of the transmissible agents, however, remains unknown; they are widely, if less than universally, referred to as 'slow viruses'. Their bizarre characteristics and behaviour are outlined on p. 291.

Not all attempts to transmit Creutzfeldt–Jakob disease to animals prove successful; Gibbs and Gajdusek (1978) have reported that cerebral tissue from 70 per cent of 122 originally ill patients had infected one or more animal species within a 3-year period.

Those animals which develop the transmitted disease show the histological pattern of a subacute spongiform encephalopathy although some variability may occur according either to the particular animal involved or possibly, as in scrapie, to a particular strain of the transmissible agent. The properties of these agents is considered in Chapter 7, but it may be briefly mentioned here that they have a different chemical make-up from conventional viruses and they are curiously difficult to destroy—indeed, as Gajdusek (1972) observed, they are better looked on as 'something new to microbiology'.

The success of the transmission experiments led to two possibilities. First, there is the risk that Creutzfeldt–Jakob disease might be transmitted from person to person. Secondly, it is conceivable that other obscure disorders and dementias might be the result of similar slow virus infections.

Case-to-case transmission of Creutzfeldt–Jakob disease In 1974 Duffy et al. reported a case of Creutzfeldt–Jakob disease which developed in a 55-year-old man 18 months after he had received a corneal transplant from a patient who had died after a short-lived dementing illness with myoclonus and who, after autopsy, was established as having the neurohistological features of Creutzfeldt–Jakob disease. Two years later Bernoulli et al. (1977) reported two instances of the development of Creutzfeldt–Jakob disease, each occurring about 2 years after temporary stereotactic implantation of silver electrodes which had previously been inserted into the brain of a 69-year-old woman with confirmed Creutzfeldt–Jakob disease. The electrodes had been 'sterilized' after their first use, with 70% alcohol and formaldehyde vapour. The biopsy and implantation of electrodes had occurred after 45 months of her illness; in the inoculated cases, both of whom had psychomotor epilepsy and may therefore have already suffered from cerebral damage, incubation to symptom development was around 18 months. The diagnosis of Creutzfeldt–Jakob disease was confirmed after death in one and electroencephalographically in the other.

Will and Matthews (1982) have reviewed the evidence for case-to-case transmission and reported details of the neurosurgical procedures which had been carried out on several of the patients with Creutzfeldt–Jakob disease reported by Jones and Nevin in 1954, and Nevin et al., in 1960. One patient had died 19 months after an intracranial operation, and on the same list, in the same theatre and on the same day, burr holes and ventriculography had been carried out on a patient with Creutzfeldt–Jakob disease. Two other patients were also noted by Jones and Nevin (1954) to have had histories of previous intracranial operative procedures. In retrospect both were found to have been operated on in the same theatre and within 2 weeks of a patient with Creutzfeldt–Jakob disease who had burr holes made and depth electrodes inserted into the brain. Two other cases in the series were reported by Will and Matthews in which previous intracranial operations had been performed but no evidence was traced of a connection with an intracranial operation on any case of Creutzfeldt–Jakob disease.

In this same report Will and Matthews (1982) have examined the evidence in their investigations of spaciotemporal clustering and contact with familial cases. One close geographical group of three cases suggested, but failed to establish, transmission through dentistry. Two other cases have been reported of patients who developed the disease after contact with families prone to develop Creutzfeldt–Jakob disease (Brown et al., 1979; Galvez, Masters and Gajdusek, 1980). So far, however, no convincing evidence has been produced that Creutzfeldt–Jakob disease has developed after contact with a sporadic case, all the possible 'contact' transmissions having been through association with familial cases. Moreover, although small clusters of cases have been identified in various countries, such as Czechoslovakia, England, Hungary, Israel and Italy, none seems striking enough to confirm that a transmission has occurred in this way. Again, careful search of the many cases identified in France (Brown and Cathala, 1979; Brown, Cathala and Gajdusek, 1979; Brown et al., 1979) and in the USA, Chile and Japan (Masters and Gajdusek, 1982) has failed to yield evidence of clustering.

In short, there still seems no convincing evidence that anyone has contracted Creutzfeldt–Jakob disease from another person either in the community or by medical (as distinct from surgical) contact in a hospital setting.

Lastly, there is the question whether other forms of chronic cerebral disease might be the result of a slow virus infection. The possibility, foreshadowed by Gajdusek in 1977, was followed up by Gajdusek and Gibbs who widened the range of their transmission studies to include examples of Alzheimer's disease, Huntington's chorea, Pick's disease and a number of other conditions. Two hundred and twenty cases were included in the study; 78 ultimately transmitted to experimental animals (Traub et al., 1977). All but three of the 78, however, proved to have been cases of Creutzfeldt–Jakob disease.

The three exceptions nevertheless constituted a potentially important group, for two of them were examples of familial Alzheimer's disease (the third was an unexplained case of supranuclear palsy). In 1980, Goudsmit et al. reported on tissue from the same two cases and found that the initial transmission could not be reproduced. Perhaps partly because a further 17 cases of Alzheimer's disease had also proved negative 4 years after the injection, the conclusion was reached that 'the association between Alzheimer's disease and an infectious agent has not yet been demonstrated with any reasonable degree of certainty'.

Brown et al. (1982) returned to the problem and again have concluded that attempts to transmit Alzheimer's disease to animals have not 'validated a common aetiology' with the spongiform encephalopathies. In short, there is no good evidence at present that Alzheimer's disease is transmissible—even if Masters and Gajdusek (1982) hold to the view that there is enough 'indirect and circumstantial evidence' linking the disease to Creutzfeldt–Jakob—to justify further research.

Finally, tissue from none of the other dementing conditions mentioned above has so far been found to induce a spongy brain in an animal; nor has cerebral tissue taken from a person with any other neurological or psychiatric illness, organic or functional, which is not in some way linked to the spongiform encephalopathies, achieved this.

Pathological conditions associated with memory disorder and dementia

Deterioration of memory is one of the main features of dementia and is usually attributable to the widespread degeneration of cerebral tissue. There are, however, occasions in which the memory disorder is dominant and in which certain regions of the brain appear to play a particular role. One is that of the mamillary bodies and the medial thalamus; the other is the grey matter in the inferomedial parts of the temporal lobe, including the hippocampus and the parahippocampal gyrus. These two regions, which are connected by the fornix, constitute a major part of the limbic areas, named after 'the great limbic lobe of Broca' (1878).

In 1890, Korsakow (Korsakoff) reported an illness, now named after him, which he attributed to toxaemia resulting from various causes including too much alcohol. He described how 'together with the confusion, nearly always a profound disorder of the memory is observed although at times the disorder of memory occurs in pure form ... this manifests itself in an extraordinary peculiar amnesia in which the memory

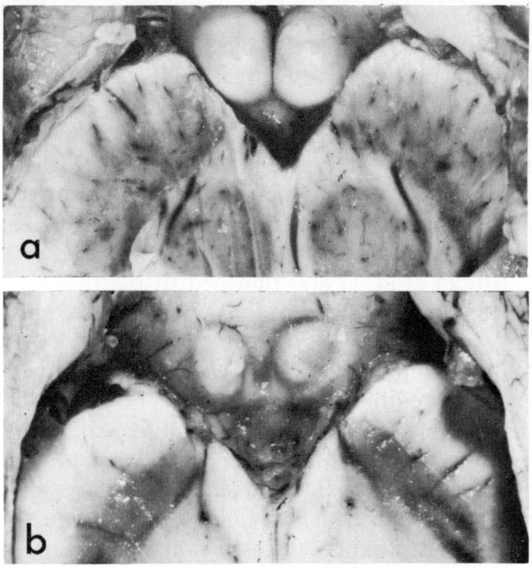

Fig. 20.31 A surface view of (**a**) normal mamillary bodies, for comparison with (**b**) the atrophied and discoloured mamillary bodies of a 'korsakovian' patient.

of recent events is chiefly disturbed, whereas the remote past was remembered fairly well'. Some 10 years before this Wernicke (1881) had identified a severe tissue reaction, now known as Wernicke's (or Gayet–Wernicke's) encephalopathy, which was centred on the periventricular grey matter in the brain of patients dying from alcoholism or from other causes. Gudden (1896) and Bonhoeffer (1897) noticed that the mamillary bodies were particularly vulnerable, and the latter hinted at a connection between the damage in this area and the Korsakoff state. This hypothesis was not generally accepted until Gamper (1928) demonstrated that, although the damage spread through the grey matter encircling the walls of the aqueduct and of the third and fourth ventricles, it was most intense in the mamillary bodies (Fig. 20.31). Gamper postulated that this lesion interfered with the pathways linking the mamillary bodies to the midbrain, thalamus and cerebral cortex, and that this interruption lay at the root of the memory disorder in the Korsakoff state. Although at first not generally accepted (Carmichael and Stern, 1931), many subsequent studies (Kant, 1933; Delay, Brion and Elisalde, 1958; Mair, Warrington and Weiskrantz, 1979) have confirmed Gamper's observations, and the illness described by Korsakow is now widely recognized to be in many, but not all, cases the result of damage to the brain caused by an attack of Wernicke's encephalopathy, which is itself attributable to the effects of alcoholism or of other disorders leading to thiamine deficiency. As described by Gamper and by Malamud and Skillicorn (1956), the mamillary bodies have nearly always been found to be the most vulnerable, and occasional cases have been reported in which no other area appeared to have been affected (Brierley, 1966). There is, nevertheless, a striking tendency for neuronal loss and gliosis to occur medially in the thalamus, and Victor, Adams and Collins (1971) have argued that the lesion in the dorsomedial nucleus is the more important factor. To add to this, Squire and Moore (1979) reported on an amnesic patient in whom CT brain scans had shown bilateral dorsal thalamic lesions. Part of the dorsomedial nucleus, moreover, is affected after prefrontal leucotomy (Meyer and Beck, 1954), and attempts were made at one time to destroy it stereotactically (Spiegel et al., 1955). Some disorder of memory had indeed been attributed to such circumscribed damage at times (see Horel (1978) for references) but it seems doubtful whether enough is known at present about the subtleties of localization to incriminate one part of the deep grey matter rather than another. The more crucial points seem to be that the damage is always bilateral and that it lies along the diencephalic sector of the limbic pathways.

Another source of pathological information comes from studying the effect of localized damage due to cerebrovascular degeneration. The medial parts of the temporal lobe are supplied mainly, but not exclusively, by branches of the posterior cerebral artery, and as early as 1899 von Bechterew had encountered a patient with gross memory disorder in whose brain bilateral softening of the inner parts of the temporal cortex was probably of vascular origin. Since then further examples have been reported by Victor et al. (1961), Van Buren and Borke (1972) and Brindley and Janota (1975). Woods, Schoene and Kneisley (1982) have added to this evidence by describing a severely amnesic patient in whose brain the medial temporooccipital region had been infarcted on the left side but the infarct on the left was limited to the hippocampus. The upshot of these studies has been a recurrent emphasis on the overriding importance to memory disorder of bilateral destruction of the hippocampal regions. Even in certain dementias, and particularly of the Alzheimer type in which memory loss is a feature, the neuronal populations in these areas is often strikingly vulnerable and it is tempting to link the clinical to the pathological phenomena.

The most striking evidence, however, of the effect on memory of damage to the temporal lobes was reported by Scoville (1954) after the resection of the inferomedial parts of the temporal lobes in several psychotic patients. He and Milner (1957) found that a severe defect in recent memory was produced by the bilateral removal of the hippocampus and parahippocampal gyrus but not by operations affecting only the uncus and the amygdaloid nucleus. Pilleri (1966) and McLardy (1970) have emphasized the importance of the parahippocampal cortex.

Petit-Dutaillis et al. (1954) removed the anterior parts, but not the hippocampi, of both temporal lobes from a patient with epilepsy. Only a transient disorder of recent memory occurred although there was a permanent retrograde amnesia covering several months. Terzian and Ore (1955) removed the entire anterior parts of both temporal lobes as well as most of the two hippocampi. 'A serious deficiency in memory' was noted as one of the effects but the main emphasis was on the resemblance of the post-operative clinical picture to the Klüver–Bucy syndrome (Gascon and Gilles, 1973).

Interference with recent memory is usual only when the medial temporal damage is bilateral, but unilateral resections may have an effect. Milner and Penfield (1955) and Serafetinides and Falconer (1962) reported that the removal of one temporal lobe was sometimes followed by a defect in recent memory although there were usually grounds to suspect that the contralateral hippocampus might have been diseased as well. Meyer and Yates (1955) and Meyer (1959) found that new verbal and auditory learning could be impaired by the removal of the dominant temporal lobe, although Blakemore and Falconer (1967) found that the defect on the auditory side tended eventually to disappear. Stepien and Sierpinski (1964) discussed the effect on memory of temporal lobe lesions. They described several epileptic patients in whom a memory disorder was associated with bilateral electroencephalographic abnormalities. After removing one lobe, however, the abnormal discharges on the unoperated side as well as the memory disorder disappeared. They postulated that unilateral lesions may interrupt normal activity throughout the brain and that their excision removes the source of irritation.

There are several other pathological conditions in which the medial parts of the temporal lobes tend to be selectively affected. One of these is the form of necrotizing encephalitis, described by van Bogaert, Radermecker and Devos (1955), in which an acute inflammatory reaction underlies the massive necrosis of much or all of both temporal lobes. The illness, in which there is often evidence of herpes simplex infection, is usually fatal within 2 weeks (Adams and Jennett, 1967). A few adults, however, survive the acute attack for months or years. At times the onset is insidious. In either case the patients are likely to be left with an incapacitating defect in recent memory or they may be demented. Rose and Symonds (1960) reported clinically on three adults with 'persistent memory defect following encephalitis'. One (case 3) who survived with gross amnesia for 17 years was found after death (Hierons, Janota and Corsellis, 1978) to have lost the medial parts of both temporal lobes as the consequence of necrotizing encephalitis (Fig. 20.32).

Not all cases of encephalitis of the limbic areas, however, are of the necrotizing type. Brierley et al. (1960) reported three patients in their 50s who had become demented over a period lasting from a few months to a year. No cause

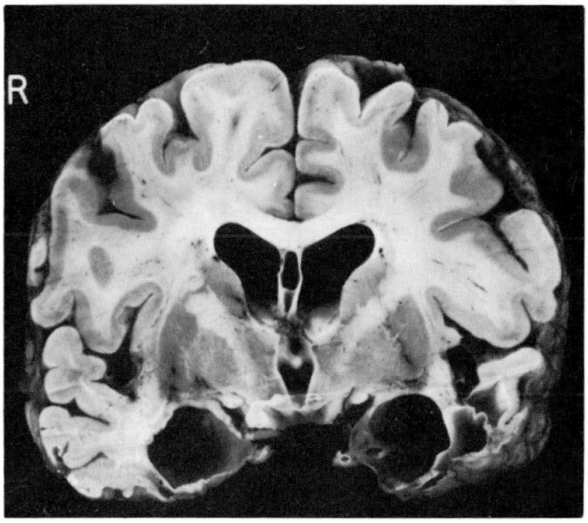

Fig. 20.32 Coronal cut through the brain of a woman who had survived, grossly amnesic, for 17 years after an attack of necrotizing encephalitis. The medial temporal matter on the right side (R) and much of the left temporal lobe have been destroyed.

for the dementia (or for the marked memory loss noted in two of the three patients) was attributed during life but the common neurohistological feature was a severe inflammatory reaction centred on the limbic grey matter. No cause was identified but in one case the presence of a secondary deposit from an unsuspected bronchial carcinoma introduced a further problem.

Limbic encephalitis and malignant disease

Patients with malignant disease, and particularly with bronchial carcinoma, are prone to become mentally ill. Sometimes the disorder is in the nature of a toxic confusional state and the brain shows no particular abnormality (Charatan and Brierley, 1956; McGovern, Miller and Robertson, 1959). Occasionally, however, dementia, or predominantly a memory disorder, may develop. This may be in the presence of other non-metastatic neurological disease, such as in the cerebellar degenerations associated with carcinoma (Brain, Daniel and Greenfield, 1951; Henson, Hoffman and Urich, 1965), or the mental deterioration may occur on its own. Corsellis, Goldberg and Norton (1968) described three patients with bronchial carcinoma in the latter category, two of whom had become demented whilst the third suffered for over 2 years from a curiously discrete loss of recent memory. Attention was drawn to several similar cases that had been reported, and Dubas et al. (1981a) have since reviewed in detail the 40 or so in the literature, as well as adding a further six. Dubas et al. (1982b) have emphasized, however, that the same condition is less often found in the absence of cancer—an observation which was previously made by Brierley et al. (1960). The brains showed perivascular round-cell infiltration, resembling an encephalitis, which was concentrated mainly on the medial temporal grey matter. Glial nodules were common and a variable degree of neuronal necrosis was seen. The appearances were usually those of a tissue reaction which was considerably more intense than that attributable to a primary neuronal degeneration and yet not as grossly destructive as that occurring in necrotizing limbic encephalitis. Henson, Hoffman and Urich (1965) and Richardson (1965) surmised that the condition might be of viral, and even of herpes simplex, origin. Some support for this was provided by Dayan, Bhatti and Gostling (1967), who reported that a fatal, and proven herpetic, encephalitis had developed in a woman several months after the removal of a uterine carcinoma. There is little direct evidence beyond this, however, to support the viral hypothesis. Similarly, metabolic and immune factors have been invoked but not identified, and both the relation of the condition to carcinoma and its aetiology remain unknown. Smith (1970) suggested that minute metastatic foci might have been overlooked, but such repeated oversight seems improbable and the curiously intense tissue reaction would remain unexplained. Henson and Urich (1982) have discussed the condition of 'limbic encephalitis' at some length within the general setting of encephalomyelitis as one of the remote effects of cancer. It should not be forgotten that dementia has been reported in association with carcinomatous infiltration of the leptomeninges (Fischer-Williams, Bosanquet and Daniel, 1955) but the amnesic features, coupled with the affective changes, are particularly noticeable in the limbic disorder.

Finally, it should be emphasized that there are many diffuse or multifocal disorders of the brain in which a variable degree of intellectual deterioration may occur. In addition to those considered in this chapter, dementia may be the sequel to infections of the nervous system, to episodes of severe cerebral ischaemia or hypoxia, and to metabolic and endocrine disturbances, whilst it may also occur in association with system degeneration and with demyelinating disease. The nature of the cerebral abnormality will then vary according to the type of illness.

In general, most patients with a progressive dementia fall into one or other of the established categories. This chapter should have shown, if nothing else, that in the present state of knowledge nosological overlap is common and drawing hard and fast lines can be less than profitable. Sometimes an abnormality is evident but its origin and its classification are not. In others it may be difficult or even impossible to find any structural abnormality. For obvious reasons, such cases tend to go unrecorded but it would be misleading to imply either that they never occur or that they are at all common.

References

Abely, X., Guirard, P. and Dechosal, J. (1958) Alzheimer of acute onset. *Annales Médico-psychologiques* **116,** 294-9.

Adam, J., Crow, T.J., Duchen, L.W., Scaravilli, F. and Spokes, E. (1982) Familial cerebral amyloidosis and spongiform encephalopathy. *Journal of Neurology, Neurosurgery and Psychiatry* **45,** 37-45.

Adams, J.H. and Jennett, W.B. (1967) Acute necrotizing encephalitis: A problem in diagnosis. *Journal of Neurology, Neurosurgery and Psychiatry* **30,** 248-60.

Akelaitis, A.J. (1944) Atrophy of basal ganglia in Pick's disease. A clinicopathologic study. *Archives of Neurology and Psychiatry* **51,** 27-34.

Albert, M.L. (1978) Subcortical dementia. In *Alzheimer's Disease, Senile Dementia and Related Disorders.* (Eds. Katzman R., Terry, R.D. and Bick, K.L.) pp. 173-180. Raven Press, New York.

Albert, M.L., Feldman, R.G. and Willis, A.L. (1974) The 'subcortical dementia' of progressive supranuclear palsy. *Journal of Neurology, Neurosurgery and Psychiatry* **37,** 121-30.

Alzheimer, A. (1898) Neuere Arbeiten über die Dementia senilis und die auf atheromatöser Gefässerkrankung basierenden Gehirhkrankheiten. *Monatsschrift für Psychiatrie und Neurologie* **3,** 101-15.

Alzheimer, A. (1907a) Ueber eine eigenartige Erkrankung der Hirnrinde. *Allgemeine Zeitschrift für Psychiatrie* **64,** 146-8.

Alzheimer, A. (19707b) Ueber eine eigenartige Erkrankung der Hirnrinde. *Zentralblatt für die gesamte Neurologie und Psychiatrie* **18,** 177-9.

Alzheimer, A. (1911) Ueber eigenartigen Krankheitsfälle des späteren Alters. *Zentralblatt für die gesamte Neurologie und Psychiatrie* **4,** 356-85.

Anderton, B.H., Breinburg, D., Downes, M.L.J., Green, P.J., Tomlinson, B.E., Ulrich, J. et al. (1982) Monoclonal antibodies show that neurofibrillary tangles and neurofilaments share antigenic determinants. *Nature* (*Lond.*) **298,** 84-6.

Arendt, T., Bigl, V., Arendt, A. and Tennstedt, A. (1983) Loss of neurons in the nucleus basalis of Meynert in Alzheimer's Disease, Paralysis Agitans and Korsakoff's Disease. *Acta Neuropathologica* **61,** 101-108.

Arregui, A., Iverson, L.L., Spokes, E.G.S. and Emson, C. (1979) Extrapyramidal diseases. In *The Molecular Basis of Neuropathology* (Eds. Davison, A.N. and Thompson, R.H.S.) pp. 345-83. Edward Arnold, London.

Averback, P. (1983) Two new lesions in Alzheimer's disease. *Lancet* **2,** 1203.

von Bagh, K. (1941) Ueber anatomische Befunde bei 30 Fällen systematischer Atrophie der Grosshirnrinde (Pickscher Krankheit) mit besonderer Berücksichtigung der Stammganglien und der langen absteigenden Leitungsbahnen. *Archiv für Psychiatrie und Nervenkrankheiten* **114,** 68-70.

Ball, M.J. (1976) Neuronal loss, neurofibrillary tangles and granulovacuolar degeneration in the hippocampus with ageing and dementia—a quantitative study. *Acta Neuropathologica* **37,** 111-18.

Ball, M.J. (1979) Topography of Pick inclusion bodies in hippocampi of demented patients. *Acta Neuropathologica* **42,** 73-80.

Ball, M.J. and Lo, P. (1977) Granulovacuolar degeneration in the ageing brain and in dementia. *Journal of Neuropathology and Experimental Neurology* **36,** 474-87.

Barbeau, A. (1973) In *Advances in Neurology*, vol. 1, *Huntington's Chorea 1872-1972* (Eds. Barbeau, A., Chase, T.N. and Paulson, G.W.). Raven Press, New York.

Barron, S.A., Jacobs, L. and Kinkel, W.R. (1976) Changes in size of normal lateral ventricles during ageing determined by computerized tomography. *Neurology* **26,** 1011-13.

von Bechterew, W.V. (1899) Demonstration eines Gehirns mit Zerstörung der vorderen und inneren Theile der Hirnrinde beider Schläfenlappen. *Zentralblatt für die gesamte Neurologie und Psychiatrie* **19,** 990-1.

Beck, E., Daniel, P.M., Alpers, M., Gajdusek, D.C. and Gibbs, C.J. Jr (1966) Experimental kuru in chimpanzees: a pathological report. *Lancet* **2,** 1056-9.

Beck, E., Matthews, W.B., Stevens, D.L., Alpers, M.P., Asher, D.M., Gajdusek, D.C. and Gibbs, C.J. Jr (1969) Creutzfeldt-Jakob disease. The neuropathology of a transmission experiment. *Brain* **92,** 699-716.

Bell, J. (1934) Huntington's chorea. In *Treasury of Human Inheritance*, vol. 4, *Nervous Diseases and Muscular Dystrophies.* Cambridge University Press, Cambridge.

Benirsche, K. and Höfnagel, D. (1961) Clinical conditions with a normal chromosome complement. *Human Chromosome Newsletter* **4,** 4.

Berlin, L. (1949) Presenile sclerosis (Alzheimer's disease with features resembling Pick's disease). *Archives of Neurology and Psychiatry* **61,** 369-84.

Bernheimer, H., Birkmayer, W., Hornykiewicz, O., Jellinger, K. and Seitelberger, F. (1973) Brain dopamine and the syndromes of Parkinson and Huntington—clinical, morphological and neurochemical correlations. *Journal of the Neurological Sciences* **20,** 415-55.

Bernoulli, C., Siegfried, J., Baumgartner, G., Regli,

F., Rabinowicz, T., Gajdusek, D.C. and Gibbs, C.J. Jr (1977) Danger of accidental person-to-person transmission of Creutzfeldt-Jakob disease by surgery. *Lancet* **1,** 478-9.

Bielschowsky, M. (1932) In *Cytology and Cellular Pathology of the Nervous System*, vol. 3 (Ed. Penfield, W.). Hoeber, New York.

Binswanger, O. (1894) Die Abgrenzung der allgemeinen progressiven Paralyse. *Berliner klinische Wochenschrift* **31,** 1103-5, 1137-9, 1180-6.

Bird, E.D. (1976a) Normal glutamic acid decarboxylase activity in kidney tissue from patients with Huntington's disease. *Journal of Neurochemistry* **27,** 1555-7.

Bird, E.D. (1976b) Biochemical studies on gamma-aminobutyric acid metabolism in Hungton's chorea. In *Biochemistry and Neurology* (Eds. Bradford, H.F. and Marsden, C.D.), pp. 83-92. Academic Press, New York.

Bird, E.D. (1978) The brain in Huntington's chorea. (Editorial) *Psychological Medicine* **8,** 357-60.

Bird, E.D., Caro, A.J. and Pilling, J.B. (1974) A sex related factor in the inheritance of Huntington's chorea. *Annals of Human Genetics* **37,** 255-60.

Bird, E.D. and Iversen, L.L. (1974) Huntington's chorea—postmortem measurement of glutamic acid decarboxylase, choline acetyltransferase and dopamine in basal ganglia. *Brain* **97,** 457-72.

Bird, E.D. and Iversen, L.L. (1976) Neurochemical findings in Huntington's chorea. In *Essays in Neurochemistry and Neuropharmacology* (Eds. Youdim, M.B.H., Lovenberg, W., Sharman, D.F. and Lagnado, J.R.), pp. 177-93. Wiley, New York.

Bird, E.D., MacKay, A.V.P. and Rayner, C. (1973) Reduced glutamic acid decarboxylase activity in postmortem brain in Huntington's chorea. *Lancet* **1,** 1090-2.

Birse, S.H. and Tom, M.I. (1960) Incidence of cerebral infarction associated with ruptured intracerebral aneurysms. *Neurology* **10,** 101-6.

Bittenbender, J.B. and Quadfasel, F.A. (1962) Rigid and akinetic forms of Huntington's chorea. *Archives of Neurology* **7,** 275-88.

Blakemore, C.B. and Falconer, M.A. (1967) Long-term effects of anterior temporal lobectomy on certain cognitive functions. *Journal of Neurology, Neurosurgery and Psychiatry* **30,** 364-7.

Blessed, G., Tomlinson, B.E. and Roth, M. (1968) The association between quantitative measures of dementia and of senile change in the cerebral grey matter of elderly subjects. *British Journal of Psychiatry* **114,** 797-811.

Blocq, P. and Marinesco, G. (1892) Sur lés lesions et la pathogénie de l'épilepsie dite essentielle. *Semaine Médicale* **12,** 445-6.

Boellaard, J.W. and Schlote, W. (1980) Subakute spongiforme Encephalopathie mit multiformer Plaquebildung. 'Eigenartige familiär-hereditäre Krankheit des Zentralnervensystems (spino-cerebellare Atrophie mit Demenz, Plaques und Plaqueähnlichen im Kleinund Grosshirn' (Gerstmann, Sträussler, Scheinker). *Acta Neuropathologica* **49,** 205-12.

van Bogaert, L., Radermecker, J. and Devos, J. (1955) Sur une observation mortelle d'encéphalite aiguë nécrosante. *Revue Neurologique* **92,** 329-56.

Boller, F., Mizutani, T., Roessmann, U. and Gambetti, P. (1980) Parkinson's disease, dementia and Alzheimer disease: clinicopathological correlations. *Annals of Neurology* **7,** 329-35.

Bolt, J.M.W. (1970) Huntington's chorea in the west of Scotland. *British Journal of Psychiatry* **116,** 259-70.

Bondareff, W., Mountjoy, C.J. and Roth, M. (1982) Loss of neurons of origin of the adrenergic projection to cerebral cortex (nucleus locus ceruleus) in senile dementia. *Neurology* **32,** 164-8.

Bonfiglio, F. (1908) Die speciali reperti in un case di probabile sifilide cerebrale. *Rivista Sperimentale di Freniatriae e Medicina Legale delle Alienazioni Mentale* **34,** 196-206.

Bonhoeffer, K. (1897) Klinische und anatomische Beiträge zur Kenntnis der Alkoholdelirien. *Monatsschrift für Psychiatrie und Neurologie* **1,** 229-51.

Boudin, G., Pépin, P. and Milhaud, M. (1965) Maladie de Creutzfeldt-Jakob à symptomatologie cérébelleuse dominante. (Etude anatomoclinique d'un cas). *Revue Neurologique* **113,** 73-5.

Bowen, D.M. (1981) Alzheimer's disease. In *The Molecular Basis of Neuropathology* (Eds. Davison, A.N. and Thompson, R.H.S.), pp. 649-65. Edward Arnold, London.

Bowen, D.M., Smith, C.B., White, P. and Davison, A.N. (1976) Neurotransmitter-related enzymes and indices of hypoxia in senile dementia and other abiotrophies. *Brain* **99,** 459-96.

Bowen, D.M., Smith, C.B., White, P., Flack, R.H.A., Carrasco, L.H., Gedye, J.L. and Davison, A.N. (1977) Chemical pathology of the organic dementias. *Brain* **100,** 427-53.

Brain, W.R., Daniel, P.M. and Greenfield, J.G. (1951). Sub-acute cortical cerebellar degeneration and its relation to carcinoma. *Journal of Neurology, Neurosurgery and Psychiatry* **14,** 59-75.

Brandenburg, W. and Hallervorden, I. (1954) Dementia pugilistica mit anatomischen Befund. *Virchows Archiv für pathologische Anatomie und Physiologie und für klinische Medizin* **325,** 680-709.

von Braunmühl, A. (1928) Zur Histopathologie der umschriebenen Grosshirnatrophie (Picksche Krankheit). *Virchows Archiv für pathologische Anatomie und Physiologie und für klinische Medizin* **270,** 448-86.

von Braünmuhl, A. (1931) Neue Gesichtspunkte zum Problem der senilen Plaques. *Zeitschrift für die gesamte Neurologie und Psychiatrie* **133,** 391–441.

Brierley, J.B. (1966) The Neuropathology of Amnesic States. In *Amnesia* (Eds. Whitty, C.W.M. and Zangwill, O.), pp. 150–80. Butterworths, London.

Brierley, J.B., Corsellis, J.A.N., Hierons, R. and Nevin, S. (1960) Subacute encephalitis of later adult life, mainly affecting the limbic areas. *Brain* **83,** 357–68.

Brindley, G.S. and Janota, I. (1975) Observations on cortical blindness and on vascular lesions that cause loss of recent memory. *Journal of Neurology, Neurosurgery and Psychiatry* **5,** 459–64.

Brizzee, K.R., Ordy, J.M. and Kaack, B. (1974). Early appearance and regional differences in intraneuronal and extraneuronal lipofuscin accumulation with age in the brain of a non-human primate (*Macaca mulatta*). *Journal of Gerontology* **29,** 366–81.

Broca, P. (1878) Anatomie comparée des circonvolutions cérébrales. *Revue d'Anthropologie*, series 3 **1,** 385–455.

Brody, H. (1955) Organization of the cerebral cortex. III. A study of aging in the human cerebral cortex. *Journal of Comparative Neurology* **102,** 511–56.

Brody, H. (1960) The deposition of aging pigment in the human cerebral cortex. *Journal of Gerontology* **15,** 258–61.

Brody, H. (1976) An examination of cerebral cortex and brain stem aging. In *Aging*, vol. 3: *Neurobiology of Aging* (Ed. Terry, R.D. and Gershon, S.), pp. 177–83, Raven Press, New York.

Brothers, C.R.D. (1949) The history and incidence of Huntington's chorea in Tasmania. *Proceedings of the Royal Australasian College of Physicians* **4,** 48–50.

Brown, P. and Cathala, F. (1979) Creutzfeldt-Jakob disease in France. I. Retrospective study of the Paris area during the ten-year period 1968–1977. *Annals of Neurology* **6,** 189–92.

Brown, P., Cathala, F. and Gajdusek, D.C. (1979a) Creutzfeldt-Jakob disease in France. III. Epidemiological study of 170 patients dying during the decade 1968–1977. *Annals of Neurology* **6,** 438–46.

Brown, P., Cathala, F., Sadowsky, D. and Gajdusek, D.C. (1979) Creutzfeldt-Jakob disease in France. II. Clinical characteristics of 124 consecutive verified cases during the decade 1968–1977. *Annals of Neurology* **6,** 430–7.

Brown, P., Salazar, A.M., Gibbs, C.J. Jr. and Gajdusek, D.C. (1982) Alzheimer's Disease and Transmissible Virus Dementia (Creutzfeldt-Jakob Disease). *Annals of the New York Academy of Sciences* **396,** 131–143.

Brownell, B. and Oppenheimer, D. (1965) An ataxic form of presenile polioencephalopathy (Creutzfeldt-Jakob disease). *Journal of Neurology, Neurosurgery and Psychiatry* **28,** 350–61.

Bruce, M.E., Dickinson, A.G. and Fraser, H. (1976) Cerebral amyloidosis in scrapie in the mouse: effect of agent strain and mouse genotype. *Neuropathology and Applied Neurobiology* **2,** 471–8.

Bruce, M.E. and Fraser, A.H. (1975) Amyloid plaques in the brains of mice infected with scrapie: morphological variations and staining properties. *Neuropathology and Applied Neurobiology* **1,** 189–202.

Brun, A. and Englund, E. (1981) Regional pattern of degeneration in Alzheimer's disease: neuronal loss and histopathological grading. *Histopathology* **5,** 549–64.

Bruyn, G.W. (1967) The Westphal variant and juvenile type of Huntington's chorea. In *Progress in Neurogenetics* (Eds. Barbeau, A. and Brunette, J.R.), pp. 666–73. Excerpta Medica Foundation, Amsterdam.

Bruyn, G.W. (1973) Neuropathological changes in Huntington's chorea. In *Advances in Neurology*, vol. 1, *Huntington's Chorea 1872–1972* (Eds. Barbeau, A., Chase, T.N. and Paulson, G.W.), pp. 399–403. Raven Press, New York.

Bruyn, G.W., Bots, A.A.M. and Dom, R. (1979) Huntington's chorea: current neuropathological status. In *Advances in Neurology*, vol. 23, *Huntington's Disease* (Eds. Chase, T.N., Wexler, N.S. and Barbeau, A.), pp. 83–93. Raven Press, New York.

Buell, S.J. and Coleman, P.D. (1979) Dendritic growth in the aged brain and failure of growth in senile dementia. *Science* **206,** 854–6.

Bugiani, O., Salvarini, S., Perdelli, F., Mancardi, G.D. and Leonardi, A. (1978) Nerve cell loss with ageing in the putamen. *European Neurology* **17,** 286–91.

Burns, B.D. (1958) *The Mammalian Cerebral Cortex*. Edward Arnold, London.

Campbell, A.M.G., Corner, B., Norman, R.M. and Urich, H. (1961) The rigid form of Huntington's disease. *Journal of Neurology, Neurosurgery and Psychiatry* **24,** 71–7.

Candy, J.M., Perry, R.H., Perry, E.K., Irving, D., Blessed, G., Fairbaird, A.F. and Tomlinson, B.E. (1983) Pathological changes in the nucleus of Meynert in Alzheimer's and Parkinson's disease. *Journal of the Neurological Sciences* **54,** 277–89.

Caplan, L.R. and Schoene, W.C. (1978). Clinical features of subcortical arteriosclerotic encephalopathy (Binswanger's disease). *Neurology* **28,** 1206–15.

Carmichael, E.A. and Stern, R.D. (1931) Korsakow's syndrome: its histopathology. *Brain* **54,** 189–213.

Castaigne, P., Escourolle, R. and Gray, E. (1976)

Chorée de Huntington et atrophie cérébelleuse (à propos d'une observation anatomoclinique). *Revue Neurologique* **132,** 233–40.

Castaigne, P., Lhermitte, F., Buge, A., Escourolle, R., Hauw, J.J. and Lyon-Caen, O. (1981) Paramedian and thalamic mid-brain infarcts. Clinical and neuropathological study. *Annals of Neurology* **10,** 127–48.

Celesia, G.G. and Wanamaker, W.M. (1972) Psychiatric disturbances in Parkinson's disease. *Diseases of the Nervous System* **33,** 577–83.

Charatan, F.B. and Brierley, J.B. (1956) Mental disorder associated with primary lung carcinoma. *British Medical Journal* **2,** 765–8.

Chase, T.N., Wexler, N.S. and Barbeau, A. (Eds.) (1979) *Advances in Neurology*, vol. 23, *Huntington's Disease*. Raven Press, New York.

Chou, S.M., Payne, W.N., Gibbs, C.J. Jr and Gajdusek, D.C. (1980) Transmission and scanning electron microscopy of spongiform change in Creutzfeldt–Jakob disease. *Brain* **103,** 885–904.

Claude, H. and Cuel, J. (1939) Démence pré-sénile post-traumatique après fracture du crâne. Considérations médico-légales. *Annales de Médecine Légale, de Criminologie, de Police Scientifique et de Toxicologie* **19,** 173–84.

Cobb, S. (1965) Brain size. *Archives of Neurology* **12,** 555–61.

Coblenz, J.M., Mattis, S., Zingesser, L.H., Kasoff, S.S., Wiesniewski, H.M. and Katzman, R. (1973) Presenile dementia. *Archives of Neurology* **29,** 299.

Constantinidis, J. (1978) Is Alzheimer's disease a major form of senile dementia? Clinical, anatomical and genetic data. In *Aging*, vol. 7, *Alzheimer's Disease, Senile Dementia and Related Disorder* (Eds. Katzman, H., Terry, R.D. and Bick, K.L.), pp. 15–25. Raven Press, New York.

Constantinidis, J., Garrone, G. and de Ajuriaguerra, J. (1962) L'hérédité des démences de l'âge avancé. *Encéphale* **51,** 301–44.

Constantinidis, J. and Tissot, R. (1967) Lésions neurofibrillaires d'Alzheimer généralisées sans plaques séniles. *Archives Suisses de Neurologie, Neurochirurgie et de Psychiatrie* **100,** 117–30.

Cook, R.H., Schneck, A. and Clark, D.B. (1981) Twins with Alzheimer's disease. Archives of Neurology **38,** 300–301.

Cornwell, G.G. and Westermark, P. (1980) Senile amyloidosis: a protein manifestation of the ageing process. *Journal of Clinical Pathology* **33,** 1146–52.

Corsellis, J.A.N. (1951) Sub-acute sclerosing leucoencephalitis: clinical and pathological report of two cases. *Journal of Mental Science* **97,** 570–83.

Corsellis, J.A.N. (1962) *Mental Illness and the Ageing Brain*. Oxford University Press, London.

Corsellis, J.A.N. (1976) Ageing and the dementias. In *Greenfield's Neuropathology*, 3rd ed (Eds. Blackwood, W.B. and Corsellis, J.A.N.), pp. 796–849. Edward Arnold, London.

Corsellis, J.A.N. and Brierley, J.B. (1954) An unusual type of pre-senile dementia (atypical Alzheimer's disease with amyloid vascular change). *Brain* **77,** 571–87.

Corsellis, J.A.N. and Brierley, J.B. (1959) Observations on the pathology of insidious dementia following head injury. *Journal of Mental Science* **105,** 714–20.

Corsellis, J.A.N., Bruton, C.J. and Freeman-Browne, D. (1973) The aftermath of boxing. *Psychological Medicine* **3,** 270–303.

Corsellis, J.A.N. and Evans, P.H. (1965) The relation of stenosis of the extracranial cerebral arteries to mental disorder and cerebral degeneration in old age. In *Proceedings of Vth International Congress of Neuropathology*, Excerpta Medica International Congress Series No. 100. Elsevier, Amsterdam.

Corsellis, J.A.N., Goldberg, G.J. and Norton, A.R. (1968) 'Limbic encephalitis' and its association with carcinoma. *Brain* **91,** 481–96.

Crapper, D.R., Krishnan, S.S. and Quittkat, S. (1976) Aluminium, neurofibrillary degeneration and Alzheimer's disease. *Brain* **99,** 67–80.

Crapper, D.R., Quittkat, S. and De Boni, U. (1979) Altered chromatin conformation in Alzheimer's disease. *Brain* **102,** 483–95.

Crapper-McLachlan, D.R. and De Boni, U. (1980) Aetiologic factors in senile dementia of Alzheimer type. In *Aging*, vol. 13, *Aging of the Brain and Dementia* (Eds. Amaducci, L., Davison, A.N. and Antuono, P.), pp. 173–81. Raven Press, New York.

Creutzfeldt, H.G. (1921) Über eine eigenartige Erkrankung des Zentralnervensystems. In *Histologische und histopathologische Arbeiten über die Grosshirnrinde*, Suppl. vol. 6 (Eds. Nissl, F. and Alzheimer, A.), pp. 1–48. Gustav Fisher, Jena.

Crezee, P. (1949) Pick's disease aggravated by cranial trauma: case. *Nederlandsch Tijdschrift voor Geneeskunde* **93,** 2871–6.

Crompton, M.R. (1964) Cerebral infarction following the rupture of cerebral berry aneurysms. *Brain* **87,** 263–79.

Cross, R.B. (1982) Demonstration of neurofibrillary tangles in paraffin sections: a quick and simple method using a modification of Palmgren's method. *Medical Laboratory Sciences* **39,** 67–9.

Cummings, J.L. and Duchen, L.W. (1981) Kluver–Bucy syndrome in Pick disease: clinical and pathologic correlations. *Neurology* **31,** 1415–22.

Curran, D. (1929) Huntington's chorea without choreiform movements. *Journal of Neurology and Psychopathology* **10,** 305–10.

Davenport, C.B. (1915) Huntington's chorea in relation to heredity and eugenics. *Priceedings of the National Academy of Sciences of the USA* **1,** 283–9.

Davidson, E.A. and Robertson, E.E. (1955) Alzheimer's disease with acne rosacea in one of identical twins. *Journal of Neurology, Neurosurgery and Psychiatry* **18,** 72–7.

Davies, P. and Maloney, A.J.F. (1976) Selective loss of central cholinergic neurons in Alzheimer's disease. *Lancet* **2,** 1403.

Davis, P.J.M. and Wright, E.A. (1977) A new method for measuring cranial cavity volume and its application to the assessment of cerebral atrophy at autopsy. *Neuropathology and Applied Neurobiology* **3,** 341–58.

Davison, C. (1942) Progressive subcortical encephalopathy. *Journal of Neuropathology and Experimental Neurology* **1,** 42–8.

Davison, C. and Rabiner, A.B. (1940) Spastic pseudosclerosis (disseminated encephalomyelopathy; corticopallido degeneration). *Archives of Neurology and Psychiatry* **44,** 579–98.

Dayan, A.D. (1970) Quantitative histological studies on the aged human brain. I. Senile plaques and neurofibrillary tangles in 'normal' patients. *Annals of Neuropathology* **16,** 85–94.

Dayan, A.D. and Ball, M.J. (1973) Histometric observations on the metabolism of tangle-bearing neurons. *Neurological Sciences* **19,** 433–6.

Dayan, A.D., Bhatti, I. and Gostling, J.V.T. (1967) Encephalitis due to herpes simplex in a patient with treated carcinoma of the uterus. *Neurology* **17,** 609–13.

De Boni, U. and Crapper, R.D. (1978) Paired helical filaments of the Alzheimer type in cultured neurons. *Nature* (*Lond.*) **271,** 566–8.

De Boni, U., Otoos, S., Scott, J.W. and Crapper, D.R. (1976) Neurofibrillary degeneration induced by systemic aluminium. *Acta Neuropathologica* **35,** 285–94.

Delay, J. and Brion, S. (1962) *Les Démences Tardives.* Masson, Paris.

Delay, J., Brion, S. and Elissalde, B. (1958) Corps mamillaire et syndrome de Korsakoff. *Presse Médicale* **66,** 1849–968.

De Reuck, J., Crevits, L., De Coster, W., Sieben, G. and vander Eecken, H. (1980) Pathogenesis of Binswanger chronic progressive subcortical encephalopathy. *Neurology* **30,** 920–8.

Dewulf, A. (1925) Un cas de maladie de Pick avec lésions prédominantes dans les noyaux gris de la base du cerveau. *Journal Belge de Neurologie et de Psychiatrie* **35,** 508–21.

Dickinson, A.G., Meikel, V.M. and Fraser, H. (1968) Identification of a gene which controls the incubation period of some strains of scrapie in mice. *Journal of Comparative Pathology* **78,** 293–9.

Dickinson, A.G., Meikel, V.M. and Fraser, H. (1969) Genetic control of the concentration of ME7 scrapie agent in the brain of mice. *Journal of Comparative Pathology* **79,** 15–22.

Divry, P. (1927) Etude histo-chimique des plaques séniles. *Journal Belge de Neurologie et de Psychiatrie* **27,** 643–57.

Divry, P. (1934) De la nature de l'altération fibrillaire d'Azheimer. *Journal Belge de Neurologie et de Psychiatrie* **34,** 147–201.

Dom, R., Baro, F. and Brucher, J.M. (1973) A cytometric study of the putamen in difference types of Huntington's chorea. In *Advances in Neurology* vol. 1, *Huntington's Chorea, 1872–1972* (Eds. Barbeau, A., Chase, T.N. and Paulson, G.W.), pp. 369–85. Raven Press, New York.

Dom, R., Malfroid, M. and Baro, F. (1976) Neuropathology of Huntington's chorea: studies of the ventrobasal complex of the thalamus. *Neurology* **26,** 64–88.

Dubas, F., Gray, F., Escourolle, R. and Castaigne, P. (1982a) Polioencephalomyelites subaiguës avec cancer. Six cas anatomo-cliniques et revue de la litterature. *Revue Neurologique* **138,** 725–42.

Dubas, F., Gray, F., Henin, D., Foncin, J.F., Escourolle, R. and Castaigne, P. (1982b) Polioencephalomyelites subaiguës sans cancer. Quatre cas anatomo-cliniqes et revue de la litterature. *Revue Neurologique* **138,** 743–53.

Duckett, S. and Galle, P. (1980) Electron-microprobe studies of aluminium in the brains of cases of Alaheimer's disease and ageing patients. *Journal of Neuropathology and Experimental Neurology* **39,** 350.

Duffy, P., Wolf, J., Collins, G., DeVoe, A.G., Streeten, B. and Cowen, D. (1974) Possible person-to-person transmission of Creutzfeldt–Jakob disease. *New England Journal of Medicine* **290,** 692–3.

Dunlap, C.B. (1927) Pathologic changes in Huntington's chorea with special references to corpus striatum. *Archives of Neurology and Psychiatry* **18,** 867–943.

Emson, P.C., Rehfeld, J.F., Langevin, H. and Rossar, R. (1980) Reduction in cholecystokinin-like immunoreactivity in the basal ganglia in Huntington's disease. *Brain Research* **198,** 497–500.

English, W.H. (1942) Alzheimer's disease. *Psychiatric Quarterly* **16,** 91–106.

Enna, S.J., Bennett, J.P., Bylund, D.B., Snyder, S.H., Bird, E.D. and Iversen, L.L. (1976a) Alteration of brain neurotransmitter receptor binding in Huntington's chorea. *Brain Research* **116,** 531–7.

Enna, S.J., Bird, E.D., Bennett, J.P., Bylund, D.B., Yamamura, H.I., Iversen, L.L. and Snyder, S.N. (1976b) Huntington's chorea: changes in neurotransmitter receptors in the brain. *New England Journal of Medicine* **294,** 1305–9.

Escourelle, R. and Poirier, J. (1973) *Manual of Basic Neuropathology*. W.B. Saunders, Philadelphia.

Esquirol, E. (1838) *Des Maladies Mentales*, Part I, pp. 201–218. Brussels.

Essen-Möller, E. (1946) A family with Alzheimer's disease. *Acta Psychiatrica et Neurologica Scandinavica* **21**, 233–44.

Farnell, F.J. and Globus, J.H. (1932) Chronic progressive vascular subcortical encephalopathy. *Archives of Neurology and Psychiatry* **27**, 593–604.

Feldman, M.L. (1976) Aging changes in the morphology of cortical dendrites. In *Aging*, vol. 3, *Neurobiology of Aging* (Eds. Terry, R.D., Gershon, S.), pp. 211–27. Raven Press, New York.

Feldman, M.L. and Dowd, C. (1974) Aging in rat visual cortex: light microscopic observation on layer V pyramidal spical dendrites. *Anatomical Record* **173**, 355.

Fényes, I. (1932) Alzheimersche Fibrillenveränderung in Hirnstamm einer 28 jährigen Post-encephalitikerin. *Archiv für Psychiatrie und Nervenkrankheiten* **96**, 700–17.

Ferraro, A. (1931) The origin and formation of senile plaques. *Archives of Neurology and Psychiatry* **25**, 1042–62.

Fischer-Williams, M., Bosanquet, F.D. and Daniel, P.M. (1955) Carcinomatosis of the meninges: a report of three cases. *Brain* **78**, 42–58.

Forno, L.S. (1978) The locus ceruleus in Alzheimer's disease. *Journal of Neuropathology and Experimental Neurology* **37**, 614.

Forno, L.S. (1982) Pathology of Parkinson's disease. In *Movement Disorders* (Eds. Marsden C.D. and Fahn, S.), pp. 25–40. Butterworths, London.

Forno, L.S. and Jose, C. (1973) Huntington's chorea: a pathological study. In *Huntington's Chorea* (Eds. Barbeau, A., Chase, T.N. and Paulson, G.W.), pp. 453–70. Raven Press, New York.

Frackowiak, R.S.J., Pozzilli, C., Legg, N.J., Du Boulay, G.H., Marshall, J., Lenzi, G.L. and Jones, T. (1981) Regional cerebral oxygen supply and utilisation in dementia. *Brain* **104**, 753–78.

Freeman, W. (1933) *Neuropathology*. W.B. Saunders, Philadelphia.

Friede, R.L. (1965) Enzyme histochemical studies of senile plaques. *Journal of Neuropathology and Experimental Neurology* **24**, 477–91.

Friede, R.L. and DeJong, R.N. (1964) Neuronal enzymatic failure in Creutzfeldt–Jakob disease (a familial study). *Archives of Neurology* **10**, 181–95.

Friede, R.L. and Magee, K.R. (1962) Alzheimer's disease: presentation of a case with pathologic and enzymatic histochemical observation. *Neurology* **12**, 213–22.

Gajdusek, D.C. (1972) Spongiform virus encephalopathies. *Journal of Clinical Pathology* **25**, suppl. (Royal College of Pathologists) 6, 78–83.

Gajdusek, D.C. (1977) Unconventional viruses and the origin and disappearance of kuru. *Science* **197**, 943–60.

Gajdusek, D.C., Gibbs, C.J. and Alpers, M. (1966) Experimental transmission of a kuru-like syndrome to chimpanzees. *Nature* (*Lond.*) **209**, 794–6.

Galvez, S., Masters, C. and Gajdusek, D.C. (1980) Descriptive epidemiology of Creutzfeldt–Jakob disease in Chile. *Archives of Neurology* **37**, 11–14.

Gambetti, P., Autilio-Gambetti, L. and Shecket, G. (1981) Immunological and silver staining characteristics of neurofibrillary tangles of Alzheimer type (NFT-AT). *Journal of Neuropathology and Experimental Neurology* **30**, 317.

Gambetti, P., Velasco, M.E., Dahl, D., Bignami, A., Roessmann, U. and Sindely, S.D. (1980) Alzheimer's neurofibrillary tangles: an immuno-histochemical study. In *Aging*, vol. 13, *Aging of the Brain and Dementia* (Eds. Amaducci, L., Davison, A.N. and Antuono, P.), pp. 55–63. Raven Press, New York.

Gamper, E. (1928) Zur Frage der Polioencephalitis der chronischen Alcoholiker. Anatomische Befunde bei alcoholischen Korsakow und ihre Beziehungen zum klinischen Bild. *Deutsche Zeitschrift für Nervenheilkunde* **102**, 122–9.

Garron, D.S., Klawans, H.L. and Narin, F. (1972) Intellectual functioning of persons with idiopathic parkinsonism. *Journal of Nervous and Mental Disorders* **154**, 445–52.

Gascon, G.G. and Gilles, F. (1973) Limbic dementia. *Journal of Neurology, Neurosurgery and Psychiatry* **36**, 421–30.

Gerhard, L., Bergener, M. and Homayun, S. (1972) Vascular changes in Alzheimer's disease. *Journal of Neurology* **201**, 43–61.

Gerstmann, J., Sträussler, E. and Scheinker, I. (1936) Ueber eine eigenartige hereditär-familiäre Erkrankung des Zentralnervensystems, zugleich ein Beitrag zur Frage des vorzeitigen lokalen Alterns. *Zeitschrift für die gesamte Neurologie und Psychiatrie* **154**, 736–62.

Ghetti, B. (1980) Experimental studies on neurofibrillary degeneration. In *Aging*, vol. 13, *Aging of the Brain and Dementia.* (Eds. Amaducci, L., Davison, A.N., and Antuono, P.), pp. 183–98. Raven Press, New York.

Gibbs, C.J. Jr., Amyx, H.L., Bacote, A., Masters, C.L. and Gajdusek, D.C. (1980) *Journal of Infectious Diseases* **142**, 205–208.

Gibbs, C.J. Jr., and Gajdusek, D.C. (1978) Atypical viruses as the Cause of Sporadic, Epidemic, and Familial Chronic Diseases in Man: Slow Viruses and Human Diseases. In *Perspectives in Virology*, Vol. 10. (Ed. Pollard, M.). pp. 161–198. Raven Press, New York.

Gibbs, C.J., Gadjusek, D.C. and Amyer, H. (1979) Strain variations in the viruses of Creutzfeldt–

Jakob disease and kuru. In *Slow Transmissible Diseases of the Nervous System*, vol. 2 (Eds Prusiner, S.B. and Hadlow, W.J.), pp. 87–110. Academic Press, New York.

Gibbs, C.J. Jr, Gajdusek, D.C., Asher, D.M., Alpers, M.P., Beck, E., Daniel, P.M. and Matthews, W.B. (1968) Creutzfeldt–Jakob disease (spongiform encephalopathy): transmission to the chimpanzee. *Science* **161,** 388–9.

Gibson, P.H., Stones, M. and Tomlinson, B.E. (1976) Senile changes in the human neocortex and hippocampus compared by the use of the electron and light microscopes. *Journal of the Neurological Sciences* **27,** 389–405.

Gibson, P. and Tomlinson, B.E. (1977) The numbers of Hirano bodies in the hippocampus of normal and demented subjects with Alzheimer's disease. *Journal of the Neurological Sciences* **33,** 199–206.

Glenner, G.G., Terry, W. and Isersky, C. (1973) Amyloidosis: its nature and pathogenesis. *Seminars in Haematology* **10,** 65–86.

Gonatas, N.K., Anderson, A. and Evangelista, I. (1967) The contribution of altered synapses in the senile plaque: an electronmicroscopic study in Alzheimer's dementia. *Journal of Neuropathology and Experimental Neurology* **26,** 25–39.

Gonatas, N.K. and Gambetti, P. (1970) The pathology of the synapse in Alzheimer's disease. In *Alzheimer's Disease and Related Conditions*, Ciba Foundation Symposium (Eds. Wolstenholme, G.E.W. and O'Connor, M.), pp. 169–83. Churchill Livingstone, London.

Gonatas, N.K., Terry, R.D. and Weiss, M. (1965) Electron microscopic study in two cases of Jakob–Creutzfeldt disease. *Journal of Neuropathology and Experimental Neurology* **24,** 575–98.

Goodman, L. (1953) Alzheimer's disease: a clinicopathologic analysis of twenty-three cases with a theory on pathogenesis. *Journal of Nervous and Mental Disease* **118,** 97–130.

Goudsmit, J., Morrow, C.H., Asher, D.M., Yanagihara, R.T., Masters, C.L., Gibbs, C.J. Jr and Gajdusek, D.C. (1980) Evidence for and against the transmissibility of Alzheimer's disease. *Neurology* **30,** 945–50.

Gowers, W.R. (1902) A lecture on abiotrophy. *Lancet* **i,** 1003–7.

Grahmann, H. and Ule, G. (1957) Beitrag zur Kenntnis der chronischen cerebralen Krankheitsbilder bei Boxern. *Psychiatria et Neurologia* **134,** 261–83.

Greenfield, J.G. and Bosanquet, F.D. (1953) The brainstem lesions in Parkinsonism. *Journal of Neurology, Neurosurgery and Psychiatry* **16,** 213–26.

Griffiths, R.A., Mortimer, T.E., Oppenheimer, D.R. and Spalding, J.M.K. (1982) Congophilic angiopathy of the brain: a clinical and pathological report on two siblings. *Journal of Neurology, Neurosurgery and Psychiatry* **45,** 396–408.

Grundke-Iqbal, I., Johnson, A.B., Terry, R.D., Wisniewski, H.M. and Iqbal, K. (1979) Alzheimer neurofibrillary tangles: antiserum and immunohistological staining. *Annals of Neurology* **6,** 532–9.

Grünthal, E. (1930a) Ueber ein Brüderpaar mit Pickschen Krankheit. Eine vergleichende Untersuchung, zugleich ein Beitrag zur Kenntnis der Verursachung und des Verlaufs der Erkrankung. *Zeitschrift für die gesamte Neurologie and Psychiatrie* **129,** 350–75.

Grünthal, E. (1930b) In *Handbuch der Geistenkrankheiten*, vol. 11 (Ed. Bumke, O.), p. 638. Springer, Berlin.

Grünthal, E. and Wenger, O. (1939) Nachweis von Erblichkeit bei der Alzheimerschen Krankheit nebst Bemerkungen über den Altersvorgang im Gehirn. *Monatsschrift für Psychiatrie und Neurologie* **101,** 8–25.

Guberman, A. and Stuss, D. (1983) The syndrome of bilateral paramedian thalamic infarction. *Neurology* **33,** 540–6.

Gudden, H. (1896) Klinische und anatomische Beiträge zur Kenntnis der multiplen Alkoholneuritis. *Archiv für Psychiatrie und Nervenkrankheiten* **28,** 643–741.

Gudmundsson, G., Hallgrimmsson, J., Jónasson, Ṫ.Á. and Bjarmason, Ó. Hereditary cerebral haemorrhage with amyloidosis. *Brain* **77,** 571–87.

Hachinski, V.C., Lassen, N.A. and Marshall, J. (1974) Multi-infarct dementia—a cause of mental deterioration in the elderly. *Lancet* **2,** 207–9.

Hachinski, V.C., Iliff, L.D., Zilkha, E., du Boulay, G.H., McAllister, V.L., Marshall, J. et al. (1975) Cerebral blood flow in dementia. *Archives of Neurology* **32,** 632–7.

Hadlow, W.J. (1959) Scrapie and kuru. *Lancet* **2,** 289–90.

Hakim, A.M. and Mathiewson, G. (1979) Dementia in Parkinson disease: a neuropathologic study. *Neurology* **29,** 1209–14.

Hall, T.C., Miller, A.K.H. and Corsellis, J.A.N. (1975) Variations in the human Purkinje cell population according to age and sex. *Neuropathology and Applied Neurobiology* **1,** 267–92.

Hallervorden, J. (1933) Zur Pathogenese des postencephalitischen Parkinsonismus. *Klinische Wochenschrift* **12,** 692–5.

Hallervorden, J. (1957) In *Handbuch der speziellen Pathologischen Anatomie and Histologie* (Eds. Lubarsch, O., Henke, F. and Rössle, R.). Springer, Berlin.

Hall, T.C., Miller, A.K.H. and Corsellis, J.A.N. (1975) Variations in the human Purkinje cell population according to age and sex. *Neuropathology and Applied Neurobiology* **1,** 267–92.

Hanley, T. (1974) 'Neuronal fall-out' in the ageing brain: a critical review of the quantitative data. *Age and Ageing* **3,** 133–51.

Hare, E.H. (1959) The origin and spread of dementia paralytica. *Journal of Mental Science* **105,** 594–626.

Hatazawa, J., Ito, M., Yamaura, H. and Matsuzawa, T. (1982) Sex difference in brain atrophy during aging: a quantitative study with computed tomography. *Journal of the American Geriatric Society* **30,** 235–9.

Haug, G., Barmwater, U., Eggers, R., Fischer, D., Kuhl, S. and Sass, N.L. (1983) Anatomical changes in aging brain: morphometric analysis of the human prosenchephalon. In *Aging*, vol. 21, *Brain Aging: Neuropathology and Neuropharmacology* (Eds. Cervos-Navarro, J. and Sarkander, H.I.). Raven Press, New York.

Heathfield, K.W.G. (1967) Huntington's chorea: investigation into prevalence in the N.E. Metropolitan Regional Hospital Board area. *Brain* **90,** 814–33.

Heathfield, K.W.G. (1973) Huntington's chorea: a centenary review. *Postgraduate Medical Journal* **49,** 32–45.

Heidenhain, A. (1929) Klinische und anatomische Untersuchungen über eine eigenartige Erkrankung des Zentralnervensystems im Praesenium. *Zeitschrift für die gesamte Neurologie und Psychiatrie* **118,** 49–114.

Henderson, G., Tomlinson, B.E. and Gibson, P.H. (1980) Cell counts in human cerebral cortex in normal adults throughout life using an image analysing computer. *Journal of Neurological Science* **46,** 113–36.

Henson, R.A., Hoffman, H.L. and Urich, H. (1965) Encephalomyelitis with carcinoma. *Brain* **88,** 449–64.

Henson, R.A. and Urich, H. (1982) *Cancer and the Nervous System.* Blackwell Scientific, Oxford.

Hierons, R., Janota, I. and Corsellis, J.A.N. (1978) The late effects of necrotizing encephalitis of the temporal lobes and limbic areas: a clinico-pathological study of 10 cases. *Psychological Medicine* **8,** 21–42.

Hiley, C.R. and Bird, E.D. (1974) Decreased muscarinic receptor concentration in post-mortem brain in Huntington's chorea. *Brain Research* **80,** 355–8.

Hirano, A., Dembitzer, H.M., Kurland, L.T. and Zimmerman, H.M. (1968) The fine structure of some intraganglionic alterations. *Journal of Neuropathology and Experimental Neurology* **27,** 167–82.

Hirano, A., Malamud, N., Elizan, T.S. and Kurland, L.T. (1966) Amyotrophic lateral sclerosis and Parkinsonism–dementia complex on Guam. *Archives of Neurology* **15,** 35–51.

Hirano, A., Malamud, N. and Kurland, L.T. (1961) Parkinsonism–dementia complex, an endemic disease on the island of Guam. *Brain* **84,** 662–79.

Hirano, A., Tuazon, R. and Zimmerman, H.M. (1968) Neurofibrillary changes, granulovacuolar bodies and argentophilic globules observed in tuberous sclerosis. *Acta Neuropathologica* **11,** 257–61.

Hirano, A. and Zimmerman, H.M. (1962a) Silver impregnation of nerve cells and fibres in celloidin sections. *Archives of Neurology* **6,** 114–22.

Hirano, A. and Zimmerman, H.M. (1962b) Alzheimer's neurofibrillary changes: a topographic study. *Archives of Neurology* **7,** 227–42.

Hollander, D. (1974) The Role of Cerebral Degeneration in Mental Deterioration. MD Thesis, University of Cape Town.

Hollander, D. and Strich, S.J. (1970) Atypical Alzheimer's disease with congophilic angiopathy presenting with dementia of acute onset. In *Alzheimer's Disease and Related Conditions*, Ciba Foundation Symposium (Eds. Wolstenholme, G.E.W. and O'Connor, M.), pp. 105–24. Churchill, London.

Horel, J.A. (1978) The neuroanatomy of amnesia. *Brain* **101,** 403–45.

Horn, S. (1974) Some psychological factors in Parkinsonism. *Journal of Neurology, Neurosurgery and Psychiatry* **37,** 27–31.

Horrocks, L.A., van Rollins, M. and Yates, A.G. (1981) Lipid changes in the ageing brain. In *The Molecular Basis of Neuropathology* (Eds. Davison, A.N. and Thompson, R.H.S.), pp. 601–30. Edward Arnold, London.

Hubbard, B.M. and Anderson, J.M. (1981a) Age, senile dementia and ventricular enlargement. *Journal of Neurology, Neurosurgery and Psychiatry* **44,** 631–5.

Hubbard, B.M. and Anderson, J.M. (1981b) A quantitative study of cerebral atrophy in old age and senile dementia. *Journal of the Neurological Sciences* **50,** 135–45.

Hubbard, B.M. and Anderson, J.M. (1983) Sex difference in age-related brain atrophy. *Lancet* **1,** 1447–8.

Humphrey, T. (1944) Primitive neurons in the embryonic human central nervous system. *Journal of Comparative Neurology* **81,** 1–45.

Hunter, R., Dayan, A.D. and Wilson, J. (1972) Alzheimer's disease in one monoxygotic twin. *Journal of Neurology, Neurosurgery and Psychiatry* **35,** 707–10.

Huntington, G. (1872) On chorea. *Medical and Surgical Reporter, Philadelphia* **26,** 317–21.

Iglesias-Rozas, J.R. and Ebhardt, G. (1974) Alterations of microvasculature in progressive subcortical encephalopathy (Binswanger). In *Pathology of Cerebral Microcirculation* (Ed. Cervos-Navarro, J.), pp. 454–61. Walter de Groyter, Berlin.

Iqbal, K., Grundke-Iqbal, I., Wisniewski, H.M. and Terry, R.D. (1978) Neurofibres in Alzheimer's disease and other conditions. In *Alzheimer's Disease: Senile Dementia and Related Disorders*. (Eds. Katzman, R., Terry, R.D. and Bick, K.L.), pp. 409–20. Raven Press, New York.

Ishii, T. (1965) Distribution of Alzheimer's neurofibrillary changes in the brain stem and hypothalamus of senile dementia. *Acta Neuropathologica* **6**, 181–9.

Ishii, T. and Haga, S. (1976) Immuno-electron microscopic localization of immunoglobulin in amyloid fibrils of senile plaques. *Acta Neuropathologica* **36**, 243–9.

Jakob, A. (1921) Über eigenartige Erkrankungen des Zentralnervensystems mit bemerkenswerten anatomischen Befunden mit disseminierten Degenerationsherden. *Zeitschrift für die gesamte Neurologie und Psychiatrie* **64**, 147–228.

Jakob, A. (1923) *Die Extrapyramidalen Erkrankungen*, pp. 218–45. Springer, Berlin.

Jakob, H. (1960) Zur pathologischen Anatomie der Pickschen Krankheit. I. Vergleichende Untersuchungen über Ausdehnung und Schwerpunkte der Atrophie. *Archiv für Psychiatrie und Nervenkrankheiten* **201**, 269–97.

Jakob, H. (1961) Zur pathologischen Anatomie der Pickschen Krankheit. *Archiv für Psychiatrie und Nervenkrankheiten* **202**, 540–68.

Jakob, H. (1969) Klinisch-anatomische Aspekte bei 'reinen' Schläfenlappenfällen Pickscher Krankheit und der basale Neocortex. *Deutsche Zeitschrift für Nervenheilkunde* **196**, 20–39.

Jamada, M. and Mehraein, P. (1968) Verteilungsmuster der senilen Veränderungen im Gehirn. *Archiv für Psychiatrie und Zeitschrift für die gesamte Neurologie* **211**, 308–24.

Janota, I. (1981) Dementia, deep white matter damage and hypertension: 'Binswanger's disease'. *Psychological Medicine* **11**, 39–48.

Jellinger, K. (1976a) Neuropathological aspects of dementias resulting from abnormal blood and cerebrospinal fluid dynamics. *Acta Neurologica Belgica* **76**, 83–102.

Jellinger, K. (1976b) Cerebrovascular amyloidosis with cerebral haemorrhage. *Journal of Neurology* **214**, 195–206.

Jervis, G.A. (1948) Early senile dementia in mongoloid idiocy. *American Journal of Psychiatry* **105**, 102–6.

Jervis, G.A. (1971a) Pick's disease. In *Pathology of the Nervous System*, vol. 2 (Ed. Minckler, J.), pp. 1395–404. McGraw-Hill, New York.

Jervis, G.A. (1971b) Senile dementia. In *Pathology of the Nervous System*, vol. 2 (Ed. Minckler, J.), pp. 1379–85. McGraw-Hill, New York.

Johnson, A.B. and Blum, N.R. (1970) Nucleotide phosphatase activities associated with the tangles and plaques of Alzheimer's disease: a histochemical study of natural and experimental neurofibrillary tangles. *Journal of Neuropathology and Experimental Neurology* **29**, 463–78.

Johnson, A.B., Cohen, S.A., Said, S.I. and Terry, R.D. (1981) Neuritic plaque amyloid, microangiopathy and Alzheimer neurofibrillary tangles: do they share a common antigen? *Journal of Neuropathology and Experimental Neurology* **40**, 310.

Jones, D. and Nevin, S. (1954) Rapidly progressive cerebral degeneration (subacute vascular encephalopathy) with mental disorder, focal disturbances, and myoclonic epilepsy. *Journal of Neurology and Psychiatry* **17**, 148–59.

Kahana, E., Alter, M., Braham, J. and Sofer, D. (1974) Creutzfeldt–Jakob disease: focus among Libyan Jews in Israel. *Science* **183**, 90–1.

Kanazawa, I., Bird, E.D., O'Connell, R. and Powell, D. (1977) Evidence for a decrease in substance P content of substantia nigra in Huntington's chorea. *Brain Research* **120**, 387–92.

Kanazawa, I., Bird, E.D., Gale, J.S., Iversen, L.L., Jessell, T.M., Muramoto, O. et al. (1979) Substance P: decrease in substantia nigra and globus pallidus in Huntington's disease. In *Advances in Neurology*, vol. 23, *Huntington's Disease* (Eds. Chase, T.N., Barbeau, A. and Wexler, N.S.), pp. 495–504. Raven Press, New York.

Kant, F. (1933) Die Pseudoencephalitis Wernicke der Alkoholiker (Polioencephalitis haemorrhagica superior acuta). Ein Beitrag zur Klinik der Alkoholpsychosen. *Archiv für Psychiatrie und Nervenkrankheiten* **98**, 702–68.

Khurana, R.K. and Garcia, J.H. (1981) Autonomic dysfunction in subacute spongiform encephalopathy. *Archives of Neurology* **38**, 114–17.

Kidd, M. (1964) Alzheimer's disease. An electron microscopical study. *Brain* **87**, 307–20.

Kilpatrick, C., Burns, R. and Blumbergs, P. (1983) Identical twins with Alzheimer's disease. *Journal of Neurology, Neurosurgery and Psychiatry* **46**, 421–5.

Kirschbaum, W.R. (1924) Zwei eigenartige Erkrankungen des Zentralnervensystems nach Art der spastischen Pseudosclerose (Jakob) *Zeitschrift für die gesamte Neurologie und Psychiatrie* **92**, 175–220.

Kirschbaum, W.R. (1968) *Jakob–Creutzfeldt Disease*. Elsevier, New York.

Kishimoto, K., Nakamura, M. and Sotokawa, Y. (1959) On population genetics of Huntington's chorea in Japan. *First International Congress of Neurological Sciences*, vol. 4.

Klatzo, I., Gajdusek, D.C. and Zigas, V. (1959) Pathology of kuru. *Laboratory Investigation* **8**, 799–847.

Klatzo, I., Wisniewski, H. and Streicher, E. (1965) Experimental production of neurofibrillary degeneration. I. Light microscopic observations. *Journal of Neuropathology and Experimental Neurology* **24,** 187–99.

Konigsmark, B.W. and Murphy, E.A. (1970) Neuronal populations in the human brain. *Nature (Lond.)* **228,** 1335–6.

Korsakow, S.S. (1890) Über eine besondere Form psychischer Störung combiniert mit multipler Neuritis. *Archiv für Psychiatrie und Nervenkrankheiten* **21,** 669–709.

Kraepelin, E. (1910) Klinische Psychiatrie. In *Psychiatrie*, vol. 2, 8th edn. Barth, Leipzig.

Kreindler, A., Hornet, Th. and Appel, E. (1959) Complex forms of cerebral senility. *Rumanian Medical Review* **3,** 43–7.

Krigman, M.R., Feldman, R.G. and Bensch, K. (1965) Alzheimer's presenile dementia. A histochemical and electron microscopic study. *Excerpta Medica Section VIIIA* **19,** abstract 63.

Krücke, W. (1950) Das Zentralnervensystem bei generalisierter Paramyloidose. *Archiv für Psychiatrie und Nervenkrankheiten* **185,** 165–92.

Ladurner, G., Iliff, L.D. and Lechner, H. (1982) Clinical factors associated with dementia in ischaemic stroke. *Journal of Neurology, Neurosurgery and Psychiatry* **45,** 97–101.

Ladurner, G., Sager, W.D. and Floch (1982) Computer tomography and vascular (multi-infarct) dementia: a quantitative and qualitative investigation. *Experimental Brain Research*, Suppl. 5, *The Aging Brain* (Ed. Hoyer, S.), pp. 264–70. Springer, Berlin, Heidelberg, New York.

Lange, H., Thorner, G., Hope, A. and Schroder, K.F. (1976) Morphometric studies of the neuropathological changes in choreatic diseases. *Journal of the Neurological Sciences* **28,** 401–25.

Larsson, T., Sjögren, T. and Jacobsen, G. (1963) Senile dementia. *Acta Psychiatrica Scandinavica* **39,** suppl. 167.

Lesser, R.L., Albert, D.M., Bobowick, A.R. and O'Brien, F.H. (1979) Creutzfeldt-Jakob disease and optic atrophy. *American Journal of Ophthalmology* **87,** 317–21.

Liebermann, A., Dziatolowski, M., Coopersmith, M., Cerb, M., Goodgold, A., Lorein, J. and Goldstein, M. (1979) Dementia in Parkinson's disease. *Annals of Neurology* **6,** 355–9.

Liebers, M. (1933) Alzheimersche Krankheit mit Pickscher Atrophie der Parieto-occipitallappen. *Archiv für Psychiatrie und Nervenkrankheiten* **100,** 100–10.

Liebers, M. (1939) Alzheimersche Krankheit mit Pickscher Atrophie der Stirnlappen. *Archiv für Psychiatrie und Nervenkrankheiten* **109,** 363–70.

Lindenberg, R. (1960) Striopallidal-nigral degeneration. *Journal of Neuropathology and Experimental Neurology* **19,** 160.

Lipkin, L.E. (1959) Cytoplasmic inclusion in ganglion cells, associated with Parkinsonian states. A neurocellular change studied in 53 cases and 206 controls. *American Journal of Pathology* **35,** 1117–33.

Lishman, W.A. (1978) *Organic Psychiatry: the psychological consequences of cerebral disorder*. Blackwell Scientific, Oxford.

Liss, L. (1960) Senile brain changes. Histopathology of the ganglion cells. *Journal of Neuropathology and Experimental Neurology* **19,** 559–71.

Llena, J.F. and Hirano, A. (1979) Abundant eosinophilic rod-like structures in subacute spongiform encephalopathy. Abstract No. 86 of the 55th Annual Meeting of the American Association of Neuropathologists. *Journal of Neuropathology and Experimental Neurology* **38,** 329.

Lloyd, K.G., Dreksler, S. and Bird, E.D. (1977) Alterations in ^{3}H-GABA binding in Huntington's chorea. *Life Sciences* **21,** 747–54.

Logue, V., Durward, M., Pratt, R.T.C., Piercy, M. and Nixon, W.L.B. (1968) The quality of survival after rupture of an anterior cerebral aneurysm. *British Journal of Psychiatry* **114,** 137–60.

Loizou, L.A., Kendall, B.E. and Marshall, J. (1981) Subcortical arteriosclerotic encephalopathy: a clinical and radiological investigation. *Journal of Neurology, Neurosurgery and Psychiatry* **44,** 294–304.

Løken, A.C. and Cyvin, K. (1954) A case of juvenile amaurotic idiocy with the histological picture of Alzheimer's disease. *Journal of Neurology, Neurosurgery and Psychiatry* **71,** 211–15.

Love, S. and Duchen, L.W. (1982) Familial cerebellar ataxia with cerebrovascular amyloid. *Journal of Neurology, Neurosurgery and Psychiatry* **45,** 271–3.

Lowenberg, K. and Waggoner, R.W. (1934) Familial organic psychosis (Alzheimer's type). *Archives of Neurology and Psychiatry* **31,** 737–54.

Lüers, T. and Spatz, U.H. (1957) Pickschе Krankheit. In *Handbuch der speziellen pathologischen Anatomie und Histologie* Vol XIII 1A (Eds. Lubarsch, O., Henke, F. and Rössle, R.). pp. 614–716. Springer, Berlin.

Lund, J.C. (1860) Chorea Sti. Viti i Saetersdalen. *Beretning om Sundhedstilstanden og Medicinalforholdene in Norge* **4,** 137–8.

Lyon, I.W. (1863) Chronic hereditary chorea. *American Medical Times* **7,** 289–90.

Lyon, R.L. (1962) Huntington's chorea in the Moray Firth area. *British Medical Journal* **1,** 1301–6.

McCaughey, W.T.E. (1961) The pathologic spectrum of Huntington's chorea. *Journal of Nervous and Mental Disease* **133,** 91–103.

McDermott, J.R., Smith, A.I., Iqbal, K. and Wisniewski, H.M. (1977) Aluminium and Alzheimer's disease. *Lancet* **2,** 710–11.

McDermott, J.R., Ward, M.K., Smith, A.I., Parkinson, I.S. and Kerr, D.N.S. (1978) Brain aluminium concentrations in dialysis encephalopathy *Lancet* **1,** 901–3.

McGovern, G.P., Miller, D.H. and Robertson, D. (1959) A mental syndrome associated with lung carcinoma. *Archives of Neurology and Psychiatry* **81,** 341–7.

McLardy, T. (1970) Memory function in hippocampal gyri but not in hippocampi. *International Journal of Neuroscience* **1,** 113–18.

McMenemy, W.H. (1940) Alzheimer's disease. *Journal of Neurology and Psychiatry* **3,** 211–40.

McMenemy, W.H. (1963) The dementias and progressive diseases of the basal ganglia. In *Greenfield's Neuropathology*, pp. 520–80. Edward Arnold, London.

McMenemy, W.H., Worster-Drought, C., Flind, J. and Williams, H.G. (1939) Familial presenile dementia: report of case with clinical and pathological features of Alzheimer's disease. *Journal of Neurology and Psychiatry* **2,** 293–302.

Mair, W.G.P., Warrington, E.K. and Weiskrantz, L. (1979) Memory disorder in Korsakow's psychosis. *Brain* **102,** 749–83.

Malamud, N. (1972) Neuropathology of organic brain syndromes associated with aging. In *Advance in Behavioral Biology*, vol. 3, *Aging and the Brain* (Ed. Gaitz, F.M.), pp. 63–87. Plenum Press, New York.

Malamud, N., Haymaker, W. and Pinkerton, H. (1950) Inclusion encephalitis with clinicopathologic report of three cases. *American Journal of Pathology* **26,** 133–5.

Malamud, N., Hirano, A. and Kurland, L.T. (1961) Pathoanatomic changes in amyotrophic lateral sclerosis on Guam with reference to the occurrence of neurofibrillary changes. *Archives of Neurology* **5,** 401–15.

Malamud, N. and Skillicorn, S.A. (1956) Relationship between the Wernicke and the Korsakow syndrome. *Archives of Neurology and Psychiatry* **50,** 288–303.

Mandybur, T.I. (1975) The incidence of cerebral amyloid angiopathy in Alzheimer's disease. *Neurology* **25,** 125–6.

Mandybur, T.I., Nagpaul, A.S., Pappas, Z. and Niklowitz, W.J. (1977) Alzheimer neurofibrillary change in subacute sclerosing panencephalitis. *Annals of Neurology* **1,** 103–7.

Mann, D.M.A. (1982) Nerve cell protein metabolism and degenerative disease. *Neuropathology and Applied Neurobiology* **8,** 161–76.

Mann, D.M.A., Lincoln, J. and Yates, P.O. (1981) Changes in the noradrenaline-containing neurones of the human CNS in Alzheimer's disease. In *Biological Psychiatry* (Eds. Perris, C., Struwe, G. and Jansson, B.), pp. 969–72. Elsevier/North-Holland Biomedical Press, Amsterdam.

Mann, D.M.A., Lincoln, J., Yates, P.O., Stamp, J.E. and Toper, S. (1980) Changes in the monoamine-containing neurons of the human central nervous system in senile dementia. *British Journal of Psychiatry* **136,** 533–41.

Mann, D.M.A. and Sinclair, K.G.A. (1978) The quantitative assessment of lipofuscin pigment, cytoplasmic RNA and nucleolar volume in senile dementia. *Neuropathology and Applied Biology* **4,** 129–35.

Mann, D.M.A. and Yates, P.O. (1974) Lipoprotein pigments—their relationship to ageing in the human nervous system. I. The lipofuscin content of nerve cells. *Brain* **97,** 481–8.

Mann, D.M.A., Yates, P.O. and Barton, C.M. (1977) Cytophotometric mapping of neuronal changes in senile dementia. *Journal of Neurology, Neurosurgery and Psychiatry* **40,** 299–302.

van Mansvelt, J. (1954) *Pick's Disease. A syndrome of lobar cerebral atrophy*. Enschede, Netherlands.

Marchbanks, R.M. (1982) Biochemistry of Alzheimer's disease. *Journal of Neurochemistry* **39,** 9–15.

Marconi, G. and Piazzesi, W. (1965) Su di un caso di malattia di Alzheimer-Perusini familiare: studio generalogico e citogenetico. *Rivista di Patologia Nervosa e Mentale* **86,** 854–72.

Marinesco, G. (1911) Sur la structure des plaques dites séniles dans l'écore cérébrale des sujets agés et atteints d'affections mentales. *Comptes Rendus des Séances de la Société de Biologie et ses Filiales* **70,** 606–8.

Marsden, C.D. (1984) Neurological causes of dementia other than Alzheimer's disease. In *Handbook of Studies on Psychiatry and Old Age* (Eds. Kay, D.W.K. and Burrows, G.D.), pp. 145–67. Elsevier, Amsterdam.

Marsden, C.D. and Harrison, M.F.G. (1972) Outcome of investigations of patients with presenile dementia. *British Medical Journal* **2,** 249.

Masters, C.L. and Gajdusek, D.C. (1982) The spectrum of Creutzfeldt-Jakob disease and the virus-induced spongiform encephalopathies. In *Recent Advances in Neuropathology—2* (Eds. Smith, W.T. and Cavanagh, J.B.), pp. 139–63. Churchill Livingstone, Edinburgh.

Masters, C.L., Gajdusek, D.C. and Gibbs, C.J. Jr (1981a) Creutzfeldt-Jakob disease virus isolations from the Gerstmann-Sträussler syndrome. With an analysis of the various forms of amyloid plaque deposition in the virus-induced spongiform encephalopathies. *Brain* **104,** 559–88.

Masters, C.L., Gajdusek, D.C. and Gibbs, C.J. Jr (1981b) The familial occurrence of Creutzfeldt-Jakob disease and Alzheimer's disease. *Brain* **104,** 535–58.

Masters, C.L. and Richardson, E.P. Jr (1978) Subacute spongiform encephalopathy (Creutzfeldt-Jakob disease). The nature and progression of spongiform change. *Brain* **101,** 333–44.

Masters, C.L., Harris, J.O., Gajdusek, D.C., Gibbs, C.J. Jr, Bernoulli, C. and Asher, D.M. (1979) Creutzfeldt-Jakob disease: patterns of worldwide occurrence and the significance of familial and sporadic clustering. *Annals of Neurology* **5,** 177–88.

Matthews, W.B. (1975) Epidemiology of Creutzfeldt-Jakob disease in England and Wales. *Journal of Neurology, Neurosurgery and Psychiatry* **38,** 210–13.

Mattson, B. (1974) Clinical, genetic and pharmacological studies in Huntington's chorea. *UMEA University Dissertations*, vol. 7, pp. 21–51. UMEA, Sweden.

May, W.W., Itabishi, H.H. and DeJong, R.N. (1968) Creutzfeldt-Jakob disease. II. Clinical, pathological and genetic study of a family. *Archives of Neurology* **19,** 137–49.

Mayer, V., Orolin, D. and Mitrova, E. (1977) Cluster of Creutzfeldt-Jakob disease and presenile dementia. *Lancet* **2,** 256.

Mayeux, R. (1982) Depression and dementia in Parkinson's disease. In *Movement Disorders*, BIMR Neurology vol. 2 (Eds. Marsden, C.D. and Fahn, S.), pp. 75–95. Butterworths, London.

Mayeux, R., Stern, Y., Rosen, J. and Leventhal, J. (1981) Depression, intellectual impairment and Parkinson's disease. *Neurology* **31,** 645–50.

Mehraein, P., Yamada, M. and Tarnowska-Dziduszko, E. (1975) Quantitation studies on dendrites in Alzheimer's disease and senile dementia. In *Physiology and Pathology of Dendrites* (Ed. Kreutzberg, G.W.), pp. 453–8. Raven Press, New York.

Meyer, A. (1929) Ueber eine der amyotropischen Lateralsclerose nahestehende Erkrankung mit psychischen Störungen, zugleich ein Beitrag zur Frage der spastischen Pseudosclerose (A. Jakob) *Zeitschrift für die Gesamte Neurologie und Psychiatrie* **121,** 107–38.

Meyer, A. and Beck, E. (1954) *Prefrontal Leucotomy and Related Operations: anatomical aspects of success and failure*. Oliver and Boyd, Edinburgh.

Meyer, A., Leigh, D. and Bagg, C.E. (1954) A rare presenile dementia associated with cortical blindness (Heidenhain's syndrome). *Journal of Neurology, Neurosurgery and Psychiatry* **17,** 129–33.

Meyer, J.S. and Shaw, T. (1984) Cerebral blood flow in ageing, the dementias and depression. In *Handbook of Studies on Psychiatry and Old Age* (Eds. Kay, D.W.K. and Burrows, G.D.), pp. 439–54. Elsevier, Amsterdam.

Meyer, V. (1959) Cognitive changes following temporal lobectomy for relief of temporal lobe epilepsy. *Archives of Neurology and Psychiatry* **81,** 299–309.

Meyer, V. and Yates, A. (1955) Intellectual changes following temporal lobectomy for psychomotor epilepsy. *Journal of Neurology, Neurosurgery and Psychiatry* **18,** 42–8.

Miller, A.K.H., Alston, R.L. and Corsellis, J.A.N. (1980) Variation with age in the volumes of grey and white matter in the cerebral hemispheres of man: measurements with an image analyser. *Neuropathology and Applied Neurobiology* **6,** 119–32.

Milner, B. and Penfield, W. (1955) The effect of hippocampal lesions on recent memory. *Transactions of the American Neurological Association* **80,** 42–8.

Mizutani, T., Okumura, A., Oda, M. and Shiraki, H. (1981) Panencephalopathic type of Creutzfeldt-Jakob disease: primary involvement of the cerebral white matter. *Journal of Neurology, Neurosurgery and Psychiatry* **44,** 103–15.

Monagle, R.D. and Brody, H. (1974) The effects of age upon the main nucleus of the inferior olive in the human. *Journal of Comparative Neurology* **155,** 61–6.

Morel, F. and Wildi, E. (1952) General and cellular pathochemistry of senile and presenile apterations of the brain. In *Proceedings of First International Congress of Neuropathology*, vol. 2, 347–74. Rosenberg and Sellier, Torino.

Morel, F. and Wildi, E. (1955) Contribution à la connaissance des différentes alterations cérébrales du grande âge. *Schweizer Archiv für Neurologie und Psychiatrie* **76,** 174–223.

Morimatsu, M., Hirai, S., Muramatsu, A. and Yoshikawa, M. (1975) Senile degenerative brain lesions and dementia. *Journal of the American Geriatrics Society* **23,** 390–406.

Mountjoy, C.Q., Roth, M., Evans, N.J.R. and Evans, H.M. (1983) Cortical neuronal counts in normal elderly controls and demented patients. *Neurobiology of Aging* **4,** 1–11.

Mountjoy, C.Q., Tomlinson, B.E. and Gibson, P.H. (1982) Amyloid and senile plaques and cerebral blood vessels. A semi-quantitative investigation of a possible relationship. *Journal of the Neurological Sciences* **57,** 89–103.

Moyano, B.A. (1932) I. Enfermedad de Alzheimer. II. Atrofia de Pick. *Archivos Argentinos de Neurologia* **7,** 231–286.

Mutrux, S. (1953) Contribution á l'étude des corrélations anatomocliniques dans les démences dégénératives et les démences artérioscléreuses. *Monatsschrift für Psychiatrie und Neurologie* **125,** 19–38.

Mutrux, S. (1958) Contribution à l'étude histologique différentielle de la démence sénile et de la maladie d'Alzheimer. *Monatsschrift für Psychiatrie und Neurologie* **136,** 157–94.

Myrianthopoulos, N.C. (1966) Huntington's chorea. *Journal of Medical Genetics* **3,** 298–314.

Neugut, R.H., Neugut, A.I., Kahana, E., Stein, Z. and Alter, M. (1979) Creutzfeldt–Jakob disease: familial clustering among Libyan-born Israelis. *Neurology* **29,** 225–31.

Neumann, M.A. (1949) Pick's disease. *Journal of Neuropathology and Experimental Neurology* **8,** 255–82.

Neumann, M.A. (1960) Combined amyloid vascular changes and argyrophilic plaques in the central nervous system. *Journal of Neuropathology and Experimental Neurology* **19,** 370–82.

Neumann, M.A. (1967) Langdon Down syndrome and Alzheimer's disease. *Journal of Neuropathology and Experimental Neurology* **26,** 150.

Neumann, M.A. and Cohn, R. (1967) Progressive subcortical gliosis, a rare form of presenile dementia. *Brain* **90,** 405–18.

Nevin, S., McMenemy, W.H., Behrman, S. and Jones, D.P. (1960) Subacute spongiform encephalopathy—a subacute form of encephalopathy attributable to vascular dysfunction (spongiform cerebral atrophy). *Brain* **83,** 519–64.

Newton, R.D. (1948) Identify of Alzheimer's disease and senile dementia and their relation to senility. *Journal of Mental Science* **94,** 225–49.

Ogata, J., Budzilovich, G.N. and Cravioto, H. (1972) A study of rod-like structures (Hirano bodies) in 240 normal and pathological brains. *Acta Neuropathologica* **21,** 61–7.

Olsen, R.W., Van Ness, P.C. and Tourtellotte, W.W. (1979) Gamma-aminobutyric acid receptor binding curves for human brain regions: comparison of Huntington's disease and normal. In *Advances in Neurology*, vol. 23, *Huntington's Disease*, (Eds. Chase, T.N., Wexler, W.S. and Barbeau, A.), pp. 697–704. Raven Press, New York.

Olson, M.I. and Shaw, C. (1969) Presenile dementia and Alzheimer's disease in mongolism. *Brain* **92,** 147–56.

Olszewski, J. (1962) Subcortical arteriosclerotic encephalopathy. *World Neurology* **3,** 359–75.

Onari, K. and Spatz, H. (1926) Anatomische Beiträge zur Lehre von der Pickschen umschriebenen Grosshirnrindenatrophie (Picksche Krankheit). *Zeitschrift für die gesamte Neurologie und Psychiatrie* **101,** 470–511.

Oyanagi, S. (1979) Aging of the central nervous system and its fine structure. Neurofibrillary change and senile plaques. *Seishin Iqatu* **21,** 834–46. (quoted by Yagashita et al., 1981).

Pantelakis, S. (1954) Un type particulier d'angiopathie sénile du système nerveux central: l'angiopathie congophile. Topographie et fréquence. *Monatsschrift für Psychiatrie und Neurologie* **128,** 219–56.

Park, T.S., Kleinman, G.M. and Richardson, E.P. (1980) Creutzfeldt–Jakob disease with extensive degeneration of the white matter. *Acta Neuropathologica* **52,** 239–42.

Paula-Barbosa, M.N., Brito, R., Silva, C.A., Farin, R. and Cruz, C. (1979) Neurofibrillary changes in the cerebral cortex of a patient with SSPE. *Acta Neuropathologica* **48,** 157–60.

Peri, D.P. and Brody, A.R. (1980) Alzheimer's disease: x-ray spectrometric evidence of aluminium accumulation in neurofibrillary tangle-bearing neurons. *Science* **208,** 297–8.

Perry, E.K., Perry, R.H., Blessed, G. and Tomlinson, B.E. (1977) Neurotransmitter enzyme abnormalities in senile dementia—choline acetyltransferase and glutamic acid decarboxylase in necropsy brain tissue. *Journal of the Neurological Sciences* **34,** 247–65.

Perry, E.K., Oakley, A.E., Candy, J.M. and Perry, R.H. (1981) Properties and possible significance of substance P and insulin fibrils. *Neuroscience Letters* **25,** 321–5.

Perry, E.K., Tomlinson, B.E., Blessed, G., Perry, R.H. and Crow, T.J. (1981) Neuropathological and biochemical observations on the noradrenergic system in Alzheimer's disease. *Journal of the Neurological Sciences* **51,** 279–87.

Perry, T.L., Hansen, S. and Kloster, M. (1973) Huntington's chorea: deficiency of γ-aminobutyric acid in brain. *New England Journal of Medicine* **288,** 337–42.

Perusini, G. (1910) Über klinisch und histologisch eigenartige psychische Erkrankungen des späteren Lebensalters. *Histologische und histopathologische Arbeiten über die Grosshirnrinde* **3,** 297–359.

Petit-Dutaillis, D., Christophe, J., Pertuisset, B., Dreyfus-Brisac, C. and Blane, C. (1954) Lobectomie temporale bilatérale pour épilepsie. Evolution des perturbations fonctionelles postopératives. *Revue Neurologique* **91,** 97–108.

Pfeiffer, E. (1975) A short portable mental status questionnaire for the assessment of organic brain deficit in elderly patients. *Journal of the American Geriatric Society* **23,** 433–41.

Pick, A. (1906) Ueber einen weiteren Symptomenkomplex im Rahmen der Dementia senilis, bedingt durch umschriebene stärkere Hirnatrophie (gemischte Apraxie). *Monatsschrift für Psychiatrie und Neurologie* **19,** 97–108.

Pilleri, G. (1966) The Klüver–Bucy syndrome in man: a clinico-anatomical contribution to the function of the medial temporal lobe structures. *Psychiatria et Neurologia* **152,** 65–103.

Pleydell, M.J. (1954) Huntington's chorea in Northamptonshire. *British Medical Journal* **2,** 1121–8.

Pollack, M. and Hornabrook, R.W. (1966) The prevalence, natural history and dementia of Parkinson's disease. *Brain* **89,** 429–448.

Post, F. (1965) *The Clinical Psychiatry of Late Life.* Pergammon Press, London.

Powers, J.M. and Skeen, J.T. (1980) An immunoperoxidase study of senile plaques. *Journal of Neuropathology and Experimental Neurology* **39,** 385.

Powers, J.M. and Spicer, S.S. (1977) Histochemical similarity of senile plaque amyloid to apudamyloid. *Virchows Archiv.* A. *Pathologische Anatomie* **376,** 107–15.

Pratt, R.T.C. (1970) *The Genetics of Neurological Disorders.* Oxford University Press, London.

Radue, E.W., du Boulay, G.H., Harrison, M.J.G. and Thomas, D.J. (1978) Comparison of angiographic and CT findings between patients with multi-infarct dementia and those with dementia due to primary neuronal degeneration. *Neuroradiology* **16,** 113–15.

Raskin, N. and Ehrenberg, R. (1956) Senescence, senility and Alzheimer's disease. *American Journal of Psychiatry* **113,** 133–7.

Redlich, E. (1898) Über miliäre Sklerose der Hirnrinde bei seniler Atrophie. *Jahrbücher für Psychologie und Neurologie* **17,** 208–16.

Reich, F. (1907) Der Gehirnbefund in dem in der Sitzung des psychiatrischen Vereins zu Berlin von 18 Mai 1905 vorgestellten Fall von 'Alogie'. *Allgemeine Zeitschrift für Psychiatrie* **64,** 380–8.

Reich, F. (1927) Zur Pathogenese der circumscripten, respektive systemartigen, Hirnatrophie. *Zeitschrift für die gesamte Neurologie und Psychiatrie* **108,** 803–12.

Reid, A.H. and Maloney, A.F.J. (1974) Giant cell arteritis and arteriolitis association with amyloid angiopathy in an elderly mongol. *Acta Neuropathologica* **27,** 131–7.

Reisine, T.D., Beaumont, K., Bird, E.D., Spokes, E. and Yamamura, H.I. (1979) Huntington's disease: alterations in neurotransmitter receptor binding in the human brain. In *Advances in Neurology*, vol. 23, *Huntington's Disease* (Eds. Chase, T.N., Wexler, N.S. and Barbeau, A.), pp. 717–26. Raven Press, New York.

Reisine, T.D., Fields, J.Z., Bird, E.D., Spokes, E. and Yamamura, H.I. (1978) Characterisation of brain dopaminergic receptors in Huntington's disease. *Communications in Psychopharmacology* **2,** 79–84.

Richardson, E.P. (1965) In discussion on paper by Yahr, M.D., Duvoisin, R.C. and Cowan, D. Encephalopathy associated with carcinoma. *Transactions of the American Neurological Association* **90,** 85.

Richardson, E.P. Jr (1977) Introduction to myoclonic dementia. In *Neurological Classics in Modern Translation* (Eds. Castleman, E. and Richardson, E.P. Jr), pp. 183–4.

Robertson, E.G. (1949) Cerebral lesions due to intracranial aneurysms. *Brain* **72,** 150–85.

Robins, A.H. (1976) Depression in patients with parkinsonism. *British Journal of Psychiatry* **128,** 141–5.

Rodda, R.A. (1981) Cerebellar atrophy in Huntington's disease. *Journal of the Neurological Sciences* **50,** 147–57.

Roizin, L., Kaufman, M.A., Willson, N., Stellar, S. and Liu, J.C. (1976) Neuropathologic observations on Huntington's chorea. In *Progress in Neuropathology*, vol. 3 (Ed. Zimmerman, W.M.), pp. 447–88. Grune & Stratton, New York.

Roizin, L., Stellar, S. and Liu, J.C. (1979) Neuronal nuclear cytoplasmic changes in Huntington's chorea: electron microscope investigations. In *Advances in Neurology*, vol. 23, *Huntington's Disease* (Eds. Chase, T.N., Wexler, N.S. and Barbeau, A.), pp. 95–122. Raven Press, New York.

Ropper, A.H. and Williams, R.S. (1980) Relationships between plaques, tangles and dementia in Down's syndrome. *Neurology* **30,** 639–44.

Rose, F.C. and Symonds, C.P. (1960) Persistent memory defect following encephalitis. *Brain* **83,** 195–212.

Rosen, W.G., Terry, R.D., Fuld, P.A., Katzman, R. and Peck, A. (1980) Pathological verification of ischemic score in verification of dementias. *Annals of Neurology* **7,** 486–8.

Rosenberg, G.A., Kornfeld, M., Stovring, J. and Bicknell, J.M. (1979) Subcortical arteriosclerotic encephalopathy (Binswanger). Computerized tomography. *Neurology* **29,** 1102–6.

Roth, M. (1955) The natural history of mental disorder in old age. *Journal of Mental Science* **101,** 281–301.

Roth, M. (1971) Classification and aetiology in mental disorders of old age: some recent developments. From *Recent Developments in Psychogeriatrics. A symposium*, Special publication no. 6. published by authority of the *British Journal of Psychiatry* (Eds. Kay, D.W. and Walk, A.), pp. 1–18.

Roth, M. and Morrisey, J.D. (1952) Problems in the diagnosis and classification of mental disease in old age with a study of case material. *Journal of Mental Science* **98,** 66–80.

Roth, M., Tomlinson, B.E. and Blessed, G. (1966) Correlation between scores for dementia and counts of 'senile plaques' in cerebral grey matter of elderly subjects. *Nature* (*Lond.*) **209,** 109–10.

Rothschild, D. (1942) Neuropathological changes in arteriosclerotic psychoses and their psychiatric significance. *Archives of Neurology and Psychiatry* **48,** 417–36.

Rothschild, D. and Kasanin, J. (1936) Clinicopathologic study of Alzheimer's disease: relationship to senile condition. *Archives of Neurology and Psychiatry* **36,** 293-321.

Russell, R.W.R. (1980) Supranuclear palsy of eyelid closure. *Brain* **103,** 71-82.

Sajdel-Sulkowska, E.M., Coughlin, J.F., Staton, D.M. and Marotta, C.A. (1983) In vitro protein synthesis by messenger RNA from the Alzheimer disease brain. In *Biological Aspects of Alzheimer's Disease, Banbury Report 15.* (Ed. Katzman, R.), pp. 193-200. Cold Spring Harbor Laboratory, Cold Spring Harbor, NY.

Salazar, A.M., Masters, C.L., Gajdusek, D.C. and Gibbs, C.J. Jr (1983) Syndromes of amyotrophic lateral sclerosis and dementia: relation to transmissible Creutzfeldt-Jakob disease. *Annals of Neurology* **14,** 17-26.

Sato, Y., Ohta, M. and Tateishi, J. (1980) Experimental transmission of human subacute spongiform encephalopathy to small rodents. II. Ultrastructural study of spongy state in the grey and white matter. *Acta Neuropathologica* **51,** 135-40.

Scheibel, A.B. (1978) Structural aspects of the aging brain: spine systems and the dendritic arbor. In *Aging*, vol. 7, *Alzheimer's Disease, Senile Dementia, and Related Disorders* (Eds. Katzman, R., Terry, R.D. and Bick, K.L.), pp. 353-73. Raven Press, New York.

Scheibel, A.B. (1979a) Aging in human motor control systems. In *Aging*, vol. 10, *Sensory Systems and Communication in the Elderly*. (Eds. Ordy, J.M. and Brizzee, K.), pp. 297-310. Raven Press, New York.

Scheibel, A.B. (1979b) The hippocampus: organisational patterns in health and senescence. *Mechanisms of Ageing and Development* **9,** 89-102.

Scheibel, M.E., Tomiyasu, U. and Scheibel, A.B. (1977) The aging human Betz cell. *Experimental Neurology* **56,** 598-609.

Schenk, V.W.D. (1955) Syndrome d'Alzheimer: étude anatomoclinique de 35 cas. *Folia Psychiatrica, Neurologica et Neurochirurgica Neerlandica* **58,** 422-37.

Schenk, V.W.D. (1959) Re-examination of a family with Pick's disease. *Annals of Human Genetics* **23,** 325-33.

Schenk, V.W.D. and van Mansvelt, J. (1955) The cortical degeneration in Pick's syndrome. A quantitative analysis. *Folia Psychiatrica, Neurologica et Neurochirurgica Neerlandica* **58,** 42-62.

Schiffer, D. (1955) Contribution à l'histologie de la maladie de Pick. *Journal für Hirnforschung* **1,** 497-515.

Schlaepfer, W.W. (1978) Deformation of isolated neurofilaments and the pathogenesis of neurofibrillary pathology. *Journal of Neuropathology and Experimental Neurology* **37,** 244-54.

Schlote, W. (1965) Die Amyloidnatur der kongophilen drusigen Entartung der Hirnarterien (Scholz) in Senium. *Acta Neuropathologica* **4,** 449-68.

Schlote, W., Boellaard, J.W., Schumm, F. and Stöhr, M. (1980) Gerstmann-Sträussler-Scheinker's disease. Electron-microscopic observations on a brain biopsy. *Acta Neuropathologica* **52,** 203-11.

Schnitzler, J.G. (1911) Zur Abgrenzung der sog. Alzheimerschen Krankheit. *Zeitschrift für die gesamte Neurologie und Psychiatrie* **7,** 34-57.

Schochet, S.S. Jr, Lampert, P.W. and Earle, K.M. (1968) Neuronal changes induced by intrathecal vincristine sulfate. *Journal of Neuropathology and Experimental Neurology* **27,** 645-58.

Schochet, S.S. and McCormick, W.F. (1972) Ultrastructure of Hirano bodies. *Acta Neuropathologica* **21,** 50-60.

Scholz, W. (1938) Studien zur Pathologie der Hirngefässe. II. Die drusige Entartung der Hirnarterien und Capillaren. *Zeitschrift für die gesamte Neurologie und Psychiatrie* **162,** 694-715.

Schottky, J. (1932) Uber präsenile Verblödungen. *Zeitschrift für die gesamte Neurologie und Psychiatrie* **140,** 333-97.

Schröder, K. (1931) Zur Klinik und Pathologie der Huntingtonschen Krankheit. *Jahrbücher für Psychologie und Neurologie* **43,** 183-201.

Schulman, S. (1956) Bilateral symmetrical degeneration of the thalamus. *Journal of Neuropathology and Experimental Neurology* **15,** 208-9.

Schwartz, P., Wolfe, K., Gier, C. and Wolf, C.E. (1967) Cerebral, cardiovascular and pancreatic insular amyloidosis in the aged. (Exhibition presented at 64th Annual meeting of American Association of Pathology and Bacteriology.)

Scoville, W.B. (1954) The limbic lobe in man. *Journal of Neurosurgery* **11,** 64-6.

Scoville, W.B. and Milner, B. (1957) Loss of recent memory after bilateral hippocampal lesions. *Journal of Neurology, Neurosurgery and Psychiatry* **20,** 11-21.

Segara, J.M., von Stockert, T.R. and Curtis, M. (1973) Thalamic dementia. In *Proceedings of the 10th International Congress of Neurology*, Barcelona, 1973 (Eds. Subirana, A. and Espadeler, J.M.), pp. 392-5. Excerpta Medica, Amsterdam.

Seitelberger, F. and Jellinger, K. (1958) Umschriebene Grosshirmatrophie bei Alzheimerischer Krankheit. *Deutsche Zeitschrift für Nervenheilkunde* **178,** 365-79.

Serafetinides, E.A. and Falconer, M.A. (1962) Some observations on memory impairment after temporal lobectomy for epilepsy. *Journal of Neurology, Neurosurgery and Psychiatry* **25,** 251-5.

Sharman, M.G., Watt, D.C., Janota, I. and Carrasco, L.H. (1979) Alzheimer's disease in a mother and identical twins. *Psychological Medicine* **9,** 771-4.

Shaw, C.M. (1979) Primary idiopathic cerebrovascular amyloidosis in a child. *Brain* **102,** 177–92.

Shibayama, H. and Kitoh, J. (1978) Electronmicroscopic structure of the Alzheimer's neurofibrillary changes in a case of atypical senile dementia. *Acta Neuropathologica* **41,** 229–34.

Shields, J. (1962) *Monozygotic Twins.* Oxford University Press, London.

Sim, M., Turner, E. and Smith, W.T. (1966) Cerebral biopsy in the investigation of presenile dementia. *British Journal of Psychiatry* **112,** 119–25, 127–33.

Simchowicz, T. (1911) Histologische Studien über die senile Demenz. *Histologische und histopathologische Arbeiten über die Grosshirnrinde* **4,** 267–444.

Sjögren, T. (1935) Vererbungsmedizinische Untersuchungen über Huntingtonsche Chorea in einer schwedischen Bauernpopulation. *Zeitschrift für menschliche Vererbungs- und Konstitutionslehre* **19,** 131–65.

Sjögren, T., Sjögren, H. and Lindgren, A. (1952) Morbus Alzheimer and morbus Pick. Genetic chemical and patho-anatomical study. *Acta Psychiatrica et Neurologica Scandinavica*, suppl. 82.

Slaby, A.E. and Wyatt, R.J. (1974) *Dementia in the Presenium.* Thomas, Springfield, Illinois.

Slater, E. and Cowie, V. (1971) *The Genetics of Mental Disorders.* Oxford University Press, London.

Smith, D.A. and Lantos, P. (1983) A case of combined Pick's disease and Alzheimer's disease. *Journal of Neurology, Neurosurgery and Psychiatry* **46,** 675–7.

Smith, W.T. (1970), The Pathology of the Organic Dementia. In *Modern Trends in Neurology—5*, pp. 96–126 (Ed. Williams, D.) Butterworths, London.

Smith, W.T., Turner, E. and Sim, M. (1966) Cerebral biopsy in the investigation of presenile dementia. II. Pathological aspects. *British Journal of Psychiatry* **112,** 127–33.

Solitaire, G.B. and Lamarche, J.B. (1966) Alzheimer's disease and senile dementia as seen in mongoloids. *Americain Journal of Mental Deficiency* **70,** 840–8.

Soniat, T.L.L. (1941) Histogenesis of senile plaques. *Archives of Neurology and Psychiatry* **46,** 101–44.

Spatz, H. (1952) La maladie de Pick, les atrophies systématisées progressives et la sénescence cérébrale prematurée localisée. In *Proceedings of First International Congress of Neuropathology*, vol. 2, 375–406. Rosenberg and Sellier, Torino.

Spiegel, E.A., Wycis, H.T., Orchinik, C.W. and Freed, H. (1955) The thalamus and temporal orientation. *Science* **121,** 771–2.

Spokes, E.G.S. (1979) An analysis of factors influencing measurements of dopamine, noradrenaline glutamate decarboxylase and choline acetylase in human post mortem brain tissue. *Brain* **102,** 333–46.

Squire, L. and Moore, R.Y. (1979) Dorsal thalamic lesion in a noted case of memory dysfunction. *Annals of Neurology* **6,** 503–6.

Sroka, H., Elizan, T.S., Yahr, M.D., Binger, A. and Mendazu, M.R. (1981) Organic mental syndrome and confusional states in Parkinson's disease. *Archives of Neurology* **38,** 339–42.

Stahl, W.L. and Swanson, P.D. (1974) Biochemical abnormalities in Huntington's chorea brains. *Neurology* **24,** 813–19.

Steele, J.C., Richardson, J.C. and Olszewski, J. (1964) Progressive supra-nuclear palsy. *Archives of Neurology* **10,** 333–59.

Stepien, L. and Sierpinski, S. (1964) Impairment of recent memory after temporal lesions in man. *Neuropsychologia* **2,** 291–303.

Stern, K. (1939) Severe dementia associated with bilateral symmetrical degeneration of the thalamus. *Brain* **62,** 157–71.

Struwe, F. (1929) Histopathologische Untersuchungen über Entstehung und Wesen der senilen Plaques. *Zeitschrift für die gesamte Neurologie und Psychiatrie* **122,** 291–307.

Surbeck, E.B. (1961) L'angiopathie Dyshorique (Morel) de l'Écorce Cérébrale. Etude Anatomoclinique et Statistique: Aspect Génétique. Thesis, Geneva.

Suzuki, K., Katxman, R. and Korey, S.R. (1965) Chemical studies on Alzheimer's disease. *Journal of Neuropathology and Experimental Neurology* **24,** 211.

Tateishi, J., Ohta, M., Koga, M., Sato, Y. and Kuroiwa, Y. (1979) Transmission of chronic spongiform encephalopathy with kuru plaques from humans to small rodents. *Annals of Neurology* **5,** 581–4.

Tellez-Nagel, I., Johnson, A.B. and Terry, R.D. (1974) Studies on brain biopsies of patients with Huntington's chorea. *Journal of Neuropathology and Experimental Neurology* **33,** 308–32.

Terry, R.D. (1963) The fine structure of neurofibrillary tangles in Alzheimer's disease. *Journal of Neuropathology and Experimental Neurology* **22,** 629–42.

Terry, R.D., Davies, P., DeTeresa, R. and Katzman, R. (1982) Are both plaques and tangles required to make it Alzheimer's disease? *Journal of Neuropathology and Experimental Neurology* **41,** 364.

Terry, R.D., Fitzgerald, C., Peck, A., Millner, J. and Farmer, P. (1977). Cortical cell counts in senile dementia. *Journal of Neuropathology and Experimental Neurology* **36,** 633.

Terry, R.D., Gonatas, N.K. and Weiss, M. (1964) Ultrastructural studies in Alzheimer's presenile dementia. *American Journal of Pathology* **44,** 269–97.

Terry, R.D., Peck, A., DeTeresa, R. and Schechter, R. (1981) Some morphometric aspects of the brain in senile dementia of the Alzheimer type. *Annals of Neurology* **10,** 184–92.

Terry, R.D. and Pena, C. (1965) Experimental production of neurofibrillary degeneration. 2. Electronmicroscopy, phosphatase histochemistry and electron probe analysis. *Journal of Neuropathology and Experimental Neurology* **24,** 200–10.

Terry, R.D. and Wisniewski, H.M. (1972) Ultrastructure of senile dementia and of experimental analogs. In *Advances in Behavioral Biology*, vol. 3, *Aging and the Brain* (Ed. Gaitz, C.M.), pp. 89–116. Plenum Press, New York.

Terzian, H. and Ore, G.D. (1955) Syndrome of Klüver and Bucy reproduced in man by bilaterial removal of the temporal lobes. *Neurology* **5,** 373–80.

Thase, M.E., Liss, L., Schmelzer, D. and Maloon, J. (1982) Clinical evaluation of dementia in Down's syndrome. *Journal of Mental Deficiency Research* **26,** 239–44.

Tomlinson, B.E. (1959) Brain changes in ruptured intracranial aneurysms. *Journal of Clinical Pathology* **12,** 391–9.

Tomlinson, B.E. (1972) Morphological brain changes in non-demented old people. In *Aging of the Central Nervous System* (Eds. von Praag, H.M. and Kalverboer, A.F.), pp. 37–57. De Ervon F. Bohn, New York.

Tomlinson, B.E. (1977) The pathology of dementia. In *Dementia*, 2nd edn (Ed. Wells, C.E.), pp. 113–80. F.A. Davis, Philadelphia.

Tomlinson, B.E. (1980) The structural and quantitative aspects of the dementias. In *Biochemistry of Dementia* (Ed. Roberts, P.J.), pp. 15–52. Wiley, Chichester.

Tomlinson, B.E., Blessed, G., Irving, D., Perry, R.H. and Bloxham, C.H. (1984) Parkinson's disease and Alzheimer's disease. The frequency of their simultaneous occurrence neuropathologically. (to be published)

Tomlinson, B.E., Blessed, G. and Roth, M. (1968) Observations on the brains of non-demented old people. *Journal of Neurological Sciences* **7,** 331–56.

Tomlinson, B.E., Blessed, G. and Roth, M. (1970) Observations on the brains of demented old people. *Journal of the Neurological Sciences* **11,** 205–42.

Tomlinson, B.E. and Henderson, G. (1976) Some quantitative cerebral findings in normal and demented old people. In *Neurobiology of Aging*, vol. 3 (Eds. Terry, R.D. and Gershon, S.), pp. 183–204. Raven Press, New York.

Tomlinson, B.E. and Irving, D. (1977) The numbers of limb motor neurons in the human lumbosacral cord throughout life. *Journal of the Neurological Sciences* **34,** 213–19.

Tomlinson, B.E., Irving, D. and Blessed, G. (1981) Cell loss in the locus ceruleus in senile dementia of Alzheimer type. *Journal of the Neurological Sciences* **49,** 419–28.

Tomlinson, B.E. and Kitchener, D. (1972) Granulovacuolar degeneration of hippocampal pyramidal cells. *Journal of Pathology* **106,** 165–85.

Tomonoga, M. (1974) Ultrastructure of Hirano bodies. *Acta Neuropathologica* **28,** 365–6.

Torack, R.M. (1975) Congophilic angiopathy complicated by surgery and massive haemorrhage. *American Journal of Pathology* **81,** 349–66.

Torack, R.M. and Lynch, R.G. (1981) Cytochemistry of brain amyloid in adult dementia. *Acta Neuropathologica* **53,** 189–96.

Traub, R., Gajdusek, D.C. and Gibbs, C.J. Jr (1977) Transmissible virus dementia: the relation of transmissible spongiform encephalopathy to Creutzfeldt–Jakob disease. In *Aging and Dementia* (Ed. Lynn Smith, W. and Kinsbourne, M.), pp. 91–172. Spectrum Publications, New York.

Uemura, E. and Hartmann, H.A. (1978). RNA content and volume of nerve cell bodies in human brains. I. Prefrontal cortex in aging and demented subjects. *Journal of Neuropathology and Experimental Neurology* **37,** 487–97.

Urechia, C., Dragomir, L. and Elekes, N. (1935) Deux cas de la maladie de Pick. Un cas de la maladie d'Alzheimer. Existe-t-il des rapports entres ces maladies? *Archives Internationales de Neurologie* **54,** 55–83.

Van Buren, J.M. and Borke, R.C. (1972) The mesial temporal substratum of memory. Anatomical study in three individuals. *Brain* **95,** 599–632.

Verhaart, W.J.C. (1936) Ueber das Vorkommen der Pickschen Krankheit und der Krankheit von Alzheimer bei den Malaien und Chinesen in Niederlandisch-Ost-Indien. *Mededelingen van Dienst der Volksgezondheid in Nederlandsch-Indië* **25,** 341–5.

Victor, M., Adams, R.D. and Collins, G.H. (1971) *The Wernicke–Korsakoff Syndrome.* Blackwell Scientific, Oxford.

Victor, M., Angevine, J.B., Mancall, E.L. and Fisher, C.M. (1961) Memory loss with lesions of hippocampal formation. *Archives of Neurology* **5,** 244–63.

Vijayashankar, N. and Brody, H. (1971) Neuronal population of the human abducens nucleus. *Anatomical Record* **169,** 447.

Vijayashankar, N. and Brody, H. (1973) The neuronal population of the nuclei of the trochlear nerve and the locus ceruleus in the human. *Anatomical Record* **172,** 421–2.

Vogt, M. (1928) Die Picksche Atrophie als Beispiel für die eunomische Form der Schichtenpathoklise. *Jahrbücher für Psychologie und Neurologie* **36,** 124–9.

Wechsler, A.F., Berity, M.A., Rosenschein, S., Friede, I. and Scheibel, A.B. (1982) Clinical, computed tomographic and histological study with Golgi impregnation observations. *Archives of Neurology* **39,** 287–90.

Weimann, W. (1921) Ueber einen atypischen präsenilen Verblödungsprozess. *Zeitschrift für die gesamte Neurologie und Psychiatrie* **23,** 355–60.

Weiner, W.J., Hitri, A., Carvey, P., Koller, W.C., Nausieda, P.A. and Klawans, H.L. (1979). ^{3}H-dopamine binding studies in guinea pig striatal membrane suggesting two distinct dopamine receptor sites. In *Advances in Neurology*, vol. 23, *Huntington's Disease* (Eds. Chase, T.N., Wexler, N.S. and Barbeau, A.), pp. 687–95. Raven Press, New York.

Weisschedel, E. (1938) Ueber eine systematische Atrophie der oberen Olive. *Archiv für Psychiatrie und Nervenkrankheiten* **108,** 219–27.

Wendt, G.G., Landzettel, I. and Solth, K. (1960) Krankheitsdauer und Lebenserwartung bei der Huntingtonschen Chorea. *Archiv für Psychiatrie und Nervenkrankheiten* **201,** 298–312.

Wendt, G.G., Landzettel, I. and Unterreiner, I. (1959) Das Erkrankungsalter bei der Huntingtonschen Chorea. *Acta Genetica et Statistica Medica* **9,** 18–32.

Wernicke, C. (1881) *Lehrbuch der Gehirnkrankheiten fur Ärzte und Studierende*. Fischer, Berlin.

Wheelan, L. (1959) Familial Alzheimer's disease. *Annals of Human Genetics* **23,** 300–10.

White, P., Hiley, C.R., Goodhardt, M.J., Carrasco, L.H., Keet, J.P., Williams, I.E.I. and Bowen, D.M. (1977) Neocortical cholinergic neurones in elderly people. *Lancet* **i,** 668–70.

Whitehouse, P.J., Price, D.L., Clark, A.W., Coyle, J.T. and DeLong, M.R. (1981) Alzheimer disease: evidence for selective loss of cholinergic neurons in the nucleus basalis. *Annals of Neurology* **10,** 122–6.

Whittier, J.E. (1963) Research on Huntington's chorea: problems of privilege and confidentiality. *Journal of Forensic Sciences* **8,** 568–75.

Wilcock, G.K. and Esiri, M.M. (1982) Plaques, tangles and dementia: a quantitative study. *Journal of the Neurological Sciences* **56,** 343–56.

Wilkinson, A. and Davies, I. (1978) The influence of age and dementia on the neurone population of the mamillary bodies. *Age and Ageing* **7,** 151–60.

Will, R.G. and Matthews, W.B. (1982) Evidence for case-to-case transmission of Creutzfeldt–Jakob disease. *Journal of Neurology, Neurosurgery and Psychiatry* **45,** 235–8.

Williams, R.S., Ferrante, R.J. and Caviness, V.S. Jr (1978) The Golgi rapid method in clinical neuropathology. The morphologic consequences of suboptimal fixation. *Journal of Neuropathology and Experimental Neurology* **37,** 13–33.

Winkelman, N.W. and Book, M.H. (1949) Asymptomatic extrapyramidal involvement in Pick's disease. *Journal of Neuropathology and Experimental Neurology* **8,** 30–42.

Wisniewski, H.M., Bruce, M.E. and Fraser, H. (1975) Infectious etiology of neuritic (senile) plaques in mice. *Science* **190,** 1108–10.

Wisniewski, H.M., Coblenz, J.M. and Terry, R.D. (1972) Pick's Disease. A clinical and ultrastructural study. *Archives of Neurology* 26, 97–108.

Wisniewski, H.M., Ghetti, B. and Terry, R.D. (1973) Neuritic (senile) plaques and filamentous changes in aged rhesus monkeys. *Journal of Neuropathology and Experimental Neurology* **32,** 566–84.

Wisniewski, H.M., Johnson, A.B., Raine, C.S., Kay, W.J. and Terry, R.D. (1970) Senile plaques and cerebral amyloidosis in aged dogs. A histochemical study. *Laboratory Investigation* **23,** 287–96.

Wisniewski, H.M., Narang, H.K., Corsellis, J.A.N. and Terry, R.D. (1976) Ultrastructural studies of the neurophil and neurofibrillary tangles in Alzheimer's disease and post-traumatic dementia. *Journal of Neuropathology and Experimental Neurology* **35,** 367.

Wisniewski, H., Narang, H.K. and Terry, R.D. (1976) Neurofibrillary tangles of paired helical filaments. *Journal of the Neurological Sciences* **27,** 173–81.

Wisniewski, H.M. and Terry, R.D. (1967) Experimental colchicine encephalopathy. I. Introduction of neurofibrillary degeneration. *Laboratory Investigation* **17,** 577–87.

Wisniewski, H., Terry, R.D. and Hirano, A. (1970) Neurofibrillary pathology. *Journal of Neuropathology and Experimental Neurology* **29,** 163–76.

Woodard, J.S. (1962) Clinico-pathologic significance of granulovacuolar degeneration in Alzheimer's disease. *Journal of Neuropathology and Experimental Neurology* **21,** 85–91.

Woodard, J.S. (1966) Alzheimer's disease in late adult life. *American Journal of Pathology* **49,** 1157–69.

Woods, B.T., Schoene, W. and Kneisley, L. (1982) Are hippocampal lesions sufficient to cause lasting amnesia? *Journal of Neurology, Neurosurgery and Psychiatry* **45,** 243–7.

Worm-Peterson, J. and Pakkenberg, H. (1968) Atherosclerosis of cerebral arteries: pathological and clinical correlations. *Journal of Gerontology* **23,** 445–9.

Worster-Drought, C. and Allen, I.M. (1929) Huntington's chorea—with report of two cases. *British Medical Journal* **2,** 1149–52.

Worster-Drought, C., Greenfield, J.G. and McMenemy, W.H. (1940) A form of familial presenile dementia with spastic paralysis. *Brain* **63,** 237–54.

Worster-Drought, C., Greenfield, J.G. and McMenemy, W.H. (1944) A form of familial presenile dementia with spastic paralysis. *Brain* **67,** 38–43.

Wright, J.R., Calkins, E., Breen, W.J., Stolte, G. and Schultz, R.T. (1969) Relationship of amyloid to aging. Review of the literature and systematic study of 83 patients from a general hospital population. *Medicine* **48,** 39–60.

Yagashita, S., Itah, Y., Wang, N. and Amano, N. (1981) Reappraisal of the fine structure of Alzheimer's neurofibrillary tangles. *Acta Neuropathologica* **54,** 239–46.

Yates, P.O. and Hutchinson, E.C. (1961) Cerebral infarction: the role of stenosis of the extracranial cerebral arteries. *Medical Research Council Special Report Series* 300.

Zeumer, H., Schonsky, B. and Sturm, K.W. (1980) Predominant white matter involvement in subcortical arteriosclerotic encephalopathy (Binswanger's disease). *Journal of Computer Assisted Tomography* **4,** 14–19.

Zeman, W. (1971) Ceroid lipofuscinosis—Batten Vogt syndrome: a model for human aging. *Advances in Gerontological Research* **3,** 147–70.

21

Muscle

D.G.F. Harriman

For many years the histopathology of skeletal muscle attracted little interest or effort. Its reactions in disease were limited, and too easily obscured by artefact. A lump of muscle hastily excised and dropped immediately into acid formalin provided a disorderly mass of hypercontracted muscle fibres, impossible to orientate. Small wonder that even 30 years ago a routine report might consist of little more than 'the muscle has lost its striations'. Only three types of muscle disease were recognised—neurogenic atrophy, muscular dystrophy and the 'very rare' polymyositis—before it was realized that muscle as highly irritable tissue had to be excised, handled and fixed with great care.

Interest revived in the 1950s when Nattrass (1954) showed that patients 'recovering' from progressive muscular dystrophy were in reality suffering from polymyositis, and the first comprehensive account of that condition by Walton and Adams (1958), based on a large material at biopsy and autopsy, revealed it to be by no means rare.

Coërs and Woolf (1959) greatly increased the value of the muscle biopsy by introducing intravital staining of the motor nerves and end-plates, but the major advances came with the introduction of histochemical methods applied to fresh-frozen sections of muscle, and of electron microscopy. The first allowed not only the demonstration of fibre types, their selective involvement in some diseases and the detection of enzyme deficiencies, but also the discovery of abnormal structure not previously detected in fixed and embedded muscle. Electron microscopy revealed detail and other unsuspected abnormalities. As a result many new myopathies have now been described, and there are no doubt others still undiscovered. The importance of a multidisciplinary approach to the investigation of muscle disease, especially clinical and biochemical, in combination with morphology cannot be emphasized too strongly.

It is useful to classify muscle diseases in two groups: *neurogenic disease* and the *myopathies* (disorders of muscle proper). The myopathies can be further divided into the primary and secondary, with intrinsic and extrinsic causes, although our ignorance of aetiology is such as to make an accurate classification impossible.

Histology

The basic structure of skeletal muscle is common to many species, but when fibre size, histochemical types and organelles are considered there is not only much variation between species but also between muscles in the same organism. To define normal muscle is therefore difficult.

The skeletal muscle cell or myofibre is a greatly elongated syncytium often stretching from the origin of a muscle to its insertion. It has many nuclei situated at the periphery of the cell close to the sarcolemma, but near its fibrous insertions the nuclei become internally placed and increasingly numerous. The tapering ends of muscle fibres are sometimes seen in a section as small round fibres ending blindly and have to be distinguished from fibres rendered atrophic by disease. Some nuclei are external to the sarcolemma (used here synonymously with plasmalemma) but indent the fibre. These are nuclei of satellite cells, or resting myoblasts, and only by electron microscopy can their true position outside the sarcolemma be shown. Muscle regeneration takes place by proliferation of these cells.

Much of the cytoplasm of the muscle fibre is occupied by myofibrils, thin cords of protein

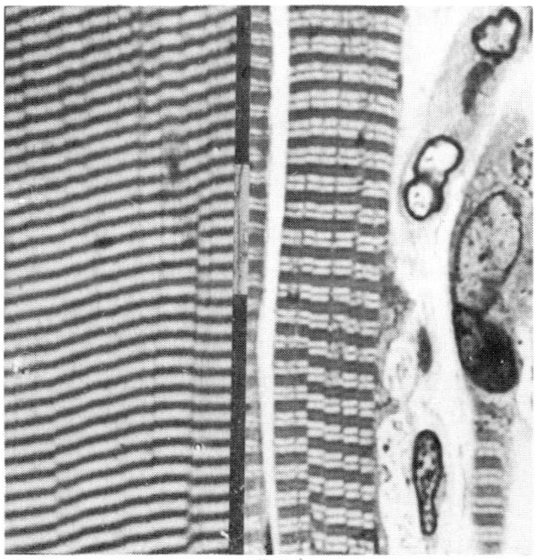

Fig. 21.1 (**a**) Part of a muscle fibre viewed by polarized light (unstained epon-embedded section). The light anisotropic A-bands alternate with the dark isotropic I-bands. × 576. (**b**) Epon-embedded muscle from a child of 3 years. The A-bands stain darkly, and the lightly stained I-bands are divided by a thin dark line, the Z-band. A *sarcomere* extends from one Z-band to the next. A myelinated subterminal axon approaches the muscle fibre from above right, running towards a motor end-plate which apparently sits on the surface of the muscle fibre, forming Doyère's eminence. Semi-thin sections. Methylene blue × 1000.

which run the entire length of the cell. They are composed of myofilaments and have an alternately light and dark banded structure, well demonstrated by polarized light and by routine staining of carefully fixed longitudinally embedded muscle. The myofibrils run in parallel with their bands in register, giving skeletal muscle its characteristic striated form (Fig. 21.1). The anisotropic (A) bands stain more darkly than the isotropic (I) bands, and a dark line, the Z-band (zwischenscheibe or intercalated plate) lies in the middle of the I-band. In transverse sections myofibrils are closely and uniformly packed, 100 or more in each fibre. The uniform 'fibrillen-struktur' pattern is seen in the vast majority of skeletal muscle fibres in man, but in much amphibian muscle and in some specialized muscles in man the myofibrils occur in clumps or 'fields' (feldenstruktur) as in extraocular muscle.

Ageing of muscle

Just as the complete range of appearances in 'normal' muscle has not yet been described, the effects of ageing also are lacking in adequate study. Papers have been published employing too few specimens from patients in whom adverse physical and environmental factors are ignored, and many do not study males and females separately, reflecting the difficulty of obtaining healthy muscle. Preliminary results (Harnden-Mayor and Harriman) in the writer's laboratory from counts and lesser diameter measurements in 72 healthy individuals aged from 40 to 74 years indicate that there is only a slight diminution in the size of fibre types in healthy old age. There is loss of type 1 and type 2b fibres in females, with relative preservation of type 2a fibres. This was not shown in males, in whom the percentage of 2a decreased after 50 years of age. The familiar picture of small fibres with accumulated nuclei in less than healthy old age must have a cause other than ageing. The muscle biopsied was always the vastus medialis, unlikely to be influenced by ageing of motor

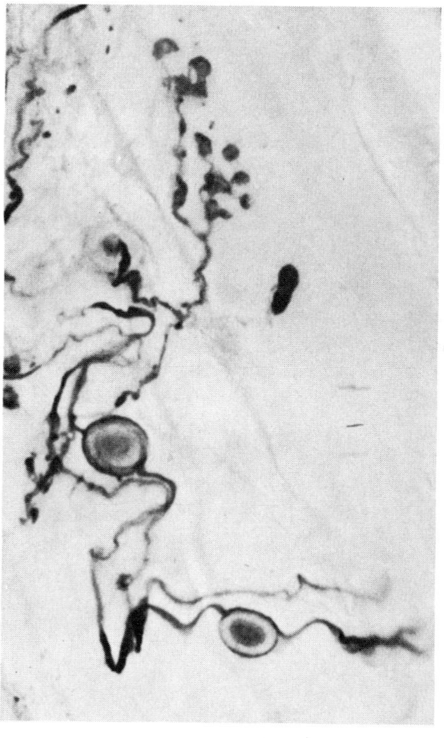

Fig. 21.2 Axonic spheres. These occur along the course of axons, especially subterminal, and usually are an ageing phenomenon. The ovoid bodies are clearly intra-axonal; they stain uniformly or concentrically. A normal end-plate is also seen. Female aged 59 years, Ekbom's syndrome for 38 years, peroneus brevis. Methylene blue × 600.

nerves, the effect of which appears first at the ends of the longest axons (Harriman, Taverner and Woolf, 1970), often as early as the age of 40. The axons contain degenerative spheres, and the muscle (Fig. 21.2) is gradually denervated. In the extensor digitorum brevis denervation may start in the second decade, but nerve entrapment may be responsible for it.

Muscle ultrastructure

The most important features to be recognized in normal muscle fibres are the constituents of the sarcomere mentioned above, the mitochondria and the sarcotubular system (Fig. 21.3). To obtain good fixation and orientation it is advisable to stretch the narrow (1 mm) muscle strip slightly

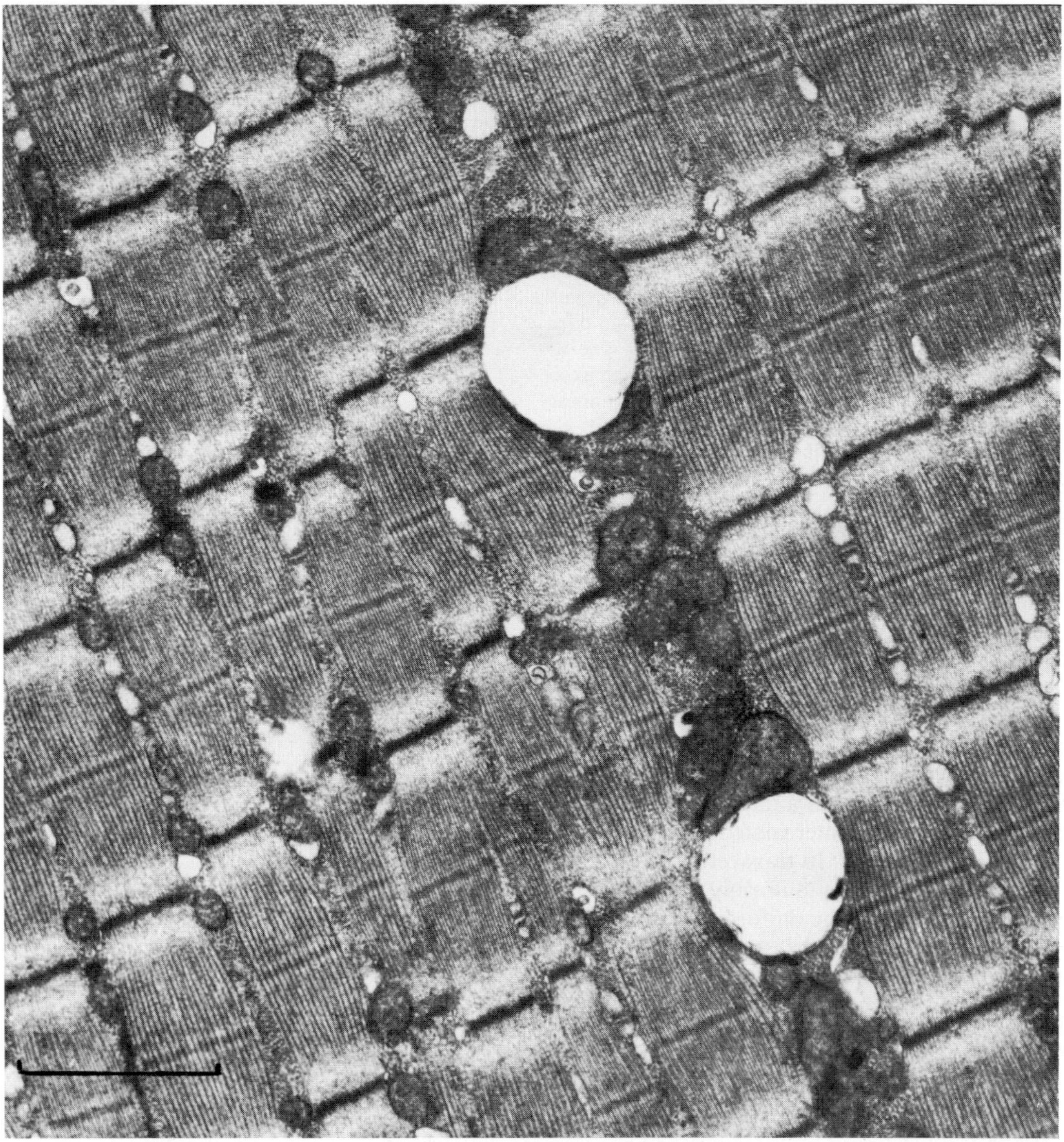

Fig. 21.3 Between the myofibrils lie a line of mitochondria or a row of elements of the sarcoplasmic reticulum. These are the triads, composed of lateral sacs on either side of a tubule. Two lipid droplets are present. The lateral sacs often contain dark material and are then less clearly seen than here. Bar = 1 μm.

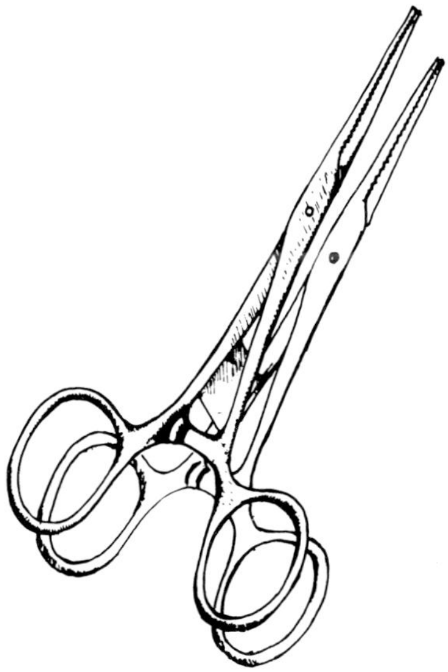

Fig. 21.4 Simple clamp used for maintaining rest length of muscle taken at biopsy. It is composed of two artery forceps united by a steel band, and permits individual control of the 'bite' at each end of the fascicle excised. Conventional muscle biopsy clamps in the form of a U or Y are more difficult to use because the bites at each extremity must be made simultaneously. Clamps are made with small or large forceps (box joints) and with different tip separations to suit the requirements for electron microscopy, for the cryostat or for paraffin embedding.

in a muscle clamp (Fig. 21.4) before placing the clamp and specimen in the fixative within a second or two. The sarcomeres are extended and the filaments clearly seen. Polyribosomes, glycogen and lipofuscin can be recognized. Mitochondria are more numerous around puberty and in athletic individuals, forming peripheral crescents; lipofuscin increases with age, but not greatly in the healthy. Glycogen should be more plentiful in type 2 fibres, but is variable in amount, and tubules may proliferate slightly in disease. The features of type 1 and type 2 fibres are not as clear cut as in histochemical preparations: type 1 fibres have more mitochondria, are more likely to contain lipid droplets, and should have less glycogen and slightly thicker Z-lines than type 2 fibres which contain more sarcoplasmic reticulum.

The ultrastructure of motor end-plates is of special importance because it alters specifically in denervation and in the myasthenic syndromes, in the latter case in a manner which cannot be recognized by light microscopy. A normal end-plate is shown in Fig. 21.5. In infancy there may be only one axonic expansion per end-plate but later more expansions develop. The sole-plates of type 1 fibres have slightly wider and shallower secondary synaptic clefts than those of type 2 fibres, in which the clefts are more numerous, longer and appear to branch. The fast-twitch type 2 fibres evidently provide a greater surface area for synaptic transmission than the slow-twitch type 1 fibres.

Muscle fibre size

Some authors measuring the lesser diameters of normal and abnormal fibres obtain figures double that of others. The reason must lie in the technique used to obtain the specimen and then to quench or fix it. The muscle strip may be rendered narrow by overstretching, or goaded into overcontraction or caused to relax gently. Most workers aim to obtain the tissue at resting length—that is, its length in the relaxed state before excision. The writer's preference is for electron microscopy specimens to be taken on a clamp with slight stretching and for specimens for frozen section and embedding to be slowly excised, kept cool at 0.4°C for 15–20 minutes to allow relaxation, and then clamped prior to quenching or fixation merely to keep the specimen straight. Specimens likely to be delayed can be placed in isotonic saline at 0–4°C but it is important to control the temperature. Frozen sections are consistent and more natural than fixed specimens, which inevitably shrink. But the latter are necessary for overview longitudinal sections, which are difficult in frozen fresh muscle.

Using these methods muscle fibres are said to vary in diameter from 8 μm at birth to 40 μm in adult life, but there is much variation between individuals and between muscles. In current work (Harnden-Mayor and Harriman) on muscle biopsies of the vastus medialis from normal healthy individuals in the fifth decade, the average fibre size range (lesser transverse diameter) is 36–74 μm. Exercise, both dynamic and isometric, has much influence on muscle fibre size. Fibre types also show wide ranges of size: type 1, 34–72 μm; type 2a, 34–82 μm. It is often stated that in females type 2b fibres are smaller than type 1; in the writer's experience this is true in only 55 per cent. In males, type 2 are larger more often (87.5 per cent).

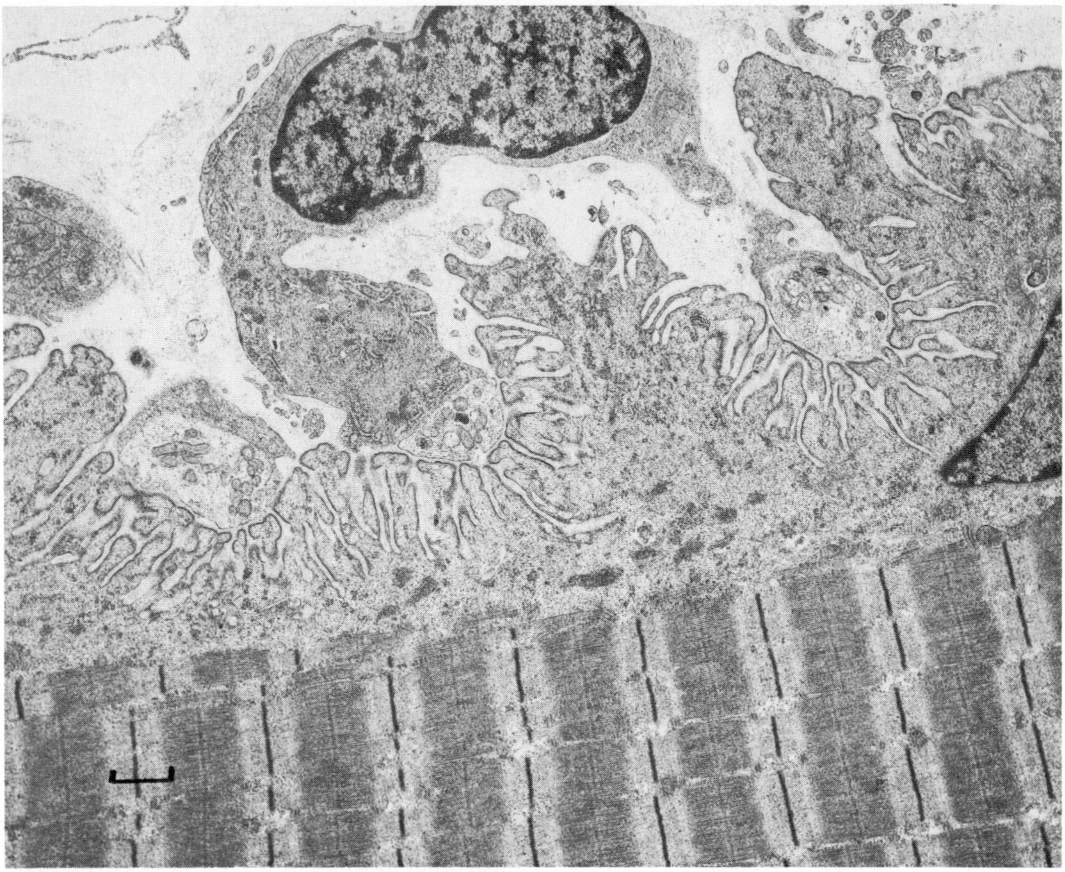

(a)

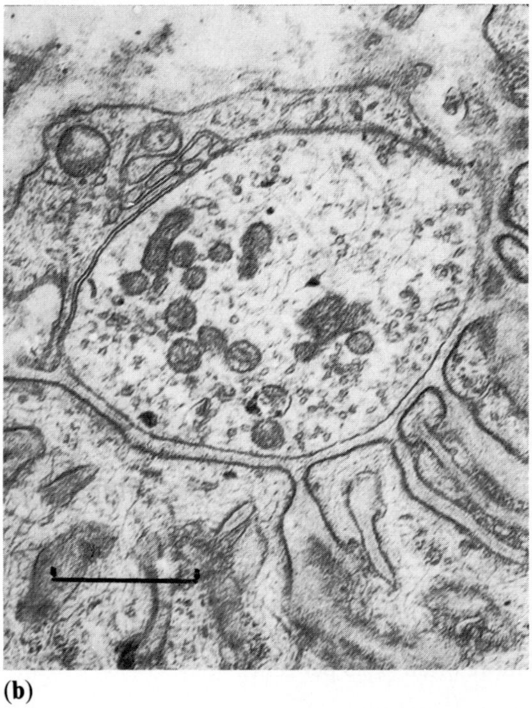

(b)

Fig. 21.5 (**a**) Motor end-plate. The darker cytoplasm of the Schwann cell covers the three axonic expansions except where these are in contact with the primary synaptic groove. Folds in the muscle surface form the secondary synaptic clefts. The axonic expansions contain variable numbers of mitochondria and synaptic vesicles, and occasional dark bodies are found in normal expansions. The sole-plate contains mitochondria and a ring of sole-plate nuclei, part of one shown on the right. Bar = 1 μm. (**b**) Axonal terminal from another end-plate showing synaptic vesicles and mitochondria. Bar = 1 μm.

Artefacts

Because of their natural irritability even to the extent of rupture, muscle fibres are liable to show artefacts unless handled with great care throughout the process of excision, quenching and fixation. Even necropsy muscle can be damaged by careless excision or undue tension especially during *post mortem* rigidity. Hypercontraction produces regular contraction bands (Fig. 21.6), and such fibres in transverse section are either

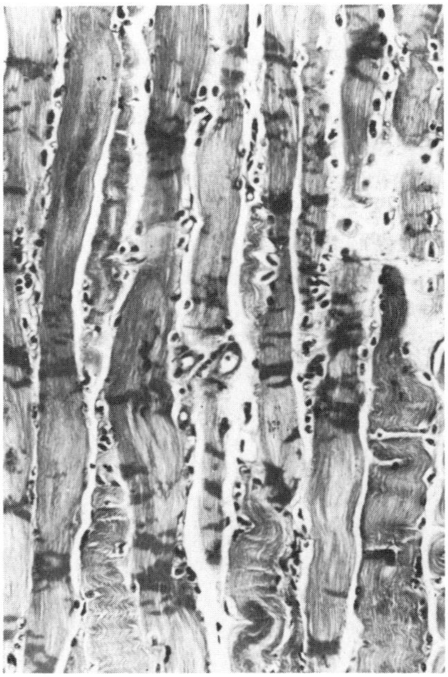

Fig. 21.6 Biopsy muscle from a female of 68 years with polyneuritis. There are numerous contraction bands due to the immersion of the specimen in fixative while still irritable. Partly denervated muscle is particularly susceptible to this artefact. H&E × 270.

swollen and hyaline or pale and granular, depending on the plane of section. The nuclei are pyknotic. When the cell membrane is torn the artefact is easily recognized, but if it is not the unwary may be deceived. Contraction bands are frequent in prematurely fixed muscle but fortunately rare in carefully quenched muscle except in Duchenne dystrophy (q.v.) and neonatal muscle. Curiously, fresh-frozen muscle cut longitudinally is more liable to gross artefact, presumably because the fibres are still capable of overcontraction when restored to room temperature after quenching and section. Contraction after section can be demonstrated by quantitative polarization (Harriman and Stocks, 1970).

There are other artefacts. One is the streaming of glycogen towards the edge of the muscle fibre to cause a crescent of intense staining. It is thought to be due to osmosis during fixation, as it is not seen in fresh frozen sections. These have their own technical pitfalls due mainly to condensation. Another life-like artefact is easily mistaken for an abnormality: the 'picture frame' fibre. It is due to rising of the edge of the fibre from the mount followed by readhesion.

Fibre types

Physiologists have long known that there are two types of twitch fibre, slow and fast, and that in many animals white muscle consists predominantly of fast-twitch and red of slow-twitch fibres. Pathologists have noted in favourable sections of fixed human muscle that even a haematoxylin and eosin preparation can show a pattern of lighter and darker fibres, but their correspondence to the physiological fibre types was not realized until histochemical strains of unfixed muscle could be performed. There are many reactions which differ in the main fibre types, but in human muscle only the ATPases are reliable for typing normal and most diseased fibres.

Muscle fibres were at first classified in two different ways depending on species, and both schemes then confusingly applied to man. In 1970 the Research Group on Neuromuscular Diseases of the World Federation of Neurology recommended two main types, types 1 and 2. Later type 2 became subdivided into 2a and 2b. These have been used by most workers on human muscle ever since, and depend solely on the staining reaction for ATPase. At a pH of 9.4, type 1 fibres are pale and type 2 dark. Preincubation at pH 4.35 reverses the reaction so that type 1 fibres are dark and type 2 fibres light; preincubation at pH 4.63 reveals two types of type 2 fibres, 2a which remain light and 2b which are intermediate in tone (Fig. 21.7). The change in reaction of individual fibres according to pH can be followed in serial sections. Type 2b fibres may be absent in normal muscle. When this appears to be the case the ATPase reactions should be repeated for confirmation, as even minor errors in pH may cause a failure to stain. Type 2c fibres have also been described (Brooke and Kaiser, 1970); they react strongly at pH 9.4 and 4.63, but

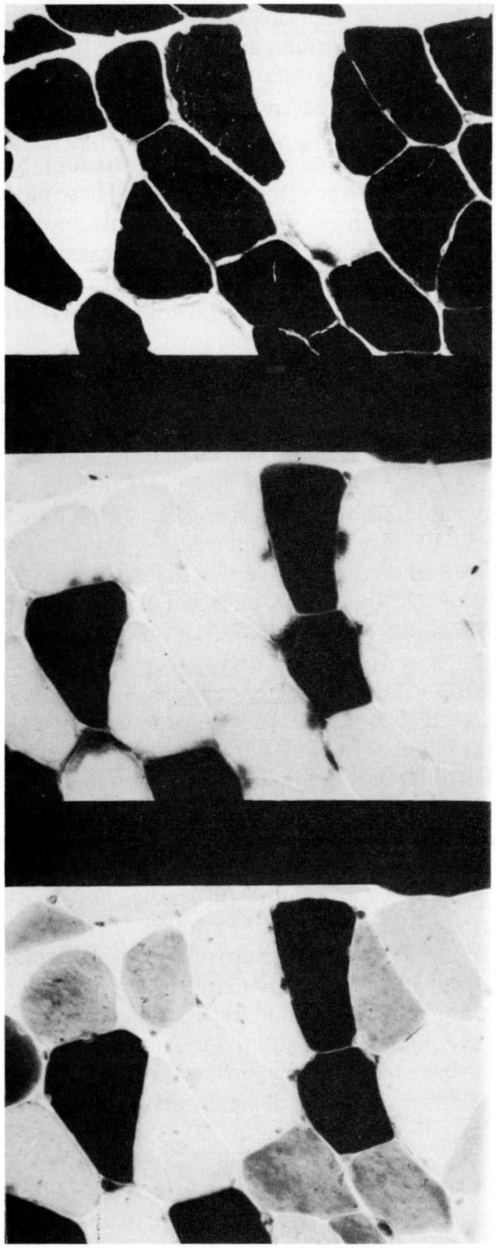

Fig. 21.7 Three serial sections are stained from above downwards for ATPase at pH 9.4, pH 4.35 and pH 4.63 respectively. At 9.4, the dark fibres are type 2 (a and b), and the light type 1. At 4.35 the reactions reverse, type 1 fibres now dark. At 4.63, type 2a fibres remain light and 2b are intermediate. ×250.

less strongly at pH 4.3. They are not often seen in normal adult human muscle but are numerous in fetal muscle and occasionally present in disease. They are thought to indicate a degree of undifferentiation such as might occur in regenerating fibres.

As papers still appear with an earlier fibre type classification of human muscle, the equivalents are as follows: type 1 (B), type 2a (C), type 2b (A).

Fibre types in animals differ in detail. Reliance for typing is placed on reactions for oxidative enzymes as well as ATPases, fibre size is taken into account, and physiological data are available to confirm the categories. One scheme consists of slow oxidative (SO), fast glycolytic (FG) and fast oxidative glycolytic (FOG) fibres. The first two are comparable to type 1 and type 2 human fibres, but the third does not occur in normal human muscle although it is sometimes considered equivalent to type 2b. When the range of speed of contraction and metabolic needs of skeletal muscle throughout the animal kingdom is remembered it is not surprising that fibre type characteristics should vary between species (Fig. 21.8).

The practical value of fibre typing in man is shown by some specific reactions of individual types. Type 1 fibres remain small in congenital fibre type disproportion, may be selectively atrophied in early neurogenic disease or undergo hypertrophy as a result of sustained exercise depending on oxidative metabolism. Type 2 fibres enlarge as a result of bouts of strenuous fast exercise requiring anaerobic glycolytic metabolism, and type 2b fibres are the first to undergo atrophy when muscles are inactive or reacting to chronic systemic disease.

Type 1 fibres are uniform in their reaction for the ATPases, but may vary to some extent when stained for NADH and in other reactions. Many have wondered whether they could be subdivided into types 1a and 1b. This was proposed by Askanas and Engel (1975) but has not gained general acceptance, probably because the reactions used to distinguish the subgroups lack contrast and are variable. Oil red O, which stains lipid droplets, provides good separation when neutral lipid is abundant but it is often virtually absent. Phosphorylase and α-glycerophosphate dehydrogenase are said to distinguish 1a and 1b fibres by a subtle difference in the staining intensity of the non-reacting fibres rather than of the stained ones. The writer can confirm that in a small series of normal biopsies stained as suggested by Askanas and Engel NADH can produce two subgroups, 1a being more darkly react-

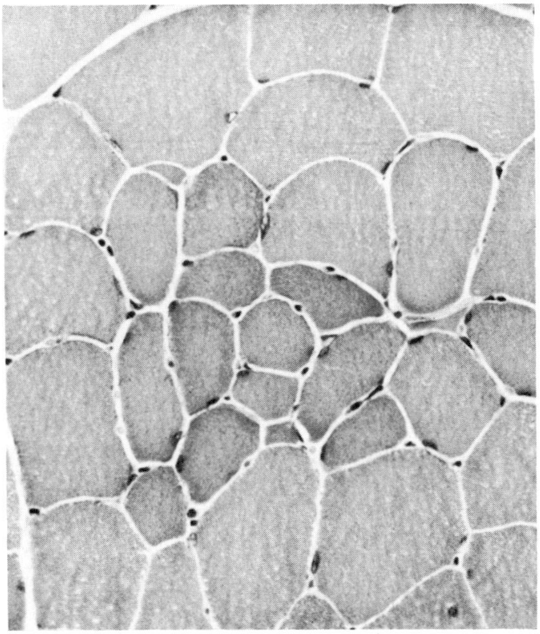

(a)

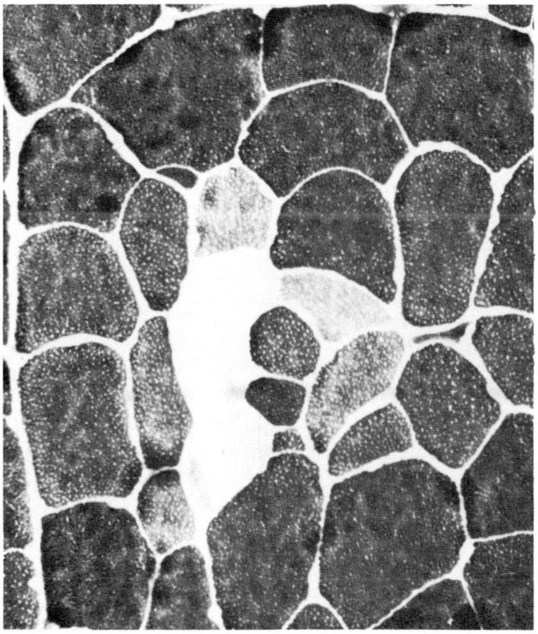

(b)

Fig. 21.8 Pig muscle. Serial sections stained with (**a**) haematoxylin and eosin, and (**b**) ATPase 9.4. The three fibre types shown cannot be assimilated into the human ATPase classification. × 300.

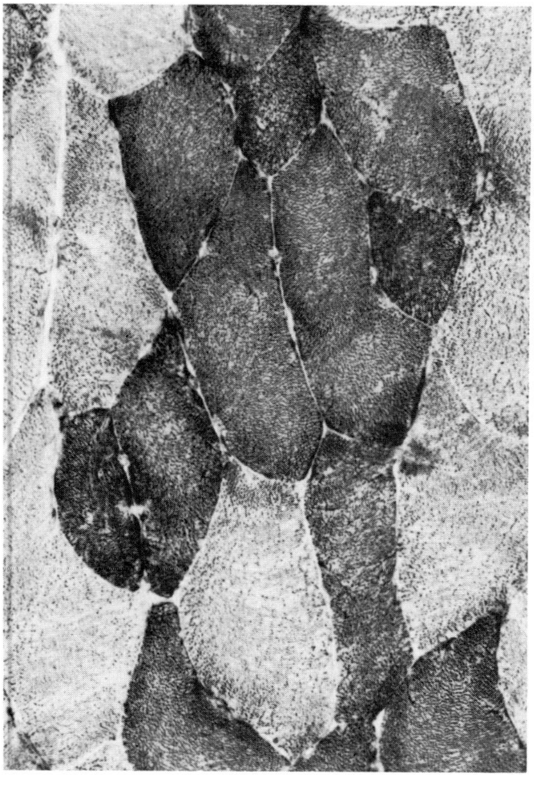

Fig. 21.9 Type 1 fibre subtypes? Normal muscle stained for NADH-TR. There are two subtypes, type 1a being darker and coarser than type 1b. In this biopsy type 1a fibres are smaller than 1b. × 300.

ing and often smaller than 1b, but only in 50 per cent.

Enough evidence has been presented to suggest that two type 1 subtypes may exist, but a more convincing and constant histochemical distinction is required (Fig. 21.9).

The distribution of fibre types. In man the two primary fibre types are normally said to be distributed at random in a checkerboard pattern, and to vary in their proportion in different muscles from 40 to 80 per cent. The checkerboard description must not be taken literally, as fibres of the same type can be distributed in small groups. The discovery that large groups of fibres of the same type indicate reinnervation following denervation led to an autopsy study of group size (Jennekens, Tomlinson and Walton, 1971) and to the conclusion that multiple groups 'enclosing' three or more fibres of the same type were abnormal. But a single cluster of even 30–40 fibres enclosing 13 fibres was not abnormal. Recent studies (Henriksson-Larsén, Lexell and Sjöstrom, 1983, Lexell et al., 1983) in which whole-muscle transverse sections taken at autopsy were cut fresh and stained have thrown doubt on whether significant grouping can be recognized at all in the usual small biopsy specimen and have re-emphasized the variation in the proportion of fibre types even in different parts of the same muscle.

The motor unit

Motor units have relevance to muscle histopathology because their enlargement in the early stages of neurogenic disease provides a sensitive clue to diagnosis. Each unit consists of an anterior horn or brain stem motor neuron and all the muscle fibres it supplies. The main axon courses to the muscle, and then branches repeatedly in nerve bundles. From these, myelinated axons fan out singly without further branching to supply skeletal muscle fibres each with a motor end-plate (Fig. 21.10). One fibre in ten may be innervated by two end-plates. The axon will innervate 100–2000 muscle fibres depending on the size of the muscle, for the largest motor units are found in the largest muscles. These figures do not apply to small specialized muscles which have a rich innervation; extraocular muscle motor units, for example, contain as few as eight fibres.

Experimental transposition of motor nerves between slow and fast muscles has demonstrated the strict control of fibre type by the innervation. A fast-twitch muscle reinnervated by a motor nerve from a slow-twitch muscle changes the first into slow-twitch almost perfectly, both physiologically and histochemically. It would therefore be expected that the fibre type content of each motor unit would be uniform. That this is likely to be true was shown by Edström and Kugelberg (1968) in the rat. Single motor nerve fibres were stimulated at low frequencies in order to deplete type 2 fibres of glycogen. Serial sections stained by PAS, phosphorylase and succinate dehydrogenase identified the fibres supplied as of uniform type. A similar uniform fibre content has been assumed in human motor units, and the mosaic

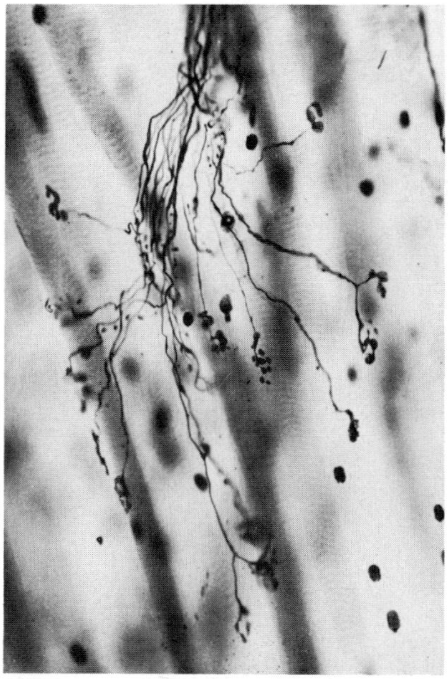

(a)

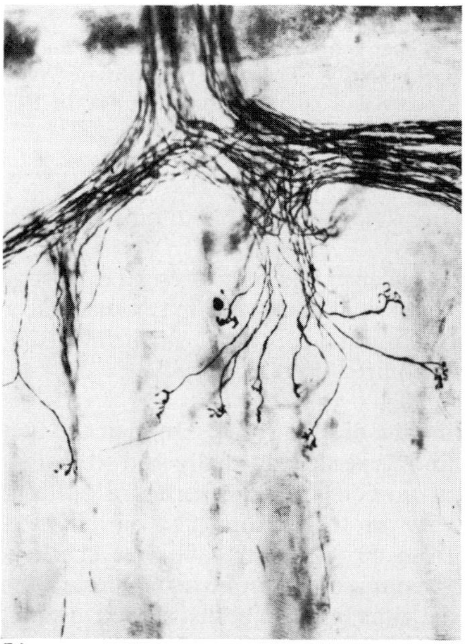

(b)

Fig. 21.10 The subterminal fibre pattern. Subterminal fibres run singly from intramuscular nerve bundles towards muscle fibres, to supply each fibre with a motor end-plate. About one fibre in ten receives two end-plates, rarely more in normal muscle. Thus normal subterminal fibres rarely branch. (**a**) Subterminal fibres in a female aged 3 years. The end-plates are formed by branching of terminal axons which form expansions. Methylene blue × 170. (**b**) Subterminal fibres and end-plates in a male aged 5 years. The end-plates are stained by silver using a block impregnation method. Expansions are present but appear smaller. de Castro × 170.

distribution of fibre types in normal muscle attributed to intermingling of units.

The motor-point muscle biopsy

The neural part of the motor unit has long been studied by motor-point muscle biopsy, a comprehensive account being given by Coërs and Woolf (1959). They showed that the earliest indication of denervation was provided not by recognizing axon degeneration but by the regenerative activity of nearby healthy subterminal fibres—showing that it is important to examine the innervation of the muscle in addition to the structure of the muscle fibres when a biopsy is being performed (see Coërs, 1982). The motor point is first located on the skin and again on the exposed muscle surface; then strips of muscle for electron microscopy, histochemistry, methylene blue injection and paraffin embedding are taken across the motor point. Coërs has always used intravital injection of 0.05% methylene blue, but the writer prefers injection of a thin fascicle immediately after excision (supravital). The results are inferior but sufficiently clear for diagnosis. The method can be capricious, especially by overstaining, so an additional strip is taken as a precaution for silver staining (see Fig. 21.10). If desired, subterminal fibres and sole-plates can be stained by combining an axon stain with cholinesterase.

Muscle spindles and other receptors

The afferent nerve supply from muscle is provided by muscle spindles, tendon organs, other receptors and free sensory nerve endings. Significant structural abnormality in spindles has been found only in myotonic dystrophy, but convincing important reactions in other conditions have not been found, probably owing to the time-consuming and difficult nature of a full examination. They are best examined at post-mortem, when small spindle-rich muscles such as the muscles of the hand and head (occipitalis) can be sampled. Extraocular muscles contain spindles near their extremities. The intrafusal muscle fibres (those

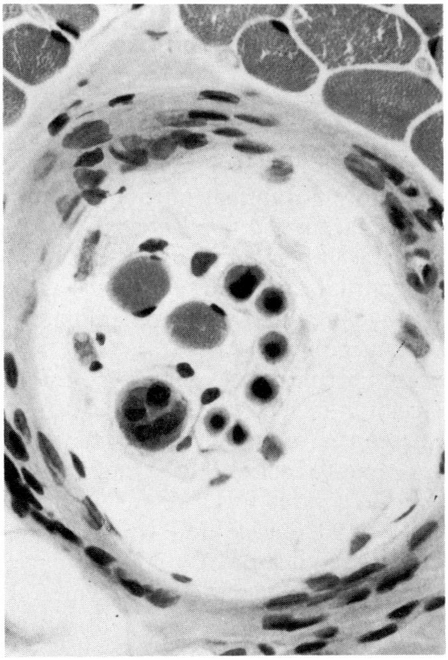

Fig. 21.11 Transverse section of a muscle spindle in the equatorial region. One of the larger 'nuclear bag' fibres contains a cluster of nuclei. The smaller nuclear chain fibres each have a central nucleus. Haematoxylin and eosin × 420.

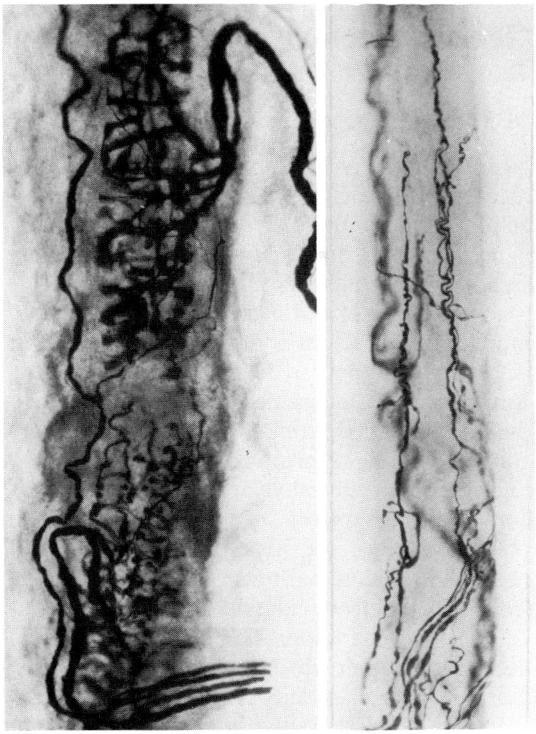

(a) **(b)**

Fig. 21.12 Muscle spindle. (**a**) Equatorial region, showing primary (coarser) and secondary sensory endings. (**b**) Polar region, with motor endings. Spindle dissected after block staining (de Castro).

within the spindle) can be studied as easily as extrafusal muscle, but a complete examination of the innervation requires painstaking dissection and removal of the intact spindle.

Spindles are small at birth, when the intrafusal fibres are of a diameter similar to the extrafusal fibres. In the adult spindles are much longer, up to 7 mm, but the intrafusal fibres remain of small diameter. The latter are of two types; larger 'nuclear bag' fibres, which contain a cluster of nuclei at their midpoint, occupying almost the entire width of the fibre and leaving little room for myofibrils; and smaller 'nuclear chain' fibres (Fig. 21.11), which have centrally placed nuclei in the middle region of the fibre, disposed in a single column. Normal spindles in man contain three to 15 intrafusal fibres, enclosed in a fibrous capsule. The capsule is quite thin in the wide equatorial part of the spindle, but it can be up to ten cells thick in the polar regions. Thickening of spindle capsules has often been reported as a pathological change by misinterpreting normal polar regions. The spindle contains a fluid which sometimes stains as a finely granular material. The innervation of the spindle is complex, comprising primary and secondary sensory endings in the equatorial region, and three types of motor junctions, trail-shaped, multiple plate and larger single plate endings all in the polar regions (Fig. 21.12). The histochemical pattern of intrafusal fibres differs from that of the extrafusal and varies in different species. The findings of different observers are conflicting and have not been fully worked out in man, in whom there seem to be two types of nuclear bag fibres—one containing combined acid-stable and alkali-stable myosin ATPase, and the other containing neither. Nuclear chain fibres are of the usual two primary fibre types.

General reactions of muscle fibres in disease

Necrosis and regeneration

Necrosis of a segment of a muscle fibre, and the regeneration that follows it, are a common reaction in neuromuscular disorders, particularly in myopathies. Clusters of regenerating fibres are seen early in Duchenne dystrophy (even in the preclinical phase) and necrosis of large areas of muscle are characteristic of infarction, and occur occasionally in polymyositis and in toxic states. But the necrosis of segments of scattered individual muscle fibres is much more frequently encountered. The segment is transformed into a finely granular, floccular or hyaline mass rarely containing fragments of myofibrils. Zenker (1864) described the hyaline or waxy type of necrosis in abdominal muscle in patients dying from typhoid fever, and it became known as Zenker's degeneration. The different forms of necrosis, however, do not appear to have any morphological specificity (Fig. 21.13).

In the initial stage the sarcolemma (plasmalemma) enclosing the necrotic segment appears intact, as does the basal lamina. Myophages invade and ingest the necrotic material, until the segment is completely filled by these cells. During this phase the sarcolemma disappears but the shape of the fibre is maintained by the inert basal lamina.

The necrosis calls forth a small number of lymphocytes, occasional polymorphs and plasma cells which lie alongside the affected fibre. It is possibly a transient phenomenon, as the number of marginated fibres is variable but usually small. It is important to distinguish them from the interstitial and diffuse collections of similar cells that predominate in inflammatory disorders such as polymyositis.

The increased permeability of the sarcolemma and its destruction in segmental necrosis permit extracellular seepage of the cytosol. The most important enzyme to escape into serum is creatine kinase (CK), which is present in large amounts in skeletal muscle and whose blood level is a sensitive indicator of muscle damage. There are also brain and heart isoenzymes of CK. The CK may rise in acute severe disease to levels of 100 000 international units. Such levels can be attained very rapidly, as in malignant hyperthermia during anaesthesia. Rhabdomyolysis, probably induced by the high temperature, develops within a matter of 2–3 hours. At postmortem large expanses of muscle may be visibly

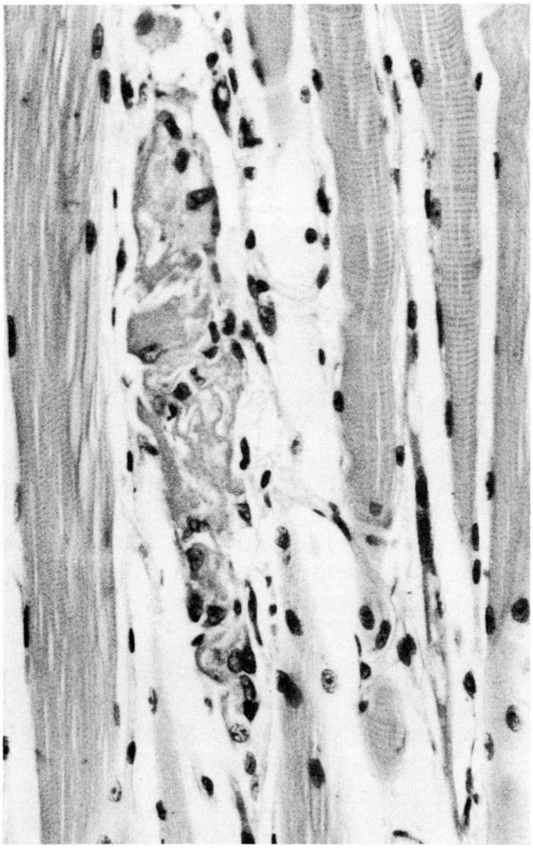

(a)

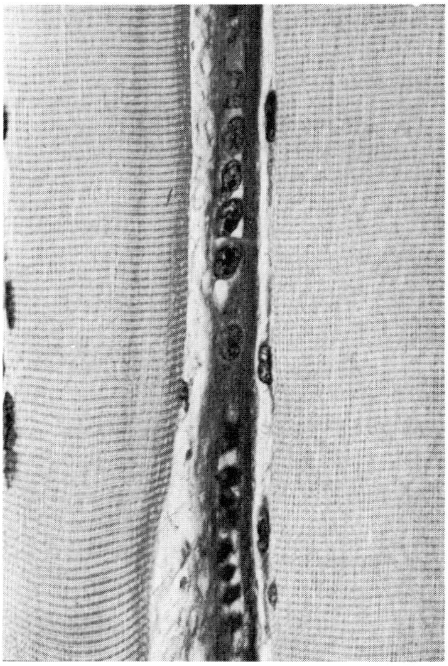

(b)

Fig. 21.13 (**a**) Segmental necrosis, invaded by myophages and lymphocytes, with commencing strap cell formation. (**b**) A basophilic regenerating fibre. Note prominent nucleoli. Haematoxylin and van Gieson × 400.

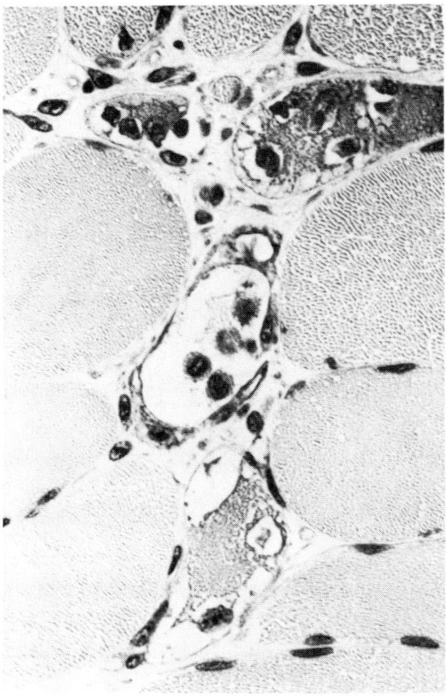

(c)

Fig. 21.14 Regenerating fibres. The fibre in the centre still contains a few myophages, but shows the early development of strap-shaped regenerating fibres on the inner surface of the sarcolemma. Regeneration is more advanced in the three other darkly staining fibres in the illustration. Haematoxylin and van Gieson × 600.

necrotic. In patients who recover, the serum CK falls quite rapidly, implying restoration of the sarcolemma. Levels may fall to a few hundred units in 1–2 days.

Regeneration of skeletal muscle fibres is complete following segmental necrosis but is inadequate in response to necrosis of large areas. In these, healing is completed by fibrosis. The regenerative reaction commences almost as soon as necrosis is established. The sarcoplasm bordering the necrotic segment becomes basophilic, an indication of RNA synthesis by polyribosomes, and subsarcolemmal nuclei enlarge and their nucleoli become prominent (see Fig. 21.13b). Occasionally the nucleoli become double or enlarge further to rectangular shapes, whilst the nuclei congregate in rows near the necrotic zone. In the past reconstitution of the necrotic segment was thought to result from 'budding' from the intact part of the fibre, but most workers now accept that the buds are in fact activated satellite cells (Mair and Tomé, 1972). These cells enlarge, filaments appear and become aligned, and the cells begin to traverse the necrotic zone in the shape of strap cells, with elongated cytoplasm and pointed apices, mingling at first with the scavenger cells. Some strap cells form a lining to the basal lamina of the fibre (Fig. 21.14). As phagocytosis of the necrotic segment is completed the muscle fibre is reconstituted by fusion of the strap cells which thereby form a new sarcolemma within the basal lamina.

Fibre splitting

Complete longitudinal splitting of the entire length of a muscle fibre is part of normal development and occurs in human muscle during the 12th to 15th week of fetal life. Unsplit fibres become less numerous, are distinctly larger than

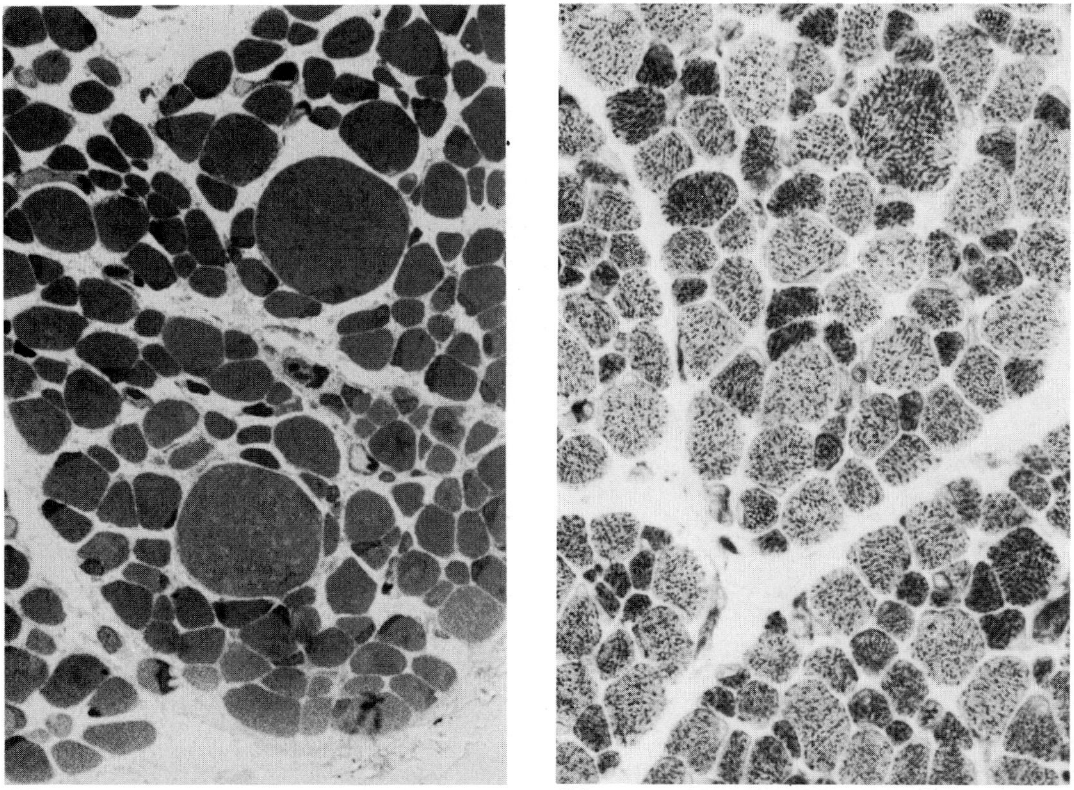

(a) **(b)**

Fig. 21.15 Wohlfart B-fibres. These large fetal fibres are more numerous after birth when there has been maturation delay, as in some hypotonic infants. In the infant muscle illustrated here the very large fibres are Wohlfart type B (fibre type 1), the smaller fibres are of type 2 and the smallest fibres are of type 1. (**a**) Semithin × 750; (**b**) NADH-TR × 470.

the small split fibres which surround them, and a few persist into early postnatal life as the B-fibres of Wohlfart (1937) (Fig. 21.15). The large fibres are of type 1 and the small numerous fibres type 2.

The splitting that occurs in human disease and in normal adult muscle differs from fetal splitting in being incomplete, involving only part of a fibre. (The only exception to this is the total longitudinal splitting of intrafusal fibres in myotonic dystrophy.) The formation of clefts within a muscle fibre, often large or hypertrophied, is not infrequent both in neuropathies and in myopathies. It may also happen in clinically normal human muscle. The clefts which form in the muscle fibre are seen in transverse section typically to enter from the surface, and in the longitudinal plane to separate the fibre segment into two parts. Complicated splits produce several fragments varying in size. Affected fibres

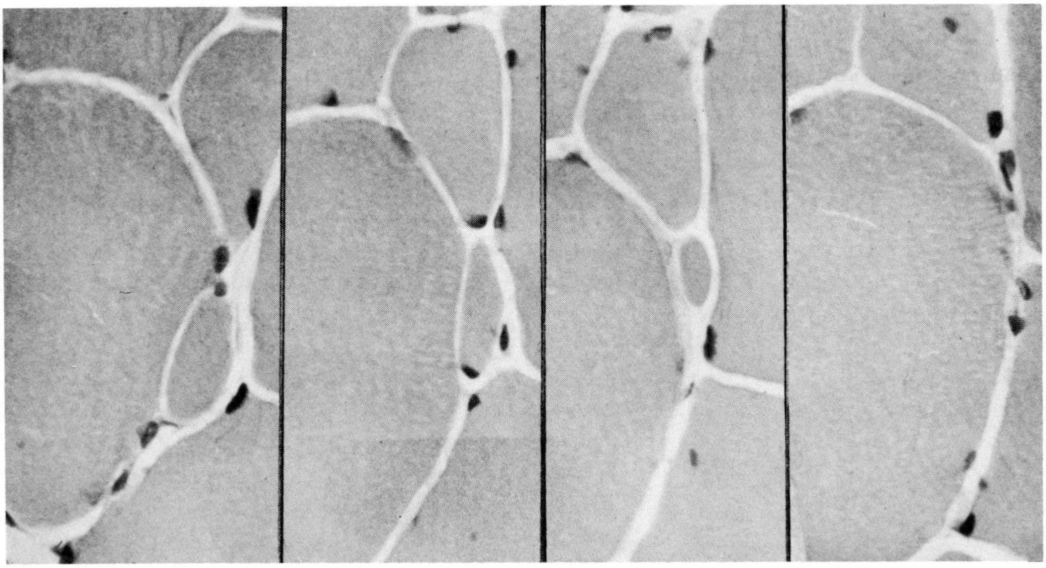

(a)

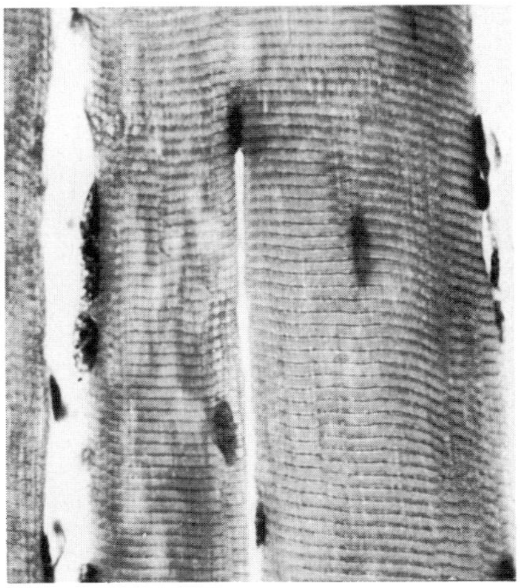

(b)

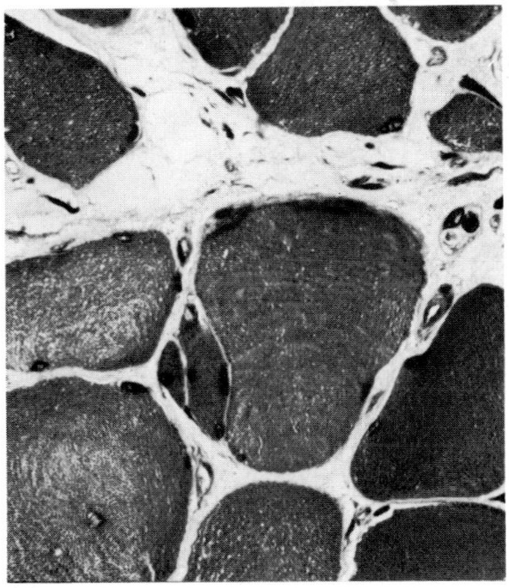

(c)

Fig. 21.16 (**a**) Small biconvex fragment of mother fibre (left), followed through by numerous serial sections to become smaller and disappear. Haematoxylin and eosin × 600. (**b**) A longitudinal split is present in the fibre, ending at an internally placed nucleus. Haematoxylin and eosin × 630. (**c**) Splitting in the central fibre alongside nuclei has separated off two crescentic segments of muscle fibre. Haematoxylin and eosin × 420.

sometimes contain an internal nucleus, close to the apex of the cleft, and this has led to the statement that splitting always occurs in pathological fibres. But the nuclear migration might equally well be induced by the split, or, if a nucleus happens to be internal, splitting could occur in its direction without being necessary for the splitting process. Sometimes small fragments of the fibre are separated off, and can be shown, by serial sections, to disappear (Fig. 21.16a). They may or may not be basophilic, shrunken and angulated. Formerly, angular fibres were thought to be specific for denervation, and have been used as the sole evidence of neurogenic disease. But they have now been found in myopathies and in small numbers in normal muscle. Splitting is sometimes simulated by a smaller fibre nestling into a larger, but three 'fibres' likely to lie within the same basal lamina and an incomplete cleft must both indicate splitting (Fig. 21.16b, c). Clefts are lined with an intact basal lamina and sarcolemma, and contain endomysium and capillaries. A capillary apparently isolated in the centre of a muscle fibre in cross-section is within the apex of a cleft.

Longitudinal sections show that splitting can also be recognized in the longitudinal plane, and confirm that it is three-dimensional and segmental. On occasions the split divides a fibre into two branches which remain separate. Splitting occurs in both main fibre types.

The pathogenesis of splitting is controversial, and several mechanisms have been proposed, such as tension on hypertrophied fibres, the need to dispose of degenerate parts of a muscle fibre (Fig. 21.17) or faulty myogenesis. Schmalbruch (1976) has proposed that myoblasts, myotubes and small myofibres enclosed by a basal lamina could fuse and become visible as a separated part of the main fibre. An ingenious method of studying splitting in dystrophic mice using serial cinematography was employed by Isaacs, Bradley and Henderson (1973), who were able to follow splits to their termination and discover that it was responsible for much of the variation of the fibre calibre in mouse dystrophy. In that

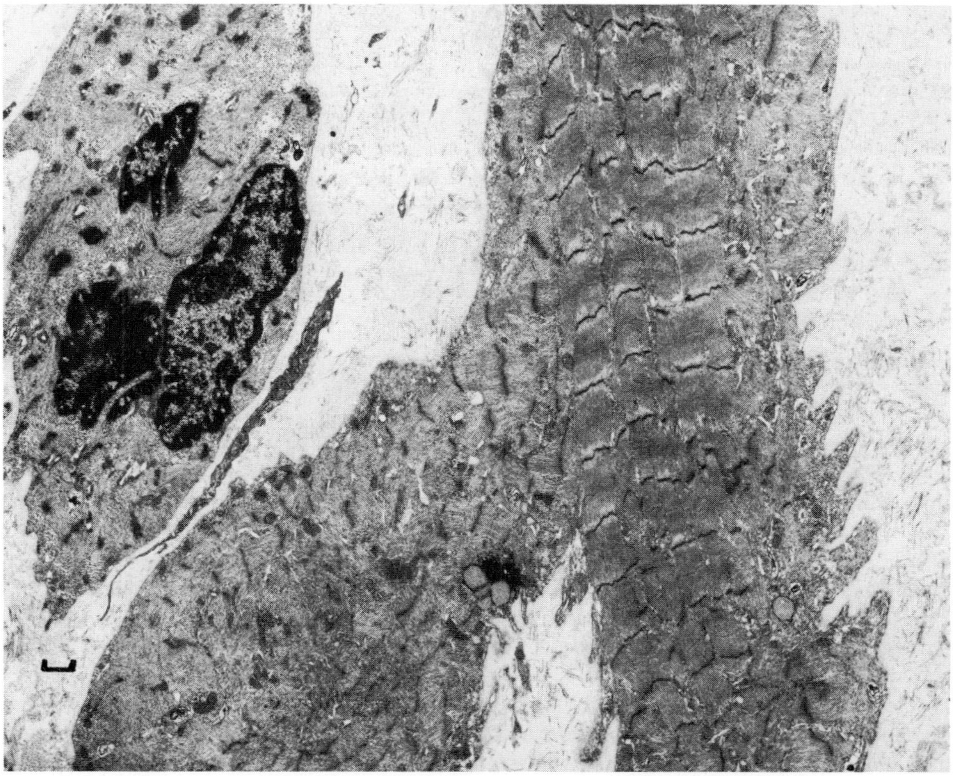

Fig. 21.17 Part of the fibre being split off shows myofibrillary disorganization. Bar = 1 μm.

disorder splitting causes branching of fibres rather than extrusion of fragments.

It is likely that no one mechanism will account for all splitting after birth. At present the most plausible seems to be the mechanism of extrusion and the effect of tension on hypertrophied or abnormal segments of muscle fibres.

Fibre atrophy

The muscle fibre atrophy which results from denervation is well known, and the muscle wasting it causes is visible to the naked eye. Disease or section of a motor nerve interrupting all its axons simultaneously should lead to a more or less equal degree of atrophy of all the muscle fibres supplied, but partial and progressive disorders of motor neurons or nerves anywhere from the spinal cord to motor end-plate result in variable atrophy.

The effect of loss of the motor nerve supply on muscle fibre structure is slow compared to loss of function. Peripheral myofibrils disintegrate, leaving intact the central myofibrils which re-

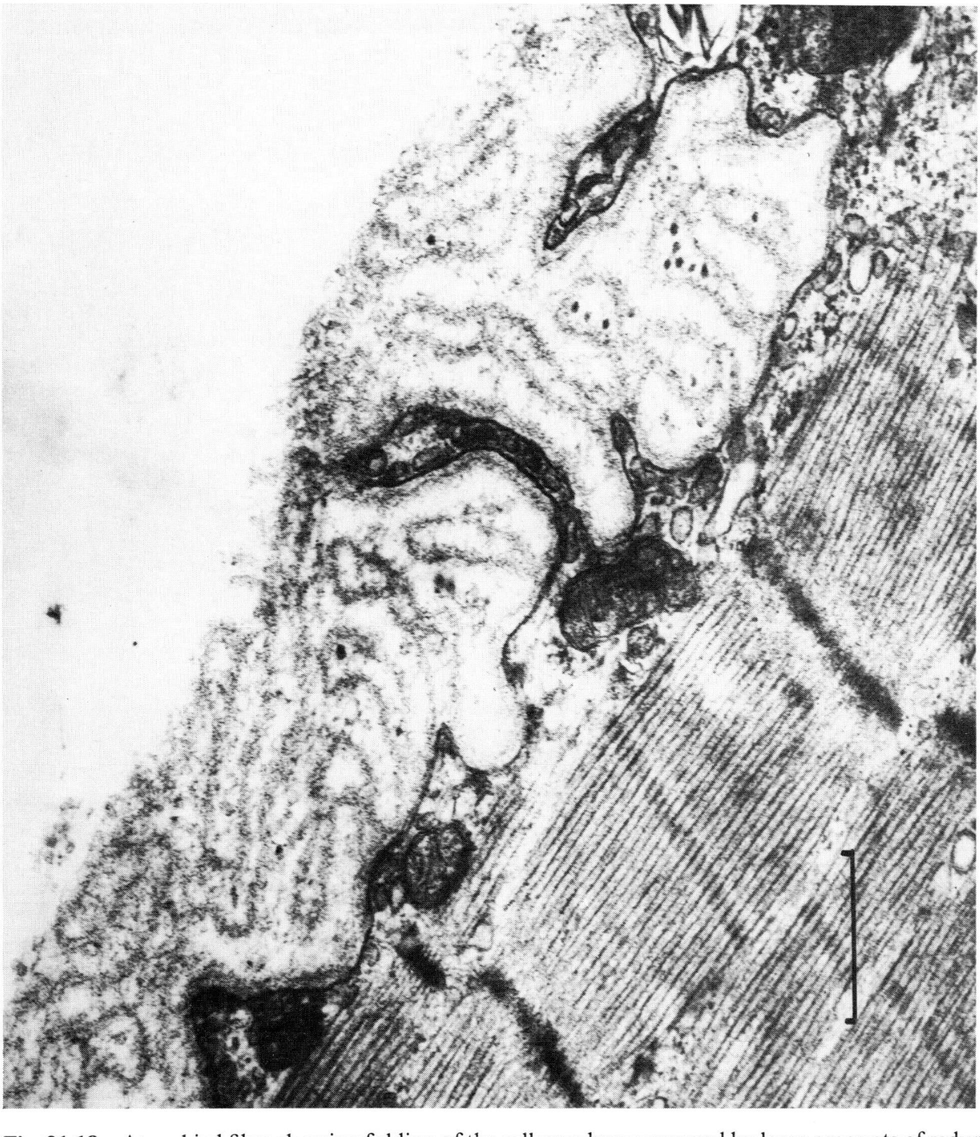

Fig. 21.18 Atrophied fibre showing folding of the cell membrane covered by large amounts of redundant basal lamina. Bar = 0.5 μm.

main aligned; the atrophied fibres are much reduced in calibre but are still striated. Nuclei may become internal, but this is not nearly so marked as in experimental denervation in small mammals. Atrophy takes 3–4 weeks to develop, but continues at a much reduced rate thereafter. In electron micrographs fibre atrophy is easily recognized by redundant folds of the basal lamina (Fig. 21.18). Atrophied fibres can be reinnervated even after prolonged denervation, but this is impossible when the remaining myofibrils disintegrate. The sarcolemma disappears, leaving groups of nuclei ('grave-stones') in connective tissue. So-called muscle giant cells are formed at the same time, when small pieces of sarcoplasm are rounded off and contain multiple nuclei. Rarely, a curious phenomenon may occur in the early reaction to denervation in certain muscles such as the diaphragm in which the denervated muscle is under tension. There is a short period during which muscle fibres enlarge before following the usual course of events.

When large groups of fibres are atrophied, whether to the same or different degrees depending on the pathogenesis, the term 'group atrophy' is employed and the pattern is diagnostic of denervation. It does not distinguish between central and peripheral nerve lesions and affects fibre types indiscriminately. When single fibres or very small groups atrophy the cause is not necessarily neurogenic, as that pattern is not infrequently seen in some myopathies such as the earlier

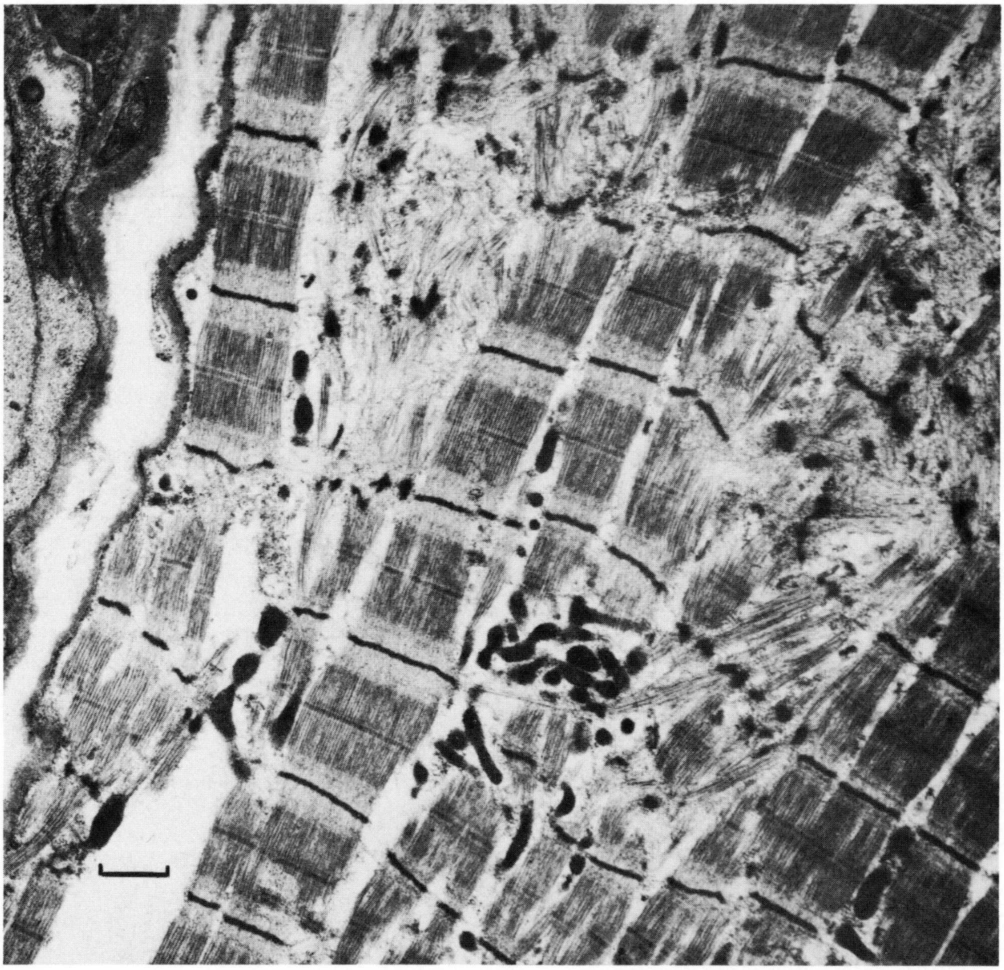

Fig. 21.19 Atrophied fibre showing undulating cell membrane and thickened basal lamina, with focal myofibrillar fragmentation. Bar = 1 μm.

stages of dystrophies and in cachectic atrophy. Thus small group atrophy is by itself insufficient for a diagnosis of neurogenic disease and must be supplemented by other feature(s) characteristic of denervation. Scattered single atrophied fibres, whether staining normally or intensely, angulated or rounded, do occur in neurogenic disease but not exclusively.

Electron microscopy of denervated fibres may show focal break-up of sarcomeres resulting in distorted fragmented Z-bands and bundles of filaments (Fig. 21.19) but more often the reduced numbers of myofibrils retain their integrity.

All small fibres are not necessarily atrophied. An apparently shrunken fibre may simply be a short extrusion produced by fibre splitting, and single very small round but otherwise normal fibres are likely to be the extremities of fibres terminating within the muscle. Finally, variably small fibres may result from denervation atrophy, but in some congenital myopathies they are small through failure to develop (e.g. type 1 fibre hypotrophy and congenital fibre type disproportion).

Ring fibres

These malformed muscle fibres, known as 'ringbinden' in the German literature, occur in both normal and pathological muscle (Fig. 21.20). These are fibres in which one or more of the outermost myofibrils turn abruptly through 90 degrees to encircle the remainder. The appearance in transverse section is that of a ring of one or more peripheral myofibrils whose striations are clearly visible formed around a core of myofibrils sectioned transversely. In longitudinal section the peripheral myofibrils may form a spiral rather than a ring, and the origin of the spiral can occasionally be seen when a myofibril runs diagonally across a fibre to reach the periphery.

In normal muscle, ring fibres are quite frequently found at tendinous insertions. They are particularly common in extraocular and pharyngeal muscle with advancing age, and single examples can occasionally be found anywhere in normal muscle.

In disease, the disorder in which they are found most often is myotonic dystrophy, especially in adults. Another feature often present in myotonic dystrophy is the sarcoplasmic mass, a peripheral area of the fibre devoid of myofibrils and faintly granular. The mass is sometimes separated from the central myofibrils by a spiralling myofibril. Other disorders in which ring fibres occur relatively often are hypothyroidism, limb girdle dystrophy and after muscle injury.

Ring fibres probably develop in several ways. Myofibrils are normally added to muscle fibres during growth, so their occasional peripheral malposition is understandable and might happen more easily where tension is exerted, namely at the insertion. They may develop as a reaction to a focal lesion in a muscle fibre, for example to a cytoplasmic body (Harriman, Sumner and Ellis, 1973), and their occurrence after trauma indicates a reaction to torn fibres.

Internal nuclei

A small proportion of normal muscle fibres contain one or perhaps two internal nuclei when sectioned transversely. The proportion probably varies from muscle to muscle. Three per cent is often given as the upper limit, but the writer has found in a survey of normal vastus medialis biopsies that absolute numbers are less important than the distribution of fibres with internal nuclei. Focal increase in internal nuclei is normal close to perimysial or epimysial seams and especially near fibrous insertions, but their presence in every fascicle in a section in an average proportion of 2 per cent or more is pathological in the vastus medialis.

In disease the number of nuclei per fibre in a transverse section can vary from one to six or more. In longitudinal section they form long or short internal rows. Relatively small numbers of internal nuclei are common in many myopathies and chronic neuropathies, and larger numbers are frequent in dystrophies which exhibit fibre hypertrophy and splitting. They occur in the later stages of polymyositis, but the most profuse numbers develop in myotonic dystrophy. A minority of patients with myotonia congenita show internal nuclei, and in severe malignant hyperthermia myopathy there may be 25 per cent (Figure 21.21c).

There is probably no single mechanism by which they develop. Figure 21.21 illustrates internal nuclei following an episode of necrosis and regeneration; this cannot be responsible for internal nuclei in myotonia, in which the disorder itself may cause the nuclear displacement and alignment.

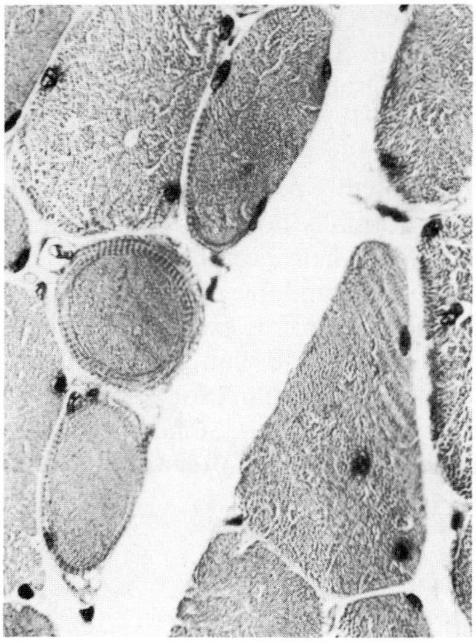

(a)

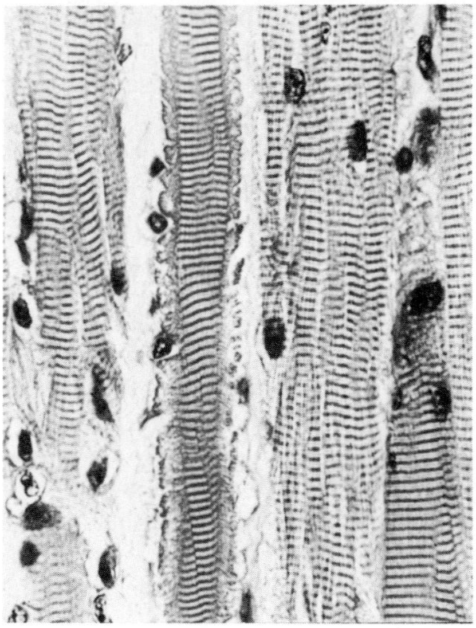

(b)

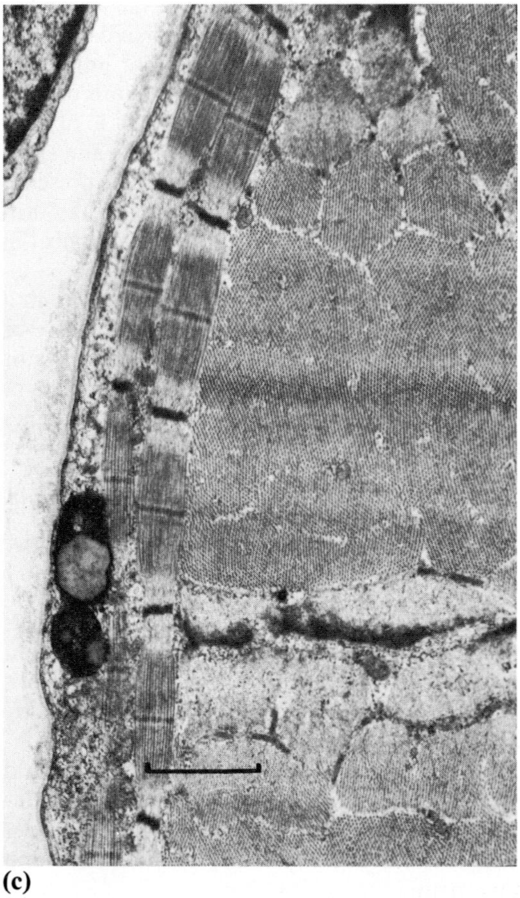

(c)

Fig. 21.20 Ring fibres. The spiral encirclement of central myofibrils by peripheral ones is seen in (**a**) transverse section and (**b**) longitudinal section. Haematoxylin and eosin × 420. (**c**) Transverse section. The two peripheral encircling myofibrils are cut longitudinally. Bar = 1 μm.

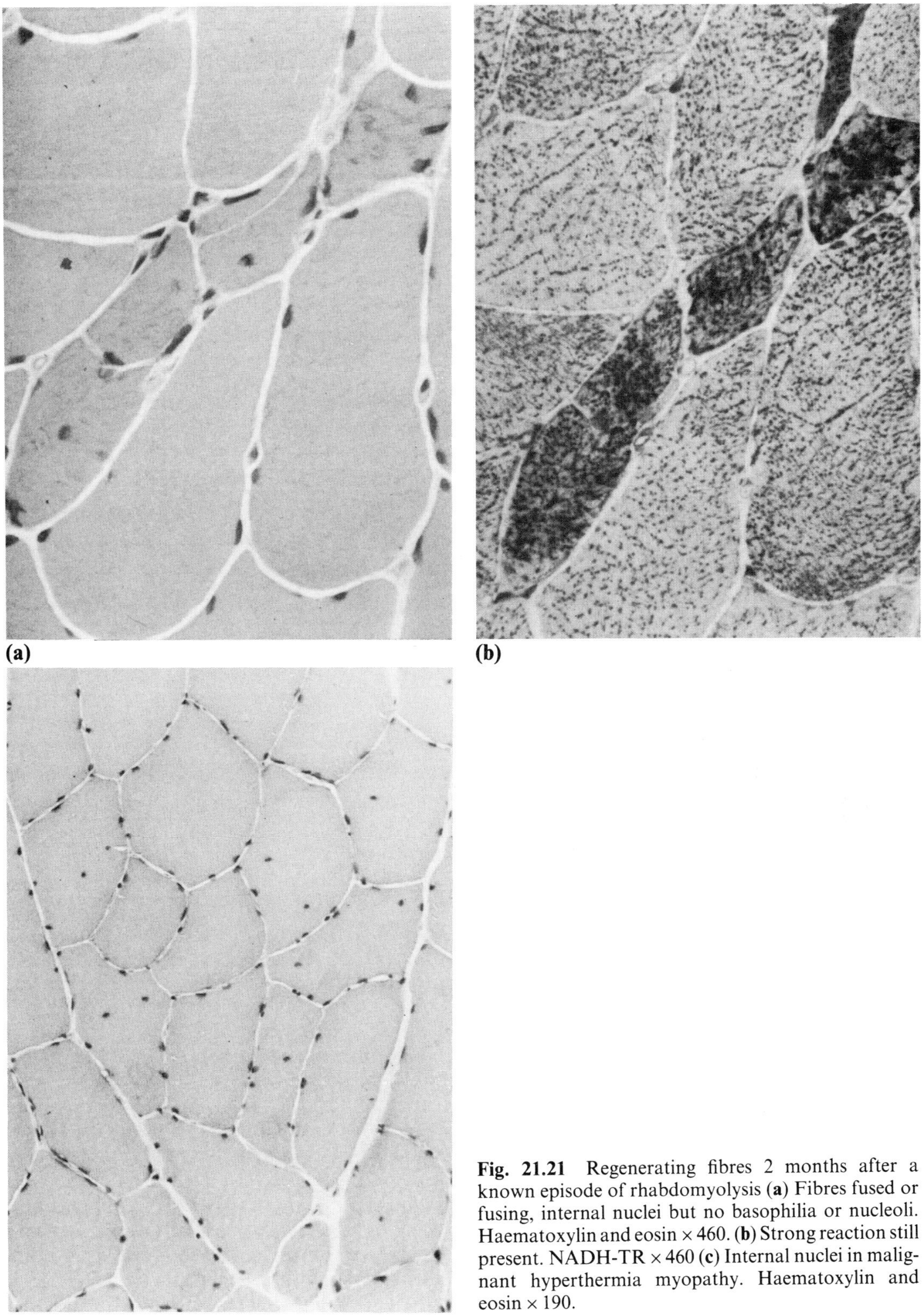

(a) (b) (c)

Fig. 21.21 Regenerating fibres 2 months after a known episode of rhabdomyolysis (**a**) Fibres fused or fusing, internal nuclei but no basophilia or nucleoli. Haematoxylin and eosin × 460. (**b**) Strong reaction still present. NADH-TR × 460 (**c**) Internal nuclei in malignant hyperthermia myopathy. Haematoxylin and eosin × 190.

Central nuclei During muscle development myotubes contain a nucleus at the centre point of the fibre, and in some congenital myopathies central nuclei may persist. The best known is centronuclear myopathy. Their presence does not exclude normally placed subsarcolemmal nuclei in the same fibre. There is obviously no difficulty in distinguishing internal from central nuclei provided both terms are used correctly. Although true central nuclei are seen in denervated muscle in the mouse, they are rare in man in neurogenic disease.

Core, target and moth-eaten fibres

Too many terms are still in use to describe different stages of a phenomenon best, and often only, seen in sections stained for oxidative enzymes (NADH-TR, succinate dehydrogenase). In one or more circumscribed areas within a fibre mitochondria disappear but myofibrils remain intact (the structured core) or undergo various stages of degeneration (unstructured core). These include shrinkage, Z-line streaming, fragmentation and coagulation. Abnormal organelles may be present such as tubular arrays and concentric laminar bodies, as well as the multivesicular bodies of autophagic origin. When the central myofibrils form an agglomerate they stain readily with trichrome dyes in frozen or paraffin sections, providing contrast between central and peripheral areas (Fig. 21.22). These lesions have at various times been called cores, targets, targetoid or core-targetoid fibres depending on their appearance, but their terminology needs to be simplified.

Cores were first described by Shy and Magee (1956). Five members in three generations of the same family, aged 2–65 years, were affected by an apparently non-progressive myopathy. In all five patients almost every muscle fibre (in paraffin sections) showed with Gomori's trichrome stain a central blue zone in contrast to the red periphery. The authors named the condition 'a new non-progressive congenital myopathy' and thought the basic lesion was a bundle of aberrant myofibrils. Unfortunately, they made one observation which has been widely misunderstood, that in longitudinal sections the fibrils in the core 'ran almost the entire length of the fibre'. This has since been taken to indicate that cores run from origin to insertion of the fibre, which might be true but difficult to demonstrate. The condition was named *central core disease* by Greenfield, Cornman and Shy (1958) on the reasonable grounds that most of the cores were central although occasionally multiple and eccentric (Fig. 21.23). Further reports which included histochemical and ultrastructural examination showed that there was much variation in the cores, that an almost universally central position was a rarity, that they could be confined to predominant type 1 fibres and that they were only occasionally seen in paraffin sections. The only reactions which invariably demonstrated cores with their characteristically sharp margins were those for oxidative enzymes. Other non-specific stains on frozen or paraffin sections tended to show them up when the centre of the core was unstructured—they then exhibited basophilia, often faint. The same could be said of the ATPase reactions which showed cores when myofibrils were disorganized. The PAS stain sometimes revealed a ring of glycogen around the cores. Lipid stains could outline the core through their ability to stain mitochondria.

Thus cores have by no means a uniform structure, and cores in different stages can be seen in the same muscle. Nor are they confined to central core disease. Their lack of specificity is shown by their appearance in some myopathies and neuropathies, and even singly in normal muscle. Their pathogenesis remains unknown although experimental tenotomy will produce them. If the spinal cord is then injured they fail to appear, suggesting that tension of the muscle has a part to play (de Reuck et al., 1982). They may also be produced by triethyl tin sulphate, and by the muscle abnormality of malignant hyperthermia.

Target fibres. Engel (1961) described fibres with three concentric zones (Fig. 21.24). The innermost zone contained compact strands of myofibrillar material, not striated but anisotropic; the middle zone was unstained in paraffin sections but showed faint striations in polarized light. In frozen sections ATPase activity was increased, oxidative activity variable but usually decreased, glycogen variable. The outer zone was provided by the normal part of the fibre. Engel believed target fibres were exclusively due to denervation and that they differed from cores which had a uniform central region and stained more darkly than the rest of the fibre. In longi-

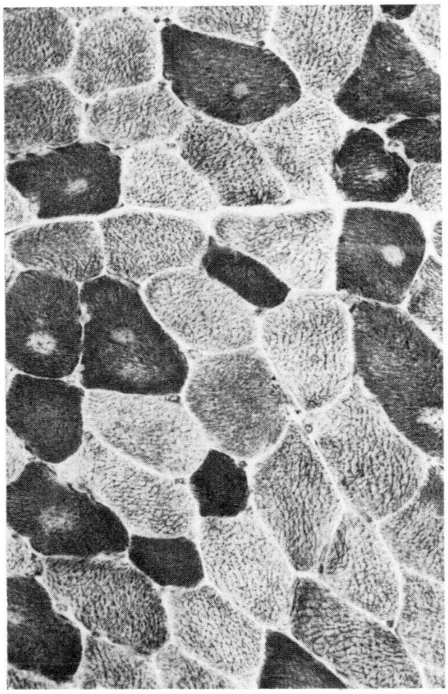

(a)

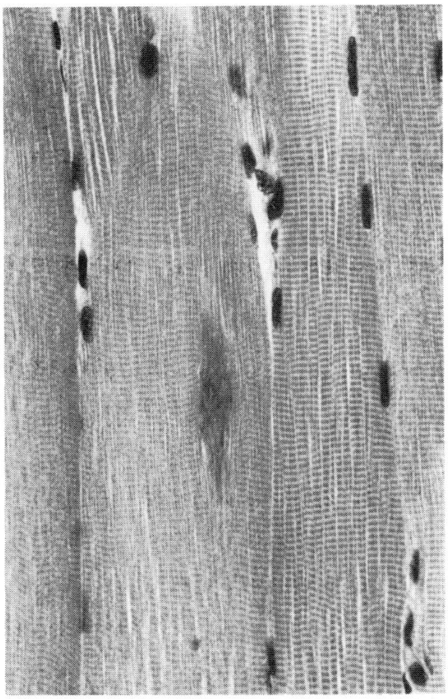

(b)

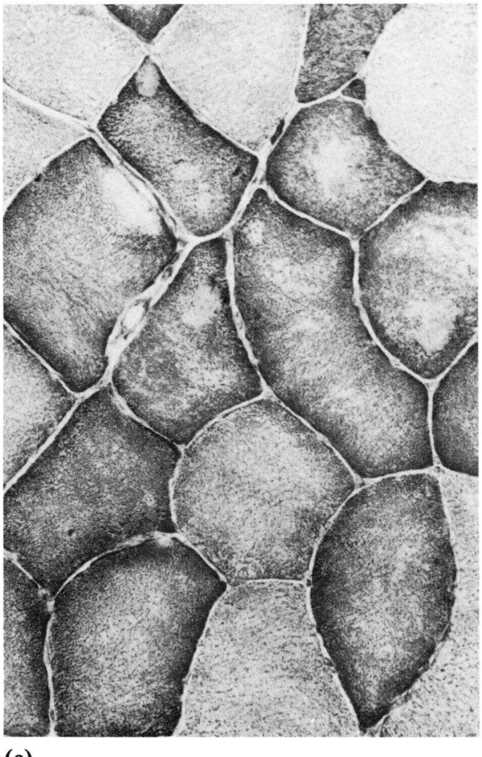

(c)

Fig. 21.22 Cores. (**a**) The well-defined clear cores are present in type 1 fibres. NADH-TR × 180. (**b**) Longitudinal section shows a core made visible by myofibrillar agglomeration. Haematoxylin and eosin × 480. (**c**) Poorly defined and irregular clear foci indicate moth-eaten fibres. Transitional forms to small cores can be recognized. NADH-TR × 300.

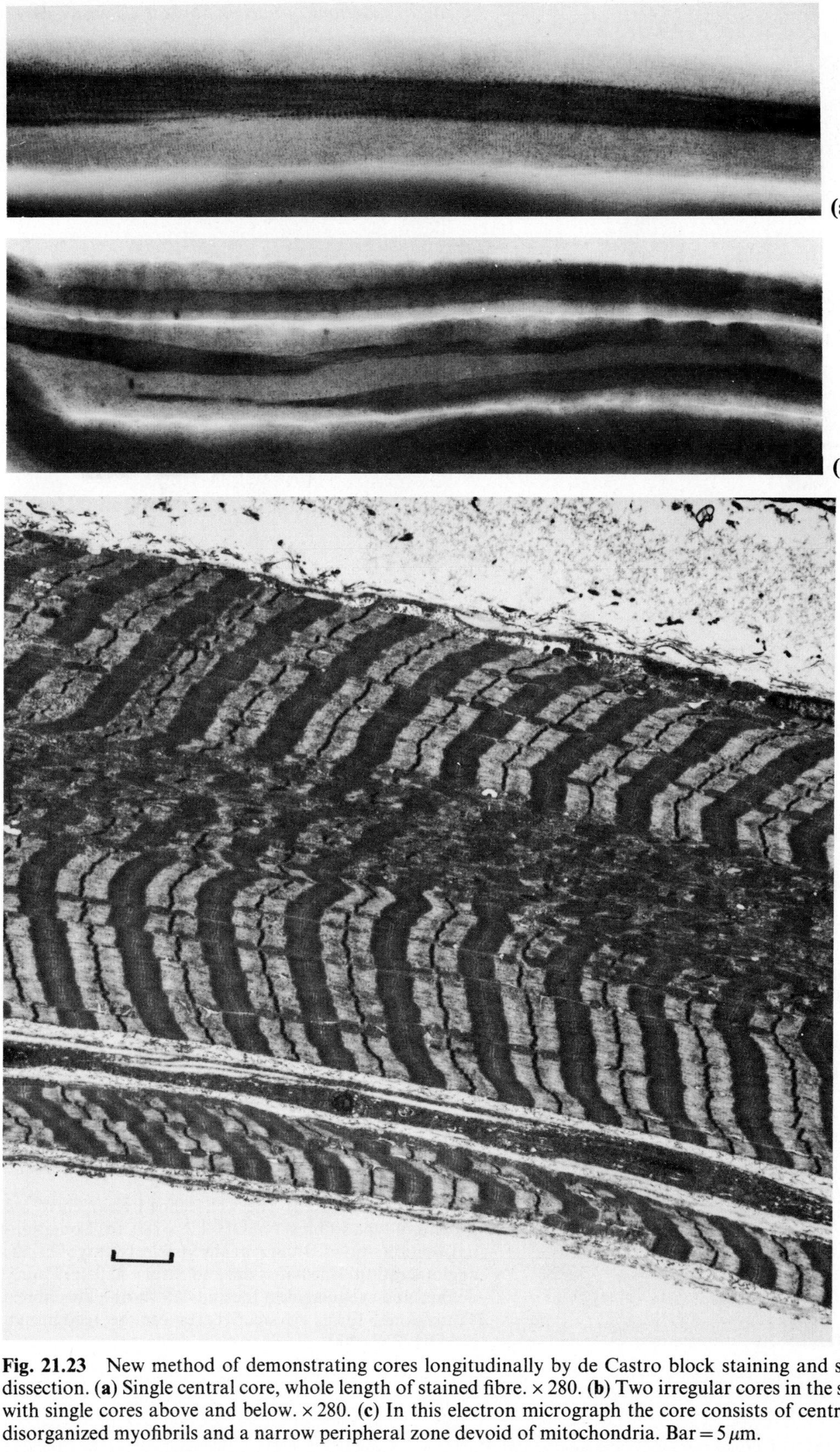

(a)

(b)

(c)

Fig. 21.23 New method of demonstrating cores longitudinally by de Castro block staining and single fibre dissection. (**a**) Single central core, whole length of stained fibre. × 280. (**b**) Two irregular cores in the same fibre, with single cores above and below. × 280. (**c**) In this electron micrograph the core consists of central mass of disorganized myofibrils and a narrow peripheral zone devoid of mitochondria. Bar = 5 μm.

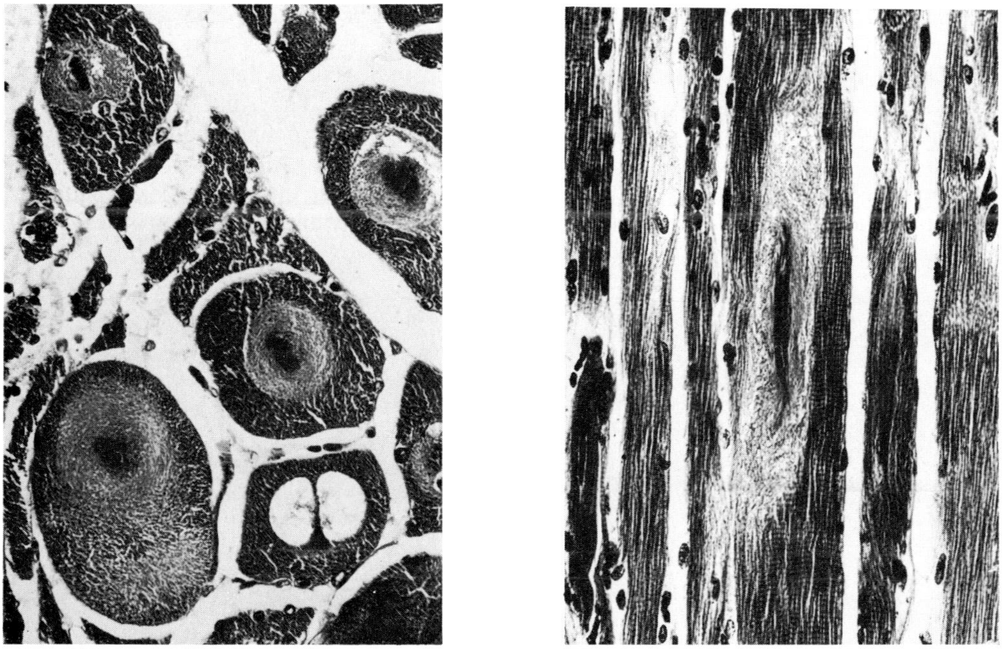

(a) **(b)**

Fig. 21.24 Target fibres seen in (**a**) cross-section and (**b**) longitudinal section. The three zones consist of a central area of coagulated myofibrils, an intermediate granular afibrillar zone and an outer ring of normal myofibrils. The target is of limited longitudinal extent. Autopsy muscle, motor neuron disease, paraffin section. PTAH × 420.

tudinal section the core had well-defined striations.

Tomonaga and Sluga (1969) found abnormality in both internal and middle zones of target fibres in electron micrographs. The central area showed myofibrillar disorganization producing electron-dense material, and the intermediate zone fragments of Z-discs and irregular disorganized myofilaments. They suspected that these were similar to cores.

There have been many reports of target fibres occurring in various myopathies; the phenomenon produced by experimental tenotomy has been called a target as often as a core, and when not conforming exactly to its definition the terms 'target-like' and 'core-targetoid' appeared. In view of the ultrastructural similarities between cores and targets, and the realization that they may both occur in the same myopathy or neuropathy, it seems likely that they represent variants of the same process. As both lack specificity, the use of the target and target-derived terms now seems superfluous. The first description of cores (or targets) was probably not by Shy and Magee, but by Farquhar Buzzard in 1905. He found in myasthenia gravis 'an appearance which is occasionally seen in conditions of very early atrophy of toxic origin. In transverse section the fibre is rounded and in the centre is a dark core surrounded by a concentric ring of lighter hue . . .'

Two other terms have been used to describe further core variations: 'multicores' and 'minicores'. Engel, Gomez and Groover (1971) reported two patients in whom many cores were small, and were due to sarcomere disruption, Z-line streaming and mitochondrial diminution or loss. Others were larger, and occasionally target fibres were produced. As there were many cores in affected fibres, he called them multicores. In each case there was type 1 fibre predominance, and cores were found in both types of fibre. Currie, Noronha and Harriman (1974) have described minicore disease in which the cores were all tiny, very numerous in the affected fibres and due to very small foci of Z-band streaming. The writer regards both conditions as variants of central core disease. Another condition has been described, 'focal loss of cross-striations', much larger than cores, but otherwise similar. Swash and Schwartz (1981), have described them in two brothers in association with the lesions of multicore disease.

Moth-eaten fibres resemble cores structurally, although they have never occurred as the only lesion in a muscle disease and given their name to a myopathy. Like cores, they involve loss of mitochondria but can be detected only in oxidative enzyme stains. They differ from a core in consisting of poorly defined patches of absent staining which appear to coalesce. A sharp edge is not produced, but the same tissue frequently contains both cores and moth-eaten fibres. Serial

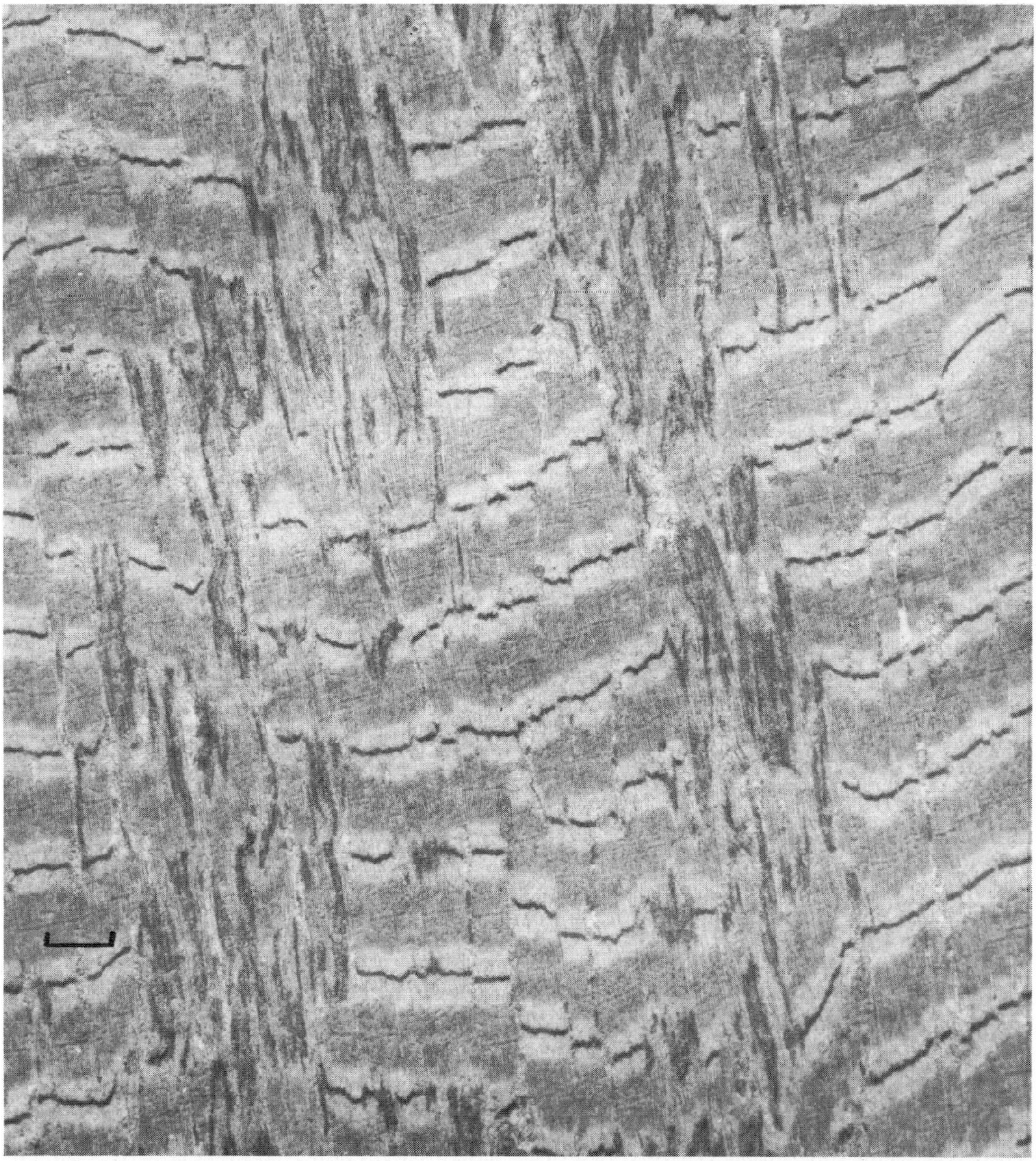

Fig. 21.25 Moth-eaten fibre. The orderly striations are disrupted by irregular Z-band streaming. Bar = 1 μm.

sections help to distinguish moth-eaten change from an artefact of staining. Electron micrographs show Z-band streaming in addition to patchy mitochondrial loss (Fig. 21.25). They are non-specific, but most often found in malignant hyperthermia myopathy.

The longitudinal extent of cores and their variants is often used to classify them. Minicores are very small in all diameters, multicores are larger, targets are relatively short and fully developed cores are at least as long as the blocks taken or fibres sampled. These differences seem not to be in essence but in severity or duration, and they do not impart any useful specificity.

Vacuoles

Vacuoles developing within muscle fibres are rare in normal muscle, and even then occur in very small numbers. In larger numbers and a variety of sizes they can be found in several myopathies, including the muscular dystrophies, polymyositis, some toxic myopathies (especially that due to chloroquine) and in some glycogenoses. In these, electron microscopy may show that the vacuoles occur because of autophagia distending lysosomal sacs to form membrane-bound structures. They differ from 'rimmed vacuoles' (p. 1072), which are not membrane-bound but often have feathery material at their edge (Fig. 21.26).

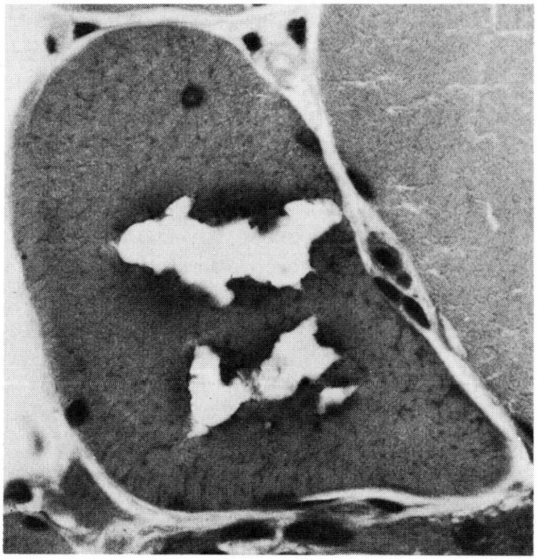

Fig. 21.26 This fibre contains two large irregular vacuoles bordered by feathery material ('rimmed' vacuoles). × 740.

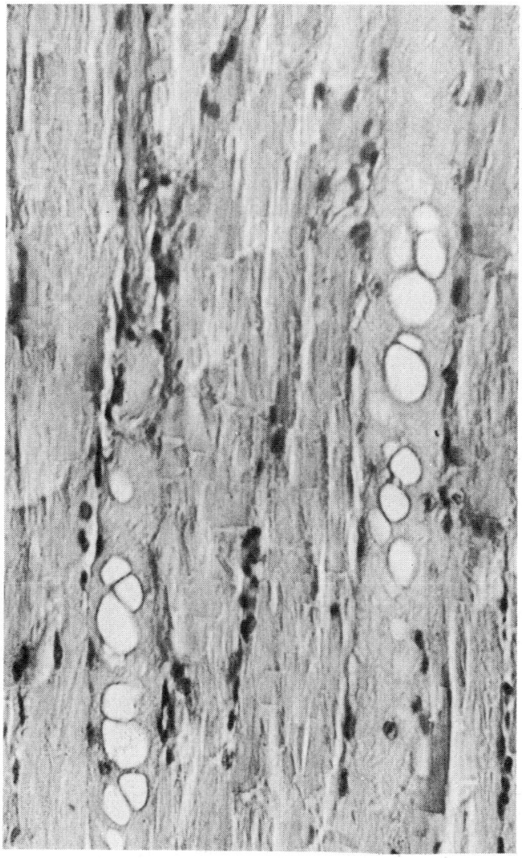

Fig. 21.27 Vacuolar myopathy induced by hypokalaemia due to diuretics, in a female of 64 years. Haematoxylin and van Gieson × 190.

Periodic paralysis induces vacuoles during an attack, which tend to disappear quickly afterwards. They also are membrane-bound, but are the results of dilatation of tubules and cisterns. Like most vacuoles they are usually empty but a little material stainable by PAS may persist within them.

'Storage' vacuoles develop when stored material such as glycogen or, occasionally, lipid is lost during processing. They are easily induced by paraffin embedding, but may occur to a lesser extent in frozen sections if they are given short fixation or if alcohol-based reagents are used. Vacuolation is also associated with the myositis of systemic lupus erythematosus. Little is known about its aetiology, but it may be due to drug therapy (Fig. 21.27).

Cytoplasmic bodies

These curious structures, which can be found singly in otherwise normal muscle, in small numbers in some myopathies and in larger numbers in cytoplasmic body myopathy, are decidedly uncommon compared to the other structural defects already mentioned. With the light microscope they show up best in Gomori-stained frozen sections as red spheres with a clear halo. With other stains they tend to be pale, but their halo makes them easily recognizable even in paraffin sections. Two or three may develop in the same fibre (Fig. 21.28). Ultrastructurally the central part is relatively dense and consists of tightly packed thin filaments. These and occasional thick filaments thinly spaced radiate haphazardly from the core within the halo. The bodies are usually found in type 2 fibres, but have been described in type 1, possibly owing to confusion with spheroid bodies, which are similar, but contain granules as well as fine filaments, and are found in type 1 fibres (Goebel et al., 1978).

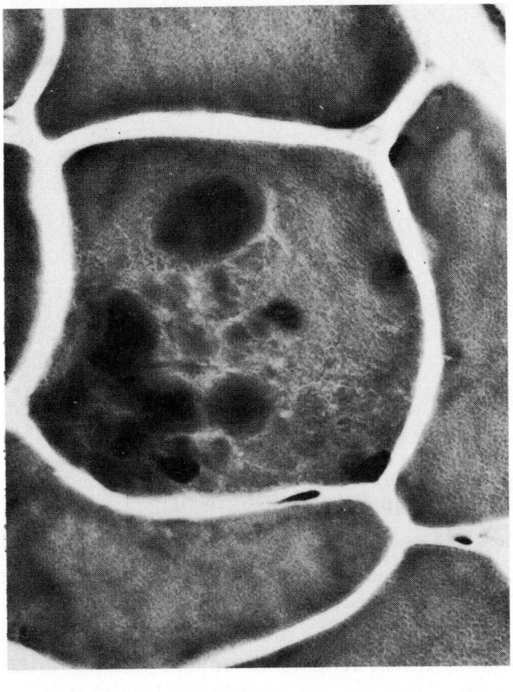

Fig. 21.28 Cytoplasmic bodies. Haematoxylin and eosin × 740.

General reactions of muscle to denervation

Group atrophy

There are many disorders involving denervation of muscle in man; in the majority, clinical examination, electromyography and nerve conduction rates provide an accurate diagnosis. Difficulties arise when the clinical course is uncharacteristic or when (pseudo-)myopathic features appear on electromyography, and a biopsy is justified.

Uncomplicated denervation produces a characteristic histopathology provided there has been time for it to develop. When neuromuscular transmission fails at the end-plate, voluntary control of contraction of the muscle fibre is immediately abolished but it takes 3–4 weeks for the inert fibre to undergo slow atrophy by disintegration of peripheral myofibrils. Cores develop in some patients, in both normal-sized and atrophic fibres. Much less commonly autophagic vacuolation is produced (Fig. 21.29). Nuclei become internal in relatively small numbers, and occasionally central. Fibre splitting is not uncommon. If the primary disease is non-progressive then all the muscle fibres controlled by the affected anterior horn cells will atrophy to a similar degree. If the motor neurons degenerate progressively then large groups of atrophied fibres (Fig. 21.30) will also be found but individual fibres will be of differing size. The atrophy will contrast with the remaining healthy muscle fibres, some of which will have undergone compensatory hypertrophy. Large group atrophy so described is of great value in diagnosis as it occurs only as a result of denervation. But end-stage neurogenic atrophy becomes indistinguishable from end-stage myopathy. Both processes leave only traces of their origin after many years, in the form of single degenerate fibres and clumps of muscle nuclei devoid of sarcoplasm in the midst of abundant fibrous and adipose tissue. Obviously such severely atrophied muscle is unsuitable for selection for biopsy.

Type grouping

If histochemical stains are applied to sections showing large group atrophy they are sometimes found to consist of atrophic fibres of the same fibre type. The apparently random distribution of fibre types is lost. The explanation lies in the

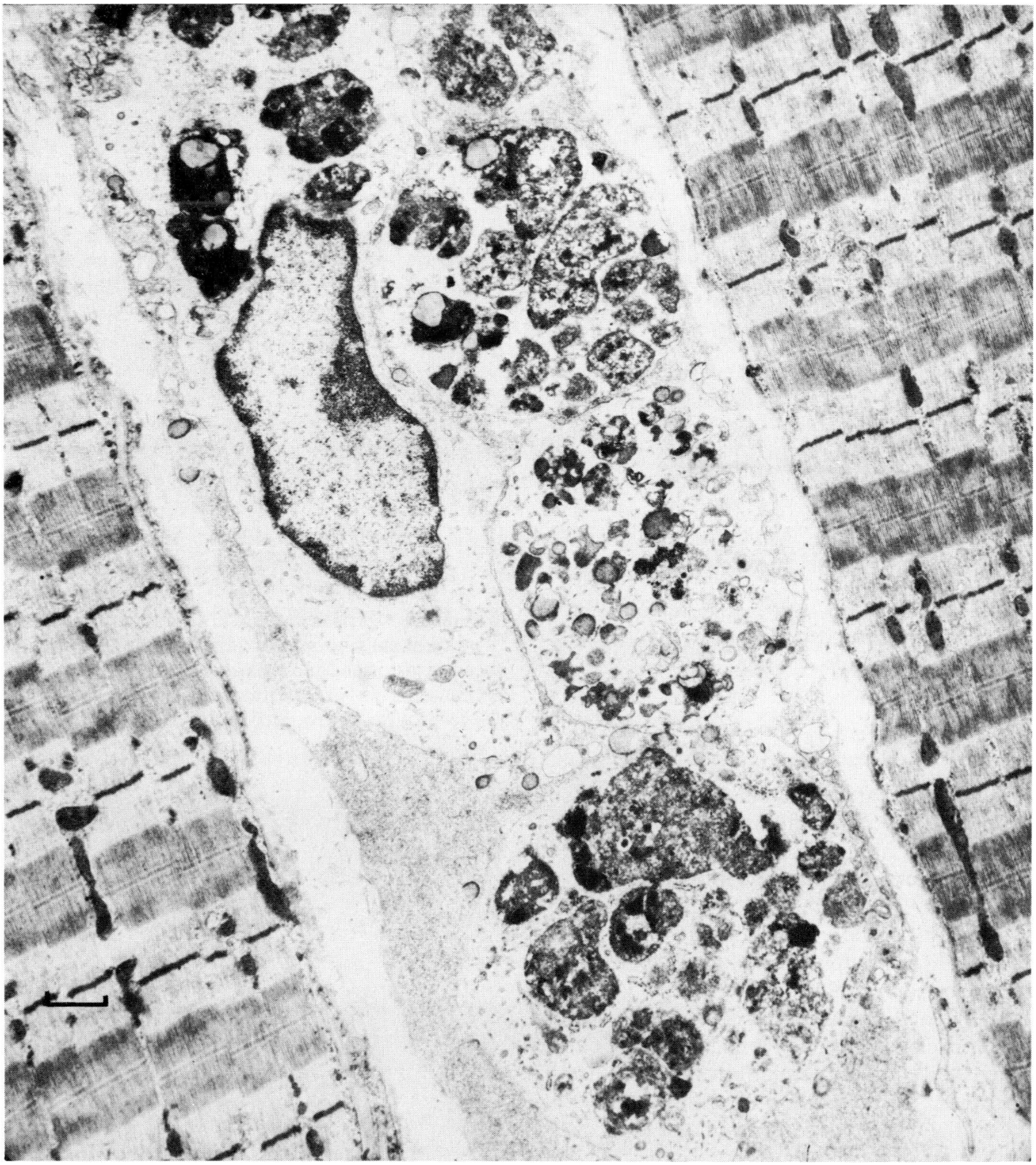

Fig. 21.29 Vacuoles containing mainly lipid degradation products as a result of denervation. Bar = 1 μm.

reaction of the motor nerves to the denervation process already described. Degeneration of a single motor neuron leads not only to the degeneration of all the branches of its axon and of its subterminal motor fibres and end-plates, but also to a rapid reaction on the part of neighbouring healthy subterminal fibres. They are stimulated to sprout from nodes of Ranvier and are attracted to the recently denervated muscle fibres whose sole-plates they reinnervate. It is a healing process, which slows the progression of the disease, but is eventually overcome. Sprouting from healthy subterminal fibres can lead to reinnervation of as many as 20 muscle fibres by a single subterminal fibre, so producing enlargement of motor units and giant potentials on elec-

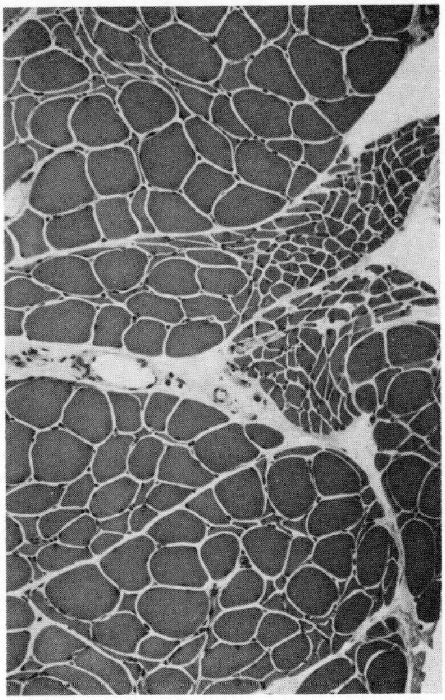

Fig. 21.30 Group atrophy. Large groups of fibres as well as single scattered fibres have been rendered small and angular by denervation. Haematoxylin and eosin × 120.

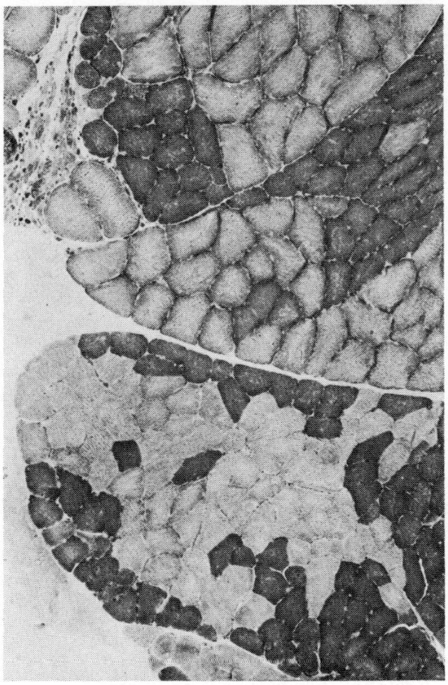

Fig. 21.31 Type grouping. Owing to collateral reinnervation, large groups of adjacent muscle fibres have been transformed into the type dictated by the reinnervating axons. The normal mosaic pattern is lost. A large group of atrophied fibres is present top left. NADH × 45.

tromyography. When the subterminal fibres of a motor unit which normally innervates type 1 fibres reinnervate type 2 muscle fibres, they convert the reinnervated fibres to their own type 1, as shown by numerous cross-innervation experiments of nerves from 'white' muscle to 'red' and vice-versa. It will result in large numbers of contiguous muscle fibres being of the same type (Fig. 21.31). Type grouping is useful as a feature diagnostic of neurogenic disease.

Very large areas of type grouping such as occur in slowly progressive chronic neuropathies like the peroneal muscular atrophies are easy to recognize, for several hundred fibres may then be of the same type interrupted by only one or two fibres of the opposite type. In the past some authors have considered, without justification, quite small type groups as diagnostic of denervation. There is considerable variation in normal individuals of fibre type predominance which can give a false impression of type grouping. The work of Lexell and colleagues (1983) shows the great variation in fibre type distribution throughout a large muscle, such as the vastus lateralis, which must be borne in mind when assessing the significance of type grouping. They found groups of about 100 fibres of the same histochemical

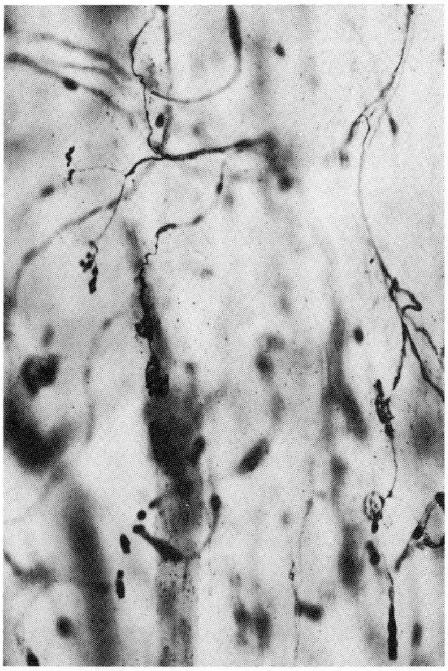

Fig. 21.32 Collateral reinnervation. Two subterminal fibres branch repeatedly, to form several end-plates each. Methylene blue × 180.

type. They do not believe that fibre types are randomly distributed, or that the usual small biopsies permit the detection of significant type grouping. Their work suggests that type grouping as an isolated finding should not be considered diagnostic of denervation unless the group numbers 100 or more. However, by examining the whole depth of the muscle their conclusion may not apply to biopsies which are by their nature confined to superficial fascicles. But the work of Lexell et al. does show that the criteria for type grouping should be re-examined in a large normal material.

The reinnervation of recently denervated muscle fibres which explains type grouping is easily recognized in a motor-point muscle biopsy. Even at a stage before type grouping or group atrophy occurs, staining of the innervation will show prominent branching of subterminal fibres and formation of new end-plates (Fig. 21.32). This process of collateral reinnervation is diagnostic of neurogenic disease. It is also detectable when type grouping and group atrophy are present, unless the latter is advanced.

The features which are diagnostic of neurogenic disease are therefore collateral reinnervation, type grouping of large groups and large group atrophy. Other findings which are useful in combination are cores (targets), internal nuclei, fibre hypertrophy and splitting. Occasionally, necrosis and regeneration, and 'pseudo-myopathic' fibre calibre variation complicate denervation.

Neurogenic diseases of muscle

Motor neuron disease (MND)

This progressive and relatively common disease, in which both upper and lower motor neurons slowly degenerate, manifests in three overlapping clinical syndromes; amyotrophic lateral sclerosis (ALS), progressive muscular atrophy and bulbar palsy. Bulbar and spinal motor neuron degeneration inevitably leads to denervation of skeletal muscle, but the third cranial nerve nuclei are usually spared.

Weakness and wasting develop in the small muscles of the hands. The disease progresses proximally. Progression of the disease is insidious but relentless; patients rarely live more than 3 years from the onset. Pyramidal tract degeneration causes for a time a characteristic increase in reflexes in the presence of muscle wasting. The disease affects those of middle age or older but has been reported, usually with atypical features, in a very few young adults. A personally studied case was that of a 24-year-old woman who died 8 months after the onset of transient blurring of vision followed by weakness of the lower limbs and impaired phonation. Severe generalized weakness of the limbs developed only terminally. At post-mortem the motor neurons throughout the spinal cord and medulla (but not higher) showed swelling and shrinkage or occasionally contained wavy bands of hyaline material or discrete inclusions without affinity for silver, lipids or aniline dyes (Fig. 21.33).

The characteristics of the cytoplasmic inclu-

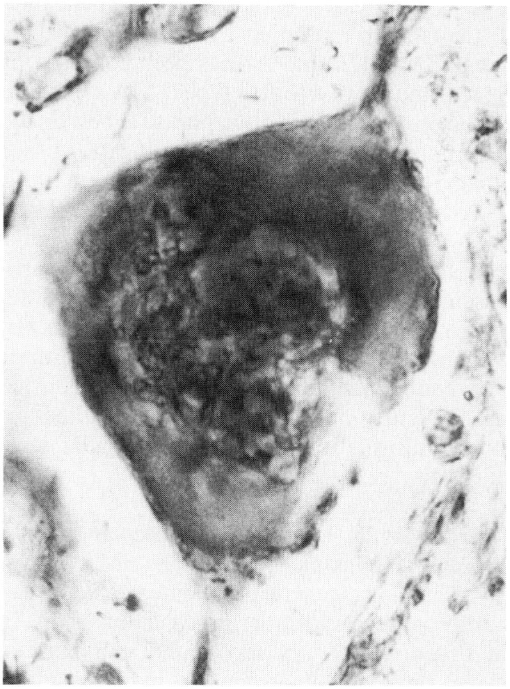

Fig. 21.33 Motor neuron disease at age 24. Unusual anterior horn cell inclusions. Holmes silver × 1130.

sions vary in the small number of cases of motor neuron disease which show them; those seen here resemble most closely the inclusions described by Schochet et al. (1969).

Muscle biopsy is indicated in only a minority of cases, and with a careful choice of muscle for biopsy (e.g. palmaris longus) collateral reinnervation and significant type grouping are found. In more rapidly progressive disease necrosis and regeneration, internal nuclei and fibre splitting are seen as well. Fully developed cores (target fibres) can be numerous but are rare in the writer's experience. If a small cutaneous nerve presents over the muscle it should be examined. When normal, it helps to confine the diagnosis to a purely motor disease.

Small darkly stained fibres of angular outline may lie within otherwise normal fascicles, but are not specific for neurogenic atrophy.

Spinal muscular atrophy

All forms of this disease resemble motor neuron disease in being due to degeneration of lower motor neurons of unknown cause, but differ in that the majority are inherited, involve proximal muscles more than distal and, except for the adult form, do not show spasticity. Classification of the spinal muscular atrophies into three types—SMA 1, 2 and 3—has been confused by the recognition of a fourth type (SMA 4), so that for the present a descriptive phrase is best added to the number. The following classification based on age of onset is acceptable: severe infantile onset spinal muscular atrophy (Werdnig–Hoffmann) (SMA type 1); intermediate spinal muscular atrophy (SMA type 2), juvenile onset spinal muscular atrophy (Kugelberg–Welander) (SMA type 3); and adult onset spinal muscular atrophy (SMA type 4). The table provided by Emery (1971) subdivides these groups and adds other rare variants; but it should be consulted for genetic information. The spinal muscular atrophies vary greatly in age of onset.

Severe infantile onset spinal muscular atrophy (Werdnig–Hoffmann disease; SMA type 1). This is genetically determined with autosomal recessive inheritance, and was one of the first diseases to be recognized as a cause of severe neonatal hypotonia. In many cases reduced fetal movements suggest that the disease begins before birth. Postnatal onset is not later than 4–6 months. As the disease progresses limb paralysis is noted, but the distinction between severe hypotonia and paralysis in an infant can be difficult. Fasciculation of the tongue is characteristic when present, and electromyography may detect fibrillation potentials. As in motor neuron disease, spinal cord anterior horn cells are predominantly affected, with occasional involvement of lower brain stem motor neurons and nearly always sparing of the third nerve nuclei. Sensory neuron and tract degeneration unsuspected clinically has been reported (Marshall and Duchen, 1975).

Degeneration in anterior horn cells is like that in the majority of cases of motor neuron disease, with ballooning or shrinkage of the perikaryon and atrophy of ventral roots.

Muscle biopsy when SMA type 1 is suspected in severe hypotonia can be misleading if practised soon after birth. At that stage fibres (apart from Wohlfart's B-fibres) are uniformly small in the normal infant, and can be mistaken for neurogenic atrophy. For the same reason, necropsy on an infant who dies early in the disease requires examination of too many rather than too few muscles as well as the central and peripheral nervous systems. The necropsy diagnosis is especially important for genetic counselling. For biopsy, one or another part of the quadriceps is suitable. The diagnosis of SMA type 1 can be sustained only if large groups of atrophied fibres are found alongside hypertrophied fibres (Fig. 21.34). In later weeks atrophied fibres can be distinguished more readily from normal ones with the growth of the infant. It has been claimed that denervated fibres in infancy are often round in outline, unlike the angular fibres of older denervated muscle. It is true enough, but normal infantile fibres are also often round.

Diagnosis at necropsy is helped by the neuronal ballooning and atrophy, but degenerating neurons may be difficult to find in the early stages. If neither neuronal nor muscle changes are found with a history of severe hypotonia, the brain must be examined for any malformation, even slight, which could give rise to secondary hypotonia.

Fibre typing does not contribute much to diagnosis in this acute form of spinal muscular atrophy. The atrophied fibres are usually of mixed types, and convincing type grouping is rarely seen. In electron micrographs of fibre atrophy, disorganization of sarcomeres, persistence of

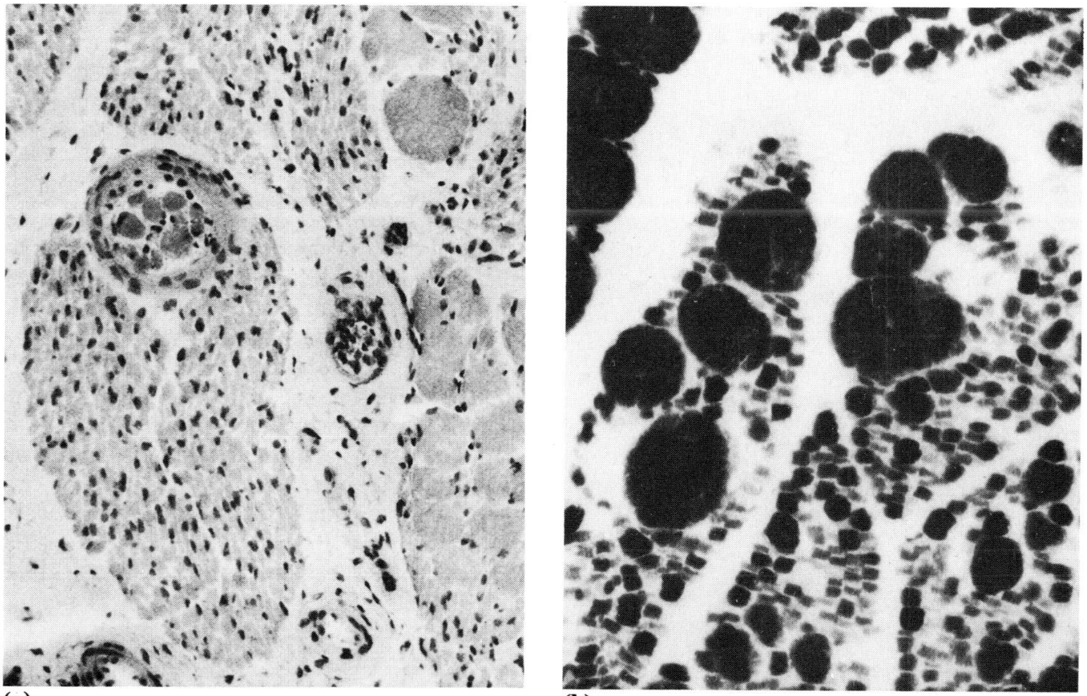

(a) **(b)**

Fig. 21.34 Spinal muscular atrophy type 1 (Werdnig–Hoffmann). (**a**) The very small fibres are atrophied in comparison with the much less numerous hypertrophied fibres. The intrafusal fibres are of normal size for age. Haematoxylin and eosin × 190. (**b**) The hypertrophied fibres are all of type 2, and the atrophied fibres mixed. ATPase pH 9.4 × 300.

filaments and increased numbers of triads are usual. The disorganization of myofibrils may result in unstructured cores recognizable in histochemical sections. The atrophy of muscle fibres gives rise to coils and folds of redundant basement membrane. Staining of the innervation shows collateral reinnervation but the writer and his colleagues have not seen it in the absence of group atrophy in SMA type 1.

Prognosis. The course of SMA type 1 is relentlessly downhill. Respiratory muscles become involved, breathing becomes rapid and death occurs in respiratory failure, often by 18 months. Survival to the age of 3 years is rare.

Genetics. Acute Werdnig–Hoffmann disease is genetically homogeneous and shows straightforward recessive inheritance (Pearn, Carter and Wilson, 1973).

Intermediate spinal muscular atrophy (SMA type 2) The onset of SMA type 2 is later than that of type 1 and altogether less severe. Nothing abnormal is noticed until after 6 months, when motor milestones are delayed. Independent running is never achieved and some may not be able to run or even sit unsupported. The CK level is sometimes moderately raised, giving rise to a suspicion of myopathy. It has been claimed that in some patients the disease becomes static, but this is not confirmed by Russman, Melchreit and Drennan (1983) in a review of 48 patients, half of whom were followed up for over 10 years. They found that all were progressive but extremely variable in duration, from a matter of months up to 30 years. Weakness and wasting tend to be generalized rather than proximal. There may be asymmetry, in contrast to the myopathies.

In their extensive genetic study of acute and chronic Werdnig–Hoffmann disease, Pearn, Carter and Wilson (1973) found a small group with dominant inheritance due probably to a mutation and responsible for most cases presenting late; but the status of the chronic group was on the whole uncertain.

At biopsy the findings are those of neurogenic

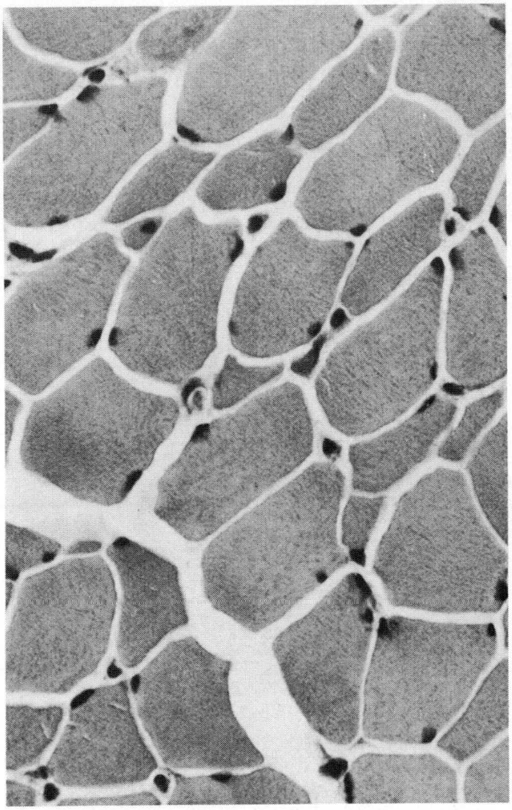

Fig. 21.35 Spinal muscular atrophy type 2. Variable pattern of fibre atrophy. Haematoxylin and eosin × 460.

disease, but there is a greater chance of finding collateral reinnervation, and a less severe group atrophy in which the degree of reduction in size of individual fibres is variable. Occasionally the whole section is composed of fibres of regularly variable size with a scattered group of three or four obviously atrophied fibres of mixed type (Fig. 21.35). It is then difficult to distinguish the pattern from that of an indolent childhood dystrophy, unless supporting evidence of denervation is available as collateral reinnervation or through electromyography. Electron microscopy helps only if the specimen is taken across the end-plate zone and end-plates are obtained showing degeneration and loss of axonic expansions and/or a covering of the sole-plate by collagen. Convincing type grouping is rarely seen.

Juvenile onset spinal muscular atrophy (Kugelberg-Welander syndrome; SMA type 3). It will not have escaped notice that the presentation of various types of spinal muscular atrophy with proximal involvement could readily give a clinical impression of muscular dystrophy rather than of neurogenic disease. This has happened especially in SMA type 3, which must often have been diagnosed as a heredofamilial syndrome of dystrophic type until the reports of Wohlfart, Fex and Eliasson (1955) and Kugelberg and Welander (1956) appeared. An autosomal recessive inheritance was described, confirmed in most cases since. The large muscles of the buttocks and thigh are involved first, less often the muscles of the upper arm. The face is usually not affected, but neck flexion and extension may become weak. A feature which causes the syndrome to simulate dystrophy more closely is pseudohypertrophy of the calves, which is noted in 25 per cent of cases, mostly males. But asymmetry of wasting can be found, which is not a feature of the dystrophies. Reflexes are usually diminished but can become exaggerated, and extensor plantar reflexes have been recorded.

It appears that the dystrophy with which SMA-3 was originally confused was Duchenne dystrophy: both could present with a disturbance of gait, proximal weakness and wasting, lumbar lordosis and pseudohypertrophy. There was often a family history. When serum CK estimations became commonplace this error was avoided, and nowadays confusion becomes more likely with one of the indolent dystrophies with onset in childhood. Electromyography may or may not be helpful. Fibrillation and the potentials characteristic of enlarged motor units can be recorded; on the other hand, small polyphasic potentials may again suggest a myopathy. CK levels are moderately raised, especially in older patients.

Muscle biopsy often provides straightforward evidence of denervation, collateral reinnervation and large group atrophy. In the earlier stages diagnosis may have to depend on innervation changes (Fig. 21.36) and type grouping. The presence of scattered single atrophic fibres, even if darkly staining and angulated, should not be relied on as evidence of neurogenic disease. Despite careful selection of muscle for biopsy the tissue obtained can be normal, emphasizing the patchy manner in which the muscle in liable to be affected. A repeat biopsy not far from the first may show denervation. The 'pseudomyopathic' pattern referred to in SMA type 2 is rare in SMA type 3.

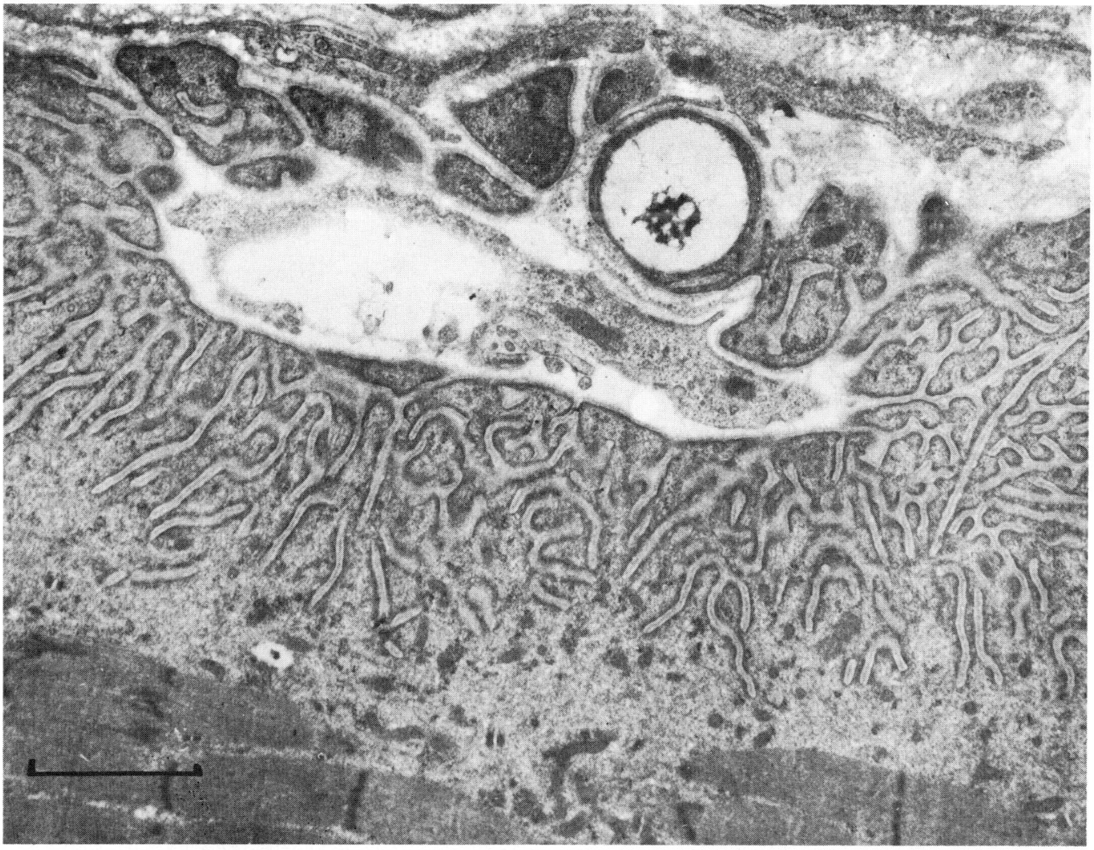

Fig. 21.36 Spinal muscular atrophy type 3 (Kugelberg–Welander). Denervated end-plate. The axonal debris is enclosed within Schwann cell cytoplasm which extends over the primary synaptic groove. Bar = 2 μm.

Adult onset spinal muscular atrophy (SMA type 4) This resembles SMA type 3 genetically and in its distribution, but is milder and the onset usually over 30. Less commonly it begins as early as 15 years. If the patient is first seen at a late stage, the biopsy may be misleading in showing features common to the end-stage of myopathies and neuropathies, with survival of scattered large fibres with internal nuclei, muscle giant cells, fibre splitting, and clumps of muscle nuclei devoid of sarcoplasm all separated by adipose and fibrous tissue (Fig. 21.37).

Other syndromes involving anterior horn cell degeneration

The spinal muscular atrophies are relatively common, but there are other rare syndromes also based on loss of anterior horn cells and presenting in juvenile or adult life. There is an autosomal recessive form of spinal muscular atrophy with a clear-cut distal distribution of weakness and wasting. A dominant form of SMA has been reported, clinically resembling facioscapulohumeral dystrophy (Fenichel, Emery and Hunt, 1967). The scapuloperoneal syndrome may have either a neurogenic or a myopathic basis.

Denervation in the peripheral neuropathies

The various forms of peripheral neuropathy are described in Chapter 18. They have in common the ability to cause neurogenic atrophy to a greater or lesser extent, even those which are clinically purely sensory. When a nerve biopsy is taken it can be advantageous to make a biopsy from a nearby muscle, especially at the motor point. The writer uses the musculocutaneous nerve above the lateral malleolus as a suitable sensory nerve for biopsy, conveniently close to the peroneus brevis or extensor digitorum longus. The muscle may be useful in showing angiitis

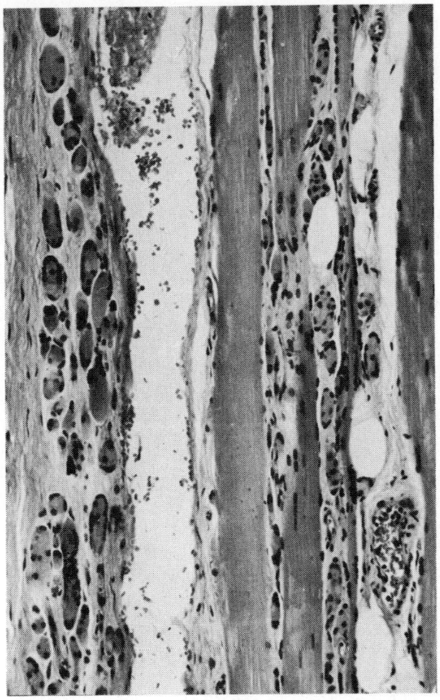

Fig. 21.37 So-called 'muscle giant cells', multinucleated fragments of sarcoplasm, occurring in neurogenic atrophy of slow progress and long duration. Haematoxylin and eosin × 110.

when it is absent from the nerve, or the intramuscular nerves may show inflammatory cell infiltration when the sensory nerve shows none. Hypertrophic neuropathy may be confined to the intramuscular nerves. For the most part, however, the muscle shows only neurogenic atrophy in its various manifestations. In addition to the common pattern of large group atrophy there is occasionally small group atrophy in which groups of three or four atrophied fibres regularly repeated alternate with larger fibres. As stated above, this pattern can be myopathic, but its presence in peripheral neuropathy shows it can equally be neurogenic, a distal pattern of neurogenic atrophy (see Fig. 21.35). In the hereditary motor and sensory neuropathies which progress very slowly, type grouping is prominent to a remarkable degree. At a late stage of slow denervation end-stage neuropathy is found. In polyneuritis, especially during the recovery phase, there may be large numbers of cores in both fibre types. It has led to the suggestion that reinnervation causes core formation. As cores develop more often in other conditions in which reinnervation plays no part, it is doubtful whether they can be so caused. As for the very early stage of polyneuritis, it is wise to avoid nerve and muscle biopsy then because both may be normal, including the innervation even when paralysis is profound.

Motor end-plates in the peripheral neuropathies are often abnormal but do not help in

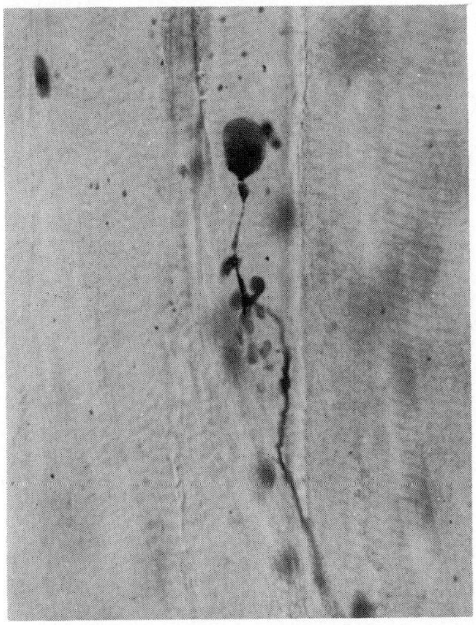

Fig. 21.38 End-plate with one large expansion which seems to be formed by fusion of smaller elements. Methylene blue × 480.

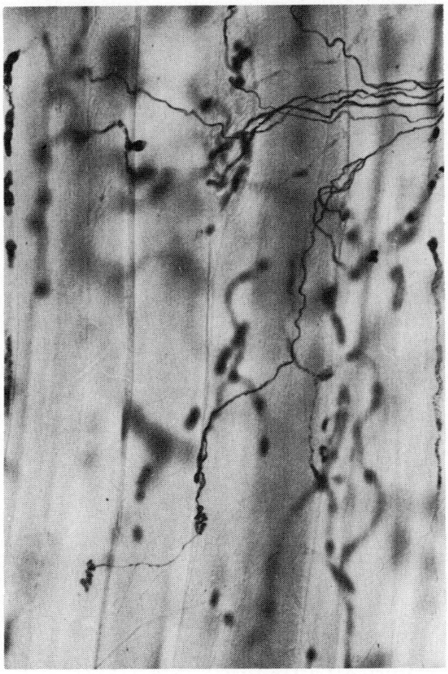

Fig. 21.39 Ultraterminal sprouting. A sprout arises from an end-plate, to form a new end-plate. Methylene blue × 180.

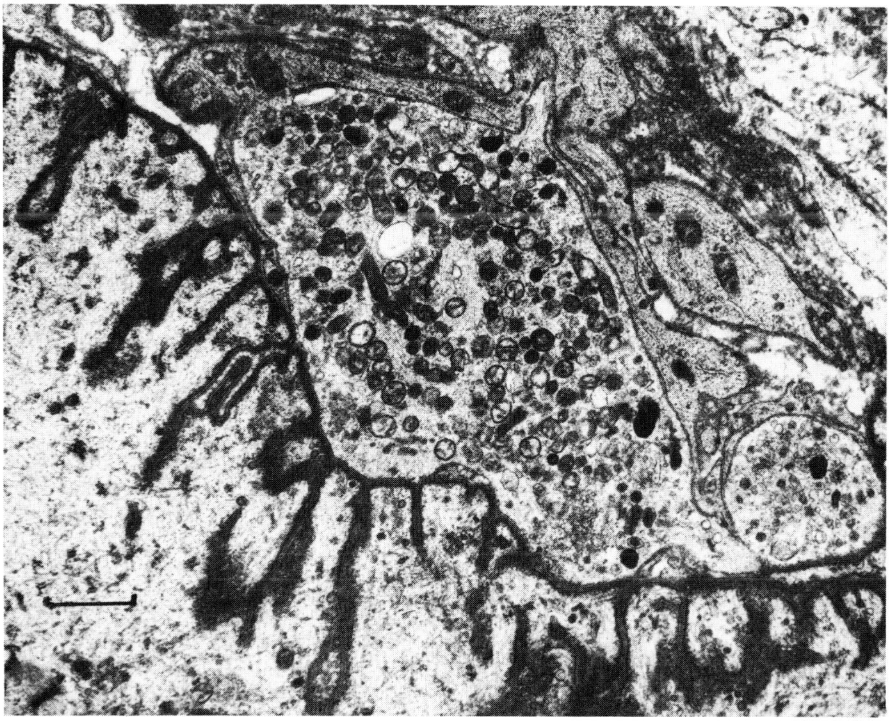

(a)

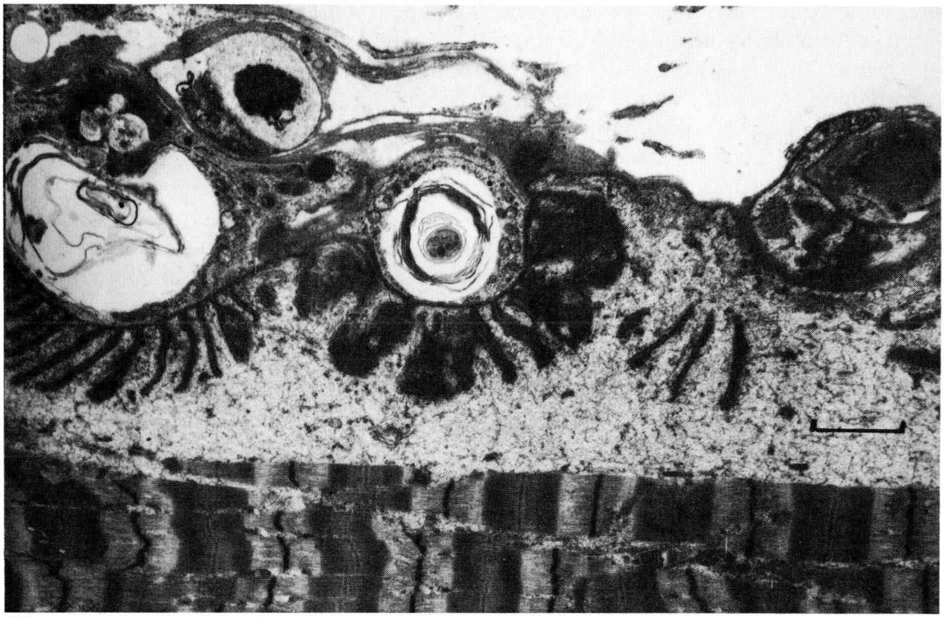

(b)

Fig. 21.40 (**a**) An axonal expansion still covering the sole-plate shows accumulation of mitochondria and dense bodies. There are very few synaptic vesicles, but more are seen in a neighbouring small expansion. Bar = 0.5 μm. (**b**) Degenerating axonic expansions. Bar = 1 μm.

diagnosis. Fusion of end-plate expansions into a single mass was originally described in diabetic neuropathy, and is commoner in that condition at an early stage of the disease than in other neuropathies (Fig. 21.38). Any neuropathy or myopathy may produce sprouting near or from end-plates, causing enlargement and deformity (Fig. 21.39). Only neuropathies produce collateral sprouting and reinnervation from the proximal parts of subterminal fibres.

Electron microscopy reveals changes involving both axonic expansions and the sole-plate. Secondary synaptic clefts may be focally or generally dilated, but not deformed or atrophied. The degeneration of axonic expansions is marked by loss of vesicles, accumulation then loss of mitochondria, formation of concentric figures and eventually the covering of the sole-plate by collagen (Fig. 21.40). The survival of denervated sole-plates as regular folds of the muscle fibre surface is remarkable, probably for as long as the parent fibre.

Poliomyelitis—chronic syndrome

A fairly regular variation of fibre calibre, which is more often seen in myopathy but can be pseudomyopathic, and the indistinguishable end-stages of chronic myopathies and neuropathies have already been mentioned. A third type of pseudomyopathy is rare, but of interest. Patients who survive acute poliomyelitis in childhood and are left with motor deficits normally remain in a static condition after the process of recovery ceases. Occasionally, 30–70 years later further weakness and wasting develop, in the most affected limb or in another. In patients who have been followed up the course of the supervening disorder is benign. Most patients are not biopsied and with electromyographic evidence the diagnosis of postpoliomyelitic denervation is made. According to Campbell, Williams and Pearce (1969) a relationship between the acute poliomyelitic episode and the late development of neurogenic atrophy was first postulated by Charcot in 1875, and many cases have been reported. Like motor neuron disease itself, it has unjustifiably been called ‘chronic poliomyelitis’. The main interest to the neuropathologist is that when a biopsy is made it may reveal changes which are normally regarded as myopathic: great variation in calibre and a few scattered small fibres, fibre splitting and regeneration. The muscle is likely to be partly replaced by fat and fibrous tissue, so the changes described will have developed in normal fascicles of a muscle whose atrophied fibres have totally disappeared. There is no reason to believe that the secondary changes are not also due to denervation, as some biopsies do reveal generally accepted neurogenic features. Its development so many years after poliomyelitis in which partial recovery implies the formation of giant motor units suggests that ageing or exhaustion of the anterior horn cells involved could be responsible.

Myasthenia gravis and other disorders of neuromuscular transmission

Abnormalities of neuromuscular transmission are conveniently classified into the presynaptic and postsynaptic. The former include the myasthenic (Eaton–Lambert) syndrome, botulism and myasthenia due to penicillamine. Postsynaptic defects occur in myasthenia gravis and in congenital and neonatal myasthenia.

The clinical features of myasthenia gravis are well known, especially the fatiguability of extra-ocular and bulbar muscle and, in severe cases, of limb and respiratory muscle. Anticholinesterase drugs are often effective. Its pathogenesis has now been clearly shown to be due to binding at acetylcholine (ACh) receptor sites of circulating antibodies (IgG) (reviewed by Simpson, 1981).

Although in most cases the clinical diagnosis of myasthenia gravis can be made on serological and neurophysiological grounds, the results may be inconclusive and a muscle biopsy is requested. Unless the biopsy is made at the motor point and motor end-plates demonstrated in detail it will not help diagnosis. The motor innervation should be stained and will show the characteristic changes of elongation of the end-plate, the terminal expansions reduced to a single line with one or two lateral sprouts (Fig. 21.41). Other end-plates show enlargement by terminal sprouting, but this is seen also in myopathies. A frequent finding is the reduction of the terminal to a single fine sprout. Whilst this happens also in peripheral neuropathies, the absence of any other evidence of denervation will suggest myasthenia. Changes in the sole-plate can be visualized only by the electron microscope but are helpful in diagnosis; blocking of ACh receptors leads to degeneration of the secondary synaptic folds, which become widened, shortened or may even disappear completely. The synaptic space

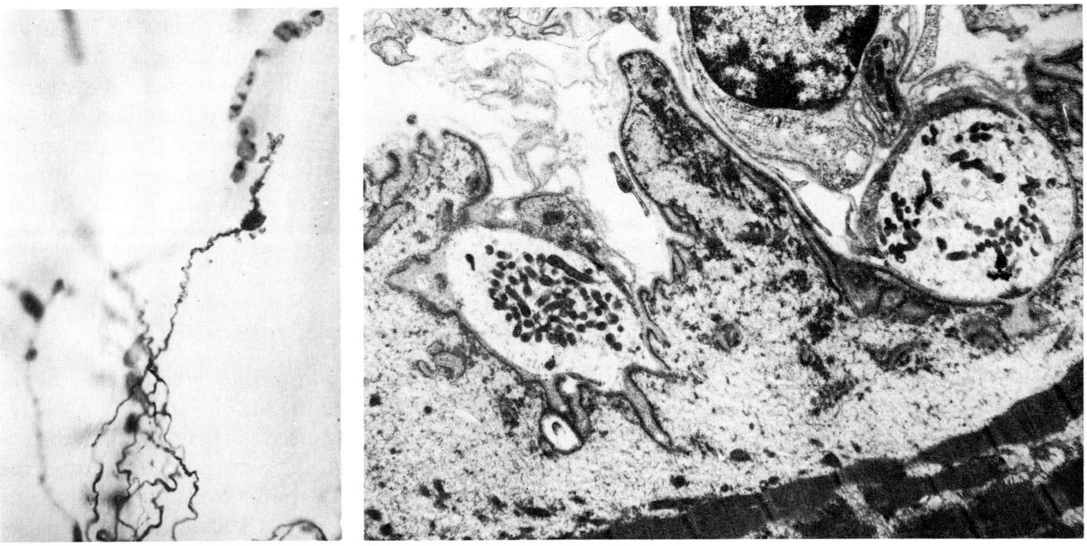

(a) **(b)**

Fig. 21.41 Myasthenia gravis. (**a**) Some end-plates become elongated and their expansions stunted and irregular. Methylene blue × 480. (**b**) The sole-plate is altered; secondary synaptic folds are reduced in number and the remainder are widened or retracted. Electron micrograph × 6200.

contains the debris of the degenerating folds. At an earlier stage the secondary synaptic folds are merely widened, but this also happens in some neuropathies. To ascertain whether it is due to myasthenia it is possible to stain the ACh receptors by an immunoperoxidase-α-bungarotoxin technique (Bender et al., 1976), staining of receptor sites being much reduced in myasthenia gravis.

Studies of intercostal end-plates using histometric methods (Santa, Engel and Lambert, 1972a) showed that, in addition to the qualitative alterations mentioned, the nerve terminal area was reduced, the postsynaptic membrane concentration also reduced but synaptic vesicles were not affected. An important observation was that patients untreated by anticholinesterases showed the same features as treated patients. The changes in man could not be ascribed to the drug treatment, despite evidence that the same drugs can cause end-plate degeneration experimentally. It is thought that end-plates of both type 1 and type 2 fibres are affected in myasthenia, but it is not always possible to identify the end-plate type.

In the majority of biopsies the muscle tissue proper is normal, but some show a variety of changes. The older literature emphasizes infiltration of the interstitial tissue by Buzzard's 'lymphorrhages', and the publication by Russell (1953) of three cases of myasthenia associated with polymyositis led to the view that cellular infiltrates were common. In fact they are comparatively infrequent, occurring only three times in 20 muscle biopsies in the writer's experience. The lymphorrhages are not as distinctive as they sound, for close examination detects plasma and other mononuclear cells in addition. When frozen section histochemistry of muscle became widely available and fibres were typed, Dubowitz and Brooke (1973) noticed atrophy of type 2 fibres in most of 6 patients, but it was unusual in being focal. The atrophy may be the result of failure of transmission at clusters of motor end-plates, and further experience suggests that type 1 fibre end-plates are also involved.

A number of patients showing permanent muscle weakness and wasting have been reported under the diagnosis of myasthenic myopathy, limb girdle myopathy, neurogenic atrophy, polyneuropathy and neuromyopathy. In some the diagnosis was made without histological evidence. The 'myopathies' can be understood if they illustrate an association with polymyositis or its sequelae, or a reaction to a neoplasm such as a thymoma. The neuropathies must be the end-result of end-plate degeneration. The most thoroughly examined cases were those reported by Brownell, Oppenheimer and Spalding (1972) in which some muscles such as those of the tongue and pharynx had been atrophied for many years. They showed obvious group atrophy but the motor innervation appeared healthy right up to end-plate level.

Myasthenic (Eaton–Lambert) syndrome

In patients over 40 with a known or cryptic carcinoma, usually of lung, there may develop recurrent muscle weakness. It differs from that of myasthenia gravis by involving proximal limb girdles but not extraocular muscles and in being overcome rather than aggravated at least for a while by exercise. Amelioration is provided by guanidine, which facilitates ACh release. It is now known that the syndrome may arise without neoplasm, and that sites other than the lung can be implicated. Histologically, the muscle is normal but in one case in which the writer examined the innervation, the end-plates by light microscopy were attenuated and linear. Ultrastructural findings made by Santa, Engel and Lambert (1972b) were the opposite of those in myasthenia gravis: the mean area of postsynaptic junctional folds and secondary synaptic clefts per nerve terminal were greatly increased. If histometrical measurements are not available, it is difficult to be sure that qualitatively one is not dealing with a normal type 2 fibre end-plate.

Penicillamine-induced myasthenia

Several drugs may induce reversible myasthenia in susceptible patients, but the commonest is D-penicillamine when used in rheumatoid arthritis. As the drug is withdrawn there is gradual recovery and ACh antibody levels previously high begin to fall. The only circumstances in which a biopsy would be required would be to distinguish between a drug-induced myasthenia not recovering as expected and an associated myasthenia gravis.

The myopathies

Disorders of muscle as opposed to those of its innervation may be classified as *primary*, in which the disease is manifested in muscle, and *secondary*, due to disease outside the neuromuscular system. There have been suggestions in the past that the muscular dystrophies, long established as diseases of muscle, might well be due to a defect of the nervous system—bearing in mind that abnormalities in the nervous system are sometimes demonstrated as associated conditions—but these suggestsions require more compelling evidence.

Primary myopathies

The muscular dystrophies

The term 'dystrophy' has been used for genetically determined diseases of muscle for many years, but that term has not been given to the recently discovered inherited congenital myopathies. These have specific structural defects and are known by their morphological abnormality (e.g. 'rod body'). 'Dystrophy' thus has a special connotation when applied to muscle, unlike its use in other systems where only an abnormality of growth is implied.

Duchenne dystrophy

This is the most severe of the muscular dystrophies. It is X-linked, occurring only in boys and transmitted by female carriers. The mutation rate is high, causing difficulty in diagnosis in individual cases. One-third of patients have a previous family history, one-third are new mutants and one-third are born to previously undetected, probably mutant, carriers. It was first described as 'pseudohypertrophic paralysis' by the French neurologist Duchenne de Boulogne (1806–1875) who has ever been known by his place of birth. The first signs of the disease are not immediately postnatal but appear at the age of 4 or 5 years. An awkward gait or tendency to trip and fall are first noticed, followed by proximal weakness. The calf muscles are nearly always enlarged and the quadriceps atrophied. Less commonly other muscles are enlarged, such as the deltoids and spinati; one of Duchenne's patients was drawn as an infant Hercules but this

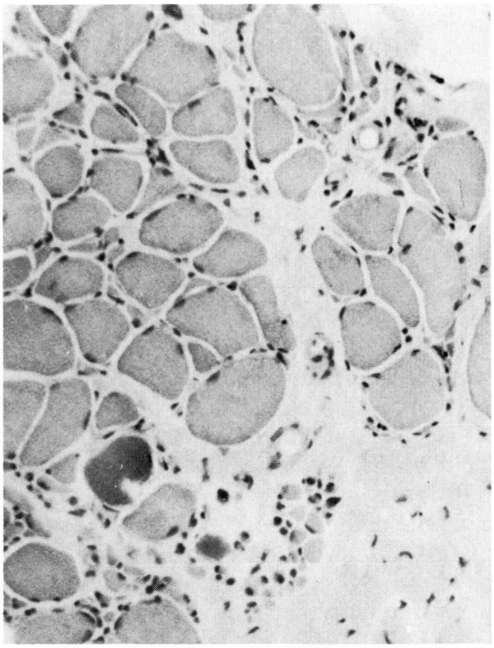

(a)

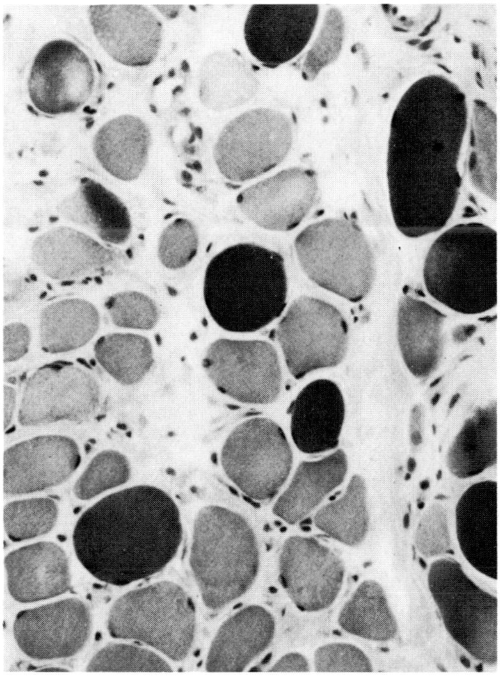

(b)

Fig. 21.42 Duchenne dystrophy. Boy aged 7 years. (**a**) Vastus medialis. Characteristic groups of small regenerating fibres, variation, hyaline hypercontracted fibres, fibrosis, slight cellular infiltration. Haematoxylin and eosin × 190. (**b**) Peroneus brevis (clinically unimpaired). Shows less variation, more hyaline fibres and virtually no regeneration. Haematoxylin and eosin × 190.

presentation is distinctly rare. Muscles are symmetrically affected on clinical examination, but biopsy of clinically normal muscles may show changes (Fig. 21.42). When the disease is established the child shows Gowers' sign, typically having to climb up his legs when asked to get up from the floor. This is no longer considered specific for Duchenne dystrophy, but merely indicates proximal lower limb weakness.

The nature of the earliest change in muscle is not known with certainty. A biopsy of an enlarged muscle showing little else than fibre enlargement suggests that the first change is hypertrophy, but studies on boys in the preclinical phase show fibre necrosis and regeneration as an early finding. Most biopsies on enlarged muscles have been performed on the gastrocnemius, revealing advanced myopathic changes and replacement by excess fibrous tissue and fat. Such muscles are weak, and designated as pseudohypertrophic rather than hypertrophic.

Histopathology. By the time a biopsy is requested there are definite clinical signs and the muscle most often chosen is the quadriceps. Invariably there is surprise at the severity of the proximal muscle involvement in a boy who may still be able to run. The muscle is unduly firm and reddish-grey, or even white; it reacts sluggishly to electrical stimulation. Transverse sections show a random variation in fibre size from hypertrophied to small round forms. Here and there are large fibre outlines, some dark irrespective of the stain and others pale (Fig. 21.43). Fibres with internal nuclei occur but are not numerous, and there is little fibre splitting. Many fibres are round in outline. Groups of small basophilic-regenerating fibres with prominent nuclei and nucleoli are frequent. Occasional necrosis and regeneration occur also in fibres of normal size. The fascicles are separated by thick seams of fibrous tissue and variable amounts of adipose tissue. Within fascicles there is the beginning of fibrous thickening of the endomysium.

Longitudinal sections indicate the origin of the dark and light fibres. They are hypercontracted fibres with alternate dark and light zones, the dark ones larger in diameter. These constitute a

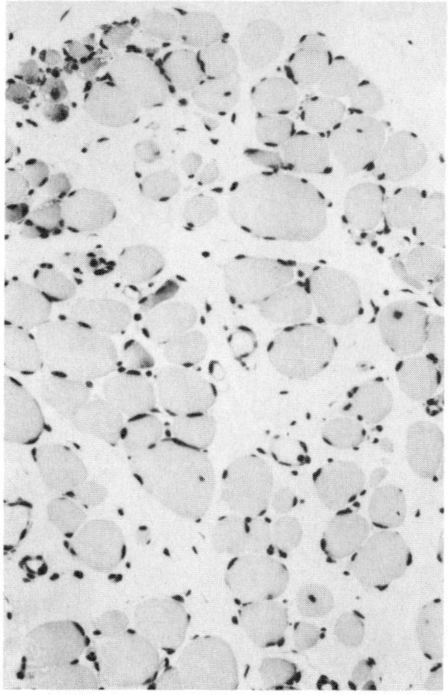

Fig. 21.43 Duchenne dystrophy. There is variation in fibre size, fibrosis, and a cluster of small basophilic regenerating fibres top left. Haematoxylin and eosin × 180.

well-known artefact, but always abundant in early Duchenne dystrophy despite the strictest precautions. They suggest that dystrophic muscle in this condition suffers from a defect which renders it particularly fragile. The regenerating fibres are also seen to better advantage in longitudinal sections. Some are identical with those in other diseases; others are attenuated and darkened as if affected by degeneration during the course of regeneration. Segmental necrosis followed by phagocytosis and regeneration are seen, often accompanied by scanty lymphocytic and plasma cell infiltration. Rarely, the infiltrates are large, like those in polymyositis, but can usually be seen to remain in the vicinity of a necrotic fibre.

Histochemical stains show that the disorder affects both main fibre types. Many workers report that the fibres are often imperfectly differentiated and so difficult to type, which is in agreement with the author's experience. Regenerating fibres stain variably according to their age. Other quite non-specific findings may occur such as a few moth-eaten fibres or fibres containing excess triglyceride. The innervation in Duchenne dystrophy is not normal but does not show the collateral reinnervation characteristic of neurogenic disease. The reaction is distal, presumably to loss of end-plates when fibres degenerate. Distal parts of subterminal fibres branch to form new end-plates or to form fine sprouts, and, as in any myopathy, sprouting takes place from end-plates (ultraterminal sprouting). There is no increase in the functional terminal innervation ratio of Coërs and Woolf (1959), which is the ratio of the number of muscle fibres innervated by a given number of subterminal axons. This ratio is increased in denervation. Duchenne dystrophy is one of a small number of myopathies which involve cardiac as well as skeletal muscle. Minor abnormalities are common in the ECG, and can indicate conduction block. At autopsy, Frankel and Rosser (1976) found extensive fibrosis in the outer half of the myocardium of the obtuse margin in five cases.

The course of the disease can be followed using the plasma CK level. In the early stages, even before clinical signs appear, the level is very high and in the next few years may reach astronomical figures of 30 000–40 000 iμ/l. At this stage there is much necrosis and regeneration. Later these become less marked, and the CK readings fall to near normal levels before death in the early 20s.

Advances have been made in recent years in detecting the carrier state in suspected females, through examination of the family history, physical examination and CK serum levels. Its probability can be predicted statistically. Occasionally muscle biopsy is used, but the minor changes sometimes detected do little to add confidence to the prediction.

Aetiology. There is no consensus regarding the cause of Duchenne dystrophy, although a number of theories have been proposed. Because a nutritional myopathy in some animals can resemble Duchenne dystrophy histologically, there was a vogue for vitamin treatment especially vitamin E. It was soon realized that the observation merely showed that the histopathology of dystrophy was not unique. In similar vein an experimental ischaemia along with a vasoactive drug produced a picture very like that of Duchenne dystrophy, which then could be considered to have a vascular cause. Blood flow studies in Duchenne patients did not confirm this (Bradley et al., 1975). A hypothesis difficult to confirm or refute was proposed by McComas, Sica and Currie (1970), known as the neurogenic hypothesis. They presented electrophysiological evidence of a reduction in the number of functioning motor units early in the course of muscular dystrophy. They ascribed it to functional neuronal failure ('sick' motor neurons). The idea was rendered less acceptable although not refuted by the failure to discover any loss of motor neurons in the spinal cord at autopsy (Tomlinson, Walton and Irving, 1974).

The current hypothesis with fairly general acceptance is that of a membrane defect allowing ingress of calcium into individual cells. This has been shown histologically by Bodensteiner and Engel (1978) but it is not clear to what extent calcium entry reflects a primary or secondary disorder of the dystrophic cell.

Ultrastructure. Early hopes that ultrastructural examination of dystrophic muscle would indicate its pathogenesis were dashed, despite the opinion that breaks in the cell membrane might indicate the first event (Mokri and Engel, 1975). It was soon found that none of the changes discovered—filamentous disarray, accumulation of ribosomes, focal streaming of Z-discs, satellite cell enlargement, features of regeneration—was specific. Other changes were due to contracted segments, loss of filament detail and darkening of nuclei corresponding to the dark fibres of light microscopy, and were looked upon either as an undue susceptibility to artefact or to the initiation of necrosis. Mastaglia, Papadimitriou and Kakulas (1970) in an ultrastructural study of Duchenne dystrophy, emphasized the abnormal regeneration.

Tunisian muscular dystrophy

There have been reports of a Duchenne-like dystrophy appearing in girls, but they have been infrequent and have provoked doubts as to whether they were identical with it in all respects other than inheritance. However, several reports have arrived recently of a very large number of children of both sexes affected by a necrotizing dystrophy with autosomal recessive inheritance (Hamida, Fardeau and Attia, 1983). Most originate in Tunisia, and comprise a study of 75 children from 17 families, and of 18 from 11 families separated from the others because they were girls. Families with only boys affected were excluded. The clinical features of onset between 3 and 12 years, the pseudohypertrophy of the calves and the early marked rise in serum CK all suggested similarity to Duchenne, but the great variability in the intensity of symptoms among siblings and between families and the longer course indicated by the preservation of walking until 10–20 years of age were different. The histological examination (made in 37 children) showed less fibrosis and a 'lesser degree of type-1 fibre predominance' than in Duchenne dystrophy, and an almost complete absence of hyalinized fibres. Examination of the heart by ECG was not possible so the involvement of cardiac muscle remains unknown.

It would seem that this disease is distinct from both Duchenne dystrophy and childhood or limb girdle dystrophy in children, and can provisionally be regarded as a new entity.

Becker dystrophy (benign X-linked muscular dystrophy)

This form of muscular dystrophy resembles Duchenne dystrophy genetically, exhibiting X-linked recessive inheritance, but is a distinct en-

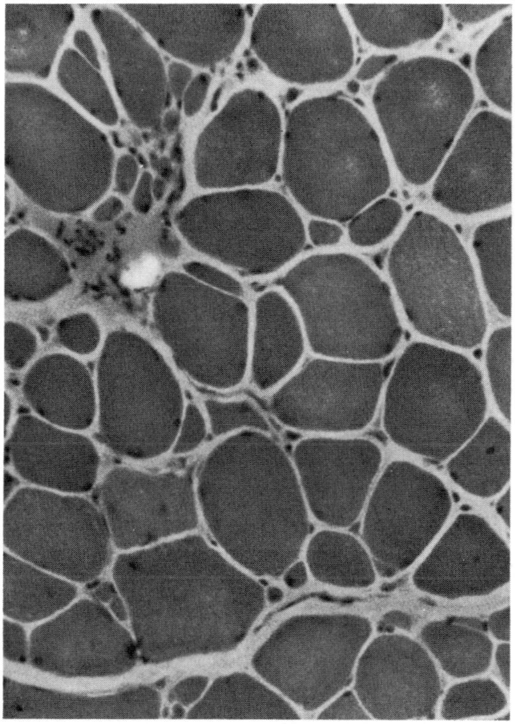

Fig. 21.44 Becker dystrophy. Male aged 14 years. Histopathology like that in Duchenne dystrophy but much less severe, age for age. Haematoxylin and eosin × 400.

tity. It begins later and its progression is slower, so the patient may remain ambulant even into the fourth decade. Pseudohypertrophy of the calves is usually present, with slight or moderate proximal weakness. It may be difficult to distinguish clinically from limb girdle dystrophy in the absence of family involvement, although there is usually no pseudohypertrophy in the latter.

Histologically the changes in Duchenne and Becker are similar but differ in intensity (Fig. 21.44). Variation in fibre calibre, relatively few internal nuclei, necrosis, groups of regenerating fibres, hyaline fibres and fibrosis are all seen, but to a lesser degree age for age. The writer and his colleagues do not confirm reports of type 1 fibre predominance in Duchenne dystrophy and its absence in Becker, or the rarity of 2b fibres in Duchenne and their presence in Becker, but believe that fibre type differentiation is not blurred in the latter as it is in Duchenne. CK levels can be very high in Becker and do not help in diagnosis. As in Duchenne dystrophy, the heart is often involved.

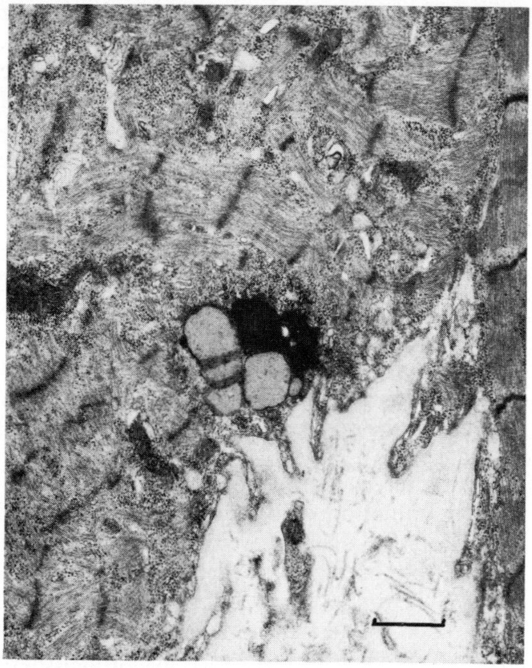

Fig. 21.45 Limb girdle dystrophy. Abnormal part of fibre splitting away from more normal part. Bar = 1 μm.

Limb girdle muscular dystrophy

Proximal wasting and weakness of slow progression, commencing in the second or third decade, with autosomal recessive inheritance are relatively rare. It is particularly rare in children in whom limb girdle dystrophy is probably overdiagnosed. The pelvic girdle is usually affected first, sometimes asymmetrically, and it affects both sexes equally. The face is not affected. Progression is slow, over 20 years or more, and may appear to cease. One personally observed male patient who had had the disease for 20 years and showed obvious wasting denied the illness completely. Eventually walking becomes impossible and the patient chair-bound. A number of different entities can produce this clinical picture, and must be excluded by a thorough examination and investigation before limb girdle dystrophy can be established. Disorders with which it may be confused include Becker dystrophy, SMA type 3 (Kugelberg–Welander) and some congenital and metabolic myopathies.

Histology. In general terms the muscle shows non-specific myopathic changes, and, as in most myopathies, diagnosis must be made by integrating clinical, electromyographical, biochemical and histological information. Some features are more prominent in limb girdle dystrophy such as internal nuclei, fibre splitting and excessive variation in fibre size (Fig. 21.45). Fibrosis does not develop until late in the disease. Ring fibres and moth-eaten fibres are not infrequent. A moderate rise in serum CK accompanies occasional necrotic and regenerating fibres. All fibre types are involved in the dystrophic process. Although groups of small fibres of the same type occur, they do not on their own justify a diagnosis of neurogenic disease. Similarly, the motor nerves react by distal sprouting only.

Ultrastructure. The findings are similar to those in other myopathies, including degenerative features, regeneration, Z-line streaming and ring fibres.

Quadriceps myopathy. A small number of cases have been reported in which wasting and weakness have clinically been confined to the quadriceps (but on electromyography abnormality is more widespread). It is inherited, but more case descriptions are required before it can be disassociated from limb girdle dystrophy.

Childhood muscular dystrophy

A childhood dystrophy almost as severe as Duchenne but occurring in both sexes especially in Tunisia has already been described. Another childhood dystrophy also of autosomal recessive inheritance has been recognized for some years, but is rare and in earlier times may have been misdiagnosed as Duchenne or Becker dystrophy. The suspicion of an entity distinct from Duchenne arose when the claim was made that Duchenne dystrophy could occur in girls. Childhood muscular dystrophy occurs in both sexes and is common in girls. The onset is between 2 and 14 years, calf hypertrophy is present in some, and the ECG is usually but not invariably normal. Weakness occurs in the same distribution as in Duchenne and in Becker dystrophy, but paresis of the lower face, deltoids and hamstrings is relatively prominent.

The histological appearances differ from Duchenne and from Tunisian dystrophy in showing much less necrosis and regeneration, less fibrosis but more internal nuclei and fibre splitting. Ring fibres are frequent. The CK level is moderately raised.

The course of the disease is more benign than that of Duchenne dystrophy, the ability to walk is maintained until over 20 years, with survival to 40–50 years. Duchenne, Becker and early limb girdle dystrophies come into the differential diagnosis.

Congenital dystrophic myopathy (congenital muscular dystrophy)

The name 'congenital dystrophic myopathy' is intended to describe a myopathy which is already established at the time of birth and must therefore begin *in utero*. Although it is one of the congenital myopathies, it is described here because of its morphological resemblance to the dystrophies. It is sometimes complicated by arthrogryposis and is one of the numerous causes of infantile hypotonia. The CK varies from normal to high. Histologically the muscle resembles that of a severe progressive dystrophy with calibre variation, occasional necrosis and regeneration, fibrosis and adiposity but unusually large numbers of small contiguous fibres which may well be surviving immature fibres. Occasionally

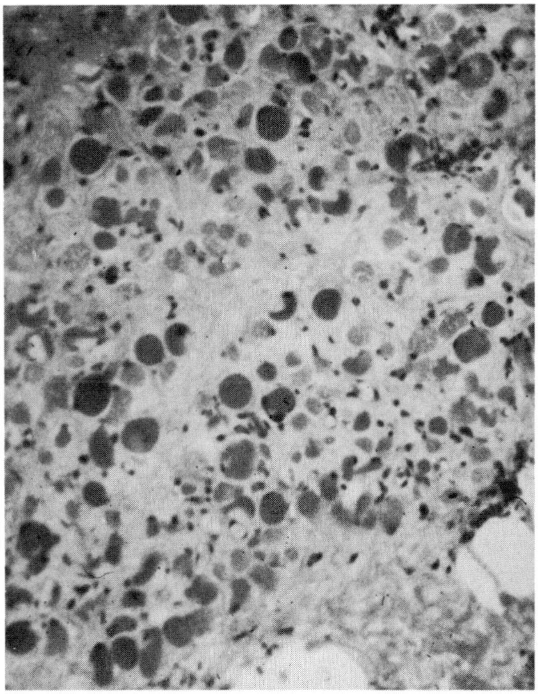

(a)

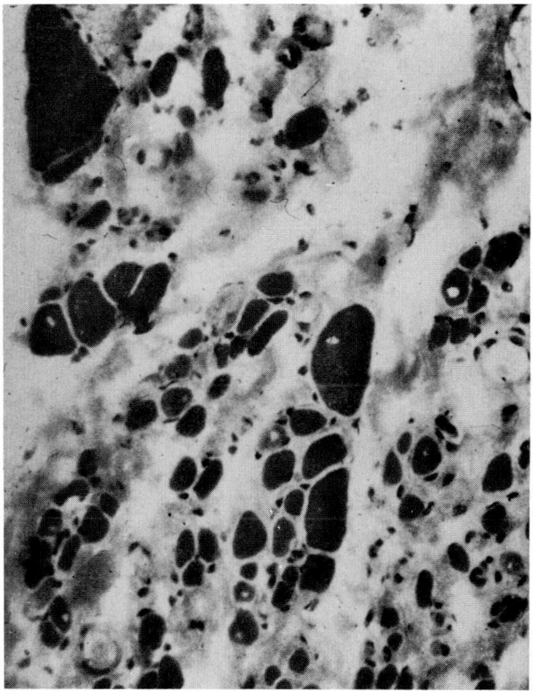

(b)

Fig. 21.46 Congenital dystrophic myopathy. (**a**) First biopsy at 8 months. (**b**) second biopsy at 5 years. Some fibres have grown, but there is little evidence of progression. Both haematoxylin and eosin × 190.

the first biopsy shows minimal changes but the characteristic picture develops later. Although many familial cases have been reported, it is not certain whether it is genetically distinct. Babies within the same family may show totally dissimilar severity. One feature frequently shown is an apparent arrest of the disease after 6 months of age. If the infant lives beyond that time there is a chance of survival with whatever improvement can be provided by remaining unaffected muscle. When the dystrophy is overcome by natural development, there results a discrepancy between clinical performance and histopathology, the former being surprisingly good despite severe muscle wasting and fibrosis. A repeat biopsy in one of the writer's patients 4 years after the first showed little change in pattern and some evidence of growth (Fig. 21.46). The arrest of the myopathy is so unlike the course of the childhood dystrophies that the term 'congenital muscular dystrophy' is best avoided.

In 1960 Fukuyama first described the association of congenital dystrophic myopathy with cerebral maldevelopment; the children were subnormal or epileptic. Since then many more examples of the Fukuyama type have been reported, particularly in Japan where it is now said to be the second most prevalent form of progressive muscular dystrophy (Fukuyama, Osawa and Suzuki, 1981). The cerebral lesion varies: microgyria, white matter gliosis and demyelination have been reported (McMenamin, Becker and Murphy, 1982). The syndrome has to be distinguished from secondary hypotonia due to a cerebral defect, in which muscle is normal or shows 2b atrophy only.

Facioscapulohumeral (FSH) muscular dystrophy (Landouzy-Dejerine dystrophy)

This relatively benign dystrophy shows autosomal dominant inheritance but there is variation of expression within families. The facial involvement may cause only weak closure of the eyes or mouth, and there may be little more than winging of the scapulae even late in life; but at the other extreme children are clinically affected from 2 years of age, and unable to walk by 20 years. Usually more muscles are affected than indicated by the name, but the deltoids when chosen for biopsy may show only minimal abnormality. In the later stages the quadriceps are affected.

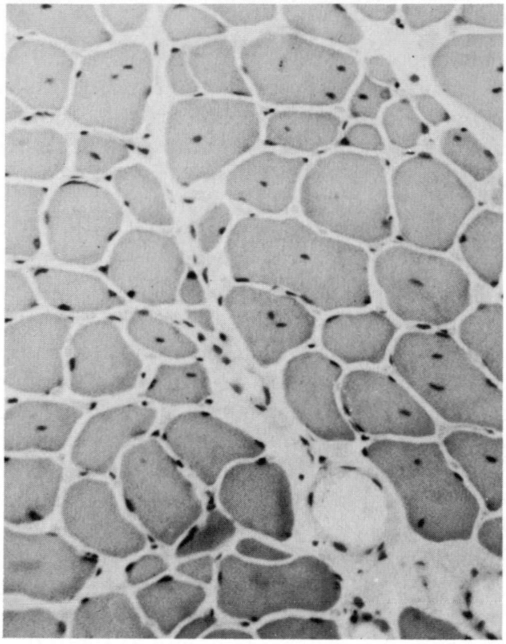

Fig. 21.47 FSH dystrophy. Numerous internal nuclei, variation in fibre calibre and splitting are shown. Haematoxylin and eosin × 190.

Serum CK varies from normal to four or five times normal. The histopathology is based on variation in fibre calibre and internal nuclei (Fig. 21.47), and eventually moderate fibrosis. Type 1 fibres show moth-eaten change and often spotted (lobulated) forms, a useful feature if not an exclusive characteristic of FSH syndrome. When the disease is relatively advanced small collections of lymphocytes are often found, but in the writer's experience they can be accounted for by degeneration. Some authors have noted profuse collections, and suspicion has been raised that polymyositis may simulate the FSH syndrome.

Other conditions which may simulate FSH syndrome are SMA type 3 (Kugelberg-Welander), the scapuloperoneal syndrome (see below), the Dreifuss type of muscular dystrophy, and mitochondrial and other congenital myopathies.

Emery-Dreifuss humeroperoneal muscular dystrophy

In 1966 Emery and Dreifuss restudied a family in which seven males in three generations were affected by a benign X-linked dystrophy. Hopkins, Jackson and Elsas (1981) reported two larger families containing 35 affected males and special investigations including muscle biopsies were performed. There were several unusual features, especially the site of contractures. The arms were bent at the elbow, the posterior cervical muscles in contracture and the Achilles tendons shortened. The biceps and triceps were affected more seriously than the deltoid (compare FSH dystrophy) and peroneal muscles affected more than the proximal. There was no pseudohypertrophy of the calves. The onset was between 5 and 15 years and progression very slow. All affected members were still able to walk, the oldest being 45. The histological picture was of varying degrees of type 1 fibre smallness compared to large type 2 fibres, slight to moderate fibrosis and internal nuclei. There was type 2 predominance in three of eight patients. One figure shows moth-eaten change in the small type 1 fibres, which were interpreted as atrophied.

Scapuloperoneal syndrome

Muscle weakness and wasting in a scapuloperoneal distribution have been observed for many years, but the diagnosis in many patients has been inconclusive because of difficulty in the interpretation of muscle biopsies. Thomas, Schott and Morgan-Hughes (1975) reported six patients with onset in early adulthood or middle age and benign progression. Two of the patients showed probable autosomal dominant inheritance. The muscle biopsies of five patients showed myopathic features of fibre calibre variation, atrophy and, sometimes, internal nuclei. At a later stage there was fibrosis and adiposity. The scapuloperoneal syndrome may also be of neurogenic origin, which is said to be commoner than the myopathic form. A variant of spinal muscular atrophy is often suggested. Further studies are required to classify this group, particularly the distinction between myopathic and pseudomyopathic histopathology.

Distal muscular dystrophy

Most dystrophies affect the proximal musculature more than the distal. A large group of cases exhibiting distal distribution, inherited as an autosomal dominant, was described in Sweden by Welander (1951). In other parts of the world distal dystrophy is rare and genetically distinct from the Welander variety (Sumner, Crawfurd and Harriman, 1971). There are no specific histological features, the pathology being that of a slowly progressive myopathy. It has to be carefully distinguished from peroneal muscular atrophy and the distal form of chronic spinal muscular atrophy (McLeod and Prineas, 1971). More recently, Edström, Thornell and Eriksson (1980) have described a dominant hereditary form of distal myopathy in which the muscle fibres contained sarcoplasmic bodies and abundant skeletin filaments.

Ocular and oculoskeletal myopathy

Extraocular muscle is peculiar in structure, differing in several aspects from skeletal muscle elsewhere. In their control of eye movements, these muscles must at times act with great speed, and at others maintain gaze for long periods by means of sustained contraction. There is a particularly rich nerve supply, the motor units containing as few as eight muscle fibres, and muscle spindles are present near the tendinous insertions. Although it has long been known that extraocular muscle fibres vary, there being three sizes of fibre, pathologists have not always been aware of this and the finding of groups of fibres of small calibre, or of groups of fibres of varying size, has led to normal extraocular muscle being described as denervated or myopathic. Ring fibres are frequent, especially in older subjects. Misdiagnosis is more frequent in biopsy specimens, especially in the tiny fragments provided at the time of corrective operations for ptosis or squint. The innervation of extraocular muscle is complex. Many fibres have a single motor endplate and others are multiply innervated like some amphibian muscle fibres. There are species differences in the organization of fibres of different sizes and types, even among mammals.

In the past few years, since histochemical methods have become available, new structural characteristics of extraocular muscle have been recognized. The situation in man has not yet been fully worked out in a sufficient number of individuals at different ages, but there appear to be three types defined by histochemical stains, each varying in size (Fig. 21.48). The three types defined by Durston (1974) in the baboon and man are recognized most easily in cryostat sections, and are coarse, fine and granular. The

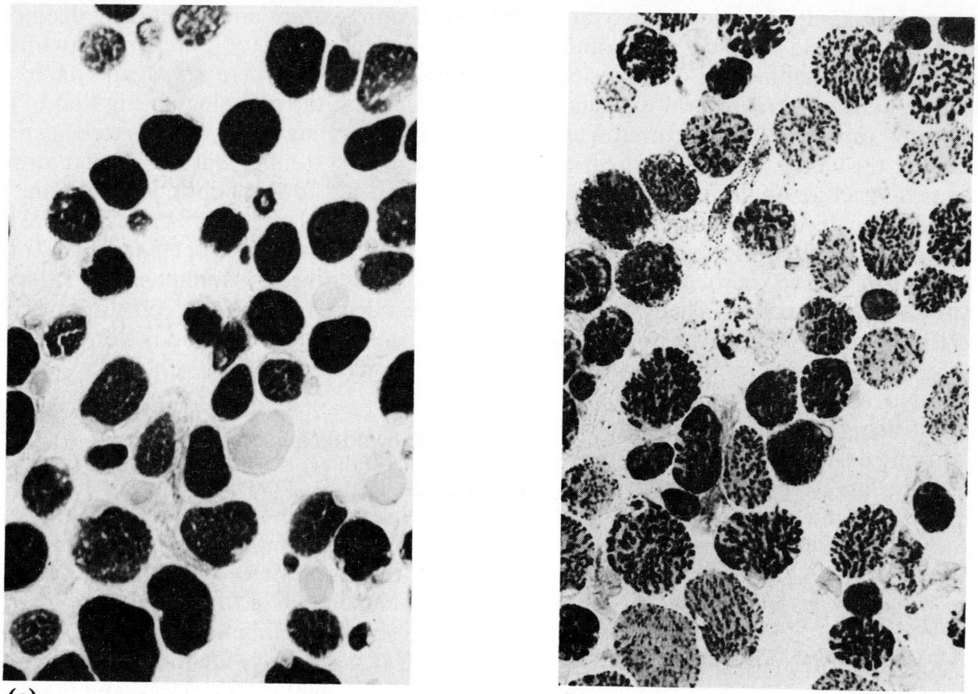

(a) **(b)**

Fig. 21.48 Extraocular muscle stained for (**a**) ATPase pH 9.4 and (**b**) NADH. The *coarse* fibres of 'Felden-struktur' pattern are shown by the ATPase stain, and react strongly with NADH. The *fine* fibres have a dense, finely stippled pattern with NADH, and react weakly for ATPase at pH 9.4. The *granular* fibres are sparsely stippled, and react strongly and uniformly with the ATPase stain. ×450.

coarse fibres correspond to those with 'felden-struktur', in which myofibrils are grouped together, the groups separated by a sparse but relatively wide intermyofibrillar network. In man these fibres have both type 1 and type 2 fibre characteristics, reacting strongly both for oxidative enzymes and for alkali-stable ATPase, and have multiple motor end-plates. The fine and granular fibres are of 'fibrillenstruktur' and resemble type 1 and type 2 fibres respectively; they are not identical with them, the fine fibres staining only moderately with oxidative enzyme stains, and the reaction of the granular fibres for phosphorylase is weak. Both fine and granular fibres have single motor end-plates.

Ocular myopathy

Patients presenting with a slow development of ptosis and limitation of ocular movements have long been described as suffering from ocular myopathy. The onset may be at any age and, although the majority are sporadic, dominant inheritance has been recognized. Some patients show undue sensitivity to curare, which may also happen in myasthenia gravis, but these patients do not respond to anticholinesterase drugs. It is doubtful whether the condition is ever confined entirely to the extraocular musculature; there may be myopathic changes in the clinically normal deltoid in patients suffering from ocular myopathy, and many patients show overt weakness elsewhere, particularly of the pharyngeal muscles (oculopharyngeal myopathy) and in the limbs (oculoskeletal or oculogeneralized myopathy). Even smooth muscle may be involved. Fortunately the histological diagnosis of ocular myopathy can usually be made by biopsy of the deltoids, biceps or triceps, as specimens from extraocular muscles are rarely obtainable and could only be minute. The changes noted are variation of fibre size, moth-eaten fibres, internal nuclei and occasional fibre type predominance, but the most characteristic are 'rimmed' vacuoles in at least a few fibres. The vacuoles are sharply defined, containing basophilic filaments at the edge, often projecting in bundles beyond and above it (see Fig. 21.26). Rimmed vacuoles occur occasionally in other disorders, but are on the whole rarely seen apart from oculoskeletal myopathy. Electron micrographs show that the vacuoles have the appearance of autophagic vacuoles of lysosomal origin and contain variegated material. Autophagic vacuoles are present in many disorders, but it is not clear why they should be rimmed under the optical microscope mainly in oculoskeletal myopathy.

Ophthalmoplegia plus (Kearns–Sayre syndrome)

Ptosis and external ocular weakness are here associated with systemic defects, such as retinitis pigmentosa, short stature, mental subnormality, deafness and defects of the conduction system of the heart. The onset is in childhood and progress is slow.

Again, arm muscle biopsies are useful, and the histopathology differs from that in oculoskeletal myopathy. Some show scattered atrophy of all

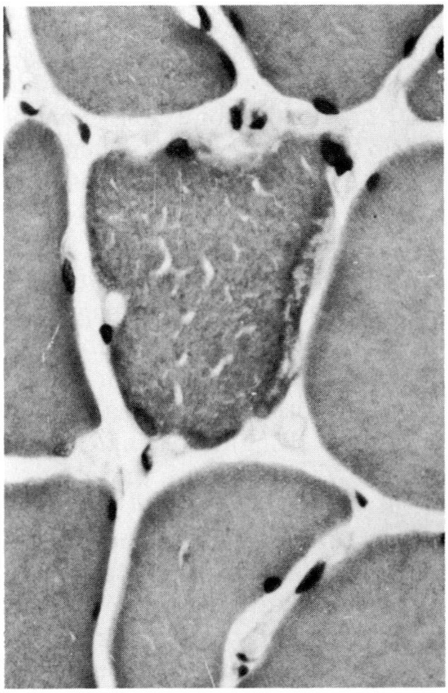

(a)

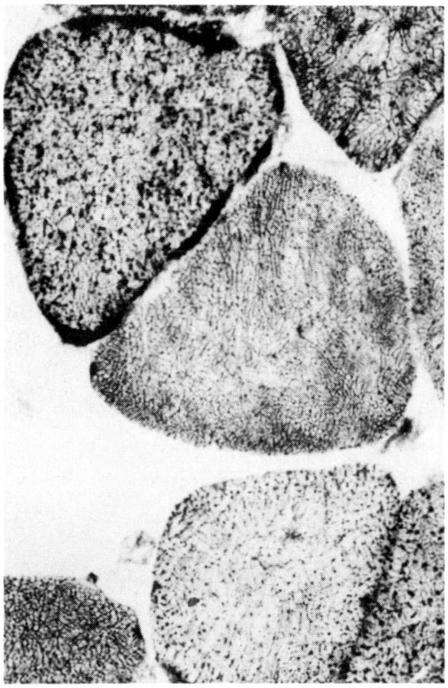

(b)

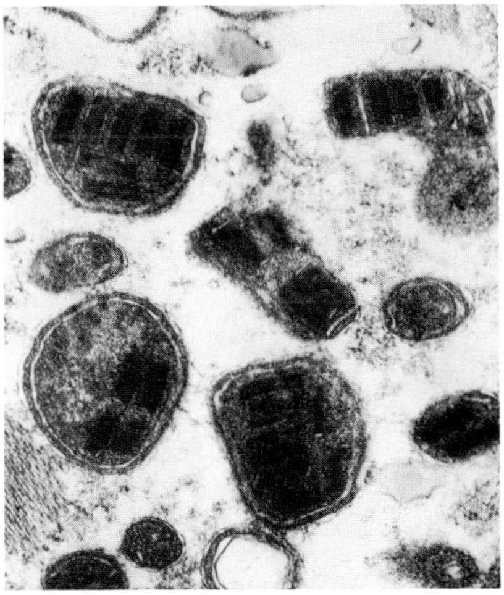

(c)

Fig. 21.49 (**a**) In 'granular' fibres the myofibrils are irregularly dispersed and basophil granules can be discerned beneath the sarcolemma. Haematoxylin and eosin × 450. (**b**) With NADH the same fibres contain excess or larger-than-normal mitochondria, dispersed and in clumps. Such fibres stain red with Gomori's method and are referred to as 'ragged-red' fibres. NADH × 450. (**c**) Abnormal mitochondria containing rectangular crystalline arrays in oculoskeletal myopathy (deltoid).

fibre types but no hypertrophy, and moth-eaten fibres are present. The main and sometimes the sole finding is of 'ragged-red' fibres, formerly called granular fibres (not to be confused with the normal granular fibres of extraocular muscle). These fibres contain large numbers of mitochondria and often lipid droplets; they separate the myofibrils, thus causing the granular appearance, and often congregate in large crescents at the periphery of the fibre. The mitochondria are often enlarged and stain more heavily than usual with NADH-TR. The peripheral mitochondrial collections generally are basophil with haematoxylin and eosin, but in the commonly used Gomori stain they are brilliantly red against the green myofibrillar background making them appear 'ragged-red'. They have to be distinguished from fibres containing mitochondria, lipid and glycogen which occur in MLG disease, first reported by Jerusalem et al. (1973) in an infant who subsequently slowly and unexpectedly recovered. Ultrastructurally the mitochondria are usually abnormal (Fig. 21.49).

Thus ophthalmoplegia plus is essentially a mitochondrial myopathy associated with diseases of other systems.

The myotonic syndromes

Dystrophia myotonica (myotonic muscular dystrophy)

This is a multisystem disorder characterized by cataract, gonadal atrophy, frontal baldness, ptosis, myocardial involvement and myopathy. There is often mental subnormality. The muscle affected, unlike most other forms of dystrophy, is predominantly distal in the limbs, but there is usually early wasting of the sternomastoids. Facial and jaw weakness produce a sagging, open mouth. The inheritance is autosomal and dominant. Although symptoms do not usually appear until the second or third decade, the occurrence of the disease in children has recently been recognized and it is yet another cause of infantile hypotonia. The course of the disease is slow, and nearly always includes a period during which myotonia occurs: this means muscle contraction persisting after the cessation of voluntary effort, so the patient is, for example, unable to relax his grip for a time, and the muscles generally feel stiff. Myotonia may disappear after a number of years, and some patients never suffer from it.

The muscle shows a number of myopathic features not individually specific but suggestive of a myotonic disorder when seen in combination (Fig. 21.50). Internal nuclei, up to six or more in a transverse section, form long internal rows in longitudinal section. Ring fibres and sarcoplasmic masses may be numerous: the latter are peripheral areas of a fibre devoid of myofibrils, sometimes separated from the myofibril column by a ring fibre and containing disintegrated myofilaments and various organelles. When the changes are not advanced, type 1 fibres show only varying degrees of atrophy, and some single small angular fibres are formed (Fig. 21.51); type

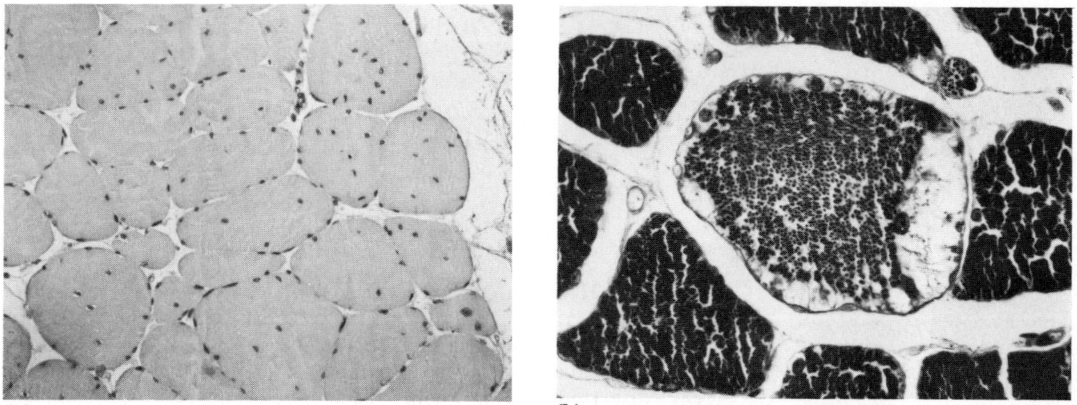

(a) (b)

Fig. 21.50 Dystrophia myotonica. (**a**) Numerous internal nuclei are present in many fibres. Haematoxylin and eosin × 180. (**b**) Myofibrils withdraw from parts of the sarcolemma to form 'sarcoplasmic masses'. PTAH × 480.

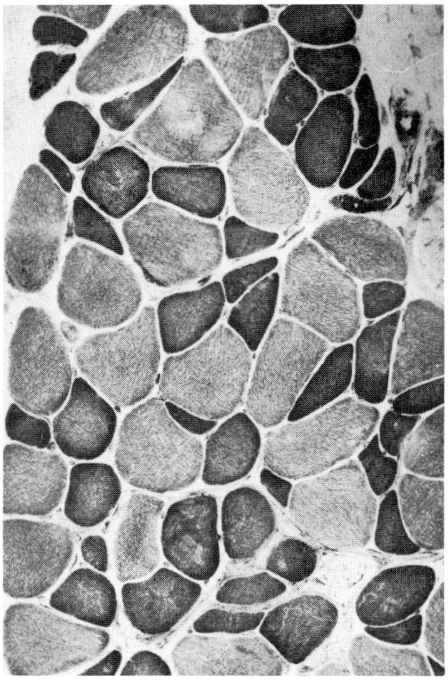

Fig. 21.51 Early stage in dystrophia myotonica with large type 2 fibres and some atrophied type 1 fibres. NADH × 110.

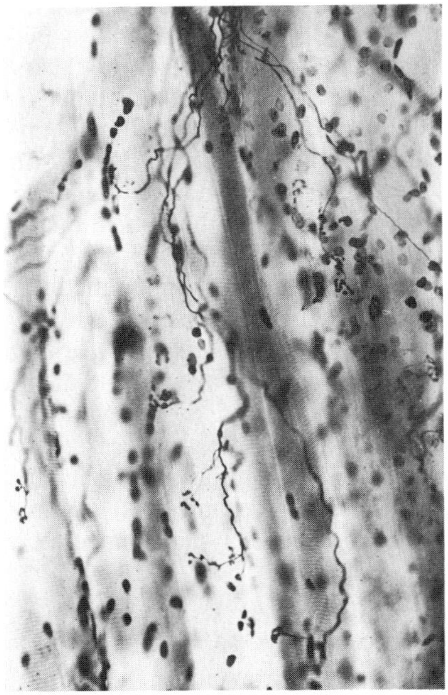

Fig. 21.52 The subterminal fibres can be followed to several large and complex end-plates, but there is no collateral reinnervation. Methylene blue × 180.

2 fibres at this stage are large or hypertrophied. At later stages the type 2 fibres are also affected by size variation. Fibre necrosis and regeneration occur, but are not usually prominent. Muscle spindles, particularly those in the more distal muscles and in advanced disease, show an interesting change (Daniel and Strich, 1964). There is a great increase in the number of intrafusal muscle fibres and so up to 60 small fibres may be found, the normal maximum in man being 14 or 15. The increase results from longitudinal fibre splitting (Swash and Fox, 1975), and is likely to be the result of abnormal tension on the spindle produced by sustained contraction. The motor end-plates are abnormal in myotonic dystrophy; some very large complexes are formed, with multiple distal sprouts, generally larger and more elaborate than in other myopathies. There is, however, no definite evidence of denervation in the form of collateral reinnervation (Fig. 21.52).

Myotonia congenita (Thomsen's disease)

This benign condition differs from myotonic dystrophy in that the clinical picture is confined to the muscles in the form of myotonia and sometimes muscle hypertrophy. The myotonia develops in infancy or at any time later, and is liable to be made worse by cold. The inheritance is usually autosomal dominant, but an autosomal recessive variant has been described in Germany. Histologically, muscle fibres are normal or large with large end-plates, but in about half there are more definite myopathic changes with internal nuclei and ring fibres. They are surpassed by the myopathy of myotonic dystrophy.

Some patients are unaware of their disease, as shown by a small number detected on biopsy for susceptibility to malignant hyperthermia (MH). They were not susceptible to MH but showed clinical and pathological features of myotonia congenita. There are three groups of patients who react paradoxically to the suxamethonium by muscle spasm instead of relaxation when used during induction of anaesthesia. The first are susceptible to MH, of which it is a common feature; the second suffer from a myotonic disorder; and the third are otherwise normal individuals who react idiosyncratically to the drug (scoline spasm).

Type 2b fibres have been reported absent in eight patients with myotonia congenita. The significance of this is uncertain, for the same absence has been noted in five out of a large series of normal biopsies. In each case the histochemical reactions were repeated with controls. In one, the 2b fibres were absent from one specimen and present in a second, suggesting that absence could be focal.

Torsion dystonia

In this disorder of central origin, voluntary effort produces continuous and slowly writhing muscle contraction. The writer has had the opportunity to biopsy a young man who suffered an episode of cerebral hypoxia and developed torsion dystonia afterwards. The muscle changes of fibre hypertrophy and numerous internal nuclei suggested that dystonia as well as the myotonic syndromes could result in muscle hypertrophy and internally displaced nuclei.

Paramyotonia congenita

Myotonia is often precipitated by cold, but when it is accompanied by attacks of weakness, both being induced by cold, the term 'paramyotonia' is used. A family comprising 157 related individuals has been described by de Jong, Slooff and van der Eerden (1973). It is inherited as an autosomal dominant trait. The muscle in one of them showed changes like those in myotonic dystrophy with the addition of vacuoles.

Periodic paralysis

This occurs in four different clinical forms, the first three usually being genetically determined and autosomal dominant, and the last sporadic. All seem to be related to the passage into and out of the muscle fibre of the cation potassium, and characteristically are associated with vacuole formation during and after attacks, some containing glycogen.

In *hypokalaemic periodic paralysis*, a healthy young adult wakens unable to move but can breathe normally, talk and smile. The attacks last for 6–24 hours, occasionally longer, and the plasma potassium is low. In *hyperkalaemic periodic paralysis* the attacks usually come on after exercise, typically after resting for 30 minutes. Most attacks are short and are over within 1–2 hours. There may be symptoms of mild myotonia, but the condition is genetically distinct from paramyotonia congenita. The serum potassium rises, and weakness occurs at levels which leave normal subjects unaffected. In severely affected members of families suffering from periodic hypo- or hyperkalaemia, a permanent myopathy ensues after several years. Histologically there is fibre necrosis and regeneration, fibre calibre variation, fibrosis and striking vacuole formation (Fig. 21.53). In the early stages or in mildly affected individuals vacuoles may not be visible with the optical microscope but electron micrographs show dilatation of the lateral sacs of the sarcoplasmic reticulum. The writer has found end-plates enlarged by terminal sprouting. In *normokalaemic periodic paralysis* the attacks are similar to those of the hyperkalaemic variety, but are more severe and of much longer duration—days or weeks. The fourth form of periodic paralysis is associated with thyrotoxicosis, is rare and is *hypokalaemic*. The thyroid disorder may not immediately be obvious.

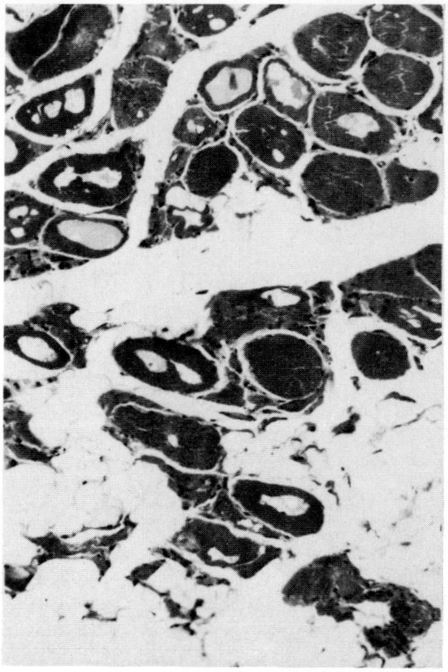

Fig. 21.53 Permanent myopathy following many years of periodic paralysis. Vacuoles are prominent and persistent. Haematoxylin and eosin × 280.

The inflammatory myopathies

All myopathies in which the principal findings are inflammatory cell infiltrates (mainly lymphocytes, plasma cells and a few polymorphs), usually accompanied by necrosis and regeneration, are grouped under this heading. Until recently most were simply referred to as polymyositis, but that term is now reserved for inflammatory conditions in which the pathogenesis is unknown or not yet fully worked out. The second group includes disorders with a recognized causative agent—bacterial, viral, protozoal etc.

Polymyositis and dermatomyositis

Polymyositis is an acquired myopathy which may occur at any age, with its highest incidence in adults of 30–60 years. Females are affected twice as often as males. The inflammatory reaction which occurs in the muscles is thought to be due to a disturbance of the immune system; lymphocytes from patients with polymyositis have been shown to be sensitized to muscle tissue. Much immunological investigation has been made, but some at least detecting epiphenomena. The consensus at present is that the reactions are cell-mediated. It has been found that the lymphocytes are predominantly T-cells, and that they are myocytotoxic. (A substantial review can be found in Mastaglia and Walton, 1982.) The routine use of immunoperoxidase reactions in polymyositis, both polyclonal and monoclonal, is helpful in distinguishing the types of infiltrating cell. A viral infection may be the initiating factor, as picorna-, myxo- and Coxsackie-virus-like particles have been seen in affected muscle, but not proven by culture. About one-fifth of adult cases are associated with a carcinoma, suggesting that a secretion or breakdown product of the tumour may then be the precipitant. Signs of the tumour may not appear until some time after the myositis, and its removal has on occasion caused remission of the muscular condition. In older patients the incidence of neoplasm is probably much higher, but a percentage figure cannot be given because of failure to distinguish polymyositis or dermatomyositis from other reactions to carcinoma such as peripheral neuropathy, carcinomatous neuromyopathy or cachectic atrophy.

Muscles are affected either symmetrically or asymmetrically by weakness, sometimes with tenderness and even swelling of muscles; the neck and trunk muscles are frequently involved and the proximal limb muscles. Rarely, the extraocular muscles are affected, sometimes exclusively but with an inflammatory reaction also in the retro-orbital fat (orbital myositis). The skin shows no changes, or there may be dusky-red patches over joints. The upper lids may have a violaceous tinge. If there are more florid changes, such as a dusky-red eruption on the face in a butterfly distribution, and on the trunk and limbs, mottled or diffuse, the condition is described as dermatomyositis; there is no clear dividing line between it and polymyositis. The course of the disease is as variable as the symptomatology, there being acute, subacute and chronic forms. The prognosis was formerly thought to be grave, although spontaneous recovery occurred in some children and probably accounted for the reports of recovery from 'muscular dystrophy' made in the earlier part of this century (Nattrass, 1954). It has been transformed in children by the use of steroids, remission and recovery being the rule, and improved in adults by steroids and immunosuppressives. Fatalities still occur, especially when the myocardium is involved. In a few patients nodular calcification (calcinosis) of subcutaneous tissues or in muscle is visible radiologically.

Histology. Two processes occur simultaneously in the muscle: interstitial inflammation, and necrosis and regeneration of muscle fibres. These are not interdependent, as one or other process can be seen alone. The inflammatory reaction occurs in the form of diffuse infiltration of muscle fascicles by lymphocytes and plasma cells (Fig. 21.54). These tend to congregate around small blood vessels, and infiltrate their adventia, but fibrinoid necrosis is rare. Occasionally the infiltrating cells include large numbers of eosinophils (eosinophil myositis), and a fruitless search is then made for parasitic infection of the muscle. In many cases there is also nodular infiltration (Fig. 21.55), lymphocytes being congregated into follicles, some of which develop germinal centres. Capillaries with prominent endothelium can usually be made out within the follicles, and some plasma cells. Segmental necrosis and regeneration are frequent: affected fibres are marginated by lymphocytes and histiocytes, and while phagocytosis is in progress lymphocytes can usually be recognized as well as histiocytes within the necrotic muscle segments (Fig. 21.56). Occasionally a large area of muscle undergoes necrosis (infarction). Sometimes large groups of small regenerating fibres are found. In the course of time, fibre calibre variation de-

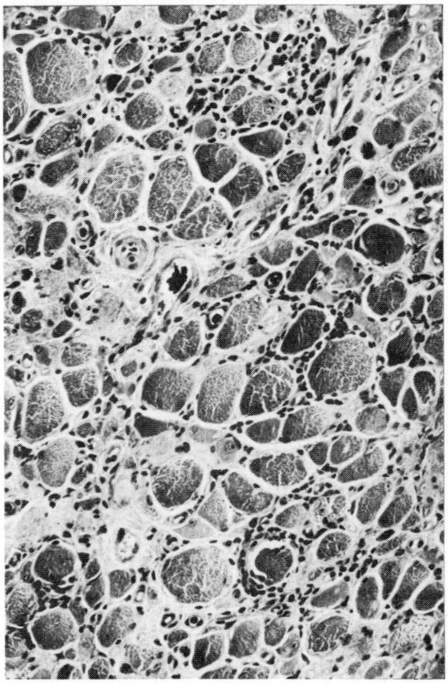

Fig. 21.54 Diffuse infiltration of lymphocytes and some plasma cells among muscle fibres of varying calibre in polymyositis. Haematoxylin and eosin × 180.

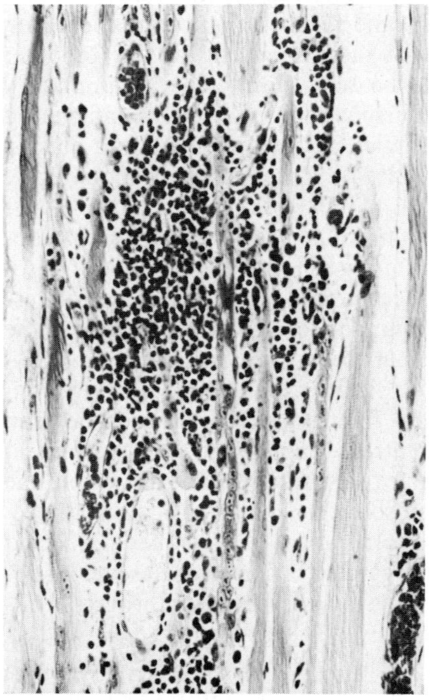

Fig. 21.55 Nodular infiltration of lymphocytes and plasma cells between normal and regenerating muscle fibres. Haematoxylin and eosin × 180.

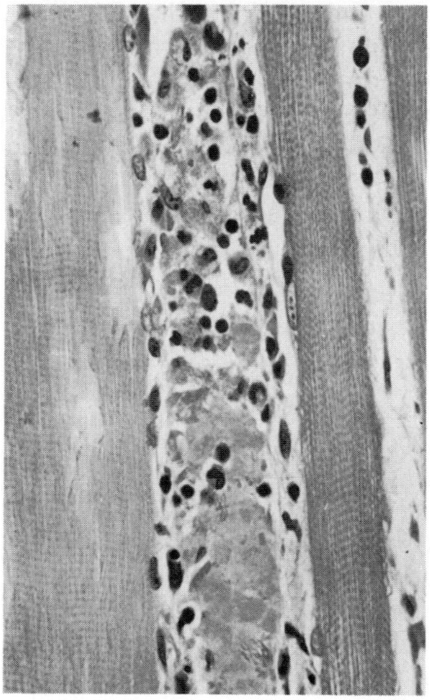

Fig. 21.56 Polymyositis. Lymphocytes accompany histiocytes in the phagocytic process. Haematoxylin and eosin × 420.

velops, and vacuolated fibres are not infrequent. As muscle fibres are destroyed, fibrosis develops. The rate of progress of the disease is reflected in the histopathology; in mild forms necrosis and cellular infiltrations are scanty, and fibrosis develops slowly (subacute and chronic polymyositis). The motor innervation generally shows deformity and sprouting from end-plates only, but in a minority the inflammatory response destroys part of the subterminal innervation, resulting in patchy collateral reinnervation. (Denervation of individual muscle fibres is thought to be responsible for the fibrillation potentials which are seen in polymyositis on electromyography.) Very rarely, calcification takes place. Amorphous deposits are formed in the epimysium or, more frequently, in the subcutaneous fat, accompanied by lymphocytic infiltration.

In *dermatomyositis* the histological changes in the skin are non-specific lymphocytic infiltrates, sometimes perivascular, and capillary congestion. Adipose tissue is similarly affected, sometimes to the extent of lipoatrophy. Calcification is commoner in adipose tissue than in muscle in both types of myositis. Muscle histopathology differs slightly. In dermatomyositis there is less infiltration of muscle fascicles by lymphocytes, and the process is more active in the epimysium. The resulting fibrous thickening of the epimysium is accompanied by atrophy of muscle fibres at the edge of fascicles (Fig. 21.57). It is seen only occasionally in polymyositis. In children, the histopathology of polymyositis and dermatomyositis is often the same as in adults. Banker and Victor (1966), however, described angiitis as a prominent feature in eight children who came to autopsy; in addition to perivascular collections of lymphocytes, there developed subintimal hyperplasia and thrombosis with consequent foci

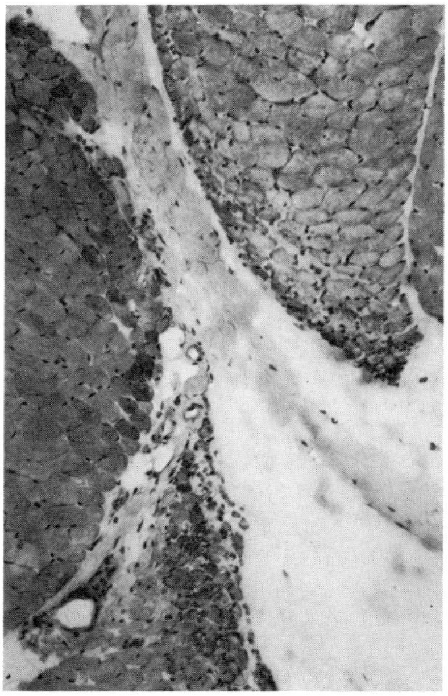

Fig. 21.57 In dermatomyositis the fibrous thickening of the epimysium is often accompanied by atrophy of muscle fibres at the edge of the fascicles. PAS × 120.

of muscular infarction. They considered childhood dermatomyositis to be a different disease. Nevertheless, the recognition of a vasculitic form at biopsy in children has been infrequent.

The diagnosis of polymyositis is made with ease when both inflammatory change and the effects of necrosis are present. An unusual diagnostic pitfall is infiltration of muscle by lymphosarcoma. Not infrequently patients with polymyositis on clinical and serological grounds, responding to treatment, show only necrosis and regeneration (necrotizing myopathy). The chronic fibrosing type of polymyositis may be indistinguishable histologically from muscular dystrophy.

Myositis fibrosa (myosclerosis)

Rarer forms of 'myositis' appear to be due to a primary proliferation of active fibroblasts, especially in the endomysium; there is no evidence of inflammation but individual muscle fibres are 'strangled' by the overgrowth. When the proliferation is massive and myogenic giant cells are produced, the term 'proliferative myositis' is used. This can also follow muscle injury. The classification of the fibromatoses of muscle is unsatisfactory, and should distinguish between those which follow polymyositis and those in which there is at no stage an inflammatory element. An example of the former occurs when polymyositis is followed by the slow proliferation of fibrocytes over 20 years or more, replacing the muscle by woody-hard fibrous tissue.

Vasculitic disease

Polymyositis may be associated with other collagen–vascular diseases. Polyarteritis nodosa (Fig. 21.58) involving many systems may affect the arteries in muscles, enabling its diagnosis by blind muscle biopsy. Sometimes it is associated with muscle weakness and wasting, and the muscle shows either polymyositis or neurogenic

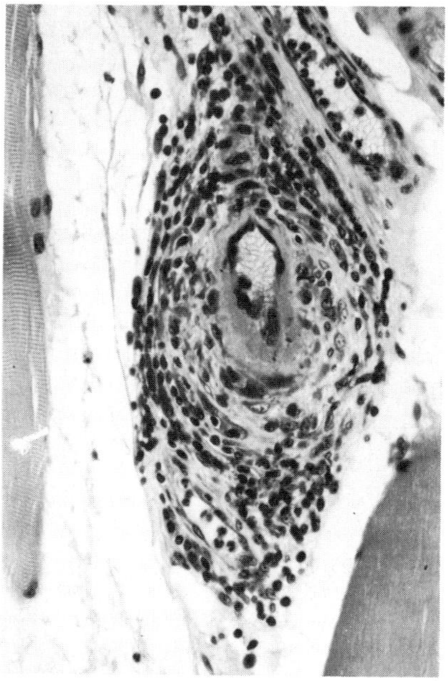

Fig. 21.58 Arteritis. A small artery shows fibrinoid necrosis of its wall and infiltration by lymphocytes and plasma cells. Haematoxylin and eosin × 280.

atrophy (due to polyarteritis affecting peripheral nerves). Small vessel angiitis may also affect muscle widely and be associated with myositis. The weakness and wasting which often develop in rheumatoid arthritis have a variety of causes acting singly or in combination: cachectic atrophy, polymyositis, arteritis and rheumatoid neuropathy. When polymyositis is found, the proportion of plasma cells is high. Muscular weakness is not common in systemic lupus erythematosus, but when muscle disorder is suspected a biopsy will show myositis. A particular feature is vacuole formation within muscle fibres, the vacuoles often enclosing an internally placed muscle nucleus. Myositis may accompany systemic sclerosis (scleroderma). The changes are predominantly in the epimysium, and thickening of small blood vessel walls is noted. It is claimed that smooth muscle is also involved in systemic sclerosis. In Sjögren's syndrome there is characteristically destruction of the ducts of the salivary and lacrimal glands, both being infiltrated by large numbers of plasma cells. A number of patients also present with muscle weakness, and show myositis with a similar predominance of plasma cell reactions.

Behçet's disease is occasionally complicated by myositis or venous infarction. One of the writer's patients showed a mild myositis at the age of 14, and years later her young son developed painful legs and a CPK of 5020. Recovery was rapid. Infarction was presumed.

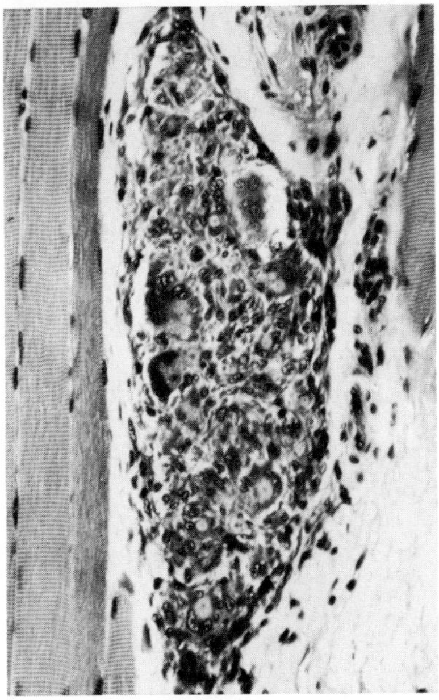

Fig. 21.59 Sarcoid granuloma in skeletal muscle, consisting of epithelioid cells, giant cells and lymphocytes. Haematoxylin and eosin × 280.

Sarcoid myopathy

Sarcoid nodules, which are sometimes palpable, are found in skeletal muscle in the majority of patients with sarcoidosis. Clinical involvement of muscle is much less frequent, but in some patients muscular weakness is the presenting feature. The muscle characteristically shows noncaseating granulomas consisting of epithelioid cells, giant cells and lymphocytes in the epimysium or within fascicles (Fig. 21.59).

Granulomatous myositis

Many still assume that this condition is a form of sarcoid myopathy, and that all granulomas in muscle are sarcoid granulomas. Coërs and Carbone (1966) reviewed the literature and found 18 cases in which muscle contained granulomas which had been assimilated into the diagnosis of sarcoid. Their own three cases, however, provided no evidence of lesions elsewhere, and they found one autopsy report in which granulomas were confined to muscle. They thought that there was a distinctive syndrome of a late myopathy in females, characterized not so much by granulomas but by a more diffuse infiltration of small epithelioid cells, in which there was no justification for the diagnosis of sarcoidosis. It is well known that there are many causes of epitheloid cell formation, and unless sarcoid can be proven it should not be used to explain granulomatous myositis. Another form of granuloma in muscle may be found in Crohn's disease.

Inclusion body myositis

Although by title this form of myositis ought to be due to a virus, its aetiology remains unknown. It differs from polymyositis by occurring chiefly in males over 60, with a relatively benign chronic course. There is little inflammation as weakness develops without pain in the limbs. It is not associated with malignancy. Histologically, two types of inclusions are seen by light microscopy—small basophil inclusions within fibres, and large acidophil hyaline bodies almost filling fibres in transverse section. On electron microscopy multilamellated bodies are found, and within nuclei masses of filamentous microtubules. These could be viral but no virus has been cultured from the muscle.

Inflammatory myopathies due to known organisms

These are due to viruses, bacteria, parasites and fungi.

Viral myositis

In influenza aching in the limbs is common, and in the postinfective phase it may become severe. Serum CK rises, and although biopsies are rare in this condition an inflammatory reaction is seen and virus has been cultured at least once from the muscle. The occurrence of myalgia after the initial infection suggests that the inflammatory response is due to an immune reaction. Infections with other viruses such as Coxsackie and echo groups may be associated with a more severe necrotizing myositis causing myoglobinuria.

Infections of muscle

Abscess in muscle is quite commonly seen in the tropics, and appears as a painful swelling in a patient with pyrexia. Often the pus is sterile. Gas gangrene occurs when anaerobic organisms such as *Clostridium welchii* invade tissue damaged by wounding or accident. Extensive necrosis and infiltration by the bacteria result with little pus initially.

Parasitic infections

The larval form of the whipworm *Trichinella spiralis* and the larva of the pork tapeworm *Taenia solium* (cysticercosis) may be found in human muscle. Biopsy of a tender muscle may reveal the organism. Cysticercosis may cause muscular pseudohypertrophy. In Chagas' disease, *Trypanosoma cruzi* invades muscle as well as other tissues and produces a polymyositis-like lesion. In toxoplasmosis, muscle may be invaded and *Toxoplasma gondii* are recognized as collections of minute pear-shaped or crescentic organisms within pseudocysts. The neighbouring tissue shows necrosis, regeneration and lymphocytic infiltration.

Amyloid myopathy

Whilst amyloid may be deposited in the interstitial tissues of muscle in secondary and especially in primary amyloidosis, massive deposition causing a myopathy is rare. Amyloid infiltration may cause pain and muscle hypertrophy.

Infantile hypotonia (the floppy baby syndrome)

It is not uncommon for infants to be floppy at birth, but it is usually transient. When it persists, and milestones are reached late, it gives cause for concern. The infant is like a rag doll, slips through the examiner's fingers easily and cannot hold its head up in the prone or supine position. A muscle biopsy may be thought necessary, and if the muscle fibres are of normal size or show no more than type 2b atrophy the baby will be suffering from benign congenital hypotonia or from secondary hypotonia due to a cerebral defect such as a malformation. A CT scan is then useful. The cause of benign congenital hypotonia is not known but carries a good prognosis, disappearing in months or, rarely, years. But there are many congenital myopathies whose presenting sign is hypotonia, and the most experienced clinicians find it difficult to detect associated weakness in the earlier stages. Even paralysis can be masked by severe hypotonia, as in SMA type 1 (Werdnig–Hoffmann). In the writer's experience about half of the infants biopsied suffer from benign congenital hypotonia or secondary ('cerebral') hypotonia and the remainder from SMA type 1 or from one of a variety of congenital myopathies. Cerebral hypotonia may precede spasticity (Little's disease).

The congenital myopathies

Many of these are the result of an error at some stage of muscle development, or are due to the onset of disease during intrauterine life. If the muscle deficit is severe and widespread, death will occur in the neonatal period, but many congenital myopathies are mild and non-progressive, and compatible with a normal life-span.

Arthrogryposis

Arthrogryposis, or arthrogryposis multiplex congenita, was at first considered to be a distinct entity caused *in utero*. Infants were born with almost immovable limbs in abnormal postures, looking as though they had been forced somehow into malposition, their 'curved joints' giving rise to the name. When muscle was examined in detail it became obvious that there was no single cause. Some showed a picture interpreted as neurogenic, although the effect on muscle of a fixed joint was not always considered. In others the picture was myopathic, therefore interpreted as congenital dystrophic myopathy. In the writer's opinion the most frequent finding is of normal muscle, the aetiology of the joint disability remaining unknown. This has been also the experience of a number of colleagues personally consulted. Although arthrogryposis occurs occasionally with other myopathies such as myotonic dystrophy and congenital fibre type disproportion, there is no condition which invariably causes it.

Central core disease

Cores (see Figs. 21.22–21.25) have already been described as structural change in muscle fibres, best seen in NADH-TR preparations as sharply defined foci of absent staining. Losses of mitochondria and of intermyofibrillar substance are responsible for the pale cores. Although non-specific, they occur most prominently in central core disease. The first case described had many single centrally placed cores, although some fibres contained up to five eccentric ones. They were well seen in paraffin sections. In subsequent cases, cores were often faint or invisible in embedded sections, explained by the variation in ultrastructure of cores. Mitochondria were always absent, but myofibrils could be normal or show various degrees of coagulation and fragmentation, making the cores universally visible.

Many cases have now been reported of this congenital myopathy which is inherited as an autosomal dominant but can be sporadic. It rarely causes hypotonia in infancy, but the disability is often slight, with mild proximal lower limb weakness and lack of progression. Increasing disability does occur in some patients, but is slight and so the disorder can be considered benign. As in some other congenital myopathies, there are not infrequently associated skeletal deformities, especially congenital dislocation of the hip.

The cores are virtually always confined to type 1 fibres, and there is almost always type 1 fibre preponderance. This can be so marked that there may be no more than two or three type 2 fibres in the section. One family has been described in which the mother had typical central core disease but two children showed type 1 preponderance without cores. The writer has seen cores increase moderately in two biopsies separated by an interval of 10 years. Another feature the writer has noticed in the biopsies, not usually reported by others although on occasion visible in illustrations, is an association with moth-eaten fibres. It is not a surpising finding in view of the ultrastructural changes which cores and moth-eaten fibres have in common. In many case reports there are no other significant changes, but on occasion variation in fibre calibre develops, including atrophic fibres. When motor end-plates are examined, and in the writer's material also, the terminal arborizations are normal apart from occasional terminal sprouting. It has been suggested that cores may be due to intrauterine denervation, but if so it takes place without collateral reinnervation.

When type 1 fibre preponderance is not present, central core disease can be confused with the myopathy of malignant hyperthermia (MH). Distinction can be helped by biopsying other affected members of the family. In central core

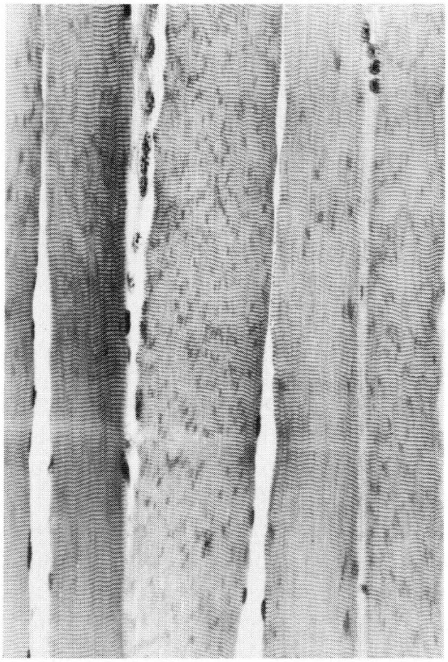

Fig. 21.60 'Minicore' disease. Some fibres shown very numerous foci of smearing of the striations. × 280.

disease the same pattern of cores will usually appear, but siblings susceptible to MH produce a variety of structural changes or none at all: they do not usually breed true in histopathology. The distinction is academic, as many (but not all) patients with central core disease are also susceptible to MH. The association is now well established, so a diagnosis of central core disease should lead to testing for susceptibility to MH.

The variants of central core disease, multicore disease and minicore disease, have already been described morphologically (Fig. 21.60). Their inheritance is usually assumed to be the same as in central core disease, but the number of cases is too few for certainty. A mild proximal myopathy greater in the lower limbs with a benign course is generally reported, but in one of the writer's patients weakness was generalized although not severe.

Rod body myopathy

This was originally and incorrectly called nemaline myopathy. The solecism was invented because it was first suspected that the tiny rods were not discrete but formed undulating threads. No one now doubts that the particles are separate, so there is no justification for retaining the term.

Most early reports were of a mild non-progressive myopathy in children, but as the number of cases grew it was realized that the involvement of muscle could be severe and extensive and a cause of death in infancy. The tiny rods and granules (Fig. 21.61) lie within fibres and can be difficult to see with haematoxylin and eosin. The Gomori stain, however, shows them up readily as red granules or tiny rods, often congregated; they have to be distinguished from mitochondria and from tubular aggregates which also stain red by Gomori in frozen sections. In paraffin sections a lightly stained PTAH is useful.

Electron microscopy depicts the rods as irregular masses of Z-band material. They are resistant to *post mortem* change and so can be recognized in *post mortem* electron micrographs.

Rods are found in any position in the cytoplasm of affected fibres but more often at the periphery. They are roughly rectangular or elongated, depending on the plane of section. In length they may reach 5 μm. In diameter they approximate to that of myofibrils, up to 1 μm. Filaments similar to actin filaments are attached to them.

Histopathology. There is no characteristic pattern for rod body myopathy. Biopsies may reveal normal fibre size apart from the presence of widely differing numbers of rods and granules, or there may be fibre calibre variation including atrophic ones. Their presence with many stains such as the ATPases is indicated by clear spaces, and serial sections are necessary to discover which fibre types are involved. They have been described in type 2 fibres only, type 1 only or in both. Post-mortem reports show that there is considerable variation from muscle to muscle or even within a muscle, so it is not wise to base prognosis on a single small biopsy. Although rod body myopathy is a distinct clinical entity, the rods are not specific; they may be found in small numbers in many other myopathies and are also formed during the disintegration of muscle fibres undergoing denervation. They were found unexpectedly in large numbers in the soleus in Adie's syndrome when searching for a neural or muscular cause for the areflexia, but their significance in that disorder is still not known (Harriman, 1970).

Clinically the disease is well defined. The very severely affected infants who die in the first year or so are in a minority. More often there is hypotonia, delayed motor development and characteristically slender muscles which are stronger than they look. The widespread distribution of muscle involvement accounts for nasal speech and facial weakness. As with other congenital myopathies, there may be skeletal abnormality including a high arched palate and scoliosis. Children are moderately disabled, and deterioration does occur. The mildest cases are those with an onset in adult life.

Initially many cases were thought to be sporadic, but sufficient families have now been reported to suggest an autosomal dominant inheritance.

Centronuclear myopathy

In this congenital myopathy the extraocular and facial muscles are affected in nearly all patients reported. Muscle involvement is generalized, so partial ophthalmoplegia and facial weakness are joined by disturbance of gait and general wasting and weakness of muscle. The condition is com-

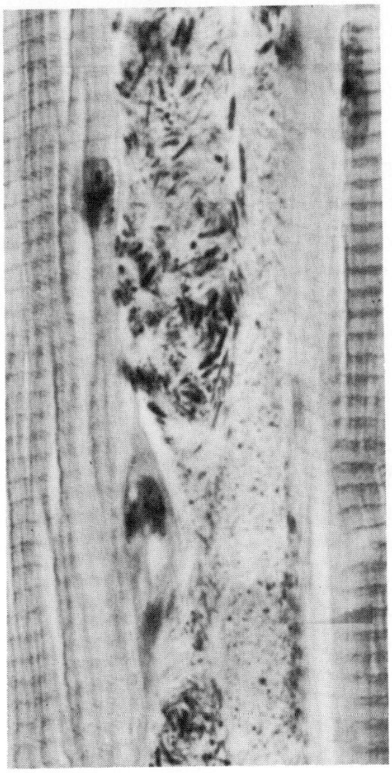

(a)

Fig. 21.61 Rod body myopathy (**a**) The rods are formed of Z-line material, and congregate as threads and granules at the edge of the muscle fibre. PTAH × 950. (**b**) The rods are composed of Z-band material with some filaments attached. Bar = 0.5 μm.

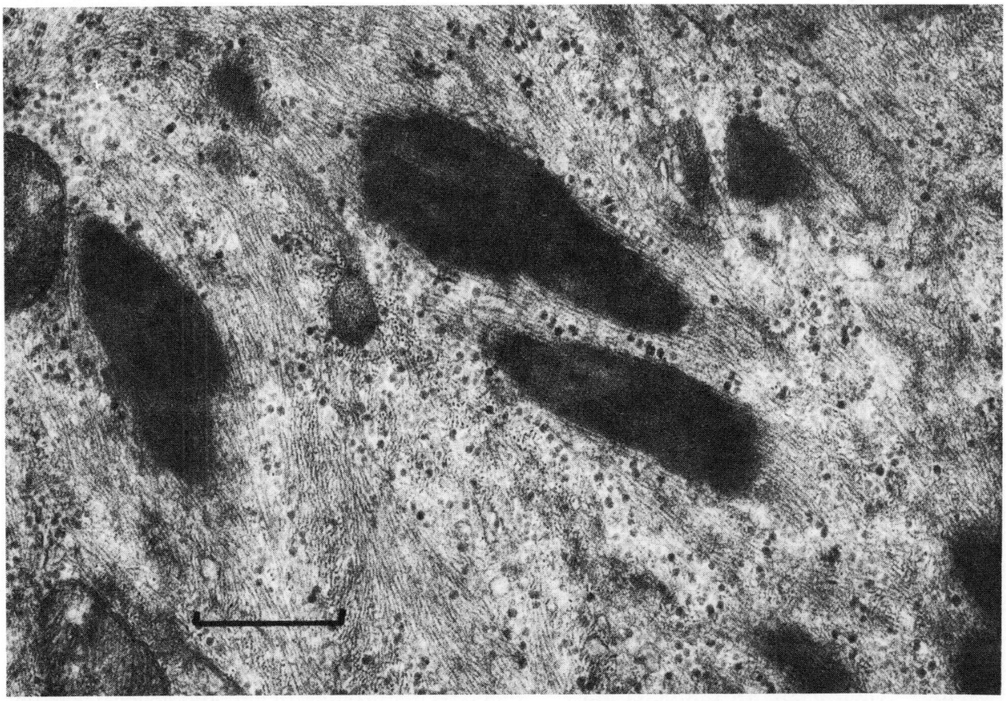

(b)

patible with a normal life-span, but a few infants have been severely affected and have died in childhood. The essential histological feature is the presence of large numbers of muscle fibres with nuclei in their exact centre as well as subsarcolemmal (Fig. 21.62). As in infants they resemble myotubes, the first report described the condition as myotubular myopathy. But many structural details are different, including size and the absence of a large perinuclear halo, so 'centronuclear' is more appropriate. In longitudinal sections the nuclei are distributed in long rows. Histochemical analysis placed patients in two groups (Harriman and Haleem, 1972): those with uniform enzyme activity; and those with two types of fibre, small and larger, corresponding roughly in enzyme reaction to type 1 and type 2 respectively.

Recognition of the disease in old age has been reported.

Congenital fibre type disproportion

This was the term devised by Dubowitz and Brooke (1973) to describe a group of children in whom type 1 fibres were universally smaller than type 2 (the mean diameters differing by at least 12 per cent). Affected children have all been floppy at birth, and show a weakness of all muscle groups, varying from mild to severe. There is a tendency to improvement after 2 years

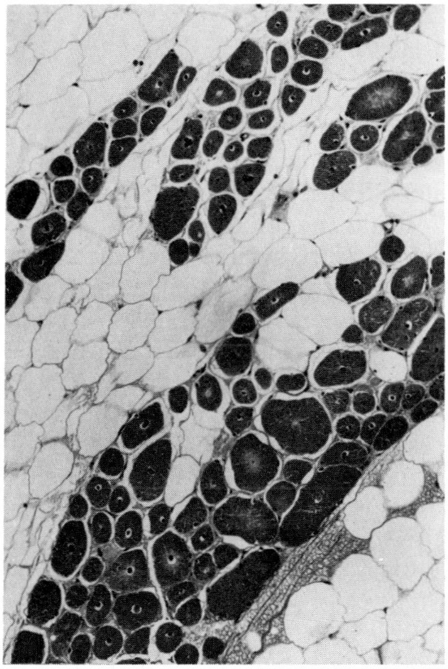

Fig. 21.62 Centronuclear myopathy. Nuclei are found in the centre of each fibre, usually enclosed by a small halo. Haematoxylin and eosin × 120.

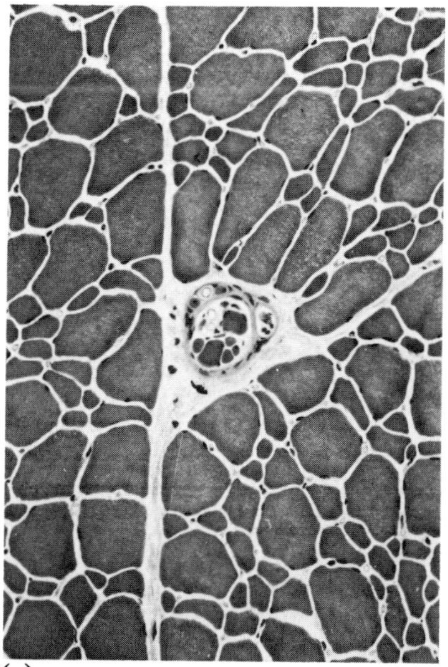

(a)

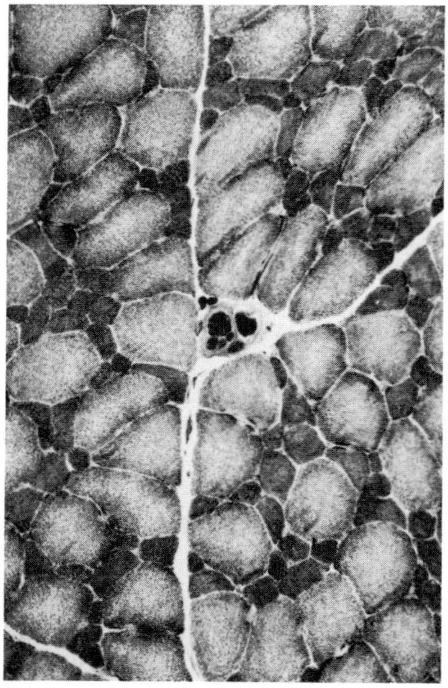

(b)

Fig. 21.63 Congenital fibre type disproportion. (**a**) There are two distinct populations of fibres—large and small. Haematoxylin and eosin × 180. (**b**) Serial section to show that the small fibres are type 1 and the large type 2. HADH × 180.

of age, although one of the writer's patients was 14 years old and still weak, with universally thin muscles. The discrepancy in size between the two fibre types can be considerable, and if histochemical stains are not applied the resulting picture with routine stains can be confused with neurogenic atrophy (Fig. 21.63). In some infants the small type 1 fibres have central nuclei, and the condition then appears to be intermediate between congenital fibre type disproportion and centronuclear myopathy. Clearly, type 1 fibres are slow in developing in this disorder, but do get larger as the child becomes older. The enlarged type 2 fibres may be a hypertrophic response.

Although Dubowitz and Brooke (1973) have laid down the relative mean diameter of the two fibre types as a result of careful measurements, it seems to the writer that a difference of 12 per cent is too modest. There have been reports of congenital fibre type disproportion developing into a benign dystrophy, suggesting that the appearance is not specific. It is very likely that specificity exists only when the disproportion is greater than 12 per cent, and needs to be reassessed.

Myopathy with tubular aggregates

Several patients have been described with features of a myopathy and tubular aggregates on biopsy (Morgan-Hughes, Mair and Lascelles, 1970), but since then the same structures have been recorded in pain on exercise, hypothyroid myopathy, in periodic paralysis with myasthenia and in normal muscle. (For details of other rare congenital myopathies, see Fardeau, 1982.)

The mitochondrial myopathies

This is a heterogeneous group of diseases associated with mitochondria abnormal in function or in appearance or both, with an early or late onset. The abnormal mitochondria are recognized on light microscopy by intense staining with NADH-TR and sometimes by enlargement. They may be accompanied by increase in intracellular lipid. The syndrome of Kearns and Sayre is a good example of a mitochondrial myopathy. For a proper assessment of each disorder biochemical investigation is essential but is not always possible. When the mitochondria are suspected to be abnormal on light microscopy their ultrastructure must be examined. They vary from showing concentric membranous whorls and loss of cristae to curious intramitochondrial regimented bars and giant forms. Abnormal mitochondria are not specific, occurring in small numbers of many muscle disorders, but when combined with ragged-red fibres they must be regarded as constituting one of the mitochondrial myopathies. Finding abnormal mitochondria in muscle arouses the suspicion that they may be affected elsewhere. The nervous system can be involved, causing epilepsy in children followed by a slowly evolving dementia.

One of the early reports elucidated the cause of the rarer hypermetabolic form of mitochondrial myopathy (Luft's disease) as loose coupling of oxidative phosphorylation. In a family a mitochondrial abnormality was discovered in which several cytochromes were absent. The primary biochemical defect was not found.

The mitochondrial myopathies are a complex group, and include metabolic disorders also classed as lipid storage disorders. A clear account has recently been published (Morgan-Hughes, 1982).

Secondary (including metabolic) myopathies

Cachectic atrophy

The commonest secondary myopathy is undoubtedly the atrophy produced by cachexia. Diseases such as chronic infections, cancer, collagen–vascular disease, various endocrinopathies and, especially, malnutrition cause wasting of every tissue in the body, and their effects are easily recognized. The effect of cachexia on muscle is to deplete it of contractile protein. Usually the cause of cachectic atrophy is obvious, and the muscle wasting and weakness produced are taken for granted. In some patients, however, wasting of muscle precedes that of other tissues, including adipose tissue, and proximal weakness develops before there is much loss of weight. This may be induced by a carcinoma, undetected until after a muscle biopsy has shown cachectic atrophy.

Type 2b fibres are reduced in size before, and to a greater extent, than type 1 and type 2a fibres. The atrophy causes sarcolemmal nuclei to congregate, and they form long rows but retain their normal subsarcolemmal position (Fig. 21.64).

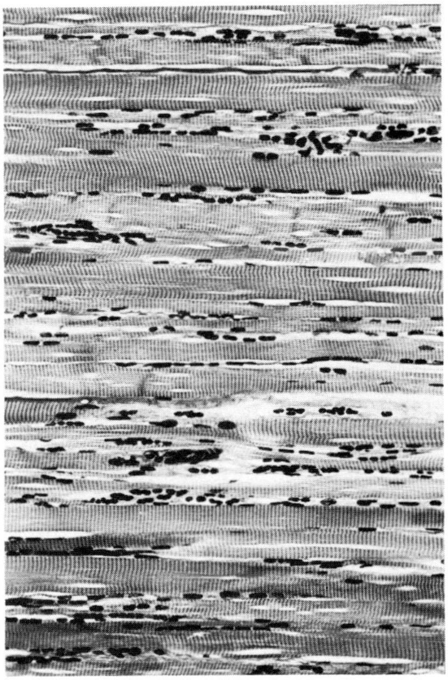

Fig. 21.64 Cachectic atrophy. The reduction in fibre size causes nuclei to congregate, retaining their subsarcolemmal position. Haematoxylin and eosin × 180.

Necrosis and regeneration are rarely seen. 'Wear and tear' lipofuscin pigments accumulate at the poles of the nuclei. The motor nerve supply remains intact, showing only minor distal sprouting until a late stage when neuropathy supervenes.

Necrotizing myopathy

This is the name given to a non-specific reaction of muscle to a variety of systemic diseases, including acute infections, collagen-vascular disease, liver disease, cancer, toxic conditions and endocrine disease. As already mentioned, Zenker (1864) described necrosis of muscle in patients dying of typhoid fever, and it is not uncommon for muscle taken at random at necropsy of patients dying of terminal infections to show necrosis and regeneration. Its pathogenesis is not understood. If it continues for some time it leads to variation in fibre calibre and fibrosis. Whatever the initiating cause, patients generally suffer from proximal weakness and, less often, wasting especially in the lower limbs. It may be a partial manifestation of polymyositis. Rarely, there is massive necrosis and widespread breakdown of muscle, leading to episodes of myoglobinuria (idiopathic rhabdomyolysis or Meyer-Betz disease). Its cause is unknown, and there is no reason to link it with collagen-vascular disease. It may also follow acute infection or unusual exertion, and is preceded by severe muscular cramps and pain. A small proportion of affected patients are found to be susceptible to malignant hyperthermia.

Carcinomatous neuromyopathy

There are many syndromes resulting from the remote effects of cancer, and one of the commonest is a mainly proximal weakness and wasting. It is usually referred to as carcinomatous neuromyopathy, because of the clinical difficulty in deciding whether the lesion is neurogenic or myogenic. The syndrome has practical importance as it may be the first sign of neoplasia. It has been stated that about half of all men with acquired myopathy aged over 50 ultimately prove to have cancer, usually in the lung. The muscles may show polymyositis, necrotizing myopathy, cachectic atrophy, a distal pattern of neurogenic disease, or a combination of these. Rarely, there is evidence of the myasthenic syndrome. The examination should obviously include the innervation.

The endocrine myopathies

Thyroid. *Hyperthyroidism* is, on rare occasions, associated with one of several dissimilar myopathies. The best known association is with myasthenia gravis. There are two forms of thyrotoxic myopathy: an acute form with necrosis, regeneration and lymphocyte collections in which extraocular muscle may be involved; and a chronic myopathy showing little but variation of fibre calibre. The least common manifestation is thyrotoxic periodic paralysis, resembling the hypokalaemic form, Rarely, tubular aggregates appear, but vacuoles are infrequent. The basic change is dilatation of the sarcoplasmic reticulum. Treatment of the primary disease is said to cause improvement, but this is unlikely once the myopathy has become permanent.

Hypothyroidism, especially if prolonged and severe, may give rise to myopathy. The muscle mass increases, possibly the result of increased mucoprotein in the connective tissue. The increase in muscle bulk and stiffness comprise

Hoffmann's syndrome (pseudomyotonia). Great variation in fibre size, vacuolation, cores, deposits of glycogen and regeneration may all be found. The CK is elevated. Mild or moderately severe myxoedema will not usually induce myopathy.

Juvenile myxoedema. At necropsy of a male aged 28 years the writer found in routine blocks crescents of a basophil material within numerous muscle fibres. They gave reactions for acid mucopolysaccharide, and strongly resembled the crescents found by Asboè-Hansen, Iversen and Wichmann (1952) in patients who had thyrotoxicosis with severe exophthalmos. Other workers were unable to find this material in muscle until it appeared in this patient. Since then the examination of chronic myxoedematous muscle has revealed on occasions deposits of glycogen. It is possible that in the course of time conversion to mucopolysaccharide could occur.

Hyperparathyroidism. Some patients present with a proximal myopathy in which the reflexes are brisk. Histological changes are mild and all the symptoms and signs remit with removal of the parathyroid tumour. Cape (1971) reported a uniform and intense staining of phosphorylase in both muscle fibre types in one patient, attributing this to activation of phosphorylase by calcium. A polyneuropathy has been reported with hyperparathyroidism, and a myopathy with hypoparathyroidism.

Acromegaly. Examination of muscle in acromegaly is comparatively rare; necropsies are few and biopsies are not required when the primary cause of unexpected muscle weakness can be treated. Those examinations which have been made have shown a remarkable variety of changes, one of which at least has been accredited to growth hormone-fibre hypertrophy. Fibre types vary in their relative proportions, and atrophic fibres develop. Electron microscopy has shown increased numbers of mitochondria, including abnormal ones. In one case there were tubular aggregates. A cardiomyopathy sometimes occurs, and the picture is complicated by neuropathies resulting from compressive hyperplasia of connective tissue.

Adrenal gland. In Addison's disease there is severe cachectic atrophy. Adrenalectomy in the treatment of Cushing's disease causes an increase of trigylceride droplets in muscle fibres. This has also been noted in untreated Cushing's disease, to be followed or accompanied by type 2b atrophy.

Hyperaldosteronism causes periodic attacks of weakness, presumably related to hypokalaemia. Histologically there are scattered small angulated fibres staining strongly with NADH.

Pituitary-ovarian axis. Stanton and Strong (1967) reported a unique myopathy in a young woman, which failed to respond to steroids but remitted twice during pregnancy. It later responded to treatment with an oestrogen and a progestogen. Histological examination showed considerable variation in fibre size.

Menopausal muscular 'dystrophy'. Although a form of limb girdle muscular dystrophy with late onset may present during the menopause, patients described under this title are generally considered to have been suffering from polymyositis. Thus there is no good evidence that the menopause may cause a myopathy.

Metabolic myopathies

The glycogenoses

Absence or deficiency of the various enzymes concerned with the degradation of glycogen to glucose lead to the accumulation of glycogen in the tissues. Not all affect muscle.

Type 2 glycogenosis is due to deficiency of acid maltase (α-1,4-glucosidase), and occurs in three forms—fatal infantile (Pompe's disease), a childhood form resembling Duchenne dystrophy and a relatively benign adult onset disease. In the infantile form hypotonia and muscle weakness are noted in the first few months of life, and the heart and liver are enlarged. In the CNS the anterior horn cells contain glycogen, and it may be present in motor nerves. Inheritance is autosomal recessive. Death usually occurs within 12 months.

As acid maltase is a lysosomal enzyme, glycogen accumulates within lysosomes and autophagic vacuoles (Fig. 21.65) and not in the cytosol. For that reason ischaemic work causes a normal rise in serum lactate. Vacuoles of various size containing PAS-positive material removable

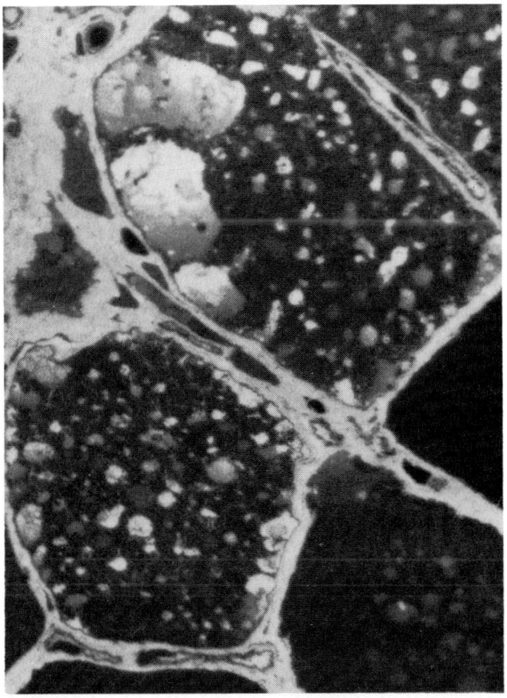

(a)

Fig. 21.65 Adult onset acid maltase deficiency. (**a**) Vacuoles of variable size in some muscle fibres. 1 μm epon section × 740. (**b**) The vacuoles contain glycogen. Bar = 1 μm.

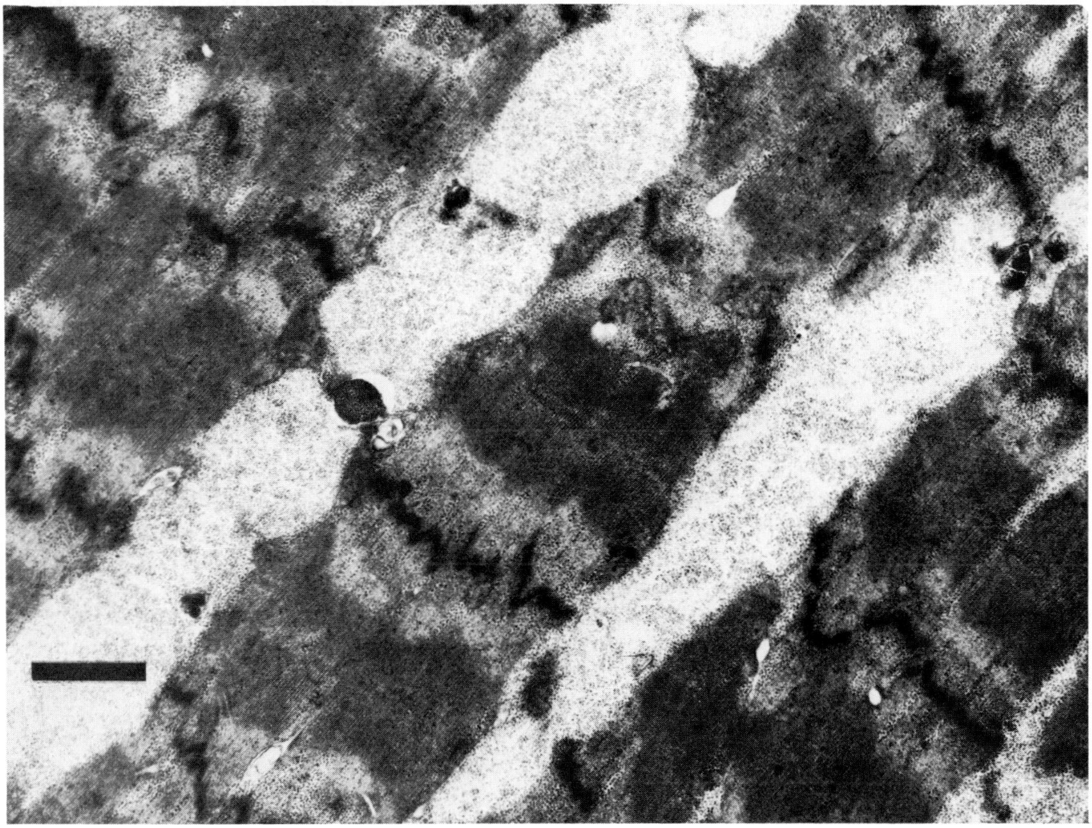

(b)

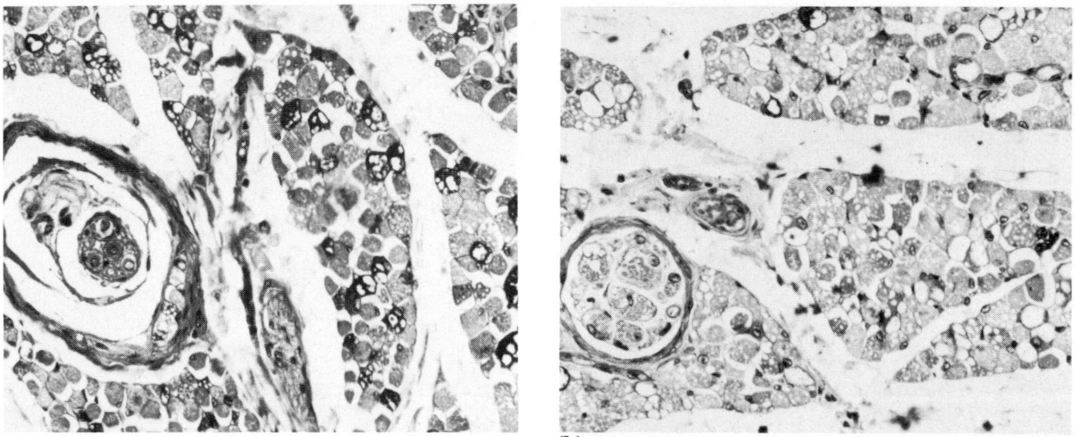

(a) (b)

Fig. 21.66 Type 2 glycogenosis. (**a**) Many fibres contain PAS-positive material. PAS × 180. (**b**) After treatment with diastase, much of the material is dissolved out, showing it to be glycogen. A small proportion persists, and gives the reactions of a mucopolysaccharide. PAS after diastase × 180.

by diastase are numerous in muscle fibres. Acid phosphatase demonstrates the enlarged lysosomes which contain the glycogen. Occasionally, diastase does not remove all the PAS-positive material. Some of it is basophil and reacts for acid mucopolysaccharide (Fig. 21.66). The cardiomyopathy is dangerous and can be the cause of death. Anaesthesia may provoke arrest in an infant not suspected to suffer from the disease.

The older children and adults who develop acid maltase deficiency show the same sort of vacuolar pattern in their muscle almost as advanced as in the infantile form. Perhaps the glycogen takes longer to accumulate. Unlike affected infants, they have some residual acid maltase activity in their muscle. Electron microscopy reveals the same membrane-bound glycogen and a lesser degree of myofibril disorganization. Again, other organs may be involved.

Type 3 glycogenosis. Muscle is as a rule only mildly affected, although this condition may present with hypotonia in infancy or chronic myopathy in adults. The liver is more seriously involved and patients may develop hypoglycaemia. The fibres contain glycogen in diffuse form in the sarcoplasm, with no suggestion of accumulation in lysosomes. The enzyme which is deficient is the debranching enzyme, amylo-1,6-glucosidase, demonstrable by liver or muscle biopsy, or in the leucocytes.

Type 5 glycogenosis (*McArdle's disease*). The first inkling of the diagnosis in this relatively mild myopathy may come from the neuropathologist, provided the histochemical series includes the stain for myophosphorylase. When this is absent the technician may think that the reaction has not worked, but repetition with a control proves the deficiency (Fig. 21.67). The disorder is restricted to striated muscle. Affected patients suffer pains in their muscles on exercise, especially in the calves, but some are able to get a 'second wind'. Usually there are no abnormal findings on clinical examination, but some develop a permanent proximal myopathy. The ischaemic exercise test shows no rise in blood lactate; this rises two to five times in normal subjects. The muscle shows no abnormality in paraffin sections, or a few fibres may carry vacuoles, chiefly subsarcolemmal. In cryostat sections glycogen may be increased diffusely in both fibre types, provided fixation of the sections is avoided and alcohol-free PAS is used. Glycogen accumulates in the cytosol and not in lysosomes. Occasionally the phosphorylase reaction may be diminished rather than absent. It is always advisable to measure the enzyme quantitatively, for its staining may be impaired by steroids and in some myopathies.

Type 7 glycogenosis (*Tarui's disease*). This is similar to McArdle's disease but the deficiency responsible is of phosphofructokinase. Venous lactate fails to rise on ischaemic exercise, and glycogen is found in the cytosol. It may be detected histochemically.

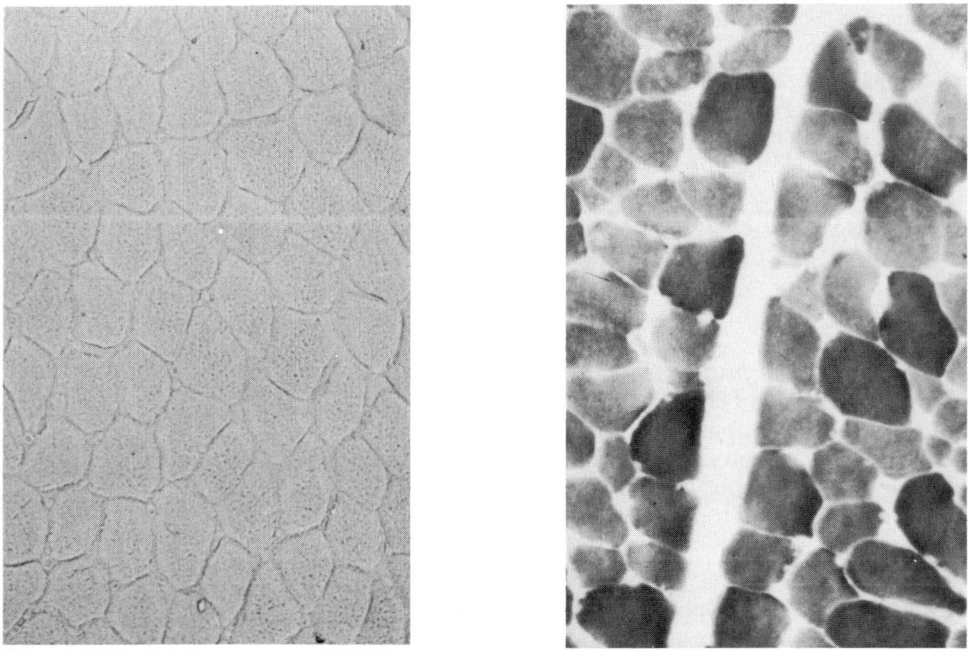

(a) (b)

Fig. 21.67 McArdle's disease. Phosphorylase reaction in (**a**) control and (**b**) patient's muscle. × 190.

Lipid storage disease

Excess lipid (triglyceride) may remain in muscle fibres in a number of conditions, especially in acute alcoholic myopathy and steroid myopathy. Rarely, a lipid myopathy has been found without apparent cause but recovering spontaneously after several years. There are, however, two muscle lipidoses in which biochemical deficiencies have been discovered in the last few years.

Carnitine palmityl acyl transferase (CPAT) deficiency

Long chain fatty acids are an important fuel for muscle, and CPAT is an enzyme in the pathway for their oxidation. CPAT deficiency therefore impairs the function of muscle, including cardiac muscle. The small number of case reports have been in children, mainly boys, in whom symptoms of muscle pain and weakness develop. Cold and exercise may precipitate rhabdomyolysis, but on occasions pain does not develop until well after the period of exercise. Muscle biopsy may show a relatively slight increase in type 1 fibre lipid, but there may be no changes at all on light or electron microscopy. Diagnosis depends on clinical history and biochemical assay. Carnitine is normal or raised in the absence of CPAT.

Carnitine deficiency

Large amounts of carnitine are present in skeletal muscle, and its function is to transport long chain fatty acids across the mitochondrial inner membrane. In deficiency, large amounts of lipid are stored in type 1 fibres. A few fibres may be atrophied in addition, which some authors have thought were denervated without other evidence. Again, diagnosis depends on biochemical assay. Clinically there is intermittent or progressive weakness, and possibly abnormal liver function tests, and renal and cardiac impairment. Carnitine deficiency is of special interest because it may be treated with oral carnitine; rapid disappearance of lipid droplets has occasionally been demonstrated. Further details are available in a useful review by Pleasure and Bonilla (1982).

Osteomalacia

Some patients with osteomalacia develop a waddling gait, and show evidence of a proximal myopathy. As in hyperparathyroidism, reflexes are preserved or even brisk, and again the myopathy is independent of calcium levels. The writer has noted some atrophic fibres with clumped nuclei, type 2 fibre atrophy and a disturbance of motor end-plates, some of which showed sprouting and others a myasthenia-like elongation and attenuation. Treatment is not always effective, so the myopathy may be due to additional factors such as disuse atrophy.

Toxic myopathies

It has been said that skeletal muscle is able to react to disease in a limited number of ways. This cannot be true when toxic myopathies are considered, for various drugs as well as venoms and other toxins may produce a focal myopathy, muscle fibrosis (from injections), acute or subacute painful proximal myopathy, hypokalaemia, inflammatory myopathy, acute rhabdomyolysis, chronic painlcss proximal myopathy, myotonia and disorders of neuromuscular transmission (Mastaglia and Argov, 1981). The list of drugs incriminated is long, including commonly used classes of drugs such as antibiotics and steroids. The effect is perhaps not surprising from cytotoxic drugs such as vincristine but in the case of others the effect is rare and may be due to individual susceptibility. Drug reactions are meant to be reported, but many are not recognized or are obscured by multiple therapy. This is illustrated by the following case. A middle-aged female patient who had been suffering from Menière's disease for many years died from unexplained renal failure. At necropsy a routine block of muscle showed widespread necrosis of some duration. Drug-induced myonecrosis was suspected, but none of the four drugs with which she had been treated had ever caused rhabdomyolysis, according to government records.

Alcoholic myopathy

Alcoholic myopathy is rare compared with alcoholic neuropathy. It occurs in two forms—acute, following a drinking bout; and chronic. The findings on biopsy are non-specific, including fibre necrosis and its sequelae, and atrophy of type 2b fibres. There may be the effects of a complicating peripheral neuropathy. The writer has examined by biopsy two well-to-do patients shortly after they suffered severe weakness following excessive drinking. In both biopsies fibres remained of normal size, but many type 1 fibres were filled with triclyceride droplets.

Steroid myopathy

Some patients on a prolonged course of steroids develop a proximal myopathy. In the earlier stages, no atrophy is observed, but muscle fibres especially of type 1 contain excess lipid in the form of triglyceride droplets. Later, type 2b atrophy develops and lipid-laden fibres are infrequent. Individual idiosyncrasy to the drug may be important, as the complication is not drug-dependent (Fig. 21.68).

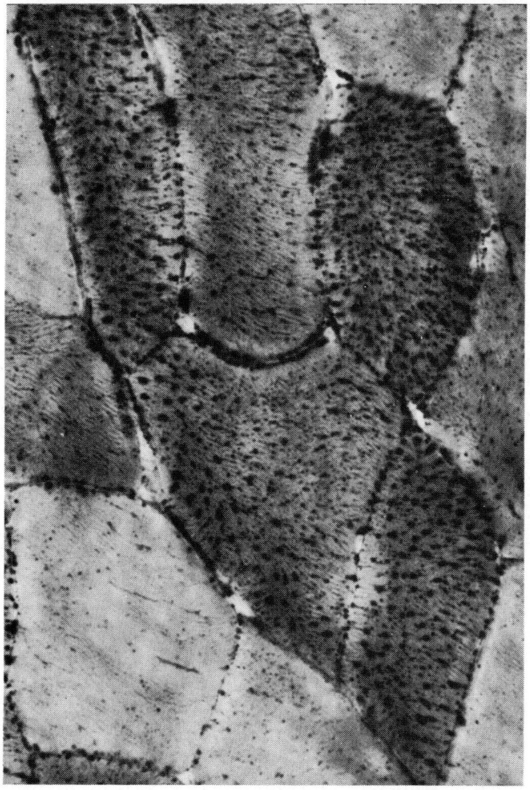

Fig. 21.68 Increase in triglyceride is liable to occur in disorders in which the utilization of lipid is impaired. It is seen here as the larger droplets in type 1 fibres, but may also occur in type 2 fibres. The grey spots are mitochondria. Paraphenylene diamine × 460.

Malignant hyperthermia (Denborough's disease)

Anaesthetic agents and muscle relaxants, especially suxamethonium and halothane, have been

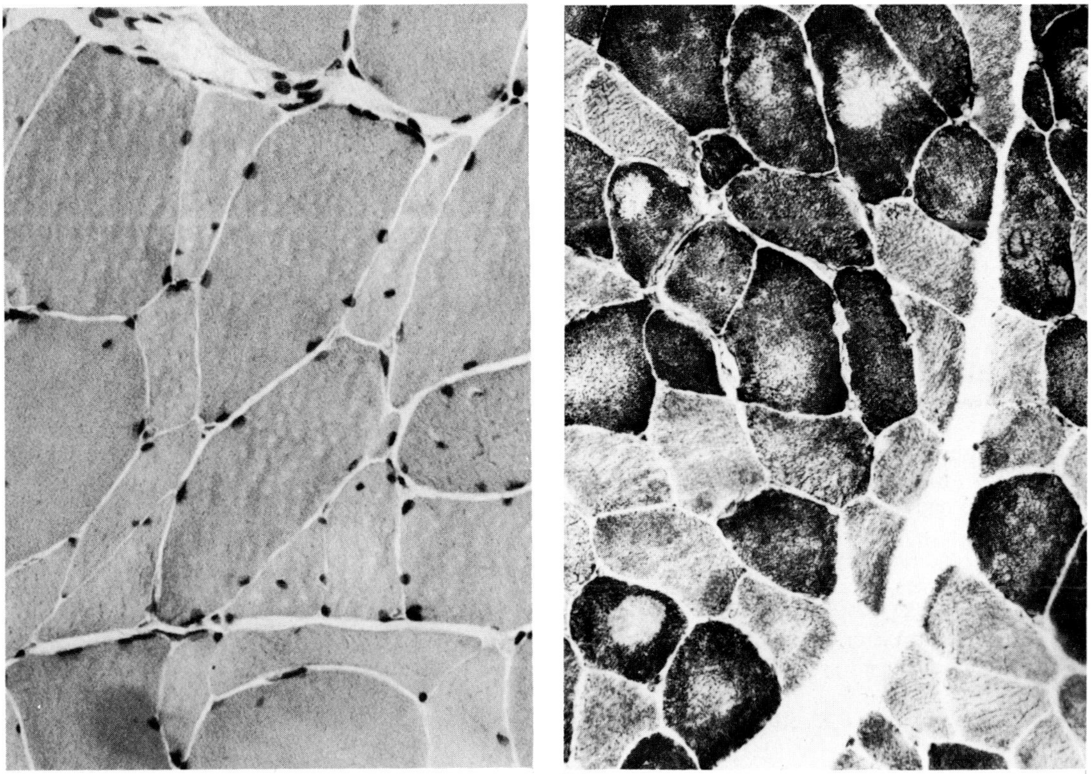

(a) **(b)**

Fig. 21.69 Malignant hyperthermia myopathy. (**a**) Fibre splitting and internal nuclei, with calibre variation. Haematoxylin and eosin × 300. (**b**) Moth-eaten and core fibres. NADH-TR × 300.

found to be responsible for this serious complication of anaesthesia, characterized by a rapid rise in temperature (to 43°C or more), often muscle rigidity, and death in over 50 per cent of cases. Susceptibility to the disorder is inherited as a dominant trait, and is associated with a muscle defect of which the patient is unaware. Patients are often of athletic build, and a few show local hypertrophy of muscles, particularly in the thighs or calves. The CK may or may not be raised.

Patients who have experienced an episode suggestive of malignant hyperthermia (MH) and, if susceptible, their parents and siblings, or the siblings of a patient who has died, must be tested for susceptibility to MH. This requires a muscle biopsy and testing of the reaction of muscle strips *in vitro* to anaesthetic and other agents. These produce a greater rise in isometric tension in susceptible than in normal muscle. At the same time muscle structure is examined. Approximately half the individuals tested are susceptible (MHS), and any future anaesthesia must avoid relaxants and the commonly used inhalational anaesthetics. The nature of the muscle defect is still not known, but is thought to cause a flow of calcium ions into the muscle fibre. A structural myopathy is not seen in the early years, and even in late adult life it is present in no more than 50 per cent. It seems likely that the changes observed—chiefly internal nuclei, fibre splitting, moth-eaten and core fibres—are secondary to the muscle defect (Fig. 21.69) (Harriman, 1982).

Ischaemia of muscle

Muscle has a rich blood supply with many collaterals and does not easily undergo infarction. However, it occurs occasionally in patients suffering from severe occlusive arterial disease of the limbs. Large foci of muscle are found to have undergone necrosis (with peripheral regeneration), or an ischaemic myopathy may occur with necrosis and regeneration of numerous scattered single muscle fibres (see Harriman, 1977). Volkmann's ischaemic contracture of muscle is a well-known but rare complication of fractures, and is thought to be the result of arterial spasm. Infarction of muscle has been reported in diabetic patients. Ischaemia is likely to be the basis of the anterior compartment or pretibial syndrome, where pain and necrosis of muscle develop after strenuous exercise, especially in athletic individuals. When patients lie without moving in a deep coma for many hours, whether from carbon monoxide hypoxia, drug abuse or some other cause, the calves may be compressed and complete or incomplete infarction ensue. The great leg arteries are not necessarily sclerotic in such cases.

References

Asboè-Hansen, G., Iversen K. and Wichmann, R. (1952) Malignant exophthalmos: muscular changes and thyrotropin content in serum. *Acta Endocrinologica* **11,** 376–99.

Askanas, V. and Engel, W.K. (1975) Distinct subtypes of type 1 fibers of human skeletal muscle. *Neurology* **25,** 879–87.

Banker, B.Q. and Victor, M. (1966) Dermatomyositis (systemic angiopathy) of childhood. *Medicine* **45,** 261–89.

Bender, A.N., Ringel, S.P., Engel, W.K., Vogel, Z. and Daniels, M.P. (1976) Immunoperoxidase localization of alpha-bungarotoxin. A new approach to myasthenia gravis. *Annals of the New York Academy of Sciences* **274,** 20–30.

Bodensteiner, J.B. and Engel, A.G. (1978) Intracellular calcium accumulation in Duchenne dystrophy and other myopathies: a study of 567,000 muscle fibers in 114 biopsies. *Neurology* **28,** 439–46.

Bradley, W.G., O'Brien, M.D., Walder, D.N., Murchison, D., Johnson, M. and Newell, D.J. (1975) Failure to confirm a vascular cause of muscular dystrophy. *Archives of Neurology* **32,** 466–73.

Brooke, M.H. and Kaiser, K.K. (1970) Muscle fibre types: how many and what kind? *Archives of Neurology* **23,** 369–79.

Brownell, B., Oppenheimer, D. and Spalding, J.M.K. (1972) Neurogenic muscle atrophy in myasthenia gravis. *Journal of Neurology, Neurosurgery and Psychiatry* **34,** 311–22.

Buzzard, E.F. (1905) The clinical history and post-mortem examination of five cases of myasthenia gravis. *Brain* **28,** 438–83.

Campbell, A.M.G., Williams, E.R. and Pearce, J. (1969) Late motor neuron degeneration following poliomyelitis. *Neurology* ***19,*** 1101–6.

Cape, C.A. (1971) Increased phosphorylase activity in muscle in hyperparathyroid disease. *Neurology* **21,** 638–41.

Coërs, C. (1982) Pathology of intramuscular nerves and nerve terminals. In *Skeletal Muscle Pathology* (Eds. Mastaglia, F.L. and Walton, J.), pp. 483–507. Churchill Livingstone, Edinburgh.

Coërs, C. and Carbone, F. (1966) La myopathie granulomateuse. *Acta Neurologica et Psychiatrica Belgica* **66,** 353–81.

Coërs, C. and Woolf, A.L. (1959) *The Innervation of Muscle. A biopsy study.* Blackwell Scientific, Oxford.

Currie, S., Noronha, M. and Harriman, D.G.F. (1974) 'Minicore' disease. *Abstracts of the IIIrd International Congress on Muscle Diseases, Newcastle upon Tyne, 1974* (Ed. Bradley, W.G.), ICS series no. 334, p. 12. Excerpta Medica, Amsterdam.

Daniel, P.M. and Strich, S.J. (1964) Abnormalities in the muscle spindles in dystrophia myotonica. *Neurology* **14,** 310–16.

Dubowitz, V. and Brooke, M.H. (1973) *Muscle Biopsy: A modern approach*, pp. 280–8. W.B. Saunders, London, Philadelphia, Toronto.

Durston, J.H. (1974) Histochemistry of primate extra-ocular muscles and the changes of denervation. *British Journal of Ophthalmology* **58,** 193–216.

Edström, L. and Kugelberg, E. (1968) Histochemical composition, distribution of fibres and fatiguability of single motor units. *Journal of Neurology, Neurosurgery and Psychiatry* **31,** 424–33.

Edström, L., Thornell, L.E. and Eriksson, A. (1980) A new type of hereditary distal myopathy with characteristic sarcoplasmic bodies and intermediate (skeletin) filaments. *Journal of the Neurological Sciences* **47,** 171–90.

Emery, A.E.H. (1971) Review: the nosology of the spinal muscular atrophies. *Journal of Medical Genetics* **8,** 481–95.

Emery, A.E.H. and Dreifuss, F.E. (1966) Unusual type of benign X-linked muscular dystrophy. *Journal of Neurology, Neurosurgery and Psychiatry* **29,** 338–42.

Engel, A.G., Gomez, M.R. and Groover, R.V. (1971) Multicore disease. A recently recognized congenital myopathy associated with multifocal degeneration of muscle fibres. *Mayo Clinic Proceedings* **46,** 666–81.

Engel, W.K. (1961) Muscle target fibres. A newly recognized sign of denervation. *Nature (London)* **191,** 389–90.

Fardeau, M. (1982) Congenital myopathies. In *Skeletal Muscle Pathology* (Eds. Mastaglia, F.L. and Walton, J.), pp. 161–203. Churchill Livingstone, Edinburgh.

Fenichel, G.M., Emery, E.S. and Hunt, P. (1967) Neurogenic atrophy simulating facioscapulohumeral dystrophy. *Archives of Neurology* **17,** 257–60.

Frankel, K.A. and Rosser, R.J. (1976) The pathology of the heart in progressive muscular dystrophy: epimyocardial fibrosis. *Human Pathology* **7,** 375–86.

Fukuyama, Y., Osawa, M. and Suzuki, H. (1981) Congenital progressive muscular dystrophy of the Fukuyama type—clinical, genetic and pathological considerations. *Brain and Development* **3,** 1–29.

Goebel, H.H., Muller, J., Gillen, H.W. and Merritt, A.D. (1978) Autosomal dominant 'spheroid body myopathy'. *Muscle and Nerve* **1,** 14–26.

Greenfield, J.G., Cornman, T. and Shy, G.M. (1958) The prognostic value of the muscle biopsy in the 'floppy infant'. *Brain* **81,** 461–84.

Hamida, M.B., Fardeau, M. and Attia, N. (1983) Severe childhood muscular dystrophy affecting both sexes and frequent in Tunisia. *Muscle and Nerve* **6,** 469–80.

Harnden-Mayor, P. and Harriman, D.G.F. (In preparation)

Harriman, D.G.F. (1970) Pathological aspects of Adie's syndrome. *Advances in Ophthalmology* **23,** 55–73.

Harriman, D.G.F. (1977) Ischaemia of peripheral nerve and muscle. *Journal of Clinical Pathology* **30,** suppl. 11, 94–104.

Harriman, D.G.F. (1982). The pathology of malignant hyperpyrexia. In *Skeletal Muscle Pathology* (Eds. Mastaglia, F.L. and Walton, J.), pp. 575–91. Churchill Livingstone, Edinburgh.

Harriman, D.G.F. and Haleem, M.A. (1972) Centronuclear myopathy in old age. *Journal of Pathology* **108,** 237–47.

Harriman, D.G.F. and Stocks, P.L. (1970) Changes in birefringence of human skeletal muscle during contraction and relaxation. *Beiträge zur Pathologie* **141,** 187–90.

Harriman, D.G.F., Sumner, D.W. and Ellis, E.R. (1973) Malignant hyperpyrexia myopathy. *Quarterly Journal of Medicine* **42,** 639–64.

Harriman, D.G.F., Taverner, D. and Woolf, A.L. (1970) Ekbom's syndrome and burning paraesthesiae. A biopsy study of vital staining and electron microscopy of the intramuscular innervation with a note on age changes in motor nerve endings in distal muscles. *Brain* **93,** 393–406.

Henriksson-Larsen, K.B., Lexell, J. and Sjöstrom, M. (1983) Distribution of different fibre types in human skeletal muscles. 1. Method for the preparation and analysis of cross-sections of whole tibialis anterior. *Histochemical Journal* **15,** 167–78.

Hopkins, L.C., Jackson, J.A. and Elsas, L.J. (1981) Emery–Dreifuss humeroperoneal muscular dystrophy: an X-linked myopathy with unusual contractures and bradycardia. *Annals of Neurology* **10,** 230–7.

Isaacs, E.R., Bradley, W.G. and Henderson, G. (1973) Longitudinal fibre splitting in muscular dystrophy: a serial cinematographic study. *Journal of Neurology, Neurosurgery and Psychiatry* **36,** 813–19.

Jennekens, F.G.I., Tomlinson, B.E. and Walton, J.N. (1971) Data on the distribution of fibre types in five human limb muscles. *Journal of the Neurological Sciences* **14,** 245–57.

Jerusalem, F., Angelini, C., Engel, A.G. and Groover, R.U. (1973) Mitochondria–lipid–glycogen (MLG) disease of muscle. A morphologically regressive congenital myopathy. *Archives of Neurology* **29,** 162–9.

de Jong, J.G.Y., Slooff, J.L. and van der Eerden, A.A.J.J. (1973) A family with paramyotonia congenita with the report of an autopsy. *Acta Neurologica Scandinavica* **49,** 480–94.

Kugelberg, E. and Welander, L. (1956) Heredo-familial juvenile muscular atrophy simulating muscular dystrophy. *Acta Neurologica Psychiatrica* **75,** 500–9.

Lexell, J., Henriksson-Larsén, K., Winblad, B. and Sjostrom, M. (1983) Distribution of different fibre types in human skeletal muscle: effects of aging studied in whole muscle cross-sections. *Muscle and Nerve* **6,** 588–95.

McComas, A.J., Sica, R.E.P. and Currie, S. (1970) Muscular dystrophy. Evidence for a neural factor. *Nature (London)* **226,** 1263–4.

McLeod, J.G. and Prineas, J.W. (1971) Distal types of chronic spinal muscular atrophy. Clinical, electrophysiological and pathological studies. *Brain* **94,** 703–14.

McMenamin, J.B., Becker, L.E. and Murphy, E.G. (1982) Fukuyama-type congenital muscular dystrophy. *Journal of Pediatrics* **101,** 580–2.

Mair, W.G.P. and Tomé, F.M.S. (1972) *Atlas of the Ultrastructure of Diseased Human Muscle.* Churchill Livingstone, Edinburgh.

Marshall, A. and Duchen, L.W. (1975) Sensory system involvement in infantile spinal muscular atrophy. *Journal of the Neurological Sciences* **26,** 349–59.

Mastaglia, F.L. and Argov, Z. (1981) Drug-induced

neuromuscular disorders in man. In *Disorders of Voluntary Muscle*, 4th edn (Ed. Walton, J.), pp. 873–906. Churchill Livingstone, Edinburgh.

Mastaglia, F.L., Papadimitriou, J.M. and Kakulas, B.A. (1970) Regeneration of muscle in Duchenne muscular dystrophy: an electron microscope study. *Journal of the Neurological Sciences* **11,** 425–44.

Mastaglia, F.L. and Walton, J. (1982). (Eds) *Skeletal Muscle Pathology*, Churchill Livingstone, Edinburgh.

Mokri, B. and Engel, A.G. (1975) Duchenne dystrophy: electron microscopic findings pointing to a basic or early abnormality in the plasma membrane of the muscle fibre. *Neurology* **25,** 1111–20.

Morgan-Hughes, J.A. (1982) Mitochondrial myopathies. In *Skeletal Muscle Pathology*. (Eds. Mastaglia, F.L. and Walton, J.) pp. 309–339. Churchill Livingstone, Edinburgh.

Morgan-Hughes, J.A., Mair, W.G.P. and Lascelles, P.T. (1970) A disorder of skeletal muscle associated with tubular aggregates. *Brain* **93,** 873–80.

Nattrass, F.J. (1954) Recovery from 'muscular dystrophy'. *Brain* **77,** 549–70.

Pearn, J.H., Carter, C.O. and Wilson, J. (1973) The genetic identity of acute infantile spinal muscular atrophy. *Brain* **96,** 463–70.

Pleasure, D. and Bonilla, E. (1982) Skeletal muscle storage diseases: myopathies resulting from errors in carbohydrate and fatty acid metabolism. In *Skeletal Muscle Pathology* (Eds. Mastaglia, F.L. and Walton, J.), pp. 340–59. Churchill Livingstone, Edinburgh.

de Reuck, J., de Coster, W., de Potter, R. and van der Eecken, H. (1982) Inhibition of the target phenomenon in tenotomized rabbit muscle by medullary lesions. *Acta Neuropathologica* **56,** 136–8.

Russell, D.S. (1953) Histological changes in the striped muscles in myasthenia gravis. *Journal of Pathology and Bacteriology* **65,** 279–89.

Russmann, B.S., Melchreit, R. and Drennan, J.C. (1983) Spinal muscular atrophy: the natural course of disease. *Muscle and Nerve* **6,** 179–81.

Santa, T., Engel, A.G. and Lambert, E.G. (1972a) Histometric study of neuromuscular junction ultrastructure. I. Myasthenia gravis. *Neurology* **22,** 71–82.

Santa, T., Engel, A.G. and Lambert, E.G. (1972b) Histometric study of neuromuscular junction ultrastructure. II. Myasthenic syndrome. *Neurology* **22,** 370–6.

Schmalbruch, H. (1976) Muscle fibre splitting and regeneration in diseased human muscle. *Neuropathology and Applied Neurobiology* **2,** 3–19.

Schochet, S.S., Hardman, J.M., Ladewig, P.P. and Earle, K.M. (1969) Intraneuronal conglomerates in sporadic neuron disease. A light and electron microscopic study. *Archives of Neurology* **20,** 548–53.

Shy, G.M. and Magee, K.R. (1956) A new congenital non-progressive myopathy. *Brain* **79,** 610–21.

Simpson, J.A. (1981) Myasthenia gravis and myasthenic syndromes. In *Disorders of Voluntary Muscle*, 4th edn (Ed. Walton, J.), pp. 585–624 Churchill Livingstone, Edinburgh.

Stanton, J.B. and Strong, J.A. (1967) Myopathy remitting in pregnancy and responding to high-storage oestrogen and progestrogen therapy. *Lancet* **2,** 275–7.

Sumner, D.W., Crawfurd, M. d'A. and Harriman, D.G.F. (1971) Distal muscular dystrophy in an English family. *Brain* **94,** 51–60.

Swash, M. and Fox, K.P. (1975) Abnormal intrafusal muscle fibres in myotonic dystrophy: a study using serial sections. *Journal of Neurology, Neurosurgery and Psychiatry* **38,** 91–9.

Swash, M. and Schwartz, M.S. (1981) Familial multicore disease with focal loss of cross-striations and ophthalmoplegia. *Journal of the Neurological Sciences* **52,** 1–10.

Thomas, P.K., Schott, G.D. and Morgan-Hughes, J.A. (1975) Adult-onset scapulo-peroneal myopathy. *Journal of Neurology, Neurosurgery and Psychiatry* **38,** 1008–15.

Tomlinson, B.E., Walton, J.N. and Irving, D. (1974) Spinal cord limb motor neurons in muscular dystrophy. *Journal of the Neurological Sciences* **22,** 305–27.

Tomonaga, M. and Sluga, E. (1969) Für ultrastruktur der 'Target-Fasern'. *Virchows Archiv. A. Pathologische Anatomie* **348,** 89–104.

Walton, J.N. and Adams, R.D. (1958) *Polymyositis.* Livingstone, Edinburgh.

Welander, L. (1951) Myopathia distalis tarda hereditaria. *Acta Medica Scandinavica* suppl. 265.

Wohlfart, G. (1937) Über das Vorkommen verschiedener Arten von Muskelfasern in der Skelett-muskulature des Menschens und einiger Säugetiere. *Acta Psychiatrica et Neurologica* suppl. 12.

Wohlfart, G., Fex, J. and Eliasson, S. (1955) Hereditary proximal spinal muscular atrophy. A clinical entity simulating muscular dystrophy. *Acta Psychiatrica Scandinavica* **30,** 395–406.

Zenker, F.A. (1864) *Ueber die Veränderungen der willkürlichen Muskeln in Typhus abdominalis.* Vogel, Leipzig.

Index

Page numbers in **heavy type** indicate illustrations

Abetalipoproteinaemia (Bassen-Kornzweig disease) 876
Abruptio placentae, causing fetal brain damage 477
Abscess, brain 243–6
  actinomycosis 325
  amoebic 304–5
  aspergillosis **325,** 326
  blastomycosis 326–7
  candidosis 327
  capsule 245, **246,** 251
  cerebrospinal fluid changes 247
  cladosporiosis 327–8
  coccidioidomycosis 328
  development 244–6, **244, 245, 246**
  intracerebral, complicating head injury 98, 118, **118**
  multilocular 245, **245**
  nocardiosis 330–1, **330**
  site of formation 244
  sources 243–4
  tuberculous 251, **253**
Abscess, epidural
  cranial 238, 246
  spinal 238–9, 246–7
Abscess, muscle 1081
Abscess, subdural 239–40, **239**
  complicating head injury 98
  histopathology 240
Acanthamoeba 305, 306–7
Acetylcholinesterase in amniotic fluid, in neural tube defects 391
Acetyl ethyl tetramethyl tetralin (AETT), neurotoxic effects 677–8
Acid maltase deficiency (glycogenosis, type 2) 548–50, **548, 549, 550**
  myopathy in 1088–90, **1089, 1090**
Acquired immunodeficiency syndrome 247
Acquired (non-wilsonian) hepatocerebral degeneration 599–602
  experimental portacaval anastomosis 601–2
  hepatic coma 600–1
  neuropathological changes 600
  peripheral nerve lesions 600
Acromegaly, 865, 1088
Acrylamide intoxication 649–51, **650,** 857
Actinomycosis 324–5
Acute idiopathic inflammatory polyneuropathy *see* Guillain-Barré syndrome
Addison's disease 772, 1088
Adenosine triphosphate (ATP), and cerebral function 126, 128
Adenoviruses
  access route 263
  acute encephalitis caused by 273
  tumour production in animals 261
Adie's syndrome, rod bodies in 1083
Adrenal gland, myopathies associated with disorders of 1088
Adrenoleucodystrophy 369–71, **371,** 872–3
Adrenomyeloneuropathy 370–1, 872–3
Ageing
  aneurysms
    miliary 213
    saccular 224
  brain in 954–8, **955, 956**
  dementia *see* Dementia and ageing
  lacunae 214–15 *see also* État lacunaire
  muscle 1027–8, **1027**
Agranular (smooth) endoplasmic reticulum 3, **4**
  peripheral axons 811
Agyria (lissencephaly) 413–15, **413, 414,** 417
Aicardi syndrome 423
Alaria americana 321
Alcoholic intoxication, acute, pathological changes 577, 1091, 1092
Alcoholism 573–9
  amblyopia 577
  central pontine myelinolysis 578–9
  cerebellar degeneration 578
  cerebral abnormalities 578
  fetal alcohol syndrome 652–3
  Marchiafava-Bignami syndrome 369, 578, **579**
  myopathy 1091, 1092
  nicotinic acid deficiency 578, 581–3
  peripheral neuropathy 856
  thiamine deficiency 573–8
  Wernicke and Korsakoff syndromes 369, 573–7, **574, 575, 576,** 1003–4, **1004**
Alder granulation 530, 537, **537,** 538, 539

Alexander type of leucodystrophy (Alexander's disease) 373–4, **373**
  Rosenthal fibres in 36, 374, **374**
Allergy in bacterial infection 236
Allocortex, and hypoxia, vulnerability to 131
Alpers' disease 477–8, 611
Alpha-fetoprotein (AFP) 390–1
Alpha-particle radiation necrosis 45
Alphaviruses 282–3
Aluminium intoxication 627–8
  and Alzheimer's disease 627–8, 979–80
Alzheimer astrocytes 596, 597, **597,** 600, 601, 606
Alzheimer's disease 952–3, 971–80
  aluminium intoxication 627–8, 979–80
  atypical cases 978–9, **978**
  brain atrophy 972–3, **972, 973**
  cortical neurons, loss of 975
  dendritic changes 975
  familial cases 977–8
  head injury, possible connection with 117, 966
  neurochemical findings 975–7
  neurofibrillary degeneration 23, **23,** 700, 961–2, **962, 963,** 971, 974, 976
    distribution 965
    Down's syndrome 23, 435
    experimental conditions 627–8, 979–80
    pathogenesis 963–5, **963, 964**
    Pick's disease, relationship to 991
    prevalence 965–6
  neuronal RNA, reduction in 975–6
  nucleolar size, reduction in 975–6
  Parkinson's disease, relationship to 705, 980–2
  plaques, neuritic (argyrophilic, senile) 973–4, **973,** 976
Amblyopia
  in alcoholism 577
  tobacco 586
Amino acid metabolism, disorders of 389, 605–6
6-Aminonicotinamide (6AN), neurotoxic effects 678
Amiodarone neuropathy 670–2, **670, 671,** 860
Ammon's horn (hippocampus) *see* Hippocampus
  sclerosis *see under* Hippocampus
Amoebiasis 304–7
Amygdaloid nucleus
  epilepsy 932, 934–7, **938,** 939
  hypoxia
    ischaemic, generalized 137
    oligmaeic, generalized 142
    vulnerability to 132
  neurofibrillary degeneration 974
Amyloid
  congophilic angiopathy 968–71, **970,** 979
  myopathy 1081
  peripheral neuropathy 865–9, **866, 867, 868**
  senile plaques containing 959–61, 969–70, 974
Amyotrophic lateral sclerosis *see* Motor neuron disease
Amyotrophies, spinal, various 735
Anaemia, pernicious 586–8
  peripheral neuropathy 587–8, 590
  subacute combined degeneration of spinal cord 587–90
Anencephaly 390–1
Aneurysms 219
  arteriovenous malformations 220, 224, 230, 431–3, **433**
  atherosclerotic fusiform 227, **228**
  bacterial 229
  berry *see* Aneurysms, saccular
  carotid-cavernous sinus 227–8, **229**
  Charcot-Bouchard (miliary) 212–13, **213,** 217
  dissecting 228
  giant 220, 226–7
  miliary (microaneurysms) 212–13, **213,** 217
  mycotic 229, 238, 246
  neoplastic 230
  saccular
    age incidence 220
    bifurcation of arteries, relationship to 222, **222,** 223, 224
    complications 224–7
    incidence 219
    macroscopical appearances 220–2, **221, 222**
    microscopical appearances 222–3, **222, 223, 224**
    pathogenesis 223–4
    predisposing factors 220
    rupture of 208, 220, 221, **221,** 225–7, 986–7
    site 219–20
    unruptured, local effects 224–5
Angiostrongyliasis 322
Anoxia 128, 143–4
  anoxic 134
Anterior compartment syndrome 1094
Anterior horn cells **2, 4**
  argyrophilic bodies **7,** 8
  chromatolysis 20–3, **20, 21**
  loss in syndromes associated with carcinoma 614
  in motor neuron disease 700 (Table), 728, **729, 730,** 733, 1055, **1055**
  in spinal muscular atrophy 1056, 1059
  in Werdnig-Hoffmann disease 735, 1056
Anterograde (wallerian) degeneration **14, 15,** 15–17
  see also wallerian degeneration
Antibodies 236–7, 262
Aorta
  aortic arch syndrome 182, **182**
  coarctation 220, 798–9
  dissecting aneurysm, neurological complications 799–800
Apallic states 115–16, 152
Apoplexy, delayed traumatic, of Bollinger 97
Aqueduct for King stenosis 435
Arachnoid cysts 242, 426–7, **426**
Arachnoid granulations, following subarachnoid haemorrhage 226, **226, 227**
Arachnoiditis
  cystic, complicating meningitis 242
  spinal 255
    progressive 242
Arboviruses
  access routes 262, 263
  biology 262, 263
  encephalitis (acute) caused by 273, 282–3
Arginosuccinic aciduria 606
Argyrophilic bodies
  in Pick's disease 24–5, **24,** 990–1
  in spinal cord **7,** 8

Arhinencephaly (holoprosencephaly) 388, 409–11, **410**
Arnold-Chiari malformation 392, 393–5, **394,** 435
Arsenic intoxication 628–9, 858–9
Artefacts 6–8, 129, 362, 419
  in muscle fibres 1031, **1031,** 1066
    in Duchenne muscular dystrophy 1031, 1066
Arterial boundary zones (border zones) **140**
    in hypoxia 132, 139–43, **140, 141**
Arterial occlusion and cerebral infarction, perinatal 470–1, **470, 471**
  in utero 475–6, **475**
Arterial vasospasm complicating saccular aneurysms 224, 225–6
Artery
  of Adamkiewicz 797
  basilar
    anatomy and physiology 157, 168
    aneurysms, atherosclerotic fusiform 227, **228**
    aneurysms, saccular 220, 221, 225
    occlusion and stenosis 168–9, **169**
  carotid, external 157
  carotid, internal 157
    aneurysms, atherosclerotic fusiform 227, **228**
    aneurysms, saccular 219, 220, **221,** 225, **229**
    occlusion and stenosis 165–7, **166**
    traumatic thrombosis 99, **99**
  cerebellar 157
    aneurysms 225
  cerebellar, anterior inferior 157
    occlusion 171
  cerebellar, posterior inferior **140,** 142, 157
    compression 66
    occlusion 171–2
  cerebellar, superior **140,** 142, 157
    compression 63, 64
    occlusion 171
  cerebral, anterior 133, 140, **140,** 157, 170
    aneurysms, bacterial and mycotic 229
    aneurysms, saccular **221, 222,** 225
    occlusion 170
  cerebral, middle 140, **140,** 157
    aneurysms, atherosclerotic fusiform 227, **228**
    aneurysms, bacterial and mycotic 229
    aneurysms, saccular 220, **221, 222,** 225
    malformations causing intracranial haemorrhage 230
    occlusion 133, 170
  cerebral, posterior 133, 140, **140,** 157
    aneurysms, bacterial and mycotic 229
    aneurysms, saccular 220, 225
    compression 63, **63,** 64
    occlusion 170
  choroidal, anterior
    compression **62,** 63, 64
    distribution 171
    occlusion 171
  communicating, anterior, aneurysms 220, **221, 223,** 225
  communicating, posterior, aneurysms 220, 225
    compression of, in raised intracranial pressure **62,** 63, **63,** 64, 66
  of Heubner 170
  innominate, occlusion 167
  medial gaps, and aneurysms 223, 224
  occlusion and stenosis 165–70, 171–2
    see also occlusion *under specifically named arteries*
  spinal 796–7
    occlusion 797–8
  subclavian, occlusion 167
  sulcal (spinal cord) 797
  vertebral
    anatomy and physiology 157, 167–8
    aneurysms, atherosclerotic fusiform 227
    aneurysms, dissecting 228
    aneurysms, saccular 220, 221, 225
    occlusion and stenosis 168–9, **168**
    traumatic rupture 99–100
  aneurysm formation 224
  in hypertension 173–4, **173,** 176, 209
Arteriosclerosis
  as a cause of parkinsonism 707
  aneurysm formation 224
  in hypertension 173–4, **173,** 176, 209
Arteriovenous malformations 431–3, **433**
  aneurysms associated with 220, 224, 230, 431–3, **433**
  intracerebral and subarachnoid haemorrhages caused by 230
  spinal cord 800–3, **801, 802**
Arteritis
  carotid, acute 182
  giant cell (temporal) 185–6, **186,** 979
  syphilitic (Heubner's) 250, 255, **256**
Arthrogryposis multiplex congenita 735, 1081–2
L-Aspartate, neurotoxic effects 679–80
Aspartylglycosaminuria 545
Aspergillosis **324, 325,** 326
Asphyxia 128
Astrocytes 27–31, **29, 30**
  Alzheimer types 596, 597, **597,** 600, 601, 606
  Bergmann type 30–1, 32, 575, 602, 612
  corpora amylacea in 36–7, **36**
  degenerative changes in 33
  fibrous 27–8, 30–1, **27, 28, 31,** 37
  functional properties 31–2, 939
  gemistocytic (reactive) 33, **34, 35,** 266, 939
  in granular ependymitis 39, **40**
  hyperplasia **31,** 33–6, **34, 35**
  hypertrophy **31,** 33–6, **34**
  hypoxia, reaction to 129
  injury and disease, reaction to 33–6, **34, 35**
  mitosis of 33, **34**
  protoplasmic 27–30, **27, 28, 31**
  reactive (gemistocytic) 33, **34, 35,** 266, 939
  Rosenthal fibres 36, 374, **374**
  senile plaque encirclement 959, **959,** 961
  subependymal 39
Ataxia 723, **723**
  Friedreich's *see* Friedreich's ataxia
  in pontocerebellar atrophy (olivopontocerebellar atrophy) 715–18, **715, 716, 717,** 726, 884
  progressive, various types 723
Ataxia-telangiectasia (Louis-Bar syndrome) 724–6, **725,** 877
Atheroma 162–5
  carotid artery, internal 165, **166**

Atheroma—*contd.*
hypertension aggravating 173
Atherosclerosis 162–5
fusiform aneurysms 227
in hypertension 209
Athetosis in diseases of basal ganglia 713
Atlantoaxial dislocation 787
Atlas, occipitalization or assimilation 785–6
Austin variant of metachromatic leucodystrophy (mucosulphatidosis) 526, 527, 528, 529, 530, 537
Autonomic nervous system
autonomic failure in system degenerations 706, 707, 718–19
autonomic neuropathy, diabetic 719, 863
hereditary sensory and autonomic neuropathies 881–2
Autoregulation of cerebral blood flow 57–8, 127, 132, 133
and hypertension 172, **172,** 176, 218–19
Axolemma, peripheral nerves 808
nodal 828–31
Axonal retraction balls 103, **104–5,** 106, 109
Axonal spheroids 610–11, 661
Axonopathies 837
central-peripheral distal 843, 857
distal 843
proximal 843
Axonotmesis 850
Axons
degeneration 12, **14, 15,** 15–17, **16**
peripheral nerves 837, 838–44, **838, 839, 840, 841, 842, 844**
injury, diffuse, in head injury *see* Diffuse axonal injury
in peripheral nerves 808–14
internodal length 819
myelin attachment zone 830–1
nodal 828–31, **828**
perinodal space 831–2
regeneration 842–3
swellings on 12
'torpedoes' 12, **12**
terminals, axonal 3, **5,** 15, **16**
Axoplasm, peripheral nerves 808, 809–11
Azide intoxication 149–150

Bacillus anthracis
cerebral oedema 237
meningitis 240
Bacterial endocarditis, aneurysm formation 229
Bacterial infections of central nervous system 236
abscess
brain 243–6, **244, 245, 246,** 247, 251, **253**
epidural, cranial 238, 246
epidural, spinal 238–9, 246–7
subdural 239–40, **239**
cerebral oedema 237
cerebrospinal fluid, changes in 246–7, 250–1
epidural suppurations and granulomas
skull 238
spine 238–9, 248
immunology 236–7
leptomeningitis *see* meningitis
meningitis 238–9, 240–3, 247, 255, 267
tuberculous 247, 248–51, **249, 250,** 267
neurosyphilis 254–8, **256, 257**
pyogenic 238–47
routes of invasion 237–8
sarcoidosis 251–4, **254**
subdural 239–40, **239**
tuberculosis 236, 247–51
'Baltic myoclonus' 940, 941
Basal ganglia, diseases of 701–13
calcification 709, **710**
definition of basal ganglia 701
hypoxia
ischaemic, generalized 136, **137**
oligaemic, generalized 142
vulnerability to 131–2
intracerebral haemorrhage in hypertension 215, **216,** 216
muscular tone and movements, disorders of, association with basal ganglia lesions 713
pallidoluysian degenerations 708
progressive supranuclear palsy 708, **709,** 966, 967, 980
striatonigral degeneration 706–7, **706**
subthalamic lesions, focal, effects of 712–13
thalamic lesions, focal, effects of 712–13
see also parkinsonism; parkinsonism-dementia complex of Gaum; Parkinson's disease
Basilar invagination or impression 786, **786**
'Basket brain' 420, 472
Bassen-Kornzweig disease (abetalipoproteinaemia) 876
Batten's disease (neuronal ceroid lipofuscinosis) 503–4, 885
adult (Kufs' disease) 504
clinical features 505
pathology 507, 511–12, **511, 512,** 885
animal models 513
chemistry 506
classification 504
clinical features 505
diagnosis 512–13
early juvenile, clinical features 505
enzymology 506
infantile
clinical features 505
pathology 506, **506,** 507–8, **507**
inheritance 505–6
juvenile
clinical features 505
pathology 507, 510–11, **510, 511**
protracted form 505
late-infantile
clinical features 505
pathology 507, 508–10, **508, 509**
Behçet's disease 295, 1080
Behr's syndrome 884
Bell's palsy, Epstein-Barr virus association 280
Beriberi 579–80
peripheral neuropathy 855–6
Betz cells 2
Alzheimer's neurofibrillary degeneration 965
Bunina bodies in 25
in Friedreich's ataxia 721

Betza cells—*contd.*
in motor neuron disease 730
Bilirubin encephalopathy 478–80, **Plate 11.1 facing p. 490**
Binswanger's disease 176, 218–19, **218,** 984, 985
Bismuth, neurological disease due to 645–6
BK virus 288–9
Blastomycosis 326–7
Blood-brain barrier 175–6, 237, 243, 263
Blood circulation, and cerebral function 127
Blood-CSF barrier 237
Blood dyscrasias causing fetal brain damage 476
Blood flow, cerebral 127
autoregulation 57–8, 127, 132, 133
and hypertension 172, **172,** 176, 218–19
cerebral oedema 75
cerebral perfusion pressure 57–8
hypertension 172, **172,** 176, 218–19
and intracranial pressure 57–8
Blood volume, intracranial, changes affecting intracranial pressure 55
Bourneville's disease *see* Tuberous sclerosis
Boutons terminaux, degeneration 15, **16**
Boxers
neuritic plaques 966
neurofibrillary tangles 23, 117, **117,** 966
punch-drunk syndrome 117, **117**
Brain abscess *see* Abscess, brain
Brain changes in ageing 954–8
Brain damage in head injury *see* Head injury, missile, *and* Head injury, non-missile
Brain damage, hypoxic *see* Hypoxia
Brain damage, perinatal
arterial occlusion and cerebral infarction 470–1, **470, 471,** 475–6, **475**
congenital heart disease 470
fetal encephalopathies of circulatory origin 474–7, **475**
haemorrhage, intracranial and intracerebral 451
cerebellar 460–1, **460**
falx and tentorial laceration 451–2, **451**
intraventricular, in full-time neonate 459–60
intraventricular, in premature infant 455–9, **455, 456**
subarachnoid 453–4, **454**
subdural 452, **452**
subependymal and intraventricular in premature infant 455–9, **455, 456**
subpial 454–5
thrombosis, sinuses and cerebral veins 452–3, **453**
hydranencephaly 420, 471–3, **472, 473,** 474, 475, 476
hydrocephalus, posthaemorrhagic 458–9
hypoglycaemia 470
hypoxic-ischaemic encephalopathies in full-term neonates 464–70, **466**
kernicterus 478–80, **Plate 11.1 facing p. 490**
leucomalacia, periventricular 132–3, 461–4, **461, 462, 463, 464**
multicystic encephalopathy 463–4, **464, 465,** 471–3, 476
polyporencephaly 463–4, **464, 465**
porencephaly 471–3, 476
pseudocysts, subependymal 473
Brain death 6, 155
Brain distortion 53–4, 58, **58**
Brain herniation 53–4, 58, **58,** 59
cerebellar tonsils **58,** 65, **65,** 66
cingulate (subfalcine) **58,** 59, **59**
circular (ring) 63, **64**
external 67
tentorial **58,** 59–63, **59, 60, 61,** 66
tentorial, reversed 66
tonsillar **58,** 65, **65,** 66
transtentorial, central 63–4, 66
transtentorial, lateral **58,** 59–63, **59, 60, 61,** 66
uncal **58,** 59–63, **59, 60, 61,** 66
Brain shift 58, 59, **59**
Brain stem
arterial blood supply 157
damage, primary, in head injury 114–15
diffuse axonal injury 100, **102,** 103–6, **103,** 115
diseases of 701
haemorrhage, intracerebral, in hypertension 216
haemorrhage and infarction, from intracranial expanding lesions 64–5, **64, 65**
hypoxia
age, influence of, on ischaemic alterations 137–8
hypoglycaemic 151
ischaemic, generalized 136, 137–8, **138**
selective vulnerability 132
'Brain stones' 709, **710, 711,** 712
Brain swelling 53, 65–6, 71
congestive 71–2, 112
head injuries 88, 100, 111–13, **112, 113**
hypoxia 155, 465
respirator brain 6, 155
Brain water, changes affecting intracranial pressure 55
Brain weight 1–2
in ageing 954–5, 957
Breakthrough hypothesis, in hypertensive encephalopathy 175–6
Brown-Vialetto-van Laere syndrome 736–7
Brucella abortus, in meningitis 240
Buckthorn poisoning 675–6
Büngner, bands of 816, 838, 840, 843
Bunina bodies 25
Bunyaviruses 282
Burkitt lymphoma, Epstein-Barr virus associated with 261
'Burning feet' syndrome 580, 584
Burst lobe in head injury 94, 95, 97, **97, 110**
Buscaino bodies 6
Buzzard's 'lymphorrhages' in myasthenia gravis 1063

Cachectic atrophy of muscle 1086–7, **1087,** 1088
Cadmium poisoning 646
Caeruloplasmin in Wilson's disease 598–9
Caisson disease 179, 180
Calcification
in basal ganglia 709, **710**
of blood vessels 709, **712**
in cerebellum 709, **711**
Canavan's type of diffuse sclerosis (spongiform leucodystrophy) 374–6, **375**
Candidosis 327, **327**
Carbon disulphide intoxication 130, 651–2, 857

Carbon monoxide intoxication 128, 131–2, 145–8, **146, 147**
fetal brain damage following maternal inhalation 476
granular atrophy of cortex 171
peripheral neuropathy 857
Carcinoma, neurological syndromes associated with 612
cerebellar cortical degeneration 612, **613**
encephalomyelitic syndromes 612–14
neuropathy 890–2, **891**
pathogenesis 614
Carcinoma, polymyositis associated with 1077
Carcinomatous neuromyopathy 1087
Cardiac arrest, hypoxic brain damage 134, **135, 136, 137, 138,** 142
Carnitine deficiency, myopathy in 1091
Carnitine palmityl acyl transferase (CPAT) deficiency, myopathy in 1091
Carotid arteritis, acute 182
Carpal tunnel syndrome 853, 865, 868, 897
Caseation necrosis in tuberculosis 236, 247–8, 250
Caudate nucleus
calcification in 709, **710**
in Huntington's chorea 993, **994,** 995
hypoxia
ischaemic, generalized 136, 137
selective vulnerability 131
in multiple system atrophy 700 (Table)
Wilson's disease 597
Cavernous angiomas 230
Cavum septi pellucidi 423, 424–5, **424**
Cavum veli interpositi 425
Cavum vergae 424–5, **425**
Cell migration, anomalies of 411
agyria (lissencephaly) 413–15, **413, 414,** 417
ectopias 411–13, **411, 412, 413**
heterotopias 411–13, **412**
pachygyria 405, 413–15, **414,** 417
polymicrogyria 415–18, **415, 416, 418,** 476
Central core disease 1046, 1049, 1082–3
Central pontine myelinolysis 368–9, **368,** 578–9
Centronuclear myopathy 1046, 1083–5, **1085,** 1086
Centrum semiovale
hypoxic damage 130, 147
myelin deficiency 463, **464**
Cerebellum
alcoholism causing degeneration 578, 715
arterial blood supply 157
in ataxia-telangiectasia (Louis-Bar syndrome) 724–6, **725**
calcification in 709, **711**
cortical degeneration (cerebello-olivary degeneration) 714–15, **714**
cortical degeneration associated with carcinoma 612, **613**
cortical dysplasia 413, 417–18, **418**
cysts 406
degenerations 713–26
see also named types under Cerebellum
ectopias 412–13
epilepsy 928, 929, **930,** 932
external granular layer, proliferation 413, **413**
in Friedreich's ataxia 719–23, **720, 721, 722**
haemorrhage
in hypertension 216
perinatal 460–1, **460**
heterotopias 412–13, **412**
hypoxia
hypoglycaemic 151
ischaemic, generalized 136, 138
oligaemic, generalized 142, **142**
selective vulnerability to 132
kuru, abnormalities in 292
late cortical cerebellar atrophy 715
malformations 402
agenesis 402–3, **402, 403**
Dandy-Walker malformation 406–8, **407**
hypoplasia 403–6, **404, 405**
Lhermitte-Duclos disease 408–9, **409**
polymicrogyria (cortical dysplasia) 413, 417–18, **418**
see also Granule cells (cerebellar); Purkinje cells
Cerebral embolism *see under* Embolism
Cerebral infarction 125, 158–9
complicating saccular aneurysms 225
hypoxia, ischaemic 133
internal carotid artery occlusion or stenosis 166–7, **167**
intracranial expanding lesions causing **62,** 63, **63,** 64–5
macroscopic appearances 159–61, **159–61, 167**
meningitis causing 242
microscopic appearances 161–2, **161, 162, 163**
midbrain and pons in expanding lesions 64–5, **64, 65**
multi-infarct dementia 174, 218–19, 953, 982–7
oral contraceptives 187–8
perinatal 470–1, **470, 471**
arterial occlusion *in utero* 475–6, **475**
pregnancy and puerperium, association with 188
subclavian artery diseases 167
transient ischaemic attacks 181
see also Stroke
Cerebral oedema *see under* Oedema
Cerebrospinal fluid
abscess, cerebral 247
changes in CNS infection 246–7, 250–1
encephalitis, values in 267 (Table)
formation and absorption 67–8
herpes simplex virus encephalitis 274
hydrocephalus 67–71
intracranial expanding lesions 58
intracranial pressure 53, 54, 55, 57
meningitis 247
tuberculous 250–1
values in 267 *including* Table 7.1
neurosyphilis 254–5
normal values 267 (Table)
Cerebrovascular resistance 127
Cestodes, infections caused by
coenurosis 318
cysticercosis 315–17, **316,** 1081
echinococcosis 317–18, **318**
Chagas' disease 313, **314,** 890, 1081
Charcot-Marie-Tooth disease 726, 734, 877
hypertrophic form **849,** 877–9, **878**

Charcot-Marie-Tooth disease—*contd.*
neuronal form 879
Chediak-Higashi disease 884
Cherry red-spot myoclonus syndrome 539–40, **540, Plate 12.1(a) facing p. 491**
Chiari malformation 392, 393–5, **393, 394,** 435
Chicken pox *see* Varicella
Chloroquine neuropathy 672–3
Cholesterol and atheroma 164–5
Cholesteryl ester storage disease 551–4
Chorea, Huntington's *see* Huntington's chorea
Chorea in diseases of basal ganglia 713
Chorea-acanthocytosis syndrome 884
Choreoathetosis in diseases of basal ganglia 708, 713
Choroid plexus, cerebrospinal fluid production 67–8, 70
Chromatolysis 20–3, **20, 21**
in pellagra 22, 581–2, **582,** 583
Chromosome abnormalities 387–8, 411
see also Down's syndrome; Trisomies
Chronic granulomatous disease 243
Chronic progressive inflammatory polyneuropathy 886
Chronic relapsing inflammatory polyneuropathy 886
Churg-Strauss syndrome (allergic granulomatosis) 895–7
Circle of Willis
anatomy 157
aneurysms, atherosclerotic fusiform 227
aneurysms, saccular 219, 221, 225
cerebral infarction 133
in hypertension 209–12
medial gaps, and aneurysms 223
Cladosporiosis 327–8
Clarke's columns *see* Thoracic nuclei
Clasmatodendrosis 33
Clioquinol, neurotoxicity 660–1
Clostridium botulinum 237
Clostridium tetani 237
Clostridium welchii in muscle infection 1081
Coarctation of aorta
complications affecting spinal cord 798–9
saccular aneurysms associated with 220
Coccidioidomycosis 328
Cochlear nerves, lesions of 723, 737
Cockayne syndrome 877
Coeliac disease, adult 607–8, **608**
Coenurosis 318
Collagen pockets in peripheral nerve fibres 816–18, **817**
Commissures and midline structures of brain, malformations of 423–5, **423, 424, 425**
Compound granular corpuscle 41
Computerized tomography
cerebral haemorrhage 208, 209, 215
cerebral oedema **68,** 74
epilepsy 922, 923
strokes 208, 209
Concussion
diffuse brain damage 115
experimental production 86, 87, 115
spinal 781
Congenital amaurotic idiocy 513
Congenital dystrophic myopathy 1069–70, **1069**
Congenital fibre type disproportion (in muscle) 1032, 1085–6, **1085**
Congenital indifference to pain 882
Congenital myopathies 1069–70, **1069,** 1081–6
Congophilic angiopathy 968–71, **969, 970,** 978–9, **978**
Connective tissue disorders, inherited, intracranial vascular disease associated with 188
Contusions, cerebral 88–93, **89, 90, 91,** 97
brain swelling adjacent to 112, **112**
contrecoup 91, 92, 93
contusion index 92
coup 91, 93
fracture 91, 92
gliding 91, **92,** 93, 107, **108**
herniation 91
intermediary coup 91–2
parasagittal 91, **92**
pathogenesis 93
structural changes **89,** 92–3, **93**
Convulsions *see* Epilepsy
Copper metabolism, disorders of
Menkes' kinky hair disease 605
Wilson's disease 596, 597, 598–9
Corpora amylacea 36–7, **36**
Corpus callosum
agenesis 388, 408, 423, **423, 424**
damage in head injury 99
diffuse axonal injury 99, **101,** 103, 106, **107**
development 423
necrosis in Marchiafava-Bignami syndrome 578, **579**
Corpus Luysii *see* Subthalamic nucleus
Corpus striatum 701, 708
ageing, changes in 957
Huntington's chorea, changes in 993–5, **994**
hypoxia, vulnerability to 131
Corticospinal tracts *see* Pyramidal tracts
Corynebacterium diphtheriae 237
Coxsackie viruses
access routes 263
aseptic meningitis 268
poliomyelitis 269
susceptibility of different cell populations to 263
Cranial nerves
damage in non-missile head injury 99
degenerations 736–7
Cranial neuritis complicating meningitis 242
Craniorhachischisis 390
Creatine kinase (CK) level in muscle damage 1036
Becker muscular dystrophy 1068
childhood muscular dystrophy 1069
congenital dystrophic myopathy 1069
Duchenne muscular dystrophy 1066
facioscapulohumeral muscular dystrophy 1070
limb girdle muscular dystrophy 1068
spinal muscular atrophy, intermediate type 1057
spinal muscular atrophy, juvenile onset 1058
Tunisian muscular dystrophy 1067
Creutzfeldt-Jakob disease 261, 289–92, 700, 726, 732, 951–2, 953, 997
clinical features 979–80
necropsy, precautions against infection 264
pathology 13, 998–1001, **999, 1001**
transmissibility 1001–3

Cri du chat syndrome 388
Crohn's disease, granuloma in muscle 1080
Crooke's hyaline change in pituitary **771,** 772
Cryoglobulinaemia 893
Cryptococcosis 328–9, **329**
Cuprizone, neurotoxic effects in animals 678–9
Curvilinear bodies in late-infantile Batten's disease
509–10, **509**
Cushing's disease, myopathy associated with 1088
Cushing's syndrome, pituitary changes in 772
Cyanide intoxication 148–9, 586, 612
experimental studies 149
Cyclopia 388, 409, 411
Cysticercosis 315–17, **316,** 1081
Cystinosis 606, 554–5, **554**
Cysts
apoplectic 216, 217
arachnoid 242, 426–7, **426**
cerebellar malformations associated with 406
in cerebral infarction 162, **164**
coenurosis 318
cysticercosis 315–17, **316**
hydatid 317–18, **318**
toxoplasma 309–11, **310**
Cytomegalovirus 262, 280
fetal malformations due to 389
latent infection 261
Cytoplasmic body myopathy 1052

Dandy-Walker malformation 406–8, **407,** 423, 435
Deafness, with pontobullar palsy 737
Decompression sickness
hyperbaric 179–80, 181
hypobaric 180
Degeneration
acquired (non-wilsonian) hepatocerebral 599–602
Alzheimer's neurofibrillary 23, **23,** 700, 961–2, **962,**
963, 971, 974, 976
distribution 965
Down's syndrome 23, 435
experimental conditions 627–8, 979–80
pathogenesis 963–5, **963, 964**
Pick's disease, relationship to 991
prevalence 965–6
anterograde **14, 15,** 15–17, 699
see also Degeneration, wallerian
axonal, central nervous system 12, **14, 15,** 15–17, **16**
axonal, peripheral 838–44, **838, 839, 840, 841, 842**
axonopathies 837
sequestration 843–4, **844**
'chain' 699, 726
granulovacuolar, in ageing and dementia 24, **24,**
966–7, **967**
linked 699, 726
myelin 12, 15–17, **17**
neuronal 11–14, 699–701
hypoxic 8–11
peripheral nerves 837–8
sites in various diseases 700 (Table)
retrograde 20, 22–3, **22**
transneuronal 18–20, **18, 19,** 699
'triggered' 700, 707–8
wallerian
central nervous system **14, 15,** 15–17, 130, **131**
peripheral 838–42, **838, 839, 840, 841, 842**
Zenker's (of muscle) 1036, 1087
Dejerine-Sottas disease 848, 877, 879–80, **880**
Dementia 951–2, 1006
causes, and their prevalence 952–4
head injury causing 117
limbic encephalitis and malignant disease 1006
paretic (general paralysis of the insane) 255, **257,**
258, 951
see also Dementia and ageing
Dementia and ageing 951–4
Binswanger's disease 218–19, **218,** 984, 985
diagnosis 954
Alzheimer's neurofibrillary degeneration *see*
under Alzheimer's disease
brain in ageing 954–8, **955,** 956
congophilic angiopathy 968–71, **969, 970,** 978–9,
978
granulovacuolar degeneration 24, **24,** 966–7, **967**
Hirano bodies 967–8
plaques, senile (argyrophilic) (neuritic) 958–61,
958, 959, **960,** 973–4, **973**
memory disorder, pathological conditions 1003–6,
1004, 1005
multi-infarct dementia 174, 218–19, 953, 982–7
Parkinson's disease 705, 980–2
'subcortical' dementia 981, 982
see also Alzheimer's disease; Huntington's chorea,
Creutzfeldt-Jakob disease; Pick's disease
Demyelination
adrenoleucodystrophy 873
alcoholic neuropathy 856
Alexander type of leucodystrophy 373–4
amiodarone poisoning 671
amyloid neuropathy 869
arsenic poisoning 629
Batten's disease 507, 509
buckthorn poisoning 676
Charcot-Marie-Tooth disease 877
classification and concept of demyelinating disease
338
Cockayne syndrome 877
conduction block, acute 850–2, **851, 852**
diabetes mellitus 862–3
encephalomyelitis, acute disseminated perivenous
341–6, **342**
giant axonal neuropathy 884
G_{M2} gangliosidosis 494
Guillain-Barré syndrome 885
hereditary pressure-sensitive neuropathy 883
histochemistry 339–40
hyperoxaluria, primary 877
intervertebral disc protrusion 791
Krabbe's disease 872
lead poisoning 859
leprosy 887
leucoencephalitis, acute haemorrhagic 346, 348
lymphoreticular proliferative disorders 892
Marchiafava-Bignami disease 369, 578, **579**
mechanisms 339–40
metachromatic leucodystrophy 527, 870–2
multiple sclerosis *see* Multiple sclerosis
myelinolysis, central pontine 368–9, 578–9
paraproteinaemia, benign 893

Demyelination—*contd.*
  periaxial 338, 341, 368
  perivascular, in acute disseminated perivenous encephalomyelitis 341, **342, 343**
  Pott's paraplegia 795
  primary 844–6
  progressive multifocal leucoencephalopathy 289, **290,** 339
  sarcoidosis 890
  secondary 846, **847**
  segmental 844–6, **845, 846**
  spongiform leucodystrophy 374–6
  tellurium poisoning 648
  'tigroid' pattern 371, **372,** 373
  vascular disease, peripheral 894, 895
  viral diseases 267
  Waldenström's macroglobulinaemia 893
  X-linked leucodystrophy 369–73
Denborough's disease *see* Malignant hyperthermia
Dendrites, loss of in ageing 957–8
Dental sepsis, brain abscess due to 244
Dentate nuclei
  calcification of 709, 711
  cerebellar hypoplasia 405
  degeneration of 708, 723
  in Friedreich's ataxia 722
  Huntington's chorea, cell loss in 995
  hypoxia
    ischaemic, generalized 136
    vulnerability to 132
Dentatopallidoluysian atrophy, neuronal degeneration, sites of 700 (Table)
Dentatorubral atrophy 941
Dentatorubropallidoluysian atrophy 708
Dermatomyositis 1077–9, **1079**
  see also Polymyositis
Diabetes insipidus, cranial 756, 758, 759, 767
  familial 760
  idiopathic 760
  pathology 760–1
  pathogenesis 759–60, **760**
  secondary 760–1
Diabetes mellitus
  autonomic neuropathy 863
  in Friedreich's ataxia 719
  peripheral nerve disorders 862–4, **863, 864**
  strokes, incidence of 158
Diastematomyelia 392, 393, 395–6
DIDMOAD syndrome 760
Diencephalic syndrome 753–4
Diffuse axonal injury 87, 100, **101, 102, 104–5,** 109
  structural abnormalities 103
    brain stem 100, **102,** 103–6, **103,** 115
    corpus callosum 99, **101,** 103, 106, **107**
    diffuse damage to axons 87, 103, 106–7, **106, 107**
  subhuman primates 107–9
  vegetative state and severe disability 116
Dimethylaminodipropionitrile (DMAPN), peripheral neuropathy 857
Diphtheritic neuropathy 861–2
Diplomyelia 392, 395–6
Disseminated sclerosis *see* Multiple sclerosis
Disulfiram neuropathy 673–4, 860
Down's syndrome 388, 406, 433–5, **434**
  aetiology 435
  Alzheimer's neurofibrillary tangles 23, 435, 708, 965
  granulovacuolar degeneration in hippocampus 967
  neuritic plaques 965
Doxorubicin toxicity 674
Dürck's malarial granuloma 307, **308**
'Dying back' process 699, 716, 720, 726, 739
Dysraphic disorders 389–96
Dyssynergia cerebellaris myoclonica 723
Dystonia musclorum deformans, and basal ganglia lesions 713
Dystrophia myotonica (myotonic muscular dystrophy) 1035, 1039, 1043, 1074–5, **1074, 1075**

Eastern equine encephalitis 282
  pathological findings 283
Eaton-Lambert syndrome (myasthenic syndrome) 612, 1062, 1064
Echinococcosis 317–18, **318**
Echinococcus granulosus 317
Echoviruses
  access routes 263
  aseptic meningitis 268
  susceptibility of different cell populations to 263
Ectopias 411–13, **411, 412, 413**
Edema *see* Oedema
Effusions, subdural, complicating meningitis 242, **243**
Elzholz body in Schwann cells 822
Embolism
  carotid arteries 165
  cerebral 177
    air, 145, 179, 181
    atheromatous 178, **178,** 180
    of cardiac origin 177–8, 179
    experimental studies 180–1
    fat 115, 178–9, **178,** 180–1
    nitrogen 179–80, 181
  septic, brain lesions caused by 229, 238, 244, 245–6
Empty sella syndrome 66, 770
Empyema, subdural 239–40, **239**
  complicating meningitis 242–3
  histopathology 240
Encephalitis
  amoebic 305, 306–7
  cerebrospinal fluid, values in 267 (Table)
  experimental allergic 273, 345–6, **345,** 348
    multiple sclerosis and acute perivenous encephalomyelitis, relationship with 366–8
  infective, acute (viral) 260–1, **265,** 273–83, **277**
    adenoviruses 273
    arboviruses 273, 282–3
    cytomegaloviruses 280
    enteroviruses 273
    Epstein-Barr virus 280
    herpes simplex 264, 266, 267, 273–8, **276, 277, 279**
    herpesvirus B (simiae) 280
    rabies 273, 280–2
    varicella-zoster virus 278–80
  necrosis (viral) 266–7, **276, 277**
  perivenous demyelinating (viral) 260, 267, 272–3, 280
  postinfectious, acute (viral) 260, 267, 272–3, 280
  postvaccinal (viral) 260, 272–3

Encephalitis—*contd.*
subacute (viral) 261, 283–93
astrocytes, reactive 266
Creutzfeldt-Jakob disease 261, 289–92
kuru 261, 289–93, **293**
measles inclusion body encephalitis in the immunosuppressed 286–8, **287**
progressive multifocal leucoencephalopathy 266, 288–9
progressive rubella panencephalitis 288
subacute sclerosing panencephalitis 261, **265,** 266, 283–6, **285**
suppurative, in brain abscess 244–5, **244**
toxoplasma 310–11
trypanosomiasis 311–15
Encephalitis lethargica 294, 705–6
neurofibrillary tangles 966
Encephalocele 391–2
anterior 391–2, **392**
occipital 391, **391**
parietal 391
Encephalofacial angiomatosis (Sturge-Weber syndrome) 431, **432**
Encephalomalacia, multicystic 474–5, 476
Encephalomyelitis, acute disseminated perivenous
classic type 341
clinical features 341
morbid anatomy 341–3, **342, 343**
multiple sclerosis and experimental allergic encephalitis, relationship with 366–8
pathogenesis 343–6, 348
pathology
recurrent cases 343
subacute and late cases 343, **344**
Encephalomyelitis, viral 260, 268–72
polioviruses causing 260, 268–70
lesions, distribution of 270
pathological findings 269–70
postinfectious
cell-mediated immune response 262
varicella-zoster virus causing 271
pathological findings 271–2, **272**
Encephalopathies, spongiform 267, 289–92, **293**
cytoplasmic vacuolation 266, 292, **293**
see also Creutzfeldt-Jakob disease; Kuru; Scrapie; Spongiform leucodystrophy
Endarteritis obliterans 182–3, **183**
in meningovascular syphilis 255
Endocrine myopathies 1087–8
Endoneurium 808, 833–4, **833,** 836
Endoplasmic reticulum in neurons 3, **4**
peripheral axons 811
Entamoeba histolytica 304, **304**
Enteroviruses 260
access routes 263
acute encephalitis caused by 273
meningitis caused by 267–8
other than polioviruses, producing poliomyelitis 269
survival in sewage 262
Enzyme assays in lysosomal storage diseases 494, 498, 502
Ependyma 27, 39
Ependymitis, granular 39, **40**
Epilepsy 921
brain damage, pathogenesis of 932–4
cerebral hypoxia producing 156, 924
convulsive treatment, pathology of 942–3
cryptogenic 921, 924–5, 927–32
lesions secondary to trauma 928, **928**
minor dysgenetic lesions 927
neuronal loss and gliosis 928–32, **931**
cytological changes and epileptogenesis 939–40
experimental studies 933–4, 939–40
genetic aspects 921–2
hemiatrophy 925, 929, 931, **931**
incidence 921, 923
incisural sclerosis 932, 933, 935
myoclonus 708, 940–2
'Baltic myoclonus' 940, 941
Lafora bodies 25, **25,** 940–1
progressive without Lafora bodies 940, 941
neuroimaging 922–3
post-traumatic 116, 924
status epilepticus 116, 156, 465, 925, 926–7, **927**
symptomatic 921, 923–5
temporal lobe 934–9, **936, 937,** 940
Epineurium 836
Epstein-Barr virus 280
Burkitt lymphoma associated with 261
Guillain-Barré syndrome 280
latent infection 261
nasopharyngeal carcinoma associated with 261
Ergotism 609
Escherichia coli, in meningitis, neonatal 240
État criblé 174, 214–15
État lacunaire 174, **174, 175,** 214–15
État marbré (status marmoratus) **463,** 467–8, **469**
Excitatory amino acid neurotoxins 679–80
Exencephaly 390
Experimental allergic neuritis
demyelination 846, **846,** 848
remyelination **848**
External ophthalmoplegia 734, 885
Extraocular muscle
myopathy 1072–3, 1077
structural characteristics 1071–2, **1072**

Fabry's disease 546–8, **547,** 874–5, **874, 875**
Familial dysautonomia 882
Familial hepatolenticular degeneration *see* Wilson's disease
Familial oculoleptomeningeal amyloidosis, intracranial vascular disease associated with 188
Familial recurrent brachial plexus neuropathy 883
Familial spastic paraplegia 699, 737–9, **738, 739**
Farber's disease (Farber's lipogranulomatosis) 550–1, 876
Fat granule cell 41
Fazio-Londe disease 736
Febrile convulsions 925–6
Ferrugination of nerve cells 13–14, **13,** 470, **470**
Fetal alcohol syndrome 652–3
Fetal encephalopathies of circulatory origin 474–7
fetal conditions
arterial occlusions *in utero* 475–6, **475**
blood dyscrasias 476
multiple pregnancies, cerebral damage 474–5

Fetal encephalopathies of—*contd.*
maternal conditions 476
inhalation of toxic gases 476–7
placenta and umbilical cord anomalies 477
Fibromuscular dysplasia 182
aneurysms associated with 182
dissecting 228
saccular 220, 223
Filarial infections 322–3
Fingerprint bodies in juvenile Batten's disease 510, 511, **511**
'Finnish snowballs' in infantile Batten's disease 508, **508**
Fistulae
arteriovenous 431–3, **433**
carotid-cavernous sinus 227–8, **229**
following head injury 100, 227
Flaviviruses 282
Floppy baby syndrome 735, 1081
see also Werdnig-Hoffmann disease
Fluorescent antibody technique in virus diseases 264
Foamy cells 41
Fabry's disease 546–7
Farber's disease 551
fucosidosis 545
gangliosidoses 496, 502
Gaucher's disease 524
mucolipidosis type I 540
mucopolysaccharidoses 536, **537**
Niemann-Pick disease 516–17, **516,** 519–20, **520**
Wolman's disease 552, 553, **553**
Foetal *see* Fetal
Folic acid deficiency 592
Framingham Study 158, 177, 208
Friedreich's ataxia 719–23
central nervous system in 700 (Table), 720–2, **721, 722**
heart in 722–3
peripheral nerves in 719–20, **720,** 884
vascular lesions in 722–3
Froin-Nonne syndrome 246
Fucosidosis 544–5
Fungal infection 324, 332
actinomycosis 324–5
aspergillosis **324, 325,** 326
blastomycosis 326–7
candidosis 327, **327**
cladosporiosis 327–8
coccidioidomycosis 328
cryptococcosis 328–9, **329**
histoplasmosis 329–30
nocardiosis 330–1, **330**
zygomycosis (mucormycosis) 331–2, **331**

Gagel type granulomas **755,** 756
Ganglia
basal *see* Basal ganglia
sensory
in ataxia-telangiectasia 724, **725**
in Friedreich's ataxia 720
sympathetic
in Parkinson's disease 705
in progressive autonomic failure 719
Gangliosides 491, 492, 493, 497
Gangliosidoses 492
G_{M1} 497
animal models 503
chemistry 497
diagnosis 502–3
enzyme histochemistry 501–2, **501**
enzymology 497–8
fetal pathology 502, **502**
pathology 498–502, **498, 499, 501,** 876
G_{M2} 492–3
animal models 497
chemistry 493–4
clinical features 493
diagnosis 496–7
enzyme defect 494
neuropathology 494–6, **494, 495, 496,** 876
G_{M3} 503
Gargoylism *see* Hurler's syndrome
Gasser cell 537
Gaucher cell 523–6, **523, 524, 525**
Gaucher's disease
animal models 526
chemistry 522–3
enzymology 523
pathology 523–6, **523, 524, 525, 876**
fetal 526
types 522
General paralysis of the insane 255, **257,** 258, 951
Geniculate bodies
hypoxia, alterations in 132
transneuronal degeneration 18, **18**
Gerstmann-Sträussler syndrome 979, 1000
'Ghost' cells 730, **730,** 735
Giant axonal neuropathy 654, 858, 884, **884**
Giant cell arteritis (temporal arteritis) 185–6, **186,** 879
Giant cell granuloma, pituitary gland involvement 765, **766**
Gigantism, cerebral 422, 423, 761
'Ginger jake paralysis' 658, 659, 859
Gitterzell (lattice cell) 41
Glial cells
microglia *see* Microglia
neuroglia (macroglia) 27
astrocytes *see* Astrocytes
ependymal cells 27, 39
oligodendroglia 27, 37–9, **37, 38**
Glial fibrillary acidic protein (GFAP) 32, 33, 36
Glial shrub formation 11, 138
Glial stars 42, **42**
Gliomesodermal reaction in hypoxia 129–30, 136, **136,** 140, **141**
Globoid cells in Krabbe's leucodystrophy 530, 532, **532,** 533, **533,** 534
Globus pallidus
calcification in 709, **710**
carbon monoxide intoxication 131–2, 146, **146**
degeneration of 708
in Friedreich's ataxia 722
Hallervorden-Spatz syndrome, pigmentation 14, 609–10
Huntington's chorea 993, 995
hypoxia
anaemic 146, **146**
hypoglycaemic 151

Globus pallidus—*contd.*
  hypoxia
    ischaemic, generalized 137
    oligaemic, generalized 142
    vulnerability to 131–2
  Wilson's disease 597
Glucose
  cerebrospinal fluid levels in meningitis 247, 250, 251
  requirements of brain 125–6, 127–8
Glue-sniffing 653, 654, 875
L-Glutamate, neurotoxic effects 679–80
Glycogenoses
  type 2 548–50, **548, 549,** 550, 1088–90, **1089, 1090**
  type 3, myopathy in 1090
  type 5, myopathy in 1090, **1091**
  type 7, myopathy in 1090
Glycosaminoglycans (GAGs) 534
Gnathostomiasis 321, 322
Gold, neurological disorders produced by 646–7, 860
Golgi apparatus 3, **4**
Golgi epithelial cells (Bergmann astrocytes) *see* Astrocytes, Bergmann type
Gowers' sign 1065
Gracile nuclei, hypoxic damage 138, **138**
Granular atrophy of cortex 170–1, **171**
Granular osmiophilic deposits (GROD) in infantile Batten's disease 508, **508**
Granule cells (cerebellar)
  cerebellar cortical degeneration 612
  coeliac disease, adult, loss in 608
  hypertrophy (Lhermitte-Duclos disease) 408–9, **409**
  hypoplasia 403
  kuru 292
  mannosidosis 543
  mercury poisoning 639
  Reye's syndrome 602
Granuloma
  aspergillosis **325,** 326
  candidosis 327
  coccidioidomycosis 328
  Dürck's malarial 307, **308**
  epidural, spinal 238–9, 248
    cerebrospinal fluid 246
  Gagel type **755,** 756
  giant cell, pituitary gland involvement 765, **766**
  histoplasmosis 330
  in muscle 1080, **1080**
  sarcoid 251–4, 1080, **1080**
  schistosomiasis 320, **320**
  tuberculous 248, 251
Granulomatosis
  allergic (Churg-Strauss syndrome) 895–7
  lymphomatoid 895–6, **895**
  Wegener's 184–5, 897
Granulomatous angiitis 188
Granulovacuolar degeneration in ageing and dementia 24, **24,** 966–7, **967**
'Grave-stones' in muscle atrophy 1042
Guam
  motor neuron disease in 733–4
  parkinsonism-dementia complex in 23, 707, 734, 965–6, 967–8
Guillain-Barré syndrome
  cell-mediated immune response 262
  chromatolysis in 22
  cytomegalovirus association 280
  Epstein-Barr virus association 280
  peripheral neuropathy 865, 885–6

Haematomas, intracranial
  in head injury 88, 94
    burst lobe 94, 95, 97, **97, 110**
    delayed 94, 97
    extradural 94, **95**
    intracerebral 94, 96–7, **97**
    intradural 94–7
    subdural 87, 94, 95–6, **96,** 97, 112, **113**
  intracerebral, in hypertension **211,** 215, 216–17
  perinatal 451–2
    cerebellar 460–1, **460**
    in falx 451, **451**
    subarachnoid 454, **454**
    subdural 452, **452,** 453
    subependymal and intraventricular 456, **456**
Haemoglobinopathies affecting nervous system 187
Haemohydrocephalus in intraventricular haemorrhage in infancy 459, **459**
Haemophilus influenzae in meningitis 240
Haemophilus pertussis 237
Haemorrhage, intracranial
  cerebral contusions 92–3
  in expanding lesions
    in midbrain and pons 64–5, **64**
    in tentorial hernia 60, **61, 62,** 64–5
  in head injury 88, 93–4, 97, 100, 113–14, **114**
Haemorrhage, intracranial, spontaneous 208
  amyloid angiopathy causing 230
  aneurysms 219–29, 230
  arteriovenous malformations 230
  blood diseases causing 230
  causes 210 (Table)
  cavernous angiomas 230
  hypertensive cerebrovascular disease 208, 209–12, **211, 212**
    aneurysms, miliary (microaneurysms) 212–13, **213,** 217
    arterial changes in malignant hypertension 214, **214**
    pathological changes in brain 214–19
  incidence 208–9
  intracerebral in hypertension 215–17, **215, 216**
    pathogenesis 217
  sites 208–9
  subarachnoid
    aneurysms, dissecting, rupture of 228
    aneurysms, saccular, rupture of 208, 220, 221, **221,** 224, 225–6
    arteriovenous malformations 230
    in head injury 94
  tumours in brain as cause of 230
Haemorrhage, intracranial and intracerebral, perinatal 451
  cerebellar 460–1, **460**
  falx and tentorial laceration 451–2, **451**
  intraventricular, in full-term neonate 459–60

Haemorrhage—*contd.*
intraventricular, in premature infant 455–9, **455, 456**
subarachnoid 453–4, **454**
subdural 452, **452**
subependymal and intraventricular in premature infant 455–9, **455, 456**
subpial 454–5
thrombosis, sinuses and cerebral veins 452–3, **453**
Haemosiderin deposition in haemorrhage 14, **211,** 215, **215,** 575
Haemosiderosis complicating hemispherectomy 14
Hallervorden-Spatz syndrome 14, 609–10, 713
Hartmannella-Acanthamoeba 305, 306–7
Hartnup disease 581
Head injury, missile 85
brain damage 118–19, **119**
depressed injury 118
epilepsy, post-traumatic 116, 924
herniation contusions 91
penetrating injury 118, **118**
perforating injury 118–19
Head injury, non-missile 85
acceleration of head as factor of 86–7, 95–6
angular 87
translational 87
brain damage 85–6
brain stem, primary damage 114–15
classification 87–8
fat embolism associated with 115
neuritic plaques 966
neurofibrillary tangles 966
brain damage, diffuse 87–8, 100
axonal injury *see* Diffuse axonal injury
brain swelling 88, 100, 111–13, **112, 113**
hypoxic 87, 100, 109–11, **110, 111,** 116
multiple small haemorrhages 88, 97, 113–14, **114**
brain damage, focal 87
contusions, cerebral *see* Contusions, cerebral
corpus callosum 99
cranial nerves 99
haemorrhage, intracranial 93–7
hypothalamus 99, **766,** 768, **768, 769**
lacerations 88
pituitary gland 99, 767–8, **766, 767, 768**
pontomedullary rent 98–9, **98,** 114
secondary to raised intracranial pressure 97–8
vascular lesions 99–100
brain damage, outcome 115
epilepsy, post-traumatic 116, 924
progressive neurological disease 116–17
severe disability and vegetative state 115–16
contact phenomena 86–7
experimental models 86–7
infection as complication of 98
scalp and skull, lesions of 88
Hemiatrophy in epilepsy 925, 929, 931, **931**
Hemiballism, lesions associated with 712
Hemispherectomy, haemosiderosis complicating 14
Hepatic coma 599, 600–1
Hepatolenticular degeneration, familial *see* Wilson's disease
'Hereditary cerebral haemorrhage with amyloidosis' 979
Hereditary motor and sensory neuropathy 877–81, 1060
type I **849,** 877–9, **878**
type II 879
type III 879–80, **880**
Hereditary neuropathies, classification 869
Hereditary pressure-sensitive neuropathy 849, **849,** 883, **883**
Hereditary sensory and autonomic neuropathies 881–2
type I 881, **881**
type II 881–2
type III 882
type IV 882
Hereditary sensory neuropathy with spastic paraplegia 882
Herniation of brain *see* Brain herniation
Heroin addiction, intracranial vascular disease associated with 188
Herpes simplex virus (HSV)
encephalitis 273–4
incidence 274
laboratory diagnosis 274–5
latent infection 275–6
necrosis 266, 267, 276–8, **276, 277**
pathogenesis 275–6
pathological findings 264, 276–8, **276, 277, 279**
latent infection 261, 275–6
serotype 1 268
serotype 2 268
susceptibility of different cell populations to 263
Herpes zoster infection 271, 280
pathological findings 271–2, **272**
Herpesvirus simiae (herpesvirus B) 262, 280
Herpesviruses 261, 273–80
access routes 262
tumour production in animals 261
Herring bodies 764
Heterotopias 411–13, **412**
Heubner's arteritis 250, 255, **256**
Hexacarbon solvents, neurotoxicity
biochemistry 656–7
clinical features 653–4
experimental studies 654–6, **655, 656,** 858, **858**
exposure 653
human pathology 654, 857, 857–8
Hexachlorophane, toxic effects 661–2
experimental studies 662–3, **662**
Hexosaminidase deficiency 492, 493, 494, 495
von Hippel-Lindau's angiomatosis 406, 430–1
Hippocampus (Ammon's horn)
epilepsy 926, 928–9, **929,** 932, 936
see also sclerosis, *below*
granulovacuolar degeneration 24, **24,** 966–7, **967**
Hirano bodies 968
hypoxia
hypoglycaemic damage 150, 151, **151**
ischaemic 135, **135,** 137, **137**
vulnerability to 131, 152, 153
memory disorders 1003, 1004–5
neurofibrillary change in Alzheimer's disease 974, **974**
sclerosis (Ammon horn sclerosis) 925, 926, 928–9, **929,** 932–5, 937–9, **937**

Hirano bodies 967–8, 1000
Histoplasmosis 329–30
Hoffmann's syndrome (pseudomyotonia) 1088
Holotelencephaly (holoprosencephaly) 388, 409–11, **410**
Homocystinuria 606
Homogenizing cell change 9–11, **11**, 129, 136
Hunger oedema 594
Hunter's syndrome 534–8, **539**, 877
Huntington's chorea 699, 701, 713, 951, 992–3
  histology 993–6, **994**
  macroscopic appearances of brain 993, **993**
  neurochemical findings 996
Hurler's syndrome 534–9, 877
  pituitary gland, abnormal deposits in 770, **770**
Hurler-Scheie syndrome 535–8
Hyaline arteriosclerosis in hypertension 173–4, **173**, 176, 209
Hydatid disease 317–18, **318**
Hydranencephaly 420, 471–3, **472, 473**, 474, 475, 476
Hydrocephalus 66, 67, 392
  active 67
  Arnold-Chiari malformation 393, **394**
  arrested 67
  cerebrospinal fluid 67–71
  communicating 55, 67, 70, 242, 393
  compensatory 67, 242
  complicating subarachnoid haemorrhage 226
  congenital 435–6
  cysticercosis causing 315, 316
  ex vacuo 67, 435, 463, 464
  external 67
  intermittent 70
  internal 67
  maternal infections producing 388–9
  meningitis causing 242, 389
  non-communicating 67, 70
  normal pressure 70–1
    idiopathic 70
  normal volume 70–1
  obstructive 55, 68, 69, 74
  occult 67
  otitic 71, 190
  pathogenesis, in man 69–70
  posthaemorrhagic, in perinatal intraventricular haemorrhage 458–9
  schizencephaly associated with 420–1
  ventricular enlargement, pathogenesis, 68–9, **68, 69**
Hydromyelia 392, 393, 395, **396**
  distinction from syringomyelia 397, 398, 401
Hygroma, subdural 97
Hyperaldosteronism, myopathy associated with 1088
Hyperammonaemia 603, 606
Hyperglycinaemia 606
Hypermyelination 849, **849**
Hyperparathyroidism, muscle disease associated with 1088
Hyperpathia 713
Hypersensitive state in bacterial infection 236
Hypertension
  cerebral circulation, pathophysiology of 172
  experimental 176–7, 219
    arterial changes 219
  intracranial 54–5, 56, 57, 71
    benign 71
  malignant 174–6, **175**, 214, **214**
  pathological changes 209
    in brain 173–7, **173, 174, 175**, 209–12, 214–19
  strokes, incidence 158
  see also Hypertensive cerebrovascular disease
Hypertensive cerebrovascular disease 208, 209–12, **211, 212**
  aneurysms, miliary (microaneurysms) 212–13, **213**, 217
  arteriolar changes in malignant hypertension 214, **214**
  pathological changes in brain 214–19
    arterial changes in experimental hypertension 219
  Binswanger disease 176, 218–19, **218**, 984, 985
  dementia, multi-infarct 174, 218–19, 953, 982–7
  hypertensive encephalopathy 174–6, 217–18
  intracerebral haemorrhage 215–17, **215, 216**
  lacunae 174, **174, 175**, 214–15
Hypertensive encephalopathy 174–6, 217–18
Hyperthyroidism, myopathies associated with 1087
Hypoglossal nuclei in motor neuron disease **728**
Hypoglycaemia 8, 128, 150–2, **150**
  experimental studies 151–2
  neonatal 470
Hypomyelination 849, **849**
Hypoparathyroidism, myopathy associated with 1088
Hypopituitarism and empty sella syndrome 770
Hypotension
  and hypoxia, oligaemic 139, 140, **140, 141**, 142–3, **142, 143**
  orthostatic (postural) 718–19
Hypothalamus 748
  anatomy 748–52, **749**
    blood supply 752
    connections **750, 751**, 752
    nuclei 749–50, **749, 750, 751**
    secretory neurons 750–2, **751**
  congenital malformations 754–5
  damage in non-missile head injury 99
  diabetes insipidus 756, 758, 759–61
  functions 752–4
    endocrine activity control 750–2, 753
    neurosecretion 750–2, 753
    vegetative functions control 753–4, **753**
  hamartoma 754–5, **754, 755**
  hypophysectomy, changes produced by 758, **758, 759**
  hypoxia 132, 137
  inflammatory diseases 755–6
  irradiation, changes produced by 758–9, **759**
  multiple sclerosis causing demyelination 758
  parkinsonism producing Lewy bodies 758
  parvicellular neurons, lesions of 761
  pituitary stalk section, changes produced by 758
  retrograde degeneration of nuclei 22–3, **22**
  scrapie causing diabetes insipidus 758
  subarachnoid haemorrhage causing lesions in 226
  traumatic lesions 99, **766**, 768, **768, 769**
  vascular lesions 756–7, **757, 768**
Hypothyroidism 865, 1087–8

Hypotonia, infantile (floppy baby syndrome) 735, 1081
see also Werdnig-Hoffmann disease
Hypoxia 125–6
anaemic 128, 145–8, **146, 147**
anoxic 128, 143–4
experimental studies 143–4
arterial boundary zones, brain damage in 132, 139–43, **140, 141**
categories 128
cerebral blood flow 127
and cerebral energy supply 127–8
complications of hypoxic brain damage 155–6
brain swelling 155, 465
epilepsy 156
no-reflow phenomenon 156
consumptive 128
definitions 111, 128
gliomesodermal reaction 129–30, 136, **136,** 140, **141**
head injury 87, 100, 109–11, **110, 111,** 116
vegetative state and severe disability 116
histotoxic 128, 148–50
hypoglycaemia causing 128, 150–2, **150**
experimental studies 151–2
hypoxic 128, 144–5
experimental studies 144–5
ischaemic 128
ischaemic, generalized 133–9
experimental studies 138–9
macroscopic appearances of brain 134–6, **135**
microscopic appearances of brain 136–8, **136, 137, 138**
ischaemic, localized 133
maturity, influence of, on brain damage 132–3
oligaemic 128, 145
generalized 139–43, **143**
localized 139
and oxygen tension 126–7
'pathoclisis' concept in brain damage distribution 152, 153
respirator brain 6, 155
selective vulnerability to 131–3, 136, 152–5
stagnant 128, 133
ischaemic 128, 133–9
oligaemic 128, 139–43, 145
structural changes resulting from 8–11, **8–11,** 128–31, **130, 131**
thresholds of ischaemia 156, 159
'vascular theory' of brain damage distribution 152–3
Hypoxic-ischaemic encephalopathies in full-term neonates 464–70, **466**
sequelae 467–70

I-cell disease 541, 877
β, β'-Iminodipropionitrile (IDPN), neurotoxic effects 680
Immunity
bacterial infection 236–7
viral infection 262
Immunoglobulins in ataxia-telangiectasia 724
Immunoperoxidase technique 6, **35,** 237, 264
fungal infections 324, **324**
measles inclusion body encephalitis in immunosuppressed 286, **287**
plaques, senile (argyrophilic) (neuritic) 974
polymyositis 1077
progressive multifocal leucoencephalopathy 289
subacute sclerosing panencephalitis **285,** 286
Inclusion bodies in viral diseases **265,** 266
measles encephalitis in immunosuppressed **287,** 288
Negri bodies 26, **26,** 266, 281–2, **281**
progressive multifocal leucoencephalopathy 289, **290**
subacute sclerosing panencephalitis 284, **285,** 286
Incrustations in ischaemic cell change 9, **10,** 11, 129, 136
infantile hypotonia (floppy baby syndrome) 735, 1081 *see also* Werdnig-Hoffmann disease
Infantile neuronal degeneration 735–6
'Infantile paralysis' 268
Infantile spinal muscular atrophy of Werdnig and Hoffmann *see* Werdnig-Hoffmann disease
Infantile subacute necrotizing encephalopathy 603–5, **604,** 885
Infarction *see* Cerebral infarction
Infectious mononucleosis 280
Inflammatory bowel disease, intracranial vascular disease as complication of 188
Inflammatory cell infiltration in viral disease 264–6, **265**
inflammatory myopathies 1076–81
Injury
astrocyte reactions 33–6
peripheral nerves 850–5
see also Head injury, missile; Head injury, non-missile
Intermediolateral columns of spinal cord 700 (Table), 718–19
Intervertebral disc protrusion 787–8
cervical disc disease 788–91
lumbar discs 792
lumbar puncture 792–3
radiography 793
spondylosis deformans 788, **789**
thoracic discs 791–2
Intracranial expanding lesions, pathology of 53–4, 58
bony changes 66–7, **66**
brain swelling 53, 65–6, 71–2, 112
external herniae 67
extracerebral lesions 65
haemorrhage and infarction in midbrain and pons 64–5, **64**
infratentorial 66
supracallosal hernia **58,** 59, **59**
supratentorial 58–66
tentorial hernia **58,** 59–63, **59, 60, 61,** 66
tonsillar hernia **58,** 65, **65,** 66
transtentorial herniation
central 63–4, 66
lateral **58,** 59–63, **59, 60, 61,** 66
Intracranial pressure
mean 54
normal 54
pressure-volume relationships 55, 56, **56**
raised *see* Raised intracranial pressure

Iron in nervous system 13–14, **13,** 470, **470**
Irradiation 42–5
  hypothalamic changes after 758–9, **759**
  intracranial vascular disease resulting from 188
  malformations induced in animal teratology 386
  peripheral nerve involvement 855
  of pituitary gland with yttrium-90 769–70, **769**
  prenatal malformations produced by 389
Ischaemia, cerebral 54, 57, 75, 128, 159
  hypertensive patients 172
  thresholds of 156, 159
Ischaemia of muscle 1093–4
Ischaemic cell change *see under* Ischaemic cell process
Ischaemic cell process 125, 129
  stages
    (i) microvacuolation 8–9, **8, 9,** 129, 136
    (ii) ischaemic cell change 9, **10,** 129, 136
    (iii) ischaemic cell change with incrustations 9, **10,** 11, 129, 136
    (iv) homogenizing cell change 9–11, **11,** 129, 136
Isoniazid (INH) toxicity 663–4, 860
  experimental studies 665–6, **664, 665, 666,** 860
Itai-itai disease 646

Jakob-Creutzfeldt disease *see* Creutzfeldt-Jakob disease
JC virus 288–9, **291**
  in progressive multifocal leucoencephalopathy 263, 288–9

Kainic acid, neurotoxic effects 679–80
Kayser-Fleischer ring 596, **596,** 598
Kearns-Sayre syndrome 885, 1073–4, **1073,** 1086
Kernicterus (bilirubin encephalopathy) 478–80, **Plate 11.1 facing p. 490**
Klinefelter's syndrome (XXY) 388
Klüver-Bucy syndrome 989, 1005
Korsakoff syndrome 573–7, **574, 575, 576,** 1003–4
Krabbe's leucodystrophy *see under* Leucodystrophies
Kufs' disease 504
  clinical features 505
  pathology 507, 511–12, **511, 512,** 885
Kugelberg-Welander disease 1056, 1058, **1059,** 1070
Kuru 261, 289–92, 951, 1001–2
  pathological findings 13, 292, **293**
Kwashiorkor 594–5

Labelled antibody techniques in viral diseases 266, 278, **279**
Lacunae 174, **174, 175,** 214–15
Lafora bodies 25, **25,** 940–1
Larva migrans 321–2
Laser irradiation, effects on brain 45
Latent infection in viral diseases 261, 271, 275–6
Lateral horns of spinal cord 718–19
Lathyrism 676–7
Lead poisoning
  inorganic lead
    clinical features 629–30
    experimental studies 630–3, **632, 634**
    exposure 629
    human pathology 630
  organic lead
    clinical features 634
    experimental studies 635–6, **635**
    exposure 634
    human pathology 634–5
  peripheral neuropathy 630, 633–4, 859
Leigh's disease (infantile subacute necrotizing encephalopathy) 603–5, **604,** 885
Leprous neuropathy 886
  borderline (dimorphous) leprosy 888–90
  lepromatous leprosy 886–7, **887, 888, 889**
  tuberculoid leprosy 887–8, **889**
Leptomeningitis *see* Meningitis
Leucodystrophies
  Alexander type 373–4, **373**
    Rosenthal fibres in 36, 374, **374**
  astrocytic reactions 34
  Krabbe's 530–1
    animal models 534
    chemistry 531
    diagnosis 534
    enzymology 531
    pathology 531–4, **532, 533,** 872
    peripheral nerve involvement 872, **873**
  metachromatic 526, 870
    animal model 530
    Austin variant 526, 527, 528, 529, 530, 537
    chemistry 526
    diagnosis 529–30
    electron microscopy 529
    enzymology 526–7
    pathology 527–9, **527, 528, 529, Plate 12.1(c) and (d) facing p. 491**
    peripheral nerve involvement **528,** 870–2, **870, 871, 872, Plate 12.1(d) facing p. 491**
    types 526
  spongiform 374–6, **375**
  X-linked 369–73
    adrenoleucodystrophy 369–71, **371,** 872–3
    adrenomyeloneuropathy 370–1, 872–3
    Pelizaeus-Merzbacher disease 371–3, **372, 373**
Leucoencephalitis, acute haemorrhagic 346
  morbid anatomy 346, **346, 347**
  pathogenesis 348
Leucomalacia, periventricular, perinatal 132–3, 461–4, **461, 462, 463, 464**
Leukaemia, peripheral nerve involvement 892
Lewy bodies
  in Alzheimer's disease 981
  in Parkinson's disease 25, **26,** 700, 702, **704,** 705, 758, 981
  in progressive autonomic failure 718–19
Lhermitte-Duclos disease 408–9, **409**
Lhermitte's sign 42
Lipid phagocytes *see* Phagocytes, lipid
Lipidosis
  in muscle 1091, 1092, **1092**
  in nervous system, drug-induced 668–72
Lipofuscin in muscle fibres 1029
Lipofuscin in neurons 2, 3, **4**
  ageing 956
  aspartylglycosaminuria 545
  Batten's disease 507, 511, 512
  Huntington's chorea 995

Lipofuscin in neurons—*contd.*
mucolipidosis type IV 542
tellurium poisoning, in experimental animals 648
Lipogranulomatosis *see* Farber's disease
Lipohyalinosis 174
Lissencephaly (agyria) 413–15, **413, 414,** 417
Listeria monocytogenes in meningitis 240
Little's disease 1081
Liver disease, neuropathological changes associated with 595
acquired (non-wilsonian) hepatocerebral degeneration 599–602
familial hepatolenticular degeneration (Wilson's disease) 595–9
peripheral neuropathy 865
'Locked in' syndrome 169, **169**
Locus ceruleus 3
in ageing 957
in Alzheimer's disease 962, 965, 976–7, 981–2
in parkinsonism-dementia complex of Guam 707
in Parkinson's disease 700 (Table), 702, 981–2
Loeffler's syndrome 321
Loiasis 322, 323
Louis-Bar syndrome (ataxia-telangiectasia) 724–6, **725,** 877
Luft's disease 1086
Lymphocytic choriomeningitis virus
access route 263
suppression of acetylcholine enzymes 263
Lymphohistiocytosis, haemophagocytic 343
Lymphoma
Burkitt's 261
in Louis-Bar syndrome 724
neuropathies related to 892
Lymphorrhages in myasthenia gravis 1063
Lysophosphatidyl choline (LPC), neurotoxic effects 680–1
Lysosomal enzyme deficiencies 491–2
light microscopy of blood films 500 (Table)
neuronal inclusion bodies 26
see also individually named lysosomal storage disorders
Lysosomes in peripheral axons 811
Lyssa bodies in rabies 282

McArdle's disease, myopathy in 1090, **1091**
Macrophages 39–40, 41
haemosiderin-containing in hypertensive intracerebral haemorrhage **211,** 215, **215**
see also Phagocytes, lipid
Malaria, cerebral 307–8, **308**
pathological comparison with acute haemorrhagic leucoencephalitis 348, **348**
Malformations of nervous system 385
aetiology 387–9
arteriovenous 431–3, **433**
experimental teratology, findings of 385–7
see also specified malformations
Malignant hyperthermia (MH) (Denborough's disease)
myopathy associated with 1036, 1075, 1082–3, 1087, 1092–3
core fibres 1093, **1093**
fibre splitting 1093, **1093**
internal nuclei in muscle fibres 1043, **1045,** 1093, **1093**
moth-eaten muscle fibres 1051, 1093, **1093**
Mamillary bodies 752
ageing 957
brain herniation 58, 63–4
epilepsy 931, **931**
hypoxia, alterations in 132, 137
memory disorders 1003–4
Wernicke and Korsakoff syndromes 573–7, **574, 575, 576,** 1003–4, **1004**
Manganese intoxication 636–7
Mannosidosis 543–4, **544**
Mantoux reaction
sarcoidosis 252
tuberculous meningitis 248
Maple syrup urine disease 606
Marchiafava-Bignami syndrome 369, 578, **579**
Marinesco bodies 25–6
Maroteaux-Lamy syndrome 534–8, **536, 537**
Maternal infections in prenatal malformations 388–9
Measles virus
access route of 262, 263
inclusion body encephalitis in immunosuppressed 286
pathological findings 286–8, **287**
latent infection 261
postinfectious encephalitis 260, 272, 273
subacute sclerosing panencephalitis 261, 283–4
pathological findings **265,** 266, 284–6, **285**
Meckel syndrome 391
Megalencephaly 422–3, **422**
Membranous cytoplasmic bodies
in G_{M1} gangliosidosis **498**
in G_{M2} gangliosidosis 495, 496, **496**
in mucolipidoses 542, **542**
in mucopolysaccharidoses 538
in Niemann-Pick disease 520, **521**
Meningiomas 65
from x-irradiation 44
Meningism 260
in rabies 280
Meningitis
aseptic 267–8, **277**
autopsy 241–2
bacterial 238–9, 240
cerebrospinal fluid values 267 (Table)
cerebrospinal fluid changes 247
complicating non-missile head injury 98
complications 242–3
fungal infection 324–8, 330, 332
histopathology 242
intrauterine 389
meningococcal 240–1, 242
neonatal 240
recurrent 243
syphilitic 255
tuberculous 247, 248–50, **249, 250**
cerebrospinal fluid in 250–1, 267 (Table)
serous 251
viral 260, 267–8, **277**
cerebrospinal fluid values 267
virus isolation 267–8

Meningocele
  cranial 391–2
  spinal 392–3
Meningococcus 237, 240–1, 242
Meningoencephalitis
  amoebic, primary 304, 305–6, **305**
  cysticercosis 315
  gnathostomiasis 322
  granulomatous, prenatal infection 389
  herpes simplex virus 278
  poliovirus and echovirus, in immunodeficient children 269
  trypanosomiasis
    African 312
    congenital 314–15
Meningomyelocele 392–3
Menkes' kinky hair disease 605
Menopausal muscular 'dystrophy' 1088
Mercury poisoning
  inorganic mercury 637, 859
  organic mercury 637–41, **638**
    experimental studies 639–40, **640,** 858
    human pathology 638–9, 859
Metabolic myopathies 1088–94
Metachromatic leucodystrophy *see* Leucodystrophies, metachromatic
Metazoal infections
  cestodes 315–18, **316, 318,** 1081
  nematodes 321–4, **321,** 1081
  trematodes 318–21, **320**
Methotrexate, toxicity 666–7
Methyl alcohol poisoning 657–8
Metronidazole, neurotoxicity 668, 860
Meyer-Betz disease 1087
Meynert, nucleus of, in Alzheimer's and Parkinson's diseases 981, 982
Micrencephaly *see* Microcephaly
Microaneurysms (miliary aneurysms) 212–13, **213,** 217
Microcephaly 421–2, **421**
  irradiation during pregnancy as cause of 389
  maternal infections causing 388, 389, 421
Microfilaments in peripheral nerves 809
Microglia 27, 39–42, **40, 41**
  in diffuse axonal injury 106, **106,** 108, 109
  hypoxia, reaction to 130
Microglial stars in viral disease **265,** 266
Microgyria 415, 476
  see also Polymicrogyria
Microtubules of peripheral nerves 809–11
Microvacuolation of neuron 8–9, **8, 9,** 129, 136
Middle ear infection
  brain abscess due to 244
  epidural tuberculosis due to 248
Migraine, intracranial vascular disease associated with 188
Minamata disease 638, 639
Minicore disease 1049, 1051, **1082,** 1083
Misonidazole, neurotoxicity 667–8, 860
Mitochondria 3, **4**
  axonal, in peripheral nerves 810–11
  in muscle 1028, **1028,** 1029
    abnormalities **1073,** 1074, 1086
Mitochondria-lipid-glycogen (MLG) disease of muscle 1074
Mitochondrial myopathy 885, **1073,** 1074, 1086
MLG disease 1074
Mongolism *see* Down's syndrome
Morquio syndrome 534–8, **537**
Morton's neuroma 853
Morular cell in trypanosomiasis 312, **312**
Mosaicism 388, 435
Motor neuron disease 699, 700 (Table), 726–33, 1055–6, **1055**
  associated diseases 733
  Bunina bodies in spinal neurons 25
  classification problems 732–3
  clinical features 727
  familial forms 734
  granulovacuolar degeneration in hippocampus 967
  in Guam 733–4
    neurofibrillary tangles 734, 966
  head injury, possible connection with 117
  muscle pathology 1055–6
  neurofibrillary tangles 966
  pathological changes 727–32, **728, 729, 732, 733**
    anterior nerve roots **727**
    neuronophagia and 'ghost cells' **730**
    pyramidal tracts 726, 730, **731, 732, 733**
    vacuolation of neurons in wobbler mouse 13, **13**
Moyamoya disease 183–4, 220
'Mucocytes' (Buscaino bodies) 6
Mucolipidoses
  Batten's disease, distinction from 512
  type I 539–41
  type II 541, **541, 542**
  type III 541
  type IV 542–3, **542, 543**
Mucopolysaccharidoses 534–5, 877
  animal models 539
  classification 534–5
  diagnosis 535, 538–9
  pathology 535–9
Mucormycosis 331–2, **331**
Mucosulphatidosis 526, 527, 528, 529, 530, 537
Multicore disease 1049, 1050, 1051, 1083
Multicystic encephalomalacia 474–5, 476
Multicystic encephalopathy, perinatal 463–4, **464, 465,** 471–3, 476
Multiple pregnancies, and fetal cerebral damage 474–5
Multiple sclerosis 349
  acute (Marburg type) 354–5, **357**
  acute perivenous encephalomyelitis and experimental allergic encephalitis, relationship with 366–8
  aetiology 359–64, **363**
  classic (Charcot type)
    clinical features 349
    clinicopathological correlations 350–2
    distribution of lesions 350, **351, 352**
    histology of lesions 352–4, **353, 354**
    morbid anatomy 349–50, **350, 351**
    remyelination 354, **356**
    shadow plaques 354, **355**
  concentric sclerosis (Balò type) 355, **359**
  early lesion 364–6
  neuromyelitis optica (Dévic type) 357–9, **360, 361**
  pathogenesis 359–64, **363**

Multiple sclerosis—*contd.*
  plaque 349–54, **351, 352, 353, 354**
    evolution and pathogenic significance 364–6, **365, 367**
    shadow plaques 354, **355**
  Schilder type 355, **358,** 359, **361**
'Multiple sulphatase' deficiency 530
Multiple system atrophy 699, 706–7, 708, 716, 718–19
  neuronal degeneration, sites of 700 (Table)
Mumps virus
  access route 263
  encephalitis (postinfectious) due to 260, 272, 273
  meningitis due to 268
  susceptibility of different cell populations to 263
Muscle
  afferent nerve receptors 1035–6
  ageing of 1027–8, **1027**
  clamp 1028–9, **1029**
  diseases, classification 1026
  histology 1026–7, **1027**
  histopathological studies, historical review 1026
  infections 1081
    parasitic 1081
  ischaemia 1093–4
  motor-point muscle biopsy 1035
  motor unit 1034–5
  spindles 1035–6, **1035**
    dystrophia myotonica, changes in 1035, 1075
    innervation **1035,** 1036
    Parkinson's disease, degenerative changes 705
  see also Muscle fibres
Muscle fibres 1026–7, **1027**
  A bands 1027, **1027**
  artefacts 1031, **1031,** 1066
  atrophy 1041–3, **1041, 1042**
    group 1042–3, 1052–5, **1054,** 1058, 1060
  axonic expansions, degeneration of, in peripheral neuropathies **1061**, 1062
  axonic spheres, in ageing **1027,** 1028
  basal lamina, in muscle atrophy **1041,** 1042, **1042**
  central nuclei 1046, 1052, 1083–5, **1085,** 1086
  cores 1046–51, **1047, 1048,** 1052, 1082–3, 1093, **1093**
    minicores 1049, 1051, **1082,** 1083
    multicores 1049, 1050, 1051, 1083
    polyneuritis, association with 1060
  cross-striation, focal loss of 1050
  cytoplasmic bodies 1052, **1052**
  denervation 1035, 1041–3, **1041, 1042,** 1078
    general reactions of muscle 1052–5
    peripheral neuropathies 1059–62, **1060, 1061**
    polymyositis 1078
    spinal muscular atrophy 1056, 1058
  Doyère's eminence **1027**
  extrafusal 1036
  giant cells, in muscle atrophy 1042, 1059, **1060**
  glycogen in 1029, 1046, 1088–90, **1089, 1090, 1091**
  'grave-stones', in muscle atrophy 1042
  group atrophy 1042–3, 1052–5, **1054,** 1058, 1060
    type grouping 1052–5, **1054**
  I bands 1027, **1027**
  internal nuclei 1042, 1043–6, **1045,** 1052, 1076
    childhood muscular dystrophy 1069
    Duchenne muscular dystrophy 1065
    dystrophia myotonica 1074, **1074**
    facioscapulohumeral muscular dystrophy 1070, **1070**
    malignant hyperthermia 1093, **1093**
    motor neuron disease 1056
    ocular myopathy 1072
  intrafusal 1035–6
    'nuclear bag' **1035,** 1036
    'nuclear chain' **1035,** 1036
  lipofuscin in 1029
  minicores 1049, 1051, **1082,** 1083
  mitochondria 1028, **1028,** 1029
    abnormalities **1073,** 1074, 1086
  moth-eaten **1047,** 1050–1, **1050**
    central core disease 1082
    Kearns-Sayre syndrome 1074
    limb girdle muscular dystrophy 1068
    malignant hyperthermia 1093, **1093**
    ocular myopathy 1072
  motor end-plates **1027,** 1034, **1034**
    dystrophia myotonica, changes in 1075
    myasthenia gravis, changes in 1062–4, **1063**
    peripheral neuropathies, changes in 1060–2, **1060**
    ultrastructure 1029, **1030**
  multicores 1049, 1050, 1051, 1083
  myofibrils 1026–7, **1027**
  myofilaments 1027, **1027**
  necrosis 1036–8, **1037,** 1043, **1045,** 1087
    muscular dystrophies 1068, 1069, 1075
    periodic paralysis 1076
    polymyositis 1077–9
    thyrotoxic myopathy 1087
  polyribosomes 1029
  'ragged red' **1073,** 1074
  regeneration 1036–8, **1037,** 1043, **1045,** 1087
    muscular dystrophies 1068, 1069, 1075
    periodic paralysis 1076
    polymyositis 1077, 1079
    thyrotoxic myopathy 1087
  reinnervation, collateral 1053–5, **1054,** 1078
    motor neuron disease 1056
    spinal muscular atrophies 1058
  ring 1043, **1044,** 1068, 1069, 1071, 1074
  sarcomere **1027,** 1029
  sarcoplasmic masses 1043, 1074, **1074**
  sarcoplasmic reticulum 1028, **1028,** 1029
  size 1029
  sole-plates 1029, **1030,** 1035, 1062
    myasthenia gravis, changes in 1062, **1063**
  splitting 1038–41, **1039, 1040,** 1052
    in childhood muscular dystrophy 1069
    in Duchenne muscular dystrophy 1065
    in dystrophia myotonica 1039, 1075
    in facioscapulohumeral muscular dystrophy **1070**
    in fetal life 1038–9, **1038**
    in malignant hyperthermia 1093, **1093**
    in motor neuron disease 1056
  sprouting of axons **1060,** 1062, 1075, **1075,** 1078, 1082
    Duchenne muscular dystrophy 1066
    myasthenia gravis 1062
  strap cells in **1037,** 1038

Muscle fibres—*contd.*
  target 1046–51, **1049**
  tubular aggregates 1086, 1087, 1088
  type disproportion, congenital 1032, 1085–6, **1085**
  type grouping in denervation 1052–5, **1054**
  types 1031–3, **1032**
    1 1027, 1029, 1031–2, **1032**
      subtypes a and b, possible existence of 1032–3, **1033**
    2 1029, 1031–2
    2a 1027, 1029, 1031–2, **1032**
    2b 1027, 1029, 1031–2, **1032**
    2c 1031–2
    in animals 1031, 1032, **1033**
    distribution 1033–4
    Wohlfart B-fibres **1038,** 1039, 1056
  ultrastructure 1028–9, **1028**
  vacuoles in 1051, **1051**
    in denervation 1052, **1053**
    glycogenosis, type 2 1088–90, **1089**
    rimmed 1051, **1051,** 1072–3
    'storage' 1051
    systemic lupus erythematosus 1051, 1080
  Z bands 1027, **1027**
Muscular atrophy 1041–3, **1041, 1042,** 1052–5, **1054,** 1058, 1060
  in ataxia-telangiectasia 724
  cachectic 1086–7, 1087, 1088
  of larynx in multiple system atrophy 719
  in motor neuron disease 726–7, 1055–6
  peroneal *see* Charcot-Marie-Tooth disease
  spinal *see* Spinal muscular atrophy
Muscular dystrophies 1064
  Becker (benign X-linked) type 1067–8, **1067**
  childhood 1069
  congenital 1069–70, **1069**
  distal 1071
  Duchenne type 1064–7, **1065, 1066,** 1069
    aetiology 1066–7
    histopathology 1065–6
    ultrastructure 1067
  Emery-Dreifuss humeroperoneal 1070–1
  facioscapulohumeral 1070, **1070**
  Fukuyama type 1070
  Landouzy-Dejerine type 1070, **1070**
  limb girdle 1068, **1068**
  myotonic 1035, 1039, 1043, 1074–5, **1074, 1075**
  Tunisian 1067, 1069
Muscular tone and movement, disorders of, association with basal ganglia lesions 713
Myasthenia, penillamine-induced 1062, 1064
Myasthenia gravis 1062–4, **1063,** 1087
  cores in muscle fibres 1049
Myasthenic syndrome (Eaton-Lambert syndrome) 612, 1062, 1064
Mycobacterium leprae 238
Mycobacterium tuberculosis 236, 247
Myelin
  attachment zone 830–1
  degeneration 12, 15–17, **17**
  formation 818–19
  oligodendroglia, relationship with 37–9, **38,** 339, **339**
  structure and chemistry 339–40, **339, 340,** 820–1
  thickness of sheath 819–20
Myelinolysis, central pontine 368–9, **368,** 578–9
Myelitis, transverse
  Epstein-Barr virus association 280
  herpesvirus B (herpesvirus simiae) causing 280
Myelocele 392–3
Myeloma, peripheral nerve involvement 892
Myelomeningocele 392–3
Myocarditis
  complicating rabies 282
  in Friedreich's ataxia 722
Myoclonus 708, 713
  see also under Epilepsy
Myopathies 1064
  primary
    congenital 1069–70, **1069,** 1081–6
    inflammatory 1076–81
    mitochondrial **1073,** 1074, 1086
    muscular dystrophies *see* Muscular dystrophies
    myotonic syndromes 1074–6
    ocular and oculoskeletal 1071–3
    ophthalmoplegia plus (Kearns-Sayre syndrome) 1034, **1073,** 1086
    scapuloperoneal syndrome 1059, 1071
  secondary 1064, 1086–94
    metabolic 1088–94
Myosclerosis 1079
Myositis
  eosinophil 1077
  fibrosa 1079
  granulomatous 1080
  inclusion body 1080–1
  orbital 1077
  proliferative 1079
  vacuolation in muscle fibres, in systemic lupus erythematosus 1051
  vasculitic disease in 1079–80
  viral 1081
  see also Dermatomyositis; Polymyositis
Myotonia congenita (Thomsen's disease) 1075–6
  internal nuclei 1043, 1075
Myotonic syndromes 1074–6
Myxoedema **771,** 772, 1088

Naegleria fowleri 305–6, **305**
Nageotte
  residual nodules of 614, 643, 720, 837, **837,** 890, **891**
  spiny bracelet of 827
Necropsy in viral disease 263–4
Necrosis
  caseation, in tuberculosis 236, 247–8, 250
  coagulative 43, 45, 161, **161**
  encephalitis, viral, acute 266–7
  herniation pressure causing 59, **59,** 60–2, **61**
  herpes simplex virus encephalitis 266, 267, 276–8, **276, 277**
  irradiation causing 42–5, **44**
  lipid phagocytes in **41,** 42
  muscle fibres 1036–8, **1037,** 1043, **1045,** 1087
    muscular dystrophies 1068, 1069, 1075
    periodic paralysis 1076
    polymyositis 1077–9
    thyrotoxic myopathy 1087

Necrosis—*contd.*
neuronal, selective, 125, 129, 131
'selective granule cell' in cerebellum 7
ultrasound causing 45
Necrotizing myopathy 1087
Negri body in rabies 26, **26,** 266, 281–2, **281**
Neisseria meningitidis 241
Nelson's syndrome, pituitary changes 772
Nematodes 321–4, **321,** 1081
Neocortex, and hypoxia, vulnerability to 131
Nephrosialidosis 540
Nerve cell *see* Neurons
Neural tube defects 389–96
Neurapraxia 850
Neurites in senile plaques **960,** 961
Neuroaxonal dystrophy 610–11
Neurofibrillary degeneration *see* Degeneration, Alzheimer's neurofibrillary
Neurofibrillary tangles
in Alzheimer's disease *see under* Alzheimer's disease
in Down's syndrome 23, 435, 708, 965
in motor neuron disease of Guam 734, 966
in parkinsonism-dementia complex of Guam 23, 700, 707
in postencephalic parkinsonism 23, 705–6, **705**
in progressive supranuclear palsy 700, 708
Neurofibromatosis 431
Neurofilaments 3, 809
Neuroglia 27
see also Astrocytes; Ependyma; Oligodendrocytes
Neurolathyrism 676–7
Neuroma, peripheral nerves 854, **854**
Morton's 853
Neuromelanin 3
Neuromuscular transmission disorders 1062–4
Neuromyelitis optica 357–9, **360, 361**
Neuronal ceroid lipofuscinosis
see Batten's disease; Kufs' disease
Neuronophagia 11, **12**
in motor neuron disease **730**
in viral disease **265,** 266, 269, **270,** 270
Neurons
Alzheimer's neurofibrillary degeneration 23, **23**
binucleated 13
chromatolysis 20–3, **20, 21**
dark (artefacts) 7, **7**
degeneration 11–14, 837–8
Alzheimer's neurofibrillary 23, **23**
granulovacuolar 24, **24**
hypoxic 8–11
peripheral nerve disorders 837–8
Pick's disease 24–5, **24**
transneuronal 18–20, **18, 19**
ferrugination 13–14, **13,** 470, **470**
hypoglycaemic damage 8, 150, **150,** 470
hypoxic damage 8–11, 128–9
inclusion bodies 23–6
'large light' cells 3
morphology 2–3, **2**
multinucleated 13
'small dark' cells 3
synapses 3, **5**
vacuolation 13, **13**
in kuru 292, **293**
viral diseases, changes caused by 266
Neuropathy, sensory
and carcinoma 614, 890–2, **891**
in Friedreich's ataxia 719–20
in pontocerebellar atrophy 718
Neurosyphilis 254
asymptomatic 254–5
congenital 258
meningovascular 254, 255, **256**
parenchymatous 254, 255–8
paretic dementia (general paralysis of the insane) 255, **257,** 258
tabes dorsalis 255–8, **256**
primary and secondary stages 254–5
Neurotmesis 850
Neurotoxic esterase (NTE) in neuropathy induced by organophosphorus compounds 660
Neurotransmitters 3–6
and astrocytes' functional role 32
Neurotubules
in neurons 3, **4**
in peripheral nerves 809–11
Nicotinic acid deficiency 578, 581–3, 856
Niemann-Pick disease 503, 513, 876
animals models 522
chemistry 515
classifications 513–14
clinical features 514–15
diagnosis 520–2
enzymology 515–16
pathology, group I 516–18
fetal 518–19
type A 516–18, **516, 517, 518**
type B 517
pathology, group II 519–20
type C **519, 520, 521**
Nissl bodies **2,** 3, **4**
in chromatolysis 20, **20,** 21, 23
in Pick's disease 989
Nitrofurantoin neuropathy 860
Nitroimidazoles, neurotoxicity 667–8
No-reflow phenomenon in hypoxia 156
Nocardiosis 330–1, **330**
Noradrenaline storage sites 3
Nuclei of neurons 2–3, **2, 4**
Nucleolus of neurons 2

Occlusion of large vessels, neuropathy related to 894
Ocular and oculoskeletal myopathy 1071–3
Oculomotor nerve, in brain herniation 60, 64
Oculopharyngeal myopathy 885
Odontoid process, separation from axis 786–7
Oedema
cerebral 55, 71, 72–5, **72,** 217
bacterial infections 237
brain swelling associated with head injuries 112, 113
cytotoxic, due to energy failure 73
cytotoxic, due to poisoning 73
effects 75
hydrostatic 73–4
hypo-osmotic 74
interstitial **68,** 74
spread and resolution 74–5

Oedema—*contd.*
cerebral—*contd.*
vasogenic 73, 75
hunger 594
spinal cord trauma 782–3
Oligaemia 128, 159
Oligodendrocytes 27, **27,** 37–9, **37, 38,** 339, **339**
hypoxia, reaction to 129–30
Oligodendroglia *see* Oligodendrocytes
Olives
in cerebello-olivary degeneration 714–15
Huntington's chorea, lesions in 995
hypoxic damage 132, 138
in olivopontocerebellar atrophy 715
transneuronal degeneration 18, **19**
Olivopontocerebellar atrophy (pontocerebellar atrophy) 699, 715–19, **715, 716, 717,** 726, 884
Onchocerciasis 322–3
'Onion bulb' formations in peripheral neuropathy 848, **849,** 862, 873
Onuf's nucleus 700 (Table), 719, 735
Opalski cells 596, **596,** 597, 598, 600
Ophthalmoplegia 718, 734, 885
Ophthalmoplegia plus (Kearns-Sayre syndrome) 1073–4, **1073,** 1086
Optic nerves and tracts
in Friedreich's ataxia 722
in other hereditary ataxias 723
Oral contraceptives and cerebral infarction 187–8
Organophosphorus compounds, toxicity 658–60, 859
Orthostatic hypotension 718–19
Osteitis deformans (Paget's disease of bone) 785
Osteolathyrism 676
Osteomalacia, myopathy in 1091–2
Osteomyelitis, infection of central nervous system 238, 239
brain abscess 243
epidural abscess, skull 238
epidural abscess, spine 238–9
Oxyachrestia 128
see also Hypoglycaemia
Oxygen cascade 126, **126**
Oxygen requirements of brain 125–7, 144
Oxygen tension 'critical' for production of brain damage 144

Pachygyria 405, 413–15, **414,** 417
Pachymeningitis 238, 239
Pachymeningitis cervicalis hypertrophica 255
Paget's disease of bone 785
Pallidoluysian degenerations 708
Pallidum *see* Globus pallidus
Pallister-Hall syndrome 754
Panenecephalitis, rubella, progressive 288
Panencephalitis, subacute sclerosing, 261, 283–4
pathological findings **265,** 266, 284–6, **285,** 966
Pantothenic acid deficiency 580–1, 855–6
Papilloedema 71, 75–6, 217
Papovaviruses 288, **291**
tumour production in animals 261, 288
Paragonimiasis 318–19
Parahippocampal gyri herniation 59–62, **60, 61, 62,** 63, **64**
Paralysis agitans *see* Parkinson's disease
Paramyotonia congenita 1076
Paramyxovirus, suppression of beta-adrenergic receptors 263
Paraproteinaemias, benign, neuropathy 893, **893**
Parkinsonism
causes 706, 707–8
idiopathic *see* Parkinson's disease
in multiple system atrophy 706–7, 716, 718
postencephalitic 23, 702, 705–6, **705,** 733
Parkinsonism-dementia complex of Guam 23, 707, 734, 965–6, 967–8
Parkinson's disease (paralysis agitans) 700–5, 952
Alzheimer's disease, relationship with 705, 980–2
autonomic failure in 718–19
dementia in 705, 980–2
head injury, possible connection with 117
Lewy bodies in 25, **26,** 702, **704,** 758
neuronal degeneration, sites of 700 (Table)
pathology 702–5, **703, 704**
'Pathoclisis' concept in hypoxic brain damage 152, 153
Pelizaeus-Merzbacher disease 371–3, **372, 373**
Pellagra 578, 581–3, **582,** 856
chromatolysis in 22, 581–2, **582,** 583
Penicillamine-induced myasthenia 1062, 1064
Perfusion pressure, cerebral 56–7, 127, 128, 132, 176, 219
Perhexiline maleate, neurotoxicity 668–70, 861
Perikaryon in neurons 2–3
Perinatal brain damage *see* Brain damage, perinatal
Perineurium 808, 834, **835,** 836
Periodic paralysis 1076
hyperkalaemic 1076
hypokalaemic 1076
normokalaemic 1076
thyrotoxic 1076, 1087
vacuoles in muscle fibres 1051, 1076, **1076**
Peripheral nerves, diseases of
axonal degeneration 838–44, **838, 839, 840, 841, 842**
axonopathies 837
sequestration 843–4, **844**
axonal regeneration 842–3
classifications 837
hereditary neuropathies 869
injuries 850
demyelinating conduction block, acute 850–2, **851, 852**
demyelination
primary 844–6
secondary 846, **847**
segmental 844–6, **845**
denervation of muscle 1059–62, **1060, 1061**
hypermyelination 849, **849**
hypertrophic neuropathy 848–9, **849**
hypomyelination 849, **849**
inflammatory neuropathies 885–90
injury
classification 850
cold 854–5
compression 853–4, **853**
crush 852, **853**
entrapment 853–4, **853**
mechanical 850–4

Peripheral nerves—*contd.*
injury—*contd.*
penetrating wounds 854
percussion 853
radiation 855
stretch 854
metabolic disorders 862–77
neuronal degeneration 837–8
neuropathies, hereditary, of unknown causation 877–85
nutritional deficiences 855–7
paraneoplastic neuropathy 890–2
remyelination 846–8, **848**
toxic neuropathies 857–62
iatrogenic 860–2
vascular 894–7
wallerian degeneration 838–42, **838, 839, 840**
retrograde effects of axon section 842
unmyelinated axons 841–2, **841, 842**
see also individually named disorders
Peripheral nerves, normal structure 807–8, **807**
axolemma 808
nodal 828–31
axon 808–9
axoplasm 808, 809–11
myelin attachment zone 830–1
nodal 828–31, **828**
transport in 809, 811–14
classification 808
fibres
myelinated 818–21
unmyelinated 816–18, **817**
mesaxon 816, 818, **822**
Schmidt-Lanterman incisures 823–6, **825,** 839
sheaths
endoneurium 808, 833–4, **833,** 836
epineurium 836
function 836
perineurium 808, 834, **835,** 836
transmission of nerve impulse 814
transport in axons 809, 811–13
anterograde, fast 812–13, 813–14
anterograde, slow 812
retrograde 813
vasculature 836–7
see also Schwann cells; Ranvier, nodes of
Perivascular cuffing in viral disease 264–6, **265,** 283, 284, 286
rabies 281
Peroneal muscular atrophy (Charcot-Marie-Tooth disease) 726, 734, **849,** 877–9, **878**
Phacomatoses 724
Phagocytes 11, **12,** 39
lipid 41–2, **41**
in cerebral infarction 162, **163**
in hypoxia 130, **130,** 131
in spinal cord traumatic lesions 783
in viral diseases 266
Phenothiazines, causing parkinsonism 707
Phenylketonuria 389, 606
Philophthalamus 321
pi granules in Schwann cells 822, 863
Pick's disease 951, 953, 978, 987–8
argyrophilic inclusions 24–5, **24,** 990–1
brain, appearances of 988–9, **988**
head injury, possible connection with 117
histology 989–91, **990**
neuronal degeneration 24–5, **24**
Pituitary gland
abnormal depositions in 770–1
adenohypophyseal cells, functional differentiation 762–3, **763**
agenesis 765
anatomy 761–4, **762**
adenohypophysis (pars distalis) 762–3
blood supply 764, **764, 765**
neurohypophysis (pars nervosa) 764, **764**
brain herniation 64
damage in head injury 99, 767–8, **766, 767**
empty sella syndrome 66, 770
endocrine conditions, pituitary changes in 771–2, **771**
hypophysitis, lymphocytic and autoimmune 765–6
hypoplasia 765
inflammatory diseases 765
in Louis-Bar syndrome 724
necrosis 768–70
ischaemic 766, **766, 767**
postpartum 766–7, **767**
radiation 769, **769**
traumatic lesions 99, 767–8, **766, 767, 769**
Pituitary-ovarian axis associated with myopathy 1088
Pituitary stalk 761, **762**
damage in head injury 99, 767, **768**
severance 766, **766,** 767–8, **767, 768**
Placenta and umbilical cord anomalies, and perinatal brain damage 477
Plaques
cerebellar, in kuru 292, **293**
multiple sclerosis *see under* Multiple sclerosis
senile (argyrophilic) (neuritic) 958–61, **958,** 959, **960,** 973–4, **973**
experimental production 979–80
Pick's disease 991
Plaques fibromyéliniques 467
Plasmodium falciparum 307
Platinum toxicity 647
Pneumococcus 237
in meningitis 240
Poliomyelitis 260, 268–70
chronic syndrome 1062
lesions, distribution of 270
motor neuron disease, association with 733
neuronophagia 269, **270,** 270
pathological findings 11, **12,** 269–70, **270**
Poliovirus 260, 261, 268
access routes 262, 263
encephalomyelitis caused by 260, 268–70
susceptibility of different cell populations to 263
Polyarteritis nodosa 184, **184,** 894–5, **895,** 1079–80, **1079**
Polycystic kidney disease, aneurysms associated with
dissecting 228
saccular 220, 223
Polycythaemia 186
Polycythaemia vera, neuropathy 892–3
Polygyria 467
Polymicrogyria 415–18, **415, 416, 418,** 476

Polymyositis 1026, 1077–9, **1078**
during menopause 1088
internal nuclei in muscle fibres 1043
vasculitic diseases associated with 1079–80, **1079**
Polyneuritis, muscle denervation 1060
Polyomavirus 288–9, **291**
transformation process 261
Polyporencephaly in infants 463–4, **464, 465**
Polysomes 3, **4**
Pompe's disease (glycogenosis type 2) 548–50, **548, 549, 550,** 1088–90
Pontine nuclei in multiple system atrophy 700 (Table), 715–18
Pontobulbar palsies 736–7
Pontocerebellar atrophy (olivopontocerebellar atrophy) 699, 706, 715–19, **715, 716, 717,** 726, 884
Pontomedullary rent in non-missile head injury 98–9, **98,** 114
Pontoneocerebellar hypoplasia 403–5, **405**
Porencephaly 419, 420, 471–3, 476
Porphyria 606–7, 876–7
Positron emission tomography 923
Posterior columns of spinal cord, degeneration of
in ataxia-telangiectasia 724
in familial spastic paraplegia 737–9, **738, 739**
in Friedreich's ataxia 720
in pontocerebellar atrophy 717–18
Postgastrectomy states inducing neuropathy 608
Postural (orthostatic) hypotension 718–19
Pott's paraplegia 794–5, **795**
Pox virus, survival 262
Precocious puberty, hypothalamic involvement 755
Pregnancy, cerebral infarction, association with 188
Presenile dementia *see* Alzheimer's disease
Pretibial syndrome 1094
Primary neuronal degenerations 699–701
Probst's bundle 423, **424**
Progressive autonomic failure 718–19
Progressive bulbar palsy *see* Motor neuron disease
Progressive cerebral degeneration in infancy (Alpers' disease) 477–8, 611
Progressive multifocal leucoencephalopathy (PML) 261, 262, 288–9, 339, 368
astrocytes, reactive 266
JC virus 263, 288–9
pathological findings 289, **290–1**
Progressive muscular atrophy *see* Motor neuron disease
Progressive rubella panencephalitis 288
Progressive subcortical gliosis 991–2
Progressive supranuclear palsy 700, 708, **709,** 966, 967, 980
Progressive systemic sclerosis, neuropathy 897
Protozoal infections
amoebiasis 304–7
malaria, cerebral 307–8, **308,** 348, **348**
toxoplasmosis 309–11, **309, 310,** 389, 756, **756,** 765, 1081
trypanosomiasis 311–15, **312, 314,** 890, 1081
Pseudoabscess, in tuberculomas 251
Pseudoaneurysms 212
Pseudocysts, subependymal 89
Pseudo-Hurler polydystrophy 541
Pseudomonas aeruginosa causing meningitis 240
Pseudomyotonia (Hoffmann's syndrome) 1088
Puerperium, cerebral infarction, association with 188
Pulseless disease 182, **182**
Punch-drunk syndrome 117, **117**
Pupil dilatation in tentorial hernia 60, 62
Purkinje (Purkyně) cells 2, **2**
Alzheimer's neurofibrillary degeneration 965
ataxia-telangiectasia, loss in 724, **725**
cerebellar cortical degeneration 714
cerebellar hypoplasia 403, **404,** 405
coeliac disease, adult 608
degeneration (torpedo formation) 12, **12,** 612, **613,** 639
homogenizing cell change 9–10
in Huntington's chorea 995
hypoxia, vulnerability to 132
kuru, abnormalities in 292
mannosidosis 543
mercury poisoning 638–9, **638**
pontocerebellar atrophy 715, 716, 718
Reye's syndrome, loss in 602
Wernicke's encephalopathy 575
Putamen
calcification in 709, **710**
in Huntington's chorea 993, **994,** 995
hypoxia
ischaemic, generalized 137, **137**
oligaemic, generalized 142
selective vulnerability 131
in multiple system atrophy 700 (Table), **706,** 716
Wilson's disease 597
Pyramidal tracts
degeneration 699, 700 (Table), 726
in familial motor neuron disease 734
in familial spastic paraplegia 737–9, **738, 739**
in Friedreich's ataxia 720, **721,** 722
in motor neuron disease 726, 730, **731, 732, 733,** 1055
in pontocerebellar atrophy 715
malformations 395–6, **396**
preservation
in pontocerebellar atrophy **716**
in Werdnig-Hoffmann disease 735, **736**
Pyridoxine deficiency 584–5, 860

Rabies 280–2
access routes of virus 262
acetylcholine receptors affected by 263, 281
dumb (paralytic) 280, 282
encephalitis
acute infective 273
postvaccinal 260, 273
furious 280
pathological findings 281–2
lyssa bodies 282
Negri bodies 26, **26,** 266, 281–2, **281**
susceptibility of different cell populations to virus 263
Radiation necrosis *see* Radionecrosis
Radionecrosis 42–5, **44**
ischaemic pathogenesis, theory of 43
Raised intracranial pressure 53–5, 77
brain damage, secondary to, in head injury 97–8

Raised intracranial pressure—*contd.*
brain swelling 53, 65–6, 71
congestive 71–2, 112
cerebrospinal fluid 53, 54, 55, 57
effects 56–8
genesis 54–6
hydrocephalus *see* Hydrocephalus
hypertension, intracranial, benign 71
intracranial expanding lesions, pathology of 53–4, 58
bony changes 66–7, **66**
brain swelling 53, 65–6, 71–2, 112
external hernia 67
extracerebral lesions 65
haemorrhage and infarction in midbrain and pons 64–5, **64**
infratentorial 66
supracallosal hernia **58,** 59, **59**
supratentorial 58–66
tentorial hernia **58,** 59–63, **59, 60, 61,** 66
tonsillar hernia **58,** 65, **65,** 66
transtentorial herniation **58,** 59–64, **59, 60, 61,** 66
oedema, cerebral 55, 71, 72–5, **72,** 217
papilloedema 71, 75–6, 217
pressure-volume relationships 55, 56, **56**
systemic sequelae 76–7
waves of 55
Ramsay Hunt syndrome 723, 941
Ranvier, nodes of 809, 819, 826–8, **827, 828, 832**
functional implications of 832–3
myelin attachment zone 830–1
nodal axon and axolemma 828–31, **828**
perinodal space 831–2
von Recklinghausen's disease 431
Red nucleus, degeneration in 700 (Table), 708
Refsum's disease 873–4, **874**
Reich granule in Schwann cells 822
Remak cells 808, 814
Remyelination
acute disseminated perivenous encephalomyelitis 346
adrenoleucodystrophy 873
amyloid neuropathy 869
Charcot-Marie-Tooth disease 877, 879
Guillain-Barré syndrome 885
Krabbe's disease 872
metachromatic leucodystrophy 870
multiple sclerosis 354, **356**
peripheral nerves, disorders of 846–8, **848**
Reovirus 282
Respiration, and cerebral function 126–7
Respirator brain 6, 155
Respiratory infections in ataxia-telangiectasia 724
Retraction balls, axonal 103, **104–5,** 106, 109, 462
Retroviruses, tumour production in animals 261
Reye's syndrome 294–5, 602–3
chickenpox complicated by 280
Rhabdomyolysis 1036–8, **1045,** 1091, 1092
idiopathic 1087
Rhabdomyoma, cardiac, in tuberous sclerosis 427, 430, **430**
Rhabdovirus 273, 280
Rheumatic fever 185
Rheumatoid arthritis
myopathy 1080
peripheral nerve involvement **896,** 897
spinal cord involvement 793–4, **793**
Rhombencephaloschisis 406
Riboflavin deficiency 583–4
Ribosomes, neuronal 3, **4**
Rich's focus 248, **249**
Riley-Day syndrome 882
River blindness 322–3
Rod body myopathy 1083, **1084**
Rod cells **41,** 42, 266, 292
general paralysis of the insane **257,** 258
hypoxia 130, 137
Rosenthal fibres 36, 374, **374**
Rough endoplasmic reticulum 3, **4**
Roussy-Lévy syndrome 723, 877
Rubella
latent infection 261
maternal, causing prenatal malformations in offspring 388–9
postinfectious encephalitis complicating 260, 272, 273
progressive panencephalitis 288
subacute sclerosing panencephalitis caused by 261
Rubidomycin toxicity 674

Sabin's non-toxoplasmic vascular encephalopathy 389
St Louis encephalitis 282
pathological findings 266, 283
Salla disease 545–6
Salmonella typhi
abscesses, epidural, spinal 238
meningitis 240
Sandhoff's disease 492, 493, 494, 495, 496
Sanfilippo's syndrome 534–8, **538,** 877, **Plate 12.1(b) facing p. 491**
Sarcoidosis (Schaumann's disease) 251–4, **254,** 756, **756, 757,** 765
myopathy 1080, **1080**
peripheral nerve involvement 890
Sarcomas, from x-irradiation 44
Satellitosis 11
'Saturday night paralysis' 850, 851
Scapuloperoneal syndrome 1059, 1071
Schaumann's disease *see* Sarcoidosis
Scheie's syndrome 534–8
Schilder's cerebral sclerosis (Schilder's disease) 355, **358**
Schistosomiasis 319–20, **320**
Schizencephalies 419–21, **419, 420**
Schmidt-Lanterman incisures 823–6, **825,** 839
Schmorl's intraosseous herniations 788
Schmorl's nodes 787–8, **795**
Schwann cells 808, 814–15, 816
development 815–16, **815**
myelin formation 818–19
periaxonal space 821
structure 821–3, **822, 823, 824**
Scrapie 289, 290–1, 1001–2
hypothalamic involvement 758
vacuolation of neurons 13
'Sea-blue histiocytes' 517, 518, 520

Seitelberger's disease 610
Selective vulnerability to hypoxia 131–3, 136, 152–5
Sella turcica
  empty sella syndrome 66, 770
  lesions in raised intracranial pressure 66
Sensory perineuritis 890
Septum pellucidum, anomalies 423, 424–5
Senile dementia *see* Dementia and ageing
Senile plaques *see under* Plaques
Sex chromatin 3
Sheehan's syndrome 767, **767**
Shigella dysenteriae 237
Shunts (in hydrocephalus), and bacterial infection of CNS 237, 238
Shy-Drager syndrome 718–19
Sialidosis
  type 1 539–40, **540, Plate 12.1(a) facing p. 491**
  type 2 539, 540
Sickle cell anemia 187
Sjögren's syndrome 897, 1080
Skull fractures 88
  contrecoup 88, 119
  contusions 93
  growing 88
Sleeping sickness 312
Slow eye movements in pontocerebellar atrophy 718
'Slow virus' 1002
Smallpox, encephalitis, postinfectious 260, 272, 273
Smooth endoplasmic reticulum in neurons 3, **4**
  peripheral axons 811
Sodium cyanate neuropathy 861
Sodium nitrite intoxication 130
Sotos' syndrome 423, 761
Spastic paraplegia, familial 699, 737–9, **738, 739**
Spatial compensation, in raised intracranial pressure 53, 58, 68
Spheroids 610–11, 661
Sphingomyelinase deficiency in Niemann-Pick disease 513–19, 520
Spina bifida 392–3
Spinal cord
  argyrophilic bodies **7,** 8
  artefactual changes 7–8
  atrophy in Friedreich's ataxia 720
  compression 784–5, 786
    bacterial infection 238, 248, 250, 795
    intervertebral disc protrusion 787–93, **789**
    Paget's disease of bone 785
    Pott's paraplegia 794–5, **795**
    rheumatoid arthritis 793–4, **793**
  diseases of spine affecting *see* Spine, diseases affecting spinal cord
  malformations 390, 392–6
  pyramidal tracts, absence and asymmetry 395–6, **396**
  traumatic lesions 779
    concussion, definition 781
    contusion, definition 781
    direct 779–80
    fracture-dislocations, cervical spine 780
    fracture-dislocations, thoracic and lumbar spine 780, **781**
    haematomyelia, definition 781
    haematorrhachis, definition 781
    indirect 780
    pathological findings 780–1; early 781–3; **782;** intermediate 783; late 783–4, **783, 784**
    spinal injuries from high-velocity missiles 780
    syringomyelia, post-traumatic 784
  vascular disorders
    anatomy 796–7
    anterior spinal artery, occlusion 797–8
    arteriovenous malformation 800–3, **801, 802**
    coarctation of aorta (adult type), neurological complications 798–9
    dissecting aneurysm of aorta, neurological complications 799–800
    posterior spinal artery, occlusion 798
    thrombophlebitis, acute 803
    thrombophlebitis, subacute and chronic 803
Spinal muscular atrophy 1056, 1059
  type 1 (severe infantile onset) (Werdnig-Hoffmann disease) 405, 699, 726, 734–7, **736, 737**
    muscle, changes in 735, 1056–7, **1057,** 1081
  type 2 (intermediate) 1056, 1057–8, **1058**
  type 3 (juvenile onset) (Kugelberg-Welander disease) 1056, 1058, **1059,** 1070
  type 4 (adult onset) 1056, 1059
Spine, diseases affecting spinal cord 784–5
  bony abnormalities in region of foramen magnum 785–7
  intervertebral disc protrusion 787–93, **789**
  osteitis deformans (Paget's disease of bone) 785
  Pott's paraplegia 794–5, **795**
  rheumatoid arthritis 793–4, **793**
Spinocerebellar tracts
  in familial spastic paraplegia 737, **739**
  in Friedreich's ataxia 720, **721**
  in motor neuron disease 730, 734
Spondylolisthesis 787
Spondylosis deformans 788, **789,** 794
Spongiform encephalopathies 267, 289–92, **293**
  cytoplasmic vacuolation 266, 292, **293**
  see also Creutzfeldt-Jakob disease; Kuru; Scrapie; Spongiform leucodystrophy
Spongiform leucodystrophy 374–6, **375**
Staphylococcal alpha-toxin 237
Staphylococcus
  brain abscess 243
  shunts (in hydrocephalus), infection of 237, 238
  subdural empyema 240
Staphylococcus albus, in shunts (in hydrocephalus treatment) 238
Staphylococcus aureus
  abscess, epidural, spinal 238
  aneurysms, bacterial 229
Status epilepticus 116, 156, 465, 925, 926–7, **927**
Status marmoratus **463,** 467–8, **469**
Status pseudoverrucosus 419
Status spongiosus 267, 292, **293,** 374–6, **375,** 999–1000
Status verrucosus 418–19
Status verrucosus simplex 419
'Steal' conditions, in arterial occlusions 167
Steroid myopathy 1091, 1092, **1092**
Stewart's syndrome 185
Strachan's syndrome 584

Streptococcus 237–8
subdural empyema 240
Streptococcus milleri, brain abscess 243
Streptococcus viridans, aneurysms, bacterial 229
Streptolysin O 237
Striatonigral degeneration 14, 706–7, **706,** 718
Stroke
computerized tomography 208, 209
dementia, multi-infarct 982–7
epidemiology 158
emboli causing 177
Framingham Study 158, 177, 208
incidence 158, 208
oral contraceptives, associated use 187–8
pregnancy and puerperium, association with 188
Strongyloidiasis 323
Strümpell's spastic paraplegia *see* Familial spastic paraplegia
Sturge-Weber syndrome 431, **432**
Subacute combined degeneration of spinal cord 587, 856
clinical features 587–8
pathology 588–90, **589**
clinical 590
Subacute myelo-optic neuropathy (SMON) 660–1
Subacute sclerosing panencephalitis (SSPE) 261, 283–4
pathological findings **265,** 266, 284–6, **285,** 966
Subclavian steal syndrome 167
Subcortical arteriosclerotic encephalopathy of Binswanger 176, 218–19, **218,** 984, 985
Substantia innominata 701, 708
in Alzheimer's disease 962
in Parkinson's disease 702
Substantia nigra 3
Alzheimer's neurofibrillary degeneration in 962, **962,** 965
Hallervorden-Spatz syndrome, discoloration in 609–10
in Huntington's chorea 993, 995
hypoxia, vulnerability to 132
in multiple system atrophy 700 (Table), 706, 716, 718
Parkinsonism-dementia complex of Guam, lesions in 707
Parkinsonism, postencephalitic, lesions in 706
Parkinson's disease, lesions in 702, **703, 704,** 951, 981, 982
in pontocerebellar atrophy 716, 718
Subthalamic nucleus
degeneration of, 708
in Friedreich's ataxia 722
hemiballism and 712
hypoxic damage 137
SV40 virus 288, 289
Sympathetic system in progressive autonomic failure 719
Synapses 3, **5**
Syringobulbia 397, 398–400, **399**
secondary degenerations 400
see also Syringomyelia
Syringomyelia 392, 393, 396–7
aetiology 401–2
pathogenesis 401–2
pathological changes 397–8, **397**
post-traumatic 784
secondary 400–1
secondary degenerations 400
symptomatology 400
'System degenerations' 699–701
transneuronal degeneration in 18, 699
Systemic lupus erythematosus (SLE) 175, 185, 897, 1051, 1080
Systemic sclerosis (scleroderma), myositis in 1080

Tabes dorsalis 255–8, **256**
Taenia multiceps 318
Taenia solium 315, 1081
Takayasu's arteritis 182, **182**
Tangier disease 875, **876**
Tanycytes 39
Tarui's disease, myopathy in 1090
Tay-Sachs disease 491, 492, 493, 494, 496
Telangiectasia in Louis-Bar syndrome 724
Tellurium toxicity 647–8
Temporal arteritis (giant cell arteritis) 185–6, **186,** 979
Thalamic syndrome, basal ganglia lesions associated with 712–13
Thalamus 701
calcification in 709, **710**
central transtentorial herniation 64, **64**
effects of lesions in 712–13
epilepsy 931, **931,** 932
Huntington's chorea 995
hypoxic damage 132, 136, 137, 142, 151
intracerebral haemorrhage, in hypertension 215, 216, **216**
in Werdnig-Hoffmann disease 735
Thalassaemia, nervous system involvement 187
Thalidomide, toxicity 674–5, 861
Thallium poisoning 641–3, 859
Thiamine deficiency 573–80, 855
experimental 580
Thomsen's disease 1075–6
internal nuclei in muscle fibres 1043, 1075
Thoracic nuclei of spinal cord 700 (Table)
in Friedreich's ataxia 720
in motor neuron disease 730, 734
Thresholds of ischaemia 156, 159
Thromboangiitis obliterans (Winiwarter-Buerger disease) 170, 171, 182, 186
Thrombosis
basilar artery 169, **169**
carotid artery
common **166**
internal 165, **166**
infarction caused by 159
veins and sinuses of brain 188
cavernous sinus 190
internal cerebral veins 190
lateral sinus 190
perinatal 452–3, **453**
primary 188–9, **189**
secondary 189–90
Thrombotic microangiopathy 187, **187**
Thrombotic thrombocytopenic purpura 186–7, **187**

Thymus in ataxia-telangiectasia 724
Thyrotoxic myopathy 1087
Tick-borne viruses 282
  pathological findings in encephalitis 283
Tin poisoning 643
  triethyl tin 643–5, **644**
  trimethyl tin 643, 645
Tobacco amblyopia 586
Tomaculous neuropathy 849, **849,** 883, **883**
Torsion dystonia 1076
Torula histolytica 328
Tourniquet paralysis 850–1, **851, 852**
Toxic myopathies 1092
Toxic oil syndrome 859–60, 890, 894
Toxocariasis 321–2, **321**
Toxoplasmosis 309–11, **309,** 389
  in adults 310–11, **310**
  congenital 311
  hypothalamic involvement 756, **756**
  muscle infection 1081
  pituitary gland involvement 765
Transfusion syndrome 474
Transient ischaemic attacks 158, 181
Transneuronal degeneration 18–20, **18, 19,** 699
Trans-synaptic degeneration 18
Trematodes 318–21
  paragonimiasis 318–19
  schistosomiasis 319–20, **320**
Treponema pallidum 237, **257**
Trichinosis 323–4, 1081
Trichlorethylene, cranial neuropathy 860
Triorthocresyl phosphate (TOCP) intoxication 658–60
Trisomies 388, 411, 435
Trypanosoma cruzi 311, 313, **314,** 315, 1081
Trypanosoma gambiense 311, 312, 313
Trypanosoma rhodesiense 311–12, 313, 315
Trypanosomiasis 311
  African 311–13, **312,** 313–14
  American (Chagas' disease) 313, **314,** 890, 1081
  congenital 313–15
Tuberculoma 248, 251
  cerebellar 251
  intracerebral 251, **252**
  meningeal 248
  supratentorial 251
Tuberculoma en plaque 248
Tuberculosis 236, 247–51
  caseation necrosis 236, 247–8, 250
  epidural 248
  miliary 248
  spinal 248
  subdural 248
  see also Meningitis, tuberculous
Tuberous sclerosis 427–30, **427, 428, 429, 430**
Tubular aggregates in muscle 1086, 1087, 1088
Tuffstone bodies 870, **871**
Tumours
  von Hippel-Lindau's angiomatosis 430–1
  syringomyelia associated with 400–1
  x-irradiation causing 43–5
Turner's syndrome (XO) 388
Twinning, and fetal brain damage 474–5
Tyrosinaemia 606

Ulegyria 415, 467, **468**
Ultrasound
  anencephaly detection 391
  brain damage due to 45
  Dandy-Walker syndrome, use in 408
Uncus
  in epilepsy 926, 934, 935, 936
  in tentorial hernia 59–60
Unverricht-Lundborg disease 940–1
Uraemic neuropathy 864–5
Uveoparotitis 251–2

Vaccinia, postinfectious encephalitis complicating 272
Vagus, dopsal nucleus of 700 (Table)
Varicella (chickenpox) 260, 271
  encephalitis (postinfectious) complicating 272, 273, 280
  Reye's syndrome complicating 280
Varicella-zoster virus 262, 278–80
  encephalomyelitis due to 271
    pathological findings 271–2, **272**
  latent infection 261
Vascular disorders of central nervous system
  aortic arch syndrome 182, **182**
  applied anatomy and physiology
    arterial blood supply 157
    venous drainage 157–8
  atheroma 162–5, **166,** 173
  atherosclerosis 162–5, 209, 227
  blood diseases 186–7, **187**
  carotid arteritis, acute 182
  cerebral embolism 177–81, **178**
  cerebral infarction 158–62, 187–8
  collagen disorders 184–5, **184**
  connective tissue inherited disorders associated with 188
  endarteritis obliterans 182–3, **183**
  epidemiology 158
  familial oculoleptomeningeal amyloidosis associated with 188
  fibromuscular dysplasia 182
  giant cell (temporal) arteritis 185–6, **186**
  granular atrophy of cortex 170–1, **171**
  granulomatous angiitis 188
  hypertension and the brain 172–7
  inflammatory bowel disease, complication of 188
  irradiation causing 188
  migraine associated with 188
  moyamoya disease 183–4, 220
  oral contraceptives and cerebral infarction 187–8
  pregnancy and puerperium associated with 188
  thromboangiitis obliterans (Winiwarter-Buerger's disease) 170, 171, 182, 186
  thrombosis of veins and sinuses of brain 188–90, **189**
  perinatal 452–3, **453**
  transient ischaemic attacks 181
  see also under Arteries; *see also* Aneurysms; Haemorrhage, intracranial

'Vascular theory' of distribution of hypoxic brain damage 152–3
Vasculitic disease affecting muscle 1079–80
Vasculitic neuropathy 894–7
Vasculomyelinopathy 307
Vasodilatation, cerebral 55, 56, 57, 112
Vasopressin 751, 753, 759
Vegetative state following head injury 115–16
Vein of Galen 158
  aneurysmal malformation 431–3, **433**
  intraventricular haemorrhage 455
Venezuelan equine encephalitis 282, 283
  pathological findings 283
Ventricles, lateral cerebral, anomalies of wall of 425–6
Vermis, cerebellar, malformations 406, **407,** 408
Vertebrobasilar circulation 157
  occlusion and stenosis 167–9
Vesicles in peripheral axons 811
Vestibular nuclei, degeneration of 700 (Table), 718–19, 722
Vincristine, toxic effects 672–3, 861
Virion, biology of 261–3
Virus diseases of central nervous system
  access routes 262–3
  biology of viruses 261–3
  encephalitis, infective, acute 260–1, **265,** 273–83, **277**
    adenoviruses 273
    arboviruses 273, 282–3
    cytomegalovirus 280
    enteroviruses 273
    Epstein-Barr virus 280
    herpes simplex virus 264, 266, 267, 273–8, **276, 277, 279**
    herpesvirus B (simiae) 280
    rabies 273, 280–2
    varicella-zoster virus 278–80
  encephalitis, postinfectious, acute (perivenous demyelinating encephalitis) 260, 272–3
  encephalitis, subacute 261, 283–93
    astrocytes, reactive 266
    Creutzfeldt-Jakob disease 261, 289–92
    kuru 261, 289–93, **293**
    measles inclusion body encephalitis in the immunosuppressed 286–8, **287**
    progressive multifocal leucoencephalopathy 266, 288–9
    progressive rubella panencephalitis 288
    subacute sclerosing panencephalitis 261, **265,** 266, 283–6, **285**
  encephalomyelitis 260, 268–72
    due to polioviruses 260, 268–70
    due to varicella-zoster virus 271–2, **272**
  latent infection 261, 271, 275–6, 733
  lytic infection 261
  macroscopical appearance 264
  meningitis 260, 267–8, **277**
    cerebrospinal fluid values 267
    virus isolation 267–8
  microscopical appearances 264–7
    astrocytes 266
    demyelination 267
    inclusion bodies **265,** 266
    inflammatory cell infiltration 264–6, **265**
    microglial cells, hyperplasia and proliferation 266
    necrosis 266–7
    neurons, changes in 266
    status spongiosus 267, 292, **293**
  necropsy 263–4
  neuronal inclusions 26, 266
  pathological features, general 264–7
  recent advances, factors influencing 260
  transformation process 261
  types 260–1
Visceral larva migrans 321
Vitamin deficiencies 573
  A 592–3
  B_2 group
    nicotinic acid 578, 581–3, 856
    pantothenic acid 580–1, 855–6
    riboflavin 583–4
  B_6 group
    and isoniazid, toxicity of 663–4
    pyridoxine 584–5, 860
  B_{12} 585–6
    in animals 590–2, **591**
    neurological disorders, causes of 586–7
    neurological effects 587–90
    peripheral neuropathy 856–7
  C (ascorbic acid) 593
  E 593–4, 857
    in animals 594, 857
  K 593
  malformations induced, in animal teratology 385
  thiamine 573–80, 855
    alcoholism associated with 573–8
    experimental 580
Volkmann's ischaemic contracture of muscle 1093–4
Vulnerability, selective, to hypoxia 131–3, 136, 152–5

Waldenström's macroglobulinaemia 187, 865, 893, **894**
Wallerian degeneration
  central nervous system **14, 15,** 15–17, 130, **131**
  peripheral 838–42, **838, 839, 840, 841, 842**
Waterhouse-Friderichsen syndrome 241
Wegener's granulomatosis 184–5, 897
Werdnig-Hoffmann disease 405, 699, 726, 734–7, **736, 737**
  muscle, changes in 735, 1056–7, **1057,** 1081
Wernicke's encephalopathy 369, 573–7, **574, 575, 576**, 1004
  haemorrhages in hypothalamus 757, **757**
West Indian, Indian and African neuromyelopathy 611–12
Western equine encephalitis 282
  pathological findings 283
Whipple's disease 609
White matter *see also* Demyelination
  Alexander's type of leucodystrophy 373–4, **373**
  carbon monoxide intoxication 146–7, **147,** 148
  cerebral infarction 160, 161, **161**
  hypoxic alterations 130–1, 146–7
  Krabbe's leucodystrophy 531–2
  metachromatic leucodystrophy 527
  motor neuron disease 730, **731, 732, 733**

White matter—*contd.*
  oedematous, reactive astrocytes in 33, 34, **34, 35**
  progressive multifocal leucoencephalopathy 289, **290–1**
  spongiform leucodystrophy 374, **375**
  X-linked leucodystrophies 370–3, **372**
Wilson's disease 595–6
  biochemistry 598–9
  copper excess in 596, 597, 598–9
  historical survey 596
  Kayser-Fleischer rings 596, **596,** 598
  Opalski cells 596, **596,** 597, 598
  pathological changes 596–8, **596, 597**
Winiwarter-Buerger's syndrome (thromboangiitis obliterans) 170, 171, 182, 186
Wohlfart B-fibres in muscles **1038,** 1039, 1056
Wolman's disease 551–4, **552, 553, 554,** 876

Xeroderma pigmentosum 877
Xeroid-lipofuscinosis 956

Yttrium-90, pituitary irradiation 769–70, **769**

Zebra bodies 530, 538, **539,** 551, 870, **872**
Zellweger's cerebrohepatorenal syndrome 412, 417, 473
Zenker's degeneration 1036, 1087
Zinc pyridinethione (ZPT), toxic effects in animals 681
Zygomycosis (mucormycosis) 331–2, **331**